Essentials of Medical-Surgical Nursing

A Nursing Process Approach

Essentials of
Medical-Surgical Nursing
A Nursing Process Approach

Edited by

BARBARA C. LONG, R.N., M.S.N.

Associate Professor Emerita of Medical-Surgical Nursing,
Frances Payne Bolton School of Nursing,
Case Western Reserve University,
Cleveland, Ohio

WILMA J. PHIPPS, R.N., Ph.D., F.A.A.N.

Professor and Chairperson of Medical-Surgical Nursing,
Frances Payne Bolton School of Nursing,
Case Western Reserve University;
Director of Medical-Surgical Nursing,
University Hospitals of Cleveland,
Cleveland, Ohio

With 625 illustrations

The C. V. Mosby Company
ST. LOUIS • TORONTO • PRINCETON   1985

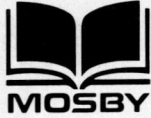

MOSBY

A TRADITION OF PUBLISHING EXCELLENCE

Editor: Julie Cardamon
Assistant editor: Bess Arends
Manuscript editors: Carol Claverie, Jan Gardner, Timothy O'Brien,
    Elaine Steinborn, Carol Wiseman
Book design: Gail Morey Hudson
Cover design: Kathleen A. Johnson
Production: Carol O'Leary, Linda R. Stalnaker, Mary Stueck
Cover photo: Four By Five, Inc.

Printed in the United States of America

The C.V. Mosby Company
11830 Westline Industrial Drive, St. Louis, Missouri 63146

Library of Congress Cataloging in Publication Data

Main entry under title:

Essentials of medical-surgical nursing.

  Bibliography: p.
  Includes index.
  1. Nursing.   2. Surgical nursing.   3. Intensive
care nursing.   I. Long, Barbara C., 1926-
II. Phipps, Wilma J., 1925-   [DNLM: 1. Nursing
Care. WY 150 E78]
RT41.E87   1985   610.73   84-18988
ISBN 0-8016-3040-1

C/VH/VH 9 8 7 6 5 4 3 2   03/A/374

Contributors

DOROTHY S. BLEVINS, R.N., M.S.N.

Associate Professor of Nursing, Kent State University, Kent, Ohio

LINDA ANNE BROSEMAN, R.N., M.S.N.

Clinical Instructor in Medical-Surgical Nursing, Frances Payne Bolton School of Nursing, Case Western Reserve University; Administrative Nurse Clinician, University Hospitals of Cleveland, Cleveland, Ohio

PATRICIA BUERGIN, R.N., B.S.N.

Senior Clinical Nurse, University Hospitals of Cleveland, Cleveland, Ohio

VIRGINIA L. CASSMEYER, R.N., M.S.N.

Ph.D. Candidate, University of Kansas, Kansas City, Missouri

BARBARA J. DALY, R.N., M.S.N., F.A.A.N.

Associate Clinical Professor of Medical-Surgical Nursing, Frances Payne Bolton School of Nursing, Case Western Reserve University; Assistant Director of Medical-Surgical Nursing, University Hospitals of Cleveland, Cleveland, Ohio

ELIZABETH CAMERON ECKSTEIN, R.N., B.S.N.

Graduate Student, Frances Payne Bolton School of Nursing, Case Western Reserve University; Formerly, Infection Control Nurse, University Hospitals of Cleveland, Cleveland, Ohio

H. FRED FARLEY, R.N., M.S.N.

Clinical Instructor in Medical-Surgical Nursing, Frances Payne Bolton School of Nursing, Case Western Reserve University; Assistant Director, Medical-Surgical Nursing, University Hospitals of Cleveland, Cleveland, Ohio

GREER GLAZER, R.N., Ph.D.

Assistant Professor of Maternity/GYN, Frances Payne Bolton School of Nursing, Case Western Reserve University; Associate in Nursing, University Hospitals of Cleveland, Cleveland, Ohio

JUDITH L. GREIG, R.N., M.S.N.

Assistant Professor of Nursing, Lakeland Community College, Mentor, Ohio

GRACE McCARTHY HARLAN, R.N., M.S.N.

Formerly, Associate Professor of Medical-Surgical Nursing, Cleveland State University, Cleveland, Ohio

ROSEMARIE HOGAN, R.N., M.S.N.

Associate Professor of Nursing, Kent State University, Kent, Ohio

MAURA A. HOPKINS, R.N., M.S.N.

Head Nurse, Intensive Care Unit, San Francisco University Hospital, San Francisco, California

BENITA C. MARTOCCHIO, R.N., Ph.D.

Associate Professor of Nursing, Frances Payne Bolton School of Nursing, Case Western Reserve University; Associate in Nursing, University Hospitals of Cleveland, Cleveland, Ohio

MARY LOU MONAHAN, R.N., M.S.N.

Nurse Clinician, University Hospitals of Cleveland; Clinical Instructor in Medical-Surgical Nursing, Frances Payne Bolton School of Nursing, Case Western Reserve University Cleveland, Ohio

PENNY O'MALLEY, R.N., B.S.N.

Director of Ambulatory Nursing Services, Cleveland Metropolitan General Hospital, Cleveland, Ohio

GAIL OSTERFIELD, R.N., M.S.N.

Assistant Professor of Nursing, Kent State University, Kent, Ohio

ELIZABETH SCHENK, R.N., M.S.N.

Clinical Supervisor, Cleveland Metropolitan General Hospital/Highland View Hospital, Cleveland, Ohio

BARBARA SOLTIS, R.N., M.S.N.

Clinical Specialist, Cleveland Metropolitan General Hospital/Highland View Hospital, Cleveland, Ohio

DOLORES VERDERBER, R.N., M.S.N.

Instructor in Gerontologic Nursing, Frances Payne Bolton School of Nursing, Case Western Reserve University; Clinical Nurse Specialist in Gerontology, Margaret Wagner House, Cleveland, Ohio

EILEEN WALSH-ESSIG, R.N., M.S.N., C.C.R.N.

Clinical Instructor in Medical-Surgical Nursing, Frances Payne Bolton School of Nursing, Case Western Reserve University; Nurse Clinician, University Hospitals of Cleveland, Cleveland, Ohio

NANCY FUGATE WOODS, R.N., Ph.D., F.A.A.N.

Professor, Department of Physiological Nursing, Director, Office for Nursing Research Facilitation, University of Washington, Seattle, Washington

E. RONALD WRIGHT, Ph.D.

Associate Professor of Microbiology, Frances Payne Bolton School of Nursing, Case Western Reserve University, Cleveland, Ohio

MAY WYKLE, R.N., Ph.D.

Associate Professor of Psychiatric Nursing, Frances Payne Bolton School of Nursing, Case Western Reserve University; Associate in Nursing, University Hospitals of Cleveland, Cleveland, Ohio

MARY A. (SANDY) WYPER, R.N., M.S.N.

Ph.D. Student; Formerly, Assistant Professor of Nursing, Frances Payne Bolton School of Nursing, Case Western Reserve University, Cleveland, Ohio

DEANNA MELTON XISTRIS, R.N., M.S.N.

Clinical Specialist in Oncology Nursing, Hematology-Oncology Associates, Inc., Stamford, Connecticut

MARGARET VETTESE ZACK, R.N., M.S.N.

Ph.D. Student; Formerly Instructor in Medical Surgical Nursing, Frances Payne Bolton School of Nursing, Case Western Reserve University, Cleveland, Ohio

Preface

Medical-surgical nursing has expanded greatly with increased promotion of health care and technologic advances. Textbooks of medical-surgical nursing have kept pace with the advances and, over the years, have increased considerably in size, serving as reference sources in addition to being textbooks. Since the publication of *Medical-Surgical Nursing: Concepts and Clinical Practice,* we have welcomed the suggestions sent us by readers. A major point of comment has been the physical size of the book and the difficulty experienced by some students in identifying the *essential* content in a limited period of time for study.

This book is an outgrowth of readers' suggestions, a book of smaller size to serve primarily as a student textbook. The format should also be useful to the graduate nurse beginning practice in acute care centers. The focus of the book is the care of *adult* persons with medical-surgical disorders. Information specific to the care of children has been omitted, since this information is more appropriately described in pediatric nursing texts.

Overview

The first three units of the book present a summary of the bases of medical-surgical nursing practice (Unit I), health promotion (Unit II), and stress and adaptation (Unit III). It is expected that students will have had at least one introductory course in nursing before beginning to use this textbook. Some chapters, such as Chapter 2, on the nursing process, and Chapter 3, on health assessment of the adult, are included to emphasize, from the student's previous courses, those aspects particularly pertinent to medical-surgical nursing practice. Health promotion is included to emphasize to the student that health promotion is an important aspect in the nursing care of adults, whether the person is well or ill.

Units IV and V focus on common occurrences in the practice of medical-surgical nursing, regardless of underlying pathologies or body systems (for example, fluid and electrolyte balance, shock, pain, infectious disease, neoplasia, chronic illness, and dying and death). The chapters on perioperative nursing focus on the *general* assessments and interventions for the person experiencing surgery. Specific care required for special types of surgical procedures is described in appropriate chapters in the latter part of the book.

The remainder of the book uses a nursing process format for the discussion of the following problem areas: sensorimotor (Unit VI), gas transport (Unit VII), metabolic and endocrine (Unit VIII), digestion and elimination (Unit IX), sexuality and reproduction (Unit X), and physiologic defense mechanisms (Unit XI). In each chapter within these units there is a brief review of the pertinent *anatomy and physiology* for quick reference by the student who will already have had an anatomy and physiology course. This is followed by essential *prevention and health education* information. The *major health problems* are then identified. Specific diseases are grouped (such as inflammatory, structural, or tumors) depending on the similarity of the required care. For each group of diseases, the focus of the discussion is on the *nursing* aspects. Medical information (etiology, signs and symptoms, and medical therapy) is summarized in tables. *Pathophysiology* is highlighted to provide the student with an understanding of assessment parameters and bases for intervention.

Assessment focuses on subjective and objective data important for the nurse to collect in the specific acute care situations. *Data analysis,* in practice, depends on the collected patient data; for the purposes of this textbook therefore we have identified some *nursing diagnoses* that *may* be present; depending on the presenting data. The nursing diagnoses identified by the National Group for the Classification of Nursing Diagnoses have been used. *Planning* for nursing care includes setting goals or outcomes of patient care, therefore *expected patient outcomes* have also been identified for special situations.

The *implementation* sections differentiate nursing actions directed toward (1) assisting with achievement of therapeutic goals, (2) assisting with comfort and activities of daily living (ADL), (3) control of environment (if pertinent), and (4) counseling and teaching. These categories are some of the major ones used in the licensure examinations. *Evaluation* is, of course, dependent on the expected patient outcomes. Some questions that may be asked during evaluation are identified for student guidance.

The final two chapters attend to selected aspects of emergency or critical care. Interventions in *emergencies or disasters* in the community are summarized. An overview of nursing care in *critical care units* is provided to give the student an overview and understanding of what the patient experiences in these units.

Features

A common difficulty experienced by students is lack of quick access to important information for the purpose of study or for preparing nursing care plans. We have addressed this difficulty by the liberal use of boxed material and by the outlining of nursing interventions. Lists of possible nursing diagnoses and expected patient outcomes should also be useful resources for the student or beginning practicing nurse. The tables providing the medical information provide a quick reference source when needed. Overall, the nursing process approach emphasizes *nursing* care rather than medical care.

Study questions have been supplied to the student for assistance in *preparing* for the reading assignment. Pedagogical aids that include suggested test questions are provided the teacher in a separate teacher's guide.

Acknowledgments

We wish to thank those persons who have assisted us in this endeavor. We appreciate the many reviewers who told us what they were looking for in a textbook and offered constructive suggestions. We are grateful for the direction and support provided by Julie Cardamon and Bess Arends of The C.V. Mosby Co. Their patience and tolerance of our efforts to meet deadlines was most helpful. Some of the illustrations for this book are the work of Kathleen Jung and Nancy Burgard. Preparation of some of the manuscript was done by Janet Mitchell and Sondra Patrizi. We also thank our many colleagues for their time, assistance and support, especially Mary Alexandra (Sandy) Wyper, Margaret Zack, Grace Harlan, Barbara Daly, and Patricia Buergin. Finally, we thank Jim Long, without whose support and patience this book would not have been possible.

Barbara C. Long
Wilma J. Phipps

Contents

UNIT I

Medical-Surgical Nursing Practice

1 Perspectives of medical-surgical nursing, 3
Barbara C. Long

2 Nursing process: a systematic approach, 10
Barbara C. Long

3 Nursing history and physical examination, 20
Barbara C. Long

4 Quality assurance in nursing, 38
Mary Lou Monahan

UNIT II

Health Promotion

5 Developmental factors affecting health of adults, 47
Dolores Verderber

6 Biologic defense mechanisms of the human body, 62
E. Ronald Wright

7 Health promotion: nutrition and exercise, 85
Barbara C. Long

UNIT III

Stress and Adaptation

8 Stress and stress management, 105
Barbara C. Long

9 Psychologic responses to stress, 113
May Wykle

UNIT IV

Common Problems Encountered in Medical-Surgical Nursing

10 Fluid and electrolyte imbalances, 133
Barbara Soltis

11 Shock, 158
Gail Osterfield

12 Pain, 174
Barbara C. Long

13 Infection control, 190
Elizabeth Cameron Eckstein

14 Cancer, 211
Margaret Vettese Zack and Rosemarie Hogan

15 Chronic illness, 258
Wilma J. Phipps, Patricia Buergin, Eleanor E. Bauwens, and Sandra Vandam Anderson

16 Dimensions of dying and death, 277
Benita C. Martocchio

UNIT V

Perioperative Nursing

17 Preoperative intervention, 291
Barbara C. Long

18 Intraoperative intervention, 303
Judith L. Greig

19 Postoperative intervention, 326
Barbara C. Long

UNIT VI

Sensorimotor Problems

20 The patient with neurologic problems, 351
Elizabeth Shenk

21 The patient with eye problems, 436
Barbara C. Long

22 The patient with ear problems, 460
Linda Anne Broseman

23 The patient with musculoskeletal disorders, 480
Grace McCarthy Harlan

Internal nonspecific defense mechanisms, 67
  Reticuloendothelial system, 68
  Blood, 68
  Interferon, 70
  Inflammatory response, 71
Specific defense mechanisms, 73
  Concept of specific immunity, 73
  Antigens and antibodies, 73
  Immune response system, 74
  Immune response, 76
Applications and implications of immune response, 81
  Immunization, 81
  Cancer immunology, 82
  Immunologic disorders, 82
  Tissue transplants, 82

7 Health promotion: nutrition and exercise, 85
Barbara C. Long

Health promotion in medical-surgical nursing practice, 85
  Factors affecting health promoting behaviors, 86
Nutrition, 86
  Relationship of nutrition to health, 86
  Assessment of nutrient intake, 88
  Data analysis and planning, 90
  Implementation, 92
Exercise, 97
  Benefits of exercise, 98
  Exercise programs, 98
  Immobility, 100

UNIT III
Stress and Adaptation

8 Stress and stress management, 105
Barbara C. Long

Adaptation, 105
Stress, 106
  Stress as a concept, 106
  Stress responses, 106
Coping, 109
Stress management, 110
  General interventions to modify physiologic responses, 110
  Stress management therapies, 110
  Problem solving, 111
  Relaxation techniques, 111

9 Psychologic responses to stress, 113
May Wykle

Anxiety, 114
  Assessment of anxiety, 114
  Interventions for anxiety, 115
  Crisis intervention, 116
Defense mechanisms, 118
  Denial, 118
  Regression, 119
Behavioral reactions to illness, 119
  Aggressive behavior, 119
  Depressed behavior, 119
  Withdrawn behavior, 120
  Suspicious behavior, 120
  Somatic behavior, 120
Alcoholism, 120
  Epidemiology, 120
  Etiology, 121
  Pathophysiology, 121
  Assessment, 122
  Intervention, 123
Drug abuse, 124
  Epidemiology, 124

Assessment, 125
Intervention, 127

UNIT IV
Common Problems Encountered in Medical-Surgical Nursing

10 Fluid and electrolyte imbalances, 133
Barbara Soltis

Basic mechanisms of fluid and electrolyte balance, 134
  Body water, 134
  Body electrolyte component, 135
  Mechanisms for fluid and electrolyte movement, 136
  Hormonal control, 136
Fluid and electrolyte imbalance, 137
  Fluid imbalances, 137
  Electrolyte imbalances, 142
Acid-base balance and imbalance, 147
  Acid-base balance, 147
  Acid-base imbalance, 148
Assessment of fluid and electrolyte balance, 151
  Patient data, 151
  Laboratory values, 152
  Additional data, 152
Management of patients with fluid and electrolyte imbalance, 153
  Prevention of fluid and electrolyte imbalance, 153
  Replacement therapy, 154
  Relief of thirst, 156

11 Shock, 158
Gail Osterfield

Etiology of shock, 158
  Hypovolemic shock, 159
  Cardiogenic shock, 159
  Vasogenic shock, 159
Pathophysiology of shock, 159
  Early stage, 159
  Later stage, 160
Organ damage in shock, 160
  Kidneys, 160
  Brain, 161
  Heart, 161
  Lungs, 161
  Gastrointestinal tract, 161
  Liver, 161
  Blood, 162
Assessment, 162
  Hemodynamic monitoring, 162
  Respiratory monitoring, 166
  Fluid and electrolyte monitoring, 167
  Neurologic monitoring, 167
  Hematologic monitoring, 167
  Other monitoring, 167
Data analysis and planning, 167
  Nursing diagnoses, 167
  Expected patient outcomes, 167
Implementation, 167
  Assisting with achievement of therapeutic goals, 167
  Maintaining comfort and rest, 171
Evaluation, 171

12 Pain, 174
Barbara C. Long

Concepts of pain, 175
  Pain experience, 175
  . Types of pain, 177
  Assessment, 180
    Acute pain, 180
    Chronic pain, 181

Data analysis and planning, 181
  Nursing diagnoses, 182
  Expected patient outcomes, 182
Medical approaches to pain control, 182
  Medications, 182
  Electrical stimulators, 183
  Neurosurgical procedures, 184
  Nerve block, 185
  Acupuncture, 185
Psychologic approaches for pain control, 185
  Behavior modification, 185
  Biofeedback and autogenic training, 185
  Hypnosis, 185
Nursing approaches for pain control, 186
  Guidelines for pain relief measures, 186
  Preventing pain, 186
  Modifying the pain stimulus, 186
  Modifying the pain response, 187
Team approach for chronic pain control, 188
  Pain clinics, 188
  Inpatient chronic pain teams, 188
Evaluation, 188

13 Infection control, 190
Elizabeth Cameron Eckstein

Historical perspective, 190
The infectious disease process, 191
  Definitions, 191
  Chain of infection, 192
  Assessment, 194
Infection control in the community, 196
  Prevention and control measures, 196
  Immunization programs, 196
Infection control in the hospital, 199
  Scope of the problem, 199
  Persons at risk, 200
  Pathogens causing nosocomial infections, 201
  Prevention and control measures, 202
Conclusion, 210

14 Cancer, 211
Margaret Vettese Zack and Rosemarie Hogan

Definition of terms, 211
Attitudes toward cancer, 212
Epidemiology, 212
  Epidemiologic variables for cancer, 212
  Nurse's role in cancer epidemiology, 214
Pathophysiology, 214
  Characteristics of malignant cells, 214
  Naming and classifying neoplasms, 218
Etiology: carcinogenesis, 218
  Host susceptibility, 218
  Environmental factors, 220
  Health practices, 221
  Viruses, 223
  Psychosocial factors, 223
  Conclusions, 223
Prevention and health education, 224
  Health teaching, 224
  Early detection and treatment, 224
  Factors that interfere with health-seeking behavior, 225
  Cancer quackery, 226
  Organizations involved in cancer education, detection,
    and rehabilitation, 226
Assessment, 228
  Subjective data, 228
  Objective data, 230
  Diagnostic studies, 230
  Nursing intervention during assessment phase, 230
Data analysis and planning, 232
Implementation, 232
  Assisting with achievement of therapeutic goals, 232

Cancer pain, 250
Psychologic support of patient and family, 252
Supportive care of the patient with cancer that is
  terminal, 253

15 Chronic illness, 258
**Wilma J. Phipps, Patricia Buergin, Eleanor E. Bauwens, and
Sandra Vandam Anderson**

Definition of acute and chronic illness, 259
Chronic illness as a force in society, 259
  Factors that influence chronic illness, 260
  Cost of disability, 261
Effects of chronic illness, 261
  Prevention of chronic illness, 262
Special needs of the chronically ill, 263
  Assessment of physical status, 263
  Intervention, 263
  Assessment of psychologic status, 263
  Assessment of social and financial status, 264
  Psychosocial considerations, 264
Rehabilitation, 265
  Teamwork and special services, 265
  Role of the nurse, 267
  Role of the patient, 268
Continuing care, 269
  Considerations for continuing care, 269
  Patterns and facilities for continuing care, 270
  Community resources, 272
Outcome criteria for the person with a chronic illness, 272
  Focus on the future, 274

16 Dimensions of dying and death, 277
Benita C. Martocchio

Societal and social dimensions, 277
  Dying and death are different, 277
  My death: your death, 277
  Age and premature death, 278
  Prolonged dying, 278
  Rights of dying persons, 278
  Good death/bad death, 279
Attitudinal dimensions, 280
  Death denial, 280
  Death defiance, 280
  Death acceptance, 281
  Desire for death, 281
Dimensions of dying persons, 281
  Chronicity of dying, 281
  Stages and phases of dying, 281
  Patterns of living-dying, 282
  Choice: a right, 283
  Role of confidant, 283
  Dying: an achievement or a failure, 284
Some family dimensions, 284
  Cohesive or disruptive force, 284
  Family control, 284
  An unreasonable situation, 284
Multifocus nursing practice considerations, 285
  Assessment, 285
  Nursing care planning, 286
  Nursing interventions, 286
  Evaluation, 287

UNIT V

Perioperative Nursing

17 Preoperative intervention, 291
Barbara C. Long

Types of Surgery, 291
  Classification, 291
  Surgical procedures, 292

Effects of surgery on the patient, 292
  Physiologic responses, 292
  Psychologic responses, 293
Informed consent, 293
Assessment, 294
  Patient knowledge, 294
  Psychologic readiness for surgery, 294
  Physiologic status, 295
Data analysis and planning, 297
  Nursing diagnoses, 297
  Expected patient outcomes, 297
Implementation, 297
  Assisting with achievement of therapeutic goals, 297
  Counseling and teaching, 298
  Assisting with comfort, 300
  Carrying out final preparation for surgery, 300
Transportation to operating room, 301

18 Intraoperative intervention, 303

Judith L. Greig

Concepts basic to operating room nursing, 303
  Perioperative nursing, 303
  Standards of perioperative nursing practice, 304
  Intraoperative patient care team members, 304
Operating room suite design, 306
Nursing practice in the operating room, 307
  Aseptic technique and infection control, 307
  Safety and protection of the patient, 311
Anesthesia, 315
  Usage, 315
  Choice, 315
  Preparation of patient for anesthesia, 316
  General anesthesia, 316
  Muscle relaxants, 320
  Regional anesthesia, 320
  Other types of anesthesia, 321
  Monitoring patient during anesthesia, 321
Termination of surgery, 323
  Dressings and drains, 323
  Documentation, 323
  Transfer of patient to recovery room, 323
Evaluation, 324

19 Postoperative intervention, 326

Barbara C. Long

Postanesthetic phase, 326
  Maintaining pulmonary ventilation, 326
  Maintaining circulation, 328
  Maintaining fluid and electrolyte balance, 329
  Maintaining safety and comfort, 329
  Discharge from recovery room, 329
Admission of patient to clinical unit, 329
  Preparation on clinical unit, 329
  Initial assessment, 329
  Data from patient's chart, 334
Data analysis and planning, 334
  Nursing diagnoses, 334
  Expected patient outcomes, 335
Implementation, 335
  Promotion of wound healing, 335
  Maintaining adequate respiration, 339
  Maintaining circulation, 340
  Maintaining fluid and electrolyte balance, 343
  Maintaining adequate nutrition, 343
  Maintaining elimination, 344
  Promoting comfort, 345
  Maintaining activity, 346
  Helping meet psychologic needs, 347
  Discharge planning, 348

UNIT VI

Sensorimotor Problems

20 The patient with neurologic problems, 351

Elizabeth Shenk

Anatomy and physiology, 351
  Neuron, 352
  Divisions of the nervous system, 354
  Sensory system pathways, 356
  Motor system pathways, 357
  Changes with aging, 357
Prevention and health education, 358
  Primary prevention: prevention of disease, 358
  Secondary prevention/early detection, 358
  Tertiary prevention/prevention of complications, 358
Common neurologic manifestations, 358
  Neurologic assessment, 359
  Headache, 361
  Neurologic pain, 367
  Increased intracranial pressure, 371
  Alterations in muscle tone and motor function, 376
  Alterations in sensory function, 382
Major health problems of the neurologic system, 385
Interference with function because of problems with
      conduction of impulses, 385
  Epilepsy or seizures, 385
  Myasthenia gravis, 390
Interference with function because of degenerative
      diseases, 393
  Multiple sclerosis, 394
  Parkinson's disease, 396
  Amyotrophic lateral sclerosis, 398
  Alzheimer's disease, 399
Interference with function because of vascular conditions,
      400
  Cerebrovascular accident, 400
Intracerebral hemorrhage, 406
Interference with function because of infection/
      inflammation, 408
  Meningitis, 408
  Encephalitis, 410
  Brain abscess, 410
  Poliomyelitis, 411
  Guillain-Barré-Strohl syndrome (polyneuritis), 411
  Neurosyphilis, 412
  Herpes zoster, 412
Interference with function because of trauma, 413
  Craniocerebral trauma, 413
  Spinal cord trauma, 417
  Peripheral nerve trauma, 422
  Trigeminal neuralgia, 424
  Bell's palsy (peripheral facial paralysis), 425
Interference with function because of tumors, 425
  Intracranial tumors, 425
  Intravertebral tumors, 433

21 The patient with eye problems, 436

Barbara C. Long

Anatomy and physiology, 436
  Anatomy of the eye, 436
  Physiology of vision, 437
Prevention and health education, 437
  Promotion of visual acuity, 438
  Promotion of eye safety, 441
  Secondary prevention, 441
Visually handicapped: blind, 442
  Impaired vision, 443
  Responses to loss of vision, 443
  Nursing activities for the newly blind, 443

Major health problems of the eye, 444
Inflammatory eye disorders, 444
Cataract, 451
Glaucoma, 453
Retinal detachment, 457

22 The patient with ear problems, 460

Linda Anne Broseman

Anatomy and physiology, 460
  External ear, 460
  Middle ear, 460
  Inner ear, 460
  Sound waves and hearing, 461
Prevention of hearing difficulties, 462
  Care of healthy ears, 462
  Prevention of ear infections, 463
  Monitoring side effects of ototoxic drugs, 463
  Monitoring noise pollution, 463
Impaired hearing: deafness, 464
  Implications of impaired hearing, 464
  Early identification of hearing loss, 464
  Classification of hearing loss, 465
  Assessment of auditory acuity, 465
  Aural rehabilitation, 468
  Communicating with the hearing-impaired person, 472
Major health problems of the ear, 473
Inflammations of the ear, 473
Otosclerosis, 475
Labyrinthine disorders, 475

23 The patient with musculoskeletal disorders, 480

Grace McCarthy Harlan

Anatomy and physiology, 480
  Components of the musculoskeletal system, 480
  Classification of joints, 482
  Physiologic changes with aging, 483
Prevention and health education, 483
  Persons at risk and risk factors, 483
Preventive health teaching, 484
  Promotion of safety, 484
Major health problems of the musculoskeletal system, 487
Inflammatory disorders, 487
  Rheumatoid arthritis, 487
  Systemic lupus erythematosus, 497
  Polymyositis (dermatomyositis), 498
  Ankylosing spondylitis, 499
Nonarticular rheumatism, 500
  Bursitis, 500
  Carpal tunnel syndrome, 501
  Dupuytren's contracture, 502
Restrictive disorders, 502
  Degenerative joint disease, 502
  Degenerative joint disease of the spine, 504
  Scoliosis, 505
Other rheumatic disorders, 507
  Gout, 507
  Bacterial arthritis, 508
Trauma, 509
  Fracture of bone and soft tissue injury, 509
  Fracture of the hip, 513

UNIT VII

Gas Transport Problems

24 The patient with nose and throat problems, 527

Linda Anne Broseman

Anatomy and physiology, 527
  Nose and sinuses, 527

  Upper throat: pharynx and tonsils, 527
  Lower throat: larynx and hypopharynx, 529
Major health problems of the nose and throat, 529
Inflammations of the nose and throat, 529
Obstructive disorders of the nose and throat, 534
Malignancies of the nose and throat, 537
  Surgery, 538

25 The patient with pulmonary problems, 543

Wilma J. Phipps

Anatomy and physiology of the respiratory tract, 543
  Pulmonary ventilation, 545
  Control of respiration, 545
  Gas exchange in the lung, 545
  Oxygen–carbon dioxide exchange, 545
Physiologic changes with aging, 548
Prevention and health education, 548
  Primary prevention: prevention of disease, 548
  Secondary prevention: early detection, 549
Major health problems of the respiratory system, 549
Restrictive pulmonary disorders, 549
  Infectious diseases of the pulmonary tract, 549
  Occupational lung diseases, 570
  Adult respiratory distress syndrome, 575
  Cancer of the lung, 576
Chest trauma, 592
  Fractures of the ribs, 592
  Paradoxical breathing, 593
  Penetrating chest wounds, 594
  Pneumothorax, 595
Obstructive lung diseases, 595
  Chronic obstructive pulmonary disease, 595
Respiratory insufficiency and respiratory failure, 612
  Epidemiology and etiology, 612
  Pathophysiology and clinical picture, 612
  Intervention, 613

26 The patient with cardiovascular problems, 626

Eileen Walsh-Essig, H. Fred Farley, and Mary A. (Sandy) Wyper

Anatomy and physiology, 626
  Basic structure of the heart, 626
  Conduction system, 628
  Cardiac cycle, 628
  Cardiac output, 630
Cardiac arrhythmias, 632
  Electrocardiogram (ECG), 632
  Cardiac monitors, 635
  Format for rhythm interpretation, 635
  Common arrhythmias, 639
  Treatment modalities, 644
Major health problems of the heart, 650
Coronary artery disease, 650
  Pathophysiology, 650
  Angina pectoris, 652
  Myocardial infarction, 656
  Cardiac surgery for myocardial ischemia, 659
Cardiogenic shock, 663
Congestive heart failure, 665
  Pulmonary edema, 673
Inflammatory heart disorders, 674
Valvular heart disease, 679
Aneurysms, 686

27 Peripheral vascular diseases, 693

Grace McCarthy Harlan and Barbara J. Daly

Anatomy and physiology, 693
  Arteries, 693
  Capillaries, 693
  Veins, 695

xvi   Detailed contents

Lymphatic system, 695
Physiologic changes with aging, 696
Prevention and health education, 696
Risk factors, 697
Counseling and teaching, 697
Major health problems of the peripheral vascular system, 698
Arterial disorders, 699
Venous and lymph disorders, 713
Thrombophlebitis, 713
Varicose veins, 717
Lymphedema, 719
Hypertension, 720

28   The patient with hematologic problems, 728
Rosemarie M. Hogan and Deanna Melton Xistris

Anatomy and physiology, 728
Components of the hematopoietic system, 728
Physiologic changes with aging, 731
Prevention and health education, 731
Major health problems related to blood and lymph systems, 732
Disorders associated with erythrocytes, 732
Anemia secondary to blood loss, 732
Anemia secondary to impaired production of RBCs: aplastic anemia, 733
Anemia secondary to increased destruction of RBCs: hemolytic anemia, 738
Anemia secondary to nutritional deficiency, 741
Erythrocytosis (polycythemia), 742
Coagulation disorders, 742
Platelet disorders—thrombocytopenia, 742
Hemophilia, 745
Disseminated intravascular coagulation, 747
Disorders associated with white blood cells, 748
Changes in number of white cells, 748
Leukemia, 748
Disorders associated with the lymph system, 752
Lymphadenopathy, 752
Lymphomas, 752

UNIT VIII

Metabolic and Endocrine Problems

29   The patient with diabetes mellitus, 759
Dorothy Blevins and Virginia L. Cassmeyer

Anatomy and physiology, 759
Hormonal regulation of blood glucose, 759
Classification of diabetes mellitus, 761
Prevention and health education, 762
Primary prevention, 762
Secondary prevention: detection of DM, 764
Pathophysiology, 765
Hyperglycemia, 765
Hyperglycemic, hyperosmolar, nonketotic coma, 765
Diabetic ketoacidosis, 767
Macrovascular changes, 767
Microvascular changes, 768
Neuropathy, 768
Lower extremity changes, 769
Assessment, 770
Subjective data, 770
Objective data, 770
Data analysis and planning, 770
Nursing diagnoses, 770
Expected patient outcomes, 770
Implementation, 770
Assisting with achievement of therapeutic goals, 770
Teaching directed toward self-care, 781
Evaluation, 788

30   The patient with endocrine problems, 791
Dorothy Blevins and Virginia L. Cassmeyer

Anatomy and physiology, 792
Pituitary gland, 792
Adrenal glands, 794
Thyroid and parathyroid glands, 794
Hormonal regulation, 795
Receptor activity, 795
Hypersecretion and hyposecretion, 795
Prevention of disease and health education, 796
Primary prevention, 796
Secondary prevention, 796
Tertiary prevention, 796
Major health problems of the endocrine system, 796
Anterior pituitary dysfunction, 797
Posterior pituitary dysfunction, 804
Adrenal gland dysfunction, 807
Parathyroid dysfunction, 816
Thyroid dysfunction, 821

31   The patient with hepatic, biliary and pancreatic problems, 832
Dorothy R. Blevins and Virginia L. Cassmeyer

Anatomy and physiology, 832
Hepatic system, 832
Biliary system, 834
Pancreatic system, 834
Prevention and health education, 835
Primary prevention, 835
Secondary prevention: detection of disease, 836
Major health problems, 839
Disorders of the liver, 839
Disorders of the biliary system, 861
Disorders of the pancreas, 867

UNIT IX

Problems of Digestion or Elimination

32   The patient with gastrointestinal problems, 875
Barbara C. Long

Anatomy and physiology, 875
Mouth and esophagus, 875
Stomach, 877
Intestines, 877
Physiologic changes with aging, 878
Prevention and health education, 878
Primary prevention: prevention of disease, 878
Secondary prevention: early detection, 878
Major health problems of the gastrointestinal system, 880
Interference with gastrointestinal motility and control, 880
Common dysfunctions, 880
Esophageal disorders, 883
Paralytic (adynamic) ileus, 889
Inflammatory disorders of the gastrointestinal system, 893
Inflammatory disorders of the mouth, 893
Acute inflammatory disorders of stomach and intestines, 895
Chronic inflammatory bowel disorders, 897
Anorectal lesions, 904
Peptic ulcer, 906
Malabsorption syndrome, 917
Obstructive disorders, 918
Intestinal obstruction, 919
Hernias, 920
Cancer of the gastrointestinal tract, 920
Cancer of the mouth, 920
Cancer of the stomach, 924
Cancer of the bowel, 927

33 The patient with urinary problems, 940

H. Fred Farley and Paula Lambrecht Miller

Anatomy, 941
Physiology, 942
  Physiologic changes with aging, 943
  Prevention and health education
Assessment of renal function, 944
  Subjective data, 945
  Objective data, 946
  Diagnostic tests, 946
Major health problems of the urinary system, 955
Congenital disorders, 955
  Pathophysiology, 956
  Assessment, 957
  Polycystic disease, 957
Inflammatory disorders, 958
  Urinary tract infections, 959
  Chemical induced nephritis, 961
  Glomerulonephritis, 961
  Chronic glomerulonephritis, 962
  Nephrotic syndrome, 964
  Pyelonephritis, 966
Vascular disorders, 967
  Renal artery stenosis, 167
  Nephrosclerosis, 968
  Diabetic nephropathy, 968
  Assessment and implementation for vascular disorders,
    968
Obstructive disorders, 968
  Renal calculi, 969
  Renal neoplasms, 974
  Benign prostatic hypertrophy, 975
  Urethral strictures, 979
  Intervention for urinary retention, 979
  Assessment, 987
  Implementation, 987
  Evaluation, 987
Urinary incontinence, 987
  Assessment, 989
  Control of urinary incontinence, 989
  Intervention related to cause, 989
  Bladder retraining, 990
  Urinary drainage for incontinence, 991
  Data analysis and planning, 992
  Nursing diagnoses, 992
  Implementation, 993
  Evaluation, 993
Trauma to the urinary tract, 993
  Data analysis and planning, 993
Renal failure, 994
  Acute renal failure, 994
  Chronic renal failure, 1000
  Medical treatment of patients with end-stage renal
    disease, 1011
  Kidney transplantation, 1020

UNIT X

Sexual and Reproductive Problems

34 Sexuality in health and illness, 1027

Nancy Fugate Woods

Sexuality and health, 1027
  Evolution of human sexuality, 1027
  Physiologic aspects of human sexuality, 1028
  Sexuality and aging, 1030
  Variations in sexual expression, 1031
Sexuality and illness, 1032
  Changes in body structure, 1032
  Changes in body function, 1033

  Effects of pharmacologic agents, 1034
  Body image changes, 1036
  Environmental restrictions, 1036
Sexual concerns, difficulties, and dysfunctions, 1037
  Sexual concerns, 1037
  Sexual difficulties, 1037
  Sexual dysfunctions, 1037
  Gender disorders, 1038
Nursing practice, 1038
  Prerequisites for intervention, 1038
  Prevention of sexual problems, 1039
  Assessment, 1040
  Promotion of sexual health, 1041

35 The patient with reproductive problems, 1044

Barbara C. Long and Greer Glazer

Anatomy and physiology, 1044
  Female genital system, 1044
  Male genital system, 1047
  Physiologic changes with aging, 1047
Prevention and health education, 1049
  Prevention of infection, 1049
  Early detection of cancer, 1049
  Health teaching related to menstruation and
    menopause, 1050
Interferences with reproduction, 1052
  Sterilization, 1052
  Infertility, 1055
Major health problems of the reproductive system, 1057
Disorders in women, 1057
  Inflammatory disorders, 1057
  Structural disorders, 1061
  Tumors, 1065
  Cancer, 1068
Disorders in men, 1073
  Inflammatory disorders, 1073
  Structural disorders, 1075
  Tumors, 1075
  Epidemiology, 1078
  Sexual transmission, 1079
  Prevention and control, 1080
  Gonorrhea, 1081
  Syphilis, 1082
  Herpes genitalis, 1083

36 The patient with problems of the breast, 1085

Barbara C. Long

Prevention and health education, 1085
  Avoidance of common breast problems, 1085
  Early detection of malignancy, 1086
Diagnostic tests for breast evaluation, 1088
  Radiographs, 1088
  Aspiration, 1088
  Breast biopsy, 1088
Benign breast disorders, 1089
Cancer of the breast, 1092
Metastatic disease, 1101

UNIT XI

Problems of Physiologic Defense Mechanisms

37 The patient with dermatologic problems, 1105

Barbara C. Long

Anatomy and physiology, 1105
  Anatomy, 1105
  Physiology, 1106
  Skin changes with aging, 1106
Psychologic effects of dermatologic problems, 1107

Prevention and health education, 1107
Major health problems of the skin, 1108
Inflammatory skin disorders, 1108
Dermatitis, 1114
Scaling papular disorders, 1117
Skin reactions from systemic diseases, 1118
  Dermatitis medicamentosa, 1118
  Erythema multiforme, 1119
  Discoid lupus erythematosus, 1119
Tumors of the skin, 1120
  Preventive measures, 1120
  Surgical removal, 1120
  Malignant melanoma, 1121
Skin disorders in blacks, 1121
  Traumatic alopecia, 1122
  Pseudofolliculitis barbae, 1122
  Keloids, 1122
Plastic surgery, 1122
  General care of the patient having plastic surgery, 1122
  Skin grafting, 1123
  Cosmetic surgery, 1125

38   The patient with burns, 1128
Penny O'Malley

Prevention and health education, 1128
  Environmental changes, 1128
  Health teaching, 1129
Pathophysiology of burns, 1129
  Classification of burns, 1129
  Pathophysiology of severe burns, 1129
Assessment, 1134
  Subjective data, 1134
  Objective data, 1135
Data analysis and planning, 1135
  Nursing diagnoses, 1135
  Expected patient outcomes, 1135
Implementation, 1135
  Prehospital emergency care, 1135
  Assisting with achievement of therapeutic goals, 1136
  Promoting comfort, 1141
  Counseling and teaching, 1141
Evaluation, 1143

39   The patient with immunologic problems, 1145
Barbara C. Long and E. Ronald Wright

Major health problems of the immune system, 1145
Immunodeficiencies, 1145
Gammopathies, 1148
  Multiple myeloma, 1149
Hypersensitivity reactions, 1149
  Type I hypersensitivities, 1149
  Type II hypersensitivities (cytotoxic), 1155
  Type III hypersensitivities (immune complex), 1157
  Type IV hypersensitivities (cell mediated), 1157
Autoimmune diseases, 1159

UNIT XII

Emergencies and Disasters

40   Problems encountered in emergencies and disasters, 1163
Barbara C. Long

Prevention of accidents, 1163
  Home, 1164
  Community, 1164
  Hospitals, 1164
Delivery of emergency care, 1165
  Community, 1165

Hospitals, 1165
Legal aspects of emergency care, 1166
Assessment, 1166
  Data collection, 1166
  Data analysis, 1167
General interventions, 1168
  Principles of management, 1168
  Psychologic support, 1169
Cardiopulmonary problems, 1169
  Airway obstruction and breathing difficulties, 1169
  Cardiopulmonary resuscitation, 1170
  Special cardiopulmonary problems, 1173
  Hemorrhage, 1174
Poisoning, 1175
Environmental injuries, 1178
  Heat, 1178
  Cold, 1178
  Radiation, 1178
Musculoskeletal injuries, 1179
  Wounds, 1179
  Fractures, 1182
Sexual assault: rape, 1183
  Rape crisis centers, 1183
  Rape trauma syndrome, 1183
  Prevention and health care, 1183
  Assessment, 1184
  Intervention, 1184
Disasters, 1185
  Effect of disasters, 1185
  Roles of nurses in disasters, 1185
  Prevention, 1186
  Assessment, 1187
  Intervention, 1187

UNIT XIII

Critical Care Nursing

41   Care of the patient in a critical care unit, 1191
Maura Hopkins

Environment in the critical care area, 1192
  Physical environment, 1192
  Psychologic environment: stress on patient and staff, 1192
Assessment of the critically ill patient, 1193
  Nursing history, 1193
  Physical examination, 1194
  Monitored data, 1194
  Baseline assessment, 1199
Interventions for the critically ill patient, 1199
  Alleviation and prevention of physiologic and physical stressors, 1199
  Alleviation and prevention of psychologic stressors, 1204
  Alleviation and prevention of social stressors for patient and family, 1206

Appendixes

A   Normal laboratory values, 1211

B   Abbreviations in common usage, 1221

C   Recommended daily dietary allowances, revised 1980, 1224

Color plates

Following p. 1102

Plates 1 to 6   The patient with dermatologic problems

Plates 7 to 12   The patient with burns

UNIT I
Medical-Surgical Nursing Practice

1 Perspectives of Medical-Surgical Nursing
2 Nursing Process: A Systematic Approach
3 Nursing History and Physical Examination
4 Quality Assurance in Nursing

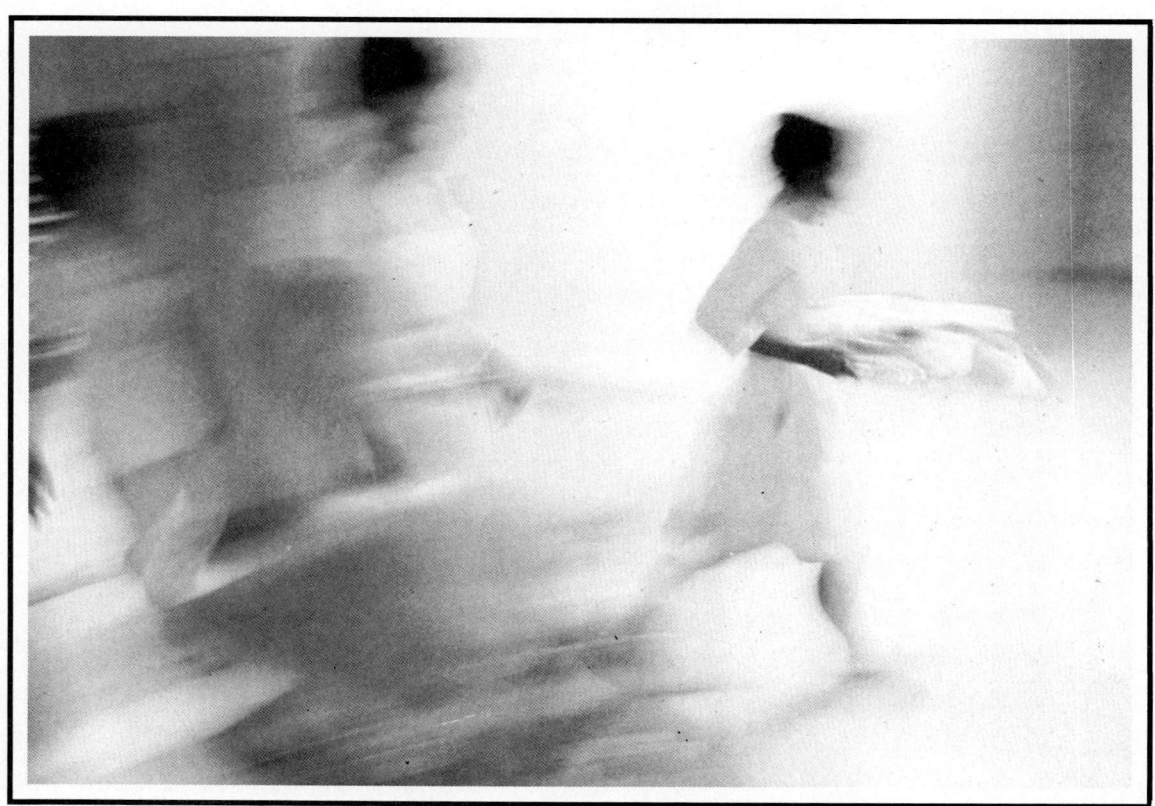

1

Perspectives of Medical-Surgical Nursing

BARBARA C. LONG

STUDY QUESTIONS

- Describe in your own words the difference between being "ill" and having a disease.

- Ask five of your patients how they feel in terms of being "ill." Compare their responses.

- Think of some practices you follow to promote health or prevent disease. Now think of any practices that are deterrents to health. How difficult would it be for you to change your behavior?

- What effect do you think there would be if the nurse smoked a cigarette when teaching a patient the ill effects of smoking?

SCOPE OF MEDICAL-SURGICAL NURSING

Medical-surgical nursing practice encompasses the nursing care of persons who are at risk for or who are experiencing pathophysiologic disorders. In most health care centers children are separated from adults because of their different needs, and the specialty practice of pediatric nursing has developed with the focus on the nursing care of children. Thus medical-surgical nursing practice has developed primarily as the nursing care of persons (1) who have attained physical/developmental maturity, (2) who are at risk for or who have expressed variations in their personal norms of physical functioning, and (3) who may require therapeutic medical or surgical intervention.

In the past the term *medical care* was the general term for the care given sick persons by professionals; it is now used to denote the care given by members of the medical profession (physicians). The trend in American society is toward a health orientation; therefore the term *health care* is the more acceptable term for the care provided by all health care professionals. The term *health care* is broader in that it includes assisting people to stay well in addition

to providing care when they are ill. The care of the sick remains a primary responsibility of health care professionals, and this care is still provided primarily in health care institutions such as acute care hospitals or long-term care centers. There is an increased use, however, of ambulatory care, primary care, and family care centers as well as other types of health care services, in part because it is more economic to keep people well than to provide care when they are sick.[4]

Nurses are one group of health care professionals. In addition to participating in health promotion, nurses are becoming more actively involved in prevention of disease and health education for persons who are at high risk for acquiring specific diseases. Health promotion, disease prevention, and care of persons with specific pathophysiologic disorders require a knowledge base of the following:

1. Health and illness
2. Factors influencing the occurrence and course of specific disorders
3. Common responses to the disorders
4. Nursing interventions that assist the person to achieve optimal health or to die with maximum comfort and dignity

HEALTH AND ILLNESS

Health and illness are complex concepts, and they are interpreted in different ways by different individuals or groups. Both health and illness are multidimensional concepts; that is to say, there are multiple aspects to be considered and multiple factors that may be of influence.

Definitions of health

During the early centuries health was defined in terms of that which was normal or natural. Therefore anything abnormal or against nature was considered not healthy and to be avoided; for example, lepers were called "unclean." Treatment of diseases consisted of amulets or spells to drive out the evil or unnatural spirits causing the abnormality. "Leeching" was a popular treatment and consisted of applying leeches (blood-sucking worms) to suck out the tainted blood. Wounds were treated by cautery to burn out the evil forces that would prevent healing. Even in more modern times, "tonics," which often included a laxative, were taken frequently by persons to stay healthy.

In later years health was defined primarily as freedom from disease. During the middle of the 20th century the concept of *mental health* was introduced, meaning the ability of the individual to cope successfully with stress in a functional manner. In 1974 the World Health Organization (WHO) defined health more broadly: complete physical, mental, and social well-being and not merely the absence of disease and infirmity. This definition introduced the concept of the subjective as well as the objective physical or behavioral responses.

The various views about health usually contain one or more of the following perspectives:

Biologic or clinical: absence of pathology
Psychologic: well-being and self-actualization
Sociologic: ability to meet social responsibilities and role functions
Adaptive: adaptation to a changing environment.

Patients and health care providers may have different views of health and may therefore be working toward different goals that may or may not be in conflict. For example, people who "feel well" and who hold the view that health is a sense of well-being may not be willing to follow-up on screening tests even when a disease may be suspected by the clinician.

Health is a dynamic, ever-changing state. It reflects the person's level of functioning in various physiologic, psychologic, and sociocultural dimensions. People can simultaneously be functioning at a high level in one aspect, such as nutrition, but at a low level in another aspect, such as oxygenation or self-esteem. Nursing is concerned with holistic health, the effect of functioning of the subcomponents on total functioning. Thus each patient is assessed in various dimensions, with consideration given for the person's overall functioning and sense of well-being. Each person presents different genetic factors and is exposed to different environmental factors. There is therefore *no one* nursing approach for all persons who are at risk for or who have a specific illness, disease, or injury. The approach used by nurses to provide care to a specific patient will depend on the pertinent factors unique to that patient.

Health promotion and prevention

The goal of nursing is to assist people to achieve optimal health, the highest level of functioning that is achievable for each person. This includes activities that promote health and prevent illness.

HEALTH PROMOTION

Health promotion refers to activities directed toward helping persons maintain or achieve a high level of functioning and feeling of well-being. The nursing activities include teaching, counseling, and motivating persons to develop life-styles that include adequate nutrition, exercise, and rest or relaxation. Persons functioning at a high level have an increased capacity to withstand physical and emotional stressors.[21] (See Chapter 7 for further information on health promotion.)

Health promotion activities are carried out whenever the opportunities occur. Thus health teaching and counseling are instituted not only with well persons but also when persons are hospitalized. For example, teaching about adequate nutrition can be done while assisting a patient to select items from a hospital menu.

PREVENTION

Prevention refers to activities directed toward protecting persons from potential or actual threats to health and the subsequent consequences.[19] In other words, prevention means inhibiting the development of disease, slowing down the progression of disease, and protecting the body from further harmful effects. There are three different levels of protection: primary, secondary, and tertiary (Table 1-1).

Primary prevention

Primary prevention includes specific protective measures against disease or trauma, such as immunizations against diphtheria or measles, environmental sanitation, and protection against occupational hazards (for example, wearing safety glasses to prevent eye injuries). Early successes in primary prevention have been the result of activities directed at preventing the occurrence of infectious diseases such as polio or smallpox through immunization and typhoid fever through purification of water. More recently dental caries have been prevented by fluoridation of water supplies.

The major health problems today are chronic diseases and accidental injuries and their sequela, both of which require modification of deeply rooted behaviors such as the use of alcohol, tobacco, and drugs; poor driving habits; and poor nutritional and exercise patterns.[17] Health promotion activities are considered a form of primary prevention.

Table 1-1. Levels of prevention

Level	Definition	Examples
Primary	Prevention of disease	Immunization, environmental sanitation, accident prevention, anticipatory counseling and guidance (for example, premarital counseling)
Secondary	Early detection and treatment of disease	Screening for tuberculosis, diabetes, glaucoma Self-breast examination or self-testes examination for cancer Outpatient mental health programs
Tertiary	Prevention of complications, rehabilitation	Prevention of complications of immobility Cardiac rehabilitation programs

Secondary prevention

Secondary prevention includes early detection and prompt intervention to stop the disease at an early stage, decrease the intensity, or prevent complications. This is accomplished by screening for diseases such as diabetes, carcinoma in situ, tuberculosis, or glaucoma. The purpose is to detect early symptoms about which the patient is unaware or lacks the knowledge, so that prompt intervention is effective for control or cure. Screening for contacts of persons with sexually transmitted diseases and treating the infected person to prevent spread of the disease are other examples of secondary prevention.

Tertiary prevention

Tertiary prevention consists of activities that prevent or limit disabilities and help restore the person with a disability to an optimal level of functioning (that is, rehabilitation). Tertiary prevention begins in the early period of recovery from an illness and includes activities such as moving and turning immobile patients to prevent respiratory complications or decubiti, encouraging leg exercises to prevent muscle weakness, and encouraging or assisting with range of motion exercises to prevent contractures.

Rehabilitation programs for persons with cardiac disease or with disabilities resulting from a cerebral vascular accident (stroke) are initiated before the patient is discharged from the hospital. Chapter 16 discusses the concept of rehabilitation in more detail. Preventive measures for specific disorders are described in the appropriate chapters of this text.

At risk status

Some persons are considered to have a greater possibility of becoming ill or acquiring a specific disease because of the presence of certain factors. These persons are considered to be *at risk* and the specific factors are termed *risk factors*. For example, a woman over age 35 with a family history of breast cancer who had her first menstrual period before age 12 and who has never had a child would be considered at high risk for developing breast cancer because several of the known risk factors for breast cancer are present. This woman may not develop breast cancer, but there is a greater than normal probability that she might.

Some risk factors, such as age and genetic factors, cannot be altered, whereas other factors, such as smoking or diet, are under the control of the person. To alter the risk factor, persons need to receive information related to the specific health threats. Persons frequently test the validity of health information by asking lay persons and professionals about the specific risks. Knowing about the risks does not always result in altered behavior, since some persons receive satisfaction from the risk behaviors and deny the risk for themselves, even in the presence of contradictory information, saying, in effect, "It won't happen to me." Frequently there is no direct causal relationship, therefore the behaviors are easy for some persons to dismiss. There are also no immediate tangible rewards for engaging in the desired behaviors. Some persons therefore deliberately choose to continue engaging in the risk behaviors.

To promote health behaviors that decrease the at risk status, people first have to receive the information. Then positive reinforcement for altering behavior is more effective than negative comments about the at risk behaviors. Group sessions (such as weight loss groups or smoker's groups) may be helpful when participants reinforce each other's positive behaviors. Finally, health care professionals should be *role models,* demonstrating the desired health behaviors.

Illness

Although the terms *illness* and *disease* are sometimes used interchangeably, the terms do not relate to the same concepts. A person with a chronic disease such as diabetes may say, "I feel well." Illness is a more abstract term than disease and is essentially the opposite of wellness. Both illness and wellness have a strong subjective component, that of feeling ill or that of feeling well. Illness implies malfunctioning, a lower level of functioning.

Humans are constantly responding and adapting to changes in the external and internal (body) environments. There are a variety of chemical, physical, biologic, and psychosocial factors in the external environment that can influence a person's functioning (Table 1-2). Defense mechanisms, either biologic (Chapter 6) or psychologic (Chapter 10), serve to protect the person from environmental factors that may cause harm. Illness results when defense mechanisms become inadequate or inappropriate.

Table 1-2. Environmental factors affecting health

Type	Examples	Possible effects
Chemical	Lead, arsenic	Poisoning
	Cholesterol	Myocardial infarction
Physical	Automobiles	Accidents
	High noise level	Deafness
	Heat	Burns, heatstroke
	Cold	Frostbite, hypothermia
	Radiation	Cancer
Biologic	Bacteria, virus, fungi	Infections
Psychosocial	Stress	Ulcers, hypertension

A relatively stable internal environment is necessary for cellular growth and functioning. The process of maintaining this relatively constant environment is the process of *homeostasis* or *dynamic equilibrium*. The term *dynamic equilibrium* is more descriptive because it implies fluctuations within a normal range rather than a static condition. Maintaining a dynamic equilibrium involves an adequate exchange of oxygen and carbon dioxide through respiration, an adequate nutrient supply to meet basal metabolic needs, and a normal balance of fluids and electrolytes. Variations above or below ranges of normal lead to illness and disease.

Disease

Diseases are specific pathologic conditions with characteristic signs and symptoms. Diseases may involve a specific organ or body part or may affect the body as a whole. Functioning of the part or body system may be impaired. The body has many integrated defense mechanisms and compensatory responses that maintain functioning for a period of time when a threat to the system occurs, but if the causative factors or stressors persist, altered structure or functioning results. Terms commonly used when discussing specific diseases are listed in the box below.

Diseases have a natural life history, usually progressing through stages. The time factor varies; acute diseases have a sudden onset and are usually of short duration, whereas chronic diseases often have a gradual or indefinite onset and have a longer duration. In the first stage of development of a disease, the *presymptomatic* or *subclinical stage,* the pathogenic changes have started to occur but there are no detectable signs or symptoms. Examples of this stage are the formation of atheromatous plaques in the coronary vessel or early malignant growth.[17] The second stage, the *clinical stage,* is characterized by the presence of signs and symptoms. It is at this stage that the person seeks help. The third stage, the *rehabilitation stage,* occurs with chronic diseases and is characterized by residual disabilities. During this stage the person must learn how to adapt to changes in life-style that result from the disability and learn how to prevent further disability.

Terminology used with disease

Acute	Disease with sudden onset and short duration
Chronic	Disease of long duration
Sign	Observable change in body function (objective)
Symptoms	Change in body function, usually expressed by the patient (subjective)
Syndrome	Cluster of signs and symptoms that collectively indicate alternate functioning
Incidence	Frequency of occurrence of a disease
Onset	Beginning of a disease
Course	Pattern of development of a disease
Duration	Length of time disease is present
Prognosis	Ultimate outcome
Morbidity	Number of persons having the disease in a given population
Mortality	Number of persons who die from the disease
Spontaneous resolution	Healing occurs with little or no treatment
Therapeutic intervention	Treatment directed toward a cure or alleviation of signs and symptoms

Illness behavior and sick role

When people perceive that they are ill, they may take action for relief of symptoms; they may decide to take no action; or they may vacillate between action and no action. Persons who decide to take action may seek help from a friend or family member, from a "folk-specialist" (someone of their cultural group who is frequently consulted about illness), from a professional such as a minister, or from a health care professional. Non-health care persons may either deal with the problems themselves or refer the patient to someone else. Often these people act as gatekeeper in helping make the decision when and from whom the sick person should seek help. Persons who perceive they are ill but take no action do so for a variety of reasons. Low income persons are more apt to seek assistance when they are ill if the health care provider or agency is within the community. Some persons know they should take action but some reason holds them back and thus they vacillate between action and no action.

Some persons are labeled as "noncompliant" because they do not follow the directions of the health care provider. Noncompliance is defined as the failure of the person to participate in carrying out the plan of care after initially indicating the intention to comply.[11] Failure to carry out an action may result from some of the same reasons as failure to seek health care rather than a deliberate action of noncompliance.

When illness becomes legitimized by the physician during the clinical stage, the patient assumes the *sick role* and is exempted from normal social roles and responsibilities as required by the type and severity of the illness. The social expectation is that the sick person will seek help and wants to get well. The sick role permits the patient to assume a dependent relationship that facilitates receiving the required health care. Many persons find the sick role undesirable and have difficulty with the enforced dependency, although they see it as necessary to

---

Selected reasons for not seeking health care

Denial that symptoms are present
Symptoms not viewed as important
Fear of consequences (for example, pain, cancer, death)
Fear of health care professionals or health care agencies
Lack of knowledge concerning which symptoms require medical care
Lack of availability of transportation
Lack of money for transportation or health care
Disabilities that hinder getting to health care agency

---

achieve the desired end, that is, wellness. They find it helpful if they are kept informed and allowed to make decisions if they are able and desire to do so. The patient is expected to relinquish the sick role and assume increasing independence during the recovery and rehabilitation stage.

MEDICAL-SURGICAL NURSING PRACTICE

Nursing actions can be divided into two types, independent and interdependent. *Independent* nursing actions are those which the nurse takes after analysis of data pertaining to those aspects of the patient's health that are amenable to nursing intervention. Providing quality care for persons at risk for or experiencing pathophysiologic disorders requires a systematic approach. In recent years the term *nursing process* has become synonymous with the systematic approach used in providing nursing care (Chapter 2).

Interdependent nursing actions are those taken by the nurse in assisting other health care professionals. Nurses are the health care professionals who have the greatest patient contact. They are therefore in a position to assist other professionals by providing additional data through monitoring and by carrying out prescribed treatments patients are unable to do for themselves. As patients are able to assume greater responsibility for their own care, *self-care activities* are promoted.

The ability to plan and implement nursing care, monitor the patient's condition, and carry out treatments effectively requires a sound knowledge base not only about people and factors pertaining to their health but also about the pathophysiologic disorders per se. The following types of knowledge about diseases can be useful in planning and providing patient care: epidemiology and etiology, pathophysiology, signs and symptoms of disease, and medical therapy.

Knowledge of epidemiologic and etiologic factors helps to identify the populations at risk. *Epidemiology* is the study of the incidence, distribution, and determinants of diseases and injuries in human populations. In other words, epidemiology is concerned with the extent of specific diseases or injuries in specific groups of people and the factors that influence that distribution.[17] *Etiology* refers to the specific causes of a disease. Most diseases have *multiple causality;* that is, there are multiple factors working and interacting together that lead to disease occurrence. This is an important point when teaching about prevention of disease, since avoidance of only one factor may not prevent disease occurrence.

Pathophysiology is the study of the effect of disease (pathology) on body organs and systems and on total body functioning. A *pathophysiologic* disorder is one in which there is altered physiologic functioning, as differentiated from a *pathopsychologic* disorder in which there is altered mental functioning. Knowledge of the physiologic effects of pathology and the nature of the compensatory or adaptive responses facilitates understanding of patient re-

---

Definitions of the nature and treatment of disease

Epidemiology	The rate and influencing factors of disease occurrence in given populations
Etiology	The cause of disease
Pathophysiology	Mechanisms and physiologic effects of disease processes
Signs and symptoms	Objective and subjective evidence of disease, including significant results of diagnostic tests
Medical therapy/treatment	Commonly used interventions by physicians directed toward cure/control of diseases, such as pharmacologic and dietary prescriptions, surgery, or radiation treatments

---

Nursing interventions for persons at risk for or who have a pathophysiologic disorder

Health restoration

Assisting with achievement of therapeutic goals
    Monitoring for signs of healing or complications
    Carrying out prescribed medical therapies that the patient is unable to do for self
    Promoting functioning of those mechanisms necessary for optimal health, for example, oxygenation, nutrition, elimination
Promoting comfort and activities of daily living (ADL)
    Promoting physical and psychologic comfort
    Assisting with ADL as necessary until self-care is possible
Modifying the environment to enhance healing and wellness
Counseling and teaching
    Promoting coping and adaptation to changes in health care
    Teaching the patient to care for self

Health maintenance

Monitoring for changes in health status
Teaching the patient and family or friends
    The nature of the illness or disease
    Signs and symptoms indicating presence of disease or complications to be reported to physician
    Health promotion activities (nutrition, activity, etc.)
    Specific preventive measures
    Rationale for medical therapies
    Name, dosage, actions, and side effects of prescribed medications
    Availability of community resources
    Need for continual monitoring or follow-up care, as necessary

sponses for the purposes of monitoring the patient's status for maladaptive responses and teaching the patient about the disease.

Knowledge of the signs and symptoms and medical therapies of common diseases facilitates monitoring for presence and course of diseases, supporting and teaching the patient, and carrying out therapies patients cannot do for themselves.

Nursing interventions

Nursing interventions for persons who are at risk for or who have pathophysiologic disorders are directed toward *restoring* optimal health and *maintaining* optimal health (see box, p. 8). Although the major focus of the care of the person who is ill may be health restoration, health maintenance interventions may be carried on concurrently to help the person maintain optimal functioning wherever possible. The interventions selected for a specific patient will be determined by the identified nursing diagnoses and the specific pathophysiologic disorders present or for which the person is at risk. Possible nursing interventions are described in appropriate chapters in this text.

REFERENCES AND SELECTED READINGS*

1. Alan, D.K., and Boldt, J.: A study of preventive health attitudes and behaviors in a family practice setting, J. Fam. Pract. **11:**77-84, 1980.
2. Alonzo, A.A.: Acute illness behavior: a conceptual exploration and specification, Soc. Sci. Med. **14A:**515-526, 1980.
3. Alonzo, A.A.: Everyday illness: a situational approach to health status deviations, Soc. Sci. Med. **13A:**397-404, 1979.
4. *American Nurses Association: Nursing: a social policy statement, No. NP-63, Kansas City, Mo., 1980, The Association.
5. Demers, R.W., and others: An explanation of the dimensions of illness behavior, J. Fam. Pract. **11:**1085-1092, 1980.
6. *Diekelmann, N.: Wellness: approaches and resources, Nurse Pract. **5:**41-44, 1980.
7. Dougherty, C.J., and Walker, V.R.: Scientific medicine, technology, and the concept of health, Ethics Sci. Med. **5:**75-81, 1978.
8. Dunn, H.L.: What high level wellness means, Health Values: Achieving High Level Wellness **1:**9-16, 1977.
9. Flynn, P.R.: Holistic health: the art and science of care, Bowie, Md., 1980, Robert J. Brady Co.
10. French, R.M.: Dynamics of health care, ed. 3, New York, 1979, McGraw-Hill Book Co.
11. Gordon, M.: Nursing diagnosis: process and application, New York, 1982, McGraw-Hill Book Co.
12. Groer, M.W., and Shekleton, M.E.: Basic pathophysiology: a conceptual approach, ed. 2, St. Louis, 1983, The C.V. Mosby Co.
13. Harris, D.M., and Guten, S.: Health-protective behavior: an exploratory study, J. Health Soc. Behav. **20:**17-29, 1979.
14. *Hover, J., and Juelsgaard, N.: The sick role reconceptualized, Nurs. Forum. **17:**407-416, 1978.
15. *Keller, M.J.: Toward a definition of health, Adv. Nurs. Sci. **4:**43-64, 1980.
16. *Macleod, A.: Illness as a deviant role: a clue to the rejection of symptoms, Nurs. Times **74:**1400-1401, 1978.
17. Mausner, J.S., and Bahn, A.K.: Epidemiology: an introductory text, Philadelphia, 1975, W.B. Saunders Co.
18. Najam, J.M.: Theories of disease causation and the concept of a general susceptibility: a review, Soc. Sci. Med. **14A:**231-237, 1980.
19. *Pender, N.J.: Health promotion in nursing practice, New York, 1982, Appleton-Century-Crofts.
20. Segall, A.: The sick role concept: understanding illness behavior, J. Health Soc. Behav. **17:**163-170, 1976.
21. *Shamansky, S.L., and Clausen, C.L.: Levels of prevention: examination of the concept, Nurs. Outlook **28:**104-108, 1980.
22. Smith, J.A.: The idea of health: a philosophical inquiry, Adv. Nurs. Sci. **3:**42-50, 1981.

---

*References preceded by an asterisk are particularly well suited for student reading.

2

Nursing Process: A Systematic Approach

BARBARA C. LONG

STUDY QUESTIONS

- What are some frameworks that can be used in medical-surgical nursing for data analysis? What framework do you now use? Is this framework adaptable for patients with medical-surgical conditions?

- Differentiate between baseline and ongoing assessment; between subjective and objective data.

- How do the different parts of a nursing diagnosis assist you in planning nursing care?

- Examine the list of nursing diagnoses identified by the National Group on Classification of Nursing Diagnosis. What use could you make of this list?

- Define what is meant by *observable patient behaviors*. Write some examples of goals written in terms of observable patient behaviors.

- Analyze the nursing activities that you carried out in your last three patient assignments in terms of action strategies (Table 2-3). Which strategies did you use? Could you have used any of the remaining strategies?

INTRODUCTION TO NURSING PROCESS

Characteristics and steps

The systematic approach used to carry out nursing's independent functions (p. 7) is frequently termed *nursing process*. It is a way of thinking and acting based on the scientific method rather than on intuition. It provides organization and direction of nursing activities, a means for predicting outcomes and evaluating results, and a method for establishing standards of nursing care. The characteristics of nursing process are listed in the box on p. 11.

Nursing process provides a framework for (1) identification of health care needs amenable to nursing care, (2) determination of patient goals (outcomes) and nursing actions, (3) implementation of nursing actions, and (4) evaluation of results of nursing actions. This systematic process is usually divided into either four or five steps; the overall process is the same regardless of the number of steps. The five-step process is as follows:

1. Assessment: collecting patient data of pertinence to nursing
2. Data analysis: using the collected data to identify the patient's health care needs that can be influenced by nursing care
3. Planning: determining priorities, patient outcomes, and specific nursing actions
4. Implementation: carrying out the planned nursing actions necessary to accomplish the defined goals
5. Evaluation: determining the extent to which the goals have been achieved

Characteristics of nursing process

Systematic	Consists of an organized series of steps
Purposeful	Has as its aim the meeting of nursing needs of the patient
Interactional	Involves interaction among nurse, patient, and significant others
Dynamic	Involves continued action and evaluation until nurse-patient relationship is terminated
Scientific	Is based on a scientific problem-solving approach; provides for identification of recurrent problems, which then initiates nursing research

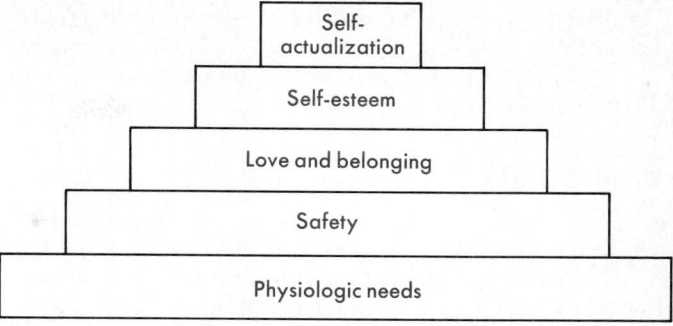

Fig. 2-1. Maslow's hierarchy of needs.

Nurses who use a four-step approach include data analysis as part of assessment; thus the four steps become assessment, planning, implementation, and evaluation.

Frameworks for data collection

Some type of framework for data collection and analysis is necessary to prevent omission of important data and to facilitate analysis and planning. Physicians and some nurses use *body systems* as a framework; for example, data that pertain specifically to the respiratory system would be collected, then analyzed to determine if there is respiratory dysfunction.

A useful framework in the practice of medical-surgical nursing is *human needs*. Maslow describes a hierarchy of needs in which physiologic needs are the most basic, followed by safety, love and belonging, self-esteem, and self-actualization (Fig. 2-1). The needs are ranked in ascending order from the needs that are basic to survival to those that focus on development of self (growth-motivated needs). In principle, the more basic needs are satisfied first. For example, a person who is having difficulty breathing (physiologic need for oxygen) will attend to that need before dealing with a feeling of loss of worth as a person (self-esteem). In most situations, however, the needs in the hierarchy exist simultaneously to different extents. Lower level needs have to be met, at least partially, before seeking gratification of higher order needs. For example, a person may omit a meal to carry out an activity that increases self-esteem. New needs usually emerge gradually except when danger is present or when the person is acutely ill.

Physiologic needs include oxygen, nutrition, elimination, activity, comfort, rest and sleep, and reproduction.

All are vital for existence or survival. (Reproduction is vital for survival of the human race.) *Oxygen* needs include everything that influences (1) taking in oxygen and eliminating carbon dioxide as carried out by the respiratory system and (2) transportation of the gases to and from the tissues as carried out by the circulatory system and its components. *Safety* (security) needs include both protection of self from psychologic threats and protection of self from the physical environment. This requires ability to see and to hear, to activate the body if threatened (neuroendocrine response), and to protect the body from invading microorganisms (immune response and intact skin).

Persons with medical-surgical disorders may also experience threats to the higher order needs of love and self-esteem. Humans have a need to relate to others in a meaningful way (*love and belonging* or *affiliation needs*). Most persons affiliate by means of long-term relationships with one or more persons (family members, close friends). A few persons can meet their belonging needs by indirect approaches, such as through creative endeavors (for example, an artist).

Self-esteem refers to the need to feel good or satisfied with oneself. This includes a feeling of confidence in oneself, of valuing oneself, and of being valued by others. Self-esteem needs are influenced by the person's ability to perceive and cope with changes in the environment. Persons with changes in their appearance (for example, facial disfigurement or amputation) or in body functions (for example, colostomy) are at higher risk of developing problems with affiliation or self-esteem. These changes can influence conscious or unconscious feelings, thoughts, and perceptions of one's body (body image).

The need for *self-actualization* (realizing one's full potential) is one that most individuals are seeking to reach throughout their lives. The need gratification is seldom reached until older age. The need to grow and develop in a meaningful way, however, is always present.

The use of human needs as a framework for nursing care consists of collecting and analyzing data that pertain to each of the need categories to determine (1) if the need is being met satisfactorily, (2) if nursing assistance is necessary to continue meeting the need (such as supporting a specific asset), or (3) if dysfunction is present that requires nursing intervention. The concept of hierarchy of needs is useful during planning of care by helping to set priorities; for example, survival needs would usually take priority over growth needs.

ASSESSMENT

The assessment process consists of collecting data about the patient that are pertinent for providing nursing care. Some of the data may be the same as those collected by other health care professionals but different use is made of the data. The sources and methods of data collection in nursing are listed in Table 2-1.

Initial assessment

Patient data are obtained by a nurse when the patient first enters the hospital or other health-care agency. This initial data base provides a basis for planning nursing care. Specific information that may be collected by patient interview or physical examination is described in Chapter 3. The extent of patient data collected initially depends on the specific circumstances. For example, fewer data would be required for a patient being admitted for a 2-day hospital stay for a hernia repair than for a patient being admitted for an expected longer hospital stay for diagnosis and treatment of a probable malignancy. Many hospitals develop an admission patient data form identifying the data pertinent to their specific patient population.

Data collected from the patient may be *subjective* or *objective* (Table 2-2). The differentiation is important. Subjective data are necessary for providing understanding of the patient's experience and sense of illness or wellbeing, but since they cannot be validated, they are subject to wide interpretation. For example, one person may describe a specific pain intensity as "severe," while another person may describe the same pain intensity as "mild." Objective data are verifiable; for example, each person palpating the same lymph node can describe it as 2 × 3 cm in size, oval shaped, and freely movable. Subjective and objective data are separated in the problem-oriented method of recording (p. 18).

Ongoing assessment

Since health is a dynamic, ever-changing state, assessment must be a continuous process; thus assessment does not end with the data collected on admission. During every nurse-patient interaction, additional data are gathered. These data are used for evaluation of already identified problems and for identification of new problems. A

Table 2-1. Methods of data collection from specific sources

Source	Method
Primary	
Patient	Interview (formal, informal), physical examination, general observations
Secondary	
Family or friends	Interactions
Patient records	Written notes of other health care professionals, nurses's notes, diagnostic reports (laboratory, x-ray films, etc.), admission record
Health team members	Interaction with other nurses, physicians, physical therapist, occupational therapist, social worker, dietitian, respiratory therapist
Literature	Consultation of textbooks (nursing, medical, pharmacologic, nutrition) and journals (nursing, medical)

Table 2-2. Types of data

Type	Definition	Methods	Examples
Subjective	Statements by the person concerning thoughts or feelings (psychologic, physical) that cannot be validated	Interview, interaction	Statements about pain, nausea, itching Statements about fears, desires, beliefs, attitudes, values
Objective	Data perceptible by the external senses that can be validated by others	Inspection, auscultation, palpation, percussion, olfaction	Vomiting, scratching, auditory breath sounds, palpable lymph nodes, breath odor

planned, organized approach is as important for ongoing assessment as it is for the initial assessement.

Observations are made of the patient and the patient's environment. *Baseline observations* establish where a patient is at any point in time and serve as a basis for future comparison. For example, an observation of warm, dry skin made in the morning is useful as a comparison when cold, moist skin is observed later in the day. Baseline observations are made early in the person's admission to the hospital, at the beginning of a time period when a particular nurse will be providing care, and whenever changes occur in the patient's condition or environment, such as a transfer to or from a special care unit.

The ability to make specific pertinent observations depends on knowledge and past experiences. A sound knowledge base facilitates making comprehensive and pertinent observations. Included in the knowledge base is information about the patient's medical diagnosis (usual cause, risk factors, usual symptoms and course, and usual medical treatment).

RECORDING PATIENT DATA

Patient data must be recorded promptly to ensure accuracy and usefulness. The initial patient data include information from the nursing history and physical examination and are recorded and used in analysis and planning of care and to provide a baseline for comparison. The method of recording the data varies with the institution and with the framework used by the nurse for col-

lecting the data. Many hospitals place portions of the patient's chart in or immediately outside the patient's room so that ongoing observations and subsequent actions can be recorded promptly.

DATA ANALYSIS

A framework for data analysis is especially important to facilitate arriving at sound conclusions from the data base. The nurse's own perspective of nursing will guide the data analysis. If the basic human needs approach is used, the data relevant to each need can be grouped and analyzed. One bit of data can influence more than one need; for example, amount of fluid intake affects nutrition, elimination, and oxygen (viscosity of secretions). The process of data analysis is illustrated in Fig. 2-2.

General conclusions

Four general conclusions can be drawn from analysis of data collected for each need:

1. Data are insufficient; more data are necessary to determine if the need is being met.
2. The need is being met by patient, family member, or other health care provider.
3. The need is being met at present, but there is a potential for future difficulty unless nursing action is taken to prevent it.
4. The need is not being met.

If the need is not being met, the decision must be made

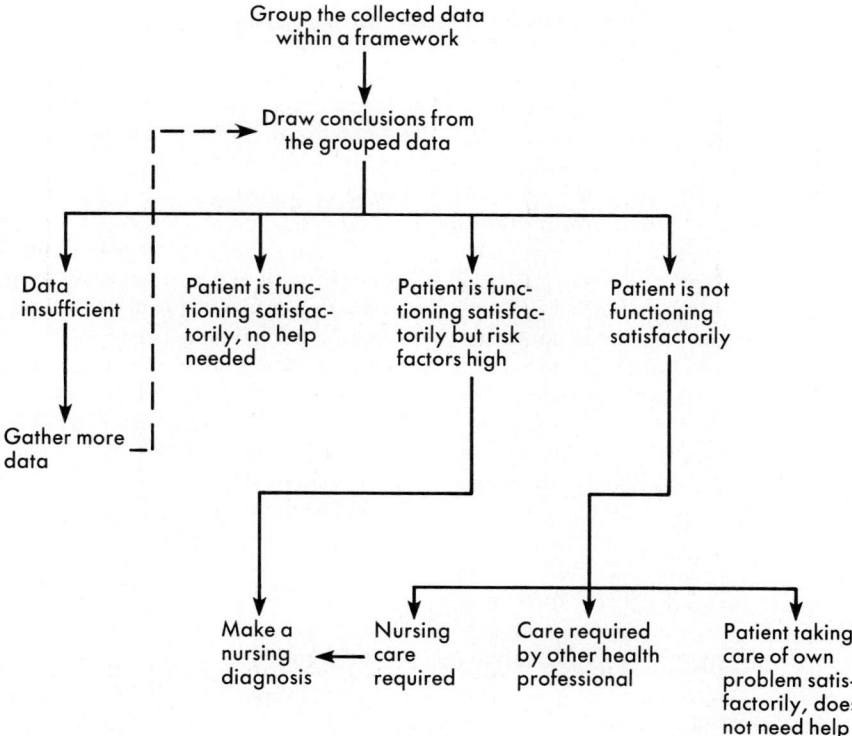

Fig. 2-2. Process of data analysis.

whether (1) the patient is already carrying out actions to meet the need and therefore no further assistance is needed, (2) action is needed that is better carried out by another health professional (nurse makes a referral), or (3) action is needed that requires nursing intervention.

Nursing diagnosis

Before nursing interventions can be planned or carried out, statements must be made that give direction to carrying out nursing care. These statements, frequently called *nursing diagnoses*, are conclusions about the patient that *indicate the need for nursing care.* Medical diagnosis require medical intervention, therefore they are not nursing diagnoses. A person with a medical diagnosis may have nursing diagnoses that relate to the disease. For example, patients with peptic ulcer frequently have a nursing diagnosis of "Pain (epigastric) related to irritation of the ulcer."

The nursing diagnoses statements are *not* limited to dysfunction (patient problems). The patient may be functioning satisfactorily in meeting a specific need but data may indicate that sufficient risk factors are present that, unless certain actions are taken, a problem may develop (that is, potential problem). Patients also may need support and assistance to help *maintain* certain practices. For example, one woman sought assistance from a nurse to help her work through her feelings about caring for her dying mother. The woman was coping satisfactorily but needed support from the nurse to maintain coping. In summary, there are three types of nursing diagnoses, *problems, potential problems,* and *health maintenance.*

A *nursing diagnosis is a succinct two-part statement that indicates (1) a pattern of patient functioning and (2) the factors that influence or are related to the functioning (etiologic factors).* It is important to include the related factors in the statement of the nursing diagnosis for a specific patient, as these factors help provide direction to the selection of pertinent nursing activities. An example of a nursing diagnosis for a specific patient is "Alteration in bowel elimination: constipation related to inactivity." To make a nursing diagnosis from collected patient data, the data must support the diagnosis. For example, with this nursing diagnosis the data base would include data supporting the altered functioning "constipation" (for example, hard dry stool, normal pattern of soft formed stool) and data supporting the etiologic factor "inactivity" (for example, 4 days postoperatively, has spent most of time sitting in a chair, walks only three times daily to door with much encouragement).

Nursing does not at this time have a classification of nursing diagnoses that are generally accepted by all nurses. Several yearly conferences have been held by a group of nurses, the National Conferences on Classification of Nursing Diagnoses,* for the purpose of identifying

*Now called North American Nursing Diagnoses Association (NANDA).

and classifying nursing diagnoses. The nursing diagnoses from the 1982 conference are listed here. The diagnostic categories will continue to be refined and validated.

PLANNING

Planning nursing care involves several steps:
1. Setting priorities when several nursing diagnoses have been identified
2. Determining goals (outcomes) of care for each nursing diagnosis
3. Selecting specific nursing actions

Setting priorities

When several nursing diagnoses have been identified, it must be determined which diagnoses take priority. One approach is the basic needs approach. Nursing diagnoses that pertain to physiologic and safety needs usually take precedence over love and belonging or self-esteem needs.

Priorities can also be determined by considering threats to the integrity of the individual. The following priority system can be used:

First	Immediate life-threatening problems (for example, lack of oxygen)
Second	Threats to physiologic or psychologic integrity for which the person is at *high risk*
Third	Threats to physiologic or psychologic integrity for which the person is at *low risk* (but which may occur if action is not taken)
Fourth	Health maintenance

This system does not deny the importance of health maintenance but emphasizes that when health problems are present, these problems are attended to first.

Goal setting

The next step in planning is to determine the goals or desired patient outcomes to be achieved. There should be *mutual nurse-patient goal setting* whenever possible so that there is congruency between what both the nurse and the patient expect as a result of nursing interventions. The role of the nurse is to facilitate the patient's recovery and future health maintenance; thus both must be moving toward the same goals.

Goals are stated as *observable patient behaviors,* that is, behavior (or signs) that can be observed in the patient if the goal is met. For example, the statement "prevent skin breakdown" is a poor goal, since it indicates nursing action and does not indicate a patient outcome to be met. The same idea stated in observable patient-outcome terms would be "skin on sacral area remains intact, no redness is observed." To evaluate whether this goal had been met, the sacral area would be inspected for signs of redness or breakdown in skin integrity.

Nursing Diagnoses accepted as of the Sixth National Conference (1982) of the North American Nursing Diagnoses Association

Activity intolerance
Airway clearance, ineffective
Anxiety
Bowel elimination, alteration in: constipation
Bowel elimination, alteration in: diarrhea
Bowel elimination, alteration in: incontinence
Breathing pattern, ineffective
Cardiac output, alteration in: decreased
Comfort, alteration in: pain
Communication, impaired verbal
Coping, ineffective individual
Coping, ineffective family: compromised
Coping, ineffective family: disabling
Coping, family: potential for growth
Diversional activity, deficit
Family process, alterations in
Fear
Fluid volume, alteration in: excess
Fluid volume deficit, actual
Fluid volume deficit, potential
Gas exchange, impaired
Grieving, anticipatory
Grieving, dysfunctional
Health maintenance, alteration in
Home maintenance management: impaired
Injury: potential for
Knowledge deficit
Mobility, impaired physical
Noncompliance
Nutrition, alteration in: less than body requirements
Nutrition, alteration in: more than body requirements
Nutrition, alteration in: potential for more than body requirements
Oral mucous membrane, alterations in
Parenting, alteration in: actual or potential
Powerlessness
Rape-trauma syndrome
Self-care deficit: feeding, bathing/hygiene, dressing/grooming, toileting
Self-concept, disturbance in: body image, self-esteem, role performance, personal identity
Sensory perceptual alteration: visual, auditory, kinesthetic, gustatory, tactile, olfactory
Sexual dysfunction
Skin integrity, impairment of: potential
Sleep pattern disturbance
Social isolation
Spiritual distress (distress of the human spirit)
Thought processes, alteration in
Tissue perfusion, alteration in: cerebral, cardiopulmonary, renal, gastrointestinal, peripheral
Urinary elimination, alteration in patterns
Violence, potential for: self-directed or directed at others

Goals are derived primarily from the first part (the pattern of functioning) of the nursing diagnosis statement

Example:

Nursing diagnosis   Decreased muscle strength (legs) related to decreased activity
Long-term goal   Leg muscles return to full baseline strength
Short-term goal   Patient raises legs 2 inches above bed against resistance within 3 days

Long-term goals describe what patient behaviors are expected for resolution of the nursing diagnosis. Short-term goals describe expected patient behaviors indicating that action is headed in the right direction toward resolution, that is, they are short steps to be achieved toward reaching the long-term goal.

Selection of nursing actions

There are usually several alternative actions that can be chosen to reach a desired outcome or goal. Selection of actions is usually guided by the second part (etiologic factors) of the nursing diagnosis. For example, different nursing actions would be selected for a nursing diagnosis of "Insomnia related to fear of surgery" than for a nursing diagnosis of "Insomnia related to persistent cough."

The action alternatives are identified and choices are made depending on the specific patient situation. Patient input is sought when feasible. When a nurse follows a preset plan of action for any given nursing diagnosis, patient care is not individualized and there is less potential for accomplishment of the desired outcomes. The determination of action alternatives is based on knowledge from experts, suggestions from the patient, observations of actions of others, suggestions from other health care providers, and the nurse's own creativity. Actions are based on scientific principles.

Selection of action is based on the following guidelines:
- The greatest possibility of success
- The least risk
- The least discomfort
- The least intrusiveness for the patient

Once the course of action has been selected, the *frequency* of action must also be determined. For example, the frequency of deep breathing and coughing exercises selected as an activity would be planned at different time intervals for different patients based on risk factors such as obesity and smoking habits identified through analysis of the data.

Plans for selected actions are *recorded* so that other persons providing nursing care may follow through, thus providing continuity of care. In some institutions these plans are called *nursing orders*.

IMPLEMENTATION

Action strategies

The nurse can assist the patient meet the goals in a number of ways (Table 2-3). The goal of nursing care is the patient's optimal health; therefore self-care is stressed to the extent possible, since it is the patient who is usually ultimately responsible for on-going health maintenance. Thus teaching, supporting, and motivating are major nursing strategies. If self-care is impossible or inappropriate, the nurse then compensates for the patient's inability by performing the actions. Monitoring is an ongoing strategy; the type and degree usually depend on the illness or disease.

Table 2-3. Action strategies for providing nursing care

Strategy	Definition	Examples of activities
Monitoring	Collecting data on an ongoing basis	Vital signs, intake and output, cardiac monitoring, assessing level of consciousness, skin turgor, urine tests
Compensating (partially or wholly)	Performing or assisting patient to perform necessary activities that patient is unable to or has difficulty performing	Assisting patient with comfort measures, ADL, carrying out prescriptive activities (medication, treatments)
Teaching	Helping patients learn what they can do to maintain or restore optimal health	Health education, methods of disease prevention, teaching skills such as dressing changes, injections, taking vital signs
Supporting	Helping patients cope with changes in life-style, environment, or new experiences	Use of empathy skills to help patient explore feelings, assistance with problem solving, facilitation of coping skills
Motivating	Providing an environment that facilitates achieving optimal health	Encouragement to carry out difficult or painful actions, health maintenance activities

Nursing activities can be directed toward different ends. One categorization that will be followed in this text is as follows:

1. *Assisting with achievement of therapeutic goals.* This category includes those activities directed toward restoration of optimal health. It includes such activities as assisting the person to carry out medical prescriptions (for example, medications, treatments), promoting nutrition and elimination, and maintaining fluid balance.
2. *Assisting with comfort and ADL.* Promotion of comfort is a major nursing activity in the care of patients with pathophysiologic disorders. In addition, some disorders limit the patient's ability to carry out ADL.
3. *Control of environment.* Some pathophysiologic conditions, such as allergies, infections, or immunosuppression, require control of environmental factors such as humidity, dust, or pathogenic organisms.
4. *Counseling and teaching.* Providing patients with support in dealing with their psychosocial needs and teaching the patient are major nursing activities for persons with pathophysiologic disorders.

Not all of the planned care is provided by the professional nurse. Some of the care may be delegated to other health-care providers working under the nurse's supervision.

Recording (documentation)

Actions that have been taken and the patient's response to the actions need to be documented. Responses to monitoring activities are most easily recorded on *flow sheets.* The flow sheets provide a means of quick comparison of a specific monitoring parameter over time. Data such as

Flow sheet

Name: Ms. Smith
Date:

Parameter observed	Third hospital day		Fourth hospital day		Fifth hospital day
	Hour				
	9 PM	11 PM	1 AM	3 AM	4 PM
Vital signs					
Blood pressure	140/100	130/100	128/98	130/100	110/80
Pulse	126	120	118	122	80
Respirations	26	24	24	22	16
Fluid intake					
Oral	Refused	120 ml OJ	Refused	150 ml	240 ml OJ
IV	—	—	—		
Protein snacks	Nauseated	Nauseated		One cheese cracker	Peanut butter crackers
Fluid output					
Urine	—	100 ml	—	200 ml	400 ml
Emesis	50 ml	—	—	100 ml	—
Other	—	—	—	—	—
Patient's behavior state	Hearing voices; moving nervously about in bed	Somewhat calmer; still having auditory hallucinations	Unchanged	Increased restlessness; visual hallucinations	Some tremulousness; embarrassed
Activity	Position changed	Up with assistance to bathroom	Turned	Turned	Up walking and in chair
Sedation	Chlordiazepoxide, 100 mg IM	—		—	—
Mouth care	Done	Done	Done	Done	Self-care
	P. Craig, R.N.	P. Craig, R.N.	J. Fugate, R.N.	N. Yates, R.N.	J. Gelein, R.N.

vital signs, fluid intake and output, activity, and urine tests are recorded as they are gathered. In some institutions these sheets subsequently become part of the patient's permanent record. In others the data are recopied onto other sheets in the permanent record. Flow sheets are used extensively in special care areas such as intensive care units, where continual monitoring of several parameters is necessary.

PROBLEM-ORIENTED RECORD

The problem-oriented system provides a means of following the progress of each identified nursing diagnosis and the patient's response to the planned interventions.

In this approach, baseline data are collected and recorded (the *database*), and a *master problem list* is developed and placed in the front of the patient's record. Each problem is numbered, and subsequent charting identifies the problem being charted by number or name. When there are data suggesting a problem but inadequate data to draw a conclusion, the symptoms are listed as the "problem" until a conclusion can be reached. Each problem is dated when identified and again when resolved. This method of documentation provides easy access to the identification, progress, and resolution of patient problems.

Narrative notes may be used for charting significant data pertaining to each problem, or a *SOAP format* may be used. In the SOAP format, the first two letters, *S* and *O*, refer to sources of the data, that is, subjective and objective data. The last two letters, *A* and *P*, refer to analysis or assessment and to plans for further action. The SOAP format can be used to record the *initial* plan and to record subsequent progress notes.

Evaluation

The last step of nursing process consists of determining whether the desired outcomes were met, analyzing the effectiveness of nursing interventions, and planning for subsequent care. The method of evaluation consists of collecting data from the patient based on the criteria established as patient goals (outcomes). Thus the more specifically the goals were stated in observable patient behaviors, the easier the task of evaluation. For example, a nursing diagnosis of "Constipation related to inadequate fluid intake" could have a goal of "Stool soft and formed." Evaluation would then consist of inspecting the stool. If it were soft and formed, the goal would be achieved and the patient's constipation would be corrected.

Some of the reasons why goals are not achieved are listed in the box below.

Once the possible reason for lack of goal achievement is identified, revisions are made and the process is repeated. As can be noted, nursing care is an ongoing and dynamic process that requires constant assessment and evaluation.

Example of a SOAP format for recording

Problem: Constipation related to inadequate fluid intake

S	"I never have problems at home; my B.M. is usually soft. It was OK 4 days ago."
O	Small hard stool past 2 days. Fluid intake averaging 900 ml/day past 3 days. Taking fluids mostly with meals.
A	Constipation is temporary. Fluid intake needs to be increased to at least 2000 ml/day
P	Evaluate patient's understanding of adequate hydration to promote normal stool. Give 240 ml fruit juice mid-AM, mid-PM, and at bedtime. Encourage patient to drink full glass of water with medications.

Possible reasons for not achieving patient goals

Data base	Incomplete; changes in data
Nursing diagnosis	Inaccurate data analysis; inaccurate statement
Goals	Unrelated to nursing diagnosis; nonspecific; unrealistic
Nursing actions	Unrelated to nursing diagnosis or goal(s); nonspecific, therefore poorly implemented; inadequate in degree of action taken

REFERENCES AND SELECTED READINGS*

1. *Aspinall, M.J.: Nursing diagnosis: the weak link, Nurs. Outlook **24**:433–437, 1976.
2. Becknell, E.P., and Smith, D.M.: System of nursing practice, Philadelphia, 1975, F.A. Davis Co.
3. Bower, F.L.: The process of planning nursing care: a theoretical model, ed. 3, St. Louis, 1982, The C.V. Mosby Co.
4. Bruce, J.: Implementation of nursing diagnosis: a nursing administrator's perspective, Nurs. Clin. North Am. **14**:509–515, 1979.
5. *Calder, M.: How we won the team's support for POMP, Nurs. 81 **11**:27–29, 1981.
6. Campbell, C.: Nursing diagnosis and intervention in nursing practice, New York, 1978, John Wiley & Sons, Inc.
7. Carnevalli, D.: Nursing care planning: diagnosis and management, ed. 3, Philadelphia, 1982, J.B. Lippincott Co.
8. *Dickie, G.L., and Bass, M.J.: Improving problem-oriented medical records through self-audit, Nurs. 80 **10**:487–490, 1980.
9. *Field, L.: The implementation of nursing diagnosis in clinical practice, Nurs. Clin. North Am. **14**:497–508, 1979.
10. Fortin, J.D., and Rabinow, J.: Legal implications of nursing diagnosis, Nurs. Clin. North Am. **14**:553–561, 1979.
11. Fredette, S., and O'Connor, K.: Nursing diagnosis in teaching and curriculum planning, Nurs. Clin. North Am. **14**:541–552, 1979.

*References preceded by an asterisk are particularly well suited for student reading.

12. *Gordon, M.: Manual of nursing diagnosis, New York, 1982, McGraw-Hill Book Co.
13. *Gordon, M.: Nursing diagnosis and the diagnostic process, Nurs. Clin. North Am. **14**:487–496, 1979.
14. *Gordon, M.: Nursing diagnosis: process and application, New York, 1982, McGraw-Hill Book Co.
15. Gordon, M., and Sweeney, M.A.: Methodological problems and issues in identifying and standardizing nursing diagnoses, Adv. Nurs. Sci. **2**:1–15, 1979.
16. Henderson, B.: Nursing diagnosis: theory and practice, Adv. Nurs. Sci. **1**:75–83, 1978.
17. Jones, P.E.: A terminology for nursing diagnoses, Adv. Nurs. Sci. **2**:65–72, 1979.
18. Kim, M.J., and Moritz, D.A., editors: Classification of nursing diagnoses: proceedings of the third and fourth national conferences, New York, 1982, McGraw-Hill Book Co.
19. *Lunney, M.: Nursing diagnosis: refining the system, Am. J. Nurs. **82**:456–459, 1982.
20. Marriner, A.: The nursing process: a scientific approach to nursing care, ed. 3, St. Louis, 1982, The C.V. Mosby Co.
21. Mayers, M.: A systematic approach to the nursing care plan, ed. 2, New York, 1978, Appleton-Century-Crofts.
22. *Mundinger, M.O., and Jauron, G.D.: Developing a nursing diagnosis, Nurs. Outlook **23**:94–98, 1975.
23. *Price, M.R.: Nursing diagnosis: making a concept come alive, Am. J. Nurs. **80**:668–671, 1980.
24. *Shoemaker, J.: How nursing diagnosis helps focus your care, RN **42**:56–61, 1979.
25. Vaughan-Wrobel, B.C., and Henderson, B.S.: The problem-oriented system in nursing, ed. 2, St. Louis, 1981, The C.V. Mosby Co.

3

Nursing History and Physical Examination

BARBARA C. LONG

STUDY QUESTIONS

- You are planning to do a nursing history and physical examination on a newly admitted patient. What would you say to the patient?

- Examine the sample nursing history guide and physical examination guide. Identify for which basic needs each item would apply. (NOTE: An item may be pertinent for more than one basic need.)

- Do a general survey of two or more young adults, middle-aged adults, and older adults. How do the data differ within and among each age group?

- Practice taking a complete nursing history with someone you do not know well. What data were difficult to obtain and for what reason? What transitional sentences were necessary to move from one topic to another?

- Practice doing a head-to-toe physical examination on a family member or friend. Were you systematic? Did it take less than 30 minutes? Write a description of your findings in each category (avoiding the use of words such as "normal").

The health status of an adult is assessed either separately or conjointly by different health care professionals. The same data may be required by different professionals but for different purposes. For example, both the physician and the nurse require data about the nature of a patient's pain. The physician uses the data for diagnosis and treatment of the conditions causing the pain; the nurse uses the data to help the patient achieve the highest degree of comfort.

Different nurses also collect and analyze different types of data, depending on their knowledge and skill level and on their specific patient population. Thus a clinical nurse specialist who has a private nursing practice will use data and assessment techniques that may be similar or different from the techniques used by the staff nurse working in an acute care hospital.

Subjective data for assessing health status are obtained by asking questions of the patient in either a formal or an informal interview. Data collected in a formal interview for the purpose of planning nursing care is called a *nursing history*. Objective data on health status may be collected by *physical examination* or by general observations.

This chapter will review the assessment methods and specific data useful for providing quality nursing care for adults experiencing pathophysiologic disorders in acute care settings. For information on more comprehensive data collection, the reader is referred to specific health assessment texts.

SUBJECTIVE DATA

Interviewing

The amount of data collected during an interview depends on the knowledge base and interviewing skill of the nurse and the openness of the patient. Interviewing skills are not intuitive but are developed with experience. A successful interview can be achieved by the following:

1. Modifying the environment to facilitate the interview
2. Listening and showing interest in the patient while simultaneously focusing on the data to be collected
3. Understanding the content base of the interview
4. Using appropriate questions to obtain the data

Guidelines for a successful interview are listed in the box below. An unsuccessful interview may occur because of factors related to the nurse or patient situation. Inability to collect data may be the result of the following factors:

1. Lack of time available to the nurse
2. Poor interviewing skills of the nurse
3. Patient condition (for example, pain, decreased consciousness)
4. Patient refusal or inability to answer questions

Guidelines for patient interviews

Modification of environment to facilitate interview

1. Provide privacy by closing door, drawing curtain, etc.
2. Facilitate patient's comfort (position of comfort, water available, etc.).
3. Sit in chair facing patient within a close distance but respecting patient's personal space (Fig. 3-1).
4. Keep environmental noises to a minimum by adjusting TV, radio, etc.
5. Ask visitors to step out of room, if applicable.

Initiation of interview

1. Introduce self.
2. Describe purpose of interview, general content, and approximate length of time.
3. Start with general nonthreatening questions to establish rapport and to demonstrate interest in patient and patient's circumstances.

Progression of interview

1. Keep questions brief and limited to a single topic.
2. Use open or closed questions, depending on the type of data sought. (Open question: "What do you drink with your supper?" Closed question: "Do you drink coffee or milk with your supper?").
3. Avoid leading questions such as "Do you have pain in your chest?" (patient may think this is expected). Instead ask, "Are you having any discomfort? Can you describe it?"
4. Use language that is easily understood by patient. Avoid awkward terms that make you feel uncomfortable (unless no other term is available that patient understands).
5. Allow sufficient time for patient to answer.
6. Use transitional statements when changing topic, for example, "We've been talking about your eating habits, now I'd like to ask you some questions about your bowel movements."
7. Keep the interview focused on data to be obtained. If patient insists on digressing to a particular topic, you can identify this but redirect the interview; for example, "I'd like to hear more about your family but perhaps we can do that later; right now I need to know more about your eating patterns."

Termination of interview

1. Summarize the major ideas offered by the patient.
2. Summarize what you will be doing with the data.
3. Thank the patient for cooperating.
4. State when you will be seeing the patient again.

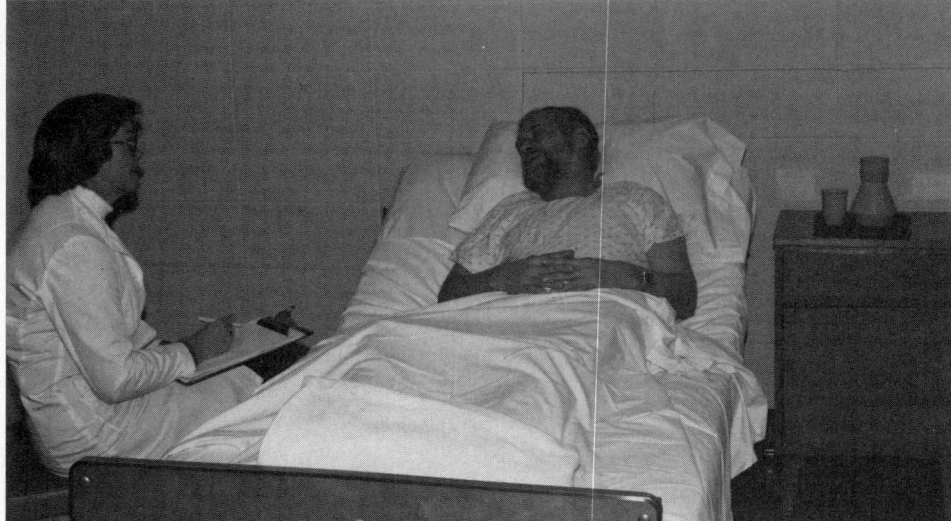

Fig. 3-1. Nurse interviewing a patient.

Nursing history

PURPOSES

If one of the goals of nursing is to assist people to maintain optimal health, a health history should be obtained by a professional nurse from all patients entering the health care system. The purpose is to obtain data for planning and implementing actions designed to strengthen positive health behaviors and to assist persons to cope with their health problems.

A comprehensive health history can be time-consuming and may not be appropriate in some acute care health centers, particularly if the patient's hospital stay will be short. Data must be collected, however, when a patient is first admitted to the health care center to identify those needs that require nursing interventions.

DATA

The nursing history may be a short (10-minute) interview to collect the immediate necessary data with additional data collected subsequently. Whenever possible, however, a more comprehensive nursing history is carried out initially to provide a data base for health teaching.

The nursing history example listed here takes approximately 30 minutes and provides data pertaining to the basic needs. The initial questions provide the nurse with the patient's perceptions of his or her health and current problems. Early in the interview data are collected about the presence of pain, since this can affect the course of the interview. The nursing history begins with data pertaining to physical functioning (physiologic and safety needs), then progresses to data pertaining to relationships with others (affiliation and sexuality), ending with data pertaining to self-esteem and self-actualization.

Sample nursing history

General information

1. Perception of present health status
2. Comparison of present with usual health status (if changed, perception of cause)
3. Medications taken regularly
4. Any allergies: food, medications, contact allergens, inhalants (describe symptoms, measures taken to avoid contact, relief measures)
5. Presence of pain/discomfort (current, past, onset, duration, characteristic, relief measures)
   - Chest pain
   - Joint or muscle problems (pain, stiffness, weakness)
   - Discomfort in extremities (pain, numbness, tingling, swelling, coldness, paleness)
   - Headaches

Sample nursing history—cont'd

Physiologic functioning

1. Prescribed activity level
2. Type and frequency of activity (recreation, exercise, work) both usual and current
3. Regular exercise routines and knowledge of benefits of activity
4. Difficulty moving about (describe difficulty and help needed, use of aids)
5. Whether tires easily with activities of daily living (ADL) or desired activity (describe)
6. Any difficulty breathing at rest (describe precipitating factors, duration, position for ease of breathing, type and effectiveness of relief measures)
7. Help needed with ADL
8. Usual hours of sleep per night for past 3 nights and if this is a change from usual pattern of sleep
9. Naps usually taken (time of day, frequency, length)
10. Feelings about quality of sleep (if poor sleep, perception of cause)
11. Aids taken to promote sleep (dose, frequency, effectiveness, length of time taken)
12. Typical day food and fluid pattern (type, amount)
13. Recent changes in amount and type of food and fluids, appetite
14. Weight, usual and current (if overweight or underweight: lifetime pattern, feelings about weight level, reasons for recent changes)
15. Patient's perception of weight level
16. Dentures (fit, comfort)
17. Problems with eating (chewing, swallowing)
18. Frequency of bowel movements (usual, recent changes)
19. Last bowel movement (time, character)
20. Aids usually taken for bowel elimination (type, frequency, effect)
21. Problems with bowel control (onset, perception of cause, effectiveness of measures taken)
22. Problems with urinary control or discomfort (onset, perception of cause)
23. Ability to see, hear, taste, smell, feel sensations (pain, heat touch) and use of corrective devices
24. Usual condition of skin and mucous membranes (dryness, cracks)
25. Frequency of colds or infections (throat, ear, bladder or kidney, boils)
26. Cough or history of coughs (productivity)
27. History of smoking or exposure to other inhalants
28. Knowledge and ability to summon help if needed (use of call cord)

Relationships with others

1. Persons or groups most helpful right now
2. Satisfaction with current role (family role, work role)
3. Self as member of a cultural or ethnic group
4. Recent changes in functioning in family, peer group
5. Living arrangements
6. Type and frequency of social activities outside home
7. Satisfaction with leisure time, hobbies, recreational pastimes
8. Anything interfering with role of mother, father, wife, husband
9. Anything (surgery, illness) changing feelings or thoughts about self as man or woman
10. Anything (illness, surgery, medications) affecting sexual function

Ideas about self

1. How do you feel right now? Is this how you usually feel?
2. What kind of person would you say you are?
3. How do you feel about yourself?
4. What do you usually do when things do not go as you plan or when things get tough?
5. Describe goals or plans for future.
6. Can you tell me about any spiritual or other beliefs and practices that are helpful to you now?
7. Is there anything else you would like to share with me that would help in your care?

Modalities of physical examination

Inspection	*Looking* at the skin and mucous membranes, body position and movements, and so on
Auscultation	*Listening* to heart, lung, and bowel sounds, blood pressure sounds
Palpation	*Feeling* or *touching* the skin to determine skin changes, enlargement of underlying structures, or presence of air or fluid
Percussion	*Tapping* an area to establish the presence of air, fluid, or dense tissue

---

OBJECTIVE DATA: PHYSICAL EXAMINATION

Modalities of physical examination

The four modalities of physical examination are inspection, auscultation, palpation, and percussion.

INSPECTION

Inspection can best be described as purposeful looking. It is the modality that yields the most information but is often performed less accurately than other modalities because of its simplicity. The key to effective inspection is *knowing what to look for.* A systematic approach to inspection is vital so that valuable data are not lost. Thoroughness is also important; all areas are examined carefully. It is especially important to examine the sacral area and to lift folds of tissue, such as under the breasts or gluteal folds. Embarrassment by the examiner or anticipated embarrassment of the patient may result in inadequate inspection. Most inspection can be carried out without special equipment, but a penlight and tongue blade are helpful aids.

AUSCULTATION

Although sounds may be heard by the unaided ear, auscultation is usually carried out with a stethoscope to enhance the examiner's ability to hear sounds coming from within the body cavity. The stethoscope is effective because it eliminates most of the sounds from the environment. Auscultation is used to obtain data about the heart, lungs, and gastrointestinal tract. Turbulent arterial blood flow can also be detected by auscultation.

PALPATION

Palpation is often used to confirm data obtained by inspection as well as to provide data concerning temperature, texture, size, consistency, discomfort, and pulsations. The backs of the fingers and hand are most sensitive to temperature; the fingertips are most sensitive to variations in texture.

Light palpation of the abdomen elicits areas of tenderness or distention. Deep palpation of the abdomen is used primarily by physicians or specially prepared nurses seeking data about organ involvement necessary to rule out a pathologic condition.

Percussion

Percussion is used less frequently in nursing practice than the other modalities. Effective percussion requires skill both in carrying out the technique and in interpreting the resultant sounds and generally elicits data more pertinent for medical diagnosis. Percussion can be used in nursing to tap the abdomen for differentiation of abdominal distention caused by gas (tympanic sound) from distention caused by fluid (dull sound).

Head-to-toe physical examination

The most common systematic approach used in a physical examination is a head-to-toe approach. This permits examining all areas in a sequential pattern to avoid omitting data. The box lists areas of assessment useful for planning nursing care of adults experiencing pathophysiologic disorders in an acute care center.

GENERAL SURVEY

General observations are made of the patient when the nurse first enters the patient's room. Items to note are the following:

State of health

Does the person look "well," that is, relaxed, in no acute distress, well-nourished, etc.
Does the person look "ill," that is, cachectic, strained facies, pale and sweating, moving with difficulty, etc.

State of awareness

Ability to respond to questions
Ability to remain alert during interview and physical examination
Oriented to person, place, and time

State of emotions

Nonverbal cues to the patient's emotional state are identified. Is the person relaxed and smiling? Restlessly pacing the floor or wringing the hands? Tearful? Listless?

Head-to-toe physical examination guide

General survey

State of health
State of awareness
State of emotions: mood, distress, grooming
Motor activity, posture, gait
Speech
Odors

General parameters

Height and weight
Vital signs
Skin parameters during inspection of each body
   area: color, turgor, moisture, temperature,
   lesions

Head

Eyes: symmetry, eyelids, conjunctiva, sclera,
   cornea, lens, pupillary reflex and accommodation,
   visual acuity, extraocular movement
Ears: external structures, external auditory canal,
   hearing acuity
Hair and scalp
Face: skin, symmetry, muscle strength of jaw, pain
   sensation
Nose: nares, vestibule
Mouth: lips, gums, teeth, mucous membranes,
   tongue, pharynx

Neck

Swallowing, position of trachea, muscle strength,
   range of motion, jugular vein distention,
   carotid pulses

Upper back and side

Inspection of skin of back and axilla
Inspection and palpation of spine
Symmetry of respiratory movement
Auscultation of lungs (posterior and lateral)

Chest

Skin turgor over sternum
Respiratory pattern
Slope of ribs
Anterior and posterior diameters
Auscultation of lung sounds (anterior)
Auscultation of heart sounds
Breast inspection

Abdomen

Inspection
Auscultation of bowel sounds
Palpation of femoral pulses

Lower back

Inspection of sacrum and buttocks

Extremities

Inspection of skin and nails
Capillary filling
Palpation for edema (legs)
Pulses: brachial and radial on arms, dorsalis pedis
   and posterior tibialis on feet
Sensation
Muscle strength
Coordination

Whole body coordination

Have poor grooming? (Unkept hair and clothing and poor personal hygiene may be observed in a depressed person.)

Motor activity, posture, gait

The general posture and activity may provide cues to such problems as fatigue (slumped posture, inactivity), dyspnea (sitting upright and trying to get breath), or pain (refusal to move, clutching a body part). The person's gait when walking may indicate weakness of one side, fear of falling (holding onto furniture), or loss of balance.

Speech

Slurring of speech, inability to articulate words, or inability to speak the language of the health-care professional may create communication problems. Difficulty with speech may be caused by problems of the central nervous system or larynx. If the patient cannot speak, does the person communicate with sign language or written materials?

Odors

Breath or body odors may result from poor personal hygiene, ingestion of certain substances such as foods or alcohol, or medical conditions such as diabetes mellitus (acetone), pulmonary infections, uremia, or liver failure.

SKIN

The skin provides a considerable amount of information about the person's state of health as well as being subject to lesions and breakdown. Data obtained on the initial physical examination provide information concerning potential for skin breakdown and a baseline of the status of existing lesions for future comparison. In the head-to-toe physical examination, the skin is examined throughout the examination whenever a specific body part is assessed. The specific observations include color, elasticity and turgor, moisture, temperature, and lesions or scars.

Color

The color of the skin depends on the amount of melanin in the cells and the blood supply (Table 3-1). Individuals differ in skin color intraracially as well as interracially. Color also varies on different skin areas of a given individual. Increased skin color is usually seen on exposed areas and in the areola of the nipples.

Lack of melanin in some skin areas may result from a genetic defect or from certain diseases such as hyperthyroidism, pernicious anemia, or adrenal cortical insufficiency. Scar tissue also lacks melanin. Areas of increased melanin often develop normally in aged persons and appear as brown patches on the skin (Fig. 3-2). A normal finding in most persons is pigmented moles. Changes in color of moles, especially to black or greenish black, should be reported to a physician for determination of possible malignancy.

Skin appears lighter with blood vessel constriction and redder with dilation, since dilated vessels are closer to the skin surface. Body areas particularly sensitive to vasodilation include a "butterfly" area across the cheeks and nose, neck, upper chest, flexor surfaces of the extremi-

Table 3-1. Skin color changes

Color	Physiology	Conditions
Redness	Vasodilation: more rapid blood flow, more oxygenated blood giving a reddish hue (erythema)	Blushing, heat, inflammation, fever, alcohol ingestion, extreme cold (below 15° C), hot flushes
Whiteness (pallor)	Vasoconstriction: slower blood flow, less blood in capillaries	Cold, fear, shock
	Partially obstructed blood flow: less blood in capillaries	Vasospasm, thrombus, narrowed vessels
	Fluid between blood vessels and skin surface	Edema
	Decreased oxygenation of blood from decreased hemoglobin	Anemia
	Loss of melanin	Vitiligo
Bluish	Deoxygenated hemoglobin (cyanosis) seen in earlobes, lips, mucous membranes of mouth, nail beds	Heart or lung disease, inadequate respiration, peripheral blood vessel obstruction
Yellow	Increased bile pigment in blood eventually distributed to skin and mucous membranes and to sclera of eye	Liver disease, obstruction of bile ducts, chronic uremia, rapid hemolysis
Brown	Increased melanin deposits: normal in brown-black races	Aging, sunburn
Dullness	Vasoconstriction in dark skin	Cold, fear, shock

ties, and genital areas. Skin and mucous membranes may also appear bluish or darker when there is an excess of deoxygenated blood (cyanosis) or yellow from an excess of serum bile (jaundice).

In dark-skinned individuals pallor is observed by the absence of the underlying red tones that normally give the brown and black skin its "glow" or "living color."[18] Brown-skinned persons will therefore appear more yellowish brown, and black-skinned persons will appear ashen gray. Generalized pallor and cyanosis may be better observed in the mucous membranes, lips, and nail beds. Erythema in the dark-skinned person is more readily observed as generalized redness of the lips.

Elasticity and turgor

Normal skin is elastic and returns to its original position after it has been stretched. It also moves freely over underlying tissue (mobility). Skin may become taut from being stretched over enlarged underlying tissue, such as that caused by fluid (edema). Loose skin over the extremities and neck results during old age because of loss of underlying subcutaneous tissue.

Turgor is the speed with which skin returns to its normal position after it has been stretched. Decreased turgor results from dehydration and is best assessed over the sternum. A fold of skin is picked up and observed for

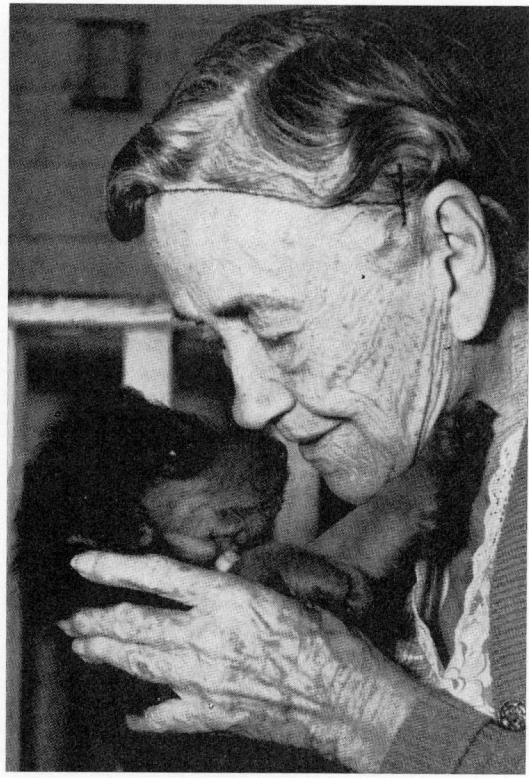

Fig. 3-2. Elderly patients have skin changes. Note discolored spots on skin and tiny raised area on this woman's eyelid. (VanDerMeid from Monkmeyer Press Photo Service.)

speed of return to normal; a delay indicates decreased turgor.

Moisture

Insensible fluid loss through the skin usually evaporates immediately, and normal skin is usually dry to the touch. Mucous membranes are normally moist and appear dry with dehydration. Increased fluid loss through the skin producing a sensation of moisture occurs when the external temperature is high, when high body temperature (fever) suddenly declines, or whenever the stress response occurs (fear, shock, etc.). The skin of the very young adult may be oily.

Temperature

Skin temperature increases with vasodilation and decreases with vasoconstriction. Vasodilation results from increased external or internal body temperature or from inflammation. Vasoconstriction results from decreased external or internal body temperature and as a result of sympathetic stimulation, as seen in the stress response. The backs of the fingers are more sensitive than the fingertips and are therefore used in the assessment of skin temperature.

Lesions

Different types of lesions may be observed on the skin (Table 3-2). Any lesions other than normal skin changes are described in terms of color, size, shape, texture, effect of pressure, arrangement and distribution over the body, and variety (presence of different types of lesions). Descriptions should be precise, and vague terms such as *small* or *medium* are avoided. Lesions may be discrete or coalesce into each other. They may occur in patches located in certain body areas or occur widely distributed in an even or uneven pattern. The use of correct medical terms when describing skin lesions facilitates communication to others.

Swelling of the skin may result from the presence of fluid in or between tissue cells or from overgrowth of tissue cells (Fig. 3-3). Fluid may appear as fluid-filled sacs on the skin surface or in the tissue. Interstitial fluid results from increased extracellular body fluid (Chapter 10) and is termed *pitting edema* because a finger pressed over the swollen tissue leaves a "pit" on the skin surface. The amount of pitting is recorded as + to + + + +, depending on the depth of the pit.

Overgrowth of tissue cells has different terms, depending on the size of the growth (Table 3–2). The term *tumor* refers to a growth over 2 cm and is not restricted to malignancy, since tumors can also be benign.

HEAD AND NECK

Eyes

The eyes are examined first after the examiner's hands have been washed. The patient is questioned about contact lenses so that a lens is not inadvertently lost during the examination of the eye.

Table 3-2. Skin lesions

Term	Description	Example
Change in color		
Macule	Flat spot less than 1 cm	Freckle
Change in cell growth		
Papule	Raised mass less than 1 cm	Measles spot
Nodule	Raised mass 1 to 2 cm	Mole
Tumor	Raised mass over 2 cm	Epithelioma
Change involving fluid		
Vesicle	Fluid-filled sac less than 1 cm	Small blister
Bulla	Fluid-filled sac more than 1 cm	Large blister
Pustule	Pus-filled sac less than 1 cm	Acne lesion
Wheal	Circumscribed raised skin containing intracellular fluid	Hives
Changes in consistence or integrity		
Plaque	Large raised surface on skin	Psoriasis
Crust	Dry exudate over a lesion	Eczema lesion
Scale	Dry exfoliation of skin cells	Psoriasis
Fissure	Crack in skin surface	Crack in corner of mouth
Ulcer	Erosion of skin surface	Decubitus ulcer
Lichenification	Leatherlike thickening of outer skin layer	Lichen planus

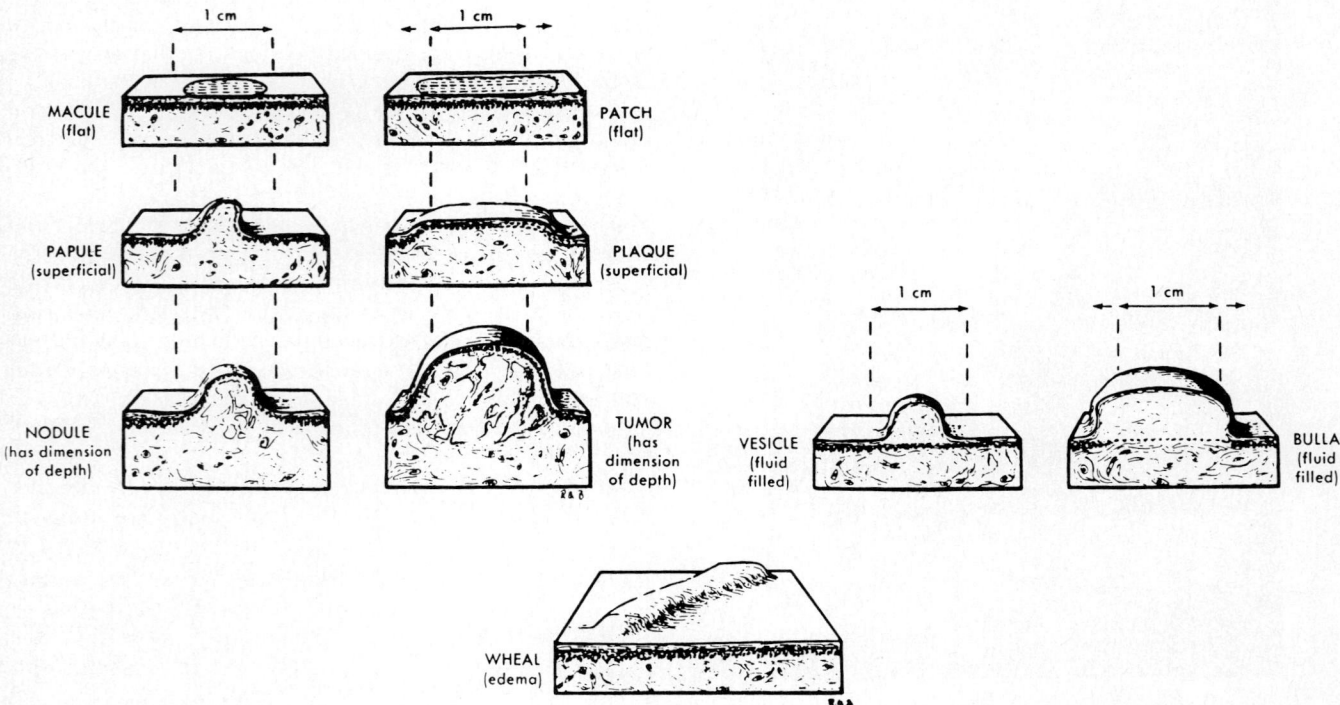

Fig. 3-3. Skin lesions. (From Stewart, W.D., Danto, J.L., and Madden, S.: Dermatology: diagnosis and treatment of cutaneous disorders, ed. 4, St. Louis, 1978, The C.V. Mosby Co.)

INSPECTION

Symmetry

Eyelids

Note position of lids to eyeballs and inspect for edema, color, lesions, and ability to close.

Drooping of lid (ptosis) may result from muscular weakness or nerve damage, edema from allergies, local inflammation, recent crying, or fluid-retaining states. Redness indicates inflammation. Failure to close may dehydrate cornea.

Conjunctiva and sclera

Examine conjunctiva by depressing the lower lid while asking the patient to look up. The normal conjunctiva is clear and the sclera is white.

Redness indicates inflammation. The sclera is yellow with jaundice.

Cornea and lens

Shine a light obliquely across eye to detect opacities of cornea and lens. Opacities will appear grayish against black pupil.

Opacities interfere with vision.

PUPILLARY REFLEX AND ACCOMMODATION

Pupils are normally equally round and reactive to light and accommodation (PERRLA).

The pupil of a false eye does not respond to light. Small fixed pupils occur with administration of opium derivative or miotic drug for glaucoma. Dilated fixed pupils occur with anticholinergic drugs, severe brain damage, or severe hypoxia.

Reaction to light

1. Ask patient to look at a distance.
2. Shine a light obliquely and quickly twice across each eye.
3. Note *direct reaction* of pupil to light and *consensual reaction* (reaction of opposite pupil).

Reaction to accommodation

1. Hold your finger about 5 to 10 cm from bridge of patient's nose.
2. Ask patient to look first at a distance, then at your finger.
3. Note pupillary constriction and convergence of the eyes when focus is on finger (near object).

VISUAL ACUITY

The ability to see is assessed both with and without glasses or contact lenses. The patient is asked to read any large print at a distance (note approximate number of feet), then small print about 35 cm (14 inches) from the face. Glasses used only for reading are not used to test far vision.

EXTRAOCULAR MOVEMENT

Test of ocular movement determines whether eyes are moving in a synchronous fashion.
Method: Have patient follow your finger in an **H** configuration (Fig. 3-4).

Asymmetry of movement may cause double vision.

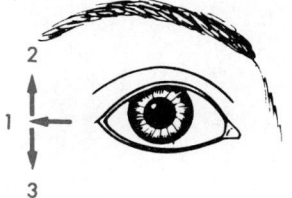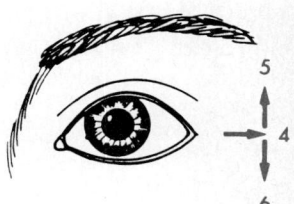

Fig. 3-4. Testing extraocular movement. The numbers indicate the sequence of motion.

Ears
INSPECTION

Inspect auricles and surrounding tissues of external ear for deformities, lumps, or skin lesions. The outer portion of external auditory canal is inspected by pulling auricle up, back, and out and using a penlight for better vision.

Ear pain, discharge, and inflammation are abnormal findings.

AUDITORY ACUITY

To estimate hearing ability, test one ear at a time. Ask the patient to occlude one ear with a finger. Stand approximately 1 to 2 feet away and whisper softly two equally accented numbers (such as 14, 25) toward the *unoccluded* ear. Repeat with the other ear. Be sure patient cannot read your lips.

Hair and scalp
HAIR

Appearance

Distribution

Attachment

Presence of lice

Lack of shine occurs with age or malnutrition.

Thin sparse hair occurs with age or malnutrition.
Alopecia (loss of hair) occurs with chemotherapy or radiation therapy.

Easily plucked hair occurs with malnutrition.

Lice may deposit tiny white ovoid nits on hair shafts, especially behind ears.

Look for presence of false eye.

SCALP

Part hair in several places and examine for dryness, scaliness of lesions.

Scaling may result from dandruff or psoriasis.

Face
SKIN

Inspect color, moisture, temperature, texture, and lesions.

SYMMETRY OF MOVEMENT

Ask patient to elevate eyebrows and forehead, frown, smile, close eyes quickly and tightly, show teeth, whistle, and blow out cheeks.

Asymmetry will be noted with weakness of the facial nerve.

MUSCLE STRENGTH OF JAW

Place both hands against jaws and ask patient to
1. Clamp jaws tightly.
2. Move jaw side to side against your hand resistance.

Muscle weakness may interfere with mastication.

PAIN SENSATION

Ask patient to close eyes. Use two safety pins (to avoid crossing of patient's eyes).
Ask patient to respond to sharp or dull pricks with pin.

Pain sensation may be lost with paralysis of the trigeminal nerve.

Nose
NARES

Inspect nares for flaring or discharge.

Flaring occurs with respiratory exertion.

SEPTUM

Using penlight, inspect nasal septum for marked deviation.

Breathing through nose may be impaired by a deviated septum.

Mouth

The mouth, like the skin, is an excellent barometer of general health, reflecting general disease and debility as well as good health. A tongue blade and penlight are necessary for inspection.

LIPS

Inspect for dryness or cracks.
Inspect for lesions.

These may occur with dehydration or malnutrition.

TEETH, GUMS, AND MUCOUS MEMBRANES

Inspect for color, moisture, lesions.

Redness or white "curd" patches occur with inflammation.

Inspect teeth for caries.
Inspect dentures for comfort and fit.

Lack of dentures or ill-fitting dentures may interfere with chewing.

PHARYNX

Depress tongue with tongue blade and ask patient to say "Ah."

Redness and discharge occur with inflammation; asymmetry with movement of soft palate may interfere with swallowing.

Touch back of throat with tongue blade to elicit gag reflex.

A decreased gag reflex (change from normal) may interfere with swallowing.

TONGUE

Inspect color, coating, and lesions.

A smooth tongue may indicate malnutrition; a thickened white patch may be a premalignant lesion.

Ask patient to move tongue up and down, and side to side.

Asymmetry of movement may indicate paralysis and interfere with eating.

Neck
TRACHEA

Inspect trachea for deviation.

Tracheal deviation may indicate neck mass, pneumothorax, pleural effusion, and atelectasis.

Place a finger on trachea and ask patient to swallow.

Decreased tracheal movement may indicate decreased ability to swallow.

MUSCLE STRENGTH

Ask patient to shrug shoulders and turn head to each side against your hands.

Assess strength of neck muscles.

RANGE OF MOTION (ROM)

Ask patient to move head through range of motion.

Decreased ROM may interfere with ADL.

JUGULAR VEIN DISTENTION

Place patient with head elevated 45 degrees. Note uppermost point of visible vein pulsation. Note level of vein pulsation above sternal angle (Fig. 3-5).

Distended neck veins (increased pressure) may result from circulatory overload or right-sided heart failure.

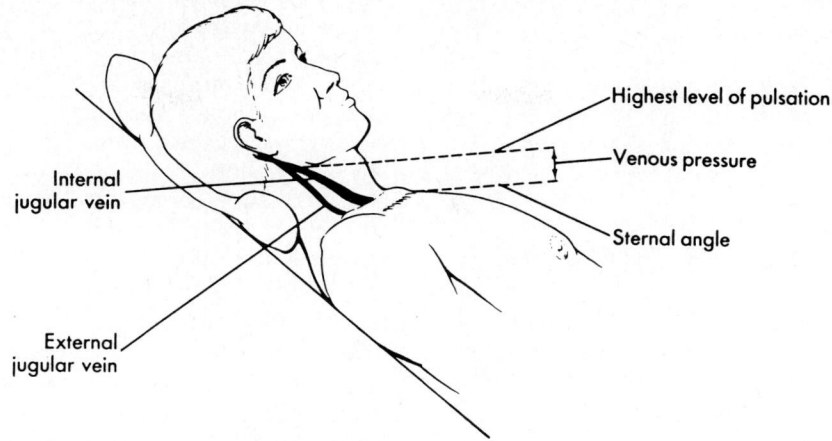

Fig. 3-5. Position of internal and external jugular veins used in measuring venous pressure.

Upper back and side

Examination of spine

Inspect back for differences in height of shoulders. Palpate length of spine with a finger on each side of spine to detect lateral curvatures.

Marked deformities may interfere with respiration or cause fatigue.

Symmetry of respiratory movement

Place both hands on lateral thorax just below scapula with thumbs at spine and fingers outstretched. Ask patient to take a deep breath. Observe and feel equal expansion of thorax.

Asymmetry suggests a lung or pleural disorder and interferes with full excursion.

Auscultation of lungs (posterior/lateral)

Auscultation of the lungs is described on p. 33.

Assess for decreased breath sounds or presence of adventitious (abnormal) sounds.

Anterior chest

Respiratory pattern

Note depth of breathing. Count rate (may also be done when counting heart rate).
Note effort of breathing.

Listen for audible breath sounds (for example, wheezing).

Very shallow breathing limits alveolar expansion. Very deep breathing indicates respiratory effort. Intercostal retraction and nasal flaring occur with labored breathing.
Audible breath sounds occur with asthma and chronic bronchitis.

Slope of ribs

Trace one intercostal space anterior to posterior.

Rib is more horizontal with emphysema.

Lung sounds

See p. 33 for auscultation of lungs anteriorly.

Same as described for posterior lungs.

Heart

Count heart rate at apex of heart. Assess rhythm.
Listen to heart sounds (see p. 34).

Describe abnormal sounds (gallops, murmurs, opening valve snaps and clicks) in terms of timing with S_1 and S_2, anatomic location, pitch, intensity, and character.

Breast inspection

The female patient is asked if she does a regular breast self-examination (BSE).

Nonperformance of BSE indicates need for patient teaching.

Abdomen

1. Inspect skin for dryness and lesions.
2. Check umbilicus for cleanliness and lesions.
3. Note contour and movements (peristaltic movements and aortic pulsations may be noted in thin persons). Measure distended abdomen with tape measure across umbilicus.
4. Listen for bowel sounds starting in right lower abdominal quadrant. If not heard in that site, listen in other quadrants.

Abdominal distention may result from fat, ascites, distended bladder, pregnancy, and tumors. Increased peristaltic waves may be seen with early intestinal obstruction.

Alterations in bowel sounds occur with diarrhea and ileus.

5. Palpate presence and strength of femoral pulses.
6. The male patient is asked if he performs a regular testicular self-examination.

Lower back

Ask patient to turn over and inspect sacrum and buttocks for redness or lesions.

Baseline data on skin of sacrum and buttocks is especially important if patient is malnourished, edematous, or on bed rest.

Extremities

NOTE: always compare right with left. Assess both legs, then both arms.

Inspection

Check size in proportion to body development.
Inspect skin (include all skin areas and skin between toes).
Check skin temperature.
Inspect nails for texture and thickness, angle of fingernail to nail base.

Nail changes seen with age and malnutrition.
Clubbing of nails seen with lung conditions (hypoxia).
Lack of blanching response or slow return of color may indicate lack of circulation to finger or toe.

Check for capillary filling: press your thumbnail against edge of patient's nail and release quickly.

Presence of pitting edema

Press finger firmly over shin, over dorsum of foot, and behind medial malleolus.

Pitting edema is caused by increased fluid in the interstitial spaces.

Pulses

Assess radial and brachial pulses in arms and dorsalis pedis and posterior tibialis pulses in feet for presence, strength, and symmetry.

Decreased pulses may suggest decreased circulation to the part.

Sensation

Test sensation by means of two safety pins (as with face), starting at fingers or toes and moving toward elbow or knee.

Areas that have decreased sensation are at high risk for injury.

Muscle strength

For legs, do straight leg raises (one at a time) against hand resistance. Place one of your hands under patient's knee and

Decreased muscle strength of legs will decrease patient's ability to ambulate and increase risk of fall.

other hand on *top* of ankle. Ask patient to lift lower leg against your resistance. Then move hand to *underneath* ankle and ask patient to lower leg against resistance (Fig. 3-6).
For arms, ask patient to grip your index and middle fingers and to first pull, then push your hands against your resistance.

Decreased muscle strength of arms may interfere with ADL.

ROM

Assess ROM of shoulders, elbows, wrists, and fingers. Assess ROM of hips, knees, and ankles.

Decreased ROM may interfere with ADL and walking.

Coordination

1. Finger coordination: Ask patient to touch thumb to each finger in rapid succession.

Awkwardness with point to point coordination may suggest motor weakness, loss of position sense, or

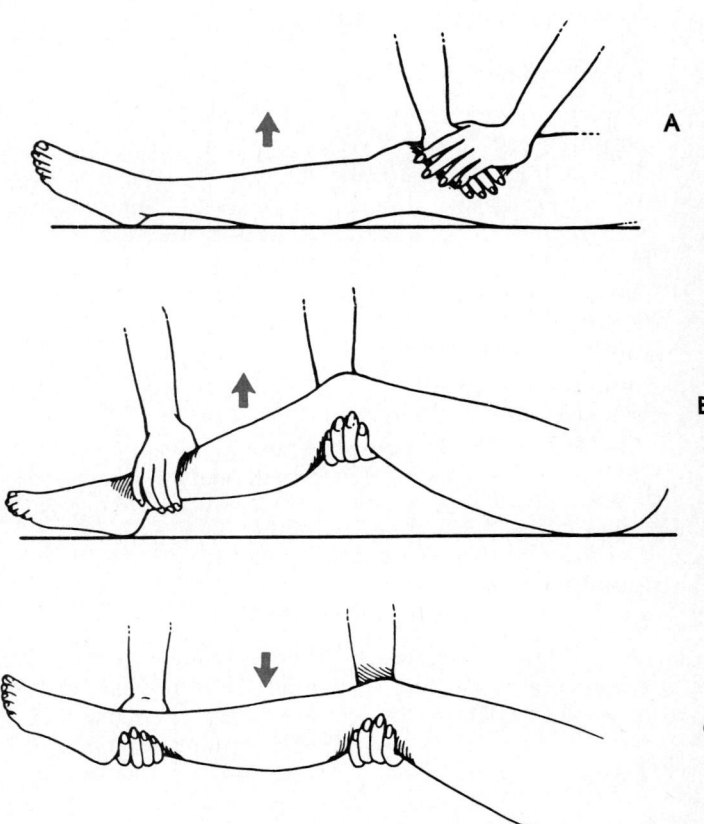

Fig. 3-6. Testing muscle strength in the legs. **A,** Straight leg raises (quadriceps). **B,** Raising lower leg against resistance (quadriceps). **C,** Pulling lower leg against resistance (hamstrings).

2. Finger-to-nose coordination: Ask patient to touch your index finger, then his/her nose several times, first with eyes open and then with eyes closed.
3. Heel-shin coordination: Ask patient to place heel on opposite shin and move heel up and down shin.

Whole body coordination
1. If patient is ambulatory, ask patient to walk across room and back to assess gait.
2. Ask patient to stand still with arms at side, first with eyes open, then with eyes closed, to assess balance (Romberg sign).

cerebellar disease. The patient may have some difficulties with ADL and have increased risk of falls.

Awkward gait and decreased balance may interfere with ambulation and increase risk of falls.

Pulmonary auscultation

Auscultation of the lungs enables a nurse to establish baseline data for identifying current and potential lung problems that require nursing interventions, such as determining the frequency for breathing exercises or the need for or effectiveness of suctioning.

BREATH SOUNDS

Breath sounds result from the movement of air through the lungs and air passages. The sounds are thought to occur as a result of two elements, the vesicular and bronchial elements. The vesicular element occurs when the walls of the alveoli separate from air entering the alveoli with inspiration. The bronchial element is a hisslike sound resulting from air flowing past the bronchi across the vocal chords.

The three types of breath sounds that can be heard are vesicular, bronchovesicular, and bronchial (Fig. 3-7). *Vesicular breath sounds* are heard over most of the lungs because of the prominence of the alveoli. The sounds are of a low pitch and have a soft rustling or swishing quality. The sound of the inspiratory phase is longer and higher

in pitch than that of the expiratory phase, which is a soft, short, low-pitched, almost inaudible sound. The relative loudness of inspiration may differ among listening sites; the sounds are usually softer at the bases of the lungs.

Bronchovesicular breath sounds are heard as auscultation approaches the main bronchi. Inspiration and expiration are loud and nearly equal in duration and intensity because of being closer to the vocal chords.

Bronchial breath sounds are *not* heard normally over any area of lung tissue, and their presence indicates consolidation or compression of lung tissue or a pleural effusion. These breath sounds are high pitched and loud; during the expiratory phase they increase in duration, pitch, and intensity.

Adventitious (abnormal) lung sounds

Adventitious lung sounds are abnormal sounds superimposed on breath sounds. There are essentially two kinds of abnormal sounds: (1) *crackles* or *rales* (rhymes with pals) caused by air flowing through *moisture* in the air passages and (2) *wheezes* or *rhonchi* caused by air flowing through *narrowed* air passages (Table 3-3). A third type of sound occurs outside the lung; a *pleural friction rub* results from the rubbing of inflamed pleura between the lung and chest wall.

General directions for pulmonary auscultation

1. Have patient seated if possible for auscultation of posterior lung fields. The female patient may be easier to auscultate anteriorly if she is lying down.
2. Use the *diaphragm* of the stethoscope. Press firmly to produce a blanched ring when the diaphragm is removed. Hold the diaphragm in such a way as to decrease extraneous sounds (fingers not touching skin and diaphragm or tubing not touching clothing or other objects).
3. Provide counter support for patient with your free hand.
4. Tell patient to (a) turn head away, (b) breathe *slightly* deeper but *not* faster, and (c) breathe through the mouth.
5. Listen in a consistent, systematic manner.
6. At each listening site (Fig. 3-8), listen for one full breath and identify:
   • Type of breath sound
   • Intensity of breath sound
   • Presence of adventitious sounds

Cardiac auscultation

Auscultation of heart sounds enables a nurse to establish baseline data for identifying current and potential cardiac problems that require nursing intervention. Cardiac auscultation also assists the nurse in evaluating a patient's progress (for example, effect of activity on heart rate) or in monitoring responses to medications (for example, quinidine or digitalis preparations).

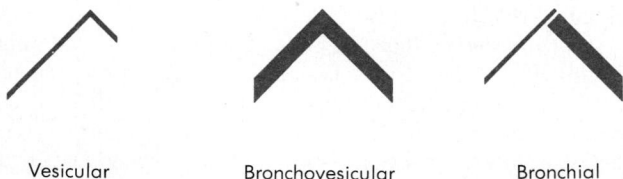

Vesicular   Bronchovesicular   Bronchial

Fig. 3-7. Schematic representation of three types of breath sounds.

Table 3-3. Abnormal (adventitious) lung sounds

Type	Physiology	Auscultation	Sound	Pathology
Crackles (rales) Fine	Air passing through secretions in *alveoli*	Heard at *end* of *inspiration*	Several hairs rubbed together between fingertips	Pneumonia, heart failure (may occur normally in elderly bedridden persons)
Medium	Air passing through secretions in *bronchioles* or *bronchi*	Heard *midway* during *inspiration*	Fizzing of carbonated drink	Later stages of pneumonia, heart failure, pulmonary edema
Coarse	Air passing through secretions in large airways, especially *trachea*	Heard at *beginning* of *inspiration*	Rough gurgling	Persons with repressed cough reflexes, unable to clear own secretions
Wheezes (rhonchi)	Air passing through narrow passages	Heard mostly during *expiration*, but may also occur with inspiration	Loud *musical* gurgling	Obstructive lung disease
Pleural friction rub	Rubbing of inflamed pleura	May occur throughout respiratory cycle, heard best at base of lung at end of expiration	Scratching, grating, rubbing	Inflamed pleura

HEART SOUNDS

The familiar "lub-dub" heard when taking an apical pulse are the first and second heart sounds (S_1 and S_2) and mark the beginning and end of each ventricular contraction; hence rate, when obtained by auscultation, is determined by counting each set of "lub-dubs" as one beat. Whether these sounds occur regularly or irregularly determines the assessment of cardiac rhythm.

The first heart sound (S_1) is the result of the closure of the atrioventricular valves (*mitral* and *tricuspid*). This sound is heard best at the apex of the heart (normally the fifth left intercostal space at the midclavicular line) (Fig. 3-9). The valves do not close at precisely the same time. However, the fact that the time difference between their closure is measured in terms of hundredths of a second and that a greater volume of sound is produced by the mitral valve generally results in only one detectable noise. Occasionally the tricuspid component may be heard along the lower left sternal border.

The second heart sound (S_2) is the result of the closure of the semilunar valves (*aortic* and *pulmonic*). This sound is usually heard best at the base of the heart in the aortic area (second right intercostal space). The aortic valve closes slightly ahead of the pulmonic valve but produces a louder sound, so S_2 is also often detected as only one sound. When auscultating in the pulmonic area (second left intercostal space) one may hear the pulmonic component of S_2 (producng what is then referred to as a *split sound*) in a phasic manner, that is, the splitting is heard for a few beats and then is absent for a few beats. This phasic appearance of a split S_2 is the result of alterations in right ventricular volume (and therefore contraction time) related to the respiratory cycle. Under normal circumstances the split S_2, if heard at all, is detected during inspiration.

Extra heart sounds

With some exceptions, the occurrence of any additional heart sounds would be considered an abnormal finding. Abnormal cardiac sounds include gallops (S_3 and S_4), murmurs, opening snaps, and clicks.

Ventricular diastolic gallop (S_3) is a faint, low-pitched sound produced by rapid ventricular filling in early diastole (Fig. 3-10). Ventricular "gallop" describes the canter of a horse, which is frequently mimicked at heart rates greater than 100 beats per minute. When this sound is present in healthy children and young adults, it is almost always a normal condition and is referred to as a physiologic S_3. An S_3 heard in an older person is usually a pathologic sign and is frequently one of the first signs of serious heart disease or cardiac decompensation as seen in congestive heart failure.

Atrial diastolic gallop (S_4) is a low-pitched sound that occurs late in diastole when atrial contractions eject blood into a noncompliant ventricle. It may be heard in such states as hypertensive cardiovascular disease, coronary artery disease (especially during an attack of angina pectoris), and aortic stenosis.

Murmurs are audible vibrations of the heart and great vessels that occur because of turbulent blood flow. They may occur either during systole or diastole or through

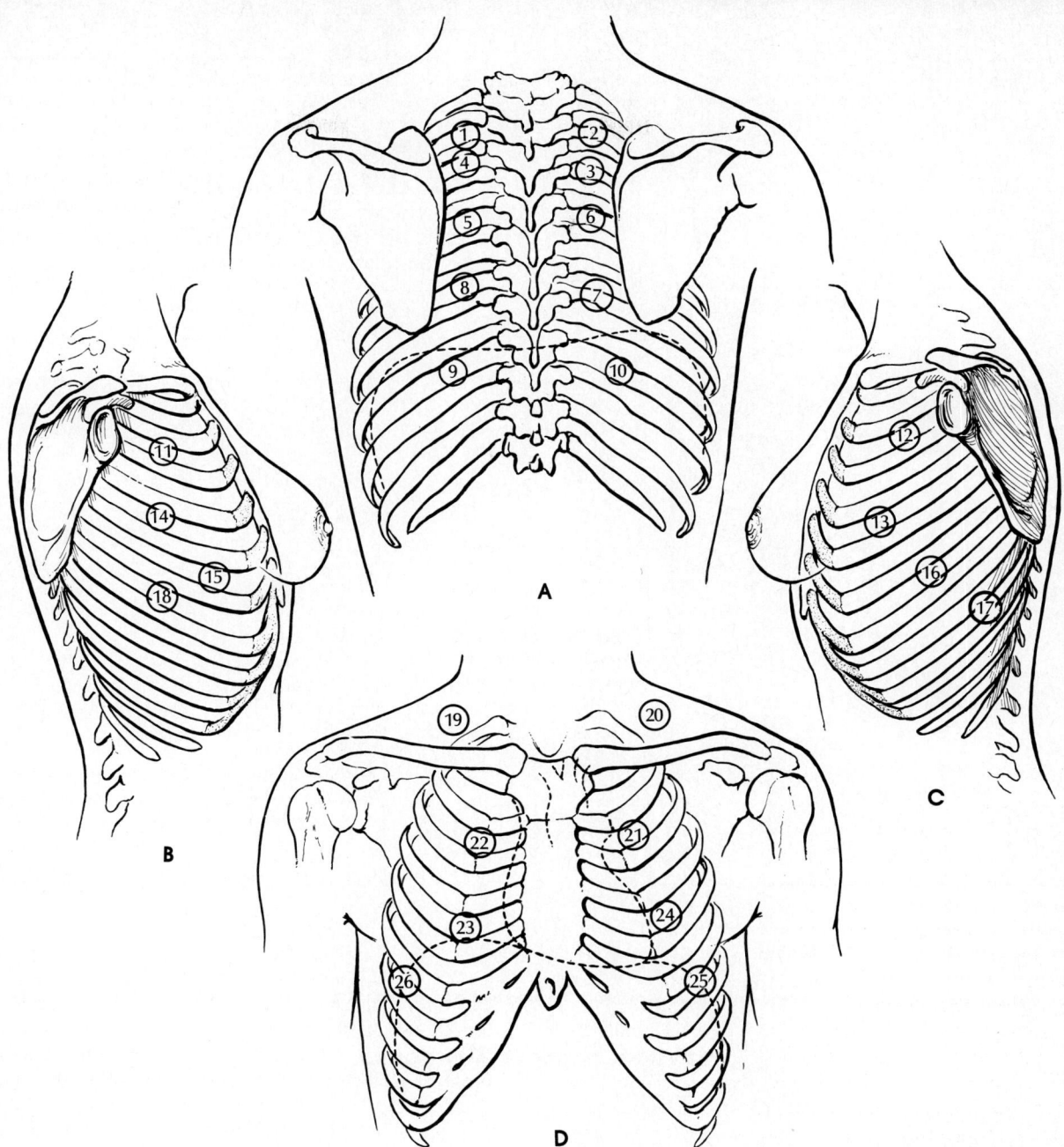

Fig. 3-8. Sites for auscultation of thorax. Numbers indicate sequence of stethoscope placement. **A,** Posterior. **B,** Right lateral. **C,** Left lateral. **D,** Anterior. (From Malasanos, L., et al.: Health assessment, ed. 2, St. Louis, 1981. The C.V. Mosby Co.)

both phases. The intensity may be faint or loud; the pitch may be high (sharp) or low (dull), and the quality is described as harsh, blowing, rumbling, or musical. Murmurs may be organic (structural cardiovascular abnormalities), functional (increased blood flow through normal structures), or physiologic.

Other sounds that may be heard include a high-pitched clicking sound heard during systole (ejection sounds) or a high-pitched snapping sound heard in early diastole (opening snap of stenosed mitral valve).

General directions for cardiac auscultation

1. Locate the landmarks for auscultation: the second and fifth intercostal spaces.
2. Start at either the mitral or aortic areas.
3. Move the stethoscope at very short intervals (inching method) along the fifth interspace to sternum, then along the left sternal border to the second left interspace, then across the sternum to the right second interspace (or vice versa) (Fig. 3-9).

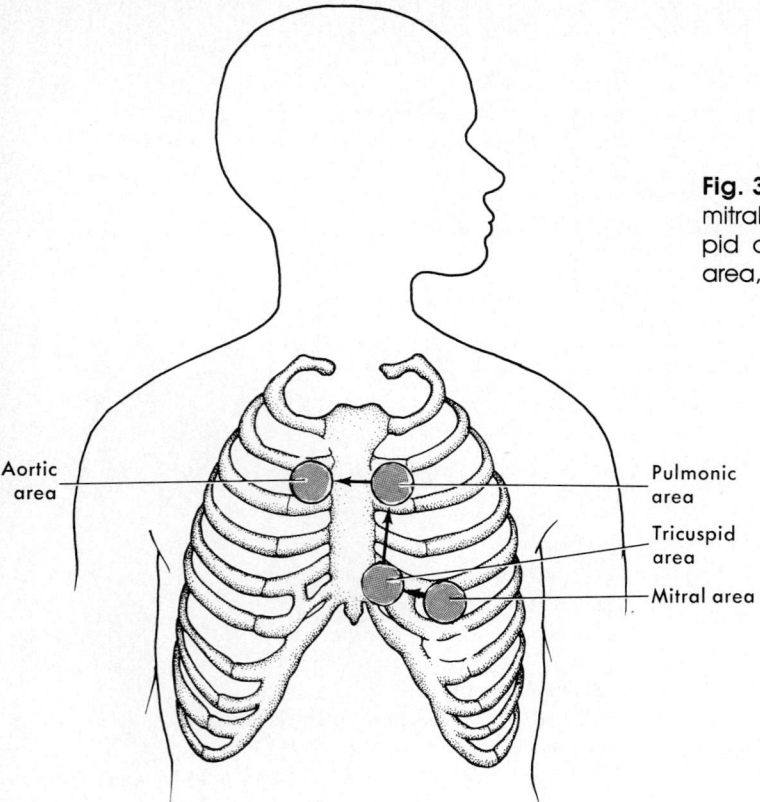

Fig. 3-9. Sequence for cardiac auscultation. Begin at the mitral area and move the stethoscope toward the tricuspid area, then up the sternal border to the pulmonic area, then across the sternum to the aortic area.

Aortic area

Pulmonic area

Tricuspid area

Mitral area

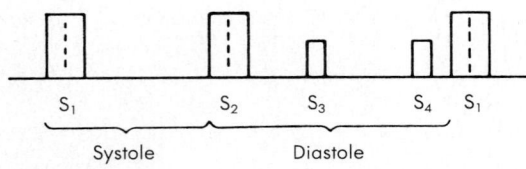

S_1 S_2 S_3 S_4 S_1

Systole   Diastole

Fig. 3-10. Location of extra heart sound during cardiac cycle.

Physical changes with aging

Loss of tissue elasticity
Loss of subcutaneous fat
Altered endocrine function (thyroid, pancreatic, estrogenic, androgenic)
Altered immune response
Alteration in bone and muscle mass
Altered sensory perception (temperature, pressure, pain, touch, taste, vision, hearing)
Respiratory changes (decreased number but increased size of alveoli, rigidity of lung tissue, decreased vital capacity, decreased cough response)
Cardiac changes (decreased cardiac output, decreased contractility, increased time for heart rate to return to normal after activity)
Vascular changes (decreased vessel elasticity, decreased blood flow to coronary arteries, liver and kidneys, decreased venous muscle tone and decreased efficiency of venous valves, decreased capillary permeability)
Gastrointestinal changes (decreased digestive enzymes, absorption, muscle tone, salivation, gag reflex)
Sleep changes (less time, changes in cycles)

4. Go through the listening sequence at least two times, first with the diaphragm for high-pitched sounds, then with the bell for low-pitched sounds. It is easier to follow the sequence three times (twice with the diaphragm listening first for normal sounds S_1 and S_2; second, for extra high-pitched sounds; and third, with the bell for extra low-pitched sounds).
5. Press firmly when using the diaphragm, but rest the bell only lightly on the skin.
6. When listening to normal heart sounds, note intensity of sounds and presence of splitting. Splitting of S_1 can be heard best at the tricuspid area and splitting of S_2 at the pulmonic area. The carotid pulse can be used to verify S_1 if needed. If splitting of S_2 is heard, note timing in relation to respiratory cycle.
7. Describe any extra sounds in terms of timing (systolic or diastolic), intensity, pitch, character, and location where heard on thorax. For example, a sound might be described as "a high-pitched, blowing, systolic murmur of medium intensity, best heard along the left sternal border."

Physical assessment changes with aging

There is great variation in the degree of change that occurs with aging when comparing one older person with another. Changes caused by aging are irreversible as contrasted with changes caused by illness, which may be reversible. The physical changes seen in older persons are not predictable and may result from the age factor alone or from other factors, such as environment (for example exposure to sun), illness, or genetic traits. Some of the changes that occur with aging are listed in the box on p. 36.

In the physical examination of an older adult, some differences may be noted that are normal variations caused by age. These variations may include some of the following:

Skin—decreased elasticity; increased wrinkles on sun-exposed areas; increased dryness with flaking and scaling; purple patches, brown spots, cherry angiomas (red); skin tags, seborrheic keratoses (greasy warts)

Hair—loss of hair, thinner, decreased luster

Face—increased facial hair on women, coarse hair on men (in ears and nose)

Eyes—decreased vision, especially for near objects; pupillary response to light may be slower; lens may look gray but have clear vision; may be opaque if cataract developing

Ears—decreased hearing, especially for high-pitched sounds; sounds may become distorted

Mouth—teeth worn, darker color; dentures common; decreased salivation

Neck—decreased range of motion, neck veins more prominent

Thorax—increased dorsal curve of thoracic spine (kyphosis); increased anterior-posterior diameter; chest expansion may be decreased; decreased size of breasts, pendulous

Abdomen—increased fat deposits in lower abdomen, weakened abdominal muscles (pot belly)

Extremities—nails: thickened (especially toes); ROM: may be decreased; muscle strength: decreased; decreased pain and touch sensation

Whole body coordination—position sense may be decreased, gait may be unsteady

REFERENCES AND SELECTED READINGS*

1. *Adler, J.: Patient assessment: abnormalities of the heart beat, Am. J. Nurs. **77**:647-672. 1977.
2. *Baer, E., McGowan, M.N., and McGivern, D.O.: How to take a health history, Am. J. Nurs. **77**:1190-1193, 1977.
3. Bates. B.: A guide to physical examination, ed. 3, Philadelphia, 1983, J.B. Lippincott Co.
4. Boyd-Monk, H.: Examining the external eye, part 1, Nurs. 80 **10**(5):58-63, 1980.
5. Boyd-Monk, H.: Examining the external eye, part 2, Nurs. 80 **10**(6):58-63, 1980.
6. Cohen, S., and Viellion, G.: Patient assessment: examining joints of the upper and lower extremities, Am. J. Nurs. **81**:763-786, 1981.
7. *Dossey, B.: Perfecting your skills for systematic patient assessment, Nurs. 79 **9**(2):42-45, 1979.
8. Ebersole, P., and Hess, P.: Toward healthy aging: human needs and nursing response, St. Louis, 1981, The C.V. Mosby Co.
9. *Eggland, E.T.: How to take a meaningful nursing history, Nurs. 77 **7**(7):22-30, 1977.
10. Froelich, R.E., and Bishop, F.M.: Clinical interviewing skills: a programmed manual for data gathering, evaluation, and patient management, ed. 3, St. Louis, 1977, The C.V. Mosby Co.
11. *Jarvis, C.M.: Perfecting physical assessment, part 1, Nurs. 77 **7**(5):28-37, 1977.
12. *Jarvis, C.M.: Perfecting physical assessment, part 2, Nurs. 77 **7**(6):38-45, 1977.
13. *Jarvis, C.M.: Perfecting physical assessment, part 3, Nurs. 77 **7**(7):44-53, 1977.
14. Mahoney, E., Verdisco, L., and Shortridge, L.: How to collect and record a health history, Philadelphia, 1976, J.B. Lippincott Co.
15. Malasanos, L., and others: Health assessment, ed. 2, St. Louis, 1981, The C.V. Mosby Co.
16. Murray, R., Huelskoetter, M.M., and O'Driscoll, D.: The nursing process in later maturity, Englewood Cliffs, N.J., 1980, Prentice-Hall, Inc.
17. Patient assessment series, 21 programmed units, New York, 1980, American Journal of Nursing Co.
18. *Roach, L.B.: Color changes in dark skin, Nurs. 77 **7**(1):48-51, 1977.
19. Thompson, J.M., and Bowers, A.C.: Clinical manual of health assessment, St. Louis, 1980, The C.V. Mosby Co.
20. *Visich, M.A.: Knowing what you hear: a guide to assessing breath and heart sounds, Nurs. 81 **11**(11):64-76, 1981.

*References preceded by an asterisk are particularly well suited for student reading.

4
Quality Assurance in Nursing

MARY LOU MONAHAN

STUDY QUESTIONS

- Identify one clinical problem and the steps you would use to assess it using the ANA model.

- Identify four nursing process standards for a patient with impaired mobility.

- Based on the current financial and regulatory environment (that is, DRG legislation), there have been a number of proposals to curtail quality assurance activities. Do you agree or disagree?

- Investigate the impact of the quality assurance program on the quality of patient care in your hospital.

Nursing is committed to professional excellence in providing the highest quality of care possible. Implicit in this commitment is the responsibility to evaluate the quality and appropriateness of that care. However, it has only been in the last decade that attempts have been made to develop an extrinsic, systematic approach to monitor and improve care. The impetus for this change has come from a variety of sources: (1) legislation, including changes in third-party reimbursement; (2) economic factors; and (3) the nursing profession itself.

First, since the passage of Medicare/Medicaid legislation in 1965, the federal government has become the largest source of third-party health care payment. Because of this increasing financial commitment, Congress and government officials at all levels are under pressure to ensure that the services rendered are necessary, that they meet professionally recognized standards of care, and that they contain costs. To establish some system of accountability for these expenditures, Congress created a system for reviewing these expenses as part of Public Law 92-603, the Social Security Amendments of 1972. This legislation established a nationwide network of professional standards review organizations (PSROs) for review of patient care financed by the federal government. Private insurance carriers such as Blue Cross also established standards for

review of the care for which they have made payment.

Second, because health care costs have assumed an increasing share of the gross national product over the past decade, there has been increased scrutiny of the components of this cost. Reviewing the cost of illness raises vital questions about the relation of quality of care to cost. For example, the principle of "high cost/low benefit" is defined by poor quality of health care in terms of overdiagnosis or overtreatment, which can lead to excessive health care expenditures even in the absence of any iatrogenic or untoward consequences. Poor quality in the form of misdiagnosis, mistreatment, or inadequate nursing care can increase mortality or morbidity, earnings loss, and therefore the costs of health problems to individuals and to society. Poor quality can also lead to increased pain and suffering and thus increase the total intangible costs of illness.

The current economic situation, with health care costs growing at an unacceptable rate, budgetary cutbacks, and the implementation of the first phase of the diagnosis-related group (DRG) reimbursement scheme in October 1983, has implications for nursing. More than ever before, the nursing profession must demonstrate the value and benefits of its service if it wishes to retain government and consumer support.

Third, the nursing profession itself places as its highest goal the delivery of quality health care. The American Nurses' Association (ANA) published *Standards of Nursing Practice*[2] in 1973 for the purpose of ensuring quality health care to the public. However, primary responsibility for implementing these standards rests with the individual nurse in the practice setting. Individual nurses must be familiar with both general and specific standards pertinent to the patient population for whom they are responsible (for example, the standards of care for the orthopedic patient). These standards identify elements of nursing care that must be met to ensure quality care and to provide a baseline for measuring that quality.

Other professional standards that apply to the nurse in the practice setting are nurse practice acts, medical practice acts, and standards set by the Joint Commission on Accreditation of Hospitals (JCAH).[14] Almost every state has a nurse practice act and a medical practice act. Both of these are external sources of standards for nursing practice. Together they define and delineate, from a legal standpoint, the content and practice of nursing.

Nurse practice acts define nursing practice and identify those activities that fall within the province of nursing. *Medical practice acts* further delineate nursing practice by defining those areas that are the exclusive province of the physician. Such exclusions limit the activities in which nurses may engage. Neither act sets actual standards for practice; rather, they define general areas of activity for both professions and establish the legal relationship of the nurse to society and to related professions.

The JCAH is a voluntary, nongovernmental organization that, since its incorporation in 1951, has established standards for operation of hospitals and other health facilities. It conducts surveys and accreditation programs to promote high-quality care and to ensure that patients receive the optimum benefits that medical science has to offer. It emphasizes organization and administration of functions for efficient patient care. Compliance with JCAH standards is recognized by issuance of certificates of accreditation.

The governing body of the JCAH, the Board of Commissioners, consists of 20 persons appointed by its four member organizations: the American College of Physicians, the American College of Surgeons, the American Hospital Association, and the American Medical Association. Currently, nursing is represented on the commission by the American Hospital Association.

JCAH accreditation is voluntary and is not the same as licensure or certification by state or local authorities. However, accreditation has come to be recognized as a benchmark of quality and is used by some regulatory agencies as one criterion for licensure or certification and by some insurance agencies as a condition for honoring reimbursement claims. In addition to its standards for organization of the nursing service department, a standard on quality of professional services was added in 1976, and delineates the characteristics of a patient care evaluation program. In 1983 this standard required a problem-focused, effective review and evaluation of the quality and appropriateness of patient care.

QUALITY ASSURANCE

Quality assurance can be described on two levels. In its strictest sense, it is a set of techniques for assuring the maintenance and improvement of standards and the efficiency and effectiveness of nursing care; more broadly, it is an effort to control nursing practice. As such, it involves relationships between nurses and consumers and between nurses and governmental bodies.

The purpose of quality assurance is always twofold. First, it determines that extent to which predetermined standards are being met by a particular nursing program. Second, these findings are used to make decisions about changes that are to be implemented by persons carrying out the program of care. Both must be in place if nursing is to ensure its accountability to the consumer. Although the specific target of each evaluation may differ depending on the information about quality that is desired, the purpose of the evaluation is always the same.

Nurses engaged in the delivery of health services cannot escape inclusion of quality assurance reviews in their practice responsibilities. Indeed, some proficiency in evaluation must be part of the modern nurse's basic repertoire.

The quality assurance process is not mysterious. Most nurses are well on their way to expertise in this area by virtue of their basic education and experience. Nurses who are expert in the care of specific patient populations, for example, patients with cardiac disease, possess the knowledge necessary to determine desired health processes and outcomes for that population. These nurses are well acquainted with the direct care processes to be used in assisting clients toward health and wellness. They are also aware of the observable changes that will occur at certain intervals in the course of healing.

Most nurses are not expert, however, in the methods used to conduct these evaluations. The following section describes the steps in the quality assurance review process.

QUALITY ASSURANCE REVIEWS
Approach to quality assurance review

A variety of techniques have been proposed to perform the quality assurance review. Presented here is the problem-solving model used by the ANA. Its eight steps include the following:
1. Identify values
2. Identify standards and criteria
3. Measure degree of attainment of standards and criteria
4. Interpret strengths and weaknesses
5. Identify possible courses of action
6. Select a course of action
7. Take action
8. Reevaluate

Each of these steps is discussed and illustrated with a clinical example (Fig. 4-1).

Topics for quality assurance reviews are generally

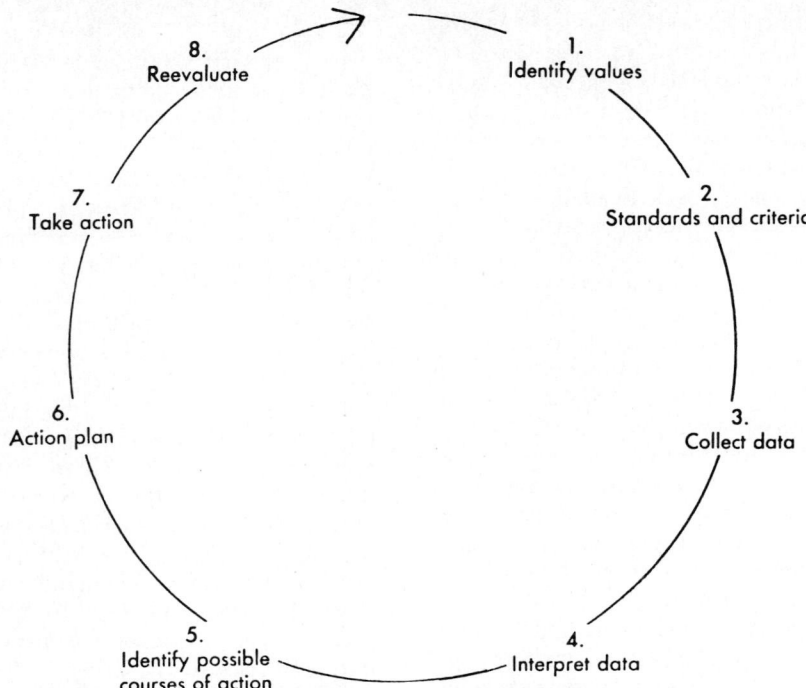

Fig. 4-1. American Nurses Association model for quality assurance review. (From American Nurses Association: Quality assurance for nursing care, Kansas City, Mo., 1976, The Association. Reprinted by permission of the American Nurses Association.)

placed in some order of priority based on their frequency and their real or potential impact on patient care. Impact is usually gauged by whether efficiency or effectiveness of patient care is affected. *Efficiency* is generally defined in terms of accomplishing a task with a minimum of resources (time, money, personnel); *effectiveness* is defined in terms of accomplishment of predetermined goals. The focus for the evaluation may be the nurse, the unit or institution, the nursing care, or a combination of the three.

If the focus of the evaluation is the nurse, it can include the actions of a single nurse or of all the nurses in a department, and any area of nursing activity can be examined. For example, is the nursing staff satisfied with the primary nursing program instituted 3 months ago? What criteria do the nursing staff use to determine the frequency of vital sign monitoring in the immediate postoperative period? Are the nursing standards for administration of intravenous therapy being adhered to?

If the nursing unit or institution is the focus of the quality assurance review, it might examine the administrative structure, the physical plant and equipment, or staffing. For example, a review could be implemented to determine whether required educational records for nurses in the critical care units are up to date. Or a review could be done in conjunction with the environmental services department to determine if there is an appropriate number of wheelchairs and IV poles and whether they are all functional.

When nursing care or a nursing care problem is the focus of the review, it is generally best to limit the scope to a certain population (for example, patients with certain diagnoses, surgical procedures, nursing care problems, or degree of illness) so that the project is manageable in terms of all the variables to be considered.

It is critical to remember that the perspective of the consumer must be considered in any evaluation. In selected instances, such as using patient outcomes or in attempting to validate patient care plans with patients themselves, consumer input is essential.

Steps in a quality assurance review

Step 1: Identify values

Before the implementation of the quality assurance model there must be an examination of the societal, professional, and individual values that guide the health care in the respective agency. The very word *quality* implies that someone somewhere has determined that certain outcomes have more value than others. As applied to nursing care, the individual nurse, nursing unit, hospital, and community will interact to influence the development of criteria to be used in the review process.

Step 2: Identify standards and criteria

A *standard* is the desirable or achievable level or range of performance of a certain criterion, or a framework against which performance is compared. An example of a standard is, "Every patient will have an admission assessment by a registered nurse." A *criterion measure* is that

Types of standards and outcomes

Patient goal Adequate pain medication to enable mobilization and pulmonary hygiene.

Structure Pain medication available and ordered by physician.

Process Nursing staff assess patient at least every 4 hours for discomfort.

Outcome Patient has adequate pain control, enabling him to ambulate, cough, and deep breathe.

variable believed to be the indicator of the quality of care, for example, "The assessment form will be completed by the admitting nurse within 8 hours of admission."

The standards for nursing practice are generally developed by clinical nursing leaders in the institution, using their professional expertise as well as professional research and literature. The standards are made operational by construction of the criterion elements. These criteria, which are the actual evaluation criteria, are generally developed by a quality assurance committee, the nursing practice committee, or some similar group.

The actual criteria that are developed can be of three types: structure, process, and outcome (see box above). *Structure criteria* describe the environmental elements, setting, and conditions within which the nurse-patient relationship occurs. It includes the philosophy and objectives of the institution; its fiscal resources, equipment, physical facilities, management structure, accreditation, and licensure; and the quality and characteristics of the professional and technical employees. Examples of structure criteria include, "Hospital beds must be 3 feet apart." "All patients must sign the required consent form

before any invasive or surgical procedure." "The current license number of each registered nurse must be on file in the main nursing office."

Process criteria describe the nature and sequence of nursing care activities. For example, process criteria might describe the nursing plan for a patient who demands pain medication every 1½ hours, although he has made a contract with his primary nurse that he will not do so. A teaching plan for a diabetic patient is another example.

Outcome criteria focus on the results of the processes of health care. Many experts consider them to be the ultimate indicators of the quality of patient care. For the patient the outcome should be measurable in terms of change in health, knowledge, or functional status.

After the criteria have been written, they must be validated, generally by "consensus among peers." The rationale for this validation step is to ensure that all criteria are correct and relevant and reflect nursing practice at the particular institution. Usually, nurses most expert in the selected clinical area are chosen to do the review.

The final step in the criteria writing process is the establishment, by the quality assurance committee and the "nurse experts," of a specific and observable level of performance for each criterion measure. For example, for the outcome criterion "Patient or significant other is able to demonstrate proper technique in insulin administration," at least 90% compliance might be expected. However, for the outcome criterion "Patient is able to apply own stoma appliance," the committee may decide that 80% compliance is appropriate, because many of the patients are elderly, are not completely independent in activities of daily living by the time of discharge, and are frequently discharged to nursing homes.

Step 3: Measure degree of attainment of standards and criteria

Multiple methods are available to collect data to assess the attainment of the standards and criteria. The degree

Outcome criteria for the person with a colostomy or ileostomy

The patient or significant other can
1. *Demonstrate how to measure the stoma for an appliance. (The stoma shrinks as healing occurs. Measure the stoma before purchasing more appliances.)*
2. *Demonstrate proper application of the appliance. (Application includes appliance removal, skin care, and reapplying an appliance.)*
3. *State plans for follow-up care.*
4. *State community resources available for obtaining permanent appliances and financial assistance, and list support groups. (Include the name of one surgical supply house, and the telephone number of the Ostomy Association, the Visiting Nurses Association, or some other home care support group.)*
5. *State need to observe stoma and skin around it for redness, bleeding, or excoriation.*
Patient or significant other has
6. *Information packet, which has been reviewed with the nurse.*

to which the actual practice exceeds, meets, or falls below the validated criteria provides the data necessary to evaluate the strengths and weaknesses of the nursing care program. Data collection methods might include questionnaires, staff interviews, patient interviews, self-assessment questionnaires, performance evaluation, utilization review, audits, patient or staff complaints, and direct observation. Whatever the method selected, the data should be easily accessible, and questions of efficiency and accuracy should be considered.

Data collected are tabulated, and the results indicate whether the percentage of yes/no responses corresponds to the previously established level of performance (percent compliance) for each criterion. If the level of performance does not achieve expectations, the criterion element has not been met.

Step 4: Interpret strengths and weaknesses

The degree to which the levels of performance have been met serves as the basis for describing the strengths

---

Quality assurance review topic: learning needs of the patient with a colostomy or ileostomy

Step 1: Identify values

Patient and family education and patient involvement in care are high priorities at this institution. Nurses on the surgical units were concerned that ostomy patients, in particular, were not receiving adequate discharge information.

Step 2: Identify criteria

The outcome criteria (written in 1980) for the person with a colostomy or ileostomy were selected as the evaluation criteria (see p. 41).

Step 3: Collect data

Charts of 30 patients with the discharge diagnosis of some type of ostomy were selected at random from patients discharged in the previous 6 months. Review of the patient record using the Outcome Criteria for the Person with a Colostomy or Ileostomy revealed incomplete teaching plans and no record of the patient having received any type of information booklets. (The rule is, "If it isn't documented, it hasn't been done.")

Step 4: Interpret data

The quality assurance committee was certain that the patients had received more information than was documented in the record. But where was such documentation to be found? It was also apparent to the committee that some of the criterion elements required updating.

Step 5: Identify possible courses of action

It was observed that the documentation system for discharge planning for these patients needed to be more efficient, yet more thorough. The surgical nursing staff suggested that the outcome criteria sheet be printed on a Nurse's Note. Another suggestion was to use a large stamp containing elements of the teaching plan, which could be checked off as completed. A group of experienced nurses was formed, who, with the assistance of the clinical nurse specialist, rewrote and assisted in the validation process for the outcome criteria.

Step 6: Write the action plan

The quality assurance committee met with the surgical nursing staff and concluded that the best choice was to have the outcome criteria overprinted on the Nurse's Notesheet. The appropriate administrative approval was obtained.

Step 7: Implement the action plan

One member of the quality assurance committee was assigned to oversee the production of the new forms. After they were obtained, the unit nursing staff took the responsibility for introducing them and explaining their purpose to the other staff members. An evaluation was planned for 4 months later.

Step 8: Reevaluate

Four months after the implementation, the surgical staff conducted a repeat review. There was 100% compliance with each criterion element.

and weaknesses of the nursing care program. However, it is essential that certain subtle factors not be overlooked before final judgments are made. Consider the following: One of the outcome criteria for a patient with a pacemaker is, "The patient or significant other is able to take a pulse." A retrospective nursing audit was done on patients with pacemakers to determine whether the outcome was being met. On nursing unit A, 95% of the patients could take their pulse, whereas on nursing unit C, only 65% of the patients could. Careful inspection of the patient data revealed that, in general, patients on unit C were older, had fewer significant others, and were frequently discharged to extended care facilities. Comparing the two units on these factors provided insights into reasons for their differences that may have been missed if the evaluator had not questioned these differences.

Step 5: Identify possible courses of action

After identifying the strengths and weaknesses, possible courses of action to correct the weaknesses are developed. The goal of the action plan is elimination of the weaknesses and reinforcement of the strengths of the existing program. Some consideration should be given to how best to motivate the nursing staff to implement the desired changes. Generally the best results will be obtained when those staff most affected by the quality assurance review are involved in the planning of subsequent courses of action.

Solutions to the identified problems can be numerous and can include administrative changes, further clinical research into the problem, continuing education, changes in practice, environmental changes, a reward system for improved compliance, or even the organization of peer pressure. Each of the possible solutions has advantages and disadvantages, and the peer group will have to weigh each one.

Step 6: Select a course of action

After examination of the alternatives, the peer group selects the course of action, based on such considerations as the identified problem, available resources, and organizational structure. How the decision is implemented will vary among institutions. For example, if it involves a nursing practice change, it may have to be reviewed by the director of nursing.

Step 7: Take action

Improving the quality of nursing care implies change, and sooner or later some action must be taken. Implementation of the selected action generally includes time frames, persons responsible for overseeing each step of the plan, and selection of a date for reevaluation. This action step is critical to the success of the quality assurance review.

Step 8: Reevaluate

After the action has been taken, the cycle begins again. If a change has been made, it must be reassessed to determine its effectiveness in improving the quality of care.

MONITORING ACTIVITIES AND INSTRUMENTS

In addition to the problem-focused quality assurance reviews, a variety of methods have been devised for ongoing assessment of the nursing care program. Some of the more frequently used methods are described here.

Incident reports

Whenever an untoward event occurs involving a patient, nurse, or visitor, an incident report must be completed. Generally these are compiled by the hospital and/or the hospital insurance carrier. Increases in certain types of incidents, such as medication errors or patient falls, would be a signal to the quality assurance committee that a review of either of these two areas may be indicated.

Nursing audit

The nursing audit compares predetermined criteria with the documentation found in the patient record. There are two types of audit: retrospective and concurrent. A *retrospective audit* is a critical examination of nursing actions, with a view toward improvement in practice. A retrospective review is done after the patient has been discharged. The reviewer has the advantage of using data from the patient's entire stay, from admission to discharge, and of evaluating the results for a large series of comparable patients. One advantage of a retrospective audit is that sometimes practitioners gain impressions from single cases in which they are personally involved. These impressions, however, may not be borne out by later systematic study of a large number of cases.

A *concurrent audit* is a critical examination of the patient's progress toward a desired health status (outcome) and patient care management activities (processes) while the care is in progress. Patient questionnaires, interviews, and observation and review of the patient record are possible sources of data for a concurrent review. Concurrent review has the advantage of providing opportunities for making changes in the ongoing care program. Retrospective and concurrent reviews each have their own advantages, and may be used singly or together in a quality assurance review.

Peer review

Nursing peer review occurs when nurses establish standards and criteria and evaluate the quality of patient care among themselves. The peer review process may be performed within a single unit or by specialty, for example, orthopedic nurses. Clinical nurse specialists also frequently have a peer review group to monitor their practice.

Patient satisfaction questionnaire

A patient satisfaction questionnaire is generally used when written data regarding a patient's perceptions of his or her hospitalization are needed, for example, by hospital management or a nurse researcher. Many hospitals routinely distribute these questionnaires to all patients and request that they complete them. Other hospitals have patient ombudsmen who visit patients, question them regarding their hospitalization experience, answer any questions they may have, and intervene in their behalf, if necessary.

Staff satisfaction surveys

Staff satisfaction surveys, either questionnaires or interviews, are used by the administration to assess general employee satisfaction or to test responses to certain program changes.

Utilization review

The utilization review program was mandated by the JCAH in 1978. Its primary goal is the appropriate allocation of hospital resources. This program does not focus primarily on nursing, but it does provide data that may require nursing involvement in a more thorough evaluation.

Infection control reports

Because nurses are involved in the direct care of patients, they may at times be included in infection surveillance and infection control programs. Even when the nursing staff is not involved directly, they should be familiar with the monthly report of nosocomial infections on their respective unit. Questions can be raised about nursing procedures and practices that may affect the infection rate on the unit.

SUMMARY

Changes in the health care sector and its financing mechanisms will undoubtedly affect quality assurance activities in the future. There is some concern that quality of health care may become secondary to the cost of that care. Properly designed and executed quality assurance activities are irreplaceable feedback devices that allow nursing to define and describe for physicians, other health professionals, and consumers the fundamental efficacy and importance of nursing care.

REFERENCES AND SELECTED READINGS*

1. American Nurses' Association: Quality assurance for nursing care, Kansas City, Mo., 1976, The Association.
2. *American Nurses' Association: Standards of nursing practice, Kansas City, Mo., 1973, The Association.
3. Bergman, R.: Evaluation of nursing care: could it make a difference? Int. J. Nurs. Stud. **19:**53-60, 1982.
4. Blake, B.: Quality assurance: an ethical responsibility, Supervisor Nurse **12:**32-38, 1981.
5. Bloch, D.: Criteria, standards, norms: crucial terms in quality assurance, J. Nurs. Adm. **7:**20-29, 1977.
6. Clinton, J., and others: Developing criterion measures of nursing care: case study of a process, J. Nurs. Adm. **7D:**41-45, 1977.
7. Davis, K.: Nursing and the health care debates, Image **15:**67, 1983.
8. Donabedian, A.: Criteria, norms and standards of quality: What do they mean? Am. J. Public Health **71:**409-412, 1981.
9. Ferguson, D., and Brunner, N.: Balancing priorities to attain quality care, Nurs. Management **13:**67-69, 1982.
10. Given, B., Given, W., and Simmoni, L.: Relationship of process of care to patient outcomes, Nurs. Res. **28:**85-93, 1979.
11. Gordon, M.: Determining study topics, Nurs. Res. **29:**83-87, 1980.
12. Griffith, N., and Megel, M.: Quality assurance: an educational approach, Nurs. Outlook **29:**670-673, 1981.
13. Howe, M.: Developing instruments for measurement of criteria: a clinical nursing perspective, Nurs. Res. **29:**100-103, 1980.
14. Joint Commission on Accreditation of Hospitals: Accreditation manual for hospitals, Chicago, 1983, The Commission.
15. *Lane, G., Cronin, K., and Peirce, A.: Teaching diploma students how to utilize the ANA quality assurance model, J. Nurs. Educ. **21**(9):42-44, 1982.
16. Marriner, A.: The research process in quality assurance, Am. J. Nurs. **79:**2158-2161, 1979.
17. *Moore, K.: What nurses learn from nursing audit, Nurs. Outlook **27:**254-258, 1979.
18. Padilla, G., and Grant, M.: Quality assurance programme for nursing, J. Adv. Nurs. **7:**135-145, 1982.
19. Phaneuf, M.: The nursing audit, ed 2, New York, 1976, Appleton-Century-Crofts.
20. *Schmadl, J.: QA examination of the concepts, Nurs. Outlook **27:**462-465, 1979.
21. Tucker, S., and others: Patient care standards, ed. 2, St. Louis, 1980, The C.V. Mosby Co.
22. Williamson, J., and others: Teaching quality assurance and cost containment in health care, San Francisco, 1982, Jossey-Bass, Inc., Publishers.

*References preceded by an asterisk are particularly well suited for student reading.

UNIT II
Health Promotion

5 Developmental Factors Affecting Health of Adults

6 Biologic Defense Mechanisms of the Human Body

7 Health Promotion: Nutrition and Exercise

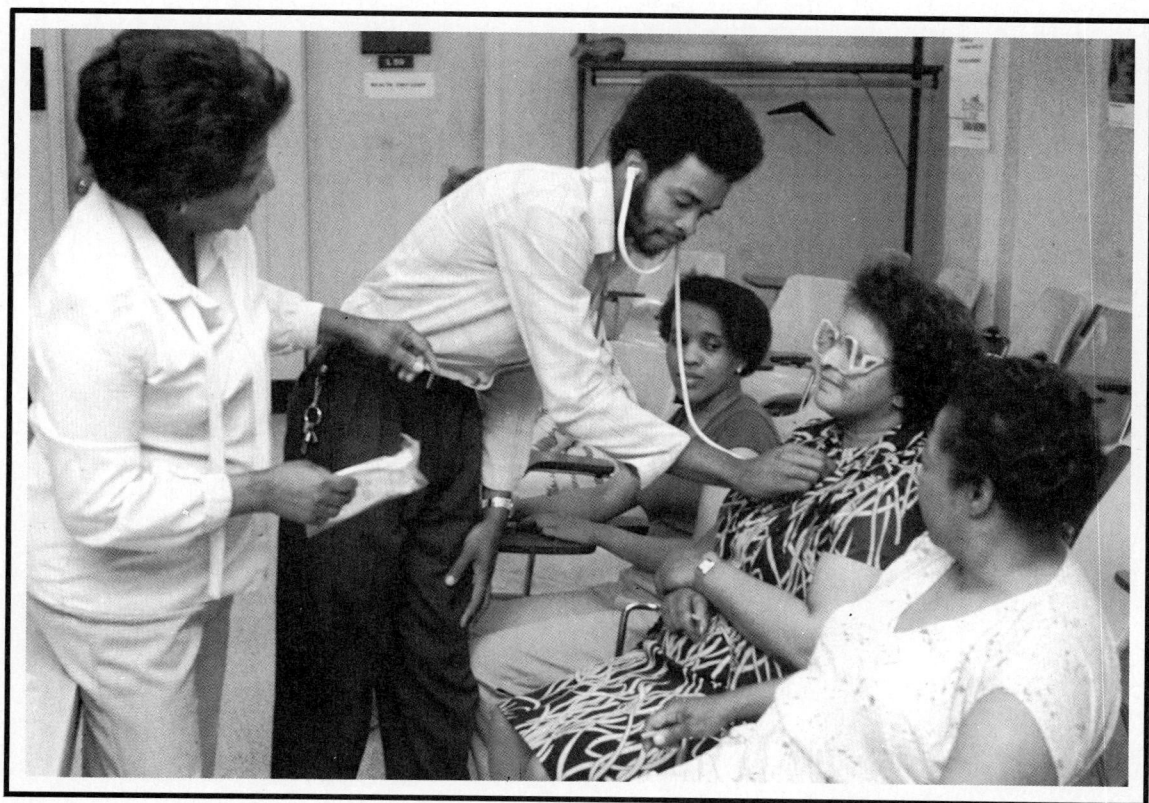

5

Developmental Factors Affecting Health of Adults

DOLORES VERDERBER

STUDY QUESTIONS

- List some of the stresses most common to persons in your own age group. How do these compare with stresses in your parents' age group?

- Talk with and observe persons in age groups other than your own. How do you and they differ in terms of physical development and major concerns in your lives?

- Review the eating patterns of an elderly person of your acquaintance; compare his or her food intake with your understanding of an adequate diet. If there are inadequacies, what are some possible reasons?

- From what you have read in newspapers and heard discussed, what would you select as major problems of elderly people in your community?

- What services are available for the elderly in your community?

Every person for whom the nurse provides care is engaged in the process of growth and development. Changes in physical and psychosocial development occur in adults as they move from young adulthood to middle adulthood and then to late adulthood. In planning nursing care, it is as important to provide for the patient's growth and development needs as it is to meet needs generated by the illness.

The number of elderly in the United States has increased steadily over the past 50 years. The growth rate of the older population has been consistently faster than that of persons younger than 65 years. At present, the number of persons 75 years of age or older is increasing at a faster rate than the number of persons older than 65 years. The number of elderly persons has increased for several reasons:

1. Decrease in infant mortality
2. Prevention and control of communicable diseases during childhood
3. Improved treatment of acute and chronic diseases in adults
4. Improvements in medical care in general

YOUNG ADULTHOOD

Young adulthood, extending from approximately 20 to 45 years, is a complex period of life, a time in which the transition from adolescence to adulthood is the primary focus. During the young adult years, energies are directed toward career fulfillment, social involvement, and the initiation and maintenance of a family.

Physical development in the young adult

1. Posture is erect, and maximum height is achieved.
2. Muscle tone and coordination are optimal.
3. Energy levels are high, and there is good control of this energy.
4. Skin is smooth and taut.
5. Tissue repair and healing occur readily.
6. Body rhythms are established.
7. Reproductive capabilities are high.

Physical development

Full growth and development are complete by the early to mid-20s, and most body systems are functioning at optimum. This includes intellectual and physical functions.

Sexuality

Sexuality is a integral part of self-concept. Competence in the area of sexuality is of prime importance during adult years. During young adulthood the body's sexual response is powerful and there is a need to find adequate and satisfactory expression. A man reaches peak sexual capacity at about 18 years of age, and a woman generally in her early 30s.

If the expression of sexual feelings is restricted, perhaps because of illness or injury, causing a felt or imagined change in body image, sexual concerns may become paramount. Nurses frequently are asked by young adults for assistance with marital or sexual problems. Unless the nurse is secure in his or her own sexual identity and has had adequate preparation to deal with such matters, patients should be referred to appropriate persons (Chapter 34).

Psychosocial development

Adulthood is often equated with maturity and is characterized by a sense of responsibility, maintenance of appropriate impulse control, ability to plan and implement realistic goals, and capacity to enter into intimate relationships.

Everyone does not arrive at young adulthood with the same level of maturity. Emotional maturity varies from person to person, as do intellectual ability and physical characteristics. In addition, an adult who appears reasonably mature under usual circumstances may, under stress, exhibit certain immature behavior, for example, become more demanding or very critical or lose his or her temper.

In Erikson's *eight ages of man,* the first adult stage is characterized by *intimacy versus isolation* (Table 5-1). Intimacy is sharing the self to form a commitment to an intense lasting relationship with another person, a cause, or a creative effort, without fear of loss of identity. Intimacy requires responsibility, impulse control, the ability to plan, and the ability to trust. The inability to develop some form of intimacy draws the person into increasing feelings of isolation, alienation, and self-absorption.

The successful resolution of this phase of the life cycle is dependent on a positive self-concept. How persons feel about themselves affects relationships as well as the choices made during this period. A person who feels adequate and competent in setting and achieving goals tends to experience positive outcomes. Negative feelings tend to foster withdrawal and the inability to mobilize resources for positive gains. When caring for the young adult, it is therefore important to assess the individual's self-perception. These data not only provide information as to motivation potential, but form a basis for nursing intervention to help increase the individual's self-esteem.

BODY IMAGE

Body image, an important aspect of self-concept, is a mental picture of the body's appearance, as well as the

Table 5-1. Psychosocial development in adulthood

Age	Erikson's eight ages of man	Maslow's hierarchy of needs
Young adulthood: 20 to 45 years	*Intimacy versus isolation* Significant objects, persons, causes	Security Love and belonging Self-esteem
Middle adulthood: 45 to 65 years	*Generativity versus stagnation* Significant persons: spouse, grandchildren, friends	Same as above
Late adulthood: 65 + years	*Integrity versus disgust, despair* Significant persons: spouse, family members, friends	Same as above Self-actualization

attitudes, emotions, and personality of the individual. At a period of life when acceptance by others is most important, and with society's emphasis on youth, beauty, and physical fitness, any alteration in body function or structure poses a threat to a positive body image. Adaptation to these alterations depends on the nature and meaning of the threat, existing coping mechanisms, and available support systems.

Nursing interventions to help someone deal with a threat to or change in body image include the following:

1. Careful assessment of the individual's perception of the condition
2. Assistance in helping the person maintain a realistic perception of the threat in relation to total self-image
3. Assistance in identifying useful coping mechanisms (Chapter 8)
4. Identification of support systems

INTELLECTUAL DEVELOPMENT

The highest overall performance on intelligence tests is achieved sometime between the late teens and late 20s. Individuals in their 30s, 40s, and 50s tend to score somewhat lower. Longitudinal evidence has shown, however, that general intelligence remains the same or increases slightly during the adult years.

DEVELOPMENTAL TASKS

The developmental tasks of early adulthood, most concretely seen in the choice of a vocation and a marriage partner, clearly involve a certain choice of life-style. Although fairly clear boundaries have been established between self and parents by this time, parental attitudes and value systems have been internalized in young adults and become part of their identity, thus affecting future life choices. Inherent in these choices is the quest for independence from family socially and economically.

Occupational choice

An occupation is much more than a set of skills and functions. It a way of life that determines much of the

---

Tasks of young adulthood

Developing a sense of social responsibility
Choosing a vocation
Establishing a life-style
Choosing a marriage partner and raising children
Establishing and maintaining a home
Forming a meaningful philosophy of life

---

environment, both physical and social, in which a person lives.[35] Occupational choice plays a significant part in further shaping the personality by providing a social system, status, roles, and life-style. The choice of an occupation often requires pursuing appropriate education, and thus educational goals and achievements become a very important part of this choice.

The women's liberation movement has exerted a significant influence on women relative to occupational choices. It is now more socially acceptable for women to choose a career goal as an alternative or as a supplement to the traditional housewife-mother role. Among married young adults there is a growing tendency to delay having children until economic and career goals are more solidified.[14] Some married women in this age group may choose to have an abortion if they become pregnant at a time that is inconvenient relative to their career or other goals.

Marital choice

Another major decision of early adulthood is whether to marry. Our society continues to support marital status among young adults. However, some choose not to marry, enjoying the independence and freedom of single living. While there may be many reasons for entering the marital relationship, marriage is generally recognized as a close and loving partnership between two people where intimacy and affection exist in a free and equal relationship, as opposed to a social institution where the man is the undisputed head of the house and the wife is the childbearer.[34]

The arrival of the first child initiates the roles of parenting. Parenthood may be experienced as a joy because a child is the product of their common bond and fulfillment of goals, or as a crisis because of required adjustments in daily routine and life-style. Preparation for parenthood has not been widespread in our society. It is therefore difficult for couples to anticipate many of the stresses of being parents and the changes required in themselves and their marital relationship.

While personality characteristics and interpersonal problems are primary sources of difficulties in adjustment to marriage and parenthood, cultural and societal variables often make these adjustments difficult. For example, the mobility of our society results in a dispersal of family members and close relatives, with less available help from these significant others in times of need and stress.

Health needs

The importance of studying growth and development lies in gaining better understanding of those physical and psychosocial variables that determine the health needs of individuals as they progress through life. The cessation of physical growth by the time a person reaches young adulthood, together with changes in life-style, requires certain alterations in physical and psychosocial needs.

NUTRITION

The young adult's nutritional needs are not the same as those of adolescents. With cessation of physical maturation there is a reduction in some nutritional requirements, such as calcium and protein, whereas an increase in some nutrients, such as vitamin B_6 and C, is necessary. In addition, young men require additional vitamin E and riboflavin, and young women need additional iron.

Nutritional problems of young adults frequently stem from the increased demands placed on them (job, home, children, economics), resulting in poor nutritional choices and habits. The nurse can help the young adult understand the importance of adequate nutrition and of adjusting schedules to allow more time for meals. An understanding of how illnesses and prolonged recovery periods can be related to inadequate nutrition is important.

EXERCISE, REST, AND SLEEP

Exercise serves several functions in the young adult. It helps to regulate appetite, release tension, aid sleep, tone body muscles, maintain cardiovascular conditioning, and retard aging. It is important that exercise should be regular and appropriate to the person's physical condition (Chapter 7).

As the demands of work, social activities, responsibilities, and educational pursuits increase, the young adult's need for adequate rest and sleep also increases, but in actuality the young adult often goes without proper rest and sleep. Although an individual can adjust to a lack of sleep for a short time, prolonged periods can contribute to altered mental and physical functions.

Health concerns

Accidents are the leading cause of death in young adults. Many injuries and illnesses require restriction of activity which presents social and economic problems.[39] Injury and illness may also necessitate some dependence, creating conflict with young adult's quest for independence.

Acute conditions such as *upper respiratory tract infections* occur more frequently in the young adult than do other acute illnesses. With young adults, the primary responsibility of the nurse is the teaching of preventive measures. Prevention is directed at supporting the body defenses and reducing susceptibility to illness. Avoiding environmental pollutants, including cigarette smoke, as much as possible, keeping alcohol intake at an acceptable level, and observing other basic health practices should be stressed.

Physiologic and psychologic changes resulting in unusual or disturbed adaptive behavior patterns occur when the young adult is unable to cope with newly acquired tasks and responsibilities. Mate selection, marriage, childbearing, college, job demands, social expectations, and independent decision making are all stressors. Stress may be a major factor in the incidence of *gastric* and *duodenal ulcers*. When stressors are perceived as overwhelming, they may result in self-destructive behavior such as *drug abuse and addiction, alcoholism,* or *suicide,* one of the leading causes of death in young adults. Nursing interventions include measures to reduce or cope with stress (Chapter 8).

MIDDLE ADULTHOOD

While the transition from young adulthood to the middle years is mostly a state of mind, rather than a dramatic body change, it is generally agreed that middle adulthood comprises those years between ages 45 and 65.

As the young adulthood phase begins to taper in the middle to late 30s our perceptions of time, productivity, self, and others begin to change. The middle years are approached with a sharpened sense of awareness as we begin to take stock of life:

Has it been fulfilling?

Am I doing what I really want to be doing?

Am I really going to accomplish my original, probably idealistic goals?

What are my goals in life from now on?

Evaluation of the quality of life already lived and the potential for the future may have a significant influence on adaptation in the succeeding years.

Physical development

The adult usually approaches this phase of life functioning at near peak efficiency. As the middle years progress, gradual physiologic changes occur:

1. Hair begins to turn gray.
2. Skin becomes dryer and less elastic.
3. Fatty tissue is redistributed regardless of diet or exercise.
4. Skeletal muscle increases in bulk until about age 50 years; no changes occur in smooth muscle.
5. Sensory changes begin to be noted:
   a. Presbyopia (decrease in near vision) results from decreased elasticity of the eyes.
   b. Auditory acuity gradually decreases.
6. Menopause occurs in women, usually between ages 40 and 55 years (Chapter 35).

Sexuality

The physical aspects of aging, together with the many pressures common to this stage of life, affect the attitudes about one's sexuality and sexual functioning.

Some adults view middle age (particularly after menopause) as lessening their physical attractiveness, thus affecting sexual interest and capacity for competent sexual functioning. This is more a psychologic phenomenon than an actual physical occurrence. Cultural influences are significant in perpetuating the idea that aging brings a decline of sexual interest and activity. Ambivalence about growing older in a youth-oriented society often breeds feelings of inadequacy relative to one's sexuality. As a result, some adults may become depressed and sexually unresponsive. Others may feel a need to retrieve that sense of youthfulness by behaving and dressing in a youthful manner or by having an affair with a younger person.

The middle-aged adult who approaches these years with self-acceptance and appreciation is apt to continue into the later years with a satisfying and fulfilling sex life.

Some of the physical changes that accompany menopause may affect the pleasure of sexual intercourse. For example, decrease in the production of vaginal lubrication caused by hormonal changes may result in some discomfort during intercourse, with a tendency to refrain from sexual activity because of discomfort. Use of a water-soluble lubricant during intercourse may be helpful.

As men age, certain social and psychologic factors influence their sexual responsiveness. Several recurrent themes relative to waning sexual responsiveness can be noted:

1. Monotony in the sexual relationship or a feeling of being taken for granted
2. Concerns with economic or career pursuits
3. Mental or physical fatigue
4. Physical or mental illness of the individual or spouse
5. Overindulgence in food or drink
6. Fear of failure[64]

Continued sexual activity contributes to quality of the sexual relationship as well as to the continuation of sexual activity into the later years.

Because of prevailing cultural attitudes about waning sexual interest in the middle years, sexual concerns are often ignored in the care and rehabilitation of the middle-aged adult. It is very important, therefore, that health care providers become knowledgeable about and sensitive to the sexual needs of patients, particularly those who experience injury or illness that restricts physical activity.

Psychosocial development

Erikson has described adaptation to middle age in terms of resolution of the crisis, *generativity* versus *stagnation* (Table 5-1). In a broad sense, generativity includes guiding the next generation, productivity, creativity, and concern for others. When this enrichment and fulfillment are not experienced, stagnation and personal impoverishment occur, to the point of isolation and preoccupation with self.[51]

INTELLECTUAL DEVELOPMENT

Contrary to some popular beliefs, mental capacity is unimpaired in the middle years. Active use of mental capacity throughout the years will contribute to mental productivity in the later years. It is therefore important that mental stimulation be provided as a part of nursing care. The middle-aged adult is encouraged to continue with involvement in activities that facilitate mental productivity.

Tasks of middle adulthood

Assisting children to become responsible adults
Coping with parent-child role transitions
Renewing and redeveloping significant relationships
Assuming responsible positions in occupation and society
Adjusting to aging and planning for retirement
Reevaluating life goals
Developing leisure activities

DEVELOPMENTAL TASKS

The psychologic and social development of the individual in the middle years is best exemplified in the various developmental tasks that are common to this stage of life. Many of these tasks involve role transitions, which may involve some alteration in self-image, life-style, values, and attitudes. This age group is at the peak in terms of productivity, wields the most power, and demonstrates the greatest social influence.

The ability to shed roles and take on new roles smoothly contributes to a creative and productive life during the middle years. With the maturation of children comes the transition of parental attitudes, values, and actions that formerly were child oriented to those more appropriate to an adult relationship. In those instances where the focus of life revolved solely around the children, the outcome of their departure from the home may be an experience of loss. What is lost is not only the grown child but all the attachments associated with the parent role, resulting in altered perceptions of self.[44]

Not only is the role transition relative to one's children complex, but the health status of one's parents is changing. Illnesses and perhaps impending death often necessitate assuming the role of parent to one's own parent(s). Decisions made regarding the care of aging parents may require changes in life-style if they come to live in the home.

During the middle years, renewal and full development of relationships can occur, and the patterns of child-centered days and of nurturing the intimate relationship of husband and wife change. The individual may enjoy the enrichment of new and renewed relationships and a new sense of freedom. If throughout previous years a couple has not developed mutual support, open communication, and awareness of each other's needs, the development of an enriching relationship may be difficult to achieve.

For some adults the middle years are a time of peak social influence, prosperity, economic success, and stability. But for some the middle years are approached with a sense of frustration and failure if goals and expectations set in earlier years have not been reached and are not attainable. The realization that the time has passed for significant achievement of status and success is often crisis producing.

Reevaluation often results in ambivalence and uncertainties associated with everyday tasks, reflecting a change in values and attitudes. The adult who previously perceived daily responsibilities as fulfilling and enjoyable may begin to complain about being trapped. It may not be the job or situation that has changed, however, but the individual.

Wives who perceive their status relative to the success of their husbands may become dissatisfied with themselves for not being involved in self-fulfilling activities. They may embark on new careers in search of self-fulfillment and satisfaction. The women's movement has contributed much to women's motivation to seek heightened self-fulfillment, satisfaction, and usefulness.

Productive use of leisure may be a source of contentment for some adults, with the exploration and development of new areas of talent, skill, and hobbies. The relationships and involvement in outside activities is demonstrative of the external orientation characteristic of this period of life. When there is a lack in the cultivation of various relationships and areas of interest, stagnation and immobilization occur. It is the mobilization of inner resources that generates the kind of creativity and productivity that facilitate continued growth throughout the remaining years.

Health needs

As individuals change, so do their health needs. Consideration of the needs of proper nutrition, rest, and exercise are most important during the middle years.

NUTRITION

Reduced energy requirements together with reduced physical activity dictate a lesser demand for calories. The middle-aged adult needs to be aware of the decreased need for calories, and the importance of lowered intake of saturated fats and cholesterol, which may contribute to obesity and atherosclerosis. The diet should contain the basic four food groups (Chapter 7), with an emphasis on protein, minerals, and vitamins; caloric intake should be based on age, body build, size, and activity.

EXERCISE AND REST

Changes in life-style may result in lack of exercise, restful sleep, and relaxation. It is important that rest and sleep be balanced with physical activity to keep the body functioning at its optimum (Chapter 7). An assessment of daily activities may give some indication as to the kind and amount of exercise necessary. Middle-aged persons should take the following precautions:

1. Before starting an exercise program, consult a physician if overweight, have a personal or family history of cardiovascular or respiratory disease, or have been leading a sedentary life-style.
2. Increase exercise gradually.
3. Exercise consistently.
4. Avoid overexertion (10 minutes after exercising, the heart rate should return to baseline status).

HEALTH ASSESSMENT

Middle-aged adults should be encouraged to have regular complete medical examinations, including rectal or proctoscopic examination. Women should have regular pelvic examinations, including a Papanicolaou test. Routine dental, vision, and hearing examinations should also be done, because periodontal disease, glaucoma, and hearing loss may be prevented or treated if detected early.

Health concerns

Motor vehicle accidents, occupation-related accidents, and falls in the home are leading causes of death in middle age. Fractures and dislocations are the leading injuries. Respiratory conditions are frequent causes of absenteeism from work. Generally, middle-aged women have more disability days from work because of respiratory and other acute disorders, whereas men have more disability days from injury.[39] The main health problems of this age group are listed below.

The close interrelationship between the physical and psychologic makeup of the human body is exemplified in menopause. How a woman reacts depends a great deal on her feelings about herself and her womanhood. If procreation and motherhood have been her major sources of self-esteem and she cannot adapt to physical changes and changing life circumstances, she may become severely depressed and require treatment. Many women adjust to menopause without difficulty (Chapter 35).

Although men do not experience the same physiologic changes as women do, they often go through a kind of psychologic "change of life." Symptoms may include fatigue, headaches, increased moodiness, impatience,

---

**Major health problems
of middle adulthood**

Cardiovascular disease
Pulmonary disease
Rheumatoid arthritis
Cancer
Diabetes
Obesity
Alcoholism
Anxiety
Depression

worry, and complaints such as indigestion, heartburn, rapid or irregular heartbeat, and insomnia. These symptoms are often related to emotional depression and anxiety, which may be associated with preoccupation with thoughts of aging, anticipation of retirement, loss of career status, and a general feeling of worthlessness.

For the middle-aged person who feels depressed, trapped, frustrated, or isolated, easily accessible escape mechanisms may include alcoholism, drug abuse, or excessive food intake. Hypochondriasis is a common symptom of the self-absorbed adult and may become a means of getting attention. The self-absorbed person is likely to demonstrate regressed, immature behavior resulting in increased dependency. Suicide is a leading cause of death among the middle aged.

Adults may experience numerous highly stressful life events. The use of a stress index, such as Holmes and Rahe's life change units (LCUs), may offer predictive value for predisposition to illness (Table 5-2). Numeric weighting is given to various life events that have a psychologic impact on an individual's life. A sum of 250 points or more within a year may indicate increased vulnerability to disease and reflect symptoms of anxiety and disorganized behavior. A sum of 350 to 400 points accumulated in a year is often associated with the onset of physical illness.

Because middle adulthood is a time when productivity, achievement, and responsibilities are dominant concerns, a crisis often results if goals and expectations are thwarted by illness or disability. The crisis may not affect just the individual but the family as well. When stress is intense, problem solving may be diminished. The nurse can be helpful at this time by assisting the patient and family to explore their concerns and by offering options and resources to assist in decision making. Independence can be fostered and maintained by facilitating the patient's participation in care planning and decision making.

LATE ADULTHOOD

Although 65 years of age is usually considered the beginning of late adulthood, or old age, tremendous individual variation exists. Age is really a sociocultural concept

Major components of aging

Biologic age	Position in time relative to potential life span.
Psychologic age	Capacity for adapting to the environment.
Social age	Role in the family, at work, and in the community, as well as interests and activities.

Table 5-2. Social readjustment rating scale (life change units)

Life event	Mean value	Life event	Mean value
Death of spouse	100	Son or daughter leaving home	29
Divorce	73	Trouble with in-laws	29
Marital separation	65	Outstanding personal achievement	28
Jail term	63	Wife beginning or stopping work	26
Death of close family member	63	Begin or end school	26
Personal injury or illness	53	Change in living conditions	25
Marriage	50	Revision of personal habits	24
Fired at work	47	Trouble with boss	23
Marital reconciliation	45	Change in work hours or conditions	20
Retirement	45	Change in residence	20
Change in health of family member	44	Change in schools	20
Pregnancy	40	Change in recreation	19
Sex difficulties	39	Change in church activities	19
Gain of new family member	39	Change in social activities	18
Business readjustment	39	Mortgage or loan less than $10,000	17
Change in financial state	38	Change in sleeping habits	16
Death of close friend	37	Change in number of family get togethers	15
Change to different line of work	36	Change in eating habits	15
Change in number of arguments with spouse	35	Vacation	13
Mortgage over $10,000	31	Christmas	12
Foreclosure of mortgage or loan	30	Minor violations of the law	11
Change in responsibilities at work	29		

From Holmes, T., and Rache, H., J. Pyschosom. Res. **11:**213, 1967.

and not wholly physiologic and chronologic. Chronologic age is related to but not identical with aging because of individual and personal variables. The three main components of the aging process are biologic age, psychologic age, and social age. Some people may be old at 45 years, whereas others are not old at 75 years.

Physical development

Biologic aging is a normal developmental process, with certain anatomic and physiologic changes. The speed with which aging occurs varies and depends on hereditary factors and the stress of life events. The genetic factor in the biologic processes determines the time of onset, the course and direction, and the time sequences of the various aging processes.

Many models of aging have been hypothesized and are generally divided into two classes: programmed aging and random deterioration. *Programmed aging* theories attribute aging to a sequential program, a biologic clock, a predetermined series of events leading to aging and eventual death. *Random deterioration* theories include interference with proper functioning of the cells resulting from error, waste products, or other biologic changes.

Biologic aging leads to some general responses in the older person. There is a gradual decline in functional ability, particularly where multisystem coordination is required. There seems to be growing evidence that some effects of aging are related to decreased effectiveness of control mechanisms in maintaining homeostasis. The elderly have increased vulnerability to pathophysiologic problems.

Cardiovascular changes that started during middle age begin to present symptoms in the older years. The heart must work harder to provide adequate oxygenation. Ischemia and infarction result if blood vessels become blocked. With prolonged standing, blood may accumulate in lower extremities, leading to decreased cerebral perfusion, dizziness, and orthostatic hypotension, and accidents may result.

Changes in the *respiratory system* and diminished defense mechanisms increase susceptibility of the lungs to congestion and infection. Chronic lung disease leads to changes in the chest configuration (barrel chest).

Changes in the *nervous system* may lead to confusion if the brain is not well oxygenated (as occurs with inactivity). Decreased sensory perception places the elderly person at high risk for injury. Loss of sense of taste and smell may lead to inadequate nutrition.

The *liver, heart, kidneys,* and other vital organs in many elderly people may have to work harder to maintain normal function, with little margin for adaptability to stress. Any additional burden may be enough to tip the balance unfavorably unless particular care is taken. Fluid and electrolyte balance may be altered, with decreased kidney function. One consequence of this change is the potentiation of the half-life of many drugs that are excreted by the kidneys. Additionally, faintness and shock may follow relatively short periods without food and fluid because of fluid and electrolyte imbalance.

Sexuality

Many younger persons falsely assume that older people have no interest in sex and lack the ability to perform sexually. Men and women of all ages are capable of sexual arousal and orgasm. Maintenance of sexual activity in old age is enhanced by consistency of sexual activity. Sexual activity may continue into the 80s and 90s (see Chapter 34). Often the aged person becomes sexually inactive only because of lack of an acceptable partner.

Physiologic changes of aging

Cardiovascular system
  Decreased elasticity of blood vessels
  Decreased cardiac output
  Possible blocking of blood vessels by fatty deposits (atherosclerosis)
  Increased peripheral vascular resistance leading to increased blood pressure
  Slowed circulation
  Decreased efficiency of valves in veins of lower extremities
Respiratory system
  Decreased elasticity of lungs and chest wall
  Decreased recoil of lungs
  Increased residual lung volume
  Decreased forced expiratory volume
  Decreased oxygen pressure (Po_2) (about 4 mm Hg/decade)
Nervous system
  Generalized loss of neurons
  Progressive decrease in weight of brain
  Decreased gag reflex
  Decreased sensory status (vision, hearing, and touch Chapters 20 to 22), taste, and smell
Musculoskeletal system
  Decreased lean muscle mass
  Increased body fat
  Decreased muscle strength
  Demineralization of bones (especially vertebrae and femur)
  Decreased joint mobility
Gastrointestinal system
  Decreased intestinal motility
  Decreased control of defecation
Urinary system
  Reduced renal blood flow
  Decreased glomerular filtration rate
  Decreased bladder muscle tone
  Decreased control of voiding

Psychosocial development

Psychologic and social development continue during maturity. Psychologic and socioeconomic concepts of aging are most important for those who work with the aged. A knowledge of the crises occurring in this stage of life is useful in assisting patients and their families in attainment of developmental tasks. These tasks are illustrative of the components of Maslow's hierarchy of needs (see Chapter 2). As these tasks demonstrate, the five levels of human need are dynamic, and an individual is frequently in the process of moving between levels. This is particularly true of the elderly person, who may have to make frequent adjustments because of health, loneliness, or other reasons.

Emotional development is reflected in Erikson's description of the mature years, *integrity versus disgust or despair*[64] (Table 5-1). The individual who looks back and perceives life to have been rich and fulfilling, with purpose and meaning, will experience a sense of satisfaction and contentment in the remaining years; otherwise, the final years will be faced with despair.

Another kind of emotional and psychologic response is seen as the elderly person looks ahead to the end of life. *Disengagement* or *withdrawal* may occur as the individual perceives the reality of being mortal.[65] This behavioral response may be initiated by the individual or by others in the social system, with the outcome being a movement away from involvement, achievement, and productivity on the part of the mature individual.[55]

Activity theorists propose that social involvement, not disengagement, facilitates successful adaptation to aging. New social roles and activities are substituted for those that were lost (work, parenting). Both activity and disengagement behaviors are seen in elderly persons to a greater or lesser degree, as determined by their personalities throughout life.

Health concerns

Multiplicity and chronicity of diseases are common among the elderly, and most patients have several chronic ailments. Some of these ailments are not particularly troublesome; most have developed slowly and usually take time to alleviate.

Elderly persons have a *decreased immune response,* with less rapid and less effective response to infections and to an increased incidence of autoimmune conditions and cancer. Complex functions that require *multisystem coordination* show the most obvious decline and require the greatest compensation and support.

Stress situations (either physiologic or psychosocial) produce more pronounced reactions in the aged and require a longer period of readjustment. When determining the stress index from life events, elderly persons are commonly found to have an accumulation of more than 350 points. Many stressful events peculiar to the older adult (and not found among those listed in Table 5-2) are listed here.

Tasks of late adulthood

Adjusting to new limitations of declining physical strength and declining health

Adjusting to retirement and change in financial status

Accepting reorganized family patterns

Adjusting to a new pattern of social and civic responsibilities

Adjusting to death of spouse and other loved ones

Establishing affiliation with one's age group

Maintaining satisfactory living arrangements

Accepting death with serenity

Major health problems of late adulthood

Heart disease

Cancer

Renal disease

Chronic obstructive pulmonary disease

Acute pulmonary disease (pneumonia, pulmonary edema)

Vascular disease (cerebrovascular accident, peripheral vascular disease)

Arthritis

Skin disorders

Accidents

Additional stressful life changes in the elderly

Loss of driver's license

Multiple relocations

Hemiplegia

Sensory deficits

Hospitalization

Institutionalization

Mechanical speech difficulties

Loss of children and friends

Dispersal of significant belongings

Incompetency proceedings

Inheritance conflicts

Birth of grandchildren

Elderly persons also have atypical presentation of illness. Pain may be less pronounced, some symptoms may be absent, or symptoms may be the opposite of what is usually seen.

COGNITIVE IMPAIRMENT

Changes in mental functioning seen in some older persons may result from several causes, 50% of which are reversible. Cognitive functioning may be impaired by acute or chronic organic brain syndromes or by depression. *Acute organic brain syndrome,* which is potentially reversible, may be caused by fluid and electrolyte imbalance, malnutrition, metabolic imbalances, toxic states, trauma, infections, decreased cardiac or renal function, drugs, or overwhelming stress.

Chronic organic brain syndromes, which include Alzheimer's disease and vascular brain disease, are irreversible. *Alzheimer's disease* (presenile dementia) is thought to be inherited and occurs in about 50% of the chronic disorders, primarily among women. It is characterized by a defect in memory and orientation, deterioration of intellectual functioning, and alterations in judgment and affect (Chapter 20). *Vascular brain disease* originates in the vascular system of the brain and may result from closure of the vessels by plaque or clots or from insufficient perfusion to the brain. The onset is abrupt, and there are periods of remission and exacerbation. During remission, personality remains intact and the person has some awareness of the problem. As the disease progresses, there is memory loss, emotional lability, and depression.

Depression is often confused with dementia and can occur with true dementia; therefore, in many elderly persons, treatable depression is not recognized. Depressed (withdrawn) behavior is discussed in Chapter 9. If there is any possibility that depression exists, the older person should receive treatment.

Many elderly persons remain alert, with good cognitive functioning, until they die at an advanced age.

Health needs and nursing interventions

The goal of medical and nursing care is to keep people functioning at the highest possible level for their age. This includes living with chronic ailments and continuing degenerative changes. The nurse who views aging as a normal, inevitable process, one requiring adjustments in living patterns but not withdrawal from life, is best prepared to work with the aging patient. A philosophy of aging is one of ever-changing life that eventually includes death.

Similarities between childhood and old age should not be assumed, because they are not valid. Even in the matter of helplessness there is no similarity. Children are in ascendance; they are developing new power daily and marking up achievements over their environment. The aged person's helplessness is infinitely more frustrating because it is increasing rather than decreasing.

Community support services for older persons	
Senior citizen centers	Social, nutritional, educational, and counseling services
Geriatric day care centers	Assistive daytime nursing care, and social, nutritional, and rehabilitative services may be available
Adult foster home care	Care in private home for the older person who is unable to live alone
Meals on Wheels	Meals delivered to the person's home
Homemaking service	Household chores, shopping, and so on
Transportation service	Arranged pickup by public transportation system
Home health service	Skilled home nursing care
Legal services	Will, settlement of estate

Necessary nursing care depends on the physiologic and anatomic changes that have taken place, the diseases that are present, and the person's emotional makeup and apparent adjustment to the particular situation. Older persons frequently talk at length about their families and the past; their conversations may give clues to interests that should be encouraged and to problems confronting them. Plans should be made to help them maintain as much independence as possible despite their limitations. Community resources are available to assist older persons maintain independence and meet their social needs.

PROMOTING SELF-WORTH

When giving nursing care to elderly patients, it is necessary to take special care to build and protect their sense of worth and feelings of adequacy:
1. Call patients by name; avoid using terms such as *grandma* or *grandpa.*
2. Face patients when speaking, and enunciate clearly to prevent embarrassment from not hearing; do not shout.
3. Give explanations clearly and slowly to prevent misunderstanding.
4. Provide written instructions for activities the patient must follow independently.

PROMOTING SELF-CARE

All persons prefer to maintain their independence and perform their own activities of daily living. For the elderly, who may see a loss of independence as a real possibility, self-care provides a sense of control of their lives.

1. Place equipment and personal supplies within easy reach
2. Provide self-help devices such as handrails in halls and bathrooms, sturdy chairs with arms, and assistive devices such as tongs for reaching and special utensils for eating, as needed.
3. Clear room of clutter to facilitate use of walkers and wheelchairs.
4. Provide *time* and equipment for personal physical care.
5. Adjust daily hospital routines whenever possible to correspond to patient's usual daily routines.

PROVIDING SKIN CARE

The skin of elderly persons is usually thin, delicate, and sensitive to pressure and trauma. The loss of subcutaneous fat and the hardening of the tiny arterioles near the surface cause the skin to wrinkle, sag, and appear sallow. Sweat glands atrophy, and the excretory function of the skin is lessened, making the skin dry and flaky and sometimes causing it to itch. Changes in skin color occur with aging. Seborrheic keratoses, lesions resembling dark, greasy warts, are common (Chapter 37).

Because the skin is likely to be very dry, daily bathing is often contraindicated. In addition to dryness, poor circulation, and low resistance, the skin readily becomes infected. Nails are often hard and scaly. A podiatrist should care for very hard nails and other conditions such as calluses and corns.

1. One or two baths a week are usually sufficient.
2. Mild glycerine soaps are usually preferred.
3. Bath oils may be used.
4. Apply lotion to dry skin areas immediately after the bath to retain moisture.
5. Soak feet and dry carefully, especially between toes.
6. Use preventive measures to protect skin of elderly patients confined to bed (for example, alternating pressure or egg crate mattress, flotation pad, sheepskin pads, frequent position changes).
7. Brush hair daily with soft-bristled brush.
8. Avoid frequent shampooing; encourage use of conditioner.

PROVIDING EYE CARE

Changes occur in the eyes with aging. There is a decrease in the conjunctival secretions, and sometimes the lower lid droops, causing the moistening fluid of the eye to be lost. Therefore, *irritation of the conjunctiva* and *tearing* are common. Smoke may be more irritating. Isotonic solution eyedrops can be ordered as a comfort measure.

An *accumulation of secretions at the inner canthus* of the eye may be present, particularly on awakening, and may be uncomfortable and unsightly. Care must be taken not to press on the eyeballs or to irritate any exposed conjunctiva when wiping the inner canthus.

Most older persons require glasses or contact lenses. These visual aids must be protected from damage or loss and need to be kept clean for best use. They also must be available; sometimes in the packing to go to the hospital, the corrective lenses are inadvertently left at home, thus curtailing the patient's mobility and ability for self-care.

The eyes of older people also accommodate more slowly to changes in light. Bright lights or sunlight may be almost unbearable; therefore blinds may need to be partially drawn. Many elderly persons see poorly in the dark; night lights are used to reduce confusion and to prevent those who get up during the night from having accidents. Cataracts, failing vision, and blindness are common in the aged (Chapter 21).

PROVIDING CARE OF MOUTH AND TEETH

The gums of elderly persons become less elastic and less vascular. They may recede from the remaining teeth, exposing areas of a tooth not covered with enamel. These areas are sensitive to injury from brushes and coarse dentrifices. In addition, diseases of the gum that may have progressed symptom free for years may cause loss of teeth. Many elderly persons have decayed, broken, or missing teeth. This leads them to avoid foods that are difficult to eat, affecting nutrition.

By 70 years of age, tooth loss is common, frequently necessitating dentures. Care of dentures and prevention of their loss are part of the general nursing care of elderly patients. Many individuals older than 65 years have oral lesions of which they are unaware. The mouth is assessed for presence of white patches (leukoplakia), irritations, and growths.

PROMOTING ACTIVITY

The feet and legs usually show the results of limitation in peripheral circulation before any other body part. It is therefore important for the older person to *exercise the feet and legs regularly,* especially during periods of decreased activity such as during hospitalization, to *avoid constriction of circulation to legs and feet,* and to *avoid injury and infections of legs and feet* (Chapter 27).

Activity promotes good systemic circulation. In the elderly person, walking or other activity helps to maintain alertness by providing the brain with more oxygen, and helps prevent constipation. Thus, unless contraindicated, elderly persons are assisted or encouraged to get out of bed and to walk, as feasible.

As the muscles become less active in age, poor posture may result. The abdomen may sag, the spine become rounded, and the chest and shoulders droop forward. Lessened elasticity of tissue tends to fix these changes. Teaching good posture and encouraging deep breathing are part of the daily nursing care of all elderly patients. Nursing interventions for the elderly patient confined to bed include the following.

1. Use a firm mattress for good body alignment.
2. Use light, warm bedcovers, tucked loosely to permit active movement in bed.
3. Use footboards to keep covers off toes and permit muscle strengthening exercises.
4. Place pillow under shoulders as well as head to permit good chest expansion.
5. Teach patient exercises to be done daily:
   a. Legs: flexion, extension, abduction, adduction
   b. Arms: cross over chest, extend over head
   c. Neck: raise head from flat position.

PROMOTING REST AND SLEEP

Elderly persons require more rest, but the rest needs to be balanced with activity.

Elderly people usually sleep lightly and intermittently, with frequent periods of waking. At home the person may get out of bed, read, wander about the house, and even prepare something to eat at odd hours. Such activity is good because it prevents excessive slowing of circulation. Some wakefulness, therefore, can be expected in the elderly patient who is hospitalized. A low bed, night lights, and adequate supervision help prevent accidents, and the nurse monitors the extent of wakefulness to ascertain that the patient does experience periods of sleep. Elderly patients, like all others, may be unable to sleep. Many sedatives, with the exclusion of chloral hydrate, may interfere with REM sleep and may cause confusion in the elderly. Altered sleep patterns that are normal in aging need to be differentiated from depression and dementia.

PROMOTING COMFORT

Protective adipose tissue under the skin disappears with age, and the volume of circulating blood, particularly to the small outer arteries, may be diminished, thus affecting the ability to withstand chilling without discomfort. Many elderly persons suffer from mild arthritis and fibrositis, which produce vague muscle and joint pains and are aggravated by chilling. Extra clothing is frequently worn; several layers of lightweight clothing are warmer than fewer heavy layers. Many elderly persons wish to wear socks and additional clothing in bed. Provision must be made to prevent drafts in the room while maintaining good air circulation.

PROMOTING NUTRITION

Many elderly people are undernourished, and for this reason a great deal of emphasis is placed on nutrition for the aged. Some causes of malnutrition are listed here. It is not unusual for the older person's diet to be high in carbohydrates and low in vitamins, minerals, and protein, especially if the person lives alone. Qualitative nutritional needs of the elderly are essentially the same as for other adults except that caloric needs diminish. Increased fiber is beneficial to the gastrointestinal system. Fluid intake is important.

Causes of malnutrition in the elderly

Acute and chronic illness
Limited financial resources
Psychologic factors such as boredom and lack of companionship while eating
Loss of teeth
Faulty eating patterns
Fads and notions regarding certain foods
Lack of energy to prepare foods
Lack of knowledge of appropriate nutrition

Some elderly persons are obese, even though undernourished. Weight reduction in the aged person should be gradual and supervised by a physician. Sudden loss of weight is poorly tolerated by many elderly persons whose vascular system has become adjusted to the excess weight. Sudden weight reduction may lead to serious consequences, including confusion associated with lowered blood pressure, exhaustion, and vasomotor collapse.

PROMOTING ELIMINATION

Motor activity of the intestinal musculature may be decreased with age, and supportive structures in the intestinal walls become weakened. Sensory perception is less acute, so the signal for bowel elimination may be missed. Constipation may occur, and in turn lead to fecal impaction. The very elderly and the somewhat confused patient may need to be reminded to go to the bathroom after meals. Measures to prevent constipation (Chapter 32) take high priority in the care of elderly persons. Any marked change in bowel habits is reported to the physician because cancer of the large bowel and diverticulosis are fairly common among this age group.

Frequency of voiding is common with aging and becomes a problem during illness. Decreased bladder muscle tone results in impairment of emptying capacity and may lead to residual urine in the bladder, with subsequent infection. Unless there is a definite contraindication to high fluid intake, the elderly patient is encouraged to take sufficient fluids to dilute urine and prevent urinary stasis. Fluids may be limited in the evening if nocturia is troublesome and interferes with sleep.

Elderly women may have relaxation of perineal structures, which may also interfere with complete emptying of the bladder. Periodic dribbling of urine suggests that the bladder is not being emptied completely. Stress incontinence also results when perineal structures are weakened.

Involutional changes in the lining of the vagina lead to lessened resistance to invasion of organisms. Mild infections with troublesome discharge are not unusual in older women. Vinegar douches are frequently prescribed. Application of cornstarch to the perineum and vaginal orifice may allay itching.

Almost all elderly men have hypertrophy of the prostate gland, which makes urination difficult. Men with severe problems in initiating the urinary stream need medical consultation.

Incontinence of urine and feces is particularly upsetting, not only to the patient and family but also to the nursing staff. Every effort is made to institute and maintain a bowel and bladder training regimen (Chapters 32 and 33).

MEETING PSYCHOSOCIAL NEEDS

Elderly patients are often lonely and appreciate just talking with others. Volunteers may provide a service by visiting with the elderly. Many patients appreciate visits with a member of the clergy. When visiting with elderly persons, it should be remembered that, although they commonly talk about events and activities in their own past, they usually are interested in the activities of young persons and of the world about them.

The need to be useful is important to all persons. There are many tasks in which even the elderly person who is ill may be able to participate. At home, the elderly may be able to help with the dishes or with meal preparation. They may be interested in crafts or making useful items. The older person may be quite slow, and great care must be taken not to show impatience, which may discourage further participation.

Elderly persons are usually aware of death as an imminent possibility and sometimes see it as a welcome event. The issue should not be avoided. If the patient shows genuine concern about death, the nurse can encourage discussion of feelings (Chapter 16). The family may also need opportunities to discuss their feelings about death.

Special precautions related to diagnosis and treatment

MEDICATIONS

Elderly persons consume disproportionately more of all kinds of drugs than do middle-aged adults because of increased frequency of illness, especially chronic illness. These drugs may not be well tolerated and may produce adverse reactions and interactions or unpredictable responses in the elderly. Age-related physiologic changes contribute to altered responses to drugs in the elderly. The effects of the medications may be altered in various ways.

Drugs have a definite place in the therapeutic regimen in the elderly, but their use must be monitored carefully. In general, *drug levels should be increased or reduced gradually,* and *the fewest possible number of drugs should be used.* If the patient is emaciated or very elderly, the use of full adult doses of drugs should be questioned.

Factors affecting drug response in the elderly

Effect	Cause
Decreased drug absorption	Decreased hydrochloric acid
	Altered gastrointestinal motility
Altered drug distribution	Storing of fat-soluble drug in fatty tissue
	Decreased serum albumin for binding of drugs
Altered drug metabolism	Decreased enzyme activity in liver
Decreased drug excretion	Decreased renal blood flow
	Decreased glomerular filtration rate
	Decreased number of functional tubules

Many elderly patients must administer medicines to themselves, and their ability to do so must be evaluated. In planning self-administration of drugs with the elderly patient, it is frequently helpful to determine when it is easiest for the person to remember to take medication. This time is usually tied to some incident of daily living, such as arising or taking meals. The use of a medication checklist may be helpful. Some persons have found it helpful to use something with compartments, such as an egg carton, with the days marked off. One dose is placed in each compartment, and it is easy to see whether the medication has been taken.

DIAGNOSTIC TESTS

Diagnostic tests should be judiciously spaced to prevent overtaxing the elderly individual. Routine preparations for various tests may need modification to prevent exhaustion or dehydration. Elderly persons may become weak or dizzy from pretest preparations such as multiple enemas or the withholding of food. Weak patients should not be left unattended on a treatment table. Persons who are dizzy are advised to sit up slowly and to remain sitting on the table for a few moments before standing. The dizziness is caused by the slow compensation of inelastic blood vessels.

Because of the rapidity with which they develop decubitus ulcers, pads should be placed under the normal curves of the back and under bony prominences in elderly patients who must lie on treatment or operating room tables for lengthy periods. If the patient is placed in the lithotomy position, both legs are placed in (and removed from) the stirrups at the same time to prevent undue pull on unresilient muscles.

SUMMARY

The kind of nursing care given the elderly may be influenced by personal attitudes toward the elderly and aging. Societal attitudes have yielded a negative stereotype of the elderly as being slow, not thinking as well as in earlier years, being mentally confused, not wanting to learn anything new, plagued by disease, dependent, behaving in a childlike manner, and burdensome to family and society. If these attitudes are also held by the nurse, the elderly person may be approached with condescending tolerance, thereby reinforcing often felt feelings of inferiority.

It is most helpful when the nurse can deal with the individual empathetically, demonstrating willingness to listen, explain, comfort, and support independent functioning. Accepting elderly individuals as they are and where they are in terms of their developmental status, and suspending youth-oriented attitudes and standards that may be inappropriate are essential elements in adequately meeting the elderly person's needs and fostering a better quality of life.

Although many of the changes discussed in this chapter require special nursing approaches, it should be emphasized that not all of these changes occur in all aging persons. Indeed many older persons are very healthy and actively engage in the world around them.

REFERENCES AND SELECTED READINGS*

1. Abdella, F.: Nursing care of the aged in the USA, J. Gerontol. Nurs. **7:**657-663, 1981.
2. Allen, M.: Drug therapy in the elderly, Am. J. Nurs. **80:**1474-1475, 1980.
3. Bahr, R.T., Sr.: Sleep-wake patterns in the aged, J. Gerontol. Nurs. **9:**534-537, 1983.
4. Birchenall, J.M., and Straight, M.E.: Care of the older adult, ed. 2, Philadelphia, 1982, J.B. Lippincott Co.
5. Burnside, I.: Nursing and the aged, ed. 2, New York, 1981, McGraw-Hill Book Co.
6. Burnside, I.: Psychosocial nursing care of the aged, ed. 2, New York, 1980, McGraw-Hill Book Co.
7. Burnside, I., editor: Working with the elderly: group processes and techniques, Boston, 1978, Duxbury Press.
8. Butler, R.N.: Why survive? Being old in America, New York, 1975, Harper & Row, Publishers.
9. Butler, R.N., and Lewis, M.I.: Aging and mental health: positive psychosocial and biomedical approaches, ed. 3, St. Louis, 1982, The C.V. Mosby Co.
10. Carotenuto, R., and Bullock, J.: Phsyiologic assessment of the gerontolgic client, Philadelphia, 1980, F.A. Davis Co.
11. Cassels, C., et al: Retirement: aspects, responses and nursing implications, J. Gerontol. Nurs. **7:**355-359, 1981.
12. Cohen, S.: Sensory changes in the elderly: a programmed instruction, Am. J. Nurs. **81:**1851-1880, 1981.
13. Dennis, K.E.: A man and a woman in the middle years, J. Gerontol. Nurs. **7:**417-422, 1981.
14. *DeVore, N.E.: Parenthood postponed, Am. J. Nurs. **83:**1160-1163, 1983.
15. Dickelman, N.L.: The young adult: the choice is health or illness, Am. J. Nurs. **75:**1272-1277, 1976.
16. Dickelman, N.L.: The middle years: a time of change, Am. J. Nurs. **75:**994-996, 1975.
17. Dickelman, N.L.: The middle years: emotional tasks of the middle adult, Am. J. Nurs. **75:**997-1001, 1975.
18. Dickelman, N.L.: Primary health care of the well adult, New York, 1977, McGraw-Hill Book Co.
19. Dresden, S.E.: The middle years: the sexually active middle adult, Am. J. Nurs. **75:**1001-1005, 1975.
20. Ebersole, P., and Hess, P.: Toward healthy aging, St. Louis, 1981, The C.V. Mosby Co.
21. Eliopoulos, C.: Gerontological nursing, New York, 1979, Harper & Row, Publishers.
22. Futrell, M., et al: Primary health care of the older adult, Boston, 1980, Duxbury Press.
23. Galloway, K.: The middle years: the change of life, Am. J. Nurs. **75:**1006-1011, 1975.
24. Hargreaves, A.G.: Life in the middle years: making the most of the middle years, Am. J. Nurs. **75:**1772-1776, 1975.
25. Havighurst, R.J.: Perspectives on health care for the elderly, J. Gerontol. Nurs. **3**(2):21-24, 1977.
26. Hazard, M.P., and Kemp, R.E.: Keeping the well elderly well, Am. J. Nurs. **83:**567-569, 1983.
27. Howells, J.G., editor: Modern perspectives in the psychiatry of middle age, New York, 1981, Brunner/Mazel, Inc.

*References preceded by an asterisk are particularly well suited for student reading.

28. Johnson, L.: The middle years: living sensibly, Am. J. Nurs. **75:**1012-1016, 1975.

29. Jury, D., and Jury, M.: Gramp, New York, 1976, Grossman Publishers.

30. Kaluger, G., and Kaluger, M.F.: Human development: the span of life, ed. 3, St. Louis, 1984, The C.V. Mosby Co.

31. Knox, A.B.: Adult development and learning, San Francisco, 1977, Jossey-Bass, Inc., Publishers.

32. Lamy, P.P.: Prescribing for the elderly, Littleton, Mass., 1980, PSG Publishing Co.

33. Lawton, M.P., et al.: Community planning for an aging society, Strousburg, Pa., 1976, Dowden, Hutchinson & Ross, Inc.

34. *Lerner, R.: Sleep loss in the aged: implications for nursing practice, J. Gerontol. Nurs. **8:**323-326, 1982.

35. Lidz, T.: The person: his and her development throughout the life cycle, rev. ed., New York, 1976, Basic Books Inc., Publishers.

36. Loether, H.J.: Problems of aging: sociological and social psychological perspectives, ed. 2, Belmont, Calif., 1975, Dickenson Publishing Co.

37. Makinodan, T., editor: Handbook of the biology of aging, New York, 1977, Van Nostrand Reinhold Co., Inc.

38. Megerle, J.S.: Surviving, Am. J. Nurs. **83:**892-894, 1983.

39. *Murray, R., and Zentner, J.: Nursing assessment and health promotion through the life span, ed. 2, Englewood Cliffs, N.J., 1979, Prentice-Hall, Inc.

40. Norman, W.H., and Scaramella, T.J., editors: Mid-life developmental and clinical issues, New York, 1980, Brunner/Mazel, Inc.

41. O'Brien, C.L.: Adult day care: a practical guide, Belmont, Calif., Wadsworth Publishing Co., Inc., Health Science Division.

42. Pacini, C.M., and Fitzpatrick, J.J.: Sleep patterns of hospitalized aged individuals, J. Gerontol. Nurs. **8:**327-332, 1982.

43. Pearson, L.J., and Kolthoff, M.E.: Geriatric clinical protocols, New York, 1979, J.B. Lippincott Co.

44. *Peplau, H.E.: Life in the middle years: mid-life crises, Am. J. Nurs. **75:**1761-1765, 1975.

45. Ramos, L.Y.: Oral hygiene of the elderly, Am. J. Nurs. **81:**1468-1469, 1981.

46. Reichel, W., editor: Clinical aspects of aging, Baltimore, 1978, Williams & Wilkins Co.

47. Rossman, I., editor: Clinical geriatrics, Philadelphia, 1977, J.B. Lippincott Co.

48. Roznoy, M.S.: The young adult: taking a sexual history, Am. J. Nurs. **76:**1279-1282, 1976.

49. Shrock, M.: Holistic assessment of the healthy aged, New York, 1980, John Wiley & Sons, Inc.

50. Schuster, C.S., and Ashburn, S.: The process of human development, Boston, 1980, Little, Brown & Co.

51. *Sheehy, G.: Passages, New York, 1976, E.P. Dutton & Co., Inc.

52. Sherwood, S., editor: Long-term care: a handbook for researchers, planners, and providers, New York, 1975, Spectrum Books.

53. Shock, N.W.: Systemic physiology and aging: introduction, Fed. Proc. **38**(2):161-162, 1979.

54. Sommers, P.P.: Life cycle nursing: health care planning for the future, J. Gerontol. Nurs. **9:**103-107, 1983.

55. *Source book on aging, ed. 2, New York, 1977, Marquis Who's Who, Inc.

56. Starr, B.D., and Goldstein, H.S.: Human behavior and development, New York, 1975, Springer Publishing Co., Inc.

57. Stevenson, J.S.: Issues and crises during middlescence, New York, 1977, Appleton-Century-Crofts.

58. Sullivan, N.S.: Vision in the elderly, J. Gerontol. Nurs. **9:**228-235, 1983.

59. Troll, L.E.: Early and middle adulthood, Monterey, Calif., 1975, Brooks/Cole Publishing Co.

60. Wolanin, M.D.: Relocation of the elderly, J. Gerontol. Nurs. **4:**47050, 1978.

61. Wolanin, M.D., and Phillips, L.R.F.: Confusion: prevention and care, St. Louis, 1981, The C.V. Mosby Co.

62. Woods, N.F.: Human sexuality in health and illness, ed 3., St. Louis, 1984, The C.V. Mosby Co.

Classic

63. Cummings, E., and Henry, W.E.: Growing old, New York, 1955, Basic Books Inc., Publishers.

64. *Erikson, E.H.: Childhood and society, ed. 2, New York, 1963, W.W. Norton & Co., Inc.

65. *Havighurst, R.J., et al.: Psychology of aging, Bethesda Conference, Public Health Rep. **70:**836-856, 1955.

66. *Schwartz, D.: The elderly ambulatory patient, New York, 1964, Macmillan Inc.

67. Shanas, E.: The health of older people, Cambridge, Mass., 1962, Harvard University Press.

68. Strehler, B.L.: Time, cells and aging, New York, 1962, Academic Press, Inc.

AUDIOVISUAL RESOURCES

Aging, Del Mar, Calif., CRM Educational Films. (Film.)

Gramp: a man ages and dies, Baltimore, Mass Media Ministries. (Filmstrip.)

Grow old along with me, New York, Focus International. (Film.)

Patient mental health, psychological growth and adjustment, Oaklawn, Ill., Westinghouse Learning Corp. (Filmstrip and audiotope.)

Peege, Princeton, N.J., Phoenix Films. (Film.)

Perspectives on aging, Costa Mesa, Calif., Concept Media.

6

Biologic Defense Mechanisms of the Human Body

E. RONALD WRIGHT

STUDY QUESTIONS

- Review the types and functions of white blood cells.

- Review the structure and function of the immune system.

- Examine an infected wound. How do the signs and symptoms reflect the inflammatory process?

- In what different ways can immunization be accomplished?

CONCEPT AND SCOPE OF BIOLOGIC DEFENSE

The human body has developed a wide variety of mechanisms designed to protect itself from the encroachment of antagonistic agents in its environment. Those agents can be *exogenous* (from outside the body), for example, foreign animal cells, parasites, microorganisms, drugs, toxins, or inorganic substances; or they may be *endogenous* (from within the body), for example, damaged or worn-out tissues and cells, obstructive agents, or neoplasms. Life as we know it could not exist without the ability to withstand and deal with these extrinsic and intrinsic onslaughts. In this chapter the array of interactive biologic mechanisms designed to provide this protection are described and the consequences of their failure or inappropriate functioning briefly discussed.

The significance for medical-surgical nursing practice of an understanding of how these mechanisms function cannot be overemphasized. Much of preventative, compensatory, and restorative nursing practice is built on the maintenance and restoration of the systems and mechanisms of these biologic functions. Knowledge of these basic structures and mechanisms helps in the understanding of the following:

1. Resistance and immunity to infectious diseases

2. Diagnosis of diseases and physiologic functions
3. Rejection of tissue transplants and reactions to transfusions
4. Adaptations in the aging process
5. Development of allergic and hypersensitivity reactions
6. Immunization against infectious diseases
7. Expression of autoimmune diseases and immunodeficiencies
8. Signs and symptoms of local and systemic inflammations
9. Development and treatment of neoplastic disease.

Concept of self versus nonself

Every human being can be regarded as a "one of a kind" collection of tissues, cells, and molecules that comprises a biologic unit of *self.* The exact nature of this unit is determined by a combination of genes inherited from one's parents, which encode for a unique array of structures and proteins that is not repeated exactly in any other individual. The only exception to this occurs in the case of identical twins. Therefore every other individual or cell or biologic product can be considered to be *nonself.* It is the function of the biologic defense mechanism of the body to recognize and protect against encroachment by nonself agents, while maintaining and supporting all that is self.

These defense mechanisms are composed of structural, chemical, cellular, special protein, and tissue elements that form an interrelated system of protection throughout the entire body. The mechanisms serve to protect self from both external and internal destructive agents by the following:

1. *Exclusion* of harmful agents from the body
2. *Recognition* of harmful agents within the body
3. *Response* designed to rid the body of the harmful agents that do gain access (Fig. 6-1)

The sources of these harmful nonself materials are generally external and include nonliving materials of the environment such as potentially harmful inorganic chemicals and compounds produced by other living organisms. The most serious external threats to biologic integrity, however, come from the living organisms that constantly surround the body. Some of these organisms pose no real threat because the mechanical, biochemical, and metabolic processes of the human body will not support them or offer them shelter. There are a myriad of living forms, on the other hand, for which the human body would be an ideal haven for growth and survival. Most of these organisms, if allowed to penetrate the body, would wreak havoc on the normal functionings of the body. The living

forms that come to mind in this regard are the organisms classified as pathogenic (disease causing). While it is true that the progress of these organisms in the body can be altered by external agents such as antibiotics, the eradication of the offending organism from the body must be accomplished by the host's own adaptive mechanisms.

In addition to protection against external agents, the defense mechanisms also protect against the accumulation of damaged or dysfunctional self material. If it were not for these processes that carry out the systematic, specific removal of damaged or worn-out cellular material, the body would become clogged with debris. Still another general function of these systems is that of recognition of the alteration of self to a potentially dangerous state. When this defense function falters, cancer results.

Scope of defense mechanisms

The array of defense mechanisms that have been adapted to protect the normal human body is formidable and complex. For the sake of orderly presentation they may be divided into *nonspecific* and *specific* mechanisms (Table 6-1). The specific and nonspecific mechanisms can be further divided on the basis of where the lines of defense are formed, that is, *external* for the mechanisms of mechanical exclusion, biochemical destruction, and microbial competition and *internal* for the physiologic reactions. The nonspecific mechanisms are nonselectively directed against *any* foreign substance. The specific mechanisms are specifically elicited by *unique* substances to which the body has *acquired* the ability to respond.

Concept of immunity

The objective of the biologic defense mechanisms is to provide the host with protection. The ultimate protection would be total resistance to encroachment or damage by an organism or agent; this is usually termed *absolute immunity*. Absence of such protective barriers is called *susceptibility*. Although generally applied to immunity from

---

Biologic defense mechanisms

Structural	Skin, mucous membranes
Chemical	pH, blood proteins
Cellular	White blood cells, phagocytes
Special proteins	Interferon, immunoglobulins
Tissue	Lymph nodes, thymus gland

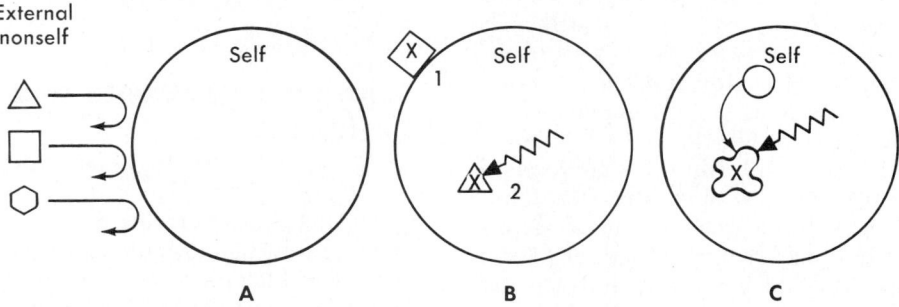

Fig. 6-1. Mechanisms of biologic defense in human body. **A,** Exclusion of external nonself. **B,** Destruction of external nonself by (1) nonspecific external mechanisms and (2) nonspecific or specific internal mechanisms. **C,** Destruction of altered self. X indicates nonspecific mechanisms; ⟿ indicates specific mechanisms.

Table 6-1. Biologic defense mechanisms

Nonspecific mechanisms	Specific mechanisms
External	
Mechanical exclusion	Immunoglobulin A
Physical structures	In mucosal secretions
Skin	In mucosal cells
Mucous membranes	
Specialized structures	
Physical actions	
Biochemical factors	
Body secretions	
pH	
Lysozyme	
Microbial antagonism	
Internal	
Reticuloendothelial system	Antigen processing by macrophages
Blood	Primary immune response
Cellular components	Humoral immune response
Fluid components	Synthesis of circulating antibodies by B cells
Opsonins	Interaction of antibodies with antigen
Complement	Cell-mediated immune response
C-reactive protein	Sensitization of T cells
Phagocytosis	Lymphokines
Inflammatory response	Combined immune response
Interferon	Secondary immune response

infectious organisms, these terms can be used to describe the relative susceptibility to encroachment by any external agent. *Nonspecific immunity* (or *innate immunity*) is provided when the external and internal nonspecific defense mechanisms serve as the barrier excluding or destroying the invading agent. *Specific immunity* protects against a single unique agent through the development of specific antibodies or response cells in the body. It is *acquired* from prior contact with that agent (antigen) or through the introduction of specifically protective antibodies or cells into the body.

The acquisition of specific immunity may result from *natural* encounter or *artificial* introduction. Immunity acquired naturally means under natural conditions, such as recovery from a disease. Immunity acquired artificially means that the antigen or protective antibodies were purposely introduced into the body (for example, by vaccination). The immunity may be an *active* or *passive*. When the antibodies are produced within the body, the immunity is active. When the protective antibodies are received from some other source, the immunity is passive. Thus when antibodies are transferred from the mother across the placenta, the child is said to have a natural passive immunity; when a vaccine is given, so that antibodies are produced within the body, the immunized individual is characterized as having an artificial active immunity. Table 6-2 summarizes the different types of specific acquired immunities.

Specific or nonspecific immunity to harmful agents is a relative state. The effects of different dosages of an infectious organism or the toxic products of such organisms in experimental studies clearly demonstrate that administration of sufficiently large numbers of an organism or high dosages of a toxin can overwhelm even the most highly immunized animal. Further, when the normal mechanisms of defense are breached, even in the highly resistant host, disease can result. Thus acquired immunity to infection is not always an absolute condition but depends on a large number of complex variables. These include not only the defense mechanisms of the host but also the dosage, route of contact, and virulence of the harmful agent.

EXTERNAL NONSPECIFIC DEFENSE MECHANISMS

Anatomic structures and mechanical actions

SKIN AND MUCOUS MEMBRANES

The first line of defense against penetration by foreign materials, including pathogenic microorganisms, is the skin. The intact skin is an extremely efficient physical barrier to harmful agents and environmental forces, such as heat, cold, and trauma. This protection is afforded by the keratinized surface cells, which provide a tough, dense, waterproof covering. Beneath this outermost layer is a dense layer of highly vascularized connective tissue (see Fig. 37-1).

Table 6-2. Types of acquired specific immunity

Type of immunity	Acquisition of immunity	Development	Duration	Protection	Example
Active Antibodies synthesized by body in response to antigenic stimulation	*Natural* Natural contact with antigen through clinical or subclinical case	Develops slowly; protective levels reached in a few weeks	Long term; often lifetime	Specific to antigen contacted	Recovery from childhood diseases (for example, chickenpox, measles, mumps)
	Artificial Immunization with antigen	Develops slowly; protective levels reached in a few weeks	Several years; extended protection with "booster" doses	Specific to antigen immunized against	Immunization with live or killed vaccines; toxoid immunization
Passive Antibodies produced in one individual are transferred to another	*Natural* Transplacental and colostral transfer from mother to child	Immediate	Temporary, to several months	All antigens to which mother has immunity	Maternal immunoglobulins in neonate
	Artificial Injection of serum from immune human or animal	Immediate	Temporary, to several weeks	All antigens to which source has immunity	Injection of pooled human gamma globulin; injection of animal hyperimmune sera

Even though some of the fatty acids derived from sebaceous gland secretions have antimicrobial activity, the environment provided by the skin does allow the growth of microorganisms on its upper layers and within hair follicles and sweat glands. For the most part these resident microorganisms are nonpathogenic; however, when these organisms gain entrance to the tissues of a host exhibiting reduced resistance, they may cause significant problems. Because even thorough scrubbing with soap and water removes only the surface organisms, the skin can never be considered sterile.

Any time the physical integrity of the skin is broken, such as in surgery, indwelling venous catheterization, or physical irritation or trauma, there is significant risk of microorganisms gaining entrance to the body. The skin must be kept relatively dry because the continued presence of moisture tends to cause maceration of the skin. Further, when essential oils are lost from the skin surface they should be supplemented by lotions to maintain the resilience and unbroken texture of the surface cells. Adequate care of the skin of the hospitalized patient is not just a luxury but a necessity for the provision of an extremely important aspect of biologic defense.

Mucous membranes protect the eye and line all body tracts that have external openings. When intact, the mucous membranes, like the skin, are basically impervious to foreign materials and microorganisms. The surfaces are covered by a viscous secretion that tends to trap and inactivate microorganisms. The mucous membrane of the respiratory tract is further protected by the surface activity of the ciliated epithelial cells, which sweep foreign material out of the tract. The mucous membranes are highly vascularized so that the internal defense mechanisms are readily available to attack any microorganisms that do gain access to the surface of these cells.

Also found in the mucosal secretions and in high concentration within the secretory mucosal cells of the respiratory and intestinal tracts are a specific class of immunoglobulins (antibodies) known as immunoglobulin A (IgA). These specific antibodies are secreted from the mucosal cells and have antibacterial, antiviral, and antitoxic properties. These antibodies serve to prevent microbial adherence and colonization of these tracts by pathogens.

SPECIALIZED STRUCTURES AND MECHANICAL FUNCTIONS

Other structures and functions of the human body that are generally taken for granted actually serve extremely important roles in defense. The filtration action of the nasal hairs serves to trap particles and microorganisms. The flushing action of saliva and urine prevents the buildup of organisms. The eyes are protected from entrance of dirt particles and organisms by the lids and lashes. Foreign material that does gain entrance to the eye tends to be washed out by tears. The constant movement of foods through the stomach and intestines prevents the buildup of organisms or toxic waste products.

Even the action of vomiting and the watery stools of diarrhea are active mechanisms of removal of harmful products from the gastrointestinal tract. Dysfunction or blockage of any of these processes means that special measures must be taken to protect against the establishment of pathogenic organisms and the buildup of toxic materials.

Biochemical factors

Many areas of the body are protected not only by mechanical barriers but also by the presence of specific antimicrobial chemicals that provide added protection.

SKIN

The acetic acid and salt concentration of perspiration is toxic to many pathogenic microorganisms. Some of the fatty acids released to the skin surface by the sebaceous glands also serve to inhibit the growth of some microorganisms.

GASTROINTESTINAL TRACT

In the stomach the acidity (approximate pH 2) of the gastric juice kills many organisms and detoxifies certain potentially toxic substances. For this reason, when gastric acidity is low, special precautions must be taken to avoid introduction of organisms through the nose and mouth. Low gastric acidity is characteristic in neonates; therefore special care should be taken in feeding and handling babies to prevent exposure to pathogens by the oral route. The upper intestine is generally freed of organisms by the action of bile and other proteolytic enzymes.

VAGINA

Vaginal secretions allow certain harmless acid-producing bacteria to colonize the vagina and create an acidic environment. This reduces the chance of the colonization of the vagina by pathogens. When either the amount or the acidity of the vaginal secretions is decreased, there is a much greater chance that a vaginal infection will develop. Because vaginal secretions are not present before puberty and are greatly decreased after menopause, young girls and older women are more prone to vaginitis. Birth control pills cause a shift in the composition and pH of the vaginal secretions, which increases the possibility of colonization of the vagina, especially by the causative agent of gonorrhea, *Neisseria gonorrhoeae.*

LYSOZYME

The most ubiquitous antimicrobial factor in the body is the enzyme lysozyme. It is capable of lysing (splitting) the bacterial cell wall of many gram-positive organisms, causing their destruction. Lysozyme is present in mucus, tears, saliva, and skin secretions and is also found in many of the internal fluids and cells of the body. Within

Table 6-3. Distribution of normal microbic flora

Region of body	Sterile areas	Nonsterile areas	Microorganisms
Skin	None	All skin	*Staphylococcus, Bacillus, Corynebacterium, Mycobacterium, Streptococcus,* transient environmental organisms
Respiratory tract	Larynx, trachea, bronchi, bronchioles, alveoli, sinuses	Nose, throat, mouth	*Staphyloccus, Candida, Streptococcus, Neisseria, Pneumococcus,* oral organisms
Gastrointestinal tract	Esophagus, stomach, upper small intestine	Esophagus and stomach (transiently), large intestine	Gram-negative rods, *Streptococcus, Bacteroides, Proteus, Clostridium, Lactobacillus*
Genitourinary tract	Cervix, uterus, fallopian tubes, ovaries, prostate gland, epididymis, testes, bladder, kidney	External genitalia, anterior urethra, vagina	Skin organisms, *Lactobacillus, Bacteroides*
Body fluids and cavities	Blood, pleural fluid, synovial fluid, spinal fluid, lymph, etc.	None	

the body it tends to work in combination with complement and other blood factors to destroy bacteria directly.

Microbial antagonism

The skin and mucosal surfaces offer varying nutritional and environmental conditions for the growth and multiplication of certain microbial cells. Although the surfaces of the body are constantly exposed to temporary contamination by organisms from the environment, most of these organisms, known as *transient flora,* do not find conditions suitable for the colonization of the body; however, many microorganisms, known as *normal microbic flora,* do colonize the skin and mucosal surfaces. Although this normal flora varies from site to site within the body and may vary in response to environmental, hygienic, and physiologic changes, it is capable of reestablishment and reflects a fairly predictable pattern. Table 6-3 provides an overview of the body areas normally colonized and shows which organisms most often make up the normal flora of the various areas.

The maintenance of this balanced microbic flora serves to make it difficult for pathogenic organisms to establish themselves on the body surfaces. Because the normal flora have a selective advantage in their environmental niche, they compete for nutrients and space. Some release antimicrobial substances to retard the growth of transient organisms seeking to occupy the same site. Such microbial interference is called *microbial antagonism.*

Most of the normal microbic flora are basically non-

pathogenic; however, some overtly pathogenic organisms, such as *Staphylococcus aureus* and *Streptococcus pyogenes,* can be part of the normal flora. The individual who harbors such organisms without demonstrating any symptoms of disease is known as a *carrier.* This carrier state is of significance because the carrier may be unknowingly shedding organisms into the environment and infecting others.

The protective effects of the normal microbic flora become most apparent when something upsets the microbic balance within the body. The use of broad-spectrum antibiotics sometimes creates such an effect. The imbalance may allow a segment of the normal flora to gain ascendency, causing adverse reactions. An example of this phenomenon is seen when certain orally administered antibiotics induce marked shifts in the normal intestinal flora, allowing organisms that are generally suppressed by the growth of competitors to thrive to an unusual degree. This imbalance may induce uncomfortable gastrointestinal tract problems or even allow gastroenteritis to develop.

INTERNAL NONSPECIFIC DEFENSE MECHANISMS

Once a foreign agent (living or nonliving) penetrates the external resistance barriers, it is met by an even more complex array of defense mechanisms, which provides for the recognition, capture, and disposal of the foreign ma-

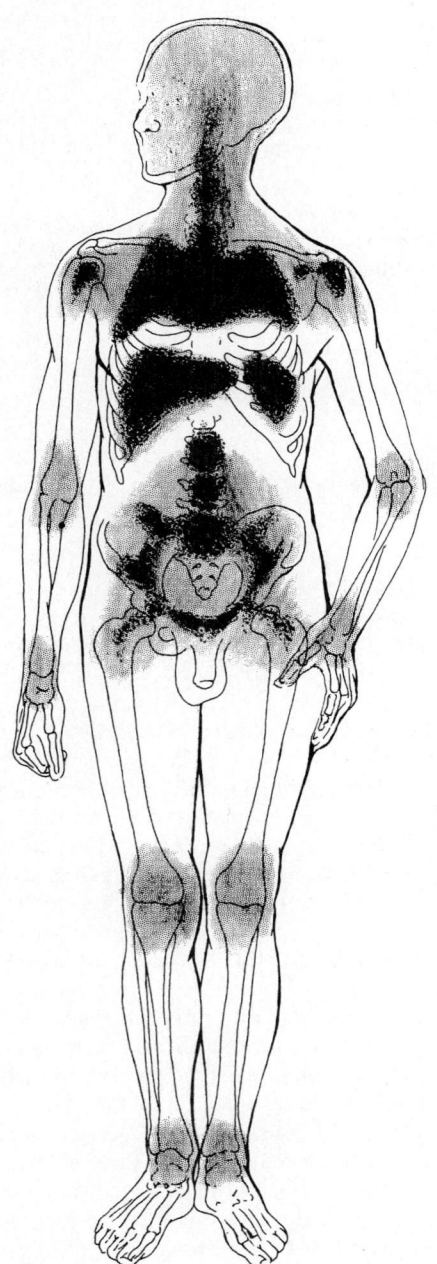

Fig. 6-2. Reticuloendothelial system. Note anatomic distribution of maximal activity in system, as indicated by black areas over body. To produce such an image certain radioactive colloidal particles are given to subject, and radiation detection techniques delineate tissue uptake. Note definition of liver, spleen, and active bone marrow in axial skeleton and proximal parts of long bones. (From Smith, A.L.: Microbiology and pathology, ed. 12, St. Louis, 1980, The C.V. Mosby Co.)

terial. The key to this process is the specific recognition and vigorous action taken against the foreign material while at the same time protecting the host tissues from extensive damage. The physiologic reactions that serve to contain and inactivate the foreign agent are carried out through interactions of cells and molecules of the blood, reticuloendothelial system, vascular system, and body tissues.

Reticuloendothelial system

The reticuloendothelial system (RES) is a widespread system of phagocytic (devouring) cells scattered throughout various body tissues (Fig. 6-2). The role of these cells is to ingest foreign particulate matter and damaged host tissues. Some of the phagocytic cells are *fixed* in a variety of tissues, such as lymphoid tissue, liver, spleen, bone marrow, lungs, and blood vessels. Within the different tissues these anchored cells have been given unique names (Table 6-4). It is the function of the fixed cells to capture and destroy foreign materials found in the fluids of their environment.

Other cells making up the reticuloendothelial network are not stationary and are called *wandering macrophages.* Depending on where they are found, they may be known as monocytes (in the bloodstream) or histiocytes (in loose connective tissues). The wandering macrophages carry out the important role of final cleanup of a damaged site in preparation for repair. The cells have the capacity to engulf and destroy virtually any type of foreign material or debris within the body. The macrophages also play an important role in the specific response mechanisms.

Blood

Blood is one of the primary sources of elements designed to provide protection against injurious agents. The blood transports these active factors to the site of an in-

Table 6-4. Distribution and names of macrophages in various tissue sites

Tissue	Macrophage
Peripheral blood	Monocyte
Loose connective tissue	Histiocyte
Liver	Kupffer's cells
Spleen and reticuloendothelial system	Wandering or fixed macrophage
Lung	Alveolar macrophage or dust cell
Granulomatous tissue	Epithelioid and giant cells
Peritoneal cavity, pleural cavity, and bone	Macrophages

jury or intrusion and through specific vascular changes concentrates these materials at the site. Both the fluid and cellular constituents of blood contain these factors.

CELLULAR COMPONENTS

The cellular components of blood that are of importance in this nonspecific response include granulocytes, lymphocytes, monocytes, and thrombocytes (platelets). The granulocytes, also referred to as polymorphonuclear leukocytes (PMNs), and the monocytes are the most important because of their phagocytic activity.

One of the key methods of nonspecific defense is the ingestion of microorganisms and other particulate matter by the phagocytic white blood cells. The phagocytes carry out the process of *phagocytosis* in several discrete steps (Fig. 6-3). Most infecting microbes are quickly and efficiently destroyed by phagocytosis; however, some pathogens exhibit methods of escape from this destruction. Some bacteria, such as strains of the streptococci and staphylococci and *Bacillus anthracis* (anthrax), actually produce factors that will kill the phagocyte. Other organisms resist ingestion or digestion. Some organisms may survive within the phagocytes or reticuloendothelial cells

and multiply there. This may lead to the transport of the organism to other sites in the body or serve as a chronic focus of continued infection.

The granulocytes can be divided on the basis of their structure and function into neutrophils, eosinophils, and basophils. The "granules" found within these cells represent discrete packets of degradative enzymes used to digest the ingested materials. The neutrophils are the most numerous in circulation and are the most efficient and responsive phagocytic cells involved in the inflammatory process. Where there is adequate blood supply to a region, the phagocytes are constantly available to move from the blood vessels to the site of injury or infection. The neutrophils and monocytes are actually attracted to the scene by chemicals released during infection or injury. This cellular response to chemical attractants is known as *chemotaxis,* and the substances released are called *chemotactic substances.*

FLUID FACTORS

The fluid portion of uncoagulated blood is called *plasma.* Some of the components of plasma provide important constituents for the internal defense mechanisms.

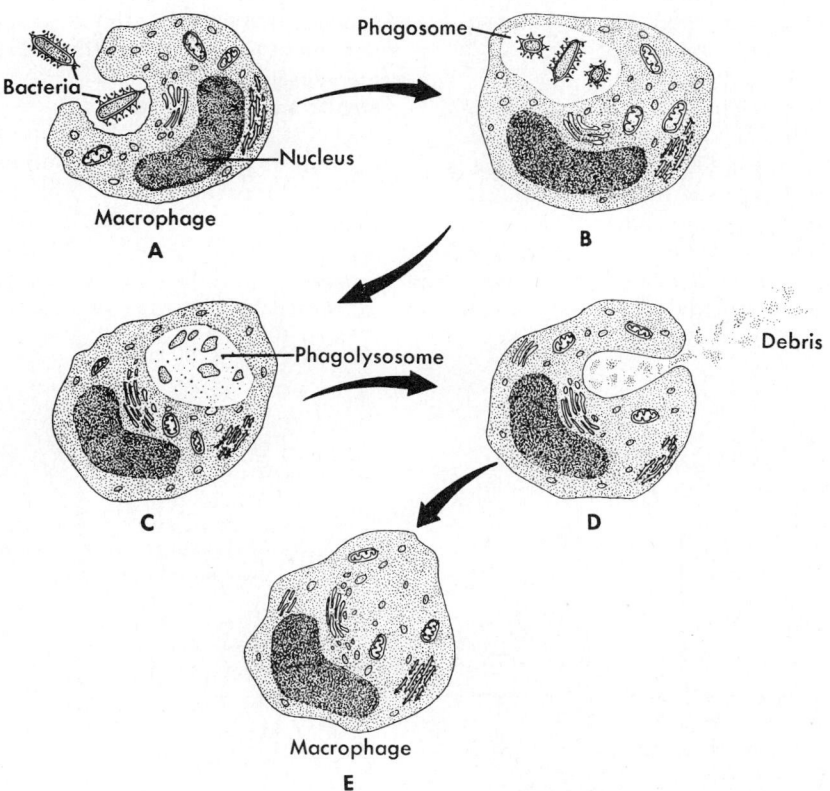

Fig. 6-3. Phagocytosis sketched in macrophage. **A,** Opsonized bacteria engulfed by phagocyte (macrophage). **B,** Phagosome formed. **C,** Phagosome becomes phagolysosome; bacteria digested. (to this point process of phagocytosis is comparable in either macrophage or neutrophil, not shown.) **D,** Debris is egested. (Neutrophil would succumb here.) **E,** Macrophage returns to resting state. (From Smith, A.L.: Microbiology and pathology, ed. 12, St. Louis, 1980, The C.V. Mosby Co.)

Plasma transports the *circulating antibodies* produced in specific response to antigenic stimulation. These antibodies, when bound to their specific antigens, enhance the ability of white blood cells to engulf the clumped and sticky antigens. The antibodies of the blood that create this coating effect are known as *opsonins.* Another plasma constituent, *fibrin,* may create a meshwork around the injured area, causing the sealing off of the area. Microorganisms may also become trapped within this meshwork, where they are more easily captured by the phagocytic cells.

One of the most important constituents of plasma is a complex series of 11 proteins known by the singular name of *complement.* The primary role of complement is to provide specific lysis (rupturing) of cell membranes. The initiation of the "complement cascade" is most often triggered by the binding of the first complement protein to complement binding antibodies that have already bound to their antigens. Thus complement serves to accentuate or complete the action of an antibody. The antibody by itself cannot produce cell lysis, but with the recruitment of complement to join in the reaction, the cell may be ruptured. However, other nonimmune substances can also activate complement. Complement is considered a nonspecific component of the plasma because it is not increased by immunization. In addition to its cytolytic effects, complement is involved in leukocyte chemotaxis, release of histamines, enhancement of phagocytosis by PMNs, viral neutralization, and bactericidal activity.

C-reactive protein is a beta globulin found in the serum of individuals with any type of severe inflammatory process. Both infectious and noninfectious inflammations elicit the formation of this protein in the plasma. The protein forms a precipitate with a consituent of the cell wall of *Streptococcus pneumoniae* known as the C polysaccharide; hence its name. The amount of C-reactive protein found in the serum is roughly proportional to the severity of the inflammation; therefore a test for this protein is useful in the diagnosis and management of hard to differentiate diseases that have a hidden inflammatory aspect, such as bacterial endocarditis, cryptic abscesses, rheumatic fever, and certain types of cancer.

Interferon

Interferon is a low molecular weight protein produced by certain virally infected cells. The protein is released into the extracellular environment, and when taken up by uninfected cells it can protect those cells from viral multiplication. This antiviral action is exerted before the antibody levels can reach protective levels. The interferons are synthesized by the cells of many different animal species, but they are species specific; that is, bovine interferon will not adequately protect human cells. In general, the product of a viral infection is the same regardless of the viral agent that initiated its formation. Therefore interferons can be described as being host specific but viral nonspecific.

Interferons are produced by cells infected with infectious viral particles, inactivated viruses, or even laboratory-synthesized double-stranded polynucleotides. Virtually all tissue cells are capable of producing interferons when properly stimulated, but the lymphocytes are the primary source of interferon in the plasma. The stimulation seems to be tied to the recognition of the "foreign" nucleic acid, which signals the infected cells to synthesize and liberate interferon for a few hours (up to about 24 hours). The interferon acts on the uninfected cells, causing them to synthesize another protein that remains within the protected cell. This protein inhibits the synthesis of the viral particle without blocking normal cell synthetic functions (Fig. 6-4). Interferon itself has no direct effect on the viral particles, nor does it interfere with the entry of the viral particle into the interferon-pro-

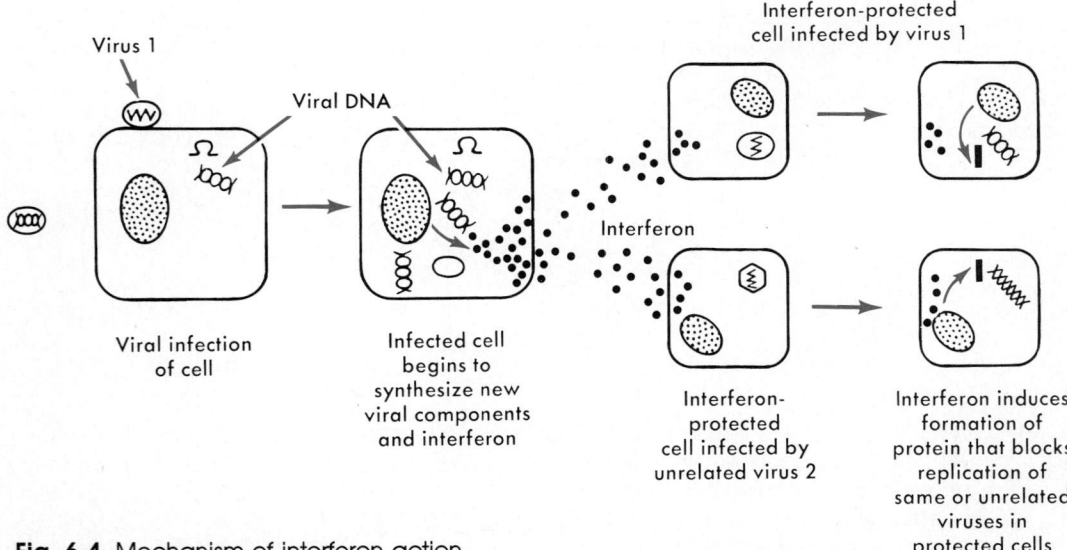

Fig. 6-4. Mechanism of interferon action.

tected cell. This interferon-mediated protection lasts only about 24 hours.

Interferon does not inhibit all viruses equally; some are more readily inhibited than others. Among the viruses that seem to be especially sensitive are the arboviruses, influenza, and smallpox viruses.

That interferon plays a significant role in the recovery from viral infections seems inescapable; however, it has never been shown conclusively that interferon is a necessary part of defense against viral infection. Because naturally occurring deficiencies have never been demonstrated, and there is no mechanism for selective inhibition in experimental animals, it is not possible to specifically evaluate the role of interferon as a defense mechanism.

Interferon has great potential as an antiviral agent because of its protective effects against a wide range of viruses and its low toxicity in the body. There are certain significant limitations to its therapeutic use, however:

1. Species specificity, which until recently meant it had to be produced in human tissue culture, which is both difficult and expensive
2. Difficulty in purification, which makes recovery of large quantities impractical
3. Lack of any effect on viral synthesis already in progress
4. Inability to deliver protective doses to susceptible host cells
5. Short duration of activity

Recent breakthroughs in genetic engineering have made it possible to produce and isolate interferon from bacteria cultures, which greatly reduces the expense and increases the availability of interferon.

Interferon has been shown to be effective in two other clinically important situations: (1) protection of patients whose immunity has been suppressed because of cancer chemotherapy, immunodeficiency disease, or organ transplant and (2) treatment of certain cancers. Interferon has been experimentally successful in protecting immunosuppressed or immunodeficient patients from viral infections by herpesvirus, cytomegalovirus, and influenza virus. Interferon, in addition to its antiviral activity, has been shown to have antitumor activity. Clinical trials with certain human cancers (osteogenic sarcomas and breast cancer) have demonstrated tumor regression after interferon therapy. Interferon may become another chemotherapeutic agent that can be used in cancer therapy.

Inflammatory response

When injury occurs in the body, all of the nonspecific and to some degree the specific defense mechanisms are directed toward localizing the effects of the injury, protecting against microbial invasion at the site, and preparing the site for repair. This process is called *inflammation*. When inflammation occurs at a particular site in the body, the suffix *-itis* is added to the site designation to indicate the pathologic state; for example, an inflammatory response on the pericardium is termed pericarditis, and of the bladder, cystitis.

The inflammatory response can be initiated by any type of injury, for example, heat, cold, irradiation, chemicals,

Table 6-5. Steps of the inflammatory response

Steps	Mediators	Outcome
1. Injury	Physical, chemical, biologic, immunologic stimulus	Cell and tissue injury
2. Vascular response a. Vascular dilation	Histamine, plasmin, serotonin, kinins, prostaglandins released or activated by injury	Dilation of vessels causing stasis of blood and margination of leukocytes
b. Fibrin clot formation	Activation of clotting mechanism	Containment of irritants
3. Fluid exudation	Histamine, kinins, prostaglandins cause opening of venule–endothelial cell junction	Fluid exudation into tissues
4. Cellular exudation a. Leukocyte exudation	Chemotactic substances released by complement activation, clot formation, and injured cells	Passage of leukocytes from blood to site of injury and accumulation there
b. Attack and engulfment of foreign materials	Neutrophils and macrophages	Removal and digestion of bacteria, foreign particles, and damaged tissues
5. Healing	Fibroblasts produce collagen fibers and tissue regeneration	Resolution of inflammation and formation of scar tissue

trauma, infection, immunologic injury, or neoplasm. Whatever the stimulus, the response of the body is the same, but the extent of the involvement of the various facets of the nonspecific response system depends on the extent and severity of the injury.

STEPS OF THE INFLAMMATORY RESPONSE

Three major physiologic responses occur in the inflammatory process: vascular response, fluid exudation, and cellular exudation (Table 6-5). The *vascular response* consists of a transitory vasoconstriction (stress response) followed immediately by vasodilation. This occurs as a result of chemical substances such as histamine or kinins released at the site of injury or invasion. The amount of blood flow to the area is thus increased *(hyperemia)*, causing redness and heat. Blood flow slows as the capillaries dilate. There is increased permeability of the capillary walls, facilitating fluid and cellular exudation. *Fluid exudation* from the capillaries into the interstitial spaces begins immediately and is most active during the first 24 hours after injury or invasion. Initially, the fluid exudate is primarily serous, but as the capillary wall becomes more permeable, protein (albumin) is lost into the interstitial spaces. This increases the colloid osmotic pressure in the interstitial spaces, which encourages more fluid exudation. The swelling of the tissue from the fluid in the interstitial spaces is called *edema* (Chapter 10). *Cellular exudation* refers to the migration of white blood cells (leukocytes) through the capillary walls into the affected tissue. An increased number of white blood cells are attracted to the vessels in the affected area as a result of chemotactic substances being released from the tissues by cell injury and complement activation. The white blood cells adhere to the capillary wall and then pass ameboid fashion through the widened endothelial junctions of the capillary wall. Neutrophils (PMNs), which make up about 60% of the circulating white blood cells, are the first leukocytes to respond, usually within the first few hours. The neutrophils ingest the bacteria and dead tissue cells *(phagocytosis);* then they die, releasing proteolytic enzymes that liquefy the dead neutrophils, dead bacteria, and other dead cells (pus). Monocytes and lymphocytes appear later. The macrophages continue the phagocytosis, and the lymphocytes play a role in the antigen-antibody response at the site.

The five cardinal symptoms of inflammation, identified many centuries ago, are redness *(rubor)* and heat *(calor)* caused by the hyperemia, swelling *(tumor)* caused by the fluid exudate, pain *(dolor)* caused by the pressure of the fluid exudate and by chemical (bradykinin) irritation of the nerve endings, and *loss of function* of the affected part caused by the swelling and pain.

CONTAINMENT OR SPREAD OF INFECTION

The inflammatory response serves to prepare the tissue for healing and to contain the spread of bacterial inva-

sion. To prevent the spread of bacteria, fibroblasts are attracted to the area and secrete fibrin, a threadlike substance that encircles the affected area to wall it off from healthy tissue. If there is interference with this walling-off process, bacteria can spread into the surrounding tissue. This explains why an abscess should not be incised and drained until it has "come to a head," or until the walling-off process is completed.

Bacteria may fail to be contained locally and spread to other parts of the body by means of the lymph system or bloodstream. If picked up by the lymph stream, the bacteria will be carried to the nearest lymph node. These nodes are located along the course of all lymph channels, and here too bacteria can be ingested and destroyed. If the bacteria are virulent enough to resist the action in the lymph nodes, leukocytes are brought in by the bloodstream to attack and engulf the bacteria in the node. The node then becomes swollen and tender because of the accumulation of phagocytes, bacteria, and destroyed lymphoid tissue. This is known as *lymphadenitis.* Swollen lymph nodes can be palpated primarily in the neck, axilla, and groin.

Moderate to severe inflammatory responses can produce generalized systemic effects. Products from the breakdown of bacteria and white blood cells can affect the temperature-regulating center in the hypothalamus and produce fever. A severe infection without accompanying fever may suggest a poor prognosis. Loss of appetite (anorexia) and fatigue may be caused by conservation of body energy needed to resist the infection. The body increases the production of white blood cells to help fight the infection, and *leukocytosis* (serum white blood cell levels >10,000/mm^3) may occur. With infection there is also an increased blood sedimentation rate; that is, when an anticoagulant is added to the blood in the laboratory, the red blood cells settle to the bottom of a test tube more rapidly than normal. This increase in the sedimentation rate is believed to be caused by an increase in fibrinogen (a blood protein essential to the healing process). The sedimentation rate is elevated during the acute inflammatory stage of infection. Its elevation is an indication that the body's defense mechanism for the repair of damaged tissue is operating. Because the sedimentation rate gradually returns to normal as tissues heal, it also is used to determine when physical activity can be safely resumed after an acute infection.

No healing will occur until inflammation has subsided and pus and dead tissue have been removed. Pus is a local accumulation of dead phagocytes, dead bacteria, and dead tissue. The bacteria most commonly causing this reaction are the staphylococci, streptococci, *Neisseria,* and *P. aeruginosa (pyocyanea).*

Inflammations can be classified as either acute or chronic. *Acute* inflammations are those characterized by a sudden onset and an increase in the fluid exudative response. *Chronic* inflammations have a slower, more insidious onset, and they are characterized by increased cellular exudation.

Some types of inflammations

Cellulitis	Inflammation involving cellular and connective tissue
Lymphadenitis	Inflammation of lymph nodes
Lymphangitis	Inflammation of lymphatic vessel
Bacteremia	Presence of bacteria in blood
Septicemia	Systemic disease associated with pathogenic microorganisms and their toxins in the blood
Abscess	Collection of pus localized by a zone of inflamed tissue
Sinus	Suppurating channel from an abscess to the surface or into a body cavity
Peritonitis	Inflammation of the peritoneum
Pleuritis	Inflammation of the pleura
Empyema	Collection of pus in a body cavity, especially the pleural cavity

---

RESOLUTION AND HEALING

After the infected area is clean, new cells are produced to fill in the space left by the injury. They may be the normal structural cells, or they may be fibrotic tissue cells known as *scar tissue*. If they are fibrotic cells, they will not function as formerly but only serve to fill in the injured area. Some body cells readily regenerate; for instance, after the bowel has healed it is almost impossible to find the injured area. The respiratory tract also regenerates its tissues readily. Liver tissue has the capacity to regenerate its tissue, but over a longer period of time. Some nerve cells are always replaced with fibrous tissue. If a large amount of tissue is destroyed, structural cells may not be replaced, regardless of the type of tissue. (See Chapter 19 for discussion of wound healing.)

SPECIFIC DEFENSE MECHANISMS

Concept of specific immunity

Nonspecific response mechanisms are often inadequate to cope with foreign agents. This is especially true when the agent is capable of multiplication and invasion of host tissues, as is the case with infectious disease microorganisms (viruses, bacteria, fungi). The body responds by activation of the specific immune response system.

The fundamental nature of the specific immune response is characterized by diversity, specificity, recognition, memory, and action. Among the most intriguing aspects of immune response is its *diversity of ability to respond* while at the same time responding with *specificity of action*. Almost any conceivable organic molecular array on the surface of a molecule has been shown to be able to induce a series of cellular events culminating in the production of *antibodies*. These antibodies combine with the inducing *antigen* by virtue of combining sites on the antibody molecule, which exhibit an extremely narrow specificity. The remainder of the antibody molecule is chemically and structurally quite similar to all other antibody molecules with distinctly different combining site specificities. *Recognition* and *memory* are two other aspects of this system that make it unique. The normal organism recognizes its own antigenic makeup and will not produce antibodies against its own antigens. This is known as *recognition of self*. At the same time, this intricate system of self-recognition must be able to recognize extremely subtle changes in its own cells when incipient tumors that differ only slightly in antigenic constitution are forming. Further, once the immune system has responded to an antigen, subsequent encounters with that antigen will produce an even more vigorous and rapid response. This response includes a wide variety of mechanisms designed to take *action* against the offending agent. Many of these actions are among the most potent biochemical and cellular reactions that the body is capable of producing, yet they are focused so discretely that the foreign agent is rapidly destroyed with a minimum of damage to the host.

Antigens and antibodies

ANTIGENS

An antigen is defined as a substance that, when introduced into an animal, elicits the formation of antibodies, or specifically sensitized cells. The antigen must be recognized as "nonself" or "foreign" material within the body. While most antigens are naturally occurring proteins of at least 10,000 molecular weight, other substances such as polysaccharides, nucleoproteins, lipoproteins, and glycoproteins may also serve as antigens. The bulk of the antigen consists of subsurface molecular structures that do not elicit an immune response but do serve as carrier for the multiple *antigenic determinants* on the surface. Most antigens have multiple antigenic determinants and are termed *multivalent antigens*; however, some molecules may be monovalent.

Certain molecules, because of their small size, cannot by themselves induce the synthesis of antibodies; however, when they are coupled with a high molecular weight carrier, they can serve as antigenic determinants. These molecules are known as *incomplete antigens*, or *haptens*. These molecules take on special significance in the consideration of hypersensitivities (allergies to low molecular weight compounds such as certain drugs and antibiotics) (Chapter 39).

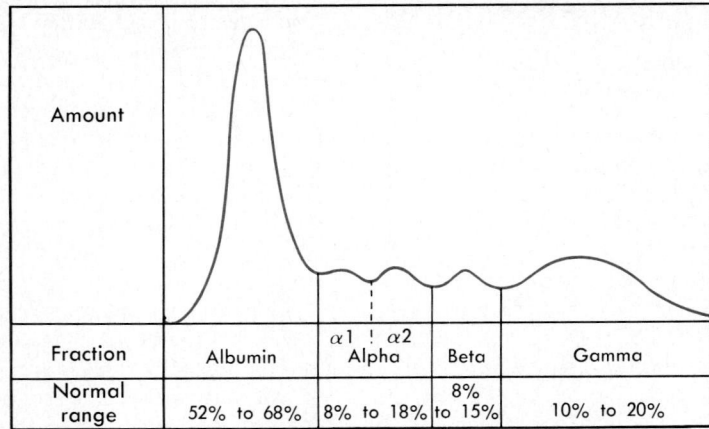

Amount					
Fraction	Albumin	α1 α2 Alpha	Beta	Gamma	
Normal range	52% to 68%	8% to 18%	8% to 15%	10% to 20%	

Fig. 6-5. Electrophoretic separation of major serum proteins. Majority of antibody activity lies within gamma globulin fraction. Gamma globulin fraction will rise with active synthesis of antibodies in response to antigenic stimulation.

ANTIBODIES

The body's response to the introduction of an antigenic substance is the production of a specific, soluble *antibody* or a sensitized (antigen reactive) lymphocyte population. The type of antigen introduced will determine the immune response: antibody synthesis, antigen-reactive lymphocyte, or a combination of both.

The circulating antibodies represent modified (that is, antigen specific) globulin proteins found in blood serum. The serum contains several distinct protein fractions, which are separable on the basis of their net electrical charge, molecular size, and molecular conformation into several fractions: albumin, alpha globulins, beta globulins, and gamma globulins (Fig. 6-5). The antibody activity of the serum is characteristically associated with the gamma globulin fraction. Those gamma globulins with the ability to bind antigens are called *immunoglobulins*.

ANTIGEN-ANTIBODY INTERACTIONS

When an immunoglobulin comes in contact with its specific antigen, there is a physical interaction between the two, causing a reversible binding of the antibody to the antigen. The affinity that the antibody has for the antigen and the avidity, or tightness, of the binding depend on the location and spatial arrangement of the antigenic determinants on the surface of the antigen and how well the antigen-combining site on the antibody molecule "fits" the antigenic determinant. Because the antigen is usually multivalent and the antibody is generally at least bivalent, the antigen molecules may be cross bound and clumped (agglutinated, precipitated) by antibody molecules (Fig. 6-6).

Within the body the binding of antibody to the antigen can have direct beneficial effects, such as detoxification of toxins, inactivation of viruses, or, coupled with complement, the direct lysis of cells. However, in most cases the antigen-antibody combination initiates and facilitates

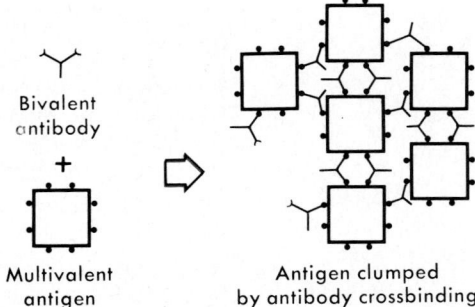

Bivalent antibody

+

Multivalent antigen

Antigen clumped by antibody crossbinding

Fig. 6-6. Clumping of multivalent antigen by its specific antibody.

the nonspecific defense mechanisms (phagocytosis, complement, inflammatory response, and so forth).

Immune response system

CELLS INVOLVED

The cells involved in the specific immune response are all derived from the original undifferentiated stem cells of the bone marrow. The stem cell has the possibility of developing into any of the blood cells of the body depending on various signals and influences. The primary cells of the immune response system develop from the lymphocytic cell population (Fig. 6-7). One population of lymphocytic cells undergoes differentiation under the influence of the thymus gland and becomes known as *thymus-dependent lymphocytes,* or *T cells.* These cells become responsible for mediating the *cell-mediated immune responses* (CMI). Another population of lymphocytes matures in the lymphoid tissues, and is referred to as *thymus-independent lymphocytes,* or *B cells.* The designation B cell comes from the fact that in the chicken, where this process was first detected, there is a single site where this differentiation occurs, the *bursa of Fabricius.* No such singular

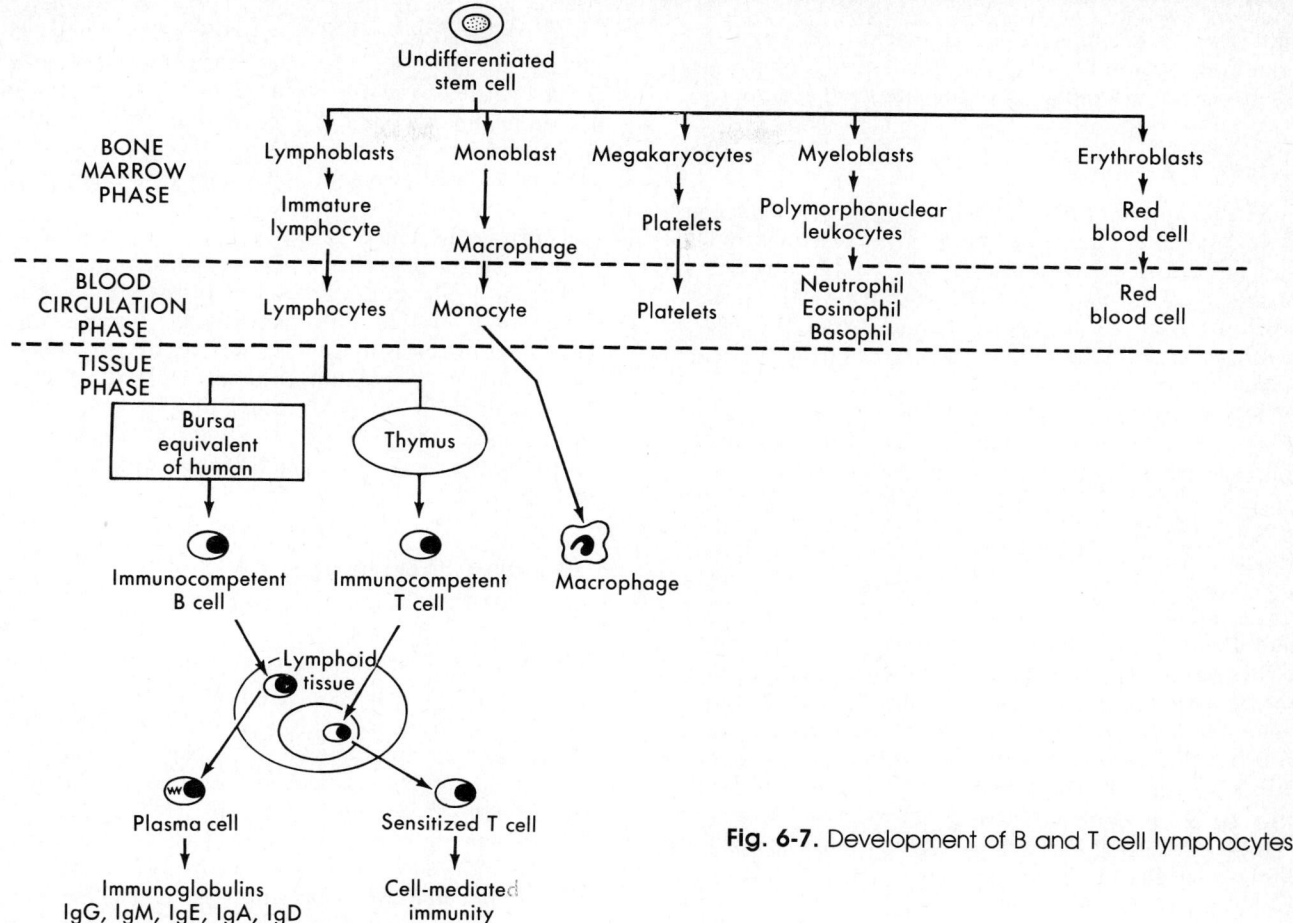

Fig. 6-7. Development of B and T cell lymphocytes.

Table 6-6. Lymphokines liberated by activated T cell lymphocytes

Lymphokine	Function
Lymphocyte-derived chemotactic factors	Chemotactic for macrophages
Lymphocytotoxins	Nonspecific lysis of cells
Macrophage inhibition-activation factors	Maintains macrophage at site and activates it
Interferon	Inhibits replication of viruses
Lymphocyte-activating factors	Activates nonsensitized lymphocytes

lymphoid organ is found in humans, but it is believed that the gut-associated lymphoid tissues, such as tonsils, Peyer's patches of the intestine, and appendix, serve as the equivalent sites in humans. The B cells are responsible for the production of the immunoglobulins and the provision of the *humoral immune response.*

The role of the lymphocytes (B or T cells) is to recognize the presence of an antigen and to initiate specific mechanisms of disposal. Just as important, the lymphocyte must recognize a component of host tissues as self and protect that tissue from immunologic reactions.

The macrophage appears to act nonspecifically, but its role in the immune response is critical. First, the macrophage seems to be responsible for initially capturing, processing, and presenting the antigen to the lympho-

cytes. Capture of the antigen occurs by phagocytosis as described earlier in this chapter. The processing of the antigen is poorly understood, but there is evidence that the macrophage digests and concentrates the antigen and then couples the antigen to RNA. This processed signal is transferred to the surface of the macrophage for presentation to lymphocytes. An antigen presented to lymphocytes in this manner triggers the series of events within the lymphocytes that leads to full immunologic response. An antigen that escapes this processing will stimulate only a weak immune response or none at all.

At the other end of the immune response the macrophage is activated to its maximum of phagocytic efficiency by the release of stimulatory, soluble substances, known as *lymphokines,* by activated lymphocytes (Table 6-6). In this way the macrophage is stimulated at the site of an immune reaction. Other of the soluble lymphokines serve to attract the macrophages to the site by chemotaxis.

ORGANS AND TISSUES INVOLVED

The organs and tissues of the specific immune response system include the central organs (bone marrow, thymus, and gut-associated lymphoid tissues) and the peripheral organs (lymph nodes, spleen, and lymphatic vessels). Within the central organs the immune response cells are synthesized and matured, whereas within the peripheral organs the mature cells are concentrated.

The *thymus* serves as the control organ of the immune system. It is the site of differentiation of the T cell lymphocytic populations and through certain soluble thymic hormones serves to regulate the overall immune system. The activity of the thymus reaches it peak in childhood, and the organ begins to shrink in size after puberty. If the thymus is removed (thymectomy) very early in the life of an animal, a severe state of immunodeficiency is induced and T cell–mediated immunity never develops. After thymectomy, a wasting disease develops, characterized by stunted growth, diarrhea, and death from massive infection by intestinal or respiratory tract normal flora. The B cell function is also reduced, pointing to a cooperative effect between the two basic systems. In the adult animal the loss of the thymus creates less severe reactions, probably because of an already functional, long-lived population of T cells.

The *lymph nodes* and *spleen* serve as the primary sites of localization of the immune response cells. The lymph node serves to filter the lymph drained from a region of tissue. The structure of the lymph node (Fig. 6-8) consists of an inner medullary and paracortical region made up primarily of T cells and an outer cortex composed of clusters, or germinal centers, of B cells known as follicles. The spleen is structured on somewhat the same pattern, with diffusely packed T cell areas and germinal centers of tightly packed B cells. In certain types of antigenic stimulation, either the T cell areas or the B cell areas will show tissue proliferation, whereas the other area remains quiescent. By the same principle, if there is a basic primary immunodeficiency of one system, the corresponding area of lymph nodes and spleen may degenerate.

During the course of the immune response reaction, within the lymph nodes there is significant proliferation of specific cells and migration of phagocytic cells to the site, which may lead to lymph node enlargement. Enlargement of the lymph nodes in a region may be the result of infection, immune disease, intrinsic neoplasm of the lymph node, or metastatic spread of malignant cells to the node. The presence of an enlarged spleen or enlarged lymph nodes is virtually always an important clinical finding.

Immune response
PRIMARY IMMUNE RESPONSE
Antigenic challenge

When an antigen is introduced into the body, it can trigger a wide or narrow spectrum of response mechanisms. The specific pattern of response depends on the amount of antigen introduced, the site of introduction, and the type of antigen introduced.

Small amounts of a noninvasive, large, particulate antigen introduced at a single body site are quickly and efficiently handled at a local site with little or no systemic involvement beyond the local lymph node. Because the inflammatory response and local lymph node can localize the spread of the antigen, the immune response may go completely unnoticed by the host organism. Larger, particulate antigens are readily cleared, but small, soluble antigens are more difficult to clear from the circulation.

Large amounts of an antigen may allow the antigen to escape from the local site by simply overwhelming the

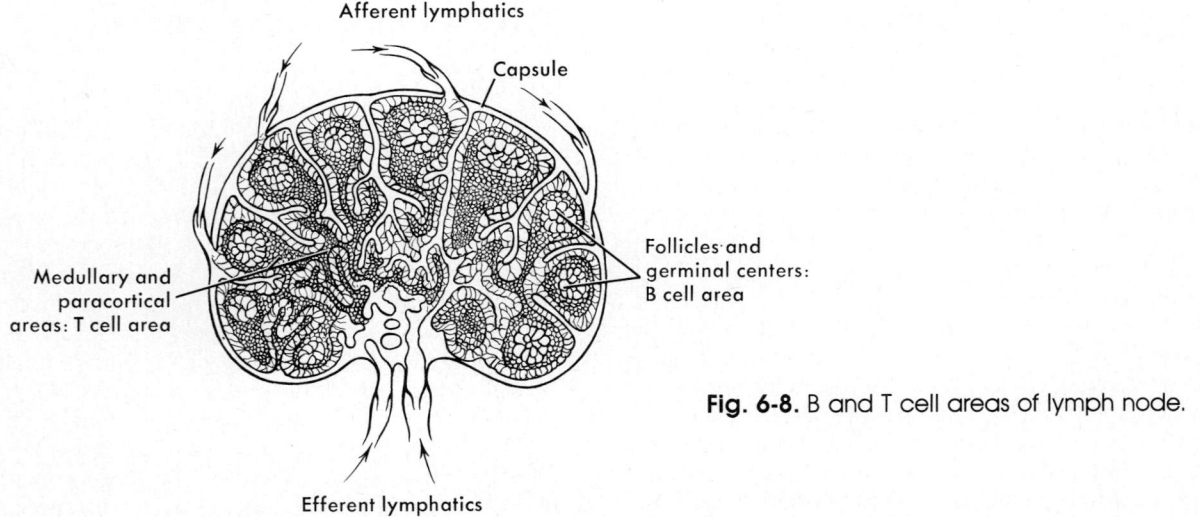

Fig. 6-8. B and T cell areas of lymph node.

local defense mechanisms. Even though the lymph nodes and reticuloendothelial organs can clear 80% to 90% of an antigen on a single pass, if the amount of the antigen is extremely large some antigen may escape the local site. An excessively large, sustained antigen dose can exhaust not only the local site but the entire reticuloendothelial system as well. This greatly reduces the body's ability to respond to even minor invasive challenges and renders the host vulnerable to secondary infections.

Highly invasive antigens (for example, bacteria such as *Staphylococcus aureus* or *Streptococcus pyogenes*) or those introduced directly into the bloodstream by blood transfusion, intravenous catheterization, or injection can immediately establish a systemic type of immune response. This is why extreme care must be exercised in the use of any type of medical procedure that could allow the introduction of organisms into the general circulation. The localization action of the immune response is critical to efficient functioning of the response.

Humoral response

When the antigen is introduced for the first time, one of three basic mechanisms of response will be elicited: a response mediated primarily by B cells, the humoral response; a response in which the T cells are primarily involved, the cell-mediated response; or a combined type of response.

If the antigen is of the type that triggers a humoral response, the first time the body is exposed to the antigen the B cell system responds with the synthesis of circulating immunoglobulins (Fig. 6-9). The encroaching antigen is phagocytosed by a lymph node macrophage or tissue-active macrophage. The macrophage processes the antigen and presents the antigenic stimulus to a B cell, which has been preprogrammed to respond to the introduced antigen. These antigen-specific B cells bear receptors on their surface, which allow them to recognize their antigenic stimulant. Only a few lymphocytes within a lymph node have the ability to respond to the antigen. The stimulated B cell then begins a process of proliferation (increase in number) and differentiation (change in structure and function). The progeny of the stimulated cell increase in number within the lymph node, forming *clones* of specifically adapted lymphocytes. With each generation of new cells within the clone, the lymphocytes become more differentiated toward a cell population ideally suited for the synthesis and release of immunoglobulin. These cells are known as *plasma cells*. With the de-

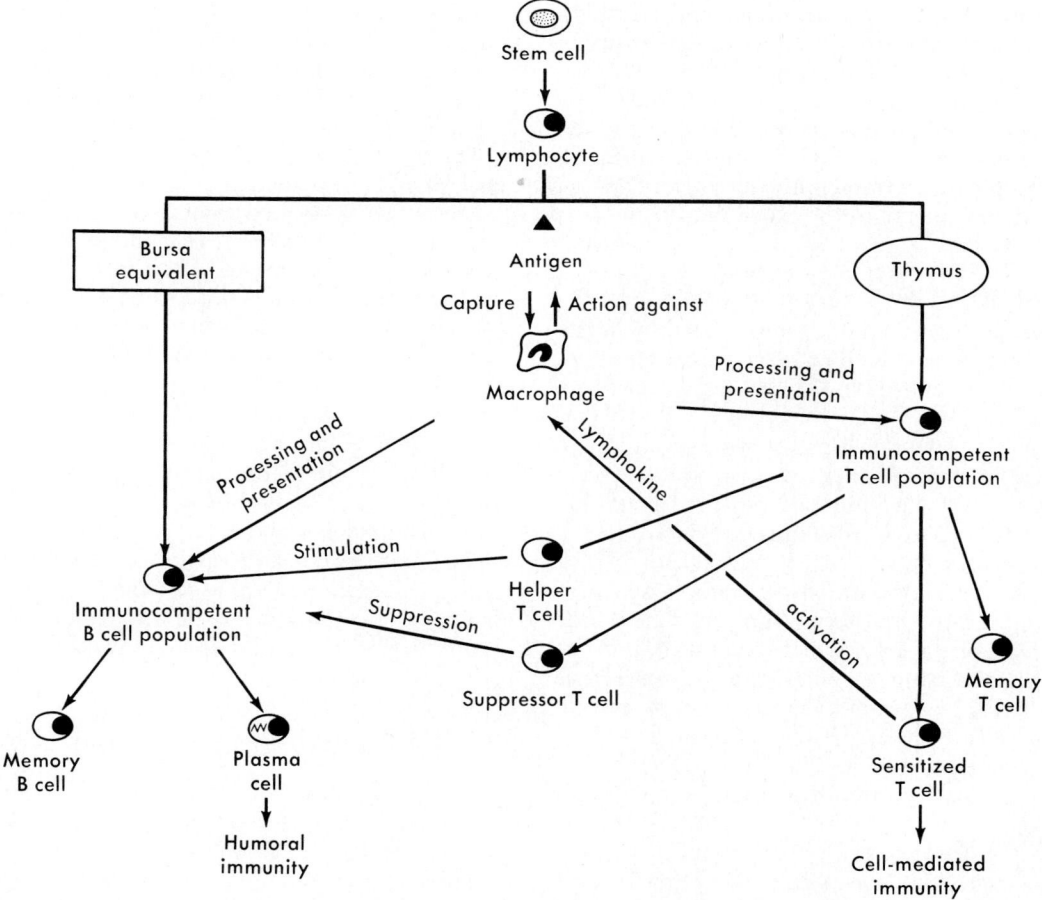

Fig. 6-9. Combined response of B and T cell systems.

velopment of this cell population in the lymph node (several days after the introduction of the antigen), antibodies can be detected in the lymph node. However, it is not until about 1 to 2 weeks after the antigenic challenge that detectable levels of specific antibodies appear in the serum. The plasma cell population of the lymph node and the levels of antibody in the blood continue to increase for another 2 to 3 weeks, and then both begin to retreat.

Two types of immunoglobulins are produced and released into the circulation. *Immunoglobulin M* (IgM or macroglobulin) is especially effective at attaching to particulate antigens such as bacterial cells and with the activation of the complement system in the serum, causes the lysis of those cells. Because IgM antibodies are so large, they cannot leave the blood vessels, so they are restricted to a role in the bloodstream.

Immunoglobulin G (IgG) makes up about 85% of the antibodies found in the serum. This immunoglobulin is smaller and can move from the blood and lymph into virtually all body fluids and can also cross the placenta from maternal circulation into fetal circulation. This class of immunoglobulin provides most of our protection against bacterial, viral, and toxic agents in the body. Usually when the term *antibody* is used, this is the type of immunoglobulin that is meant.

Some of the lymphocytes of the activated clone may become "memory cells," which are much more responsive, both in time of reaction and efficiency of antibody synthesis, to subsequent contact with the antigen.

The humoral response serves to protect the body from such agents as microbial toxins, bacteria within the extravascular spaces in the blood and on mucosal surfaces, and viruses that must pass through the circulatory system to reach their site of infection (for example, poliomyelitis virus).

Cell-mediated response

Certain antigens trigger a response mediated by T cell proliferation and reaction. A T cell that has received its antigenic stimulus is referred to as a *sensitized T cell lymphocyte* (Fig. 6-9).

The initial steps of the cell-mediated response, those involving the antigen processing by the macrophage, seem to be the same as in the humoral response. Following presentation of the antigenic stimulus to lymph node T cells, there is proliferation in the T cell domain. There is no release of circulatory antibodies; rather, activated lymphocytes are released into the circulation. These cells migrate to the site of the entrance of the antigen into the body, where the invading agent or residual antigen is found. These activated lymphocytes, along with macrophages, infiltrate the regions of the tissue and begin a direct attack on the antigen or tissue cells labeled with the antigen. The T cells participating in this direct attack are known as *killer T cells.*

To amplify the site reaction further, the sensitized lymphocytes activate the nonspecific phagocytotic cells (macrophages, PMNs, and noncommitted lymphocytes) in the region of the antigen. This is accomplished through the release of the soluble lymphokines (Table 6-6), which recruit additional cells to attack the antigenic materials.

The cell-mediated response is especially effective in protection against diseases that grow and do their damage intracellularly where the circulating immunoglobulins cannot reach them. Diseases of this type include viral and rickettsial diseases and those produced by certain chronic types of infective agents, fungal pathogens and tubercle bacillus being the most outstanding examples. One other important function of this system is the provision of *cancer cell surveillance.*

Combined immune response

Most antigens do not cause a purely humoral or purely cell-mediated response; rather, both types of response are evoked. Likewise, our protection against most harmful antigens is the result of both of these specific response systems being brought to bear on the antigen involved. In the *combined type of response,* there is an initial perturbation within the T cell areas of the lymph node. This becomes obvious within about 2 days after the introduction of the antigen. About 3 to 5 days later, the B cell areas begin to proliferate.

To mount a maximal immune response, the cooperative action of the three central cell types is necessary. The macrophage serves to capture, process, and present the antigen to immunocompetent cells of both T and B cell ancestry. The T cells aid in the direct cell-mediated response, but there also seems to be a population of T cells that serves to interact with the B cell population to control the development of an effective immune response. A *helper T cell* population cooperates with the B cells by some as yet undefined mechanism to enhance the activation and proliferation of the immunoglobulin synthesizing cells. The existence of the helper T cell explains the observation noted earlier in this chapter that the removal of the thymus from the neonate not only compromises the cell-mediated immune response but also significantly reduces the host's ability to mount a humoral immune response.

Another group of T cells also exerts an effect on the synthesis of circulating antibodies. Cells known as *suppressor T cells* may provide a negative control function over B cell clones and other T cell clones, preventing the expression of an immunologic response. Exactly how these cells suppress the function of other immunologically responsive cells is not understood, but they play an important role in turning on and off the body's response to certain antigens.

SECONDARY IMMUNE RESPONSE

As emphasized at the outset of this section, one of the touchstone characteristics of the specific response system is the ability of the system to remember prior contact with an antigen and to provide a more complete protective reaction on subsequent contact. The first contact between the immune response system and an antigen leads

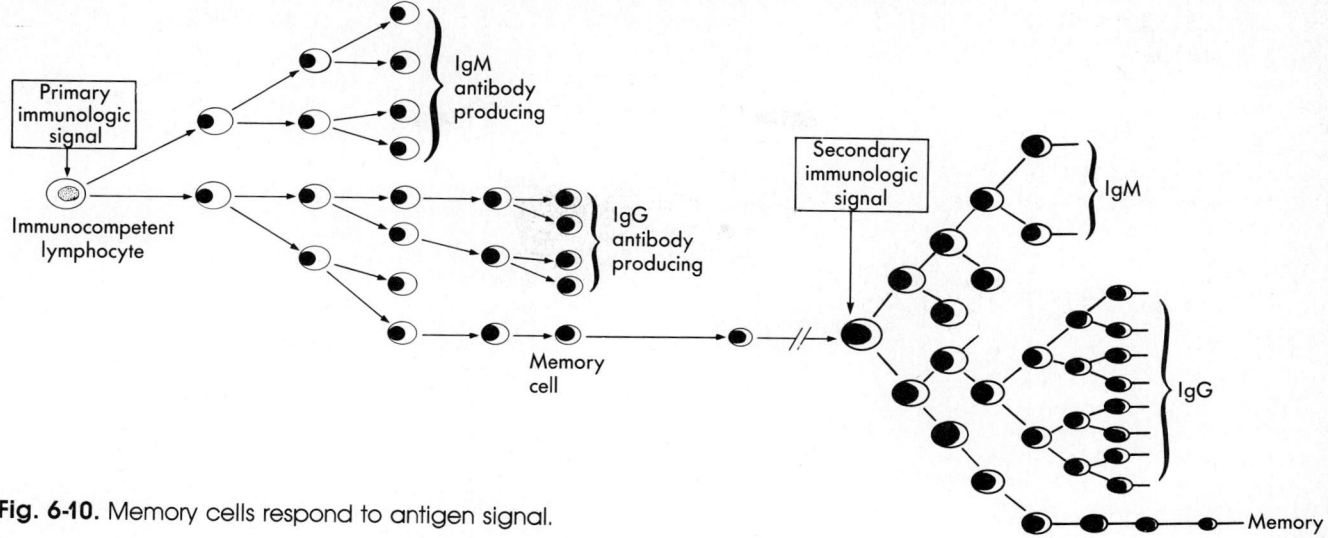

Fig. 6-10. Memory cells respond to antigen signal.

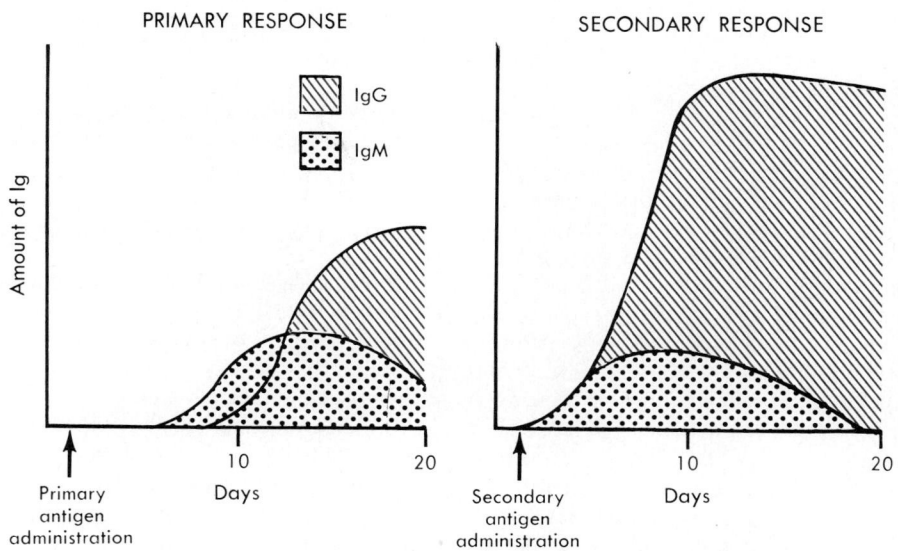

Fig. 6-11. Primary and secondary humoral responses.

to the *primary response,* the events of which have been laid out in the preceding paragraphs. When antibody synthesis is measured in a primary response, there is a significant lag time to the appearance of antibodies in the circulation (Figs. 6-10 and 6-11). Immunoglobulins of the IgM class are the first to appear, but they maintain protective levels for only a short period. Specific IgG antibodies follow and reach protective levels within 12 to 14 days, but they too fall off fairly quickly with only this initial exposure.

When the "primed" immune response system encounters the antigen again, a *secondary response* ensues, which is more rapid, of greater intensity, and longer lasting than

the primary response. This secondary response is also termed an *anamnestic response.* This "remembered" response is a characteristic of both the B and T cell systems. The prior contact with the antigen is stored in special memory cells of both cell lines. As illustrated in Fig. 6-10, the memory cells respond immediately to the antigenic signal, so that the lag time between exposure to the antigen and production of protective antibody levels is greatly reduced. This phenomenon provides the basis for active immunization and "booster" doses to maintain the protective levels of immunity. In an immunized individual the memory cells elicit the rapid response in time for the immune system to overwhelm the pathogen or toxin before it can produce its damage.

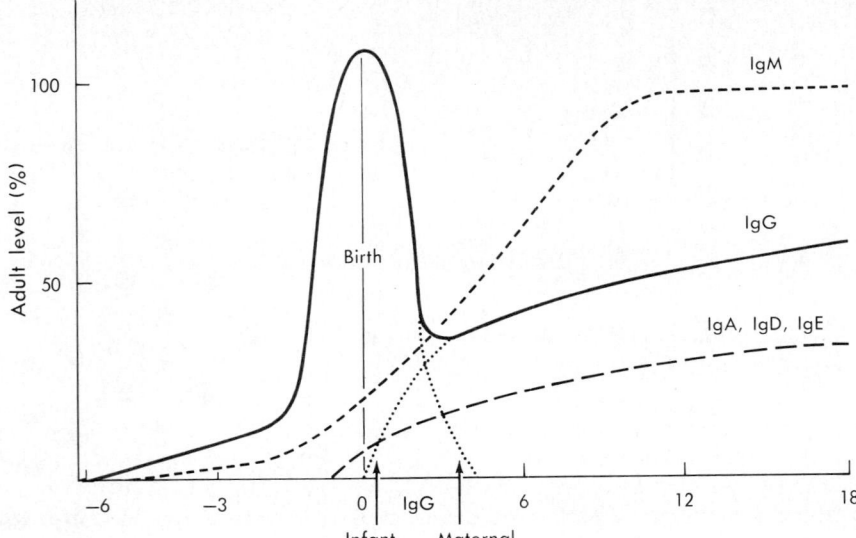

Fig. 6-12. Immunoglobulin levels in fetus and neonate.

DEVELOPMENTAL ASPECTS OF THE IMMUNE RESPONSE

Lymphoid cells first appear in the fetus as stem cells in the fetal liver at about the end of the first trimester. The lymphoid tissues of the thymus also develop fairly early in the fetus. At birth, however, the lymph nodes and spleen are still underdeveloped, but T and B cell responsiveness is fully functional. The fetus is capable of some immune response if challenged by an in utero (within the uterus) infection, such as in the case of congenital syphilis or rubella. Unless the fetus has been exposed to a congenital infection, at birth the neonate-synthesized immunoglobulin levels are low (Fig. 6-12). The child does have high levels of transplacentally acquired maternal IgG antibodies. These maternal antibodies have a half-life of about 30 days in the child, and this coupled with the increase in blood volume in the growing infant leads to a drop in the IgG levels of the blood over the first 3 months. Thereafter the rate of the child's own synthesis of IgG provides for a steady increase in the immunoglobulin concentration within the serum. IgM levels reach adult concentrations by about the age of 9 months.

Numerous studies in both animals and humans have shown that during the aging process there is a progressive loss of immunologic vigor. The prime immunologic age probably is achieved during the late teens, when virtually the full complement of immunities has been developed and the responsiveness of the system peaks. The middle years are characterized by a plateau and slowly falling curve until the later years of life, when a sharp decline in both the cell-mediated and humoral response systems becomes evident. This loss in immunologic sensitivity is associated with an increasingly less effective and more misdirected immune response. There is an increasing frequency of autoimmune disease, susceptibility to pathogenic and opportunistic microorganisms, and incidence of cancer.

DEVELOPMENT OF IMMUNE TOLERANCE

Immune tolerance is defined as the state of immunologic nonresponsiveness. By some mechanisms the body becomes tolerant to self while maintaining responsiveness to foreign materials. Evidence establishes that self-tolerance is acquired during embryonic development; however, the exact mechanisms by which it develops remain an issue. During fetal development the immune system is presented with antigens from the developing tissues; these become identified as self-antigens, so that when exposed to these antigens postnatally the individual is tolerant of them.

One proposed mechanism by which this state could be induced is known as the *clonal selection theory*. This theory states that when potentially responsive clones of B or T cells come into contact with an antigen prenatally, the responsive cell line is killed, thus eliminating the responsiveness to that antigen from the body. This produces a state of *natural tolerance*. This theory is supported by experimental data that show that by exposing experimental animals to foreign antigens in utero a tolerance to that antigen is developed; however, some antigens introduced in this manner are found to be more *tolerogenic* (capable of inducing tolerance) than others. Further, the clonal selection theory does not explain how it is possible to break tolerance in adults, as indicated in certain experimental studies or as in the case of certain of the autoimmune diseases (see Chapter 39). In some cases at least, tolerance is not the result of the total elimination of specifically reactive cells but of the blocking of expression or temporary inactivation of the responsive cells. The action of suppressor T cells or the failure of mobilization by helper T cells may play a significant role in maintaining the state of self-tolerance.

APPLICATIONS AND IMPLICATIONS OF IMMUNE RESPONSE

Immunization

Long before the mechanisms of immune response were worked out, it was recognized that recovery from certain diseases conferred protection against subsequent exposure. Dating from the days of Jenner's vaccination with cowpox exudate to protect against smallpox (1798), through the success of Pasteur with anthrax and rabies (1880s), to the present, the specific protective mechanisms of the immune system have been used to protect against serious infectious diseases.

PASSIVE IMMUNIZATION

Temporary protection, usually measured in days or at most weeks, is afforded by the acquisition of preformed antibody from another host. As the acquired antibodies are used up through binding with antigen or by being catabolized, the protection is lost.

Transplacental passive immunization occurs through the transfer of IgG antibodies from the maternal circulation across the placenta to the fetal blood. There is also some acquisition of immunoglobulins through the colostrum of the mother's milk.

Artificial passive immunization may be necessary if the individual to be immunized has suffered exposure to a serious infectious agent to which he has no immunity or if the individual's own immune system is impaired or deficient. The sources of these preformed antibodies are pooled human adult gamma globulin or heterologous (from another species) globulin fractions. Pooled human gamma globulin has been used to modify the effects of measles, particularly in premature infants, in children with primary immunodeficiencies, and in patients undergoing immunosuppressive therapies. Persons who have contact with persons with hepatitis and smallpox may also be protected by this method. It should be noted, however, that isolated gamma globulin preparations tend to form small protein aggregates, and these, if injected intravenously, could lead to severe anaphylactic reactions. For this reason the material is always administered *intramuscularly*.

The most commonly used heterologous antibody fractions are antitetanus and antidiphtheria antisera derived from horse globulins. Because these are foreign proteins, they can lead to the development of serum sickness (Chapter 39). Serum sickness is more likely to occur in individuals already primed by previous contact with horse globulin; thus multiple use of heterologous sera is to be avoided.

ACTIVE IMMUNIZATION

The objective of active immunization is to provide effective long-term immunity by establishing within the individual's body the capacity to produce effective levels of immune response and to establish a population of sensitive cells that can respond to a subsequent antigenic contact.

Immunizing agents ideally should be noninjurious to the individual being immunized. To accomplish this, the pathogenic effects must be modified while at the same time maintaining the antigenicity of the agent. Bacteria exotoxins such as those produced by the diphtheria and tetanus bacteria can be successfully detoxified by formaldehyde treatment without destroying the major antigenic determinants on the protein molecule. Such detoxified antigenic materials are called *toxoids*. The use of *killed vaccines* of viruses and bacteria can also provide a safe antigen for immunization. Killed vaccines include those for pertussis (whooping cough), typhoid, and cholera, and the Salk poliomyelitis vaccine. The protection conferred by these vaccines is generally inferior to that produced by live vaccines. A number of the most successful vaccines consist of living organisms that have been modified so that they are nonvirulent. The *attenuated life vaccines* provide excellent protection, but there is some risk in their use because of the possibility of reversion to the virulent form of the organism or the risk of their producing immunodeficiency in the individual. Live vaccines that are of importance include those for measles, mumps, and tuberculosis (BCG), and the Sabin poliomyelitis vaccine.

The provision of protective levels of residual immunity depends on the inducement of the right type of response (that is, cell mediated or humoral), in sufficient amounts, at the right place (that is, where the immune response can contact the antigen), and against the right antigenic determinants (that is, the antibodies formed produce an inactivating effect). Simply the induction of an immune response is not sufficient to provide protection. For example, the early killed virus measles vaccines elicited a splendid production of circulating antibodies against the measles virus, but protection against measles is most effectively mediated by cellular immune responses. The humoral protection did not prevent infection.

Another problem of immunization for which provision must be made is the *interference* that one antigen may have with another if the two are given simultaneously. The live virus vaccines occasionally interfere with each other; when measles and smallpox vaccines are administered at the same time, they each interfere with the development of immunity by the other. This is probably the result of interferon production. Some live virus vaccines contain more than one strain of the virus, and these can cross-inhibit. In the case of the Sabin oral polio vaccine, three separate doses are required because there are three strains within the same vaccine. With the initial dose, immunity to only one strain may develop if the strain interferes with the other two.

COMPLICATIONS OF IMMUNIZATION

Although immunization is the most successful approach to the control of many infectious diseases, there are small but still real risks involved. The development of postvaccination encephalitis or other neural autoimmune complications is a serious risk with such vaccines as those for smallpox or rabies. Children with immunodeficiencies may be overwhelmed by vaccination with live vaccine. With viral vaccines, which are produced in monkey kidney of human cell culture, there is a slight risk of the introduction of oncogenic (cancer causing) viruses. A fetus may be significantly at risk if the mother receives a live virus vaccine during pregnancy. Such vaccines as smallpox and live influenza should never be administered to a pregnant woman. It is still unclear whether the rubella virus vaccine harms the fetus, so it too should be avoided. Besides these rather serious risks, general discomfort is to be expected from some forms of immunization. The typhoid vaccine, for instance, is composed of large numbers of killed salmonella bacteria; because the endotoxic cell wall materials of these cells is a pyrogenic (fever producing) substance, fever and malaise are not uncommon sequelae. The influenza vaccines often produce febrile reactions in children.

Cancer immunology

One of the functions of the cell-mediated immune response system may be the recognition and destruction of cancer cells within the body. It is postulated that, by the same mechanisms that are operative in allograft rejection, the immune system continually protects against the establishment of tumor growths. The recognition of these cells as nonself is based on the appearance of "new" surface antigens that allow identification. A growing body of evidence supports the view that this is a vital function of the immune system. Patients in whom the cellular immune system is impaired (immunosuppressed) or defective (immunodeficient) for significant periods are at especially high risk of certain neoplastic diseases. To these data is coupled the observation that cancers are most prone to appear early in life before the immune system is fully functional or in later life as the system becomes less effective.

Cancers may become established in the body by escaping the surveillance mechanisms or by growing so rapidly that they outdistance the immune system's ability to respond. Experimentally, if a few thousand tumor cells are transferred from a cancerous animal to a noncancerous animal, the latter is capable of responding and destroying the tumor; however, if the tumor cell load is increased to several billion cells, the tumor may become established. The humoral immune system may actually serve to protect the developing cancer by producing noncytotoxic antibodies (*enhancing antibodies*) that coat the tumor cell surfaces and mask the surface from recognition by sensitized lymphocytes. As a tumor grows, it is capable of both specific and nonspecific suppression of the immune system. This further reduces the effectiveness of a response.

Some of the new surface antigens (known as *tumor-specific transplantation antigens* [TSTA]) appearing on the cancerous cell are shed into the circulation and can be immunologically detected there. Some of these antigens, such as carcinoembryonic antigen (CEA) and alpha fetoprotein (α-FP), are present during fetal development but are not expressed in the adult. Their reappearance lends support to the theory that cancer represents a dedifferentiation to a more primitive cell. These antigens, termed *oncofetal antigens* (OFA), are of some significance in early detection, diagnostic confirmation, and determination of malignant disease progress.

Some very early progress has been made in stimulating, both specifically and nonspecifically, the body's immunologic response to cancers in the hope of preventing further growth of the tumors. With further knowledge of both the cancer process and the immune response mechanisms, the possibility of using immunotherapy, immunoprophylaxis, and immunodiagnosis as specific tools against malignancies seems quite realistic.

Immunologic disorders

As expected in such an interrelated, complex system as is operative in the mechanisms providing biologic defense, there are innumerable points at which the system may malfunction. The immunologic disorders that have been characterized may result from the following:

1. Nonresponsiveness
2. Blocked responsiveness
3. Limited responsiveness
4. Misdirected responsiveness
5. Overresponsiveness

The underlying causes of the disorders may be attributed to developmental defect, infection, malignancy, trauma, metabolic state, or pharmacologic intervention. The severity of the disorders ranges from creation of a minor nuisance (for example, mild hayfever) to a life-threatening situation (for example, anaphylactic shock). The disorders may be classified into the following general categories:

1. Immunodeficiencies: deficiencies in the proper expression of the immune response system, parts of the system, or individual cell types within the system
2. Gammopathies: abnormal production of immunoglobulins
3. Hypersensitivities: exaggerated or inappropriate response to specific antigens
4. Autoimmunities: immunologic attack on self-antigens

Each of these immunologic disorders is discussed in Chapter 39.

Tissue transplants

The transfer of healthy tissues and organs from one individual to replace damaged or diseased tissues in another has been surgically possible for many years. Early attempts failed because of the rejection of the foreign cells and tissues by the body. With the growing knowledge of the immune response, the mechanisms of this rejection process became more apparent, and it is now possible to make judgments and predictions concerning the likelihood of success of transplantation. It has now become possible to control the course of the graft transfer process to favor the acceptance of the transplanted tissue.

The antigenic determinants of the tissues that lead to graft rejection are primarily found on the surface of the cells within the transplanted tissues. These antigens are known as *histocompatibility antigens* and are controlled by independently segregating genes within the chromosomal structure of the animal. They are also called *human leukocyte (HLA) antigens*. Some of the histocompatibility antigens are more antigenic than are others; thus some antigens are referred to as major and others as minor. The major transplantation antigens are those of the ABO and Rh blood groups and the HLA antigens (Chapter 39).

Graft rejection can be minimized by the use of chemical (drug) or physical (radiation) agents that nonspecifically or specifically interfere with the development of an immune response reaction against the foreign tissue. Clinically, four types of chemical immunosuppressive agents are effective in providing the transitional protection needed to promote the graft establishment (Table 6-7).

Glucocorticoids, especially prednisone, are significantly antiinflammatory and impair lymphocyte (B and T cell) activation and function. Prednisone exerts a wide spectrum of activity against all immune response and inflammatory response mechanisms. Although it suppresses the cell-mediated system to a greater degree than the humoral system, the continued high dosage needed to maintain cell-mediated suppression creates significant risks in reducing the responsiveness of the humoral system. Often lower dosages of prednisone and azathioprine are used together because they seem to act synergistically.

Table 6-7. Effect of selected drugs on the immune system

Drug	Immune system impairment	Indications for immunosuppressive therapy
Corticosteroids	Impairment of T cell function Catabolism of immunoglobulins (decreased IgG) Lymphocytopenia Type 1 hypersensitivity: vasoconstriction, eosinopenia Type 3 hypersensitivity: decreased vascular permeability Type 4 hypersensitivity: decreased macrophage function	Diseases where immune disorder is unknown Tissue and organ transplantation Autoimmune diseases
Antimetabolites (azathioprine)	Interference with RNA, DNA, and protein synthesis Depression of bone marrow and antibody reproduction Decreased primary immune response	Autoimmune diseases Tissue transplantation Dermatologic disease (pemphigus, psoriasis) Neoplasia
Alkylating agents (cyclophosphamide)	Interference with DNA, RNA, and protein synthesis Lymphocytolytic effect Suppression of primary immune response	Autoimmune disease Tissue transplantation Inflammatory disease of unknown cause
Antilymphocytic serum (ALS, ALG)	Inhibition of lymphocyte stimulation by specific antigens Inhibition of lymphocyte mobility Agglutination and lysis of lymphocytes in the presence of complement	Renal transplantation Bone marrow transplantation Autoimmune diseases
Antibiotics (actinomycin D, chloramphenicol, tetracycline, cyclosporine)	Interference with DNA-directed RNA synthesis Suppression of primary immune response Inhibition of protein synthesis	None

Antimetabolites and alkylating agents, such as azathioprine and cyclophosphamide, act nonspecifically against rapidly dividing cells within the body, and for this reason they are also used for cancer chemotherapy. They interfere with DNA synthesis and with the B and T cell systems.

A more specific immunosuppression of the T cell system is achieved with the use of *antilymphocytic serum* (ALS). ALS blocks the action of the sensitized cells in circulation while leaving the lymph node B cell system only slightly suppressed. This leaves the host with protection against the humorally protected infectious agents while providing protection against the most active rejection system.

The newest of the immunosuppressive therapeutic agents is cyclosporine (cyclosporin A), an antibiotic derived from fungi that exerts its action on the T lymphocytes. Recent success with this drug has greatly improved the prognosis after transplantation.

REFERENCES AND SELECTED READINGS*

1. Alexander, J.W., and Good, R.A.: Fundamentals of clinical immunology, Philadelphia, 1977, W.B. Saunders Co.
2. Allen, J.C.: Infection and the compromised host, Baltimore, 1976, The Williams & Wilkins Co.
3. Barrett, J.T.: Textbook of immunology: an introduction to immunochemistry and immunobiology, ed. 4, St. Louis, 1983, The C.V. Mosby Co.
4. Basten, A.: Clinical immunology in medical practice, St. Louis, 1981, The C.V. Mosby Co.
5. Buckley, C.E. III, and Roseman, J.M.: Immunity and survival, J. Am. Geriatr. Soc. **24:**241-243, 1976.
6. Burke, D.C.: The status of interferon, Sci. Am. **236:**42-43, 1977.
7. Burnet, F.M.: Immunology, aging, and cancer, San Francisco, 1976, W.H. Freeman & Co., Publishers.
8. *Dharan, M.: Immunoglobulin abnormalities, Am. J. Nurs. **76:**1626-1628, 1976.
9. Dodd, M.J.: Theoretical bases of immunotherapy, Am. J. Nurs. **79:**310-314, 1979.
10. *Donley, D.L.: Nursing the patient who is immunosuppressed, Am. J. Nurs. **76:**1619-1625, 1976.
11. Makinodan, T.: Immunobiology of aging, J. Am. Geriatr. **24:**249-251, 1976.
12. Mertz, D.H.: The mechanism of action of interferon, Cell **6:**429-432, 1975.
13. Mims, C.A.: The pathogenesis of infectious disease, New York, 1977, Acedemic Press, Inc.
14. *Nysather, J.O., Katz, A.E., and Lenth, J.L.: The immune system: its development and function, Am. J. Nurs. **76:**1614-1616, 1976.
15. Old, L.J.: Cancer immunology, Sci. Am. **235:**62-66, 1977.
16. *Rana, A.N., and Luskin, A.: Immunosuppression, autoimmunity, and hypersensitivity, Heart Lung **9:**655-659, 1980.
17. Richards, F.F., and others: On the specificity of antibodies, Science **187:**130-135, 1975.
18. Roitt, I.M.: Essential immunology, ed. 4, Oxford, England, 1981, Blackwell Scientific Publications Ltd.
19. Rose, N.R., and Friedman, H.: Manual of clinical immunology, Washington, 1976, American Society for Microbiology.
20. Sell, S.: Immunology, immunopathology, and immunity, ed. 3, New York, 1980, Harper & Row, Publishers, Inc.
21. Smith, A.L.: Microbiology and pathology, ed. 12, St. Louis, 1980, The C.V. Mosby Co.
22. Yunis, E.J., Fernandes, G., and Greenberg, L.J.: Tumor immunology, autoimmunity and aging, J. Am. Geriatr. **24:**253-256, 1976.

*References preceded by an asterisk are particularly well suited for student reading.

7

Health Promotion: Nutrition and Exercise

BARBARA C. LONG

STUDY QUESTIONS

- Make a list of foods you like best. Compare your list with a classmate's list. What are some of the reasons for the differences? Would you eliminate many of these foods if a health professional told you these would place you at high risk for X disease? What factors would influence your decision about complying or not complying?

- Write a list of your food intake over a typical day (be honest!). Compare your food intake with the daily food guide described in this chapter. Does your intake meet the recommendations? What changes, if any, would you make?

- A friend tells you that she had discovered a great discount store for buying vitamin pills so she takes 35 different vitamins a day. What problems could result?

- Compare your weight to the standard tables (do not forget to allow for the shoe heels in height). If you are 20% or more above or below the 100% level (midpoint of the range) for your height and frame, what difficulties might you experience?

- Why would it be ineffective to tell an obese person he/she should lose weight?

- Develop a teaching plan for a patient who will be giving herself total parenteral nutrition feedings at home.

- How often do you participate in 15 minutes or more of aerobic activities each week? What change, if any, would you make to meet recommendations for health promotion?

HEALTH PROMOTION IN MEDICAL-SURGICAL NURSING PRACTICE

Health promotion can be defined as activities directed toward helping persons maintain or achieve a high level of functioning and well-being. Health promotion is an integral part of nursing care for all types of patients and clients in all types of environments of care. In ambulatory care centers, health promotion assumes a major focus. In acute care centers the major focus is assisting patients to regain their health (illness care). However, health care must also be considered, that is, that which is healthy must be maintained.

Health promotion strengthens the person's capacity to withstand physical and emotional stress.[41] Thus the person who is in an excellent nutritional state, has good physical endurance, and copes well with stress is at less risk of developing a pathophysiologic disorder and has resources to use in regaining optimal functioning more quickly if illness or disease does occur.

Factors affecting health promoting behaviors

Why do some persons take actions that promote a high level of functioning, whereas others do not? Pender[36] has identified factors that (1) affect the individual's perceptions, (2) modify behaviors, and (3) influence the likelihood of health-promoting actions.

INDIVIDUAL PERCEPTIONS

Motivation to participate in health-promoting behaviors is influenced by the person's perceptions about health and perceptions about self:

1. Perceptions about health
   a. Value placed on health by the person
   b. Desire for the highest achievable health level vs that for maintaining status quo
   c. Evaluation of present health status
   d. Perceived benefits of health-promoting behaviors
2. Perceptions about self
   a. Perceived control over own behavior (internal vs external control)
   b. Desire for mastery of the environment
   c. Self-concept
   d. Self-esteem

Thus persons who do not value health or see a need to improve their health status, who are not self-motivated, or who have a poor self-concept are less likely to engage in health-promoting behaviors. Nursing approaches in these situations include helping these persons identify their values and explore feelings about themselves with emphasis placed on identifying strengths. Helping these persons set their own goals (thus exerting internal control) will greatly enhance the likelihood of achieving desired behaviors.

MODIFYING FACTORS

Pender[36] has identified three categories of modifying factors: demographic (age, sex, ethnicity, education, income), interpersonal, and situational variables. The specific effect of demographic variables on health-promoting behaviors is not clearly established and requires further research.

The major interpersonal factors influencing health-promoting behaviors are the influence of family or friends and the family patterns of health care. Persons more likely to participate are those who have support for the health-promoting behaviors from family or friends and who have been raised in a family in which health-promoting behaviors are valued. Health teaching is enhanced when the patient's support persons are included in the teaching.

Situational factors include the availability of opportunities to engage in health-promoting behaviors. For example, facilitation of a nutritionally balanced weight control program is enhanced by the availability of fruits and vegetables rather than vending machines with candy and potato chips. Nurses can assist patients to explore alternative ways of achieving their goals.

LIKELIHOOD OF HEALTH-PROMOTING ACTIONS

The probability that a person will engage in health-promoting actions is influenced by actual or perceived barriers to action, such as cost, time, or ability, and the presence of cues to action.[36] Nursing approaches include assisting the person to differentiate between perceived and actual barriers and to promote behaviors directed toward overcoming actual barriers.

Cues to action include hearing about activities that promote health either in interactions with others or through the mass media. Nurses can participate in health teaching of patients or by encouraging patients to read, to listen to radio, or to watch television programs that emphasize health promotion. Nurses also need to be instrumental in the development of these health-teaching tools.

Since health promotion is an integral part of the care of persons with pathophysiologic disorders, promotion of nutrition and exercise will be discussed further in this chapter. Stress management is discussed in Chapter 8.

NUTRITION

Relationship of nutrition to health

Good nutritional status exists when the necessary nutrients (protein, fat, carbohydrate, minerals, vitamins, and water) are consumed in sufficient amounts and are used appropriately by the body to meet needs regardless of age, sex, life-style, or state of health. All persons need the same nutrients throughout life.

All nutrients are equally important, although they are not required in equal amounts. The nutrients providing energy (protein, fats, carbohydrates) and water are required in much larger quantities than vitamins that regulate body processes. The differences in the quantities of various nutrients required by an individual are much greater than the change in amounts of any one nutrient over the life cycle. The amounts of required nutrients vary in predictable patterns. Growth, basal metabolic needs, and physical activity are the major factors responsible for changing nutrient needs. Disease, trauma, variations in metabolism (normal or abnormal), medications, and treatments can also affect needs.

NUTRITIONAL DEFICITS

When nutritional supplies are limited, growth, function, or reproduction may be impaired. Since the body exists in a state of dynamic equilibrium, anabolism (tissue building) and catabolism (tissue breakdown) are continuous. Muscles, organs, bones, fat, and blood participate in

---

Essential nutrients required for health

Water
Protein (essential amino acids)

Isoleucine	Phenylalanine
Leucine	(tyrosine)
Lysine	Threonine
Methionine	Tryptophan
(cystine)	Valine

Carbohydrate: starches, sugars, fiber
Fat: linoleic acid and arachidonic acid (poly-
unsaturated)
Minerals

Calcium	Manganese
Chloride	Molybdenum
Chromium	Phosphorus
Copper	Potassium
Fluorine	Selenium
Iodine	Sodium
Iron	Zinc
Magnesium	

Vitamins

Vitamin A	Biotin
Vitamin B_6	Folacin
Vitamin B_{12}	Niacin
Vitamin C	Pantothenic acid
Vitamin D	Riboflavin
Vitamin E	Thiamin
Vitamin K	

Effects of good nutrition

Growth and development of tissues/organs
Source of energy for metabolic processes and
physical activity
Tissue healing and repair
Resistance to infection

---

mitted to continue long enough, classic deficiency diseases, such as scurvy, beriberi, and pellagra, will result from depletions of vitamin C, thiamin, B complex vitamins, and niacin. If untreated, progressive depletion results in death.

An insufficient intake of calories and proteins containing the essential amino acids may result from inadequate diet (seen in low-income populations) or be associated with some pathologic disorders, such as diseases of the gastrointestinal tract that interfere with intake or absorption of nutrients, or with malignancies that interfere with appetite or increase the use of nutrients. Protein may be lost through body fluids, such as fluid loss from diarrhea or removal of ascitic fluid from the abdominal cavity. Persons with severe protein-calorie malnutrition heal slowly, because there are no resources available for use in tissue building. In addition to protein and calories, vitamins B, C, and K are necessary for tissue healing and clot formation.

Malnutrition increases susceptibility to infection by decreasing the availability of nitrogen and amino acids necessary for production of white blood cells and fibroblasts, which are necessary to counteract an invasion of microorganisms. Infection, in turn, increases the body's need for nutrients that are already depleted. Thus a severely malnourished person may die from a severe infection that would not be fatal to a well-nourished person. The immune response is also impaired by nutritional deficits. Protein-calorie malnutrition is related to a decrease in thymic activity with a reduction in T cell activity (Chapter 6) and with changes in metabolic activity that interfere with phagocytosis of bacteria by white blood cells. Lack of vitamin B_6 and pantothenic acid depresses antibody formation.

NUTRITIONAL EXCESS

Nutritional excesses can also produce malnutrition. Mechanisms tend to protect the body by accumulating reserves or, for some nutrients, by increasing the rate of excretion from the body or decreasing efficiency of absorption. When excesses are large or prolonged, increased concentrations of nutrients and alterations in enzyme activities and levels of metabolites develop.

Over time, clinical signs and symptoms develop. The most common example of this type of malnutrition in the U.S. population is obesity. Consumption of energy-yielding compounds (for example, protein, fat, carbohydrate, and alcohol) in amounts greater than needed for energy expenditure results in storage of energy as body fat. Eventually these stores of body fat become large enough to affect body functions, physical mobility, and health. Obese persons have a greater risk of osteoarthritis, diabetes mellitus, cardiovascular disease, and hypertension.

Excesses of cholesterol and triglycerides in the circulating blood are associated with atherosclerosis and coronary artery disease. These excesses may result from an increased intake of saturated fatty acids associated with increased production by the liver. A high intake of dietary

the constant exchange of materials, with some tissues more active than others. There is some loss of nutrients; therefore replacement from food is necessary throughout life. Periods of growth increase requirements for nutrients and energy.

Homeostatic mechanisms tend to protect the body against minor or temporary changes in nutrient status as nutrient reserves are mobilized to meet needs. With nutrient deficits, adaptations occur to conserve body resources. For example, when energy supplies are limited, physical activity and then basal metabolism are reduced. Over time, however, there is gradual nutrient loss in the tissues when a deficit is present. If this process is per-

cholesterol will increase the blood cholesterol level; however, the liver normally compensates for the high intake level by synthesizing less cholesterol and converting more cholesterol into bile acids. This compensatory mechanism is altered in some persons, perhaps as a result of genetic factors, and it is these persons specifically who are at a higher risk for atherosclerosis. Most persons in the United States ingest more fat than is needed; therefore health education should include teaching the substitution of complex carbohydrates for some fats and use of unsaturated rather than saturated fats.

Some persons have an unsupported intuitive feeling that nutrient supplements are essential.[46] Response to these supplements occurs only when persons have been relatively nutrition deficient, have been eating foods marginal in nutrient value, and when the supplement provides the specific nutrient or nutrients that are deficient. There is a point beyond which supplementation does not help the person and may actually cause harm. Continued intake of vitamins and minerals at levels from 10 to 100 times the recommended daily allowance (RDA) is associated with chronic toxicity.

Assessment of nutrient intake

To assess nutritional status, it is necessary to determine the supply of available nutrients, the sources available for metabolic processes, body size, and physical signs. Data are obtained primarily by patient interview, by observing the patient's general appearance, and by physical examination.

SUBJECTIVE DATA

Interviewing for the purpose of collecting data is discussed in Chapter 3. Data to be collected to determine nutritional status are described here.

Initial nutrition history

Food intake
   Typical day food/fluid pattern (type, amount)
   Recent changes in amount and type of intake
   Recent changes in appetite
Eating ability
   Dentures (fit, comfort)
   Problems with chewing or swallowing
Weight
   Usual and current weight
   Patient's perception of weight level
   If overweight/underweight: lifetime patterns, feelings about weight, reasons for recent change
Food supplements, medications, drugs (types, duration)

Food intake

When collecting data about nutrition, it is especially important to phrase the questions so that patients describe what they typically do eat rather than what they think they should. For example, the question, "Do you usually drink orange juice for breakfast?" implies (1) that breakfast is a desirable or expected behavior and (2) that orange juice is essential. Thus the patient may answer, "Yes," believing that is the expected answer, when in fact neither orange juice nor breakfast is usually eaten. A better approach is to say, "Tell me what you typically eat and drink in a day. What do you usually eat or drink first?" Questioning should elicit a picture of total food consumption for a day including all snacks. Designation by meals or snacks is not really necessary and may bias answers by implying value judgments.

Identification of amount consumed is as important as the type of food. Often people find this difficult to estimate. Persons familiar with cooking may be able to estimate in terms of tablespoons or cups. For the hospitalized patient the equipment or portions on the tray can be used as a basis for comparison.

Changes in appetite or in the amount or type of food or fluids ingested may be the result of illness (for exam-

---

Effect of some drugs on nutritional status

Aspirin	Malabsorption of folate Excretion of vitamin C
Barbiturates	Malabsorption of thiamin, vitamin B$_{12}$ Excretion of vitamin C
Corticosteroids	Malabsorption of calcium, zinc, phosphorus
Hydralazine	Excretion of pyridoxine
Methotrexate	Malabsorption of vitamin B$_{12}$, folate, fat
Mineral oil	Malabsorption of fat-soluble vitamins, calcium, phosphorus
Neomycin	Malabsorption of major nutrients
Oral contraceptives	Possible decreased absorption of vitamin C, B complex vitamins, magnesium, zinc
Penicillin	Loss of potassium
Tetracycline	Malabsorption of calcium, iron, magnesium, pyridoxine Excretion of vitamin C, riboflavin, niacin, folic acid
Thiazides	Excretion of potassium, magnesium, zinc, riboflavin

Table 7-1. Height and weight tables for adults with desirable weights for persons age 25 and over

Men					Women				
Height		Small frame (lb)	Medium frame (lb)	Large frame (lb)	Height		Small frame (lb)	Medium frame (lb)	Large frame (lb)
Feet	Inches				Feet	Inches			
5	2	128-134	131-141	138-150	4	10	102-111	109-121	118-131
5	3	130-136	133-143	140-153	4	11	103-113	111-123	120-134
5	4	132-138	135-145	142-156	5	0	104-115	113-126	122-137
5	5	134-140	137-148	144-160	5	1	106-118	115-129	125-140
5	6	136-142	139-151	146-164	5	2	108-121	118-132	128-143
5	7	138-145	142-154	149-168	5	3	111-124	121-135	131-147
5	8	140-148	145-157	152-172	5	4	114-127	124-138	134-151
5	9	142-151	148-160	155-176	5	5	117-130	127-141	137-155
5	10	144-154	151-163	158-180	5	6	120-133	130-144	140-159
5	11	146-157	154-166	161-184	5	7	123-136	133-147	143-163
6	0	149-160	157-170	164-188	5	8	126-139	136-150	146-167
6	1	152-164	160-174	168-192	5	9	129-142	139-153	149-170
6	2	155-168	164-178	172-197	5	10	132-145	142-156	152-173
6	3	158-172	167-182	176-202	5	11	135-148	145-159	155-176
6	4	162-176	171-187	181-207	6	0	138-151	148-162	158-179

Weights at ages 25-59 based on lowest mortality. Weight in pounds according to frame (in indoor clothing weighing 5 pounds, shoes with 1-inch heels). | Weights at ages 25-59 based on lowest mortality. Weight in pounds according to frame (in indoor clothing weighing 3 pounds, shoes with 1-inch heels).

Metropolitan Life Insurance Co., New York, 1983.

ple, anorexia, nausea, vomiting, or pain), self-imposed dietary regimens, or emotional or physical stress.

Medications

Some medications may affect nutritional status if taken over a period of time. Conversely, food can interfere with absorption of oral medications.

Drugs are absorbed more readily if the gastrointestinal tract is free of food. Drugs taken with water when the stomach is empty move rapidly into the small intestines, where much drug absorption takes place. Fatty foods delay gastric emptying for as long as 2 hours; therefore drugs that are absorbed in the small intestine have delayed absorption if taken with a meal high in fats. Food particularly delays the absorption of antimicrobial drugs, specifically the tetracyclines, the penicillins, and the sul-

fonamides. However, medications that have a gastric irritant effect may be enhanced if taken with food.

Drugs that are normally slightly acidic, such as aspirin or barbiturates, usually ionize and are absorbed in the stomach. If the stomach pH is increased, such as by milk or antacids, the rate and extent of absorption of these drugs will be decreased. Alteration in stomach acidity may also break down the protective coating of spansules or enteric-coated tablets, resulting in premature release of contents.[3] Acidic liquids, such as lemon, pineapple, or cranberry juices or dry ginger ale may inactivate acid-unstable drugs, such as ampicillin, penicillin G potassium, cloxacillin, and erythromycin.

Food components can interact with oral medication by the chemical or physical binding of one substance on another, thus interfering with absorption of either the food component or the drug. Tetracycline becomes bound with calcium, aluminum, or magnesium ions when taken with milk or antacids. This decreases absorption of tetracycline. Foods containing tyramine (cheeses, wines) may interact with monoamine oxidase (MAO) inhibitors, such as phenelzine (Nardil) or tranylcypromine (Parnate), which are depressants, causing hypertensive reactions.

Additional data

If nutritional intake is identified as inadequate, additional data will facilitate analysis and planning:
1. Food and fluid likes and dislikes
2. Financial resources
3. Facilities and ability for purchasing, storing, and preparing food
4. Problems with prescribed diets.

Medications to be taken with food

Aminophylline
Chlorothiazide (Diuril)
Ferrous sulfate
Indomethacin (Indocin)
Metronidazole (Flagyl)

Nitrofurantoin (Macrodantin)
Phenylbutazone (Butazolidin)
Phenytoin (Dilantin)
Prednisolone
Reserpine (Serpasil)
Triamterene (Dyrenium)

OBJECTIVE DATA

Height and weight

Height and weight are easily measured and are important data to obtain and use. The most reliable weight measurement is in the morning after voiding and before eating or drinking fluids. The patient's weight and height are compared with a table of recommended values (Table 7-1). One quick estimate for body frame size is to measure the person's wrist.

A useful item is the weight of the adult at 25 years of age and the person's perception of desirable body weight. The first provides data about a good weight for the person (if not obese at 25), and the second helps predict the person's response to attempts to change weight.

Physical examination data

The time elapsing between the lack of nutrient supply and the actual appearance of clinical signs that are obvious on physical examination can be as little as a week or as long as several years. Data from the head-to-toe physical examination (p. 25) that may suggest malnutrition include the following:

Hair:	lack of shine, easily plucked
Eyes:	pale conjunctiva, fissures at corner of eyelids
Lips:	redness, edema, fissures at corners of lips
Tongue:	swollen, smooth, raw, enlarged papillae
Teeth:	cavities, loose or missing teeth
Gums:	bleeding gums
Skin:	lack of subcutaneous fat, dryness, petechiae
Nails:	brittle, ridged
Muscles:	decreased muscle tone

Data analysis and planning

ANALYSIS OF FOOD INTAKE

Food guides developed to help people choose the kinds and amounts of food to eat for health can be used for rapid evaluation of adequacy of the diet eaten at home or food intake in the hospital. There are many different food guides, since to be effective they must be devised for a specific country or culture and feature the foods readily available and acceptable to the people being evaluated.

Wrist sizes for estimating body frame: medium size

Less than 5 feet 2 inches	5½ to 5¾ inches
5 feet 2 inches to 5 feet 5 inches	6 to 6¼ inches
More than 5 feet 5 inches	6¼ to 6½ inches

Table 7-2. Daily food guide

Food group (servings/day)	Amount/serving	Nutrients supplied
Milk 2	1 c milk 40 g (1½ oz) cheese 1¾ c ice cream 1 c yogurt	Protein, calcium, phosphorus, riboflavin, other vitamins and minerals (except iron and vitamin C)
Meat protein 2	60 to 75 g (2 to 3 oz) lean meat, poultry, fish 1 egg ½ c beans, peas, lentils 4 Tbsp peanut butter	Protein, fat, B complex vitamins, (plant products lack B_{12})
Vegetables/fruits 4 or more total		
1 dark green or deep yellow at least every other day	½ c broccoli, kale, carrots, squash, spinach, sweet potatoes, turnip or mustard greens, apricots, canteloupe, pumpkin	Vitamin A
1/day (vitamin C sources)	½ c citrus fruits/juices, cabbage, broccoli, brussels sprouts, peppers, strawberries, tomatoes	Vitamin C
2 to 3/day (other)	½ c medium potato or apple, other vegetables or fruits	All fruits/vegetables: vitamins, minerals (low sodium), fiber
Bread/cereal 4 (whole grain or enriched)	1 slice bread 30 g (1 oz) dry cereal ½ to ¾ c cooked cereal, rice, pasta	Complex carbohydrates, protein, iron, thiamin, riboflavin, niacin

A daily food guide used in the United States is shown in Table 7-2. The guide groups staple food items rich in protein, vitamins, and minerals into four major classes according to their major nutrient contributions. Recommendations are made for the number and size of servings to be selected from each food group. One can evaluate a diet quickly by checking to see if the recommended types of food and servings are included in the usual dietary pattern.

Since foods are mixtures of nutrients, the protein, vi-

tamin, and mineral requirements are substantially met when the daily intake includes the recommended servings from each group. The calorie level of the basic diet is low, but it is approximately sufficient for adult basal metabolism. Adequacy of energy intake is best judged by evaluation of body weight. In this method of evaluation, fats, oils, and sweets are not tabulated, since they provide primarily energy.

Each food group contributes particular nutrients to the total diet. The absence of any one food group from the

---

Assessment of a diet history

45-year-old woman with obesity and hypertension; meals eaten at home

7:00 AM
1 c cooked oatmeal
2 tsp sugar
1 c skim milk (fortified)
3 c coffee, plain

10:15 AM
2 c coffee, plain

1:00 PM
Sandwich
  2 slices white bread, enriched
  ½ tsp margarine
  ½ tsp mayonnaise
  60 g (2 oz) meatloaf or luncheon meat
4 cookies (fig bars, gingersnaps)
3 c coffee, plain

4:00 PM
7 cookies
½ c unsweetened fruit (canned, frozen, or fresh)
2 c tea, plain

10:00 PM
8 soda crackers
60 g (2 oz) American cheese
360 ml (12 oz) cola (sweet)
½ c homemade bread-and-butter pickles

Midnight
2 aspirin
1 c tea, plain

Assessment

Food group	Servings	Evaluation
Milk		Choice from milk group adequate. Meat intake low. Fruit and
Skim milk	1	vegetable intake low; choice of items rich in vitamin C or A
Cheese	1	happenstance. Bread intake is 6 servings. Intake of sweets,
Meat-protein		particularly cookies, high. Use of pickles and soda crackers
Meatloaf	1	questionable, since patient reports that low-sodium diet was
Fruits, vegetables		prescribed for her several years ago.
Fruit	1	Dietitian was asked to check caloric value. Intake is 1500 to 1600
Vegetable	1	calories/day, which includes 800 calories from basic food items;
Bread, cereal		remainder from sweets and fat. Protein levels adequate, although
Oatmeal	2	source of protein could be improved.
Bread, enriched	2	
Crackers	2	
Sweets		
Cookies	11	
Cola (360 ml [12 oz])		
Pickles, cucumber		
Fats		
Margarine		
Mayonnaise		

To the reader: Identify nutritional risks for this person; identify appropriate interventions and behavioral goals for her.

diet or particular types of food should alert the nurse that the patient has a potential nutrition problem. The box on p. 91 is an example of an analysis of food intake using the daily food guide.

The daily food guide can also be used for evaluating vegetarian diets. Many people are vegetarians and their reasons vary (for example, religion, food cost, philosophy). The diets vary as well. Generally the lacto-ovovegetarian (includes milk products and eggs) diet is nutritionally sound when a variety of foods is included. Persons on more restricted vegetarian (vegan) diets should be considered at nutritional risk and candidates for more detailed study (refer to dietitian). One potential problem with the vegan diet is vitamin B_{12} insufficiency unless fortified cereal or a dietary supplement is taken. The young adult who has changed to a vegan diet may use body stores of B_{12} for a time (a 5-year store is possible), but is at potential risk, especially if intake of folacin in vegetables is high, masking the signs of megaloblastic anemia.

NURSING DIAGNOSES

Possible nursing diagnoses based on collected data include:

Knowledge deficit
Alteration in nutrition: potential for more than body requirements
Alteration in nutrition: more than body requirements
Alteration in nutrition: less than body requirements

Implementation
TEACHING

Good nutrition can be promoted by giving positive reinforcement for selection of balanced meals from hospital menus. Teaching patients with specific knowledge deficits includes identification of the patient's motivation to learn. Patients with extensive lack of knowledge about food preparation, particularly with ways of preparing nutritionally balanced meals at low cost, may require the services of a dietitian.

The daily food guide (Table 7-2) is a useful tool for teaching persons a method of evaluating their own food intake. The dietitian may be helpful in developing a specific food guide for persons whose cultural patterns or personal preferences (for example, vegetarians) do not fit the standard food guides.

Persons who have been prescribed a dietary modification may need interpretation of the rationale for the diet and assistance in planning acceptable meals using the prescribed dietary plan. The dietitian usually initiates the discussion of a new home-going diet, but the nurse serves as interpreter to the patient by providing explanations

Types of diet modifications

Protein	Increased with losses from tissue catabolism, bleeding, exudates
	Decreased for chronic renal failure or hepatic coma
	Elimination of specific proteins (for example, allergies or malabsorption of gluten)
Fats	Increased to provide essential calories in concentrated form
	Decreased for pain with gallbladder disease
	Modified for disorders of digestion or absorption, lipid metabolism, or to alter serum lipid levels
Carbohydrates	Increased for weight gain
	Decreased for weight loss or diabetes mellitus
	Changed from simple to complex carbohydrates in diabetes mellitus
	Elimination of specific carbohydrates with disorders of carbohydrate intolerance (for example, lactase deficiency)
Vitamins	Increased for vitamin deficiency
	Provided in an alternate form to enhance absorption or use
Minerals	Sodium restriction with hypertension, fluid retention, kidney disease
	Potassium and calcium increased or decreased for lack or excess
	Provided by prescription for deficiency
Liquid, soft, pureed	Postoperative, diseases of gastrointestinal tract, difficulty with chewing or swallowing
Elimination diets	Food allergies

about the diet and feedback on how to make changes in current dietary patterns to meet the dietary prescription. Since the patients are the ones who must implement the dietary changes, they need to internalize the need for a behavior change. This takes active participation in all phases of the learning process. The person who does the cooking (if not the patient) also needs to be involved in the learning process. Dietary changes are more likely to be implemented if the changes can be easily adjusted to the family's usual meal plans.

FACILITATING WEIGHT LOSS

Etiology of obesity

Obesity is a major health problem in the United States. The incidence of cardiovascular disease, hypertension, diabetes mellitus, and gallbladder disease is high among obese persons.

Obesity is defined as 20% or greater over the established height and weight standards (Table 7-1). *Morbid obesity* is generally defined as 45 kg (100 lb) above the standard. Persons in an overweight category (up to 20% above the standard) who are gaining weight have a potential for malnutrition. The fat cells of obese people contain more fat than do those of lean persons and the number of fat cells may increase in adulthood. In general, obesity results from an increased caloric intake and a decreased energy output.

There are many genetic, psychologic, and social factors that influence the development of obesity. Although "fatness" seems to occur in some families, much of this may be a result of learned eating behaviors of high caloric foods rather than genetically influenced.

Weight reduction

Obesity exists in two forms: adult onset (hypertrophic) and lifelong (hyperplastic-hypertrophic). Persons with adult-onset obesity (middle-aged spread) have a fixed number of fat cells, but each cell contains excessive fat. These persons respond well to weight-reduction regimens. Persons with lifelong obesity not only have excessive fat in each cell, but also have more fat cells and generally respond poorly to weight reduction regimens. Persons who become massively obese are usually of the lifelong type.

Without behavior modification, over 90% of obese persons who successfully lose weight either through dietary or medical therapy return to or surpass their original weight within 5 years.[25] Medical therapies include (1) wiring the jaws shut and maintaining nutrition with a specially prepared liquid diet; (2) intestinal bypass surgery in which a large part of the jejunum and ileum are bypassed, thus decreasing the amount of intestinal absorption; or (3) gastric stapling in which the stomach is made smaller by stapling across most of one portion, thus allowing only a small amount of food to be ingested at one time. Problems result with these medical therapies over and above the lack of long-term success.

Behavior modification consists of changing the pattern of eating and exercising. This is accomplished by self-action over a period of time by the following:

1. Setting own goals
2. Self-monitoring
3. Developing a personal reward system
4. Obtaining positive feedback
5. Developing a new self-concept of "thinness"
6. Developing and implementing an activity program

Self-control is important in learning to change eating habits to facilitate weight loss and to maintain desirable body weight. Setting one's own goals and developing a personal reward system can facilitate motivation to participate in the desirable behaviors. Self-monitoring by means of planning the menus and keeping food diaries increases the person's awareness of the foods consumed. (Many persons are unaware of the number of calories consumed, especially by "nibbling.")

Reinforcement from others is a major factor in the success of a weight control program. The effectiveness of weight control groups, such as Weight Watchers, is based on this concept.

Exercise is an essential component of any weight control program. It promotes expenditure of energy and makes body appearance more pleasing to the person and thus desirable to maintain. It is important that the exer-

---

Factors influencing obesity

Genetic	Heavy bone structure, large muscle mass
Psychologic	Pleasure associated with eating
	Emotional problems (for example, grief, stress, or boredom)
	Interpersonal problems with family, friends, or co-workers
Sociologic	Learned behaviors of overeating or eating high caloric foods
	Reinforcement from others to eat large amounts of high caloric foods
Environmental	Easy availability of high caloric "junk" foods
	Availability of money to spend on high caloric foods

cise program be agreeable to the person so that it becomes a pattern of behavior to be continued throughout life.

Persons consuming high levels of calories before weight-reduction therapy are likely to be successful in achieving rapid weight loss, because the calorie deficit between need and the recommended diet is large. Men have a reputation for being more cooperative than women because they lose weight more rapidly. If both a man and a woman are instructed to adhere to a 1000-calorie intake, the man should lose at a faster rate not because he is more cooperative, but because his calorie deficit is larger.

Rapid weight loss is usually the result of loss of fluid rather than fat. Thus after an initial successful loss of weight on a weight-control diet, a plateau is reached when weight appears to remain constant or decrease only slightly. This can be discouraging to the person who is following the prescribed approach. Reinforcement to continue the regimen is usually needed at this point.

Fad diets should generally be avoided, although they usually induce rapid weight loss in a relatively easy way. However, there will be a loss of nutrients (marked protein catabolism with losses of nitrogen, phosphorus, calcium, potassium, sodium, and water). Weight then returns to the original level after termination of the diet, because the person's general pattern of eating has not been changed.

In summary, maintenance of weight loss is not usually achieved by participation in fad diets or medical therapies, but by a change in eating behaviors and increase in energy expenditure. This requires a long period of time and considerable involvement by the person with support from others. The nurse in an acute care setting cannot achieve this goal; however, the nurse can identify those persons who are obese, explore with them their perceptions and desires about their weight level, and provide support and guidance about ways to begin a weight control program.

FACILITATING WEIGHT GAIN

Etiology of underweight

Underweight is defined as more than 20% below the accepted weight standards. Weight loss is often the first sign of ill health. Loss may be mild or severe, insignificant or serious. It may be caused by

1. Inadequate calorie intake
2. Problems in digestion or absorption
3. Abnormalities in metabolism
4. Excretion of nutrients before they can be used
5. Failure to increase calorie intake when physical activity is increased

Anorexia (lack of appetite) is a mental state, a desire not to eat whether hunger is present or not. A number of factors may contribute to anorexia.

Encouraging food intake

Persons with inadequate nutrition stores need encouragement to eat, although forced feeding may lead to frus-

---

Factors influencing anorexia

Offensive sights or smells
Past experiences with foods
Pattern of behavior when coping with stress
Poor oral hygiene
Inflammatory disorders
Nausea or vomiting
Edema or decreased muscle tone of gastrointestinal tract
Liver failure
Abdominal distention
Increased blood temperature (heat, fever)
Drugs (amphetamines)

Formulas for tube feedings

Blended	Foods liquefied with a blender
	Generally well tolerated
	Relatively inexpensive
Milk-based	Mixtures of egg, milk, sugar, skim milk powder, and protein hydrolysates
	May cause diarrhea
Elemental	Synthetic low-residue mixtures of amino acids, sugars, vitamins, and minerals
	Expensive
	Require monitoring of blood glucose and electrolytes

---

tration or nausea and vomiting. Motivating a person with anorexia to eat can be a challenge. Interventions that can correct the cause will lead to improved appetite. Determining the person's likes and dislikes, providing an environment conducive to eating, and providing several small meals rather than three large meals a day may facilitate an adequate nutrition intake.

TUBE FEEDINGS

A nutritionally balanced fluid can be given through a nasogastric tube for patients who are unable to eat but for whom peristalsis is still present. The feedings should be well-tolerated (no vomiting, diarrhea, constipation, or distention), easily prepared, and reasonable in cost. Three types of formulas are common: blended, milk-based, or elemental formulas.

Guidelines for tube feedings

1. Place patient in sitting position both during and for 30 minutes after feeding if possible (use left side-lying position if patient cannot sit up).
2. Check placement of tube in stomach by inserting 15 to 20 cc air in tube and listening with stethoscope over abdomen (left upper quadrant).
3. Aspirate gastric contents before giving feeding. Hold feeding and notify physician if 60 ml or more of previous feeding are aspirated.
4. Keep feedings refrigerated until ready to use.
5. Give feeding at a slow constant rate through gavage drainage system or continuous drip.
6. Give small amount of water before and after feeding to flush tube.
7. Monitor patient for signs of dehydration (thirst, low urinary output, decreased skin turgor) or intolerance to feeding (diarrhea, vomiting, abdominal cramping).
8. Give water between feedings based on patient's needs.

Guidelines for total parenteral nutrition

1. Maintain strict aseptic technique
2. Prevent air from entering tubing
   a. Tape all connections of the system
   b. Cover insertion site with an air-occlusive dressing (dressing covered by adhesive tape)
   c. When changing tubing
      (1) Have patient lying down
      (2) Make tube change rapidly
      (3) Ask patient to perform Valsalva maneuver (forced air against closed glottis) while tube is disconnected
   d. Monitor and report signs of air embolism (chest pain, cough, dyspnea)
   e. If air embolism occurs, place patient on left side in a Trendelenburg (head down) position and notify physician
3. Maintain fluid and electrolyte balance
   a. Maintain a continuous uniform infusion rate
      (1) Use an automatic alarm monitoring system
      (2) Check drip rate every 30 to 60 minutes if no automatic system is used
   b. If rate is too *slow*
      (1) Return rate to established setting
      (2) If established rate does not resume, ask patient to change position
      (3) If filter is blocked, change the tubing
      (4) Monitor and report to physician signs of hypoglycemia (pallor, diaphoresis, tachycardia, trembling, hunger, or behavioral changes)
   c. If rate is too *fast*
      (1) Slow infusion to prescribed rate
      (2) Monitor for signs of overhydration (neck vein distention or cough)
      (3) Monitor for signs of hyperglycemia (sugar in urine)
   d. Monitor daily weights and intake and output
   e. Monitor serum electrolytes level, glucose level, and BUN level
4. Encourage ambulation and activities of daily living
5. Promote comfort
   a. Provide for good oral hygiene
   b. Provide emotional support to enhance coping
6. Monitor for sensitivity reactions (headache, fever, myalgia, chills, nausea and vomiting, rash, vasodilation, abdominal pain) and for signs of infection (fever)

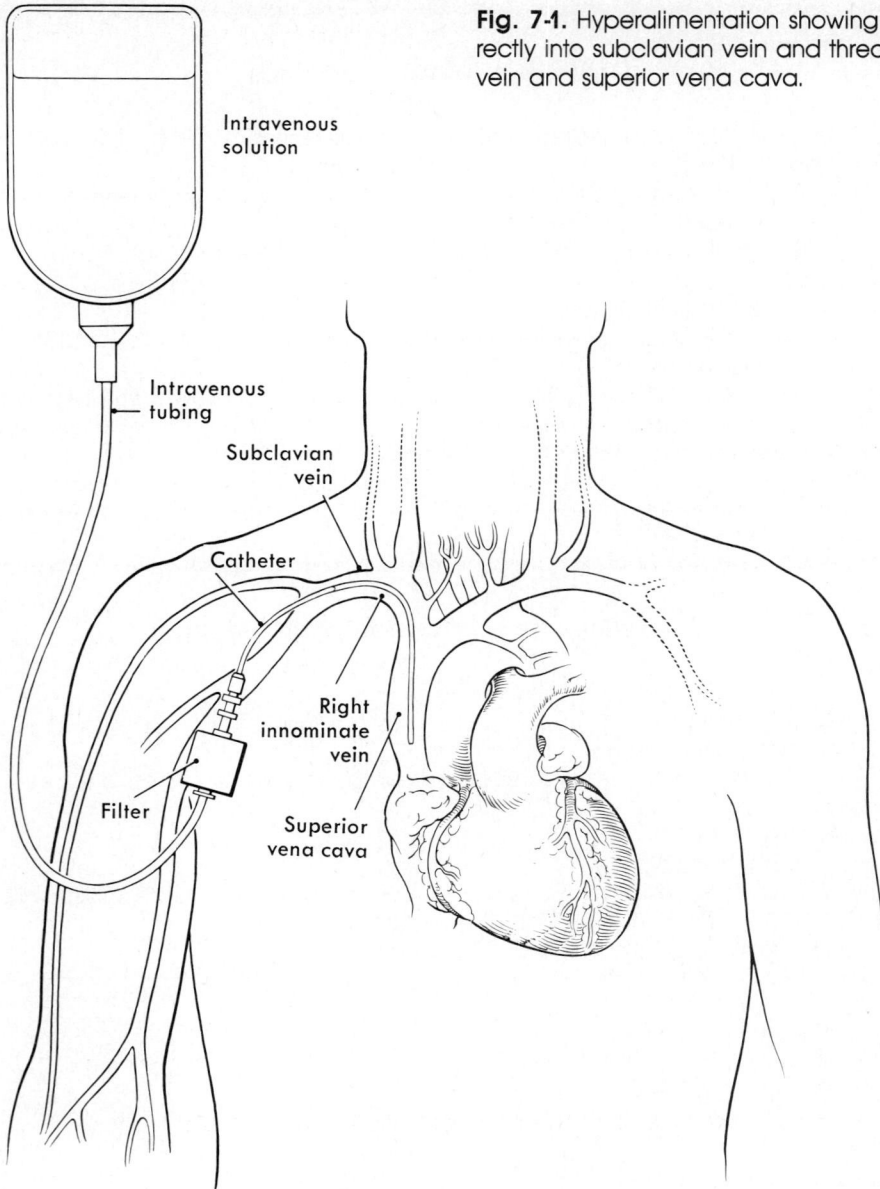

Intravenous
solution

Intravenous
tubing

Subclavian
vein

Catheter

Right
innominate
vein

Filter

Superior
vena cava

Fig. 7-1. Hyperalimentation showing catheter placed directly into subclavian vein and threaded into innominate vein and superior vena cava.

Rapid or forced feedings of large volumes or excessively concentrated mixtures, especially with insufficient water, increase the danger of dehydration. A patient with an inadequate swallowing reflex may aspirate if vomiting occurs; therefore suctioning equipment must be readily available at the bedside in this situation. A patient with a cuffed endotracheal or tracheostomy tube in place is never left alone while fluids are being given by tube feeding. Guidelines for giving tube feedings are listed on p. 95.

TOTAL PARENTERAL NUTRITION

Total parenteral nutrition (TPN), also known as parenteral hyperalimentation, is a method of giving concentrated solutions intravenously to maintain protein synthesis. Indications for this therapy are (1) major gas-

trointestinal diseases, fistulas, or inflammatory diseases; (2) extensive negative nitrogen balance, such as occurs with major body burns, extensive wounds, or cachexia; and (3) gastrointestinal side effects from radiation therapy.

Technique

An intracatheter is inserted either into the subclavian vein through the chest wall (Fig. 7-1) or into the basilic vein in the antecubital fossa and then threaded through to the superior vena cava. The large amount of blood in the superior vena cava helps to dilute the highly concentrated solution rapidly and thus prevent phlebitis or vein occlusion.

A Broviac or Hickman catheter may be used in place of a standard intracatheter. These catheters are designed so that the end of the catheter can be capped between infusions. At the completion of an infusion, the catheter is filled with heparinized saline solution to prevent clotting and is capped until the next infusion.

The catheter is secured with one suture and covered by an air-occlusive dressing. The infusion is started with a standard intravenous fluid (5% dextrose) until a radiograph confirms the location of the catheter tip in the superior vena cava.

Solutions

The composition of the infusate varies. The basic nutrient solution usually contains 20% to 50% glucose (to meet energy needs so that the amino acids are used for protein synthesis rather than for energy), as well as amino acids, minerals, electrolytes, and vitamins. The commercial preparations are relatively trouble free, but some patients do experience sensitivity reactions or fluid and electrolyte imbalances. Prepared solutions must be kept refrigerated and should be warmed to room temperature just before infusion. Solutions should not be hung for longer than a 12-hour period.

Nursing interventions

Nursing care centers on prevention of infection and air embolism, maintenance of fluid and electrolyte balance, and promotion of activity and comfort. Dressing changes are carried out under aseptic technique. Some medical centers have a hyperalimentation team, and one nurse changes the dressings for all patients to ensure consistency of technique and to reduce the chance of infection. If a dressing becomes wet, it is changed immediately to prevent transmission of bacteria by capillary action. The dressing should be air occlusive. Patients who experience itching under the dressing are cautioned not to scratch or disturb the dressing.

The possibility of air embolism is greater with use of the superior vena cava than with a peripheral vein, because the decreased venous pressure as the blood approaches the heart can cause air to be sucked into the tubing. Filters are useful for trapping air as well as bacteria.

Patients may have many fears and concerns about being fed by intravenous fluids over a long period of time. They should have an understanding of what is occurring and the reason for the frequent dressing changes. If food is not permitted orally, the patient may need aid in coping with stress incurred by the smell of food or watching others eat. If receiving TPN over a long period of time, they may be concerned about regaining taste or normal eating patterns. Being fed only by tube, even though temporary, may create stress from a change in body image.

EXERCISE

A large number of American adults live a sedentary life-style, although there has been a positive trend toward increased exercise in recent years. Most people are aware that activity or mobility is necessary for carrying out tasks

---

Benefits of aerobic exercise

Sense of well-being
Enhanced coping with stress
Decreased anxiety or depression
More restful sleep
Maintenance of physiologic functioning at optimum level
Enhanced weight control
Decreased risk factors for coronary artery disease
Better control of hypertension and diabetes mellitus
Assistance with reduction of addictive behavior (for example, smoking, overeating, or drinking)

Physiologic effects of exercise

1. Musculoskeletal system
   a. Maintains muscle strength
   b. Maintains joint flexibility
   c. Maintains endurance (tolerance to continue an activity)
2. Neurosensory system
   a. Maintains coordination
   b. Maintains orientation to environment
3. Circulatory system
   a. Maintains a more constant average work load on heart
   b. Maintains normal blood pressure regulatory adjustment to transient position changes
   c. Promotes venous return through contraction of muscles
4. Respiratory system
   a. Contributes to ease of breathing
   b. Provides stimulus to deep breathing and aeration of alveoli
   c. Provides movement of secretions
5. Gastrointestinal system
   a. Maintains elimination through muscle activity and visceral reflex patterns
   b. Encourages the person to heed defecation reflex
6. Urinary system
   a. Promotes urine formation
   b. Promotes complete emptying of bladder

Table 7-3. Target pulse rates with exercise

Category	Pulse target zone	Pulse return after exercise
Healthy active adults	70% to 85% of maximum heart rate (220 minus age)	Less than 120 in 5 min Less than 100 in 10 min
Obese, low physical conditioning	50% to 60% of maximum heart rate	Baseline level in 10 min
Cardiac disease, following bed rest	No more than 20 beats above baseline	Baseline level in 5 min

of daily living. The need for exercise (activity that requires physical exertion) as a part of one's life-style is less commonly understood or accepted. The topic of exercise is value laden. Persons who do not value exercise as a means of maintaining optimal health often find excuses for not participating in a planned exercise program on an on-going basis. Exercise does imply effort; if exercise is not valued, the effort will not be taken.

Why is it important for the nurse caring for patients in an acute care center to consider the concept of exercise? Understanding the effects of exercise will assist the nurse in promoting exercise for the hospitalized patient and encouraging all persons to be as active as possible within their limitations and capabilities.

Benefits of exercise

A program of regular exercise can have both psychologic and physiologic benefits. A physically fit person also generally has greater endurance and faster recovery time (return to resting rate), which contribute to more rapid recovery from illness.

Exercise is important regardless of age. Some elderly persons believe they are too old to begin an active fitness program, but these programs are possible even for persons with chronic illness. The fitness program is individually planned and based on the person's interests, capabilities, and limitations.

Physically, exercise enhances cardiovascular fitness, endurance, muscle strength, flexibility, and weight control. It has positive effects on the musculoskeletal, neurosensory, circulatory, respiratory, gastrointestinal and urinary systems.

Exercise programs

CLASSIFICATION OF EXERCISE

Exercises may be classified as aerobic or anaerobic. *Aerobic* exercises are those activities that are supported by aerobic metabolism (the breakdown of carbohydrates and fats to carbon dioxide and water in the presence of oxygen, that is, the Krebs cycle). Aerobic exercises are characterized by activities that involve large muscle groups and that are performed in a rhythmic and continuous nature for more than 15 minutes. Examples of aerobic exercises include brisk walking, jogging, bicycling,

swimming, skating, cross-country skiing, and aerobic dancing.

Anaerobic exercises involve anaerobic metabolism (the breakdown of glucose to lactic acid in the absence of oxygen). This occurs with high-intensity activities in which the available oxygen is used up and the anaerobic pathways are then used to provide the necessary additional energy. Anaerobic types of exercises include weight lifting and competitive sports, such as football, soccer, basketball, baseball, volleyball, and hockey. Greater benefits to overall physical fitness and well-being are achieved with aerobic rather than with anaerobic exercises.

RECOMMENDATIONS FOR PHYSICAL FITNESS PROGRAMS

Persons with a personal or family history of cardiovascular disease or who are over 35 years of age should have a physical examination before beginning an exercise program. A program is then planned on the basis of the person's tolerance and interests (it should be enjoyable).

Tolerance is evaluated by assessing pulse rate (Table 7-3). For example, a healthy active 50-year-old person should aim at maintaining a pulse rate during exercise of 70% to 85% of 170 beats per minute (220 minus 50), that is, within a range of 119 to 145. The pulse is then assessed for the time it takes to return to normal. Tolerance to activity of hospitalized patients who are starting to ambulate (aerobic exercise) after inactivity is assessed in the same manner; that is, the pulse rate should not increase greater than 20 beats per minute over the patient's baseline pulse rate and should return to baseline level within 5 minutes after ambulating.

Exercising should be done on a regular basis a minimum of two to three times per week. All persons should start each exercise period with deep diaphragmatic breathing and stretching exercises. Duration of the exercise period, which depends on the person's conditioning, is usually about 15 to 60 minutes per period. The exercises should be performed at just under the anaerobic threshold (identified by a tightness or "burning" sensation in the muscles and shortness of breath). It is best to start out slowly and gradually extend the program as conditioning improves. If the pulse target zone is exceeded or if the recovery period is extended, the exercise is too strenuous. With inactivity there is a loss of 20% conditioning within 2 to 3 weeks and up to 50% loss by one month.[7]

Table 7-4. Complications of immobility

System	Physiologic effect	Dysfunction/pathology	Nursing intervention (preventive)
Cardiovascular	Pooling of venous blood in legs Decreased venous return to heart Decreased cardiac output	Thrombophlebitis Pulmonary embolus Postural hypotension Decreased tolerance for activity when initiated	Range of motion: active and passive Isometric exercises of legs Turn frequently Avoid pressure on major blood vessels Slow mobilization
Respiratory	Pooling of secretions from decreased movement Decreased stimulation to cough Decreased depth of ventilation	Hypostatic pneumonia Atelectasis	Turn and move frequently Active range of motion Deep breathing and coughing
Gastrointestinal	Decreased peristalsis Change in eating/drinking habits Change in position to eliminate (bedpan)	Constipation	Increase fluid intake Good dietary intake of fiber foods Active movement in bed Use of stool softener or suppositories
Urinary	Increased calcium from bone destruction Alkaline urine Urinary stasis	Urinary calculi Urinary retention Urinary tract infection	Increase fluid intake Decrease calcium intake Use commode rather than bedpan if possible
Musculoskeletal	Muscle atrophy and shortening Fibrosis or bony ankylosis of joints Loss of bone matrix with release of calcium	Muscle weakness Contractures Osteoporosis	Active range of motion Isometric and isotonic exercises Positioning of joints to facilitate use
Neurologic	Decreased stimuli	Decreased orientation	Social contacts Diversionary materials
Skin	Friction, pressure or shearing forces Decreased circulation from pressure Break in skin integrity Maceration from perspiration or urinary incontinence	Abrasions Decubitus ulcers	Frequent assessment Protection of vulnerable areas (foam or alternating pressure mattresses, sheepskin, flotation pads, elbow or heel pads) Turn frequently

TYPES OF EXERCISES

Isometric exercises

With isometric exercises, opposing muscles are contracted, thus increasing the tone of the muscle fibers but not changing muscle length or moving the joints. The purpose of these exercises is to maintain muscle strength and tone. There is very little effect on cardiovascular or respiratory conditioning, although isometric exercises may not be easily tolerated by persons with coronary artery disease. Examples of isometric exercises for hospitalized patients are quadriceps-setting exercises and gluteal sets (p. 299) to maintain muscle strength in the thighs and buttocks for walking.

Persons doing isometric exercises should be taught to exhale while exerting effort. Many persons tend to hold their breath while bearing down (Valsalva maneuver). This increases intrathoracic pressure, causing a decrease in venous return to the heart. When the breath is then released, the intrathoracic pressure decreases, causing a large surge of blood return to the heart and increasing the cardiac work load. Exhaling while exerting effort can prevent the Valsalva effect.

Isotonic exercises

With isotonic exercises, muscle length changes and joint movements occur. There is less muscle tension than with isometric exercises. Isotonic exercises maintain and increase muscle strength. Aerobic exercises are one form of isotonic exercises. Isotonic exercises for the hospitalized patient include moving and turning in bed, ambulating, and moving arms and legs against light resistance.

Immobility

Immobility may be accompanied by a number of complications that can involve any or all of the major systems of the body (Table 7-4). It is important that those caring for the patient whose mobility is impaired be aware of these potential complications and be skilled in interventions designed to help prevent them. The patient is encouraged to be as active as possible within the activity limitations by moving and turning in bed and by carrying out active range of motion, isometric, and isotonic exercises.

REFERENCES AND SELECTED READINGS*

1. Abramson, E.F.: Behavioral approaches to weight control, New York, 1977, Springer Publishing Co., Inc.
2. Anderson, M.A., Aker, S.N., and Hickman, R.O.: The double lumen Hickman catheter, Am. J. Nurs. **82:**272-273, 1982.
3. *Black, C.D., Popovich, N.G., and Black, M.C.: Drug interactions in the GI tract, Am. J. Nurs. **77:**1426-1429, 1977.
4. *Borgen, L.: Total parenteral nutrition in adults, Am. J. Nurs. **78:**224-228, 1978.
5. Briggs, G.M., and Calloway, D.H.: Bogert's nutrition and physical fitness, ed. 10, Philadelphia, 1979, W.B. Saunders Co.
6. *Caly, J.C.: Helping people eat for health: assessing adult's nutrition, Am. J. Nurs. **77:**1605-1609, 1977.
7. *Cantu, R.C.: Toward fitness: guided exercise for those with health problems, New York, 1980, Human Sciences Press, Inc.
8. Cantu, R.C.: Health maintenance through physical conditioning, Littleton, Mass., 1981, PSG Publishing Co., Inc.
9. Cooper, K.H.: The aerobics way, New York, 1977, M. Evans & Co., Inc.
10. Cornacchia, H.J., and Barrett, S.: Consumer health: a guide to intelligent decisions, ed. 3, St. Louis, 1985, The C.V. Mosby Co.
11. Ebersole, P., and Hess, P.: Toward healthy aging: human needs and nursing response, St. Louis, 1981, The C.V. Mosby Co.
12. Englert, D.M., and Dudrick, S.J.: Principles of intravenous hyperalimentation, AORN J. **25:**1253-1267, 1977.
13. Feldtman, R.W., and Andrassy, R.J.: Meeting exceptional nutritional needs; total parenteral nutrition, Postgrad. Med. **64**(8):64-77, 1978.
14. *Friedman, B.J., and Knight, K.: Running for life, health, and pleasure, Am. J. Nurs. **78:**602–607, 1978.
15. Getchell, B.: Physical fitness: a way of life, ed. 2, New York, 1979, John Wiley & Sons, Inc.
16. Goodhart, R.S., and Shils, M.E.: Modern nutrition in health and disease, ed. 6, Philadelphia, 1980, Lea & Febiger.
17. *Gordon, M.: Assessing activity tolerance, Am. J. Nurs. **76:**72-75, 1976.
18. Griggs, B.A., and Hoppe, M.C.: Update: nasogastric tube feedings, Am. J. Nurs. **79:**481-485, 1979.
19. Healthy people, the Surgeon General's report on health promotion and disease prevention, Pub. no. 79-55071, Washington, D.C., 1979, Public Health Service—U.S. Department of Health, Education, and Welfare.
20. Hedlin, A.: Exercise: how the body responds, Can. Nurse **76**(4):33-35, 1980.
21. Herbert, V.: Nutrition cultism: facts and fiction, Philadelphia, 1980, George F. Stickley Co.
22. *Hirschberg, G., and others: Promoting patient mobility, Nurs. 77 **7**(5):42-46, 1977.

*References preceded by an asterisk are particularly well suited for student reading.

23. Hunt, S.M., Froff, J.L., and Holbrook, J.M.: Nutrition: principles and clinical practice, New York, 1980, John Wiley & Sons, Inc.

24. Hutchison, M.M.: Administration of fat emulsions, Am. J. Nurs. **82**:275-277, 1982.

25. Kaye, D., and Rose, L.: Fundamentals of internal medicine, St. Louis, 1983, The C.V. Mosby Co.

26. *Kornguth, M.L.: When your client has a weight problem: nursing management, Am. J. Nurs. **81**:553-554, 1981.

27. Krause, M.V., and Mahan, L.K.: Food, nutrition, and diet therapy, ed. 6, Philadelphia, 1979, W.B. Saunders Co.

28. March, D.C.: Handbook: interaction of selected drugs with nutritional status in man, Chicago, 1976, American Dietetic Association.

29. Mechanic, D., and Cleary, C.: Factors associated with the maintenance of positive health behavior, Prev. Med. **9**:805-814, 1980.

30. Michel, L., Serrano, A., and Malt, R.A.: Current concepts: nutritional support of hospitalized patients, N. Engl. J. Med. **304**:1147-1152, 1981.

31. Miller, B.K.: Jejunoileal bypass: a drastic weight control measure, Am. J. Nurs. **81**:564-568, 1981.

32. *Mojzisik, C.M., and Martin, E.W. Jr.: Gastric partitioning-the latest surgical means to control morbid obesity, Am. J. Nurs. **81**:569–572, 1981.

33. Murray, R.B., Huelskoetter, M.M., and O'Driscoll, D.L.: The nursing process in later maturity, Englewood Cliffs, N.J., 1980, Prentice-Hall International, Inc.

34. Nehme, A., and Nehme, E.: Nutritional support of the hospitalized patient: the team concept, JAMA **243**:1906-1908, 1980.

35. Overeaters anonymous, Am. J. Nurs. **81**:560-563, 1981.

36. *Pender, N.J.: Health promotion in nursing practice, Norwalk, Conn., 1982, Appleton-Century-Crofts.

37. Pollock, M.L.: Exercise: a preventive prescription, J. Sch. Health, **49**:215-219, 1979.

38. *Pratt, M.A.: Physical exercise: a special need in long term care, J. Gerontol. Nurs. **4**(5):38-42, 1978.

39. Ragg, K.E.: Exercise: a misused factor in weight control, J. Sch. Health **49**:459-461, 1979.

40. Shepard, R.J.: Physical activity and aging, Chicago, 1978, Year Book Medical Publishers, Inc.

41. *Shamansky, S.L., and Clausen, C.L.: Levels of prevention: examination of the concept, Nurs. Outlook **28**:104-108, 1980.

42. Shannon, B.M., and Parks, S.C.: Fast foods, a perspective on their nutritional impact, J. Am. Diet. Assoc. **76**:242-247, 1980.

43. Stefee, P.: Malnutrition in hospitalized patients, JAMA **244**:2630-2635, 1980.

44. Van Italie, T.B., and Kral, J.G.: The dilemma of morbid obesity, JAMA **246**:999-1003, 1981.

45. White, J.H., and Schroeder, M.A.: When your client has a weight problem: nursing assessment, Am. J. Nurs. **81**:550-563, 1981.

46. *Willett, W., and others: Vitamin supplement use among registered nurses, Am. J. Clin. Nutr. **34**:1121-1125, 1981.

47. Williams, S.R.: Nutrition and diet therapy, ed. 4, St. Louis, 1981, The C.V. Mosby Co.

48. *Young, C.: Exercise: how to use it to decrease complications in immobilized patients, Nurs. 75 **5**(3):81-82, 1975.

Classic

49. Cooper, K.H.: Aerobics, New York, 1972, Bantam Books, Inc.

UNIT III
Stress and Adaptation

8   Stress and Stress Management
9   Psychologic Responses to Stress

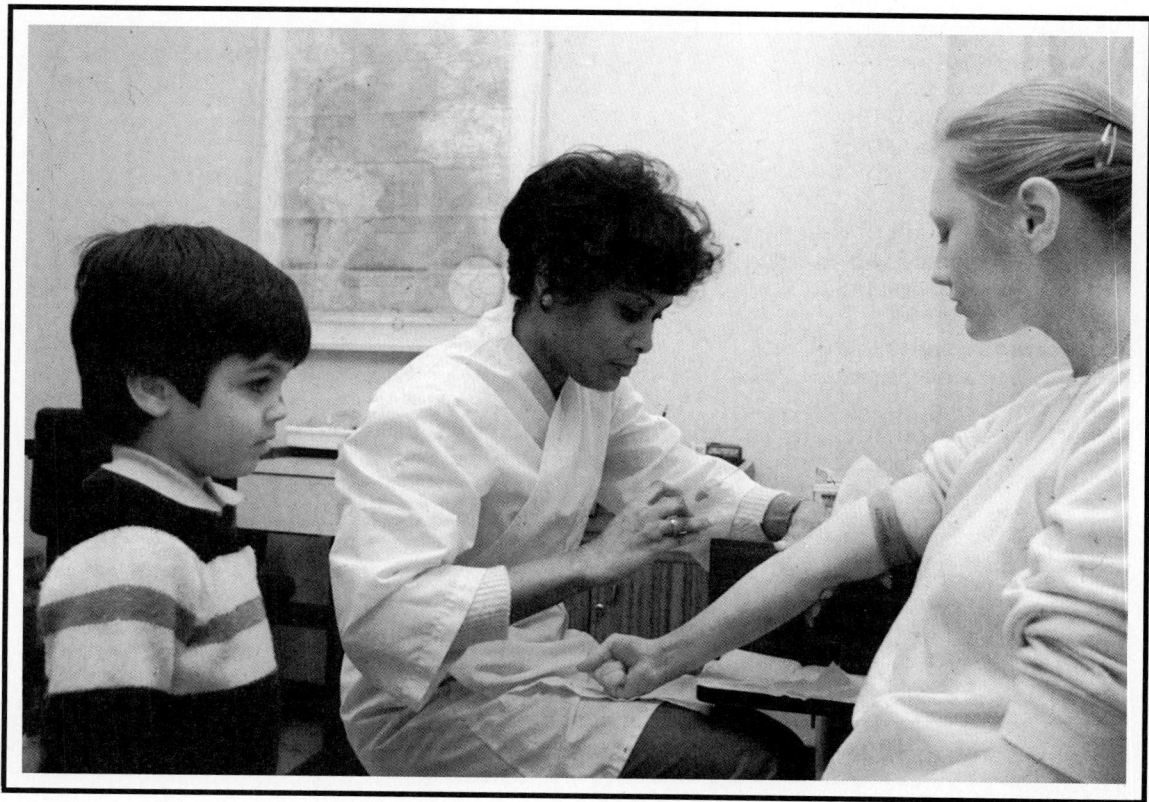

8

Stress and Stress Management

BARBARA C. LONG

STUDY QUESTIONS

- Differentiate among the terms *stress, stressor,* and *eustress.*

- Should you try to lead a life that is free from stress? Explain.

- Think back over several situations when you were experiencing stress.
   What type of physical symptoms did you experience?
   What is the physiologic reason for each symptom that you experienced?
   Were the symptoms always the same? If not, state why.

- In what way(s) do you cope with stress? What other coping strategies might be useful for you?

- Try one or both of the relaxation techniques described in this chapter.
   Describe the sensations experienced during relaxation.
   How did you feel after completing the exercise?
   What types of difficulties did you have in carrying out the relaxation exercises?
   Identify a patient situation from your experience where you think relaxation exercises might have been a useful nursing intervention.

Promotion of health involves activities that facilitate a sense of well-being. This implies a feeling of "ease," which is accomplished in part by coping effectively with internal or external stressors.

Many pathophysiologic disorders that are stress-related can be exacerbated by inadequate techniques for coping with stress. Nurses can help patients learn how to cope with stress in a positive manner and thus prevent or diminish the effects of stress. This chapter will discuss concepts of adaptation and stress, responses to stress, and stress management.

ADAPTATION

Humans can be conceptualized as open systems that respond to stimuli from the internal and external envi-

---

Selected stress-related disorders

Hypertension
Angina pectoris
Myocardial infarction
Hyperthyroidism
Bronchial asthma
Allergies
Peptic ulcer
Ulcerative colitis
Headaches
Insomnia
Alcoholism

ronments. This process of interaction can be termed *adaptation*. In this context, adaptation has neither positive nor negative values. However, many prefer to use the term in a positive sense, to mean the process of interaction with the environment that promotes dynamic equilibrium (homeostasis) and growth. The process that leads to inadequate functioning is then termed *maladaptation*.

Human beings adapt biologically, psychologically, and socially. The goal of biologic adaptation is survival or stability of internal processes. The body has numerous physiologic feedback loops and compensatory mechanisms that help to maintain body processes within the ranges of normal, which facilitate optimal functioning. When the ability to maintain this equilibrium is lost, pathophysiologic disorders result.

Psychologic adaptation is directed toward preservation of self-identity and self-esteem. The person adapting in this mode is mentally healthy, whereas maladaptation leads to mental illness. Social adaptation depends on the sociocultural expectations of the society of which the person is a member. A maladaptive or socially deviant behavior in one society may be acceptable in another.

STRESS

Stress as a concept

The term *stress* has been used for many years to denote mental strain, for example, the comment, "He's under stress." Selye was the first to use the term in a biologic context, that is, the nonspecific response of the body to a variety of noxious stimuli.[15] He termed the stimulus a *stressor*. The stressor may be a stimulus from the internal or external environment, and it places a demand on the system, disrupting the dynamic equilibrium. The stressor may produce a biologic or a behavioral response.

The stress or tension that results from the stressor may have either negative or positive results or both. For example, a person may experience pain (a stressor). The pain may cause anorexia, which may lead to nutrient imbalance and inactivity, which may lead to the side effects of immobility. These are negative results. On the other hand, the presence of pain may guide the person to seek medical intervention. This may lead to removal of the underlying condition causing the pain, a positive result.

Stress is not necessarily something to be avoided, and in fact a certain amount of normal stress (*eustress*) is considered necessary for adaptation. For example, microorganisms can upset cellular function, leading to disequilibrium and death. However, exposure to microorganisms in limited numbers or of decreased strength can help the body develop mechanisms to defend against subsequent exposures. Similarly, exposure to psychologic stressors in everyday living helps develop useful coping methods that facilitate dealing with new stressors. Coping with biologic or psychosocial stressors in an adaptive manner facilitates optimal functioning and growth. Maladaption leads to dysfunction and pathophysiologic or psychopathologic disorders.

Stress responses

FACTORS INFLUENCING STRESS RESPONSES

A given stressor may cause one person to respond adaptively, a second person to respond maladaptively, and a third person to respond neutrally (that is, little response). The following factors can influence the type of response:

1. Stimulus characteristics
   a. Intensity
   b. Duration
   c. Number
2. Personal characteristics
   a. Meaning of stressor to person
   b. Availability of resources and coping responses
   c. Health status

Stimulus characteristics

A stimulus of low intensity may not be a stressor if the body can deal with it automatically, without disturbing the equilibrium. In general, the greater the intensity of the stimulus, the greater the probability of a stress response.

A sudden, intense stimulus will generally produce a more marked response than a stimulus that develops gradually. The insidious onset often gives the person time to develop coping responses that may not be present with the acute onset. On the other hand, a persistent stressor may deplete the person's energy and eventually exhaust the resources available for coping.

The number of stimuli present at a given time will also affect response. The common phrase "the straw that broke the camel's back" describes the concept by which a specific stimulus may have no effect by itself, but may precipitate a stress response when combined with numerous other stressors.

Personal characteristics

The meaning of the stressor for the individual is one of the major factors influencing the stress response. Stressors creating a change that is viewed negatively have a high probability of an increased response. For example, a woman who places great value on her body as a means of personal and sexual gratification will likely experience a greater response to removal of a breast than a woman who places little significance on her bodily appearance.

The individual's perception of the stressor (and hence the meaning that is interpreted) is influenced by cognitive ability, verbal skills, past experiences, interpersonal relationships, support person's responses, and feelings of control. A sense of control over the stressor helps to decrease the response. For example, patients who know in advance some measures to decrease postoperative pain (that is, have control over the pain) will usually adapt more effectively in the postoperative period. Persons who have developed a repertoire of coping skills can select one that will facilitate adaptation to a new stressor. Thus persons who have had to cope with numerous intense stressors in the past are often able to cope effectively when crises occur.

When health status is poor, less energy is available to

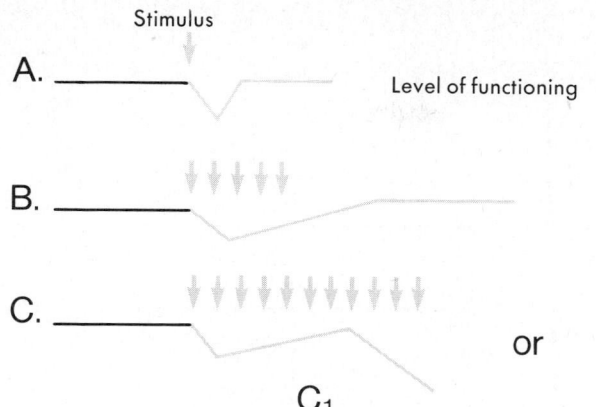

Stimulus

A. _____

Level of functioning

B. _____ ↓↓↓↓↓

C. _____ ↓↓↓↓↓↓↓↓↓↓↓

or

C_1

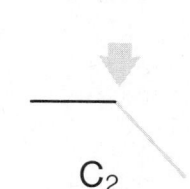

_____

C_2

Fig. 8-1. General adaptation syndrome. **A,** Alarm reaction with return to prestressed level. **B,** Continued application of stimulus leads to resistance stage; return to prestressed level may occur when stimulus is removed. **C,** Depletion of resources with continued stimuli or strong damaging stimulus leads to exhaustion.

deal with environmental stimuli, and responses to stressors may be affected. Nutritional deficits especially place the person at higher risk of maladaptive responses (see Chapter 7).

INTEGRATED PSYCHOBIOLOGIC RESPONSE

People respond to stress as a unified whole, that is, compensatory or defense mechanisms are initiated to help the individual cope with the stress biologically and psychologically. Some of the evoked responses will be biologic, others will be behavioral, and both frequently occur simultaneously. For example, anxiety can cause sweaty palms, pale skin, and frequent voiding as well as decreased attention span, decreased ability to follow directions, or immobility. For the purpose of study, it is easier to separate physiologic responses from behavioral responses. This chapter will focus on the general responses to stressors, the physiologic responses, and modes of stress management. Chapter 9 focuses on specific behavioral responses with integration of physiologic responses.

GENERAL ADAPTATION SYNDROME

A small locally applied stimulus may result in a *local adaptation syndrome* (LAS). The inflammatory process (Chapter 6) is an example of LAS. Moderate to severe stressors will cause a *general adaptation syndrome* (GAS). The GAS proposed by Selye as a response of individuals to stress consists of 3 stages: alarm reaction, resistance, and exhaustion. The first two stages are repeated continuously throughout life as persons encounter stressors. The exhaustion stage occurs when resistance cannot be sustained, and altered functioning then results.

Alarm reaction stage

During the initial alarm stage (shock), the "fight or flight" response is initiated. The individual prepares to counteract the stressor or remove himself or herself from the stressor. If the shock is too severe, a "freeze" response occurs; the person is overwhelmed by the stressor and cannot fight or flee. During the alarm reaction stage, the neuroendocrine mechanisms are activated. If the

compensatory mechanisms are sufficient to deal with stressor, the individual returns to the prestressed level (Fig. 8-1, A).

Resistance stage

Continual and prolonged application of the stressor leads to the resistance stage. During this stage, there is continued adrenocortical activity to facilitate adaptation. Energy is required to maintain a high level of resistance. If the stressor is maintained a sufficient time, stress-related pathophysiologic disorders (p. 105) may result. If adaptation is successful and the stressor removed, the person may return to the prestressed level (Fig. 8-1, B).

Exhaustion stage

If the original stressor is so damaging that it is impossible for the defense mechanisms to be effective or if the stressor is not removed and energy to maintain resistance is depleted, the exhaustion stage occurs (Fig. 8-1, C). Examples of extreme stress situations are arterial bleeding, pressure on the hypothalamus, overwhelming infection, blockage of a major branch of the coronary artery, or sudden death of a spouse. Presenting symptoms may include those seen in the initial shock phase. Unless the primary biologic condition can be controlled promptly, death may ensue. Overwhelming psychologic stressors may also lead to mental dysfunction or death.

NEUROENDOCRINE RESPONSE TO STRESS

The hypothalamus responds to stimuli from the peripheral receptors or cerebral cortex by activating two different mechanisms, the sympathetic-adrenal medullary mechanism and the anterior pituitary-adrenocortical mechanism (Fig. 8-2).

The first mechanism, the *sympathetic-adrenal medullary mechanism,* suppresses functions that are nonessential for life and augments those that facilitate overcoming or escaping the stressful situation. Impulses are conducted from the hypothalamus to the sympathetic centers in the thoracolumbar segments of the autonomic nervous effectors to prepare the body for "fight or flight." An adequate blood supply to the brain and heart is maintained, and

Fig. 8-2. Physiologic response to stress.

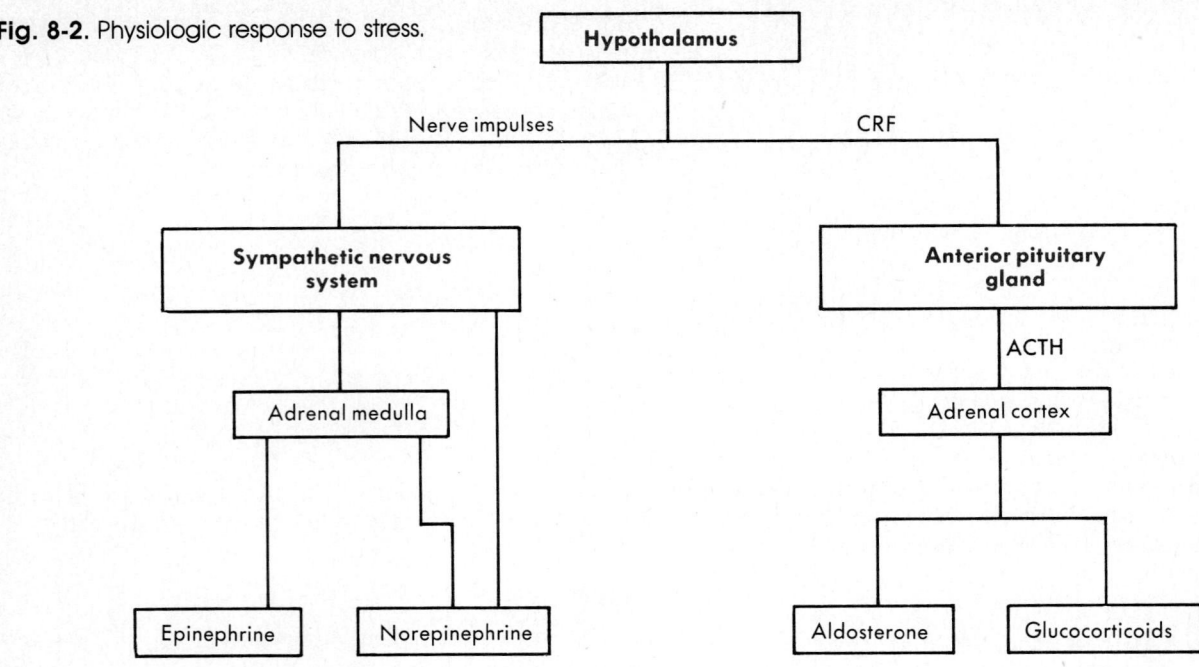

Effects of sympathetic-adrenal medullary mechanisms

Eye	Pupillary dilation
Heart	Increased rate, contractility and cardiac output
Blood vessels	
Coronary, brain, lungs	Dilated
Skin, mucosa, renal, abdominal viscera	Constricted
Lungs	Relaxation of bronchial muscles, decreased secretions
Gastrointestinal tract	Decreased motility and secretions
Pancreas	Decreased secretion
Liver	Glycogenolysis, gluconeogenesis
Urinary bladder	Relaxed
Glands; salivary, sweat	Increased secretion
Skin	Piloerection (goose bumps)

the blood supply to the skeletal muscles is increased. Provision is made to maintain the body's water, electrolyte, and temperature balances and to supply extra energy. To achieve these responses, the adrenergic fibers (sympathetic) of the autonomic nervous system are stimulated to produce a chemical called norepinephrine, and the adrenal *medulla* secretes norepinephrine and epinephrine. The effects of the sympathetic-adrenal medullary mechanism are listed above.

The second mechanism, the *anterior pituitary-adrenocortical mechanism,* is not activated by nerve impulses but by a neurosecretion called corticotropin-releasing factor (CRF). This chemical is produced in the hypothalamus and released into the pituitary portal veins. CRF stimulates the pituitary gland to increase the amount of adrenocorticotropic hormone (ACTH) released, which in turn

causes an outpouring of adrenocorticosteroid hormones. The effects of the adrenal cortical hormones, aldosterone, and the glucocorticoids are to maintain fluid and electrolyte balance, provide for emergency energy and materials for repair, and stabilize the internal environment.

ASSESSMENT OF PHYSIOLOGIC STRESS RESPONSE

The signs and symptoms seen in the presence of major stressors are caused by both the stressors and the neural and hormonal activation of body responses. In addition, muscle wasting will occur in long-term stress situations secondary to increased protein breakdown and decreased protein synthesis. In times of minor stressors or danger the body's response may be minimal or so short lived as not to produce any symptoms.

Effects of adrenal cortical hormones

Aldosterone

Maintenance of fluid and electrolyte balance
  Reabsorption of sodium and water
  Excretion of potassium, ammonium, and magnesium

Glucocorticoids

Provision of emergency fuel and repair materials
  Protein catabolism
  Release of glucose from liver and muscle glycogen
  Gluconeogenesis
  Glycogen synthesis
Stabilization of internal environment
  Reabsorption of sodium and excretion of potassium
  Increased ability of skeletal muscle to contract and delay fatigue
  Stabilization of lysosome membranes in cells
  Increased oxygen transport
  Decreased lactic acidosis
  Increased microcirculatory flow

Physiologic signs and symptoms of stress

Skin	Pale or ashen, moist
Pupils	Dilated
Pulse	Increased rate and strength
Respirations	Deeper; may or may not be faster
Body temperature	Slightly increased
Gastrointestinal tract	Nausea, constipation
Urinary tract	Frequency of urination with moderate stress; oliguria with severe stress
Motor system	Restlessness, frequent hand movements with moderate stress; immobility with severe stress

Table 8-1. Types of coping strategies

Category	Examples
Action	Taking walks, washing floors, gardening
Cognitive	Problem solving
Intrapsychic	Religion, activities to search for meaning of stress
Interpersonal	Use of support persons, talking it over with someone
Emotional	Use of defense mechanisms, such as denial

COPING

Coping refers to processes or skills that individuals use to deal with events, circumstances, or situations that are out of the ordinary. Coping strategies are overall plans of action for overcoming stressors.[1] Thus coping is a general behavioral response to stress.

People cope with stressors in one or more ways (see Table 8-1). Actions to cope with stress may be adaptive or maladaptive, depending on the achieved level of functioning. (See Chapter 9 for a discussion of defense mechanisms.) Some persons respond to most stressors in one characteristic mode; however, this limits their ability for adaptation when new stressors occur. For example, persons who generally respond to stressors by physical activity are severely hampered when an illness (stressor) that decreases physical mobility occurs. Persons who have developed several coping strategies are better able to cope effectively with new stressors.

There is no one specific or best way to cope with any given situation. What is useful to one individual may be inappropriate for another. The nature of the stressor, the state of development of the individual, the social and cultural environment, and the physical and interpersonal resources available all influence the style and effectiveness of coping strategies.

In nursing, as in other helping relationships, it is most useful to assist a person to cope in ways that are congruent with previously established styles. Stress management includes reinforcing existing appropriate coping mechanisms and helping the person explore alternative strategies if existing coping mechanisms are inappropriate. Data must therefore be collected to identify the person's usual coping strategies.

One method is by asking the question, "What do you usually do when things don't go as you plan or when things get tough?" Weisman[21] suggests seven simple questions that may obtain a great deal of information about coping strategies:

1. What problems, if any, do you see this illness creating?
2. How do you plan to deal with them?
3. When faced with a problem you must do something about, what do you do?
4. How does it usually work out?
5. To whom do you turn when you need help?
6. What has happened in the past when you have asked for help?
7. What kinds of problems usually tend to get you upset or down?

These questions establish perception of the current problem, present and usual ways of dealing with problems, sources and responses to help, and recurrent problems that affect coping.

STRESS MANAGEMENT

General interventions to modify physiologic responses

Any hospitalized patient may show signs and symptoms associated with the body's response to stressors because of the stress of illness or the fears associated with the illness. Without an understanding of the body's mechanisms for handling stressors, nursing actions may impede rather than complement or supplement the protective mechanisms. It should be remembered that the purpose of the initial response to stressors is to help the person escape the stress-producing situation or to mobilize all defenses to resist it.

SUPPORT OF PROTECTIVE MECHANISMS

Nursing measures designed to support the protective mechanisms are necessary. Rest is absolutely essential with severe stress to maintain an energy supply for metabolic functions essential to life. The patient is kept comfortably warm but never overly warm, because overheating causes vasodilation and counteracts the arteriolar constriction necessary to ensure an adequate blood supply to the vital organs.

PREVENTION OF ADDITIONAL PHYSICAL OR EMOTIONAL STRESS

Although patients may be able to cope with one stress-producing situation, they may not be able to adapt to further stressors. Special care must be taken to prevent further trauma, superimposed infection, anxiety, or fear. Extraordinary thoughtfulness is necessary, because the patient is likely to be very alert. Anxiety-producing conversations with the patient or in the vicinity of the patient are to be avoided. Noise, bright lights, and disturbances should be kept to a minimum. Pain should be alleviated as much as possible.

RELIEF OF DISCOMFORT

Even minor stress reactions cause annoying discomforts such as backache, generalized muscle tension, and headache. These discomforts can act as additional stressors, and comfort measures such as back rubs, position changes, and back support to relax the muscles are indicated. During severe stress, oral food and fluids may need to be withheld until nausea subsides and gastrointestinal tract activity returns to normal.

Stress management therapies

Some approaches to stress management require special training or equipment. Stress management therapists help persons design and implement a structured program of change to enable the individual to control and deal more effectively with stress. Some of the therapies include the following:

1. *Biofeedback:* learning voluntary control over autonomically regulated body functions
2. *Behavioral change programs:* behavioral conditioning to eliminate a specific stress-related behavior, such as smoking or overeating
3. *Systematic desensitization:* providing specific stressful stimuli (such as those related to phobias) in increasing doses while the individual acquires relaxation skills
4. *Autogenic training:* teaching cognitive behavior change together with physiologic behavior change through passive concentration

Nurses can help patients prevent or minimize the effects of stress by assisting in (1) identifying existing or potential stressors, (2) recognizing the effectiveness of responses to stressors, (3) developing and testing new behaviors such as problem solving, and (4) learning ways to minimize the effects of stress, such as by deep breathing or relaxation exercises.

Problem solving

Some persons solve problems in a haphazard manner. Problem solving can be a means for coping with stress and is more effective if the problem-solving steps are consciously followed. The steps include the following:

1. Gathering data
2. Identifying the problem (or effect of stressor)
3. Identifying factors affecting the problem or stressor
4. Determining goals
5. Exploring alternative ways and consequences of the actions to achieve the goals
6. Implementing action
7. Evaluating effectiveness of actions

If the stressor has been identified, the nurse first assists the patient to explore feelings and reactions associated with the stressor. Often persons are not consciously aware of what they are experiencing and therefore may select inappropriate actions. Persons vary in their ability to identify problems and in their desire to discuss personal feelings, although it is widely accepted that talking does help. If the patient is pushed indiscriminately to talk about problems, the relationship will become superficial and mechanical. The identification of the consequences of actions is often omitted but is an important component if problem solving is to be effective.

Problem solving reduces ambiguity and feelings of loss of control. Persons who do not generally employ conscious problem solving as a means of coping with stressors may benefit from learning about problem solving as a strategy for coping with stress.

Relaxation techniques

Relaxation exercises are developed from the concept that stress with anxiety does not and cannot exist when the muscles of the body are relaxed. Relaxation exercises do not "cure" stress but do help to minimize effects of stress and give the person a sense of control. A daily program of relaxation exercises has been shown to have an effect on physiologic responses to stress (for example, lowering of elevated blood pressure or elevated blood sugars) and in psychologic responses to stress (for example, decreased level of anxiety). They are also helpful on a short-term basis when anxiety is present.

There are four basic components of relaxation techniques:

1. *Quiet environment:* deleting all possible noise and distractions
2. *Comfortable position:* sitting with no undue muscle tension
3. *Passive attitude:* emptying all thoughts from the conscious mind
4. *Mental device:* focusing on a sound, word, phrase, mental image, object, or breathing pattern to shift the mind from logical, externally oriented thoughts

The important factor is that the person empties the mind of all thoughts and concentrates on the mental device. It is natural for the mind to wander. When this occurs, the person simply redirects the mind back to the mental device. Each relaxation session should take approximately 20 minutes.

There are several approaches to performing relaxation exercises. Two approaches that can be carried out by nursing instructions to patients, without use of special equipment and without physician's orders, are *progressive relaxation* and *Benson's relaxation response.*

Progressive relaxation consists of tensing and relaxing muscle groups and focusing on the feelings of relaxation. The systematic application of progressive relaxation has three major effects, which are as follows:

1. Muscle groups are relaxed more and more with each practice.
2. Each of the major muscle groups is relaxed one after the other. As a new muscle group is added, the previously relaxed portions also relax.
3. More total body relaxation is experienced as the person moves into the relaxation phase. The relaxed state is maintained beyond the relaxation period.[6]

Progressive relaxation

1. Assume a comfortable position in a quiet room
2. Begin by focusing on easy breathing
3. Tense specific muscle groups (see step 5) for 5 to 7 seconds, then relax quickly
4. Concentrate for 10 seconds on the sensations of the relaxed muscles
5. Follow a sequence, repeating each muscle group, tensing two or three times:
   a. Hand and arm: clench fist, pull elbow tightly to sides (dominant arm first)
   b. Face: wrinkle forehead, close eyes tightly, wrinkle nose, purse lips, smile with teeth tightly clenched
   c. Neck: pull chin to chest
   d. Trunk: pull shoulder blades together, tighten stomach and buttocks
   e. Leg and foot: push down with leg, point toes upward (dorsiflexion); dominant leg first
6. Repeat process in any areas in which increased tension has been identified

Benson's relaxation response omits the muscle tensing. It is particularly helpful for muscle relaxation in patients who are experiencing pain or discomfort. It is important to remain with the patient to coach and encourage the relaxation.

Benson's relaxation response

1. Assume a comfortable sitting position in a quiet room
2. Close eyes
3. Relax body muscles (that is, "let go")
4. Concentrate on breathing. Repeat a word or sound such as "one" or "um-m" after each exhalation
5. Continue for about 20 minutes
6. Open eyes
7. Take time to adjust to surroundings before moving

REFERENCES AND SELECTED READINGS*

1. Antonovsky, A.: Health, stress and coping, San Francisco, 1979, Jersey-Bass Publishers.
2. Benson, H.: The relaxation response, New York, 1975, William Morrow & Co., Inc.
3. *Breedon, S.A., and Kondo, C.: Using biofeedback to reduce tension, Am. J. Nurs. **75:**2010-2012, 1975.
4. Byrne, M.L., and Thompson, L.F.: Key concepts for the study and practice of nursing, ed. 2, St. Louis, 1978, The C.V. Mosby Co.
5. Carlson, C.E., editor: Behavioral concepts and nursing interventions, ed. 2, Philadelphia, 1978, W.B. Saunders Co.
6. *Curtis, J., and Detert, R.: How to relax, Palo Alto, Calif., 1981, Mayfield Publishing Co.
7. Ebersole, P., and Hess, P.: Toward healthy aging: human needs and nursing response, St. Louis, 1981, The C.V. Mosby Co.
8. *Jasmin, S.A., Hill, L., and Smith, N.: Keeping your delicate balance: the art of managing stress, Nurs. 81 **11**(6):52-57, 1981.
9. Marcinek, M.B.: Stress in the surgical patient, Am. J. Nurs. **77:**1809-1811, 1977.
10. Morris, C.L.: Relaxation therapy in a clinic, Am. J. Nurs. **79:**1958-1959, 1979.
11. O'Flynn-Comiskey, A.I.: The type A individual, Am. J. Nurs. **79:**1956-1958, 1979.
12. Pender, N.J.: Health promotion in nursing practice, Norwalk, Conn. 1982, Appleton-Century-Crofts.
13. *Richter, J.M., and Sloan, R.: A relaxation technique, Am. J. Nurs. **79:**1960-1964, 1979.
14. Selye, H.: Stress without distress, New York, 1975, New American Library.
15. Selye, H.: The stress of life (revised edition), New York, 1976, McGraw-Hill Book Co.
16. Shontz, F.: The psychological aspects of physical illness and disability, New York, 1975, Macmillan Publishing Co., Inc.
17. *Smith, M.J.T., and Selye, H.: Reducing the negative effects of stress, Am. J. Nurs. **79:**1953-1955, 1979.
18. *Stephenson, C.: Stress in critically ill patients, Am. J. Nurs. **77:**1806-1808, 1977.
19. *Stewart, E.: To lessen pain: relaxation and rhythmic breathing, Am. J. Nurs. **76:**958-959, 1976.
20. Sutterly, D.C., and Donnelly, G.S.: Stress management, Top. Clin. Nurs. **1**(1):1-104, 1979.
21. *Weisman, A.: Coping with cancer, New York, 1979, McGraw-Hill Book Co.

---

*References preceded by an asterisk are particularly well suited for student reading.

9

Psychologic Responses to Stress

MAY WYKLE

STUDY QUESTIONS

- What physical signs have you experienced when you have felt anxious (such as before a major examination)?

- Study the behavior of several selected patients on your hospital unit. What impression do you receive of their mental health from observing their posture, facial appearance, grooming, and relationships with others?

- What resources are available in your community for rehabilitation of alcoholics and drug addicts?

Humans are social beings, and one of their basic needs is to feel secure and accepted by others in a social group. An individual's entire life comprises a series of adjustments to meet biologic and emotional needs in socially acceptable ways. Human behavior is characterized by a powerful tendency to repeat itself, especially if the behavior is rewarded; therefore it is essential that health care professionals possess a thorough knowledge of human behavior and factors that influence it. An awareness of what shapes patients' behavior, how to manage stress, and how behavior affects others increases care givers' effectiveness in implementing nursing interventions.

Personality refers to all that a person is, feels, and does, either consciously or unconsciously, as manifested in interactions with the environment. Behavior is an expression of personality and is defined as all the activity of which a human being is capable. It is a person's never-ending attempt at adjustment to the environment and is determined by the stress of unmet needs. Thus according to the humanists, all behavior is motivated, purposeful, and meaningful.

Behavior is the manner in which an organism responds to a need. Once the need is gratified, the organism changes its behavior. Unmet needs create frustration, which leads to increased anxiety. This anxiety is then demonstrated through behavior. If the behavior is such

that anxiety is resolved in an acceptable manner to the person and to others in the environment, it is termed *adaptive*. Persons who display adaptive behavior are those who make appropriate use of their coping mechanisms and do not exhibit symptoms of psychologic disturbance. Those with maladaptive behavior are at the other end of the spectrum (Fig. 9-1); their psychiatric symptoms are a way to deal with increased stress.

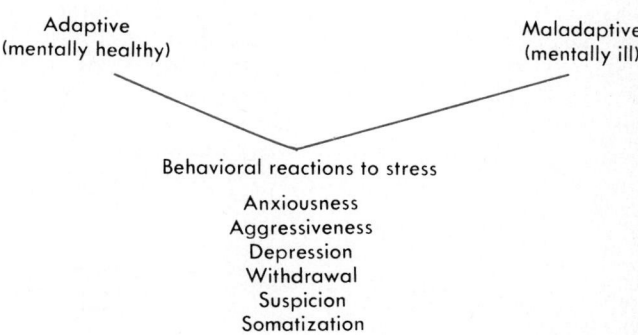

Fig. 9-1. Behavioral responses of persons experiencing anxiety from stress such as illness range from behavior that is adaptive to that which is maladaptive.

113

ANXIETY

Anxiety is a psychologic response to stress with both physiologic and psychologic components. Anxiety is a feeling of tension, dread, and uneasiness, the source of which is unknown or unrecognized.[51] Anxiety stems from the frustration of unmet needs, which lead to a state of disequilibrium in the individual. The resulting tension is manifested as anxiety states. States of anxiety are the behavior manifestations of the need-tension experience. Since anxiety is an energy that cannot be seen, it is only implied by the individual's actions. This state of anxiousness manifested by behavioral changes is communicated interpersonally.

Assessment of anxiety

Anxiety is manifested in different levels ranging from mild to severe.[51] Although the ego attempts to deal with anxiety through the use of defense mechanisms, certain amounts of anxiety are reflected in behaviors resulting from a discharge of energy necessary to restore equilibrium of the individual. These responses range from behavior that is adaptive to behavior that is considered by our social standards to be maladaptive (Fig. 9-2). The type of behavioral reactions that occur is influenced by psychosociocultural factors, basic personality development, past experiences, values, and economic status.

Levels of anxiety

Level	Behavior patterns
Mild anxiety	Alertness
	Quick eye movements
	Increased hearing ability
	Increased awareness
Moderate anxiety	Decreased awareness of environmental details
	Focus on selected aspects of self (or illness)
Severe anxiety	Disturbances in thought patterns
	Incongruency of thoughts, feelings, and actions
Panic	Distorted perceptions of environment
	Inability to see or understand situation
	Unpredictable responses
	Random motor activity

Signs of anxiety

Appearance

Increased muscle tension (rigidity)
Skin blanches, pales
Increased perspiration, clammy skin
Fatigue
Increased small motor activity (for example, restlessness, tremor)

Behavior

Decreased attention span
Decreased ability to follow directions
Increased acting out
Increased somatizing
Increased immobility

Conversation

Increased number of questions
Constant seeking of reassurance
Frequent shifting of topics of conversation
Describes fears with sense of helplessness
Avoids focusing on feelings
Focuses on equipment or procedures

Physiologic signs mediated through autonomic nervous system

Increased heart rate
Increased rate or depth of respirations
Rapid extreme shifts in body temperature, blood pressure, menstrual flow
Diarrhea
Urinary urgency
Dryness of mouth
Decreased appetite
Increased perspiration
Dilation of pupils

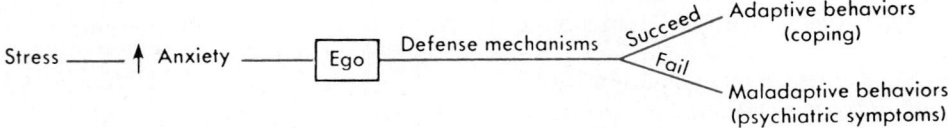

Fig. 9-2. When increased anxiety occurs from stress such as illness, the ego attempts to decrease anxiety by means of defense mechanisms. If these mechanisms fail, the ego resorts to psychiatric symptoms (maladaptive behaviors) as a means of coping.

Persons can vacillate among the several levels of anxiety. The level of anxiety engendered and its manifestations depend on the person's maturity, understanding of need tension, level of self-esteem, and coping mechanisms.

In assessing a patient, the nurse observes appearance, behavior, and the conversation for signs of anxiety. The conclusion that the patient is demonstrating anxious behavior can be made when several of the signs of anxiety are present. With mild anxiety the signs are fewer and less prominent, and it is important to validate the conclusion with the patient. Mild anxiety heightens the use of capacities, whereas severe anxiety and panic states severely paralyze or overwork capacities. Signs of anxiety are therefore more overt in persons who are experiencing severe anxiety or panic.

Interventions for anxiety

Since anxiety is felt empathetically and communicated interpersonally, it is imperative that the nurse take steps to lower a patient's anxiety level. If anxiety is not reduced, other patients and staff are caught up in the tension. Recognition of the effects that the patient's anxiety is having on the nurse, followed by problem-solving steps to reduce anxiety in self, in turn helps to reduce some of the patient's anxiety.

The type of intervention used by the nurse depends on the patient's anxiety level and includes explanations, exploration of feelings, and intervention for severe anxiety. Since the capacity to tolerate stress varies among individuals, nursing intervention is geared toward support of the person's coping mechanisms, which prevent further escalation of anxiety.

EXPLANATIONS

Structure decreases anxiety and is helpful for the person experiencing mild or moderate anxiety. Explanations are one method of providing structure. Each new experience should be explained to patients and, if possible, related to familiar experiences. The higher the level of anxiety, the more simple should be the explanations.

If patients are to have treatments or tests they need to be given some idea of what will be done, the preparation involved, and the reasons why the procedure is necessary. To remove the water pitcher and inform patients that they cannot have any more water until after the x-ray examination can generate many anxious thoughts: "What x-ray examination?" "I wonder when it is?" "What will it be like?" "It must be something special if I can't have any water." Lack of knowledge as a cause of anxiety reflects the nurse's lack of consideration for the patient's rights as an individual.

Explanations should be given in the patient's own terms at appropriate times and repeated as necessary. If the patient is very anxious, repeated explanation may be necessary, since extreme anxiety reduces intellectual function. It is useless to give detailed explanations to patients who are severely anxious or sedated or to those who

have high temperatures or severe pain. Repetition is often required for older persons and children because they may have short memory spans.

Time spent in giving explanations to relatives is not wasted. Not only does it relieve their anxieties, which may be transmitted to the patient, but it also saves having to untangle misinformation. Often the family is helpful in interpreting necessary instructions to the patient in a manner that the patient understands and accepts.

EXPLORATION OF FEELINGS

In most instances a large part of the nurse's work is to encourage patients to express anxieties, to help patients see the universality of fear in their situation, to help them seek outlets for their fears and tensions, and to allay these negative feelings whenever possible. Nurses provide opportunities for the patient to talk, but they should not probe. There is a difference between prying into a patient's thoughts and beliefs and eliciting information that will aid in the understanding of behavior and in planning for care. Without seeming unduly curious, one can usually find some topic of personal interest to the patient that will provide an opening. A picture on the bedside table may create such an example. Nurses who listen with sincere interest and without making judgments about the patient may begin to gain insight into the patient as a person. And more important, the patient may begin to speak about personal fears.

As soon as the patient begins to talk about feelings, the nurse should proceed with conversation, taking cues from what the patient offers. The nurse who feels inadequate or anxious may cut off the conversation. For instance, if a patient says, "You know, I don't think I'll ever get to see my little boy again," a common response is "Oh, don't say that, certainly you will; you're going to be all right." The patient may very well not be all right. Would it not be better to respond, "What makes you feel this way?" Such a response helps the patient explore the subject and leaves opportunity for the patient to examine this concern. The nurse who is willing to listen to patients, to be guided by their reactions, and to work with them rather than to make decisions for them will give them needed emotional support. Solving patients' problems for them, even if it were possible, is not the aim of nursing. Indeed it would tend to make patients less healthy psychologically.

The art of meaningful communication involves more than just listening; it includes moving the conversation so that the patient's attempts to communicate are assisted. Observing the patient for facial changes and general body movements provides opportunities for the nurse to discover from the individual the full meaning of the situation. For example, consider the patient who sucks in air while talking. The mouth becomes drier and drier as the tongue seems to stick in the mouth. These patients are not at ease and show anxiety even though their words may be quite innocuous. A simple statement such as, "Your mouth seems very dry. Would a glass of water help?" allows the nurse to clarify observations. Such an approach gives the patient a chance to tell what is being experienced, and to gain understanding by talking about it.

The nurse helps patients examine those problems that they are able to bring into awareness. Underlying problems should be handled by people trained in psychotherapy. A nurse needs to be able to recognize normal anxiety reactions and to report exaggerated reactions that may indicate the need for psychiatric referral.

INTERVENTION FOR SEVERE ANXIETY

When any patient's anxiety increases to a high level, the nurse may need to sit with the patient. The nurse's very presence is often reassuring. If possible, the patient is helped to recognize the anxiety by the nurse asking, "Are you uncomfortable?" or "What are you feeling?" In severe anxiety and panic, being there is most important, and touch may be used as a means of reassurance. Some severely anxious persons, however, view touching as an intrusion of their personal boundary, and the nurse needs to keep this in mind. When the patient is able to talk, the nurse helps the patient to describe what is happening, what has happened, and what is expected to happen.

Crisis intervention

Awareness of what occurs during a crisis helps the nurse understand the accompanying behavior. When the ego is met with overwhelming anxiety created by biologic, physiologic, or social threats to the self, a crisis ensues. The ego is not able to cope successfully with the sudden disequilibrium, and the person needs assistance to use the situation as a growth experience.

A crisis occurs when a person is unable to use customary methods of coping when faced for a time with what seems to be an unsurmountable obstacle to an important life goal. A period of disorganization ensues, a period of upset during which many abortive attempts at solutions are made.

PHASES OF CRISIS

Shontz describes several phases or stages that occur during crisis.[25] These stages are similar to the stages of death and dying as described by Kübler-Ross.

1. *Initial impact.* During this phase the client experiences shock and depersonalization as reality is clearly perceived. Functioning is organized and automatic with individual centering and docility.

2. *Realization.* In the second phase there is a collapse of the existing self-structure. Reality seems overwhelming, and the person experiences high anxiety, panic, and helplessness. There is inability to plan, reason, or understand the situation.

3. *Defensive retreat.* The third phase is one of regression in which there is an attempt to establish previous identity, to return to better times. There is an avoidance of reality, and denial and wishful thinking may ensue to

relieve the anxiety. When challenged, the ego reacts with anger and the person may experience rage and disorientation. Thinking is situation-bound, and there is a resistance to change.

4. *Acknowledgment.* This is the "yes" stage: "It has happened to me." The individual experiences depression and self-depreciation. Reality imposes itself again and looms large in relating the event to one's life. Without intervention the client may become more disorganized, depressed, and suicidal.

5. *Adaptation.* This is the stage when change occurs if help is adequate. New identity appears along with hope and renewed sense of personal worth. There is a subsequent decrease in anxiety and an increase in satisfaction as a result of the stabilization and reorganization. Functional improvement is noted without actual change in disability status.

The model just offered is a useful approach for explaining what a person experiences during an illness crisis, even though reactions to crisis are individual. People are not equally vulnerable to all categories of stress, but there is thought to be some commonality in the reactions. Knowledge about the commonalities can facilitate plans for nursing intervention.

INTERVENTION

The essential element of crisis intervention is the intensive nature of support required to help the ego maintain its integrity and its ability to use coping mechanisms. Crisis, according to Caplan,[35] is self-limiting. Early intervention can prevent maladaptive behavior, and the individual can emerge a stronger person. Acute illness or catastrophic illness often precipitates a crisis reaction. The outcome of a crisis is governed by the kind of interaction that takes place between the individual and key figures in the environment during the time of crisis.

Often because of changes in society, previous guidelines for behavior in stressful situations render the individual helpless. In crisis the individual is helped to find ways to facilitate efforts to enlarge on the experience. A state of disequilibrium produces a felt need to reduce anxiety. The following balancing factors have been identified as being necessary to resolve the problem and to avert crisis:

1. A realistic perception of the event
2. Adequate situational support (staff and family)
3. Adequate coping mechanisms[1]

When one or more of these balancing factors are absent, the result is an increase in anxiety, with immobilization and an inability to avert the crisis (Fig. 9-3).

In crisis, help should be immediate. Staying with the person, talking through the situation, and encouraging catharsis facilitate recognition and expression of feelings and subsequent relief of guilt. Strengthening of coping mechanisms is crucial in preventing the formation of symptoms. Personal growth is facilitated by using problem-solving skills and a hierarchy of needs framework to help the person set priorities.

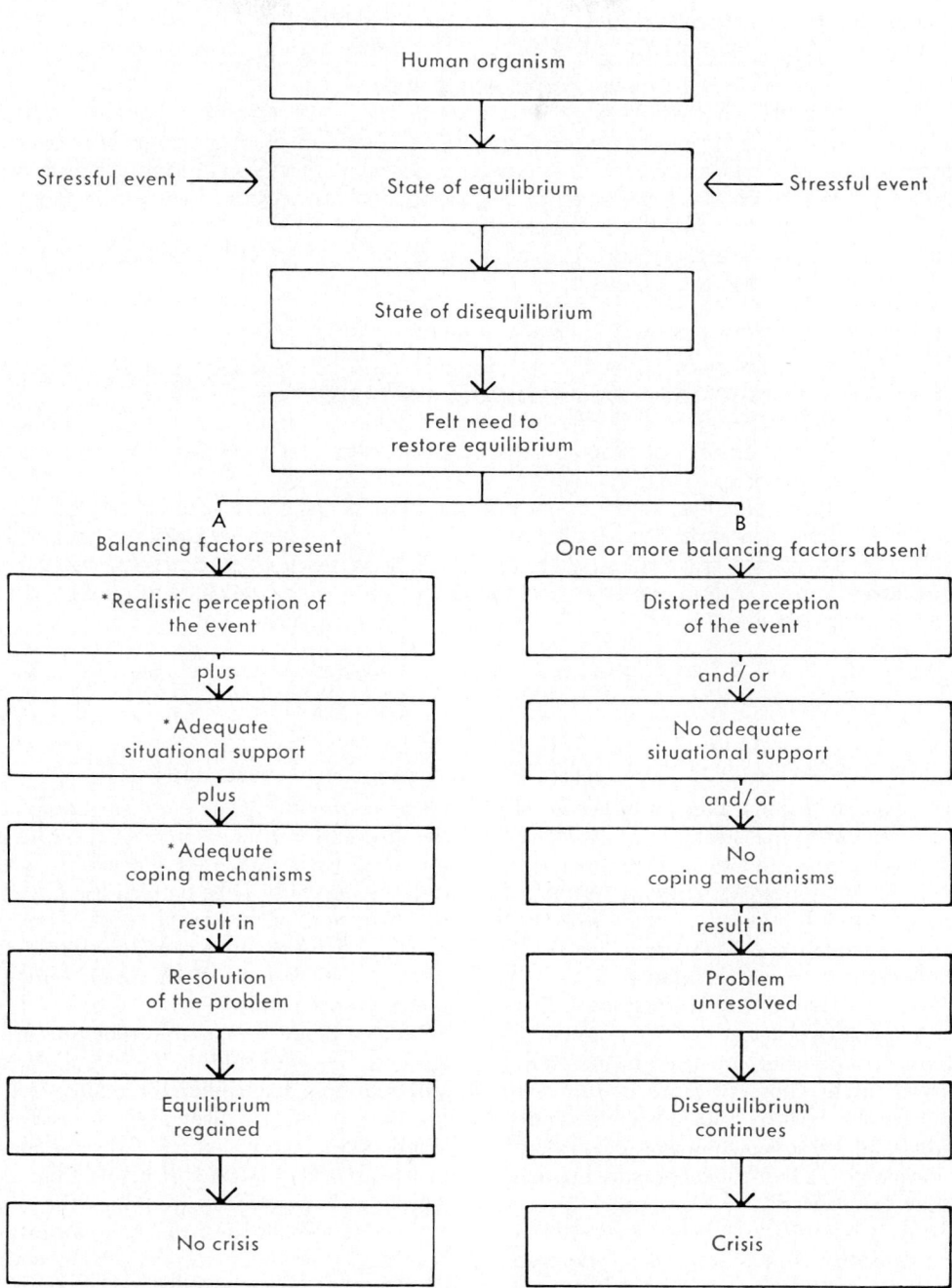

* Balancing factors.

Fig. 9-3. Paradigm: effect of balancing factors in stressful event. (From Aguilera, D.C., and Messick, J.M.: Crisis intervention: theory and methodology, ed. 4, St. Louis, 1981, The C.V. Mosby Co.)

Defense mechanisms

Higher level: less primitive mechanisms

Repression	Ideas painful to consciousness are forced into the unconscious
Suppression	Thoughts or desires are consciously inhibited
Sublimation	Energy of repressed tendencies is transformed and directed to socially acceptable goals
Identification	Person assumes the personal qualities or elements of the personality of another
Compensation	Person makes up, covers up, or disguises real or fancied inadequacies in another area
Displacement	An emotion is transferred or displaced from its original object to a more acceptable substitute that is less threatening
Rationalization	Plausible explanations are given to account for a belief or behavior motivated from unconscious sources

Lower level: more primitive mechanisms

Denial	The disavowal of intolerable thoughts, feelings, or wishes; person refutes external elements of reality that are unpleasant or painful
Regression	Person reverts to a pattern of behavior belonging to an earlier stage of development
Conversion	Painful emotional experience is repressed and later is expressed in the form of a physical symptom
Projection	That which is emotionally unacceptable within the self is rejected and attributed to others
Introjection	Person absorbs the emotional attitudes, wishes, ideals, or personality of others into oneself; the aspirations and self restraints of others are incorporated into the personality
Reaction formation	Person adopts attitudes and behavior that are opposites of the impulses to which the individual is reacting

---

DEFENSE MECHANISMS

Defense mechanisms are unconscious processes used by individuals in adjustment to life stresses. They evolve during personality development and serve to protect the personality, satisfy emotional needs, maintain harmony between conflicting tendencies, and reduce the tension of anxiety by modifying reality to make it more acceptable. Defense mechanisms are compromise solutions.

There are two levels of defense mechanisms: those that are considered more primitive and those that are of a higher level. Defense mechanisms are used by mentally healthy people as well as by those who are neurotic or psychotic. In the mentally healthy the mechanisms are used less frequently and those mechanisms of a more primitive kind are avoided. Defense mechanisms become pathologic when they are overused.

A defense mechanism is effective when it succeeds in easing intrapsychic tensions. When lower level defense mechanisms fail, a more pathologic process evolves, and the person exhibits psychiatric symptoms. All defense mechanisms are unconscious with the exception of suppression. Two defense mechanisms, denial and repression, that are frequently manifested by the hospitalized patient are discussed in more detail.

Denial

One of the defense mechanisms used frequently in dealing with the stress of illness is denial. This mecha-

nism occurs during the early stages of crisis after the initial stressful impact. Denial of the illness helps the person deal with increased tension by protecting the ego (self) from reality. The pattern used by the person is similar to games played by children when they close their eyes and believe no one can see them. "It's not there because I don't see it." That which cannot be perceived is therefore not painful.

During denial intolerable thoughts are disowned. The ego gets rid of unwelcome facts (such as an illness) while still retaining its faculty for reality testing. The person manifests denial by disowning any body changes. For example, patients with coronary disease may deny they have had heart attacks and will blame their discomfort on indigestion. Patients may even deny the severity of the pain and act as though the pain were not present.

Denial works well for the person who has been independent and has a self-image of a strong, self-made individual or who views sickness as a sign of weakness. Denial can be complete or partial and includes a "splitting" of thoughts, feelings, and actions; for example, the patient may own the thoughts but deny the feelings.

INTERVENTION FOR DENIAL

Intervention for denial is vital if improvement in the physiologic condition of patients depends on their gaining some awareness of the seriousness of the illness or at least enough insight so that they can participate in nursing care. At one time it was believed necessary to confront the patient's denial; however, *direct* attack usually makes the patient more defensive. Patients will give up the need to deny once they feel supported by others and the anxiety is lessened. Denial, although a more primitive mechanism, can be very useful to the person in the face of sudden crisis. Patients should be given reasons for their needed cooperation, but the nurse does not dwell on the patients' dependency or fearfulness. Patients need not agree that the treatment procedures are necessary for them, but neither can their participation cause any harm.

Limits are set firmly but kindly when denial behavior interferes with treatment. Persons experiencing denial need control over those routines not vital to their care and need reassurance that it is all right to ask for help because the nurse is there for assistance. Nursing care is given in a manner that emphasizes the patient's worth as a human being although in a dependent state. When patients get enough support and reassurance, they will be able to give up some of the denial and face reality.

Regression

Regression is a defense mechanism often seen in persons who are ill, since regression facilitates acceptance of the patient role. The ego is acted on rather than acting. Regression makes a dependency relationship possible because of the individual's reversion to behavior patterns of an earlier level of development. Illness necessitates patients placing themselves in the hands of competent others. They often become self-centered and concerned only with their own needs and interests. These interests focus on what is happening to the person and on their acceptance or rejection by care givers. Often regression is a help to patients in that it promotes conservation of energy.

BEHAVIORAL REACTIONS TO ILLNESS

It is essential that nurses not underestimate the psychosocial aspects of health care. Emotional stress may accentuate physical symptoms in patients. Because of this effect alone, nurses need to have a working knowledge of the dynamics of behavioral responses to illness.

Illness stimulates certain kinds of behavior based on the person's previous adjustment patterns, degree of physical impairment, abruptness of illness onset, prognosis, and meaning of the part of the body affected. All illness is a threat to self and evokes some anxiety, but an acute illness can create a crisis situation for the patient. A necessary part of total care therefore is to support the person's adaptive behaviors and prevent further decompensation.

Many persons are able with the added support from health professionals to maintain behavior within the adaptive range when subjected to the stress of illness. For support to be provided and for the ego to achieve balance, the person's coping mechanisms and dependency needs are assessed. By reinforcing existing coping mechanisms that are appropriate to the reduction of anxiety and by supporting problem-solving skills, the nurse can draw on the inherent strengths of the person.

The five behaviors presented in this section are all adaptive behaviors that are normal reactions to illness, both acute and chronic (Fig 9-1). Anxiety behavior is discussed on p. 114. Intervention is aimed at preventing further disintegration and crisis.

Aggressive behavior

Whenever there is a threat to self-concept, such as occurs with illness, individuals may respond by aggression, a way that makes them feel less helpless and more powerful. Aggression is another way of handling anxiety. People are often angry at the loss of health status and question what is happening. They become irritable and uncooperative and may project their anger onto the staff and become demanding. It is important that staff accept patients' hostility without retaliation and that patients not be made to feel guilty. Limits should be set and the patient's demands anticipated. Expression of anger in socially acceptable ways prevents anger from being turned inward, causing depression. Patients should be given reasonable control of their environment and the opportunity to participate in planning and implementing their own care.

Depressed behavior

Depression is a normal response to illness, once the illness has been accepted. In making an assessment of the person who is depressed, the nurse needs to be aware of the following clinical signs of depression:
1. Decreased interaction with others
2. Lack of interest in activities or environment
3. Voiced concern about illness and amount of required care
4. Expressed wish for or concerns about dying
5. Dependent behavior
6. Decreased activity
7. Complaints of weakness or fatigue

Intervention requires that the nurse approach the patient in a serious mood, conveying through actions and communication an understanding of what the patient must feel. The nurse helps the patient express feelings and conveys acceptance of the right to feel sad. When patients show signs of readiness, they are helped to focus on interested areas outside the illness. These patients may need to talk about activities that they were involved in before hospitalization. This is particularly true for persons who have chronic illnesses. It is important to *listen* to the person who is depressed complain about problems so that the anger may be turned outward.

DEPENDENCY

Dependency, a common behavior of the depressed patient, is a reaction that may follow the stage of accepting an illness. Patients readily place themselves in the hands of others. While dependency is a form of regression, it is also a part of learning to trust. These patients do not want to do much for themselves and accept total care, although they may not demand it. Supportive care is indicated in the early stages with gradual advancement from doing *for* the patient to doing *with* the patient, and then facilitating patient self-care. Thus patients return gradually to helping themselves.

Overdependency exists when the patient shows physical readiness to progress but prefers to remain dependent. Nurses need to assess the difference through deliberate observation and then set limits kindly on those nursing interventions that continue to promote the dependency. Appropriate interventions at this time include the use of saturation (that is, anticipating and meeting patient needs before the patient requests them), along with helping patients develop cognitive awareness of their physical ability to do more for themselves. The nurse also makes it clear that patients will not be abandoned and that support in the form of the presence of a member of the nursing staff will be available as they do more for themselves.

Withdrawn behavior

Withdrawn patients usually do not pose as many problems and are apt to be labeled "good" patients. They demand little from others and thus may be overlooked. Withdrawn patients regress more easily to earlier levels of behavior at which they can accept the patient role. Withdrawn patients need gentle encouragement to talk, to express feelings, and to relate to the staff. Spending time sitting with these patients, often in silence, does much to increase their sense of self-worth.

Suspicious behavior

Suspicious patients have difficulty with trust and may have had previous experiences in which they learned to distrust care givers. They are often suspicious of staff, the routines, the medicine, and the procedures. They need to talk about these concerns but should not be forced to do so. It is imperative that staff keep promises made to these patients and avoid an overzealous approach. Explanations of procedures and establishment of expected routines are helpful. Whispering and talking about patients within their field of hearing are avoided as the communication may be misinterpreted.

Somatic behavior

A familiar reaction to illness is one that can be labeled flight into illness. Patients somatize their concerns; that is, they have learned to express anxiety through complaints about a variety of physical symptoms. They may be preoccupied with bodily functions and feelings of pain. Vague complaints of backache, headache, or fatigue are expressed to legitimize the attention needed. Support and

acceptance by allowing patients to talk about their symptoms with some limit setting will decrease the anxiety.

Staff often become angry at patients who use somatic behavior because of the vague symptomatic complaints and because staff members feel "caught" if they "play down" the symptoms, since there is always the possibility that the complaints are truly connected with an illness. Guilt on the part of staff prevails for some time if a complaining patient who was ignored is diagnosed as having a physical illness. It is wise for the staff to accept all symptoms and report them. Time spent with these patients, listening to their complaints and using a saturation technique helps lessen this behavior.

ALCOHOLISM

Alcoholism is a disease that involves the whole person and can be defined as a physiologic dependence on alcohol as a result of excessive use. It is a progressive, primary, chronic, and very often fatal disease that compounds the problems of a person experiencing other health disorders. Alcoholism is a treatable illness, and, when treated early, chances for recovery are good. The problem of alcoholism has received national attention, and extensive treatment programs have been established. Significant changes in the identification and treatment of alcoholism point toward advances that are having an important impact on this major health problem.

Epidemiology

Alcoholism is the third major health problem in this country and is on the increase.[10] Conservative estimates are that 90 million people use alcohol and about 10 million people are afflicted with alcoholism. Alcoholism is defined as a continuing problem that affects a person's life, family, work, and social activities. One out of every 10 Americans who drink is likely to experience symptoms of alcoholism. Further, drinking has increased at an alarming rate among adolescents, particularly girls. Three out of 16 high school students reportedly are moderate to heavy drinkers.

Alcoholism is widely distributed among all social classes and is considered a familial disease, since a history of alcoholism in the family suggests a high potential for the disease.

Of all deaths in this country 10% are alcohol related, as are 80% of all suicides. From 25% to 30% of all patients in the medical-surgical units of general hospitals are suffering from alcohol-related problems. Industries lose at least $10 billion yearly because of alcoholism. This figure includes the cost of time lost, misjudgments, spoiled materials, broken machines, and other factors. Many companies have special programs for the treatment and rehabilitation of employees with alcoholism. Recent court rulings have declared that the alcoholic individual is sick and entitled to medical treatment, not imprisonment. Unfortunately, there are not enough facilities to treat the alcoholic, and treatment is often long, expensive and unsuccessful.

Etiology

There is a lack of agreement over the etiology of alcoholism, although several theories have been proposed. The genetic theory is particulary interesting, since alcoholism tends to occur in families. Psychodynamic theories call attention to the regressive aspects of alcoholism and define the alcoholic as a passive-dependent personality. The behaviorists believe that alcoholism is a learned behavior that continues because it is rewarded; alcoholic consumption continues because it decreases anxiety. Other theories of alcoholism include allergic responses, cultural influences, central nervous system (CNS) pathology, nutritional deficiencies, and endocrine dysfunctions. There are insufficient data to support any one theory, and it is likely that the root of alcoholism is *multicausal*.

Alcoholics have been classified empirically into the following three groups:
1. Persons whose alcoholism is a symptom of mental disease
2. Persons for whom alcohol is a physiologic poison
3. Alcoholics who develop from social drinkers

Persons who develop alcoholism from social drinking may appear well-adjusted until some trouble arises to cause excessive drinking, and they then may drift slowly and unwillingly into alcoholism. The alcoholic person is likely to be basically insecure and unable to face realities without difficulty. Alcohol may become a means of escaping the demands of life. Persons who are becoming alcoholics tend to be untruthful about their drinking and defend themselves by rationalizations and pretenses.

Pathophysiology

Although alcohol is rarely thought of as a drug because of its social acceptance, it does belong to the category of anesthetics and has the same risks when abused as all other addictive drugs.

Absorption of alcohol is accelerated by increased alcohol concentrations and an empty stomach. After absorption, alcohol is distributed equally throughout body fluids, passing across all membranes. Blood alcohol levels depend on the amount ingested and the size of the individual. Most laws designate blood alcohol serum levels of 100 mg/100 ml (0.10%) as the legal limit for driving a motor vehicle. High blood alcohol levels have increasingly more serious effects.

Alcohol also has a diuretic effect, partly because of the increased amount of fluids ingested. Increased amounts of electrolytes, particularly potassium, magnesium, and zinc, may be excreted in the urine of the heavy drinker. Prolonged use of alcohol has a toxic effect on the intestinal mucosa, resulting in decreased absorption of thiamin, folic acid, and vitamin B_{12}.

Alcohol is not converted to glycogen, so it cannot be stored; it provides calories but no minerals or vitamins (Fig. 9-4). One ounce (30 ml) of alcohol provides about 200 kcal. About 5% of the alcohol is excreted through perspiration and urine, but the majority is metabolized in the liver at a rate of about 10 g/hour. The excess remains in the bloodstream where it acts as a depressant and an anesthetic, which in turn slows down cellular metabolism. The anesthetic action of alcohol can have serious consequences. The margin of safety for the person anesthetized by alcohol is very small. Unless stimulants are given or the alcohol is removed from the stomach, and attention is paid to respiratory function, death may occur.

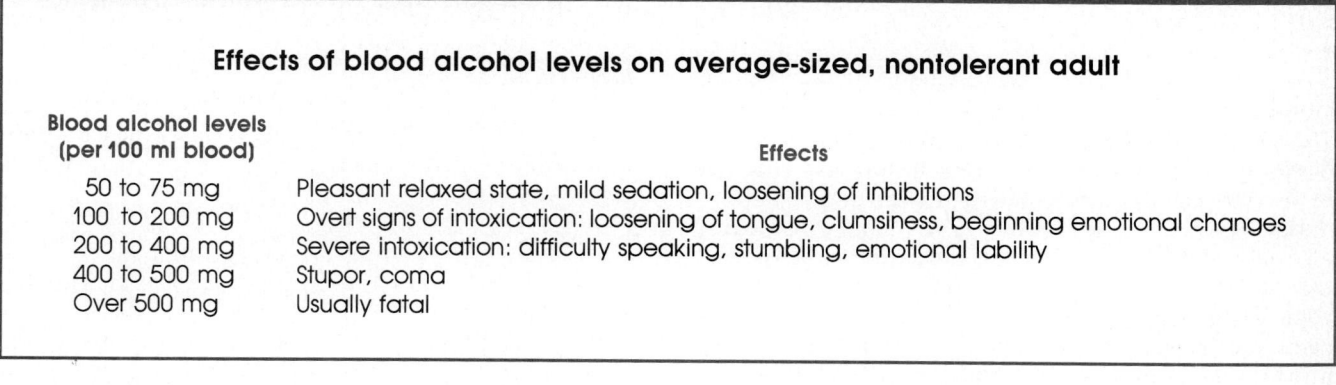

Effects of blood alcohol levels on average-sized, nontolerant adult

Blood alcohol levels (per 100 ml blood)	Effects
50 to 75 mg	Pleasant relaxed state, mild sedation, loosening of inhibitions
100 to 200 mg	Overt signs of intoxication: loosening of tongue, clumsiness, beginning emotional changes
200 to 400 mg	Severe intoxication: difficulty speaking, stumbling, emotional lability
400 to 500 mg	Stupor, coma
Over 500 mg	Usually fatal

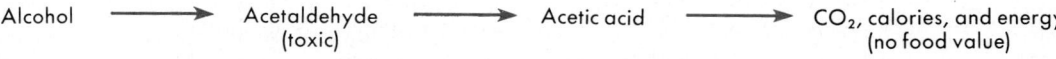

Alcohol ⟶ Acetaldehyde (toxic) ⟶ Acetic acid ⟶ CO_2, calories, and energy (no food value)

Fig. 9-4. Metabolism of alcohol.

Assessment

Alcoholism has been described as alcohol dependence[2] and has all the qualities of substance abuse and substance dependence. Alcoholism may involve physiologic, psychologic, and social dysfunction, showing a pattern of pathologic alcohol use. The National Council on Alcoholism[36] divides alcoholism into a major and minor criteria system and outlines the development of alcoholism on two tracks as follows:

Major criteria

Track I: *Physiologic*
1. Withdrawal syndrome
2. Tolerance
3. Blackout periods
Clinical
1. Alcoholic hepatitis
2. Laennec's cirrhosis
3. Wernicke-Korsakoff syndrome

Track II: *Behavioral, psychologic, attitudinal*
1. Drinking despite medical contraindications
2. Drinking despite social contraindications
3. Subjective complaint of loss of control

Minor criteria

Track I: *Physiologic and clinical*
1. Odor of alcohol on breath
2. Alcohol facies
3. Abnormal liver function test
4. Blood-alcohol level over 300 mg/100 ml at any time

Track II: *Behavioral*
1. Gulping drinks
2. Morning drinking
3. Missing work
4. Frequent automobile accidents
Psychologic and attitudinal
1. Frequent talk about drinking
2. Drinking to release stress
3. Spouse complains about drinking
4. Family disruption

Heinemann and Estes[14] discuss problems involved with assessment of the patient with alcohol problems. They developed a comprehensive nursing history tool that can be used by nurses for assessment of alcoholism.

Habitual drunkenness is the main symptom of the disease of alcoholism. Usually alcoholism develops slowly, over a period of 10 to 20 years, until the persons reach a point where they "drink to live and live to drink." At this point they tend to be irritable and unreasonable. They may lack judgment and develop physical as well as mental ailments.

MALNUTRITION

The true alcoholic is more interested in alcohol than in food. Persons who drink a great deal may get as much as a third of their daily intake of calories from alcohol, and alcoholics may get more calories from alcohol than from any other source. When they obtain the alcohol they wish, they may be too intoxicated to eat or they may have no appetite for normal food. Alcohol is also the most common cause of acute gastritis that results in severe vomiting, which contributes to poor nutrition. Malnutrition may therefore contribute greatly to the alcoholic's physical and mental decline. Alcoholics may be in a general state of poor health with vitamin deficiency, anemia, liver changes, and debility. Resistance to infectious disease is low, and contact with infection is likely during severe bouts of drinking. Consequently, alcoholics are often admitted to the hospital with infectious diseases such as pneumonia or tuberculosis. Cirrhosis of the liver occurs often in persons who are alcoholic, and it is believed that the cause is primarily malnutrition—a lack of protein and perhaps other food constituents that are not contained in alcohol.

POLYNEUROPATHY

Many alcoholics have neurologic symptoms (polyneuropathy) that may include severe pain in the legs and arms and burning of the soles of the feet. Foot drop and wrist drop may develop, and walking and use of the hands may be seriously limited or made impossible. Many alcoholics develop pellagra with its characteristic skin changes of redness, dryness, scaling, and edema. Both pellagra and polyneuropathy are caused by vitamin deficiency and are treated with massive doses of vitamin B complex. Weakening of the heart muscle and resultant heart enlargement ("beer heart") is believed to be caused largely by vitamin deficiency. Symptoms of acute heart failure may bring the patient to the hospital.

Disorders associated with alcoholism	
Hepatic	Alcoholic hepatitis, Laennec's cirrhosis, fatty liver
Gastrointestinal	Gastritis, pancreatitis, duodenal ulcers, malabsorption syndromes, cancer of mouth and esophagus
Neurologic	Peripheral neuropathy, Wernicke-Korsakoff's syndrome, organic brain disease
Cardiovascular, hematologic	Cardiomyopathy, hypertension, familial type IV hyperlipidemia, hypoglycemia, anemia, hyperuricemia
Musculoskeletal	Skeletal myopathies
Immunologic	Increased susceptibility to infections

PERSONALITY CHANGES

Chronic alcoholics often exhibit personality changes and general deterioration of thinking processes. They may be emotionally unstable, suspicious, quick to take offense, and unpredictable in social and related situations. Serious impairment of memory may occur. Severe tremor, visual hallucinations, and loss of memory may develop even if nutrition has been adequate.

Any hospitalized patient who is not known to be an alcoholic but who does not respond normally to preoperative medication, to anesthetics, or to sedatives should be observed carefully for signs of alcoholism. Alcoholic patients usually require large doses of sedatives and anesthetic agents for effect and are likely to be overly excited and active as they react from anesthesia. The most apparent signs of chronic alcoholism that may be noted by the nurse are a tremor that is worse in the morning and morning nausea. These patients feel "jittery," and if alcohol is available, they will have one or two drinks to "steady the nerves" before eating.

Intervention
CARE OF HOSPITALIZED ALCOHOLIC PERSONS

Alcohol may be prescribed for alcoholic patients during their hospitalization, particularly during an acute illness when reaction to deprivation is severe. However, close observation is necessary because even the patient receiving alcohol as prescribed may be extremely resourceful in obtaining an additional supply. If a patient appears to be obtaining unauthorized alcohol, the physician is notified, since additional alcohol may interfere with the medical regimen. Any alcoholic patient admitted to the hospital for an acute medical-surgical condition is observed closely for signs of impending delirium tremens. Early treatment may prevent the development of an acute psychosis.

Regardless of the circumstances surrounding hospitalization, alcoholic patients often feel hopeless, guilty, and apprehensive. If their physical ailment is related directly to alcoholism, they are usually quite ill before they consent to be hospitalized. Often they wish to talk to someone, but the person must be one who seems to accept them as they are and to understand their problems. Nurses providing care to alcoholic patients need to be calm and willing to listen. They should not appear critical of the patients or offer specific advice but should try to make the patients feel that they are ill and that help is available. Patients are more likely to be able to accept help if they feel that they still have their self-respect.

ALCOHOL WITHDRAWAL

Persons with a physical dependence on alcohol experience varying symptoms ranging from mild tremors to severe agitation and hallucinations (delirium tremens) when alcohol intake is withheld. The type and severity of symptoms depend on several factors. Alcoholics at higher risk of experiencing severe withdrawal symptoms are older aged persons, those who have had previous convulsive seizures or delirium tremens with withdrawal, and those with coexisting acute illnesses or nutritional deficiencies. The amount of alcohol consumed and the duration of the drinking episode also influence the severity of withdrawal symptoms.

Tremors may be observed 6 to 48 hours after withdrawal of alcohol and persist for 3 to 5 days. The hands are involved first, but the tremors may become generalized with involvement of the extremities, tongue, and trunk. Chlordiazepoxide (Librium) is useful in reducing tremors without affecting the ability to eat and drink.

Seizure disorders may occur 12 to 24 hours after abstinence. Usually auras do not precede the grand mal seizures, but postictal stupor usually follows them. Dilantin is of questionable value in controlling seizures. Chlordiazepoxide may be helpful, and measures are taken to protect the patient's safety.

Delirium tremens, an acute alcoholic psychosis, is more rare and usually occurs 3 to 4 days after abstinence. It can occur when the confirmed alcoholic is denied a regular supply of alcohol, or it may develop when the patient

---

Terms used to describe responses to drugs/alcohol

Tolerance	Decreased susceptibility to effects because of long-term ingestion of drug/alcohol
Behavioral tolerance	Few changes in social behavior or activities despite ingestion of large amounts of drug/alcohol
Pharmacologic tolerance	Adaptive metabolic changes despite ingestion of large amounts of drug/alcohol
Cross tolerance	Decreased sensitivity to other drugs as a result of tolerance to drug/alcohol
Dependence	Need to continue use of drug/alcohol to prevent symptoms
Physical dependence	Withdrawal symptoms occur when the drug/alcohol is withheld
Psychologic dependence	Person feels the need to take the drug/alcohol to prevent occurrence of symptoms
Cross dependence	Suppression of abstinence symptoms by withdrawal of another drug

is taking alcohol regularly. It may follow injury, infectious disease, anesthesia, or surgery and may develop in patients who have not revealed their alcoholic status to the physician. Delirium tremens is a serious mental illness and may cause the death of the patient. Signs of acute alcoholic psychosis include severe uncontrollable shaking and hallucinations. These patients often say that they see insects on the wall and that rats or mice are on the bed and sometimes that they are biting. They become extremely restless and apprehensive and perspire freely; sometimes true panic occurs. The treatment consists of tranquilizing drugs such as chlordiazepoxide; sedatives such as paraldehyde given rectally, intramuscularly, or orally; and a high-caloric and high-vitamin diet that may have to be given by nasogastric tube. The patient must be protected from physical injury and observed carefully for signs of cardiac failure. Corticosteroids may be given. Recovery usually takes from 1 to 2 weeks.

REHABILITATION

It is only when alcoholic patients truly desire and seek help with their alcohol problem that treatment is useful. The nurse frequently is the person present at the time patients are most ready for help—when they have "reached the bottom" and are suffering from the embarrassment and discomfort of a physical misfortune brought on by drinking. It may be at this time that they are a little more ready to face reality than they have been for some time in the recent past. Nurses' attitudes toward patients and their knowledge of facilities for treatment of alcoholism may be crucial to the life of patients and their families.

The objective of all treatment is to induce patients to stop drinking alcohol. When alcoholics do stop drinking, they can *never take one single drink* on any occasion without serious danger of relapsing. They are never considered cured, and abstinence is their major course. Sedatives and tranquilizers may be administered until they recover from the nervous agitation and insomnia caused by the withdrawal of alcohol. Vitamins and a diet high in calories, proteins, and carbohydrates may be prescribed to improve nutrition and to help overcome weakness and fatigue. Thiamin, 100 to 200 mg IM or IV; folic acid, 1 to 5 mg IM or orally; magnesium sulfate; and vitamin K may be given.

Both group and individual psychotherapy may be helpful to alcoholics in overcoming the desire to drink.

DISULFIRAM

Disulfiram (Antabuse) is an effective deterrent to drinking and is useful as an adjunct to the treatment of alcoholism. In combination with alcohol, disulfiram produces unpleasant physical side effects; thus it serves to weaken the alcoholic person's urge to take the first drink. Used as part of a total treatment program, disulfiram allows the alcoholic to remain sober while undergoing psychotherapy and social and vocational rehabilitation.

Disulfiram interferes with the breakdown of alcohol, causing a buildup of acetaldehyde in the patient's blood. This excessive buildup occurs rapidly, causing the person to experience extremely unpleasant side effects such as flushing, nausea, a sense of suffocation, and difficulty in breathing. This reaction is dangerous in that it could be fatal if the individual continues to drink. Because of the potential severity of the drug's effect, disulfiram should be administered under careful supervision. Both the alcoholic patient and family members should be fully informed of the risks involved and informed that disulfiram potentiates the toxic effects of alcohol.

Disulfiram is not recommended for alcoholic individuals who have serious mental illness, heart disease, liver impairment, diabetes, or epilepsy. It is eliminated slowly. It remains in the body at least 72 hours and one fifth of a dose has been reported to remain by the end of a week. It is important to warn patients not to resume drinking immediately after stopping the medication. While disulfiram has been used as an effective medicine in many cases, its effectiveness depends on the patient's motivation as well as other treatment modalities.

COMMUNITY RESOURCES

Because alcoholism is a major health concern, nurses need to be aware of community efforts and resources for its treatment. Alcoholic persons in the community who are seeking help should be directed by the nurse to sources of help. Most facilities do not require a physician's referral; patients may come themselves. When the person is hospitalized, the nurse works with the physician and social worker before discharge for referral to community sources.

Alcoholics Anonymous (AA) is a group of self-acknowledged alcoholics whose aims are to stay sober and to help other alcoholics gain sobriety through total abstinence. There are AA groups that hold regular meetings in most communities. These self-help groups are open to anyone who has a problem with alcohol, and there are no charges involved. Local AA groups are listed in the telephone directory for each community. A phone call at any hour will bring an AA member to see the alcoholic person desiring help. Some communities have subgroups of AA that meet regularly; these include Al Anon for relatives and friends of alcoholics and Alateen for children of alcoholics. These groups are supportive and educational for family and friends of the alcoholic individual. AA has a high rate of success for its members.

DRUG ABUSE

Epidemiology

In recent years drug abuse has risen sharply. There are no reliable statistics on drug abusers, and experts disagree as to what actually constitutes drug abuse. Some would include repeated use of any drug, while others limit it to those drugs that used repeatedly lead to habituation or addiction.

While there is no general agreement on a definition for

Table 9-1 Effects of mind-altering drugs

Drug	Tolerance	Physical dependence	Psychologic dependence
CNS depressants			
Narcotics	High	High	High
Barbiturates	Moderate	High	High
Glutethimide (Doriden)	Moderate	High	High
Methaqualone (Quaalude, Sopor)	Moderate	High	High
Tranquilizers	Moderate	Moderate	High
CNS stimulants			
Amphetamine	High	Low to moderate	High
Cocaine	Low	Low to moderate	High
Hallucinogens			
LSD	Moderate	None	Moderate
Mescaline	Low	None	Moderate
Phencyclidine (PCP, angel dust)	Low	None	Low
Cannabis			
Marijuana	Low	None	Moderate

drug addiction, the World Health Organization has suggested the following:

Drug addiction is a state of periodic or chronic intoxication produced by the repeated consumption of a drug (natural or synthetic). Its characteristics include an overpowering desire or need (compulsion) to continue taking the drug or to obtain it by any means; a tendency to increase the dose; a psychological and gradually a physical dependence on the effects of the drug; and a detrimental effect on the individual and on society.*

Drug traffic has particularly increased among adolescents and young adults, and drugs are readily available on most elementary and secondary school and college campuses. The use of marijuana is widespread. There is much controversy as to whether it is addicting; many experts say that it is not but may lead to use of "hard" drugs. There have been many reports of actual psychotic episodes following the use of drugs such as LSD (lysergic acid diethylamide) or other hallucinogenic drugs such as peyote or mescaline. It must be remembered that the drug user may have an underlying personality problem that is aggravated by the drug, not necessarily caused by it.

There is uncertainty as to the extent of the narcotic problem because many narcotic users are not known. Heroin is the narcotic frequently used by American addicts today. There are many reported cases of children aged 12 years and under who admit to heroin addiction. There has been a shift toward younger addicts and an increase in the percentage of whites using heroin. Cocaine, a CNS stimulant, is in more frequent use than heroin. Drugs commonly taken in an attempt to "get high" include barbiturates, sedatives, amphetamines,

synthetic analgesics, and cough syrups. The tolerance and dependence effects of mind-altering drugs that are frequently abused are listed in Table 9-1.

The use of drugs is not limited to any socioeconomic group. The problem has long existed in the ghetto, and today it has spread to the affluent suburbs and homes of middle-class Americans. Increased social pressures, the stresses of puberty, the search for self, frustration, and even boredom can lead adolescents to try drugs as they seek something to ease the pain of growing up.

One of the obstacles to early detection and treatment of addiction is the reluctance of parents to admit that their son or daughter is a drug user. Even members of the health professions "overlook" the often obvious symptoms of drug addiction or, having confronted the user, fail to report their findings to the parents or authorities. The incidence of drug addiction is high also among health care professionals, probably because drugs are more available to them than to other groups of people. Occasionally a patient who must be given narcotics to control pain over a long period becomes an addict. It is rare, however, that addiction develops in those given narcotics for real pain, and nurses should not let fear of the development of addiction keep them from administering prescribed narcotics to patients hospitalized and in severe pain.

Assessment

Early indications of drug use vary with the individual but frequently include the following:
1. Abrupt changes in behavior; mood swings
2. Loss of interest in school, sports, and social or other activities
3. Frequent talking and reading about drugs
4. Loss of appetite

*From Expert Committee on Addiction-Producing Drugs: Seventh report, Technical report series no. 116, Geneva, 1957, World Health Organization.

Table 9-2. Acute intoxication and withdrawal of mind-altering drugs

| Drug group | Acute intoxication | | Withdrawal symptoms |
	Symptoms	Treatment	
Narcotics	Respiratory depression, bradycardia, hypotension, cold clammy skin, decreased body temperature; deep sleep, stupor, or coma; pinpoint pupils	Maintain ventilation, provide oxygen Give narcotic antagonist: naloxone (Narcan) 0.4 mg IV Monitor vital signs every 15 to 30 min until patient is conscious Treat for shock	(Not life threatening) Early: restlessness, irritability, drug craving, yawning, lacrimation, diaphoresis, rhinorrhea; followed by "yen" sleep (intense desire to sleep; sleeps restlessly) Later: awakens with more severe symptoms, nausea, vomiting, anorexia, abdominal cramps, bone and muscle pain, tremors, piloerection ("gooseflesh")
Other CNS depressants	Same as narcotics (above)	Lavage if recent oral ingestion Maintain ventilation, provide oxygen Monitor vital signs every 15 to 30 min until patient is conscious Position patient side-lying or prone, not supine Treat for shock Hemodialysis for renal shutdown	(May be life threatening) Insomnia, restlessness, tremors, anorexia, followed by convulsions, and symptoms similar to delirium tremens (confusion, visual and auditory hallucinations), fever, dehydration
CNS stimulants	Labile cardiovascular symptoms (flushing or pallor, pulse and blood pressure changes, arrhythmias), hyperpyrexia, mental disturbances (agitation, paranoia, hallucinations), convulsions, circulatory collapse	Give chlorpromazine, 25 to 50 mg IM Provide a quiet environment Orient patient to reality Monitor vital signs until stable	(Withdrawal is not severe) Somnolence, apathy, irritability, depression, fatigue
Hallucinogens	Physiologic toxicity low at doses that produce strong psychologic effects Acute panic reaction ("bad trip") may lead to suicide "Flashback" episodes Prolonged psychotic disorders (paranoia, depression) Phencyclidine: CNS depression or stimulation may lead to death	Provide quiet, supportive environment and constant attention Give diazepam (Valium), 2 to 10 mg IM for severe anxiety	No evidence of withdrawal symptoms
Cannabis	Adverse reactions infrequent Simple depression, paranoid ideation, confusion, disorientation, hallucinations	Provide support and reassurance Give tranquilizer for agitation	(Withdrawal symptoms rare) Insomnia, anorexia

5. Increased thirst
6. Constipation

When the drug is actually present in the body, the user may seem drowsy or inebriated and be unconcerned about painful stimuli; the pupils of the eyes may be constricted.

After persons have developed a tolerance, they may appear quite normal, converse easily, and carry on activities. Constipation and appetite loss persist, and the person may look undernourished. If the person has been "mainlining" (injecting the drug directly into the vein), needle marks, scars, or small scabs can be seen on the hands and forearms or the instep. Addicts often wear long sleeves to hide such marks. However, many other veins are used as points of entry to conceal addiction, including such inconspicuous areas as the dorsal vein of the penis or the conjunctival artery of the eyelid.

Persons who are drug abusers may develop toxic effects from high doses taken accidentally or in efforts to achieve desired mind-altering effects, especially when tolerance to lower doses develop (Table 9-2). Physical and psychologic symptoms result from withdrawal of the drug. Complete withdrawal of the drug without the substitution of another drug is called "cold turkey" and is a very uncomfortable physical and psychologic condition that may last up to 3 days. Because of the fear of withdrawal or the reluctance to give up the drug experience, addicts often resort to clever ways of smuggling drugs into the hospital. This may occur in spite of the desire to give up drugs.

Because of the expense involved, users often sell their belongings or steal to get the money to buy a "fix." Each day drug abuse in the United States costs the economy millions of dollars. Property loss through crimes connected with drugs can be extensive. The disappearance of such items as radios, watches, jewelry, and other similar objects from the home should arouse the suspicion of parents and friends.

Intervention

In the United States, the addiction to narcotics has been considered a crime ever since the passage of the Harrison Narcotic Act in 1914. The general belief of the Council on Mental Health of the American Medical Association is that narcotic addiction should be considered and treated as an illness. The present methods of treating narcotic addicts are not satisfactory, and the incidence of relapse is high.

There are two federal narcotics hospitals, one in Lexington, Kentucky, and the other in Fort Worth, Texas. Most of the patients in these institutions are there by court order and have little motivation for giving up drugs. Treatment is conservative. More than 90% of these patients return to heroin use. There is much controversy as to the merits of the various programs. Financial problems are serious, and there is much competition for the limited available funds.

Although patients receiving treatment for drug addiction usually are housed in special units of psychiatric facilities, medical-surgical units may have patients who are drug addicts. The drug addict may develop any of the medical-surgical ailments that any other person may have. Because of their poor nutritional state, many addicts have lowered resistance to disease and infection. Their use of contaminated syringes and needles often causes hepatitis.

Drug addicts, in an attempt to get drugs, may seek admission to a general hospital. They may complain of severe pain such as that from renal colic or back strain, since these are disorders for which narcotics often are given even before a specific diagnosis is made. Thus complaints of the drug addict stem from either acute drug toxicity or an abstinence syndrome. These persons need to learn new ways of handling stress and to learn to develop satisfying interpersonal relationships. Education is an important part of their management.[24]

METHADONE MAINTENANCE PROGRAM

One approach to the treatment of narcotic addiction is the methadone maintenance program. Methadone is a synthetic drug, and the average narcotic user's daily dose is inexpensive. The drug is given legally as a part of a rehabilitation program that includes group or individual therapy or both. Methadone reduces the severity of the heroin withdrawal, and the user can often maintain employment while undergoing treatment. Methadone itself is addictive and must be tapered off or the user may continue the habit the rest of his/her life. Because this drug is easily available through legal channels and permits the person to work, methadone advocates feel its use is essentially the same as that of the diabetic taking insulin or that of persons on maintenance doses of other drugs such as steroids or digitalis.

RESIDENTIAL COMMUNITIES

One of the most effective means of treatment to evolve recently is the use of residential communities. Synanon, founded in California, has several chapters across the country. Other centers include the Phoenix and Horizon Houses (New York), Marathon House (Rhode Island-Massachusetts area), and Gateway House (Chicago). Such centers are usually listed in local telephone directories, and the organizations often have literature for distribution and provide speakers for groups.*

The treatment in such communities consists of helping individuals through the withdrawal state and then attempting to help them increase self-understanding and to change their life pattern. Therapy is provided by the group. Rules of the community are strict, and breaking them results in severe consequences. The programs range in length from 18 to 36 months. Many addicts stay in the community after they no longer use the drug and help to rehabilitate other addicts. This provides support, and a good number of former users can "stay clean." Of those who leave the community, many return to drug use.

---

*Additional information on drug abuse can be obtained from the National Clearinghouse for Drug Abuse Information (NCDAI), P.O. Box 1909, Rockville, MD 20850.

REFERENCES AND SELECTED READINGS*

1. *Aguilera, D.C., and Messick, J.M.: Crisis intervention: theory and methodology, ed. 4, St. Louis, 1981, The C.V. Mosby Co.
2. American Psychiatric Association: Diagnostic and statistical manual of mental disorders, ed. 3, Washington, D.C., 1980, The American Psychiatric Association.
3. Bahra, R.: The potential for suicide, Am. J. Nurs. **75:**1782-1788, 1975.
4. Bailey, D., and Dryer, S.: Therapeutic approaches to the care of the mentally ill, Philadelphia, 1977, F.A. Davis Co.
5. Burgess, A., and Lazare, A.: Community mental health, Englewood Cliffs, N.J., 1976, Prentice-Hall, Inc.
6. Carlson, C.E.: Behavioral concepts and nursing interventions, ed. 2, Philadelphia, 1978, W.B. Saunders Co.
7. Corsini, R.: Current psychotherapies, Itasca, Ill., 1978, Peacock Publishers, Inc.
8. *DeGennaro, M., Hymen, R., Cranwell, A., and Mansky, P.: Antidepressant drug therapy, Am. J. Nurs. **81:**1304-1308, 1981.
9. *Ditzler, J.: Rehabilitation for alcoholics, Am. J. Nurs. **76:**1772-1775, 1976.
10. Haber, J., et al.: Comprehensive psychiatric nursing, New York, 1982, McGraw-Hill Book Co.
11. *Harris, E.: Antipsychotic medications, Am. J. Nurs. **81:**1316-1328, 1981.
12. *Harris, E.: Mental status assessment, Am. J. Nurs. **81:**1493-1518, 1981.
13. *Harris, E.: Sedative and hypnotic drugs, Am. J. Nurs. **81:**1329-1334, 1981.
14. *Heinemann, E., and Estes, N.: Assessing alcoholic patients, Am. J. Nurs. **76:**785-789, 1976.
15. Lambert, V.A., and Lambert, C.E.: The impact of physical illness and related mental health concepts, Englewood Cliffs, N.J., 1979, Prentice-Hall, Inc.
16. Lancaster, J.: Community mental health nursing, St. Louis, 1980, The C.V. Mosby Co.
17. *Lewis, L.W.: The hidden alcoholic: a nursing dilemma, Nurs. 75 **5**(7):20-30, 1975.
18. Manfredo, L., and Krampetz, S.: Psychiatric nursing, Philadelphia, 1977, F.A. Davis Co.
19. Mereness, D., and Taylor, C.: Essentials of psychiatric nursing, ed. 10, St. Louis, 1978, The C.V. Mosby Co.
20. Pasquali, E.A., Alesi, E.G., Arnold, H.M., and DeBasio, N.: Mental health nursing: a bio-psycho-cultural approach, St. Louis, 1981, The C.V. Mosby Co.
21. Payton, C.R.: Substance abuse and mental health, Pub. Health Reports **96**(1):20-26, 1981.
22. Reynold, J.L., and Logsdon, J.B.: Assessing your patient's mental status, Nurs. 79 **9**(8):27-32, 1979.
23. Rogers, J.A., and Cohen, S.: Helping depressed patients in general nursing practice (Programmed instruction) Am. J. Nurs. **77:**1007-1038, 1977.
24. Rosenbaum, C., and Beebe, J.: Psychiatric treatment: crisis clinic, consultation, New York, 1975, McGraw-Hill Book Co.
25. *Shontz, F.: The psychological aspects of physical illness and disability, New York, 1975, Macmillan Publishing Co., Inc.
26. Simmons, J.A.: The nurse-client relationship in mental health nursing, Philadelphia, 1976, W.B. Saunders Co.
27. Snyder, J.C., and Wilson, M.F.: Elements of psychological assessment, Am. J. Nurs. **77:**235-239, 1977.
28. Strain, S.: Psychological care of the medically ill, New York, 1975, Appleton-Century-Crofts.
29. Topalis, M., and Aguilera, D.: Psychiatric nursing, ed. 7, St. Louis, 1978, The C.V. Mosby Co.
30. U.S. Department of Health, Education and Welfare: Meeting America's needs, alcohol, drug abuse and mental health administration, Washington, D.C., 1975, U.S. Government Printing Office.
31. Wilson, H., and Kneisl, C.: Psychiatric nursing, Menlo Park, Calif. 1982, Addison-Wesley Co.
32. Wykle, M.: Emotional responses in health and illness. In Phipps, W., Long, B., and Woods, N.: Medical-surgical nursing: concepts and clinical practice, ed. 2, St. Louis, 1983, The C.V. Mosby Co.

Classic

33. Bowles, C.: Children of alcoholic parents, Am. J. Nurs. **68:**1062-1064, 1968.
34. Burd, S., and Marshall, M.: Some clinical approaches to psychiatric nursing, New York, 1963, Macmillan Publishing Co., Inc.
35. Caplan, G.: Principles of preventative psychiatry, New York, 1964, Basic Books, Inc., Publishers.
36. Criteria Committee, National Council on Alcoholism: Criteria for the diagnosis of alcoholism, Am. J. Psych. **129:**127-135, 1972.
37. Erickson, E.H.: Childhood and society, New York, 1963, W.W. Norton and Co., Inc.
38. *Estes, N.J.: Counseling the wife of an alcoholic spouse, Am. J. Nurs. **74:**1251-1255, 1974.
39. Faberow, N., and Schneidman, E.: The cry for help, New York, 1961, McGraw-Hill Book Co.
40. Gerrein, J.R., and Rosenberg, C.M.: Disulfiram maintenance in outpatient treatment of alcoholism, Arch. Gen. Psych. **28:**798-801, 1973.
41. Janis, I.: Psychological stress: psychoanalytical behavioral studies of surgical patients, New York, 1958, John Wiley & Sons, Inc.
42. Kaufman, R., and Levy, S.: Overdose treatment, JAMA **227:**411-413, 1974.
43. Kids and heroin: the adolescent epidemic, Time Magazine, March 16, 1970, pp. 16-25.
44. Kübler-Ross, E.: On death and dying, London, 1969, Collier-Macmillan Co.
45. Maslow, A.H.: Toward a psychology of being, New York, 1968, D. Van Nostrand Co.
46. Mueller, J.F.: Treatment for the alcoholic, cursing or nursing, Am. J. Nurs. **74:**245-247, 1974.
47. Nelson, K.: The nurse in a methadone maintenance program, Am. J. Nurs. **73:**870-874, 1973.
48. Peplau, H.: Interpersonal techniques: the crux of psychiatric nursing, Am. J. Nurs. **62:**111-116, 1962.

---

*References preceded by an asterisk are particularly well suited for student reading.

49. Peplau, H.: A working definition of anxiety. In Burd, S., and Marshall, M., editors: Some clinical approaches to psychiatric nursing, New York, 1963, Macmillan Publishing Co., Inc.

50. Rappaport, L.: The state of crisis: some theoretical considerations, Chicago, 1972, The University of Chicago Press.

51. *Robinson, L.: Liaison nursing: psychological approach to total care, Philadelphia, 1974, F.A. Davis Co.

52. Schwartz, L.H., and Schwartz, J.F.: The psychodynamics of patient care, Englewood Cliffs, N.J., 1972, Prentice-Hall, Inc.

53. Thomas, B.: Clues to patients' behavior, Am. J. Nurs. **63:**100-102, 1963.

54. Umscheid, Sr. T.: With suicidal patients caring for is caring about, Am. J. Nurs. **67:**1230-1232, 1967.

55. Wilner, D., and Kassebaum, G.: Narcotics, New York, 1965, McGraw-Hill Book Co.

UNIT IV
Common Problems Encountered in Medical-Surgical Nursing

10   Fluid and Electrolyte Imbalances

11   Shock

12   Pain

13   Infection Control

14   Cancer

15   Chronic Illness

16   Dimensions of Dying and Death

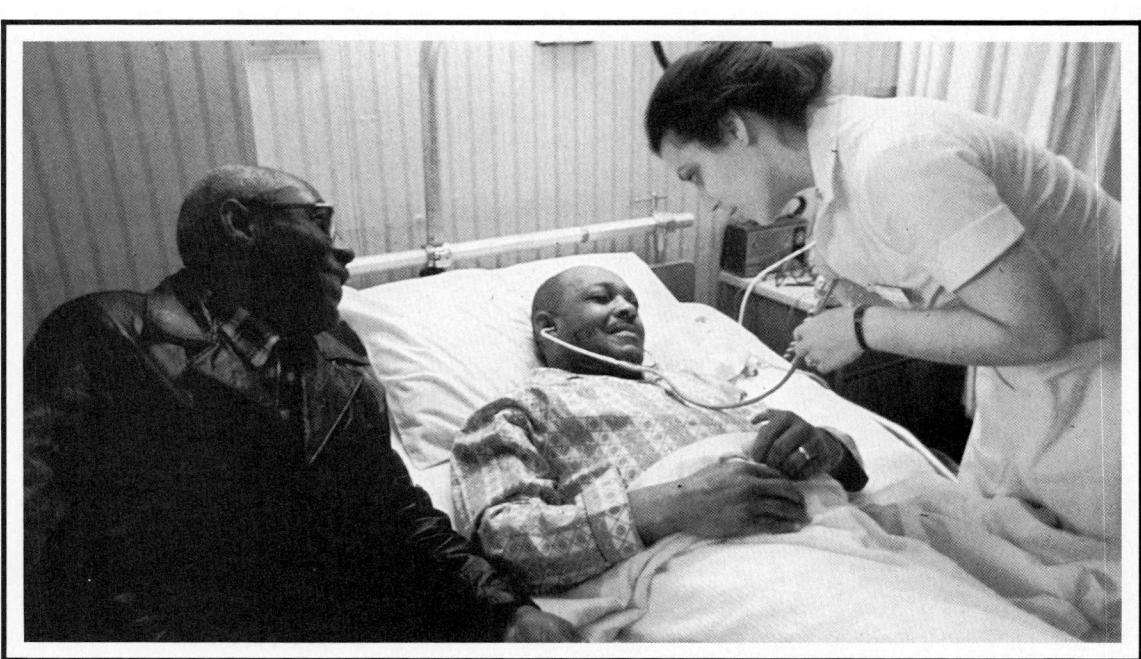

10

Fluid and Electrolyte Imbalances

BARBARA SOLTIS

STUDY QUESTIONS

- Review the sources and actions of the hormones aldosterone, antidiuretic hormone, and parathormone.

- Review methods of giving fluids intravenously (in your fundamentals text or procedure manual).

- What happens when a 5% salt solution is placed in a container in which it is separated by a semipermeable membrane from a 1% salt solution?

- What happens if a solution containing a protein such as gelatin is separated by a semipermeable membrane from water?

- What happens to the extra salt and water you consume when eating a ham dinner?

- If you (or a close friend) have recently had severe vomiting, diarrhea, or high fever, what symptoms did you observe that might indicate a fluid or electrolyte imbalance?

- Examine the laboratory values on the chart of an acutely ill patient. What values are suggestive of a fluid or electrolyte imbalance? What symptoms did the patient demonstrate?

The "internal environment" is a term used to describe body water and the constituent electrolytes and other dissolved substances that sustain all the physiologic processes that maintain life. The amount and distribution of water in the various body compartments, as well as the type and amount of electrolytes and nonelectrolytes dissolved in the water, are kept in an extremely delicate balance by a number of control mechanisms. These mechanisms are so effective that normal values have been established for all constituents of the internal environment in healthy individuals. Knowledge of these normal values is used for detection and correction of imbalances that occur during illness.

The assessment and maintenance of a patient's fluid and electrolyte balance is a major nursing responsibility. This chapter describes some basic information about water and electrolytes in the body and the causes and effects of common fluid and electrolyte imbalances. The last part of the chapter discusses nursing measures employed to prevent, identify, and alleviate these imbalances and to relieve discomfort.

BASIC MECHANISMS OF FLUID AND ELECTROLYTE BALANCE

Body water

A large percentage of body weight is composed of water containing dissolved particles of organic and inorganic substances vital to life. A newborn infant's weight is approximately 75% water, whereas a young adult male's is about 60% and a female's 50% (Fig. 10-1). The percentage of body weight that is water gradually declines with age. Since fat contains little water, the more obese an individual is, the smaller the percentage of weight that is water. Both obese and aged persons have increased risk of morbidity and mortality in situations involving fluid loss because they have less fluid reserve on which to draw.

FLUID DISTRIBUTION

Water is distributed throughout the body but is described as being contained in the following three compartments: intracellular, interstitial, and intravascular. Functionally the fluids in the three compartments are considered as two fluids, intracellular and extracellular (which includes both the interstitial and intravascular) (Table 10-1). The largest percentage of body water is lo-

cated in the billions of individual body cells (Fig. 10-2). Gastrointestinal (GI) secretions, urine, sweat, and exudates are considered extracellular water because when they are lost in large amounts, extracellular volume decreases severely.

FLUID BALANCE

Body fluid is constantly being lost and must be replaced for normal processes to continue. With an average daily intake of food and liquids, the healthy body easily maintains compartmental balance. The body receives water from ingested food and fluids and through metabolism of both foodstuffs and body tissues. Solid foods, such as meat and vegetables, contain 60% to 90% water. Table 10-2 shows the approximate daily intake for an average adult. Note that the normal daily replacement of water equals the normal daily loss. Easily measurable intake (liquid) and easily measurable output (urine) are also approximately equal. These figures therefore serve as guides for determining normal fluid balance and emphasize the great need for recording patient fluid intake and output accurately.

Two vital processes demand continual expenditure of water: the removal of body heat by vaporization of water through the skin and lungs, and the excretion of urea and

Table 10-1. Body fluid distribution

Compartment	Description	Fluid
Intracellular	Fluid within cells	Intracellular fluid (ICF)
Extracellular	Fluid outside cells	Extracellular fluid (ECF)
Intravascular	Fluid within blood vessels	Plasma
Interstitial	Fluid in tissues (between cells or in body spaces)	Examples: interstitial fluid, lymph, cerebrospinal fluid, intraocular fluid, GI secretions, urine, sweat, exudates

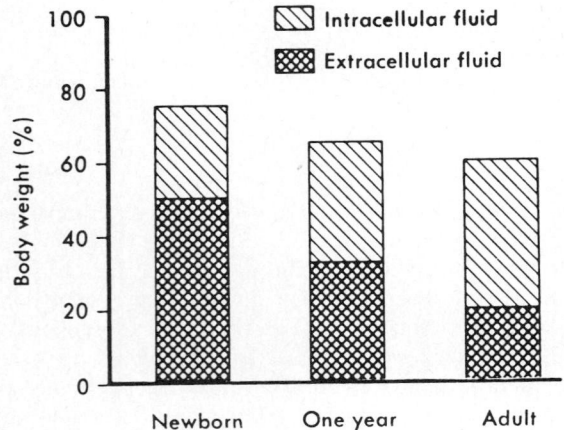

Fig. 10-1. In newborn more than half of total body fluid is extracellular. As the child grows, proportions gradually approximate adult levels.

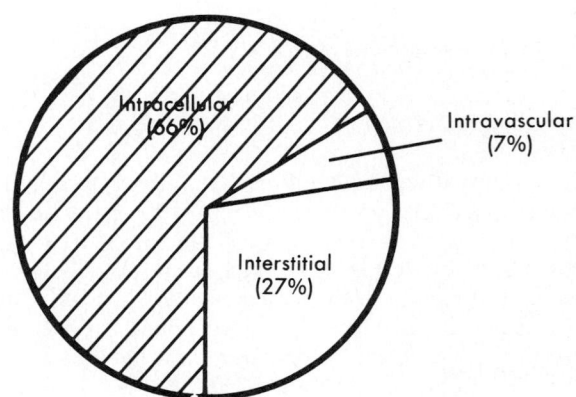

Fig. 10-2. Volumes of body fluids in each fluid compartment.

other metabolic wastes by the kidneys. The volume of water used in these processes varies greatly with external influences such as temperature and humidity.

Body electrolyte component
TYPES OF BODY ELECTROLYTES

All body fluids contain chemical compounds. Chemical compounds in solution may be classified as electrolytes or nonelectrolytes on the basis of their ability to conduct an electric current in solution. Electrolytes in solution break up into charged particles called *ions*. Sodium chloride in solution exists as positively charged sodium ions, Na^+, and negatively charged chloride ions, Cl^-. Positively charged ions are called *cations*. Negatively charged ions are called *anions*. Proteins are special types of charged molecules. They have a charge that is dependent on the pH of the body fluids. At normal plasma pH (7.4) the proteins exist with a net negative charge. Nonelectrolytes such as urea, dextrose, and creatine remain molecularly intact and are essentially uncharged.

Electrolytes account for most of the osmotic pressure of the body fluids, are important in the maintenance of acid-base balance, and help to control body water volume.

DISTRIBUTION OF BODY ELECTROLYTES

The three fluid compartments contain similar electrolytes, but the concentration of the electrolytes in each compartment varies markedly (Table 10-3). Electrolytes move between compartments but most of the exchange occurs between *interstitial* and *intravascular* fluids.

Differences in individual ion concentrations occur in various *extracellular* fluids. For instance, gastric secretion is acid; hence the concentration of hydrogen ions is high. Pancreatic secretion, on the other hand, is more alkaline than plasma and contains a high concentration of bicarbonate. Gastric and pancreatic secretions and bile all contain high concentrations of sodium ions. Knowing the common electrolytes found in various body fluids is helpful in preventing depletion of necessary substances and in noting early signs of imbalance.

ELECTROLYTE BALANCE

In health the ratio of cations to anions in each of the body fluids and the concentration of the various ions in these fluids are relatively constant. Dietary intake and, in some instances intravenous infusions, are the routes by which an individual obtains a supply of electrolytes to replace daily losses and to keep the body in electrolyte balance. Electrolyte loss is mainly through the kidneys, with smaller losses through the skin and lungs and relatively minimal losses through the bowel. The kidneys selectively excrete certain electrolytes, retaining those needed for normal body fluid composition. Hormonal influences affect the kidneys' selective function. For example, the adrenocortical hormone aldosterone, favors sodium reabsorption and the excretion of postassium.

Table 10-2. Normal fluid intake and loss in an adult eating 2500 calories per day (approximate figures)

Intake		Output	
Route	Amount of gain (ml)	Route	Amount of loss (ml)
Water in food	1000	Skin	500
Water from oxidation	300	Lungs	350
Water as liquid	1200	Feces	150
		Kidney	1500
TOTAL	2500	TOTAL	2500

Table 10-3. Normal electrolyte content of body fluids*

Electrolytes (anions and cations)	Extracellular		Intracellular (mEq/L)
	Intravascular (mEq/L)	Interstitial (mEq/L)	
Sodium (Na^+)	142	146	15
Potassium (K^+)	5	5	150
Calcium (Ca^{++})	5	3	2
Magnesium (Mg^{++})	2	1	27
Chloride (Cl^-)	102	114	1
Bicarbonate (HCO_3^-)	27	30	10
Protein ($Prot^-$)	16	1	63
Phosphate ($HPO_4^=$)	2	2	100
Sulfate ($SO_4^=$)	1	1	20
Organic acids	5	8	0

*Note that the electrolyte level of the intravascular and interstitial fluids (extracellular) is approximately the same and that sodium and chloride contents are markedly higher in these fluids, whereas potassium, phosphate, and protein contents are markedly higher in intracellular fluid.

Mechanisms for fluid and electrolyte movement

Fluids, electrolytes, gases, and small molecules move freely through the semipermeable membranes that separate compartments. This movement occurs constantly as oxygen and nutrients are carried to cells and wastes are removed from cells by the blood. In spite of the constant movement of water and dissolved particles *(solutes)* back and forth, the actual amount of water and concentration of solutes in each compartment remain relatively unchanged when the body is functioning normally. The mechanisms by which water and solutes move are osmosis, diffusion, and filtration.

OSMOSIS

Osmosis is the movement of a *solvent* (water) through a membrane from an area of lower concentration of solute to an area of higher concentration (Fig. 10-3). The water moves to dilute the more highly concentrated solution until an equilibrium is reached on both sides of the membrane. The concentration of solute in any one compartment is called *osmotic pressure* or *osmolality* and is determined by the total number of dissolved particles per unit of solvent.

Because of their large size, protein molecules normally have little movement between compartments. Their presence, especially in the intravascular fluid, creates a pressure called *colloid osmotic* or *oncotic* pressure, which functions to hold water within the compartment.

DIFFUSION

Diffusion is the movement of a *solute* from an area of greater concentration to an area of lesser concentration (Fig. 10-4). This is known as *movement along a concentration gradient*. Diffusion includes dispersion of solute throughout the fluid within a compartment as well as movement of the solute through a membrane that separates two compartments until its concentration is equal on both sides of the membrane. The semipermeable walls of blood vessels and cells contain tiny pores through which small molecules and electrolytes diffuse freely.

Large molecules such as glucose are too large to pass through membrane pores and are assisted in crossing the membrane by *carrier substances;* this process is *facilitated diffusion.*

FILTRATION

Filtration pressure is another means by which water and diffusible particles are moved through a membrane. Movement occurs because the weight or pressure of the fluid is greater on one side of the membrane than on the other. Filtration pressure is discussed later in this chapter in relation to normal exchange of water and solutes across capillary membranes (p. 140).

Hormonal control

Three hormones play a particularly vital role in maintaining fluid and electrolyte balance as follows:
1. Antidiuretic hormone (ADH)
   a. Is produced in the hypothalamus and stored and released from the posterior pituitary gland
   b. Acts on the renal tubules to retain water and to decrease urinary output
2. Aldosterone
   a. Is secreted by the adrenal cortex
   b. Acts on the renal tubules to reabsorb sodium and to excrete potassium
   c. Increases circulatory volume by reabsorbing water along with sodium
3. Parathormone
   a. Produced by the parathyroid glands

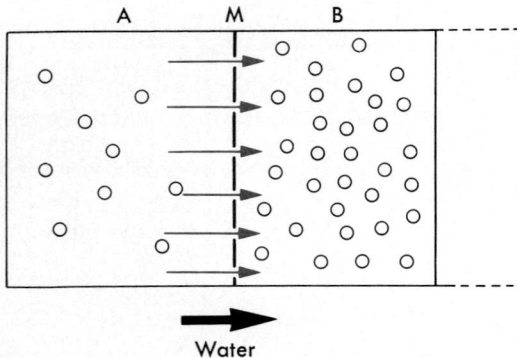

Fig. 10-3. Osmosis: water moves from area of less solute concentration *(A)* through a membrane *(M)* to area of great solute concentrations *(B)* until concentration of solute on both sides of the membrane is equal. Compartment *B* will have to expand (as shown by dotted lines) to accept the additional water.

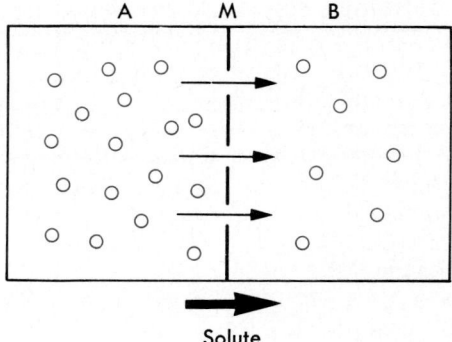

Fig. 10-4. Diffusion: Solute moves through membrane *(M)* from area of greater concentration *(A)* to area of lesser concentration *(B)* until concentration on both sides is equal.

b. Promotes absorption of calcium from the intestine

c. Promotes release of calcium from bone

d. Increases the excretion of phosphate ions by the kidneys

Table 10-4 lists the factors that stimulate or inhibit release of these hormones.

FLUID AND ELECTROLYTE IMBALANCE

Almost all medical-surgical conditions threaten fluid and electrolyte balance. There may be deficits or excesses of water or of any electrolyte. Actually several imbalances occur simultaneously because of the interrelationship of body fluids and their electrolytes. For clarity, imbalances of body fluid and of each ion are considered separately.

Fluid imbalances

Tonicity is a term used to compare the osmolality of a solution to the normal osmolality of body fluids. As previously mentioned, osmolality is determined by the total number of particles dissolved in a unit of solvent. The osmolality of body fluid is measured in milliosmols or thousandths of an osmol because the number of particles in solution is relatively small. Normal osmolality of body fluids is approximately 300 mOsm/L. Solutions relate to normal osmolality in the following ways:

1. *Isotonic:* same osmolality as body fluids
2. *Hypotonic:* less osmolality than body fluids
3. *Hypertonic:* greater osmolality than body fluids

When the body gains or loses fluid in excess of normal fluid balance, the intercompartmental fluid movement that occurs depends on whether the extracellular fluid

Table 10-4. Factors influencing hormone release and effects on fluid and electrolyte balance

Hormone	Factors promoting or inhibiting hormone release	Effect
Aldosterone	*Promotes hormone release* Increased serum potassium Decreased serum sodium Decreased circulating volume	Reabsorption of sodium and water: increased circulating volume, hypertension Excretion of potassium: hypokalemia Excretion of hydrogen ions: alkalosis
	Inhibits hormone release Increased serum sodium Decreased serum potassium Increased circulating volume Spironolactone (diuretic)	Excretion of sodium and water: decreased circulating volume, hypotension Potassium retention; hyperkalemia Retention of hydrogen ions: acidosis
Antidiuretic hormone (ADH)	*Promotes hormone release* Hypertonic plasma Low circulating volume Pain, stress Drugs: narcotics, anesthetics	Reabsorption of water in renal tubules
	Inhibits hormone release Hypotonic plasma Increased circulating volume Alcohol ingestion	Blocking of water reabsorption: loss of water via kidneys
Parathormone	*Promotes hormone release* Decreased serum calcium	Loss of calcium from bone Increased absorption of calcium from GI tract Decreased renal excretion of calcium, increased excretion of phosphate
	Inhibits hormone release Increased serum calcium Increased calcium and vitamin D in diet	Decreased absorption of calcium from GI tract Increased renal excretion of calcium, decreased loss of phosphate

Table 10-5. Fluid imbalances

Fluid imbalance	Pathophysiology	Signs and symptoms	Medical therapy
Isotonic fluid deficit	Decreased body water and electrolytes; extracellular fluid remains isotonic but volume decreases	Hypotension, increased pulse and respirations, cool skin, delayed vein filling, shock, decreased urinary output	Replacement of water and sodium: oral intake of salty fluids; IV of normal saline
Hypertonic fluid deficit	Decreased body water more than decreased electrolytes; water moves out of cells to dilute extracellular fluid (cellular dehydration)	Thirst; skin flushed, dry, poor turgor; dry coated tongue; increased body temperature; increased hemoglobin and hematocrit levels; apprehension, restlessness	Water taken orally, if possible; IV of 5% dextrose in water; additional water given with tube feedings
Hypotonic fluid excess (Water intoxication)	Excess body water without excess electrolytes; water moves into cells causing cells to swell	Behavior changes, confusion, incoordination; sudden weight gain; warm moist skin; lethergy, convulsions	Water restriction; for severe signs: 3% to 5% sodium chloride IV
Isotonic fluid excess (edema)	Excess body water and sodium; excess fluid moves into extracellular spaces	Edema of dependent body parts: pitting over bony prominences; swollen, tight, shiny skin Pulmonary edema: dyspnea; wheezing cough with frothy sputum; cyanosis	Elevation of dependent part; treatment of underlying condition; diuretics, reduced salt intake; treatment of pulmonary edema

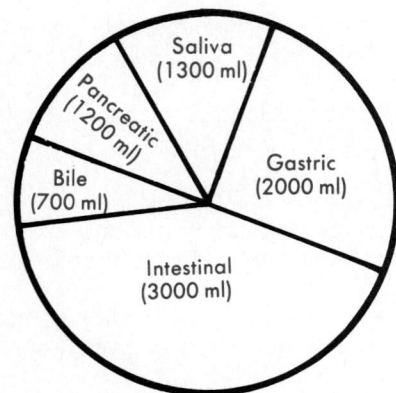

Fig. 10-5. Fluid volume of gastrointestinal secretions.

Losses of fluid and electrolytes

Skin: diaphoresis, oozing from severe wounds or burns
GI tract: profuse salivation, vomiting, diarrhea, GI drainage, enemas
Kidneys: diuretics, polyuria
Hemorrhage
Trapping of fluids: wound swelling, edema, ascites, intestinal obstruction

becomes hypertonic or hypotonic or remains isotonic. The effects of different types of fluid imbalances are illustrated in Table 10-5.

FLUID LOSS

There are a number of ways in which body fluids and electrolytes contained therein are lost or made unavailable for normal fluid and electrolyte balance. The GI tract secretes approximately 8 L of fluid daily (Fig. 10-5), therefore large amounts of fluid may be lost through the GI tract. Loss of both water and solutes leads to *isotonic* fluid deficit with resulting circulatory collapse. Loss of water in excess of solutes leads to a *hypertonic* fluid deficit with resulting dehydration.

Isotonic fluid deficit

Sodium ions constitute most of the osmolality of *extracellular* fluid. If both water and sodium are lost, the result is isotonic fluid loss; the extracellular fluid becomes depleted, and there is a decrease in circulating blood volume (Table 10-5). The body attempts to maintain circulation vital to tissue perfusion by initiating several compensatory mechanisms to preserve adequate circulating volume. If adequate blood volume cannot be maintained by these mechanisms, cardiac output is decreased and blood pressure drops. If volume depletion occurs rapidly, shock may ensue.

Isotonic loss can result from hemorrhage, profuse diaphoresis, and large losses of GI fluids. Treatment is directed toward replacing both fluids and electrolytes.

If plasma proteins are lost from the body, as occurs in hemorrhage, or if they are shifted from the blood to the interstitial fluid, as occurs in burns, the blood volume drops rapidly because fluid from interstitial spaces cannot be mobilized to maintain it, and shock follows. Whole blood, plasma, or plasma expanders usually must be given to these patients to replace the protein loss before extensive fluid therapy is effective.

Hypertonic fluid deficit

When water is lost from the body in excess of sodium and other electrolytes or when water intake is inadequate to replace normal losses, the extracellular fluid becomes hypertonic (Table 10-5). Water moves out of the cells by osmosis to dilute the extracellular compartment and cellular *dehydration* results. As both extracellular and intracellular fluids decrease, cell function is impaired because food, oxygen, and waste products are inadequately diffused.

When solutes are taken in without sufficient water, such as occurs when high-protein tube feedings are given, the extracellular fluid becomes hypertonic. The kidneys attempt to remove excess solute by excreting large amounts of urine; this is known as *osmotic diuresis*.

Dehydration may be encountered in patients who have dysphagia (difficulty swallowing), are unaware that they are thirsty (confused, disoriented), hyperventilate excessively, or have severe diarrhea or diabetes insipidus. Treatment consists of water replacement. Intravenous infusion of 5% dextrose in water is given to the patient who cannot take oral fluids. Water is given along with or between tube feedings.

FLUID EXCESS

Fluid that is retained in the body in excess of normal is termed overhydration. There may be an excess of water without an increase in electrolytes (hypotonic fluid excess) or an increase in both water and electrolytes (isotonic fluid excess).

Hypotonic fluid excess (water intoxication)

If there is an excess of water without an increase in sodium or protein, water enters the cells through osmosis, causing them to swell. This is referred to as *water intoxication* (dilution syndrome) (Table 10-5). This form of overhydration can occur when the water intake is greater than the kidney's ability to excrete it.

Compensating mechanisms resulting from decreased circulatory volume

Mechanism 1

1. Decreased intravascular fluid increases the plasma colloid osmotic pressure.
2. Interstitial fluid is pulled back into the blood vessel to equalize pressure (Starling's law of the capillaries, p. 141).
3. Blood volume is increased.

Mechanism 2

1. Bloodflow through kidneys is decreased because of the decreased blood volume.
2. Aldosterone is released from adrenal cortex resulting in sodium retention and potassium excretion.
3. Sodium retention increases the reabsorption of water because of osmolality.
4. Urinary excretion is decreased and extracellular fluid is increased.
5. Blood volume is increased.

Water excess can occur in the following situations:
1. Excess secretion of ADH as seen in acute stress such as trauma, surgery, pain, fear, acute infections, anesthetics, analgesics (morphine, meperidine), and cerebral lesions
2. Low renal bloodflows, as seen in congestive heart failure, cirrhosis of the liver, acute renal insufficiency, and Addison's disease
3. Large amount of water given rectally as occurs with repeated enemas
4. Frequent and continuous amounts of water taken orally, especially in the seriously ill patient who drinks sodium-free liquids rather than eating solid foods
5. Absorption of irrigating fluids during transurethral resection of the prostate

The signs and symptoms of acute water intoxication result from the swelling of cells, especially in the brain, and may develop rapidly and dramatically. The patient usually recovers with careful water restriction. If convulsions or coma occur or if serum sodium is below 110 mEq/L, rapid treatment is necessary and may be accomplished by infusion of a small amount of 3% or 5% sodium chloride solution intravenously.

Isotonic fluid excess (edema)

If there is an excess of body water with a concomitant increase in sodium (isotonic fluid), the excess fluid is retained in the *extracellular* compartment and leads to the formation of edema (Table 10-5). *Edema* is the accumulation of fluid in the interstitial spaces. In normal tissue there is a negative interstitial fluid pressure, and cells are held in close approximation to facilitate the exchange of gases, nutrients, and waste products between the cells and capillaries. If fluid accumulates in the interstitial space and is not removed, either by direct return to the blood vessel or through the lymph system, a positive interstitial fluid pressure develops, and cells are pushed farther apart. If a finger is pressed over an edematous area, the indentation made by the finger may remain briefly as the fluid is pushed to another area; this is called *pitting edema*. Fluid refills the interstitial space in the "pit" area within a few seconds.

In the healthy individual, edema does not develop immediately with the initial inflow of fluid into the interstitial spaces because of the body's compensatory mechanisms, that is, the existing negative interstitial fluid pressure and the removal by the lymph system of excess fluids and proteins that accumulate in the interstitial spaces.

Capillary dynamics

A review of normal capillary dynamics aids in understanding the various factors that can cause edema to develop. There are two types of pressures that influence the flow of fluid across a capillary membrane: *fluid pressure*

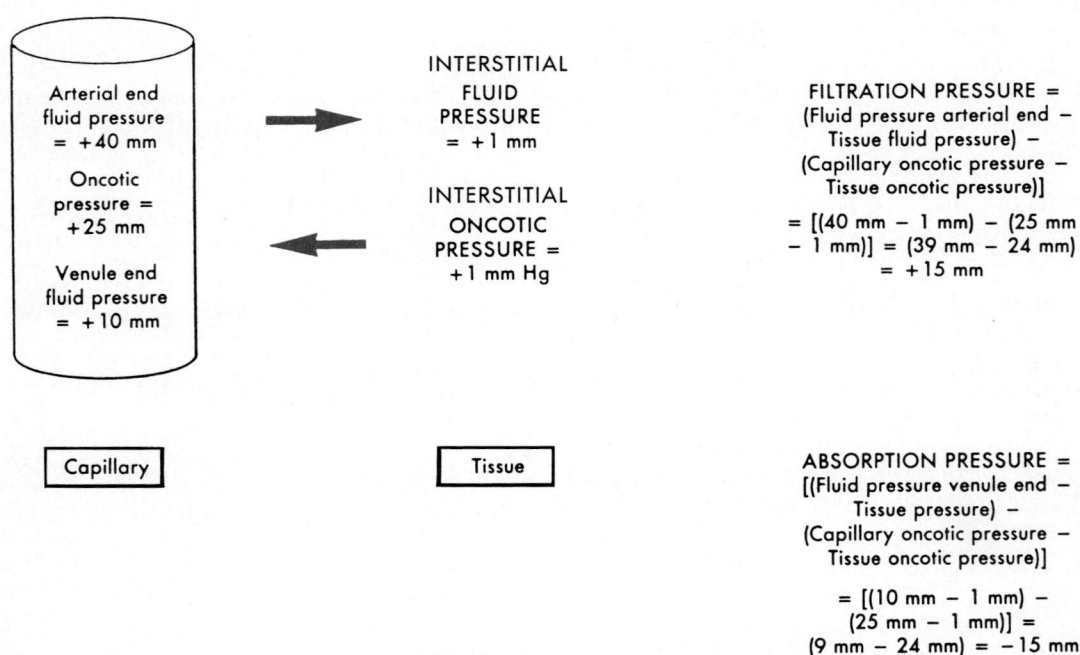

Fig. 10-6. Starling's law of capillaries. An equilibrium exists between forces filtering fluid out of capillary and forces absorbing fluid back into capillary. Note that fluid pressure within capillary is greaten than fluid pressure in tissue. This differential (fluid pressure gradient) serves as a filtering force. Note also that oncotic pressure (colloid osmotic pressure) is greater within capillary. This serves as an absorbing force.

(pressure resulting from the hydrostatic force of fluid) and *colloid osmotic pressure* or *oncotic* pressure (pressure resulting from the presence of proteins that do not diffuse across the membrane wall). Fluid pressure within the capillary is much greater than fluid pressure in the interstitial space; therefore, this force *filters* fluid out of the capillary. Since there are a larger number of proteins in plasma than in interstitial fluid, the oncotic pressure within the capillary serves as a force to *absorb* fluid back into the capillary.

According to Starling's "law of the capillaries," pressures that promote movement of fluid *out* of the capillary are greatest at the *arteriole* end, while pressures promoting fluid movement back *into* the capillary are greatest at the *venule* end. An exchange of fluid occurs across the capillary membrane but an overall equilibrium between the forces filtering fluid out of the capillary and the forces absorbing fluid back into the capillary (Fig. 10-6).

Pathophysiology of edema

Edema was defined as an accumulation of fluid in the interstitial spaces creating a positive fluid pressure. Thus edema can be produced by the following:
1. Increase in capillary fluid pressure
2. Decrease in capillary oncotic pressure
3. Increase in interstitial oncotic pressure (Table 10-6)

The same mechanisms that create edema in the interstitial spaces can create fluid collection in *potential fluid spaces*. These are spaces between two membranes that normally contain only traces of fluid. The main potential fluid spaces are intrapleural (lung and chest wall), pericardial (heart and pericardial sac), peritoneal (intestines and abdominal wall), and joint spaces. Large amounts of fluid also collect in areas of trauma, burn, and surgical wounds. When fluid is abnormally accumulated in any of these places, the condition is referred to as *third-spacing* of fluids. The symptoms of fluid collection in these spaces are usually caused by the pressure of the collected fluid against adjoining organs or structures. Large amounts of fluid may collect in the peritoneal space (*ascites*). This fluid is high in protein and electrolytes. Accumulation of large amounts of fluid in all body tissue is called *anasarca*.

Overloading of vascular system

A major cause of increased capillary fluid pressure is overloading of the vascular system. This overloading results in an increase in the hydrostatic pressure of the blood, in turn resulting in generalized tissue edema. More important, if the increase in hydrostatic pressure is great enough to push large amounts of fluid into the alveoli of the lungs, it rapidly leads to death from "drowning" in one's own fluids (pulmonary edema). The hydrostatic pressure in the pulmonary vessels normally is much lower than that in the general circulation, and therefore any increase is reflected rapidly in the lungs.

Table 10-6. Causes of edema according to underlying physiologic mechanism

Fluid pressure	Oncotic pressure
Increased capillary fluid pressure	**Decreased capillary oncotic pressure**
Increased venous pressure	*Loss of serum protein*
Vein obstruction	Burns, draining wounds, fistulas
Varicose veins	Hemorrhage
Thrombophlebitis	Nephrotic syndrome
Pressure on veins from casts, tight bandages, or garters	Chronic diarrhea
Increased total volume with decreased cardiac output	*Decreased intake of protein*
Congestive heart failure	Malnutrition
Fluid overloading	Kwashiorkor
Sodium and water retention: increased aldosterone from:	*Decreased production of albumin*
Decreased renal blood flow	Liver disease
Congestive heart failure	
Renal failure	**Increased interstitial oncotic pressure**
Increased production of aldosterone	*Increased capillary permeability to protein*
Cushing's syndrome	Burns
Aldosterone added to system	Inflammatory reactions
Corticosteroid therapy	Trauma
Inability to destroy aldosterone	Infections
Cirrhosis of liver	Allergic reactions (hives)
	Blocked lymphatics: decreased removal of tissue fluid and protein
	Malignant diseases
	Surgical removal of lymph nodes
	Elephantiasis

Overloading of the vascular system may be caused by giving too much fluid within a short period of time to a person who cannot dispose of the surplus because of circulatory or renal disease. *Elderly* people tolerate increases in blood volume poorly, since, with inelastic vessels, only relatively small increases in volume are needed to markedly increase hydrostatic pressure. Monitoring the central venous pressure is one method used to determine if overloading is occurring.

Overloading the vascular system also may be caused by increasing the oncotic (pull) pressure of the intravascular fluid by giving proteins so rapidly that the body cannot dispose of those which are in excess of its need. This overloading causes fluids to be pulled into the intravascular compartment from other body fluid compartments. The blood volume increases rapidly, neutralizing the oncotic pressure but increasing the hydrostatic pressure of the vascular system and the oncotic pressure of the interstitial fluid compartment. Fluid is then pushed into the tissues. Overloading is a danger when fluids such as plasma, plasma expanders, albumin, or blood are given to any patient regardless of age or state of health.

Physiology of therapy

Edema is often treated with diuretics. Some diuretics, such as the thiazides, block sodium reabsorption and consequently water reabsorption by the renal tubules. Other diuretic agents are partially or completely unabsorbable by the renal tubules and tend to carry sodium and water with them into the urine. When diuretics are given, a large amount of fluid is lost from the vascular compartment, increasing its oncotic pressure and causing fluid to be pulled back into it from the tissues. Potassium is usually lost along with sodium and water.

Reducing the salt intake also may reduce edema because the remaining supply of sodium seems to be needed to maintain the isotonicity of the blood and therefore is not available for holding water. If edema is caused by venous stasis, elevating dependent body parts and applying supportive stockings promote venous return.

Electrolyte imbalances

Serum electrolytes are measured in milliequivalents per liter (mEq/L), indicating the chemical combining activity of an electrolyte. For example, 1 mEq of the cation sodium is available to combine with 1 mEq of an anion such as chloride or bicarbonate. The concentration of cations in blood serum or plasma is the same as the concentration of anions when expressed in terms of milliequivalents. This is more useful than measuring electrolytes in milligrams per 100 ml, which is only an indication of the amount of an electrolyte by weight and thus gives no information about the relationship between cations and anions. No single electrolyte can be out of balance without causing some others to be out of balance.

Sodium, potassium, and calcium are all essential for the *passage of nerve impulses.* Whenever the concentrations of any of these cations are increased or decreased in body fluids, the increase or decrease is reflected in the stimulation of muscles by nerves. The muscles may become weak and atonic because of inadequate stimulation, or they may become somewhat spastic because of excess stimulation. For example, a decrease in calcium concentration in body fluids causes the stimulus to be increased and results in muscle spasms. GI and cardiac symptoms, so often produced by electrolyte imbalances, result in part from changes in neural stimulation on the muscles of these systems.

With cation imbalances, the *distribution of body fluids* is frequently upset. Abnormal collections of fluid probably cause some of the GI symptoms such as nausea, vomiting, and diarrhea. Decreased amounts may cause anorexia, dyspepsia, and constipation. It is thought that edema of cerebral tissues may be responsible for headache, convulsions, and coma.

SODIUM

Sodium deficit

The normal concentration of sodium in the blood is 138 to 145 mEq/L. A low sodium level in the blood (*hyponatremia*) can indicate either a deficit of sodium or an excess of water. Whenever sodium is lost from the body fluids, the fluids become hypotonic. Sodium loss from the intravascular compartment, therefore, causes fluid from the blood to diffuse into the interstitial spaces. As a result, sodium in the interstitial fluid is diluted. In response to this reduction of the sodium concentration in the extracellular fluid, potassium moves out of the intracellular fluid. Therefore the patient with sodium imbalance is also likely to have a potassium imbalance.

Causes and symptoms of sodium deficit

Causes	Symptoms
Loss of GI fluids	Headache
Vomiting	Muscle weakness
Diarrhea	Fatigue
GI or biliary drainage	Apathy
	Postural hypotension
Fistulas	Nausea/vomiting
	Abdominal cramps
Loss through skin	
Diaphoresis	*Severe prolonged deficit*
Large open lesions (burns)	Shock
	Mental confusion
Shifting of body fluids	Coma
Massive edema	
Ascites	
Burns	
Small bowel obstruction	

Sodium depletion results most often from the loss of GI secretions. It can also occur from losses through the skin and in the shifting of body fluids so that the sodium is not accessible for use.

Anyone who is perspiring profusely because of environmental conditions, exercise, or fever is losing large amounts of both sodium and water. If salt is not replaced with water, such as by drinking salty fluids, water intoxication occurs.

Sodium excess

A serum sodium level greater than 145 mEq/L is known as *hypernatremia*. There are actually two kinds of sodium excess, edema and hypernatremia. When there is a sodium and water excess, edema exists; when there is an excess of sodium in relation to water in the extracellular compartment, hypernatremia exists. As seen in Table 10-7, hypernatremia does not necessarily indicate an excess of total body sodium.

If fluids are markedly limited or if excess salt is taken into the body and retained because of poor renal function, sodium may be concentrated in body fluids. Excess intravascular sodium causes fluid to be withdrawn from interstitial spaces. Extracellular fluids become hypertonic and draw water from the cells, causing cellular dehydration. If fluids are not given to dilute the sodium and if excretion of sodium is not increased, severe fluid and electrolyte disturbances occur, causing manic excitement, tachycardia, and eventual death.

POTASSIUM

Potassium is the major cation of the cells. During the formation of new tissue *(anabolism)* or when glucose is converted to glycogen, potassium enters the cell. With tissue breakdown *(catabolism)*, potassium leaves the cell. This occurs with trauma, dehydration, or starvation. The normal serum level of potassium is 3.5 to 5.0 mEq/L.

Potassium deficit

A serum potassium level below 3.5 mEq/L is known as *hypokalemia*. The body's mechanism for conserving potassium is not as effective as that for conserving sodium, and the kidneys may excrete potassium even when the body needs it. Whenever sodium is being retained in the body through reabsorption by the kidney tubules, potassium is excreted. Thus whenever aldosterone secretion is increased, such as in stress, potassium is excreted. Potas-

---

Causes and symptoms of hypokalemia

Causes	Symptoms
Decreased potassium intake	Muscle weakness
Increased potassium loss	Anorexia, nausea/vomiting
Increased aldosterone activity	Diminished deep tendon reflexes, lethargy
GI losses	Cardiac arrhythmias
Potassium-losing diuretics	ECG changes
Loss from cells as in trauma, burns	*Severe or prolonged deficit*
Conditions causing very large urine output	Flaccid paralysis
Potassium shift into cells	Kidney damage
Treatment of acidosis	Paralytic ileus
Metabolic alkalosis	Cardiac/respiratory arrest

Table 10-7. Comparison of serum sodium levels with total body sodium*

Condition	Serum sodium	Total body sodium
Prolonged sweating	Low (hyponatremia)	Low
Diuretics and low sodium diets	Low	Low
Addison's disease	Low	Low
Edema (cardiac, renal, hepatic disease)	Low or normal	High
Excretion of dilute urine, early stages of gastrointestinal sodium loss	Normal	Low
Excess oral or IV sodium intake	High (hypernatremia)	High
Water and sodium loss with water loss > sodium loss	High	Low

*Note that a low or high serum level does not necessarily correspond with total body sodium.

sium depletion, therefore, is common in many diseases and injuries and during therapy such as surgery. Potassium may also be lost through the urine as a result of certain diuretics such as the thiazides and furosemide (Lasix).

The patient who has a balanced diet withheld for several days, is dehydrated, or is given large amounts of parenteral fluids with no replacement of potassium develops potassium depletion. Dilution of extracellular potassium by the administration of 5% dextrose without potassium supplements and potassium loss caused by catabolism of body proteins account for many electrolyte imbalances in the postoperative patient.

The practice of giving multiple enemas is becoming less common because it is now known that some of the enema fluid is absorbed and dilutes the potassium in the interstitial compartment, upsetting the balance between compartments. Solutions for hypertonic enemas may damage cells in the bowel mucosa, causing potassium loss.

Potassium has a direct effect on cardiac and skeletal muscle function. The patient with potassium deficit shows characteristic electrocardiographic changes of flattened or inverted T waves with a prolonged Q-T interval (see Chapter 26). The most striking symptom of hypokalemia is muscle weakness. Digitalis toxicity can occur in patients taking digitalis if they develop hypokalemia. With severe hypokalemia, the patient may die unless potassium is administered promptly.

The safest way to administer potassium is orally. Fresh fruits (especially oranges and bananas) or foods high in protein are good sources of potassium. A potassium salt may be prescribed orally; if given in liquid form, it should be given in fruit or vegetable juice or chilled to increase palatability. When potassium is given intravenously, the rate of flow must be monitored closely to prevent hyper-

kalemia and atrial arrest. The usual rate of infusion should not exceed 20 mEq of potassium per hour.

Potassium excess

A serum potassium level greater than 5.0 mEq/L is termed *hyperkalemia*. This condition does not occur as frequently as hypokalemia, especially if renal function is normal.

As previously stated, whenever there is severe tissue damage, potassium is released from the cells into the extracellular fluids. Since shock usually accompanies this damage, renal function is reduced, and a high blood potassium level results. There is great danger in giving extra potassium to any patient with poor renal function. If the patient is dehydrated or has lost vascular fluid, glucose and water or plasma expanders usually are given until renal function returns. Untreated adrenal insufficiency also is a contraindication for giving potassium.

The patient with hyperkalemia develops spasticity of muscles because of their overstimulation by nerve impulses. The patient complains of nausea, colic, diarrhea, and skeletal muscle spasms. The muscles later become weak because overstimulation produces an accumulation of lactic acid and because potassium is lost from the muscle cells.

If the condition is not controlled, overstimulation of the cardiac muscle causes the heartbeat to become irregular and eventually stop. ECG evidence of potassium elevation includes tall, peaked, symmetric, or tented T waves with a short Q-T interval. As the blood potassium level increases further, the QRS spreads and atrial arrest occurs.

If the patient who has hyperkalemia needs a blood transfusion, *fresh* blood must be used. Cells in blood that has been kept for several days tend to release potassium

---

Foods rich in potassium

Fruits (including juices)	Vegetables*	Protein foods	Beverages
Apricots	Asparagus	Beef	Cocoa
Bananas	Dried beans	Chicken	Cola drinks
Grapefruit	Broccoli	Liver	Dry, instant tea
Melon	Cabbage	Pork	and coffee
Canteloupe	Carrots	Veal	
Honeydew	Celery	Turkey	
Dried fruits	Mushrooms	Milk	
Figs, dates, raisins	Dried peas	Nuts, peanut	
Oranges	Potatoes	butter	
	White, sweet		
	Spinach		
	Squash		

*Most raw vegetables contain potassium, much of which is lost in cooking.

during storage. A transfusion of stored blood may further increase the patient's serum potassium level.

When hyperkalemia occurs, the patient is allowed nothing orally, and infusion of 10% glucose with 50 units of insulin is often given to induce transfer of potassium from the serum to the intracellular fluid. If the patient is in a state of acidosis (p. 149), correction of the situation results in movement of potassium back to the cell.

Kayexalate, a cation exchange resin, can be given orally or rectally. It results in the release of sodium and binding of potassium, with the potassium then excreted in the stool. If the patient is in renal failure or if the serum potassium is dangerously high, hemodialysis is necessary. The patient is placed on absolute bed rest until the potassium blood level is returned to normal.

CALCIUM

There is a considerable amount of calcium in the human body, most of it located in the bony skeleton and a small amount dissolved in body fluids. Serum calcium level must be maintained at a level of 4.5 to 5.8 mEq/L to maintain vital functions of neuromuscular irritability and blood clotting. Calcium is present in the blood in two forms, free ionized calcium and calcium bound to protein. Only ionized calcium is physiologically active. Both parathyroid hormone and vitamin D are necessary for normal absorption of calcium from the GI tract, for reabsorption of calcium from bone to maintain the normal serum cal-cium level, and for prevention of excess calcium loss in urine.

Calcium deficit

A decrease in serum calcium level below 4.5 mEq/L is termed *hypocalcemia*. Some conditions lead to excessive calcium binding, such as the infusion of large amounts of blood containing citrate (citrate binds calcium) and alkalosis (more calcium is bound in an alkaline medium). When these conditions are present, the patient begins to show signs of calcium deficit, because, although the total amount of blood calcium is not changed, there is less physiologically active (unbound, ionized) calcium available.

Patients with pancreatic disease or disease of the small intestine may fail to absorb calcium from the GI tract, and they may excrete abnormally large amounts of calcium in the feces, thus reducing the blood level of calcium. Hypocalcemia may also occur during the diuretic phase of acute renal failure as calcium is excreted.

The patient with a calcium deficiency usually first complains of numbness and tingling of the nose, ears, fingers, and toes. If calcium is not given at this time, painful muscular spasms, especially of the feet and hands (carpopedal spasm), muscle twitching, and convulsions may follow (*tetany*). There are two tests used to elicit signs of calcium deficiency as follows:

1. Trousseau's sign
   a. Constrict the circulation of the arm by grasping the wrist or inflating a blood pressure cuff

---

Causes and symptoms of hyperkalemia

Causes

Potassium intake in excess of kidney's ability to
    excrete (parenteral or oral)
Renal failure
Adrenal insufficiency
Potassium enters bloodstream, from injured cells
    with extensive trauma
Metabolic acidosis

Symptoms

Nausea, vomiting
Diarrhea, colic
Cardiac arrhythmias
ECG changes
Numbness, tingling
*Severe or prolonged excess**
Flaccid paralysis
Cardiac arrest
Anuria

Causes and symptoms of hypocalcemia

Causes

Excess binding of calcium ions
    Large amount of citrated blood
    Alkalosis
Dietary deficiency of calcium
Chronic renal failure
Draining intestinal fistulas
Deficiency of parathyroid hormone or vitamin D
Increased magnesium

Symptoms

Osteoporosis, pathologic fractures
Tingling around nose, mouth, fingers
Muscle spasms (later tetany)
Nausea, vomiting,
Diarrhea
Cardiac arrhythmias, cardiac arrest
Calcium deposits in body tissues

---

*Prolonged potassium excess results in symptoms similar to those of hypokalemia.

b. Positive sign of serious calcium deficit—hand goes into a position of palmar flexion
2. Chvostek's sign
   a. Tap the face lightly over the facial nerve (just below the temple)
   b. Positive sign of calcium deficit—facial muscle twitching

The specific treatment for a low blood level of calcium is the administration of calcium gluconate or calcium chloride orally or intravenously.

Calcium excess

A serum calcium level above 5.8 mEq/L is called *hypercalcemia*. It may be caused by calcium leaving the bone and concentrating in the ECF (as seen in bone diseases or with prolonged immobilization) or by increased intake and absorption of calcium.

Normal retention of calcium in the bones is believed to be caused by the pressure exerted on bones by active movement or exercise. When a large amount of calcium accumulates in the extracellular fluid and passes through the kidneys, calcium can precipitate and form stones (calculi), a not infrequent complication of immobilization. Calcium precipitates more readily in alkaline solution. This can be a problem in a urinary tract infection, which increases the alkalinity of the urine.

Treatment for hypercalcemia is removal of the cause. Intravenous saline and a diuretic (furosemide) may be given to promote renal excretion of the calcium. Oral or intravenous phosphate may also be given, since calcium is excreted when phosphorus serum levels are increased.

Nursing responsibilities for the person with hypercalcemia include the following:
1. Active exercises for immobilized persons
2. Increased fluid intake (3000-4000 ml/day) for both high-risk persons and those with hypercalcemia
3. Prevention of urinary tract infection
4. Gentle handling to prevent pathologic fractures.

MAGNESIUM

The normal serum magnesium level is within the range of 1.5 to 2.5 mEq/L. About 50% of magnesium is located in bones, 5% in ECF, and the remaining 45% within the cells. It functions in the activation of enzymatic reactions, especially in carbohydrate metabolism. Magnesium has a sedative effect on the CNS similar to that of calcium. High serum levels result in vasodilation and lowering of blood pressure; this rarely occurs except with kidney failure.

Metabolically, magnesium is closely interrelated with both calcium and potassium. In the presence of a large amount of calcium in the GI tract, calcium is absorbed in preference to magnesium, and the magnesium is excreted. Conversely, low calcium levels increase magnesium absorption. The kidneys effectively conserve magnesium when intake is low.

Causes and symptoms of hypercalcemia

Causes

Loss from bone
Immobilization
Metastatic bone cancer
Multiple myeloma

Excess intake
Dietary
Antacids containing calcium

Increased absorption
Increased parathyroid hormone
Increased vitamin D

Symptoms

Thirst, polyuria
Renal stones
Decreased deep tendon reflexes
Lethargy, coma
Cardiac arrhythmias, cardiac arrest
Decreased muscle tone
Decreased GI motility

Causes and symptoms of hypomagnesemia

Causes

Decreased intake
    Prolonged malnutrition
    Starvation
Impaired absorption from GI tract
    Alcoholism
    Hypercalcemia
    Diarrhea
    Draining intestinal fistulas
Conditions causing large losses of urine

Symptoms

Mental changes
    Agitation, depression, confusion
    Paresthesias
    Tremors
    Ataxia
    Cramps, spasticity, tetany
    Tachycardia
Hypotension
Arrhythmias

Magnesium deficit

Hypomagnesemia is a serum magnesium level below 1.5 mEq/L. It may be caused by impaired absorption from the GI tract, excess loss through the kidneys, or prolonged malnutrition states.

A low serum magnesium level leads to increased neuromuscular irritability. Hypomagnesemia is usually manifested by behavioral and neurologic symptoms such as confusion, hallucination, convulsions, increased reflexes, muscle spasms, and parasthesias.

Nursing responsibilities for the person with hypomagnesemia include the following:
1. Encouraging foods high in magnesium (fruits, green vegetables, whole grain cereals, milk, meats, and nuts)
2. Careful observation and supervision of the patient who is confused or hallucinating
3. Providing for patient safety if convulsions occur

Magnesium excess

Hypermagnesemia is a serum magnesium level greater than 2.5 mEq/L. The action of magnesium is on the myoneural junction where a high magnesium level blocks acetylcholine release, decreasing the excitability of the muscle cells. Hypermagnesemia rarely develops unless there is renal failure, although it has been identified in diabetic ketoacidosis where there is severe water loss. In persons with renal failure, frequent use of magnesium-containing antacids or cathartics can cause toxicity. The vasodilating effect of magnesium is accentuated in hypermagnesemia and can lead to hypotension. There may be loss of deep tendon reflexes, respiratory depression, and cardiac arrest.

Correction of the underlying cause corrects magnesium excess. If renal failure is present, dialysis is necessary. Intravenous calcium gluconate may be a useful temporary treatment, since calcium has an antagonistic effect on magnesium.

ACID-BASE BALANCE AND IMBALANCE

Acid-base balance

BUFFER SYSTEM

Cells are sensitive to changes in the pH (hydrogen ion concentration) of body fluids. The maintenance of a stable pH of body fluids is essential to life. Normal body fluid is slightly alkaline (pH 7.35 to 7.45) and is maintained in a relatively stable condition by buffer systems in the body.

A *buffer* is a substance that can act as a chemical sponge, either soaking up or releasing hydrogen ions so that the pH remains relatively stable. The main buffer systems of the ECF are hemoglobin, protein, and the carbonic acid-bicarbonate system. The latter is the most important clinically. Two types of carbonate are present in body fluids—carbonic acid (H_2CO_3) and bicarbonate (HCO_3^-). The ability of the body to keep the pH of body

fluids within normal limits relies essentially on maintenance of the normal ratio of *one part of carbonic acid to 20 parts of bicarbonate* (Fig. 10-7).

Carbonic acid concentration is controlled by the lungs, because if carbon dioxide is retained in large amounts, more is available to combine with water to form carbonic acid in the following chemical reaction:

$$CO_2 + H_2O—H_2CO_3$$

The amount of carbon dioxide expelled is varied by the rate and depth of respiration.

Bicarbonate concentration is controlled by the *kidneys,* which selectively retain or excrete bicarbonate, depending on body needs.

LABORATORY TESTS

Information about a patient's acid-base status is obtained by testing a sample of arterial blood (arterial blood gas) for the following values:
1. pH (normal 7.35-7.45): measure of hydrogen ion concentration.
2. P_{CO_2} (normal 40 mm Hg): partial pressure of carbon dioxide.
3. Bicarbonate (normal 27 mEq/L): sometimes reported as carbon dioxide content, which is a measure of all carbon dioxide dissolved in the blood as carbonic acid and bicarbonate. The approximate bicarbonate can be determined by subtracting 1 mEq/L from the carbon dioxide content.

The P_{O_2}, partial pressure of oxygen, is also measured and indicates how well the patient is obtaining oxygen, but does not indicate the acid-base status.

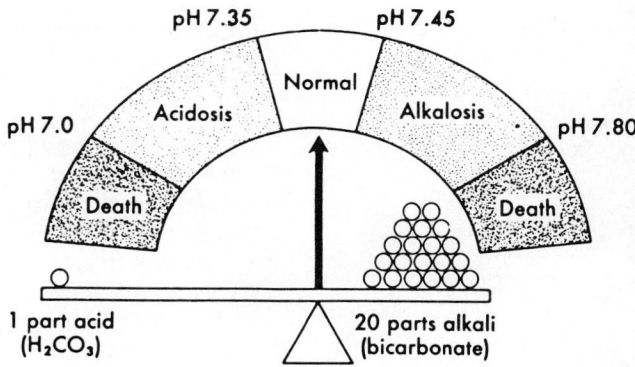

Fig. 10-7. Note that relationship of 1 part carbonic acid to 20 parts bicarbonate will maintain hydrogen ion concentration (pH) within normal limits. Increase in H_2Co_3 or decrease in HCO_3 will cause acidosis; similarly, decrease in H_2CO_3 or increase in HCO_3 will cause alkalosis. (Redrawn from Abbott Laboratories: Fluid and electrolytes, North Chicago, Ill., 1970, Abbott Laboratories.)

Acid-base imbalance

When the buffer systems are unable to maintain the hydrogen ion concentration (pH) of the blood within the normal range, the blood becomes more acid (*acidosis*) or more basic (*alkalosis*). If the pH of the blood drops below 6.8 or rises above 8.0, death usually ensues (Fig. 10-7). Carbonic acid (PCO_2) excess or deficit is referred to as *respiratory* acidosis or alkalosis, whereas base bicarbonate change is called *metabolic* acidosis or alkalosis. Changes in laboratory values are illustrated in Table 10-8.

Maintenance of the 20:1 ratio of bicarbonate to carbonic acid is crucial to keeping serum pH within the nor-

mal range. Actual amounts of both bicarbonate and carbonic acid may vary, but the pH remains normal as long as the 20:1 ratio exists. For example, if the PCO_2 indicator of carbonic acid rises, the bicarbonate rises to keep the normal ratio between these two substances intact. This effort of the body to maintain normal pH when acidosis or alkalosis occurs is known as *compensation*.

There are two other compensatory mechanisms besides the buffer systems. The first is the action of hydrogen ions on the respiratory center in the medulla to *increase or decrease rate and depth of breathing*. As a result, carbon dioxide is removed rapidly or retained to a greater extent in the blood. This decreases or increases carbonic acid content.

Table 10-8. Serum levels of pH, PCO_2, HCO_3^- seen in acidosis and alkalosis

| | Metabolic levels | | Respiratory levels | |
	Acidosis	Alkalosis	Acidosis	Alkalosis
Serum pH	Decreased below 7.35	Increases above 7.45	Decreases below 7.35	Increases above 7.45
PCO_2	Normal Begins to decrease to less than 40 mm Hg to compensate	Normal Begins to increase to more than 40 mm Hg to compensate	Increases above 40 mm Hg (because of excessive retention of carbon dioxide)	Decreases below 40 mm Hg (result of excessive loss o carbon dioxide)
HCO_3^-	Decreases below 27 mEq/L	Increases above 27 mEq/L	Normal Increases to more than 27 mEq/L to compensate	Normal Decreases to less than 27 mEq/L to compensate
Urine pH	Less than 6.0	More than 7.0	Less than 6.0	More than 7.0

Table 10-9. Types of acid-base disturbances and compensatory mechanisms

Disturbance	Physiologic causes	Method of compensation
Respiratory acidosis	Carbonic acid excess: lungs not removing sufficient CO_2 (hypoventilation)	Bicarbonate production by kidneys increased; bicarbonate retained and chloride excreted instead by kidneys; secretion and excretion of hydrogen ions in urine increased
Respiratory alkalosis	Carbonic acid deficit: lungs removing too much CO_2 (hyperventilation)	Kidneys increase excretion of bicarbonate ions
Metabolic acidosis	Bicarbonate deficit: retention of acid metabolites, diabetic ketoacidosis, excess acid intake (salicylate poisoning), or loss of bicarbonate	Increased rate and depth of respiration cause increased excretion of CO_2 by lungs; formation of bicarbonate ions in the kidneys increased
Metabolic alkalosis	Bicarbonate excess: excess intake (sodium bicarbonate, carbonated drinks) or retention of bicarbonate Potassium depletion Loss of acid	Rate and depth of respiration decreased; lungs retain more CO_2; kidneys excrete bicarbonate

The second mechanism is the *excretion of an acid or alkaline urine by the kidneys.* In acidosis the kidney reabsorbs bicarbonate and excretes hydrogen ions with nonbicarbonate ions or as ammonia (NH_4). The reverse occurs with alkalosis (Table 10-9). When conditions leading to acid-base imbalances occur, the compensatory mechanisms are not completely effective. Normal pH can only be attained by correction of the underlying cause.

The major effect of acidosis is depression of the CNS as evidenced by disorientation followed by coma. *Alkalosis* is characterized by overexcitability of the nervous system, and the muscles may go into a state of tetany and convulsions. Acid-base imbalances always produce an imbalance of the body's electrolytes as well; therefore, symptoms of these imbalances also occur.

BICARBONATE DEFICIT (METABOLIC ACIDOSIS)

When acid production or addition of acid by ingestion exceeds acid loss, bicarbonates attempt to buffer the acid load; but the bicarbonate supply soon becomes depleted and a bicarbonate deficit, metabolic acidosis, results (Table 10-9). Bicarbonate may also become depeleted by losses of large amounts of alkaline secretions, such as intestinal secretions.

Increased acid production occurs during the development of ketoacidosis, uremic acidosis, or lactic acidosis. In *ketoacidosis,* glucose either cannot be used or is not available for oxidation. The body compensates for this by using body fat for energy, thus producing abnormal amounts of ketone bodies, which are fatty acids. Ketoac-

idosis also develops whenever a person does not eat sufficient food to meet daily needs and body fat must be burned for energy. It is the reason why extremely low-carbohydrate or high-protein—zero-carbohydrate reduction diets are criticized by nutrition experts.

Lactic acidosis results when lactic acid is produced in large quantities by anerobic oxygenation, such as occurs with shock. *Uremic acidosis* results from the inability of the failing kidney to excrete the acid end products of metabolism.

Hyperkalemia may result during metabolic acidosis; as the hydrogen ion concentration of the extracellular fluid increases, hydrogen moves into the cell and potassium moves out into the bloodstream.

The patient in acidosis becomes hyperpneic and has deep, periodic breathing. Hyperventilation represents an attempt to blow off carbon dioxide and to lower the P_{CO_2}, thus compensating for the acidosis. If the condition is untreated, disorientation, stupor, coma, and death occur.

Metabolic acidosis is controlled by giving an intravenous solution of sodium bicarbonate or sodium lactate. Sodium bicarbonate sometimes is given orally if it can be retained. Treatment of the condition precipitating the acidosis is then instituted.

BICARBONATE EXCESS (METABOLIC ALKALOSIS)

When acid loss is greater than acid production, there is a loss of hydrogen ions from body fluids and bicarbonate excess (metabolic alkalosis) exists. An excess may also occur with an excessive intake of sodium bicarbonate or other alkaline salt, especially if renal function is impaired.

Loss of potassium can also lead to metabolic alkalosis. When potassium is lost from the body, hydrogen ions

---

Causes and effects of metabolic acidosis

Causes

Increased acid production
    Ketoacidosis (uncontrolled diabetes mellitus, starvation)
    Uremic acidosis (kidney failure)
    Lactic acidosis (shock, respiratory or cardiac arrest)
Increased acid ingestion
    Salicylates, ethanol, ethylene glycol
Loss of bicarbonate
    Severe diarrhea
    Intestinal fistulas

Effects

Hyperventilation
    Weakness
    Hyperkalemia
    Disorientation
    Coma

Causes and effects of metabolic alkalosis

Causes

Loss of stomach acid
    Gastric suctioning
    Persistent vomiting
Excess alkali intake
Loss of potassium
Biliary drainage
Intestinal fistulas
Diarrhea

Effects

Numbness, tingling of extremities
Hypertonic muscles, tetany
Bradycardia
Depressed respirations

move into the cells to replace the lost potassium, leaving a decreased hydrogen ion concentration in the extracellular fluid, that is, metabolic alkalosis.

In metabolic alkalosis, breathing becomes depressed in an effort to conserve carbon dioxide for combination with hydrogen ions in the blood to raise the blood level of carbonic acid (Table 10-9).

Treatment consists of administration of sodium chloride or ammonium chloride. If the condition is associated with a loss of sodium chloride, potassium must be restored because it is lost with the sodium.

CARBONIC ACID EXCESS (RESPIRATORY ACIDOSIS)

Any condition that decreases the rate of pulmonary ventilation increases the concentration of dissolved carbon dioxide and hydrogen ions and results in a build-up of carbonic acid known as respiratory acidosis. The excess of carbon dioxide (hypercapnia) can cause *carbon dioxide narcosis*. In this condition carbon dioxide levels are so high that they no longer stimulate respirations but depress them. Associated with the decreased respiratory rate are lack of oxygen and hypoxia. During respiratory acidosis, potassium moves out of the cells, producing hyperkalemia. Ventricular fibrillation may occur if the blood potassium levels are greatly increased.

Treatment is aimed at increasing the excursion of the lungs to improve the exchange of carbon dioxide and oxygen. This objective is accomplished by using positive pressure breathing and bronchodilators to assist the patient in exhaling carbon dioxide. Because the respiratory center is narcotized by increased amounts of carbon dioxide, the lowered oxygen tension of the blood maintains respiration. For this reason, oxygen is never given to patients with carbon dioxide narcosis, and low flow oxygen is used when a patient has an impaired ability to exhale carbon dioxide normally.

CARBONIC ACID DEFICIT (RESPIRATORY ALKALOSIS)

Excessive pulmonary ventilation decreases hydrogen ion concentration and the formation of carbonic acid, leading to respiratory alkalosis. A common cause of respiratory alkalosis is *hyperventilation*. A person who hyperventilates blows off large amounts of carbon dioxide.

Respiratory alkalosis can be prevented in a person who is hyperventilating by administering a few whiffs of carbon dioxide or by having the person breathe into a paper bag and then rebreathe the exhaled carbon dioxide. Care should be taken in adjusting mechanical respirators so the patient does not breathe too deeply or too rapidly.

The patient may complain of lightheadedness and numbness or tingling of the fingers and toes. If the alkalosis becomes more severe, tetany and convulsions may be present. Serum potassium levels will decrease because potassium moves into the cells as hydrogen ions move out in an attempt to correct the alkalosis.

Treating the underlying condition usually effectively resolves respiratory alkalosis. Respiratory alkalosis becomes especially dangerous when it leads to cardiac arrhythmias caused partly by a decreased serum potassium level. If tetany is present, calcium gluconate is given intravenously. Renal function must be maintained to promote renal compensation of the alkalosis.

Causes and effects of respiratory acidosis

Causes

Damage to respiratory center in medulla
Depression of respiratory center by drugs (narcotics)
Obstruction of respiratory passages: pneumonia, chronic bronchitis
Loss of lung surface for ventilation
    Atelectasis
    Pneumothorax
    Emphysema
Weakness of respiratory muscles

Effects

Rapid breathing
Visual disturbances
Confusion
Drowsiness
Headache
Coma

Causes and effects of respiratory alkalosis

Causes

Hyperventilation syndrome (caused by anxiety, hysteria)
Hyperventilation caused by:
    Fever
    Hypoxia
Pulmonary disorders
CNS lesions
Excess assisted ventilation

Effects

Paresthesias: numbness and tingling around mouth and in extremities
Inability to concentrate
Blurred vision
Dry mouth
Coma

ASSESSMENT OF FLUID AND ELECTROLYTE BALANCE

Patient data

The nurse should be familiar with signs and symptoms of fluid and electrolyte disturbances. Since these symptoms are frequently subtle, it is necessary to have a high degree of sensitivity to the possibility of occurrence in certain persons, as in the following:

1. Has an illness of a type that usually disrupts fluid and electrolyte balance
2. Has medical-surgical treatments that result in imbalances
3. Has considerable limitation of food and fluid intake
4. Sustains significant loss of body fluids

With knowledge of conditions that put an individual at risk and by making careful ongoing assessments, the nurse can prevent or detect imbalances before they become severe.

Table 10-10. Data supporting fluid and electrolyte imbalances

	Signs and symptoms	Imbalance
Change in mental status	Irritable, restless	Sodium or potassium excess
	Confusion, lethargy	Sodium or calcium excess or deficit
		Hypotonic fluid excess
		Isotonic fluid deficit
Head/neck	Dry sticky mucous membranes	Sodium excess
	Facial puffiness (edema)	Isotonic fluid excess
	Distended neck veins	Isotonic fluid excess
	Thirst, dry mucous membranes, longitudinal furrows on tongue	Isotonic fluid deficit
	Flat neck veins in supine position	Isotonic fluid deficit
Temperature	Increase	Water loss, sodium excess
	Decrease	Fluid excess
GI	Absent bowel sounds (ileus)	Potassium deficit
	Anorexia, nausea, vomiting	Fluid excess or deficit
		Potassium excess or deficit
		Calcium excess
Circulation	Increased blood pressure	Increased circulatory volume
		Magnesium deficit
	Decreased blood pressure	Decreased circulatory volume
		Magnesium excess
	Increased pulse, slow vein filling	Potassium excess or deficit
		Isotonic fluid deficit
	Bounding pulse	Increased circulating volume
		Potassium excess or deficit
	Weak, irregular pulse Cardiac arrhythmias	Potassium excess or deficit
Respiration	Dyspnea, orthopnea, moist breath sounds	Isotonic fluid excess
	Decreased rate	Magnesium excess
Skin	Pale, cool extremities (without edema)	Decreased circulating volume
	Pitting edema	Isotonic fluid excess
	Poor turgor (test over sternum)	Fluid deficit, sodium excess
	Dryness in groin, axillae	Isotonic fluid deficit
	Flushed dry skin	Sodium excess
Neuromuscular	Numbness, tingling around mouth, fingers, toes	Calcium deficit
	Increased irritability, muscle spasms	Calcium deficit
	Muscle weakness, paralysis	Potassium deficit
	Decreased muscle tone, decreased deep tendon reflexes	Magnesium deficit
	Abdominal cramps	Potassium excess

Subjective data include thirst, headache, pain, nausea, dyspnea, and orthopnea. The time of origin and a description of symptoms are noted. *Objective* data, as noted in Table 10-10, can be compared to the baseline assessment obtained at the time of the patient's initial contact with health care providers.

Laboratory values

Laboratory determinations of serum levels of the specific electrolytes help in making decisions concerning electrolyte excesses or deficits. When electrolyte disturbances develop slowly, symptoms may not be pronounced, and the problem may be detected only by a determination of the electrolyte concentration in the patient's blood. Serum pH and PCO_2 levels help in identifying acid-base balances (Table 10-8). When there is excess water hemodilution occurs, and the hemoglobin and hematocrit levels are decreased. With excessive fluid loss, there is hemoconcentration, and the hematocrit and BUN levels are increased.

Additional data

Important data to be considered in assessing fluid balances are comparison of fluid intake to output and changes in patient weight. Acutely ill medical patients and patients undergoing major surgery need to have their fluid intake and output and daily weight closely monitored. The practice of totaling the fluid intake and output every shift or every 24 hours provides additional data for determining whether or not the patient has a fluid imbalance.

FLUID INTAKE

The intake record should show the type and amount of all fluids the patient has received and the route by which these were administered. This includes fluids given orally, parenterally, rectally, or fluids administered by tubes and retained by the patient. Foods that are eaten in a semisolid state but are basically liquid, such as gelatin or ice cream are recorded as fluids. Ice chips are recorded by dividing the amount of chips by one half (60 ml of ice chips would equal 30 ml water). Patients may receive a considerable amount of fluid intake through the frequent sucking of ice chips.

FLUID OUTPUT

Urinary output

Urinary output is recorded as to time and amount of each voiding to help evaluate renal function. If renal function is a major concern, such as in the patient with shock, an indwelling catheter is used so the amount of urine can be recorded every hour and fluid intake regulated accordingly.

Wound drainage

Any drainage from a catheter draining a wound is measured and the amount and character of the drainage is recorded. If there is excessive drainage on dressings, it may be necessary to weigh the dressings. Fluid loss equals the difference between the wet weight and dry weight of the dressing.

GI drainage

Electrolytes are lost in large amounts with vomiting, diarrhea, and gastric and intestinal drainage. The amount and kind vary according to the type of GI fluid lost. For determination of the amount and type of fluid replacement, vomitus, GI drainage, and liquid stools are measured as accurately as possible and are described as to consistency, color, and odor (Table 10-11). Fluid used to irrigate nasogastric tubes is subtracted from total drainage before it is recorded.

Other output

Fluid aspirated from any body cavity, such as the abdomen or pleural spaces, must be measured. This fluid contains not only electrolytes but also proteins.

Diaphoresis is difficult to measure. If the clothing and linen become saturated, there may be as much as 1000 ml of fluid lost in perspiration. Dry and wet weights may be taken to get a more accurate measure of the amount of fluid loss.

DAILY WEIGHT

The daily weight record is often the best way to determine the onset of dehydration or of the accumulation of fluid either as generalized edema or as "hidden" fluid in body cavities. *An increase of 1 kg in weight is equal to the retention of 1 L of fluid.* If the weight record is to be useful, the patient must be weighed on the same scale and

Table 10-11. GI output

Type of fluid	Consistency	Color	Odor
Gastric	Watery	Pale yellow-green	Sour Fruity odor with metabolic acidosis
Biliary	Thicker than gastric	Bright yellow to dark green	Acrid odor and bitter taste
Intestinal	Thick	Dark green to brown	Fecal

at the same hour each day and must be wearing the same amount of clothing. Usually weights are taken in the early morning before the patient has eaten or defecated but after voiding.

URINE SPECIFIC GRAVITY

The specific gravity of urine is a measure of the density (amount of solutes) in a sample of urine compared with the density of pure water (which is 1.000). Normal range for urine specific gravity is approximately 1.003 to 1.030. A person with renal impairment excretes a small amount of dilute urine (low specific gravity) because of the inability of the kidneys to concentrate solutes in the urine.

MANAGEMENT OF PATIENTS WITH FLUID AND ELECTROLYTE IMBALANCE

Important nursing functions include prevention of fluid and electrolyte imbalance, assessment of patients to recognize and report early signs of imbalance, planning and carrying out actions related to therapy to correct the condition, and relief of symptoms.

Prevention of fluid and electrolyte imbalance

Unless preventive measures are employed, many medical-surgical conditions and therapies may lead to fluid and electrolyte imbalance. There are some frequently encountered situations in which attention to preventive aspects may lessen the possibility of the development of serious imbalance.

Determination of fluid balance from urine specific gravity

Fluid deficit: small urine volume with high specific gravity
Fluid excess: large urine volume with low specific gravity

Persons at risk for fluid deficit

Aphasic	Dysphagic
Catatonic	Weak
Confused	Receiving tube feedings
Disoriented	

PREVENTION OF INADEQUATE FLUID INTAKE

Any patient who is unable to ask for fluids, to identify a need for fluid, or to swallow easily may develop a fluid deficit. The fluid intake of these patients is monitored, and specific plans are made to offer fluids at regular intervals.

PREVENTION OF IMBALANCES FROM GI FLUID LOSS

Vomiting and diarrhea

Vomiting and diarrhea are common symptoms of many illnesses. Sodium and some potassium are lost in vomiting and diarrhea, whereas chloride is lost only from vomitus. As soon as fluids are tolerated, the patient may be served salty broth and tea or another fluid high in potassium to replace the losses. Dry salty crackers often are tolerated when fluids are not and can be used to replace sodium. These measures often keep the patient from feeling weak and exhausted.

Draining fistulas

A patient with a draining fistula from any portion of the GI tract loses sodium, calcium, and some potassium, and dietary supplements are needed. Extra milk can replace all the losses if tolerated by the patient. The Vitamin D in the milk enables the body to use the calcium contained. A person with a permanent fistulous opening, such as an ileostomy, needs to be especially careful to supplement sodium and potassium when vomiting, diarrhea, or fever adds to the already unusually large loss of electrolytes.

Nasogastric drainage

Routine intravenous replacement usually is adequate to compensate for losses through nasogastric drainage, unless the patient has been sucking many ice chips or has had the tube irrigated frequently with water. Both of these practices, although they seem to be harmless because the fluid is removed immediately through the aspiration apparatus, stimulate the secretion of gastric juices. Aspiration of gastric juices of the stomach at rest may lead to loss of electrolytes and fluid. If irrigation of the tube is necessary, normal saline is used.

Enemas

Repeated enemas may result in water intoxication and potassium loss. If there is an order for enemas until the returns are clear, it is best not to give more than three enemas at one time without consulting the physician. If an elderly person living at home complains of pronounced weakness without apparent cause, the person is asked whether cathartics or enemas are being taken. If so, stopping this practice, eating foods with high potassium content, and increasing fluid intake may relieve the symptoms. Methods to combat constipation without taking laxatives or frequent enemas are then taught.

PREVENTION OF EXCESSIVE FLUID LOSS FROM SKIN, LUNGS, KIDNEYS

Diaphoresis

Excessive diaphoresis may result from heat, strenuous exercise, or fever. Even the healthy person who is perspiring profusely needs extra salt in the diet and should drink extra fluids. Some salty fluids are needed by the patient with a fever. Patients on salt-restricted diets and those with draining fistulas are especially likely to suffer from sodium depletion and should increase their salt intake slightly when perspiring profusely.

Diuretics

Diuretics are administered to encourage excretion of sodium and water in excess of body needs. However, potassium, which may not be in excess, is also lost with the increased urinary output. The patient receiving diuretics is encouraged to eat foods that are *high in potassium but low in sodium*. Good sources are bananas and other fresh fruits (see box, p. 144).

Diuretics such as the thiazides may eventually cause sodium depletion; therefore, the person receiving extensive diuretic treatment is taught to observe for symptoms indicating sodium depletion (p. 142) and to report these symptoms to the physician. Table 10-12 lists some commonly used diuretics.

Renal or circulatory impairments

Any patient with renal or circulatory impairment, as may occur in shock, cardiac failure, renal insufficiency, or constriction of blood vessels because of disease, may develop a fluid and electrolyte imbalance. Common imbalances include the following:

1. Edema from sodium and water retention
2. Hyperkalemia
3. Hyponatremia
4. Acidosis from inadequate tissue oxygenation
5. Overhydration

These patients are instructed to avoid taking too much food containing sodium, potassium, or bicarbonate. They should not drink carbonated beverages. The nurse must be especially aware of overhydration whenever intravenous fluids are being given in these situations.

Respiratory impairments

Patients with diseases such as emphysema that limit lung excursion and therefore limit gaseous exchange should not take carbonated beverages or bicarbonate of soda. These substances tend to make the blood more alkaline than normal, and respiration is depressed in an effort to correct this imbalance. Depression of respiration is highly undesirable for these patients. Early recognition and treatment of chronic lung disease may help prevent acid-base imbalances.

Replacement therapy

Fluids may be replaced by various routes as follows: orally (preferred route), by intravenous infusion, or by tube feedings (see Chapter 7).

SPACING OF FLUIDS

Fluids given by any route should be spaced throughout a 24-hour period. Not only does this practice help to maintain normal body fluid levels, but it also provides for better regulation of the electrolyte balance by the kidneys and prevents the end products of metabolism and toxic materials from being excreted in concentrated form. In this way the danger of renal damage, formation of calculi, and irritation of the lower urinary tract are reduced. In

Table 10-12. Possible fluid and electrolyte imbalances of common diuretics

Generic name	Trade name	Possible effect
Thiazides		
Chlorothiazide	Diuril	Hyponatremia, hypochloremia, hypokalemia, decreased extracellular volume, hyperglycemia, hyperuricemia, decreased calcium excretion
Hydrochlorothiazide	HydroDiuril	
Potent diuretics		
Furosemide	Lasix	Hyponatremia, hypokalemia, decreased ECF, hyperuricemia, hypocalcemia, hypomagnesemia, hypochloremia, alkalosis
Ethacrynic acid	Edecrin	
Potassium saving		
Spironolactone	Aldactone	Hyperkalemia, hyponatremia, decreased ECF, acidosis
Triamterene	Dyrenium	
Osmotic agent		
Mannitol	Osmitrol	Hyponatremia, hypochloremia, increased ECF, water intoxication if renal excretion is not adequate

addition, fluid spacing prevents overloading of the circulation.

CONCENTRATION OF FLUIDS

Infusing concentrated solutions rapidly and in large amounts into the alimentary tract causes the blood volume to drop because large amounts of fluid are needed to dilute the substance. If the circulating volume becomes considerably depleted, irreversible shock can result. The "dumping syndrome", which sometimes occurs after gastric resection, is caused by this abnormal shift of fluid. Concentrated solutions sometimes are given intentionally to reduce cerebral edema.

Concentrated intravenous solutions of sugar or protein should also be given slowly in small amounts because of the need for fluids for dilution. Hypertonic saline solution may cause fluid to diffuse from the tissues to equalize the concentration of salt in the intravascular compartment. The superior vena cava is the preferred site for infusions of hypertonic solutions, such as parenteral hyperalimentation because of the rapid dilution by the larger amount of blood at this site. If any of these concentrated solutions flows too rapidly into the vascular system, pulmonary edema can develop.

ORAL INTAKE

Adults who have no circulatory or renal malfunction usually need between 1500 and 3000 ml/day of fluid, depending on the amount of food consumed. Patients who have anorexia and are not eating well require more fluid to maintain a fluid balance. Medical prescriptions for fluid restriction are usualy given for patients who have fluid excess (edema or water intoxication) or whose kidneys are not functioning well.

A medical prescription may be given to the patient to "force fluids" or the nurse may make the decision that a large intake of fluids is desirable, such as for prevention of urinary stasis with its subsequent complications. No standard amount can be stated since the amount required depends on the following:

1. Size of the patient
2. Patient's circulatory and renal status
3. Amount of food intake
4. Amount of fluid loss (if appropriate)

It must be remembered that people with small or inelastic vascular systems become overhydrated easily. If the person has had a large portion of the body such as a limb removed either by surgery or trauma, the person's size is thereby decreased. If there is a question concerning the amount of fluids to encourage a patient to drink, the physician should be consulted.

PARENTERAL FLUIDS

Type of fluid

The nurse needs to know the common solutions used parenterally (Table 10-13). Some of the reasons for giving the more common intravenous solutions are listed here. Potassium chloride may be added to maintain normal intake of potassium and to replace losses. Ascorbic acid and vitamin B (Solu-B) may be added for nutritional purposes.

Whole blood, plasma, concentrated albumin, or plasma volume expanders can be given to substitute for blood protein loss and are used to establish normal blood volume and prevent shock. *Dextran* is the most generally accepted plasma volume expander. It increases the oncotic pressure of the blood, thus increasing the reabsorption of fluid from instertitial spaces. This creates an increase in plasma volume. *Low-molecular dextran* decreases the viscosity of the blood, allowing greater blood flow through the capillaries; thus it is useful in treating cardiogenic, hemorrhagic, or septic shock. It may cause prolonged bleeding time and should not be used if renal disease with severe oliguria or anuria is present. The patient is moni-

Table 10-13. Solutions for intravenous use

	Contents of solutions								
	Cations (mEq/L)					Anions (mEq/L)			
Type of solution	Na^+	K^+	Ca^{++}	Mg^{++}	NH_4^+	Cl^-	HCO_3^- lactate	PO_4^-	Glucose (g/L)
5% Dextrose in water									50
10% Dextrose in water									100
Normal saline (0.9%)	154					154			
3% Saline	513					513			
Ringer's solution	147	4	4			155			
5% Dextrose in Ringer's lactate	130	4	3			109	28		50
Ringer's lactate	130	4	3			109	28		
Ammonium chloride (0.9%)					170	170			
Sodium lactate ⅙ molar	167						167		
5% Dextrose in 0.2% saline	34					34			50
5% Dextrose in 0.45% saline	77					77			50

Usages of common intravenous solutions

Dextrose
  5% in water   Maintenance therapy when sodium not desirable
  5% in saline (0.9%, 0.45%, 0.2%)   Maintenance therapy depending on desired amount of sodium
Sodium chloride (0.9%)   For large losses of sodium, as in loss of GI fluids, burns
One-sixth molar lactate   Replacement of sodium but not chloride
Ringer's lactate   Balanced solution containing several electrolytes

---

tored for signs of anaphylactic reaction (apprehension, dyspnea, wheezing, respirations, tightness of chest, itching, hypotension) when dextran is being given.

Intravenous fluids containing electrolytes should be run slowly to allow the body to regulate their use. The patient is monitored for signs of intoxication (excess of fluids or electrolytes) and satisfactory urinary output. Increased serum potassium (hyperkalemia) can be particularly dangerous, since it may cause cardiac arrest. Renal failure and untreated adrenal insufficiency are contraindications for the use of potassium. Many physicians do not start intravenous therapy until chemical analyses of the blood have been reported for the day.

Amount and rate of administration

The administration rate of fluids usually is ordered by the physician and depends on the patient's illness, the kind of fluid given, and the patient's size and age. Approximately 30 ml/kg body weight is needed to meet daily fluid requirements. Fever increases water needs by about 15% for each 1 degree Centigrade rise in a patient's body temperature.[7] If there has been an acute illness resulting in a significant fluid deficit, fluid is replaced at the rate of 1000 ml/kg loss in weight. The physician calculates water needs based on the amount needed to replace losses and the amount required to meet daily needs.

The usual rate for replacement of fluid loss is 3 ml/ min; it is rarely run at a rate faster than 4 ml/min. If fluids are given continuously or if they are given when there is impaired renal or cardiac function, they are rarely run faster than 2 ml/min. Intravenous infusions that are run at too rapid a rate (sometimes seen when an infusion is "speeded up" to complete the treatment at a specified time) may result in overloading and pulmonary edema. At the first signs of increased blood volume (p. 141) in any patient receiving an intravenous infusion, the rate of flow is reduced and the physician notified.

Relief of thirst

Thirst, the first and most insistent sign of dehydration, sometimes causes the patient more misery than surgery or the symptoms of a disease. It may develop even when fluids have been withheld only for a number of hours. If fluid is being withheld intentionally, thirst often is made more bearable by explaining to patients why fluid is withheld and when they can expect to receive some.

Thirst usually is relieved rather readily by taking fluids. If fluids cannot be taken orally, the administration of fluids parenterally usually gives relief. It is often helpful to explain to the patient who is receiving an infusion that the procedure will soon provide some relief from thirst.

Mouth care allays some of the discomfort from thirst and may need to be repeated every hour. If patients can be trusted not to swallow, they may be given ice chips, which are held in the mouth and then spit out. Hard candies often give relief, even though they also must be expelled. The chewing of gum helps some patients.

Pronounced and continued thirst, despite the administration of fluids, is not normal and is reported. In the patient recently returned from surgery, this kind of thirst may indicate internal hemorrhage, elevation of temperature, or some other untoward development. Thirst may also be an indication of hypercalcemia or the onset of diabetes mellitus.

REFERENCES AND SELECTED READINGS*

1. Aspinwall, M.J.: A simplified guide to managing patients with hyponatremia, Nurs. 78 **8**(12):32-35.
2. Cardin, S.: Acid-base balance in the patient with respiratory disease, Nurs. Clin. North Am. **15**(3):593–601, 1980.
3. Daly, B.J.: Intensive care nursing, St. Louis, 1979, The C.V. Mosby Co.
4. *Felver, L.: Understanding the electrolyte maze, Am. J. Nurs. **80**:1591-1599, 1980.
5. Friedman, F.B.: Clinical controversies: can we really trust those I & Os? RN **45**(4):52-3, 118-120, 1982.
6. Goldberg, P.B.: Medications that contain sodium, Geriatr. Nurs. **1**:204-205, 1980.
7. *Golberger, E.: A primer of water, electrolytes and acid-base syndromes, ed. 6, Philadelphia, 1980, Lea & Febiger.
8. Guyton, A.C.: Textbook of medical physiology, ed. 6, Philadelphia, 1981, W.B. Saunders Co.
9. Haughney, E., and Sica, F.: Diuretics, how safe can you make them? Nurs. 77 **7**(2):34-39, 1977.
10. Kee, J.L.: Fluids and electrolytes with clinical applications (programmed approach), ed. 3, New York, 1982, John Wiley & Sons, Inc.
11. Kemp, G., and Kemp, D.: Diuretics, Am. J. Nurs. **78**:1007-1010, 1978.
12. Keithley, J.K., and Fraulini, K.E.: What's behind that I.V. line? Nurs. 82 **12**(3):33-45.
13. *Kubo, W., and others: Fluid and electrolyte problems of tube-fed patients, Am. J. Nurs. **76**:912-916, 1976.
14. Lane, G., and Peirce, A.G.: When persistence pays off: resolving the mystery of an unexplained electrolyte imbalance, Nurs. 82 **12**(1):44-47, 1982.
15. Managing special patients' fluids and electrolytes, Nurs. 82 **12**(11):111-113, 1982.
16. Manzi, C.: Edema, how to tell if it's a danger signal, Nurs. 77 **7**(4):66-70, 1977.
17. McFadden, E.A., Zaloga, G.P., and Chernow, B.: Hypocalcemia: a medical emergency, Am. J. Nurs. **83**:226-231, 1983.
18. *Metabolic acid-base disorders: chemistry and physiology (programmed instruction), I, Am. J. Nurs. **77**:1619-1650, 1977.
19. *Metabolic acid-base disorders: physiology abnormalities and nursing actions (programmed instruction) II, Am. J. Nurs. **78**:87-108, 1978.
20. *Metabolic acid-base disorders: clinical and laboratory findings (programmed instruction), III, Am. J. Nurs. **78**:443-460, 1978.
21. Metheny, N.: Preoperative fluid balance assessment, AORN J. **33**:51-56, 1981.
22. *Metheny, N., and Snively, W.D.: Nurses' handbook of fluid balance, ed. 3, Philadelphia, 1979, J.B. Lippincott Co.
23. Metheny, N., and Snively, W.D.: Perioperative fluids and electrolytes, Am. J. Nurs. **78**:840-845, 1978.
24. Menezel, L.K.: Clinical problems of electrolyte balance, Nurs. Clin. North Am. **15**(3):559-576, 1980.
25. Menezel, L,K.: Clinical problems of fluid balance, Nurs. Clin. North Am. **15**(3):549-558, 1980.
26. Nursing skillbook: monitoring fluid and electrolytes precisely, Horsham, Pa., 1978, Intermed Communications, Inc.
27. Plumer, A.L.: Principles and practice of intravenous therapy, ed. 3, Boston, 1982, Little, Brown & Co.
28. Quinlan, M.: Beyond electrolytes: solving the mysteries of calcium imbalance: an action guide, RN **45**(11):50-54, 1982.
29. Rando, J.T.: Fluid and electrolyte management of the adult surgical patient, AANA J. **50**:49-54, 1982.
30. Sabiston, D.C., editor: Davis-Christopher textbook of surgery, ed. 12, Philadelphia, 1981, W.B. Saunders Co.
31. Todd, B.: Drugs and the elderly: when the patient has a potassium deficiency, Geriatr. Nurs. **2**:373-376, 1981.
32. *Tripp, A.: Hyper and hypocalcemia, Am. J. Nurs. **76**:1142-1145, 1976.
33. Weldy, N.J.: Body fluids and electrolytes (programmed instruction), ed. 3, St. Louis, 1980, The C.V. Mosby Co.
34. Williams, S.R.: Nutrition and diet therapy, ed. 3, St. Louis, 1980, The C.V. Mosby Co.
35. Wright, T.R., and Murray, M.: Potassium problems: which patient's in danger? RN **45**(6):56-62, 1982.
36. Wyngaarden, J.B., and Smith, L.H.: Textbook of medicine, ed. 16, Philadelphia, 1982, W.B. Saunders Co.
36. Zerwekh, J.V.: The dehydration question, Nurs. 83 **13**(1):47-51, 1983.

---

*References preceded by an asterisk are particularly well suited for student reading.

11
Shock

GAIL OSTERFIELD

STUDY QUESTIONS

- Review the effects of the sympathetic nervous system on blood vessels of the heart, brain, and peripheral vessels.

- Review the physiologic requirements for the maintenance of adequate blood pressure.

- Explain physiologically why a person who has suffered severe injuries should not be covered by blankets on a warm day at the scene of an accident.

- Review in your physiology text the difference between alpha receptors and beta receptors.

- Review in your pharmacology text the actions and effects of adrenergic drugs.

Shock is a syndrome characterized by hypoperfusion of body tissues. Any condition that prevents cells from receiving an adequate blood supply can interfere with their metabolism and produce shock.

Blood flow is dependent on pressure changes within the vascular compartment. Blood flows from areas of greater pressure to areas of lesser pressure. In the systemic circulation, the mean pressure is highest in the aorta, where the blood leaves the left ventricle, and lowest in the right atrium. In order for the necessary pressure gradients to exist so that blood can flow, the following three factors are necessary:

1. An adequate amount of blood for the heart to pump around the body
2. Ability of the heart to pump blood
3. Blood vessels with good tone, able to constrict and dilate to maintain normal pressure.

Shock results from the disruption of one or more of these factors.

ETIOLOGY OF SHOCK

Shock may be classified as hypovolemic, cardiogenic, or vasogenic.

Types of shock

Hypovolemic	Shock, from loss of fluid from vascular system (through blood loss or fluid loss)
Cardiogenic	Shock, from inability of heart to pump blood to tissues (decreased cardiac output)
Vasogenic	Shock, from massive vasodilation (from interference with sympathetic nervous system or effects of histamine or toxins)

Hypovolemic shock

Hypovolemic shock is the most common type of shock. Any condition that reduces the *volume* within the vascular compartment by 15% to 25% can result in hypovolemic shock.[33] Common causes include the following:

1. Excessive blood loss: trauma (most common cause), gastrointestinal bleeding, coagulation disorders, surgery
2. Loss of body fluids other than blood: excessive diuresis (diabetic ketoacidosis or other hyperosmolar states, plasma loss from burns, fluid loss from excessive vomiting or diarrhea
3. Movement of fluid into another body space (third space), for example, bowel obstruction (up to 5 or 10 L may collect in bowel) or peritonitis (4 to 6 L may collect in peritoneal cavity within 24 hours).

Cardiogenic shock

Cardiogenic shock results from the inability of the heart to pump blood sufficiently to perfuse the cells of the body. When stroke volume falls initially, cardiac output may be maintained by an increase in heart rate (Chapter 26); however, an increase in the heart rate may further damage the heart. As the heart rate increases, the period of diastole shortens and the period of systole remains relatively constant. Because the coronary arteries fill during diastole, their filling time is reduced. The heart works for longer periods and requires more oxygen and nutrients. Thus, tachycardia can both increase the oxygen need of the heart and decrease its oxygen supply.

Although cardiogenic shock may be caused by various cardiac conditions including cardiac tamponade, restrictive pericarditis, pulmonary embolism, severe valvular disease, or arrhythmias, the most common cause by far is myocardial infarction. Studies have shown that in most patients who die from cardiogenic shock, at least 40% of the left ventricle was damaged by a recent infarction or by a recent infarction plus a previous scar.[37] In spite of improvements in managing cardiogenic shock, the mortality still remains above 80%. (Additional information on cardiogenic shock is given in Chapter 26).

Vasogenic shock

Vasogenic shock is caused by massive dilation of the blood vessels, resulting in disproportion between the size of the vascular space and the amount of blood contained. As arterial blood pressure falls, there is a decrease in the difference between arterial and venous pressures. Because blood flow is dependent on pressure differences, blood flow decreases. Blood pools in the blood vessels, resulting in decreased venous return to the heart. Cardiac output falls, and blood pressure decreases even further.

Initially in vasogenic shock, the extremities are warm because of vasodilation. However, as cardiac output decreases and tissue perfusion is reduced, compensatory vasoconstriction occurs.

Loss of vascular tone may result from a number of conditions. *Neurogenic shock* results from interference with the sympathetic nervous system, which helps maintain vasomotor tone. Spinal cord injury, spinal anesthesia, and rarely, brain damage are among the causes. *Anaphylactic shock* occurs when there is massive dilation of the blood vessels from the direct effect on the vessels of a substance such as histamine. Histamine, released by mast cells and basophils, has a powerful dilating effect on blood vessels, particularly capillaries. The endothelial cells that line the capillaries separate and expose the basement membrane, which is permeable to fluid and plasma proteins, resulting in hypovolemia.[30]

Septic shock, another form of vasogenic shock, may result from various infections, including those caused by both gram-positive and gram-negative bacteria, viruses, and fungi, although it most commonly results from gram-negative bacterial infections. The primary sites of infection are the urinary tract, respiratory tract, or blood. Organisms that ordinarily dwell in the gastrointestinal tract may cause sepsis and shock if they enter the bloodstream.

Conditions that predispose to septic shock include the following:

1. Age, both very young and very old
2. Immunosuppressive and steroid therapy
3. Chronic disease of the immune system
4. Urologic or gastrointestinal tract surgery.

Elderly men are particularly susceptible to septic shock because of the high incidence of prostatic hypertrophy in this group. They are more likely to develop urinary tract infections and to have urologic surgical procedures.

The mechanism by which septic shock occurs is not completely understood. Some believe that early in sepsis, fluid leaks out of the vascular system, and the resultant shock is simply a form of hypovolemic shock.[3] Others see the primary cause as faulty cellular metabolism from the direct effect of the toxin.[14] Although the early pathophysiology of septic shock is not completely understood, it is known that when some organisms enter the bloodstream, they are destroyed by the immune system and a toxin is released. This toxin, in some way, causes the characteristic symptoms of early septic shock (increased cardiac output, peripheral vasodilation, skin flushing, hyperthermia, increased renal output, and respiratory alkalosis.)[35] As septic shock progresses and cardiac output decreases, it resembles other types of shock, with low urinary output, vasoconstriction, and cool moist skin.

PATHOPHYSIOLOGY OF SHOCK
Early stage

In the early stage of shock the body responds to hypoperfusion as it would to any other stressor. The heart beats faster and stronger, sending more blood to the tissues. The kidneys retain fluid, and fluid shifts from the tissues into the bloodstream, so more fluid is available to maintain intravascular pressure. More oxygen is available to the tissues as a result of hyperventilation. Blood pres-

---

Major pathophysiologic changes in shock

Change	Effect
Early stage (compensatory stage)	
Increased epinephrine and norepinephrine	Increased cardiac output to send more blood to tissue
Increased glucocorticoids and mineralocorticoids	Sodium and fluid retention to increase intravascular volume
Hypoxemia	Hyperventilation: provides more oxygen to tissues; may cause respiratory alkalosis
Decreased capillary fluid pressure	Fluid shifts from interstitial to intravascular space to increase vascular volume
Later stage (noncompensatory stage)	
Decreased blood flow to heart	Impaired cardiac pumping ability (decreased cardiac output); blood pressure decreases
Anaerobic metabolism	Acidosis; decreased ATP; failure of cellular N^+-K^+ pump (K^+ leaves cell, Na^+ and water enter cell); cellular damage
Arteriolar dilation but venule constriction	Fluid shift from intravascular to interstitial space
Decreased blood flow to kidney	Decreased kidney function (oliguria or anuria, retention of nitrogenous waste products)

---

sure may be normal or even elevated at this stage. This early stage of shock is often referred to as the *compensatory stage* of shock. If the condition that precipitated the shock is corrected at this time, the patient will probably recover.

Later stage

If the primary problem is not or cannot be corrected in the early stage, shock will progress. During this next stage of shock, the compensatory mechanisms begin to fail, and they begin to have an adverse effect. In spite of the vasoconstriction, the blood pressure begins to fall. Adequate blood flow to the heart may not be maintained, resulting in impaired pumping ability and an even further reduction in cardiac output. The ischemic pancreas releases a substance called myocardial depressant factor (MDF), which further impairs the heart's pumping ability. The brain may suffer from insufficient blood flow, resulting in lethargy and stupor.

Cells in organs with vasoconstriction do not receive sufficient oxygen, and *anaerobic metabolism begins*. In the absence of oxygen, cells produce energy very inefficiently. In anaerobic metabolism, only 2 moles of adenosine triphosphate (ATP) are produced for each mole of glucose metabolized, whereas in the presence of oxygen 38 moles of ATP are produced for each mole of glucose. In addition, lactic acid cannot be further metabolized in the absence of oxygen. Thus anaerobic metabolism results in energy deficiency and acidosis. Without enough energy the sodium-potassium pump fails. Potassium leaves the cell, and sodium, along with water, enters the cell. Various organelles within the cell may be damaged. Lyso-

somes in the cell contain digestive substances within their walls to aid in phagocytosis of foreign substances. If the walls of the lysosomes are damaged, digestive substances can spill into the cell and destroy it. These lysosomal enzymes then come in contact with adjoining cells and cause further damage.[20] Cellular death results in organ death. The kidneys cease to function: oliguria or anuria develop: the serum blood urea nitrogen level and creatinine clearance increase.

Acid metabolites cause dilation of the arterioles, but the venules remain constricted. This causes an increase in the hydrostatic pressure within the capillaries, and fluid shifts from the capillaries into the interstitial space. This is the opposite of what happens during the compensatory stage. Hypovolemia is further intensified.

Shock is a dynamic process, with shock itself causing further shock.[21] At some point a cycle begins that cannot be interrupted, and an *irreversible* stage of shock develops. Even if the primary problem is corrected and good supportive care is given at this time, the patient will die. It is not known, however, the exact point at which irreversible shock is reached. Regardless of the symptoms present, all efforts should be made to reverse the progression of shock.

ORGAN DAMAGE IN SHOCK
Kidneys

The kidneys contain about 2,400,000 nephrons, each of which is capable of forming urine. Each nephron is composed of a glomerulus, made up of capillaries and the collecting tubules (Chapter 33). Under normal conditions the pressure within the glomerulus is sufficiently high to force fluid out of the capillaries into the collecting chamber. When the systolic pressure falls below 70 mm Hg, glomerular filtration ceases and the body is unable to rid itself of fluid and nitrogenous wastes.

The tubules, which are perfused by the peritubular capillaries, suffer from the lack of oxygen and nutrients. Acute tubular necrosis develops. The tubular epithelial cells slough and block the tubules, causing loss of function of the nephron.

The kidneys often are affected in the early stage of shock, even before systolic blood pressure falls, because the renal vessels respond to sympathetic stimulation and constrict. A decrease in urinary output is often an early sign of shock.

Brain

The brain is not affected early in shock. Because it does not contain alpha adrenergic receptors, its vessels do not constrict in response to the increased levels of epinephrine and norepinephrine, and blood is shunted to the brain (and heart) at the expense of the other organs. As shock progresses and compensatory mechanisms fail, the brain does suffer inadequate perfusion. As cerebral hypoxia occurs, restlessness and anxiety, followed by lethargy and coma may be seen. Cerebral function may also be altered by the increasing acidosis and the accumulation of toxic substances.

Heart

Although deterioration of cardiac function is a primary problem only in cardiogenic shock, the heart eventually is affected in all types of shock. As cited earlier, in the early stage of shock the heart is spared. As shock increases, the pumping ability of the heart is affected and cardiac output decreases (p. 160). As the heart muscle becomes increasingly hypoxic, it begins to show disturbances of electrical activity. Most dysrhythmias have a detrimental affect on cardiac output, and some may be fatal. In the later stages of shock, deterioration of myocardial function is probably the most important factor in the further progression of shock.[21]

Lungs

The effect of shock on the lungs has only been more recently determined. During the Viet Nam War, many victims of traumatic shock survived the early complications because of the use of massive blood transfusions and renal dialysis. The effect of shock on the lungs surfaced as a later complication. The pulmonary condition that results from hypoperfusion of the lungs has been known by a number of names, including shock-lung, white lung, and Da Nang lung. It is now generally known as adult respiratory distress syndrome (ARDS) (Chapter 25).

ARDS can result from any condition that causes hypoperfusion of the lungs, but is seen most commonly with traumatic or septic shock.[32] It is characterized by increased permeability of the pulmonary capillaries to proteins and water, resulting in noncardiac pulmonary edema. Type 2 pneumocytes are destroyed, impairing the production of surfactant that normally prevents collapse of the alveoli. Alveoli either become filled with fluid or collapse, and lungs become stiff.

In the early stages, hypoxemia results from impaired gas exchange, and hyperventilation occurs, resulting in hypocapnea and respiratory alkalosis. Platelet aggregation in the pulmonary capillaries further damages the lungs. Hypoxemia persists despite administration of increasing amounts of oxygen. As shock progresses, ventilation is impaired and carbon dioxide is retained. Respiratory acidosis results. As hypoxemia increases, platelet aggregation increases, and a destructive cycle is initiated.

Gastrointestinal tract

Sympathetic stimulation, which occurs early in shock, causes vasoconstriction and therefore decreased blood supply to the organs of the gastrointestinal tract. Bowel function decreases, and paralytic ileus may result. If the blood supply is severely impaired for a length of time, necrosis of the intestinal mucosa may occur. Microorganisms normally found in the bowel lyse and release endotoxins when they are attacked by the leukocytes in the blood. Shock, from whatever cause, will now also have a septic component. The gastric mucosa commonly ulcerates when it becomes ischemic, which may result in occult bleeding or massive hemorrhage.

Liver

Sympathetic stimulation causes vasoconstriction in the liver. In the early stages of shock this can be beneficial. Normally the liver is capable of storing large amounts of blood in its veins. With vasoconstriction it can release up to 350 ml blood into the general circulation, resulting in improved cardiac output. With continued sympathetic stimulation and decreased blood flow, liver tissue is affected. In septic shock there is an increase in oxygen uptake and a decrease in energy production in the liver. All types of shock affect the metabolic functions of the liver including the excretion of bile and cholesterol, gluconeogenesis, detoxification, and protein synthesis.[28]

The sinusoids of the liver are lined with Kupffer cells, which are part of the reticuloendothelial system (RES). These cells are very powerful phagocytes and destroy the many bacteria from the colon that reach the liver by way of the portal system. Normally, very few bacteria get past the RES. With the destruction of the RES, bacteria enter the general circulation and produce toxins, which under normal circumstances would be detoxified by the liver. The liver can no longer perform this function, and overwhelming infection and toxicity result.

Parameters for assessing status of patient in shock

Hemodynamic monitoring

Blood pressure (cuff and/or intraarterial)
Pulse
Central venous pressure
Pulmonary artery pressure
Pulmonary wedge pressure
Cardiac output
Electrocardiogram

Respiratory monitoring

Respiratory rate, depth
Breath sounds
Blood gases
   pH
   Po_2
   Pco_2
Percent saturation

Fluid and electrolyte monitoring

Serum electrolytes
Blood lactate and
   pyruvate levels
Intake
   By mouth
   Intravenous
   Nasogastric
   Irrigation solutions
   Solution in medications
Output
   Urinary
   Gastrointestinal tract
   Sweating
   Dressings
Weight
Serum creatinine level
Blood urea nitrogen level
Serum and urinary
   osmolality
Urinary specific gravity

Neurologic monitoring

Alertness
Orientation
Confusion

Hematologic monitoring

Erythrocytes
Hematocrit and hemoglobin
   levels
Leukocytes
Platelets
Prothrombin and partial
   thromboplastin times
Clotting time

Other monitoring

Bowel sounds
Skin temperature

Blood

Disseminated intravascular coagulation (DIC) (Chapter 28) can be a cause or a result of shock. It is characterized by intravascular clotting, resulting in the formation of microthrombi in the capillaries. Some of the factors that activate clotting factors in the blood are acidosis, stagnation, and procoagulant substances such as bacterial toxins.[25] Acidosis and stagnation of blood are present in all types of shock, and bacterial toxins are found in septic shock. As clotting occurs in the capillaries, clotting factors in the rest of the body become depleted. Hemorrhage may then occur from incisions, punctures, the gastrointestinal tract, and other sites. A vicious cycle ensues. Intravascular clotting results in even further decrease in tissue perfusion and acidosis. The hemorrhage caused by DIC decreases the cardiac output even further and worsens tissue perfusion. The mortality in patients with DIC in association with infection and shock is 50% to 60%.[17]

ASSESSMENT

The signs and symptoms of shock are summarized in Table 11-1. There are few observable signs in the early stage; the patient may be restless and the pulse and respiratory rates may be increased. Cool, clammy skin, decreased blood pressure, and lethargy or unconsciousness are signs of the later stage. The status of patients in shock is monitored by various methods.

Hemodynamic monitoring

Hemodynamic alterations are often the first sign of the onset of shock. The patient's hemodynamic status can be assessed at various levels (Fig. 11-1).

VITAL SIGNS

Vital signs are assessed frequently. In the early stages of shock the pulse is usually increased. As shock progresses, the pulse becomes quite rapid and difficult to palpate. Irregularities in the pulse may develop as cardiac dysrhythmias occur.

Early in shock the blood pressure may be normal or even elevated because of compensatory vasoconstriction. Blood pressure can be heard without difficulty at this stage. As shock progresses, the blood pressure may be difficult to auscultate, and it may be possible to obtain the systolic pressure by palpation. If intraarterial pressure monitoring is not instituted, Doppler ultrasound (Chapter 27) may be helpful in obtaining the blood pressure.

Venous pulsation in the neck is noted. Both the external and internal jugular veins should be examined. Generally, the external jugular vein is easier to see, but in some patients with heart disease the external jugular veins are occluded by fibrosis or are absent.[18] Normally, venous pulsations are visible when the patient is lying flat but not when the head is elevated to 45 degrees (Fig. 11-2). Flat neck veins, when the patient is in a horizontal position, often indicate hypovolemia, common in most types of shock.

Table 11-1. Comparison of signs and symptoms in early and late shock by body system

	Early shock	Late shock
Respiratory system	Hyperventilation; ↑ minute volume; ↓ Pco_2; normal Po_2	Respirations shallow; breath sounds may suggest congestion; ↑ Pco_2; ↓ Po_2
Cardiovascular system	Blood pressure normal to slightly lowered; ↑ diastolic pressure; ↓ pulse pressure; cardiac output normal; tachycardia; mild vasoconstriction in hypovolemic and cardiogenic shock	↓ Blood pressure; ↓ cardiac output; tachycardia continues; vasoconstriction worsens in hypovolemic, cardiogenic, and septic shock
Renal system	Normal to slightly depressed urine output; ↑ urine osmolality; ↓ urine sodium concentration	Oliguria or complete renal shutdown; buildup of waste products
Acid-base balance	Respiratory alkalosis	Metabolic acidosis; respiratory acidosis
Vascular compartment	Fluids shift from interstitial space to vascular compartment; thirst	Fluids shift from vascular space to interstitial and intracellular space, causing edema
Skin	Minimal to no changes in hypovolemic and cardiogenic shock; warm, flushed skin in neurogenic, vasogenic, and septic shock	Cool, clammy skin in hypovolemic, cardiogenic, and septic shock; cool and mottled skin in neurogenic and vasogenic shock
Hematologic system	Release of red blood cells from bone marrow to increase vascular volume; platelet aggregation	Disseminated intravascular coagulation
Mental-neurologic system	Restless; alert; confused	Lethargic; unconsciousness
Gastrointestinal-hepatic system	No obvious changes	Perfusion decreases and bowel sounds may be diminished

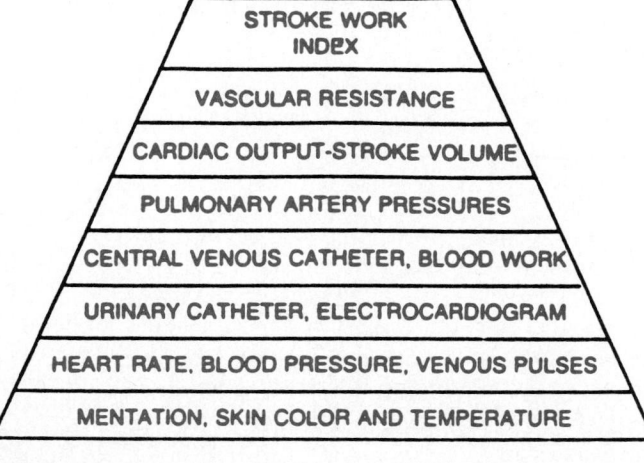

Fig. 11-1. Levels of hemodynamic monitoring. (From El-lerbe, S.: Fluid and blood component therapy in the critically ill and injured, New York, 1981, Churchill Livingstone, p. 35.)

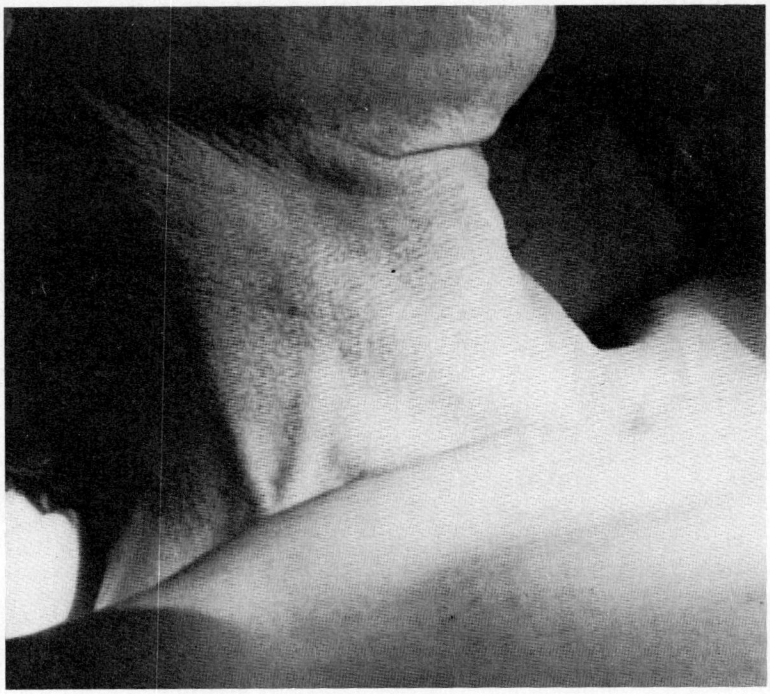

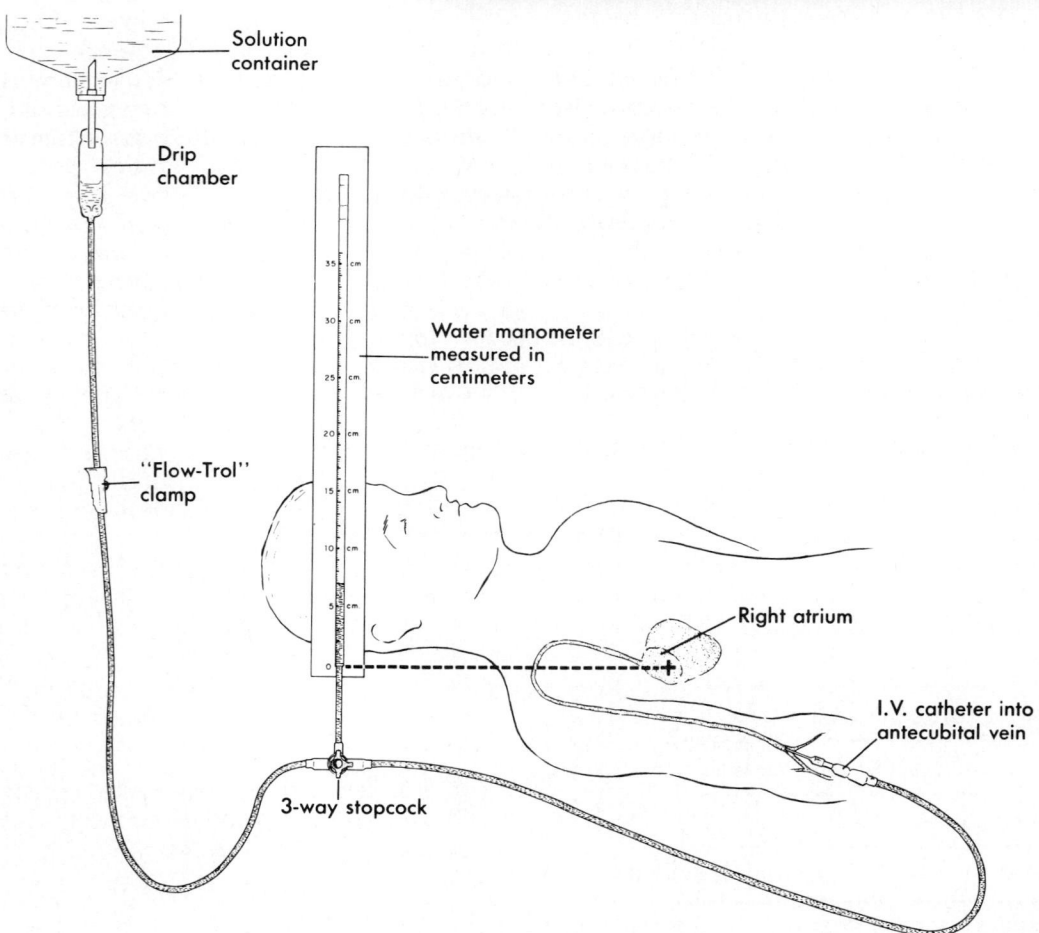

Fig. 11-2. Distended external jugular neck vein of a patient with right-sided heart failure. (From Daily, E.K., and Schroeder, J.: Techniques in bedside hemodynamic monitoring, ed. 2, St. Louis, 1981, The C.V. Mosby Co.)

Fig. 11-3. Measurement of central venous pressure (CVP) using water manometer. Zero point on manometer is at level of midright atrium, and CVP reading is 7 cm of water.

CENTRAL VENOUS PRESSURE

Central venous pressure (CVP) is a more accurate means of determining the fluid status of a patient in shock. CVP measures right ventricular filling pressure, which reflects venous return to the heart. CVP monitoring is most valuable in assessing status in patients with absolute or relative hypovolemia, including those with vasogenic, neurogenic, and hypovolemic shock. It is less valuable in assessment in patients with cardiogenic shock, who may have intravascular fluid excess.

To obtain an accurate CVP reading, a catheter is inserted into a major vein and threaded through the superior vena cava into the right atrium. The catheter is attached by a three-way stopcock to an intravenous infusion and a water manometer (Fig. 11-3). The intravenous solution (usually 5% glucose in water) is allowed to drip slowly into the vein to keep the vein open. When a reading is to be taken, the stopcock is opened to the manometer and the manometer is filled with the intravenous solution. The stopcock is then turned to the venous opening (the patient). The fluid level in the manometer should fluctuate with each respiration. The fluid is allowed to stabilize before a reading is taken, and the highest level of the fluid fluctuating in the column is used for the CVP reading. As soon as the reading is taken, the stopcock is turned to the solution position, and the infusion is continued.

For the CVP reading to be accurate, the patient must be relaxed; and the zero point of the manometer must always be at the level of the right atrium, which in most people is level with the midaxillary line. If the patient cannot be flat in bed, the zero point on the manometer is adjusted to the level of the right atrium in a sitting position. Any change in the patient's position requires that the zero point be reset. The initial CVP reading and the position that the patient was in when it was taken should be recorded, because these will serve as a baseline for comparison with subsequent readings. The patient should be placed in the same position for each reading, since even a slight change in position alters the CVP.

The normal values for CVP will vary with the use of different equipment; however, a range of 5 cm to 15 cm water is acceptable. It is important to note that a change or a trend in the CVP is more important than the actual numeric value.

Central venous catheters can also be used to obtain blood samples, to assess venous oxygen saturation determinations, and to administer fluids. The catheter insertion site should be kept scrupulously clean to minimize the possibility of phlebitis. Patient movement is not restricted as long as the catheter and tubing are secured adequately and intravenous flow is maintained.

PULMONARY ARTERY PRESSURES

The status of the left side of the heart can best be evaluated by the measurement of *pulmonary artery pressure*

(PAP) and *pulmonary capillary wedge pressure* (PCWP). These pressures are measured with a special balloon-tipped (Swan-Ganz) catheter (see Fig. 26-27). The catheter is inserted into a vein, usually the subclavian, and advanced to the atrium. The balloon is inflated and carried by the blood flow into the right ventricle and then to the pulmonary artery. The balloon is then deflated and the tip of the catheter is left in the pulmonary artery. The other end of the catheter is connected to low-compliance tubing, which in turn is connected to a transducer. The transducer converts the pressure that it senses through the catheter to an electrical signal, which is displayed on a monitor. Thus the pressure in the pulmonary artery can be monitored continuously. A continuous flush system usually is used to maintain patency of the catheter.

In individuals without lung or pulmonary vascular disease, PAP is a good indicator of how well the left side of the heart is functioning. Pressure changes in the left ventricle are reflected in the left atrium and back to the pulmonary artery. If there is any disease in the lungs, however, as frequently occurs in shock, the PAP does not accurately reflect left ventricular pressure. In this case the PCWP should be obtained. By inflating the balloon, which is near the tip of the catheter, the pulmonary artery can be occluded. This blocks communication between the pressure in the pulmonary artery and the lumen of the catheter, allowing for pressure that is ahead of the occluded artery to be transmitted through the catheter. The PCWP is identical to the left atrial pressure.

It is extremely important that the balloon does not remain inflated for an extended period, because blood flow to the lung would be impaired and a pulmonary infarction could result. Pulmonary infarction could also result if the catheter were advanced too far into the pulmonary vasculature, thereby interfering with blood supply. The nurse providing care in this situation must be able to recognize the difference between the waveforms of PAP and PCWP.

INTRAARTERIAL MONITORING

Intraarterial monitoring is usually instituted along with pulmonary artery pressure monitoring. A catheter is inserted into a radial, brachial, or femoral artery and attached to a transducer in much the same way as the pulmonary artery catheter (Fig. 11-4). Because this is a high-pressure system, hemorrhage is a possible complication, and the insertion and connections in the system must be monitored frequently. The extremity distal to the insertion site must be monitored for signs of arterial occlusion (color, temperature, movement, presence or absence of pulses, and pain). It is essential that sterile technique be maintained during insertion of the catheter and during dressing changes. A patient who is ill enough to require hemodynamic monitoring has little reserve to fight infection.

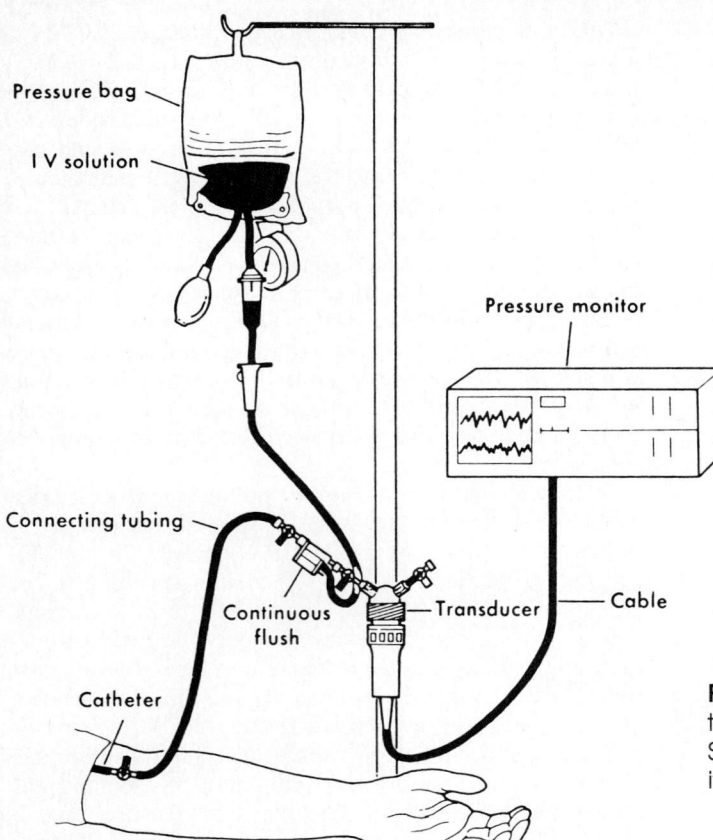

Pressure bag

I V solution

Pressure monitor

Connecting tubing

Continuous flush

Transducer

Cable

Catheter

Fig. 11-4. Connections between intraarterial catheter, transducer, monitor, and fluid. (From Daily, E.K., and Schroeder, J.: Techniques in bedside hemodynamic monitoring, ed. 3, St. Louis, 1985, The C.V. Mosby Co.)

CARDIAC OUTPUT AND CARDIAC INDEX MONITORING

Some pulmonary artery catheters allow for cardiac output and cardiac index to be monitored at the bedside. Such catheters have a port through which fluid can be injected into the right atrium. A thermistor is located at the tip of the catheter and attached to a wire that runs through the catheter and is attached to a cardiac output computer. Iced saline solution is injected into the right atrium. The solution travels with the blood into the pulmonary artery. The thermistor senses the extent of temperature change, and from this data the computer is able to calculate cardiac output.

Respiratory monitoring

As cited earlier (p. 161), hypoperfusion of the lungs, common in shock, may result in adult respiratory distress syndrome (ARDS). This may be suspected very early in the course of the disease from changes in the patient's mentation. There may be minor changes in orientation, unusual interpersonal exchanges, and mood changes.[6] The patient is observed for *cough* and *dyspnea,* which develop as ARDS progresses. Changes in respiratory rate and in the color of the mucous membranes and skin are important indicators of pulmonary status. Breath sounds

are auscultated. Early in the course of the disease the lungs may be clear, but as ARDS progresses, rales and rhonchi may be heard.

If the patient is receiving mechanical ventilation, the amount of pressure required to deliver a specific tidal volume is noted. As the lungs become increasingly stiff, the pressure required to deliver the volume increases. With ARDS, the pulmonary artery pressure may rise, although the pulmonary capillary wedge pressure remains normal.[22]

Arterial blood gases may provide valuable information and are monitored as indicated depending on the patient's condition. Characteristically with ARDS, the PaO_2 falls, in spite of ventilation with increasing amounts of oxygen, because of physiologic shunting of blood through the lungs to the left side of the heart. Shunting occurs because many alveoli are either collapsed or filled with fluid, and diffusion cannot occur. In the earlier stages of ARDS, when a sufficient number of alveoli are functioning, the $PaCO_2$ is usually normal or more likely low because of the rapid diffusion of CO_2 and of hyperventilation that results from hypoxia. However, as the number of functioning alveoli decreases, the $PaCO_2$ increases.

Arterial blood gas determinations are also used to assess the acid-base balance of the patient in shock. In the early stages of shock, mild respiratory alkalosis is common, from hyperventilation that is part of the stress response. As shock progresses and tissues become progressively hypoxemic, anaerobic metabolism takes place and metabolic acidosis occurs. In the advanced stages of shock, when respirations decrease and ARDS becomes progressively worse, respiratory acidosis may also develop.

Fluid and electrolyte monitoring

The urinary output and the CVP most accurately reflect fluid status. An indwelling urinary catheter is usually inserted, and the urine output is measured hourly. Other output, such as gastrointestinal drainage, wound exudate, or perspiration, is measured or estimated as accurately as possible. Body weight often gives a more accurate assessment of fluid changes than the measurement of intake and output; however, this can be an inaccurate determinant of intravascular volume when "third spacing" of fluid occurs. Noting the presence of edema, auscultating the chest for the presence of fluid, and measuring the abdominal girth for the development of ascites are means of assessing fluid collection in the third spaces.

In the early stages of shock, the serum potassium concentration may be abnormally low as a result of increased levels of aldosterone in response to stress. However, as shock progresses the serum K^+ level may become abnormally high as damaged cells release K^+. As urinary output falls, the body is unable to eliminate the excess amounts of K^+ that are accumulating in the serum. If K^+ is administered in the early stage of shock, it is extremely important that the urinary output and serum electrolytes be monitored frequently.

The concentration of other serum electrolytes may be abnormal as a result of acid-base abnormalities, altered renal function, or fluid therapy. Serum enzymes may be elevated because of ischemia and damage to the heart, liver, and pancreas.

Neurologic monitoring

In shock, the brain may be adversely affected by hypoxia, acid-base imbalance, or toxins. Often, subtle changes in mentation are the earliest signs of cerebral hypoxia. The patient is observed for increasing restlessness. Sedation should not be given until the patient's status has been assessed further and it has been determined that the restlessness does not have an organic cause. In the late stages, when perfusion of the brain is severely impaired, loss of consciousness occurs. Vital signs and arterial blood gas determinations can aid in assessing the cause of subtle neurologic changes.

Hematologic monitoring

The hemoglobin and hematocrit levels are valuable tools for assessing blood loss in hypovolemic shock secondary to hemorrhage. It must be remembered, however, that the hemoglobin and hematocrit levels do not drop immediately with loss of an excessive amount of blood, because plasma is lost along with the blood cells. The blood that remains in the intravascular compartment initially will have a normal concentration of RBCs. Because the kidneys retain water in response to blood loss, the blood becomes more dilute and there is a decrease in the hemoglobin and hematocrit concentrations.

Patients in shock are assessed for the development of DIC. The nurse may be the first to observe that the patient is bleeding for an excessively long time after a venipuncture, or that blood is oozing from an incision. If DIC is suspected, laboratory studies are initiated; clotting factors (including fibrinogen and platelet counts) are decreased, prothrombin time and partial thromboplastin time (aPTT) are prolonged, and fibrin degradation products are increased.

Other monitoring

Abdominal assessment is important in the patient in shock. Decreased blood flow to the intestines may result in decreased peristalsis or paralytic ileus (Chapter 32). Decreased or absent bowel sounds are noted. Gastric drainage and stools are assessed for occult blood because of the high incidence of gastrointestinal tract bleeding with shock.

DATA ANALYSIS AND PLANNING
Nursing diagnoses

Although there will be some variation according to the individual patient's symptoms and stage of shock, the following nursing diagnoses are appropriate in most patients in shock:

Decreased cardiac output
Alterations in tissue perfusion
Fluid volume deficit
Impaired gas exchange
Activity intolerance
Potential for injury
Potential impairment of skin integrity
Anxiety

Expected patient outcomes

1. The patient's tissue perfusion, cellular oxygenation, and cellular metabolism will improve.
2. The patient will have decreased metabolic needs.
3. The patient will be free of avoidable injuries.
4. The patient and significant others will be free of avoidable anxiety.

IMPLEMENTATION
Assisting with achievement of therapeutic goals

Treatment of shock will vary to some extent, depending on the cause. The cause of the shock must be treated first. Blood must be given if the patient has hemorrhage; antibiotics are given if an infection is present; and epinephrine is given if anaphylaxis has occurred. All types of shock have enough in common, however, that there are some common forms of treatment. In most types of shock, fluid replacement is the first therapeutic measure to be instituted, followed by administration of vasoactive drugs.

ASSISTING WITH FLUID REPLACEMENT

The need to administer fluids to the patient with hypovolemic shock is obvious. At times, fluid replacement is the only therapy needed in this type of shock. Vasogenic and septic shock are accompanied by hypovolemia because fluid is leaking out of the capillaries. Fluids are always part of the treatment. What is less obvious is that patients with cardiogenic shock *may* also require fluid therapy, although many may require fluid *restriction* or removal of fluid. Before fluid therapy is instituted for cardiogenic shock, a pulmonary artery catheter is inserted and the pulmonary end diastolic pressure measured. If the pressure is less than 20 mm Hg, fluid therapy may be beneficial.[2]

Various fluids may be given to the patient in shock. It is generally agreed that the patient who has sustained a large blood loss will require blood replacement. There is a great deal of disagreement concerning what other types of fluids should be used to treat shock. There are both advantages and disadvantages to all types of resuscitative fluids, including blood.

Administration of whole blood

The administration of whole blood has the obvious advantage of increasing the oxygen-carrying capacity of the blood. It also has many disadvantages (transmission of diseases, transfusion reactions, cost) (Chapter 39). If massive transfusions are given, additional problems may result. Because blood for transfusion contains an anticoagulant to prevent it from clotting while it is being stored, the patient who receives large amounts of blood may develop clotting defects. Stored blood is also deficient in platelets and other clotting factors. Massive transfusions of cold blood can result in hypothermia, which can cause cardiac arrhythmias.

Stored blood also contains some debris resulting from the aggregation of platelets, leukocytes, and fibrin. It is believed that some of this debris is able to pass through standard blood filters and is eventually filtered out of the blood by the pulmonary capillaries. This probably causes little difficulty in the patient who receives only a few units of blood, but it is likely to cause a problem for the patient who receives massive transfusions. It is recommended by some that microfilters be used when large quantities of blood are transfused.[15]

The pH in stored blood is lower than in normal blood. The added anticoagulant makes the blood more acid. Also, because blood is stored in an airtight bag, the metabolism that continues is anaerobic, and the end products are lactic and pyruvic acid. With all of its disadvantages, until a blood substitute is available for general use, blood must be given to maintain relatively normal hemoglobin and hematocrit levels.[10]

Some patients who are losing large amounts of blood may be given transfusions with their own blood, collected from the bleeding site with special equipment. Autotransfusion has been used in patients bleeding massively from an uncontaminated wound as well as in patients who bleed excessively during surgery. While it does eliminate transfusion reactions and hepatitis associated with blood transfusions, it is not without risks. The most common complications of autotransfusion are hemolysis resulting in renal failure, coagulopathy, embolization of debris, and sepsis.[43] Its main use is in patients who are bleeding so rapidly that the supply of stored blood is becoming depleted.

Other types of fluid therapy

Other fluids given are classified either as crystalloid or colloid solutions (see Table 11-2). Controversy exists concerning which should be used. Those who favor the use of crystalloid solutions believe these are better able to restore and maintain urinary output.[14] Some believe that colloid solutions should be given because they remain in the intravascular compartment where the fluid is needed.[36] Still others believe that a proper mixture of the two types of solution should be given.

Regardless of the type of fluid that the patient receives, the nurse must carefully monitor the rate at which it is

Table 11-2. Fluids used for replacement therapy in shock

Type	Examples	Comments
Blood	Whole blood Packed cells	Problems result with massive transfusions (clotting defects, acidosis, transfusion reactions, ARDS)
Crystalloid solutions	Ringer's lactate Normal saline	More efficient in restoring extravascular fluid loss Restore and maintain urinary output
Colloid solutions	Plasma Albumin Dextran Hydroxyethyl starch (HES)	Restore intravascular fluid volume

Vasoactive drugs commonly used to treat shock

Mixed alpha and beta adrenergic drugs

Norepinephrine (Levophed)	Positive inotropic and chronotropic effects
	Vasoconstrictor
Metaraminol (Aramine)	Similar to norepinephrine, slightly less potent but longer acting
Epinephrine (Adrenalin)	Positive inotropic and chronotropic effects
	Decreased vascular resistance at low dosage
	Vasoconstriction at higher dosage
	(Used in anaphylactic shock)
Dopamine (Intropin)	Low dosage: positive chronotropic effect, dilation of renal vessels
	Higher dosage: positive inotropic effect; vasoconstriction
Dobutamine (Dobutrex)	Positive inotropic effect
	Vasodilator
	(Used in cardiogenic shock)

Beta adrenergic drugs

Isoproterenol (Isuprel)	Positive inotropic and chronotropic effects
	Vasodilator

Vasodilators

Nitroprusside (Nipride)	Vasodilator
	No effect on heart
	(Used primarily in combination with other drugs)

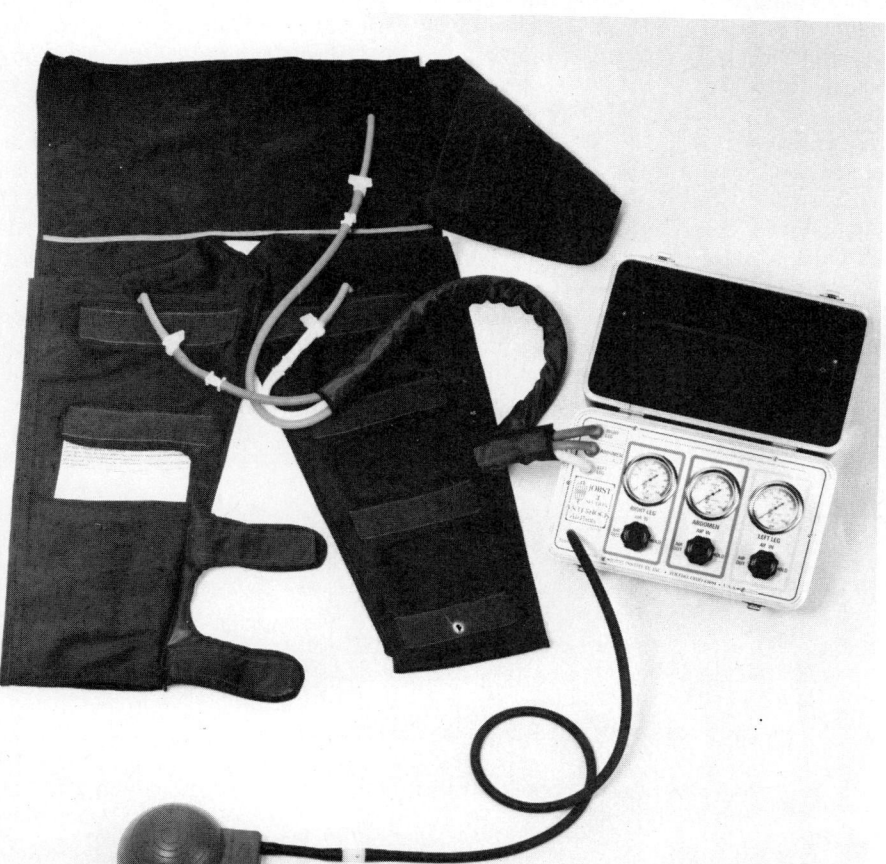

Fig. 11-5. Military antishock trousers (MAST) with inflation device and manometers. (Courtesy The Jobst Institute, Inc., Toledo Ohio; From Burrell, L.O., and Burrell, A.L.: Critical care, St. Louis, 1982, The C.V. Mosby Co.)

administered. The patient is assessed frequently for signs of hypovolemia or fluid overload (Chapter 10). Neck veins are observed for distention, and lungs are auscultated for signs of fluid (rales, rhonchi).

Fluid redistribution

Another way in which fluid resuscitation may be accomplished is by the use of the MAST suit (Military Anti-Shock Trousers). The suit consists of three inflatable parts, one for each leg and one for abdomen (Fig. 11-5). When inflated, the trousers "autotransfuse" the upper circulation with up to 2 L blood from the lower extremities, redirecting blood to the heart, lungs, and brain.[43] The trousers also increase peripheral resistance, which helps compensate for decreased blood volume. If there is bleeding in the lower extremities, the MAST suit helps to control bleeding by tamponade (counterpressure). The suit is used as a temporary measure until adequate fluid can be administered. When the suit is to be removed, it must be deflated gradually to prevent a sudden fall in peripheral resistance and a return of shock.

ASSISTING WITH DRUG THERAPY

If fluid therapy alone is not sufficient to reverse the shock state, vasoactive drugs may be given. Most vasoactive drugs are catecholamines, which stimulate alpha or beta receptors in the body. Generally, stimulation of alpha receptors causes vasoconstriction, and stimulation of beta receptors causes vasodilation. Stimulation of beta receptors also causes the heart to increase its rate (chronotropic effect) and strength of contraction (inotropic effect). The abdominal viscera, skin, and muscles respond primarily to the alpha effects of the catecholamines.

Mixed alpha and beta adrenergic drugs are used most commonly. In the past, drugs that caused vasoconstriction were used primarily because they enhanced the body's normal compensatory mechanisms. One problem was that the compensatory mechanisms themselves can have an adverse effect on the body. As blood is shunted away from the kidneys to perfuse the heart and brain, renal perfusion decreases and renal failure may result. In addition, bowel necrosis may develop, and the ischemic pancreas may begin to produce myocardial depressant factor. The ischemic liver can no longer perform its important functions.

Vasodilator drugs have been used to counteract the adverse effects of the body's compensatory mechanisms. They decrease the amount of pressure against which the heart has to pump, and thereby have the effect of increasing cardiac output without increasing the work load and oxygen need of the heart. *Fluid therapy must be given along with vasodilator drugs,* or the decrease in peripheral resistance can cause a decrease in venous return, thereby decreasing cardiac output. Cardiac output must be maintained when vasodilators are given, or the heart and brain may be poorly perfused. The drug selected will depend to some extent on the cause of shock and how far shock has progressed.

Combinations of drugs may be given. Dopamine and nitroprusside may be given together to increase cardiac output by combining the inotropic effect of dopamine with the decreased peripheral resistance effected by nitroprusside. For these two drugs to work together effectively, adequate fluid must be administered.[42] Low-dose dopamine may be given for its effect on renal and mesenteric perfusion along with dobutamine for its inotropic effect.

Patients receiving vasoactive drugs require very careful monitoring. Ideally, intraarterial and pulmonary pressure monitoring should be instituted. If the blood pressure is being measured by both cuff and intraarterial line, the two readings may vary. It is imperative that everyone working with the patient use the same measurements in adjusting the rate of drug infusion.

Steroids are often administered to patients in shock; however, their use is controversial. Many benefits from their use have been suggested, the most important of which is stabilization of lysosomal membranes, thereby preventing the leak of destructive enzymes.[28] The clinical success related to their use has been variable, as has the incidence of complications.[40] Other drugs are being used experimentally at present and may become accepted therapeutic agents in the future; these include calcium chan-

---

Care of patients receiving vasoactive drugs

1. Monitor blood pressure every 5 to 15 minutes at the beginning of the infusion and every 15 minutes thereafter to maintain a *mean* blood pressure at prescribed level (usually 80 mm Hg).
2. Drug must be diluted in a compatible solution and administered slowly by intravenous pump (for control).
3. Observe peripheral site of infusion (if used) frequently for signs of infiltration (necrosis and sloughing of tissues may occur with infiltration).
4. If infiltration occurs, infiltrate area around site with norepinephrine blocker (Regitine) as prescribed.
5. Monitor urinary output.
6. When discontinuing drug infusion, taper infusion slowly while continuing to monitor blood pressure every 15 minutes.

nel blockers,[24] Naloxone (a beta endorphin antagonist),[26] and energy substrates.[15]

ASSISTING WITH CARDIAC SUPPORT

When the left ventricle becomes severely impaired, as in cardiogenic shock or in the late stages of any type of shock, its function may be augmented by the use of the intraaortic balloon pump (Chapter 26). A balloon-tipped catheter is inserted into the aorta by way of the femoral artery. The catheter is attached to a machine that inflates and deflates the balloon in synchrony with the patient's cardiac cycle. During systole the balloon is deflated as the heart pumps blood into the aorta. During diastole the balloon inflates, enhancing blood flow to the heart, which is perfused during diastole, and to the rest of the body. During the next period of systole, the balloon deflates again, leaving a space in the aorta that must be filled. This causes a reduction in resistance, which allows the heart to eject a large quantity of blood with less effort than would normally be required.

Complications are not uncommon with use of the balloon pump. The most common complication is vascular insufficiency of the extremity distal to the insertion site. Frequent assessments are made of the pulses, color, temperature, movement, and sensation of the extremity, and any abnormality is reported immediately. Infection may occur with this procedure, as with any invasive procedure; therefore, the patient's temperature is also monitored.

The use of the intraaortic balloon is a temporary measure used to enhance cardiac output only until the heart is able to function adequately on its own.

ASSISTING WITH RESPIRATORY SUPPORT

Most patients in shock have some degree of hypoxemia. Oxygen is usually administered because tissues are already suffering from oxygen deprivation from poor blood flow. Because the energy system of the body is impaired, the muscles used in ventilation may not function adequately and breathing may have to be assisted. If symptoms of ARDS develop, positive end expiratory pressure (PEEP) may have to be used. Positive pressure at the end of expiration prevents surfactant-deficient alveoli from collapsing, resulting in atelectasis. Coughing and deep breathing are important, if the patient is able. If the patient is too weak to cough or if an endotracheal tube is in place, suctioning is necessary to keep the airway free of excessive secretions. Meticulous mouth care is necessary while the endotracheal tube is in place, because the mouth remains open and swallowing may be difficult.

PREVENTING INJURIES

In the early stages of shock, the patient may exhibit restlessness, which may then progress to confusion. During this time, injury is likely to occur if preventive measures are not taken. If the patient attempts to remove or disconnect lifesaving equipment, soft restraints may have to be applied.

Infections are very common in patients who are in shock, because of the many invasive procedures that are performed. Some potential sources of infection are indwelling catheters, arterial lines, pulmonary artery catheters, intravenous lines, endotracheal tubes, surgical incisions, and traumatic wounds. Meticulous sterile technique must be used with endotracheal suctioning, dressing changes, tubing changes, and urinary catheter care. Patients who are receiving steroids or who have experienced excessive blood loss are at increased risk for developing infection.

Complications of immobility must be prevented. It is not uncommon for the patient in shock to remain in one position for an extended period because of the constant activity that is occurring at the patient's bedside. This immobility can predispose the patient to thrombi, pneumonia, and decubitus ulcers.

Maintaining comfort and rest

The patient should be kept as comfortable as possible. In the past, patients in shock were kept in the Trendelenberg position (head down), but this is no longer recommended. It is usually suggested that the patient remain flat, with the legs elevated if necessary. If a patient in shock has difficulty breathing, a small pillow may be used to elevate the head slightly.

Rest is important. All nonessential activities should be eliminated, because activity increases the body's need for oxygen and nutrients, substances already deficient in the cells of the patient in shock.

Ambient temperature should be kept at a comfortable level. Excessive warmth increases the metabolic rate of the tissues, thereby increasing their oxygen need. Excessive coolness may cause the blood to flow even more sluggishly through the microcirculation, enhancing the formation of microthrombi. Patients with an endotracheal tube in place or who are very lethargic may not be able to express how they feel. Covers should be used according to the room temperature.

Both the conscious patient and the family will probably experience considerable anxiety. The nurse should remain calm and explain all interventions whenever possible. It may be necessary to repeat explanations frequently to both patient and family, because anxiety can interfere with their ability to comprehend and to remember.

EVALUATION

Evaluation is based on expected patient outcomes and may include the following:

The patient's tissue perfusion, cellular oxygenation, and cellular metabolism will return to normal.

Is the patient's mean blood pressure >80 mm Hg?

Is the pulse rate between 60 and 100 beats per minute and regular?

Is the cardiac index 3.5 ± 0.7 L/min/m^2?

Is the CVP >6 and <15 cm water?
Is the PCWP between 10 and 20 mm Hg?
Is the urinary output >30 ml/hr?
Is the serum potassium concentration between 3.8 and 5.0 mEq/L?
Is the serum sodium concentration between 136 and 142 mEq/L?
Is the BUN level between 8 and 25 mg/dl?
Is the serum creatinine clearance between 0.6 and 1.2 mg/dl?
Is the serum lactic acid level <1.9 mEq/L?
Is the patient's temperature within the normal range?
Is the patient's skin warm and dry? Are mucous membranes pink?
Is the patient's mental status the same as it was prior to the onset of shock?
Are respirations regular and between 16 and 22 per minute?
Are breath sounds clear?
Are blood gas values within normal limits?
  PO_2 80 to 100 mm Hg
  PCO_2 35 to 45 mm Hg
  HCO_3 22 to 26 mEq/L
  pH 7.35 to 7.45
  O_2 saturation $\geq$95%
Is the hemoglobin 12 gm/dl or greater?
Is the hematocrit 38% to 54%?
Is the platelet count $\geq$200,000?
Are all coagulation factors within the normal range?
Is the leukocyte count between 4500 and 11,000/ mm^3?

The patient will have decreased metabolic needs.
Is the patient comfortably warm?
Is the patient free of discomfort?

The patient will be free of avoidable injuries.
Is the patient free of nosocomial infections?
Is the patient free of self-inflicted injuries, such as abrasions?
Is the patient free of complications of immobility?

The patient and significant others will be free of avoidable anxiety.
Have they received explanations of all interventions?
Have they been informed of the patient's status?
Are they able to verbalize fears and feelings?
Are they free of signs of anxiety?

REFERENCES AND SELECTED READINGS*

1. Armstrong, P., and Baigrie, R.: Hemodynamic monitoring in critically ill patients, Heart Lung **9**:1060-1062, 1980.
2. *Barrow, J.J.: Shock demands drugs—but which one's best for your patient? Nurs. 82 **12**(2):34-41, 1982.
3. *Blaisdell, W.F.: Anaphylactic shock. In Perry, A.G., and Potter, P.A.: Shock: comprehensive nursing management, St. Louis, 1983, The C.V. Mosby Co.
4. Brinkmeyer, S.D.: Fluid resuscitation: an overview, J. Am. Osteopath. Assoc. **82**:326-330, 1983.
5. Chaudry, I.H., and Baue, A.E.: The use of substrates and energy in the treatment of shock, Adv. Shock Res. **3**:27-46, 1980.
6. *Cline, B.A., and Fischer, M.L.: ARDS means emergency, Nurs. 82 **12**(2):63-67, 1982.
7. Clough, D.H., and Higgins, P.: Discrepancies in estimating blood loss, Am. J. Nurs. **81**:331-333, 1981.
8. Corpening, J.T.: Colloid vs crystalloid fluid resuscitation in shock and injury. In Ellerbe, S.: Fluid and blood component therapy in critically ill and injured, New York, 1981, Churchill Livingstone.
9. Daily, E., and Schroeder, J.: Techniques in bedside hemodynamic monitoring, ed. 2, St. Louis, 1981, The C.V. Mosby Co.
10. Demling, R.H., and Nerlich, M.: Hypovolemic shock resuscitation: an update. In Collins, J.A., et al.: Massive transfusion in surgery and trauma, Prog. Clin. Biol. Res. **108**:30-35, 1982.
11. *Denny, M.: Septic shock, JEN **3**:19-23, 1977.
12. DeSantis, D., et al.: Delayed appearance of a circulating myocardial depressant factor in burn patients, Ann. Emerg. Med. **10**:22-24, 1981.
13. Elenbass, R.: Anaphylactic shock, Crit. Care Q. **2**:85-90, 1980.
14. Ellenbogen, C.: Treatment priorities for septic shock, Am. Fam. Physician **25**:163-167, 1982.
15. *Ellerbe, S.: Fluid and blood component therapy in the critically ill and injured, New York, 1981, Churchill-Livingstone.
16. Eskridge, R.: Septic shock, Crit. Care Q. **2**:55-76, 1980.
17. Feinstein, D.I.: Diagnosis and management of disseminated intravascular coagulation: the role of heparin therapy, Blood **60**:284-287, 1982.
18. Fowler, N.O.: Examination of the heart: inspection and palpation of venous and arterial pulses, New York, 1978, American Heart Association.

*References preceded by an asterisk are particularly well suited for student reading.

19. Glover, J.L., and Broadie, T.A.: Intraoperative autotransfusion. In Collins, J.A., et al.: Massive transfusion in surgery and trauma, Prog. Clin. Biol. Res. **108:**160-165, 1982.

20. Goldstein, I.M.: Lysosomes and their relation to the cell in shock. *In* Symposium on the cell in shock, April 25-25, 1975, Kalamazoo, 1975, The Upjohn Co.

21. Guyton, A.C.: Textbook of medical physiology, ed. 6, Philadelphia, 1981, W.B. Saunders Co.

22. Hardaway, R.M.: Pulmonary artery pressure vs pulmonary capillary wedge pressure and central venous pressure in shock, Resuscitation **10:**47-56, 1982.

23. *Hathaway, R.: Hemodynamic monitoring in shock, JEN **3:**37-43, 1977.

24. Hess, M.L., et al.: Improved myocardial hemodynamic and cellular function with calcium channel blockade (Verapamil) during canine hemorrhagic shock, Circ. Shock **10:**119-130, 1983.

25. Hudak, C.M., Lehr, T., and Gallo, B.M.: Critical care nursing, Philadelphia, 1982, J.B. Lippincott Co.

26. Isoyama, T., et al.: Effects of naloxone and morphine in hemorrhagic shock, Circ. Shock **10:**119-130, 1982.

27. Karliner, J.S., and Gregorates, G.: Coronary care, New York, 1981, Churchill Livingstone.

28. Lefer, A.M., and Schumer, W.: Molecular and cellular aspects of shock and trauma, Prog. Clin. Biol. Res. **111:**144-145, 1983.

29. Metheny, N.: The insterstitial (third space) phenomenon, NITA **6:**251-254, 1983.

30. *Myers, J.L.: Introduction to complications of shock. *In* Perry, A.G., and Potter, P.A.: Shock: comprehensive nursing management, St. Louis, 1983, The C.V. Mosby Co.

31. *Muray, J., and Smallwood, J.: CVP monitoring, Nurs. 77 **7**(1):42-47, 1977.

32. Nicholson, D.P.: Corticosteroids in the treatment of septic shock and the adult respiratory distress syndrome, Med. Clin. North Am. **67:**717-723, 1983.

33. *Niedringhaus, L.: Hypovolemic shock. *In* Perry, A.G., and Potter, P.A.: Shock: comprehensive nursing management, St. Louis, 1983, The C.V. Mosby Co.

34. *Park, G.: Cardiogenic shock, Crit. Care Q. **2:**43-54, 1980.

35. *Perry, A.G., and Potter, P.A.: Shock: comprehensive nursing management, St. Louis, 1983, The C.V. Mosby Co.

36. Pinsky, M.R.: Cause-specific management of shock, Postgrad. Med. **73:**127-149, 1983.

37. Rackley, C.E.: Critical care cardiology, Philadelphia, 1981, F.A. Davis Co.

38. Reed, L.: Intraaortic balloon pump, AORN J **23:**995-1001, 1976.

39. Riede, U., Sandritter, W., and Mittermayer, C.: Circulatory shock: a review, Pathology **13:**299-311, 1981.

40. Schumer, W.: Controversy in shock research: the role of steroids in septic shock, Circ. Shock **8:**667-682, 1981.

41. Schuster, H., and others: The influence of disseminated intravascular coagulation on renal function after experimental hemorrhagic shock, Resuscitation **8:**3-28, 1980.

42. *Shearer, J.K., and Caldwell, M.: Use of sodium nitroprusside and dopamine hydrochloride in the postoperative cardiac patient, Heart Lung **8:**302-307, 1979.

43. Shine, K.I., et al.: Aspects of the management of shock, Am. Coll. Phys. **93:**723-734, 1980.

44. *Spinella, J.: Clinical assessment of the shock patient, JEN **5:**34-45, 1979.

45. Tilkian, S.M., Conover, M.B., and Tilkian, A.G.: Clinical implications of laboratory tests, St. Louis, 1979, The C.V. Mosby Co.

46. *Visalli, F., and Evans, P.: The Swan-Ganz catheter: a program for teaching safe, effective care, Nurs. 81 **11**(1):42-47, 1981.

47. *Wilson, R., and Wilson, J.: Physiology, diagnosis, and treatment of shock, JEN **3:**11-26, 1977.

12
Pain

BARBARA C. LONG

STUDY QUESTIONS

- Review your notes on the nervous system. How are impulses carried to and from the brain? What anatomic terms describe nerve pathways?

- Review the analgesic drugs. What are the main classifications? Review the therapeutic benefits and potential hazards of each.

- Differentiate pain tolerance and pain threshold, and drug tolerance, drug dependence, and drug addiction.

- How does acute pain differ from chronic pain? Why is it important to make this differentiation?

- Which type of data, subjective or objective, is more valid in diagnosing pain? Explain.

- If a patient has moderate or severe acute pain, should the prescribed narcotic be delayed because of concern for addiction? Explain.

- Collect subjective and objective data on two of your patients who are experiencing pain, using the assessment parameters described in this chapter. What are the similarities and differences in their experience with pain? What specific factors are involved? How would your nursing interventions differ?

Pain is experienced to one degree or another by all persons. It is, however, a very individualized experience. It has never been satisfactorily defined or understood. It is an unpleasant feeling, entirely subjective, that only the person experiencing it can describe or evaluate. It can be evoked by a multiplicity of stimuli, but the reaction to it cannot be measured objectively. Pain is a learned experience that is influenced by the entire life situation of each person.

Pain accompanies many pathophysiologic disorders as well as some therapies. It is a sensation that is frequently feared by persons undergoing surgery. Although many persons with cancer do *not* experience it, pain is one of the major concerns people have about cancer.

Relief of pain and discomfort is a major nursing intervention and one that requires skill in both the art and science of nursing. It requires knowledge about concepts related to pain, data collection, and useful therapies. It also requires sensitivity and empathy—an effort on the part of the nurse to try to understand what the patient is experiencing and to communicate understanding and caring. It requires that the nurse use a systematic approach (nursing process) with the patient in pain. Too often when a patient states that he or she has pain, medication is given without valid assessment and evaluation, resulting in undermedication, overmedication, or medication when other interventions would be more effective.

CONCEPTS OF PAIN

Pain experience

The pain experience is influenced by the meaning of the pain for the patient, pain threshold, pain perception, and reaction to pain.

MEANING OF PAIN

Pain has different meanings for each person, which may differ for the same person at different times. In general, most persons view pain as a negative experience, although it may also have some positive aspects.

Numerous factors influence the meaning of pain for an individual, including age, sex, sociocultural background, environment, and past or present experiences. For example, two women may be experiencing pain from a fractured leg. The 75-year-old woman who lives alone and has few social contacts might interpret the pain on the basis of fear of aging and long-term loss of mobility that could interfere with activities of daily living. The 25-year-old secretary might interpret the pain as an expected nuisance, with the realization that healing will occur and she can get back to work soon.

PAIN TOLERANCE

Pain tolerance refers to the *intensity of the pain that a person is willing to endure before seeking relief*. A high tolerance means that considerable pain is endured before relief is sought. Pain tolerance varies among individuals. Some persons maintain a relatively stable pattern of pain tolerance; others have different levels of tolerance depending on the situation.[20] Numerous factors can affect pain tolerance.

American society tends to reward high tolerance to pain, as evidenced by phrases such as "Grin and bear it" and "Bite the bullet." Persons with high tolerance may, however, refuse measures to relieve pain, even when continued pain may delay recovery. Other persons may demand pain medication for what the nurse perceives as only minor pain. Both of these situations may create problems for the nursing staff. It is important that health practitioners *not* make value judgments about how much pain a patient "should" or "should not" endure. It is often expected that men should tolerate pain more than women. Each person is different, and each person's tolerance to pain is part of that person's total pain experience. Each person is also entitled to refuse or receive relief measures without censure.[20]

PERCEPTION OF PAIN

Physiology of pain

Stimuli causing pain may be of chemical, thermal, electrical, or mechanical origin. Nerve receptors respond to the stimuli and transmit the impulses by two types of fibers (fast myelinated A-delta fibers and slow unmyelinated C fibers) to the posterior horn (gray matter) of the spinal cord (Fig. 12-1). Within the cord, the impulses are transmitted to the white matter on the opposite side, from which they ascend by the lateral spinothalamic tract to the thalamus. Impulses are then sent to the cerebral cortex (where perception takes place) by way of the corticothalamic tracts.

Descending pain pathways from the brain are of two types. One pathway, which descends from the brainstem reticular formation and ends in the posterior horn of the spinal cord, has the ability to *inhibit pain transmission* (by means of neurotransmitters resembling naturally occurring opiates called *endorphins*). The second pathway sends signals from the cortex through the spinal cord to the muscles to initiate action.

Factors that influence pain perception

Pain perception may be altered by factors affecting stimulation of nerve receptors, transmission of the impulses, receptivity of the cortex, and interpretation in the cortex (see box, p. 176).

Selected meanings of pain

Harm or damage
Complication, such as infection
New illness
Recurrence of illness
Fatal disease
Increasing disability
Loss of mobility
Aging
Healing
Necessary for cure
Punishment for sins
Challenge
Appreciation for suffering of others
Something to be tolerated
Release from unwanted responsibilities

Factors that influence pain tolerance

Increase tolerance	Decrease tolerance
Alcohol	Fatigue
Drugs	Anger
Hypnosis	Boredom
Warmth	Anxiety
Rubbing	Persistent pain
Distraction	Illness
Faith	
Strong beliefs	

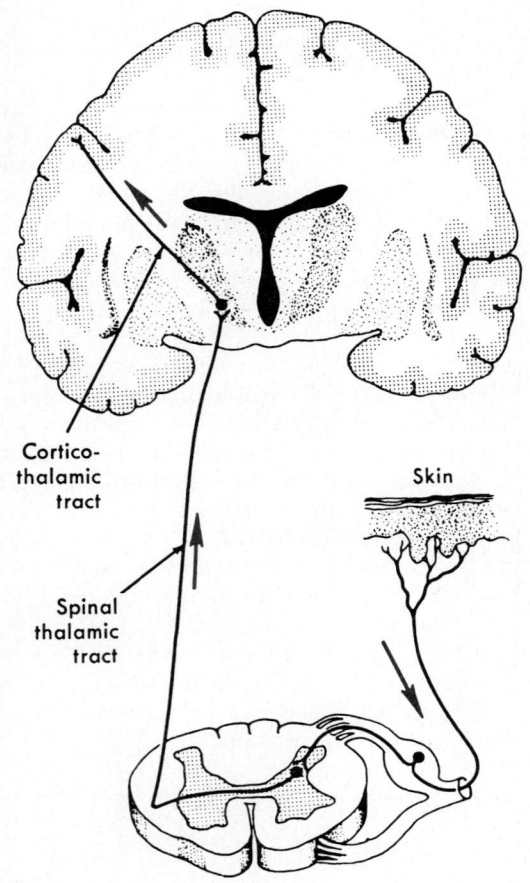

Cortico-
thalamic
tract

Skin

Spinal
thalamic
tract

Fig. 12-1. Pathways of pain transmission to cortex.

Factors that influence pain perception

Stimulation of nerve receptors

Increased number of stimuli
Increased duration of the stimulus

Alteration of transmission

Damage to nerve endings
Inflammation, tumors, or injuries to spinal cord

Receptivity of cortex

Inflammation, degenerative changes of brain
Depression of brain function
Anesthesia

Interpretation in cerebral cortex

Childhood training
Past experience with pain
Cultural values
Religious beliefs
Physical and mental health
Knowledge and understanding
Attention and distraction
Fear, anxiety, tension
Fatigue
State of consciousness

Table 12-1. Factors affecting pain transmission based on the gate control theory

	Close gate (block transmission)	Open gate (permit transmission)
Fibers	Impulses transmitted by large fast myelinated A-delta fibers	Impulses transmitted by slow unmyelinated C fibers
	Stimulation of unaffected skin areas (for example, massage)	Stimulation of affected skin areas (for example, sunburned skin)
Brainstem (descending pathway)	Endorphin effect	No endorphin effect
	Sufficient or maximum sensory input (for example, distraction)	Insufficient sensory input (for example, monotony)
Cortex	Past experiences	Past experiences
	Feelings of pain control	Anxiety

Pain *threshold* refers to the *intensity of the stimulus necessary for the person to perceive pain*. As with other pain characteristics, the pain threshold varies among and within individuals. Inflammation of the skin or tissues lowers the pain threshold. For example, a sunburned back is hyperalgesic (has increased sensitivity to pain); a light touch on a sunburned back may produce intense pain.

Damage to nerve endings can block the pain sensation at its origin. For example, persons with third-degree burns may have no sensation of pain despite the severity of the injury because of destruction of nerve endings.

Elderly persons may fail to perceive tissue damage that normally would cause pain and thus alert a younger person. Atrophy of nerve endings, degenerative changes in the pain-bearing pathways, and decreased alertness may reduce the perception of pain in the elderly, and more stimulation may be required to evoke a response.

Theory of pain transmission

Numerous theories have been proposed over the years to explain pain transmission. The most commonly accepted theory is the *gate control theory* proposed by Melzak and Wall. This theory suggests that transmission of pain impulses can be controlled by a gating mechanism that, when open, permits the pain impulses to be transmitted, but which can be partially or totally closed to inhibit some or all of the impulse transmission.

According to the theory, pain transmission can be influenced by three factors:
1. Effect of impulses transmitted over the two types of pain nerve fibers (A-delta and C fibers) to the spinal cord
2. Effect of impulses from the brainstem
3. Effect of impulses from the cortex.

Stimuli traveling over the large fibers may block those from the slow fibers (Table 12-1). Endorphins are present in the brainstem and in the substantia gelatinosa (gray matter in the dorsal horn of the spinal cord, where pain fibers synapse). The endorphins have morphinelike action that inhibits pain transmission. The cortex may either inhibit or facilitate pain transmission, depending on variables such as thoughts, attitudes, past experiences. For example, believing that a pain will be controlled will usually result in less pain perception than believing that pain will not be relieved.

REACTION TO PAIN

People respond to pain in different ways. Some may be fearful, apprehensive, and anxious, while others are tolerant and optimistic. Some weep, moan, scream, beg for relief or help, threaten to destroy themselves, thrash about in bed, or move about aimlessly when in severe pain; others lie quietly in bed and may only close their eyes, grit their teeth, bite their lips, clench their hands, or perspire profusely when experiencing pain.

Some people, by training and example, are taught to endure severe pain without reacting outwardly. Persons

---

Factors that influence reaction to pain

Meaning of pain to individual
Degree of pain perception
Past experience
Cultural values
Social expectations
Physical and mental health
Parental attitudes toward pain
Setting in which pain occurs
Fear, anxiety
Usual way of responding to stressors
Age

---

from cultures in which health teaching and disease prevention are emphasized tend to accept pain as a warning to seek help, and expect that the cause of pain will be found and cured.

Numerous factors influence reaction to pain. One cannot predict how any given person will respond, and value judgments should not be made concerning how a patient responds. It is very important to some persons to respond to pain in ways that are part of their sociocultural values.

Types of pain
GENERAL TYPES OF PAIN

There are two types of pain syndromes: acute and chronic. Unfortunately, a number of health care professionals provide care for the person experiencing chronic pain as though it were acute pain. There are many differences between acute and chronic pain (Table 12-2), and the approaches to pain relief are usually different, although some of the same techniques may be used.

Acute pain

Acute pain lasts no longer than 6 months. It is essentially a transient episode and informs the person that something is wrong. There is usually sudden onset from a perceived cause, and the painful areas can generally be well identified.

Acute pain is characterized by increased muscle tension and anxiety, both of which may contribute to increased perception of pain (Fig. 12-2). If the pain is moderate or severe, there are overt physiologic and behavioral signs that facilitate assessment of the pain. The person usually seeks pain relief.

Chronic pain

Pain that persists longer than 6 months is classified as chronic pain. Either the source of the pain is unknown or the pain cannot be eliminated. The pain sensation often becomes more diffuse, so that it is difficult for the person to identify a specific pain site. The pain may have

Table 12-2. Comparison of acute and chronic pain

Characteristic	Acute pain	Chronic pain
Experience	An event	A situation, state of existence
Source	External agent or internal disease	Unknown or cannot be changed or treatment is prolonged or ineffective
Onset	Usually sudden	May be sudden or develop insidiously
Duration	Transient (up to 6 months)	Prolonged (months to years)
Pain identification	Pain vs. nonpain areas generally well identified	Pain vs. nonpain areas less easily differentiated; intensity becomes more difficult to evaluate (change in sensations)
Clinical signs	Typical response pattern with more visible signs	Response patterns vary; fewer overt signs (adaptation)
Meaning	Meaningful (informs person something is wrong)	Meaningless; person looks for meanings
Pattern	Self-limiting or readily corrected	Continuous or intermittent; intensity may vary or remain constant
Course	Suffering usually decreases over time	Suffering usually increases over time
Actions	Leads to actions to relieve pain	Leads to actions to modify pain experience
Prognosis	Likelihood of eventual complete relief	Complete relief usually not possible

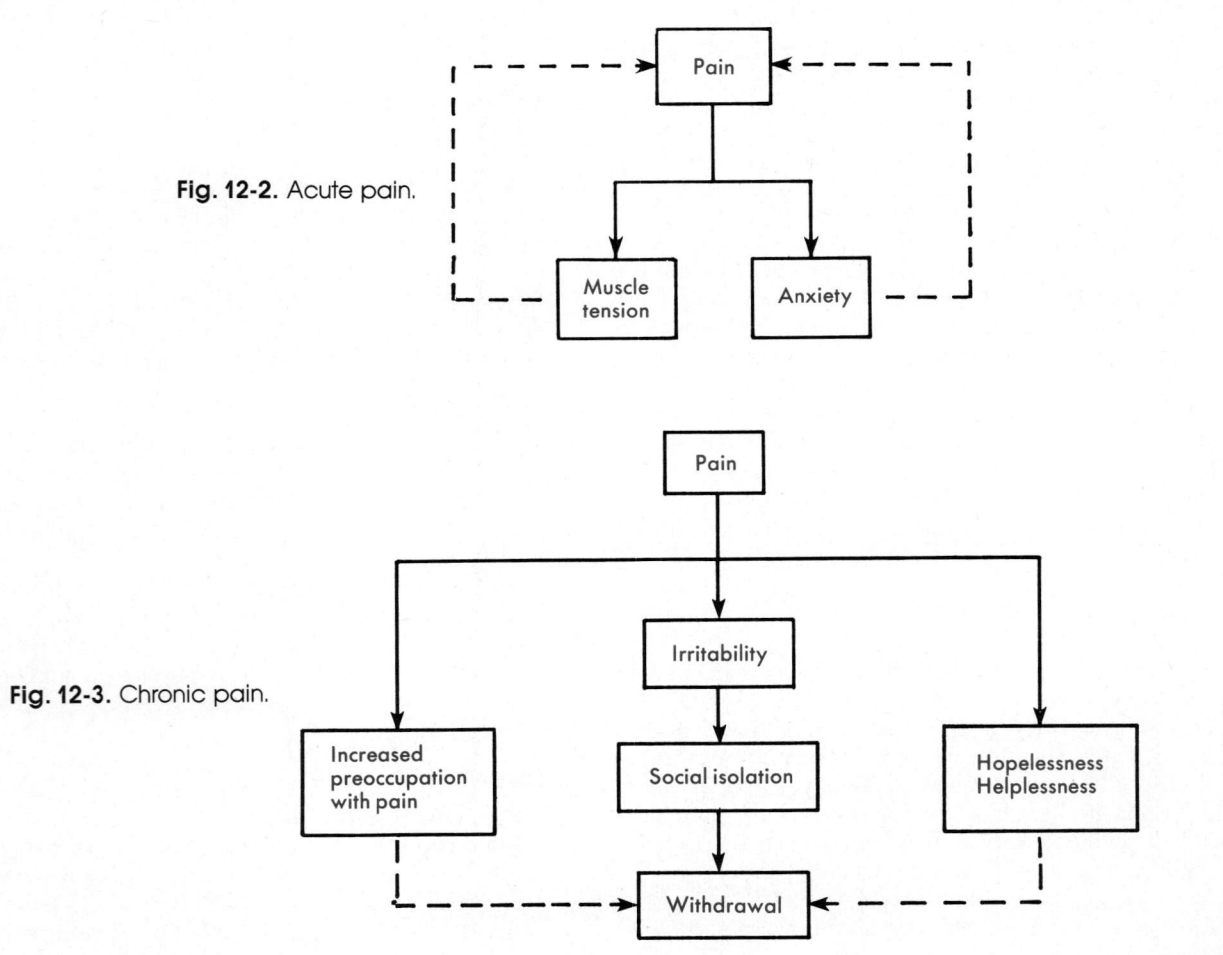

Fig. 12-2. Acute pain.

Fig. 12-3. Chronic pain.

originally been acute pain but persisted (for example, third-degree burns), or the onset may be so insidious that the person cannot state specifically when it was first experienced.

There are different types of chronic pain. *Intermittent* chronic pain occurs only at specific periods; at other times the person is pain free (migraine headaches). *Persistent* pain is always present, although there may be periods when pain is more or less intense (as seen with low back pain). One form of persistent pain may increase in frequency because of the pathologic condition (pain from incurable cancer). (Cancer pain is discussed in Chapter 14.)

Chronic pain is characterized by irritability (often compounded by insomnia), which leads to decreasing interests and isolation from friends and family. Added to that is the centering of the persons's life on the pain experience, with increasing feelings of helplessness and hopelessness as the pain persists. Ultimately the person withdraws from social interactions (Fig. 12-3).

The patient's world centers on ways to modify the pain experience. Some patients go from one physician to another seeking pain relief, which takes time, effort, and money. Even as they seek relief, they often lose faith in the ability of anyone to help them. The lack of continuity of care augments the problems. Physicians themselves may feel helpless when the patient continues to complain of pain. Tender loving care (TLC) which is appropriate for acute pain is *destructive* for chronic pain, because it reinforces the patient role. Acceptance without emphasis on the chronic pain is more effective. The development of pain clinics and inpatient teams has led to successful control of chronic pain for some (but not all) persons with chronic pain.

SPECIFIC TYPES OF PAIN

Pain from specific sites

Pain may originate in the skin, subcutaneous tissue, muscles, or bones (*somatic pain*) or in body organs (*visceral pain*).

Referred pain

Referred pain is felt in areas other than those stimulated. It may occur when stimulation is not perceived in the primary area. For example, the person experiencing a heart attack may complain only of pain radiating down the left arm when in fact the tissue damage is occurring in the myocardium.

Referred pain seems to occur most often with damage or injury to visceral organs, and the pain is referred to cutaneous surfaces (Fig. 12-4). The exact physiologic mechanism that occurs in referred pain is not clearly understood but may relate in part to the lack of sensory nerve endings near visceral organs. The cutaneous pat-

---

Characteristics of somatic and visceral pain

Somatic pain

May be sharp, pricking, burning, or dull

Superficial pain (skin, subcutaneous tissue) is well localized

Deep pain (muscle, bone) is often more poorly localized and may be accompanied by nausea, diaphoresis, and blood pressure changes

Visceral pain

May be sharp, dull and aching, or cramping

Is poorly localized

May be associated with nausea, diaphoresis, and blood pressure changes

Is caused by distention, ischemia, spasms, or chemical irritants but not by cutting

May initiate contractions of adjacent muscles (such as the abdominal wall, causing abdominal rigidity)

May be referred to other areas.

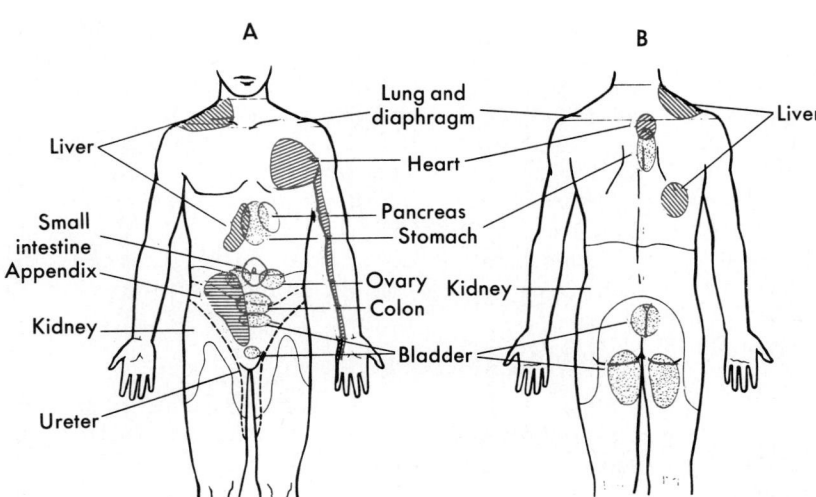

Fig. 12-4. Referred pain. **A,** Front. **B,** Back.

tern of various referred pains is fairly constant and frequently seen in practice. The nurse should be able to recognize the possibility of visceral organ disease in patients with appropriate complaints of cutaneous pain.

Psychogenic pain

Psychogenic pain is pain for which no physical findings exist; that is, it appears to originate in the person's mind. A sensation is perceived by the person as "pain," and it can be just as intense as pain originating from physical stimuli. Pure psychogenic pain, that is, pain with absolutely no physiologic basis, is rare. More often what is called psychogenic pain is pain that appears to have a greater psychologic basis than apparent physical basis.[20] In some instances pain that has been labelled as psychogenic pain is discovered later to have a strong physical basis not previously identified.

Phantom limb pain

Phantom limb pain is pain or discomfort perceived by the individual to be occurring in an extremity that has been amputated. It is more likely to develop in persons who experienced pain before amputation, and may persist long after healing has occurred. The phenomenon of phantom limb pain is poorly understood, and therefore treatment is not very effective.

Neurologic pain

Pain in the neurologic system occurs in different forms. *Neuralgia* is sharp, spasmlike pain along the course of one or more nerves. Two common areas of neuralgia are the trigeminal nerve in the face and the sciatic nerve in the lower trunk. *Causalgia,* a form of neuralgia, is severe burning pain associated with injury to a peripheral nerve in the extremities. The patient may go to great lengths to protect against irritating stimuli (which may be something as simple as the noise of a plane overhead).

ASSESSMENT

Acute pain

When a patient states having pain or asks for pain medication, it is important to make a rapid assessment, collecting both subjective and objective data before taking any actions. Omission of assessment may lead to inadequate pain relief. Consider the example of a young woman who, after pelvic surgery, was crying loudly and demanding pain medication, which was given to her without assessment of the pain. No relief was obtained from the medication. When an assessment was finally made, it was discovered that she had a full bladder of which she was unaware. After she voided, the pain disappeared.

SUBJECTIVE DATA

Data that is useful to obtain *before* pain is anticipated is the patient's expectations for pain relief from health

---

Subjective data for assessment of acute pain

Occurrence: new or recurrent
Onset and duration
Site
Intensity
Quality (dull or sharp)
Patient's perception of cause
Effectiveness of previous relief measures

Pain scale

0—No pain*	0—No pain	0—No pain
1— Mild pain	1— Mild pain	1—Slight pain
2—Discomfort	2—Moderate pain	2—Moderate pain
3—Distressing	3—Severe pain	3—Severe pain
4—Horrible	4—As bad as it could be	
5—Excruciating		

*McGill Pain Scale.

---

care providers. Many persons are unaware of their expected role in speaking out when they have pain or discomfort. Some patients think they will be considered "complainers" or "bad patients" if they state that they are experiencing discomfort. In this situation, an explanation is given of the subjective nature of pain and the need for patient input to facilitate selection of effective pain relief measures.

The best assessment of pain is the patient's own evaluation.

Pain *intensity* can be determined by various means. One way is to ask the patient to describe the pain or discomfort. Another method is to ask the patient to describe the severity of the pain or discomfort using a pain scale. The pain scale score can be recorded on a flow chart to provide ongoing assessment of progression of the pain. A third approach is to ask the patient to mark an **X** on a visual analog scale (Fig. 12-5).

When acute pain has subsided, further data can be collected about the *meaning* of pain for the person.

OBJECTIVE DATA

Objective data assists the nurse in identifying possible pain or discomfort in a person who has not reported pain and in helping to clarify the subjective response.

Objective signs of pain are of two types: physiologic and

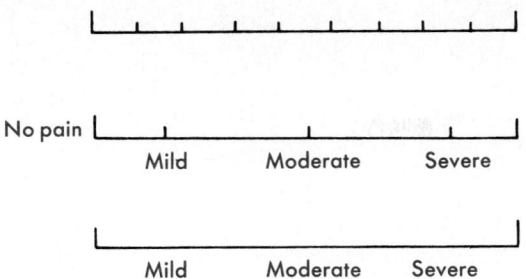

Fig. 12-5. Visual analog pain scales. Person marks line describing intensity of pain.

Physiologic signs accompanying pain

Pulse: increased rate
Respirations: increased depth and frequency
Blood pressure: increased systolic and diastolic
Diaphoresis
Pallor
Dilated pupils
Muscle tension (face, body)
Nausea and vomiting (if pain severe)

---

behavioral. *Physiologic* signs of pain result from activation of the sympathetic nervous system. With very severe acute pain, neurogenic shock may result from the stressful insult to the system.

Common *behavioral* manifestations of pain include holding the body rigid, moving restlessly, frowning, gritting teeth, clenching fists, crying, and moaning. The behavioral signs are not specific to pain; therefore, if the observable data suggest that pain may be present, subjective data must be elicited to validate the assumption.

Sometimes the patient's subjective response differs from the objective signs. For example, the patient may request an analgesic, a back rub, or other measure to relieve pain, but when the nurse arrives to carry out the request, the patient is found to be asleep. It is possible that the patient is exhausted from the pain and thus falls asleep, but the sleeping may be totally unrelated to the continuing presence of pain. It is important to reiterate that pain is what the patient says it is, and although objective data may assist in confirming the existence of pain, the diagnosis cannot be made solely on the basis of the objective data.

Chronic pain

SUBJECTIVE DATA

Long-term pain requires a much more in-depth assessment of the pain syndrome. Hospitals or pain clinics that use a team approach in providing care to the person with chronic pain often develop their own pain history form or questionnaire (see references 20, 31, and 32 for examples). This history may be collected by one or more health team members, and the data are used by one or more health team givers. Types of data collected may include the following:
1. Demographic data
2. Sociocultural data
3. History of the pain pattern from time of onset
4. Factors perceived to increase or decrease the pain
5. Effects of the pain on the person's life-style
6. Meaning of the pain for the person
7. Effects of the patient's pain on other family members or friends
8. Measures used in the past and present for pain relief.

OBJECTIVE DATA

Physiologic signs of pain *may be absent* in the person with chronic pain because of the body's compensatory mechanisms. Although there is adaptation to the pain stimuli, the pain persists. The absence of physiologic signs, therefore, does not indicate absence of pain. Prolonged pain, however, may create changes in the person's appearance over time, perhaps as a result of decreased appetite or lack of interest in appearance because of fatigue or depression.

Behavioral responses to chronic pain are varied and unique to the individual. Here, also, there may be few overt signs to indicate the presence of pain. If the person is extremely depressed because of the ongoing pain, withdrawal behaviors may be noted.

DATA ANALYSIS AND PLANNING

The need to assess the person with pain is ongoing, yet the nurse must begin to plan an approach to the person and the pain, particularly acute pain. The nurse is able to function independently with many interventions, but careful planning with other members of the health care team should ensure that all have the same patient outcomes or goals in mind.

One aspect of the treatment plan that is often forgotten or omitted is the incorporation of measures the patient thinks may help relieve the pain, even if these measures are different from those usually carried out in that institution. Without encouragement, the patient may hesitate to mention these possible remedies, for example, nonprescription liniments, special applications of heat and cold, unusual positioning, or favorite homemade foods or drinks. If there are no contraindications to the remedy the patient wishes to try, the health care team may consider using it before trying other relief measures.

In some situations it may be appropriate for the patient to help plan the use of pain relief measures. For example, the patient may wish to receive parenteral analgesics at bedtime to improve sleep and to receive a less potent medication that causes less drowsiness before family members visit.

Planning for the same health care team members to care for the patient regularly should result in a more consistent approach and plan of care. Between the small group of health care team members and the patient, a plan of care can be developed in which the patient's decisions are honored, and a daily routine can be devised that will reduce anxiety and frustration about constant changes. This plan should include, if appropriate, such items as specified hours for analgesic administration before uncomfortable procedures, specified blocks of time for rest or napping, and coordination between various departments, such as physical therapy and occupational therapy. For some patients fatigue is a great problem, so regular visits to off-unit departments should be interspersed with rest periods; for other patients the most beneficial plan includes ensuring that they go directly from one department to the next so that time is not wasted getting in and out of bed or performing other painful maneuvers.

Nursing diagnoses

If pain is present for which specific nursing interventions may be effective, a nursing diagnosis is made of "Alteration in comfort: pain (specify location)." Pain may also be an etiologic factor for other nursing diagnoses such as the following:

Ineffective breathing pattern related to pain in chest or abdomen
Anxiety related to increasing pain
Impaired physical mobility related to pain
Self-care deficit related to pain
Sexual dysfunction related to pain
Sleep pattern disturbance related to pain

Expected patient outcomes

1. The patient states that comfort is improved.
2. If pain is still present when patient is discharged, the patient or significant other can:
   a. Describe general measures for pain relief (for example, exercises)
   b. Explain prescribed medications (actions, dosages, frequency, side effects)
   c. Describe when to seek medical assistance if pain is not relieved as expected
3. The person with chronic pain can:
   a. State plans to participate in ongoing therapies
   b. State plans for increasing independence in activities of daily living.

MEDICAL APPROACHES TO PAIN CONTROL

Medications

Medications can relieve pain in various ways. Any medication given to treat the cause of pain will decrease the pain. Pain can also be relieved by interfering with the transmission of the stimulus to alter perception and by decreasing cortical response to the pain. Some drugs, such as narcotics, will affect both perception and response.

MEDICATIONS TO RELIEVE CAUSE OF PAIN

Some common causes of pain are smooth muscle spasms, impaired circulation, and inflammation. Any drugs, such as antibiotics, given to treat the underlying condition will, in the long run, decrease the pain. *Smooth muscle relaxants* include propantheline bromide (Pro-Banthine) and drugs of the belladonna group, such as atropine. For example, belladonna and opium (B & O) suppositories are effective in relieving bladder spasms after prostatectomy.

If pain is caused by *impaired circulation,* drugs that dilate the blood vessels, such as papaverine hydrochloride or nitroglycerin, may do more good than analgesic drugs.

Anti-inflammatory drugs decrease pain by decreasing the inflammatory response. Steroids have anti-inflammatory action. Nonsteroidal anti-inflammatory agents, such as indomethacin (Indocin), fenoprofen calcium (Nalfon), and ibuprofen (Motrin), are often given to relieve pain related to inflammation of the joints, such as arthritis. Phenylbutazone (Butazolidine) has the same properties but is usually given for short-term effect, such as for acute bursitis, because of major side effects of long-term therapy.

COUNTERIRRITANTS

Some drugs effectively relieve local pain by producing counterirritation (stimulation of the large A-delta fibers). Examples of counterirritants include ointments containing methyl salicylate (oil of wintergreen) or ethyl aminobenzoate, and oil of cloves (for toothache).

NONNARCOTIC ANALGESICS

The two most commonly used non-narcotic analgesics for mild to moderate pain are aspirin and acetaminophen. Aspirin has analgesic, antiinflammatory, and antipyretic effects, and synergistic effect when given with codeine. Aspirin is especially helpful for relief of headache, muscle aches, and arthritic pain.

Acetaminophen (Tylenol, Datril) has analgesic and antipyretic effect but no anti-inflammatory effect; therefore it is not given for arthritic pain. It has fewer side effects than aspirin but can cause severe liver damage if used indiscriminately. It is often prescribed when aspirin is contraindicated.

NARCOTICS

The opiates are most widely recognized and used for control of moderate to severe pain. Morphine and codeine are examples of opium alkaloids commonly used. Synthetic narcotic drugs such as meperidine hydrochloride

(Demerol) and methadone hydrochloride (Dolophine) are also widely used. They affect both the perception and reaction to pain.

The effects of narcotics vary with the physiologic state of the patient. The very young and the very old are sensitive to the effects of narcotics and require smaller doses to obtain relief from pain. A person of any age may be more depressed physically and emotionally by narcotics during the early morning hours (1:00 to 6:00 AM) than at any other time of the day and should be watched carefully for untoward effects.

Narcotics can cause lowering of the blood pressure and general depression of vital functions, including respiratory depression, bradycardia, and drowsiness. Some of these reactions can be advantageous; for example, with hemorrhage some lowering of blood pressure may be desireable. Hypotension may be a disadvantage in the debilitated patient, who may go into shock from an excessive dosage of a drug. The narcotics are less likely to cause shock if the patient is up and moving about and taking food and fluids, because these activities tend to maintain the blood pressure at a safe level.

Concern for addiction

Narcotics are frequently underprescribed by physicians and underadministered by nurses because of concern for addiction. It is important to differentiate tolerance, dependence, and addiction.

Drug tolerance creates a problem in terms of pain relief

Drug effects

Tolerance	Larger doses are needed to produce desired effects
Dependence	Need to continue use of drug to prevent symptoms
Addiction	Behavioral pattern of compulsive drug use, obtaining drug at any cost

---

over time when the stimulus persists or increases. This is a physiologic response. Physical dependency, appearance of physiologic withdrawal symptoms, may occur if a narcotic is *suddenly* discontinued when a person has been receiving it for a week or more. This *rarely happens,* because as pain decreases the dosage is gradually tapered, and no symptoms are experienced. Physical dependency and drug tolerance are involuntary behaviors.

Persons receiving narcotics for relief of severe pain rarely develop addiction, which is a voluntary behavior. Fewer that 1% of all narcotic addicts in the United States become addicted during hospitalization.[20] Persons more likely to become addicted are those who seek the narcotic for the feeling of well-being it provides rather than for relief of pain.

Persons with moderate to severe acute pain should not be denied full pain control with narcotics. Control of *acute pain* is best achieved by giving smaller doses more frequently (such as 6 to 10 mg morphine sulfate every 3 to 4 hours). Relief of *cancer pain* is best achieved by giving larger doses less frequently (such as 10 to 25 mg morphine sulfate every 6 hours). The use of narcotics for relief of *persistent chronic pain* (other than for cancer) is controversial. In general, efforts are made to reduce narcotic intake and to substitute other pain relievers.

OTHER DRUGS FOR PAIN RELIEF

Sedatives and tranquilizers are sometimes prescribed for pain. These drugs do *not* have analgesic effect but may permit relaxation and decrease anxiety and thus prevent potentiation of pain. The drugs may permit the patient to sleep and thus be better able to cope with the pain; the drugs do not relieve the pain.

In some persons sedatives and tranquilizers may lead to disorientation and agitation, which can increase the pain and decrease the patient's ability to cope. Treating pain with analgesics is the more effective and preferred method.

Electrical stimulators

The purpose of electrical stimulators is to modify the pain stimulus by blocking or changing the painful stimu-

---

Methods of electrical stimulation for pain control

Transcutaneous electrical nerve stimulator (TENS)	Manually controlled stimulation of specific pain areas through externally placed electrodes
Percutaneous implanted spinal cord epidural stimulator (PISCES)	Stimulation by an external transistorized receiver of leads inserted percutaneously in epidural space of spinal column
Dorsal column stimulator	Stimulation by a transistorized receiver, implanted surgically in an infraclavicular or abdominal skin pouch, of electrodes surgically implanted on dorsum of spinal cord

lus with stimulation perceived as less painful. The success of this approach, used for *chronic pain,* is thought to be explained by the gate control theory of pain transmission, that is, blockage of pain stimulus by stimulation of the large sensory fibers.

Several methods may be used. The transcutaneous electrical nerve stimulator (TENS) is a noninvasive procedure, useful in persons who cannot tolerate more extensive procedures or as a temporary method to determine effectiveness of electrical stimulation before initiating more permanent methods. Success with this device may come only after repeated trials with various electrode placements of battery-box manipulations. The nurse may be very valuable in encouraging patients and assisting them to make these small manipulations.

The PISCES is less intrusive than the dorsal column stimulator; local anesthesia is used while the leads are implanted. The dorsal column stimulator is surgically implanted. Postoperative care after dorsal column stimulator implantation includes that following laminectomy, with monitoring for infection and leakage of cerebrospinal fluid (Chapter 23).

Neurosurgical procedures

Constant relentless chronic pain that cannot be controlled by analgesics (intractable pain) may be reduced or eliminated by one of various neurosurgical procedures (see Table 12-3 and Fig. 12-6). Other forms of pain control are usually attempted before neurosurgical procedures.

Table 12-3. Neurosurgical procedures for pain control

Procedure	Method	Use
Neurectomy	Severing of nerve fibers from the cell body	Trigeminal neuralgia (fifth nerve resection); incapacitating dysmenorrhea (presacral neurectomy)
Rhizotomy	Resection of posterior nerve root before it enters spinal cord	Severe pain in upper trunk (for example, lung cancer)
Cordotomy	Severing of ascending anterolateral pain-conducting pathways of spinal cord	Severe pain of lower body (for example, pelvic cancer)
Sympathectomy	Excision or destruction of one or more sympathetic ganglia or nerves	Pain secondary to vascular insufficiency of extremities (for example, Raynaud's disease)

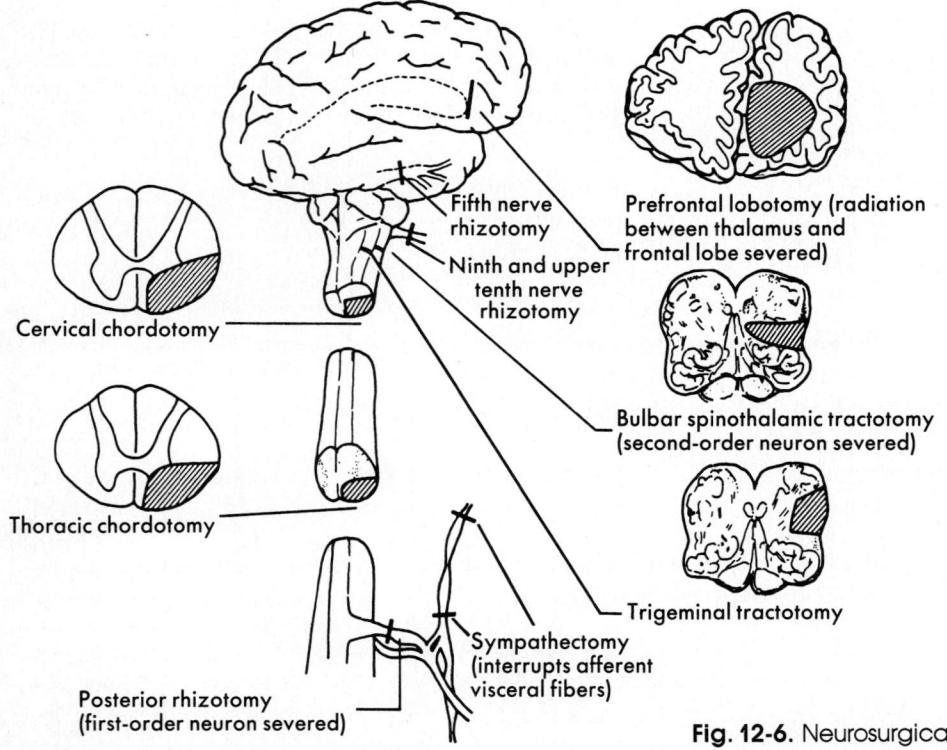

Fifth nerve rhizotomy

Ninth and upper tenth nerve rhizotomy

Cervical chordotomy

Thoracic chordotomy

Posterior rhizotomy (first-order neuron severed)

Sympathectomy (interrupts afferent visceral fibers)

Trigeminal tractotomy

Bulbar spinothalamic tractotomy (second-order neuron severed)

Prefrontal lobotomy (radiation between thalamus and frontal lobe severed)

Fig. 12-6. Neurosurgical procedures for pain relief.

Neurectomy has limitations in that peripheral nerves may regenerate. Both rhizotomy and cordotomy require laminectomy. Rhizotomy interferes with the ability to perceive heat and cold; therefore, protection from extremes in temperature is important for prevention of injury. The advantages of cordotomy include a wide sense of analgesia below the surgical site while preserving other sensory and motor functions. After surgery there may be temporary leg weakness and loss of bowel and bladder control from edema of the spinal cord; these usually disappear within 2 weeks. If quadriceps setting exercises are begun in the early postoperative period, walking will be less difficult.

Pain pathways in the brain may also be interrupted (tractotomy, thalamotomy, lobotomy). These surgical procedures have complications and are usually reserved as a final solution for patients with intractable pain, usually from malignant invasion of cranial or facial structures. Lobotomy usually results in a change in personality.

Nerve block

A nerve block involves the injection of substances such as local anesthetics or neurolytic agents (for example, alcohol or phenol) close to nerves to block the conduction of impulses over the nerves. Nerve blocks are frequently used for the symptomatic relief of pain. They are used to treat chronic pain associated with peripheral vascular disease, trigeminal neuralgia, causalgia, and cancer.

A nerve block may be unsuccessful because of difficulty in locating the correct nerve fiber or because of the complexity of the pain. Because the nerve fibers, ganglia, and roots contain other fibers than those for pain, and because some of the injected agents may leak out of the injection site and affect other nerves, the nerve block usually produces some other type of neurologic deficit.

Acupuncture

Acupuncture is an ancient form of disease treatment that can be used for pain relief. Only recently has the method been used in Western countries. Small needles are skillfully inserted and manipulated at specific body points, depending on the type and location of pain. The gate control theory provides the best explanation for the success of acupuncture: the local stimulation of large-diameter fibers by the needles "closes the gate" to pain. It is not known to what extent the psyche and the power of suggestion contribute to the effectiveness of this therapy. Nursing intervention includes careful client assessment and teaching.

PSYCHOLOGIC APPROACHES FOR PAIN CONTROL

Behavior modification

Behavior modification consists of a planned change in the way a person behaves by means of rewarding desired behavior and ignoring undesirable behavior. Forms of behavior modification are used unconsciously all the time: a young boy "throwing a tantrum" may be ignored, but as his behavior becomes more appropriate his mother may reward him with her time and attention.

Behavior modification may be useful for persons with chronic pain. For example, one protocol for patients with chronic low back pain is to set a limit of 10 minutes daily for discussion of their pain experiences (with the exception of data-gathering interviews). Pain medications are given on a regular schedule to dissociate the feelings of pain with inappropriate use (reward) of analgesics or other unhealthy behaviors. The medication can be refused, but no additional or stronger medication is given except acetaminophen or aspirin. The patient is praised for participating in desired activities.

In using behavioral methods in altering pain-associated behavior or in encouraging patient activities, success will occur only with a consistent approach on the part of the health care team. While patients should always be praised for their efforts to comply with or assist with treatment regimens, a true behavior modification program requires careful analysis of patient behavior and the development of a specific and comprehensive treatment plan.[12]

Biofeedback and autogenic training

Some persons are able to alter their body functions through mental concentration. In biofeedback training a machine that monitors brain wave activity (electroencephalograph [EEG]) is used. The individual concentrates on slowing his or her brain wave activity to rates at which pain and distress are unlikely to cause discomfort (that is, complete relaxation). It may take many months of regular practice to achieve the desired level of control. The nurse can be very helpful in encouraging and praising the person's efforts.[38]

In autogenic training the same type of self-regulation is used to alter various autonomic nervous system functions, such as pulse, blood pressure, and muscle tension. Practiced use of transcendental meditation and other methods of concentration and self-control may achieve the same degree of autoregulation without the use of sophisticated physiologic monitoring equipment.

Hypnosis

Hypnosis may be used in the treatment of various conditions, particularly when these conditions are aggravated by tension and stress. Individuals are helped to alter their perception of pain through the acceptance of positive suggestions made to the subconscious. Many persons are able to learn self-hypnosis. Individuals vary in their suggestibility and readiness to try this approach. The nurse's most helpful role may be to support the patient's desire to make hypnotism work.

NURSING APPROACHES FOR PAIN CONTROL

Specific nursing interventions for pain relief include those related to preventing pain, modifying the stimulus, and modifying the response to pain. General guidelines for pain relief are listed here.

Guidelines for pain relief measures

1. *Preparation for painful experiences*
   Prepare patients for what to expect in terms of discomfort and measures of pain control *before* pain occurs, whenever possible (such as before painful tests or treatments). Intensity and duration of pain are decreased because of decreased anxiety and the patient's sense of control.
2. *Preventive approach*
   Use pain relief measures *before* pain becomes moderate or severe. The more severe the pain the less the possibility of relief.
3. *Placebo response*
   Use methods that employ a placebo response, that is, some relief from discomfort not related specifically to the applied pain relief method. If the person expects relief from the pain, anxiety and muscle tension will decrease, and decreased pain is experienced. This can be accomplished by suggestion ("This should help you feel better") or by using methods the patient believes will work.
4. *Patient's ability or will to participate*
   Consider the patient's ability or will to be active or passive in using pain relief measures.[20] Decreased ability results from severe pain, fatigue, sedation, or unconsciousness. Decreased will occurs with some persons with chronic pain who have experienced numerous failures in pain relief.
5. *Varying pain relief measures*
   Use more than one type of pain relief measure when appropriate. For example, give an analgesic, rub the patient's back, and then offer some distraction; or combine an analgesic with relaxation response.
6. *Introducing new pain relief measures*
   Introduce a new method in combination with known effective methods. Some measures, such as distraction or relaxation, require practice; do not discard the new method until after several tries.
7. *Giving analgesics*
   a. Give analgesics before pain becomes severe.
   b. Determine which patients are at high risk for developing pain and assess them frequently for presence of increasing pain.
   c. Consider giving narcotics for a limited time (for example, 24 to 48 hours) on a regular basis rather than as needed when acute severe pain is anticipated, such as after some general surgical procedures.
   d. If the medication will be given "as needed," instruct the patient to report the presence of developing or recurrent pain.
   e. Use the parenteral route in acute intermittent pain to provide immediate, short-term relief.
   f. Use the oral route, when possible, in chronic unfluctuating pain to provide more sustained relief.[14]
   g. Report signs of undermedication to the physician (patient who watches the clock, waiting for the next dose, or patient who states having pain before next dose is due).
   h. When a variable analgesic dose and time schedule is prescribed, avoid the roller coaster effect (using wide variations in dose and timing), providing inconsistent pain relief.
   i. Assess and record the effectiveness of analgesics given.

Preventing pain

Although in many instances pain cannot be prevented, it is often possible to avoid additional pain when pain is already present. For example, when moving the body or an extremity, supporting the trunk or extremity will prevent increasing the pain by unilateral pulling on muscles, joints, and ligaments. Interventions include the following:

1. Using a turning sheet for patients with severe neck, back, or general trunk pain
2. Placing a pillow under a painful joint when helping a patient change position
3. Supporting limbs at the joints rather than the muscle bellies when handling an extremity
4. Using special beds (Stryker frame, Foster bed, CircOlectric bed) for patients with severe general or trunk pain
5. Avoiding bumping or moving the bed suddenly.

Modifying the pain stimulus

CUTANEOUS STIMULATION

Cutaneous stimulation innervates the large A-delta fibers to block the pain stimuli across the small C fibers. Methods of cutaneous stimulation include the following:

1. Lightly rubbing the affected area
2. Back rub
3. Application of heat or cold
4. Whirlpool massage.

REDUCTION OF NOISE AND VISUAL STIMULI

The patient may experience sensory overload. If nurses could stand still for 5 minutes in the patient's environment and watch and listen, they might understand that some patients are simply bombarded with noise and visual stimulation. If these are problems, it may be possible to change the environment. Changes include the following:

1. Move the patient to a quieter room away from the center of activity.
2. Dim any bright lights; pull shades if sunlight is intense.
3. Keep verbal interactions at a minimum when pain is severe.

4. Keep television or radio at a reasonable level but not loud.
5. Control the number of persons entering the patient's room according to patient's wishes.

REDUCTION OF SOCIAL ISOLATION

When external stimuli are decreased too much, the patient may lack distraction from the pain stimuli; thus pain perception is increased. Social isolation may occur for a variety of reasons: the serious nature of a patient's disease may necessitate being in a private room for an extended period; hospitalization far away from home may mean few family members and friends can visit; extended periods of hospitalization may result in friends losing interest in visiting; or the patient may complain so much that no one cares to visit to hear the monologue repeated.

Each of these causes of isolation may have a different solution. In any event, careful assessment may indicate that social isolation is a problem for the patient. Before determining the plan for addressing this problem, the patient should be consulted about the desire and need to alter the present situation. Possible nursing interventions include the following:
1. Placing the patient with a compatible roommate
2. Planning for frequent contacts with health team members
3. Facilitating visits by family and friends
4. Assisting patient to be as comfortable as possible during visits by family or friends.

THERAPEUTIC TOUCH

A less traditional therapy, that of therapeutic touch, may be helpful to patients in pain. The rationale for the success of therapeutic touch is not clearly understood. The nurse undergoes a brief period of meditation before coming in contact with the patient. During this period the nurse quiets his or her internal energy levels and then touches the patient and transmits the healing energies. Few nurses are trained in the use of therapeutic touch as described. It does seem to be helpful for some patients and some kinds of pain.

DISTRACTION AND RELAXATION EXERCISES

Patients can be taught to modify their sensory input to control pain by activities that promote distraction or relaxation.

Distraction

Distraction interferes with the pain stimulus, thereby modifying the awareness of the pain. Mild or moderate pain can be modified by focusing on activity in the environment. A very quiet environment providing little or no sensory input can actually intensify the pain experience because the individual has nothing to focus on but the painful stimulus.

Severe pain requires more active participation by the individual in an effort to block out the painful stimulus.

This can be enhanced by involving two or more sensory modalities, such as vision, hearing, touch, or movement. The distracters must be powerful enough to involve the individual's total interest without resulting in fatigue. Pain of long duration requires a variety of meaningful distracters. Methods of distraction include the following:
1. Playing games, watching television
2. Talking with someone
3. Listening to favorite music
4. Rhythmic breathing
5. Focusing on an object

Waking-imagined analgesia

Waking-imagined analgesia is defined as imagining a pleasant situation when a noxious stimulus is applied.[20] This intervention is similar to distraction except that the person concentrates on trying to relive the sensations that occurred during a previous pleasant experience rather than on enumerating the events that took place. Only a small percentage of the population in pain can use this method of analgesia; more can derive benefit from distraction alone.

Relaxation

Full relaxation decreases muscle tension and fatigue that usually accompanies pain. It also helps to decrease anxiety, thereby preventing augmentation of the pain stimulus. Carrying out relaxation techniques also serves as a form of distraction.

Not all persons with severe pain are able to achieve sufficient relaxation to have an effect on decreasing the pain sensation. Relaxation exercises may be especially beneficial for persons with chronic pain to help reduce stress that exacerbates the pain and to help the person achieve a sense of control, of being better able to cope with the pain.

There are numerous forms of relaxation techniques. Two techniques, Progressive Relaxation and Benson's Relaxation Response, are described in Chapter 8. Success with a relaxation technique requires practice and encouragement.

Modifying the pain response

EXPLANATION OF THE PROBLEM

As a result of nursing assessment, it may become clear that the patient's response to pain is really the manifestation of a lack of knowledge about the cause of the pain. Sometimes a simple explanation about what is causing the pain and how long it will last is all that is necessary. Understanding that pain or discomfort is to be expected may relieve anxiety or help the patient to alter expectations and be better prepared for what will happen. In all cases, an explanation that includes information about pain is given before each diagnostic test.

DECREASING ANXIETY

Because anxiety increases pain, measures taken to decrease anxiety may help to decrease pain (see Chapter 9 for a discussion of anxiety). Interventions for the patient with pain include the following:

1. Maintain a calm, quiet manner.
2. Help the patient explore concerns related to the pain (meaning of pain for the patient).
3. Respect the patient's response to pain, even if it differs considerably from what the nurse expects.
4. Hold the patient's hand, if appropriate.
5. Arrange for someone to be with the patient if the patient fears being alone.
6. Talk with family or close friends and help them to allay their anxieties so these are not transmitted to the patient.
7. Teach the family and close friends ways in which they can help the patient, such as massage, encouraging the patient to use distraction or relaxation techniques, or supporting painful parts when moving. People often feel helpless when observing a loved one in pain.

TEAM APPROACH FOR CHRONIC PAIN CONTROL

In recent years knowledge of the nature of chronic pain and the need for coordinated efforts of different health care professionals have resulted in the establishment of pain clinics and inpatient pain teams for control of chronic pain.

Pain clinics

Most pain clinics use a team approach that includes physicians (internists, dolorologists [pain specialists], surgeons, psychiatrists), nurses, physical and occupational therapists, social workers, psychologists, vocational rehabilitation counselors, and appropriate others. Each pain clinic is organized differently and places greater emphasis on different aspects of pain relief. Usual approaches to pain relief include the following:

1. Behavior modification (with patient's approval)
2. Medications: pain cocktail given at a scheduled time (not pain related) with decreasing amounts of medication
3. Exercise and activity prescriptions
4. Family training to support planned goals/activities.

The responsibility of the nurse varies depending on the available team members and may include patient assessment, documentation of observations, creating and maintaining a therapeutic milieu, providing emotional support for patient and family, and patient teaching. Nurses who work in pain clinics must be skilled in nurse-client interactions, be knowledgeable about the mechanisms of pain and the effectiveness of various treatment modalities, and possess patience and understanding as they assist patients to reach their goals.

Inpatient chronic pain teams

Persons with chronic persistent pain are sometimes admitted to a hospital for evaluation or initiation of treatment by a multidisciplinary health team similar to that in a pain clinic. One example is a team for evaluation and treatment of chronic back pain. Each team member participates in the evaluation individually and collectively and in team conferences to develop a specific treatment plan. The culmination of the hospitalization is a discharge conference with the patient and family members in which future treatment plans and recommendations are presented and discussed.

Protocols are developed for the approach to be used in control of the chronic pain; all persons providing patient care during the hospitalization need to become familiar with the protocols so that a consistent approach is used for pain control. For example, protocols for control of chronic back pain in one large medical center include an initial immobilization phase in which patients are placed in pelvic traction and instructed to move as little as possible (for example, eat in side-lying position). This phase is followed by a mobilization phase in which the patients are encouraged to be active (for example, walk to physical therapy and to the cafeteria for meals and make their own beds). The type of nursing care is therefore different depending on which phase is being implemented.

Nursing responsibilities include patient assessment, documenting observations, carrying out phase-related activities, carrying out designated behavior modification modalities, and patient teaching.

EVALUATION

Evaluation is an important component that is often forgotten in the care of the patient with pain. It is vital that the effectiveness of the interventions be assessed to determine whether the interventions should be continued, modified, replaced with another intervention, or discontinued. The essential questions in acute pain are as follows:

Does the patient still have pain?

If so, how does it compare with the pain experienced before the intervention?

If it is better but still present, should the same intervention(s) be continued unchanged or modified?

Should new interventions be added?

If it is not better, was sufficient data obtained in the initial assessment to determine the cause of pain?

Is there new data to indicate a different diagnosis?

What are the patient's thoughts about the continuing pain and the modes of intervention?

Assessment of pain relief

0—No relief
1—Slight relief
2—Moderate relief
3—Considerable relief
4—Complete relief, no pain

One method of assessing the extent of *pain relief* is to ask the patient to rate the pain relief on a scale of 0 to 4. The answers can be documented on a flow chart to provide an ongoing assessment of effectiveness of pain relief. The essential questions for chronic pain are as follows:

To what extent is the patient participating in the planned therapeutic program?

What is the patient's assessment of present pain?

Pain teams often have special evaluation guidelines specific to their patient population and treatment goals.

REFERENCES AND SELECTED READINGS*

1. *Armstrong, M.D.: Current concepts in pain, AORN J 32:383-390, 1980.
2. Barrett-Griesemer, P., Meisel, S., and Rate, R.: A guide to headaches—and how to relieve them, Nurs. '81 11(4):50-57, 1981.
3. *Beyerman, K.: Flawed perceptions about pain, Am. J. Nurs. 81:302-304, 1982.
4. Boguslawski, M.: Therapeutic touch: a facilitator of pain relief, Top. Clin. Nurs. 2:27-37, 1980.
5. Booker, J.E.: Pain: it's all in your head (or is it?), Nurs. '82 12(3):46-51, 1982.
6. Boyer, M.W.: Continuous drip morphine, Am. J. Nurs. 82:786-790, 1982.
7. Coyle, N.: Analgesics at the bedside, Am. J. Nurs. 79:1554-1557, 1979.
8. *Cummings, D.: Stopping chronic pain before it starts, Nurs. '81 11(1):60-63, 1981.
9. *Davitz, L.J., Sameshima, Y., and Davitz, J.: Suffering as viewed in six different cultures, Am. J. Nurs. 76:1296-1297, 1976.
10. *Donovan, M.I: Relaxation with guided imagery: a useful technique, Cancer Nurs. 3:27-32, 1980.
11. *Fagerhaugh, S.Y., and Strauss, A.: How to manage your patient's pain . . . and how not to, Nurs. '80 10(2):44-47, 1980.
12. *Fordyce, W.E.: Behavioral methods for chronic pain and illness, St. Louis, 1976, The C.V. Mosby Co.
13. Gramse, C.A.: Dorsal column stimulation, Am. J. Nurs. 78:1022-1025, 1978.
14. *Heidrich, G., and Perry, S.: Helping the patient in pain, Am. J. Nurs. 82:1828-1833, 1982.
15. *Holderby, R.A.: Conscious suggestion: using talk to manage pain, Nurs. '81 11(5):44-46, 1981.
16. *Jacox, A.K.: Assessing pain, Am. J. Nurs. 79:895-900, 1979.
17. Jacox, A.K. editor: Pain: a sourcebook for nurses and other professionals, Boston, 1978, Little, Brown & Co.
18. Johnson, M.: Pain: how do you know it's there and what do you do? Nurs. '76 6(9):48-50, 1976.
19. McCaffery, M.: How to relieve your patient's pain: fast and effectively . . . with oral analgesics, Nurs. '80 10(11):58-63, 1980.
20. *McCaffery, M.: Nursing management of the patient with pain, ed. 2, Philadelphia, 1979, J.B. Lippincott Co.
21. *McCaffery, M.: Patients shouldn't have to suffer: how to relieve pain with injectable narcotics, Nurs. '80 10(10):34-39, 1980.
22. *McCaffery, M.: Relieving pain with noninvasive techniques, Nurs. '80 10(12):54-57, 1980.
23. *McCaffery, M.: Understanding your patient's pain, Nurs. '80 10(9):26-31, 1980.
24. *McCaffery, M.: Undertreatment of acute pain with narcotics, Am. J. Nurs. 76:1586-1591, 1976.
25. *McCaffery, M.: When your patient's still in pain, don't just do something, sit there, Nurs. '81 11(6):58-61, 1981.
26. McCaffery, M.: Would you administer placebos for pain? Nurs. '82 12(2):80-85, 1982.
27. McDonnell, D.E.: TENS in treating chronic pain, AORN J 32:401-410, 1980.
28. *McGuire, L.: A short simple tool for assessing your patient's pain, Nurs. '81 11(3):48-49, 1981.
29. *McGuire, L., Dizard, S., and Panayotoff, K.: Managing pain: in the young patient . . . in the elderly patient, Nurs. '82 12(8):52-57, 1982.
30. *McMahon, M.A., and Miller, Sr. P.: Pain response: the influence of psycho-social-cultural factors, Nurs. Forum 17(1):58-71, 1978.
31. *Meissner, J.E.: McGill-Melzaek pain questionnaire, Nurs. 80 10(1):50-51, 1980.
32. *Melzack, R.: The McGill pain questionnaire: major properties and scoring methods, Pain 1:277-299, 1975.
33. *Meyer, T.M.: TENS: relieving pain through electricity, Nurs. 82 12(9):57-59, 1982.
34. O'Conner, A.B., editor: Nursing: patients in pain, New York, 1979, American Journal of Nursing Co.
35. Perry, S.W., and Heidrich, G.: Placebo response: myth and matter, Am. J. Nurs. 81:722-725, 1981.
36. Rogers, A.G.: Pharmacology of analgesics, J. Neurosurg. Nurs. 10:180-184, 1978.
37. Schmitt, M.: The nature of pain, Nurs. Clin. North Am. 12:621-629, 1977.
38. *Shealy, C.N.: The pain game, Millbrae, Calif., 1976, Celestial Arts.
39. Silman, J.: The management of pain: reference guide to analgesics, Am. J. Nurs. 79:74-78, 1979.
40. Sternback, R.A., editor: The psychology of pain, New York, 1978, Raven Press.
41. *Storlie, F.: Pointers for assessing pain, Nurs. '78 8(5):37-39, 1978.
42. Terzian, M.P.: Neurosurgical intervention for the management of chronic interactable pain, Top. Clin. Nurs. 2:75-78, 1980.
43. Valentine, A.S., Steckel, S., and Weintraub, M.: Pain relief for cancer patients, Am. J. Nurs. 78:2054–2056, 1978.
44. *West, B.A.: Understanding endorphins: our natural pain relief system, Nurs. '81 11(2):50-53, 1981.
45. *Wilson, R.W., and Elmassian, B.J.: Endorphins, Am. J. Nurs. 81:722-725, 1981.
46. Wolf, Z.R.: Pain theories: an overview, Top. Clin. Nurs. 2:9-18, 1980.
47. Wright, Z.: From I.V. to P.O.: titrating your patient's pain medication, Nurs. 81 11(7):38-43, 1981.

*References preceded by an asterisk are particularly well suited for student reading.

13

Infection Control

ELIZABETH CAMERON ECKSTEIN

STUDY QUESTIONS

- List six factors that put a hospitalized patient at risk of developing an infection.

- Define the following terms: (1) active immunity, (2) active acquired immunity, (3) passive immunity, and (4) herd immunity.

- What is the danger of giving antibodies in horse serum? What is the procedure that should be followed before injecting this type of solution?

- Plan a teaching program to encourage susceptible persons to obtain influenza immunization.

- What is the most common nosocomial infection? What measures could nurses take to reduce the incidence of this nosocomial infection?

HISTORICAL PERSPECTIVE

Infection control has become a recognized discipline only in the last decade, although the principles governing it have been in existence for some time. In the middle of the nineteenth century Semmelweiss, an obstetrician in Vienna, demonstrated the significance of hand washing in combating the transmission of infection. He showed that when the students and physicians were required to wash their hands and rinse them in a chlorinated lime solution before a delivery, the incidence of puerperal fever decreased markedly. The idea that hand washing alone could prevent the spread of disease met with much opposition by his colleagues. Better acceptance came after Pasteur, Lister, and Koch developed the germ theory of disease and related asepsis to the prevention of the spread of disease. At about the same time, Nightingale made significant contributions to sanitation and isolation practices. From this evolved an era in which medical asepsis was practiced more by ritual than with the true understanding of the scientific principles on which it was based.

A turning point came during World War II when the sulfonamides and penicillin were first used successfully to treat infections. As new antibiotics were developed, a false sense of security developed about infection control. It soon became apparent, however, that antibiotics were not the sole answer to infection control. Organisms, once well controlled by antibiotics, demonstrated the ability to develop resistant strains. In the late 1950s and the 1960s outbreaks of pencillin-resistant *Staphylococcus aureus* infections were common, and gram-negative organisms such as *Pseudomonas,* which were previously considered nonpathogenic (incapable of producing disease), were suddenly implicated as the cause of infections acquired in the hospital. Along with drug resistance and the emergence of newly recognized pathogens came an increase in the number of persons at risk for secondary infections. An increase in life expectancy, the use of immunosuppressive agents, and an increase in the use of invasive procedures to diagnose and treat disease all increased the risk of infection in certain persons.

The rise in the number of hospital infections made apparent the need to examine preventive and control measures, including a reemphasis on aseptic techniques. In 1970 an international conference to address the problem of hospital-acquired infections was held in Atlanta. As a result, the Centers for Disease Control (CDC) in Atlanta set forth guidelines for prevention and control of infections in hospitals. The CDC is constantly updating and revising its recommendations based on epidemiologic studies and research findings. The American Hospital Association (AHA) and the Joint Commission on Accreditation of Hospitals (JCAH), a major private accrediting agency, looked at the ethical and economic issues concerning hospital-acquired (nosocomial) infections and established standards for programs in infection control. The purpose of these programs was to decrease morbidity and mortality of infections as well as to reduce the cost of infections that could have been prevented. Consumer awareness of the problem also contributed to the attention given the issue of infection control. In the early 1970s only 10% of U.S. hospitals had infection surveillance and control programs, while by the end of the decade nearly all had them.

The field of infection control is a challenging one, with the identification of new pathogens (for example, *Legionella pneumophila*) and advances in research uncovering new information that may change current thinking and

practices. Infection control practitioners (ICPs) serve as a valuable resource, since they interact with virtually every department in a hospital as they survey for infections and teach staff how to prevent and control infection. The ICP is an important link between personnel from various hospital departments. When there is a question or problem regarding infection control, the ICP should be called on without hesitation.

This chapter presents an overview of the role of the nurse in the prevention and control of infection. For further information regarding a specific infectious disease, the reader should consult the chapter in which the site of the disease is discussed, for example, Chapter 31 for hepatitis, Chapter 25 for tuberculosis, and so on.

THE INFECTIOUS DISEASE PROCESS

Definitions

There are a number of definitions that are useful when describing certain conditions related to the infectious disease process. These are presented in Table 13-1.

Table 13-1. Selected definitions related to the infectious disease process

Term	Definition
Pathogen	Microorganism or substance capable of producing disease
Pathogenicity	Capability of a pathogen to infect and produce disease; determined by ability to survive and multiply outside host, virulence, dose, host specificity, and resistance of host
Invasiveness	Injury to host as a result of presence and spread of pathogen through body tissues
Toxigenicity	Injury to host as a result of effects to host of toxins produced by pathogen
Incubation period	Period of time after pathogen enters host and before clinical symptoms of infection appear
Infection	Presence in the body of a pathogen that multiplies and produces effects injurious to the host
Apparent (symptomatic, clinical)	Clinical signs and symptoms present
Inapparent (asymptomatic, subclinical)	No perceivable signs or symptoms present
Acute	Rapid onset, immediate host response, severe symptoms, and usually short course
Chronic	Insidious onset, delayed host response, mild symptoms, and long course
Latent	Pathogen ever-present in host, symptoms present only intermittently, often in response to a stimulus; pathogen dormant at other times
Localized	Focal point of symptoms or injury
Generalized	Systemic, whole body involvement
Superinfection	New infection by a pathogen different from one that caused initial infection
Colonization	Presence of pathogenic microorganisms in or on a host that do not produce injury or incite an injurious body response
Normal flora	Presence of nonpathogenic microorganisms that normally reside in various body locations without invasion or harm (May become pathogenic if introduced into an area in which they do not normally reside.)
Contamination	Presence of pathogenic microorganisms on inanimate objects or in substances

The question of whether a person has an infection or colonization can be difficult to answer. What is important to realize is that persons who are colonized, as well as infected persons, can easily serve as a source of infection to themselves and to others who are at risk.

Chain of infection

Essential to appropriate intervention in the prevention and control of infection is an understanding of the infectious disease process. All infectious diseases occur as a result of a sequence of events (Fig. 13-1). These events involve (1) a causative agent, (2) a reservoir, (3) a portal of exit, (4) a mode of transmission, (5) a portal of entry, and (6) a susceptible host.

First there must be a *causative agent,* or pathogen. This can be a bacterium, virus, fungus, rickettsia, protozoon, or helminth (worm). The causative agent exists in a *reservoir.* The reservoir can be animate (human or animal) or inanimate (soil, water, intravenous solutions, or equipment). Human reservoirs can be either persons with an acute clinical infection or persons who are asymptomatic *carriers,* who harbor the infectious agent but do not develop the infection. Carriers can (1) *be incubating* the agent before the onset of signs and symptoms, (2) have an *inapparent infection (subclinical),* (3) be in the *convalescent stage* of an infection, or (4) be *chronic carriers* of the agent. Viral hepatitis B is an example of an infectious disease that can be transmitted by human carriers in all

of these stages. Often the reservoir for an agent responsible for an outbreak of an infection is not readily apparent and, in fact, may never be identified. If the process of infection is well understood, however, appropriate and effective control measures can be instituted even though the original source of the causative agent is not known.

The agent must have a *portal of exit* from the reservoir. If the reservoir is human, the exit can be (1) the respiratory tract, (2) the gastrointestinal tract, (3) the genitourinary tract, (4) the skin or mucous membranes, (5) the blood, or (6) across the placenta.

Once the agent has left the reservoir, it needs a *mode of transmission* to a host. There are four modes of transmission: contact, airborne, vehicle, and vector. These modes and examples of how infection is spread by each mode are explained in the upper box on p. 193.

After the infectious agent has been transmitted to a host, it must gain entry into the host. The *portals of entry* are similar to the modes of exit from the human reservoir and include the respiratory tract, the gastrointestinal tract, the genitourinary tract, the skin or mucous membranes, the blood, and across the placenta.

The final step in the process after the inoculation of the host is the maturation and multiplication of the infectious agent. Entry of an infectious agent into a host does not mean that the agent will proliferate and cause infection. Infection depends on the dose and virulence of the agent and the *susceptibility of the host.* The healthy human body is extremely resistant to infection; however, when

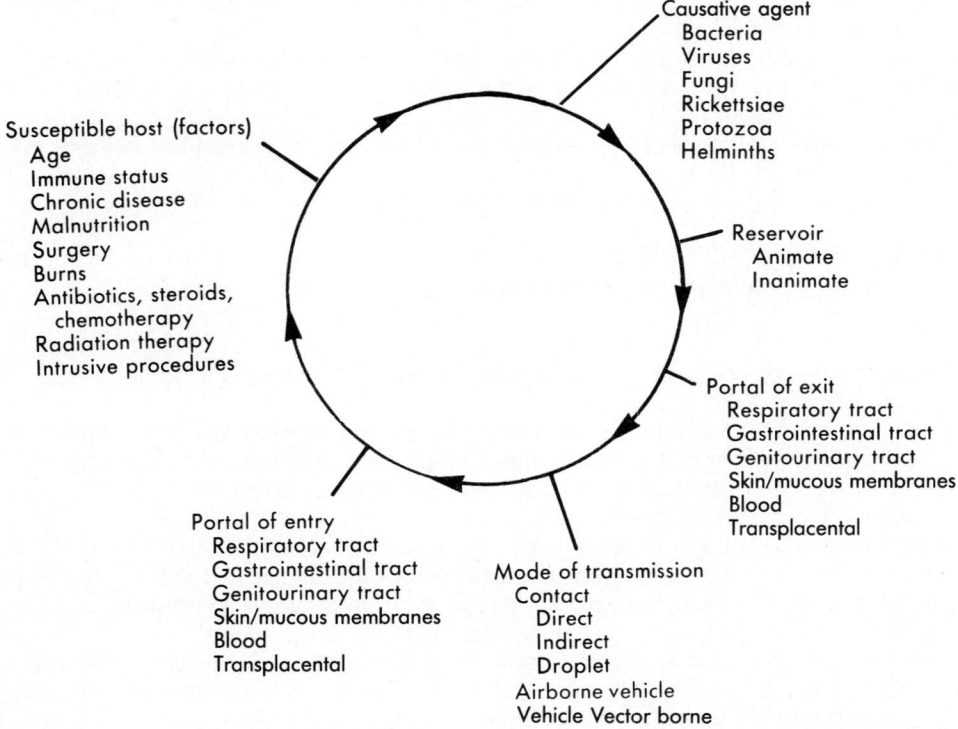

Fig. 13-1. The infectious disease process.

the basic biologic defense mechanisms of the body are compromised, an infectious organism has a much greater chance of causing an infection. Chapter 6 deals with many of the factors of biologic defense exhibited by the host to prevent infection and injury. Some of the factors that affect host susceptibility to infection appear in the second box below.

From the preceding it is evident that no one factor alone is responsible for an infection. Rather, there are a number of variables—the *agent*, the *environment*, and the *host*—that determine the outcome and to which prevention and control measures are directed. To intervene effectively in the infectious disease process it is important that all of these concepts be understood.

Examples of modes of transmission of infection

Mode	Example
Contact	
Direct	
Source to host	Gonorrhea
	Syphilis
Indirect	
Source to intermediate object to host	Animate: person touches contaminated material, does not wash hands, and carries organism on hands to susceptible host
	Inanimate: intermediate object is a *fomite*, that is, contaminated tissues, silverware, with which host comes in contact
Droplet (large particles)	
Reservoir expels droplets of infection in air and host breathes in droplets	Meningococcal meningitis, influenza
Airborne	
Droplet nuclei (1 to 5 μm in size) Reservoir of infection expels droplet nuclei in air and host breathes them in	Chickenpox (varicella), tuberculosis
Vehicle	
Contaminated inanimate vehicle serves as intermediary agent to multiple hosts	Contaminated food, water, intravenous fluids can cause salmonellosis, hepatitis B
Vector	
Source to animate intermediary to host	Source bites infected persons and then bites host Mosquitos (malaria), ticks (Rocky Mountain fever)

Factors affecting host susceptibility to infection

Age	Young and old—most susceptible
Impaired immune status	Chronic diseases: cancer, diabetes, endstage renal disease
	Immunosuppressive therapy: radiation or immunosuppressive drugs
Therapeutic treatments	Antibiotics, chemotherapy for cancer, steroids
Surgery	
Burns	
Poor nutritional status	
Invasive procedures	Intravenous catheters, chest tubes, or urinary catheters

Signs and symptoms of infection

Localized infections

Subjective complaints

1. Pain
2. Tenderness
3. Warmth
4. Redness
5. Swelling
6. Itching

Objective findings

1. Edema, redness, warmth of area
2. Exudate or drainage that is bloody, serous, cloudy, clear, creamy, or purulent

Respiratory infections

1. Sore throat
2. Rhinitis
3. Congestion
4. Cough
5. Sputum
6. Chest pain
7. Shortness of breath

1. Fever
2. Increased pulse rate
3. Elevated white blood cell count
4. Positive throat culture
5. Positive x-ray findings
6. Positive sputum culture
7. Abnormal breath sounds

Gastrointestinal infection

1. Nausea
2. Vomiting
3. Diarrhea
4. Anorexia
5. Abdominal cramps
6. Distention

1. Fever
2. Increased pulse rate
3. Elevated white blood cell count
4. Positive guaiac test
5. Abnormal bowel sounds

Genitourinary infection

1. Dysuria
2. Frequency
3. Urgency
4. Hematuria
5. Purulent or foul discharge
6. Flank or pelvic pain

1. Fever
2. Elevated white blood cell count
3. Positive urine culture

Generalized infections

Subjective complaints

1. Fatigue
2. Malaise
3. Weakness
4. Headache
5. Light-headedness
6. Congestion
7. Muscle aches
8. Joint pain
9. Decreased appetite

Objective findings

1. Fever
2. Increased pulse rate
3. Hypotension
4. Altered mental status
5. Shock
6. Confusion
7. Convulsions
8. Jaundice (in some infections)
9. WBC may be elevated

Assessment

The incubation period for an infection is variable, depending on the condition of the host. However, it is often predictable and diagnostically significant. The establishment of an infection within the human body leads to a number of specific and generalized manifestations. The exact signs and symptoms elicited in the host depend on the agent responsible for the infection and the site of the infection. (For details on host response to specific infectious disease, see the particular chapter that discusses the disease site.) Recognition of the patient with a suspected infection is a crucial step in initiating early prevention and control measures. There are some general subjective, objective, and diagnostic findings that can alert the nurse to suspect an infection, even if the causative agent is not known. These are summarized here.

The normal WBC count in blood is 5000 to 10,000 WBC/mm.[3] With the presence of a serious infection the number of WBCs rises above 10,000/mm^3 in response to the infectious inflammation. Leukocyte values between 10,000 and 20,000 are considered slightly elevated; 20,000 to 40,000 moderately elevated; and greater than 40,000 greatly elevated. In a few infectious diseases the number of WBCs in circulation actually drops, which is also a significant piece of diagnostic data.

Five types of mature WBCs are found in circulation: neutrophils, eosinophils, basophils, lymphocytes, and monocytes. Each type of WBC plays a more or less specific role in body defense (Chapter 6); therefore different diseases produce different reactions among the white cell populations in the blood. These changes in patterns of distribution are detected not just by counting the total number of WBCs in a stained blood smear but also by classifying them according to morphology and calculating the relative percentage of each cell type present. This type of count is known as a differential count. The differential count may provide information that can be correlated with other clinical data to help diagnose a situation. Table 13-2 provides some general correlations between leukocyte response and infectious diseases.

None of the signs and symptoms present in localized or generalized infections are diagnostic in themselves. Many can be demonstrated by other disease processes. They can, however, serve as helpful clues in the diagnosis of a suspected infectious process.

DIAGNOSTIC TESTS

Diagnostic tests are important in the diagnosis of an infection. Examples of some of the diagnostic tests used to obtain data are given here.

Specimens for microbiologic testing are perhaps the most frequently ordered when an infection is suspected.

Proper collection and handling of laboratory specimens are essential to ensure accurate laboratory results. Inappropriate collection or handling of specimens may lead to unnecessary delays in test results or to inaccurate results, thus affecting the therapy given to the patient. When an infection is suspected, cultures are taken of the suspected

---

Diagnostic tests to help detect the presence of infection

Bacterial, viral, and fungal cultures, gram stain
Blood counts
Skin tests
Radiologic tests
Gallium scans
Ultrasound examinations
CT scan

---

site. If the patient has a fever and the site of infection is unknown, cultures are commonly taken of the blood, urine, sputum, and any other possible sites of infection. This may include spinal fluid cultures, aspirates of body fluid, or intravenous catheter tips. *It is imperative that these cultures be obtained before the initiation of antibiotic therapy whenever possible, since antibiotics can suppress any bacteria that are present and give inaccurate or false-negative culture results.* Cultures should be obtained in a manner that avoids contamination. Aseptic preparation of the site to be cultured, observance of aseptic technique, and placing specimens in an appropriate container are crucial factors to be observed in ensuring the best sample. Once obtained, the specimen must be properly stored and transported promptly to the laboratory. Each institution should have guidelines for the proper method for collecting and handling specimens for the laboratory (Table 13-3).

Table 13-2. White blood cell response to infections

Leukocyte response	Associated infectious process
Increase in neutrophils (neutrophilia)	Usual in a large number of acute local and systemic infections caused by bacteria (especially pyogenic bacteria), rickettsia, some viruses, and a few protozoa
Decrease in neutrophils (neutropenia)	Frequent in salmonellosis, brucellosis, whooping cough, overwhelming bacterial infections, influenza, infectious mononucleosis, infectious hepatitis, mumps, rubella, rubeola, and some rickettsial and protozoan diseases
Increase in eosinophils (eosinophilia)	Frequent in allergic reactions, chronic skin disease, helminthic infections, and scarlet fever
Increase in lymphocytes (lymphocytosis)	Frequent in chickenpox, mumps, measles, infectious mononucleosis, influenza, whooping cough, syphilis, ruberculosis, salmonellosis, viral hepatitis, and viral pneumonia; sometimes in convalescence from acute bacterial infection
Increase in monocytes (monocytosis)	Common in tuberculosis, chickenpox, brucellosis, mumps, syphilis, and certain rickettsial diseases; may occur in certain viral and protozoan diseases and in convalescent phase of acute bacterial infections

Table 13-3. General guidelines for specimen collection

Objective:

To obtain specimen containing infecting pathogen that is free of contamination

Method:

1. Wash hands.
2. Prepare site aseptically.
3. Collect specimen using aseptic technique; wear gloves if appropriate; avoid coughing, sneezing, or talking.
4. Obtain adequate amount of specimen.
5. Collect and transport in sterile container appropriate for type of specimen.
6. Label requisition with patient's name, location, date and time of collection, type of specimen, how obtained (clean void or catheter urine), test requested, and current antibiotic therapy.
7. Store properly and transport promptly to laboratory.
8. Keep record of test.

Interpretation of laboratory results is sometimes difficult. Certain body sites have bacteria known as normal flora, which reside there in a commensalistic (intimate) relationship with the host. These bacteria do not cause infection in the normal host. The skin, upper respiratory tract, vagina, urethra, and bowel are examples of body sites in which normal bacterial flora can be found. The bacteria found vary from site to site, and knowing the normal flora is helpful in discerning the significance of laboratory culture results. A *Clinician's Dictionary Guide to Bacteria and Fungi*[16] is an excellent publication that lists in detail the normal flora of various sites. It must be emphasized that laboratory results alone cannot be used to make diagnostic and therapeutic decisions. Rather, they are used in conjunction with the clinical status of the patient to make appropriate diagnostic and therapeutic decisions.

Knowledge about the infectious disease process and about how to recognize or suspect an infectious process is vital to the prevention and control of infectious diseases in both community and hospital settings. Each component of the process must be understood for appropriate assessment of real or potential infection risks. The nurse can then intervene to minimize or eliminate that risk. Prevention and control of disease are addressed in the remainder of this chapter.

INFECTION CONTROL IN THE COMMUNITY

An infectious disease is termed a communicable disease when it is highly transmissible to other persons. Smallpox is an example of a communicable disease that through cooperative efforts worldwide, has been successfully eradicated. The methods used to eradicate smallpox throughout the world can serve as a model of how to eliminate other communicable diseases. The eradication of smallpox also demonstrates the importance of accurate reporting of communicable diseases to the proper authorities so that appropriate prevention and control measures can be instituted.

The community health nurse plays a vital role in the collection of data, surveillance activities, immunization programs, education, and other control measures. Physicians and health care facilities have a responsibility to report communicable diseases promptly to the health department. Health agencies in the community can use the reported data to determine potential or real problems, to identify the causative agent and hopefully its source, and to identify the population at risk. A method to control the problem, care for the exposed, and protect the population at risk can then be devised and implemented.

Prevention and control measures

One method of prevention and control of disease in the community involves environmental control measures such as sanitation techniques that ensure a pure water supply and proper disposal of sewage and other potentially infectious materials. These measures have been legislated into building codes, state laws, and federal regulations. Similarly, there are regulations regarding health practices in institutions that handle, package, and prepare foods. Another example of an environmental control measure is the spraying of a designated area to kill mosquitos, which are implicated in the spread of viral encephalitis. Spraying usually is done only after an outbreak has been identified.

Depending on the communicable disease, care of exposed persons and protection of the population at risk for contracting the disease may entail prophylaxis, immunization, or only careful monitoring of new cases. Often, simple adherence to basic principles of hygiene is sufficient. Determination of additional required measures should be made by the local or state health department. Attempts are made to reach those at risk and inform them of the preventive measures. Education of the public is a key component of these efforts.

In the United States there has been a marked reduction in recent years in the incidence of infectious diseases, such as measles, whooping cough, and poliomyelitis, which can be prevented by immunization. Concern is being expressed, however, about the decrease in the number of children presently being immunized, despite the fact that these immunizations can often be obtained free of cost. Additionally, concern is being expressed that federal monies used to support local immunization efforts may be reduced to such a level that free immunizations will no longer be equally available in all 50 states. Infections formerly seen only in children are now being seen more frequently in adults because of the failure of the population to develop acquired immunity during early childhood.

A more recent concern because of air travel is the elimination of the barriers of time and distance and the possibility of a person with an infectious disease being brought from a remote area of the world to a major population center where the disease can be readily spread to a susceptible public.

The dramatic control of several infectious diseases has been caused by the development and use of a variety of *inactivated vaccines* and *live attenuated antigens*. The potential for eradication of common infectious diseases brings with it major responsibilities for public health agencies, physicians, and nurses. Ways must be found not only to carry out planned programs of immunization, but also to educate the public to the hazards of apathy and failure to maintain proper levels of immunization. Continued progress in control and eradication requires that there be commitment to continue to add to knowledge about immunization patterns, to evaluate effectiveness and risks of antigens used, and to monitor the levels of protection present in a population.

Immunization programs

Immunization programs have played and continue to play a primary role in the control of infectious disease throughout the world. The body can be stimulated to produce antibodies against some specific diseases without actually having the disease *(active artificial immunity)*. Temporary protection sometimes can be provided by injecting antibodies produced by other persons or other animals into the bloodstream of a human being *(passive artificial immunity)*.

Recommendations concerning current immunization schedules are found in the *Red Book* published by the Committee on Infectious Diseases of The American Academy of Pediatrics and in *Morbidity and Mortality Weekly Reports,* which present recommendations of the United States Public Health Service's Advisory Committee on Immunization Practices (ACIP). The reader should refer to these resources when there are questions about proper immunization practices, prophylaxis, interruption in immunization schedules, or adverse reactions and side effects. A summary of active and passive immunization appears below.

ACTIVE IMMUNIZATION

If 90% of the population is protected against organisms that require continued passage through human beings to

---

Immunization

Active

Produce own antibodies after being inoculated with a vaccine

Passive

Injected with antibodies produced by other persons or animals (horse, cow, rabbit)

Active artificial immunity

Vaccine made from attenuated or dead organisms or modified toxins of the organisms; protection is temporary and is called *artificial passive acquired immunity*

Vaccines available

Usually given when person has been exposed to disease and has no immunity to it

Smallpox (eliminated from world by vaccination)
Diphtheria
Tetanus
Pertussis
Measles (rubella)
Influenza
Mumps
Poliomyelitis
Typhoid
Pneumococcal pneumomia

---

reproduce and live, the disease caused by the organism can be virtually eliminated because there are too few susceptible hosts for organism spread. Smallpox has been eliminated from the world in this way. This type of protection of a group is called *herd immunity.* It is ineffectual, however, against organisms such as tetanus bacilli that can exist indefinitely (in the soil), and in this instance each person must be immunized to be protected. If the disease is one not prevalent in the environment, such as diphtheria in the United States, or is not spread from person to person by direct contact, such as tetanus, the inoculation must be repeated at regular intervals to maintain protection. This inoculation is called a *booster dose,* and usually one tenth of the original inoculating dose is sufficient.

An inoculation often causes a local tissue response. Symptoms of inflammation (redness, tenderness, swelling, sometimes ulcerations) appear at the site of the injection, and symptoms of widespread tissue involvement (slight febrile reactions, general malaise, muscle aching) for 1 or 2 days are not uncommon. The initial inoculation produces delayed symptoms because the immune response system must become sensitized to the antigen. There usually is an accelerated and less servere systemic reaction to subsequent inoculations because the immune response is stimulated at once. The local reaction also is less severe than that which occurs following the initial inoculation because the organisms have less opportunity to produce inflammation.

Active artificial immunization against many bacilli and viruses is now available. All persons should be encouraged to avail themselves of the protection advised by health officials in their local area. They also should be advised to keep a permanent record of the date of each immunization.

Primary immunization schedules

In the United States, the ACIP recommends that all children be immunized against diphtheria, pertussis, (whooping cough), and tetanus (DPT); measles, mumps, and rubella (MMR); and poliomyelitis (OPV) (Table 13–4). Children who have not been immunized as infants can be immunized at any age. All susceptible children, adolescents, and adults should be immunized unless contraindicated.

Routine vaccination against smallpox is no longer recommended by the CDC, since the side effects and complications of the vaccine are greater than the danger of acquiring the disease. The vaccine is indicated only for laboratory workers who are directly involved with smallpox or closely related orthopox viruses.

At the present time, immunization against typhoid fever is recommended only when there is exposure to a typhoid carrier in the household, when there is an outbreak to typhoid in a community, or for travelers to countries where typhoid is endemic (always present).

Immunization to protect against other diseases is given on a selective basis; that is, groups at a high risk are immunized. Hepatitis B vaccine is an excellent example

Table 13-4. Recommended schedule for active immunization of normal infants and children (See individual ACIP recommendations for details)

Recommended age	Vaccine(s)	Comments
2 months	DTP-1, OPV-1	Can be given earlier in endemic areas
4 months	DTP-2, OPV-2	6-week to 2-month interval desired between OPV doses to avoid interference
6 months	DTP-3	An additional dose of OPV at this time is optional in areas with a high risk of polio exposure
15 months	MMR	
18 months	DTP-4, OPV-3	Completion of primary series
4–6 years	DTP-5, OPV-4	Preferably at or before school entry
14–16 years	Td*	Repeat every 10 years throughout life

From Morbid. Mortal. Week. Rep. **32**(1):4, 1983.
*Adult tetanus toxoid and diphtheria toxoid in combination; contains same dose of tetanus toxoid as DTP or DT and a reduced dose of diphtheria toxoid.

of a vaccine that is only recommended for persons at high risk of acquiring the virus, such as dentists, hemodialysis personnel, and people who have frequent contact with blood and blood products.

Because of the prevalence of *influenza* and its potential for causing death, the ACIP recommends immunization against influenza for all individuals at increased risk of adverse consequences from infection of the lower respiratory tract. This includes persons over 60 years of age and persons over 2 years of age who have chronic cardiac, respiratory, metabolic, or renal disease or diseases that impair the person's immune system.

The use of pneumococcal vaccine against *Streptococcus pneumoniae* is under investigation. There is not yet enough data for the ACIP to formulate formal recommendations about the routine use of the vaccine for immunization in the general population. It is currently being administered to adults and children over 2 years of age with chronic illnesses who are at increased risk of complications associated with pneumonoccal infections. A single dose is given only once. The duration of protection is unknown. Further investigation of the use of vaccines for protection against other bacterial infections is under way and could offer promise in improving immune defenses in immunocompromised patients.

PASSIVE IMMUNIZATION

Passive immunization usually is reserved for situations in which the disease would be detrimental to the person. For example, it is rarely given to prevent a disease such as chickenpox or mumps in children because they are at an optimal age for the body to respond immunologically with minimal inflammatory response. On the other hand, an adult exposed to the same diseases often would be given antibodies because adults may have a severe pathologic response. Immunization is given to all age groups exposed to pathogens that cause serious diseases such as hepatitis, poliomyelitis, diphtheria, tetanus, or rabies. Antivenins, which are given to people bitten by poisonous snakes or black widow spiders, are other examples of passive immunologic products.

Products used for passive immunization may be specific to the disease. Antitoxins and immune animal and human sera are examples. These materials contain elevated levels of immune globulins, which can specifically detoxify the toxin, neutralize the virus, or inactivate the bacterium. The whole blood of a patient who has recently recovered from a disease against which antibodies are produced also may be used. Antitoxins are available for diphtheria, tetanus, botulism, gas gangrene, and the venom of snakes. *Immune animal serum* is available against rabies; *human immune serum* is available for mumps, measles, pertussis, poliomyelitis, and tetanus.

Immune serum globulin (ISG), or gamma globulin (γ-globulin), is an antibody-rich fraction of pooled plasma from normal donors. The rationale for pooling plasma is that someone among the donors will have had the diseases and will have developed antibodies against them. The *globulin fraction* of the plasma carries the antibodies, and because it is known not to transmit the virus of hepatitis, it is considered safe to use. Because of occasional side effects, it is now recommended that the use of immune serum globulin be limited to those disorders in which its efficacy has been definitely established. These are measles prophylaxis or modification, viral hepatitis type A prophylaxis or modification, and immune deficiency diseases. Immune serum globulin is considered to be of *questionable value* in the following situations: (1) prevention of rubella in the first trimester of pregnancy, (2) prevention or modification of varicella in certain high-risk patients, (3) prevention or modification of viral hepatitis type B (serum hepatitis) after accidental inoculation, and (4) life-threatening bacterial infections.

Special human immune serum globulins are derived from the sera of persons previously immunized or convalescing from specific diseases. Tetanus immune globulin (human) is of value in prophylaxis and treatment of tetanus in persons who have not received prior immunization. Pertussis immune globulin (human) and mumps immune globulin (human) are of uncertain or unproved value in the prevention and treatment of pertussis and mumps, respectively. Hepatitis B immune globulin (human) is available for prophylaxis after exposure to hepatitis B. Zoster immune globulin (human) is available for restricted use for prophylaxis against chickenpox.

NURSING RESPONSIBILITIES IN IMMUNIZATION

The greatest responsibility of the nurse in immunization programs is to teach the public the advantages of immunization and encourage widespread participation in programs recommended by the local public health officer.

Teaching

In teaching it is advisable to provide the public with the following information: against what disease protection is being given, why immunization is desirable, and when booster doses should be obtained. The relative safety of the immunization and the advantages of immunization early in life should be stressed.

The nurse is responsible for assessing persons before immunization because there are some contraindications to receiving certain immunizing substances. Those that are prepared in chicken or duck embryos may cause an allergic reaction in persons who are allergic to eggs. Many people are allergic to horse serum, and substances containing horse serum, such as tetanus antitoxin, should never be given unless a small amount of the substance has been injected intradermally (a sensitivity test) and after 20 minutes produces no "hive" reaction about the injection site. *Active immunologic products* should not be given while a person has a cold or other infection because the inflammatory reaction from the immunization will be greater than usual.

Live attenuated virus vaccines should not be given to persons with alterations in their immune status, since virus replication after administration may be unchecked in these individuals. OPV viruses are excreted by the recipient of the vaccine and are communicable to other persons, so individuals who live with an immunocompromised person should not receive OPV. If a person has a febrile illness, it is usually best to wait until recovery before vaccination is given. Pregnant women should not receive *live attenuated virus* vaccines because of the theoretical risk to the fetus. Live attenuated virus vaccines should not be given at the same time as passive immunization, since passively acquired antibodies can interfere with the response to live attenuated virus vaccines.[14]

Before leaving the clinic, the person or family members should be instructed as to the expected effects of an inoculation and told to contact the physician or to report to a hospital emergency room if any other symptoms develop.

The person is cautioned not to scratch any lesion produced by an inoculation. If a severe local reaction with redness, swelling, and tenderness occurs, the physician may order the application of hot, wet dressings. If the lesion is open, these dressings should be sterile.

When antitoxins, antisera, or antivenins are given, the patient is kept under observation for 20 to 30 minutes. Symptoms of severe allergic response usually will appear within that period of time.

Persons employed in health care facilities should maintain their immune status against poliomyelitis, diphtheria, and tetanus. Persons with negative tuberculin tests should be retested every 6 months, and those with positive tuberculin tests should have a yearly chest x-ray film taken. Persons working in dialysis units and blood processing areas (laboratories, blood banks) need to guard against infection with hepatitis B virus.

Home care

Persons with communicable diseases are frequently cared for at home. The community health nurse is often asked to teach family members how to care for the patient and how to protect family members, friends, and neighbors. The same principles apply in the home as in the hospital. It must be emphasized that the extent of the care measure depends on the communicable disease involved. The local health department should be consulted for full information regarding specific communicable diseases.

The person who is discharged from the hospital with an infection that may be apparent or incubating at the time of discharge is also a public health concern. This person should be cared for similarly to those with known infections using the guidelines already mentioned. Likewise, the person who is admitted to the hospital from the community with an infection poses a potential problem in the hospital as well. This person can serve as a source of infection to other patients and personnel and it would be best to treat such a person at home, if possible. The special problems the nurse encounters in controlling *hospital-acquired infections* will be the focus of the remainder of this chapter.

INFECTION CONTROL IN THE HOSPITAL
Scope of the problem

A *nosocomial* infection is one that is not present or incubating at the time a person is admitted to the hospital but develops after admission. A *community-acquired infection* is one that is present or incubating at the time of admission to the hospital. The nurse should be aware of the problem of nosocomial infections; their effects on patient morbidity, mortality, and increased hospital costs; as well as the legal aspects concerning them. The nurse also should be knowledgeable about the types of infections seen most often, the common pathogens and how they are transmitted, factors that predispose a patient to a nosocomial infection, how to recognize persons at risk of infection, and the prevention and control measures necessary to decrease the incidence of nosocomial infections.

At least 2 million persons, or about 5% of all patients admitted to U.S. hospitals each year, develop nosocomial infections. In addition to the considerable morbidity and mortality caused by these infections, their diagnoses and treatment (including additional days of hospitalization) cost more than $1 billion per year.[17] The JCAH requires that those institutions seeking accreditation have a program of infection control centered around monitoring (1) patients with infections, (2) patient care practices, (3) antibiotic usage, (4) health of personnel, and (5) the environment of the institution. The AHA and the CDC have developed guidelines for the prevention and control of infectious diseases for use in patient care centers. Because of these external forces, as well as to provide the best possible care for their patients, hospitals are recognizing the need to increase infection surveillance and to upgrade programs to prevent nosocomial infections.

As seen in Table 13-5, the incidence of nosocomial infections varies with the type of hospital, and this can be attributed to differences in the size of hospitals, the severity of illness in the patient population, the susceptibility of the patient population, and the number of personnel who have hands-on contact with the patients. The patient with the greatest-risk of developing a nosocomial infection is one with a chronic illness, a prolonged hospital stay, and the most direct contact with various hospital personnel (that is, physicians, students, nurses, or therapists). These factors hold true not only for variations of infection rates from institution to institution, but also for variations in infection rates within an institution. Certain patient care areas are considered to be *high-risk areas* for developing nosocomial infections. These areas understandably are those that care for patients who have decreased host defenses or in whom invasive procedures and devices are common. Areas generally considered to be high risk are (1) intensive care units (including neonatal units), (2) burn units, (3) dialysis units, and (4) oncology units. The infection rate in these areas may be well over 20%.

Persons at risk

The nurse needs to be able to recognize those patients who are at the greatest risk of a nosocomial infection. Some of the factors that predispose a person to infection are mentioned on p. 193. Probably the single most important factor predisposing a patient to acquiring a nosocomial infection is the severity of the patient's underlying disease.

A patient admitted to the hospital with an infection may develop during the hospitalization a *superinfection* with another organism. Often this superinfection is with a more virulent or drug-resistant organism. For example, a patient admitted with a leg ulcer infected with *Staphylococcus aureus* may develop further infection (not colonization) with *Pseudomonas aeruginosa*. Furthermore, if this infection progresses to involve the bloodstream, then a *secondary bacteremia* has occurred. Infection can occur secondary to (1) an existing infection, (2) an underlying disease process, or (3) an anatomic defect that may be causing obstruction. An example of this is the man who has benign prostate hypertrophy (BPH) and who develops a urinary tract infection secondary to the obstruction caused by the BPH.

Table 13-5. Nosocomial infection rates by category of hospital

Category of hospital	Percent of patients with nosocomial infections*
Community	2.5
Community-teaching	3.1
Federal	3.7
Municipal or county	4.1
University	4.4
All hospitals	3.3

From Centers for Disease Control: National nosocomial infections study report: Annual summary, 1979, Atlanta, 1982, The Centers.
*Rate per 100 patient discharges.

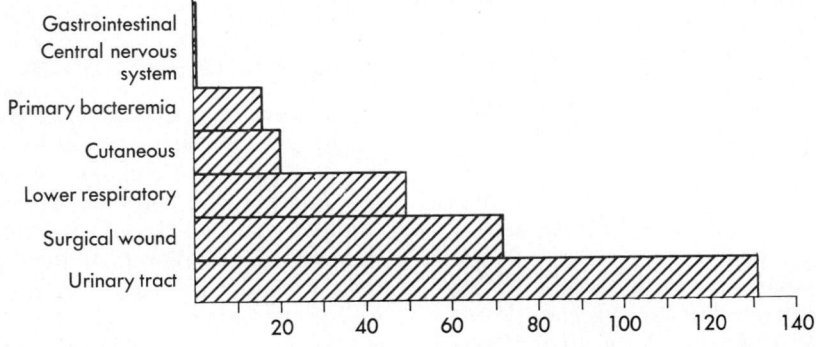

Fig. 13-2. Nosocomial infection rates per 10,000 patients discharged by site of infection. (From Centers for Disease Control: National nosocomial infections study report. Annual summary 1979, Issued March 1982, U.S. Department of Health and Human Services.)

The most common site for a nosocomial infection is the urinary tract; 75% of these infections are related to instrumentation, including indwelling urinary catheters, catheterizations, and urologic procedures. Infected surgical wounds, followed by lower respiratory tract infections, and then bloodstream infections (some associated with the use of intravascular lines) are the next most frequently encountered types of nosocomial infections. Together these sites account for about 85% of all nosocomial infections (Fig. 13-2).

Pathogens causing nosocomial infections

The different types of pathogens commonly responsible for nosocomial infections and their most common reservoirs are listed in Table 13-6). In the past 2 decades there has been a decline in the number of nosocomial infections caused by gram-positive bacteria, especially staphylococci and streptococci; however, *S. aureus* is still the single most common organism causing nosocomial surgical wound infections. At the same time, there has been an increase in the incidence of nosocomial infection caused by gram-negative bacteria, particularly members of the family Enterobacteriaceae and the genus *Pseudomonas,* which now cause 60% to 65% of all nosocomial infections. These gram-negative organisms collectively are responsible for nearly all nosocomial urinary tract infections, 70% of the bacteremias, and the majority of respiratory tract and surgical wound infections. *P. aeru-*

ginosa is present throughout the hospital environment, especially where there is a persistent presence of water (in sinks, irrigating solutions, or nebulizers). Patients who are receiving antibiotic therapy, who are immunedeficient, or who are subject to invasive procedures are particularly susceptible to infections by these organisms. Antibiotic drug resistance can present a serious problem when treating these patients.

Serratia marcescens and *Serratia liquefaciens* are gram-negative organisms that are being seen with increased frequency in nosocomial infections. The reservoirs for these organisms are soil and water, and they are found in the hospital in similar reservoirs as *Pseudomonas.* Previously thought to be nonpathogenic, *S. marcescens* was used because of its red pigmentation to mark air flow and settling patterns of bacteria. It is now recognized as a pathogen that can cause severe infection in a susceptible host. One problem with *Serratia* organisms has been their ability to rapidly develop resistance to antibiotics. This can have devastating consequences in an intensive care or burn unit when an outbreak occurs. Because its mode of transmission is through direct or indirect contact on the hands of personnel or on contaminated articles, good hand-washing and aseptic techniques are the most effective measures to prevent outbreaks of infection.

Candida albicans is a yeastlike fungus that can cause infection, especially in immunocompromised patients or in patients receiving antibiotics. These patients have a decrease in their normal flora, which provides a niche for the *Candida* organism's to settle in and proliferate. Anti-

Table 13-6. Common reservoirs of some pathogens

Pathogen	Common reservoir
Gram-positive cocci	
Staphlococcus aureus	Anterior nares, skin (especially hands) of human carriers, contaminated objects
Group A *Streptococcus*	Nose and throat of human carriers, GI tract of humans
Enterococcus	
Gram-negative rods	
Escherichia, Klebsiella, Enterobacter, Proteus, Salmonella, Serratia, Pseudomonas, Providencia	GI tract, food, water, soil, contaminated solutions and objects, other infected patients
Anaerobes	
Clostridium	Soil, contaminated environment
Bacteroides	Oropharynx, bowel
Fungi	
Candida albicans	Normal flora in some people, contaminated environment
Viruses	
Varicella	Human carriers
Herpes	Human carriers
Rubella	Human carriers
Hepatitis B	Human carriers, contaminated objects
Poliomyelitis	Human carriers, contaminated food, water and environment

biotics suppress bacterial growth but do not affect fungal growth; special antifungal agents are necessary to control these infections unless there is a return of the normal flora following discontinuance of the antibiotics.

Prevention and control measures

In the hospital there are many potential sources of infection, including patients, personnel, visitors, equipment, and linen. The patient may become infected with organisms from either the external environment (*exogenous*) or, as is often seen in the severely immunocompromised host, from their own internal organisms (*endogenous*). Virtually any microorganism can be a potential pathogen to the immunocompromised patient. Most of the causative organisms are present in the external environment of the patient and are introduced into the body through direct contact or contaminated materials. In many instances nosocomial infections could be prevented by strict aseptic technique when giving care to the patient and by using greater restraint in the use of invasive procedures and antibiotics. A summary of some of the prevention and control measures are presented in the box

below. The reader is referred to the CDC manual of *Guidelines for the Prevention and Control of Nosocomial Infections* for greater detail.

PREVENTION OF URINARY TRACT INFECTIONS

As mentioned previously, *urinary tract infections* (UTIs) are the most common nosocomial infections seen in the hospital. The majority of these infections are associated with catheterization and instrumentation of the urinary tract. Urinary catheters should be used only when absolutely necessary. If a catheter must be used, it should be discontinued as soon as medically feasible, since the longer the catheter is in place, the greater the risk of developing an infection. As small a catheter as possible should be used to minimize urethral trauma.

Strict aseptic technique is necessary when inserting the catheter to prevent transmission of bacteria into the bladder. Bacteria that are present around the catheter-meatal junction can also be transmitted on the tip of the catheter into the bladder along the thin layer of mucus that surrounds the catheter in the urethra. For this reason, the catheter should be securely anchored to prevent

---

Prevention of and control measures for nosocomial infections

Control of external environment (exogenous sources of infection)
Health care providers

1. In good health—not care for patients when ill
2. Keep immunizations current
3. Practice effective hand washing between each patient, after handling contaminated material, before handling sterile equipment and supplies
   a. If skin dry, rough, broken—seek appropriate attention
   b. If active herpes simplex infection of hand (herpetic whitlow)—do not give direct patient care until lesion healed

Housekeeping and sanitation

1. Bed linens not shaken in air or thrown on floor
2. Proper disposal of wastes—solid and liquid
3. Proper cleaning and sterilization of contaminated articles
4. Proper ventilation for adequate air exchanges
   a. Modern hospitals—patients' rooms under negative pressure
   b. Negative pressure keeps air from patients' rooms from moving into hallways
5. Proper mopping and damp dusting to remove dust and other environmental reservoirs of infection

Control of internal environment (endogenous sources of infection)

1. Preventive measures aimed at increasing patient's defense mechanisms and thus reducing risk of infection
   a. Teach patient about good nutrition
   b. Teach patient about personal hygiene, especially hand washing
2. Be aware that normal flora of patient can be disrupted when patient is receiving antibiotics or chemotherapy and colonization may occur
   a. Give antibiotics on time as scheduled
   b. Teach patient about appropriate use of antibiotics and dangers of taking them when not prescribed by physician

it from moving in and out of the urethra. Movement of the catheter can track bacteria into the urethra and up into the bladder along the mucous sheath. Furthermore, the catheter-meatal junction should be kept clean; the patient incontinent of stool can pose a problem in this regard. In some institutions antiseptic agents are used to cleanse the meatus and antimicrobial agents are applied around the catheter-meatal junction. *Both of these practices are considered controversial.* Good hand-washing techniques by personnel, cleansing of the patient's meatal area with soap and water, and proper anchoring of the catheter are considered to be effective ways to reduce the incidence of UTIs in patients with indwelling catheters.

Another portal of entry for bacteria is through the distal catheter–proximal drainage tube junction. Every time the system is disconnected there is an increased risk of introducing bacteria into the system. For this reason a sterile closed drainage system should be maintained. The tubing should be kept from kinking and obstruction. Bladder irrigations should not be a routine practice. If irrigation is necessary, a sterile disposable syringe and sterile solution should be used, and the catheter-tubing junction should be disinfected before disconnection. If frequent irrigations are necessary, as in patients who have had a transurethral prostatectomy (TURP) in which blood clots are common, a three-way catheter drainage system with continuous bladder irrigation is recommended. In this way a closed system is maintained. Urine specimens should be obtained from the rubber portal on the drainage tubing (Fig. 33-17). The portal should be cleansed with an antiseptic before insertion of the sterile needle into the portal.

Another portal of entry of bacteria into the system is through the collection bag. The bag should be kept below the bladder level at all times to prevent reflux of urine into the bladder. It also should be kept off the floor and the emptying spout should be cleansed with an antiseptic before and after the urine is emptied from the bag. The container used to collect the urine from the bag must be used for only one patient; it should not be shared between patients. Catheters should not be changed on a routine basis. Rather, they should be replaced only when they become obstructed, requiring frequent irrigations, or when concretions are detected in the tubing, which can lead to obstructed flow. A final control measure in preventing nosocomial UTIs is to place patients with urinary catheters in separate rooms. This is helpful in preventing cross-infection between patients.

PREVENTION OF SURGICAL WOUND INFECTIONS

Surgical wounds often are inoculated with bacteria at the time of surgery. To minimize the risk, proper preoperative preparation should include preparation of the site with an antiseptic agent and shaving of hair around the site only when it will interfere with the surgical procedure. Shaving of hair should be done as close to the time of surgery as possible. During surgery, the most important factor is observance of strict asepsis by all. The operating room nurse is responsible for maintaining surgical asepsis during surgery. On the patient care units nurses continue to play vital roles in ensuring that aseptic technique is maintained by all who have contact with the patient's wound or dressing. Again, hand washing is the major measure to prevent nosocomial surgical wound infections. Appropriate use of antibiotics both preoperatively and postoperatively is also a concern because of their effect on the patient's own flora.

PREVENTION OF RESPIRATORY TRACT INFECTIONS

Pneumonia is the most common nosocomial infection of the lower respiratory tract. Preventive measures include proper maintenance and decontamination of respiratory therapy equipment and respiratory assistive devices. Special attention should be given to nebulizers, which contain moisture and are ideal reservoirs for organisms, especially gram-negative organisms such as *Pseudomonas* and *Serratia*. The patient who has a tracheostomy or is intubated is at great risk because these tubes bypass the patient's normal oropharyngeal defense mechanisms. Suctioning should be performed using aseptic technique and sterile irrigants (Chapter 25). Inappropriate use of antibiotics should be avoided to minimize oropharyngeal colonization with pathogens that could be aspirated and lead to pneumonia. Patients should be taught the importance of pulmonary toilet and should be instructed how to cough, take deep breaths, and use respiratory therapy equipment properly. Debilitated patients should be protected from the hazards of aspiration, especially while eating.

PREVENTION OF BACTEREMIAS

Many blood infections (bacteremias) occur secondary to infections at another site; thus prevention may depend a great deal on control of the underlying infection. Some bacteremias are the result of the use of intravascular devices and systems. The sources of infection in these instances are the hands of personnel, the patient's skin, or infusions that are contaminated either from mishandling by hospital personnel or, less commonly, at the time of manufacture. Intravenous and intraarterial catheters should be inserted under aseptic conditions, and catheter insertion sites should be cared for aseptically. A sterile dressing should cover the insertion site. The insertion site is inspected frequently for any sign of infection, such as redness, swelling, exudate, purulence, or warmth. The patient may also complain of pain at the site. Peripheral catheters should be changed every 48 to 72 hours or more often if there is a complication such as infiltration or phlebitis. The catheter is secured to prevent in-and-out movement and tracking of bacteria into the cannula site. Aseptic technique should be followed when mixing and adding drugs, changing the infusion, or manipulating connections or stopcocks. It is recommended that the tubing be changed every 48 hours (24 to 48 hours for hyperalimentation). Before hanging a solution, the nurse should check it for turbidity and particulate matter and for leaks in the system. Solutions should be discarded after 24 hours. Hyperalimentation solutions require special adherence to these practices, since they are composed of nutrients that are an excellent culture media for organisms. *Candida* infections are commonly seen in patients receiving hyperalimentation, particularly those who are immunocompromised.

PROTECTION BY ISOLATION

When a person is admitted to the hospital with an infection or develops a nosocomial infection, other patients and personnel should be protected against possible infection from this person. This is accomplished by isolation. In planning care the nurse determines the site of the infection and the characteristics of the pathogen involved in deciding whether isolation is indicated and, if so, what type is required. Factors that affect the decision include the virulence of the organism and its mode of transmission. The nurse must correlate the clinical status of the patient with the laboratory results to ascertain whether the patient has an infection or is merely colonized. This facilitates making an intelligent decision about the appropriate isolation measures.

The CDC recently revised the guidelines for isolation precautions in hospitals. Two systems are offered for use by an institution, one based on categories of isolation, the other based on disease-specific isolation precautions. An institution is advised to choose only one of these systems and to adapt it to meet the specific needs of the institution. The major categories of isolation are (1) strict, (2) contact, (3) respiratory, (4) tuberculosis (acid-fast bacilli [AFB]), (5) enteric, (6) drainage/secretion, and (7) blood/body fluids. The recommended specifications and examples of diseases for which the category is used are presented in Table 13-7. Because protective isolation has not been shown to reduce the risk of infection in compromised patients, the CDC no longer includes it as a separate category. Adherence to good hand washing and aseptic techniques is emphasized.

General principles of isolation

Some general principles apply regardless of the type of isolation. Gowns, gloves, and masks should be used only once and then discarded in an appropriate receptacle before leaving the patient's room. Clean gowns, gloves, and masks are kept on a table or cart outside the door of the contaminated room. Hands must be washed before and after patient contact, even when gloves are a required part of the isolation procedure. Masks become ineffective when they are moist and therefore should never be reused. They should be worn over the nose and mouth and should not hang around the neck and then be reused. Contaminated articles should be placed in an impervious clean bag in the contaminated area, closed securely, placed into a second clean bag outside the contaminated area, sealed, and labeled "contaminated." Mattresses and pillows should be covered with impervious plastic.

Text continued on p. 210.

Table 13-7. Category-specific isolation precautions

Strict isolation

Strict isolation is designed to prevent transmission of highly contagious or virulent infections that may be spread by both air and contact.

Specifications for strict isolation

1. Private room is indicated; door should be kept closed. In general, patients infected with the same organism may share a room.
2. Masks are indicated for all persons entering the room.
3. Gowns are indicated for all persons entering the room.
4. Gloves are indicated for all persons entering the room.
5. Hands must be washed after touching the patient or potentially contaminated articles and before taking care of another patient.
6. Articles contaminated with infective material should be discarded or bagged and labeled before being sent for decontamination and reprocessing.

Diseases requiring strict isolation

Diphtheria, pharyngeal
Lassa fever and other viral hemorrhagic fevers, such as Marburg virus disease*
Plague, pneumonic
Smallpox*
Varicella (chickenpox)
Zoster, localized in immunocompromised patient or disseminated

From Garner, J.S., and Simmons, B.T.: CDC guidelines: nosocomial infections, Infect. Control **4**:261-283, 1983.
*A private room with special ventilation is indicated.

Table 13-7. Category-specific isolation precautions—cont'd

Contact isolation

Contact isolation is designed to prevent transmission of highly transmissible or epidemiologically important infections (or colonization) that do not warrant Strict isolation. All diseases or conditions included in this category are spread primarily by close or direct contact. Thus masks, gowns, and gloves are recommended for anyone in close or direct contact with any patient who has an infection (or colonization) included in this category. For individual diseases or conditions, however, one or more of these three barriers may not be indicated. For example, masks and gloves are not generally indicated for care of infants and young children with acute viral respiratory infections, gowns are not generally indicated for gonococcal conjunctivitis in newborns, and masks are not generally indicated for care of patients infected with multiply resistant microorganisms, except those with pneumonia. Therefore some degree of "overisolation" may occur in this category.

Specifications for contact isolation

1. Private room is indicated. In general, patients infected with the same organism may share a room. During outbreaks, infants and young children with the same respiratory clinical syndrome may share a room.
2. Masks are indicated for those who come close to the patient.
3. Gowns are indicated if soiling is likely.
4. Gloves are indicated for touching infective material.
5. Hands must be washed after touching the patient or potentially contaminated articles and before taking care of another patient.
6. Articles contaminated with infective material should be discarded or bagged and labeled before being sent for decontamination and reprocessing.

Diseases or conditions requiring contact isolation

Acute respiratory infections in infants and young children, including croup, colds, bronchitis, and bronchiolitis caused by respiratory syncytial virus, adenovirus, coronavirus, influenza viruses, parainfluenza viruses, and rhinovirus
Conjunctivitis, gonococcal, in newborns
Diphtheria, cutaneous
Endometritis, group A *Streptococcus*
Furunculosis, staphylococcal, in newborns
Herpes simplex, disseminated, severe primary or neonatal
Impetigo
Influenza, in infants and young children
Multiply resistant bacteria, infection of colonization (any site) with any of the following:
1. Gram-negative bacilli resistant to all aminoglycosides that are tested (in general, such organisms should be resistant to gentamicin, tobramycin, and amikacin for these special precautions to be indicated)
2. *Staphylococcus aureus* resistant to methicillin (or nafcillin or oxacillin if they are used instead of methicillin for testing)
3. *Pneumococcus* resistant to penicillin
4. *Haemophilus influenzae* resistant to ampicillin (beta lactamase positive) and chloramphenicol
5. Other resistant bacteria may be included if they are judged by the infection control team to be of special clinical and epidemiologic significance.
Pediculosis
Pharyngitis, infectious, in infants and young children
Pneumonia, viral in infants and young children
Pneumonia, *Staphylococcus aureus* or group A *Streptococcus*
Rabies
Rubella, congenital and other
Scabies
Scalded skin syndrome, staphylococcal (Ritter's disease)
Skin, wound, or burn infection, major (draining and not covered by dressing or dressing does not adequately contain the purulent material) including those infected with *Staphylococcus aureus* or group A *Streptococcus*
Vaccinia (generalized and progressive eczema vaccinatum)

Continued.

Table 13-7. Category-specific isolation precautions—cont'd

Respiratory isolation

Respiratory isolation is designed to prevent transmission of infectious diseases primarily over short distances through the air (droplet transmission). Direct and indirect contact transmission occurs with some infections in this isolation category but is infrequent.

Specifications for respiratory isolation

1. Private room is indicated. In general, patients infected with the same organism may share a room.
2. Masks are indicated for those who come close to the patient.
3. Gowns are not indicated.
4. Gloves are not indicated.
5. Hands must be washed after touching the patient or potentially contaminated articles and before taking care of another patient.
6. Articles contaminated with infective material should be discarded or bagged and labeled before being sent for decontamination and reprocessing.

Diseases requiring respiratory isolation

Epiglottitis, *Haemophilus influenzae*
Erythema infectiosum
Measles
Meningitis
   Haemophilus influenzae, known or suspected
   Meningococcal, known or suspected
Meningococcal pneumonia
Meningococcemia
Mumps
Pertussis (whooping cough)
Pneumonia, *Haemophilus influenzae,* in children (any age)

Tuberculosis isolation (AFB isolation)

Tuberculosis isolation (AFB isolation) is an isolation category for patients with pulmonary tuberculosis who have a positive sputum smear or a chest x-ray film that strongly suggests current (active) tuberculosis. Laryngeal tuberculosis is also included in this isolation category. In general, infants and young children with pulmonary tuberculosis do not require isolation precautions because they rarely cough, and their bronchial secretions contain few AFB, compared with adults with pulmonary tuberculosis. On the instruction card, this category is called AFB isolation to protect the patient's privacy.

Specifications for tuberculosis isolation (AFB isolation)

1. Private room with special ventilation is indicated; door should be kept closed. In general, patients infected with the same organism may share a room.
2. Masks are indicated only if the patient is coughing and does not reliably cover mouth.
3. Gowns are indicated only if needed to prevent gross contamination of clothing.
4. Gloves are not indicated.
5. Hands must be washed after touching the patient or potentially contaminated articles and before taking care of another patient.
6. Articles are rarely involved in transmission of tuberculosis. However, articles should be thoroughly cleaned and disinfected, or discarded.

Table 13-7. Category-specific isolation precautions—cont'd

Enteric precautions

Enteric precautions are designed to prevent infections that are transmitted by direct or indirect contact with feces. Hepatitis A is included in this category because it is spread through feces, although the disease is much less likely to be transmitted after the onset of jaundice. Most infections in this category primarily cause gastrointestinal symptoms, but some do not. For example, feces from patients infected with "poliovirus" and coxsackieviruses are infective, but these infections do not usually cause prominent gastrointestinal symptoms.

Specifications for enteric precautions

1. Private room is indicated if patient hygiene is poor. A patient with poor hygiene does not wash hands after touching infective material, contaminates the environment with infective material, or shares contaminated articles with other patients. In general, patients infected with the same organism may share a room.
2. Masks are not indicated.
3. Gowns are indicated if soiling is likely.
4. Gloves are indicated if touching infective material.
5. Hands must be washed after touching the patient or potentially contaminated articles and before taking care of another patient.
6. Articles contaminated with infective material should be discarded or bagged and labeled before being sent for decontamination and reprocessing.

Diseases requiring enteric precautions

Amebic dysentery
Cholera
Coxsackievirus disease
Diarrhea, acute illness with suspected infectious etiology
Echovirus disease
Encephalitis (unless known not be caused by enteroviruses)
Enterocolitis caused by *Clostridium difficile* or *Straphylococcus aureus*
Enteroviral infection
Gastroenteritis caused by
  Campylobacter species
  Cryptosporidium species
  Dientamoeba fragilis
  Escherichia coli (enterotoxic, enteropathogenic, or enteroinvasive)
  Giardia lamblia
  Salmonella species
  Shigella species
  Vibrio parahaemolyticus
  Viruses—including Norwalk agent and rotavirus
  Yersinia enterocolitica
  Unknown etiology but presumed to be an infectious agent
Hand, foot, and mouth disease
Hepatitis, viral, type A
Herpangina
Meningitis, viral (unless known not be caused by enteroviruses)
Necrotizing enterocolitis
Pleurodynia
Poliomyelitis
Typhoid fever *(Salmonella typhi)*
Viral pericarditis, myocarditis, or meningitis (unless known not to be caused by enteroviruses)

Continued.

Table 13-7. Category-specific isolation precautions—cont'd

Drainage/secretion precautions

Drainage/secretion precautions are designed to prevent infections that are transmitted by direct or indirect contact with purulent material or drainage from an infected body site. This newly created isolation category includes many infections formerly included in wound and skin precautions and discharge (lesion), and secretion (oral) precautions, which have been discontinued. Infectious diseases included in this category are those which result in the production of infective purulent material, drainage, or secretions, unless the disease is included in another isolation category that requires more rigorous precautions. For example, minor or limited skin, wound, or burn infections are included in this category, but major skin, wound, or burn infections are included in contact isolation.

Specifications for drainage/secretion precautions

1. Private room is not indicated.
2. Masks are not indicated.
3. Gowns are indicated if soiling is likely.
4. Gloves are indicated for touching infective material.
5. Hands must be washed after touching the patient or potentially contaminated articles and before taking care of another patient.
6. Articles contaminated with infective material should be discarded or bagged and labeled before being sent for decontamination and reprocessing.

Diseases requiring drainage/secretion precautions

Abscess, minor or limited
Burn infection, minor or limited
Conjunctivitis
Decubitus ulcer, infected, minor or limited
Skin infection, minor or limited
Wound infection, minor or limited

These infections are included in this category provided they are *not* 1) caused by multiple resistant microorganisms, 2) major (draining and not covered by a dressing or dressing does not adequately contain the drainage) skin, wound, or burn infections, including those caused by *Staphylococcus aureus* or group A *Streptococcus,* or 3) gonococcal eye infections in newborns. See contact isolation if the infection is one of these three.

Table 13-7. Category-specific isolation precautions—cont'd

Blood/body fluid precautions

Blood/body fluid precautions are designed to prevent infections that are transmitted by direct or indirect contact with infective blood or body fluids. Infectious diseases included in this category are those which result in the production of infective blood or body fluids, unless the disease is included in another isolation category that requires more rigorous precautions, for example, strict isolation. For some diseases included in this category, such as malaria, only blood is infective; for other diseases, such as hepatitis B (including antigen carriers), blood and body fluids, such as saliva or semen, are infective.

Specifications for blood/body fluid precautions

1. Private room is indicated if patient hygiene is poor. A patient with poor hygiene does not wash hands after touching infective material, contaminates the environment with infective material, or shares contaminated articles with other patients. In general, patients infected with the same organism may share a room.
2. Masks are not indicated.
3. Gowns are indicated if soiling of clothing with blood or body fluids is likely.
4. Gloves are indicated for touching blood or body fluids.
5. Hands must be washed immediately if they are potentially contaminated with blood or body fluids and before taking care of another patient.
6. Articles contaminated with blood or body fluids should be discarded or bagged and labeled before being sent for decontamination and reprocessing.
7. Care should be taken to avoid needle-stick injuries. Used needles should not be recapped or bent; they should be placed in a prominently labeled, puncture-resistant container designated specifically for such disposal.
8. Blood spills should be cleaned up promptly with a solution of 5.25% sodium hypochlorite diluted 1:10 with water.

Diseases requiring blood/body fluid precautions

Acquired immunodeficiency syndrome (AIDS)
Arthropod-borne viral fevers (for example, dengue, yellow fever, and Colorado tick fever)
Babesiosis
Creutzfeldt-Jakob disease
Hepatitis B (including HB_sAg antigen carrier)
Hepatitis, non-A, non-B
Leptospirosis
Malaria
Rat-bite fever
Relapsing fever
Syphilis, primary and secondary with skin and mucous membrane lesions

CONCLUSION

The goals of infection control should be to keep the institution as germ free as possible, to control the sources of contamination, to prevent transmission of infectious agents, and to protect those at risk of acquiring infection. All personnel have a responsibility to help attain these goals. The importance of proper hand washing cannot be overemphasized. Personnel should also use the infection control nurse, the hospital epidemiologist, and the infection control committee in their institutions to address problems concerning any of the many aspects of infection control.

REFERENCES AND SELECTED READINGS

1. Albert, R.K., and Condie, F.: Handwashing patterns in medical intensive care unit, N. Engl. J. Med. **304:**1465-1466, 1981.
2. American Academy of Pediatrics: Report of the Committee on the Control of Infectious Diseases, ed. 19, Evanston, Ill., 1982, The Academy.
3. American Hospital Association: Infection control in the hospital, ed. 4, Chicago, 1979, The Association.
4. American Public Health Association: Control of communicable disease in man, ed. 13, New York, 1981, The Association.
5. Band, J.D., and Maki, D.G.: Safety of changing intravenous delivery systems at intervals longer than 24 hours, Ann. Intern. Med. **91:**173, 1979.
6. Barrett-Conner, E., and others: Epidemiology for the infection control nurse, St. Louis, 1978, The C.V. Mosby Co.
7. Bennett, J.V., and Brachman, P.S., editors: Hospital infections, Boston, 1979, Little, Brown & Co.
8. *Bond, G.B.: Infection control: *Serratia*—an endemic hospital resident, Am. J. Nurs. **81:**2183-2186, 1981.
9. Buxton, J., and others: Contamination of intravenous infusion fluid: effects of changing administration sets, Ann. Intern. Med. **90:**764, 1979.
10. Castle, M.: Hospital infection control, New York, 1980, John Wiley & Sons, Inc.
11. Centers for Disease Control: AIDS—precautions for health care workers and allied professionals, Morbid. Mortal. Week. Rep. **32:**1983.
12. Centers for Disease Control: Hepatitis B vaccine, Morbid. Mortal. Week Rep. **31:**317, 1982.
13. Centers for Disease Control: National nosocomial infections study report, Atlanta, annual summary 1979 issued 1982, U.S. Department of Health and Human Services.
14. Centers for Disease Control: Recommendation of the Immunization Practices Advisory Committee (ACIP): diphtheria, tetanus, and pertussis: guidelines for vaccine prophylaxis and other preventive measures, Morbid. Mortal. Week Rep. **30:**392, 1981.
15. Centers for Disease Control: Recommendation of the Immunization Practices Advisory Committee (ACIP): general recommendations on immunization, Morbid. Mortal. Week. Rep. **32:**1-8, 13-17, 1983.
16. A clinician's dictionary guide to bacteria and fungi, ed. 4, Indianapolis, 1981, Eli Lilly Co.
17. Dixon, R.E., editor: Nosocomial infections, New York, 1981, Yorke Medical Books.
18. Dixon, R.E.: Nosocomial respiratory infections, Infect. Control **4:**376-381, 1983.
19. Farke, B.F., Kaiser, D.L., and Wenzel, R.P.: Relationship between surgical volume and incidence of postoperative wound infection, N. Engl. J. Med. **305:**200-204, 1981.
20. *Fernsebner, B.: Antimicrobial therapy for surgical patients, AORN J. **36:**479-486, 1982.
21. *Fernsebner, B.: Patients at risk for nosocomial infections, AORN J. **38:**613-620, 1983.
22. Garibaldi, R.A., and others: Meatal colonization and catheter-associated bacteremia, N. Engl. J. Med. **303:**316-318, 1980.
23. Hawley, H.B.: Bacterial infection from intravascular monitoring devices, Infect. Control. **4:**399-401, 1983.
24. Infection control: topics in clinical nursing, vol. 1, no. 2, Germantown, Md., 1979, Aspen Systems Corp.
25. *Jenner, E.A.: Catheterization and urinary tract infection: preventing catheter associated urinary tract infections, Nurs. 83 **2**(suppl.): 1-3, 1983.
26. *Jenner, E.A.: Infection control in hospital and community. Identification of the infected patient, Nurs. 83 **19**(suppl.): 1-3, 1983.
27. *Kaye, W.: Catheter and infusion-related sepsis: the nature of the problem and its prevention, Heart Lung **11:**221-228, 1982.
28. *Knittle, M.A., Eitzman, D.V., and Baer, H.: Role of hand contamination of personnel in epidemiology of gram negative nosocomial infections, J. Pediatr. **86:**433-437, 1976.
29. Kunin, C.: Detection, prevention, and management of urinary tract infections, ed. 3, Philadelphia, 1979, Lea & Febiger.
30. Labet, C., and Roderick, M.: Infection control in the use of intravascular devices, Crit. Care Q. **3:**67-80, 1981.
31. *Moore, M., and Abbott, N.K.: Can handwashing practices be changed, Am. J. Nurs. **80:**80, 1980.
32. *O'Donnell, J.: Antibiotic prophylaxis in surgical infection, Heart Lung **12:**20-22, 1983.
33. *Seal, D.V., and Ward, K.: Catheterization and urinary tract infection: basic techniques for aseptic catheterization of the urinary tract, Nurs. 83 **2:**5-6, 1983.
34. Symposium on Infection Control, Nurs. Clin. North Am. **15**(4): entire issue, 1980.
35. *Taylor, L.J.: Infection control in the hospital and the community: prevention of the spread of infection, Nurs. 83 **2**(suppl.): 3-4, 1983.
36. Youmans, G.P.: The biological and clinical basis of infectious diseases, ed. 2, Philadelphia, 1980, W.B. Saunders Co.

*References preceded by an asterisk are particularly well suited for student reading.

14

Cancer

MARGARET VETTESE ZACK and ROSEMARIE HOGAN

STUDY QUESTIONS

- Review the differences between isolation for infectious disease and protective (reverse) isolation.

- If you have a family member who has had cancer, did the person know the diagnosis? What were the person's reactions to the illness? What was the family reaction?

- What might be some possible reasons why the person with cancer might hesitate to share the diagnosis with other persons? What effects might witholding this information incur?

- Review the chart of a patient with a diagnosis of cancer. What has been the patient's psychologic response to the illness? What have been the psychologic and physiologic responses to therapy? What measures could be taken to assist the patient to cope?

- What resources are available in your community to provide assistance for the person with cancer?

Cancer was recognized in ancient times by skilled observers who gave it its name (from the Latin *Cancri,* crab) because it stretched out in many directions like the legs of a crab. It would be preferable if the image of the crab, suggested by Hippocrates for superficial cancer in the advanced stages, could be dropped, because it maintains a legend of incurability. Forms of cancer are found in plants and in humans and other animals. The term is somewhat general and is used interchangeably with *malignant tumor* and *malignant neoplasm.*[89]

One of the least understood facts about cancer is that the name designates more than 200 diseases that have in common the production of abnormal cells that do not obey the laws of normal tissue growth.[69] Therefore cancer should never be looked on as a disease entity but only as a traditional term that describes a neoplastic process.

DEFINITION OF TERMS

The term *neoplasm* comes from the Greek word meaning *new growth* or *new formation.* Normally, cell division is an orderly process with a distinct purpose of organism development or replacement of destroyed or injured cells. When cells divide without such a distinct purpose, they form neoplasms, sometimes referred to as *tumors.* Strictly speaking, a tumor is a swelling caused by any number of conditions, for example, inflammation or trauma. However, the terms *neoplasm* and *tumor* often are used interchangeably.

Oncology, a term used in association with the treatment and study of cancer is the study of tumors (from the Greek *onkos,* mass). Neoplasms are classified broadly by distinguishing between those which are "benign" and those which are "malignant." A *malignant* neoplasm (that is, a cancer) will cause death if it is not controlled. A *benign* neoplasm usually will not cause death unless by its location it interferes with vital functions.[65]

ATTITUDES TOWARD CANCER

Cancer has become one of the more curable chronic diseases[19]. Progress is evidenced by people's knowledge about the disease and the means to prevent it, more sophisticated diagnostic techniques revealing more cancers in the early curable stages, and improved methods of treating cancer, particularly with radiotherapy and chemotherapy.

Despite this progress, few diseases cause greater feelings of anxiety and apprehension. A diagnosis of cancer still may carry with it a social stigma. In many ways, cancer has replaced tuberculosis as a metaphor for contemporary social ills—dirty, deadly, setting the "victim" apart.[77] The myths surrounding malignant disease, often focusing on incurability, help foster feelings of hopelessness and dread.

Nurses may also have the same negative attitudes that exist in society. For this reason it is extremely important that all nurses examine their own feelings about cancer and try to work them through, both by increasing their knowledge of the diseases and treatments and by discussing feelings openly with members of the health team. Nurses who have worked through their feelings are more able to be of assistance to patients and their families than nurses who have not done so.

The nurse's role in helping cancer patients is broad in scope and area of influence. The nurse must have correct knowledge of prevention, control, and treatment of cancer and be able to apply this information in a variety of settings. Teaching about cancer is not limited to the hospital or clinic setting but takes place in industry, at PTA meetings, and at other public forums. In addition to teaching about prevention, the nurse has an active role in treatment and control programs in all settings in which clients are found. Clients and their families look to the nurse for assistance and guidance in all phases of illness from detection to terminal care.

To be effective as a helping person, the nurse must be aware of the emotional impact that the diagnosis of cancer has on the patient and family, because this emotional response affects every aspect of nursing care. Cancer nursing is a challenge to the creativity, skill, and commitment of the nurse.

EPIDEMIOLOGY

Cancer is a disease that is universal in scope. It has existed since the beginning of history and affects humans wherever they live and whatever their race, color, level of culture, and material progress.[2]

Cancer ranks second to heart disease as the cause of death in the United States, but significant progress has been made in prevention and treatment. In the early 1900s few cancer patients had any hope of long-term survival. By the 1960s, 1 in 3 was alive at least 5 years after treatment. Today about 320,000 Americans, or 3 out of 8 cancer patients, will be saved, a gain of 40,000 persons in 1 year.[1] This success can be attributed to the following:

1. Diagnosis of more cancers in the early, localized stage
2. Treatment of more patients within 4 months of diagnosis
3. Development of new diagnostic and treatment modalities, especially chemotherapy

Despite these advances, it was estimated that about 145,000 persons would probably die in 1983 who might have been saved by earlier diagnosis and prompt treatment. There has been a steady rise in the age-adjusted national death rate for cancer, from 143/100,000 population in 1930 to 176/100,000 in 1978. ("Age-adjusted" denotes a method used to make valid statistical comparisons by assuming the same age distribution among different groups being compared.) The major cause of the increased death rate has been cancer of the lung. Death rates for other major sites are leveling off or declining in some cases.

Epidemiologic variables for cancer

Although, in general, cancer shows no respect for economic or social status, there are some variations with regard to sex, site, age, race, and geographic location.

SEX AND SITE

The average incidence of cancer is similar in both sexes. Overall survival rates (proportion of people alive 5 years after diagnosis) for some cancers have increased, such as those for cervical cancer. Rates for most other cancers have leveled off in the past 25 years. The average cancer mortality in developed countries is higher for men than for women.

Twenty-five year trends in age-adjusted cancer death rates per 100,000 population (1951 to 1953 and 1976 to 1978) indicated the following:

1. For both sexes
   a. Steady decrease in cancer of the liver and stomach
   b. Steady increase in cancer of the lung caused by cigarette smoking
   c. Steady increase, then leveling off, in cancer of the pancreas
2. For males
   a. Steady, slight increase in cancer of the kidney
3. For females
   a. Steady decrease in cancer of the uterus
   b. Noticeable decrease in cancer of the bladder and colorectal cancer.[1]

Fig. 14-1 compares cancer incidence and deaths by site and sex.

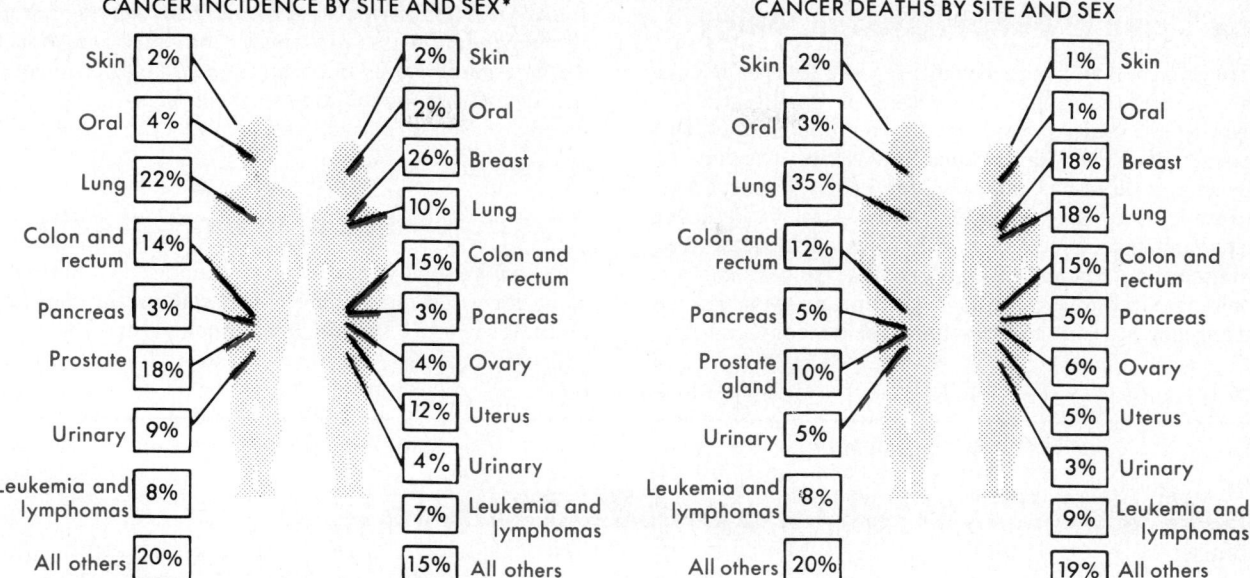

CANCER INCIDENCE BY SITE AND SEX*

Skin 2% | 2% Skin
Oral 4% | 2% Oral
Lung 22% | 26% Breast
Colon and rectum 14% | 10% Lung
Pancreas 3% | 15% Colon and rectum
Prostate 18% | 3% Pancreas
Urinary 9% | 4% Ovary
Leukemia and lymphomas 8% | 12% Uterus
All others 20% | 4% Urinary
| 7% Leukemia and lymphomas
| 15% All others

CANCER DEATHS BY SITE AND SEX

Skin 2% | 1% Skin
Oral 3% | 1% Oral
Lung 35% | 18% Breast
Colon and rectum 12% | 18% Lung
Pancreas 5% | 15% Colon and rectum
Prostate gland 10% | 5% Pancreas
Urinary 5% | 6% Ovary
Leukemia and lymphomas 8% | 5% Uterus
All others 20% | 3% Urinary
| 9% Leukemia and lymphomas
| 19% All others

*Excluding nonmelanoma skin cancer and carcinoma in situ of uterine cervix.

Fig. 14-1. Comparison of cancer incidence and deaths by site and sex (1984 estimates). (From American Cancer Society: 1984 Cancer facts and figures, New York, 1983, The Society.)

AGE

Although more than half of the deaths from cancer occur in persons over 65 years of age, cancer is the leading cause of death in women between 30 and 54 years of age, and more children aged 3 to 14 years die of cancer than any other disease. However, mortality among children with cancer has declined.[1]

RACE

Cancer incidence and mortality are higher for blacks than for whites. Blacks have shown significantly higher increases in cancer of the lung, colorectum, prostate, and esophagus. Esophageal cancer has declined in whites but has risen rapidly in blacks of both sexes. Although invasive cervical cancer has declined in women of both races, the incidence in black women is still more than twice that in white women. Endometrial cancer is the one cancer for which the incidence rate in white women is double that in black women.[1]

Most differences in the cancer rates of black and white populations are attributed to environmental and social factors rather than to inherent biologic characteristics. One American Cancer Society survey showed that urban blacks tend to be less knowledgeable about warning signals and less apt to seek medical care if symptoms do occur. These blacks also tended to underestimate the prevalence of cancer and the choices of cure. Increased risk of exposure to industrial carcinogens and limited educational opportunities among those in the lower socio-

economic group also may be contributing factors, because a higher percentage of blacks are in the lower socioeconomic group.[1]

GEOGRAPHIC FACTORS

There is no place or country on earth that is free of cancer, although differences in the geographic distribution of cancer occur.[69,73]

1. The cancer incidence in Chile is less than 100/100,000 population. The U.S. rate is 175/100,000 population. Great Britain has the highest rate with more than 250/100,000 population.
2. Scotland has the highest cancer mortality, and Thailand has the lowest.
3. Primary cancer of the liver is common in Indonesia and parts of Africa and Asia but rare in other regions.
4. Cancer of the breast is more common in the United States and Western Europe than it is in Japan.
5. Ugandans, Nigerians, and South African blacks are at lower risk for cancer of the lung, stomach, large intestine, uterus, and kidney.

Genetic differences between populations may contribute to international variations. However, observations of what happens to cancer incidence when people migrate from one country to another show that environmental (for example, air pollution) and cultural (for example, diet) factors play a more important role than genetic differences in the rate changes that occur.[13]

Nurse's role in cancer epidemiology

Cancer is not only a threat to life, but its cost in loss of income and disruption of the lives of families cannot be estimated. Nurses must be in the forefront of the thousands of health professionals who are working to eradicate the disease. Cancer epidemiologic research has contributed to cancer prevention and control by identifying epidemiologic trends that can be used to determine individuals and groups at high risk for cancer. Nurses can play a vital role in cancer prevention by assessing people's cancer risks and teaching them about environ-

mental and personal carcinogenic risk factors, including recommendations for prevention and early detection. Table 14-1 summarizes important epidemiologic aspects and risk factors for the six major cancer sites.

PATHOPHYSIOLOGY

Characteristics of malignant cells

Normal tissue contains large numbers of mature cells of uniform size and shape. Each cell contains a nucleus of uniform size. Within each nucleus are the chromo-

Table 14-1. Risk and epidemiology for six major cancer sites

Site	Estimated new cases 1983*	Estimated deaths 1983*	Risk factors	Comments
Breast	115,000	38,000	Over age 50, personal or family history of breast cancer, never had children, first child after age 30	Leading cause of death from cancer in women
Colorectum	126,000	58,000	Personal or family history of colon and rectum cancer, personal or family history of polyps in colon or rectum, ulcerative colitis, diet high in beef and/or deficient in fiber content	Considered a highly curable disease when digital and proctoscopic examinations are included in routine check-ups
Lung	135,000	117,000	Heavy cigarette smoking, history of smoking 20 or more years, exposure to certain industrial substances such as asbestos, particularly for those who smoke	Leading cause of cancer death among men, and rising mortality among women
Mouth	27,000	9,200	Heavy smoking and drinking, use of chewing tobacco	Many more lives could be saved, because the mouth is easily accessible to visual examination by physicians and dentists
Skin	17,000†	7,000	Excessive exposure to the sun, fair complexion, occupational exposure to coal tar, pitch, creosote, arsenic compounds and radium	Readily detected by observation and diagnosed by simple biopsy
Uterus	55,000‡	10,000	Cervical cancer: early age at first intercourse, multiple sex partners. Endometrial cancer: history of infertility, failure of ovulation, prolonged estrogen therapy, late menopause, combination of diabetes, high blood pressure, and obesity	Uterine cancer mortality has declined 70% during past 40 years with wider use of Pap test; post-menopausal women with abnormal bleeding should be checked

*American Cancer Society, 1983 Cancer facts and figures, New York, 1982, The Society.
†Estimated new cases of nonmelanoma skin cancer about 400,000.
‡If carcinoma in situ is included, cases total 99,000.

somes, a specific number for the species, and within each chromosome is deoxyribonucleic acid (DNA). DNA is a giant molecule whose chemical composition controls the characteristics of ribonucleic acid (RNA), which is found both in the nucleoli of cells and in the cytoplasm of the cell itself and which regulates cell growth and function. When ovum and sperm unite, the DNA and RNA within the chromosomes of each will govern the differentiation and future course of the trillions of cells that finally develop to form the adult organism. In the development of various organs and parts of the body, cells undergo differentiation in size, appearance, and arrangement; thus the

histologist or the pathologist can look at a piece of prepared tissue through a microscope and know the portion of the body from which it came.

Some abnormal changes in cell growth are malignant growths. Other types of cellular growths are benign. Benign (nonmalignant) neoplasms involve cellular proliferation of adult or mature cells growing slowly in an orderly manner in a capsule. These tumors do not invade surrounding tissue but may cause harm through pressure on vital structures within an enclosed structure such as the skull. Benign tumors remain localized, do not metastasize (spread), and do not recur after they are completely removed (see Table 14-2).

Table 14-2. Characteristics of benign and malignant neoplasms

Characteristics	Benign	Malignant
Cell characteristics	Cells resemble normal cells of the tissue from which the tumor originated	Cells often bear little resemblance to the normal cells of the tissue from which they arose; there is both anaplasia and pleomorphism (assumption of two or more different forms)
Mode of growth	Tumor grows by expansion and does not infiltrate the surrounding tissues; encapsulated	Grows at the periphery and sends out processes that infiltrate and destroy the surrounding tissues
Rate of growth	Rate of growth is usually slow	Rate of growth is usually relatively rapid and is dependent upon level of differentiation; the more anaplastic the tumor the more rapid the rate of growth
Metastasis	Does not spread by metastasis	Gains access to the blood and lymph channels and metastasizes to other areas of the body
Recurrence	Does not recur when removed	Tends to recur when removed
General effects	Is usually a localized phenomenon that does not cause generalized effects unless by location it interferes with vital functions	Often causes generalized effects such as anemia, weakness, and weight loss
Destruction of tissue	Does not usually cause tissue damage unless location interferes with blood flow	Often causes extensive tissue damage as the tumor outgrows its blood supply or encroaches on blood flow to the area; may also produce substances that cause cell damage
Ability to cause death	Does not usually cause death unless its location interferes with vital functions	Will usually cause death unless growth can be controlled

From Porth, C.: Pathophysiology: concepts of altered health states, Philadelphia, 1982, J.B. Lippincott Co.

A malignant cell is one in which the basic structure and activity have become deranged in a manner that is unknown and from a cause or causes that are still poorly understood. It is believed, however, that the basic process involves a disturbance in the regulatory functions of DNA. It is known that the DNA molecule is affected by radiation in certain instances, and it is speculated that it may be affected by other factors as well.

In the neoplastic cell, normal restraints on growth are defective. It is believed that malignant neoplasms occur as the result of faulty mechanisms inside the cell nucleus.[9]

DNA, the permanent genetic material in nuclear chromosomes, contains information necessary for cell replication, the chemical code for cell growth and development. To convey this information, RNA serves as a messenger. Any small change in DNA (mutation) causes a distortion of biologic information, which results in the affected cells running wild. Malignant neoplasm is the result.[9] The malignant cells lose the normal specialized function of the normal cell or may take on new characteristics and functions.

A characteristic of malignant cells that can be observed through a microscope is *loss of differentiation,* or loss of likeness to the original cell (parent tissue) from which the tumor growth originated. This loss of differentiation is called *anaplasia,* and its extent is a determining factor in the degree of malignancy of the tumor.

Anaplasia is characterized by alterations in intracellular macromolecular synthesis and intercellular relationships and associations. Two types of anaplasia have been identified. In positional or organizational anaplasia, the usual distinct histologic patterns in tissues are altered. In cytologic anaplasia, there is increased or altered nucleic acid synthesis in growing tissues.[64] Anaplasia is one of the most reliable indicators of malignancy. It is seen only in cancers and does not appear in benign neoplasms.

Other characteristics of malignant cells that can be seen through a microscope are the presence of nuclei of various sizes, many of which contain unusually large amounts of chromatin, and the presence of mitotic figures (cells in the process of division), which denotes rapid and disorderly division of cells. The proportion of cells actively proliferating in malignant tumors is generally greater than that of normal cells.

Malignant tumors have no enclosing capsule; thus they invade adjacent or surrounding tissue, including lymph and blood vessels, through which they may spread to distant parts of the body to set up new tumors *(metastases)*. Unless completely removed or destroyed, they tend to recur after treatment, and their continued presence causes death by replacing normal cells and by other means not fully understood. Characteristics of malignant cells are summarized in box below.

GROWTH OF MALIGNANT NEOPLASMS

The term *neoplasm* has been defined as a relatively autonomous growth of tissues, the term *autonomy* meaning that a malignant tumor is not subject to the "rules and regulations" that govern cells and cell interaction of the healthy individual. This autonomy is relative in that the tumor is not completely independent of the tissue from which it arose.

There are considerable differences in the rate of growth of malignant tumors. Occasionally, one grows so slowly that it can be removed completely after a long period of time. This characteristic probably accounts for the good results obtained in a few circumstances even when treatment has been delayed. No physician, however, ever relies on this possibility to justify delay in treatment. Occasionally, a malignant tumor grows slowly for a long time and then undergoes change, and the rate of growth increases enormously.

SPREAD OF CANCER

The rate of growth of a malignant neoplasm determines its capacity to spread. Cancer may spread by direct extension, by gravitational metastasis, or by metastatic spread.

Direct extension or invasion

Direct extension or invasion of neighboring tissue produces the typical local effects of ulcerating, bulky, hem-

---

Characteristics of malignant cells

1. Nuclei are larger and irregular in shape.
2. DNA is coarsely distributed and tends to appear near nuclear membrane.
3. Nucleoli are large, usually increased in number, and contain more chromatin than usual.
4. Mitosis is increased and atypical in appearance.
5. Abnormal multipolar mitoses and multinucleated cells may appear.
6. Cytoplasm is comparatively scanty and stains more deeply than normal cytoplasm (greater RNA concentration).
7. Cells vary in size from normal cells.
8. Surface characteristics of cells related to the cell membrane are altered: loss of contact inhibition, failure to form intracellular junctions, and impaired cell-to-cell communication.

orrhagic masses or indurative, fibrosing lesions with tissue fixation, distortion of the structure, and the pitting of the skin seen in some breast cancer. Infection may accompany this local infiltration. Because of local spread, any cancer excision must include a margin of surrounding tissues to ensure removal of all malignant cells.

Gravitational metastasis and seeding

Gravitational metastasis involves the erosion of cancer cells into body cavities and their dropping onto the serous membrane lining the cavity. The pathway is determined by gravity or movements of the body. A tumor may penetrate the wall of the stomach and its cells implant on the surfaces of the peritoneal cavity. In the peritoneal cavity, cells tend to gravitate to the pelvis. Cells from neoplasm of the pleura of the thoracic cavity may "drop" to the diaphragm. Cancer cells can also be implanted by the surgeon into the operative area, causing metastatic lesions (mechanical transplantation).

Metastatic spread

Metastatic spread occurs when   cer cells invade vascular or lymphatic channels and travel to distant parts of the body where implantation occurs. In *lymph vessels,* cells may detach and become emboli, which lodge in the regional lymph nodes that receive their drainage from the tumor site. Spread continues to the next group of nodes and into the other organs. Cells also may gain access to the bloodstream by way of the thoracic duct.

Vascular embolism of malignant cells may occur through the veins or arteries to various parts of the body depending on the vascular drainage of the organs involved. The liver is a common metastatic site for cancers originating in the gastrointestinal tract, pancreas, and spleen because of routing through the portal vein before entering the general circulation. Because venous blood travels through the lungs, this is another common site for secondary growth via the venous system. Cancer cells in the arterial system frequently form secondary neoplasms in the bone and the brain, especially if the primary site is in the lungs, where cancer cells can gain direct access to the left heart and systemic circulation.

In metastatic spread, there is almost always a high degree of histologic, cytologic, and functional similarity between the primary cancer and these metastases. Consequently, the type of cell and the probable site of the primary tumor can be identified from the morphology of the metastasis. In addition, metastases usually mimic the primary tumor in the formation of cell products and secretions.

Table 14-3. Names of neoplasms

Tissue type	Benign	Malignant
Epithelium		
Skin and mucous membrane	Papilloma	Squamous cell carcinoma
Glands	Adenoma	Adenocarcinoma
Connective tissue		
Fibrous	Fibroma	Fibrosarcoma
Adipose	Lipoma	Liposarcoma
Cartilage	Chrondroma	Chondrosarcoma
Bone	Osteoma	Osteosarcoma
Blood vessels	Hemangioma	Hemangiosarcoma
Lymph vessels	Lymphangioma	Lymphangiosarcoma
Muscle tissue		
Smooth muscle	Leiomyoma	Leiomyosarcoma
Striated muscle	Rhabdomyoma	Rhabodmyosarcoma
Nerve tissue		
Nerve fiber end sheath	Neuroma	Neurogenic sarcoma
Ganglion cells	Ganglioneuroma	Neuroblastoma
Glia cells	Astrocytoma	Gliobastoma multiforme
Hematopoietic tissue		
Plasma cells		Multiple myeloma
Lymphoid		Lymphatic leukemia
Miscellaneous		
Placenta	Hydatiform mole	Chorioepithelioma (choriocarcinoma)

Histologic grading

G1   Well-differentiated grade
G2   Moderately well-differentiated grade
G3, G4   Poorly to very poorly differentiated grade

TNM staging classification system

Tumor

T0	No evidence of primary tumor
TIS	Carcinoma in situ
T1, T2, T3, T4	Ascending degrees of tumor size and involvement

Nodes

N0	No regional nodes demonstrably abnormal
N1a, N2a	Demonstrable regional lymph nodes, metastasis not suspected
N1a, N2b, N3	Demonstrable regional lymph nodes; metastasis suspected
Nx	Regional nodes cannot be assessed clinically

Metastasis

M0	No evidence of distant metastasis
M1, M2, M3	Ascending degrees of metastatic involvement of the host including distant nodes

Naming and classifying neoplasms

Tumors derive their names from the parent tissue or the tissue type from which the growth originated (Table 14-3). In general, the names of benign tumors carry the suffix *-oma* following the name of the parent tissue, for example, *neuroma* or *fibroma*. Malignant tumors generally are of two types, those of epithelial and those of mesenchymal (connective tissue) origin. The term *carcinoma* denotes a malignant tumor of epithelial cells, and the term *sarcoma* denotes a malignant tumor of connective tissue cells. Hematopoietic or blood-forming tissues are involved in malignant processes that are disseminated from the beginning, in contrast to solid tumors that initially are confined to a specific tissue or organ.

Tumors containing embryonic elements of all three primary germ layers, such as hair, teeth, and so on; are called *teratomas*. These are usually benign and often are found in the ovaries.

Some malignant tumors are known by the names of the scientists who first described them, for example, Hodgkin's disease and Wilm's tumor. Other types of malignant neoplasms occur with a wide variety of seemingly unrelated names. The diversity in naming malignant neoplasms reflects the complexities involved in identifying and classifying the many forms of cancer. However, a system of naming and classifying tumors is necessary to facilitate communication among researchers and health professionals.

There are two methods for classifying cancers: *grading* according to histologic criteria and *staging* according to the extent of the spread of the disease. Tumors may be graded by roman or arabic numerals into four grades; the higher the grade, the worse the prognosis.[89] A grade 1 tumor is the most differentiated (more like the parent tissue) and therefore the least malignant; whereas grade 4 is the least differentiated (more unlike the parent tissue) and has a high degree of malignancy. These classifications are useful to the physician in knowing whether the tumor may be expected to respond to radiation treatment as well as in planning all other aspects of the patient's treatment. Usually, malignant tissue is slightly more sensitive to irradiation than normal tissue.

Determination of the extent of the spread of cancer (staging) and the site of the original tumor is vital for planning therapy. The International Union Against Cancer has devised the TNM system of classification: *T*, tumor; *N*, regional lymph nodes; *M*, distant metastases.

Adding a number to the letters (for example T1, T2, N1, N2) indicates the extent of the malignancy. This system provides a type of shorthand notation to describe the particular tumor. The purpose of the TNM system is to define categories for all cases and also allow subsequent and more detailed information to be added. A TNM classification has been identified for major cancer sites, and the choice of treatment depends on the clinical TNM stage, both for the primary tumor and the lymph nodes.

ETIOLOGY: CARCINOGENESIS

The factors that contribute to the development of cancer are many and at present are not fully understood; however, certain health practices are known to decrease the possibility that cancer may occur. Since cancer is not a single disease entity, it is not likely that there is a single cause. Cancer probably occurs as the result of the interaction of many risk factors or because of long-term exposure to a single carcinogenic agent. Factors involved in carcinogenesis include host susceptibility, environmental carcinogens, habits and customs, and viruses.

Host susceptibility

GENETIC FACTORS

Studies of genetic factors have focused on specific cancer sites and the disease in general. Chromosomes have

Some carcinogenic factors

Host susceptibility

Genetic factors
   Cancer family syndrome (CFS)
   Familial polyposis of colon
   Multiple endocrine adenomatosis (MEA)
   Retinoblastoma
Hormonal factors
   Estrogens
Precancerous lesions
   Polyps of colon and rectum
   Pigmented moles
   Cervical dysplasia
   Paget's bone disease
   Senile keratosis
   Xeroderma pigmentosum
Chronic irritation
   Coal tars and products in industry
   Sunlight overexposure
   Restrictive clothing
   Chronic use of laxatives
Immunologic factors
   Early childhood and old age
   Immunodeficiency disease
   Immunosuppressive therapy

Viruses

Herpesvirus hominis (HSV-2)—cervical cancer
Epstein-Barr virus—Burkitt's lymphoma

Psychosocial factors

Stressful life changes
Depression
Low social support and high need

Environmental factors

Ionizing radiation
   Radiographs
   Radioisotopes
Chemical pollutants
   Polycyclic hydrocarbons (soot, tar, pitch, mineral oils)
   Arsenic compounds
   Asbestos
   Aromatic amines
   Chromium compounds
   Benzol
   Nitrosamines (meat preservatives)
   Nitrates (food additives)
   Aflatoxin 13 (mold on nuts and grains)
   Vinyl chloride
   Diethylstilbestrol (DES)
   Red dyes (food coloring)
   Sweeteners (cyclamates and saccharin)

Health practices

Smoking
Nutrition
   Diets high in refined foods and low in roughage (colon cancer)
   Smoked foods ingestion
   High caloric intake
   Vitamin A, B (riboflavin), and C deficient diets
Alcohol
Sexual practices
   First coitus at an early age
   Multiple sex partners
   Uncircumcised sex partners

been studied to find evidence of the genetic origin of cancer. Chromosomal abnormalities associated with neoplasia may consist of extra or missing chromosomes or the presence of abnormal chromosomes. The question is whether these changes are the cause or the effect of cancer.

A second indication of genetic origin is that cancer cells are a population of cells descendant from a single cell of origin (clones). Future generations of cancer cells are always malignant; they inherit and pass on the trait.

Finally, there is a possibility that cancer arises from an innate genetic inability, possibly a defect in mitotic regulation. Theoretically, in normal cells mitosis is either inhibited or induced by diffusible substances. The repressor substances are called chalones. Cancer cells may fail to be regulated by the chalones either because the chalones may not be secreted, or if they are, they fail to respond.[25]

Familial polyposis of the colon, a precursor of cancer, is indisputably hereditary. There is also a high incidence of breast cancer in a vertical line of descent, such as from mother to daughter. Risk of breast cancer in the first-degree relatives of a patient is five times that of the general population. Heredity in some way seems to be connected with bronchogenic cancer. It seems to interact with cigarette smoking to cause a synergistic effect.[41]

In general, inherited cancers are a direct expression of an inherited defect, but these syndromes are rare and account for only a small percentage of familial cancer.[53] Studies have shown that the pattern of inheritance is not usually that of single mendelian gene, and it is still not known whether the incidences of many specific cancers are a result of a combination of genetic and environmental factors.

HORMONAL FACTORS

Hormones do not appear to be primary carcinogens, but rather they seem to influence carcinogenesis in the following three ways:

1. By a preparative action on the target tissues, making them susceptible to the carcinogenic agent
2. By a "permissive" influence of carcinogenesis allowing the process to progress
3. By a conditioning effect on the tumor

Hormones are capable of restraining or enhancing growth of tumors that have developed.[60] Hormone therapy (p. 244) and some surgical therapies (hypophysectomy and oophorectomy) are based on this fact.

There is evidence that tissues that are endocrine responsive (for example, breasts, endometrium and prostate) do not develop cancer unless they are stimulated by their growth-promoting hormones. Estrogens have been associated with cancers such as adenocarcinoma of the vagina, hepatic tumors, breast tumors, and uterine cancer.[49]

In addition to tissue stimulation by the hormone, carcinogenesis may be determined by the length of time of the hormonal effect. The longer the preparative influence of the hormone, the greater the chance of cancer development.

PRECANCEROUS LESIONS

Certain benign lesions and tumors have a tendency toward malignant change. These cancers are preventable if minor precursor conditions are treated carefully. Precancerous lesions are a large and heterogeneous group. In some cancer is inevitable, whereas in others the risk is so low that medical management disregards the cancer risk. For example, the risk of cancer is high in xeroderma pigmentosa, a rare skin disease, but low in leukoplakia (white patches) of the mucous membranes, especially of the oral cavity, larynx, and vulva.[68]

CHRONIC IRRITATION

It is also known that cancer may follow chronic irritation of any part of the body. There are many ways to prevent irritation that may lead to cancer. Effort is being made in industry to protect workers from coal-tar products known to contain carcinogens. Masks and gloves are recommended in some instances, and workers are urged to wash their hands and arms thoroughly to remove all irritating substances at the end of the day's work. Occupational health nurses participate in intensive educational programs to help workers understand the need for carrying out company rules that may help prevent cancer.

Prolonged exposure to wind, dirt, and sun may also lead to skin cancer. Skin cancer of the face and hands is particularly common among outdoor workers who have fair complexions and who do not protect themselves from exposure.

Any kind of chronic irritation to the skin should be avoided, and moles that are in locations where they may be irritated by clothing should be removed. Shoelaces, shoetops, girdles, brassieres, and shirt collars are examples of clothing that may be a source of chronic irritation. Glasses, earrings, dental plates, and pipes that are in repeated contact with skin and mucous membrane may contribute to cancer. Cancer of the mouth is sometimes associated with rough jagged teeth and the constant irritation of tobacco smoke. Indiscriminate use of laxatives is believed to have possible carcinogenic effects on the large bowel.

IMMUNOLOGIC FACTORS

It may be possible that failure of the normal immune mechanism may predispose to certain cancers. The change from normal to malignant cells is relatively common. These new cells are antigenically different and are recognized as such by the body's immune system. If the immune response is initiated, the malignant cell will be destroyed. That a kind of immune surveillance system may exist is suggested by the following evidence:

1. The two peaks of high incidence of tumors in humans are in early childhood and old age.
2. Individuals with rare immunodeficiency diseases in which there is a defect in cellular immunity have increased evidence of tumor development.
3. Individuals receiving immunosuppressive drugs to prevent organ transplant rejection have an increased evidence of neoplasia.[33]

Cancer itself appears to suppress the immune response early in the disease as well as late in its progression. It has not been definitely established that cancer develops because of failure in immune surveillance, and at present there is not enough data to make a strong case.[54] (The role of the immune system and cancer therapy is discussed later in this chapter and in Chapter 6.)

Environmental factors

It has been estimated that 70% to 90% of human cancers result from environmental factors and that we have the knowledge to prevent 30% to 40% of cancers in the United States. Occupational exposure causes 1% to 5% of human cancer, and the Environmental Protection Agency indicates that as many as 50,000 chemical substances, *excluding* pharmaceutical and food additives in common use, are carcinogenic.[73]

There are several types of chemical and physical carcinogens (cancer-producing substances). Various carcinogens may have an additive or enhancing effect on one another, and even small amounts of these substances in the environment may constitute a hazard. Carcinogens act on different organs depending on the portal of entry and the distribution in the body.

IONIZING RADIATION

Radiographs and radium may cure cancer, but in other cases they cause it. Ionizing radiation consists of electromagnetic waves or material particles that have sufficient energy to ionize atoms or molecules (that is, remove electrons from them) and thereby alter their chemical behavior. In adequate amounts, it destroys the cells.

Every living thing from the beginning of time has been exposed to small amounts of radiation from the sun and from certain natural elements in the earth, such as uranium, that emit gamma rays (γ-rays) in the process of their decay. This is called natural background radiation. No problem regarding radiation existed until after 1895, when the Roentgen ray (x-ray) machine was developed and became widely used in diagnosis of disease. The development of this machine was followed by the discovery of radium and the use of both radium and radiographs for treatment of diseases such as cancer. With developments in the field of nuclear energy, it has been possible to produce radioactive isotopes of a number of the elements, although only a few of them, such as gold, iodine, cobalt, and phosphorus, have medical application at the present time. The problem of overexposure and possible harm to patients and to personnel caring for them has increased greatly with the increased use of radiographs in diagnosis and treatment and the more recent use of radioisotopes in diagnosis and treatment. Also, radiation-producing substances are being used to greater extents in the work and home environments.

No one really knows how much exposure to radiation is safe for persons working with patients and for patients having repeated radiographs taken for various purposes. Relatively small amounts of exposure have produced serious damage in experimental animals, but humans have not lived through enough generations of relatively high exposure for conclusive evidence of safe levels to be obtained. It is reasonable to assume that the less exposure one has the better. This does not mean that a patient receiving radiation treatment should not receive adequate nursing care. There are ways to protect persons from exposure, and hospitals are required to have protective procedures and guidelines for persons who care for patients receiving radiation therapy. Nurses should be familiar with the procedures used in the institution in which they are employed.

The ionizing effect of radiation on the body cells remains, so that exposure is cumulative throughout life. Exposure of the entire body enormously increases the amount of radiation received. For this reason all of the body except the part being treated is protected from exposure when relatively high doses are given for therapeutic purposes.

The amount of exposure the patient receives from a series of radiographs taken for diagnostic purposes depends on the machine used and the technical skill involved. Usually, the fluoroscopic examination entails more exposure than radiography. To prevent excessive exposure with fluoroscopy, physicians allow time for their eyes to accommodate to the darkened room so that the patient can be observed with a lower intensity of the machine. The exposure of the average nurse working in a hospital and occasionally assisting a patient while a radiograph is taken is almost negligible.

Badges are worn by persons whose daily work exposes them to radiation. The badge, which contains photographic film capable of absorbing radiation, is developed each month. A darkening or blackening of the film indicates excessive exposure. Personnel who are becoming overexposed are removed, at least temporarily, from direct contact with radiation.

Because of the possible danger to the fetus, particularly between the second and sixth weeks of life, radiographs are seldom taken of pregnant women. Also, pregnant women usually are not employed in radiology departments or in caring for patients who are receiving radioactive materials internally.

CHEMICAL POLLUTANTS

Air pollution has been blamed for the rising cancer incidence in the twentieth century. Ten polycyclic aromatic hydrocarbons have been recognized as carcinogenic.[89] Tar and pitch and their derivatives as well as mineral oils containing aromatic hydrocarbons were discovered to be carcinogenic many years ago. Bladder cancer from aromatic amines is an occupational disease of workers in the rubber industry. The risk of contacting lung cancer is 15 to 30 times greater among those exposed to chromium compounds. Other common occupational cancers are respiratory cancers from asbestos and leukemia resulting from long-term inhalation of benzol.

A liver carcinogen, aflatoxin 13, has been isolated from a common mold that grows on peanuts, soybeans, fruit, some meats, and mild and cheddar cheese. A rare form of vaginal cancer in young women has been linked to the ingestion by their mothers of diethylstilbestrol (DES) prescribed to prevent spontaneous abortion.

In 1969 cyclamates, which were widely used as sugar substitutes, were banned when experimental studies revealed that in high doses they could produce cancer of the bladder in mice. Saccharin has also been identified as being carcinogenic in a study of rats, and the Food and Drug Administration has recommended that it not be used as an artificial sweetener. The use of some hair dyes has also been implicated in cancer.

Health practices
SMOKING

There is now no question that the rise in lung cancer during the past 70 years can be attributed to the increased use of cigarettes. The American Cancer Society estimates that cigarette smoking is responsible for 83% of lung cancer cases among men and 43% among women—more than 75% overall. Those who smoke two or more packs of cigarettes a day have lung cancer mortality 15 to 25 times greater than nonsmokers, according to the 1982 Surgeon General's Report.[1] In the past, more men than women smoked, and men smoked more heavily; however, the gap has been narrowing. The rise in the number of women smokers has captured the attention of cigarette manufacturers, who have increased their advertising efforts in this direction, to the point of designing cigarettes expressly for women.

Smoking accounts for about 25% of all cancers (for example, mouth, pharynx, larynx, esophagus, pancreas, and bladder) and is also linked to heart disease, gastric ulcers, chronic bronchitis and emphysema.[1] If smoking is discontinued, even after a habit of 30 years, there is a decrease in the evidence of lung cancer. Not smoking for 10 to 15 years reduces the risk of cancer to equal that of a person who has never smoked.[69,87]

The American Cancer Society recently reported a steady decline in the proportion of adult smokers in the United States. Overall, by 1980 the percentage of men and women smokers in the population had dropped to 32%. There are more than 33 million ex-smokers now living in the U.S. Of these, 95% quit on their own, without the aid of any organized program. However, for smokers who need more intensive assistance and group support, smoking cessation clinics are available in most communities.[1]

After the release of the Surgeon General's Report on Smoking and Health in 1964, the National Interagency Council on Smoking and Health was formed. This group, composed of 27 public and private health, educational, and youth organizations, has as its major objective combating smoking as a health hazard. Several of these participating organizations have produced films and other educational materials that are available to schools, organizations, and individuals. Assistance in securing films and other materials can be obtained from the Library, National Clearinghouse for Smoking and Health, Public Health Service.* One of the main concerns of the Interagency Council is how to convince young people not to start smoking. The American Lung Association† produced a film, *Breathing Easy,* especially for the preteen group. Antismoking education drives in schools are conducted through school courses, assemblies, and exhibits.

Many smokers have switched to brands of cigarettes with filters that reduce the tar and nicotine (T/N) exposure. Although low T/N smokers may find it easier to quit smoking and the lung cancer mortality is reduced somewhat, many people only smoke *more* of filtered cigarettes, resulting in no reduced lung cancer risk. In addition, certain filtered brands have been found to deliver more carbon monoxide than those without filters.[1,69]

Switching from a cigarette to a pipe or cigar also may reduce the risk of lung cancer but not the risk of cancer of the lips, pharynx, and esophagus. The smoke from pipes and cigars contains the same amount of tar and nicotine as cigarettes. It simply is not inhaled.[69]

The question of hazards for nonsmokers who breathe the smoke of others' cigarettes is not resolved, but recent studies have aroused concern. Two studies have shown increased risk of lung cancer among wives of cigarette smokers; however, another study found little, if any, risk

for "passive smokers." The American Cancer Society's new Cancer Prevention Study II is including an assessment of the cancer risk among passive smokers.[1]

Nurses have a responsibility, both as well-informed citizens and as professional persons, to be aware of the most recent antismoking programs and to interpret them to the public. One of the best ways for nurses to do this would be to stop smoking themselves. Although there are no figures available on the number of nurses who have stopped smoking, the American Cancer Society estimates that 50,000 physicians have done so.

NUTRITION

Nutritional habits are increasingly being investigated and implicated in the etiology of cancer. A high incidence of cancer of the colon occurs in populations whose diet is high in refined food and low in nonabsorbable cellulose "roughage" or fiber. Evidence indicates that there is a low incidence of colonic carcinoma among persons who eat a largely vegetarian diet that has relatively few animal products[34,75] and is especially low in fats.[87] Breast cancer appears to be associated with a diet high in animal fat, but the precise relationship has not been identified.[48]

Other factors in the daily diet may be responsible for cancer. These are not only specific carcinogenic agents but also certain nutritional deficiencies. Breast and colon cancers have also been correlated with nutritional deficits, especially with vitamins A, B (riboflavin), and C, although these may play an indirect role.[24] Ingestion of smoked foods, which contain benzopyrene, has been correlated with an increased incidence of stomach cancer. Some epidemiologic and experimental evidence suggests that high caloric intake may lead to cancer and calorie deprivation may prevent it. Obesity may increase the risk of endometrial cancer.[48]

Some foods may protect against cancer. The food additives butylated hydroxyanisole (BHA) and butylated hydroxytoluene (BHT) seem to inhibit cancer. Although reports are conflicting, some investigators believe vitamins A, B, and C actually have anticancer effects. The *Lactobacillus bulgaris* and *Streptococcus thermophilus* microorganisms found in yogurt have been found to inhibit tumor cell proliferation.[24]

Many food substances contain additives, contaminants, and naturally appearing substances such as aflatoxin, which may be carcinogenic. Food additives being studied include food dyes, flavoring agents, and antimicrobial preservatives such as sodium and potassium nitrite and nitrate. Although some potential carcinogens are present in the diet, the time trends do not indicate that additives now in use are significant in the etiology of cancer. The present government policy is to keep the levels of potential carcinogenic agents in food as low as feasible, recognizing that it is almost impossible to state with absolute certainty that any ingested chemical is safe.[34]

The U.S. Delaney amendment to the Federal Food, Drug and Cosmetic Act requires that no substance producing tumors in experimental animals should be permit-

---

*5401 Westbord Ave., Bethesda, MD 20016
†1740 Broadway, New York, NY 10019

ted in food for human beings. The problem is that effects from ingesting carcinogenic agents may not be seen for decades because of the long latency periods. Childhood exposure, particularly, may provide the time for cancer to appear.[24]

ALCOHOL

There is a significant association between high alcohol intake and cancer of the mouth, pharynx, larynx, and esophagus. However, alcoholism is often associated with smoking and with vitamin and dietary deficiencies, whose roles in the etiology of cancer are not known. It is speculated that alcohol and nutritional deficiencies enhance carcinogenesis by increasing the metabolic activities of specific tobacco carcinogens.[24] Tumors of the involved sites occur with greater frequency in men, blacks, lower socioeconomic groups, increasingly urbanized societies, and the elderly.[72]

SEXUAL PRACTICES

Carcinoma of the uterine cervix is less common in virgins than in married women. It is higher in those who have first coitus at an early age, who have an early first marriage, and who have had multiple sex partners. Cervical cancer is more frequent in women who have had multiple pregnancies, but this factor decreases in importance when the groups of women compared started their sex life at the same age. The development of cancer seems to be connected with coitus rather than pregnancy.

Carcinoma of the penis is virtually unknown among circumcised men. The means by which circumcision provides protection is not clear, but it is probably related to better hygiene. There is also a lower incidence of cancer of the uterine cervix in women whose sexual partner has been circumcised and in cultures in which the men, even though not circumcised, have a high standard of genital hygiene.[90]

The correlation with sexual experience and breast cancer is the reverse of that for the uterine cervix. Breast cancer patients have usually been married and become pregnant later in life. Lactation may provide some protection against breast cancer, since women who have breast-fed their infants show a lower incidence of breast malignancy. Cancer of the breast is reported to be unknown among Eskimo women and to be relatively rare among Japanese women; both cultures practice breast-feeding.

Viruses

There is strong evidence from animal studies that viruses play an important role in carcinogenesis, but evidence for viral etiology of human cancers is much less convincing. The strongest evidence of a causal relationship to cancer in humans is from studies of the DNA Epstein-Barr virus (EBV), a human virus known to be the etiologic agent of infectious mononucleosis and suspected in Burkitt's lymphoma and nasopharyngeal cancer.

However, a positive serum test for EBV antibody (indicating past exposure) has been found in healthy adults, suggesting that other factors need to be involved to develop cancer.[69,83]

Cervical cancer may result from a virus introduced into the cervix during sexual intercourse. This virus may be a member of the herpes group, *herpesvirus hominis* (HSV-2). Carriers of HSV-2 in the population are generally uncircumcised males with poor personal hygiene.[86]

Even if the evidence of viral etiology were more conclusive, consideration needs to be given to the question of whether the virus is transmitted horizontally, from host to host, or vertically, from generation to generation via the viral chromosome. In addition, successful immunization against a virus would require the following :

1. Suppression of the genetic expression of the virus
2. Sufficiently high incidence of the type of cancer to justify the cost of immunization
3. Consideration of previous natural exposure to the virus
4. Consideration of the effects of the immunization on any other etiologic factors that may be linked to the occurrence of the cancer[83]

The viruses found in animal tumors indicate that viruses may act individually or as co-carcinogens in causing malignancy in humans.[86] The question is no longer, however, whether viruses have a role in the cause of cancer but when they will be definitely implicated and whether one or many will be involved.

Psychosocial factors

Stressors such as life changes, loss of a significant other, and personality variables have been suggested as etiologic factors in the development of cancer. Some researchers believe that stress alters the body's immune system, making a person more susceptible to cancer. Depression has also been linked to cancer deaths by causing changes in immune mechanisms.

Social support in the form of institutions, family, and friends also may be an important variable. The individual with low social support and high need may be at a higher risk for developing cancer. In addition, lack of social support may adversely affect coping responses to therapy and to the illness. At the present time, however, how one defines the nature of social support and the degree to which it is present or lacking is unclear.

Conclusions

Carcinogenesis is a dynamic process that is influenced by many independent and poorly defined variables. The initial molecular changes are irreversible, but they may not be expressed when cooperative conditions are absent. Changes in these conditions may alter the carcinogenic process, resulting in either acceleration, inhibition, or even reversal of the process. Etiologic agents may be co-carcinogens. A genetic predisposition for a "weak" immune system along with a viral infection may lead to cancer, or oncogenic viruses may act as suppressants of the immune system. Chemical carcinogens may activate latent viral genes or inhibit the immune system's effectiveness in destroying cancer cells.

Nurses have a vital role to play in communicating to the public the factors involved in carcinogenesis. They can clarify misconceptions as well as do health teaching so that known carcinogenic practices may be eliminated. They can also set an example of good health practices for the general public, perhaps a more difficult role. As knowledgeable and concerned citizens, nurses must be initiators and supporters of efforts to have carcinogens removed from the environment.

PREVENTION AND HEALTH EDUCATION

Health teaching

The American public is more widely read and informed about health problems than ever before. Health-seeking behavior and a desire to be more knowledgeable about health problems are indicated by the frequency of articles about topics such as cancer in the lay press. The topic of cancer is also discussed more openly than ever before. Nurses have a major responsibility in the prevention of cancer. Because of their knowledge about the disease and their opportunity for contact with the public in the inpatient and outpatient setting, nurses have the opportunity to teach about cancer and to help motivate patients to seek treatment.

Case finding is a responsibility of all nurses. The nurse must be able to (1) counsel and direct patients to the proper sources of help, (2) have information about those

conditions that are known to predispose individuals to the development of the disease, and (3) educate the public about these factors. In addition, the nurse must be sensitive to the needs of patients who may be afraid and embarrassed when confronted with the possibility of cancer.

Since prevention of cancer is a primary goal of health professionals, the nurse must be aware of and able to communicate to others the importance of good health habits and the importance of avoiding conditions that predispose to cancer.

Early detection and treatment

The approach to early detection of cancer is worldwide. General criteria for cancer screening and testing programs have been drawn up by the epidemiology section of the American Public Health Association, and these criteria have been adapted by the World Health Organization. Multiphasic screening and a periodic health examination are being accepted by the public. In some cases diagnosis can be made months before the development of symptoms causes the person to seek care.[70]

Cancer detection is expensive. Education of the public often includes convincing them that a periodic health examination is a sound investment. Some cities have cancer detection centers where a complete physical examination including chest radiograph, Papanicolaou smear, breast examination, proctoscopy, urinalysis, and blood count are performed for a moderate fee. Nurses should be aware of clinics in their area where persons needing such resources may be referred.

The American Cancer Society has revised its guidelines for cancer-related checkups to provide essentially

Table 14-4. Guidelines for cancer related checkups*

Test or examination	Sex	Age (yr)	Recommendation
Papanicolaou test	Female	Over 20; under 20 if sexually active	q 3 yr after two initial negative tests 1 yr apart
Pelvic examination	Female	20-40	q 3 yr
		Over 40 or at menopause	Yearly
Endometrial tissue sample	Female	At menopause if high risk	High risk: history of infertility, obesity, failure of ovulation, abnormal uterine bleeding, estrogen therapy
Breast self-examination	Female	Over 20	Monthly
Breast physical examination	Female	20-40	q 3 yr
		Over 40	Yearly
Mammogram	Female	35-40	One baseline mammogram
		40-50	q 1-2 yrs
		Over 50	Yearly
Stool guaiac slide test	Male and female	Over 50	Yearly
Digital rectal examination	Male and female	Over 40	Yearly
Sigmoidoscopic examination	Male and female	Over 50	q 3-5 yrs after two initial negative examinations 1 yr apart

*American Cancer Society recommendations, 1980.

the same benefits with greatly reduced cost, risk, and inconvenience. Protocols for the early detection of cancer in asymptomatic persons are listed in Table 14-4. In general, persons over 20 years of age should have a cancer-related health checkup every 3 years, and those over 40 years old should have one every year. These checkups should also involve health counseling including information about personal cancer risk factors.[31] Women should request that the Pap test (Papanicolaou stain) be done if it was inadvertently overlooked by the health care provider. The Pap test still is one of the best means of preventing death from cervical cancer.

Early detection of cancer can decrease mortality. The guidelines of the American Cancer Society have been developed for people *without* symptoms; however, those who have any signs or symptoms suggestive of cancer should report them immediately to a physician. The nurse must know and be able to explain the significance of the American Cancer Society's seven warning signals and seven safeguards. It should be emphasized that any of these signs should be investigated medically, but their occurrence does not necessarily mean that the person has cancer.

All persons should know the most common sites of cancer. In women these are the breast, uterus (cervix), and colorectum (Fig. 14-1). Women should be taught to examine their breasts each month immediately after the menstrual period or, for postmenopausal women, on a designated day each month. Such self-examination is a much better method of detecting early breast cancer than an annual physical examination (see Chapter 36). Women of all ages should know the importance of reporting any abnormal vaginal bleeding or other discharge occurring between menstrual periods or after menopause. (Further information about cancer of specific organs can be found in appropriate chapters of this text.)

Testicular cancer accounts for only 1% of all male cancer, but it is the commonest carcinoma in the 15- to 35-year-old age group.[21] Men, especially those in this young population, should be taught testicular self-examination (see Chapter 35). Testicular cancer, if diagnosed early, has an excellent chance for cure if treated with surgery and/or radiation therapy.

Two common misconceptions that lead the person to ignore symptoms should be corrected. The first is a belief that a disease as serious as cancer must be accompanied by weight loss. Weight loss is usually a late symptom of cancer, yet the person often remarks, "I wasn't losing weight so I thought nothing serious could be wrong." Another reason for neglect of cancer is that it may not cause pain, and again the person believes the absence of pain means that the indisposition is minor. It must be repeatedly emphasized to the public that pain is not an early sign of cancer and that cancer often is far advanced before pain occurs.

Nurses also have a role in prevention and early detection of genetic cancer. They systematically obtain family cancer histories, teach about health maintenance, and do genetic counseling.[53] They may be involved in centralized familial cancer registries analogous to the monitoring of communicable diseases by health departments. Familial cancer registries would be helpful in pooling data on suspected cancer-prone families, as well as in disseminating current methods of surveillance and management of the conditions.[51]

In addition to being knowledgeable about measures for prevention and early detection of cancer, nurses must be aware of current therapeutic modalities and their rationales. Because of lack of information, misinformation, or fear of the effects of treatment, persons may put off seeking help. Clearly presented information about therapy will help to allay anxiety and confusion.

Cancer's seven warning signals

Change in bowel or bladder habits
A sore that does not heal
Unusual bleeding or discharge
Thickening or lump in breast or elsewhere
Indigestion or difficulty in swallowing
Obvious change in wart or mole
Nagging cough or hoarseness

Cancer's seven safeguards

Lung: Don't smoke cigarettes.
Colorectum: Have a proctoscopic exam as part of a regular checkup after age 40.
Breast: Practice monthly breast self-examination.
Uterus: Have a Pap test as part of a regular checkup.
Skin: Avoid overexposure to the sun.
Oral: Have a regular mouth examination by physician or dentist.
Complete body: Have an overall physical checkup annually or at 3-year intervals, depending on age.

Factors that interfere with health-seeking behaviors

Even though there is more widespread knowledge of cancer, a more positive attitude toward the disease is essential if individuals are to follow good health practices and seek help when warning signs of cancer are noted. The public underestimates the incidence of cancer although they are aware of and concerned about it. This suggests that defense mechanisms are at work. The public does not view the conventional types of therapy as optimal, although they have a high level of awareness of cancer's warning signals. Less-educated people and men in general are less likely to have physical examinations.[66] These are all factors that may interfere with health-seeking behaviors.

Unfortunately, anxiety and fear may immobilize the individual. Despite all the public announcements that have been made in the last few decades, there are still people who think of cancer as a disgraceful disease that must be hidden from others. Cancer is talked about in whispers by some people who look on it as a punishment for past sins, a shameful disease, or a disgrace to the family. This attitude stems partly from the fact that cancer in its terminal stages may be a painful and demoralizing disease that is sometimes accompanied by body odor and other signs of physical debility that are deeply etched on the consciousness of friends and relatives. Actually, there is no characteristic odor of cancer, although diseased tissue that breaks down and becomes infected with odor-producing organisms will be as unpleasant as any other infected wound. The essential point—so often missed by the public—is that this tragic situation is by and large an unusual one.

Some people fear cancer and shun persons who have the disease because they believe it is contagious. Scientific speculation on the possibility that a virus may be the cause has added to this fear. At this time, there is no conclusive evidence that cancer can be spread among humans in a way similar to the spread of infectious diseases, and absolute proof of the specific role of viruses in human malignancy is still not available.

The positive aspects of cancer care should be emphasized. It is estimated that approximately one third of the persons for whom a diagnosis is made are cured by medical treatment. Another one third could perhaps be cured by medical treatment if the cancer is diagnosed early enough. Only a third have cancer occurring in locations in which the disease advanced beyond permanent medical aid before sufficient signs appear to warn the patient of trouble. In spite of these facts, some persons think it is useless to report symptoms early, since they believe that if they do have cancer they cannot be cured. It can only be hoped that the recent publicity given to well-known persons who have been treated for cancer will help overcome some of these beliefs. If nothing else, the open discussion of the diagnosis and treatment in all types of media should result in a better informed public than ever before.

Cancer quackery

Fatal delay in seeking medical care may occur because of the patient's reliance on a "quick, painless cure." Despite public education and efforts of the medical profession to control extravagant claims of a few unethical practitioners, cancer quackery still exists, feeding on the ignorance and fear of the cancer patient and family.[2,79]

Quacks rely on testimonials of people they have "cured." Books and testimonials in magazines may be so appealingly written that the reader gets the impression that the content is factual and accurate. Electronic gadgets, dietary regimens, and various drugs and enzymes have all been purported to cure cancer.

Two drugs still available mostly outside the United States are krebiozen and Laetrile, a substance derived from apricot kernels. Use of Laetrile for cancer therapy has been outlawed by the FDA, whose regulations prohibit the transportation of Laetrile across state lines. In response to active lobbying by various groups, however, 11 states in 1977 passed legislation legalizing use of Laetrile within their borders. The American Cancer Society and the American Medical Association do not recommend use of Laetrile or krebiozen, since neither drug has been scientifically demonstrated to result in objective benefit to the person or show evidence that metastatic growth has been controlled.

In 1979 the National Cancer Institute (NCI) announced that it would sponsor human testing of Laetrile. In 1981 investigators reported that the drug was a failure as a cancer treatment based on a study of 156 patients at four medical centers. These patients had advanced cancer, usually of the lung, breast, colon, and rectum, that could not be treated by standard methods. In addition to intravenous and oral administration of the drug, the patients received the metabolic program prescribed: vitamins, pancreatic enzymes, and a diet containing fresh fruits, vegetables, and whole grains. Within 1 month cancer had progressed in 50% of the patients and cancer had progressed in 3 months in 90%. Only one fifth were alive after 8 months, findings comparable to no therapy at all.

Laetrile advocates state that the drug was not pure Laetrile and charge that the study was designed to discredit Laetrile. However, NCI stated that the drug was structurally the same as that used in Mexico's Laetrile clinics. The tragedy in the use of these drugs is the false security the treatment gives to patients. The security results in delay in seeking medical care until it is too late.[93]

Federal legislation is aimed at controlling quackery, and the FDA has published a booklet, *The Big Quack Attack: Medical Devices*, that describes various methods of quackery and directs consumers where to report complaints regarding practitioners of these methods.*

Organizations involved in cancer education, detection, and rehabilitation

FEDERAL ORGANIZATIONS

Federal recognition of the need to give intensive assistance to educational programs in cancer began in 1926 when Congress proclaimed April of each year as National Cancer Control Month. In 1937 the National Cancer Institute was created within the National Institutes of Health. This institute, with generous support from the federal government, conducts an extensive program of research in the field of cancer.

---

*FDA Office of Public Affairs, Rockville, MD 20857.

Cancer patients may also obtain help from both Medicare and Medicaid. The Community Services Administration provides services through state agencies such as Welfare and Aging or by direct grants. The Rehabilitation Services Administration will arrange and pay for services that help the cancer patient return to productive living.[2] With the passage of the National Cancer Act of 1971, impetus was given for the development of Cancer Clinical Research Centers. The goal was to translate research results into medical practice so that no one will be denied professional advice and care because of lack of facilities and knowledge. These centers combine research capability, demonstration of recent techniques and therapy, and community outreach programs.

Nurses can be articulate speakers for the cause of cancer care and cure, since they are intimately aware of the effects of cancer in threat to life and cost in dollars, disrupted lives, and human suffering. Nurses must asser-

Organizations and programs offering services to the cancer patient and the family

Organization	General description
National organizations and affiliates	
American Cancer Society* 777 Third Ave. New York, NY. 10017	Voluntary organization offering programs of cancer research, education, and patient service and rehabilitation.
CanSurmount	Composed of patient, family member, trained volunteer (also a cancer patient), health professional. Volunteers visit hospitals and homes.
I Can Cope	Addresses the educational and psychological needs of people with cancer.
International Association of Laryngectomees	Voluntary umbrella organization of 225 local clubs (varying names) that promote and support total rehabilitation program. Volunteers visit hospitals.
Reach to Recovery (Breast Cancer)	Provides rehabilitation support for women who have had mastectomies. Volunteers visit hospitals.
Cancer Information Service	Telephone information and referral service supplemented by printed materials.
The Concern for Dying 250 W. 57th St. New York, N.Y. 10019	Nonprofit educational organization distributes the living will, a document that records patient wishes concerning treatment.
Leukemia Society of America 211 E. 43rd St. New York, N.Y. 10017	Offers financial assistance and consultation services for referrals to other means of local support to cancer patients with leukemia and allied disorders.
Make Today Count P.O. Box 303 Burlington, Iowa 52601	More than 200 chapters comprising patients and family members, with the general goal of living each day as fully and completely as possible.
The National Hospice Organization 301 Tower, Suite 506 301 Maple Ave. W. Vienna, Va. 22181	Membership organization consisting of groups providing or preparing to provide hospice care; institutions concerned with care of the terminally ill and their families.
United Cancer Council, Inc. 1803 N. Meridian St. Indianapolis, Ind. 46202	Federation of voluntary cancer agencies that seeks the control of cancer through a three-point program of service, education, and research. Agencies are funded by the United Way of Giving.
United Ostomy Association 1111 Wilshire Blvd. Los Angeles, Ca. 90017	Nonprofit organization with more than 500 chapters in United States and Canada. General goal is to provide ostomy patients with mutual aid, moral support, and education. Members visit hospitals.

From Rosenbaum, E.: Living with cancer, St. Louis, 1982, The C.V. Mosby Co.
*For information on the following programs, contact the American Cancer Society.
†Direct services in tristate metropolitan areas of New York, New Jersey, and Connecticut.

Continued.

**Organizations and programs offering services to the
cancer patient and the family—cont'd**

Organization	General description
Regional organizations and programs	
Cancer Call PAC (People Against Cancer)	Emotional support telephone service; volunteers are recovered cancer patients and family members.
American Cancer Society 37 S. Wabash Ave. Chicago, Ill. 60603	
Cancer Care, Inc., of the National Cancer Foundation† One Park Ave. New York, N.Y. 10016	Voluntary social service agency providing professional counseling and planning to patients with advanced cancer and their families.
TOUCH, Coordinator, Cancer Control Program University of Alabama in Birmingham 104 Old Hillman Bldg. Birmingham, Ala. 35294	General goal is to provide assistance to cancer patients and their families in forming realistic, positive attitudes toward cancer and its treatment.
Psychosocial Counseling Service UCLA-Jonsson Comprehensive Cancer Center 1100 Glendon Ave. Suite 844 Los Angeles, Ca. 90024	Telephone counseling service directed to psychosocial needs of patients and care givers.

---

tively express to their representatives in government the importance of a combined effort to eradicate cancer.

NATIONAL AND REGIONAL ORGANIZATIONS

The nurse should know of other sources of information and help for persons who have cancer. Organizations and programs offering services to the cancer patient and the family are listed in box on pp. 227-228.

ASSESSMENT

Subjective data

The physician obtains a careful medical history inquiring into family history to determine those with a familial tendency for cancer, social history, marital and sex history, habits, occupation, and past medical history, since all may provide valuable clues to the presence of cancer.

It is especially important that the nurse obtain baseline data in relation to the cancer patient's health and health habits, since the treatment of cancer often involves complex changes in the patient's ability to meet psychologic, physiologic, and sociologic health needs. By careful collection of data the nurse can plan and carry out the complex nursing care that may be needed by the patient with cancer.

KNOWLEDGE OF DIAGNOSIS

Some initial data are needed to plan care. The first important question to be answered is whether the patient knows the diagnosis. This information should be recorded on the nursing care plan and discussed with other health team members. This will ensure that the person does not receive different answers to the same questions from the health care providers. Some hospitals have partially overcome this problem by having regular meetings of all the members of the professional staff at which the information given to each patient is reviewed. If meetings of this type are not being held, nurses should take the initiative in planning such a meeting.

The nurse should also elicit from both the patient and the physician what the patient has been told. Because of anxiety and the need for denial to protect the ego, the patient may have only heard part of the information given by the physician or have misinterpreted the information. The nurse can identify any discrepancies to plan care on the basis of the patient's perceptions of the illness.

Members of the medical profession differ in their opinions as to whether the patient with cancer should be told the diagnosis. The decision is usually made by the physician after consultation with the patient's family. The present trend is toward telling patients they have cancer. When patients are not informed, the reasons seem to be related much more to the physician's own attitudes and emotional reactions than to concern about patients' reactions. The nurse may help by discussing with the physician the reactions of the patient and the feelings expressed. It is the nurse's responsibility and sometimes a challenge to work effectively for the ultimate benefit of the patient within the seeming limitation it may impose.

Many spiritual advisers recommend telling the truth. Some persons, however, may not want to know the diagnosis and may ask and then answer their own questions negatively. Some do not ask for the diagnosis because they do not wish to have confirmed what they already suspect. Some insist on knowing the diagnosis and are preoccupied with every detail of their progress and treatment in a detached but completely abnormal fashion. Finally, there are some who wish to know the facts and who can accept them in a realistic way when given an opportunity to discuss their feelings with others. Some physicians prepare the patient over a period of time and tell the complete truth when they feel the patient is ready to accept it.

It is also important to determine how long the patient has known the diagnosis. The patient who has just been told may be going through the initial grief reactions. The person who has known for many years may have made a realistic adaptation and may see cancer as a chronic disease and not as a death sentence. The nurse should ascertain from the physician whether the cancer has already metastasized and, if so, whether the patient is aware of this fact. Responses of the patient with metastatic cancer will be different from those of the patient who can be more hopeful of a cure.

COPING SKILLS

Coping skills should be identified, for in no other disease are the person's inner resources and those of friends and families tested to a greater degree. Some persons cope by directly verbalizing fears and seeking support from others, while other persons are less direct. Some deal with problems with a problem-solving approach, while others try to avoid dealing with the problem.

The patient's and family's interpersonal, physical, and financial resources must be determined. What kind of support can be expected from the family? The financial burden the patient anticipates because of the therapy may affect the reaction to the disease.

PSYCHOLOGIC RESPONSE TO CANCER

Once the diagnosis of cancer has been made, the patient and family may be overwhelmed and immobilized. As one patient stated, "I cried all day Saturday, Sunday, and Monday. My daughter and my husband wanted to help but they didn't know what to do or say. I know my daughter was scared that she'd get cancer, too." Not all patients can openly express their feelings. Consequently, the nurse may have difficulty gathering data in order to assess and plan intervention. Some individuals are stoic, feeling it is a sign of weakness to display their psychologic

devastation in public. The nurse must be alert for subtle cues that may indicate that intervention is needed.

Grief

The general psychologic responses to a diagnosis of cancer are those accompanying the grieving process (see Chapter 16). The patient and family may go through a period of denial, during which there may be a delay in beginning therapy. Anxiety, depression, regressive behavior, and anger may all be manifested (see Chapter 9).

To many the diagnosis of cancer signifies the end of life itself, the ultimate loss. Nurses must be careful that they do not communicate any negative reactions to cancer. Beginning practitioners must look at their own attitudes toward the disease.

Guilt

Guilt is also a frequent psychologic response. Cancer patients may feel that the disease is punishment for actions of their past life. They may also feel guilty if they have delayed seeking treatment.

Sense of isolation

Perhaps one of the most prevalent reactions described by patients with cancer is a sense of isolation, of being cut off from those persons and things that are important to them. Patients with cancer may report that there is a gradual break in relationships. In some cases the isolation is patient initiated, in others it may result from actions of significant others because of their negative attitude toward the disease. Perhaps the most profound isolation is psychologic isolation, an inability to relate to and derive comfort from others, the feeling of being alone in a crowd.

Sexual disequilibrium

Nurses must be comfortable with their own sexuality and sensitive to the patients' responses, which may indicate that sexual tension is present.

Cancer is particularly destructive to the sexual relationship. It may so occupy the patient's life that all energy is directed to the illness. Sexual roles change. There may be fear that sexual activity may either cause the cancer to spread or that the well partner may "catch" it. Treatment modalities that affect the genital organs may cause sexual dysfunction, and the psychologic responses of anxiety, anger, depression, and body image disturbance may do violence to the sexual relationship[35] (see Chapter 34).

Fantasies of death and dying

Some patients report that they are overwhelmed with fantasies of death and dying. Most patients are more concerned about the process of dying, fearing pain, mutilation, and deterioration in both their physiologic and psychologic status, than with death itself. Patients may be open about their fantasizing, but they are more apt to communicate this in less obvious ways. Patients may focus their attention and discussion on the suffering and

portant in determining whether patients will continue diagnostic examination, treatment, or repeated follow-up care after discharge. The care they receive in the hospital may shape their attitudes toward the disease and may determine whether they can return home and either care for themselves or be cared for by the family. An important nursing function in the care of patients with cancer is building up faith in the physician and in the clinic or the medical center where care is received. The patient needs to feel certain that everything possible is being done and that new measures will be tried if there is any promise whatsoever of their being helpful.

Many patients must undergo extensive diagnostic examinations and surgery in large medical centers a long distance from their homes. Some patients have reported that, although they were confident that they were in "good medical hands," such confidence did not make up for the feelings that they were not always known as individuals. They needed desperately to feel that at least one person knew and understood them. Some patients experience near panic at the thought of their loved ones coming to visit and being unable to locate them. In most instances it is best for the patient to be accompanied by a relative or a close friend. It should also be recognized that even a patient in familiar surroundings may feel very much alone when awaiting diagnostic tests or surgical treatment for known or suspected cancer.

Both patient and family need something to help pass the time during the period of diagnostic tests and treatment and between steps of treatment such as surgery or x-ray therapy. Psychologic relief may sometimes come from keeping occupied with usual daily activities. Anxious relatives also receive satisfaction from doing things that the patient would do, if possible, thus preserving parts of cherished routines.

Members of the family often need direction in their activity when they have just learned that a loved one has cancer. They may need to talk over immediate and long-term plans with someone not close to the family situation. The nurse can sometimes be this listening person. At other times the family can best be served by a social caseworker, who will help them talk through and think through a course of action.

DATA ANALYSIS AND PLANNING

A sound personal philosophy and an objective, positive attitude toward the disease based on knowledge will help the nurse who is caring for the patient with cancer. The nurse should be able to give support and hope to the patient and family or friends.

The following four principles should be considered by the nurse when planning nursing interventions that are patient centered:

1. Persons have a right to be part of the treatment team.
2. Persons have the right to choose the desired degree of privacy or communication.
3. The nurse must respect the coping mechanisms of patients who are trying to maintain themselves through a difficult illness.
4. The nurse must remember not to give the appearance of hurrying, thus blocking communications.

The plan of care that a nurse develops for a patient with cancer needs to be individualized to reflect problems unique to a particular disease, treatment regimen, or the personality and life situation of the patient. Table 14-6 provides guidelines for data analysis and planning by listing common problem areas, nursing diagnoses, and expected outcomes for the patient and family. The section that follows will detail the nursing interventions for the patient experiencing one or more of the four treatment modalities and for the patient with chronic pain and cancer that is terminal.

IMPLEMENTATION

Assisting with achievement of therapeutic goals

Often several physicians are involved in determining the appropriate treatment for cancer. The medical team decides on the choice of treatment on the basis of the biologic characteristics of the tumor, its clinical stage (p. 218), and the condition of the patient. The histologic type of the tumor is particularly important in determining the treatment to be used.

Therapy may be curative (removal of all traces of the disease from the body) or palliative (directed only toward relieving symptoms). At the present time there are four major forms of treatment: surgery, radiotherapy, chemotherapy, and immunotherapy. The latter is the newest form of treatment for cancer. Combinations of the four treatment modalities are often employed to achieve the best result for each patient.

SURGERY

Surgery, the oldest method of treating cancer, may be either curative or palliative. The best treatment for cancer at present is complete surgical removal of all malignant tissues before metastasis occurs. Surgery must often be extensive and may require adjustments beyond those needed in many other conditions. There may not be time to accustom oneself gradually to the idea of surgery and the effect it can have on one's body and life-style. The individual often faces the prospect of mutilating surgery with only the hope that it will cure the cancer and be lifesaving. Concern about what will happen to the family may be utmost in the patient's mind. Obviously, the patient and family need empathy and understanding as they attempt to accept the recommendation for immediate surgery.

The operative procedures used to treat various types of cancer are discussed in the appropriate chapters of this book.

Table 14-6. Guidelines for data analysis and planning for patients with cancer

Problem area*	Possible nursing diagnoses	Expected patient outcomes*

Coping	Anxiety
	Coping, ineffective individual
	Coping, ineffective family (specify)
	Family processes, alterations in
	Fear (specify)
	Grieving (specify)
	    Anticipatory
	    Dysfunctional
	Powerlessness
	Self-concept, disturbance in: body image, self-esteem, role performance, personal identity
	Social isolation
	Spiritual distress
		Within a level consistent with physical, psychosocial, and spiritual capacities and their value system, the person and family:
		1. Use appropriate resources for support in coping
		2. Communicate feelings about living with cancer
		3. Participate in care and ongoing decision making
		4. Identify alternative resources when present coping strategies do not provide support
		5. State accomplishable goals

Comfort	Comfort, alteration in: pain Sleep pattern disturbance	The person and family: 1. Report alterations in comfort level 2. Identify measures to modify psychosocial, environmental, and physical factors that influence comfort and enhance the continuance of valued activities and relationships 3. State the source of pain, the treatment, and the expected outcome of proposed intervention 4. Describe appropriate interventions for potential or predictable problems of pain and sleep managment program
Nutrition	Nutrition, alterations in: less than body requirements	1. Identify foods that are tolerated and those that cause discomfort or aversion 2. State measures that enhance food intake and retention 3. Select appropriate dietary alternative to provide sufficient nutrients when usual foods are not tolerated 4. State methods of modifying consistency, flavor, or amounts of nutrients to ensure adequate nutrient intake 5. State dietary modifications compatible with cultural, social, and ethnic practices 6. State foods and fluids that provide optimal comfort during the terminal stage of illness

*From Oncology Nursing Society and American Nurses Association Division on Medical-Surgical Nursing Practice: Outcome standards for cancer nursing practice, Kansas City, Mo., 1979, American Nurses Association.

Continued.

Table 14-6. Guidelines for data analysis and planning for patients with cancer—cont'd

Problem area*	Possible nursing diagnoses	Expected patient outcomes*
Protective mechanisms (immune, hematopoietic, integumentary, and sensorimotor systems)	Fluid volume deficit Injury, potential for (specify) Knowledge deficit Oral mucous membrane, alterations in Skin integrity, impairment of	1. List measures to prevent skin breakdown, mucosal trauma, infection, and bleeding 2. Identify signs and symptoms of infection, bleeding, and sensorimotor dysfunction 3. Contact an appropriate health team member when initial signs and symptoms of infection, bleeding, or sensorimotor dysfunction occur 4. State measures to manage infection, bleeding, or sensorimotor dysfunction
Mobility	Mobility, impaired physical	1. State the cause of the immobility, the treatment, and the outcome of treatment 2. Describe an appropriate management plan to optimally integrate the alteration in mobility into life-style 3. Describe optimal levels of activities of daily living in keeping with disease state and treatment 4. Identify health services and community resources available for managing changes in mobility 5. Use measures to aid or improve mobility 6. Demonstrate measures to prevent complications of decreased mobility
Elimination	Bowel elimination, alterations in: constipation Bowel elimination, alterations in: diarrhea Urinary elimination, alteration in patterns of	1. State appropriate actions if changes in elimination patterns occur 2. Describe the relationship between adequate elimination and physiologic integrity 3. Identify and manage factors that may affect elimination, such as diet, stress, physical activity, and neurogenic conditions 4. Develop a plan for managing an altered elimination route within personal life-style
Sexuality	Sexual dysfunction	1. Client and partner identify potential or actual alterations in perception of sexuality or sexual function 2. Client and partner identify alternate methods of expressing sexuality

Table 14-6. Guidelines for data analysis and planning for patients with cancer—cont'd

Problem area	Possible nursing diagnoses	Expected patient outcomes
Ventilation	Respiratory function, alterations in Airway clearance, ineffective Breathing patterns, ineffective Gas exchange, impaired	1. State plans for daily activity that demonstrate maximum conservation of energy 2. List measures to reduce or modify pulmonary irritants from the environment, such as smoke, dry air, powders, and aerosols 3. Describe the effect of environmental extremes on ventilatory function and oxygen use 4. State effective measures to maintain a patent airway 5. Identify reasons for altered ventilation, such as decreased hemoglobin, infection, anxiety, effusion, and obstructed airway 6. Identify an appropriate plan of action should altered ventilation occur 7. Develop a plan for managing an altered airway

RADIOTHERAPY

Radiotherapy, or the use of radiation in the treatment of disease, has been used in the treatment of cancer for about 80 years. The principal radiation agents are: (1) x-ray, which consists of electromagnetic radiation produced by waves of electrical energy traveling at a very high speed; (2) radium, which is a radioactive isotope occurring freely in nature; and (3) the artificially induced radioactive isotopes produced by bombarding the isotopes of elements with highly energized particles in a cyclotron. The most common sources of radiation for external beam therapy are the linear accelerator, the cobalt-60 teletherapy machines, and the betatron. These machines produce radiation of varying types of energy, which control the depth of penetration of the x-rays into tissues.

Radiotherapy is effective in curing cancer in some instances; in other instances it controls the growth of cancer cells for a time. Because it may deter the growth of cancer cells, it may relieve pain even when extension of the disease is such that cure is impossible.

Principle underlying radiotherapy

Radiotherapy is based on the fact that rapidly reproducing malignant cells are more sensitive to radiation than are normal cells. Therapeutic doses of radiotherapy are calculated to destroy or delay the growth of malignant cells without destroying normal tissue. Rotation of either the target site in the patient or the radiation beam makes it possible to deliver a high total dose to the tumor while at the same time only part of the dose reaches the noncancerous tissue surrounding it.

The radiation used medically consists of alpha- (α-), beta- (β-), and gamma- (γ-) rays (Fig. 14-2). α- and β-rays cannot pass through the skin. γ-Rays, however, have been found to penetrate several inches of lead, although lead shielding offers a considerable degree of protection. X-rays, which are similar to γ-rays, require lead protection.

Radiation can be delivered to the patient *externally* by exposure to rays, such as from an x-ray machine or from cobalt 60, or *internally*, either by placing radioactive material such as radium within the tissues or body cavity (sealed internal radiation) or by administering the materials intravenously or orally so that they are distributed throughout the body (unsealed internal radiation).

Protection of health workers from radiation hazards

Radiation delivered externally (including x-rays) can do harm to persons working with the patient *only during* the time that the patient is being treated. This is true also of the radiation from some radioactive substances used for other methods of treatment. Patients with internal radiation who emit γ-rays, however, may expose other persons to radiation for varying periods of time, and the time one can be exposed safely to the patient is important in planning care. The time interval required for the radioactive substance to be half dissipated is called its *half-life* (Table 14-7). This period varies extremely widely, but as the end of the half-life is reached, danger from exposure decreases.

There are three ways by which exposure to radiation

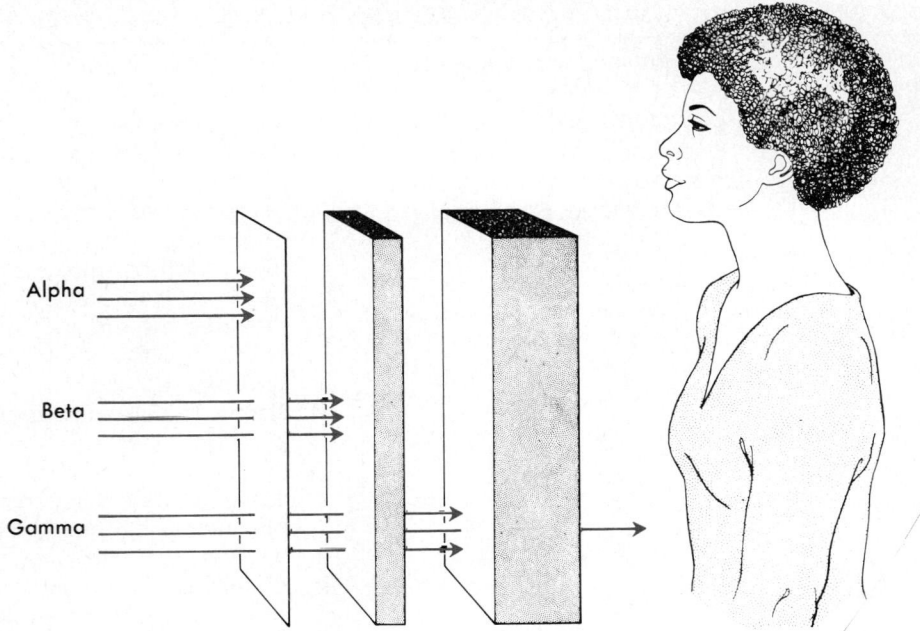

Fig. 14-2. Relative penetrating power of three types of radiation. (From Bouchard-Kurtz, R., and Speese-Owens, N.: Nursing care of the cancer patient, ed. 4, St. Louis, 1981, The C.V. Mosby Co.)

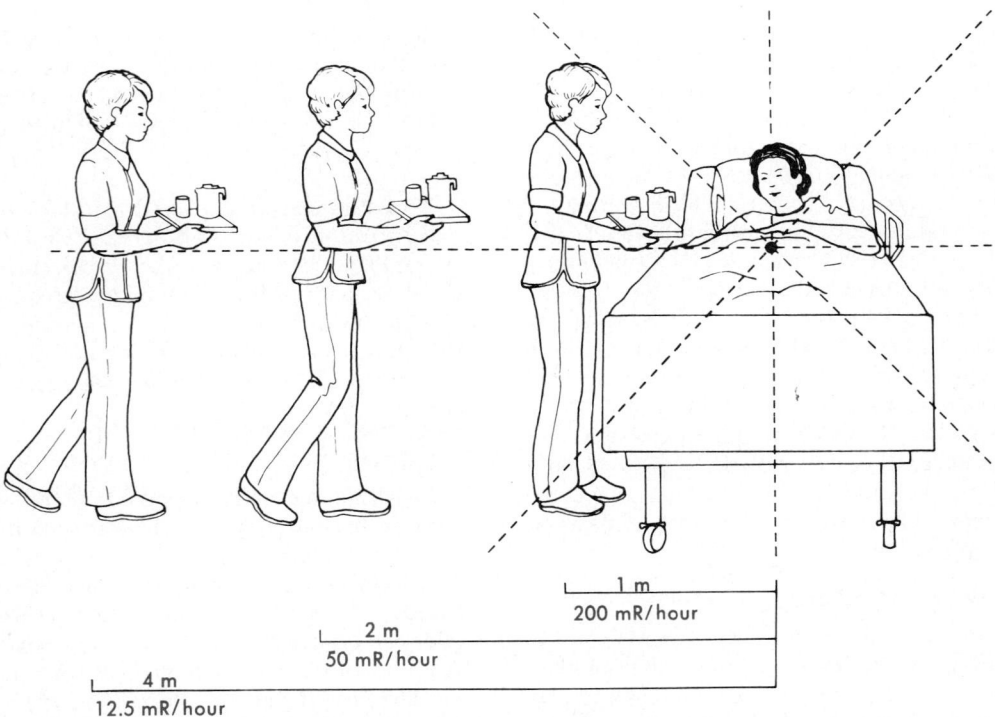

1 m
200 mR/hour

2 m
50 mR/hour

4 m
12.5 mR/hour

Fig. 14-3. Nurse nearest source of radioactivity (patient) is exposed to more radioactivity. (Adapted from Bouchard-Kurtz, R., and Speese-Owens, N.: Nursing care of the cancer patient, ed. 4, St. Louis, 1981, The C.V. Mosby Co.)

can be controlled: *time, distance,* and *shielding.* All emanations are subject to the physical law of inverse-square. For example, a person who stands 2 meters away from the source of radiation receives only one fourth as much exposure as when standing only 1 meter away. At 4 meters, only one sixteenth of the exposure will be received. Therefore increasing the distance from the emanations decreases the exposure (Fig. 14-3). When a patient such as an infant must be held for x-ray treatment, the nurse or person who holds the patient must be careful to keep at arm's length or as far away as possible and to avoid having any body part in the direct path of the rays. *Lead-lined gloves and a lead apron, which act as a shield to reduce exposure, should be worn by anyone who attends patients during x-ray treatment or during examination by fluoroscopy.*

When the nurse knows the kind of substance used, the kind and amount of rays it emits, its half-life, and its exact location in the patient and considers these facts in relation to control of exposure, safe and adequate care for the patient can be planned.

Nurses wishing to know about radioactive substances can obtain information from the Division of Radiological Health of the Public Health Service or from their state health department. Several drug companies also publish pamphlets that contain helpful information. In cities with large medical facilities a radiation physicist may be consulted.

External radiotherapy
Preparation of the patient

Teaching the patient and family is an important aspect of care. Orientation programs, information booklets, and weekly group sessions for patients and families are useful methods of communicating information. In group meetings, topics such as scheduling, whom to see for assistance with special problems, or care of the skin are discussed. There is an opportunity to discuss fears and misconceptions about radiation and cancer. Both inpatients and outpatients can attend.

Patients who are to receive radiation therapy should know that they will be attended by radiotherapists who will be stationed outside the treatment room and who will observe the treatment and be in communication at all times. The patient must often lie absolutely still for a period of time, a very tiring experience. There is no pain associated with radiation therapy.

Procedure

In giving treatment, rays can be directed at the tumor from several different angles so that normal tissue receives a minimum of exposure. The areas through which rays pass are known as *ports.* Different ports may be used on different days, or the position may be changed at intervals during a daily treatment so that only a certain amount is given through each of several ports. The patient may be placed on a rotating device such as a rotating chair so that although the tumor mass receives the full dose of radiation, skin areas receive less exposure.

In medical centers, where hyperbaric oxygen chambers are available, patients may receive radiation therapy while receiving hyperbaric oxygen. The rationale for this combined therapy is that malignant cells, in which the oxygen tension is increased, are more susceptible to the effects of radiation. At the same time the sensitivity of normal cells to the radiation effects is not increased.[37]

Early reaction

When radiation therapy is used, some degree of radiation reaction may occur. Early reactions include blanching or erythema of the skin and mucous membranes, possibly progressing to dry or moist desquamation. If the mucosa of the mouth, pharynx, bladder, or rectum is affected, there may be pain, inhibition of the normal secretions, and impairment of functions.

When treatment is directed toward abdominal organs or any deep tissues there is almost always some skin reaction. There may be itching, tingling, burning, oozing, or sloughing of the skin. The term *burn* should never be used in referring to this reaction, since it implies incorrect dosage. Reddening may occur on or about the tenth day, and the skin may turn a dark plum color after about 3 weeks. The skin may also become dry and inelastic and may crack easily.

Gastrointestinal reactions to radiation therapy are more common when treatment includes some part of the gastrointestinal tract or when the ports lie over this system. The patient may have nausea, vomiting, anorexia, malaise, and diarrhea. This difficulty is usually not discussed with the patient before treatment is started because it is thought that the power of suggestion may contribute to symptoms. Almost all patients who receive moderate or large doses of radiation, however, have these symptoms in varying degrees.

Radiation therapy also causes depression of the hematopoietic system and in turn a low white blood cell count, predisposing the patient to infection. Sloughing of tissue and subsequent hemorrhages are complications that must be considered when radiation is used in any form. Hemorrhage is not mentioned to the patient, but ambulatory patients are told that they should call the physician at once should any sloughing of tissue occur.

Late reaction

Effects of radiation may be apparent months or years after therapy. Genital tissue, muscles, and kidneys may be affected, resulting in painful radionecrosis.[90] Radiation causes destruction of fine vasculature, and the skin may show signs of atrophy (thinning and blanching), pigmentation, and telangiectasis. If there is severe vascular damage or if there are other complications that require further surgery, the irradiated tissues may fail to heal.

Nursing care of patients receiving external radiation

Nursing care is directed toward preventing skin breakdown, decreasing gastrointestinal upset, and preventing infection. The area to be treated is usually outlined by the radiologist at the time of the first treatment. Occasionally, a small tattoo mark is used instead of the conspicuous skin markings when treatment is given to exposed parts of the body. Marks must not be washed off until the treatment is completed, because they are important guides to the radiologist (Fig. 14-4). Medicated substances that may contain heavy metals such as zinc are not permitted on the skin until

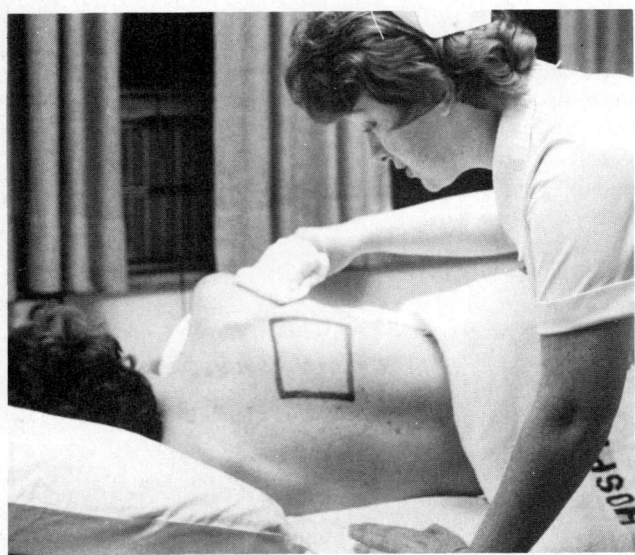

Fig. 14-4. When bath is given care must be taken not to remove skin markings used to guide radiologist in giving x-ray treatments.

the series of treatments is completed, because they may increase the radiation dosage.

If the radiation dosage has been high and blanching or discoloration of the skin has resulted, the patient may be advised to avoid exposure to temperature changes for several years. The patient may have to take much cooler baths or showers than formerly and may have to avoid sunbathing or any other extreme of temperature. If x-ray treatments have been given to a woman's face, she must be cautioned regarding the use of cosmetics to cover discolored skin. They may contain heavy, irritating oils and should not be used until consultation with the physician.

When treatment must be given to any part of the head, patients may ask about the possibility of loss of hair. Whether hair will return after falling out depends on the amount of radiation received. Attractive scarves and wigs are useful for patients with alopecia or when returning hair is too thin.

Internal radiotherapy

Internal radiation may be delivered by sealed or unsealed methods. In either type special precautions may be necessary, depending on the amount of radioactive material used, its location, and the kind of rays being emitted (Table 14-7). Special precautions may be taken if more than a tracer diagnostic dose has been given. Hospitals in which therapeutic doses of radioactive isotopes are administered are required to have a radiation safety officer. Quite often this person is a physicist. The radiation

---

Nursing care of patients receiving external radiation

1. *Preventing skin breakdown*
   a. Skin preparation: cleansing, alcohol rub
   b. Care must be taken *not* to remove skin markings used to guide radiologist
   c. Vegetable fat or oil may be ordered to protect the affected skin
   d. Medicated solutions, ointments, or powders that may contain heavy metals such as zinc are *not* permitted on the skin
   e. Consult radiologist about skin care for local radiation reactions; do *not* remove crusts
   f. Keep dressings loose; use nonirritating tape and avoid pulling on affected skin
   g. Teach patient to avoid constricting clothing or friction of any kind on exposed skin
   h. Teach patient to avoid excesses of heat and cold to affected skin surfaces.
2. *Decreasing gastrointestinal upset*
   a. Advise resting before and after meals to control nausea and vomiting
   b. Breakfast is usually the best tolerated meal of the day
   c. Suggest frequent small meals during the day
   d. Sour beverages and effervescent liquids may relieve nausea
   e. Suggest high-protein, high-carbohydrate, fat-free, low-residue diet to prevent nausea and vomiting; low-roughage diet for diarrhea
   f. Administer palliative medications, as ordered.
3. *Preventing infection*
   a. Teach patient to avoid persons with upper respiratory infections
   b. Use protective isolation if white blood count is low
   c. Administer antibiotic drugs, as ordered

safety officer determines the precautions to be observed in each situation. Most hospitals have printed instruction sheets stating the precautions to be followed for each substance used. Personnel should be fully acquainted with all precautions and should be supervised in carrying them out. Generally, the patient will be placed in a single room or in a double room with another patient who is also receiving radiation therapy. A radiation precaution sign should be placed on the door to the patient's room, and visitors should be restricted.

Sealed internal radiotherapy

Brachytherapy is used to deliver a concentrated dose of radiation directly to the malignant lesion or tumor area. Usually this involves insertion of radioactive substances within hollow cavities or within tissues. The radioactive isotopes commonly used are cobalt 60, iridium 192, iodine 125, phosphorus 32, cesium 137, gold 198, and radium 226.[82] These radioactive substances may be used in the form of molds, plaques, needles, wires, special applicators, or ribbons that are carefully placed and left in position for a specified length of time (Fig. 14-5). Emanations from the radioactive substances may also be sealed in tiny gold tubes (seeds) and left indefinitely within the tissues into which they are inserted (Fig. 14-6). The half-life of the seeds is much less than that of the substances from which their emanations come.

A fairly common site for the implantation of seeds is the mouth. Plaques and molds also are used for lesions in the mouth. Sealed internal radiation also is used widely in treatment of cancer of the cervix.

PREVENTION OF RADIATION HAZARD. Safe practice for the nurse caring for a patient receiving sealed internal radiotherapy depends on the principles of time, distance, and shielding (p. 237). Radioactive materials for sealed internal therapy usually are kept in a lead-lined container in the radiology department and are inserted into the patient in the operating room. They should never be touched with bare hands. A pair of forceps should be kept in the patient's room for handling in case the radioactive implant becomes dislodged.

Sealed radioactive material is often reused. On removal from a patient the radioactive material should be cleansed using the precautions just described and returned to the radiology department in a lead-lined container at once so that it may be safe from accidental handling or loss. Even if it is not to be reused, it is returned in a lead-lined container. To prevent accidental loss in cleansing, radioactive material is cleansed in a basin of water instead of in an open sink. If a brush must be used, it must be grasped with forceps so that close contact with the material is avoided.

Exposure is sometimes termed *external* in that it can occur only by direct exposure to the encased radioactive substance. It cannot result from contact with linen, vomitus, or urine or from touching the patient. Knowing where the radioactive material is implanted helps the nurse to plan activities of care. If, for example, the substance is in the patient's mouth, there is less exposure if one stands toward the foot of the bed. If it is in the uterus or bladder, standing at the head of the bed is safer.

Table 14-7. Characteristics and uses of some commonly used radioactive agents

Radiation source	Half-life (where applicable)	Rays emitted	Appearance or form	Method of administration
X-ray	—	γ	Invisible rays	X-ray machine
Radium	1600 yr	α β γ	In needles, plaques, molds	Interstitial (needles) Intracavitary (plaques, mold)
Radon	4 days	α β γ (low intensity)	In seeds, needles	Interstitial (seeds, needles)
Cesium (^{137}Cs)	33 yrs	β γ	In needles, capsules	Interstitial (needles) Intracavitary (capsules)
Cobalt (^{60}Co)	5 yr	β γ	External (cobalt unit) Internal (needles, seeds, molds)	Machine (teletherapy) Interstitial (needles, seeds)
Iodine (^{131}I)	8 days	β γ (low intensity)	Clear liquid	By mouth
Phosphorus (^{32}P)	14 days	β	Clear liquid	By mouth, intracavitary, intravenous
Gold (^{198}Au)	3 days	β γ	Purple liquid	Intracavitary
Iridium (^{192}Ir)	74 days	β γ (low intensity)	In needles, wires, seeds	Interstitial
Yttrium (^{90}Y)	3 days	β	Beads, needles	Interstitial

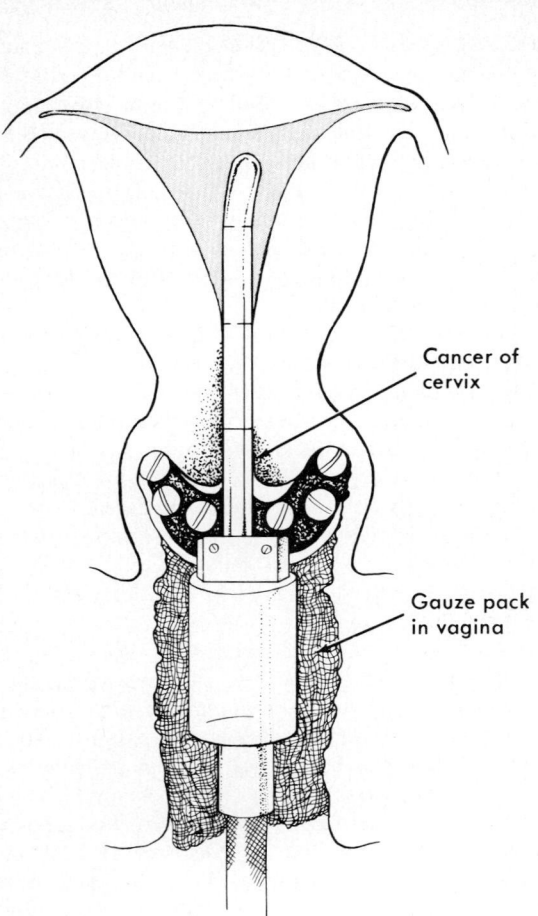

Fig. 14-5. Ernst applicator in place for treatment of cancer of cervix. Note gauze packing in vagina to help maintain applicator in position.

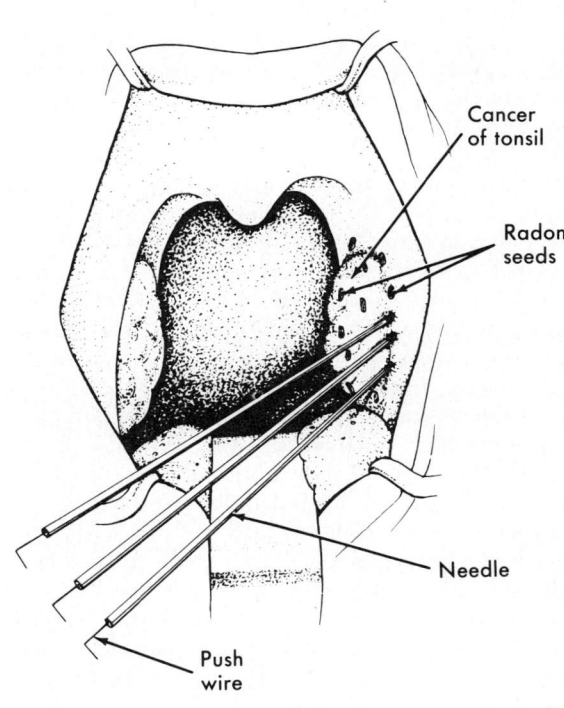

Fig. 14-6. Radium emanations may be sealed in tiny gold tubes (radon seeds) and left indefinitely within tissue into which they are inserted. Schema shows insertion into tonsil.

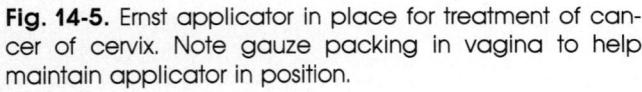

Table 14-8. Special precautions for unsealed internal radiotherapy

Substance or object	Radioactive element	Precautions
Urine	Iodine (^{131}I)	Urine emptied directly into lead-lined container. *All* urine must be collected (amount of radioactivity determines when patient may be removed from isolation). Urine in lead-lined container is stored in radioisotope laboratory until it can be safely disposed of.
Linen	Iodine (^{131}I)	Monitor with Geiger counter for contamination; if contaminated, place in special container marked "Radioactive" and send to radioisotope laboratory.
Equipment	Phosphorus (^{32}P) Gold (^{198}Au)	
Vomitus	Phosphorus (^{32}P)	Place vomitus in lead-lined container and send to radioisotope laboratory.
Wound drainage	Phosphorus (^{32}P) Gold (^{198}Au)	Place dressings in lead-lined container and send to radioisotope laboratory.

Unsealed internal radiotherapy

Unsealed internal radiation is delivered to the patient by mouth as an "atomic cocktail" or as a liquid instilled into a body cavity. Exposure for persons caring for the patient can result from direct contact with emanations from the substance in the patient (external exposure) or from contact with the patient's discharges that contain the radioactive substances (internal exposure). It may be inhaled, ingested, or absorbed through the skin. The exposure varies with each of the substances used, and safety for the nurse and others caring for the patient depends on a thorough knowledge of the substance used and its action within the body. If only tracer doses (very small amounts) of radioactive substances are used, as for diagnostic purposes, no precautions are necessary.

PREVENTION OF RADIATION HAZARDS. Special precautions that need to be taken when using radioactive iodine, phosphorus, or gold are listed in Table 14-8. With radioactive iodine, small amounts will be present in sputum, vomitus, perspiration, or feces, but special precautions are needed *only for urine*. The nurse should know the approved hospital procedure to safely dispose of any urine spilled on the floor.

No linen or equipment is removed from the room until it is monitored with a Geiger-Muller counter for contamination. Paper dishes are usually used and then burned. If the nurse's skin should become contaminated, it should be washed thoroughly with soap and water and then monitored. If contamination remains, washing should be continued until monitoring shows that additional cleansing is not necessary.

When the patient is removed from isolation, all equipment is monitored and carefully scrubbed by attendants who have been instructed in safe methods by persons who are in charge of the administration of the radioactive substances. It is then remonitored. The room is aired until monitoring shows that radioactivity is negligible and that the room is safe for any other patient. Airing takes at least 24 hours.

Nursing intervention for patients receiving internal radiotherapy

Nursing interventions consist of teaching the patient, decreasing patient isolation, and promoting comfort. The

---

Nursing care of patients receiving internal radiotherapy

1. Teach routine and reasons for precautions
2. Decrease isolation by providing radio or television for outside contact and encouraging permissible interaction with nursing staff
3. Plan trips into room to include several tasks
4. Promote comfort: complete bath before treatment, clean bed linens, turn sheet, pillow positioning

---

patient should know that isolation is temporary, that the restrictions will be removed on a certain day, and that members of the nursing staff will be available but that they will work quickly and will remain in the room only long enough to carry out essential activities. The patient can assist in notifying family and friends about the restriction on visitors and how long it will last. The patient should also know how the radioactive substance is eliminated to lessen worry about being a danger to others, particularly after therapy is concluded.

Trips made in haste into the patient's room are disturbing psychologically, because they imply that the patient is not acceptable to others. The nurse who plans thoughtfully might deliver a letter, fresh water, and the newspaper and make pertinent observations in less time than the one who plans less well and must make several trips into the patient's room.

CHEMOTHERAPY

Advances in knowledge of cancer growth and chemotherapeutic agents have led to concomitant advances in cancer treatment. Improvement in overall survival and longer disease-free intervals can be directly ascribed to the use of chemotherapeutic agents, particularly in combination chemotherapy regimens and as adjuvant therapy.

Benefits of chemotherapy

Chemotherapy is potentially curative in gestational choriocarcinoma, acute lymphocytic leukemia (ALL), Ewing's sarcoma, advanced Hodgkin's disease, diffuse histiocytic lymphoma, Burkitt's lymphoma, testicular cancer, and ovarian cancer. Prolonged disease-free or controlled intervals may be achieved by chemotherapy in the treatment of several non-Hodgkin's lymphomas, multiple myeloma, breast cancer and oat cell carcinoma of the lung. In other advanced malignancies, such as colorectal carcinoma, chemotherapy rarely produces a complete response and only a few such patients experience an increased survival time. In the treatment of chronic myelogenous leukemia (CML) and chronic lymphocytic leukemia (CLL), although the duration of life may not be prolonged, the quality of life may be enhanced by chemotherapy because of control of symptoms. Patients and families may be told that incurable does not mean untreatable or uncontrollable.

In the care of an individual patient with cancer, the expected benefit of chemotherapy (cure, control, or palliation) should be known by the physician, nurse, and patient. This allows for realistic goal setting by the care givers, patients, and family. Such background also provides a perspective from which to view side effects. The potential for cure, prolonged disease-free survival, or reduction of symptoms is a benefit that most often outweighs the risk and discomfort of short-term toxicity and side effects. Conditions in which risk may outweigh benefits include overt or occult infections, bleeding dyscrasias, bone marrow depression, severe metabolic disturbances, renal or liver dysfunction, and pregnancy.

Adjuvant chemotherapy refers to chemotherapy administered after surgical removal of all known cancer present in the body. It is aimed at the destruction of micrometastases thought likely to be present but too small to be detected by current diagnostic techniques. Left untreated, the micrometastases have a high potential for tumor growth and cancer recurrence. With the use of chemotherapy at a time when the malignant cell population is small and likely to be susceptible, complete tumor cell eradication is possible. The goal is cure.

Adjuvant chemotherapy is now generally considered to be indicated after mastectomy in all women with involved axillary lymph nodes at the time of surgery and it has demonstrated a significant decrease in recurrence rates and prolonged disease-free intervals. Adjuvant chemotherapy also appears to be beneficial in osteogenic sarcoma and Wilms' tumor. Evidence is currently equivocal regarding its benefit in other malignancies, such as colon cancer and malignant melanoma. The precise role of adjuvant chemotherapy will be more clearly delineated during the next decade, but it is already established as one of the major recent developments in health care.

A feeling of well-being and knowledge that all diagnostic tests are negative for cancer understandably may cause the patient to question the need for adjuvant therapy. This is emphasized when side effects are experienced. A sensitivity to these feelings, coupled with the knowledge of the expected benefit of therapy, is the basis for both patient teaching and the supportive encouragement often needed for continued therapy.

Despite an intellectual understanding of the benefits of chemotherapy, it is sometimes difficult for a nurse to maintain an appropriately optimistic and realistic outlook if all one sees are those patients who did not respond to or are no longer responsive to therapy, manifest severe toxicity, or are dying. The practitioner must take into account the setting in which patients are seen. Hospital-based nurses tend to see patients at the time of diagnosis, when they are critically ill, or during the final days of life. The public health nurse may see the patient at comparable points of illness while providing nursing care in the home. Discussion between the nurse and primary physician, contact with the outpatient clinic, and readmission to the same nursing unit are useful ways of acquiring a more complete picture of an individual's response to treatment. Such positive experiences are a means of nurturing one's own beliefs in therapy so that a realistic and at times very optimistic approach to caring for, supporting, and teaching the chemotherapy patient exists.

Pathophysiologic principles of chemotherapy

Normal and malignant cells progress through various phases in the cell cycle as they replicate. Cancer chemotherapy is based on the action of certain drugs that create changes in the cell cycle phases and interrupt cell growth and replication. They specifically do this by disrupting production of essential enzymes, damaging structural proteins, and inhibiting DNA, RNA, and protein synthesis or direct interaction with DNA.

Drugs such as antimetabolites and *Vinca* alkaloids that are effective during a particular point of the cell cycle are said to be *cell cycle specific*. Drugs that are active throughout the cell cycle *(cell cycle nonspecific)* include the alkylating agents, antibiotics, and steroid hormones. Combinations of cycle-specific and cycle-nonspecific drugs have proved useful in constructing treatment regimens.

One major factor that influences the response of a cancer to chemotherapy is the fraction of tumor cells in replication at a given time, a percentage that varies among different tumors, individual patients, and at different times in the same patient. Malignancies with high growth fractions (proportion of cells in active cycle) and short cell cycle time (for example, leukemia) are most vulnerable to chemotherapy.[38]

Cell population growth

The concept of cell population growth recognizes the fact that the population of both normal cells and cancer cells contains more dividing cells when the overall cell population is small and fewer dividing cells when the overall cell population is large.[32] This relates to chemotherapy in that the choice of drug differs for large, slow-growing tumors as opposed to small tumors whose cell population is likely to be more rapidly proliferating. The latter, because of their sensitivity to interference with DNA, are susceptible to phase-specific drugs whereas the large, slow-growing tumor is more likely to respond to phase-nonspecific drugs.

Log cell kill hypothesis

The log cell kill hypothesis states that any dose of a chemotherapy drug will destroy only a fraction of the malignant cells.[32] Treatment must be repeated multiple times to eradicate the cancer. Moreover, clinical symptoms disappear before all malignant cells are destroyed so that treatment must often be continued even when all apparent evidence of disease has disappeared.

Chemotherapeutic agents

Drugs may be classified as alkylating agents, antimetabolites, plant *(Vinca)* alkaloids, antibiotics, and hormones (Table 14-9).

Alkylating agents

The alkylating agents are cell cycle nonspecific and act against already formed nucleic acids by cross-linking DNA strands, thereby preventing DNA replication and the transcription of RNA.

Antimetabolites

The antimetabolites act by interfering with the synthesis of chromosomal nucleic acid. Antimetabolites are analogues of normal metabolites and block the enzyme necessary for synthesis of essential factors or are incorporated into the DNA or RNA and thus prevent replication. Most antimetabolites are pyrimidine analogues, purine analogues, or folic acid antagonists and are, in general, cycle specific.

Table 14-9. Agents used in cancer chemotherapy*

Agent	Mechanism of action	Major toxic manifestations
Alkylating agents		
Chlorambucil (Leukeran) Melphalan (Alkeran) Cyclophosphamide (Cytoxan) Busulfan (Myleran)	Interfere with DNA replication by attacking DNA synthesis throughout cell cycle (cell cycle nonspecific)	Bone marrow depression with leukopenia, thrombocytopenia, and bleeding; cyclophosphamide may cause alopecia and hemorrhagic cystitis
Antimetabolites		
Methotrexate (MTX) 6-Mercaptopurine (6-MP) 5-Fluorouracil (5-FU) Cytarabine (Cytosar)	Structural analogs of essential metabolites and therefore interfere with synthesis of these metabolites (cell cycle specific)	Bone marrow depression, oral and gastrointestinal ulceration
Antibiotics		
Doxorubicin (Adriamycin) Bleomycin (Blenoxane) Dactinomycin (Cosmegan) Daunomycin (Daunorubicin) Mithramycin (Mithracin) Mitomycin (Mutamycin)	Interfere with DNA or RNA synthesis, varying with the drug (cell cycle nonspecific)	Stomatitis, gastrointestinal disturbances, and bone marrow depression Doxorubicin causes cardiac toxicity at cumulative doses over 500 mg/m² Bleomycin can cause alopecia and pulmonary fibrosis, but only minimal bone marrow depression
Plant alkaloids		
Vinblastine (Velban) Vincristine (Oncovin)	Interfere with mitosis (cell cycle specific)	Alopecia, areflexia, bone marrow depression Neurotoxicity with ataxia and impaired fine motor skills, constipation and paralytic ileus
Steroid hormones		
Androgens (Neo-Hombreol) Estrogens (DES) Progestins (Depoprovera) Adrenocorticosteroids (Prednisone)	Alter the host environment for cell growth (cell cycle nonspecific)	Specific for the actions of the hormone

Adapted from Porth, C.: Pathophysiology: concepts of altered health states, Philadelphia, 1982, J.B. Lippincott Co.

Vinca *alkaloids*

Vincristine sulfate and vinblastine sulfate are plant alkaloids that act as mitotic inhibitors. These agents exert their cytotoxic effect by binding to proteins within the cells. The *Vinca* alkaloids are cell cycle specific. Although these two agents are similar in composition, mechanism of action, and metabolism, their antitumor spectrum, dose, and clinical toxicity differ.

Antibiotics

Those antibiotics that demonstrate antitumor activity appear to affect either the function or synthesis of the nucleic acids. In addition, antimitotic and cell surface ef-

fects may be caused by these agents. The cytotoxic antibiotics are cell cycle nonspecific agents.

Steroids

The corticosteroids are produced by the adrenal cortex and include mineralocorticoids and glucocorticoids. It is the glucocorticoids that, in addition to their use in numerous nonmalignant diseases, are effective in the treatment of many neoplastic disorders. In some malignancies (for example, lymphomas, breast cancer, multiple myeloma, acute lymphocytic leukemia, and chronic lymphocytic leukemia) steroids exert a direct antitumor effect. Steroids are also able to reduce edema and inflammation around a tumor and therefore are useful for symptom relief. There are many side effects associated with long-term steroid use, most notably a compromised immunologic response to infection, osteoporosis, and a cushingoid syndrome. Steroids in cancer treatment regimens are often given intermittently and for short periods of time and are not often associated with the debilitating side effects associated with chronic, long-term use. Patients often describe an improved sense of well-being and an increased appetite while receiving prednisone. With completion of a prescribed course of therapy, a brief period of fatigue, malaise, and emotional lability may be experienced.

Hormones

Hormonal alteration may be a desired therapeutic goal when tumor growth is directly influenced by certain hormones. The mechanism whereby the steroid hormones stimulate or inhibit cellular growth is not clear; an important mechanism may be interference or alteration at the cell membrane.

Estrogen receptor assays are now routinely done at the time of mastectomy for breast cancer. This technique has made it possible to evaluate the ability of a breast tumor to bind estrogen and thus project the probable sensitivity of the tumor to hormonal therapy.

Combination chemotherapy

Increased knowledge of how specific cytotoxic drugs exert their effect and of the potential for the emergence of tumor cells resistant to a specific therapy, similar to antibiotic resistance, has led to the use of combination chemotherapy. Combination chemotherapy demonstrates a therapeutic effect superior to a single agent therapy for many cancers. Drugs considered for combination chemotherapy are those that (1) are active when used alone, (2) have different mechanisms of action, (3) have a biochemical basis for possible synergism, (4) do not produce toxicity in the same organs, and (5) produce toxicity at different times after administration.[44] Repeated brief courses of drug therapy are given to reduce immunosuppressive effects.

Dose calculations

The dosage range for a particular drug is determined at the time of clinical trial and regimen development. Given these guidelines, the dosage for a specific individual must be calculated before starting therapy. Although some regimens may still prescribe milligrams per kilogram, drug doses are usually stated in terms of body surface area, and therefore, the doses are given in milligrams per square meter (sqm).[41] An individual's height and weight are used to determine body surface, therefore it is very important that height and weight be measured *accurately.*

Methods of administration of chemotherapeutic agents

The route of administration is based on the metabolism and absorption of a given drug. The route of choice is that which will deliver the optimal amount of drug to the tumor. Chemotherapeutic agents are given orally, intravenously, intramuscularly, intraarterially, and by local instillation (that is; intrapleurally and intrathecally). If tumor cells are in an area that drugs cannot reach, cancer cells will survive with a consequent increase in disease recurrence. An example is the sanctuary effect afforded leukemic cells by the meninges in patients with acute lymphocytic leukemia. For this reason, local instillation of chemotherapy via an Ommaya cerebrospinal reservoir or intrathecally (directly into the spinal fluid by lumbar puncture) is used to treat tumor cells present in the CNS.

Before administering a cytotoxic drug, the clinician consults a reference for usual dosage, acceptable routes of administration, and any precautions that should be taken for that particular drug. Since protocols may deviate from drug manufacturers' guidelines, discussion with the prescribing physician may also be indicated.

Oral administration

Many cytotoxic drugs are given in pill form. Since these may be prescribed on a daily basis to be taken at home, careful instructions need to be given to patients. Areas to be discussed include the importance of taking the drug as prescribed, the relationship to meals, fluid intake, and the use of an antiemetic.

Intravenous administration

The clinician must know specific properties for each drug to be administered. Of particular importance is the identification of those drugs that are vesicant (produce blisters). If infiltration and extravasation occur, extensive tissue damage and necrosis may result. Nitrogen mustard, doxorubicin (Adriamycin), vincristine, and vinblastine are the principal vesicant drugs. The intravenous site is evaluated before the administration of these drugs. If *any* suspicion of an infiltration or leak exists, the site is changed. Most often, vesicant drugs are given via the side arm of a running IV. If extravasation occurs, immediate action is taken to minimize damage. Guidelines vary but may include the administration of methylprednisolone (Solu-Medrol) or sodium bicarbonate to the area of infiltration and the intermittent application of ice for a 24-hour period.

For patients with poor venous access, an indwelling Hickman catheter (Fig. 14-7) may be used for chemotherapy administration.[8,16] Aside from the daily care of dressing changes to the insertion site and the flushing of the line with a heparin solution, the presence of the catheter requires little attention by the patient.

Perfusion

Regional and isolation perfusion is a means of delivering a high dosage of a drug directly to a tumor. This is accomplished by the placement of a catheter into an artery that provides the blood supply to the area being treated. By this method, a high percentage of the drug is delivered because it is not diluted in the general circulation.

Fig. 14-7. Placement of a Hickman catheter through chest incision between right nipple and sternum through cephalic vein into superior vena cava at entrance to right atrium.

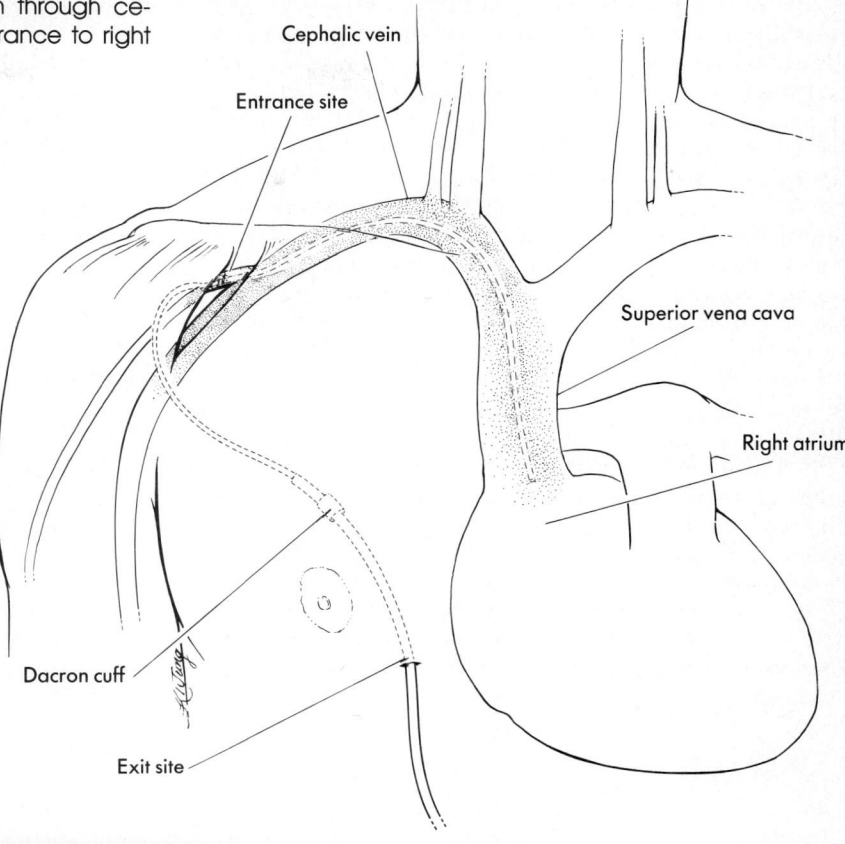

Cephalic vein

Entrance site

Superior vena cava

Right atrium

Dacron cuff

Exit site

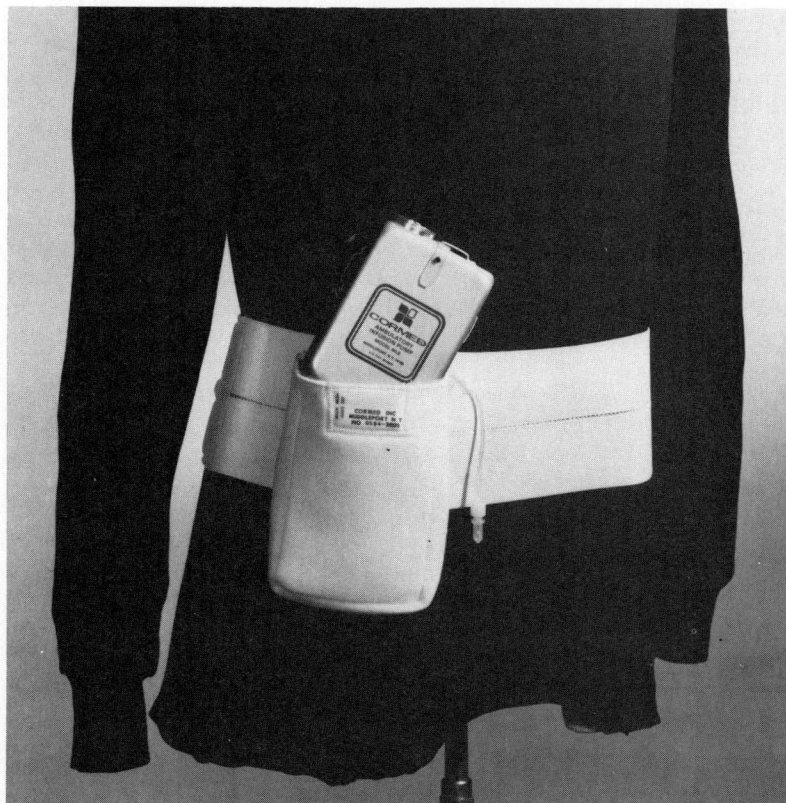

Fig. 14-8. Lightweight, battery-operated infusion pump for ambulatory patient. Flow rate is adjustable. Power pack operates for 7 days before needing recharging. (Courtesy CORMED, Inc., Middleport, N.Y.)

Intraarterial perfusion is used occasionally for cancers of the head and neck and of the liver, and as adjuvant chemotherapy with radiotherapy for advanced cancer of the cervix. Because infusions may be continuous for long periods of time (several hours to days), the patient may be restricted in activity. However, intraarterial perfusion can be accomplished in ambulatory patients by means of a portable infusion pump (Fig. 14-8). Aspects of nursing care include assessment of the catheter insertion site, care of the line to maintain placement and prevent infection, and observation for bleeding. Outpatients need careful and detailed instruction so that these same criteria can be maintained in the home. Hospital nurses involved in the discharge planning of such patients need to ensure that the community-based nurse also be informed of these details.

Side effects and nursing intervention

Some degree of injury to normal cells often occurs with treatment by chemotherapeutic agents. The basis for normal cells being affected is their rate of proliferation. Many normal tissues have a high proliferation capacity, in some instances exceeding that of malignant disease. It is these rapidly proliferating tissues (the bone marrow, gastrointestinal epithelium, and hair follicles) that bear the brunt of the toxic effects of many of the cytotoxic drugs.

Bone marrow suppression

Recognition of the bone marrow suppressive (myelosuppressive) potential of the chemotherapeutic agents is critical to the care of patients receiving chemotherapy. It is the major life-threatening toxicity associated with chemotherapy. Frequent blood counts are done to monitor this toxicity, and astute attention must be given to the results of the white blood count, platelet count, and hemoglobin, with appropriate modification of drug dosage. Patients who have received previous chemotherapy or radiation therapy, particularly to areas of bone marrow reserve (sternum, hips, or pelvis) may have an increased sensitivity to myelosuppression. Blood counts are done before the administration of chemotherapy and at regular intervals to assess the predictable lowest point, which varies with the drugs used. Nursing care of patients with neutropenia, thrombocytonpenia, and anemia are discussed in Chapter 28.

Infection

The prevention of infection is of utmost importance in the care and teaching of the cancer patient. Body areas with high potential for infection should be inspected daily. The *skin and mucous membranes,* especially the mouth, axillae, and perineal areas, are infection prone. Assessment of the *respiratory tract* is also important to identify early signs of respiratory infection. Patients are susceptible to middle-ear infections, sinusitis, and pharyngitis. Pneumonia is especially prevalent in patients with leukemia and in elderly persons. Families of patients are instructed not to visit if they have colds.

Injections are usually avoided. Aseptic technique must be scrupulously maintained during intravenous infusions and dressing changes. In preventing all types of infection, good medical asepsis and especially careful hand washing by the medical and nursing staff are important.

USE OF PATIENT ISOLATION. If the white blood count is low, reverse isolation may be ordered to prevent infection. Reverse isolation is not usually effective unless life islands or laminar airflow units are used. The *life island* consists of a special large plastic canopy placed around and over the patient's bed. All equipment is sterilized and the air is filtered to remove airborne bacteria. Objects are passed in and out through locks irradiated by ultraviolet light. Patient contact is through arm-length gloves built into the side of the canopy.

Laminar airflow units are rooms that have a constant flow of purified air flowing across the width and breadth of the room (Fig. 14-9). Anyone in the room remains downstream from the patient. If the patient must be touched, a mask, cap, and gown are worn. The advantage of the laminar airflow room is that it is large and allows more freedom of movement than the life island.

One problem with any type of isolation is that the patient may experience sensory deprivation and social isolation. In addition, when reverse isolation is terminated, the patient may feel unsafe, vulnerable, and angry because of removal from the protected environment.

Gastrointestinal effects

Changes in bowel habits commonly occur but usually do not require intervention. If diarrhea becomes marked or persists, an antidiarrheal medication such as diphenoxylate with atropine (Lomotil) may be prescribed. Persons receiving vincristine are assessed for signs of paralytic ileus and are instructed to report constipation.

Stomatitis, an inflammation of the mucous membranes of the oral cavity, may range from an erythema of the oral mucosa to mild or severe ulceration. Methotrexate, 5-fluorouracil, doxorubicin, dactinomycin, and bleomycin are the chemotherapeutic drugs most frequently associated with stomatitis. Patients may also develop a superimposed *Candida* infection of the mouth and esophagus, and oral nystatin is usually prescribed. Good mouth care is encouraged.

NAUSEA AND VOMITING. Nausea and vomiting are among the most uncomfortable and distressing side effects of chemotherapy. For the ambulatory patient, nausea may interfere with the ability to continue daily work. Persistent vomiting may result in fluid and electrolyte imbalance, general weakness, and weight loss. Decline of nutritional status renders the patient more susceptible to infection and perhaps less able to tolerate therapy. Such physiologic symptoms can accompany or precipitate psychologic responses that might include depression and withdrawal. Every effort must be made to minimize chemotherapy-induced nausea and vomiting. The onset and duration vary greatly among patients and with the drug given.

Antiemetics vary in success. Tetrahydrocannibinol

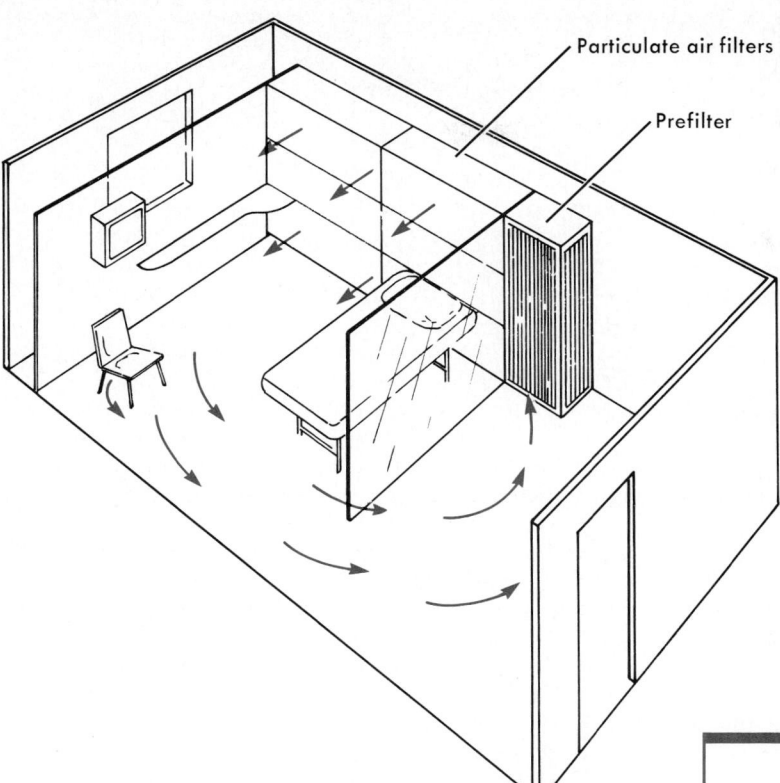

Particulate air filters

Prefilter

Fig. 14-9. In laminar airflow units constant flow of purified air flows across width and breadth of room. (From American Cancer Society: Proceedings of the National Conference on Cancer Nursing, New York, 1973, The Society.)

(THC) taken in pill form produces an antiemetic effect in some patients who have not benefited from the commonly prescribed prochlorperazine (Compazine). Timing of food and fluid intake in relation to treatment is often ascertained by the patient, as are the types of foods that are best tolerated. Relaxation techniques are useful for some patients.

Alopecia

Alopecia (loss of hair) may occur by two mechanisms. If the hair roots are atrophied, alopecia occurs readily. The hair either falls out spontaneously or by hair combing, often in large clumps. If the hair shaft is constricted because of atrophy or necrosis, the hair will break off very near the scalp. The root remains in the scalp and a patchy, thinning pattern of hair loss occurs.[41] Hair loss may occur on other parts of the body in addition to the scalp. Loss of leg, arm, and facial hair is seen less often, although loss of eyebrows and eyelashes may occur.

The pattern and extent of hair loss cannot be accurately predicted for a given patient. When the treatment is given with a drug known to cause alopecia, the patient needs to be told that severe hair loss can begin within a few days or weeks of treatment and that partial or complete baldness can quickly ensue. *Drug-induced alopecia is never permanent.* Occasionally, hair growth may return while chemotherapy treatment continues. Given this perspective, coupled with the goal of disease control or cure, most patients tolerate the hair loss with minimal distress, although it is common and normal that some feelings are expressed about the hair loss.

Drugs commonly causing alopecia

Bleomycin	ICRF-159
Cyclophosphamide	Hydroxyurea
Dactinomycin	Mitomycin
Daunomycin hydrochloride	VP-16-213
Doxorubicin hydrochloride	Vinblastine
5-Fluorouracil	Vincristine

From Knopf, M., et al.: Cancer chemotherapy treatment and care, New Haven, Conn., 1979, Yale Comprehensive Cancer Center.

Drugs not causing alopecia

5-Azacytidine	Melphalan
Busulfan	Mercaptopurine
Carmustine	Mithramycin
Chlorambucil	Nitrogen mustard
Cis-platinum	Procarbazine
Cytarabine	Semustine
Dacarbazine	Streptozotocin
Ftorafur	Triazinate
Hexamethylmelamine	Zinostatin
Lomustine	

From Knopf, M., et al.: Cancer chemotherapy treatment and care, New Haven, Conn. 1979, Yale Comprehensive Cancer Center.

Nursing care of patients receiving chemotherapy

Bone marrow suppression or infection

1. Check blood counts
2. Assess infection-prone areas daily to identify early signs of infection
3. Maintain medical asepsis through careful handwashing
4. Maintain intact skin and mucous membranes
   a. Teach avoidance of bumping and breaking skin
   b. Maintain aseptic technique during IV infusion and dressing changes
   c. Keep fingernails short
   d. Teach good perineal hygiene
   e. Teach avoidance of excessive friction and importance of vaginal lubrication
   f. Teach avoidance of anal intercourse
   g. No enemas, rectal medications, or rectal thermometers
   h. Encourage fastidious oral hygiene with a soft toothbrush
   i. Inspect mouth daily for ulcers and white patches
   j. Use lubricants to prevent drying and cracking of lips
5. Maintain optimal respiratory function
   a. Assess for early signs of respiratory infection
   b. Instruct family/friends not to visit if they have colds
6. Maintain reverse isolation if ordered

Gastrointestinal effects: stomatitis, nausea, vomiting

1. Administer oral nystatin, as ordered
2. Use a rinse and lidocaine before meals to lubricate and provide an analgesic effect
3. Use a cleansing rinse of plain water or dilute hydrogen peroxide after meals
4. Administer antiemetic as ordered
5. Determine from patient best time for food and fluid intake in relation to treatment
6. Teach relaxation techniques and imagery, if appropriate

Alopecia

1. Explain that drug-induced alopecia is not permanent
2. Allow expression of feelings about hair loss
3. Scalp tourniquets or scalp hypothermia via ice pack may be ordered to minimize hair loss with some agents (for example, vincristine, adriamycin)

Effects on skin

Inspect administration site for signs of infiltration or extravasation

Organ toxicities

1. Assess signs and symptoms of liver dysfunction (see Chapter 31)
2. Monitor cardiac status (arrhythmias, congestive heart failure) (see Chapter 26)
3. Assess signs and symptoms of pulmonary toxicity (see Chapter 25)

Urinary effects: hemorrhagic cystitis, renal toxicity

1. Maintain hydration by encouraging drinking of large amounts of fluid (if receiving cyclophosphamide)
2. Monitor renal function: check serum creatinine or creatinine clearance (with cisplatin or streptozotocin)

Sterility

1. Assess knowledge of known and possible effects on fertility
2. Provide birth control and reproductive counseling, as appropriate

Effects on skin

Vesicant drugs may cause severe tissue necrosis if infiltration should occur. Other skin reactions that might occur are hyperpigmentation, nail changes, and an increased sensitivity to the sun (photosensitivity).

Organ toxicities

Liver toxicity is uncommon but may occur. There may be a transient increase in liver enzymes. Alteration in liver function has been associated with Ara-C, methotrexate, and 6-mercaptopurine. *Cardiac* status is carefully monitored in patients receiving doxorubicin. A baseline echocardiogram is usually done before beginning treatment and at regular intervals while therapy continues. Two forms of cardiac damage may occur: arrhythmias, most commonly associated with a preexisting cardiac disease, and a delayed moderate to severe congestive heart failure.[44] Other drugs associated with some potential for cardiac toxicity are daunorubicin (Daunomycin) and high-dose cyclophosphamide (Cytoxan). *Pulmonary* toxicity may occur with methotrexate and some of the alkylating agents. The most common cause of chemotherapy-induced pulmonary toxicity is bleomycin. Pulmonary fibrosis can occur and may be irreversible. Each time bleomycin is administered, the pulmonary status of the patient is assessed by auscultation and questioning regarding the presence of cough or shortness of breath.

Urinary effects

Hemorrhagic cystitis occurs in about 10% of patients being treated with cyclophosphamide but rarely occurs with other agents.[38] Patients receiving cyclophosphamide are encouraged to drink a large amount of fluid to minimize this effect. Taking the cyclophosphamide early in the day may also be of some benefit. Renal toxicity is associated with several drugs, but most notably with cisplatin and streptozotocin. Before the administration of each dose of these drugs renal function is evaluated by either a serum creatinine or a 24-hour urine collection for creatinine clearance.

Sterility

Cancer chemotherapy reaches the reproductive organs at dose levels similar to those achieved at the site of the target tumor. The potential exists for a disruptive effect on genetic and fetal development.[56] It is recognized that chemotherapy, particularly some of the alkylating agents, may cause transient or permanent sterility. Patients on chemotherapy need to be informed of the known and possible effects on fertility. Birth control and reproductive counseling need to be factors included in patient teaching. If a nurse does not feel comfortable or qualified to discuss the topic, resources useful to the patient and spouse should be identified. Sperm banking before the initiation of therapy offers male patients the option of future conception. Following completion of chemotherapy, conception and the birth of normal, healthy children are possibilities for couples. It is customary to recommend that procreation be avoided until at least 18 months after completion of treatment.

IMMUNOTHERAPY

Pathophysiology

The role of immunotherapy in the prevention and treatment of cancer is being studied. Many scientists believe cancer occurs in the body more frequently than once in a lifetime; however, in most cases clinical evidence of the disease is not apparent. It is postulated that there is a natural immunity against the development of the disease and that cancer cells are destroyed almost as quickly as they develop.[93] Studies of cancer show that when the normal cell becomes malignant, it often undergoes biochemical changes resulting in formation of new cellular antigens that cause an immune response. Clinical malignancy may occur as a result of failure in the immunologic surveillance system of the body.

The immune response has two major components. The first, or *cellular immune response* (see Chapter 6), produces lymphocytes capable of destroying tumor cells on contact. These lymphocytes (T cells) undergo division and are released into the bloodstream when stimulated by an antigen. In addition to destroying cancer cells on contact, T cells may release cytotoxins, which cause holes in the cell membrane, eventually resulting in lysis or death of the malignant cell.

The second component of the immune response is *antibody production* resulting from activation of lymphocytes (B cells). When stimulated by antigens, B cells proliferate and differentiate into plasma cells, which are the major source of antibody production.

Approaches used in immunotherapy

There are three major approaches to immunotherapy for cancer: nonspecific immunotherapy, specific immunotherapy, and transfer of tumor immunity (Table 14-10). The ultimate goal of immunotherapy is to immunize patients effectively against their own tumors. A perhaps more utopian goal is prophylactic immunization.

At the present time, the immune response can handle only a limited number of tumor cells, up to 10 million. After a growth to 100 million cells, the immune response is not capable of preventing further growth. Once the cancer is large, it cannot be totally controlled by the immune system, so immunotherapy cannot be the primary mode of cancer therapy at the present time. It is used after surgery, radiotherapy, and chemotherapy have removed the bulk of the tumor.

Much is yet to be learned about the immunology of cancers. The number of cancers once thought to be immunogenic and responsive to immunotherapy is less than originally supposed. If cancer vaccines are developed, they will be effective in tumors caused by viruses, and these are probably limited in number. Even if a cancer-carrying virus is isolated, it must be attenuated so it can be given safely.

Complications of immunotherapy

Some complications of immunotherapy may occur. Intratumor injection of bacillus Calmette Guérin (BCG) vaccine has resulted in fever, chills, localized abcesses,

Table 14-10. Approaches used in immunotherapy

Type of approach	Method	Substance used
Nonspecific immunotherapy	Use of substances that increase the general immune capacity of the host	Bacillus Calmette Guérin *Corynebacterium parvum*
Specific immunotherapy	Use of substances antigenically related to the tumor or its products	1. Killed tumor cells from patient or patient with similar tumor 2. Altered tumor cells (more immunogenic) 3. Antigen extracted from tumor cells
Transfer of tumor immunity	Use of specific immune substances	1. Lymphocytes from another tumor patient 2. Immune RNA 3. Transfer factor

and draining sinuses. Regional lymphadenitis, systemic infections, anaphylactic reactions, malaise, and influenza-like reactions may also occur. There has been some evidence of liver dysfunction, although the incidence is low.

Interferons

Interferons are a family of secretory glycoproteins produced by leukocytes in response to viral infections or to other stimuli. Interferons induce cellular resistance to a broad spectrum of viruses and are a first line of defense against viral infections. In addition, they may protect against intracellular parasites, neoplastic changes in cells, and the tumor growth itself. They appear to have an inhibitory effect on DNA synthesis and cell growth and may suppress the tumor directly.[54]

All nucleated cells are capable of interferon production, which can be induced by many natural and synthetic agents. Exogenous interferon is induced in cells that are either propagated or maintained in cultures, secreted into the culture medium, concentrated, and purified to give a preparation that can be injected. The cost of large-scale production of interferon has hampered its use for therapy. Biologically active synthetic interferon has been manufactured by gene-cloning technique, which may reduce the high cost of treatment.

Interferon's antitumor effect develops from its ability to augment natural killer (NK) cell activity, which is the spontaneous killing of tumor cells by lymphocytes from an animal or person not previously sensitized by tumor cells. Interferon appears to convert inactive lymphocytes into cytotoxic NK cells. Second, it enhances cytotoxicity of monocytes and of antibody-related mechanisms. In addition, human cancer patients have decreased amounts of NK activity, and in most patients this is enhanced for a short time by administration of BCG, which stimulates interferon production.[3]

Leukocyte interferon given systemically results in little or no toxicity. Some patients who have responded were resistant to other therapy. At the present time interferon is being used in treatment of melanoma, multiple myeloma, breast carcinoma, prostatic cancer, laryngeal papilloma, and osteogenic sarcoma. Data about final tumor response and possible long-term side effects of interferon are unknown. Precise doses, dose timing, immune effects, and coordination with other types of treatment must be identified before interferon's role in cancer therapy can be delineated.

Nursing intervention for persons receiving interferon therapy include monitoring for side effects: fever, local discomfort at the injection site, and minimal nausea and vomiting. Acetaminophen (Tylenol) is given for discomfort and antiemetics for nausea and vomiting. At some centers nurses teach the patients to give their own intravenous injections.[52] Nurses must be careful not to raise false hopes in patients who may view interferon as a last-resort therapy.

Cancer pain

Pain is one of the most feared effects of cancer, although, contrary to popular belief, it is frequently the last symptom to appear. Even in terminal stages, 60% of persons with cancer will experience mild or no pain. The etiology of cancer pain is complex since it has physical, psychologic, social, and spiritual aspects.

STAGES OF CANCER PAIN

Three stages of cancer pain have been described: early, intermediate, and late. Early pain usually occurs after initial surgery for diagnosis or treatment and usually subsides after the third day; thus this pain is an acute episode, that is, short term and temporary.

Intermediate-stage pain results from postoperative contraction of scars and nerve entrapment or from cancer recurrence or metastasis. This pain may subside or may be controlled by palliative therapy such as radiation, chemotherapy, neurosurgery, and analgesics. Therapy itself may initiate the pain.[67]

Late-stage pain occurs in terminal cancer when therapy no longer controls the disease. This pain is chronic, may slowly increase in intensity, and at times may be intractable. Severe chronic pain occurs in only about 20% of patients who die from cancer.[45]

PATHOPHYSIOLOGY

Malignant neoplasms cause pain by five physiologic changes: bone destruction, obstruction of lumens (viscera or vessels), peripheral nerve involvement, pressure of growing tumors causing ischemia or distention, and inflammation, infection, or necrosis of the tissue.

Bone destruction with infraction (fractures without displacement) is the most frequent cause of pain, usually resulting from metastatic lesions. Bone destruction may cause increased sensitivity over the area or sharp, continuous pain.

Obstruction of a viscus, such as in the gastrointestinal or genitourinary tract, causes severe, colicky, crampy-type pain. Visceral pain is dull, diffuse, and poorly localized. Obstruction of an artery, vein, or lymphatic vessel may initiate arterial ischemia, venous engorgement, or edema. This pain is dull, diffuse, and aching.

Infiltration or compression of peripheral nerves or nerve plexuses causes continuous, sharp or stabbing pain sometimes accompanied by hyperesthesia or paresthesia.

Infiltration or distention of the integument, fascia, or tissue initiates a severe localized pain that is dull and aching, increasing in intensity as tumor size increases. An example of this is the pain resulting from distention of the abdomen by ascites or the stretching of the skin by carcinoma of the neck.

Finally, inflammation, infection, and necrosis of the tissue itself may cause pain by producing either pressure or ischemia. Chemical mediators of pain are present during inflammation and necrosis.

PSYCHOSOCIAL ASPECTS

The psychologic component of cancer pain is associated with the patient's perception of the threat and stress of cancer and varies from individual to individual. Three categories of stressors have been identified: injury or threat of injury as a result of the cancer, loss or threat of loss (body part or death), and frustration of drives as a result of disabilities from the cancer per se or from the effect of therapies. Patients may respond with depression, decreased self-esteem, hostility, and irritability.

The sociologic effects include decreased interaction and participation in activities of daily living. There is decreased productivity characterized by absenteeism from work, economic problems, and deterioration in family relationships. The spiritual effects of pain are evidenced by loss of hope and trust and an overwhelming feeling of despair, rejection, and sense of isolation.

Side effects of cancer pain include fatigue, sleepless-ness, anorexia, and decreased movement followed by the complications of immobility, namely, muscle weakness, decubiti, contractures, and respiratory dysfunction.

INTERVENTION

Medical therapy in early-stage pain focuses on therapy directed at the cancer per se. Late-stage pain is treated symptomatically by analgesia, neurosurgery, and nerve blocks. Surgical procedures to relieve the pain include simple intercostal nerve block where feasible, surgical section of posterior sensory roots adjacent to the spinal cord, and spinothalamic tractotomy (interruption of pain- and temperature-conducting tracts). Dorsal column stimulators and transcutaneous electrical stimulators (see Chapter 12) may be helpful in selected cases.

Cancer pain, as with other types of severe pain, may occupy the patient's entire attention and, unless treated vigorously, may demoralize the patient and interfere with eating, resting, or sleeping. Interventions are directed toward helping the patient live as normal a life as possible and cope with the pain. Pain tolerance is increased when the patient's energy is preserved for enjoyable activities. General comfort measures to promote rest and sleep, good body positioning, and nutrition may do much to increase the patient's pain tolerance. Teaching patients conscious muscle relaxation during which they systematically contract and relax muscle groups throughout the body may decrease pain resulting from muscle tenseness as well as anxiety associated with the pain (see Chapter 12).

Diversionary activities help decrease the patient's perception of the pain by distraction. These activities may be physical (work, walking, rocking, swimming), social, or mental (watching television, reading, crafts). Some patients find imagery (waking-imagined analgesia) helpful. Others may try to separate the pain from their bodies thereby "quieting the mind by letting the body drop away."[67]

Medications

Drugs may be the one significant method that alleviates the pain of cancer. Aspirin is the most effective single analgesic for mild to moderate pain.[45] There is an additive and perhaps synergistic effect between aspirin and codeine; therefore combinations of these drugs are useful in moderate acute pain and in chronic aching pain.

In severe chronic cancer pain the narcotics, with the exception of codeine and oxycodone, are the most effective. Although there are no significant differences among the various drugs in potency or side effects, there are significant differences in the duration of action. Those with long duration of action are preferred for relief of chronic cancer pain. Tolerance and dependence in these drugs are less common with cancer pain than when the narcotics are used for acute pain.[45]

There are three important principles in adminstration of narcotics. The first is that the optimal dose must be determined, and initial pain control may require seemingly large doses of the narcotics. The second principle is to start with a dose that is too high rather than one that is too low since the person may become anxious if there is no analgesia despite analgesic administration. This anxiety may exacerbate the pain. The third and most important principle is that the narcotic must be *administered regularly,* not prn. Each dose must be given before the previous dose loses effect. Prevention of pain recurrence usually requires less analgesia than treatment of pain after it has recurred.

Oral administration is preferred. Parenteral therapy produces higher initial serum and tissue levels of the narcotic, but the oral doses are as effective as parenteral doses in maintaining drug levels in the body. Intramuscular and subcutaneous injections are more difficult to administer and are painful to patients with marked muscle wasting. In addition, parenteral administration may make the patient dependent on others for drug administration.[64]

Analgesic drug "cocktails," such as Brompton's cocktail mixture, have become more widely used. This liquid commonly contains morphine, cocaine, alcohol, syrup, and chloroform water. In countries where it is legal, heroin may be substituted for morphine, although a controlled double blind study has shown morphine to be as effective as heroin. More recently, at St. Christopher's Hospice in London, directed by Dr. Cicely Saunders, simple aqueous solutions of morphine are being used as the primary analgesic. Dr. Saunders, a pioneer in symptomatic care of patients with advanced cancer, no longer advocates use of heroin or Brompton's cocktail over simple narcotic analgesics that are available in the United States.[45]

Phenothiazines are the principal adjunct drug given to control severe chronic cancer pain. They are effective as antiemetics and also have an antianxiety effect.

Nurses provide the psychologic and social support necessary to help the cancer patient cope with severe pain. Administration of analgesics over the 24-hour period and explanations of the physiologic and pharmacologic effects of the drugs can be very helpful to patients and their families (see Chapter 12).

Psychologic support of patient and family

Cancer nursing demands not only caring *for* the patient but also caring *about* the patient, who may be angry, depressed, and perhaps physically unattractive because of the effects of the disease or its treatment. Communication is vital in meeting the needs of the cancer patient and the family. Validating assumptions and assisting patients to describe, clarify, and identify reasons for feelings are important to promote communications. In addition, the nurse must try to make explanations clear and uncomplicated. Getting feedback from the patient is one way to ensure that the message has been received.

NURSING INTERVENTIONS TO HELP THE PATIENT COPE

Since the threat to life and the potential for other losses are great for patients with cancer, they need especially to have their existing coping mechanisms supported or to receive support if coping mechanisms are inadequate to meet their needs.

Each patient's reaction to cancer is unique, so there can be no easy formula for care. The nurse must be able to work with and accept patient's behavior and coping style. Avoidance of false reassurance and pat answers that block communication will contribute to patient comfort. Openness, honesty, and creativity of the nurse are essential. The nurse reinforces patients' hope but is careful to avoid giving false hope, which can be more devastating than none at all. At times patients may need to deny their illness, while at other times they may want to talk about it.

Trusting patients' resilience and their will to try and helping them live as fully as possible are all appropriate interventions. When patients complain, perhaps the best response is, "Tell me how you feel. Perhaps we can do something about it." Self-esteem is maintained by fostering patients' independence, even if this only involves taking part in decision making about the care to be given.

Persons working with these patients must have confidence in themselves and the ability to suspend their own concerns, needs, and desires to concentrate on patients' problems. To do this one must be able to tolerate a high level of anxiety and to look at problems on both a feeling (affective) and a thinking (cognitive) level.

Listening carefully and attentively to concerns of patients helps to calm fears. In addition, nurses who are knowledgeable about cancer, who can answer questions and clear up misconceptions, help promote the patient's psychologic well-being.

NURSING INTERVENTIONS TO HELP THE FAMILY COPE

The interventions that help the patient cope are also important in helping the family cope. The nurse must get to know them and their reactions. They may feel guilty, helpless, and angry, just as the patient does. Letting them know that their feelings are normal may increase their comfort. Families should not be pushed into responsibilities that they cannot handle. Some want to participate in care, others are overwhelmed by the disease and are afraid to or may not want to help. Their feelings need to be respected.

Teaching the family is a major responsibility. They should be reminded not to cut the patient off from family activities and concerns. If possible, the patient should be included in family decision making and planning. In their desire to help their loved ones, families may unintentionally contribute to the patient's sense of isolation by shielding him or her from family concerns.

INTERDISCIPLINARY APPROACH TO CARE

The skills of many members of the health team may be required to meet the needs of the cancer patient. Clear, concise communication of ideas about care and the planned interventions is essential for coordination, continuity, and integration of care. Team conferences are helpful in promoting the sharing of expertise. The social worker, occupational therapist, minister, and psychologist may all be needed to contribute to the patient's well-being. The nurse, who spends the most time with the patient, may be the first to recognize that the patient and family could benefit from the services of health team members.

Rehabilitation of the cancer patient to an optimal level of functioning through the efforts of many health team members results in a more satisfying life for the patient and the family. Often the community health nurse is called on to give care, teach, counsel, and support the patient and family after discharge.

Supportive care of the patient with cancer that is terminal

PLANNING CARE

When all possible surgery and maximal radiation therapy have failed to control the spread of cancer, the patient and family have many special problems. They need encouragement and help in living as normally as possible, in planning for the late stages of the patient's illness, and in adjusting to death and its implications for the family.

Before nurses can help the patient and family, they must have developed a mature philosophy that allows acceptance of death as an eventual reality for everyone. This philosophy is not acquired overnight. The nurse needs the opportunity to discuss feelings about caring for the patient whose death is imminent, since the nurse's attitude toward death and suffering will affect the ability to plan and give care to the patient with advanced cancer. (See Chapter 16 for discussion of death and dying.)

No one can say with certainty when death will come. The patient may ask about the length of time remaining, but no absolute answer can be given. Physicians may have made a statement to the patient about life expectancy. The nursing staff should know what the patient has been told, since the patient's willingness to participate in self-care and attitude toward the illness may be influenced by perception of life expectancy.

Planning, doing, and achieving are the best way to prevent the hopelessness and despair that may overwhelm the patient. Every effort must be put forth to meet the patient's physiologic needs so that higher order psychologic needs may be expressed. The patient who is in pain or feels "dirty" will have difficulty expressing concerns and fears.

Other factors to consider in planning care are the personality of the patient, feelings about death and illness, and the reactions of those significant others whose opinion the patient values. The goal of nursing care should be to relieve physical, mental, and spiritual distress. The most common nursing diagnoses for the patient with cancer that is terminal are listed in box below.

PLANNING FOR HOME CARE

At least half of all deaths from cancer occur in the patients' homes. Planning for home care of the patient without completely disrupting the rest of the family takes the concerted efforts of many people. Patients must always be consulted, and their wishes should be respected in the early stages of the disease. In the final stages they may be too ill to be bothered or concerned with making decisions. The physician, the social worker, and the nurse must work together with the local community agencies, such as the American Cancer Society, to ensure continuity of care from the hospital to the home. The principles governing suitability for home care are similar to those for any patient receiving home care, although the patient with cancer may not live as long as many others with chronic long-term illnesses. Medical and nursing supervision must be available; it must be possible for required care to be given; both patient and family must want the patient home; and home facilities must be suitable. Rehabilitation teams may also be sent into the home to help the patient and family.

The growth of the *hospice* concept, a place where patients may come for short or long periods for nursing care and then return to their homes as their condition warrants, is exciting. The hospice tries to maintain a homelike setting while

---

Nursing diagnoses for the patient with cancer that is terminal

Bowel elimination, alterations in: constipation
Comfort, alterations in: pain
Family processes, alterations in
Fear (specify)
Grieving (specify)
    Anticipatory
    Dysfunctional
Nutrition, alterations in: less than body requirements
Oral mucous membranes, alterations in
Powerlessness
Respiratory function, alterations in: airway clearance
Self-care defect: bathing/hygiene
Skin integrity, impairment of
Social isolation

relieving the family of the emotional and physical burden of constant care. Hospice programs provide medical, social, and psychologic support for patients and their families so that dying can be truly dignified.

The hospice concept may also be implemented by home care for the patient with the inpatient facility as a backup for home care. If a family wishes to go away on a trip, for example, the patient may request to stay in the hospice. The ultimate goal of the hospice is for the family to develop its ability to give care; thus the relationship of the hospice to the family becomes primarily one of consultation and referral. The family is aided in remaining the patient's primary support system.

Hospice staff are multidisciplinary and are employed and evaluated based on their interests and abilities to care for the terminally ill person. The focus of activities is care rather than cure, with an emphasis on symptom control. Actions are identified to help the patient and family deal with their chief concerns.

NURSING INTERVENTION TO MEET PSYCHOLOGIC NEEDS OF PATIENTS WITH ADVANCED STAGES OF CANCER

Avoiding false hope

Occasionally, there is a mistake in diagnosis or the disease is in some way arrested for a long time. If the patient assumes that one of these occurrences may take place, the nurse should not suggest facing probable reality. The nurse must, however, avoid encouraging false hopes. Many patients accept their prognosis philosophically, with the hope that a cure for cancer will be found before their disease is far advanced. Some patients are better able to accept the situation if their religious faith can be strengthened. Some patients and their families find it helpful to live each day as fully as possible without looking too far ahead. Sometimes patients with cancer have few symptoms and are able to carry on quite well until shortly before death.

Nurses also must be careful that they do not experience false hope. The inability to fulfill the hope to sustain life may make it more difficult for nurses to accept the patient's death and they may see themselves as having failed.[23]

Encouraging social and vocational activities

Patients with advanced cancer should resume their regular work if they can possibly do so, for work makes them feel as though they are still an active part of their group and worthy of the approval of others. It was said many centuries ago that employment is a person's best physician, and this concept applies particularly to persons whose existence is seriously threatened by cancer. Social activities and all experiences associated with normal family life should be continued whenever possible. There is probably no greater service the nurse can give to patients with uncontrollable cancer than to help them continue their everyday lives in any way possible. Family members often need guidance in seeing the patient's need to live as

normally as possible. Sometimes the patient appears almost unduly concerned with the details of some aspect of the immediate treatment and almost oblivious to the entire problem. Such a patient senses that success with the immediate treatment is the only way to remain up and about or to carry on at that time.

Decreasing fear of helplessness

Patients may be haunted by fear of brain involvement, loss of mental faculties, and the possibility that they may become completely helpless and dependent on others. By these fears they express a basic human wish: the wish to leave the world with as much dignity as possible. The nurse should urge the patient and family to discuss such fears with the physician. The patient may feel that the physician is too busy and that questions are too trivial to justify the use of the physician's time. Some questions, however, are not trivial at all, and a satisfactory answer to them adds tremendously to the patient's peace of mind. Metastasis to the brain in persons who have other metastases is somewhat rare, and some patients suffer more from fear of damage to the brain than is justified. The patient should know that good general hygiene, good nutrition, being up and about for part of each day, and doing deep-breathing exercises with attention to posture all help to prevent helplessness. A positive approach to all problems certainly shortens the time of helplessness and makes the patient more content.

NURSING INTERVENTIONS TO MEET PHYSIOLOGIC NEEDS OF PATIENTS WITH ADVANCED STAGES OF CANCER

Increasing comfort

Giving good nursing care to the patient with advanced cancer is challenging. Promoting the patient's comfort should be high on the list of goals. Nursing measures that increase rest and sleep and reduce pain will help maintain the patient's physical and psychologic well-being.

Maintaining nutrition

Cachexia is a frequent problem. Anorexia may accompany therapy, and the increased protein needs of the body resulting from tumor growth may be difficult to meet. Mealtimes should be incorporated with family visiting, or patients can eat together if possible. A high-protein diet enhances the response from therapy, and an adequate intake of calories spares protein for cell building. Because chewing may be difficult, food should be cut in small pieces and creamed or combined with cooked vegetables, rice, or noodles. Meat may also be ground or used as a base for soups or stews. Fish, cottage cheese, and eggs are also good sources of protein.

Intravenous hyperalimentation (total parenteral nutrition [TPN]) may be used as an adjunct to therapy. Studies have found that this did not stimulate tumor growth and that it often resulted in a return of immune system competence, a decrease in sepsis, wound healing, and an increase in response to chemotherapy.[15]

Maintaining elimination

Diarrhea may be a problem, but constipation is more likely. If the patient is receiving narcotics, especially opium derivatives, peristalsis is decreased. Patients receiving the plant alkaloid vincristine (Oncovin) may develop neurotoxicity, causing a high fecal impaction. Increasing the intake of roughage and fluids in the diet, maintaining activity, and using stool softeners may be helpful. Enemas and laxatives may be necessary.

Maintaining personal hygiene

Careful and meticulous hygiene is essential. Careful bathing and attention to skin, hair, and clothing will all promote self-esteem in the patient. Odors from body exudates, draining wounds, and incontinence may occur. Soiled dressings and bed linen are changed immediately. Judicious use of deodorizers is helpful, but deodorizers do not take the place of good hygiene.

Preventing the effects of immobility

Pressure sores may be a severe problem. The combination of inactivity, poor nutrition, and incontinence seen in patients with advanced cancer predisposes them to skin breakdown. Maintaining the patient's activity by getting him or her out of bed as much as possible will prevent pressure and also promote the patient's joint mobility and muscle strength.

Teaching the patient and family

The nurse is involved in teaching during most interactions with the patient and family. Careful explanations about care and sensitivity to what the patient thinks and feels about the disease contribute to the nurse's effectiveness in promoting change in the patient's behavior. When possible, self-care activities should be emphasized. Maintaining the patient's independence whenever possible should be the goal while recognizing that the time may come when dependence is necessary.

REFERENCES AND SELECTED READINGS*

1. American Cancer Society: 1983 Cancer facts and figures, New York, 1981, The Society.
2. American Cancer Society: A cancer source book for nurses, New York, 1975, The Society.
3. At year's end: what's new with interferon, JAMA **242:**2829-2830, 1979.
4. Baird, S.B.: Economic realities in the treatment and care of the cancer patient, Top. Clin. Nurs. **2:**67-80, 1981.
5. Barlock, A., Howser, D., and Hubbard, S.: Nursing management of adriamycin extravasation, Am. J. Nurs. **79:**94-96, 1979.
6. *Bersani, G., and Carl, W.: Oral care for cancer patients, Am. J. Nurs. **83:**533-536, 1983.
7. *Bjeletich, J., and Hickman, R.: The Hickman indwelling catheter, Am. J. Nurs. **80:**62-65, 1980.
8. Blumberg, F., Flaherty, M., and Lewis, J.: Cancer in the adult. In Coping with cancer, Bethesda, Md., 1980, National Cancer Institute.
9. Bouchard-Kurtz, R.E., and Speese-Owens, N.F.: Nursing care of the cancer patient, ed. 4, St. Louis, 1981, The C.V. Mosby Co.
10. Buckingham, R.: Hospice care in the United States: the process begins, Omega **13:**159-171, 1982.
11. *Bullough, B.: Nurses are teachers and support persons for breast cancer patients, Cancer Nurs. **4:**221-225, 1982.
12. *Buehler, J.A.: What contributes to hope in the cancer patient, Am. J. Nurs. **75:**1353-1356, 1975.
13. Cairns, J.: The cancer problem, Sci. Amer. **233:**64-69, 1975.
14. Carpenito, L.J.: Nursing diagnosis: application to clinical practice, Philadelphia, 1983, J.B. Lippincott Co.
15. Copeland, E.N., Van Eys, J., and Shils, M.: Nutrition and cancer, New York, 1978, American Cancer Society.
16. Crowley, M., and Baker, M.: Preparing nurses for Hickman catheter care: a self-learning module, Oncol. Nurs. Forum **7**(4):17-19, 1980.
17. *Daeffler, R.: Oral hygiene measures for patients with cancer, Cancer Nurs. **3:**347-355, 1980.
18. Daniels, F.J.: Sunlight. In Schottenfeld, D.: Cancer epidemiology and prevention, Springfield, Ill., 1975, Charles C Thomas, Publisher.
19. DeVita, V., Jr., Hellman, S., and Rosenberg, S.A.: Cancer principles and practice of oncology, Philadelphia, 1981, J.B. Lippincott Co.
20. Donovan, M.I., and Pierce, S.G.: Cancer care nursing, New York, 1976, Appleton-Century-Crofts.
21. Drasga, R.E., Einhorn, L.H., and Williams, S.D.: The chemotherapy of testicular cancer, CA **32:**66-77, 1982.
22. Drugs and dosages: interferon, Occup. Health Nurs. **8**(5):47-51, 1980.
23. *Duncan, S., and Rodney, P.: Hope: a negative force, Can. Nurs. **74**(11):22-23, 1978.
24. Fagin, C., and Dubin, L.: Causes of cancer, Cancer Nurs. **2:**435-441, 1979.

---

*References preceded by an asterisk are particularly well suited for student reading.

25. Fisher, B., et al.: Ten year follow-up of patients with carcinoma of the breast, Surg. Gynecol. Obstet. **140:**528-534, 1975.

26. Fortner, J., and Pahnke, L.: A new method for long-term intrahepatic chemotherapy, Surg. Gynecol. Obstet. **143:** 979-980, 1976.

27. Golden, S., et al.: Chemotherapy and you: a guide to self-help during treatment, NIH pub. no. 80-1136, Washington, D.C., 1978, National Institute of Health.

28. Goodman, L., and Gilman, A.: Pharmacological basis of therapeutics, ed. 6, New York, 1980, Macmillan Publishing Co., Inc.

29. Greenfield, L.D., and Herman, M.W.: Radiation safety precautions with ^{131}Iodine therapy, Cancer Nurs. **1:**379-384, 1978.

30. *Groer, M., and Pierce, M.: Guarding against cancer's hidden killer: anorexia-cachexia, Nurs. 81 **11**(6):39-43, 1981.

31. Guidelines for the cancer-related check-up, CA **30:**195-196, 1980.

32. Haskell, C.: Cancer treatment, Philadelphia, 1980. W.B. Saunders Co.

33. Herrman, C.S.: Immunology: the method to our madness, Cancer Nurs. **2:**359-363, 1979.

34. Higginson, J., Terracini, B., and Agthe, C.: Nutrition and cancer: ingestion of foodborne carcinogens. In Schottenfield, D.: Cancer epidemiology and prevention, Springfield, Ill., 1975, Charles C. Thomas, Publisher.

35. *Hogan, R.: Human sexuality: a nursing perspective, New York, 1980, Appleton-Century-Crofts.

36. Holland, J.: Understanding the cancer patient, CA **30:**135-139, 1980.

37. Horton, J., and Hill, G.J.: Clinical oncology, Philadelphia, 1977, W.B. Saunders Co.

38. Kaempfle, S.: The effects of cancer chemotherapy on reproduction: a review of the literature, Oncol. Nurs. Forum **8:**11-18, 1981.

39. *Kelly, P.P., and Tinsley, C.: Planning care for the patient receiving external radiation, Am. J. Nurs. **81:**338-342, 1981.

40. Kennedy, M., et al.: Chemotherapy related nausea and vomiting: a survey to identify problems and interventions, Oncol. Nurs. Forum **8:**19-22, 1981.

41. Knopf, M., et al.: Cancer chemotherapy treatment and care, New Haven, Conn., 1979, Yale Comprehensive Cancer Center.

42. Knudson, A.G.: Genetic differences in human tumors. In Becker, F.F.: Cancer: a comprehensive treatise, New York, 1977, American Cancer Society.

43. *Koren, M.D.: Cancer immunotherapy: what, why, when, how? Nurs. 81 **11**(1):34-41, 1981.

44. Krakoff, I.: Cancer chemotherapeutic agents, New York, 1977, American Cancer Society.

45. Krim, M.: Toward tumor therapy with interferons. I. Interferons's production and properties, Blood **55:**711-721, 1980.

46. Krim, M.: Toward tumor therapy with interferons. II. Interferons's in vivo effects, Blood **56:**875-882, 1980.

47. *Kripman, A.G.: Drug therapy and cancer pain, Cancer Nurs. **3:**39-46, 1980.

48. LaFortune, S., and Gloriant, F.S.: Nursing diagnoses in cancer chemotherapy: in theory and practice, Am. J. Nurs. **81:**2013-2022, 1981.

49. Lippsett, M.B.: Interaction of drugs, hormones, and nutrition in the causes of cancer. In Proceedings of the American Cancer Society and National Cancer Institute's National Conference on Nutrition in Cancer, New York, 1979, American Cancer Society.

50. *Lovejoy, N.: Preventing hair loss during adriamycin therapy, Cancer Nurs. **2:**117-120, 1979.

51. Lynch, H.T., et al.: Hereditary cancer: ascertainment and management, CA **29:**216-229, 1979.

52. McAdams, C.W.: Interferon: the penicillin of the future, Am. J. Nurs. **80:**714-718, 1980.

53. *McGuire, D.B.: Familial cancer and the role of the nurse, Cancer Nurs. **2:**443-451, 1979.

54. McKhann, C.: Cancer immunotherapy: a realistic appraisal, CA **30:**286-293, 1980.

55. McKhann, C.: Immunotherapy of cancer. In Gottlieb, A.A., Plescia, P.J., and Bishop, D.H.: Fundamental aspects of neoplasia, New York, 1975, Springer-Verlag New York, Inc.

56. McKhann, C., and Yarlott, M.A.: Tumor immunology, CA **25;**187-197, 1975.

57. Morton, D.L., et al.: Response to active immunotherapy of malignant melanomas. In Gottlieb, A.A., Plescia, P.J., and Bishop, D.H.: Fundamental aspects of neoplasia, New York, 1975, Springer-Verlag New York Inc.

58. *Mundinger, M.: Nursing diagnosis for cancer patients, Cancer Nurs. **1:**3-9, 1978.

59. Murawski, B.J., Penman, D., and Schmitt, M.: Social support in health and illness, Cancer Nurs. **1:**365-371, 1978.

60. Newell, G.R.: Prologue: the national cancer plan and its relationship to basic research. In Gottlieb, A.A., Plescia, P.J., and Bishop, D.H.: Fundamental aspects of neoplasia, New York, 1975, Springer-Verlag New York.

61. *Northouse, L.L.: Living with cancer, Am. J. Nurs. **81:**960-962, 1981.

62. Nutrition for patients receiving chemotherapy and radiation treatment, New York, 1978, American Cancer Society.

63. Oberst, M.T.: Priorities in cancer nursing research, Cancer Nurs. **1:**281-290, 1978.

64. Pitot, H.C.: Fundamentals of oncology, New York, 1978, Marcel Dekker, Inc.

65. Porth, C.: Pathophysiology: concepts of altered health states, Philadelphia, 1982, J.B. Lippincott Co.

66. Public attitudes toward cancer and cancer tests, New York, 1980, American Cancer Society.

67. *Rankin, M.: The progressive pain of cancer, Top. Clin. Nurs. **2:**59-73, 1980.

68. Rosai, J., and Ackerman, L.V.: The pathology of tumors. I. Precancerous and pseudomalignant lesions, CA **28:**331-342, 1978.

69. Rosenbaum, E.H.: Living with cancer, St. Louis, 1982, The C.V. Mosby Co.

70. Sackett, D.: Periodic examination of patients at rest. In Schottenfeld, D., editor: Cancer epidemiology and prevention. Springfield, Ill., 1975, Charles C. Thomas, Publisher.

71. Schmale, A.H.: Psychologic aspects of anorexia. In Proceedings of the American Cancer Society and National Cancer Institute's National Conference on Nutrition in Cancer, New York, 1978, American Cancer Society.

72. Schottenfeld, D.: Alcohol as a co-factor in the etiology of cancer. In Proceedings of the American Cancer Society and National Cancer Institute's National Conference on Nutrition in Cancer, New York 1978, American Cancer Society.

73. Schottenfeld, D., and Haas, J.F.: Carcinogens in the workplace, CA **29:**144-168, 1979.

74. *Schreier, A.M., and Lavenia, J.: The nurse's role in nutritional management of radiotherapy patients, Nurs. Clin. North Am. **12:**173-183, 1977.

75. Shills, M.E.: Nutrition and cancer: dietary deficiency and modifications. In Schottenfeld, D.: Cancer epidemiology and prevention, Springfield, Ill., 1975, Charles C. Thomas, Publisher.

76. Shinkin, M.B.: Reporting on cancer research, CA **25:**105-106, 1975.

77. Sontag, S.: Illness as a metaphor, New York, 1977, Farrar, Straus and Giroux, Inc.

78. Steel, J.F.: Nursing looks at pain. In Proceedings of Second National Conference on Cancer Nursing, New York, 1977, American Cancer Society.

79. Unproven methods of cancer management: cancer quackery, CA **25:**66-71, 1975.

80. Upton, A.C.: Low level radiation, New York, 1979, American Cancer Society.

81. Van Scoy-Masher, M.: Chemotherapy: a manual for patients and families, Cancer Nurs. **1:**234-240, 1978.

82. *Varricchio, C.G.: The patient on radiation therapy, Am. J. Nurs. **81:**334-337, 1981.

83. Vredevoe, D., et al.: Concepts of oncology nursing, Englewood Cliffs, N.J., 1981, Prentice-Hall, Inc.

84. Warren, B.: Adjuvant chemotherapy for breast disease: the nurse's role, Cancer Nurs. **2:**32-37, 1979.

85. *Welch, D.A.: Assessment of nausea and vomiting in cancer patients undergoing external beam radiotherapy, Cancer Nurs. **3:**365-371, 1980.

86. Winters, W.D., and Morton, D.L.: Immunobiology. In Schottenfeld, D.: Cancer epidemiology and prevention, Springfield Ill., 1975, Charles C.Thomas, Publisher.

87. Wynger, E.L., and Mabuch, K.: Tobacco and cancer epidemiology and prevention. In Schottenfeld, D.: Cancer epidemiology and prevention, Springfield, Ill., 1975, Charles C. Thomas, Publisher.

Classic

88. Boeker, E.H., editor: Symposium on radiation uses and hazards, Nurs. Clin. North Am. **2:**1-113, 1967.

89. Committee on Professional Education of International Union Against Cancer, editors: Clinical oncology: a manual for students and doctors, New York, 1973, Springer-Verlag New York, Inc.

90. George, M.M.: Long-term care of the patient with cancer, Nurs. Clin. North Am. **8:**623-631, 1973.

91. Hughes, J., and Ryser, P.: Chemical carcinogenesis, CA **24:**351-360, 1974.

92. Isler, C.: Cancer quackery, RN **37;**55-59, 1974.

93. Silverstein, M.J., and Morton, D.L.: Cancer immunotherapy, Am. J. Nurs. **73:**1178-1181, 1973.

15

Chronic Illness

WILMA J. PHIPPS, PATRICIA BUERGIN, ELEANOR E. BAUWENS,
and SANDRA VANDAM ANDERSON

STUDY QUESTIONS

- What types of patients do you think are most in need of rehabilitation? Outline the rehabilitation needs of a patient you are now caring for or have cared for in the past.

- What proportion of the patients on the hospital unit to which you are assigned have a chronic illness as either their primary or secondary diagnosis? What proportion has more than one chronic health problem? What age group is affected most by more than one chronic health problem?

- What resources are available in your community for the care of the chronically ill? Are the facilities adequate for the number of persons needing care? How are these facilities supported financially?

- From what you have learned in anatomy, outline in detail the physical movements necessary to rise from a sitting position in a chair to a standing position. Describe how you would assist a patient to stand while allowing him or her to be as independent as possible.

Prevention and control of chronic disease constitute one of the major health problems in the United States today. In the past the impact of chronic diseases on individuals, families, and communities has been overlooked. Recently, there has been an increasing awareness in the United States of great pockets of unmet needs among people with long-term health problems. These individuals have needs that extend beyond the strictly medical. Their problems demand the use of multiple sources of help and care. In many cases the coping capacities of chronically ill individuals are reduced because of advancing age, serious functional impairment and disability, and limited personal, social, and financial resources.

Chronic disease is not an entity in itself but an umbrella term that encompasses long-lasting diseases, which

are often associated with some degree of disability. Each chronic illness is unique and has a different impact on the individual, family, and community. Nevertheless, common problems and complications that accompany the various chronic health problems can be studied in general to help the nurse understand and care for individuals with specific long-term illnesses.

The incidence and prevalence of chronic diseases have increased since the beginning of the twentieth century. This increase has been brought about by a number of developments including decreased mortality from infectious diseases, improved sanitation, and the development of effective vaccines and mass immunizations. Today only 1% of people who die before age 75 in the United States die from infectious diseases. Although the mortality from infectious diseases declined between 1900 and 1980, the proportions of deaths from major chronic diseases such as heart disease, cancer, and stroke have increased more than 250%.[28] According to the surgeon general's report, 80% of the over-65 population has one or more chronic illnesses.[28] Since the late 1960s, declining mortality from heart disease (particularly ischemic heart disease) and cerebrovascular diseases has contributed to increased longevity. In fact, 1977 was the first year in which cardiovascular causes were responsible for less than 50% of all deaths in the United States.[27] Longevity of the total U.S. population has increased by 3.1 years since 1970, compared with a gain of 0.8 year in the sixties. This gain in longevity is undoubtedly the result of self-help measures by individuals.

DEFINITION OF ACUTE AND CHRONIC ILLNESS

An *acute illness* is one caused by a disease that produces symptoms and signs soon after exposure to the cause, that runs a short course, and from which there is usually a full recovery or an abrupt termination in death. Acute illness may become chronic. For example, a common cold may develop into chronic sinusitis. A *chronic illness* is one caused by disease that produces symptoms and signs within a variable period of time, that runs a long course, and from which there is only partial recovery. The Commission on Chronic Illness defines chronic illness as any impairment or deviation from normal that has one or more of the characteristics listed in the box below.

The symptoms and general reactions caused by chronic disease may subside with proper treatment and care. The period during which the disease is controlled and symptoms are not obvious is known as a *remission*. However, at a future time the disease may become active again with recurrence of pronounced symptoms. This is known as an *exacerbation* of the disease.

Acute exacerbations of chronic disease often cause the patient to seek medical attention and may lead to hospitalization. The needs of a patient who has an acute illness may be very different from those of the patient with an acute exacerbation of a chronic disease. For example,

---

Characteristics of chronic illnesses

One or more of the following is present with an *illness* or impairment that

Is permanent.

Leaves residual disability.

Is caused by nonreversible pathologic alteration.

Requires a long period of supervision, observation, or care.

---

a young person may enter the hospital with complaints of fever, chest pain, shortness of breath, fatigue, and a productive cough. If the diagnosis is pneumonia, the patient usually can be assured of recovery after a period of rest and a course of antibiotic treatment. However, if the diagnosis is rheumatic heart disease and if the patient is being admitted to the hospital for the third, fourth, or fifth time, the reassurance needed will not be so definite, clear-cut, or easy to give. In such a case it is necessary to begin planning care that will extend beyond the period of hospitalization, taking into consideration many aspects of the patient's total life situation. The concerns of the patient who has repeated attacks of illness will be very different from the concerns of the one who has a short-term illness.

Further, the needs of patients who are admitted to the hospital with an acute illness but who also have an underlying chronic condition must not be overlooked. For example, elderly patients who enter the general hospital with pneumonia may receive treatment for the pneumonia and recover from their illness. However, they may still be hampered by the arteriosclerotic heart disease and arthritis that they have had for years. Also these two chronic conditions may have been aggravated by the acute infection, or the return to former activity may be hindered by joint stiffness resulting from the enforced bed rest and inactivity. Consideration of a patient's several diagnoses can help in preventing new problems associated with the chronic illness.

Neither completely well nor acutely ill, the individual with chronic disease must make daily adjustments in living. Strauss[23] has listed some problems surrounding chronic illness: (1) preventing and managing medical crises as they occur, (2) controlling symptoms, (3) following a prescribed regimen and managing attendant problems, (4) normalizing interactions with others, (5) adjusting to recurrent patterns in the disease course, and (6) arranging payment for treatment. Emotional, social, and economic implications of chronic illness will be discussed later in this chapter.

CHRONIC ILLNESS AS A FORCE IN SOCIETY

According to the National Health Survey, 80 million people have one or more chronic conditions. The National Health Survey list of chronic diseases includes asthma, allergy, tuberculosis, bronchitis, emphysema, sinusitis, rheumatic fever, arteriosclerosis, hypertension, heart disease, cerebrovascular accident and other vascular conditions, hemorrhoids, gallbladder or liver disease, diabetes mellitus, thyroid disease, epilepsy or convulsions, spinal disease, cancer, chronic dermatosis, and hernia.

Many of these specific illnesses cause a limitation of activity, which affects the life-style of the chronically ill. One of the trends that has been documented is that the impact of acute illness has seemed to diminish, whereas the burden of chronic health problems and related disability has increased. Limitation of activity is a measure of long-term disability resulting from chronic health problems or impairment and is defined as the inability to carry on the major activity for one's age group, such as cooking, keeping house, going to school, or going to work.[17] Approximately 15% of the population experience some limitations in their activities, whereas almost half of the persons over 65 years of age are limited in their activities by one or more chronic conditions. Some activity limitations are associated with mental disabilities, but most are the result of physical handicaps caused by heart conditions and arthritis. Since chronic disability increases in direct proportion to age, persons over 65 years of age are most prone to severe chronic disability.[10]

The inability to work or to move about influences greatly the kind of medical treatment and health supervision needed by persons who have a chronic illness. Some persons only need periodic medical examination and perhaps continuing treatment with medications; others may require complete physical care. Some have a disease that progresses very slowly without remissions, while others may have episodes of acute illness and then seem comparatively well for a time. Each person requires a thorough assessment to determine the stage of the illness, the course the illness is likely to take, the type of care needed, and the method by which that care will be delivered if the individual is to be helped appropriately.

Factors that influence chronic illness

AGE

Different age groups have different kinds of experience with acute and chronic diseases. The young are more likely to experience short, intense, acute conditions that are quickly over. The elderly are more likely to have long, drawn-out chronic diseases; nevertheless, it is true that anyone can have either an acute or a chronic disease at any age. Chronic illness and disability may date from birth (e.g., spina bifida with neurologic damage), or it may originate in childhood, adolescence, or early adult life (e.g., multiple sclerosis, rheumatoid arthritis). Table 15-1 depicts the prevalence of selected chronic conditions by age groups for selected years from 1970 to 1977.

Because of strides made in pediatric medicine, children who 30 years ago would have died from diseases such as cystic fibrosis are now living longer. The reduction in death rates among the younger age groups has allowed a higher percentage of the population to reach the age of greatest risk from chronic diseases. Cancer develops far more frequently in older people. Because the average age of our population continues to rise, one out of four people now alive will eventually contract cancer.[3]

Much remains to be learned about interactions of the normal, pathologic, and physiologic changes of aging with various diseases. A common question that is asked is "When does aging end and illness begin?" Differences found in age groups or changes found in individuals as they age represent normal aging; that is, a universal, intrinsic process of growth and development that is inevitable, irreversible, unpreventable, but ultimately detrimental. Even though aging, a normal process, is distinct from chronic disease, a pathologic process, chronic illness is often concomitant with aging. The problems of aging and chronic disease are influenced in major ways by each other; for example, the social problems confronting the aged are strongly influenced by the presence and severity of chronic disabilities. Remissions and exacerbations are possibilities with chronic illness; they are not with aging.

Table 15-1. Prevalence of selected chronic conditions, 1970 to 1977*

Condition	17 to 44 years		45 to 64 years		65 years and older		All ages	
	A†	B‡	A	B	A	B	A	B
Arthritis (1976)	45.5	13.1	255.8	18.3	436.6	25.5	116.7	20.3
Asthma (1970)	26.0	17.0	33.0	19.0	36.0	27.0	30.0	17.0
Cerebrovascular diseases (1972)	NA§	NA	12.0	NA	48.0	NA	8.0	22.0
Diabetes (1975)	9.4	23.5	50.3	30.3	83.0	34.4	22.9	30.6
Emphysema (1970)	NA	NA	14.0	NA	32.0	NA	7.0	45.0
Heart conditions (1972)	25.0	22.0	89.0	46.0	199.0	52.0	50.0	42.0
Major extremity missing (1977)	0.8	56.3	3.1	61.9	6.2	73.2	1.7	65.9
Vision impairment, severe (1977)	1.2	42.7	6.0	36.4	44.5	35.5	6.6	37.0

*From National Center for Health Statistics, Division of Health Interview Statistics; data from the Health Interview Survey.
†Per 1000 persons.
‡Percent resulting in limitation of activity.
§NA, Not available.

CULTURAL VALUES

Western culture tends to be cure oriented, therefore, health care for acute conditions is often more valued than is health care for the chronically ill. In contrast to the exciting aspects of sophisticated and mechanical technology, caring for chronically ill persons is often considered boring. The continual struggle to cope with day-to-day living soon becomes tedious for ill persons, their families, and health professionals. The rewards of treating chronic illness cannot be measured by a cure but by the prevention of complications and by helping individuals function at their optimal level.

The cultural context has many symbolic meanings, beliefs, and values that health professionals need to understand to meet individual's health needs. Some individuals may view their chronic disease as a form of punishment from God. Thus they may experience a sense of guilt. Individuals who view their chronic disease as a "leper phenomenon" may experience a sense of social rejection. Others may see their chronic illness as a destructive force without meaning or simply as a physical response of their body. Appreciation of the person's beliefs and behavior in the context of his or her cultural heritage rather than denial of the cultural influence increases understanding between the health professional and the chronically ill person. Differences need not imply deviance. It is possible to introduce health practices in a manner congruent with the individual's cultural values.

RACE AND ETHNICITY

Race or ethnic group membership is a factor that influences chronic health problems. Race-specific rates measure the association between disease occurrence and race. Data on specific conditions indicate not only that some problems are more prevalent among nonwhites (blacks, American Indians, and Asiatics), but also that nonwhites fail to receive necessary care. For example, nonwhites are more than three times more likely to die of hypertension than whites of the same age group.[13] They are also more likely to die from other conditions resulting from untreated hypertension. For example, nonwhites face a 60% higher risk of dying of cerebrovascular disease than do whites and are almost four times as likely to die of hypertensive heart disease. They are also twice as likely as whites to die from diabetes and four times as likely to die of chronic kidney disease.

Ethnic and racial factors can help identify individuals at risk for various chronic diseases. For example, after 45 years of age nonwhite women in the United States have an incidence of diabetes about twice that of whites. Pima Indians in Arizona have a 50% incidence of diabetes among those 35 years of age and older. This is 10 times higher than the incidence of diabetes for the same age group in the United States.[13]

Cost of disability

Each chronically ill person and family are subjected to great personal and emotional losses that must be dealt with—loss of self-esteem, loss of status within the family, loss of independence, feelings of rejection, and feelings of helplessness are only a few. These can be more devastating than economic deprivation, which is a constant problem.

The economic cost to the patient and family is considerable. The cost of hospitalization rises yearly. Frequent or extended hospitalization and medical expenses can be ruinous if the patient is inadequately insured or if he or she is unable to qualify for insurance programs. Many are forced to seek public assistance merely to survive. Placement in quality nursing homes is frequently financially impossible for patients or their families to manage. The cost of medications to control or maintain a patient's health status may require a major portion of the family budget. Additional expenses may include special diets and equipment, home modifications (e.g., ramps or widening of doors for wheelchairs), transportation, and support services provided by homemakers, day or live-in attendants, or nurses.

The ability of the individual family to pay its own way is determined in part by which member of the family becomes disabled. Studies show that if the wife is disabled, the family suffers less economic deprivation than if the husband is disabled. However, three fourths of the chronically ill persons unable to carry on their major activity are men.[19]

Some financial assistance is provided by Medicare. This federally administered program provides hospital and medical insurance protection for individuals 65 years of age and over as well as for people under 65 who are disabled and eligible for Social Security benefits. The Social Security Administration in 1972 was mandated by Congress to finance treatment for individuals with chronic kidney disease. An original estimate for the program was an annual cost of approximately $250 million; however, at the end of 4 years, the cost was double that amount. The estimated cost of the program by 1983, approximately 10 years after the start of the program, is $2.7 billion per year.[20]

In considering the cost of disability to the community, it must be realized that most individuals who are unable to work must be supported by others, either from private or from public funds. There are 3 million adults between the ages of 18 and 64 years who are unable to work because of chronic disabilities. There are an additional 9.4 million who are partially limited in their ability to work.[19]

EFFECTS OF CHRONIC ILLNESS

The effects of chronic illness on individuals and their families are numerous and varied. The first impact of the disability may nearly immobilize them. Time must be provided them to talk through their concerns and fears before they can be expected to begin coping with their new situation.

Marked changes often take place, and are often required to take place, in family living as a result of chronic illness. Some families may find themselves drawn closer together. Other families may drift apart, the individual members being incapable of helping one another. At times, chronic illness may threaten an individual's basic emotional stability, and the whole situation may be unbearable to others. Sometimes the individual's emotional needs may not have been apparent to the family early in the illness, but when such needs grow obvious, relatives feel inadequate to cope with the situation. The length of illness, periodic hospitalizations, and increased financial, emotional, and social burdens are stressors that threaten the family's integrity.

Many persons struggle on their own to assume the full financial burden of the illness and consequently expose other members of the family to lower standards of nutrition, housing, and care. Many times relatives move in with one another, arguments develop, and family ties are strained or broken. Public assistance may be acceptable to some families, whereas others find it impossible to accept.

Chronic illness imposes additional problems of learning how to cope with restrictions on activities of daily living, how to prevent or identify medical crises that occur, and how to carry out treatment regimens as delineated by the health care provider. Family members also need to learn about the restrictions, not only to be of assistance to the chronically ill person, but also because their own activity patterns may be disrupted by the person's activities.

Since chronic illness may have periods of exacerbation when symptoms become more acute and medical crises may occur, patients and family members need to know which symptoms must be reported to the health care provider as well as the time interval for reporting these symptoms. They also need to know how to contact the provider and what measures to take if a medical crisis occurs. For example, the person who has a history of myocardial infarction as well as family members must know what to do if the person experiences severe chest pain. Should the person be taken immediately to a hospital emergency room or should the physician be contacted first? Patient and family should plan in advance the sequence of actions to take during a medical crisis, depending on the nature and extent of the presenting symptoms.

Persons with chronic illness are often labeled as "compliant" or "noncompliant" in carrying out regimens prescribed for them. There are many factors that influence the person's ability or motivation to carry out the prescribed regimen. If the person does not carry out the regimen (noncompliant), it does not necessarily mean that the individual is refusing to do so deliberately, although this may sometimes occur. One reason for noncompliance may be lack of knowledge of the importance of doing what is required because learning the appropriate regimen never occurred. The person may have been "told" the reason for the regimen, but he or she may not have perceived it or have internalized it. In many situations, however, there are other more influential factors for noncompliance: (1) time-consuming activities, (2) difficult techniques to learn or carry out, (3) presence of side effects, (4) expense, (5) visibility to others, (6) inefficient

as perceived by clients, or (7) social isolation.[23] Social and cultural patterns will also affect compliance.

Conflicts occur within the family structure when one family member recognizes the importance of carrying out the prescribed regimen but another does not. For example, a wife may see the need for continuing checkups and medication for her husband's hypertension, whereas he may perceive this as a needless expense since he feels well and has no symptoms. Persons vary from time to time in the extent of compliance. Individuals who are not hospitalized are their own health care agents and they (or their significant others) determine the actions that are taken.

Coping mechanisms that have been developed should not be tampered with unless, based on a thorough understanding of the situation, viable and more appropriate alternatives can be proposed. If the goal of maintaining the chronically ill person in the optimal state of health is being interfered with by the individual's or the family's attitudes or capacities, a change in those attitudes or capacities is necessary, but it must be a change that is mutually acceptable.

Prevention of chronic illness

Because chronic disease evolves over time and pathologic changes may become irreversible, the goal is to detect risk factors as early as possible.

Generally, prevention means inhibiting the development of a disease before it occurs. The term includes several levels of prevention to interrupt or slow the progression of disease (see box below).

Chronically ill persons and their families require long-term care. The nursing profession has been concerned with chronic health problems and the challenge involved in providing long-term nursing care to chronically ill individuals and their families.

Levels of prevention

Primary

Health promotion
Specific protection against diseases

Secondary

Early detection of disease
Prompt intervention to halt progression of disease

Tertiary

Rehabilitation (appropriate to the stage of disability)
Prevent further complications
Restore optimal functioning as much as possible

The American Academy of Nursing has made the following statement regarding long-term care:

Long-term care is the provision of that range of services—physical, psychological, spiritual, and social, including socioeconomic—needed to help people attain, maintain, or regain their optimal level of functioning. It includes health maintenance throughout the life span as well as care during acute and protracted illness and disability. Such care is the legitimate province of nurses who now are making social contributions through health teaching and promotion, prevention of illness, and rehabilitation.[2]

In the past nursing has followed the general pattern of providing health services by placing the emphasis on acute and episodic care rather than on health promotion and health maintenance. However, there is an emerging consensus among the health community that the health strategy must be changed dramatically to emphasize the prevention of disease. In the same vein, the American Academy of Nursing has proposed that "nursing assume major responsibility for health promotion, maintenance, and teaching within the context of its definition of long-term care."[2]

SPECIAL NEEDS OF THE CHRONICALLY ILL

Before a plan of care can be devised for the chronically ill person, a thorough assessment of needs and capabilities must be carried out. Included in such an assessment are the individual's physical, psychologic, social, and financial status.

Assessment of physical status

Since medical diagnoses do not accurately reflect the physical status and functioning of the chronically ill person, the use of a profile system or assessment tool may be instituted as a guide for those working with the patient. One such tool[34] provides a guide for grading the patient in six different categories: (1) physical condition including cardiovascular, pulmonary, GI, genitourinary, endocrine, or cerebrovascular disorders; (2) upper extremities, structure and function, including the shoulder girdle and cervical and upper dorsal spine; (3) lower extremities, structure and function, including the pelvis and lower dorsal and lumbar sacral spine; (4) sensory components relating to speech, vision, and hearing; (5) excretory function, including the bowels and bladder; and (6) mental and emotional status. The ability of the person to carry out activities of daily living (for example, dressing, feeding, bathing, brushing teeth, combing hair, toileting, and moving from place to place) specifically need to be assessed. The completed assessment should indicate in what areas the patient has difficulty and the extent of that difficulty. Such a guide can be used in planning care, both immediate and long term, and will be useful in assisting the individual and the family to make realistic plans for care. Since a chronic condition is not static, reassessment should be carried out at regular intervals whether there is improvement or regression.

Intervention

The first focus in intervention for the chronically ill person is on prevention and reduction of disability and on enabling the person to remain a socially functioning individual in every respect. Some of the disability seen among the chronically ill might have been prevented if prompt, aggressive, suitable medical and nursing care had been available at the onset of the illness. Many of the difficulties that limit the chronically ill may not have been caused by the disease itself but may have developed because of immobility during the acute phase of the illness.

Keeping the person's body in good alignment, maintaining joint range and strength, and preventing decubitus ulcers are physical measures that must constantly be borne in mind. (For further information see Chapter 23.) A careful plan of rest and activity helps preserve physical resources and makes the day purposeful. If assistance is needed, it should be given until the persons can manage the activity by themselves or until an alternative method of management can be taught.

Second, recognizing what is meaningful to the individual is a primary step toward helping develop self-care. Physical needs become of paramount importance to chronically ill persons. Meeting these physical needs provides a way to convey to such individuals an interest in their progress and welfare. Helping them to take their own baths, to attend to toilet needs, and to groom themselves can give some sense of accomplishment and help them maintain their self-respect. Helping them to be dressed appropriately promotes a sense of wellness. Success in performing portions of their own self-care may be stimulating enough to strengthen the persons' motivation so that they and their families may make amazing strides in thinking through and working out future problems themselves. For their planning to be realistic and ultimately functional, all health care personnel must teach chronically ill persons the total physiologic ramifications of their disability as well as methods of coping with those ramifications.

Persons who are in their homes or in substitute homes should be encouraged to dress in regular, comfortable street clothing rather than in pajamas or gowns. Visitors coming into the home and members of the family who constantly see such individuals dressed in bedclothes think of them as sick and are reminded of their illness. Seeing them dressed as they ordinarily would be helps to maintain normal attitudes, relationships, and expectations.

Assessment of psychologic status

Assessment of the individual's psychologic needs and capabilities includes determining attitudes and stage of adaptation to the illness, feelings concerning how illness affects the family or significant others, and the person's own goals in regard to living with an illness.[31] For example, individuals who are almost totally helpless as a result of an accidental spinal cord injury may seem to have no interest in learning ways to help themselves. Their families may react in the same manner and be of little help to them. Both the individuals and their families need interest and support from professional persons as they learn to cope with the change in their life situations.

Feelings of anxiety, frustration, irritability, bitterness, and guilt may be expressed by some chronically ill persons who face unending pain and loss of economic and social security. Some persons become hypochondriacal, obsessed with their health problems, and spend much of each day thinking about what will happen and what to do. Guilt may result from being unable to work and support oneself or from the belief, as a result of a search for some purpose or reason for the affliction, that one must deserve the suffering.

Assessment of social and financial status

Social and financial status must be considered, as they relate specifically to the kind of support and resources available to the individuals in meeting their goals. It would be unrealistic, for example, to plan for a hydraulic bathtub chair if the patient could not afford it, family members were unavailable to help operate it, or the patient's apartment manager would not permit it to be installed. Alternative methods of helping the patient to take a tub bath would have to be explored.

The social assessment includes living arrangements, family roles, support of significant others, cultural and social group memberships, education, and vocational and avocational activities. The data collected through the performance of this kind of thorough assessment should make it possible to devise a plan of care directed toward the accomplishment of attainable goals that are mutually acceptable to the patient, the family, and the caregivers.

Psychosocial considerations

The care of chronically ill persons requires alertness of feeling, seeing, and hearing. Continued warmth and interest are necessary to the well-being of any chronically ill person. Very often it is a relationship based on an understanding of these requirements that helps the individual to become highly motivated. It may be taxing to listen to the same questions and to say the same things day after day, but the nature of chronic illness may require this attention, and the manner in which responses are given will convey warmth and interest. The world of chronically ill persons, whether they are in the hospital or elsewhere, becomes narrowed and circumscribed. They treasure and are interested in those things and those people who are close to them. Their conversations may be largely about themselves, their immediate environment, a few close objects, and the persons who are close to them. Al-

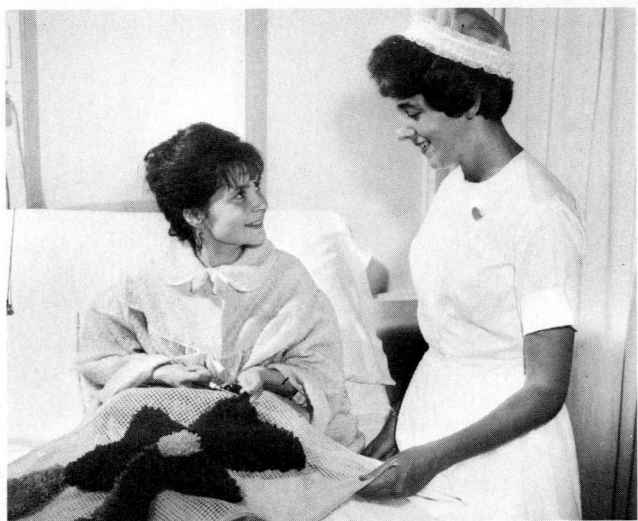

Fig. 15-1. Occupational therapy provides patient with purposeful activity. Interest shown by nurse encourages patient to complete project.

though they may be confined to bed and to their room, others can keep them up-to-date on outside news. Depending on their level of adaptation to their illness, they may welcome hearing about outside events, or they may not be able to think beyond themselves. When they reach the stage of being able to look beyond themselves, newspapers, magazines, radio, television, or creating something with their own hands (Fig. 15-1) may help to keep up their interest in others and in outside events.

Coping skills may be challenged by persistent, ongoing problems such as chronic pain, recurring medical expenses, or continuing difficulties in carrying out activities of daily living. Usual coping methods may become impossible; for example, a person who usually copes by expending energy in physical activity may become unable to do so. The person who usually copes by discussing problems with family members will need to find an alternative method if family communication patterns break down. The person can be helped to identify usual coping methods and to explore alternative approaches when necessary (see Chapter 9).

It is important to recognize that chronically ill persons or their families may suffer from unresolved sadness known as chronic grief. Chronic grief may be defined as accumulated or prolonged grief. Chronic grief extends over long periods of time with permanent characteristics in a large number of sufferers. It carries with it a potential for decreased functioning. The causes are varied, and new waves of grief are constantly triggered. One example is that of the mother of the retarded child who has accepted her situation and is coping well, but over and over is faced with unattainable goals, repeated frustrations, and an uncertain future. Another example is grief caused by the losses associated with aging: youth, dreams, jobs, hair, friends, family, health, visual acuity, social role, money, body parts, and mobility. Each loss is accompanied by grief, which builds on previous grief like bricks placed by the mason creating a wall. In chronic grief the patient may be faced with repeated acute episodes. These episodes may coincide with exacerbation of the condition, facing a new limitation, or meeting new indignities. Each new episode requires a renewed struggle back and forth through the various stages of grief.[23]

The nurse can assist by listening and helping the person explore feelings and the content related to these feelings. Since the grief is ongoing, family members can also be helped to identify their feelings and to strengthen the communication patterns within the family structure for mutual support of its members.

Nurses who work with chronically ill persons need to be able to distinguish between their own values, standards, and goals and those of the patient. In day-to-day contact with individuals who are making little or no progress, it is tempting to make plans for their future because of a sincere interest in helping them. This is particularly true when the patient's age is similar to one's own. There may be a feeling that something must be done to speed progress. One may become frustrated by the feeling of wanting to do something or wanting to see some marked change. However, it must be recognized that management of chronically ill persons requires a slow-moving, persistent pace with possibly little or no change for a long time. The person's physical and mental condition must be maintained at its present level or improved, and effort must be made to further progress and to encourage the family's adaptation to the patient's condition. Eagerness and readiness to progress will be determining factors for the future. The "doing" in the care of the chronically ill person is not always an active, physical "doing" with the hands. Many times the maintenance of a positive approach and attitude and a demonstration of real interest are the greatest help to the patient. Teaching patients to perform activities related to their own care independently rather than performing those activities for them may also lead to progress.

Health care personnel must also be prepared to provide care for those patients whose disease will follow a course of progressive disability, for example, multiple sclerosis or rheumatoid arthritis. In these instances, goals of care must be modified to retard the downhill progression of disability rather than to achieve maintenance or improvement of physical status. Helping the patient and family cope with progressive deterioration and, in some cases, eventual death is a demanding task. Those who wish additional information relating to this aspect of care are referred to the literature treating this subject.[23,31]

Success in learning to adjust to living with a disability depends on the person's premorbid personality, total life experience, and premorbid family relationships, as well as the current behavior and motivation the person presents. Certainly, some rehabilitation can occur in any health agency; nevertheless, the greater the number of rehabilitation disciplines that can be made available as needed to individuals, the greater is their chance of achieving their highest potential. The rehabilitative process, as with any form of education, is involved as deeply in the motives and purposes of the teacher as in those of the learner.[38]

Persons with a disability, whether it is obvious to others or unrecognizable, should not be viewed from the standpoint of their disability alone. Usually the greatest need is for comprehensive health services and continuing care. Comprehensive care is that which is provided to patients according to their needs in an appropriate, continuous, and dynamic pattern. Accommodating the plan of care to the needs and goals of individul patients rather than to those of the providers of care is the essence of comprehensive care.

REHABILITATION

Rehabilitation is the process of assisting the individual with a handicap to realize his or her particular goals, physically, mentally, socially, and economically. As such, "rehabilitation" is an active concept and must be clearly differentiated from the concept of "maintenance" care. Following a thorough assessment of patients' disabilities and capabilities, assumptions can be made regarding the potential for improving their condition. If improvement can be made, patients are candidates for rehabilitation. If improvement cannot be made, care is directed toward maintaining the current condition, that is, preventing further disability. The process of rehabilitation can be viewed more appropriately as patient education rather than patient "care." It must be remembered, however, that the rehabilitation of every patient reaches an end point; that is, a point at which no further progress is possible. At that point, the focus of care reverts to that of maintenance.

The purpose or extent of rehabilitation ranges from employment or reemployment for the handicapped person to the more limited achievement of developing the ability to provide his or her own daily care. This latter accomplishment can be just as important to the individual as earning money and may represent that person's greatest life achievement. This might be true, for example, for a person who was born with a severe physical handicap such as cerebral palsy.

Teamwork and special services

The number of professional people required to assist the patient and family with rehabilitations varies. Most often the patient, the family, the physician, and the nurse can work out a practical plan. If a patient's problems are complex, other members may be added to the team. Typically, such a team consists of a physician, nurse, social worker, vocational counselor, psychologist, speech pathologist, occupational and physical therapists, and a caseworker from the patient's social agency. Teamwork requires that members of the team be able to use their special knowledge and skill and understand the value of their contribution to the patient's care. In addition, team members need some understanding of each other's professional functions and contributions. One of the cooperative efforts of the involved team members is to meet regularly to thoroughly evaluate patients and their abilities. Based on this assessment, each patient and the team devise a plan to foster readjustment, compensation, and the learning of new ways of managing self-care and living. In Fig. 15-2 some of the members of a team review a patient's rehabilitation program.

Persons with complex problems of rehabilitation may need to receive care at specialized centers for rehabilitation or they may receive care at home combined with visits to day rehabilitation centers. The variety of specialized centers includes teaching and research centers (centers located in and operated by hospitals and medical schools), community centers with facilities for inpatients, community out-patient centers, insurance centers, and vocational rehabilitation centers. In addition to centers that provide multiple services for the physical disabled, there are specialized centers for rehabilitation of the blind, deaf, mentally ill, and mentally retarded. Most centers offer a wide range of services that usually fall into the following three areas:

Physical
    Physical, nursing, and medical evaluation
    Physical therapy
    Occupational therapy
    Speech therapy
    Medical and nursing supervision of appropriate activities
Psychosocial
    Evaluation
    Personal counseling
    Social service
    Psychometrics
    Psychiatric service
    Recreational therapy
Vocational
    Work evaluation
    Vocational counseling
    Prevocational experience
    Industrial fitness of programs
    Trial employment in sheltered workshops
    Vocational training
    Terminal employment in sheltered workshops
    Placement

There are several advantages for patients participating in organized programs for rehabilitation. They have an opportunity to see and be with others who have similar or more extensive disabilities. Often they progress more rapidly when they realize that others have similar difficulties and are overcoming them. Group therapy often arouses a competitive spirit, and a formerly reluctant person may become willing and diligent. On the other hand, all personnel need to be alert to those patients who have had the opposite reaction. Patients who see others advance in activity while they either do not improve or progress very slowly may become so discouraged that they give up trying.

On a rehabilitation unit, activities are scaled so that individuals can see their own progress in comparison with their beginning abilities. Patients may take an active interest in keeping their own scores. After a program of therapy has been planned and is scheduled as to time of day, patients can help to keep themselves on the schedule

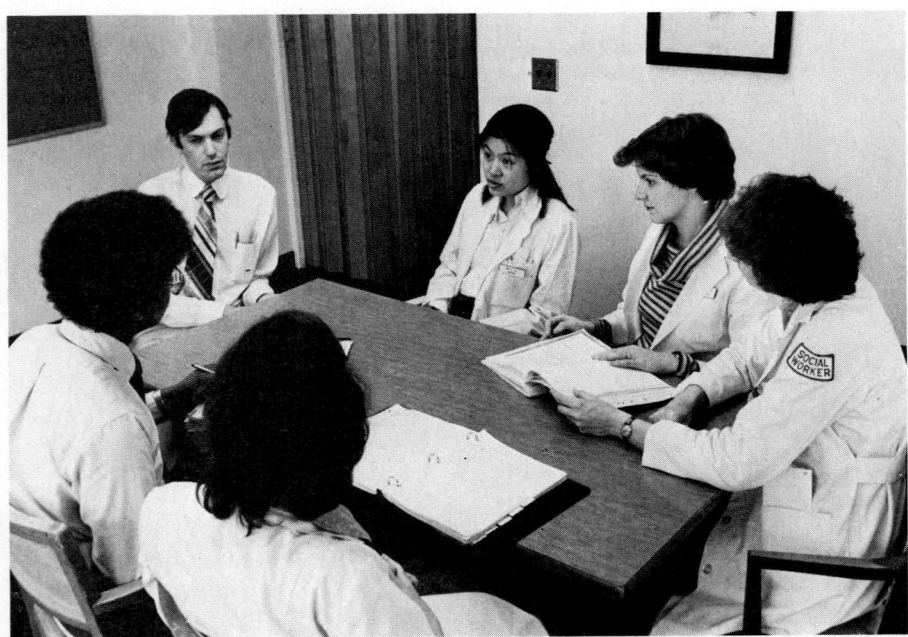

Fig. 15-2. Team approach to rehabilitation is essential. Here, physicians, nurse, physical therapist, and social worker review a patient's program and progress.

by having a copy of it at the bedside. Individuals can then be helped to gradually assume more and more responsibility for getting themselves ready for scheduled activities. In addition, a master plan of activities for all patients on the unit can be a useful device for nurses, physicians, and therapists. The plan can be kept in a central place on the unit and should list name, activity, and time of activity for each patient. This type of plan is helpful, too, when a patient's progress is to be reevaluated.

A public program for vocational rehabilitation has been serving the nation since 1920. The program involves a partnership between the state and the federal governments. Services for disabled persons are provided by state divisions of vocational rehabilitation. The federal government, through the Social and Rehabilitation Service (SRS), administers grants-in-aid and provides technical assistance and national leadership for the program. Opportunities and services are available in each of the 50 states, the District of Columbia, and Puerto Rico. All persons of working age with a substantial job handicap resulting from either physical or mental impairment are eligible for help or assistance. The purpose of this service is to preserve, develop, or restore the ability of disabled persons to earn their own livings. The individual services offered are medical care, counseling and guidance, training, and job finding. All 50 states have separate rehabilitation programs for the blind. Application for such services can be made to the SRS or to the agency in the state for serving the blind.

Role of the nurse

The concepts of comprehensive nursing care and rehabilitation can be considered synonymous. Helping the patient and the family to help themselves is an integral part of nursing care. Nurses who work with patients who have disabilities have two major responsibilities: (1) to see that disability from disease is limited as much as possible and (2) to see that a rehabilitation program is planned and implemented. Details of the nursing responsibilities are listed below.

Nursing responsibilities

I. Limit disability from disease as much as possible.
  A. Prevent complications
    1. Early recognition of symptoms of patient's condition worsening.
      a. Review signs and symptoms and pathology of the chronic illness so as to recognize changes
      b. Review signs and symptoms of complications frequently associated with the chronic illness, that is, infection
    2. Prevent deformities
      a. Maintain proper body alignment
      b. Position limbs to prevent contractures
      c. Turn frequently, keep skin clean and dry to prevent skin breakdown
      d. Provide adequate nutrition
      e. Provide adequate fluid intake to maintain bladder and bowel program
      f. Take precautions to prevent infection
II. Plan and implement a rehabilitation program appropriate to the patient.
  A. Determine patient's own goals for rehabilitation
  B. Plan appropriate nursing interventions based on mutually agreed upon goals
      Early in rehabilitation nurse may have to assume total responsibility for assisting with activities of daily living (ADL), bathing, intake of food and fluids, bowel and bladder programs, maintaining skin integrity, turning patient, and so on.
  C. Plan nursing interventions that encourage patient to assume responsibility for own ADL as soon as possible
    1. Set short-term goals with patient
    2. Goals should be realistic and attainable
    3. Reinforce patient's progress (no matter how small) with positive feedback
    4. Work with other members of the rehabilitation team in providing a consistent, coordinated rehabilitation plan
    5. Keep patient's significant others informed of patient's progress so they can give positive feedback to patient
    6. Reassess goals periodically and set new goals as possible
    7. Teach patient, family, and, if necessary, the employer about patient's limitations and rehabilitative expectations

One of the most important aspects of giving continuing care to a patient with a disability is the nurse's own attitude, perseverance, and expectations. Improvement may be slow, and patients may reach a "plateau" in their progress. Such a time can be critical for patients because they may become discouraged and not wish to continue with their program of care. Realistic encouragement can often sustain patients so that they will not regress until some improvement is noted.

Patients in a rehabilitation program must often learn and practice special physical techniques to strengthen muscles and to improve mobility. Such measures as physical exercise to improve walking, activities to improve self-care abilities, and the use of prostheses require the special knowledge and skills of physical and occupational therapists. To be effective in the rehabilitation process, nurses must have an understanding of the techniques used by the various therapists so that they can plan and work cooperatively with them in caring for the patient. This knowledge is also used to help the patient employ appropriate techniques in carrying out activities of daily living (ADL).

Role of the patient

The most important contributions to patients' rehabilitation are made by the patients themselves. The patient, the nurse, the physician, the social worker, the occupational therapist (Fig. 15-3), and sometimes others planning together can arrive at the best plans for the future, but the patient's attitudes, acceptance, and direction of motivation are the most important considerations. If the patient cannot adjust to the disability, whatever it may be and however extensive it may be, attempts at rehabilitation usually are hindered. Patients are the persons who really make the decisions, and they change at their own

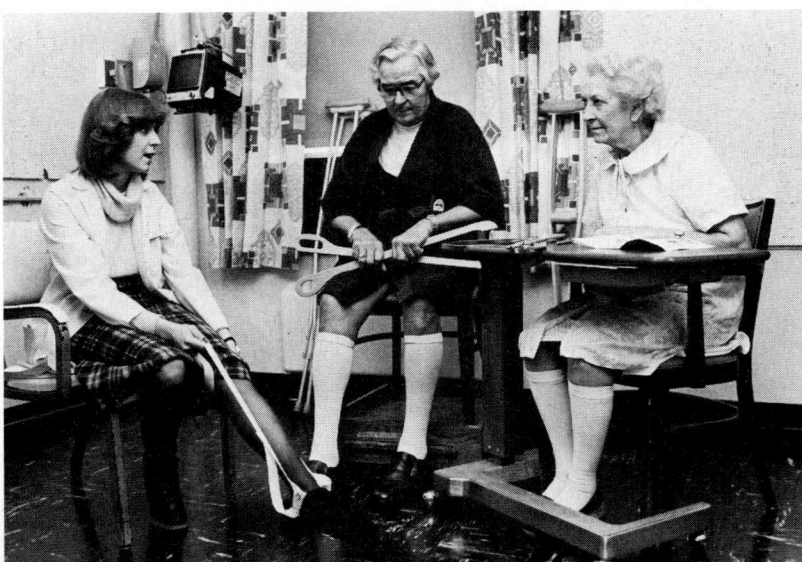

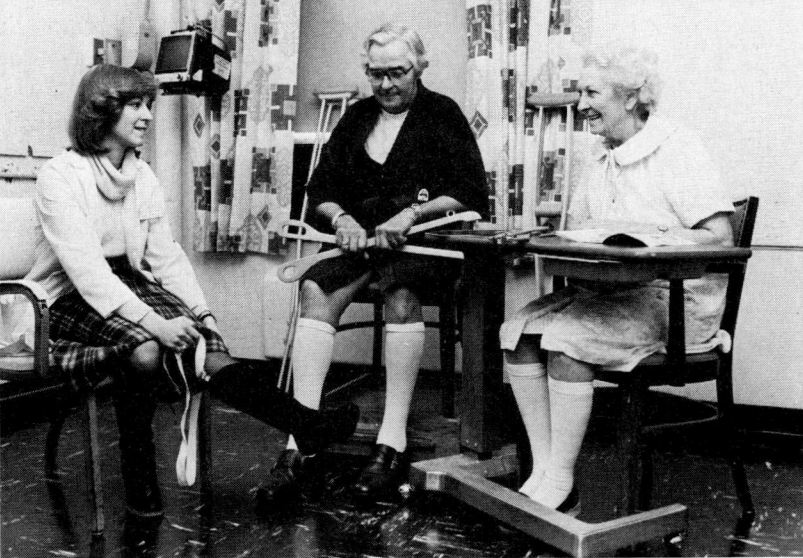

Fig. 15-3. Occupational therapist is concerned with helping patients make necessary adaptations in activities of daily living to permit independent functioning. Here the occupational therapist demonstrates the use of a stocking aid that to the delight of the patients really works.

pace. If they are agreeable to suggestions but make little or no effort to try them, one should question if they really have accepted them.

Self-care is encouraged within existing limitations. The patient's behavior from day to day can be the first indication of the direction of positive motivation. For example, if the patient makes every effort to resume normal daily activities such as feeding, bathing, and dressing, one can be quite certain that this is a person with a sincere desire to be independent. As patients become ready for more advanced activities such as ambulation and work in the occupational therapy shop, they need continuing genuine interest and support (Figs. 15-3 and 15-4). As obstacles present themselves, patients may be able to accept them and eventually overcome them. Patients who are truly motivated toward helping themselves never seem to give up, finding ways of accomplishing activities that professional personnel might believe impossible. Each person working with the chronically ill has seen that many times life has meaning for the individual even though it may not be readily apparent to others. However, there are some patients who, when faced with an added burden, cannot accept it and give up trying. Guidance and support for the families of such patients become tremendously important. Health care personnel who understand these attitudes and behaviors can help make life more satisfying for the chronically ill person and can positively influence the behaviors of the family, professional co-workers, and the public.

CONTINUING CARE
Considerations for continuing care

Traditionally, health care professionals have assumed responsibility for the patient's well-being within the hospital and little to no responsibility for the client and family in the home setting. This dichotomy between health care in the home and hospital facility in the case of chronically ill individuals interferes with a smooth transition from hospital to home. The major portion of health care for persons with chronic illnesses takes place in the home; thus there needs to be ongoing communications between the client and health professionals. Strauss[23] advocates that sick people participate more in their care within health facilities and that health care professionals play a larger role in aiding chronically sick people and their families to cope with their problems at home.

Most persons with a chronic or long-term illness can care for themselves or be cared for at home, and most actually prefer to be at home, where family and friends are close by and where they can still participate in family life. Many chronically ill persons require health care supervision at home. The arrangements that can be made vary greatly and depend on the needs of the individual and the facilities available. Many persons are ambulatory and, during remissions, are able to visit their local clinic. Others manage with visits from their personal physicians and with periodic workups in the physician's office. The assistance of a home health nurse or aide who goes into the home may also be necessary. Many chronically ill persons with disabilities also visit special rehabilitation units of hospitals or outpatient centers for daily or periodic instruction and practice in physical skills and job training.

Nurses from voluntary and official health agencies help the chronically ill in their homes. Nurses who visit the home to assist the individual or family members to accomplish daily care need to understand the patient. Chronically ill persons are often misjudged by even the closest members of the family because of blinding emotional ties or lack of knowledge and understanding. Families need to be helped to understand the limitations and necessary restrictions on the patients. Hopefully this process will have begun while the patient was hospitalized, but it will need to continue in the home setting.

The benefits and the necessity of self-care as a valid part of the health care system are receiving new recognition. Although the main impetus for this recognition has come from consumers, health care providers are increasingly incorporating self-care into the delivery of primary care. One definition of self-care is "an action taken by the consumer or patient to reduce to the degree possible, incremental debilitation resulting from chronic disease."[32] The increasing prevalence and importance of chronic illness as a principal cause of disability and death place greater demands on the client and family for involvement in self-care.

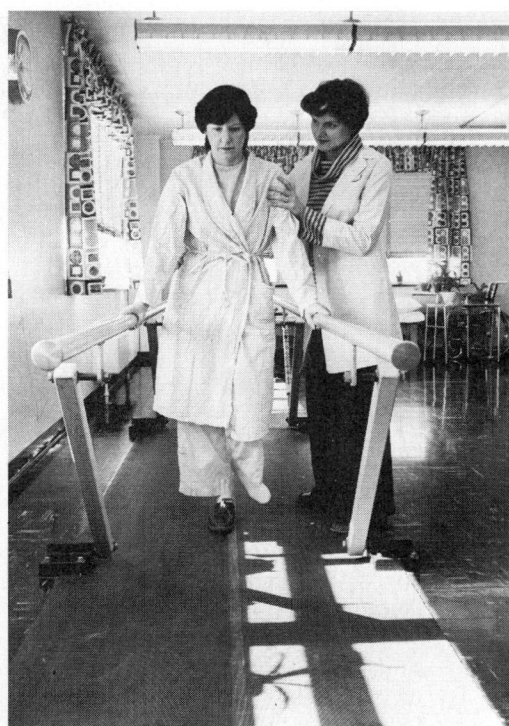

Fig. 15-4. Physical therapist begins patient's ambulation training by teaching her to walk with the support of parallel bars. The patient wears no shoe on her left foot to remind her not to bear weight on it.

Self-help groups are associated with self-care. These groups may or may not include the guidance of health care providers. They provide social support to their members through the creation of a caring community, and they increase members' coping skills through the sharing of information, experiences, and problem solutions. Examples of self-help groups include those for women who have had mastectomies and those for individuals who have colostomies, diabetes, or obesity. There are now self-help groups or clubs for patients with a variety of conditions. Nurses should learn what groups are available to patients in their community. A telephone call to a health agency such as the American Cancer Society, American Heart Association, or American Lung Association can elicit information about clubs available to patients who have the specific condition served by the agency.

In some hospitals nurses have been instrumental in setting up support groups for families of patients with chronic health problems.

It can be expected that more support groups, both those for patients and those for families, will be developing in the near future. Some of the impetus for these groups can be traced to changes in health care reimbursement. With the move to prospective reimbursement and the use of Diagnosis Related Groups (DRGs) as a basis for reimbursement for patients whose care is being paid for with federal dollars (Medicare and Medicaid), the need for such groups will increase. It is anticipated that prospective reimbursement will result in shorter hospital stays for both acute and chronic illnesses. As a result, patients and their families will need to be better prepared to care for the patient in the home since patients will be sent home sooner than in the past and their needs for continuing care will be greater.

Patterns and facilities for continuing care

It is impossible to include here all of the many facilities that provide continuing care. Only those programs that have been developed or emphasized recently will be covered. It must also be noted that each of the programs that will be mentioned has its own criteria for acceptance of patients for the services it renders. Before application for service is made, a determination of the individual patient's eligibility for that service must be carried out.

AMBULATORY CARE

The term *ambulatory care* is used interchangeably with *outpatient care* and refers to first contact health care services as well as to continuing contact services in settings that do not require overnight stays. There has been a marked increase in the use of ambulatory care facilities because of the increase in chronic illness and the increase in cost of inpatient services. A good ambulatory care service constitutes one of the most important elements of the hospital's contribution to community health. There is a trend toward development of ambulatory care facilities in neighborhood health centers to assist the disabled, the aged, or the disadvantaged person obtain needed health care. An ambulatory care center usually provides long-term follow-up care needed by the person with a chronic illness, in addition to preventive health care, diagnostic workups, and treatment of acute illnesses for which hospitalization is unnecessary.

HOME CARE

Before the 1940s the home was the place where medical treatment was given. Well-to-do persons rarely thought of going into a hospital, and they received the services of a private physician in their own home. The family was responsible for the day-to-day care. Poor families were among the first persons to use hospitals. The philosophy of home care can be traced as far back as 1796, when the Boston Dispensary provided medical care to the sick poor in their homes. One of the first institutions to study and demonstrate the advantages of continuous medical care for patients at home was University Hospital in Syracuse, New York, in 1940. By 1950, 16 New York City hospitals were offering this service. In 1959 the Commission on Chronic Illness defined care of the aged and disabled as one of the foremost national health problems and recommended the development of home nursing care as an alternative to institutionalization.

One of the most obvious reasons for the development of home care programs was to provide care to patients with long-term illnesses who did not need the around-the-clock services of an institution and yet who were too ill to go to an outpatient center. Caring for patients at home is what the individual and the family often want, and it also releases hospital beds for use by acutely ill patients.

Frequently the issue arises as to who should pay for home health services and who should be reimbursed for health care provided. The American Nurses Association's (ANA's) position is that reimbursement systems should foster care of individuals in their homes based on the following premises[4]:
1. Home care is humane and respectful of the dignity and integrity of the individual.
2. Home care or care within the community can be less costly than institutional care.
3. Nursing care is the primary element in home care.
4. Payment systems for home care should recognize nurses as the major providers of home care, and as such their services should be reimbursed on their own authority.

Home care is not the solution for all patients. For those living in smaller dwellings, adequate space for the patient and other members of the family may be at a premium. The choice of home care, independent living center, or institutional care will depend largely on the desires of the patient and the family. Despite many inconveniences some families wish to have the patient with them. The family's understanding of the patient and their ability to assist one another will make a great difference in choosing between home care or other living arrangements. Not only may space be inadequate, but many times it is impossible to have a member of the family in attendance with the patient during the day. Members of the family who work cannot afford to sacrifice jobs to stay with the patient. However, many families find it easier financially to have the patient at home and are able to make satisfactory arrangements even though the facilities are limited.

Many communities now provide portable meals (Meals-on-Wheels) for homebound persons. Most programs provide one hot meal daily and unheated food for at least one other meal. The cost differs widely and depends on the services offered, such as special diets, and on the sponsorship of the plan. Volunteer groups frequently act as delivery messengers. The local public health nursing service usually participates actively in the plan by selecting suitable patients and by being a resource for the workers who encounter health problems on their "rounds." This service alone often makes it possible for a chronically ill or aged person to remain at home.

HOME HEALTH AIDE SERVICES

Home health aide services have developed with the increased use of home care plans and particularly since Medicare plans came into existence. The greater number of persons eligible for home health aide services under Medicare has spurred the growth of such services, not because the services were not needed before, but because the cost of such services would have been prohibitive for most of the persons who needed them. Home health aides, who provide actual physical care to the patient, are being trained in many states and are assigned to home care through a central office that coordinates plans of care, often in collaboration with community health nursing agencies. The community health nurse assists by evaluating the home situation and the patient's need for physical personal care. Consequently, the community health nurse supervises the home health aide in the provision of continuing care.

With the emphasis on shorter hospital stays, a number of proprietary agencies have entered the home health care field. These agencies provide a variety of health care services for a fee. Increasingly, insurance companies are reimbursing for these services since it is cheaper to provide care to the patient in his or her own home than in the hospital. Some hospitals are developing their own health care programs in response to the changes in length of stay and in reimbursement. Changes in home health care are occurring very rapidly and nurses will need to keep abreast of changes in their own communities.

HOMEMAKER SERVICES

Homemaker services also have developed with the increased use of home care plans. These services are increasingly in demand in many communities and may be sponsored by a public or voluntary health or welfare agency. Homemakers provide service to families with children and to the person who is convalescing, aged, or acutely or chronically ill. Homemakers are trained to assist in homes where the responsible family manager is temporarily unable to perform his or her usual responsibilities because of illness or absence.

DAY CARE CENTERS

In a number of communities some nursing homes are expanding their facilities and services to include day care centers. There are a great number of chronically ill persons who are able to live with their families, but who require 24-hour attendance. Often the caretaker in the family has to work 8 hours a day. Homemaker or home health aide services are generally not available 8 hours a day, 5 days a week. Day care centers fill this gap in care by providing a place where the chronically ill person can be looked after on a daily basis. Nursing services, physical and occupational therapy, recreational facilities, meals, and in some instances, transportation to and from the center are provided. This kind of service may allow a person to remain at home with the family rather than have to resort to fulltime institutional care.

INDEPENDENT LIVING CENTERS

Some persons with chronic illnesses may be unable to cope with the demands of maintaining a home but wish to live as independently as possible. There are a variety of options available in some communities that range from living units where persons cook their own meals but are provided with maintenance of the living unit to assisted living units where persons can have their own physical living area but are assisted with activities of daily living, as necessary. Living units in such centers are designed with such features as hand rails for support in ambulation or wide doors to facilitate passage of wheelchairs.

INSTITUTIONAL RESOURCES

Many patients and families have to resort to institutional care for the patient because their own facilities are not suitable, no member of the family can be in attendance during the day, community alternatives are not available, or the kind of care needed by the patient requires close professional supervision. A large or a limited selection of outside facilities may be available, depending on the community. These include chronic disease hospitals, skilled care facilities, convalescent homes, rest homes, homes for the aged, and nursing homes. The patient's potential for rehabilitation, need for maintenance care, or the level of physical disability are factors that will determine eligibility for placement in any of these facilities.

FOSTER HOMES

Care in foster homes is a relatively new service that is now being widely used in many communities. Carefully selected families volunteer to take chronically ill persons into their own homes and provide the nonprofessional care that is needed. The family is paid either by the patient or the patient's family, from public funds, or by some social agency. The plan is primarily for those patients who have no family and cannot live alone, but who neither desire nor need institutional care.

Community resources

Nurses must know the community resources available to patients to interpret to them and their families what resources they may be able to obtain, the types of service from which they may benefit, and what kinds of referrals they need for obtaining those services (see list of community resources). When care is to be continued beyond the hospital setting, the hospital nurse should clearly communicate to the continuing care agency data pertinent to the care of the patient to provide continuity in the transfer of services. Teamwork and continuity are the keys to successful rehabilitation and management services for patients, and they must be practiced at all stages of care if patients are to realize their fullest potential.

There has been an increasing interest in providing programs for the chronically ill and in assisting chronically ill or disabled persons to assume a more active role in their communities. Volunteer workers may assist patients, both in hospitals and in homes (Fig. 15-5). Institutions receiving federal funds are required to make aids such as ramps available to individuals who are unable to climb stairs or who are in wheelchairs. With the development of structural changes that facilitate mobility, some persons with physical limitations are becoming more actively involved in local activities and associations. Nurses can assist by supporting the further development

of these structural changes in all community buildings and by encouraging the participation of chronically ill persons in community activities of interest. Various kinds of information may be obtained from national organizations involved with chronic illness and disability. Many of these agencies have services available in the community. Programs, facilities, and legislation of this nature reflect an increasing awareness on the part of the public of the difficulties that are faced by the chronically ill or disabled (see box on pp. 273-274).

OUTCOME CRITERIA FOR THE PERSON WITH A CHRONIC ILLNESS

Discharge outcomes for specific chronic diseases are discussed in the chapters dealing with those diseases. However, it may be stated on a general basis that on discharge from the hospital patients with a chronic disease or their family members should be able to perform the following:

1. Demonstrate or explain those measures that must be taken to avoid further preventable disability.
2. Demonstrate or explain those self-care activities of which they are capable.
3. Identify those activities for which help is needed.
4. Explain who will be available to help them with those activities and on what basis that help will be available.
5. Explain what community resources are available to them for help and how they may obtain that help.
6. Discuss in reasonable detail their plans for follow-up care and reevaluation.

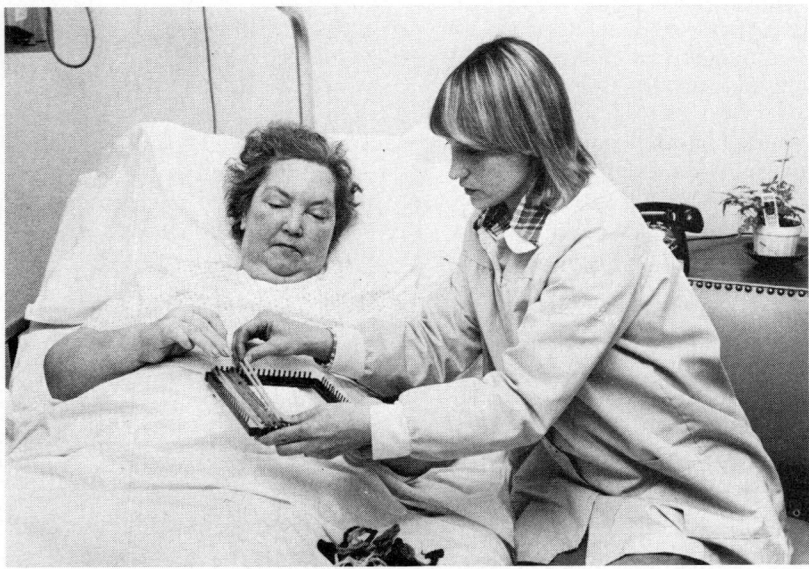

Fig. 15-5. Volunteers can actively involve patients in activities that provide diversion as well as a sense of accomplishment. Nurses often provide assistance or encouragement for completion of projects.

Community resources involved in chronic health problems

Various kinds of information may be obtained by writing these national organizations. In addition, services of the various agencies are usually available at the local level.

General

American Association of Diabetes Education
3553 W. Peterson Ave.
Chicago, IL 60659

American Association of Retired Persons
1909 K St., N.W.
Washington, DC 20006

American Cancer Society
777 3rd Ave.
New York, NY 10017

American Diabetes Association
1 W. 48th St.
New York, NY 10020

American Heart Association
44 E. 23rd St.
New York, NY 10010

American Lung Association
1740 Broadway
New York, NY 10019

American Parkinson Disease Association
147 E. 50th St.
New York, NY 10022

Arthritis Foundation
221 Park Ave. S.
New York, NY 10003

Leukemia Society of America, Inc.
211 E. 43rd St.
New York, NY 10017

Mental Health Materials Center
419 Park Ave. S.
New York, NY 10016

Muscular Dystrophy Association, Inc.
810 7th Ave.
New York, NY 10019

National Aid to Retarded Citizens (formerly N.A.R. Children)
2709 E. St.
Arlington, TX 76011

National Association for Visually Handicapped
305 E. 24th St.
New York, NY 10010

National Asthma Center
875 Avenue of the the Americas
New York, NY 10001

National Council on the Aging
1828 L. St. NW
Washington, DC 20036

National Kidney Foundation
116 E. 27th St.
New York, NY 10016

National Multiple Sclerosis Society
205 E. 42nd St.
New York, NY 10017

Nutrition Foundation, Inc.
489 5th Ave.
New York, NY 10017

Stroke Clubs of America
805 12th St.
Galveston, TX 77550

United Ostomy Association
1111 Wilshire Blvd.
Los Angeles, CA 90017

Rehabilitation

American Coalition of Citizens with Disabilities
1346 Connecticut Ave. N.W., Rm. 817
Washington, DC 20036

Architectural and Transportation Barriers Compliance Board
330 C St. W.W., Rm. 1010
Washington, DC 20201

Closer Look, National Information Center for the Handicapped
Box 1492
Washington, DC 20013

Mainstream, Inc.
1200 15th St., N.W., Rm. 403
Washington, DC 20005

Continued.

Community resources involved in chronic health problems—cont'd

Rehabilitation—cont'd

National Center for a Barrier-free Environment
8401 Connecticut Ave.
Washington, DC 20015

National Center for Law and the Handicapped
1235 N. Eddy St.
South Bend, IN 46617

National Congress of Organizations of the Physically
   Handicapped
7611 Oakland Ave.
Minneapolis, MN 55432

National Paraplegia Foundation
333 N. Michigan Ave.
Chicago, IL 60601

Paralyzed Veterans of America
7315 Wisconsin Ave. N.W.
Washington, DC 20014

President's Committee on Employment of the
   Handicapped
111 20th St. N.W., Rm. 636
Washington, DC 20210

Prevention/wellness

American Association of Fitness Directors in Business
   and Industry
President's Council on Physical Fitness and Sports
Room 3030
400 Sixth Ave. S.W.
Washington, DC 20201

Bureau of Health Education
Centers for Disease Control
Atlanta, GA 30333

Center for Health Promotion
American Hospital Association
840 N. Lake Shore Dr.
Chicago, IL 60611

Know Your Body Project
American Health Foundation
320 East 43rd St.
New York, NY 10017

Society of Prospective Medicine
Department of Family Medicine
University of South Florida
12901 North 30th St.
Tampa, FL 33612

Well Aware About Health
University of Arizona Health Sciences Center
P.O. Box 43338
Tucson, AZ 85733

Wellness Associates
42 Miller Ave.
Mill Valley, CA 94941

Wholistic Health Center
137 S. Garfield Ave.
Hinsdale, IL 60521

Focus on the future

Five measurable and achievable national goals for public health action have been identified in the 1979 surgeon general's report.[28] These goals include one major goal for each major age group in our society. The time frame for the achievement of these goals is between now and 1990. The goals are concerned with the major health problems and the preventable risks for diseases throughout the life span. These goals and their realtionship to chronic health problems follow:

1. *To continues to improve infant health and, by 1990, to reduce infant mortality by at least 35%, to fewer than 9 deaths per 1000 live births.* The two principal threats to infant survival and good health are low birth weight and congenital disorders, including birth defects. Low birth weight may be associated with long-term health problems such as mental retardation, cerebral palsy, and other con-

ditions that impede growth and development. Many birth defects, including congenital disorders, mental retardation, and genetic diseases are immediate serious hazards to infants. Many others, if not diagnosed and treated immediately after birth or during the first year of life, can affect health and well-being in the later years.

2. *To improve child health, foster optimal childhood development, and, by 1990, to reduce deaths among people aged 1 to 14 years by at least 20%, to fewer than 34 per 100,000.* The major cause of death among children is accidents, followed by cancer, birth defects, influenza and pneumonia, and homicide. But not all health problems are reflected in mortality figures. Habits and attitudes developed during childhood can lead to adult disease and disability. As many as 40% of school children ages 11 to 14 are estimated to already have one or more of the risk factors associated with heart disease: overweight, high

blood pressure, high blood cholesterol, cigarette smoking, poor physical fitness, or diabetes.

3. *To improve the health and health habits of adolescents and young adults and, by 1990, to reduce deaths among people aged 15 to 24 by at least 20%, to fewer than 9.3 per 100,000.* Despite improvements in health over the past 75 years, death rates for adolescents and young adults are increasing. The principal health problems of this age group include violent death and injury, sexually transmitted diseases, alcohol and drug abuse, and emotional problems. Young men are at particular risk, since their death rate is almost three times that of young women. Although chronic diseases are not among the major causes of death at this period of life, the life-styles and behavioral patterns that are shaped during these years may determine later susceptibility to chronic diseases.

4. *To improve the health of adults, and, by 1990, to reduce deaths among people aged 25 to 64 by at least 25%, to fewer than 400 per 100,000.* The leading causes of death in this age group are heart disease, cancer, stroke, and cirrhosis of the liver. Accidents are a prominent problem for the younger members of this group, but overall the chronic diseases predominate. In addition to causes of death, disability from mental illness presents a major health problem. More than one third of all deaths in this group are caused by cardiovascular diseases, principally coronary artery disease and stroke. However, such deaths have declined in recent years and account for most of the recent decreases in mortality.

5. *To improve the health and quality of life for older adults and, by 1990, to reduce the average annual number of days of restricted activity due to acute and chronic conditions by 20%, to fewer than 30 days per year for people aged 65 and over.* Today there are 24 million people aged 65 years and over in the United States, accounting for 11% of the population. This group is the fastest growing segment of the population. By the year 2030 there will be more than 50 million Americans in the over-65 group, and they will represent nearly 17% of the population. The leading causes of death for this age group are heart disease, cancer, stroke, influenza, and pneumonia. The long-term goal of a health-promotion and disease-prevention strategy for older people must be not only to achieve further increases in longevity but also to allow such individuals to seek independent and rewarding lives in older age, unlimited by the many health problems that are within their capacity to control.

Even though it is possible to identify health goals for a nation, it is far more difficult to carry them out so that the effect is noticeable to the individual seeking health care.

The challenge of providing health care to all people includes the challenge to promote the full participation of individuals with physical and mental disabilities. The United Nations proclaimed 1981 as the International Year of Disabled Persons (IYDP). The United States Council for the IYDP has worked to strengthen public understanding of the needs and contributions of 35 million people. The council has defined the following long-term national goals of and for the disabled:

1. Expanded educational opportunities
2. Improved access to housing, buildings, and transportation
3. Greater opportunity for employment
4. Broader recreational, social, and cultural activities
5. Expanded and strengthened rehabilitation programs and facilities
6. Increased biomedical research aimed at conquering major disabling conditions
7. Reduced incidence of disability through accident and disease prevention
8. Increased application of technology on behalf of persons with disabilities
9. Expanded international exchange of information and experience to benefit the disabled everywhere

The commitment of health care providers must be not only to find ways to help the disabled and other chronically ill individuals cope with chronic health problems but also to educate individuals in the prevention of disease and the promotion of health.

REFERENCES AND SELECTED READINGS*
Contemporary

1. Albee, G.: In Curtis, N., editor: Self help reporter, 3(4):Sept.-Oct. 1977.
2. American Academy of Nursing: Long-term care: some issues for nursing, Kansas City, Mo., 1976, American Nurses Association.
3. American Cancer Society: 1983 Cancer facts and figures, New York, 1982, The American Cancer Society.
4. American Nurses Association: A national policy for health care: principles and positions, 1977, American Nurses Association.
5. *Anderson, S.V., and Bauwens, E.E.: Chronic health problems: concepts and application, St. Louis, 1981, The C.V. Mosby Co.
6. Boroch, R.M.: Elements of rehabilitation in nursing, St. Louis, 1976, The C.V. Mosby Co.
7. Expectation of life in the United States at a new high, Stat. Bull. **61**(4):13-15, 1980.
8. Hirschberg, G.G., Lewis, L., and Vaughn, P.: Rehabilitation: a manual for the care of the physically disabled and elderly, ed.2, Philadelphia, 1976, J.B. Lippincott Co.
9. Kalisch, P.A., and Kalisch, B.J.: Nursing involvement in the health planning process, DHEW pub. no. (HRA) 78-25, Hyattsville, Md., 1977, U.S. Department of Health, Education, and Welfare.
10. Kottke, F., Stilwell, G.K., and Lehman, J.: Krusen's handbook of physical medicine and rehabilitation, ed. 3, Philadelphia, 1982, W.B. Saunders Co.
11. Lawson, B.A.: Chronic illness in the school aged child: effects on the total family. In Anderson, S.V., and Bauwens, E.E.: Chronic health problems: concepts and application, St. Louis, 1981, The C.V. Mosby Co.
12. Lekowitz, B.: Health differentials between white and nonwhite Americans, Washington, D.C., 1977, U.S. Government Printing Office.

---

*References preceded by an asterisk are particularly well suited for student reading.

13. *Leslie, F.M.: Nursing diagnosis: use in long-term care, Am. J. Nurs. **81:**1012-1014, 1981.

14. *Martin, N., Holt, N.B., and Hicks, D.: Comprehensive rehabilitation nursing, New York, 1981, McGraw-Hill Book Co.

15. Morris, R., editor: Allocating health resources for the aged and disabled, Lexington, Mass., 1981, Lexington Books.

16. National Center for Health Statistics: State estimates of disability and utilization of medical services: United States, 1974-76, DHEW pub. no. (PHS) 78-1241, Washington, D.C., 1978, U.S. Government Printing Office.

17. Public Health Service: Vital and health statistics—current estimates from the Health Interview Survey (1981). U.S. Department of Health, Education and Welfare, series 10, no. 141, Rockville, Md., Sept. 1981.

18. Public Health Service: Vital and health statistics—health characteristics of persons with chronic activity limitations (1979), U.S. Department of Health and Human Services, series 10, no. 137, Rockville, Md., Oct. 1981.

19. Rettig, R.A.: End-stage renal disease and the cost of medical technology. In Altman, S.H., and Blendon, R.J., editors.; Medical technology: the culprit behind health care costs? DHEW pub. no. PHS-79-3216, Washington, D.C., 1979, U.S. Government Printing Office.

20. Rush, H.: Rehabilitation medicine, ed. 4, St. Louis, 1977, The C.V. Mosby Co.

21. Sternberg, F.U., editor: the care of the geriatric patient, ed. 6, St. Louis, 1983, The C.V. Mosby Co.

22. Stewart, J.E.: Home health care, St. Louis, 1979, The C.V. Mosby Co.

23. Strauss, A.L.: Chronic illness and the quality of life, St. Louis, 1975, The C.V. Mosby Co.

24. Stryker, R.: Rehabilitative aspects of acute and chronic nursing care, ed. 2, 1977, Philadelphia, W.B. Saunders Co.

25. Thom, A.: Home health care agencies in the 1980s, Home Health Care Serv. Q. **3:**5-24, 1982.

26. U.S. Congress, House Committee on Interstate and Foreign Commerce: National Health Promotion and Disease Prevention Act, 1976.

27. U.S. Department of Health, Education and Welfare: Final mortality statistics, 1977, DHEW pub. no. PHS-79-1120, Washington, D.C., 1979, U.S. Government Printing Office.

28. U.S. Department of Health, Education and Welfare: Healthy people: surgeon general's report on health promotion and disease prevention, Washington, D.C., 1979, U.S. Government Printing Office.

29. *Wright, B.A.: Value-laden beliefs and principles for rehabilitation, Rehabil. Lit. **42:**266-269, 1981.

Classic

30. Christopherson, V.A.: Role modifications of the disabled male, Am. J. Nurs. **68:**290-293, 1968.

31. Crate, M.: Nursing functions in adaptation to chronic illness, Am. J. Nurs. **65:**72-76, 1965.

32. *Martin, N., King, R., and Suchinski, J. The nurse therapist in the rehabilitation setting, Am. J. Nurs. **70:**1694-1697, 1970.

33. *Palmer, I.S., editor: Nursing in long-term illness, Nurs. Clin. N. Am. **5:**1-84, 1970.

34. Moskowitz, E., and McCann, C.B.: Classification of disability in the chronically ill and aging, J. Chronic Dis. **5:**342-346, 1957.

35. Olson, E.V., editor: The hazards of immobility, Am. J. Nurs. **67:**780-797, 1967.

36. *Riffe, K.L., editor, The patient with long-term illness, Nurs. Clin. N. Am. **8:**571-681, 1973.

37. *Sorensen, K., and Amis, D.B.: Understanding the world of the chronically ill, Am. J. Nurs. **67:**811-817, 1967.

38. Talbot, H.S.: A concept of rehabilitation, Rehabil. Lit. **22:**358-359, 1961.

16

Dimensions of Dying and Death

BENITA C. MARTOCCHIO

STUDY QUESTIONS

- What is the difference between dying and death?

- Do you think nurses respond differently to the death of a child as compared to that of an elderly person? What are some of the reasons?

- What resources are available in your community for assistance in the care of terminally ill persons?

Despite the amazing advances of science, technology, and nursing and medical knowledge, people die. Dying is and will continue to be a part of living. It is difficult to think of dying as a part of living. It is easier to think of living at one end of a continuum and dying at the other; however, living and dying are *not* the opposite ends of a continuum. They are *not* the opposite sides of the same coin; they are the same coin.

If we are to care successfully for dying persons and their families, we must simultaneously think living even as we think dying. Since there is no word in the English language that incorporates both, as you read this chapter, think living as you read dying. Think about it: you interact with a *living* person who is known to be dying. You identify with the suffering and the sorrows of living persons as they live their dying.

It is the purpose of this chapter to share understandings and to offer guidelines to assist in caring for persons who are living while dying and to assist their family members who are sharing the experience. There are guidelines for caring for dying persons, but there are no recipes, nor should there be. There are great variations in how people live their living. It should come as no great surprise then that there are great variations in how people live while dying. The best way to learn to care for dying persons and their families is to observe and to grow to understand the process and all its dimensions.

SOCIETAL AND SOCIAL DIMENSIONS

Dying and death are different

Dying is different than death. *Dying,* a part of living, is a *process*—the process of coming to an end. *Death,* the permanent cessation of all vital functions, the end of human life, is an *event* and a *state.* The event is the moment of death; the state is that of being dead.[7]

Both dying and death have unique aspects that evoke fears, anxieties, and uncertainties. Some aspects of dying, such as physical and emotional pain, the loss of others, the inability to function in familiar ways, may occur under other circumstances (for example, illness, retirement, relocation) and therefore are not unique to dying. The unique aspect of dying is that it ends in death. Death is a unique event. People have no prior experiences to help them to understand what it means to be dead. Questions surface: Can a dead person think? Can they have feelings? What is it like to be dead? Is there another life? Where will they go?

My death: your death

The very thought of dying and its endpoint, death, evokes feelings of fear, anxiety, and uncertainty.[5,6] The knowledge that death is imminent or probable within a predicted period of time adds reality to these feelings. As a result, feelings of persons facing imminent death are experienced in a different way than those of healthy persons who are speculating about what it is like to be dying. Healthy persons speak of death in the abstract; they talk about the death of another or project it into the distant future. People cannot imagine the actual end of their own lives on earth. The fact that they can continue to think about others who have died causes them to conceive a continuity beyond death. Casual comments such as, "We all have to die some day," "We are all dying from the time we are born," or "Everyone has to die of something," reflect what Freud called "unconscious immortality." In other words, we have an unconscious but strong belief in our own immortality. Others die but we live.

The unconscious belief in our own immortality is neither good nor bad; it just is. The casual comments just stated are neither good nor bad in and of themselves. They offer little in the way of understanding or support, however, when made to a dying person or to their families. The statements are usually in response to the discomfort we feel when someone tells us that death is imminent. Hearing of someone else's dying or death forces us to face our own finiteness. For a brief moment we glance more directly at the possibility of "my" death rather than "your" death. In such instances we may quickly respond to the news of someone's dying. "Everyone has to die of something" or "We are all dying from the time we are born," to dispel our own anxiety or discomfort. A more understanding response might be "I'm sorry to hear that."

Views toward dying and death vary considerably depending on whether the discussion is about *my* death or *your* death or if the discussion is about a member of my family or your family.

Even when we are discussing hypothetic situations, our closeness to dying or to a dying person can influence our views and our responses. The same data are seen differently from different perspectives. We can use age as a common factor and consider how our responses may change. For example, *my* father is 75 years old, and *your* father is 75 years old. When death appears imminent, our thoughts may vary depending on the referent of *my* or *your* father. For example, *my* father is still young; *your* father has lived a long and a good life.

It is important to identify the referent under discussion whether we are talking in theoretic terms or about practical situations. In other words, from whose perspective are we evaluating the situation, my perspective, your perspective, the patient's perspective, or a family member's perspective?

Lack of recognition of different perspectives leads to poor communication, faulty nursing judgments, and inappropriate nursing interventions.

Age and premature death

There was a time when people did not make a connection between aging, loss of bodily functioning, or general progressive debilitation and dying. For example, primitive people believed that if there were no accidents or magically induced illnesses, no one would die.

The expectations of living have changed as life expectancies have changed. During the Roman period, life expectancy was 20 years and increased to about 35 during the Middle Ages. By the late 1800's Americans could anticipate living 50 years; few persons lived into their 60's or 70's. In contemporary American life, people not only anticipate living more than 70 years, they expect to do so as active functioning individuals.

Any age is too young to die. In contemporary society, death is perceived as unnecessary, premature, and clinically unnecessary. The concept of clinical death is well entrenched.[4] People do not die of natural causes or of old age. They die while receiving treatment for a recognized diagnosed clinical problem, for example, heart disease, stroke, disseminated intravascular coagulation (DIC), or total body failure. As a consequence, many deaths can be interpreted as avoidable, unnecessary, and premature.

If death is always interpreted as avoidable, unnecessary, or premature, it follows that someone must be blamed. Who can we blame—the physician, the hospital, society? Perhaps we blame the person who died for not getting help sooner, for surely if they had sought help sooner they would not have died. It is this interpretation of death as always being avoidable that contributes to conflict and guilt. People die; death is a part of living. We can give the best care we know and people will die. In fact sometimes the very mechanisms that save lives create dilemmas by prolonging life or, perhaps, dying.

Prolonged dying

Just as there is concern over premature death, there is concern over prolonged dying. Through modern technology we have become adept at maintaining life in the desperately ill person. Unfortunately, at times the same techniques used to maintain life during temporary crises, create dilemmas related to what constitutes life. When are we prolonging dying rather than life? Our ability to prolong dying leads to many moral and ethical issues related to life (What is quality of life?) and to death (What is the definition of death?).

Tension rises as there are disagreements over whether modern therapies should be continued or discontinued. Questions are raised about the rights of dying persons.

Rights of dying persons

Some consumers are demanding that dying and death no longer be hidden behind closed doors. As a consequence, there is a movement to recognize that dying persons have rights. These rights have been identified and, in some cases, written.[1,2]

One right of dying persons is the right to know they are seriously ill and that they may die. The assumption is that if persons know they are seriously ill and that they may die, they will have more control over what happens to them. They can participate in decisions about their care and can complete unfinished business.

Another right is to die in an atmosphere of hopefulness. Persons have a right to die in peace and dignity unencumbered by tubes and machines and surrounded by loved ones. They have a right to privacy. Dying persons are entitled to be cared for by sensitive, caring, knowledgable people who attempt to understand them and their loved ones. They are entitled to die as free from pain or other discomforts as is possible. Comfort contributes to dying with dignity.

THE LIVING WILL

The concern that patients be allowed to die with dignity has led to the development of the living will. The living will is a document that is directed toward any individual who may become responsible for the person's health, welfare, or affairs. It may be directed toward the person's family, lawyer, clergyperson, or physician or representatives of any medical facility in which the person may be.

Living wills generally request that under conditions when (1) the individual can no longer take part in decisions about his or her own future, and (2) there is no reasonable expectation for recovery, the individual be allowed to die and not be kept alive through use of artificial or extraordinary means. Most wills also request that the person be kept free of suffering and pain although the medications may hasten the moment of death.

At the present time, living wills are not legally enforceable in all states. In addition, there are many questions related to the conditions under which a living will can or should be honored. What is important for purposes of this chapter is that a living will can help care givers and family members to know what the dying person's wishes were, at least at the time of the writing.

Copies of living wills are usually given to family members, physicians, the person's attorney, and a member of the clergy. People are advised to sign and date them, at least yearly. The wills are more likely to be honored if they are written or signed immediately before the person's becoming unable to express his or her own wishes about dying care.

A sharing of philosophy of life and desires related to the process of dying with loved ones and primary health care providers is perhaps a more effective way of assuring death with dignity or what has been referred to as a "Good Death."

Good death/bad death

Many nurses, and in fact people in general, express concern over dying with dignity or dying a "good" death. Is there such a thing as a "good death?" There is no one "good" death but many. There is no one right way to die; just as there is no proper way to die.

The question of what constitutes a good death is as difficult to answer as it is easy to ask. There are as many views about what constitutes a good death as there are

---

Example of a living will

To my family, my physician, my lawyer, my clergyman
To any medical facility in whose care I happen to be
To any individual who may become responsible for my health, welfare, or affairs

Death is as much a reality as birth, growth, maturity, and old age; it is the one certainty of life. If the time comes when I, (Name), can no longer take part in decisions for my own future, let this statement stand as an expression of my wishes, while I am still of sound mind.

If the situation should arise in which there is no reasonable expectation of my recovery from physical or mental disability, I request that I be allowed to die and not be kept alive by artificial means or "heroic measures." I do not fear death itself as much as the indignities of deterioration, dependence, mental incapacity, and hopeless pain. I, therefore, ask that medication be mercifully administered to me to alleviate suffering even though this may hasten the moment of death.

This request is made after careful consideration. I hope you who care for me will feel morally bound to follow its mandate. I recognize that this appears to place a heavy responsibility on you, but it is with the intention of relieving you of such responsibility and of placing it on myself in accordance with my strong convictions, that this statement is made.

_____ (Signature)

Witnessed
Copies to: (names of persons)

people. To die as one lived; to die without pain; to die in the company of loved ones are all answers.

There are many ways to die well. A good death involves individual perceptions of the living-dying process as well as shared observations of the death event. A death is more likely to be labeled as good when dying is viewed as a part of living and not as a separate phenomenon. A good death also is associated with the way all persons involved interact with each other preceding and during the event. The death is more likely to be seen as good if there is harmony than if there is conflict.

Sometimes nurses refer to deaths as normal or abnormal. Normal deaths are seen as good deaths. Deaths are perceived as normal or good when most or all persons involved perceive that all was done that could be done, that the actions were appropriate and accepted by most persons involved. In these instances there is a sense of loss, but the loss is accompanied by a sense of fulfillment and closure.

Nurses label deaths as bad or abnormal when there is conflict over the type of treatment, the length of treatment, and when there are bad feelings about a lack of honesty, especially with family members.

One can see that whether a death is seen as good or bad does not always have to do entirely with the way the person died. Sometimes it has to do with who is present and how they interpret what is happening in the situation. People's attitudes toward dying influence how they interpret the situation and how they act and interact with others.

ATTITUDINAL DIMENSIONS

Death denial, death defiance, death desire, and death acceptance are four prevailing societal attitudes toward death. As these general attitudes are discussed, it is important to remember that there are no pure attitudes that exist in all situations. (Remember the differences in responses with *my* death and *your* death.)

The descriptions of these societal attitudes is based on responses and actions of many people. They may be reflected in each of us but should not be directly applied or expected from any of us. Recognition of the prevailing attitudes helps us to understand the process of dying and serves as a guide when interacting with others. If we are aware there are basic differences in attitudes, we may recognize the differences and accept them for what they are. In doing so many conflicts among health professionals can be avoided. More importantly, a recognition of the attitudinal bases of all persons in the situation enhances communication and thus patient care. It is quality care for dying persons and family members that must remain our constant goal.

No attitude is good or bad. They are only different. Our attitudes may enhance or distract depending on the situation and how the attitude is manifested. In other words, our attitudes are reflected in our behavior. If we recognize our own attitudes toward dying and death in a particular situation, we may better understand why we feel the way we do and why we are acting the way we are. Just as importantly, if we recognize the attitudinal stance of others in the situation, we may better understand their perspectives and behavior.

Recognition and understanding of another person's perspective may not always lead to mutual agreement, but it can contribute to understanding and to decreased conflict in decision making. These attitudes will be explored briefly in the following sections.

Death denial

Western society has been described as a death denying society.[11] Many people avoid the subject of dying and death. We may speak of mass deaths, but speaking of individuals' dying or death has been described as a taboo topic. Health professionals, particularly physicians have been described as avoiding talking to patients about their dying.[12] Persons, whether health professionals or family members, maintain a death-denying stance and often justify their stance by expressing the belief that they are "protecting" the dying person.

In taking a death-denying stance, we are protecting someone. The question is, *who* are we protecting? In most situations, we protect ourselves. Consciously or unconsciously, we weigh the impact on ourselves of acting or of not acting. If we become involved in conversation about "hard things" like dying, then we must be prepared for a reaction or response. It is the reaction or response we usually fear. Even a lack of overt reaction is a response. The following questions arise in our minds:

What will happen to us?

Will the other person shout, cry, become angry?

Will the family become angry?

Will the physician become angry?

Will I know what to do or say?

What if they do not react at all?

In nursing, speaking of a death–denying attitude has taken on a negative connotation, but remember, no attitude is good or bad—it just is. For example, a death–denying attitude may contribute to a lack of open communication about dying, but it may also contribute to continuing care in bleak situations. This latter situation may also be an example of death defiance.

Death defiance

Defiance of death is a part of the Judeo-Christian heritage. Throughout the ages people have fought for causes or ideologies, despite knowing that they might die in the attempt. The attitude is reflected in hospitals, especially in critical care units or during emergency situations. The cause is to save a life; the battle is with death.

Although it is not the staff who die in the battle, they are open to loss. If the patient dies, the staff lives with the sense of a battle lost. Moreover, they face once again the finiteness of their own lives and the inevitability of death, despite modern technology.

Death defiance is helpful as we fight for life; it is not

helpful when we do not also attend to the realities of the situation.

Death acceptance

Death acceptance is viewing death as a normal, natural, and integral part of living. Becker,[11] a prominent philosopher, defined the resignation to and acceptance of our limited existence as the central task for achieving maturity. With this acceptance, death becomes the conclusion of life's plan. It sounds so simple. It calms the fears and pains of dying, of facing our own immortality. But like the other attitudes toward death, this attitude is not a panacea. In fact, Schneidman[10] helps us to regain our perspective when he points out how romantic this attitude can be.

Death acceptance is for some the ultimate achievement of maturation, a form of self-actualization. The maturation is the dying persons'; it is not an attitude to be forced on them by others.

Remember, the worth of the attitude is in the effectiveness of its use for dying persons. It is not to be judged as a static good or bad phenomenon in and of itself.

Desire for death

The fourth attitude, the desire for death, is more common in our society than people generally know or like to admit. People may desire their own death or the death of others.

Many circumstances give rise to the desire to die or for someone else to die. One major reason is the search for relief from misery. Misery takes many forms; pain, loneliness, disability, fear, uncertainty, and economic and emotional crises are but a few.

There are other reasons contributing to the desire to die. Most are associated with a relief from misery but are expressed in a different way. Some persons search for reunion with loved ones. Still others look forward to death as a last phase in the fulfillment of life.

Recognition of how people express their desire to die is important. In many instances the expression of the desire to die is the dying person's or family member's way of confirming their recognition that death is inevitable within a predictable period of time in the near future.

DIMENSIONS OF DYING PERSONS

Confirmation that death—the event—may occur in the near future rather than in the distant future raises another question. Who is the dying person?

Thus far we have discussed dying and death in somewhat global terms. Now let us turn more directly to discussing dying persons and their characteristics.

Chronicity of dying

The nature of dying has changed. Because of modern therapies and technology, patterns of illness have shifted from acute infectious diseases to chronic conditions; as a result, dying has become a chronic process. With the exception of some acute problems such as myocardial infarction, severe infections, and fatal accidents, most dying persons experience chronic problems with multiple pathophysiologic alterations. These alterations are usually permanent and result in disability with a need to adjust to loss and to accommodate to change. The multiple series of loss can affect the person's behavioral responses and ability to cope.

Dying takes on the characteristics of chronic illness. Dying persons, just as other chronically ill persons, express feelings of being socially displaced or isolated. They grieve over the loss of former activities and abilities. They express sorrow over the continued loss of friends, business associates, and acquaintances. They talk of being alive and yet not able to live. They are expected to be present rather than future oriented.

Persons may be healthy and yet viewed as chronically ill or dying. Whenever the anticipated life span is *perceived as shortened,* a person may be viewed as chronically ill or dying and treated accordingly. With increasing age, the anticipated life remaining is shortened, and adjustments may be made regarding allocation of time, effort, and resources. Some elderly persons are perceived and perceive themselves as not having enough time left to make future oriented plans or decisions. The same perception is associated with some persons with diagnoses associated with dying and disability, such as cancer, stroke, and multiple sclerosis. Unfortunately, some people may perceive themselves or be perceived by others as not deserving services or not being worthy of the efforts of others, since they will not live long enough.

Thus dying persons may be displaced, isolated individuals, not allowed to live their living. Furthermore, the chronicity of their dying may force them into experiencing a social death while they are functionally and biologically very much alive.

Many factors contribute to promoting social dying long before the event of death; these factors will be discussed.

Stages and phases of dying

Kübler-Ross[14] has been credited as the first person to describe a series of stages through which people pass in response to their dying.

Kübler-Ross' stages of dying

Shock and disbelief
Denial
Anger
Bargaining
Depression
Acceptance

Physicians and nurse scientists, family members, and dying persons have challenged the accuracy and more importantly the usefulness of the stages of dying.

Weisman[17] identified no well-defined behavioral responses typical of individual persons facing death. He believed the notion of stages of dying was artificial and suggested changing phases of dying instead. Schultz and Aderman[16] also disagreed with Kübler-Ross' stages of dying. They found that each dying person adapted a specific way of responding and maintained that pattern until death.

Three phases of dying—acute, chronic living-dying, and terminal—were proposed by Pattison (1977) as clinically useful for understanding the behaviors accompanying dying.

A dying person's wife, who lovingly cared for her husband throughout his long illness and dying, stated her disillusionment in the following way:

I've had it; I just can't take it anymore. He's unconscious; he just lies there. That's not him. It's a terrible thing, I just can't stand to look at him anymore. It's terrible that Kübler-Ross makes it sound so easy. Well, she surely oversimplified things. I never knew it was going to be anything like this . . . She doesn't tell you anything about the way it's really going to be.[17]

This and the following statement by Jory Graham,[3] a well-known journalist and person dying with cancer, is certainly something to think about.

Dr. Elisabeth Kübler-Ross, who popularized the erroneous idea that people die in stages, taught that step I of the dying process was denial and isolation, and emphasized denial in a way I do not understand. I remember one of her students (a therapist) showing me a film of an interview with a dying patient. Suddenly she leaned forward and said, "Watch, watch his denial." I was shocked. Why should therapists be so hell-bent on pinning down examples of denial? That seemed unnecessarily pejorative to me. Furthermore, if one stresses denial, it becomes exceedingly difficult to understand that for some individuals denial has a far more positive quality: hope.

The challenges to the stages do not mean Kübler-Ross had no contribution to make. It means that just as with the attitudes discussed previously, the stages offer us some ideas of how *some people may respond, not how all people will respond or should respond.*

The stages and phases of dying are sensitizing schemes to help us in being open to assessing what is "going on" in a situation so that we may understand it better. Our ultimate goal is quality care for dying persons and their families. Understanding, observation, and assessment assist in determining appropriate intervention to better achieve that goal.

Patterns of living-dying

Another tool to help understand the nature of dying is the patterns of living-dying described by Martocchio,[7,8] and confirmed by Dufault.[6]

The four major patterns and their various combinations are based on the clinical courses of dying patients. They describe what has occurred, not what will occur. In other words, they are descriptive *not* predictive. They are useful for understanding the variations of behavior among dying persons. They also demonstrate the futility of expecting persons to pass through a series of stages of behavior in any fixed sequence.

PEAKS AND VALLEYS PATTERN

The pattern of peaks and valleys is characterized by a period of greater health (peaks) and periods of crises (valleys). Dying persons refer to the peaks as "hopeful highs" and the valleys as "terrible or depressing lows." Although there are times of greater health, the overall course is downward to the event of death. Many hospitalizations and many moments of increased expectation and dashed hopes are associated with the experience of dying in this pattern. Yet dashed hopes may be revived by recalling valleys that gave rise to peaks.

The uncertainties are great; fluctuations in behavior are to be expected as goals and plans change. Difficulties in planning and in adjustment are to be expected.

DESCENDING PLATEAUS PATTERN

The pattern of descending plateaus is characterized by an unpredictable number of progressive degenerative steps with plateaus (periods of stable health) lasting an indeterminate period of time. Again, the overall general course is downward. People do not return to their former level of health or functioning after each crisis. Like the peaks and valleys pattern, the course if fraught with uncertainty or whether another crisis will occur and cause more debilitation.

This pattern is associated with expressions of futility and anger. Dying persons and family grieve the loss of functional ability after concerted rehabilitative efforts to maintain or regain abilities.

DOWNWARD SLOPES PATTERN

The downward slopes pattern, the third pattern, is characterized by a consistent, persistent, easily discernible downward course. Unlike the other patterns, death is expected within a predictable period of time measured in hours or days. In most instances, the dying person loses consciousness, and there is little time to prepare family members for the death of their loved one.

GRADUAL SLANTS PATTERN

The fourth pattern of living-dying, gradual slants, is characterized by an ebb of life, gradually and almost imperceptibly culminating in death. Generally these persons experience a debilitating bodily insult from which there is little recovery. In many instances the person is no longer conscious and life is maintained by life support systems, such as respirators.

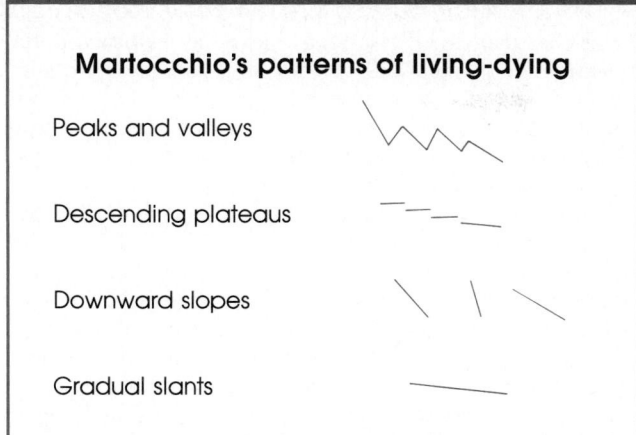

Martocchio's patterns of living-dying

Peaks and valleys

Descending plateaus

Downward slopes

Gradual slants

This pattern is associated with many of the following questions:

When should life support systems be discontinued?

Where should these persons be cared for?

Who should be repsonsible for their care?

In reality, many combinations of the four patterns may occur in one person's experience of living-dying. For example, a person's pattern may change from peaks and valleys to a downward slope, or from a downward slope to a gradual slant.

Choice: a right

Choice is the act of selecting from options. The question is not whether dying persons should be told their fate, but whether they are given the opportunity *to know* or *not to know*. All persons eventually learn of their fate. The circumstances under which they learn and the approach of the persons giving the information are of great importance.

Dying persons describe a system of filtering out or listening to that which they wish to know or to realize. They tell us of how they listen to or look at the facts initially but do not hear them or see them until later. People allow the facts to permeate their minds at their own pace. Dying people, or any person facing an extreme crisis, can describe reaching an emotional readiness when they suddenly hear or see the facts and wonder how long they have been there. Sometimes facts have to be introduced more than once by various people and in various ways. Sometimes patients look for confirmation of what they heard or what they saw—of what they think they know.

The person who recognizes that death is imminent but is not allowed to talk about it or is locked behind an impermeable wall of silence with no way to escape to the comfort of loving arms or to the closeness of a relationship with a loved one. No one should be condemned to such total isolation. No rationalization or self-protection exists to support such punishment of dying persons or their loved ones.

How does this happen? Fear is probably the greatest cause. Families and health care providers blunder into subterfuge and into tragedy. No one anticipates all the lies that will be needed to support the first lie. No one anticipates the energy that will be spent futilely guarding the secret that all know.

Whether the dying person is cared for at home or in the hospital, it is difficult to live a lie 24 hours a day. Television, magazines, and even visits from clergy become a major threat. What if the clergy member should tell? What is there is a program on TV or an article in the journal and the patient figures it out? Even friends and uninformed health professionals constitute a new threat. The impermeable wall grows wider with each added threat until it surrounds and isolates everyone.

What of the tremendous hurt and anger when the truth becomes recognized, and it eventually will become recognized. Would the person have chosen to live differently during the time that can never be returned? What of the confidence the person may have had in the nurses, physicians, and health system? Will the trust be regained or does the person now have to cope with feelings toward dying and inconsolable feelings of loss and injustice toward those who were expected to be trusted and helpful?

There are patients who sincerely choose not to see or to hear, who choose not to know. If that is their *informed choice*, then it is not appropriate to push them to know that which they do not wish to see or to hear. To force them to see or hear that which they wish to deny is as cruel and as inhumane as the conspiracy of silence. The refusal of the patient to know or to discuss the facts creates its own set of problems.

Role of confidant

Nurses can introduce the element of choice by fulfilling the need for a confidant who will initiate and allow honest talk. The role of confidant is a necessary but not an easy role. Talking of dying is not easy and periods of awkwardness and expressions of fear are inevitable.

Dying persons look to the confidant for honesty and acceptance as they search for understanding of their state. They are not searching for pity, consolation, or sympathy. They are uncomfortable with the pity and helplessness that they see in the eyes of others.

They look to the confidant to voice their deepest fears. We do not voice such fears to business associates; we cannot expect casual friends to understand. We do not reveal our most terrible anxieties to those we love; we protect them from our panic. There are great risks to seeking information about that which we most dread; what we dread most might be confirmed. There is also the superstition that lurks in our minds, that what is said might happen or come true; therefore, if we do not talk about it, it will not happen. The result is silence and fear.

The role of confidant is primarily to listen and to reassure as the dying person grapples with the experience of dying. The confidant can help to make the period of shifting from living to dying a time for deepening feelings of closeness; a time for reinforcing family relationships; a time to say what needs to be done and said.

Dying: an achievement or a failure

The use made of dying is a factor that influences the dying person's behavior. Although most dying people express resentment, fear, or sorrow over the major changes in their lives forced on them by their progressive debilitation, some view dying as an achievement, others as a scapegoat.[7]

Some persons, especially those with a prolonged course of living with dying, focus on living their dying so as to die well. They speak about their dying to selected people and at selected times.

People who see dying well as an achievement are sometimes described by health professionals as denying or defying death. These people recognize their dying but choose therapy or choose to go home and participate in their customary activities. If you listen carefully to what they tell you, you will see that they intend to live their dying the way they wish, and thus from their own perspective they die well. These persons seem to do more than adjust and accommodate. They rise to an unseen challenge and in so doing expand their living rather than extend their dying.

A minority of persons may perceive dying as a personal failure or attribute it to external forces. They dwell on all they could have accomplished were it not for their illness. They usually exude a sense of powerlessness and futility and express overt anger. Others with the same perception appear depressed, helpless, and resigned to their situation.

Remember that how people perceive their dying may change throughout the course of their dying. Do not expect attitudes to remain static any more than you expect physical capabilities to remain static. Dying encompasses the whole person; it is an emotional, behavioral, and physical process.

SOME FAMILY DIMENSIONS

Thus far we have focused on the dying person, but the impact of the knowledge that death is imminent extends beyond the dying person to their families, social groups, and the society in which they live.

The reality is that it is difficult to cope with dying. The very thought that you may not see the person that you love much longer is terrifying. Yet complete debilitation of a loved one is not an acceptable alternative. How many of us have experienced witnessing a loved one become less and less functional physically and emotionally? How does it feel to have your husband of 50 or more years accuse you of treating him cruelly, when, in fact you are bathing him and tending to his needs? What is the impact on family who are miles away and concerned about things such as proper care?

Cohesive or disruptive force

The experience of dying may serve as a cohesive force in some families and a disruptive force in others. In general, families who have responded to stresses or crises as a unified force in the past will offer each other strength and support. For familes who have strained relationships, the dying experience may promote further strain.

Family members generally express remorse over the fact that a family member had to come face-to-face with death before they realized how much they needed each other or cared for each other. The recognition, without assistance in learning how to make the relationships grow, will not necessarily lead to greater social and emotional solidarity.[6]

Family control

Dying persons, at times, use their dying to control the behaviors of family members. Exertion of control may be to the benefit of family members but in many instances the control is for self-gain. When dying persons use dying as a means of control for self-gain or as a weapon, the result is anger, resentment, and perhaps retaliation by family members.[6] The retaliation is usually by not visiting, by not phoning, or by visiting for only short periods. It is an attempt to protect themselves from the tyranny of the dying person even while they wish to be close and loving.

The problem becomes more grave for family members and dying person alike if the dying person is being cared for at home. The dying person usually recognizes the antagonism of family members but may interpret it as inappropriate, since, after all, they are dying. More frequently, the dying person may feel rejected and unloved and may not understand that their family loves them but not the behaviors they are displaying.

Family members may recognize their own behavior as a response to the dying person's manipulation, but at the same time they feel guilty about their responses because the other person is dying and they do care. The problem is best addressed openly and honestly but it is usually difficult to resolve. It is difficult to deal with expressions of anger, resentment, and of long-term depression under the best of circumstances. They are almost impossible to deal with when one person is dying. Such behavior usually denotes an inability to cope with the realities of what may be perceived as an unreasonable and unresolvable situation.

An unreasonable situation

American society has yet to resolve its discomfort with the concept of death. Biomedical technologic advances continue to shift the locus of dying to the institution, while at the same time the hospice movement has begun to deinstitutionalize dying. The effect of the latter is that more and more persons are encouraged to die in the privacy of their homes surrounded by family.

Dying at home, cared for by family, may fulfill many

Factors to consider in home care of the dying

Who will be the caretakers?
Who will relieve the caretakers?
How is the home arranged?
Are the doors large enough to accommodate wheelchairs?
Can rooms be arranged to accommodate commodes or other necessary equipment?
Would a hospital bed or other hospital equipment be helpful?
Are the people in the home prepared for the changes they must make in their own life styles?
Was the decision made as a family?

---

of the romantic ideas we have surrounding dying, but it takes proper, careful, advanced planning. In many instances, two major factors are considered: the economic situation and the dying person's wishes. These factors are extremely important, but there are other important factors to be considered.

When all factors are not discussed in advance, family members may be ill-prepared to deal with the most simple tasks. They may not know how to change an occupied bed. They may be concerned about how, what, or even whether to feed the dying person. Nurses choose to become nurses and have been educated to nurse. Family members are expected suddenly to assume nursing responsibilities which they neither desire nor are prepared to do, for example, change dressings, irrigate wounds, and administer medications.

When families are asked to do more than they believe they can accomplish, especially when they do not have readily available assistance, they may feel trapped in an unreasonable situation. Feelings of entrapment lead to anger, frustration, depression, fear, and despair.

Family members who are prepared to care for dying persons in the home need planned times for their own social activities, as well as for grocery shopping and other necessities. Visitors and other family members as well as the dying person need help in actively supporting the caretaker. Time off and credit for what they are doing are two ways to offer support. Nurses can help people to realize that caretakers, like others in the situation, are grieving. They share the guilt, fatigue, and depression of the crisis. They cannot be expected to remain cheerful, supportive, and compassionate, and to cope and assist others in coping without the assistance of others.

Interestingly enough, the same feelings of entrapment are expressed by nurses and physicians when they have higher expectations than they can achieve or when others place demands on them that the nurses or physicians interpret as outrageous.

MULTIFOCUS NURSING PRACTICE CONSIDERATIONS

Nursing care of the dying includes multiple clients and multiple processes.

Focus of nursing practice in care of the dying

Clients	The dying person
	The family and significant others
	The nurse
Processes	Dying
	Grieving

Dying persons and their families and friends may or may not experience the dying process and the grieving process simultaneously. Dying people may grieve the loss of physical function, the loss of past abilities, the ultimate loss of life, and separation from all they know and love. Significant others grieve over the potential loss of the loved one, the hurt they feel, and the emptiness they anticipate.

Although each person's experiences of dying and grieving are unique and personal, there are some similarities. Knowledge of the uniqueness of the perceived experience coupled with knowledge of some expected common responses assist nurses in assessing each situation, planning care, intervening, and evaluating both the plan of care and the interventions for dying people and their families and friends.

Nurses who do not consider family members as well as the dying person as the focus of their care will not achieve quality of care for the dying person.

Assessment

Nursing assessment is an ongoing process throughout the term of the dying person-family-nurse relationship. It will continue and become the family-nurse relationship at the death of the patient. A thorough initial assessment with direct input from the dying person and significant others provides the basis for relationships. Assessment parameters are listed in the top right hand box on p. 286.

Nursing assessment: input from dying person and significant others

General perception of each individual

Awareness of clinical diagnosis and prognosis
Philosophy of living while dying
Expected physiologic and behavioral changes
Past experiences with major illness or crises
Shared experiences with major illnesses or crises

Perceived strengths, desires, and hopes

Personal abilities and coping techniques
Personal support systems
Availability of resources
Beliefs, religious convictions, cultural views of dying, death, and bereavement
Past experiences with death
Expectations about care, dying, use of life supports (present and future)

Timing planned nursing interventions

Times for physical care
Social interaction times
Times for privacy for family members and patient
Quiet times alone for reflection, grieving, or rest
Times for reassessment
Times for group planning and evaluation

Plans for nurse's health maintenance

Time commitments
Support from other professionals or own significant others
Considerations of actual or potential value conflicts and means of dealing with conflicts

---

Nursing assessment: input from nurse

Beliefs, values, attitudes, responses
Support systems: personal and professional
Expertise including incorporating others in care

Another important aspect of nursing assessment is that of the nurses own personal responses, beliefs, and attitudes in each individual situation involving dying persons and their families.

Nursing care planning

As with assessment, planning is a joint venture. Successful planning incorporates the goals of the family and the dying person as well as goals of nurses and other health care providers.

The expertise of the nurse is of special importance in anticipating the dying person's various needs as his/her physical state declines. This expertise is needed to identify the neighbors, church groups, and family members who may serve as support persons and to help them to know when and how they may be of assistance to the dying person and to each other. These persons can participate with the nurses in planning the timing of nursing interventions and identifying alternative interventions.

Nurses need to plan for their own health maintenance. This planning is done in relation to each individual situation involving a dying person or the significant others of dying persons.

The care of dying persons and their families is best accomplished by a team of care givers. Planning care, therefore, includes obtaining input from and relying on and listening to others in the situation, if comprehensive care is to be achieved.

Nursing interventions

The nursing needs of dying individuals are the nursing needs of living individuals. The range of activities are as broad as for any diverse population of patients, family, and significant others. Nursing intervention may occur in a variety of settings—at home or in various institutional settings.

Direct physical care is a major part of caring for dying persons. Maintenance of comfort, both physical and emotional, is of the essence. Teaching others involved in direct care the maintenance of comfort allows their participation and promotes their feelings of competence and well-being.

Health teaching may include teaching such measures as breathing exercises, relaxation techniques, and coping strategies to the significant others for use throughout their grieving process. Teaching how dying persons may use medication for comfort, while dispeling expressed fears of patient addiction may help patient and family alike. There is recognition and respect for cultural differences and fears about addiction. Addiction in dying persons is improbable and in the last days of living, inconsequential.

Another nursing responsibility is to be well-informed about organized support systems, agencies, and independent resources within the community and to be prepared

---

Evaluation methods in the care of dying persons

Care of patient and significant others

Observation of responses to interventions
Discussion of goals and how they have been achieved
Discussion of alternative methods to achieve goals more effectively
Mutual evaluation of continued appropriateness of goals
Mutual identification of new or revised goals and means to achieve these goals

Preestablished nursing evaluation systems

Formal and informal peer review of goals and interventions
    Open discussion of problems
    Venting of feelings
    Sharing of positive responses
Specific criteria developed by groups of nurses involved in caring for dying persons

---

to assist patients and their families in contacting and using these resources. Inquiries related to the many alternative modes of care for dying persons, such as hospice care, other forms of home care, nursing home care, other forms of institutional care, should be answered openly and honestly. If the nurse cannot answer the patient or family's questions, they should be referred to those who can supply the answers.

Nursing intervention may include participation in resuscitative efforts and the maintenance of dying patients on life-support systems. Along with direct patient care in these circumstances, nurses are responsible for communicating with and supporting family members or for assuring that someone is providing this service.

In essence, nurses assist patients and families in maintaining control over their individual lives as much as is possible to ensure dignity and self-esteem. This control is accomplished through the actions discussed above.

If nurses are to care effectively for patients and families, they need to maintain their own well-being. Planned sessions, within the confines of confidentiality, to discuss thoughts and feelings about a particular situation may be helpful. Recognition that others, health professionals, volunteers, and family members, have much to contribute and are as committed and concerned about the patient's welfare is of importance.

Withdrawal from a situation may be necessary in some rare situations, but should occur only when other nursing personnel are available to maintain the care of the patient and significant others.

Evaluation

Each nurse is responsible for evaluating his or her own practice as it relates to each situation. Comfort and satisfaction of the patient may be used as criteria. Nursing intervention may be evaluated through a preestablished evaluation system. Use of these systems contribute to the development and feelings of well-being of nurses by affording support in the decision process.

At the conclusion of a nurse-patient relationship that includes the death of the patient, a nurse will experience a loss. Evaluation of his or her contribution to the relationship gains importance, especially for each nurse's well-being. Recognition of specific successful interventions and contributions leads to feelings of achievement and success. Lack of this recognition may lead to perceiving consecutive losses as a sign of failure.

Peer support is most beneficial to nurses caring for dying persons. Peer support may be accomplished through formal and informal groups. In addition to groups, one-to-one interactions with a trusted peer or personal significant other may alleviate some of the stress related to working with dying persons. More importantly, such relationships serve as an appropriate avenue for recognizing and reinforcing the inherent rewards of providing nursing care for people who are living their dying and those who are sharing the experience.

REFERENCES AND SELECTED READINGS*

1. Curtin, L.: The mask of euthanasia, ed. 2, Cincinnati, 1976, Nurses Concerned For Life, Inc.
2. Donovan, M.L., and Pierce, S.G.: Cancer care nursing, New York, 1976, Appleton-Century-Crofts.
3. *Graham, J.: In the company of others, New York, 1982, Harcourt Brace Jovanovich, Publishers.
4. Illich, I.: Medical nemesis: the expropriation of health, New York, 1976, Pantheon Books.
5. *Kalish, R.A.: Death and dying in a social context. In Binstock, R.H., and Shanes, E., editors: Handbook of aging, New York, 1976, Van Nostrand Reinhold Co.
6. *Martocchio, B.C., and Dufault, Sr. K.: Dying: a part of living. In Diamond, M., editor: Advances in geriatrics: long term nursing, vol. l, New York, 1983, Pro Scientia, Inc.
7. *Martocchio, B.C.: Living while dying, Bowie, M., 1982, Robert J. Brady Co.
8. Martocchio, B.C.: The social processes surrounding the dying person, Unpublished doctoral dissertation, Cleveland, 1975, Case Western Reserve University.
9. Pattison, E.M.: The experience of dying, Englewood Cliffs, N.J., 1977, Prentice Hall, Inc.
10. *Schneidman, E.S.: Voices of death, New York, 1980, Harper & Row Publishers, Inc.

---

*References preceded by an asterisk are particularly well suited to student reading.

Classic

11. *Becker, E.: The denial of death, Riverside, N.J., 1973, Free Press.
12. *Feifel, H.: The functions and attitudes toward death: death and dying, attitudes of patient and doctor, New York, 1965, Group for Advancement of Psychiatry.
13. Harrington, A.: The immortalist, New York, 1969, Random House, Inc.
14. *Kübler-Ross, E.: On death and dying, New York, 1969, Macmillan Co.
15. Schneidman, E.S.: On the deromantization of death, Am. J. Psycho. **25:**4-17, 1971.
16. *Schultz, R., and Aderman, D.: Clinical research and stages of dying, Omega **7:**137-143, 1974.
17. *Weisman, A.D.: The realization of death: a guide for psychological autopsy, New York, 1974, J. Aronson.

UNIT V
Perioperative Nursing

17 Preoperative Intervention
18 Intraoperative Intervention
19 Postoperative Intervention

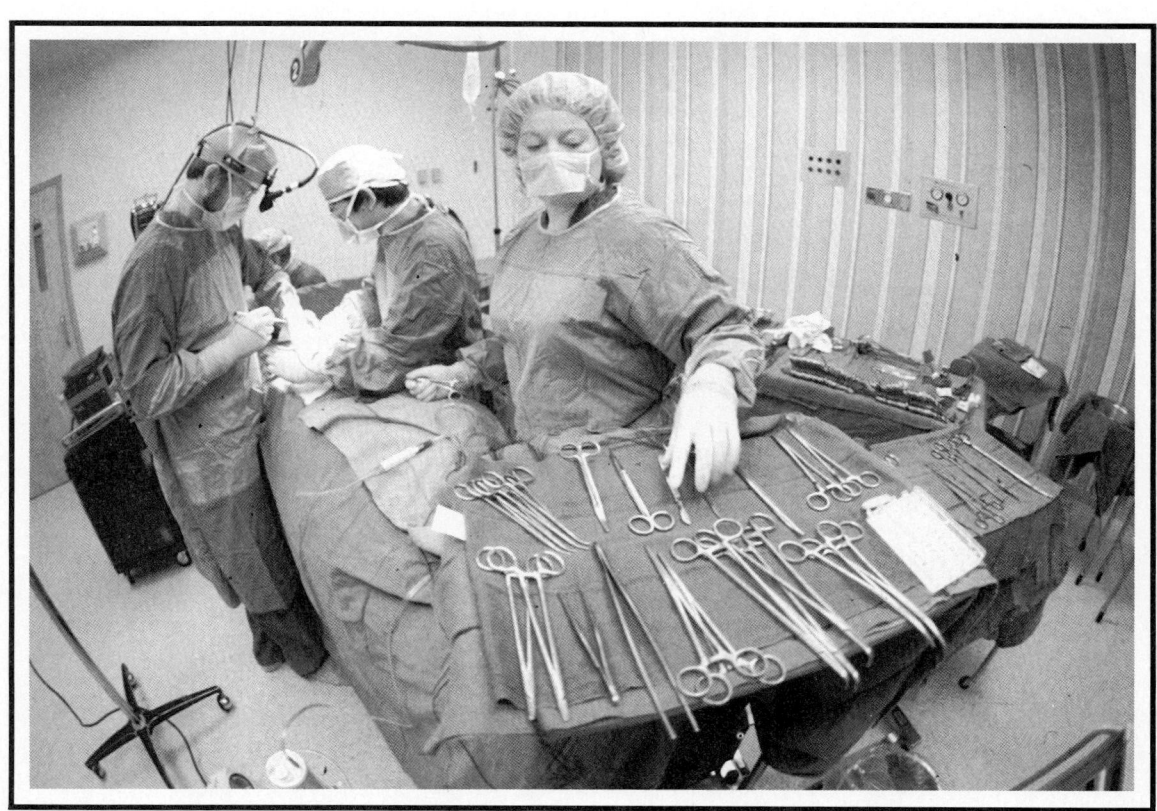

17

Preoperative Intervention

BARBARA C. LONG

STUDY QUESTIONS

- What general reactions do you believe you would have if told you must have immediate general surgery? What questions would you want answered? Compare and contrast your reaction and questions with those of a classmate.

- Review the physiologic response of stress (Chapter 8) and the psychologic responses to stress (Chapter 9). Which of these responses could occur with the anticipation of surgery?

- Examine the charts of several patients on your clinical unit who have had surgery as to the following:
  Do the preoperative notes provide data concerning the patient's psychologic readiness for or concerns about surgery?
  Was any preoperative teaching carried out?
  What were some of the preoperative medications given?

Surgery is one of the major modes of medical therapy. It is a stressful experience as it involves a threat to body integrity and sometimes a threat to life itself. Pain frequently occurs. The nurse is in a position of assisting the person to cope with the stressors, to seek relief from the pain, and to return to optimal functioning.

The surgical (perioperative) experience can be divided into three stages: preoperative, intraoperative, and postoperative. The next three chapters discuss knowledge basic to the care of the patient during each of the three stages.

TYPES OF SURGERY

Classification

Surgeries may be classified in several ways, such as by location, extent, or purpose of the surgery.

LOCATION

Surgery may be performed externally or internally. In *external surgery* the skin or underlying tissues are readily accessible to the surgeon. External surgery has disadvantages; it may result in scarring or disfiguration that may be readily visible, leading to great concern and distress for some patients. *Plastic surgery* is an example of external surgery and is directed toward reconstruction and repair of deformed tissues. *Internal surgery* involves penetration of the body. The scars of internal surgery may not be visible but may lead to complications such as adhesions. Surgery of major internal organs may lead to decreased function if sufficient tissue is removed.

Surgery may also be classified by location of body parts or systems, such as cardiovascular surgery, chest surgery, neurologic surgery, and so on. Information specific to these types of surgery are described elsewhere in the text.

Table 17-1. Purposes of surgery

Type of surgery	Reason performed	Examples
Diagnostic	Determine cause of symptoms	Biopsy, exploratory laparotomy
Curative	Removal of diseased part	Appendectomy
Restorative	Strengthen weakened areas	Herniorrhaphy
	Correct deformities	Mitral valve replacement
	Rejoin a separated area	Bone pinning
Palliative	Relieve symptoms without curing disease	Sympathectomy
Cosmetic	Improve appearance	Plastic surgery

EXTENT

Surgery may be classified as minor or major. *Minor surgery* is simple surgery that presents little risk of life. It may be performed in a surgeon's office, a clinic, or an outpatient or inpatient surgical suite. Many minor surgeries are performed with the patient under local anesthesia, but general anesthesia may also be used. Although the operation is termed "minor," it is frequently not viewed as a minor episode by the patient and may evoke fears and concerns.

Major surgery is usually performed under general anesthesia in an inpatient surgical suite. It is more serious than minor surgery and may involve risk of life. There is a trend toward an increased number of surgical procedures being performed in hospital ambulatory centers in which persons are admitted to the center on the morning of surgery, remain there for their immediate postoperative care, and are then discharged to their homes before the end of the day. Some major surgical procedures, such as herniorrhaphy, are now being performed in this manner.

PURPOSE

There are several purposes for performing surgery (Table 17-1). The surgeon explains the method and purpose for the proposed surgery to the patient and family. Because the preoperative period is often a time of increased anxiety for the patient or family, they may not perceive or understand the reason for the surgery and may require further clarification, which the nurse can provide.

Surgical procedures

Most surgical procedures are given names that describe the site of the surgery and the type of surgery performed. Some surgeries, however, carry the name of the surgeon who developed the technique, such as the Heineke-Mikulicz procedure (widening of the pyloric opening of the stomach).

Common surgical suffixes

-ectomy	Removal of an organ or gland
-rrhapy	Suturing or stitching
-ostomy	Providing an opening (stoma)
-otomy	Cutting into
-plasty	Plastic repair
-scopy	Looking into

EFFECTS OF SURGERY ON THE PATIENT

Surgery is a potential or actual threat to a person's integrity and thus may produce both physiologic and psychologic stress reactions. The physiologic stress reaction is directly related to the extent of the surgery, that is, the more extensive the surgery, the greater the physiologic response. The psychologic response, however, is not directly related. A relatively minor surgical procedure, such as removal of a cyst from the face, may evoke a greater psychologic response than removal of an organ such as the spleen because of the former's potential for scarring. Removal of the uterus, however, may evoke a greater response than would removal of the spleen. This is because of the implications and values attached to the uterus.

Physiologic responses

Major surgery is a stressor to the body and evokes a neuroendocrine response. The response, which consists of sympathetic nervous system and hormonal responses (Table 17-2), serves to protect the body from the threat of injury. When the stress to the system is severe or if blood loss is excessive, the body's compensatory mechanisms are overwhelmed, and shock is the result. Certain types of anesthesia used may also contribute to shock formation.

Metabolic responses also occur. Carbohydrates and fats

Table 17-2. Effects of physiologic responses to surgery

Response	Positive effect	Negative effect
Sympathetic nervous system		
Vasoconstriction	Maintain blood pressure, adequate bloodflow to heart and brain	
Increased cardiac output	Maintain blood pressure	
Decreased GI activity		Anorexia, gas pains, constipation
Hormonal		
Increased glucocorticoid secretion (adrenal cortex)		
Sodium retention	Increased blood volume	Potassium loss
Protein and fat catabolism	Increased energy, amino acids available for healing	Weight loss
Increased platelet production	Prevent bleeding through clotting	Possible thrombus formation
Increased ADH secretion (posterior pituitary)	Increased blood volume	Possible fluid overload

---

Fears related to surgery

General

Fear of unknown
Loss of control
Loss of love from significant others
Threat to sexuality

Specific

Diagnosis of malignancy
Anesthesia
Dying
Pain
Disfigurement
Permanent limitation

---

are metabolized to produce energy. Body proteins are broken down to provide a supply of the amino acids used to build new tissues. Those amino acids that are not used are broken down to nitrogen end products, such as urea, and excreted. This leads to a *negative nitrogen balance;* that is, nitrogen loss exceeds nitrogen intake. All of these factors lead to weight loss after major surgery. A high protein intake is necessary for restoration of needed proteins for healing and for restoration of optimal functioning.

Psychologic responses

Persons differ in the way they perceive the meaning of surgery, and thus they respond in different ways. There are, however, some common fears and concerns. Some of the fears underlying preoperative anxiety are elusive, and the person may not be able to identify the cause. Others are more specific.

Fear of the unknown is most common. If the diagnosis is uncertain, fear of malignancy is frequent, regardless of the probability of occurrence. Fears concerning anesthesia are usually related to dying, "going to sleep and never waking up." Some persons are concerned about what they will say when they are awakening from anesthesia; if they do speak, their words often make little sense. Fears concerning pain, disfigurement, or permanent disability may be realistic or may be influenced by myths, lack of information, or lurid stories told by friends. The patient may also have other concerns related to hospitalization, such as job security, loss of income, and care of family.

Persons with anxiety so high that they cannot talk about and begin to cope with their anxiety before surgery frequently experience difficulty in the postoperative period. They are more apt to be angry, resentful, confused, or depressed. They are also more vulnerable to psychotic reactions than are persons with lower levels of anxiety.

Lack of any emotional response to surgery may indicate denial; this precludes dealing with and coping with the anxiety before surgery. A moderate amount of anxiety enables the individual to identify and begin to cope with feelings. These persons usually experience a smoother postoperative course.

INFORMED CONSENT

Written permission must be obtained from the patient for each operation performed and is usually obtained for major diagnostic procedures, such as a thoracentesis, cystoscopy, bronchoscopy, and so on, that involve entering a body cavity. The consent implies that the patient has been provided with the knowledge necessary to understand (1) the nature of the procedure to be performed, (2) the available options, and (3) the risks associated with each option. Signed permission protects the patient from undergoing unauthorized surgery and protects the surgeon and hospital against claims of unauthorized surgery or that the patient was unaware of the risks involved. Persons who cannot write their names may sign by making a "mark," which must be witnessed by two persons.

The physician is usually responsible for explaining the surgery, options, and risks, but the nurse is responsible for seeing that the consent form has been signed and witnessed before the patient is sent to surgery. Sometimes patients wish to talk to a close family member or friend before signing the operative permit. This is a serious step for some patients, and they may need support as they work through the decision-making process. Patients may refuse to undergo a procedure; it is their right to do so.

When a patient is a minor or is incompetent, a legal guardian signs for the patient. An incompetent person is one who is intoxicated or who is incapable of understanding (mentally deficient or metally ill). "Emancipated minors," persons who are married or earning their own livelihood and retaining their earnings, can sign their own permit. The signature of the spouse of a married minor is also acceptable. Parenthood alone does not emancipate a minor. Consent for a procedure on the child of an unwed minor parent must be obtained from an adult who is next of kin to the unwed parent.

In an emergency situation, the surgeon may operate without written permission if the patient is unable to sign, is a minor, or is incompetent. Every effort is made, however, to contact a family member or guardian. Consent in the form of a telephone call or telegram is permissible in this situation.

ASSESSMENT

Data is collected in the preoperative period to identify the patient's (1) knowledge of events that will occur, (2) psychologic readiness for surgery, and (3) physiologic status before surgery.

Patient knowledge

A major nursing strategy in the preoperative period is teaching the patient about forthcoming events and exercises that can be used in the postoperative period to decrease the potential for complications. Before teaching can take place, it must be determined what the patient knows. Suggested subjective data to collect is listed in the box below.

Psychologic readiness for surgery

The degree of anxiety experienced by the patient needs to be assessed. Most surgeons will cancel surgery for a patient who is extremely anxious. Both subjective and objective data are collected to assess the anxiety.

SUBJECTIVE DATA

1. Concerns or fears about proposed surgery
2. Usual coping methods
3. Religion and its meaning for patient
4. Family and close friends
   a. Geographic distance
   b. Perception of family and friends as source of support
5. Changes in sleep patterns
6. Increased urinary frequency

OBJECTIVE DATA

1. Speech patterns
   a. Repetition of themes
   b. Change of topic
   c. Avoidance of topics related to feelings
2. Degree of interaction with others
3. Physical changes
   a. Increased pulse and respiratory rate
   b. Excessive hand movements
   c. Clammy hands
   d. Restlessness

If the collected data indicate that the patient is severely anxious or if the patient describes a fear of dying while in surgery, this information is reported to the physician for further evaluation.

Assessment of teaching needs

1. Past surgical experience (type, nature, interval)
2. Understanding of proposed surgery (site, type of surgery)
3. Knowledge of preoperative events (diagnostic tests, surgical preparation)
4. Knowledge of postoperative events (recovery room, postoperative routines, probable interventions such as intravenous therapy)
5. Knowledge of exercises to be carried out postoperatively (deep breathing and coughing, leg exercises).

Physiologic status

Data are collected in the preoperative period concerning the patient's physiologic status to obtain baseline data for comparison in the intraoperative and postoperative phases and to identify potential postoperative problems requiring preoperative intervention. Admission histories and physical examinations by the physician and nurse are good sources of pertinent data. The physician may order special tests (Table 17-3) to detect the presence of diseases that may affect the perioperative course. Patients often need explanations concerning the necessity for the sometimes numerous tests.

Assessment data pertinent to nursing care are listed here.

Senses	Ability to see and hear, use of aids
Language	Ability to understand English, speech clarity
Respiration	Respiratory rate
	Ease and symmetry of respirations
	Presence and character of lung sounds
	Ability to use diaphragmatic breathing
	Degree of chest expansion
	Presence of upper respiratory tract infection
	Smoking habit
Circulation	Pulse rate, rhythm, and strength
	Heart sounds
	Circulation in extremities (skin color and temperature, capillary refill, strength of peripheral pulses)
Nutrition	Weight to height ratio
	Presence of nausea or vomiting

	Signs of dehydration (decreased skin turgor, dry mucous membranes, high hematocrit level)
Elimination	History of chronic constipation
	Last bowel movement
	Diarrhea
	Signs of urinary tract infection (urgency, frequency, burning with urination)
	Difficulty initiating stream
Activity	General muscle strength (arms, legs)
	Limitations to walking, sitting, moving in bed
Comfort	Presence of discomforts
	Perceptions of expected discomforts from surgery
	Knowledge of medication routines
	Expectations regarding alleviation of postoperative pain

INTERPRETATION OF PHYSIOLOGIC DATA

Ability to communicate

Data relating to the senses and language indicate the patient's ability to understand directions and to receive support during the perioperative experience. Deficits need to be communicated with the operating room staff.

Oxygenation

Respiratory data is especially important for determining the person's ability to expand the lungs, the risk for postoperative atelectasis or pneumonia, and the ability to carry out deep breathing exercises. Circulatory data is particularly important when the patient is elderly or is

Table 17-3. Preoperative tests to establish baselines and detect presence of diseases that can affect patient responses in intraoperative or postoperative phases

System	Test	Disease or condition
Respiratory	Chest radiograph	Tuberculosis or other pulmonary disease
	Vital capacity	
	Pulmonary function	Tuberculosis, chronic obstructive lung disease, bronchitis, asthma
	Blood gas studies	
Circulatory	Electrocardiogram	Cardiac arrhythmias, myocardial damage
	Blood studies	
	WBC and differential	Chronic infection
	RBC, hemoglobin, hematocrit	Anemia
	Electrolytes	Electrolyte imbalances
	Platelet count, bleeding and clotting times, prothrombin	Liver disease, blood dyscrasias
	Typing and cross-matching	Compatibility for transfusion
	Blood volume	Heart disease
Renal	Urine studies	
	Bacteria	Urinary tract infection
	Albumin, specific gravity	Kidney disease
	Blood studies	
	Creatine, BUN, NPN, electrolytes	Kidney disease
Metabolic	Blood sugar, urine sugar, acetone	Diabetes mellitus
		Starvation

undergoing vascular or heart surgery. Persons with chronic lung, heart, or peripheral vascular disease may experience more difficulties with tissue oxygenation in the postoperative period.

Nutrition

The height to weight ratio indicates whether the patient is overweight or underweight (see Chapter 7). Fluid and electrolyte imbalances occur with dehydration and prolonged vomiting and diarrhea.

Undernourished persons already have diminished reserves of carbohydrates and fats. Body proteins will be used to provide the necessary energy requirement to maintain metabolic functioning of cells. Nitrogen imbalances will be greater than normal and less protein will be available for healing. Wound healing becomes considerably delayed in undernourished persons, and wound separation and infection may occur. If surgery is not an emergency, it is delayed until the patient's nutritional status is improved.

The *obese* person presents numerous risks during the surgical experience. The organs are enlarged and excessive demands are placed on the cardiovascular system. Fatty tissue lacks circulation so wounds heal more slowly. Obese persons have greater difficulty expanding their chests, moving in bed, and walking.

Elimination

Decreased activity after surgery predisposes a patient to constipation. Persons with a history of chronic constipation have a higher risk for developing constipation postoperatively.

Activity

Mobility and ambulation are important activities in the postoperative period for preventing postoperative complications. The patient's ability to move and walk preoperatively will determine actions that must be taken to enhance maximum mobility.

Comfort

Many persons are not aware of the hospital's routines or the nursing staff's expectations regarding the giving of medications for postoperative pain. The routines need to be clarified with the patient to prevent misunderstandings.

ELDERLY PERSONS' RESPONSE TO SURGERY

The ability of the elderly patient to tolerate surgery depends on the extent of physiologic changes that have occurred with the aging process, the duration of the surgical procedure, and the presence of one or more chronic diseases. Elderly persons vary greatly in the extent to which physiologic changes occur. The changes that affect responses to surgery are cardiovascular, renal, pulmonary, and musculoskeletal.

The greater the number of changes present, the greater the potential for the development of a postopera-

---

Risk of surgeries in elderly persons

Lower risk

Elective
Away from diaphragm
Not involving infections
Permitting early mobility
Requiring minimal narcotics

Higher risk

Thoracic
Radical head and neck
Closure of wound dehiscence
Perforated ulcer
Colostomy following obstruction

Surgical risks with obesity

Respiratory complications
Vital signs fluctuations
Wound separation and infection
Incisional hernias
Thrombophlebitis

Potential postoperative complications in elderly persons

Decreased circulation	Shock, wound infection, thrombophlebitis
Decreased kidney function	Prolonged response to anesthesia, fluid and electrolyte imbalances (especially over-hydration)
Decreased respiratory function	Atelectasis, pneumonia
Decreased mobility	Atelectasis, pneumonia, thrombophlebitis, constipation or fecal impaction

tive complication. Heart rate changes in the elderly occur more slowly than in younger persons; therefore, the pulse rate *may not* be a good index in assessment of shock, and a longer period of time may be necessary to wait for pulse stabilization after activity.

The duration of the surgical experience can affect the response of elderly persons to surgery. Surgery of short duration is more easily tolerated. Presence of chronic diseases such as pulmonary, cardiac, or CNS disease limits the elderly person by prolonging recovery or by increasing the risk of mortality. Certain types of surgery present low or high risks for elderly persons.[8]

DATA ANALYSIS AND PLANNING

Nursing diagnoses

After collecting the assessment data the nurse identifies nursing diagnoses based on specific patient data. Possible nursing diagnoses might include the following:

Anxiety
Fear of death, disfigurement
Knowledge deficit
Potential injury

Expected patient outcomes

Expected patient outcomes might include the following:

1. Demonstrates no more than moderate anxiety.
2. Can explain (if conscious) the surgery to be performed and has signed the operative consent form (consent on chart).
3. Can explain sequence of events and physical activities expected in the early postoperative period (turning, deep breathing and coughing)
4. Has had a baseline assessment and current vital signs taken and charted.
5. Has had any significant physical or psychologic changes reported to the surgeon.
6. Is wearing a legible identification band, which has been checked.
7. Is not wearing nail polish, hairpins or wigs, dentures, or jewelry. (Articles have been stored for safekeeping.)
8. Has voided.
9. Has received preanesthetic medication as ordered.

IMPLEMENTATION

Assisting with achievement of therapeutic goals

MEDICAL INTERVENTIONS: CORRECTION OF EXISTING DEFICIENCIES

Postoperative complications can be minimized if existing medical conditions are treated or are under good control before surgery. Measures to treat wound infections are carried out before secondary closure or skin grafting.

Dehydration from vomiting and diarrhea is treated with parenteral fluids to reestablish fluid and electrolyte balance.

Patients with chronic diseases should be at their optimal health level before surgery. The undernourished patient is placed on a high-protein, high-carbohydrate diet rich in vitamins B_1, C, and K. Supplementary vitamins may be ordered. If an oral diet is poorly tolerated or poorly absorbed, total parenteral nutrition (TPN) will be initiated. The obese patient is placed on a weight-reducing diet. Both the undernourished and the obese patient should understand the rationale for the diets. They may need considerable support and encouragement to maintain the diets.

Patients with chronic obstructive pulmonary disease (COPD) are frequently placed on vigorous respiratory therapy to ensure maximal ventilation and to decrease postoperative respiratory complications. This therapy usually includes postural drainage, aerosol inhalations, and antibiotics. Smoking is discouraged for all patients preoperatively and especially for patients with lung disease. Diabetes mellitus should be under good control.

PREOPERATIVE PREPARATION

Diet

Except in bowel surgery for which patients may be placed on a low residue diet, a regular diet is permitted the day before surgery, but no food is allowed 8 hours before surgery. Fluids are usually withheld at least 4 hours before surgery. Presence of food or fluids in the stomach increases the possibility of aspiration of gastric contents should the patient vomit while under anesthesia. This can lead to aspiration pneumonia. If it should be discovered that the patient has consumed food or fluids when ordered "nothing by mouth" (NPO), the surgeon should be notified, since this may necessitate rescheduling the surgical procedure. If a local or spinal anesthetic is planned, a light meal may be permitted.

Patients who are dehydrated will usually have parenteral fluids initiated before surgery. If it is anticipated that the patient may have decreased peristalsis after surgery (as a result of anesthesia or manipulation of the abdominal viscera), a nasogastric tube may be inserted before surgery.

Bowel preparation

Enemas are usually given preoperatively only for surgery of the GI tract or of the pelvic, perineal, or perianal areas. If a preoperative enema is ineffectual, it may be repeated. The purpose of the preoperative enema is to prevent injury to the colon and to provide better visualization of the surgical area.

If enemas are to be given until the returns are clear, it is important to remember that fluid excess and potassium deficits can occur with repeated enemas. It is common practice to check with the physician if returns are not clear after the third enema. One method is to give up to three enemas the evening before surgery, and then if the returns are still not clear to repeat the enemas the following morning. Repeated enemas are very tiring for the patient and may irritate rectal and bowel mucosa. If antibiotic enemas are ordered for the purpose of decreasing intestinal bacteria before intestinal surgery, synthesis of vitamin K by the intestinal bacteria may be inhibited. Supplementary vitamin K may be given to prevent bleeding after surgery.

Skin preparation

The purpose of preoperative skin preparation is to free the operative site of as many microorganisms as possible. In many instances showering well with hexachlorophene soap will suffice. In certain types of surgery, such as orthopedic implants where infections can lead to dysfunction, a special cleansing routine is prescribed. No soap, alcohol, or alcohol-based solutions should be used in conjunction with hexachlorophene solutions as these substances decrease the antiseptic properties of hexachlorophene.

Hair is removed from the surgical site because microorganisms cling to the hair. A depilatory may be used if the skin is not sensitive to the depilatory. Shaving of the hair may be ordered either the night before or immediately before surgery. A sharp disposable razor is used with good lighting. Shaving must be *against the grain* of the hair shaft for a closer shave. The skin should not be scratched or nicked since microorganisms can harbor in broken skin surfaces.

Shaving of hair on certain areas of the body may have a special meaning for some persons. These areas include face, head, and pubic area. If the entire head is to be shaved, it is frequently carried out after the patient has been anesthetized. The eyebrows are not shaved. Pubic hair is shaved only when necessary, the regrowth of this hair is uncomfortable to many patients.

Some hospitals have specified procedures delineating the size of the area to be shaved. The surgeon usually specifies which of the areas is to be shaved. An area larger than the anticipated incision is shaved to permit flexibility in location and size of incision.

Counseling and teaching

PSYCHOLOGIC PREPARATION FOR SURGERY

Both patient and family need opportunities to discuss their concerns and fears about the forthcoming surgery. The assessment of the patient's psychologic readiness for surgery provides the nurse with data about the patient's specific fears or concerns.

Having opportunities to talk with a supportive, knowledgeable individual helps persons begin to identify the reasons for their anxiety and to marshal coping responses. It is helpful for the nurse to plan for a quiet unhurried time to sit down with the person and give an opportunity to ask questions and to talk about concerns. Touch is often a helpful form of communication, sending the message, "I care," and some persons will talk more readily while receiving a back rub. Knowing that a nurse is interested and cares helps to reduce anxiety. If the person

knows also that anxiety is a normal reaction to the threat of surgery, it may help to remove the often self-imposed expectation, "I shouldn't be nervous."

Loss of control is one of the fears associated with surgery. Allowing persons to participate in decision making in regard to their own care, when feasible, helps them partially meet the need for control. Identifying and carrying out measures to help the patient meet physical needs in the preoperative phase may help provide a feeling of security about having postoperative needs met and thus allay some anxiety.

Teaching is an important function of the nurse in the preoperative phase and helps to allay anxiety when the patient knows what to expect. Also if persons are to move toward self-care and independence, they need to know early the what, why, and how of activities that will help them regain an optimal level of functioning after surgery. Waiting until the patient has sufficiently recovered from the insult of surgery before teaching is started means a considerable loss of time, and learning may be less effective. In addition, the patient may be discharged before teaching is completed.

EXPLANATION OF EVENTS

Fear of the unknown can be decreased by an understanding of the events that will occur. The amount of information to give preoperatively depends on the background, interest, and stress level of the patient and the family. A good rule to follow is to ask patients what they would like to know about forthcoming surgery and to base responses on the types of questions asked. Simple explanations are indicated for persons under considerable stress or those with severe pain. A highly anxious person may not take in and remember information given. Information helpful for preoperative patients is listed in the box below.

Helpful information for preoperative patients

Preoperative tests—reason, preparation
Preoperative routines
Transfer to operating room (time, checking procedures)
Recovery room
    Place where patient will awaken
    Frequent monitoring of vital signs
    Return to room when vital signs stable
Probable postoperative therapies
    Need for increased mobility as soon as possible
    Need to keep respiratory passages clear
    Anticipated treatments (for example, I.V.)
    Pain medication routines (timing sequence, "as needed" {p.r.n.} status)

DEEP BREATHING AND COUGHING EXERCISES

Some persons are at high risk for developing postoperative pulmonary complications such as atelectasis or pneumonia (see box below). These persons need to carry out deep breathing and coughing exercises in the early postoperative period. Waiting until after surgery to teach these persons how to carry out the exercises decreases the effectiveness of the outcome, since anesthesia and pain will decrease the ability to retain information.

The person needs to know how to perform diaphragmatic breathing, as this increases lung expansion by permitting the diaphragm to descend fully. Many males normally breathe diaphragmatically, whereas few females do. With diaphragmatic breathing, the abdomen *rises with inspiration* and *falls with expiration*. The nurses assesses the person's normal breathing pattern by placing a hand lightly on the person's abdomen and asking the person to take a deep breath. If diaphragmatic breathing does not occur naturally, the person can be taught to inspire deeply while pushing the abdomen up against the hand.

The method for deep breathing and coughing exercises is listed as follows.

1. Lie in semi-Fowler's or high Fowler's position with knees flexed to relax abdomen and allow full chest expansion.
2. Place a hand lightly on the abdomen.
3. Breathe in slowly through nose letting chest expand and feeling abdomen rise against hand.
4. Hold breath for 3 seconds.
5. Exhale slowly through pursed lips (abdomen contracts with inspiration).
6. Inhale and exhale 3 more times. *Following last inspiration cough forcefully* to expel any secretions.
7. Rest.
8. Repeat steps 3 through 7 two more times.

If thoracic or high abdominal incisions are present, the person can "splint" the incision with a pillow during coughing to relieve stress or pull on the incision.

LEG EXERCISES

Venous stasis in the postoperative period may lead to thrombophlebitis (blood clot). Persons at high risk include those who (1) will have decreased mobility after surgery, (2) have a history of decreased peripheral circulation, or (3) experience cardiovascular or pelvic surgery. These patients will need to carry out exercises postoperatively to prevent venous stasis in the legs. Tightening and relaxing leg muscles (see the box below) help to "pump" the blood along the veins. Valves in the veins prevent back flow of blood.

Persons who will be on bed rest for several days after surgery will need to exercise the legs to maintain muscle tone to facilitate ambulation at a later date. These persons need to learn to carry out quadriceps drills and gluteal tightening exercises.

MOBILITY

Moving and turning in bed help to prevent pulmonary and circulatory complications, prevent decubiti, stimulate peristalsis, and decrease pain. During the preoperative period, persons can be taught how to use the side rails effectively for turning and how to sit up on the side of the bed with the least amount of pull on the incision.

Postoperative leg exercises

Muscle pump exercises
1. Contract calf and thigh muscles
2. Relax leg muscles
3. Rest
4. Repeat at least 10 times

Quadriceps drill
1. Bend knees with foot flat on bed
2. Straighten leg on bed
3. Lift heel, pressing back of knee against bed
4. Repeat at least 5 times

Gluteal tightening exercises
1. Pinch buttocks together
2. Attempt to move leg to side of bed
3. Relax
4. Repeat at least 5 times

High-risk factors: pulmonary complications

Inhalant anesthesia
Thoracic surgery
Upper abdominal surgery
Smoking
Chronic lung disease

Tight abdominal binders
Body casts
Obesity
Elderly

Decreasing incisional pull when sitting up on side of bed

1. Move to edge of bed
2. Raise head of bed to high Fowler's position
3. Drop feet over side of bed
4. Push up to sitting position with hand closest to edge of bed

Assisting with comfort

Anxiety often causes sleeplessness and restlessness. If the patient is extremely restless, a tranquilizer may be given for 1 to 2 days before surgery. Ambulation is encouraged before surgery to give the patient a feeling of well-being, to stimulate circulation and ventilation, and to maintain muscle tone. Fatigue is to be avoided, and patients with chronic illnesses may need planned periods of rest.

The person should be permitted to sleep on the morning of surgery for as long as possible and to rest undisturbed until shortly before administration of preanesthetic medication. Many persons therefore prefer to take their bath or shower the evening before surgery rather than in the morning. The person who has bathed the night before is given an opportunity to wash hands and face and to perform mouth care. The person is reminded that he or she should not swallow water if fluids by mouth are not permitted.

Comfort also implies readiness for surgery and that the patient is able to marshal effective coping mechanisms. Family are advised to arrive at least 1 hour before the scheduled time for surgery. The patient should have an opportunity to have last-minute questions answered. Explanations for last-minute routines are given if this was not done previously. If the surgery is to be delayed even for a short time, both the person and family should be informed.

Carrying out final preparation for surgery

PREVENTION OF INJURY

Measures taken to protect the patient from errors of identification or injury include the following:
1. Check identification band for secureness and legibility
2. Remove hair pins and wigs; protect hair with a cap
3. Remove jewelry; wedding ring may be taped to finger
4. Remove nail polish (for assessment of circulation during surgery)
5. Remove contact lenses and store in proper container
6. Remove any prostheses (dentures, false eyes, and so on); store prostheses in a safe place
7. Leave hearing aid in place if patient is unable to hear without the aid (inform operating room nurse)
8. Apply antiembolic stockings if patient is at high risk for thromboembolism or shock (elderly, marked varicosities, pelvic surgery, time-consuming surgery)
9. Have patient empty bladder immediately before receiving preanesthetic medication.

PREANESTHETIC MEDICATION

A sedative is usually ordered the night before surgery to ensure a full night's sleep. If additional sedation or medication for pain is given during the night, it must be given at least 4 hours before the preanesthetic medication.

Preanesthetic medications, commonly referred to as *premedication,* are given when the patient is "on call" for the operating room (usually about 45 to 90 minutes before surgery is anticipated). Preanesthetic medications are given to decrease anxiety, to provide a smoother induction and maintenance of anesthesia, and to diminish undesirable reflexes during emergence from anesthesia.

The effects of commonly used preanesthetic medications are listed in Table 17-4. Adults frequently receive a combination of drugs. Dosages may be decreased in the elderly.

Any delay in giving the medication should be reported to the anesthesiologist. All preoperative routines should be completed before the preanesthetic medication is given. The patient should remain in bed following administration of the medication to promote maximum effect and to prevent falls from dizziness. One major desired effect is decreased anxiety. It must be reemphasized that psychologic preparation of the patient for surgery is the most effective approach to help allay anxiety. Studies have shown that the administration of preanesthetic medication without any attempt at psychologic preparation may render the patient drowsy but does not reduce anxiety.

RECORDING

A check-off list that includes the final preparations is often used. A final nurse's note is written listing the times the patient voided, when the patient leaves for surgery, and any final pertinent remarks regarding the patient's condition and emotional response. Presence of any handicaps such as blindness or deafness should be noted for use by the surgical staff.

Before the patient leaves for surgery the chart is checked for completeness as to the following:
1. Skin preparation done and checked by nurse
2. Vital signs (temperature, pulse, respiration, blood pressure) charted
3. Premedication charted
4. Regular medication charted
5. Weight and height recorded (for use by anesthesiologist)
6. Operative permit signed, witnessed, and attached to chart
7. All recent laboratory, radiographic, and ECG reports attached to chart.

Table 17-4. Commonly used preanesthetic medications

Drug	Desired effects	Undesired effects
Sedative-hypnotics		
Pentobarbital sodium (Nembutal)	Reduces anxiety, promotes relaxation and sleep	May cause excitement or confusion in elderly persons or in those with severe pain
Secobarbital sodium (Seconal)	Same as above	Same as above
Flurazepam hydrochloride (Dalmane)	Promotes relaxation and sleep	
Chloral hydrate	Same as for flurazepam	
Narcotics		
Morphine sulfate	Reduces anxiety, promotes relaxation, decreases preoperative pain, decreases amount of anesthetic needed	Depresses respiration, circulation, and gastric motility; may cause nausea and vomiting
Meperidine hydrochloride (Demerol)	Same as for morphine sulfate	Same as for morphine sulfate
Tranquilizers		
Promethazine hydrochloride (Phenergan)	Reduces anxiety, antiemetic	Postoperative hypotension
Chlorpromazine (Thorazine)	Same as for promethazine hydrochloride	Same as for promethazine hydrochloride
Neuroleptanalgesic agent		
Fentanyl and droperidol (Innovar)	General quiescence, state of indifference, decreased motor activity, analgesia, antiemetic	Respiratory depression, muscle rigidity, hypotension
Vagolytic agents		
Atropine sulfate	Decreased secretions, prevention of laryngospasms	Excessive dryness of mouth, tachycardia
Scopolamine hydrochloride (Hyoscine)	Decreases secretions, amnesia, state of indifference, sedation	Excessive dryness of mouth

TRANSPORTATION TO OPERATING ROOM

Personnel transporting the patient bring the stretcher from the operating room and identify themselves to the nurse. The unit nurse assigned to prepare the patient for surgery checks the patient record, accompanies the transportation attendant to the patient's bedside, checks the patient's identification band, and signs the patient identification form. This form is usually then attached to the stretcher. Patients should be protected from drafts. Since the operating room is kept cool, cotton blankets are used to keep the patient warm.

The patient's family or close friends are provided with the following information:

1. Where to wait until patient returns to the unit
2. Availability of coffee shop, cafeteria, and so on
3. Expected time intervals
   a. Patient is sent to surgery 45 to 60 minutes before surgery actually commences
   b. Surgery may be delayed if the previous surgery took longer than anticipated
   c. Patient will be sent to a post-anesthesia room (recovery room) after surgery for varying periods of time
4. Method of receiving information when surgery is completed
5. Visit by surgeon after surgery (if this is the policy)
6. What to expect when patient returns from surgery (condition, special equipment, and so on)

REFERENCES AND SELECTED READINGS*

1. American College of Surgeons' Committee on Pre- and Post-operative Care: Manual of preoperative and postoperative care, ed. 3, Philadelphia, 1983, W.B. Saunders Co.
2. Bastasaraswathi, K., and El-Etr, A.A.: Preoperative evaluation of drug history, AORN J. **23:**616-620, 1976.
3. Bernstein, A.H.: Current status of the law of consent to treatment, Hospitals **53**(3):83-85, 1979.
4. *Besch, L.B.: Informed consent: a patient's right, Nurs. Outlook **27:**33-35, 1979.
5. Caranasos, G.J.: Drug reactions and interactions in the patient undergoing surgery, Med. Clin. N. Am. **63:**1245-1256, 1979.
6. Copeland, W.M.: Informed consent and the OR nurse, AORN J. **29:**928-944, 1979.
7. *Dziurbejko, M.M., and Larkin, J.C.: Including the family in preoperative teaching, Am. J. Nurs. **78:**1892-1894, 1978.
8. Feigal, D.W., and Blaisdell, F.W.: The estimation of surgical risks, Med. Clin. N. Am. **63:**1131-1143, 1979.
9. Felton, G., and others: Preoperative nursing intervention with the patient for surgery: outcomes of three alternative approaches, Int. J. Nurs. Stud. **13:**83-96, 1976.
10. *Greenwood, B.S.: Check out your patient's presurgery fears, Nurs. 82 **12**(7):34-35, 1982.
11. *Gruendemann, B.: The impact of surgery on body image, Nurs. Clin. N. Am. **10:**635-643, 1975.
12. Guerra, F., and Aldrete, J.A., editors: Emotional and psychological responses to anesthesia and surgery, New York, 1980, Grune & Stratton, Inc.
13. Hoopes, N.M., and others: An approach to preoperative visits, AORN J. **26:**1048-1091, 1977.
14. *Laird, M.: Techniques for teaching pre- and postoperative patients, Am. J. Nurs. **75:**1338-1340, 1975.
15. *Lyons, M.L.: What priority do you give preop teaching? Nurs. 77 **7**(1):12-14, 1977.
16. *Marcinek, M.B.: Stress in the surgical patient, Am. J. Nurs. **77:**1809-1811, 1977.
17. Metheny, N., and Snively, W.D., Jr.: Perioperative fluids and electrolytes, Am. J. Nurs. **78:**840-845, 1978.
18. *Saylor, D.: Understanding presurgical anxiety, AORN J. **22:**624-636, 1975.
19. Schumann, D.: Preoperative measures to promote wound healing Nurs. Clin. N. Am. **14:**683-699, 1979.
20. *Silva, M.C.: Preoperative teaching for spouses, AORN J. **27:**1081-1086, 1978.
21. Strauss, R.J., and others: Operative risks of obese patients: nursing care, AORN J. **25:**1053-1057, 1977.
22. *Wilson, W.: Routine shaving and wound infection, AORN J. **28:**762-770, 1978.

*References preceded by an asterisk are particularly well suited for student reading.

18

Intraoperative Intervention

JUDITH L. GREIG

STUDY QUESTIONS

- Review the chart of several patients who have experienced major surgery:
  What kinds of anesthetics were administered and by what method?
  What observations should have been made of the patient in the early postoperative period based on the anesthetic given?
  Is there documentation of nursing care given (actions taken to meet identified needs)?

- If you were to observe your patient's surgical procedure in the surgical suite, what actions would you need to take to protect the patient's safety (such as wearing apparel or your body positions when close to operating team members)?

Each surgical patient is unique, and therefore surgery on each is a unique experience. Patients bring with them to the operating suite a unique set of feelings and values that must be considered in planning nursing care during the intraoperative period.

The operating room nurse functions as the patient's advocate during surgery. This role has been viewed in the past as being entirely technical in nature. One cannot deny that an operating room nurse must possess knowledge of skills, procedures, instruments, and supplies to function as an effective team member. All of operating room nursing, however, is not technical, and the integration of nursing process into this arena of care has become the accepted standard for operating room nurses. These nurses are responsible for providing a safe, caring, and efficient environment in which the surgical team can function to provide the best outcome for each patient.

CONCEPTS BASIC TO OPERATING ROOM NURSING

Perioperative nursing

The perioperative role of the operating room (O.R.) nurse consists of nursing activities performed by the professional operating room nurse during the preoperative, intraoperative, and postoperative phases of the patient's surgical experience (Fig. 18-1). The extent of activities depends on the nurse's knowledge and skill, varying from a basic competency level to a level of excellence.

Each phase of this role begins and ends at an appointed time in the chain of events involved in surgical intervention; and each includes a variety of nursing activities that can be performed using nursing process. The *preoperative phase* begins when the decision for surgical intervention is made and ends when the patient is transferred to the operating room table. The scope of nursing activities involved can be as broad as beginning assessment of the patient in the clinic or at home through a preoperative interview or as limited as doing a preoperative assessment in the holding area of the surgical suite.

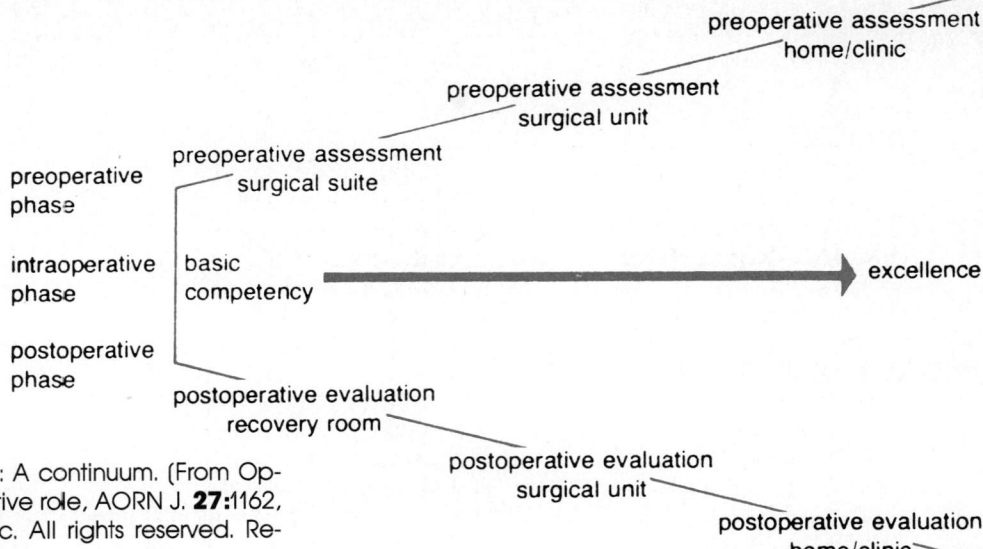

Fig. 18-1. The perioperative role: A continuum. (From Operating room nursing: perioperative role, AORN J. **27**:1162, 1978 Copyright © by AORN, Inc. All rights reserved. Reprinted by permission.)

The *intraoperative phase* begins when the patient is transferred to the operating table and ends with transfer to the recovery area. Again the activities performed by the nurse can be as broad as recognizing the patient's potential for skin breakdown in certain areas and taking special precautions or as limited as simply positioning the patient on the table according to the basic principles of good body alignment.

The *postoperative phase* begins with admission of the patient to the recovery area and ends with a follow-up evaluation. The scope of care could be as broad as seeing the patient at home or in a clinic setting or as limited as the nurse communicating pertinent information relative to the patient's surgery to personnel in the recovery area. Table 18-1 illustrates a sample list of nursing activities in the three phases of perioperative nursing.

The practice of perioperative nursing is envisioned as a goal for care given by operating room nurses. The role has been developed through the efforts of the Association of Operating Room Nurses (AORN), a voluntary organization of registered nurses concerned with the care of patients before, during, and after surgery. By practicing the perioperative role, the O.R. nurse brings together traditional and extended nursing activities during the intraoperative period with the more recently developed preoperative and postoperative assessment, teaching, and evaluation functions, thus integrating both technical and professional functions.

Standards of perioperative nursing practice

Standards have been developed to guide the practice of operating room nursing.[6] These standards are based on nursing process and serve as a model to measure the quality of patient care delivered. The standards include all aspects of nursing process (assessment, planning, implementation, and evaluation) pertinent to the planned surgical intervention.

Standards of care and the use of nursing process during the intraoperative period are viewed as paving the way for nurses in the operating room to expand knowledge, to increase sensitivity to individuals' needs, and to be accountable to patients as consumers. This is also a means to provide continuity of care in an integrated manner using preoperative assessment, intraoperative intervention, and postoperative evaluation.

Intraoperative patient care team members

OPERATING TEAM

The intraoperative patient care team members are commonly subdivided into two basic categories, scrubbed sterile members and nonsterile members.

The *scrubbed sterile* team members usually include the following:

1. Primary surgeon
2. Assistants to the surgeon (may vary in number and qualifications; however, most medical staff bylaws state, "A qualified physician shall assist during all major operations."[12])
3. Scrub nurse or technician

The *nonsterile* team members may include the following:

1. Anesthesiologist or anesthetist
2. Circulating nurse
3. Others (technicians to operate complicated monitoring devices or equipment such as the heart-lung machine, biomedical engineers, pathologist if a frozen tissue section is necessary, and so on)

Table 18-1. Examples of activities in the perioperative role*

Preoperative phase	Intraoperative phase	Postoperative phase
Preoperative assessment	*Maintenance of safety*	*Communication of intraoperative information*
Home/clinic	1. assures that the sponge, needle, and instrument counts are correct	1. gives patient's name
1. initiates initial preoperative assessment	2. positions the patient	2. states type of surgery performed
2. plans teaching methods appropriate to patient's needs	a. functional alignment	3. provides contributing intraoperative factors, ie, drain, catheters
3. involves family in interview	b. exposure of surgical site	4. states physical limitations
Surgical unit	c. maintenance of position throughout procedure	5. states impairments resulting from surgery
1. completes preoperative assessment	3. applies grounding device to patient	6. reports patient's preoperative level of consciousness
2. coordinates patient teaching with other nursing staff	4. provides physical support	7. communicates necessary equipment needs
3. explains phases in perioperative period and expectations	*Physiological monitoring*	*Postoperative evaluation*
4. develops a plan of care	1. calculates effects on patient of excessive fluid loss	Recovery area
Surgical suite	2. distinguishes normal from abnormal cardiopulmonary data	1. determines patient's immediate response to surgical intervention
1. assesses patient's level of consciousness	3. reports changes in patient's pulse, respirations, temperature, and blood pressure	Surgical unit
2. reviews chart	*Psychological monitoring* (prior to induction and if patient conscious)	1. evaluates effectiveness of nursing care in the OR
3. identifies patient	1. provides emotional support to patient	2. determines patient's level of satisfaction with care given during perioperative period
4. verifies surgical site	2. continues to assess patient's emotional status	3. evaluates products used on patient in the OR
Planning	3. communicates patient's emotional status to other appropriate members of the health care team	4. determines patient's psychological status
1. determines a plan of care	*Nursing management*	5. assists with discharge planning
Psychological support	1. provides physical safety for the patient	Home/clinic
1. tells patient what is happening	2. maintains aseptic, controlled environment	1. seeks patient's perception of surgery in terms of the effects of anesthetic agents, impact on body image, distortion, immobilization
2. determines psychological status	3. effectively manages human resources	2. determines family's perceptions of surgery
3. gives prior warning of noxious stimuli		
4. stands near/touches patient during procedures/induction		
5. communicates patient's emotional status to other appropriate members of the health care team		

*From AORN, Inc.: Operating room nursing: perioperative role, AORN J. **27**:1164, 1978. Copyright © by AORN, Inc. all rights reserved. Reprinted by permission.

SCRUB NURSE

Nursing responsibilities in the operating room are commonly divided into the roles of scrub nurse and circulating nurse. The scrub nurse may or may not be a nurse, as this role can be carried out by a registered nurse, practical or vocational nurse, or a trained technician. Scrub nurse activities may include the following:

1. Preparing sterile supplies and equipment needed for the operation
2. Assisting the surgeon and surgical assistants during the procedure
3. Teaching new personnel, if qualified to do so
4. Assisting in accounting for needles, scalpel blades, sponges, and instruments used during the pro-

cedure, using the established "count" procedure

To carry out these activities effectively the scrub nurse must possess thorough knowledge of aseptic technique, manual skill and dexterity, physical stamina, the ability to work under pressure, and a sincere concern for accuracy and accountability in performing in a manner consistent with optimal patient care.

CIRCULATING NURSE

The circulating nurse plays a role in the overall management of the operating room. This person is vital to the effective flow of patient care before, during, and after the surgical procedure. Although the surgeon is in charge of the operative site, the circulating nurse is relied on to coordinate all activities of the room and to manage the nursing care required for the patient. The circulating nurse is often the one team member who is in a position to have an overall picture of patient care needs and to be the patient's advocate. Consistent with such responsibility, it is considered vital to the perioperative role that this individual be minimally prepared as a registered professional nurse.

Circulating nurse activities may include the following:

1. Assessing, planning, implementing, and evaluating nursing activities to meet individual patient needs.
2. Creating and maintaining a safe and comfortable environment for the patient. This often involves diligent observation for breaks in aseptic technique and initiation of appropriate measures to correct the situation.
3. Providing assistance to any team member as necessary (directing and anticipating the performance and needs of the scrub nurse and providing extra supplies and equipment as needed to any team member).
4. Maintaining communication between team members in the operating room and any necessary contact with other health care professionals and patient's family.
5. Identifying any potential environmental dangers or traumatic situations involving the patient or team members and taking appropriate action to correct or assist with the problem.

ALLIED PERSONNEL

There are a number of other persons who function in an indirect relationship in contributing to the needs of each surgical patient. These persons may include clerical personnel, blood bank employees, laboratory technicians, nursing assistants, pharmacists, central service employees, pathologists, radiologists, and laundry personnel.

OPERATING ROOM SUITE DESIGN

The design of an operating room suite offers a challenge to the planning team to optimize efficiency by creating realistic traffic and work flow patterns for patients, personnel, and supplies. Designs also need to allow for flexibility for future needs. Since no one plan meets all hospitals' requirements, each O.R. suite is designed on an individual basis to meet projected and specific community needs.

Specific traffic patterns are determined dependent on the entrances and exits for both personnel and materials. Traffic control can be aided by designating a 4-zone concept.

Infection control practices that are related to design may include but are not limited to the following:

1. Walls that are smooth and easily washable
2. Cabinets that are recessed to facilitate cleaning
3. No windows
4. Sliding doors (as opposed to swinging doors) decrease air turbulence
5. Presence of adequate air filtration system
6. Ceiling mounted lighting units on a single post as opposed to lights on tracks. (Ceiling light tracks are not readily accessible for cleaning, and handles are likely to become contaminated.)
7. Disposal systems for contaminated equipment should be uniform for all cases.

Temperature and humidity are also important design factors. High relative humidity should be maintained. Moisture provides a relatively conductive medium, allowing static to leak to earth as fast as it is generated. Temperature is purposely cool to deter bacterial growth. The combination of increased humidity and decreased temperature is also desirable for maintaining the patient's exposed tissue.

A *communication system* is a vital link to summon routine or emergency assistance or to relay appropriate information to and from the operating room team. An intercom system is commonly used, but team members must be aware of the type of information that is shared over an intercom if the patient is awake. Call light systems outside the operating room door may be used to summon selected persons such as orderlies or housekeeping personnel.

Operating room zones

Protective	Locker rooms, lounges, offices, patient receiving areas
Clean	Clean storage areas, scrub areas, recovery room
Sterile	Operating rooms, storage of sterile supplies
Dirty	Disposal area for all used materials

NURSING PRACTICE IN THE OPERATING ROOM

Aseptic technique and infection control

Aseptic technique is the foundation on which modern surgery is based. Asepsis means the absence of any infectious agents; therefore, aseptic technique is aimed at eliminating microorganisms present in the surgical environment. This also includes those microorganisms living harmlessly on the body surface or within, which must be prevented from reaching the open wound to allow healing by first intention.

Principles of bacteriology and microbiology are applied in developing infection control programs to be followed by all operating room personnel. Such programs involve specific guidelines for O.R. attire, for sterilization and packaging of supplies, for scrubbing, for gowning and gloving, and for methods of housekeeping.

When following infection control principles, self-discipline and a "surgical conscience" are imperative. A surgical conscience may be described as a Surgical Golden Rule, that is, "Do unto the patient as you would have others do unto you."[12] This implies that the nurse takes appropriate action to rectify any break in technique whether the person is alone or observed by others. Thus the nurse must be as conscientious about monitoring his or her own technique as when observing other team members.

BASIC RULES OF SURGICAL ASEPSIS

Definite rules must be adhered to during surgery to create and maintain a sterile field with a well-defined margin of safety for the patient. Strict adherence to these rules eliminates or minimizes possible contamination.

1. Only sterile materials may be used within a sterile field. If there is any doubt about the sterility of an item, it is considered unsterile.
2. Gowns of scrubbed team members are considered sterile in the *front from shoulder to waist level and sleeves to 2 inches above the elbow*. Unsterile areas of gowns are shoulders, neckline, axillary region, and back. Scrubbed persons should not allow their hands or any sterile item to fall below waist or tabletop level.
3. Draped tables are considered to be sterile on top surface only. Any item that extends over the table edge is considered contaminated and cannot be brought back up to tabletop level.
4. Sterile surfaces should contact only other sterile areas. Unsterile team members must avoid reaching over a sterile field. Scrubbed persons should stay close to the sterile field, and if they change positions, they should turn back to back or face to face.
5. Edges of any sterile package or container are considered unsterile. Sterile boundaries are not always well defined, therefore the following rules are accepted guidelines:
   a. Cap edges of a bottle of sterile solution are considered contaminated once the cap is removed.

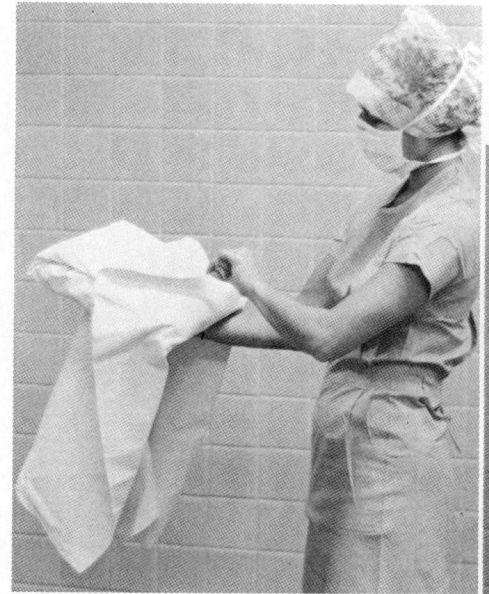
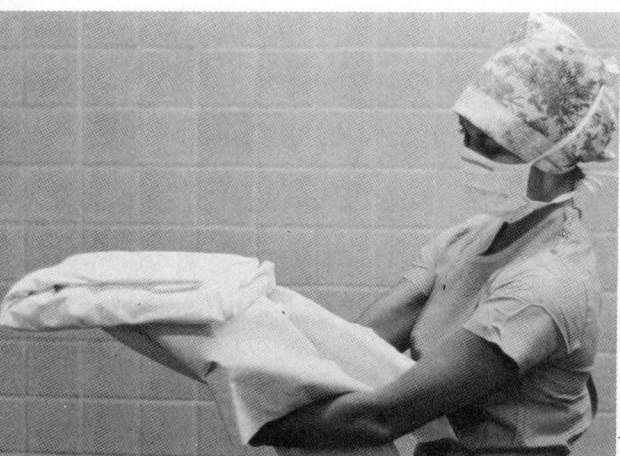

Fig. 18-2. A, When opening sterile package, circulating nurse opens corner nearest body last to avoid potential contamination of inner pack. **B,** To prevent unsterile corners of outer wrapper from touching scrub nurse or sterile field, circulating nurse draws back corners of opened wrapper when presenting inner package. (From Gruendemann, B.J., and Meeker, M.H.: Alexander's care of the patient in surgery, St. Louis, 1983, The C.V. Mosby Co.)

Since the cap cannot be replaced without contaminating the pouring edges, the sterility of the bottle contents is no longer certain and the remainder is discarded.

b. Package wrappers are usually considered to have a 1-inch safety margin around the edge. The flap ends are secured in the hand of the person opening them to avoid dangling the flap ends loosely (Fig. 18-2).

c. Peel-back packages should not be torn open but rather pulled back to expose sterile contents. The inner edge of the heat seal is considered to be the boundary between sterile and unsterile.

6. The sterile field should be created as close to the time it is going to be used as possible. The degree of contamination is proportional to the length of time items are left uncovered. Sterile areas are kept continuously in view, and once supplies are opened, someone must remain in the room to ensure sterility.

7. Sterile barriers that have been permeated are considered contaminated. Filtration of airborne microorganisms through materials (as when an item is dropped on the floor), passage of liquids through materials, and undetected holes are modes of contamination.

O.R. ATTIRE AND PERSONNEL HEALTH HABITS

Adherence to proper practices regarding the attire worn by health care workers within the operating room greatly lessens the risk of them serving as potential sources of infection for the patient. It is known that large quantities of bacteria are present in the nose and mouth, on the skin, and on the wearing apparel of persons who enter the operating room. For this reason, areas must be provided for staff members to remove personal attire, to put on appropriate O.R. attire, and to enter the operating room suite directly without passing through a contaminated area.

Daily body hygiene practices and clean hair also help prevent wound infections. Hair is a fertile source of bacteria, and other body areas may shed bacteria and dead cells into an open wound. Policy should prevent personnel who have active infections of any kind or who are known to be carriers of infection from entering the operating room suite.

Uniform

Street clothes should not be worn in restricted areas of the surgical suite. There should be a visible line beyond which no one may go without proper attire (Fig. 18-3). Clean operating room apparel made of fabric that meets the National Fire Protection Association standards should be available to anyone requiring entrance into restricted areas. Scrub pants with close fitting cuffs are superior to scrub dresses; such cuffs prevent the liberation of bacteria from the perineal and thigh area. Shirts are tucked inside pants to prevent accidental contact with sterile

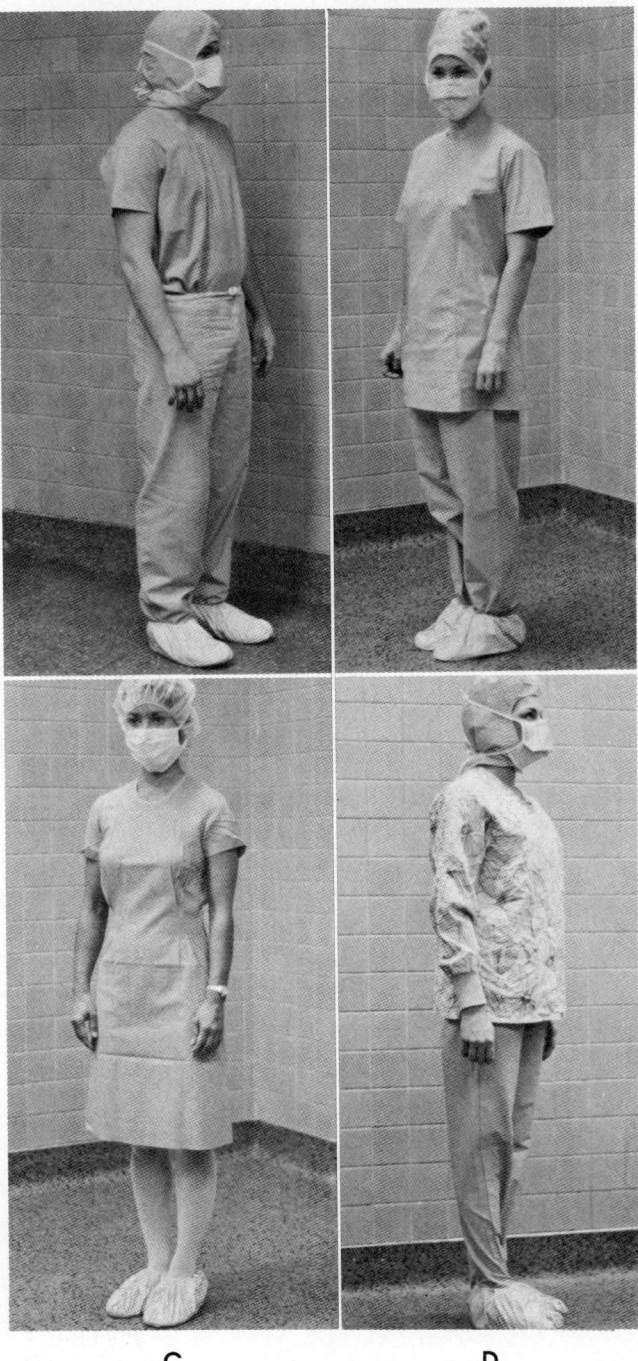

Fig. 18-3. Proper operating room attire. **A,** Scrub top should be tucked into pants or, **B,** should conform to waist to reduce dispersal of bacteria. Ankle closures on scrub pants ensure containment of potential contaminants. **C,** Scrub dress should be secured at waist. Advocates of scrub dresses believe that bacteria can be contained as effectively with panty hose as with pantsuits. **D,** Warm-up jacket worn over scrub suit provides maximum coverage of skin. (From Gruendemann, B.J. and Meeker, M.H.: Alexander's care of the patient in surgery, St. Louis, 1983, The C.V. Mosby Co.)

areas and to contain skin shedding. It is also recommended that nonsterile team members wear long-sleeved warm-up jackets to prevent shedding from bare arms. If scrub dresses are worn, they are secured at the waist and panty hose are worn to reduce bacterial shedding. Operating room attire that becomes visibly soiled or wet is changed, and all O.R. apparel is laundered by the hospital laundering facilities.

Head coverings

All possible head and facial hair, including sideburns and neckline are completely covered before donning other O.R. attire. This prevents the possibility of hair or dandruff being shed onto the scrub suit. Caps should be flame resistant, provide comfort, and fit snugly. Cleanliness of homemade caps is debatable; if they are used, it is recommended that they be laundered by hospital facilities. Disposable head coverings are discarded in designated containers before the person leaves the operating room suite.

Masks

All personnel should wear disposable high filtration masks in specified restricted areas of the surgical suite. The mask must completely cover the mouth and nose and be secured so as to allow no venting to occur at the sides. This prevents droplets from the oro- or nasopharynx from being expelled into the surgical environment. Masks must also be handled properly during and after use. Masks should be either on or off and not dropped loosely around the neck; if allowed to dangle, bacteria that have been filtered onto the mask will become dry and airborne. When masks are removed, only the strings are touched to reduce contamination of the hands from the nasopharyngeal area. Masks are changed between cases and more often if they become moist during a long case.

Shoe coverings

All persons entering the restricted areas of the surgical suite should wear shoe covers. When the same shoes are worn in the O.R. for successive operations, they will have a very high bacterial count and a potential for cross-infection.

Shoe covers must be conductive in areas where static spark is a hazard, and conductivity is checked when entering the restricted area and at intervals throughout the tour of duty. Care must be taken to make sure that the black carbon strip is placed inside the shoe between the sock or hose in good contact with the inner sole to provide conductivity or an electrical ground for the wearer.

Shoe covers are removed when leaving restricted areas, and clean ones are reapplied on returning. This prevents cross-contamination with other areas of the hospital. In the interest of safety, clogs, sandals, and tennis shoes should not be worn in the operating room. Clogs can be a hazard when a person tries to move quickly, and if sharp objects are accidentally dropped, sandals and tennis shoes provide little protection.

Other considerations

Additional considerations in relation to O.R. attire may address the amount and type of jewelry that may be worn. Dangling necklaces and earrings may fall into the sterile field. Excessive rings or rings with sharp stones interfere with good handwashing technique as well as possibly injuring patient during transfers.

No operating attire, including surgical uniforms, caps, and shoe covers, should be worn outside the surgical suite as this creates a two-way hazard. Any contaminants coming in contact with the operating room team members can become airborne and find susceptible hosts outside the surgical suite. Conversely, bacteria present outside the suite may be carried back on O.R. attire. If this practice is not feasible, head and shoe coverings are removed and the scrub clothes are covered by a clean, buttoned lab coat when a person leaves the suite. On return, the scrub clothes are changed.

Scrubbing, gowning, and gloving

Only personnel who are free of upper respiratory infections and skin problems should scrub. Abrasions and cuts tend to ooze serum that may serve as a medium for bacterial growth.

The major objective of the surgical scrub is to reduce the microbial skin count as much as possible and to leave an antimicrobial residue on the skin to prevent regrowth. This is achieved by mechanically cleansing the hands and lower arms to remove skin oil, dirt, and microbes.

The exact procedure to be followed and the selection of materials used may differ among hospitals. The most frequently used antimicrobial agents include povidone-iodine, hexachlorophene, and chlorhexidene gluconate. When scrubbing, it is recommended that light friction be applied as opposed to hard scrubbing. This will produce dilation of blood vessels with better circulation, which helps recondition the skin; on the other hand, scrubbing with harsh bristles can cause desquamation of the dermis. The use of synthetic disposable sponges in place of brushes has become popular, however, reusable or disposable nylon brushes have been shown to be equally effective.

The actual scrub procedure may be based on the "time method" or the "anatomic brush-stroke method." Both methods are effective if properly carried out. The time method involves scrubbing the fingers, hands, and arms for an allotted period of time for each area. The brush-stroke method prescribes a number of brush strokes to be applied lengthwise with the brush or sponge for each surface of the fingers, hands, and arms. There is no difference in microbial reduction whether the scrub is of 5 or 10 minutes in duration. The same scrub procedure should be used consistently, whether it is the first or last scrub of the day.

Before beginning the surgical scrub, the hands are inspected for cuts or skin problems. Nails should be short to avoid glove puncture, and no polish is preferred to prevent a harbor for microbes. The head covering is adjusted to ensure that all hair is contained, and a fresh mask should be properly applied. (Surgical scrub guidelines are described in the box below.)

After the scrub, the team member is ready to put on sterile gown and gloves. The procedure for gowning and gloving may vary, depending on the type of materials used (linen or disposable) and gown design, and whether the gloving will be done by self or by another team member. Sterile gloves may be applied using an open or closed method. The closed method is usually preferred, since bare skin on the hands and wrists are not exposed during the process. (For detailed discussion on the procedures, see references 12 and 28.)

Surgical scrub guidelines

Suggested action

1. Remove all hand jewelry. Make last minute adjustments of head covering, mask, and eyeglasses.

2. Adjust water to a comfortable warm temperature. (Most scrub sinks have automatic or knee controls for water flow.)

3. Wet hands and forearms and apply antimicrobial soap or detergent into palms via foot control. Rub palmar surfaces together and add water as needed to make a lather.

4. Using friction, wash the hands and arms thoroughly to a level at least 2 inches above the elbow. The amount of time required may vary with the cleansing agent used and the amount of soil present.

5. Hands and arms should be rinsed thoroughly, being careful to keep the hands higher than elbows. Avoid splashing water onto clothing.

6. A sterile brush or sponge (either prepackaged or from a dispenser) should be obtained. A metal or plastic nail cleaner should be included and used to clean under the fingernails while hands are held under running water.

7. An antimicrobial agent should be applied to the brush or sponge if not already impregnated. Starting at the fingertips, the nails and subungual area should be scrubbed vigorously with the brush held perpendicular to them. All sides of each finger are scrubbed, followed by the back and palm of the hand.

8. The arms are scrubbed on each side with a circular motion to 2 inches above the elbow. (The time spent in steps 7 and 8 may be established by setting a time limit for the scrubbing of one part after another or by counting a particular number of strokes for each side of each part.)

9. The hands and arms are rinsed thoroughly with the brush being discarded into the proper container. Hands and arms are held up in front of the body with elbows slightly flexed as the person enters the operating room.

Rationale

1. Jewelry harbors microorganisms and also serves as a potential source of foreign bodies in the operative wound.

2. Warm water has a lower surface tension than cold, which is believed to enhance cleansing action.

3. Detergents and soaps lower surface tension of water and emulsify oil.

4. Microbes are removed by physical, mechanical separation as well as chemical antisepsis. By washing one handbreadth above contaminated areas, recontamination of hands and forearms during rinsing and drying is more readily avoided.

5. This allows water to run off at the elbow and prevents contaminated water from above the elbow from running down onto scrubbed hands. If the scrub attire becomes wet, the moisture may cause contamination of the sterile gown by wicking action.

6. Special attention should be given to the subungual space where microbes can accumulate. Orangewood sticks should not be used because they cannot be sterilized properly afterwards.

7. and 8. Hospital policy should be established, and the procedure posted in the scrub area. The individual's conscientious attention to detail is of utmost importance.

9. Rinse procedure should be followed as in step 5. Same rationale applies.

Safety and protection of the patient

ADMITTING PATIENT TO THE OPERATING ROOM AREA

Most hospitals have an established procedure for admission into the holding area of the O.R. suite. The holding area is ideally a quiet, restful area where patients can gain optimum benefit from any premedication they have received. This is also an area where patients may feel terribly alone. They now come face to face with their impending surgery. Separation from family members has become a reality, and any fears the patient might have are likely to resurface.

The professional nurse's first goal is to establish a meaningful relationship with the patient. The nurse greeting the patient can decrease the patient's apprehension by a friendly introduction and by talking to the patient in a positive manner. The patient is told that the circulating nurse will be in constant attendance once the patient is admitted to the surgical room, and an explanation is given of what is being done in preparation for the surgery. If the nurse treats the patient with respect and warmth, answering any questions, and seeing to the patient's comfort at the time, much will be accomplished toward instilling security and confidence in the entire O.R. team. Any necessary delays are explained to the patient and also relayed to the waiting family.

The circulating nurse also has a number of important observations to make when admitting the patient to the operating room.

1. Ask the patient to state his or her name, the operative procedure to be done, and the site of the operation, if pertinent.
2. Check the patient's name and hospital number on the chart and compare it with the name and number on the patient's identification band.
3. Check for a signature on the operative permit and determine if properly signed, dated, and witnessed. The procedure on the permit must agree with the scheduled procedure.
4. Review the chart, checking for the following:
   a. The medical history and physical examination results, which must be completed before surgery begins
   b. Laboratory reports and x-rays (abnormalities are reported to the surgeon and anesthesiologist)
   c. Availability of blood if the patient was typed and crossmatched
   d. Allergies and any previous reactions to anesthesia or transfusions
5. Check for jewelry, wigs, contact lenses, prostheses, dentures, and objects in the mouth.
6. Observe the patient for any signs of adverse effects to preoperative medication and ask patient if anything has been taken by mouth if an NPO order was written.

TRANSFERRING AND POSITIONING PATIENT FOR SURGERY

Based on the scheduled procedure and the surgeon's preferences, the circulating nurse should be able to anticipate the basic patient position required. The final responsibility for the position of the patient on the O.R. table is one shared by the nurse, surgeon, and anesthesiologist. During the preoperative assessment, the patient's height, weight, and individual health problems that may relate to safe transfer and positioning have been determined and recorded.

No matter what position is to be assumed, good positioning is important to the following:

1. To adequately expose the operative area
2. To make the patient accessible for induction of anesthesia and administration of intravenous solutions or drugs
3. To minimize interference with circulation as a result of pressure on a body part
4. To provide protection from injury to nerves as a result of improper positioning of arms, hands, legs, or feet
5. To provide for the maintenance of respiratory function by avoiding pressure on the chest to allow for adequate ventilation of the lungs and by holding the jaw forward to keep it from dropping on the chest
6. To provide for patient's privacy by proper draping and avoiding unnecessary exposure

Specific nursing care planning may involve deciding the appropriate method of transfer, determining equipment and positioning aids needed, and if additional personnel will be needed to carry out the plan safely. Implementation of the plan includes certain safety measures, which may include the following:

1. The O.R. table and transfer cart are securely locked
2. A physician assumes responsibility for movement of an unsplinted fracture
3. All muscles, nerves, and bony prominences are positioned or padded to avoid injury
4. Heavily sedated patients and the elderly are moved slowly and gently to prevent shearing forces on the skin and to allow the circulatory system to adjust
5. Care is taken to see that no tubings (for example, intravenous, lines, urinary catheters) are dislodged or obstructed
6. Restraints are placed snugly over a blanket covering the patient, avoiding contact with the skin. Straps should not interfere with circulation or exert pressure on nerves or bony prominences
7. Sterile tables are positioned high enough to prevent any pressure on the patient's body
8. Sterile team members are reminded not to lean on any part of the patient.

The patient may be positioned on the operating room table in a number of different positions (Table 18-2 and Figs. 18-4 and 18-5). Whatever the position, special at-

Table 18-2. Commonly used operative patient positions

Position	Description	Comments
Supine	Flat on back with arms at side, palms down, legs straight with feet slightly separated (Fig. 18-4, A)	Most commonly used position, used for hernia repair, exploratory laparotomy, cholecystectomy, gastric and bowel resection, and mastoidectomy.
Prone	Patient lies on abdomen with face turned to one side, arms at side with palms pronated, elbows slightly flexed; feet elevated on pillow to prevent plantar flexion (Fig. 18-4, B)	Patient is anesthesized in supine position, then placed prone; used for surgery on back, spine, and rectal area.
Trendelenburg	Head and body are lowered into a head-down position and held in place with padded shoulder braces; knees are flexed by "breaking" table (Fig. 18-4, C)	Respiratory excursion is decreased from upward movement of viscera; used for surgery on lower abdomen and pelvis
Reverse Trendelenburg	Head is elevated and feet lowered	Used for biliary surgery
Lithotomy	Patient lies on back with buttocks to edge of table; thighs and legs are placed in stirrups simultaneously to prevent muscle injury; head and arms are secured to prevent injury (Fig. 18-5, A)	Used for perineal, rectal, and vaginal surgery; elastic wraps may be used on legs to prevent thrombus formation
Lateral	Patient lies on side; table may be "bent" in middle (Fig. 18-5, B)	Used for renal surgery

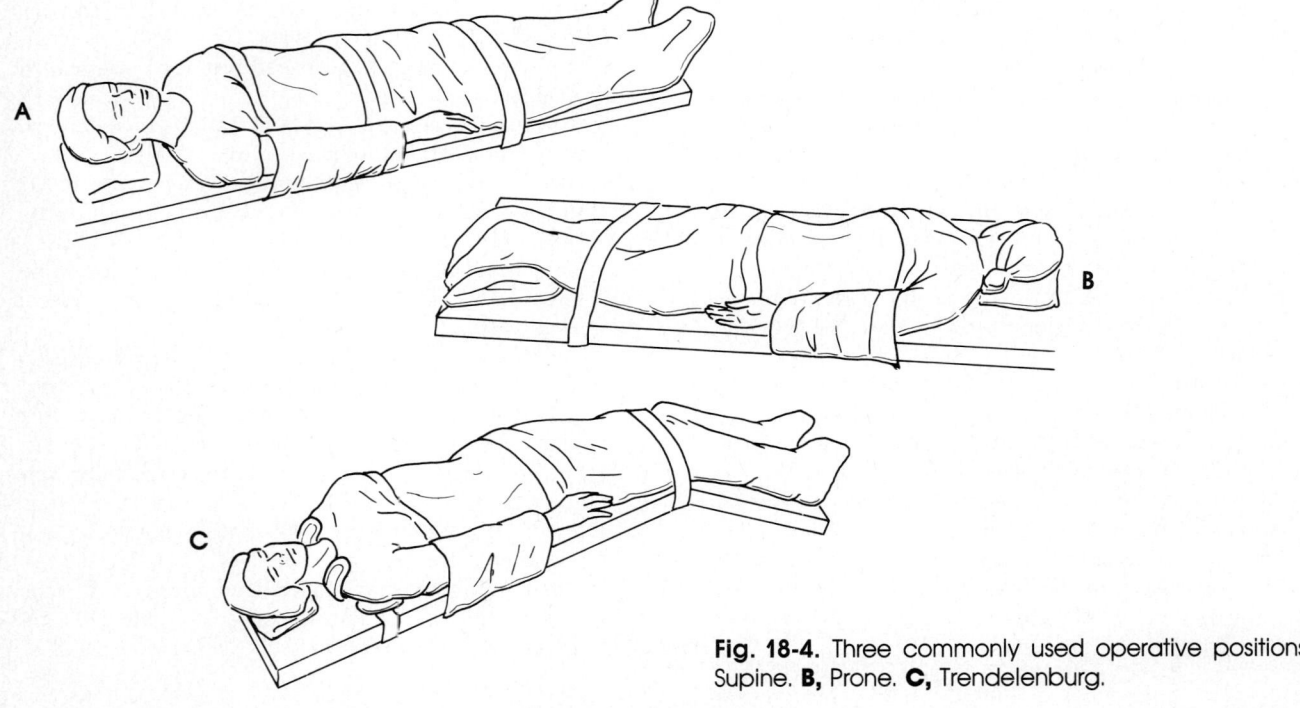

Fig. 18-4. Three commonly used operative positions. **A,** Supine. **B,** Prone. **C,** Trendelenburg.

tention is given to prevent injury to the patient's arms and legs and to prevent pressure on any one given area.

One major problem that may occur is the pooling of blood in dependent areas. Sudden shifting of blood when the supine position is reassumed following surgery may place a strain on the cardiovascular system with a precipitous drop in blood pressure. For this reason, the patient is always returned *slowly* from the operative positon to the supine position. Elderly persons and persons with preexisting cardiovascular problems are at high risk and are monitored carefully.

SKIN CLEANSING AND PREPARATION

The purpose of preoperative skin preparation is to establish an operative site as free as possible from dirt, skin oils, and transient microbes, as well as reducing the resident microbial count to as low as possible. This should be accomplished in the shortest period of time with the least amount of tissue irritation. If the skin "prep" is to be done while the patient is awake, the nurse explains the procedure to the patient, providing for comfort and minimizing exposure.

Removal of hair from the operative site should only be done as necessary and as near the time of surgery as possible. Alternatives for hair removal include a depilatory, electric clippers, and shaving with a razor. Studies have revealed that differences in wound infection rates are higher for patients shaved preoperatively than for patients with no preoperative shave or on whom a depilatory is used.[19] If a shave is ordered, it should be done by a per-

son who has demonstrated skill in the procedure to avoid nicking and cutting the skin. Such skin breaks can allow cutaneous bacteria to proliferate and increase the chances of infection.

After hair is removed, the operative site is prepared with an antimicrobial agent(s). The agent used, the method of application, and the exposure time of the skin to the agent is determined by institutional policy and the surgeon's preference. Criteria used in selection of the agent include the following:

1. Spectrum of activity (gram-positive or gram-negative organisms, activity in presence of blood or pus)
2. Speed of action
3. Potential for skin irritation and sensitivity
4. Flammability characteristics (especially if electrosurgery will be used)
5. Possible incompatibility or inactivation by alcohol, soap, detergent, or organic matter

Supplies used for the final skin preparation are arranged on a separate sterile table. The scrub begins at the proposed incision line and proceeds to the periphery of the area involved. A soiled sponge is never brought back over a scrubbed area. Open wounds and body orifices are prepared last, even when these areas are the proposed incision line.

STERILE DRAPING

The purpose of draping is to create a sterile field around the operative site. An effective barrier eliminates the passage of microorganisms between sterile and non-

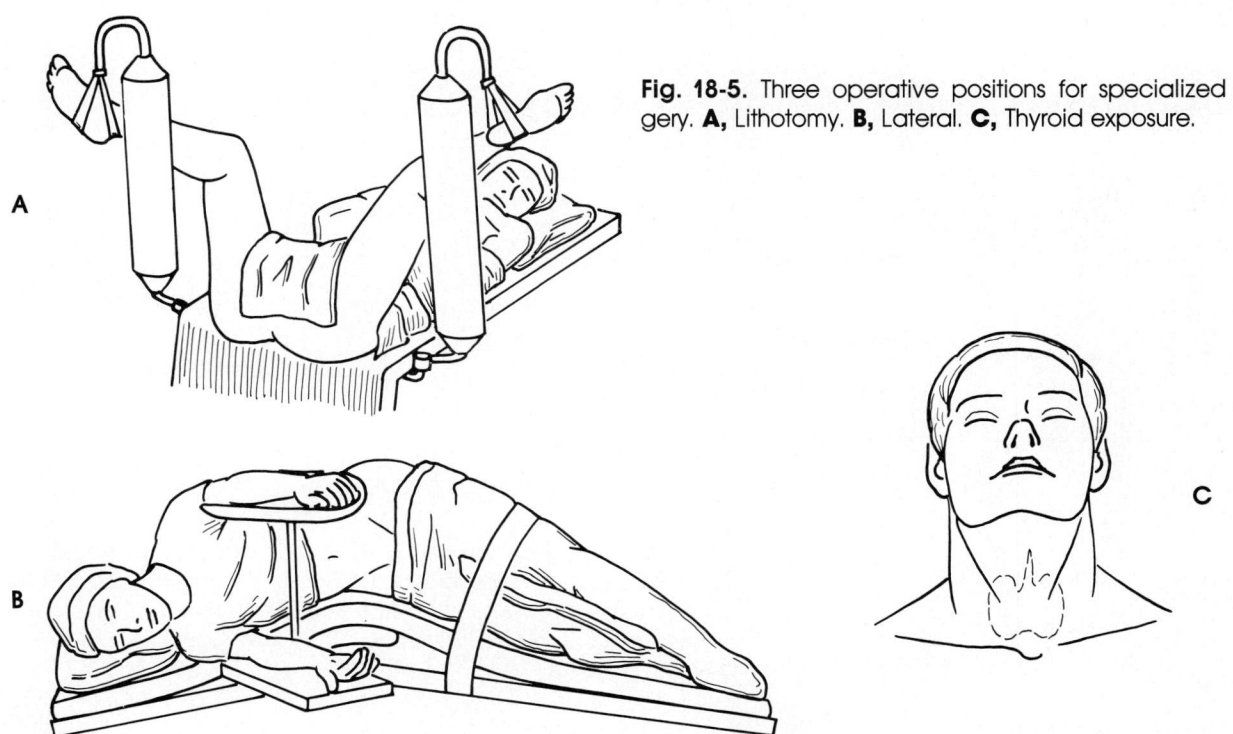

Fig. 18-5. Three operative positions for specialized surgery. **A,** Lithotomy. **B,** Lateral. **C,** Thyroid exposure.

Table 18-3. Types of anesthesia

Type	Action and effect	Method of administration	Definition
General	Blocks awareness centers in brain; produces unconsciousness, body relaxation, loss of sensation	Inhalation	Vapors from liquids and gases under pressure, administered through a tube and/or mask
		Intravenous	Drug given directly into vein, usually used for induction
Regional	Inhibition of excitatory process in nerve endings or fibers; analgesia over a specific body area with consciousness retained	Nerve block	Injection of drug to anesthetize an isolated nerve
		Intravenous regional block with tourniquet (Bier block)	Injection of drug intravenously into an extremity
		Field block	Series of injections of drug into tissues surrounding the operative site
		Spinal (intrathecal)	Injection of drug into subarachnoid space of spinal cord (Fig. 18-6)
		Epidural	Injection into space surrounding dura mater without breaking dural membrane
Local	Blocks transmission of nerve impulses at site of action; analgesia over limited tissue area with consciousness retained	Topical	Drug applied directly to surface, mucous membrane, or open wound
		Infiltration	Injection of drug into tissue at site of incision

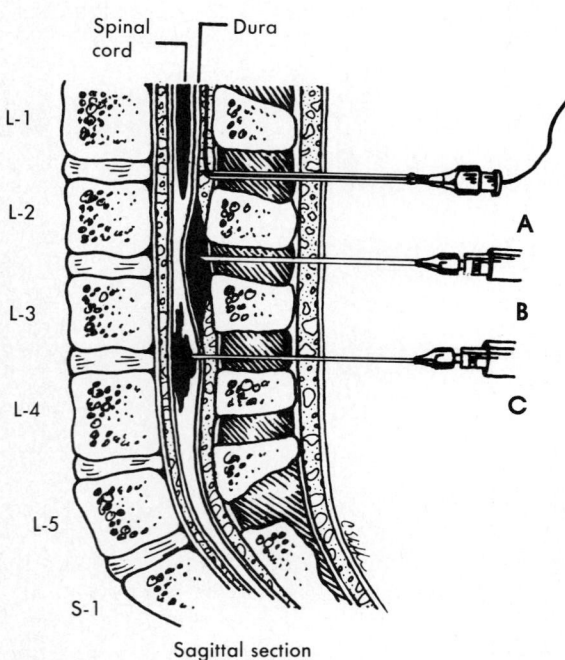

Spinal cord   Dura

L-1

L-2

A

L-3

B

L-4

C

L-5

S-1

Sagittal section

Fig. 18-6. Position of needles and injection sites. **A,** Epidural catheters. **B,** Epidural anesthesia. **C,** Spinal anesthesia. (From Gruendemann, B.J. and Meeker, M.A.: Alexander's care of the patient in surgery, ed. 7, St. Louis, 1983, the C.V. Mosby Co.)

Table 18-3. Types of anesthesia—cont'd

Type	Action and effect	Method of administration	Definition
Hypoanesthesia	Artificially induced passive state of consciousness in which there is increased amenability to suggestions and commands, reduced awareness, and restricted attentiveness	Hypnosis	Induction of the anesthetic state by hypnosis; may be combined with use of small dose of IV anesthetic or muscle relaxant
Acupuncture	Blocks painful stimuli by "gate control theory" and by stimulating release of endorphins with consciousness retained	Use of needles or surface electrodes	Needles or electrodes are connected to an electronic machine that creates current flow between these electrodes

sterile areas and leaves a minimal area of skin exposed.

Towels or self-adhering plastic sheeting are commonly used to drape the area immediately surrounding the operative site. Towels may be made of cotton muslin or synthetic disposable materials. If muslin is used the towels are held in place with towel clips, while synthetics may have their own self-adherent edge. Sterile, waterproof, antistatic, plastic sheeting, commonly referred to as an "incise drape," has an adhesive backing that is applied to dry skin. The skin incision is made through the plastic, preventing skin excretions and bacteria from coming in contact with the wound.

Various other sizes of draping sheets are used to cover the areas above and below the operative area. The patient and the operating table are covered with sterile drapes in such a manner as to allow exposure of the surgical site and isolation of the area of the surgical wound. Fenestrated sheets are available with openings of different sizes and shapes. Several reusable and disposable materials are available; they are not equally impermeable to moisture over time, and this is considered during draping.

ANESTHESIA

Usage

Anesthetics must be administered by an experienced person who has been trained in the administration of anesthetic agents. Although surgical nurses do not administer anesthetic agents, they may be called on to assist the physician in doing so on the clinical unit or in a specialized area of the hospital such as the emergency room. It is essential for the nurse to have an understanding of drug interactions, of the preanesthetic preparation of the patient, and of the effects of anesthetic agents given dur-

---

Effects of anesthesia

Amnesia	Loss of memory
Analgesia	Insensibility to pain
Hypnosis	Artificially produced sleep
Relaxation	Rendering a part of the body less firm or rigid

---

ing the operative phase to provide effective nursing care in the postoperative period.

The effects of anesthesia are listed in the box above. Anesthetic agents may be given to produce unconsciousness (general anesthesia) or to produce loss of sensation in specific body areas (regional anesthesia). "Local" anesthesia can be considered a form of regional anesthesia (Table 18-3). Hypoanesthesia (usually hypnosis) is rarely used, and acupuncture, although commonly carried out in Oriental countries, is seldom used.

Choice

The choice of anesthetic is based on many factors: the physical condition and age of the patient; the presence of coexisting diseases; the type, site, and duration of the operation; and the personal preferences of the anesthetist. The anesthesiologist evaluates each patient carefully and selects the anesthetic agents best suited for that individual. An apprehensive patient may not respond well to a regional anesthetic.

Preparation of patient for anesthesia

Patients have many anxieties related to anesthesia. Most anxieties can be dispelled if the patient and family are well informed about the anesthetic selected for use and the care taken by the physician and nurse in assessing the patient's physical condition. The patient is encouraged to discuss any questions or concerns about the anesthetic with either the anesthesiologist or the surgeon.

The patient can be assured that there will be close surveillance during anesthesia and in the immediate postoperative period. Very few patients talk while under anesthesia, and what is said is usually unintelligible so that talking need not be of great concern to the patient. Persistent anxiety on the part of the patient regarding the anesthetic should be discussed with the surgeon and the anesthesiologist.

Fears related to anesthesia

Going to sleep and not waking up
Fear of the unknown
Effectiveness of the anesthetic
Pain during the surgical procedure
Postoperative nausea and vomiting
Talking, revealing personal information while anesthetized
Mask over face

A premedication is commonly ordered to assist in sedating the patient, and if necessary, in drying secretions that may interfere with safe deliverance of a general anesthetic. This is usually administered before the patient's arrival in the operating room suite but may be given there in an emergency situation.

After the patient is transferred to the operating room table, an intravenous infusion is started and any necessary noninvasive monitoring equipment is connected (for example, electrocardiogram leads, blood pressure cuff, stethoscope, and so on. The desired anesthesia will then be administered.

It is very important that the circulating nurse remain near the patient during induction of the anesthetic. The nurse may be called on to protect the patient physically if an untoward reaction occurs. It is possible for the patient to become excited and to move excessively, requiring additional restraint to prevent self-injury. Stimulation of the patient in the form of noise or moving body parts is avoided as this may cause vomiting, retching, or laryngospasm, which in turn may lead to hypoxia. If this occurs, the anesthesiologist may require the nurses' assistance with suctioning equipment and with observing the monitors. Emotional support can be very inmportant, and simply holding the patient's hand has been reported by many to be a great comfort.

General anesthesia

General anesthesia is produced by inhalation or by injection into the bloodstream of anesthetic drugs. Certain drugs that produce general anesthesia when administered

Table 18-4. Comparison of selected anesthetic agents

Name	Method of administration	Advantages	Disadvantages	Special postoperative care
Nitrous oxide	Inhalation	Rapid induction and recovery; nonirritating; nonflammable but supports combustion	Possible hypoxia with excessive amounts	Monitor for signs of hypoxia
Halothane (Fluothane)	Inhalation	Rapid induction; low incidence of postoperative nausea or vomiting; nonirritating; nonflammable	Shivering with emergence; circulatory-respiratory depressant	Monitor vital signs closely
Methoxyflurane (Penthrane)	Inhalation	Decreased need for analgesics in immediate postoperative period; nonflammable	Prolonged induction; renal toxicity (dose dependent); postoperative nausea or vomiting	Position to prevent aspiration if vomiting occurs
Enflurane (Ethrane)	Inhalation	Rapid induction and recovery; some muscle relaxation on its own; nonflammable	Circulatory/respiratory depression (dose dependent); expensive; shivering with emergence	Monitor vital signs frequently

Table 18-4. Comparison of selected anesthetic agents—cont'd

Name	Method of administration	Advantages	Disadvantages	Special postoperative care
Cyclopropane	Inhalation	Rapid induction; adequate muscle relaxation	Highly flammable; possible cardiac irritability and arrhythmias; emergence excitement; postoperative nausea, vomiting, headache	Monitor pulse frequently for irregularities; position to prevent aspiration with vomiting
Isoflurane (Forane)	Inhalation	Smooth and rapid introduction; good muscle relaxant; nonirritating; cardiovascular stability	Expensive	Hypotension may occur
Ether	Inhalation	Inexpensive; good muscle relaxation; decreased need for postoperative analgesia	Irritating to mucous membranes; prolongation of anesthesia; postoperative nausea or vomiting; flammable	Supervise constantly in early postoperative period; position to prevent aspiration; suction if large amounts of mucus present; inspect face and eyes for blistering or irritation
Thiopental sodium (Pentothal Sodium)	IV	Rapid smooth induction and recovery	Laryngospasm with stimulation of larynx; respiratory depression with high doses; blood pressure may drop suddenly	Monitor for signs of stridor, neck tissue retraction, cyanosis; monitor vital signs for ↓ respiratory depth or ↓ blood pressure
Droperidol and fentanyl	IV	Rapid smooth induction and recovery; nontoxic to liver, kidneys, or heart; less analgesia required postoperatively	Hypoventilation	Monitor for ↓ respiratory rate or depth; decrease postoperative narcotics to one third to one fourth usual dose
Ketamine	IV	Profound analgesia with no loss of consciousness; amnesia for surgical event	Unpleasant dreams in early postoperative period and sometimes later; does not block visceral pain	Maintain quiet environment postoperatively
Procaine Cocaine Tetracaine Dibucaine Lidocaine Carbocaine Bupivacaine Chloroprocaine	Tissue injection (local); spray	No loss of consciousness	CNS stimulation or seizures; cardiac depression; absorbed into bloodstream	Monitor for excitability, twitching, pulse, or blood pressure changes, pallor, respiratory difficulty

Table 18-5. Stages and planes of ether anesthesia and selected central nervous system effects*

Central nervous system effects	Stage 1	Stage 2	Stage 3 planes 1	2	3	4	Stage 4
Consciousness	Maintained Analgesia Euphoria Some distortion of perceptions Variable amnesia	Lost	Absent	Absent	Absent	Absent	Absent
Respiration	No alteration or increased rate with some irregularity	Rapid, irregular	Regular	Regular but expirations longer than inspirations	Diaphragmatic	Thoracic ceased Diaphragmatic depressed	No respiratory movement Respiratory paralysis
Skeletal muscles	Normal tone	Tone increased	Small muscles relaxed	Large muscles relaxed	Complete relaxation	Complete relaxation	Diaphragm paralyzed
Eyes							
Pupils	Reaction to light	Dilated	Constriction	Mid-dilation	None	Dilated	Dilated
Movements	Unchanged	Increased	Increased	None	None	None	None
Tear secretion				Decreased	Decreased	Absent	
Reflexes							
Lid	Present	Present	Absent	Absent	Absent	Absent	Absent
Corneal	Present	Present	Present	Absent	Absent	Absent	Absent
Pharyngeal or "gag"			Absent				
Laryngeal				Absent			
Cough					Absent in large bronchi	Absent in small bronchi	
Heart rate	Unchanged	Increased	Decreased	Normal	Decreased	Decreased	
Blood pressure	Unchanged	Increased	Normal				Decreased
Venous pressure		Increased	Unchanged				Increased

*From Nahn, A.B., Barkin, R.L., and Oestreich, S.J.K.: Pharmacology in nursing, ed. 15, St. Louis, 1982, The C.V. Mosby Co.

intravenously, such as thiopental sodium (Pentothal sodium), are used to put the patient to sleep and are almost always supplemented with other agents to produce surgical anesthesia.

Frequently a combination of inhalation anesthetic agents such as nitrous oxide and oxygen may be used with muscle relaxants and narcotics. This form of combined drug administration is referred to as *balanced anesthesia*. The combination of drug effects provides analgesia, hypnosis, and adequate muscular relaxation as well as sleep. The choice of agents (Table 18-4) depends on the anesthesiologist's judgment and the individual patient's needs.

General anesthesia affects all the physiologic systems of the body to some degree. It chiefly affects the central nervous, respiratory, and circulatory systems. The anesthesiologist judges the depth of anesthesia by the changes produced in these systems. These changes are observed by monitoring heart rate (with stethoscope and ECG), blood pressure, and respiratory rate.

STAGES OF GENERAL ANESTHESIA

The stages of anesthesia may vary, depending on the drug used, the rapidity of induction, and the skill of the anesthesiologist. Since current practice is to induce anesthesia with a rapid-acting intravenously administered drug before inhalation anesthesia, a rapid transition through the early stages may occur. The classic, distinct stages are best seen when diethyl ether is used. All stages will not be observable with all anesthetics (Table 18-5). Characteristics of each stage are listed in box below.

INHALATION ANESTHESIA

Inhalation anesthesia is produced by having the patient inhale the vapors of certain liquids or gases. Oxygen is always given with these anesthetic agents. The gas mixture may be administered by mask or into the lungs through an endotracheal tube inserted into the trachea. The use of endotracheal intubation ensures an airway can be maintained when the chest wall is open. The endotracheal tube may have a balloon that is inflated after insertion. The balloon fills the tracheal space, lessening the chance of aspiration of gastric contents. Regardless of the skill of the anesthesiologist, an endotracheal tube cannot help causing some irritation to the trachea and subse-

quent edema. If it is difficult to intubate the patient, which may occur because of anatomic differences, it is not uncommon for the patient to complain of a sore, irritated throat postoperatively.

Some of the more common inhalant anesthetics are described in Table 18-4. The use of *nitrous oxide* is limited because it cannot be administered alone in adequate concentrations to produce deep muscle relaxation. The effect of nitrous oxide is additive with other anesthetics and is used extensively as an adjunct to halothane, enflurane, and methoxyflurane. Its greatest use is an agent for induction and as a component of balanced anesthesia for prolonged or complicated surgery. In low concentrations, nitrous oxide may provide adequate anesthesia for intraabdominal procedures in patients who are in profound shock, debilitated, or who are critically ill and cannot tolerate other anesthetic agents.

Cyclopropane quickly produces unconsciousness and adequate relaxation for most abdominal surgery. Emergence excitement is common. During the administration of this gas, extreme care must be taken to prevent the production of any electric charge that might cause it to be ignited.

Halothane (Fluothane) is easily inhaled and is usually administered through special vaporizers with nitrous oxide and oxygen. It is nonirritating, and laryngospasm is infrequent. Halothane does not provide adequate muscle relaxation, and a separate muscle relaxant must be used. It is contraindicated in patients with hepatic or biliary disease.

Isoflurane (Forane) is a relatively new anesthetic that many anesthesiologists believe will eventually become widely used. It is a depressant anesthetic similar to halothane. It provides adequate muscle relaxation and induction is smooth and rapid.

Ether is seldom used in the United States today because of its flammability and disagreeable side effects. Because it does have a wider margin of safety with minimal effects on the cardiovascular system, it may be used in areas of the world where sophisticated monitoring equipment is unavailable.

INTRAVENOUS ANESTHESIA

Thiopental sodium (Pentothal sodium) is the drug used most frequently for induction of anesthesia. It produces

---

Stages of anesthesia

Stage I	Extends from beginning of administration of anesthetic to beginning of loss of consciousness
Stage II	Extends from loss of consciousness to loss of eyelid reflexes; often called the stage of *excitement or delirium*
Stage III	Extends from loss of eyelid reflex to cessation of respiratory effort; called stage of *surgical anesthesia*. Patient is unconscious; muscles are relaxed; reflexes are abolished
Stage IV	Stage of *overdose* or danger; death will follow if anesthetic is not immediately discontinued.

Care of patient during prolonged hypothermia

1. Prepare patient for procedure
2. Give complete bath before procedure; protect skin with a thin coating of emollient
3. Insert indwelling catheter (if ordered) for monitoring urinary output
4. Monitor patient
   a. Monitor vital signs for sudden increases or decreases or rapid fluctuations
   b. Note shivering and give prescribed medication (usually chlorpromazine hydrochloride)
   c. Observe skin for signs of pressure, edema, discoloration
5. Turn patient every 2 hours and maintain good body alignment
6. Provide fluids and nutrients as ordered (usually by intravenous or tube feedings)
7. Provide good oral hygiene
8. Cleanse and protect eyes if corneal reflexes and eye secretions are decreased
9. When hypothermia is terminated:
   a. Apply blankets to rewarm patient
   b. Monitor return of normal body temperature and remove blankets as necessary

Monitoring methods during anesthesia

Arterial blood pressure	
Indirect method (sphygmomanometer)	Used in all situations
	Automatic equipment available
	Arm is protected from injury
Direct method (arterial catheter)	Catheter usually inserted percutaneously in radial artery
	Used for continuous monitoring in complex procedures and for induced hypotension
Stethoscopy	Stethoscope taped to chest
	Pressure sensitive units may be placed in esophagus
	Units are attached to anesthesiologists ear by indwelling earpiece
Electrocardiogram	Usually consists of a screen and a print-out system
	Chest and extremity electrodes used
	Other electrosurgical equipment may affect ECG recordings
Arterial blood gases	For evaluation of acid-base status and pulmonary gas exchange
Central venous pressure	For evaluation of overall circulatory status
	Serves as a guide during blood and fluid administration
	Aids in preventing too rapid fluid replacement that could lead to pulmonary edema
Estimation of blood loss	Weighing of blood-soaked sponges (dry weight subtracted from wet weight)
	Measurement of blood in suction systems
	Estimation of blood on drapes and team members' gowns
Body temperature	Thermistor inserted in esophagus or rectum
	Identification of events that are preceded by hypo- or hyperpyrexia
Urinary output	Hourly measurement from indwelling urinary catheter
	Evaluation of blood volume and fluid administration

INDUCED HYPOTENSION

Hypotension may be induced for the purpose of decreasing bleeding at the operative site in selected instances such as radical head and neck or pelvic surgery. Hypotension can be induced by deep anesthesia with an inhalant anesthetic such as halothane or by an intravenous anesthetic that affects the autonomic nervous system. Vital signs are monitored closely in the early postoperative period.

Monitoring patient during anesthesia

MONITORING METHODS

During surgery requiring anesthesia the patient's body is subjected to a variety of stressors. Potent drugs, required body positions, aggravation of preexisting disease processes, and bleeding may all contribute to situations that interfere with respiration and circulation and contribute to altered physiology.

Many devices are now available to augment the measurement of patient's responses to these stressors. Most of this equipment is expensive, takes up extra space in the operating room, and may constitute an electrical safety hazard. Involved personnel must still use skills of looking, listening, and palpating, even when sophisticated monitoring equipment is in use (see box, p. 322).

A variety of other monitoring devices may be used depending on the complexity of the procedure being performed and the physical condition of the patient. Computers are being used more extensively in monitoring and processing patient data and greater use of the computer is envisioned in the future.

ELECTRICAL SAFETY HAZARDS

Monitoring of patient safety during anesthesia must also take into consideration electrical safety hazards. The operating room is an area containing many potential life threatening and mechanically injurious situations related to electrical shock, burns, fire, and explosions. It is imperative that team members have up to date knowledge of the equipment and supplies most often involved in such incidents.

Federal regulations govern the marketing and safety standards of electronic devices used in operating rooms, and the Joint Commission on Accreditation of Hospitals has standards that must be met. The most significant hazards, however, are inadequately trained personnel, malfunctioning equipment caused by improper maintenance, inappropriate design of operating room suites, and inappropriate surveillance by team members.

TERMINATION OF SURGERY

One of the most crucial periods for the surgical patient is the immediate postoperative phase after surgery has been completed and the patient is transferred to the appropriate recovery area. During this period, the operating room nurse may be involved in a variety of activities related to providing effective patient care.

Dressings and drains

The circulating nurse will assist in the application of the outer layer of any necessary dressings. Dressings are used to protect the wound from trauma and contamination, to absorb drainage, and to support or immobilize the incisional area. Pressure dressings may be applied to aid in minimizing edema and to assist with hemostasis.

A wide variety of gauzes, pads, and tapes are available for use. The type used will depend on the area of the body involved, the amount of drainage anticipated, and the pressure that is necessary. Montgomery straps may be used if frequent dressing changes or wound inspections are anticipated. In some instances the application of a splint or cast will be required.

Some surgeons prefer that the wound be covered with a transparent spray dressing. This commonly stays on for 3 to 6 days and may either peel off or be removed with solvent. This type of dressing is particularly suitable for areas where gauze dressings could become contaminated with urine or feces.

Other surgeons prefer that the wound be left uncovered and open to the air to allow the incisional area to heal with the aid of air and light. It also allows for easy observation, prevents possible tape reactions, and increases comfort and maneuverability for certain patients.

A variety of drains may also be inserted at the time of surgery (see Chapter 19). Drains are used to expedite the removal of air and fluids such as blood, serum, bile, and pus from the involved site. The type and exact location of the drains are recorded and reported to the recovery room nurses.

Documentation

Written documentation is important for communicating to other health team members the nursing actions that were performed in the intraoperative period and the patient outcomes. If the perioperative role is to be effectively implemented, operating room nurses must be accountable by documenting what they do.

Some facilities have the operating room nurse document information on the same form used for all nursing notes. Others have found it more expedient to develop a separate form that combines a checklist format along with areas for narrative comments.

Transfer of patient to recovery room

After appropriate dressings have been applied, the circulating nurse checks to see that the patient is clean. A clean gown and blanket are applied.

Special care must be taken in moving the patient from the operating room table to the recovery stretcher or bed. At least four people are usually required to transfer the unconscious patient safely while keeping the body in proper alignment. Care must be taken not to allow the patient to slip between the table and the stretcher and that no body tissues have shearing forces applied to them. Arms and legs must be carefully supported and IV sites splinted to prevent dislodging the needle. The anesthesiologist protects the head and neck from injury during the transfer. A patient lifting frame or roller device is very helpful when moving heavy patients.

6. Drapes are applied in a manner that provides minimal skin exposure and maximal skin protection from infection.
7. The person receives proper monitoring while receiving anesthesia and until completion of transfer to recovery area.
8. Documentation includes presence of drains and actions taken to meet identified needs.

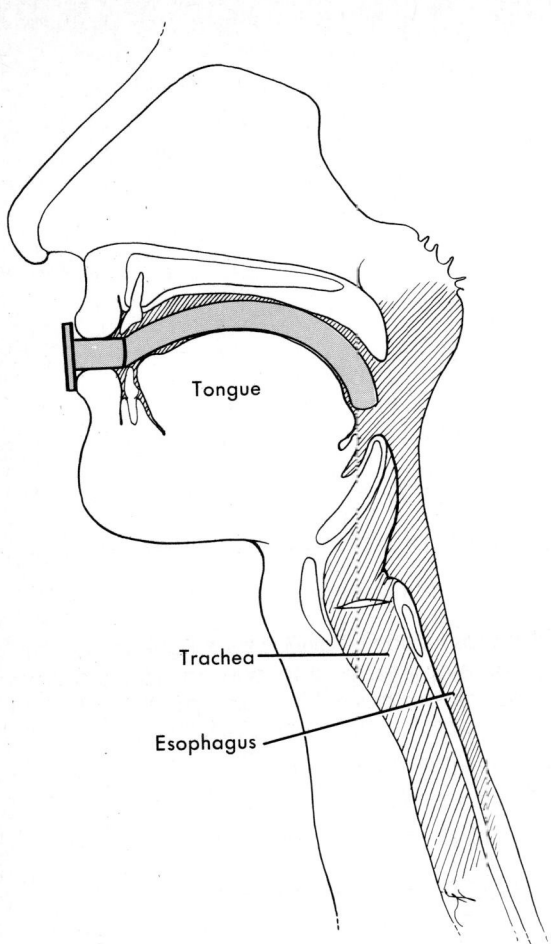

Fig. 19-2. Airway in place to prevent tongue from falling back against pharynx and blocking airway.

can be enhanced by oxygen therapy and breathing exercises.

Oxygen therapy

Oxygen is usually given postoperatively because after anesthesia almost all patients have decreased pulmonary expansion and areas of atelectasis, both of which result in hypoxemia. Oxygen is administered by nasal cannula or catheter, disposable face mask or shield, or endotracheal or tracheostomy tube if one is in place. Patients with thoracic or upper abdominal incisions or with preexisting pulmonary disease may be given oxygen for several hours or even into the next day.

Breathing exercises

Deep-breathing exercises are started as soon as the patient is conscious and able to follow directions. Considerable encouragement and repetition of directions are needed because of amnesia related to the anesthetic. If the patient is unconscious or will not breathe deeply when stimulated, the nurse can hyperventilate the lungs passively using a breathing bag and mask.

Possible causes of postoperative shock

Moving patient from operating table to bed
Jarring patient (bed) during transport
Reactions to drugs and anesthesia
Loss of blood and other body fluids
Cardiac arrhythmias
Cardiac failure
Inadequate ventilation
Pain
Residual sympathectomy from conductive anesthesia

Maintaining circulation

Hypotension and cardiac arrhythmias are the most common cardiovascular complications in the immediate postanesthetic period. Early recognition and management of these complications before they become serious enough to diminish cardiac output depend on frequent assessment of the patient's vital signs.

The blood pressure, pulse, and respirations are usually taken every 15 minutes until stable, then every half hour for 2 hours, and then every 4 hours until ordered otherwise. In many hospitals the monitoring of vital signs every 15 minutes extends for as long as the patient is in the recovery room and for at least 1 hour after leaving the recovery room. The rate, volume, and rhythm of the pulse are carefully observed and the character and rate of respiration are noted.

HYPOTENSION

Many factors can cause circulatory changes that result in lowering of blood pressure in the postoperative patient. A mild decrease in blood pressure from the normal preoperative range is not uncommon during the early postoperative period. It is usually well tolerated in healthy patients and does not require treatment. Shock, however, must be prevented because the brain, heart, kidneys, and other vital organs do not tolerate long periods of hypoxemia. Measures to control shock are immediately instituted when signs of shock occur (Chapter 11).

CARDIAC ARRHYTHMIAS

Hypoxemia and hypercapnia are common causes of postoperative cardiac arrhythmias, especially premature beats and sinus tachycardia. These arrhythmias often can be suppressed by adequate ventilation. Other common causes of postoperative cardiac arrhythmias include pain, hypovolemia, gastric distention, and acidosis. Significant arrhythmias are treated by attention to the underlying cause when possible. Antiarrhythmic drugs may be prescribed (Chapter 26).

Maintaining fluid and electrolyte balance

In most patients admitted to the recovery room administration of intravenous fluids is the immediate postoperative means of maintaining fluid and electrolyte balance. Careful monitoring of the intravenous fluids is essential to ensure adequacy of replacement and prevention of fluid overload (Chapter 10).

Maintaining safety and comfort

PREVENTING INJURY

After anesthesia, side rails on the stretcher or bed are generally raised and are left so until the patient is fully awake. The patient is turned frequently and placed in good body alignment to prevent nerve damage from pressure and muscle and joint strain from lying in one position for a long time.

PROMOTING PHYSICAL COMFORT

Incisional pain is a common complaint after surgery, and from the patient's point of view it is probably the most significant postoperative complication. In the immediate postanesthetic period, narcotic analgesics are given for pain when warranted, but this should be done with the realization that pronounced depression of the respiratory, circulatory, or central nervous system may follow. Because the patient generally has not completely recovered from the effects of the anesthetic, the first postoperative dose of a narcotic is usually reduced to about *one half* the dose to be received after full recovery from anesthesia. Pain medication for restlessness is given only after it has been determined that the restlessness is not a result of hypoxia.

PROMOTING PSYCHOLOGIC COMFORT

The immediate postanesthetic period is often frightening for the patient. Psychologic support is imperative for physical as well as emotional well-being. While awakening from anesthesia, the patient needs frequent orientation to place and reassurance of not being alone. The patient also needs to know that the operation is over and that recovery from anesthesia is satisfactory. Careful explanations of procedures being carried out are given even when it appears that the patient is not alert. The need for privacy is considered at all times. Patients who receive this type of support frequently recover from anesthesia faster, with fewer complications and less incisional pain.

Discharge from recovery room

Patients are discharged from the recovery room when the following criteria have been met:
1. Vital signs are stable and indicate adequate respiratory and circulatory function.

> ### Preparing room for patient's return from surgery
>
> 1. Make an open surgical bed to facilitate easy transfer of patient.
> 2. Provide sufficient covers (patient may feel cold).
> 3. Clear a passageway to the bed.
> 4. Provide necessary equipment
>   a. Intravenous pole
>   b. Sphygmomanometer
>   c. Any special equipment as designated by recovery room nurse.

2. Patient is awake or easily aroused and can call for assistance if needed.
3. Postsurgical complications have been thoroughly evaluated and are under control.
4. After regional anesthesia, motor and partial sensory functions have returned to all anesthetized areas.

Acutely ill patients who require further close supervision are transferred to an intensive care unit. Most patients are transferred to a clinical unit. The unit is notified to expect the patient, and all pertinent information concerning the patient's status is communicated to the nurse who will continue to provide postoperative nursing care. The recovery room nurse writes a discharge summary note before the patient leaves the recovery room.

ADMISSION OF PATIENT TO CLINICAL UNIT

Preparation on clinical unit

The patient's room is prepared and the family is notified of the expected return.

Most surgeons discuss the results of the operation with the family immediately after surgery and also visit the patient to describe briefly what was found and to provide reassurance. The family is frequently highly anxious concerning the patient's condition and may not perceive or understand all that the surgeon tells them. Patients frequently experience periods of amnesia during the hours when they first regain consciousness and may not remember what they have been told. The nurse needs to know what information was given to the patient and family to be able to answer their questions. The family also needs to know what to expect when the patient returns to the unit.

Initial assessment

As soon as the patient is positioned on the bed in the clinical unit, the nurse makes a rapid assessment of the patient's condition.

Table 19-1. Some causes of vital sign changes in early postoperative phase

Vital sign	Increase	Decrease
Temperature	Stress reaction (low-grade fever)	Cold operating room and recovery room
Pulse rate	Jarring during transfer Shock, hemorrhage Hypoventilation Acute gastric dilation Pain Anxiety Cardiac arrythmias	Digitalis overdose Cardiac arrhythmias
Respiratory rate	Hypoventilation: poor positioning, tight chest or upper abdominal dressing, obesity, gastric dilation	Drugs: anesthetics, narcotics, sedatives
Blood pressure	Anxiety ($\uparrow$ systolic) Pain	Jarring during transfer Severe pain Cardiac arrhythmias Shock: fluid loss, hemorrhage, acute gastric dilation

---

Patient assessment on return from recovery room

Respiratory status	Patency of airway Respirations: depth, rate, character Breath sounds: presence, character
Circulatory status	Pulse, blood pressure, temperature Skin color, temperature Capillary filling
Neurologic status	Level of consciousness
Dressing	Presence of drainage Presence of tubes to be connected to drainage systems
Comfort	Presence of pain, nausea, vomiting Patient positioned for comfort and to facilitate ventilation
Safety	Necessity for side rails Call cord within reach
Equipment	Monitors connected and functioning Intravenous fluids: rate, amount in bag, patency of tubing Drainage systems (e.g., nasogastric, chest, urinary): type, patency of tubing, connection of appropriate container, character and amount of drainage

---

SUBJECTIVE DATA

The patient is asked for symptoms of discomfort after having been transferred to the bed and positioned in supportive body alignment. This gives the nurse a quick indication of the level of alertness as well as symptoms of discomfort. An indirect question such as, "How do you feel?" will elicit data concerning nausea or pain without focusing on a specific area where there may be no discomfort. There is frequently an increase in pain perception at this time because of the movement from stretcher to bed. It is important to seek specific data concerning location, onset, and change in pain intensity and not to assume that the pain is incisional.

Nausea occurs less frequently postoperatively with the use of newer anesthetics. There is greater possibility of nausea when the stomach has been manipulated extensively during the surgical procedure or if considerable amounts of narcotics have been administered. The emesis basin should be easily available but not in sight if vomiting is a possibility.

OBJECTIVE DATA

Respiratory status

Respirations may be increased or decreased (see Table 19-1). If hypoventilation is present, oxygen may be given if a nasal catheter is in place.

Very noisy respirations may be heard without the aid of a stethoscope. Noisy respirations may be caused by airway obstruction from the tongue falling back against the pharynx or from secretions. The patient with noisy respirations should be assisted to cough and then positioned side-lying if possible. Suctioning may be indicated if coughing does not clear the airway.

If respirations are not noisy, the lungs are auscultated to establish a baseline for future comparison and to identify adventitious sounds (Chapter 3). Absent breath sounds indicate hypoventilation of the lobe (Table 19-1). Coarse rales indicate secretions in air passages. Presence of adventitious sounds indicates the need for energetic ventilatory exercises. Deep-breathing and coughing measures are instituted immediately in all patients who have had general anesthesia (Chapter 17).

Circulatory status

The pulse, blood pressure, skin color and temperature, and capillary filling are assessed (Table 19-1). Signs of shock or hemorrhage are reported immediately to the surgeon. Hypotensive changes may be related to shock, although other signs of shock usually occur before changes in blood pressure. The skin often feels cool to the touch after surgery as a result of coolness of the surgical suites, hypovolemia from blood loss, or vasoconstriction from stress. Restlessness is an early sign of shock.

After surgery of the extremities, local circulation is assessed by the presence and strength of peripheral pulses *distal* to the operative site or plaster cast. If the dressing is too tight it should be loosened, if permissible, or reported at once to the physician.

Level of consciousness

Level of consciousness can be ascertained by asking the patient to respond to simple questions or commands. Variations in consciousness level from alertness to drowsiness will be observed. If the patient is not easily aroused, these data are compared with the patient's consciousness status at the time of discharge from the recovery room. A decrease in consciousness level may indicate shock (from jarring motions during the transfer) and should be reported to the surgeon at once along with any other pertinent data.

Dressing

The entire dressing is inspected with the covers pulled back or the patient turned as necessary. A dressing applied to the side, such as after kidney surgery, may appear dry on the top visible area if the patient is supine but may have excess drainage on the lower portion as a result of gravity. Excess drainage is reported immediately.

Whenever it is anticipated that fluid may collect in a body area postoperatively, leading to delay in healing, the surgeon usually inserts a tube or drain (Table 19-2) to permit escape of the fluid. One end of the tube or drain is placed in or near the organ or cavity to be drained, and the other end is passed through the body wall, either through a separate "stab wound" or through the incision.

After most types of surgery, usually the surgeon changes the dressing for the first time. If small amounts of unexpected drainage are observed, especially bright red drainage, the area can be outlined with a pen on the dressing so that the rate of drainage can be easily determined. Dressings that *cannot* be changed by the nurse are reinforced with dry dressings if drainage penetrates the outer layer; this prevents bacterial contamination by capillary action through the wet dressings. If these additional dressings become wet, they are removed and replaced with new dressings, leaving the original dressing intact. Dressings that *can* be changed by the nurse are changed as often as necessary to prevent maceration of the skin and to promote patient comfort.

Body position

The patient is placed in a position of comfort and one that facilitates good ventilation. Except after spinal anesthesia or in certain types of eye surgery or neurosurgery when the bed must remain flat, most patients prefer the head of the bed slightly elevated. The patient who is not very alert needs to be placed in a position of good alignment. There should be no strain on the area surrounding the incision. Pillows should *not* exert pressure on the popliteal area (behind the knee), because this leads to venous obstruction.

ASSESSMENT OF FLUID LINES

Fluids may be ordered to be given intravenously or instilled in body cavities for irrigation, such as in the bladder. The contents of the fluid containers, the patency of the tubing, and the rate of fluid adimistration are checked. Fluids are usually given intravenously at rates ranging from minimal (to keep the line open, K/O) to 3 ml/min. If the rate is > 3 ml/min, and if the physician's order sheet is not available in the patient's room, the rate should be slowed, the order checked immediately, and the rate adjusted appropriately. Rate of administration varies with the amount of fluid lost, size and age of the patient, and the underlying illness (Chapter 10). The patient and family should be instructed early concerning permissibility of fluids taken orally.

Drainage from tubes can be accomplished by either gravity or suction (Table 19-3). All tubing is connected to the drainage receptacle and checked for patency. The amount of fluid in each receptacle is marked on the receptacle and recorded as baseline for future comparison.

SAFETY

Bed siderails are kept raised until the patient is fully awake and responding or to prevent the heavily medicated patient from falling. The patient is instructed early re-

Table 19-2. Surgical tubes and drains

Type	Purpose	Examples	Comments
Tubes	Prevent blockage of drainage Drain an area by suction	T-tube (Fig. 19-3) Abramson all-purpose tube (Fig. 19-4) Saratoga sump tube (Fig. 19-4)	Connect to drainage system as ordered
Drains	Drain an area by gravity	Penrose drain (Fig. 19-5) Cigarette drain (Fig. 19-5)	Use a safety pin to prevent drain from sliding back into abdomen Encase outer end of drain in a dressing

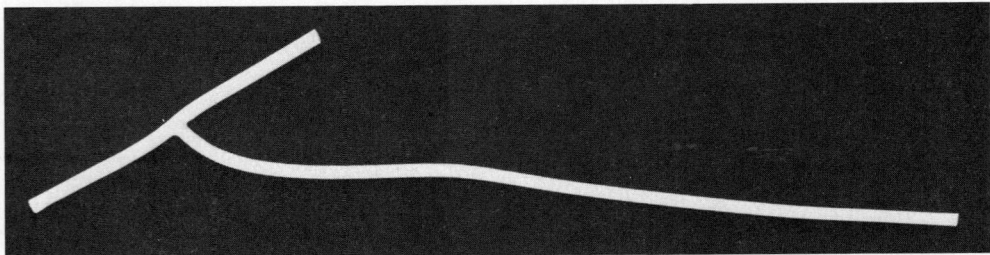

Fig. 19-3. T tube for draining common bile duct.

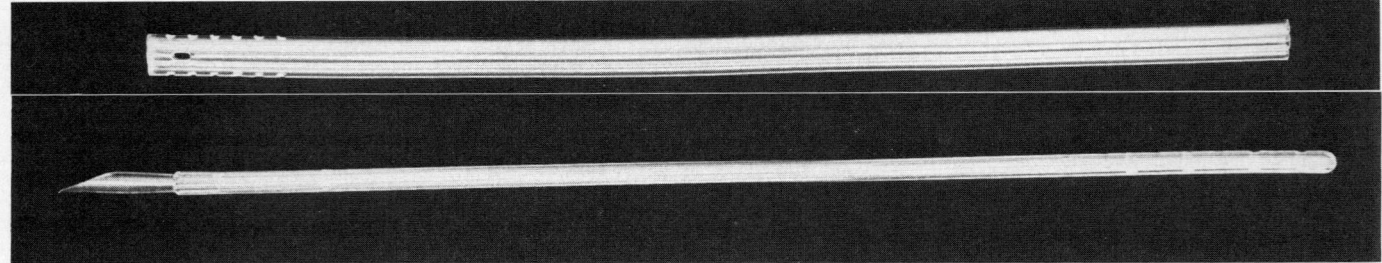

Fig. 19-4. Surgical drain tubes. *Top,* Abramson all-purpose drain has three lumens: for aspiration, irrigation, and instillation. *Bottom,* Saratoga sump drain has a tube within a tube for low-pressure suction.

Fig. 19-5. Wound drains. *Top,* Penrose drain. *Bottom,* Cigarette drain.

Table 19-3. Drainage systems

Tube	System
Nasogastric tube	
Levine tube	Intermittent low electric suction
Sump tube	Constant low electric suction
Urinary catheter	Gravity urinary drainage system
Chest tube	Waterseal drainage system (gravity or suction)
Incisional tubes	Low negative pressure: Hemovac (Fig. 19-6), Jackson-Pratt (Fig. 19-7), or low constant electric suction

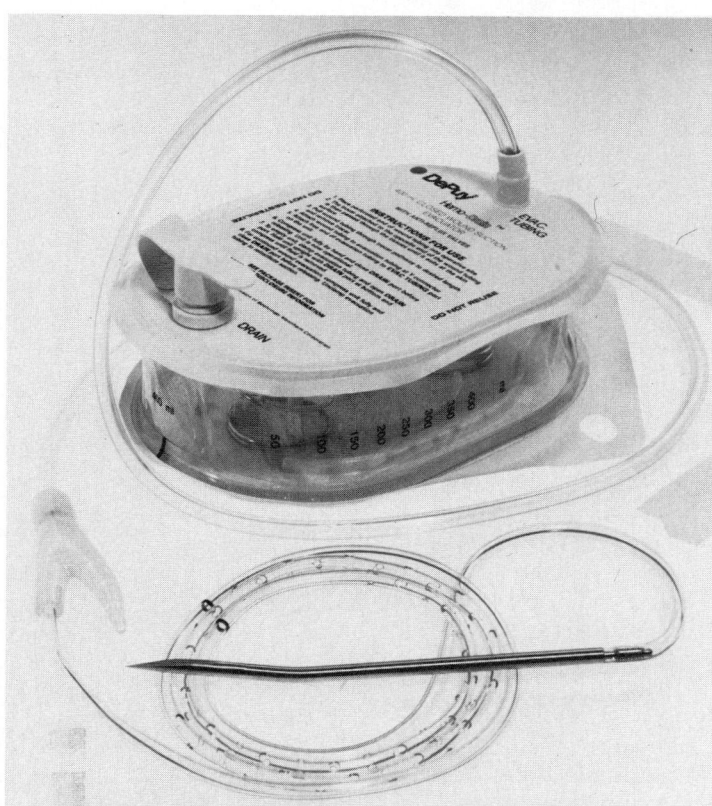

Fig. 19-6. Hemo-drain for low-suction wound drainage. Unit is compressed, then drain cap closed. Inner spring expands slowly, creating suction through tube. (Courtesy De Puy, Warsaw, Ind.)

Fig. 19-7. Jackson-Pratt wound suction apparatus. After emptying through spout, reservoir bulb is kept compressed until spout is closed. Slow expansion of bulb creates low-pressure suction.

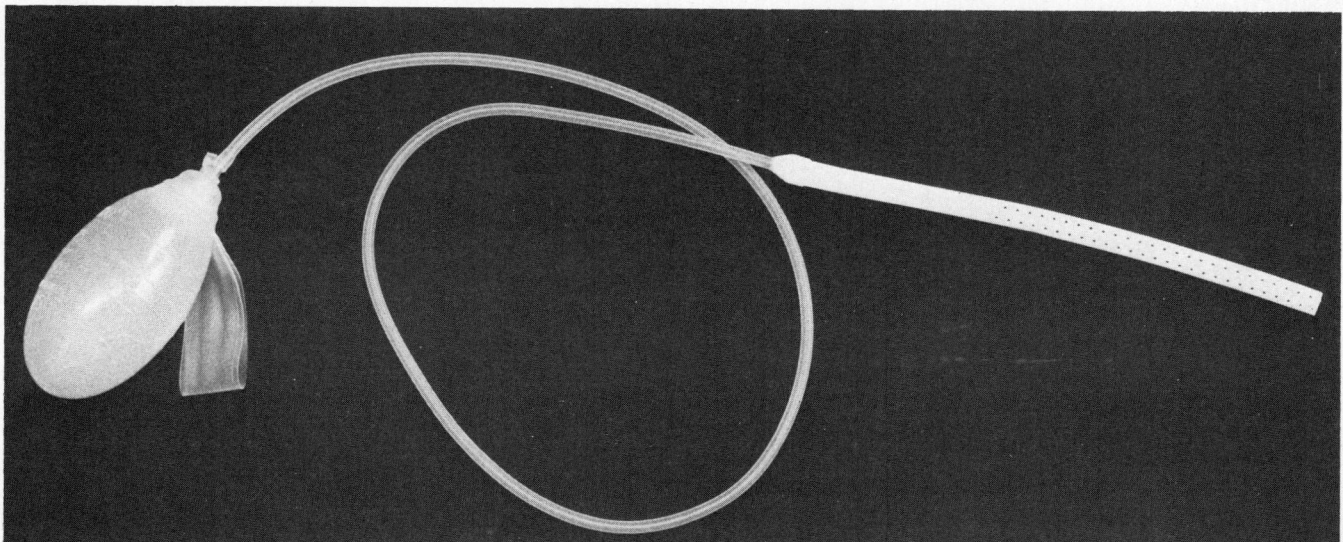

garding permissibility of ambulation and the need to call for assistance for initial attempts. The call cord should be easily accessible to the patient.

FAMILY MEMBERS

If family members are present in the room when the patient returns, they may be asked to step outside until the patient has been transferred and assessed. Before leaving the patient, the nurse invites the family to return, explains equipment, and describes the patient's state of awareness and comfort. Family members who understand what is occurring can offer support to the patient. Explanations should be simple but concrete and accurate.

Data from patient's chart

After the patient has been assessed and positioned comfortably and safely, the nurse gathers additional data from the patient's chart (Table 19-4) before planning and initiating general postoperative care.

DATA ANALYSIS AND PLANNING

The collected data are recorded in the nursing admission notes and used to identify the specific needs of the patient in the postoperative period. The preoperative condition of the patient, type of surgery performed, and strengths and resources of the patient are determining factors in postoperative discomfort or complications. In planning the patient's care the nurse uses previously collected data, present data, knowledge of factors related to specific types of surgery (as illustrated in succeeding chapters of this text), and specific postoperative needs and possible postoperative complications.

Nursing diagnoses

Some common nursing diagnoses for the postoperative patient include the following:

Breathing pattern: ineffective
Potential tissue perfusion: alteration, peripheral
Potential fluid volume: excess
Nutrition, alteration in: less than body
   requirement
Urinary elimination: urinary retention
Bowel elimination, alteration in: constipation
Comfort, alteration in: pain, nausea, hiccoughs
Potential impaired mobility
Potential for injury
Knowledge deficit
Anxiety

Table 19-4. Chart data useful in planning postoperative care

Data	Direction for action/interpretation
Surgeon's orders	
Activity	Extent permissible
Fluids, food	Intravenous: type, amount, rate
	Oral: type
Medications	Type and frequency of medications to be taken as needed
	Medications to be started immediately
Other orders	Special orders to be carried out depending on type of surgery
Surgical notes	
Postoperative diagnosis	Interpretation to patient/family
Type of surgery	Special nursing interventions
	Interpretations to patient/family
Anesthetic	
Inhalant	Need for deep-breathing measures
Muscle relaxants	Assessment of respiratory distress
Spinal	Supine position postoperatively; headache may occur
Estimated blood loss (EBL) and fluid replacement	Potential for fluid and electrolyte imbalance or transfusion reactions
Drains	Possible drainage on dressing
Recovery room notes	
Vital signs before transfer	Identification of changes related to transfer
Patient progress	Identification of persistent problems
Medications given	Times when drugs given and patient response
Urinary output	Status of renal function or urine retention

Expected patient outcomes

1. No injury occurs during hospitalization.
2. The incision heals normally without infection.
3. No avoidable complications (atelectasis, pneumonia, thrombophlebitis) occur.
4. Elimination patterns are reestablished.
5. The person carries out activities of daily living at an optimal level, although fatigue may still be present.
6. The person has an opportunity to explore individual concerns.
7. At discharge the person or significant other can explain:
   a. Treatments to be carried out at home, if any.
   b. Medications to be taken at home (name, dosage, frequency, side effects).
   c. Any dietary changes required by the surgery.
   d. Activity limits incurred by the surgery and any exercise programs to be carried out at home.
   e. When and where to go for follow-up care by the surgeon.

IMPLEMENTATION

Promotion of wound healing

PATHOPHYSIOLOGY OF WOUND HEALING

Result of wound healing

Wounds may heal by *regeneration* of the tissue or by *scar* formation. Injured cells that have the capacity to regenerate (Fig. 19-8) will do so if the underlying structure has not been destroyed. Muscle and nerve cells rarely undergo mitotic division and are unable to regenerate. When muscle cells are injured, satisfactory performance may result by hypertrophy of marginal cells. Nerve cells in the central nervous system do not regenerate. In the peripheral nervous system there is no regeneration if the cell body is destroyed; however, if the axon is injured there is partial degeneration of the axon, followed by regeneration.

In a typical surgical incision, muscle tissue is cut into. Although the epithelial cells regenerate over the scar tissue, the epithelial layer is so thin that the scar tissue is visible.

Types of wound healing

Tissue may heal by primary, secondary, or tertiary intention (Fig. 19-9).

Primary intention

All layers of the wound are closely approximated by suturing. If not infected, they heal quickly with minimum scarring.

Secondary intention

Ulcers with edges that cannot be sutured heal by filling the area in from the bottom. The wounds are open, with increased chance of infection, and heal slowly with considerable scarring.

Tertiary intention

The wound is sutured several days after wounding. The wound is more contaminated than with primary intention, so scarring is greater.

Process of wound healing

Regardless of the type of wound healing, the process is the same. The difference is in length of time for each

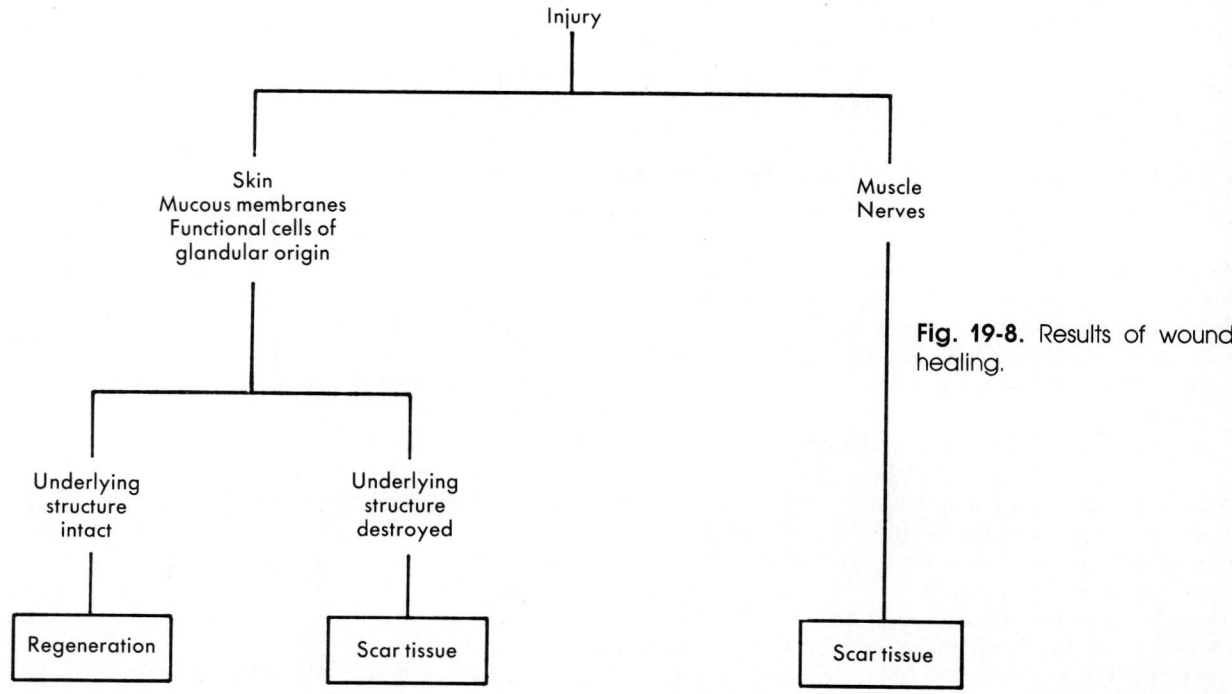

Fig. 19-8. Results of wound healing.

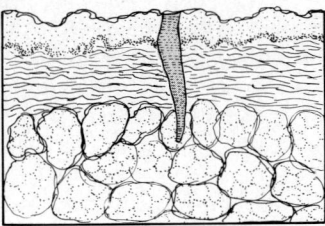 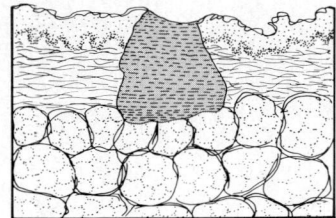 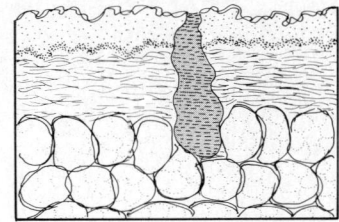

Fig. 19-9. Types of wound healing; primary, secondary, and tertiary intention.

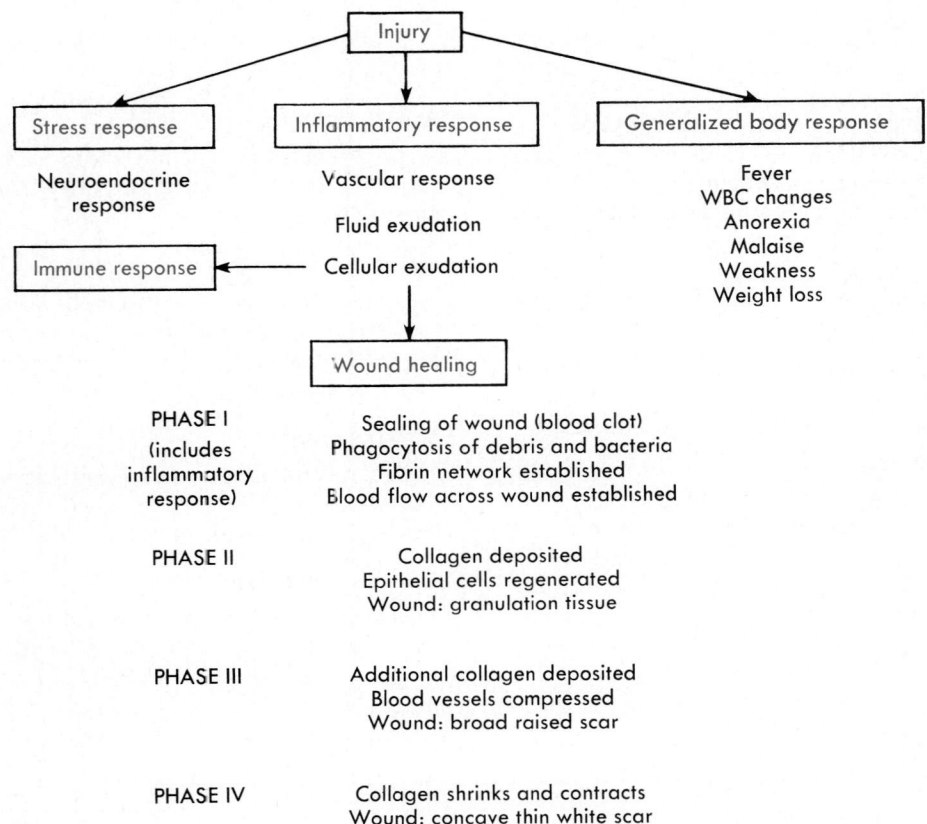

Fig. 19-10. Response of body to injury.

phase of healing and the extent of granulation tissue formed. When there is injury to tissue, two major responses occur: the stress response (Chapter 8) and the inflammatory response (Chapter 6). The inflammatory response serves to prepare the tissue so that wound healing can take place (Fig. 19-10).

In *phase I* of wound healing, leukocytes (white blood cells) ingest bacteria and debris. Fibrin is deposited throughout the clot that fills the wound, and new blood vessels develop across the wound using the fibrin threads as a framework. A thin layer of epithelial cells migrate across the wound and help to seal the wound. The wound strength is low but sutured wounds will hold together if sutured correctly. After major surgery the patient looks and feels ill during this first phase, which lasts 3 days.

Phase II lasts from 3 to 14 days after surgery. The leukocytes start disappearing and the space begins to fill with *collagen*, a white protein fiber. All layers of epithelial cells are completely regenerated in about 1 week. The new tissue is a highly vascular connective tissue, reddish from the numerous blood vessels, and is called *granulation tissue*. If scraped, this tissue will bleed readily. The patient begins to look and feel better.

The collagen that is deposited will provide good support for the wound in 6 to 7 days. Thus, sutures are often removed about this time, depending on the site and extent of surgery. Commonly used skin sutures include black silk, fine wire, metal skin clips, and metal staples (Fig. 19-11).

During *phase III* collagen continues to be deposited.

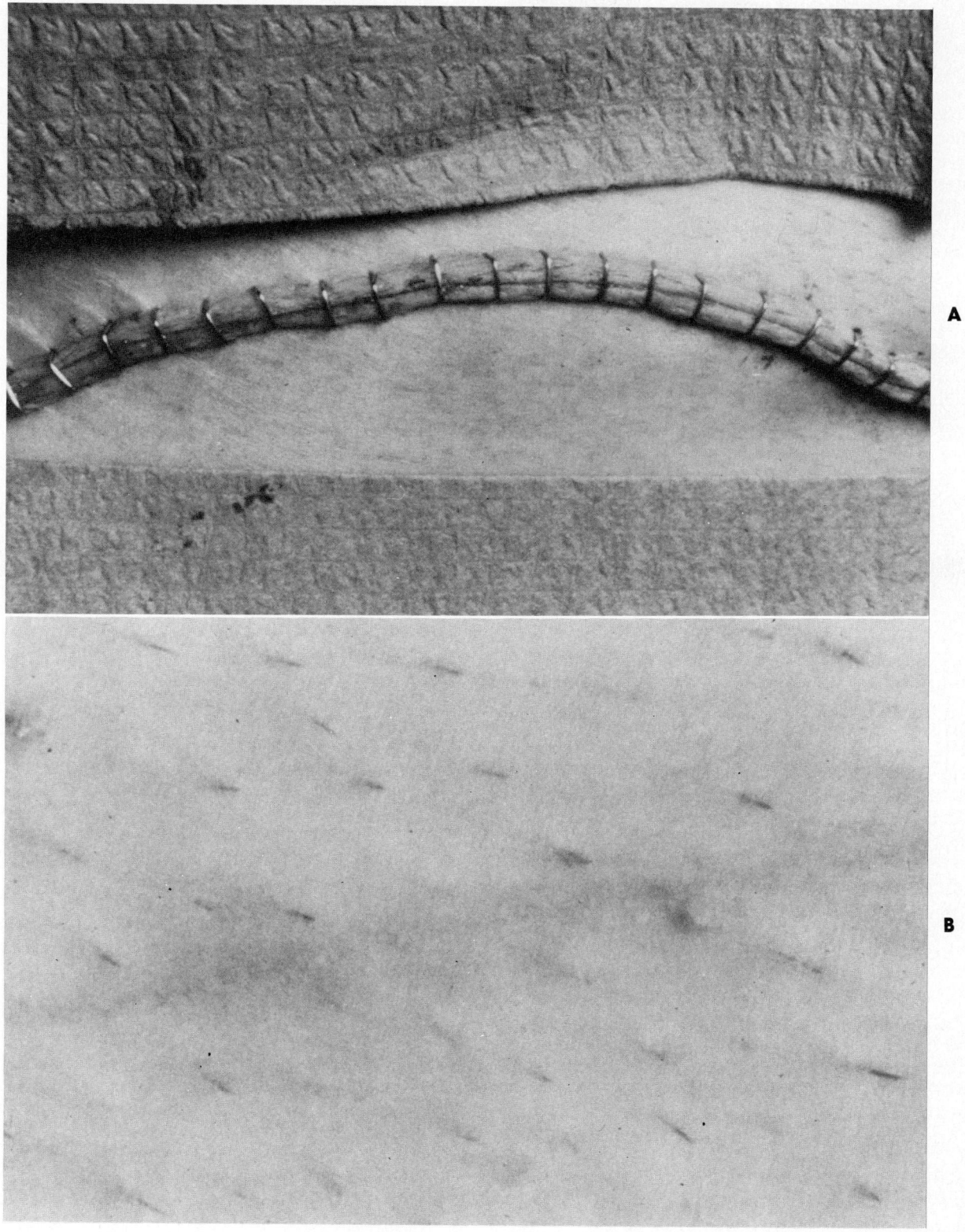

Fig. 19-11. Skin staples used for wound closures. **A,** Immediately after surgery. Note staples grasping only superficia layer of skin. **B,** Same site 6 months later. (Courtesy Ethicon, Inc., Somerville, N.J.)

This compresses the new blood vessels, and blood flow decreases. The wound now looks like a broad pinkish raised scar. During this phase, which lasts from about the second to the sixth week after surgery, the patient should avoid heavy use of the affected muscles.

The final phase, *phase IV*, lasts for several months after surgery. The patient may complain of itching around the wound. Although collagen continues to be deposited during this time, there is shrinkage and contraction of the wound. If the wound is near a joint, contractures may occur. Because of the shrinkage the wound becomes a concave thin white line. Scar tissue is acellular, avascular collagen tissue. It will not tan with sunlight nor sweat or produce hair.

INTERVENTIONS TO PROMOTE HEALING

1. Promote intake of foods high in protein and vitamin C. Protein is needed for the formation of collagen. Vitamin C also facilitates collagen formation and helps maintain the integrity of the capillary walls.
2. Carry out measures to increase circulation (p. 340). Healing requires that the necessary cells to fight infection and nutrients be brought to the wound and that the debris and dead cells be removed.
3. Avoid antiinflammatory drugs (such as steroids) when healing is desired; inflammation is a desired part of the healing process.
4. Prevent infection that delays healing:
    a. Change soiled wet dressings immediately
    b. Use strict aseptic technique when changing dressings
    c. Cover moist dressings with a dry sterile cover.
5. Irrigate contaminated wounds well to remove foreign substances that create an excessive inflammatory reaction and infection, which delay healing.
6. Maintain suction of wound catheters. Fluid remaining in a wound space delays healing.

WOUND DEHISCENCE AND EVISCERATION

Pathophysiology

Wound *dehiscence* (disruption) is partial to complete separation of the wound edges. Wound *evisceration* is protrusion of abdominal viscera through the incision and onto the abdominal wall (Fig. 19-12).

Wound separation can be avoided in many cases by good nutrition and by prevention of infection and postoperative pulmonary complications. Persons with obesity, cachexia, multiple trauma, or malignancy are at higher risk for developing wound separation.

Assessment

The patient may complain of a "giving" sensation at the incision or a feeling of wetness. If evisceration has occurred and a loop of bowel is obstructed, the patient will complain of severe pain at the incision. On inspection the dressing will be found to be saturated with clear pink drainage. The wound edges may be partially or entirely separated, and loops of intestine may be lying on the abdominal wall. Signs of shock may be present.

Intervention

1. Notify physician.
2. Put patient in bed in low Fowler's position.
3. Tell patient to lie quietly and not cough, eat, or drink until seen by the physician.
4. Cover protruding viscera with a dressing moistened with warm sterile saline solution.
5. Remain with the patient until the physician arrives if evisceration is present.

The treatment for wound dehiscence or evisceration is immediate closure of the wound under local or general anesthesia. If the patient is in shock, the preanesthetic medication may be omitted. Convalescence is usually prolonged, although the wound usually heals surprisingly well after secondary closure.

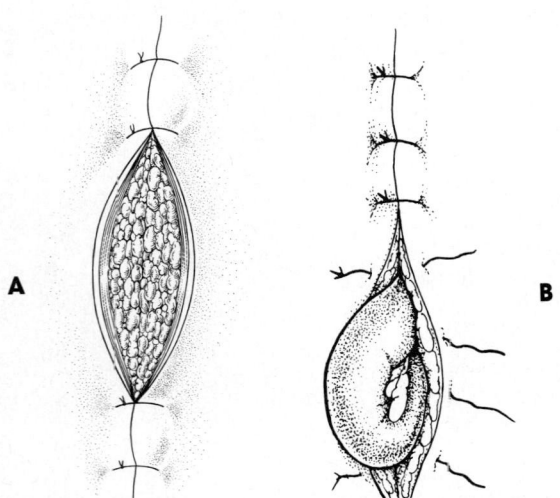

Fig. 19-12. A, Wound dehiscence. Wound edges are partially separated. **B,** Wound evisceration. Viscera protrude through incision.

Maintaining adequate respiration

PATHOPHYSIOLOGY

Postoperative patients are at high risk for developing pulmonary complications (Table 19-5). The pulmonary complications are often preventable by nursing management. The most common respiratory complications are atelectasis and hypostatic pneumonia.

In *atelectasis* a bronchiole becomes blocked by secretions and the distal alveoli collapse as the existing air is absorbed, producing hypoventilation. A major bronchus or many small bronchioles may be involved. The latter situation is frequently undetected because there are few symptoms. The extent of atelectasis is determined by the site of the blockage; if the main stem bronchus to one lung is blocked, that *lung* will be atelectatic. If a bronchus to a lobe is blocked, that *lobe* will atelectatic.

Hypostatic pneumonia is inflammation of the lung from stasis of secretions. Both atelectasis and hypostatic pneumonia decrease oxygenation, prolong recovery, and add to the patient's discomfort.

ASSESSMENT

The patient is assessed frequently during the first 24 to 48 hours after an inhalant anesthetic, depending on the number of risk factors present. A person at high risk may need to be assessed as often as every hour. Assessment includes monitoring respirations and chest expansion, auscultating the lungs, evaluating the productiveness of the cough, and observing for signs of atelectasis and pneumonia (see upper box on p. 340.)

INTERVENTION

After general anesthesia most patients will need to ventilate their lungs well *at least* every 1 to 2 hours during the first postoperative day, and then every 3 to 4 hours while awake for several days if not active. The decision for the type and frequency of preventive respiratory measures is based on each patient's risk factors and hour-by-hour and day-by-day response. Measures effective in increasing ventilation in one patient may be less effective in another.

Table 19-5. Risk factors in development of postoperative pulmonary complications

Risk factors	Effect
Increased respiratory secretions	
Smoking	Irritation of lining of tracheobronchial passages
Intubation	Decreased ciliary action to remove secretions
Inhalant anesthetics	Secretions will block bronchial passages or alveoli
Chronic lung disease	
Upper respiratory infection	
Dry sticky secretions	
Chronic lung disease	Difficult to cough up secretions
Dehydration	Secretions will block bronchial passages
Decreased thorax expansion	
Pain (chest, upper abdomen)	Lung does not expand fully, resulting in hypoventilation of alveoli
Obesity	
Age	
Tight binders or casts	
Skeletal abnormalities (for example, scoliosis)	
Decreased diaphragm mobility	
Abdominal distention	Decreased lung expansion, leading to hypoventilation
Surgery of chest or upper abdomen	
Muscle relaxants	
Neurologic deficit	
Depression of respiratory center	
Sedatives	Depressed respirations result in hypoventilation
Narcotics	
Acid-base imbalance	
Aspiration of gastric contents	
Vomiting	Causes aspiration pneumonia

Ventilatory measures

A number of ventilatory maneuvers (Table 19-6) can be used in the postoperative period to prevent atelectasis by inflating the alveoli as fully as possible. Once the alveoli are fully inflated, they will remain open for at least 1 hour. The two most effective ventilatory maneuvers that lead to maximum alveolar inflation are the yawn and the incentive spirometer (Fig. 19-13).

Positioning and turning

If the patient lies in one position with continuous pressure from body weight against the chest wall, proper ventilation and drainage of secretions on that side of the chest are not possible and atelectasis can develop (Fig. 19-14). Turning and changing of position frequently (at least every 2 to 3 hours) provide for better ventilation of the lungs. The patient should be encouraged to help in the turning. Alternating the height of the bed is useful: high Fowler's position facilitates diaphragm movement; low Fowler's or a flat position facilitates drainage and expectoration of respiratory secretions.

Maintaining circulation

PATHOPHYSIOLOGY

Thrombophlebitis, which results from venous stasis, is a preventable postoperative complication in many situations. Platelets adhere to the venous wall, especially at bifurcation of vessels, with resultant thrombus formation (Fig. 19-15). Venous stasis occurs postoperatively for a number of reasons (see box on p. 342).

ASSESSMENT

If a patient complains of any discomfort in a leg, examine the leg (with gentle palpation) for redness and tenderness along the course of a vein if a superficial vein is involved or for tenderness and edema if a deep vein is involved. There is usually pain on dorsiflexion of the foot (Homan's sign), and fever.

PREVENTION

1. Use elastic stockings, both in and out of bed, in patients at high risk.
2. Teach patient to avoid sitting for long periods (pres-

Signs of postoperative pulmonary dysfunction

Hypoventilation	Rapid shallow respirations
	Absent or diminished breath sounds in lower lobes
	Decreased chest expansion
Increased secretions in airways	Rales heard on auscultation
	Nonproductive cough
Atelectasis	Signs may be absent
	Fever, increased pulse and respirations; dyspnea, cyanosis, and shock if a large bronchus is blocked
Hypostatic pneumonia	Fever, dyspnea, chest pain, cough productive of mucopurulent sputum

---

Guidelines for using ventilatory maneuvers in postoperative patients

1. Schedule ventilatory maneuvers 30 minutes after narcotic is given, if possible — Facilitates patient cooperation
2. Place patient in high Fowler's position, if permitted — Facilitates diaphragm and chest expansion
3. Auscultate lungs — Baseline assessment
4. Suggest patient take three to five normal breaths between each deep inspiration — Prevents dizziness from hyperventilation
5. After patient takes three to five deep breaths, ask patient to cough *deeply* — Removes loosened secretions; shallow cough is ineffective and causes fatigue
6. Splint chest or abdominal incision with towel, small pillow, or hand before cough, if necessary — Prevents additional pain and muscle strain; provides support to incision to encourage deep cough
7. Auscultate lung — Comparison with baseline for evaluation of effectiveness

Table 19-6. Common postoperative ventilatory maneuvers

Manuever	Method	Comments
Yawn	Inhale deeply with mouth open (yawn), hold breath for 3 seconds, exhale	Easy to do; good deep breath when yawn occurs
Incentive spirometer	Breathe in through mouthpiece as deeply as possible, hold breath 3 seconds, exhale; work toward increasing inspiratory effort	Promotes sustained maximal inspiration; requires minimal instruction; avoid using at mealtimes (may cause nausea)
Deep breathing	Inhale deeply through nose using diaphragm (abdomen rises), exhale slowly through pursed lips	Effectiveness depends on depth of respirations; patients with chest or abdominal incisions tend to limit depth; patients need encouragement
Blow bottles	Blow in tube with one deep breath to push water from one bottle to the other	Increases alveolar pressure by prolonging expiration against resistance; uses Valsalva maneuver, therefore avoid use with known cardiac disease

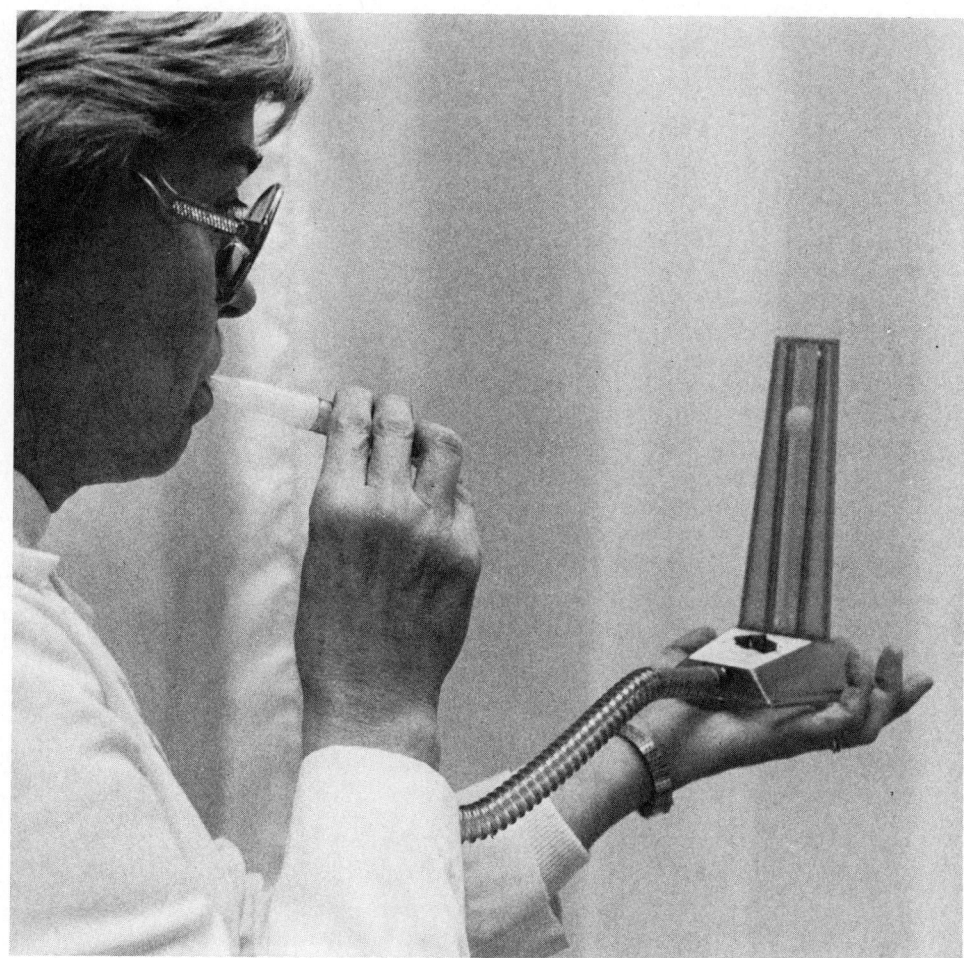

Fig. 19-13. Incentive spirometer. Ball rising with inspiration is a visual cue for patient. Ball remains up as patient holds breath for 3 seconds.

Risk factors for postoperative thrombophlebitis	
Intrinsic factors	Older age, obesity, malnutrition, contraceptive use
Pathologic condition	Malignancy, congestive heart failure, history of previous deep-vein thrombosis, polycythemia
Type of surgery	Pelvic, abdominal, thoracic; fracture of hip or lower extremity
Effects of surgery	Anesthesia, shock, decreased mobility
	Prolonged sitting with legs crossed
	Pressure on popliteal area
	Tight dressings or cast on lower extremities

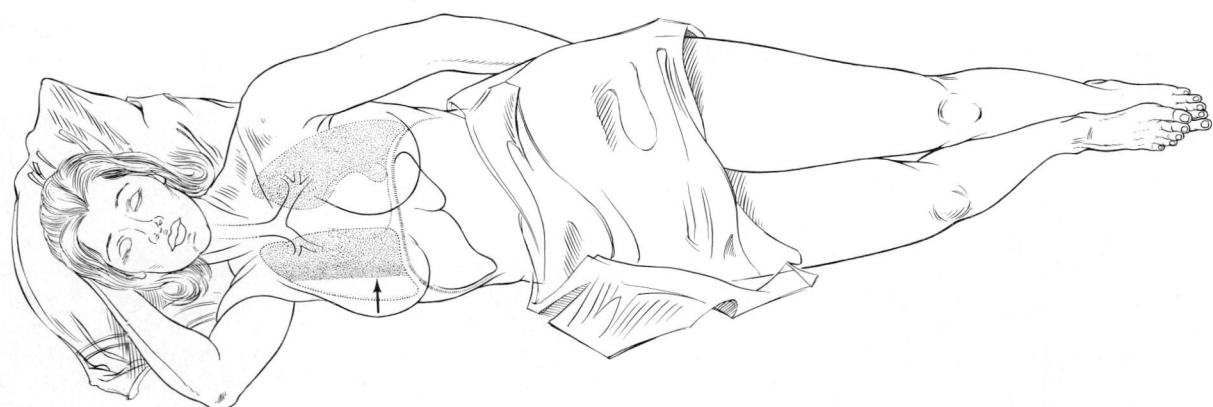

Fig. 19-14. Gravity will facilitate drainage of secretions from upper lung. In lower lung next to bed, secretions will pool in alveoli as a result of gravity and decreased chest expansion. Frequent turning will facilitate drainage from both lungs.

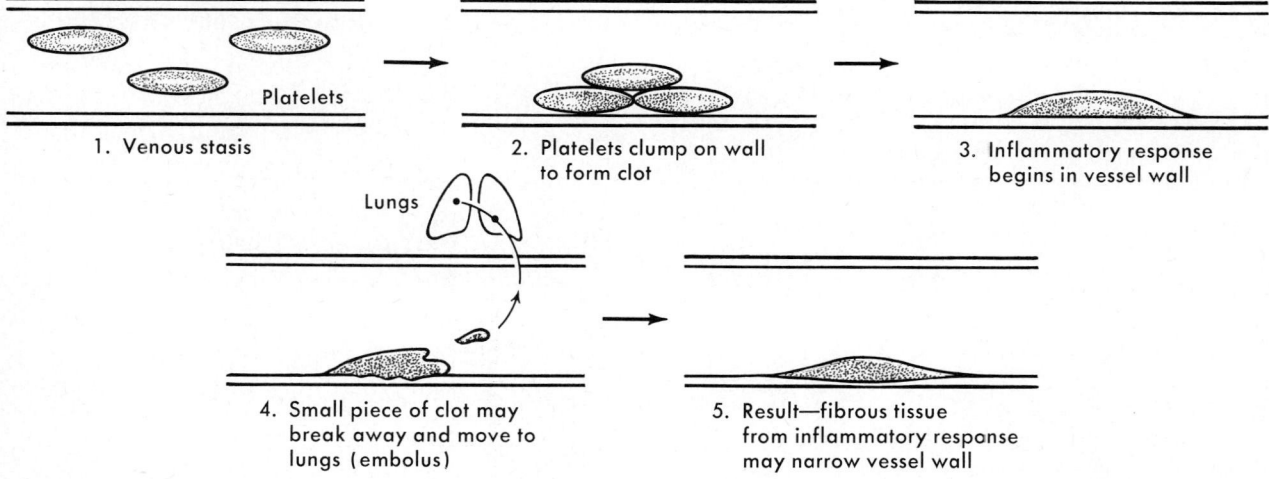

Fig. 19-15. Diagram illustrating formation of thrombus on wall of vein following venous stasis resulting in narrowing of blood vessel.

sure on popliteal area) and to elevate feet on a stool when sitting.

3. Avoid any pressure on popliteal area (for example, pillow under knee).
4. Avoid leg massage postoperatively.
5. Teach and encourage leg exercises (Chapter 17) for the inactive patient.
6. Encourage early ambulation.

INTERVENTION

The care of the patient with thrombophlebitis is discussed in Chapter 27. At the first sign of possible thrombophlebitis, ask the patient to return to bed and notify the physician. Rest, heat, elastic bandages, and anticoagulant therapy are usually prescribed. Monitor the patient for signs of pulmonary embolus (chest pain, dyspnea).

Maintaining fluid and electrolyte balance

PATHOPHYSIOLOGY

Fluid is lost during surgery through blood loss and increased insensible fluid loss through the lungs and skin. During the surgical procedure the blood loss is estimated and fluids are replaced intravenously.

For at least the first 24 to 48 hours after surgery, fluids are retained by the body because of the stimulation of antidiuretic hormone (ADH), as part of the stress response to trauma and the effect of anesthesia. During surgery there is also renal vasoconstriction and increased aldosterone activity, leading to increased sodium retention and subsequent water retention. *Overhydration* can occur with vigorous fluid replacement, especially in very small or elderly persons. Both water intoxication and pulmonary edema can occur, depending on the type and amount of fluids given. (For further information on fluid overload, see Chapter 10.)

Sodium and potassium depletion can occur in the postoperative patient from the loss of blood or body fluids during surgery or the loss of gastrointestinal secretions by vomiting and through nasogastric tubes. Potassium is also lost during catabolism (tissue breakdown), especially after severe trauma or crush injuries. Loss of gastric secretions can result in chloride loss, producing metabolic alkalosis.

ASSESSMENT

Monitor for signs of fluid overload, particularly in small or elderly persons:

1. Behavior: change in behavior, confusion
2. Skin: warm, moist
3. Neck: distended neck veins
4. Respiration: dyspnea, cough, moist breath sounds
5. Anorexia, nausea, vomiting
6. Fatigue
7. Weight gain (weigh high-risk patients)

INTERVENTION

Intravenous administration of fluids is monitored carefully so that fluids are given evenly over the entire 24 hours. (For further information on intravenous fluids, see Chapter 10.) If signs of fluid overload appear, slow the intravenous fluid to a keep-open rate and notify physician.

Fluids are started orally as soon as peristalsis is present. Sips of water are offered first to see if fluids can be tolerated. Some persons better tolerate sucking on ice chips. Ice chips must be recorded as fluid intake (two parts ice equal one part water). As soon as the patient can tolerate drinking fluids, the physician discontinues the intravenous fluid administrations.

Maintaining adequate nutrition

PATHOPHYSIOLOGY

Convalescence after surgery can be shortened if protein deficiency does not develop. The best way to supply essential foods is orally. Weight loss usually occurs after surgery as a result of catabolism, nutrients used for healing, and inadequate caloric intake while receiving fluids intravenously. A gradual loss of about 0.15 to 0.25 kg (⅓ to ½ lb) per day indicates tissue loss. Rapid weight loss indicates *fluid* loss: rapid weight gain indicates fluid retention.

Two food substances of special importance in wound healing are protein and vitamin C (p. 338). During catabolism in the early postoperative period, a negative nitrogen balance occurs; more nitrogen is lost than is taken in. Nitrogen is an essential constituent of amino acids, the building blocks of proteins. Protein intake is necessary to restore nitrogen balance and to provide the necessary amino acids for anabolism. Vitamin C is stored only in small amounts in the tissues, so must be supplied daily from an external source.

ASSESSMENT

1. *Weigh* the patient in whom weight loss may present a problem, that is, the person who is severely undernourished or receiving feedings intravenously for ≥1 week.
2. Monitor *meal trays* to identify those persons who are not eating foods high in protein and vitamin C.

INTERVENTION

1. Encourage and teach postoperative patients to eat foods high in protein and vitamin C.
2. Do not force food if patient is anorexic. Instead, offer frequent small amounts of food or high protein, high calorie liquids (such as milkshakes or eggnogs).
3. Encourage activity to improve desire to eat.
4. Discuss with underweight persons their plans for obtaining the desired nutrients after discharge.

Maintaining elimination

URINE ELIMINATION

Pathophysiology

A patient who is well hydrated usually voids within 6 to 8 hours after surgery. Although 2000 to 3000 ml solution usually is given intravenously on the day of surgery, the first voiding may be ≤ 200 ml, and the total urinary output for the day may be < 1500 ml. The small amount of urinary output results from the loss of body fluid during surgery, increased insensible fluid loss, vomiting, and increased secretion of antidiuretic hormone. As body functions stabilize, fluid and electrolyte balance returns to normal in about 48 hours.

Urinary retention, or the inability to void, may occur in the early postoperative period for several reasons. *Urinary tract infections* may occur in patients who must have prolonged bed rest after surgery, have a history of urinary tract infections, have had pelvic surgery, or have indwelling catheters.

Assessment

1. Monitor urinary output until output equals fluid intake.
2. If patient does not void sufficiently, especially within 6 to 8 hours after surgery, assess for urinary retention (suprapubic distention, sensation of full bladder, suprapubic discomfort).
3. If patient complains of frequency of urination with burning, check body temperature, send a clean voided urine specimen to laboratory for culture and sensitivity (if protocols permit), and notify physician.

Intervention

If urinary retention is present, carry out measures to facilitate voiding (Chapter 33). Catheterization may be delayed longer than the usual 8 hours postoperatively in the hope that the patient will void normally. Bethanechol chloride (Urecholine) may be ordered by the physician for acute postoperative urine retention, and may be given orally or subcutaneously but not by intramuscular injection because this may induce circulatory collapse.

If the bladder must be catheterized repeatedly after surgery, an indwelling catheter may be inserted. Fluids are then encouraged up to 3000 ml, unless contraindicated, to prevent urinary stasis.

BOWEL ELIMINATION

Pathophysiology

Peristalsis will be decreased for at least 24 hours after abdominal or pelvic surgery and for several days after surgery of the gastrointestinal tract. No bowel movement can occur when peristalsis is absent or markedly decreased. *Constipation* occurs frequently after major surgery for several reasons. A bowel movement may be intentionally delayed after burns of the buttocks or extensive rectal surgery (by administration of paregoric orally) to prevent additional trauma.

Assessment

1. Monitor daily for bowel movement. If absent, ask if patient is passing flatus.
2. After abdominal surgery, record signs of returning peristalsis (bowel sounds, passing flatus).
3. Examine stool for amount and consistency; small dry hard stool indicates constipation.
4. Assess for potential constipation:
   a. Narcotics given frequently or in high doses
   b. Inactivity
   c. Fluid intake < 1200 ml/day
   d. Previous history of constipation.

Intervention

1. Institute measures to *prevent* constipation for the first 2 or 3 days after major surgery:
   a. Facilitate fluid intake of 2000 to 3000 ml/day
   b. Encourage maximal activity within prescribed limits
   c. Provide bathroom privileges as early as possible.
2. If no bowel movement within 3 or 4 days after surgery:
   a. Give prune juice, if permissible and desirable
   b. Consult physician about a laxative order. A hypertonic (Fleet) enema or small soapsuds enema may be necessary if laxative is ineffective
   c. Encourage intake of foods high in fiber, if permissible.

Causes of postoperative urinary retention

Recumbent position
Nervous tension
Anesthetic; decreased bladder sensation and ability to void
Narcotic: decreased bladder sensation
Pelvic surgery: interference with innervation of bladder muscles, and local edema

---

Causes of postoperative constipation

Neuroendocrine response to stress (decreased gastrointestinal motility)
Anesthetic agents
Narcotics
Inactivity
Decreased intake of high-fiber foods

Promoting comfort

The major discomforts after surgery are nausea and vomiting, abdominal distention and gas pains, and incisional pain.

NAUSEA AND VOMITING

Nausea and vomiting, which occur less frequently with the newer anesthetic agents, may be related to a number of factors. Persistent postoperative vomiting is usually a symptom of pyloric obstruction, intestinal obstruction, or peritonitis. Vomiting tires the patient, puts strain on the incision, and causes excessive loss of fluids and electrolytes. Choking while vomiting may lead to aspiration pneumonia.

Interventions for the person who is experiencing nausea and vomiting include:

1. Side-lying position to prevent aspiration
2. No food or fluids until vomiting subsides
3. Sips of fluid (ice chips, ginger ale, hot tea) or dry solid food (crackers) after vomiting subsides
4. Frequent oral care
5. Prescribed antiemetics given parenterally.

ABDOMINAL DISTENTION AND GAS PAINS

Pathophysiology

Postoperative *distention* results from accumulation of nonabsorbable gas in the intestines caused by a reaction to the handling of the bowel during surgery, by swallowing of air during recovery from anesthesia or attempts to overcome nausea, and by passing of gases from the bloodstream to the atonic portion of the bowel. Distention will persist until the tone of the bowel returns to normal and peristalsis resumes. It is experienced to some degree by most patients after abdominal and renal surgery.

Gas pains are caused by contractions of the unaffected portions of the bowel in an attempt to move the accumulated gas through the intestinal tract.

Assessment

If the patient complains of diffuse or cramping abdominal pain, monitor the following:

1. Measurement of abdominal girth with tape measure to determine degree of distention
2. Percussion of distended abdomen for drumlike (tympanic) sounds
3. Presence of signs of shock from acute gastric dilation.

Intervention

If the stomach is distended, the fluid and gas can be aspirated with a nasogastric tube. General distention or gas pains from sluggish intestinal peristalsis can be relieved by passage of flatus. Useful measures include:

1. Ambulation (most effective method)
2. Rectal tube for 20 minutes every four hours as necessary
3. Heat to the abdomen (heating pad or hot water bottle), most effective if used with a rectal tube
4. Prescribed enema.

PAIN

Pathophysiology

Pain is common after nearly all types of surgical procedures in which there has been cutting, pulling, or manipulation of tissues and organs. It may result from stimulation of nerve endings by chemical substances released at the time of surgery or from tissue ischemia caused by interference of blood supply to the part, such as by pressure, muscle spasm, or edema. After surgery other factors can add to the sensation of pain, such as infections, distention, muscle spasms surrounding the incisional area, and tight dressings or casts.

Postoperative pain usually lasts 24 to 48 hours but may continue longer depending on the extent of the surgery, the pain threshold of the patient, and response to pain (Chapter 12). The presence of pain can prolong convalescence because it may interfere with return to activity.

Assessment

When the patient complains of pain in the postoperative period, do not assume that the pain is incisional. It is important to try to ascertain the possible cause of the

---

Causes of postoperative vomiting

Anesthetic agent
Narcotic
Abdominal distention (fluid, gas)
Pain
Electrolyte imbalances
Drug idiosyncrasies

Common postoperative pain syndromes

Pain with fever
Pain with vomiting and abdominal distention
Suprapubic discomfort
Pain with coldness or numbness to part
Wound infection
Gas collecting in intestinal tract
Full bladder
Decreased circulation from tight dressing or cast or from venous stasis

pain. Subjective data include origin, area involved, nature of the pain, and possible cause from the patient's point of view. Objective data include observation of facial expressions, body position, activity, muscle rigidity, and pulse rate. If the patient is experiencing severe pain, the assessment should be made gently and quickly but thoroughly.

Intervention

It is often impossible to prevent postoperative pain, but it can be minimized so that the patient is relatively comfortable. Patients who have had adequate preoperative instructions and who have confidence in the surgeon, in the nurse, and in the outcome of the surgery usually have less postoperative pain than apprehensive patients because they have less tension. Measures to reduce anxiety and apprehension will also help reduce pain. Relief of pain may encourage the patient to move and breathe more deeply, thus preventing postoperative complications, which cause more pain.

If the cause of pain is determined to be other than incisional, measures are taken to relieve the cause. Emptying a full bladder can relieve what was thought to be pain from a lower abdominal incision. Elevation of a part may relieve venous stasis. Loosening of a tight bandage, if permissible, will relieve ischemic pain.

Incisional pain can be relieved by nursing measures and by analgesics.

1. Encourage patient to move in bed or to ambulate, to decrease pain from muscle tension and increase circulation to the part.
2. Move the injured part as a whole; for example, move trunk as one unit.
3. Support an injured limb during a move (a pillow is a useful support).
4. Teach patient to use siderails in moving to decrease incisional pull.
5. Teach relaxation and distraction techniques, if suitable (Chapter 8).

6. Give medications according to the guidelines for acute pain (Chapter 12)
   a. Narcotics are usually required on a regular basis for 12 to 48 hours after major surgery
   b. Patients receiving meperidine hydrochloride (Demerol) are monitored for signs of orthostatic hypotension (dizziness, fainting, rapid pulse) during ambulation
   c. Non-narcotics may provide relief after 48 to 72 hours following major surgery.

Maintaining activity

PATHOPHYSIOLOGY

Early ambulation has been a significant factor in hastening postoperative recovery and preventing postoperative complications. Numerous benefits are derived from the exercise of getting in and out of bed and walking during the early postoperative period (Fig. 19-16). Ambulation is usually contraindicated when there is a severe infection or thombophlebitis.

ASSESSMENT

Before assisting the patient to ambulate for the first few times after major surgery, an assessment is made of the patient's level of alertness to follow directions, cardiovascular status, and motor status:

1. Level of alertness: ask patient simple questions or to follow simple commands
2. Cardiovascular status
   a. Assess pulse and respiratory rate and depth while supine, then after sitting
   b. Observe skin color for pallor while sitting
   c. Note complaints of dizziness when sitting
3. Motor status
   a. Assess muscle strength of legs (Chapter 3)
   b. Assess sitting ability:
      (1) Assist patient to sitting position on side of bed

Effects of early postoperative ambulation

Increased rate and depth of breathing	Prevention of atelectasis and hypostatic pneumonia
	Increased mental alertness from increased oxygenation to brain
Increased circulation	Nutrients required for healing are more available to wound
	Prevention of thrombophlebitis
	Increased kidney function
	Decreased pain
Increased micturition	Prevention of urinary retention
Increased metabolism	Prevention of loss of muscle tone
	Restoration of nitrogen balance
Increased peristalsis	Promotion of expulsion of flatus
	Prevention of abdominal distention and gas pains
	Prevention of constipation

(2) Ask patient to maintain an erect position while being gently pushed sideways.

It is also important to know of any limitations to ambulation present preoperatively. The patient with arthritis or arteriosclerosis may take longer to move and to adjust to standing and walking. The patient who used a walker preoperatively will need assistance for a longer time before progressing to using the walker again.

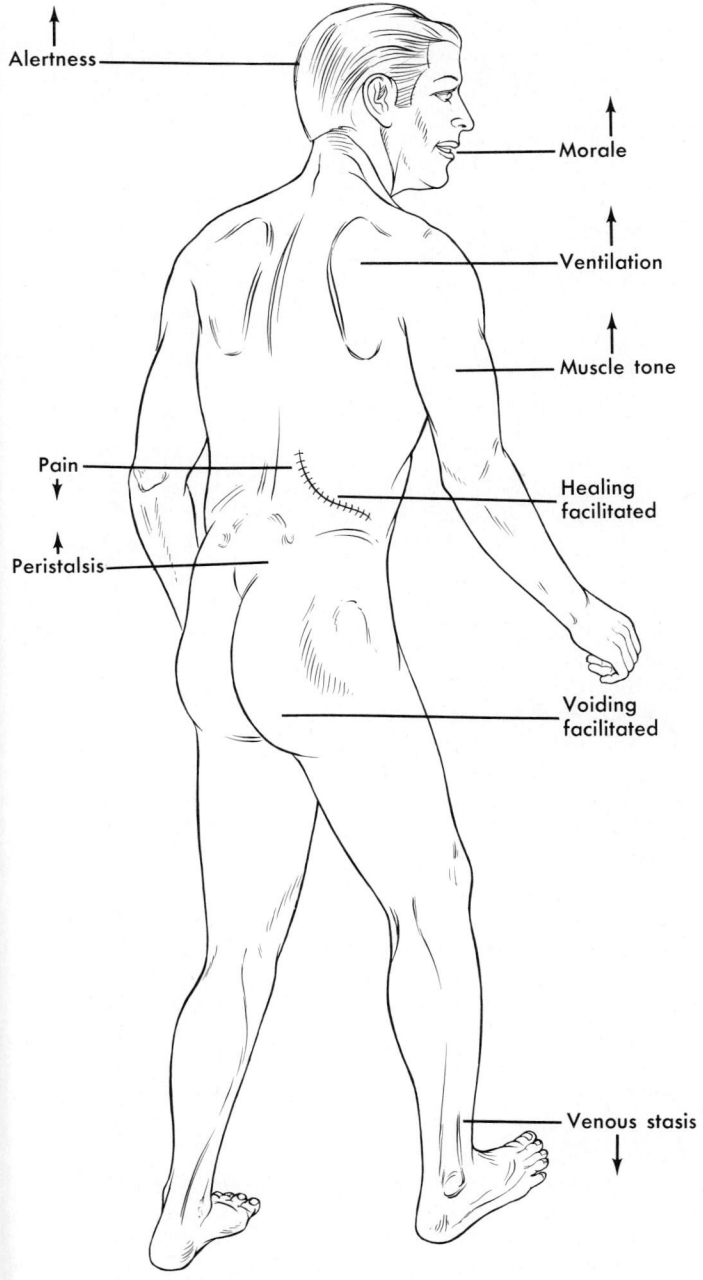

Alertness

Morale

Ventilation

Muscle tone

Pain

Healing facilitated

Peristalsis

Voiding facilitated

Venous stasis

Fig. 19-16. Benefits from early postoperative ambulation.

INTERVENTION

1. Encourage muscle strengthening exercises prior to ambulation
   a. Bend knees, lower knees, press back of knees hard against bed
   b. Alternately contract and relax calf and thigh muscles 10 times using the following cycle: contract, relax, rest.
2. Have patient sit on side of bed (legs dangling) to become accustomed to upright position before ambulating the first time. Be sure *pulse has stabilized* (returned to baseline) before ambulation is attempted.
3. Adjust tubings prior to ambulation
   a. Clamp off nasogastric tube until patient has ambulated, then reconnect
   b. Keep urinary tube connected to drainage bag; carry bag or pin bag to inside of robe
   c. Attach intravenous bag to a movable pole.
4. Use two people to assist a weak patient receiving intravenous fluids to ambulate
5. Encourage patient to walk farther at each ambulation.

The word *ambulate* means to move from place to place, to walk. Sitting in a chair is not considered ambulation. After ambulating, the patient may sit in a chair if permitted, but should be advised to stand and walk at intervals and to elevate the legs while sitting to prevent venous pooling in the extremities. Sitting in a chair for long periods is to be avoided.

Helping meet psychologic needs

PSYCHOLOGIC FACTORS

Some of the concerns that were present preoperatively may continue into the postoperative period. These concerns fall into essentially three categories: concerns specific to the surgery performed, concerns over loss of a body part, and concerns about the future. Future concerns include those related to changes in sexuality, economic status, prognosis, or permanent effects. Sexuality may be threatened by enforced absence from home or by a specific surgical procedure. Sexual concerns may center around the effect of the surgery on the spouse or parent relationship or on sexual performance itself.

ASSESSMENT

Anxieties will be expressed in many different ways. It must be remembered that expressions such as anger, resentfulness, crying, excessive joking, inappropriate laughter, or withdrawal may all be signs of anxiety and are often seen in the postoperative period. Some of these feelings may be projected against the surgeon, nurse, housekeeping aide, food, and such.

INTERVENTION

Sitting down and talking with surgical patients about their concerns is as important a nursing action in many instances as any of the physical activities. Time must be planned for this. If a specific concern is expected, such as sexual functioning after a perineal prostatectomy, the topic may have to be introduced by the nurse who has established rapport with the patient in order to let the patient know that it is permissible to talk about it.

Discharge planning

As a result of early resumption of ambulation and a nutritious diet, most patients regain their strength rapidly; the average hospital stay after major surgery is 3 to 8 days. During this time the patient and family should be prepared for any care that must be given at home, and any necessary arrangements for convalescent care should be completed several days before discharge. Patients are helped to become as self-sufficient as possible before being discharged so they do not have to depend any more than necessary on the assistance of relatives and friends.

If dressings are needed, the patient may be given a 48-hour supply to take home unless a family member has already obtained them. The patient and family must know where in the community they can get dressings and other needed materials. A community health nurse is a useful resource person when treatment of almost any kind is to be provided at home.

On discharge the patient is given an appointment for a follow-up examination in the surgeon's office or clinic. This appointment is usually for 1 to 2 weeks after discharge. The patient should understand the importance of returning for the medical examination (which is usually included in the surgeon's operating fee).

With modern surgical techniques the wound is usually healing well by the time of discharge from the hospital. Therefore the convalescent period usually is relatively short, and most patients may return to their usual activities and occupation within 2 to 4 weeks. Normal activities should be resumed gradually. Driving is usually permitted 2 weeks after major surgery, but the patient should avoid any heavy lifting, pushing, or pulling for at least 6 weeks.

REFERENCES AND SELECTED READINGS*

1. Alexander, J.W., editor: Symposium on surgical infection, Surg. Clin. North Am. **60:**1-240, 1980.
2. American College of Surgeons: Manual of pre- and postoperative care, ed. 3, Philadelphia, 1983, W.B. Saunders Co.
3. *Baker, P.J.: Postoperative atelectasis, Nurs. Dig. **5:**42-47, 1977.
4. *Blackwell, A., and Blackwell, W.: Relieving gas pains, Am. J. Nurs. **75:**1474-1475, 1975.
5. Bushong, M.E.: Principles of postanesthetic management: criteria for patient discharge, Curr. Rev. Recovery Room Nurses **1:**73-80, 1979.
6. *Cahill, C.A.: Yawn maneuver to prevent atelectasis, AORN J **27:**1000-1007, 1978.
7. Cooper, D.M., and Schumann, D.: Postsurgical nursing as an adjunct to wound healing, Nurs. Clin. North Am. **14:**713-726, 1979.
8. *Croushore, T.M.: Postoperative assessment: the key to avoiding the most common nursing mistakes, Nurs. 79 **9**(4):46, 1979.
9. *Cullen, D.J.: Recovery room complications, AORN J **26:**746-763, 1977.
10. *Flynn, M.E.: Influencing repair and recovery, Am. J. Nurs. **82:**1550-1558, 1982.
11. *Flynn, M.E., and Rovee, D.T.: Promoting wound healing, Am. J. Nurs. **82:**1543-1549, 1982.
12. Friedman, J.: Ventilatory function in the recovery room, Curr. Rev. Recovery Room Nurses **1:**57-64, 1979.
13. *Garrett, J.: Oliguria in postoperative patients, Nurs. Clin. North Am. **10:**59-67, 1975.
14. Gelman, S.: The recovery room care of the patient with spinal, epidural, and other regional blocks, Curr. Rev. Recovery Room Nurses **2:**81-83, 1980.
15. *Gordon, M.: Assessing activity tolerance, Am. J. Nurs. **76:**72-76, 1976.
16. *Greenwood, B.S.: The before and after of good postoperative pulmonary care, Nurs. 82 **12**(12):68-69, 1982.
17. Harman, E., and Lillington, G.: Pulmonary risk factors in surgery, Med. Clin. North Am. **63:**1289-1298, 1979.
18. Hercules, P.R.: Nursing in the postoperative care unit: a review, AORN J **26:**1042-1052, 1987.
19. *Johnston, M.: Outcome criteria to evaluate postoperative respiratory status, Am. J. Nurs. **75:**1474-1475, 1975.
20. *Keithley, J.K.: A unified approach to assessment of the surgical patient, Am. J. Nurs. **82:**612-614, 1982.
21. *McConnell, E.A.: After surgery, Nurs. 77 **7**(3):32-39, 1977.
22. *McConnell, E.A.: Toward complication-free recoveries for your surgical patient, I, R.N. **43**(6):30-33, 1980; II, R.N. **43**(7):34-38, 1980.
23. *Metheny, N., and Snively, W.D., Jr.: Perioperative fluid and electrolytes, Am. J. Nurs. **78:**840-845, 1978.
24. *Mitchell, M.A.: An RR experience: as nurse and patient saw it, R.N. **38:**46-47, 1975.
25. O'Byrne, C.: Clinical detection and management of postoperative wound sepsis, Nurs. Clin. North Am. **14:**727-742, 1979.
26. *Patras, A.Z.: The operation's over but the danger is not, Nurs. 82 **12**(9):50-56, 1982.
27. *Postoperative complications: how to help the patient when everything goes wrong, Nurs. 81 **11**(3):50-55, 1981.
28. *Robusto, N.: Advising patients on sex surgery, AORN J **32:**55-61, 1980.
29. *Schumann, D.: How to help wound healing in your abdominal surgery patient, Nurs. 80 **10**(4):34-40, 1980.
30. *Smith, B.J.: Safeguarding your patient after anesthesia, Nurs. 78 **8**(10):53-56, 1978.
31. Symposium on postoperative nursing care, Nurs. Clin. North Am. **10:**1-67, 1975.
32. *Weaver, T.E.: New life for lungs . . . through incentive spirometers, Nurs. 81 **11**(2):54-58, 1981.
33. Webb, G.E.: Hyper- and hypotension in the recovery room, AORN J **26:**546-574, 1977.

*References preceded by an asterisk are particularly well suited for student reading.

UNIT VI
Sensorimotor Problems

20   The Patient with Neurologic Problems
21   The Patient with Eye Problems
22   The Patient with Ear Problems
23   The Patient with Musculoskeletal Problems

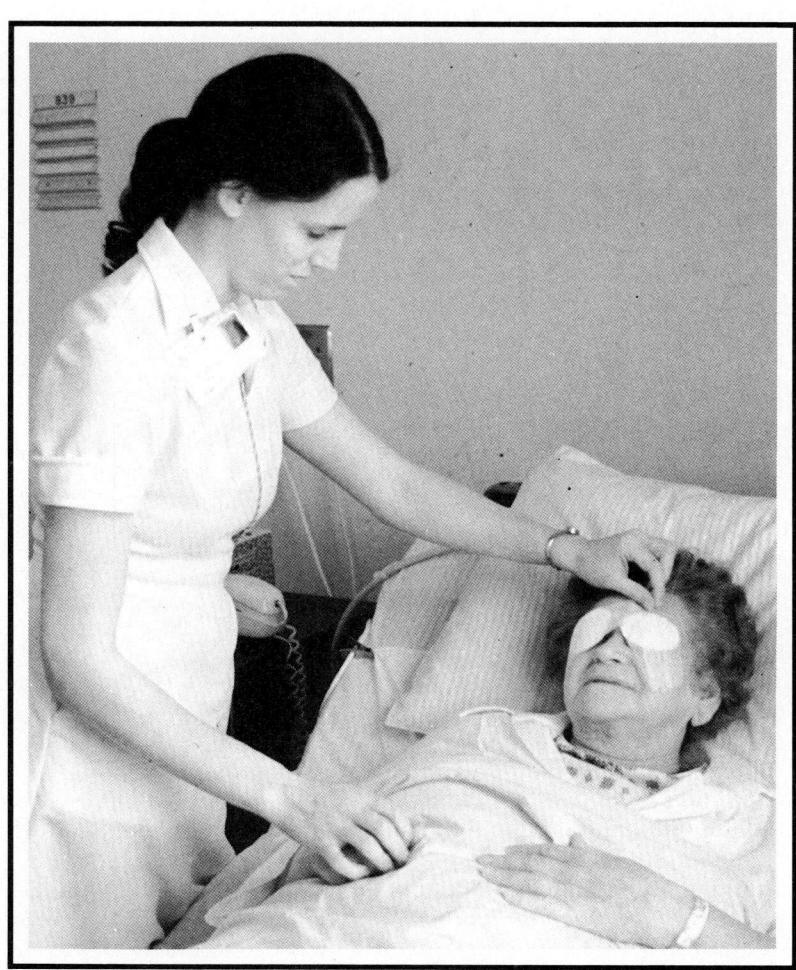

20

The Patient with Neurologic Problems

ELIZABETH SCHENK

STUDY QUESTIONS

- What four functions does the nervous system accomplish?

- Where are the speech centers located in the brain?

- What structures are located in the brainstem and what are the functions of each?

- What are the two major conducting arteries in the brain and what areas do they supply?

- What are the normal characteristics of cerebrospinal fluid?

- What are the six major components of the neurologic examination?

- Define the following terms:
  Paresthesia
  Hyperalgesia
  Hypoalgesia
  Analgesia
  Dysesthesia
  Referred pain
  Causalgia
  Local pain

ANATOMY AND PHYSIOLOGY

The application of the nursing process to patients with neurologic problems requires knowledge of the structure and function of the nervous system. The nervous system works as an electrical conductance system. It coordinates and controls all activities of the body. These activities can be divided into the following four kinds of functions:

1. Receiving information (stimuli) from the internal and external environment over sensory (afferent) pathways

2. Communicating information between distant parts of the body (periphery) and the central nervous system

3. Computing or processing the information received at various reflex (spinal cord) and conscious (higher brain) levels to determine responses appropriate to existing situations

4. Transmitting information rapidly over varied motor (efferent) pathways to organs for body action control or modification

Neuron

The basic structural and functional unit of the nervous system is the *neuron*. It is a highly specialized and differentiated cell, but it has all the basic biologic and biochemical properties of other body cells. The neuron consists of a *cell body* (soma) with two extensions: *dendrites*, which receive information from axon terminals at special sites called *synapses*, and *axons*, which transmit information away from the cell body to adjacent neurons. A cell membrane encloses the outer boundary of the soma, dendrite, and axon (Fig. 20-1).

Collections of neurons are connected in complex ways. The connection determines what each collection of neurons is capable of doing. The neurons are organized into circuits, some of which are simple and made up of relatively few neurons and others that are very complicated. A single neuron may be a part of several different neurologic circuits and thus may have a role in several functions.

Many of the important functional properties of the neuron lie within the *cell membrane*. The membrane is permeable to oxygen, carbon dioxide, and certain inorganic ions, and it is impermeable to organic compounds (proteins) and other inorganic ions. The characteristic of the membrane is called *differential permeability*.

The neuron also can be characterized by the property

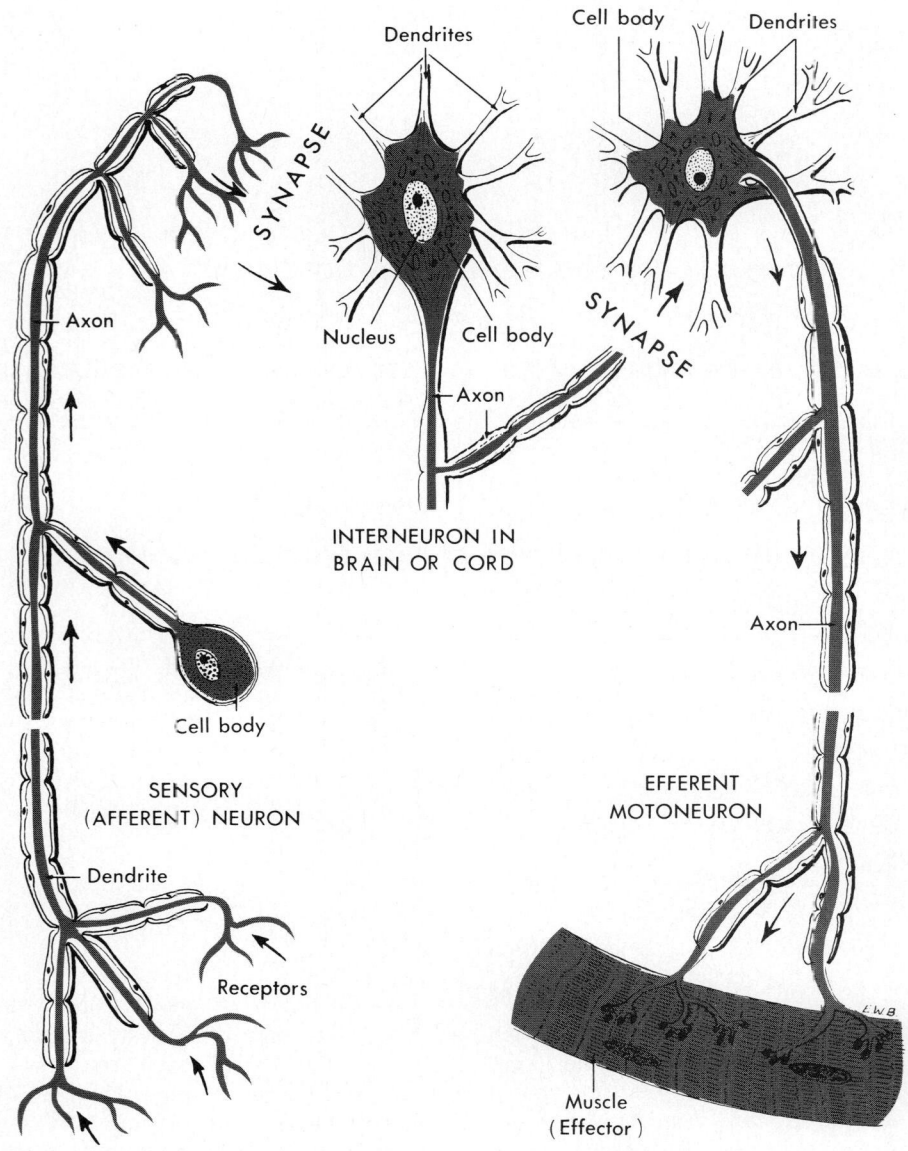

Fig. 20-1. Diagram of structure of three kinds of neurons. Note that each neuron has three parts: a cell body and two types of extensions, dendrite(s), and an axon. Arrows indicate direction of impulse conduction. (From Anthony, C.P., and Thibodeau, G.D.: Textbook of anatomy and physiology, ed. 11, St. Louis, 1983, The C.V. Mosby Co.)

of *excitability*. Excitability means that the resting potential of neurons is unstable under certain conditions, as when the membrane of the neuron is stimulated. This unstable condition gives rise to *action potentials*. Action potentials can only arise from excitable cells. All nervous system functions occur from the phenomenon of the action potential (Fig. 20-2).

ACTION POTENTIAL

Two phases occur within the action potential—*depolarization* (positive state) and *repolarization* (return to the more normal resting potential). When an action potential is generated it proceeds automatically to completion regardless of the type of stimulus that started the depolarization. This means that a strong stimulus does not cause a larger action potential. The action potential also spreads over the entire membrane without a decrease in velocity. The velocity is related to the size of the axon (velocity is higher with a larger diameter) and whether myelin is present.

Myelin is an excellent insulator of axons. The myelin sheath is deposited around the axons by Schwann's cells, and this layer may be as thick as the axon itself. Myelin prevents almost all ion flow across the axon and its membrane. However, at distances of approximately 1 mm, the sheath is interrupted by *nodes of Ranvier*. At these small, uninsulated areas, ions can flow easily between the extracellular fluid and the axon.

The presence of myelin causes such fibers to be called *large fibers;* those without myelin are called *small fibers*. Large fibers have a greater conduction velocity because (1) the jumping effect allows depolarization to proceed quickly and (2) energy is conserved, since only the nodes depolarize. Large fibers appear white because of the myelin; the *white matter* of the nervous system is made up of myelinated fibers.

Many action potentials of neurons originate in a receptor neuron where internal and external stimuli are normally received. A receptor is like a transducer and can change one form of energy into another form. A receptor, however, responds or depolarizes to *only one* type of stimulus. For example, the retina of the eye responds only to the stimulus of light, which is converted to electrical energy and travels over the optic nerves to the visual cortices for perception.

SYNAPSES

Neurons make contact with one another at sites called *synapses*. Transmission that occurs across a synapse is a chemical process. The end of the axon contains a chemical substance that is released by the action potential. The substance diffuses across the synapse to the adjacent cell membrane. *Synaptic transmission* is both *excitatory* and *inhibitory* in nature (inhibitory means that the membrane of the dendrite becomes hyperpolarized because of the release of the neurotransmitter). Whether a neuron fires is

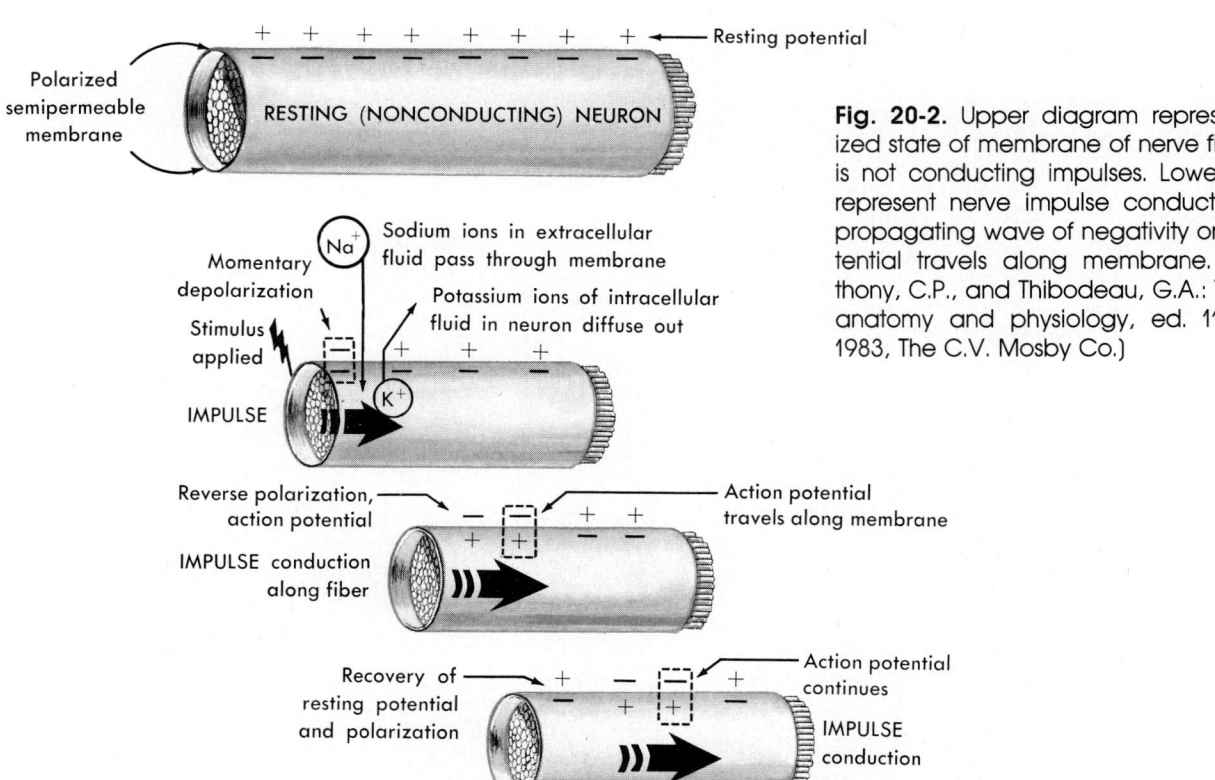

Fig. 20-2. Upper diagram represents polarized state of membrane of nerve fiber when it is not conducting impulses. Lower diagrams represent nerve impulse conduction: a self-propagating wave of negativity or action potential travels along membrane. (From Anthony, C.P., and Thibodeau, G.A.: Textbook of anatomy and physiology, ed. 11, St. Louis, 1983, The C.V. Mosby Co.)

dependent on the sum of the excitatory and inhibitory inputs. Chemicals allowing excitatory transmission are *acetylcholine, norepinephrine, dopamine,* and *serotonin.* Those inhibiting transmissions are *gamma aminobutyric acid (GABA)* in brain tissue and *glycine* in the spinal cord.

Divisions of the nervous system

Macroscopically, the nervous system has two major divisions. These are the *central nervous system* and the *peripheral nervous system.*

CENTRAL NERVOUS SYSTEM

The central nervous system (CNS) is made up of collections of neurons and their connections into the brain and spinal cord. Areas of the brain and spinal cord are distinguished where cell bodies are concentrated into *nuclei* and groups of axons run in *tracts* that interconnect the parts. The brain and spinal cord are structurally continuous. The brain is housed in the skull and the spinal cord in the vertebral column.

The brain (encephalon) is divided grossly into three main areas, which are as follows:
1. The cerebrum
2. The brainstem
3. The cerebellum
Each of these areas carries out unique functions.

Cerebrum

The cerebrum of each hemisphere (right and left) is composed of four major lobes, the *frontal, parietal, temporal,* and *occipital.* The cortex of the cerebrum, which is approximately ¼ inch thick, contains over 14 billion neurons. It receives and analyzes all impulses, controls voluntary movement, and stores knowledge of all impulses received. Each cerebral lobe, named for the overlying cranial bone, carries out specific functions such as general sensation, perception, special senses perception, and speech (Fig. 20-3).

Deep within the cerebrum are the *basal ganglia.* These are masses of gray matter (cell bodies) and include the caudate nucleus, putamen, and globa pallidus. The basal ganglia function as part of the extrapyramidal system and control postural adjustment and gross voluntary movements.

One function of the cerebrum deserves special men-

Specific functions of cerebral cortexes

Frontal cortex	Conceptualization
	Abstraction
	Judgment formation
	Motor ability
	Ability to write words
Parietal cortex	Highest integrative and co-ordinating center for perception and interpretation of sensory information
	Ability to recognize body parts
	Left versus right
Temporal cortex	Memory storage
	Auditory integration
Occipital cortex	Visual center
	Understanding of written material

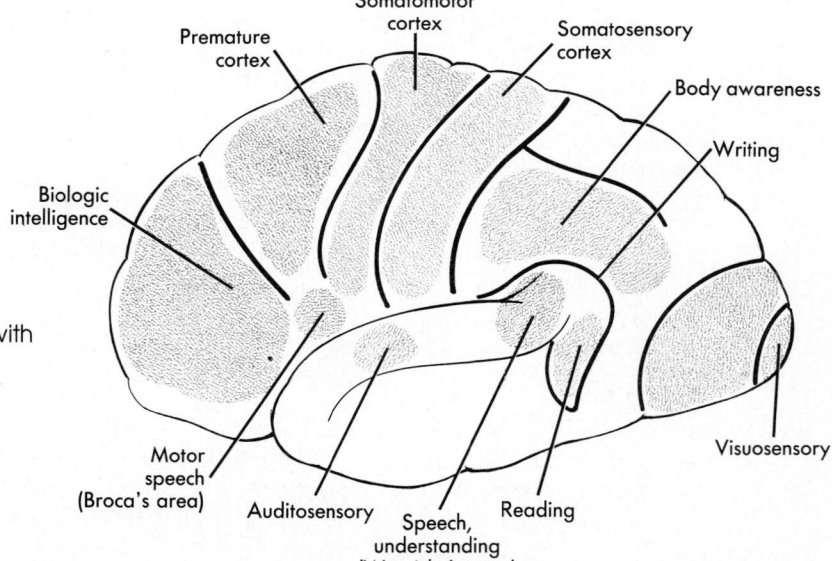

Fig. 20-3. Lateral view of cerebral cortex with identification of major cortical areas.

Premature cortex
Somatomotor cortex
Somatosensory cortex
Body awareness
Writing
Biologic intelligence
Motor speech (Broca's area)
Auditosensory
Speech, understanding (Wernicke's area)
Reading
Visuosensory

tion—that of speech. Speech is a function of the dominant hemisphere, which is on the left side of the brain for all right-handed people as well as most left-handed people. The two identified speech centers are Broca's area and Wernicke's area. *Broca's area* is in the frontal lobe adjacent to the motor cortex and controls verbal, expressive speech. *Wernicke's area* is in the posterior part of the temporal lobe and may extend to adjacent parts of the parietal lobe. It is responsible for reception and understanding of language. An area in the frontal lobe governs ability to write words, and an area in the occipital lobe controls ability to understand written material.

Brainstem

The *brainstem* lies deep in the center of the hemisphere and connects with the spinal cord at the level of the medulla. It carries all nerve fibers passing between the brain hemisphere and the spinal cord; additionally, all cranial nerves except cranial nerve I arise from it. Several structures are contained in the brainstem. These include the diencephalon, the midbrain, the pons, and the medulla oblongata. The specific functions of each of the structures located in the brainstem are listed in the box below.

Brainstem functions

Diencephalon (thalamus and hypothalamus)

Receives sensory impulses (pain, temperature, and touch)
Acts as relay station
Controls pain threshold
Acts in synthesis of vasopressor and oxytocin
Helps maintain wakeful state
Controls temperature
Generates emotional response

Midbrain

Motor movement
Relay of impulses
Postural reflex patterns
Auditory reflexes
Righting reflex
Some control of vision

Pons

Pneumotaxic center (rhythmicity of respirations)
Connection between medulla, midbrain, and cerebellum

Medulla

Cardiac, vasomotor, and respiratory center
Center for cough, swallowing, hiccuping
Role in reticular activating system

Of special importance is the core of tissue that extends throughout the entire brainstem called the *reticular formation*. This interconnecting network of cells is the integrating center for respiration, cardiac function, motor systems, and states of consciousness. Stimulating these cells leads to wakefulness, and decreasing stimulation results in sleepiness (as in anoxia caused by increased intracranial pressure).

Cerebellum

The cerebellum is located below the posterior cerebrum. It controls skeletal muscles to produce coordinated movement, equilibrium, and erect posture. It acts with the cerebrum to coordinate muscle activity and produce skilled movement. Voluntary movements can proceed without the cerebellum, but they are clumsy and incoordinated (as in *asynergia* and *cerebellar ataxia*). The cerebellum receives both sensory and motor impulses, and it can detect errors in muscle synergy and adjust muscular control within the body.

Spinal cord

The spinal cord includes H-shaped central gray matter (cell bodies) surrounded by white matter composed of ascending and descending tracts. The spinal cord serves as a passageway for conducting information to and from the brain and the periphery. It also is the site of reflex pathways. Reflexes do not require relay to the brain level for action—they are an example of the simplest neural circuit. A reflex action consists of a specific stereotyped motor response to an adequate sensory stimulus. The response may involve skeletal muscle movement. A reflex may involve only one spinal cord level, or it may involve more spinal cord levels (segmental reflex). One example of the simple reflex arc is the knee jerk.

Circulation of the brain

The arterial system of the brain includes the larger conducting arteries and the penetrating smaller vessels that enter the brain at right angles after branching off from the conducting vessels. The smaller vessels supply nutrients to the neurons. The conducting arteries and the areas they supply are as follows:
1. Internal carotid arteries
   a. Most of the cerebral hemispheres
   b. Basal ganglia
   c. Upper two thirds of the diencephalon
2. Vertebral arteries
   a. Brainstem
   b. Lower one third of the diencephalon
   c. Cerebellum
   d. Occipital lobe

The two systems anastomose at the *circle of Willis*. This allows compensation for alterations in cerebral blood flow and blood pressure.

Circulation to the brain has several unique characteristics. Systemic circulation favors the CNS overall, balancing parts to assure a constant supply of nutrients (glucose and oxygen) to the brain. The brain is also able to autoregulate its blood flow to respond to changes in intraluminal pressure. In the presence of increasing blood pressure, cerebral vessels constrict, while they dilate when blood pressure falls. Vasodilation also occurs with elevated carbon dioxide content, hypoxia, and an elevated hydrogen ion concentration.

Cerebral veins have no valves. All veins of the brain terminate in dural sinuses. They empty into the superior vena cava via the jugular vein.

Cerebrospinal fluid

Cerebrospinal fluid is found in the ventricles of the brain, in the central canal of the spinal cord, and in the subarachnoid space. It serves as a fluid cushion for the tissue of the nervous system and helps support the weight of the brain. The cerebrospinal fluid is formed in the vessels of the choroid plexus. After circulating around the brain and spinal cord, the fluid returns to the brain and is absorbed through the arachnoid villi. The cerebrospinal fluid then enters the venous system and follows the pathway through the jugular vein to the superior vena cava into systemic circulation.

Normally there are up to 8 lymphocytes/ml of spinal fluid. An increase in the number of cells may indicate an infection, such as tuberculosis or a viral infection. Bacterial infections such as tuberculous meningitis often lower the blood sugar level as well as the chloride levels. Spinal fluid protein is increased in the presence of degenerative disease and/or brain tumor. Blood in the spinal fluid indicates hemorrhage from somewhere in the ventricular system.

Meninges

The coverings of the nervous tissue in the brain and spinal cord are called the meninges. These coverings help support, protect, and nourish the vital tissues below. The outermost is the *dura mater.* It is a very touch membrane with two layers. One of these meningeal layers sends four

processes deep into the brain. These processes form fibrous compartments for protection of the brain. The *arachnoid* is a delicate membrane that lies beneath the dura and closely covers the brain. Projections called *arachnoid villi* extend into the overlying dura. The innermost of the meninges is the *pia mater,* which is a vascular membrane with many minute plexuses of blood vessels. The same three meninges are also found in the spinal cord.

Three potential spaces are associated with the meninges. These are as follows:
1. Extradural (external to the dura)
2. Subdural (between the dura and the arachnoid)
3. Subarachnoid (between the arachnoid and pia mater)

PERIPHERAL NERVOUS SYSTEM

The peripheral nervous system (PNS) is basically a set of common channels located outside the CNS. Peripheral nerves are individual nerves or bundles of nerves that are either motor, sensory, or "mixed" (both sensory and motor fibers) in nature. The peripheral nervous system consists of 12 pairs of cranial nerves, which carry impulses to and from the brain, and 31 pairs of spinal nerves, which carry impulses to and from the spinal cord.

Peripheral nerves that transmit information toward the CNS are *afferent* or sensory in nature, and peripheral nerves that transmit information away from the CNS are *efferent* or motor in nature. In the peripheral nervous system the motor and sensory nerves usually travel together but separate at the cord level into a *posterior* or *sensory root* and an *anterior* or *motor root.*

The peripheral nervous system is divided into the *somatic and autonomic nervous systems.* The somatic nervous system innervates skeletal (striated) muscles. Fibers of axons liberate the neurotransmitter *acetylcholine* at skeletal muscle cells—this produces an action potential and movement.

AUTONOMIC NERVOUS SYSTEM

Body functions regulated by the *autonomic nervous system* include those of the cardiovascular, respiratory, and endocrine systems. Regulatory efforts have the goal of preserving homeostasis. Fibers of the autonomic nervous system synapse once after leaving the CNS at a site called the *ganglion.* The neurotransmitter is *acetylcholine.* The autonomic nervous system can be subdivided into the *sympathetic nervous system* and the *parasympathetic nervous system.* The sympathetic system functions to maintain homeostasis and to provide defense against stressors. The parasympathetic system conserves and restores regulatory functions.

Sensory system pathways

Stimulation of receptor neurons in the body is the first step in sensation. These receptor neurons provide the brain with information about the internal and external

---

Normal characteristics of cerebrospinal fluid

Specific gravity	1.007
pH	7.35 to 7.45
Chloride	120 to 130 mEq/L
Glucose	65 mg/100 ml
Pressure	50 to 200 mm water
Total volume	80 to 200 ml (15 ml in ventricles)
Total protein	15 to 45 mg/100 ml (lumbar)
	10 to 25 mg/100 ml (cisternal)
	5 to 15 mg/100 ml (ventricular)
Gamma globulin	6% to 13% of total protein

environments. The general sensory system includes the following:

1. Receptor neurons, which respond to specific stimuli
2. Posterior roots of the peripheral or afferent sensory nerves, which carry nerve impulses (action potentials) toward the CNS
3. Ascending or sensory tracts within the spinal cord and brain
4. Sensory area of the cerebral cortex, in which stimuli are perceived and interpreted

Motor system pathways

Once sensation has been perceived by the brain, corrective action or response is initiated. This action is conveyed by the descending motor pathways, which include the *corticospinal (pyramidal) tracts,* the *extrapyramidal system,* and the *cerebellar system.* The corticospinal system is primarily concerned with skilled, voluntary movement of skeletal muscle. Fibers that combine to form the corticospinal tracts arise from the upper motor neurons, which are located in most areas of the cerebral cortex.

After fibers leave the cerebral cortex they travel to the medulla, in which the majority of fibers *decussate* (cross over) to the opposite side. These fibers eventually synapse with the anterior horn cells, which are in the spinal cord and the motor nuclei in the brainstem. These cells are the *lower motor neurons* and are the final communication pathway with muscles via the myoneural junction (Fig. 20-4).

The extrapyramidal tracts provide separate pathways between the cortex, the basal ganglia, the brainstem, and the spinal cord. These include all descending motor pathways other than the corticospinal tracts, and they are named for their points of origin and termination. Generally, the extrapyramidal tracts help maintain muscle tone and control of gross autonomic skeletal muscle movement.

Visceral efferent pathways from the spinal cord control the action of involuntary or smooth muscles located within the walls of hollow organs, tubes, the heart, and glands.

Changes with aging

Studies have shown that the nervous system does change with aging. The effect of these changes is variable. The brain itself significantly *decreases in weight* with aging, along with a substantial loss of neurons. These changes occur most often in the sixth decade. In addition, there is both a significant *reduction of cerebral blood flow* and a *decrease in brain metabolism.*

The aged may also experience an altered *sleep/wakefulness ratio* and a *decreased ability to regulate body temperature.* These suggest changes in the function of the hypothalamus in the aging.

The control of the autonomic nervous system over various functions of the body is unpredictable and labile in the elderly, but some changes do occur. Additionally, sensory and motor conduction *decreases in velocity of nerve impulses* occur with aging, sensory conduction decreasing faster than motor. This occurs especially in peripheral nerves.

It is important for the nurse to realize that normal changes that occur with aging in the nervous system can-

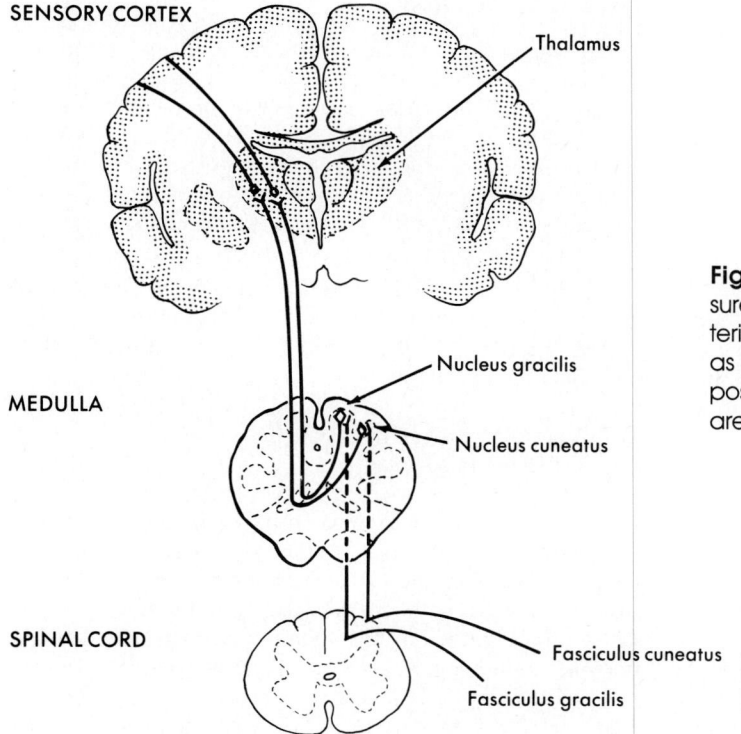

SENSORY CORTEX

Thalamus

MEDULLA

Nucleus gracilis

Nucleus cuneatus

SPINAL CORD

Fasciculus cuneatus

Fasciculus gracilis

Posterior columns

Fig. 20-4. Pathways for fine touch, deep touch and pressure, vibration, and proprioception. Note how stimuli entering through dorsal root (posterior) travel on same side as posterior columns to medulla, where they cross to opposite side, ascend to thalamus, and end in somesthetic area where perception occurs.

not be equated with senility, Alzheimer's disease, or organic brain disease. These conditions occur in a small number of older persons, and many reach advanced ages without any deterioration in the ability to think.

PREVENTION AND HEALTH EDUCATION

Problems that occur in the nervous system can have devastating results. These results often have impact on almost every body system and produce changes that are chronic and debilitating. Problems in other body systems, if discovered and treated in a timely fashion, can have much more satisfactory results than those in the nervous system.

Primary prevention: prevention of disease

Many of the problems of the nervous system have no known cause and thus cannot be prevented. For other problems, however, preventive measures can be emphasized. Neurologic problems can be divided into several main categories as follows.

PROBLEMS RESULTING FROM VASCULAR DISEASE

Neurovascular diseases can at times be prevented, or their results can at least be minimized. Many of the cerebrovascular diseases are thought to occur more frequently as a result of the presence of certain risk factors. These same factors also increase the risk of cardiac disease:
1. Cigarette smoking
2. Hypertension
3. Hypercholesterolemia
4. Obesity
5. Stress-related occupations and a hectic pace of life

PROBLEMS RESULTING FROM METASTASIS

Cigarette smoking has been identified as a major cause of lung cancer. This is significant to the nervous system, because neoplasms of the lung often metastasize to the brain. In fact, a significant number of lung malignancies are discovered subsequent to signs and symptoms of brain metastasis.

PROBLEMS RESULTING FROM TRAUMA

Some actions can play an important role in preventing head injuries and spinal cord injuries. Factors that can influence the outcome are as follows:
1. Use of seat belts in automobiles
2. Use of helmets while riding motorcycles or snowmobiles
3. Practice of firearm safety—keeping guns away from children
4. Minimal use of drugs and alcohol
5. Not driving after drinking or taking of drugs
6. Safe use of motor vehicles—no showing off or speeding
7. Use of precautions while swimming and especially not diving into shallow water

Secondary prevention/early detection

Early detection of neurologic diseases often is difficult. Many initial symptoms are so vague that it is easy to deny or minimize their importance. Also, some changes may occur over such a long period of time that adaption to them occurs. Certain warning symptoms can be found in such vague patterns that patients may be thought at first to be suffering from hysteria. The symptoms that are significant include the following:
1. Headaches that first occur after middle age or change in character, especially ones that are worse in the morning or awaken a person from sleep
2. Clumsiness or loss of function in an extremity
3. Changes in visual acuity
4. Any new or worsened seizure activity
5. Numbness or tingling in one or more extremities
6. Pain that is neurologic in nature
7. Galactorrhea
8. Cessation of menses

Tertiary prevention/prevention of complications

It is important to mention the issue of tertiary prevention for the patient with neurologic dysfunction. Unfortunately, many of these patients are prone to iatrogenic complications as well as functional disabilities. These occur secondary to the neurologic problems and include contractures, decubiti, and eye damage, as well as other hazards of immobility.[70] It is extremely important for the nurse working with these types of patients to be aware of rehabilitative concepts and apply them in the nursing care. Many patients with neurologic dysfunctions may also benefit from formal inpatient rehabilitative care after the acute hospitalization.

COMMON NEUROLOGIC MANIFESTATIONS

The practice of neurologic nursing is concerned with problems of the nervous system that have a variety of causes. Whatever the cause, various symptoms occur, at times related to both organic and functional causes. Because of the nature of the anatomy and physiology of the nervous system, *organic lesions or trauma result in clinical manifestations related to the site affected, regardless of the underlying pathologic condition.* Other manifestations result not from the damaged site itself, but from other parts of the nervous system that are affected by the damaged site. One example of this is a lack of control or regulation. The nurse must realize that patients with neurologic problems may have to make significant changes in life-style and adaptation. The psyche and the body are one in the person; often there is no clear-cut distinction of symptoms. A person is an open system in which many subsystems interplay.

In this section, we will discuss neurologic manifestations resulting from alterations in neurologic function and structure that are common to many pathologic conditions. A brief review of neurologic assessment is helpful in this discussion.

Neurologic assessment

Complete neurologic assessment is usually performed in phases and is dependent on the condition of the patient and the urgency in collecting the data. It includes a history and neurologic examination. The reader is referred to Chapter 3 for a discussion of assessment.

Neurologic examination of the conscious adult includes physical examination of the following:
1. Mental status
   a. Level of consciousness
   b. Orientation
   c. Mood and behavior
   d. Knowledge
   e. Vocabulary
   f. Memory
2. Cranial nerve function (Table 20-1)
3. Language and speech
4. Meningeal signs
5. Sensory status
   a. Touch
   b. Pain
   c. Temperature
   d. Proprioception
6. Motor status
   a. Gait and stance
   b. Muscle strength
   c. Muscle tone
   d. Coordination
   e. Involuntary movements
   f. Muscle stretch reflexes

Table 20-1. Assessment of cranial nerve function

Nerve	Function	Assessments
Olfactory (I)	Sensory—smell	Identification of odors
Optic (II)	Sensory—vision	Visual acuity; inspection of fundi; determination of visual fields
Oculomotor (III)	Motor—pupil constriction, elevation of upper eyelid, extraocular movements	Tested together for extraocular movements; also pupil reflex for CNIII
Trochlear (IV)	Motor—downward/inward eye movements	
Trigeminal (V)	Motor—jaw movement; Sensory facial sensation	Jaw strength; facial sensation; corneal reflex
Abducens (VI)	Motor—lateral eye movements	
Facial (VII)	Motor—facial muscles; Sensory taste on anterior two thirds of tongue	Facial movements; identification of tastes
Acoustic (VIII)	Hearing—cochlear division; Balance—vestibular division	Whisper; caloric test
Glossopharyngeal (IX)	Sensory—pharynx and posterior tongue, with taste	Identification of tastes
	Motor—pharynx; Sensory—pharynx and larynx; Motor—palate, pharynx and larynx	Gag reflex; uvula motion; soft palate movement; hoarseness
Vagus (X)		
Spinal accessory (XI)	Motor—stemocleidomastoid, upper part of trapezius	Shoulder and neck motion
Hypoglossal (XII)	Motor—tongue	Tongue motion

Adapted from Bates, B.: A guide to physical examination, ed. 2, Philadelphia, 1979, J.B. Lippincott Co.

Table 20-2. Comparison of migraine, cluster, and tension headaches

Type	Onset	Frequency	Duration	Nature	Prodromal symptoms/associated symptoms	Treatment
Migraine headaches	Occur at any age Strongly hereditary More common in women than men	Episodic, tend to occur with stress or life crisis	Hours to days	Occur slowly; pain becomes severe, with one side of head affected more than other	Prodromal: visual field defects, confusion, paresthesias Associated: nausea, vomiting, chills, fatigue, irritability, sweating, edema	Ergotamine tartrate Inderal Nonnarcotic analgesics Relaxation techniques
Cluster headaches	Early adulthood; precipitated by alcohol or nitrates More common in older men	Episodes clustered together in quick succession for few days or weeks with remissions that last for months	Few minutes to few hours	Pain intense: throbbing, deep, often unilateral; begin in infraorbital region and spread to head and neck	Prodromal: uncommon Associated: flushing, tearing of eyes, nasal stuffiness, sweating swelling of temporal vessels	Narcotic analgesics during acute phase, often intramuscularly
Tension headaches (muscle contraction)	Often in adolescence; related to tension or anxiety No family history	Episodic; vary with stress	Variable, can be constant	Dull, constant, uncommon aggravating pain; vary in intensity; usually bilateral and involve neck and shoulders; pain may be poorly defined	Prodromal: uncommon Associated: sustained contraction of head and neck muscles	Nonnarcotic analgesics Relaxation techniques Amitriptyline (Elavil)

More detailed descriptions of selected portions of the examination will be covered in specific parts of this chapter. The reader is also referred to a neurologic nursing text for additional information.

Headache

Headache is a common symptom experienced by many patients. It can result from many pathologic processes, and its significance also is variable. *The source of recurring headache should be determined through careful physical examination with appropriate neurologic assessment.* Persons have been known to self-treat headaches for months, believing them to be nothing to worry about, only to learn later that the pain was caused by a more serious problem such as a brain tumor. Because of the site of some tumors in the brain, headache may be the only symptom for many months.

PATHOPHYSIOLOGY

Headache may have many causes. Some of these are as follows:
1. Expanding masses such as neoplasms
2. Intracranial bleeding
3. Inflammation of the meninges as in meningitis
4. Other infections of the brain and spinal cord
5. Head trauma
6. Cerebral hypoxia
7. Dilation of the cerebral blood vessels
8. Psychologic factors such as stress
9. Systemic disease including eye, ear, and sinus problems

The exact pathophysiology of head pain is not known. Although the skull and brain tissues are not capable of sensory pain, pain arises from the scalp and its blood vessels and muscles, from the dura mater and its venous sinuses, and from the blood vessels at the base of the brain. Blood vessels dilate and become congested with blood. The pain is also thought to be the result of tension that occurs with stretching of these tissues, as well as from sustained contraction of extracranial skeletal muscles around the face, scalp, and cervical areas. In one type of headache, *migraine headache,* chemical changes in and around the cranial blood vessel walls appear to play a role in causation.

Headaches can be divided into three categories, as follows:
1. Vascular
2. Tension
3. Combination of the two

See Table 20-2 for details about and comparison of three specific types of headache.

ASSESSMENT

Both subjective and objective data are important in determining more about the cause and nature of the headache.

Subjective data

1. Patient's understanding of headache and possible causes
2. Awareness of any precipitating factors such as stress
3. Measures that relieve symptoms, including medications
4. Location, frequency, pattern, and character of head pain, including site of return, time of day, and intervals between headaches
5. Initial onset of headache
6. Presence of any prodromal symptoms
7. Presence of associated symptoms
8. Family history of headaches (especially important with migraine)
9. Situations that make headache worse

Objective data

1. Behavior: signs indicating stress or anxiety or pain
2. Change in ability to carry on daily activities
3. Abnormalities on physical assessment part of neurologic examination
4. Temperature

Information about the patient's understanding of the nature and precipitating factors is helpful for planning necessary teaching. It is not unusual for the patient to manifest little objective data in the presence of subjective complaints.

Headache pain may be made worse by stress or tension. Knowledge of the patient's perception of the effect of stress on the symptoms is important in planning for measures that relieve or reduce effects of stress.

Migraine headaches are unusual in that there are prodromal signs and symptoms that occur before the acute attack. These may include the following:
1. Visual field defects
2. Confusion
3. Paresthesias
4. Paralysis in rare cases

During the actual attack, signs and symptoms may include nausea, vomiting, sensitivity to light, chilliness, fatigue, irritability, sweating, edema, and other autonomic signs.

In assessing headache there are several key points to consider. These include the following:
1. Localized type of head pain is usually associated with migraine headaches or an organic disorder.
2. Generalized headache is usually related to psychologic causes or the presence of increased intracranial pressure.
3. Migraine headaches may change from one side of the head to the other.
4. Headaches that occur with increased intracranial pressure usually are present on awakening and may awaken the person from sleep.
5. Sinus headaches typically occur early in the morning and increase in intensity as the day progresses.
6. Many headaches are related to stress.
7. Pain described as dull, nagging, aggravating, and

ever present often occurs with psychogenic head-aches.

8. Organically caused pain tends to be constant and progressive in nature.
9. Migraine headaches may be associated with menstruation.
10. Headaches may be precipitated by eating foods containing monosodium glutamate or sodium nitrate as well as by alcohol.
11. A family history of headache is important, especially with migraine headaches.
12. Sleeping too long, fasting, or inhaling toxic fumes in work situations with inadequate ventilation can cause headaches.
13. Oral contraceptives may make migraine headaches worse.
14. Any secondary gains that patients receive from headaches must be assessed.

DIAGNOSTIC TESTS

It is important to evaluate headaches that are not slight and transient. Usual testing includes a neurologic examination including a CT scan. The CT scan is becoming more available as a way to easily and safely detect abnormalities in the CNS. It has replaced many invasive and painful procedures that neurologic patients previously were subjected to during a diagnostic workup.

A lumbar puncture may also be performed. A lumbar puncture is not done, however, if there is evidence of increased intracranial pressure or if a brain tumor is suspected, since the quick reduction in pressure produced by removal of the spinal fluid may cause brain herniation. In this situation a CT scan must be done first. The box outlines the procedure for lumbar puncture.

At times, because of anatomic abnormalities or other causes, a lumbar puncture may not be possible. At these times a cisternal puncture may be attempted. The cister-

---

Computed tomography (EMI, CT, or CAT scan)

Purpose
Detection of cerebral and spinal cord pathology using a technique of scanning without radioisotopes.

Preparation of patient
1. No special physical preparation
2. Patient teaching
   a. Explain procedure
   b. Time: Approximately 20 to 30 minutes for CT scan without contrast medium; 60 minutes if scans with and without contrast medium are done.
   c. Sensation: Procedure is painless, except for slight discomfort when IV is started for injection of contrast medium. Also, there is some discomfort in lying still and possible feelings of claustrophobia as a result of head being positioned in head holder.
   d. Patient must maintain motionless position until scan is completed.
3. If contrast medium is used, history of allergy to iodine (seafood) is determined before medium is given.

Procedure
1. Patient lies supine with the head positioned within a rubber head-holder to prevent air gaps between the machine and scalp.
2. Head is scanned in two planes simultaneously and at various angles. Each image s a specific layer of brain tissue.
3. The computer calculates tissue absorption in contiguous layers of brain tissue ard displays a printout. Selected photographs of the printouts are taken.
4. Tumor densities are compared with the normal brain tissue. (Tumors, infarctions, bone displacement, and the ventricles are well visualized).
5. If a contrast study is desired, the patient receives the contrast medium and the scanning process is repeated.

After procedure
1. No adverse effects except the risk of transient increased intracranial pressure in patients with masses or other brain pathology.
2. Plan period of rest as needed for the patient.

Lumbar puncture

Purpose

To obtain cerebrospinal fluid (CSF) for examination or relief of pressure.

Preparation of patient

1. Usually a permit is signed by patient or family member.
2. Occasionally sedation is given before procedure.
3. Patient teaching
   a. Explain procedure.
   b. Time: approximately 10 to 15 minutes.
   c. Sensation: slight pain and pressure may be felt as the dura is entered. A sharp shooting pain down one leg may be experienced, caused by the needle coming close to a nerve.
   d. Other: Remind patient to lie still and not to move suddenly.

Procedure

1. Patient is usually positioned on the side with both knees and head flexed at an acute angle to allow maximum lumbar flexion and separation of interspinous spaces. Occasionally patients may be positioned sitting up and leaning over the bedside table.
2. Local anesthetic is usually used to anesthetize the lumbar area.
3. Under strict aseptic technique the needle is inserted below the level of the spinal cord at the L4-L5 or L5-S1 interspace (Fig. 20-5).
4. Inner needle is removed to allow drainage and measurement of spinal fluid.
5. Level of fluid column in manometer used to measure pressure is read.
6. Fluid is collected for various tests or to relieve pressure. Occasionally the first specimen of spinal fluid contains blood from slight bleeding at the site of puncture. This specimen should not be sent for cell count.
7. *Queckenstedt's test* may be performed to test for subarachnoid block. The jugular veins are compressed for 10 seconds, first on one side, then on the other side, and then on both sides at the same time. Any change in spinal fluid pressure during the compression is noted.
8. Needle is withdrawn.

After procedure

1. Patient lies flat in bed for several hours
2. Site of puncture should be observed for any leakage of CSF.
3. Headache is fairly common and is thought to be caused by the loss of spinal fluid through the dura mater. The sharpness and size of the needle, the skill of the physician, whether the patient lies flat, and the patient's emotional state may determine if a headache occurs.
4. Headaches are usually treated with bed rest, analgesics, and ice applied to the head.

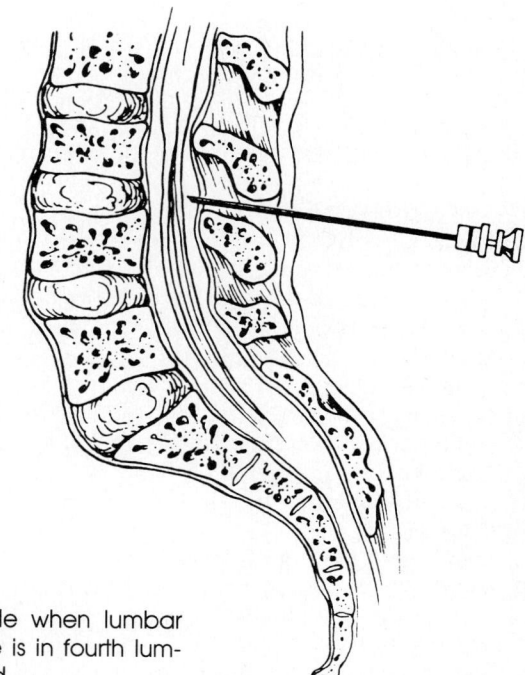

Fig. 20-5. Position and angle of needle when lumbar puncture is performed. Note that needle is in fourth lumbar interspace below level of spinal cord.

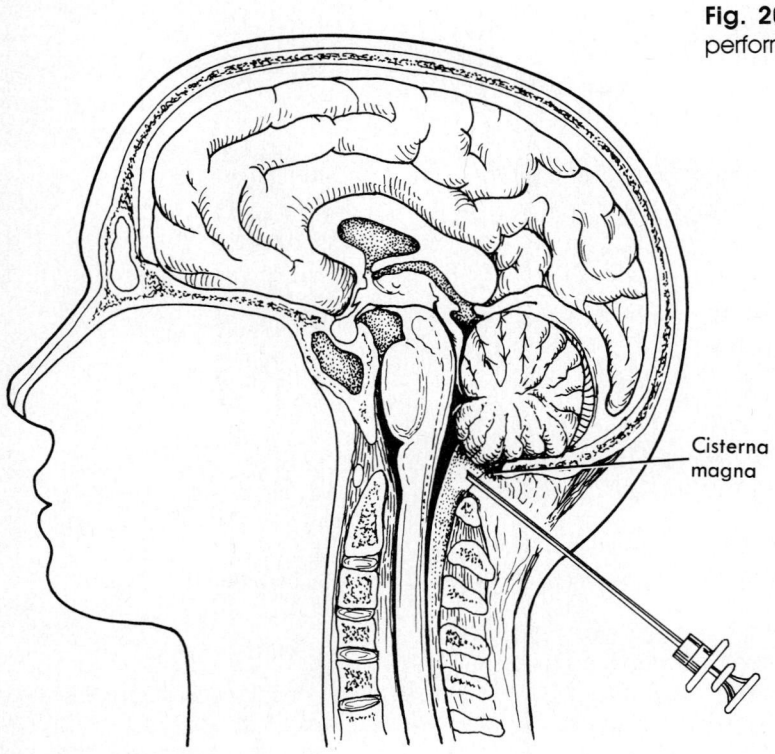

Fig. 20-6. Position of needle when cisternal puncture is performed. Note needle length and short bevel.

Cisterna
magna

Cisternal puncture

Purpose
To obtain CSF for examination, or for instillation of contrast medium for diagnostic studies

Preparation of patient
1. Usually a permit for surgery is signed.
2. Back of patient's neck may be shaved.
3. Procedure is performed in the patient's bed or in treatment room.
4. Patient is positioned in a side-lying position at the edge of the bed or treatment table with the head bent forward.
5. Patient teaching
   a. Same as for lumbar puncture.
   b. Procedure may be more frightening to the patient because of the close proximity of the procedure to the brain.

Procedure
1. Same as for lumbar puncture except for different site (between C1 and base of skull).
2. Head of patient should be held firmly during procedure so it does not rotate.

After procedure
1. Patient is observed immediately for dyspnea, apnea, or cyanosis.
2. Headache occurs less frequently than with lumbar puncture.

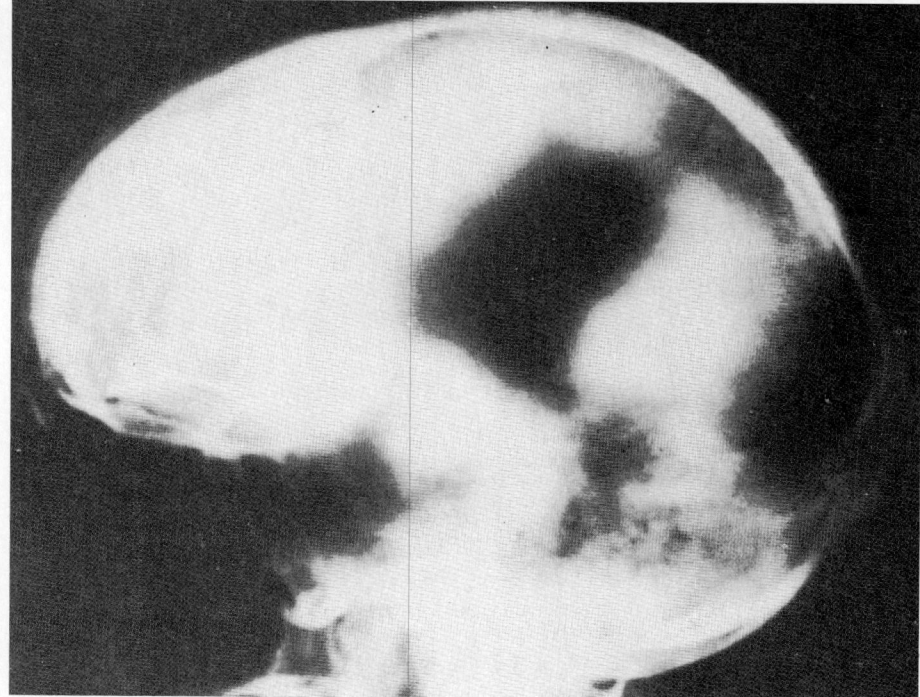

Fig. 20-7. Radioisotope brain scan. Intracranial mass (brain tumor) is seen in two dark areas (parietal and occipital) of scan where abnormal uptake of ^{197}Hg-tagged chlormerodrin accumulated. (Courtesy Abbas M. Rejali, M.D., Department of Radiology, Case Western Reserve University, Cleveland, Ohio.)

Brain scan

Purpose
Detection of cerebral pathology using radioactive isotopes and a scanner.

Preparation of patient
1. No physical preparation of patient.
2. When mercury is used as the isotope indicator, a mercurial diuretic (meralluride [Mercuhydrin]) is administered several hours before the procedure. This allows a greater concentration of radioactive mercury to be circulated to brain tissue, since melluride minimizes the uptake of mercury by the kidneys.
3. Patient teaching
   a. Explain procedure.
   b. Time: approximately 45 minutes for the actual scan.
   c. Sensation: minimal discomfort associated with the IV administration of the radioactive iosotope. Some patients may find it uncomfortable to lie still for the scan.

Procedure
1. Patient is injected with radioisotope (mercury or sodium pertechnetate Tc 99m)
2. While patient lies still, usually in supine position, scanner is passed over head. This picks up concentrated areas of uptake. Several scans are taken.

After procedure
1. No adverse effects.
2. Plan period of rest as needed for the patient.

nal puncture is made between the first cervical vertebra and the base of the skull (Fig. 20-6). See the box on p. 365 for a description of this procedure.

Other tests that may be done include a brain scan (Fig. 20-7) and plain skull films.

The skull x-ray films will demonstrate bony abnormality as well as congenital changes, but will not yield the information that more sophisticated procedures do.

DATA ANALYSIS AND PLANNING

Nursing diagnoses

Possible nursing diagnoses for the person with a headache include the following:

Alteration in comfort: pain
Anticipatory grieving
Ineffective individual coping
Knowledge deficit
Sleep pattern disturbance

EXPECTED PATIENT OUTCOMES

Expected patient outcomes for the patient with headache include the following:

1. Headache pain is decreased.
2. Patient can carry on ADL.
3. Patient can explain prescribed medication (dosage, action, side effects, and frequency).
4. Patient can identify any factors that trigger headaches.
5. Patient can demonstrate prescribed relaxation techniques.
6. Patient can explain the importance of continuing medical supervision for chronic headache.
7. Patient can explain the danger of continued use of over-the-counter drugs for chronic, recurring headache.

IMPLEMENTATION

Assisting with achievement of therapeutic goals
Medications

Treatment for headache often includes the use of selected medications. These will be described in terms of their use for migraine, cluster, and tension headaches.

MIGRAINE HEADACHES. *Acetylsalicylic acid* (aspirin) is seldom effective for classic migraine, but may be helpful after the headache has developed. *Ergotamine tartrate* preparations taken early in the attack may prevent the headache from developing. These drugs are the treatments of choice in migraine, and their success in relieving the headache is often considered diagnostic of migraine. Ergotamine tartrate preparations act by constricting cerebral blood vessel walls, thus reducing cerebral blood flow. It may be administered orally, sublingually, or rectally in 2 to 4 mg dosages. It is also available for injection in 0.25 to 0.5 mg dosages. Ergot preparations are also available in combination with other drugs such as *caffeine, phenobarbital,* and *belladonna*. Ergot

preparations have the side effects of nausea, vomiting, numbness and tingling, muscle pain, and changes in heart rate. They also stimulate uterine smooth muscle, so they cannot be taken by pregnant women. Other drugs that may be substituted include nonnarcotic analgesics, such as *phenacetin, acetaminophen,* or *propoxyphene (Darvon),* as well as narcotics, such as *codeine. Propranolol hydrochloride (Inderal)* has been used to prevent migraine headaches with limited success.

CLUSTER HEADACHES. Because the pain associated with cluster headaches is so severe, narcotic analgesics are often prescribed during the acute attack. Often these must be administered intramuscularly for optimal relief.

Patients with cluster headaches usually feel fine between attacks, so no analgesia is needed during these times.

TENSION HEADACHES. The nonnarcotic analgesics are often prescribed for tension headaches. These include acetaminophen, propoxyphene, phenacetin, and acetylsalicylic acid. Narcotic analgesics such as codeine may be prescribed along with diazepam (Valium) for relief of tension. It is far better, however, to counsel the patient to develop other ways to relieve the headache.

Promotion of rest and relaxation

Since stress and emotional upsets may precipitate some headaches and make others worse, measures are taken to facilitate relaxation and rest. Relaxation techniques (Chapter 8), planned sleeping hours, and rest periods as needed may prove helpful. Because alcohol has been found to be significant in causing cluster headaches, it should not be used as a way to relieve tension.

Some patients who have tension headaches have found relaxation by regular physical exercise to be helpful.

Psychotherapy

Patients with chronic headaches may respond to psychotherapy. It may be used to help the patient develop awareness of stressors as well as to deal with feelings about being the victim of headache pain.

Assisting with comfort and ADL

Other treatments that have been found to be helpful with headache include cold packs applied to the forehead or base of the brain. Pressure applied to the temporal and carotid arteries may be helpful depending on the cause of the headache. Patients who are experiencing migraine headaches, especially, may be most comfortable lying in a dark room with minimal auditory stimulation.

Identification of triggering factors

Discovery of triggering factors associated with severe recurring headaches will need to be made through ongoing assessment of the person's personality, habits, and ADL. Clues may be obtained from seeking information about the person's goals and aspirations, work habits, family relationships, coping mechanisms, and relaxation patterns. The person may be asked to keep a diary of activities and the occurrence of headaches as well as the nature of the headache and how they were treated.

Teaching for the patient with headache

1. Avoid factors found to increase headache.
2. Use relaxation measures (such as biofeedback) when emotional tension is present.
3. Maintain regular sleep patterns.
4. Take medication as ordered—be aware of their side effects, and report these to physician.
5. Follow up with medical care as indicated.
6. Allow others to assist with activities during headaches.
7. Structure home and work environment to keep stressors at a reasonable level.

Types of pain sensation

Paresthesia	Abnormal sensation
Hyperalgesia	Increased pain sensation
Hypoalgesia	Decreased pain sensation
Analgesia	Blocked pain sensation
Dysesthesia	Pain sensation caused by stimulus that normally would not be painful
Referred pain	Pain that occurs in a site other than its origin
Causalgia	Intense, continuous, burning pain
Local pain	Occurring as a result of direct stimulation of pain receptors

---

Triggering factors may include the following:
1. Fatigue
2. Alcohol
3. Stress
4. Climatic changes
5. Hunger
6. Menstruation

Teaching

Teaching is an important part of nursing care of the patient with head pain. The above box lists appropriate teaching activities.

EVALUATION

Evaluation of headaches is based on the nursing outcomes and should be done in conjunction with the patient. Questions to ask include the following:
1. Is the use of medication within medical guidelines?
2. Is the patient keeping follow-up appointments?
3. Is the patient functioning optimally?
4. Is the patient following medical advice?

Neurologic pain

PATHOPHYSIOLOGY

Neurologic pain other than headache is commonly seen in nursing. It is sometimes difficult to distinguish between pain produced by lesions within the nervous system that cause objective sensory abnormalities and peripherally produced, somatic pain in a distant organ. Although in practice pain may be viewed from the standpoint of neural transmission, the transmission of pain impulses is not fully understood. Neurologic pain may arise from lesions involving peripheral cutaneous nerves, the sensory nerve roots, the thalamus, and the central pain tract (spinothalamic) at some level (Fig. 20-8). Pain receptors are not adaptable. Pain impulses continue at the same rate as long as the stimulus is present. They are specific for pain only. Pain receptors can be activated by:

1. Cellular damage
2. Certain chemicals such as histamine
3. Heat
4. Ischemia
5. Muscle spasms
6. Sensations of heat, cold, and itching that go beyond a specific level of intensity

Pain that is described as unbearable and does not respond to treatment is classified as *intractable*. It is chronic and often disabling.

ASSESSMENT

Both subjective and objective data are important to assess in the patient with neurologic pain. Again, it should be remembered that pain is highly subjective, and there may not be a great deal of objective data to accompany the subjective complaints.

Subjective data

1. Patient's understanding of the pain
2. Any precipitating factors
3. Measures that relieve symptoms, including medication
4. Site, frequency, and nature of pain
5. Usual coping patterns when under stress
6. Presence of associated symptoms
7. Measures that make pain worse

Objective data

1. Behavior: signs indicating pain or stress
2. Change in ability to carry out ADL
3. Muscle weakness or wasting
4. Vasomotor responses (flushing, and so on)
5. Spinal reflexes and sensory examination

The quality of pain and its distribution are important factors to assess. Pain may vary from mild to excruciating. Terms with which the nurse should be familiar with include those listed in box above.

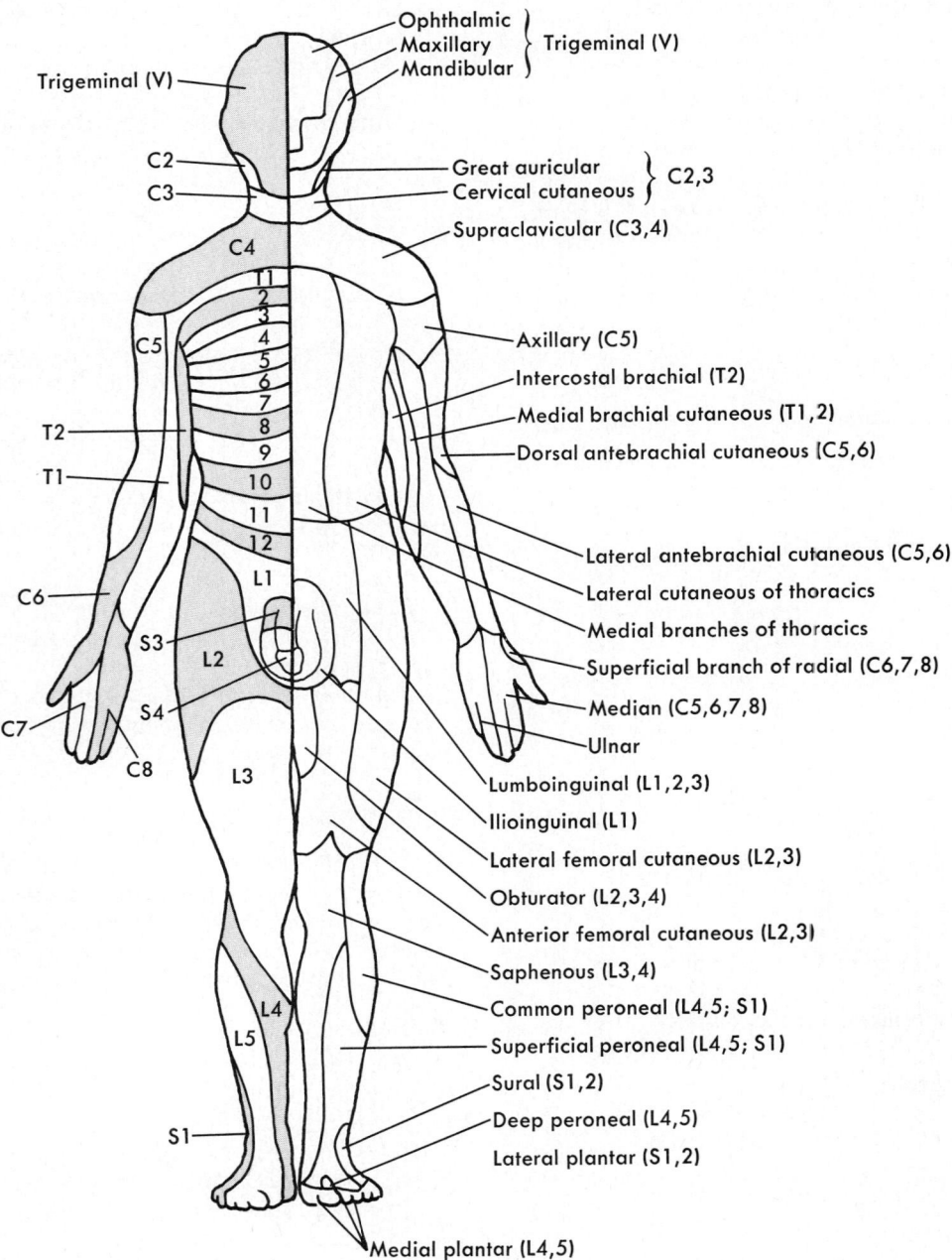

Fig. 20-8. Peripheral distribution of sensory nerve fibers, anterior view. Right, distribution of cutaneous nerves. Left, dermatomes (shaded) or segmental distribution of cutaneous nerves.

Site of problem and resulting neurologic pain

Site of problem	Results	Characteristics of pain
Peripheral cutaneous nerves	Pain usually limited to anatomic area supplied by affected nerve or nerves	Often described as burning sensation, but can be described as sharp or dull and aching. Pain may be constant or permanent. Often described as severe. Also called local pain
Root pain	Limited to dermatomes supplied by affected sensory nerve roots (pain from lesion arising from deep somatic and visceral stimulus may radiate beyond dermatomes) (Fig. 20-8)	Aggravated by anything that causes direct or indirect movement of spinal cord (sneezing, coughing, or straining)
Central lesion within thalamus	Pain confined to contralateral side of body	Pain described as burning, pulling, and swelling Often aggravated by emotional stress and fatigue Influenced by cutaneous stimulation
Central spinothalamic tract	Pain sensation distributed to level of tract involved Hemisection of spinal cord produces loss of pain and temperature sensation on contralateral side at a level one or two segments below injury	May be similar to thalamic pain, but less disturbing

As stated earlier, neurologic pain may arise from lesions involving peripheral cutaneous nerves, the sensory nerve roots (posterior), the thalamus, and the central pain tract. Each of these sources produces characteristic pain.

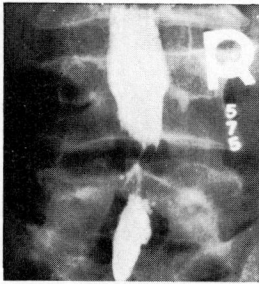

Fig. 20-9. Myelogram showing almost complete block in interspace between fourth and fifth lumbar vertebrae. (From Moseley, H.F., editor: Textbook of surgery, ed 3. St. Louis, 1959, The C.V. Mosby Co.)

Diagnostic tests

It is extremely difficult to evaluate pain objectively. Electrical stimulation may be attempted to define the pain to a greater extent. The person with intractable pain may undergo psychologic testing as part of the workup. Tests to rule out causes of the pain may be indicated. One such test is the myelogram. This is commonly done when back pain is present (Fig. 20-9).

DATA ANALYSIS AND PLANNING
Nursing diagnoses

Possible nursing diagnoses for the person with neurologic pain include the following:
Alteration in comfort: pain
Impaired physical mobility
Ineffective individual coping
Knowledge deficit
Sleep pattern disturbance

Myelogram (metrizamide and Pantopaque)

Purpose

To identify lesions in the intradural or extradural compartments of the spinal canal by observing the flow of radiopaque dye through the subarachnoid space.

Preparation of patient

1. Permit must be signed.
2. If metrizamide dye is to be used the patient should not take the following drugs for 24 to 48 hours before the test:
   a. Phenothiazines
   b. Tricyclic antidepressants
   c. CNS stimulants
   d. Amphetamines
3. With metrizamide dye, fluids are encouraged.
4. Lower extremity strength and sensation should be assessed for baseline.
5. Patient teaching
   a. Explain procedure.
   b. Time: approximately 2 hours.
   c. Sensation: slight pain and pressure may be felt as dura is entered. Some patients find varied positions they must assume during procedure uncomfortable.

Procedure

1. Patient is usually positioned on the side with both knees and head flexed at an acute angle to allow maximum lumbar flexion and separation of interspinous spaces. Cisternal puncture may also be done (Fig. 20-6).
2. Local anesthetic is used to anesthetize the puncture site.
3. Under strict aseptic technique needle is inserted at L4-L5 or L5-S1 or cisternally.
4. Inner needle is removed to allow drainage, measurement of pressure, and collection of specimens.
5. Dye is instilled and needle removed.
6. Patient is turned to varied positions to visualize the spinal cord while fluoroscopic and radiologic films are taken.
7. After the procedure is completed, Pantopaque dye is removed via another lumbar puncture. Leaving it in would cause serious irritation to the meninges.
8. Metrizamide dye is water soluble and does not need to be removed.
9. With metrizamide dye the patient usually undergoes a CT scan of the spinal cord 4 to 6 hours after the myelogram.

After procedure

1. Pantopaque myelogram
   a. Patient lies flat in bed overnight.
   b. Site of puncture should be observed for leakage of CSF.
   c. Headache is fairly common.
   d. Strength and sensation of lower extremities should be assessed.
2. Metrizamide
   a. Patient's head and thorax must remain elevated 30° to 50° for at least 8 hours and then elevated at least 30° for 24 hours.
   b. Fluids are encouraged.
   c. Common side effects include nausea, vomiting, seizures (peak time of risk is 4 to 8 hours after procedure), and some nonspecific behavior changes.
   d. Strength and sensation of lower extremities should be assessed after procedure.
   e. Site of puncture should be assessed for leakage of CSF.
   f. Avoid drugs previously listed—they lower seizure threshold. (When nausea occurs after a metrizamide myelogram, prochlorperazine [Compazine] cannot be used. Drugs that may be used include benzquinamide [Emete-Con.]])
   g. The advantages of metrizamide outweigh the risks. It is less viscous than iodine-based dye and therefore permits better visualization of smaller areas.

Expected patient outcomes

Expected patient outcomes for the patient with neuro-logic pain include the following:
1. Pain is decreased
2. Patient can
   a. Better carry on ADL
   b. Demonstrate physical methods that can be used for pain control
   c. Describe positioning methods and their relationship to pain
   d. Explain the relationship between pain and emotional upsets
   e. State the plan for follow-up care
   f. Explain medication to be taken at home (dosage, action, side effects, and frequency)
   g. Explain how to manage sleep and rest patterns

IMPLEMENTATION

Assisting with achievement of therapeutic goals
Medications

Treatment for patients with neurological pain may include the use of medications. These often include the nonnarcotic analgesics—acetaminophen, propoxyphene (Darvon), phenacetin, and acetylsalicylic acid. Narcotic analgesics such as codeine may be prescribed along with diazepam (Valium) or amitriptyline hydrochloride (Elavil). The emphasis should be on helping the patient learn other measures to control pain.

Promotion of rest and relaxation

As with headache, stress and emotional upsets may precipitate neurologic pain or make it worse. Rest and relaxation should be facilitated. Relaxation techniques, planned sleeping hours, and rest periods throughout the day may be helpful. Relaxation techniques used include biofeedback and meditation.

Some patients with pain, especially pain defined as intractable, may respond well to psychotherapy. It can help the patient develop awareness of stressors and how they influence the perception of pain.

Assisting with comfort and ADL

Patients experiencing neurologic pain may be extremely uncomfortable. The nurse should help the patient attain a position of comfort. For example, the patient with root pain should avoid movements that cause direct or indirect movement of the spinal cord. Significant nursing activities include the following:
1. Patient should not lie in a horizontal plane for long periods, as this causes tension or traction on the thoracic and sacral nerve roots.
2. Sitting may help to relieve tension on the nerve roots.
3. When moving a person with root pain, sharp flexion of the neck and extension of the legs should be avoided as much as possible.
4. Straining during bowel movements can intensify pain—stool softeners are often indicated.

The identification of any triggering factors of neuro-

Teaching for the patient with neurologic pain

1. Avoid factors that increase pain
2. Use relaxation measures such as biofeedback and meditation when emotional tension is present
3. Maintain regular rest and sleep pattern
4. Take medication as prescribed
5. Be aware of physical methods of controlling pain (such as positioning) and use them
6. Follow up with medical care as indicated
7. Structure home and work environment to keep stressors at a minimum

---

logic pain is important. This can be done by a thorough assessment of personality, habits, and ADL. The person may be asked to keep a diary of ADL and the occurrence of the pain.

SURGERY

In cases of intractable pain that does not respond to medical and nursing actions, surgery may be necessary. The surgeries that are used include the following:
1. Nerve block
2. Neurectomy
3. Rhizotomy
4. Cordotomy

Electrical stimulation may also be used in cases of recurring pain. See Chapter 18 for a description of the varied surgeries and treatment.

Teaching

Teaching is an important part of nursing care for the patient with neurologic pain. Appropriate teaching activities are listed in box below.

EVALUATION

Evaluation of the patient with peripheral nerve or intractable neurologic pain considers how the person is functioning in spite of the pain. Questions to consider include the following:
1. Is the use of medications within guidelines?
2. Is the patient following up with appointments?
3. Is the patient able to carry on normal functions?
4. Is the patient cooperating with medical advice?
5. Is the patient using physical methods to control the pain in a correct way?

Increased intracranial pressure

PATHOPHYSIOLOGY

Increased intracranial pressure is a complex manifestation that is the consequence of multiple neurologic conditions. It often occurs suddenly and requires surgical intervention.

The contents of the skull, or cranial contents, are brain tissue, vascular tissue, and cerebrospinal fluid. Any increase in the volume of one of the cranial contents results in increased intracranial pressure, because the cranial vault is rigid, closed, and nonexpandable. Specific causes of increased intracranial pressure are listed in box below.

An increase in any one of the cranial contents is usually accompanied by a reciprocal change in the volume of one of the others. Brain tissue cannot expand without serious effects in the flow and amount of cerebrospinal fluid and cerebral circulation. Space-occupying lesions displace and distort the brain and vacular tissues as pressure increases. The buildup of pressure may occur slowly (days or weeks) or rapidly, depending on the cause. At first, one hemisphere of the brain will be more involved, but eventually both hemispheres will be affected.

As pressure increases within the cranial cavity it is at first compensated for by venous compression and cerebrospinal displacement. As the pressure continues to rise, the cerebral blood flow decreases and inadequate perfusion occurs. This inadequate perfusion initiates a vicious cycle causing the Pco_2 to increase and the Po_2 and the pH to fall. These changes cause vasodilation and cerebral edema. The edema further increases the intracranial pressure, causing increased compression of neural tissue and an even greater increase in intracranial pressure.

When the pressure exceeds the brain's ability to compensate, the only escape for the relief of pressure is for the brain to be displaced caudally or herniated downward. As a result of herniation, the brainstem is compressed at variable levels, which in turn compresses the vasomotor center, the posterior cerebral artery, the oculomotor nerve, the corticospinal nerve pathway, and the fibers of the ascending reticular activating system (Fig. 20-10). The life-sustaining mechanisms of consciousness, blood pressure, pulse, respiration, and temperature regulation fail.

ASSESSMENT

Subjective data

1. Patient's understanding of condition
2. Presence of visual changes: diplopia or blurred vision
3. Ability to think
4. Presence of pain, especially headache
5. Ability to carry on daily activities
6. Presence of nausea

The patient with increased intracranial pressure may complain of a headache. It is thought to result from venous congestion and the tension in the intracranial blood vessels as the cerebral pressure rises. The location and duration of the headache should be elicited from the patient. Headache that occurs with increased intracranial pressure usually increases in intensity with coughing, straining, or stooping. Headache is usually present in the early morning and may awaken the patient from sleep.

Objective data

1. Level of consciousness
2. Pupillary signs
3. Vital signs
4. Focal motor or sensory signs
5. Presence of vomiting or hiccuping
6. Eye changes including papilledema
7. Speech patterns

The detection of increased intracranial pressure must occur early when it is still reversible and before the stage of decompensation. The ability to make accurate observations, to interpret observations intelligently, and to record observations carefully is the most important part of nursing care for patients with increased intracranial pressure.

Level of consciousness

A decreasing level of consciousness is an early sign of internal herniation. Any change in the level of consciousness is one of the most important observations for the nurse to make, report, and record. In describing a person's level of consciousness it is important to describe the patient's behavior—not just label it. Description of levels of consciousness is presented in box on page 373.

Another way to standardize objective observations of the loss of consciousness is with the Glasgow Coma Scale.[25] It was developed in 1974 and its use is becoming more widespread. The scale consists of the three following parts:

1. Assessment of eye opening
2. Best motor response
3. Verbal response

The stronger the stimulus needed to obtain a response,

> ## Causes of increased intracranial pressure
>
> **Space-occupying lesions that increase tissue volume**
> Cerebral contusions
> Hematomas
> Infarctions
> Abscesses
> Intracranial tumors
>
> **Cerebrospinal problems**
> Increase in production of cerebrospinal fluid
> Blockage in ventricular system
> Decreased absorption of cerebrospinal fluid
>
> **Cerebral edema**
> Use of contrast dye that changes homeostasis of brain
> Overhydration with hypotonic solution
> Aftereffects of trauma to brain

the lower the score assigned to the part. The number value assigned to each parameter is added to yield an objective score. The score for normal persons is 14. The lowest possible score is 3. Any score of 7 or less is commonly accepted as a definition of coma.

Pupillary signs

Pupil responses are controlled by cranial nerve III (the oculomotor nerve). This nerve carries sensory, motor, and parasympathetic fibers as well as sympathetic fibers. As the brain herniates, the oculomotor nerve is com-

---

Levels of consciousness

Loss of ability to abstract	Inattentiveness, slowed thinking, difficult to arouse
Confusion	Disorientation, inability to follow simple commands
Stupor	Responds to verbal commands with moaning or groaning, if at all
Semicomatose	Loss of ability to cooperate, responds only to pain—response may range from purposeful to decerebrate or decorticate
Comatose	Loss of ability to respond to any external stimuli and loss of all brain functions[12]

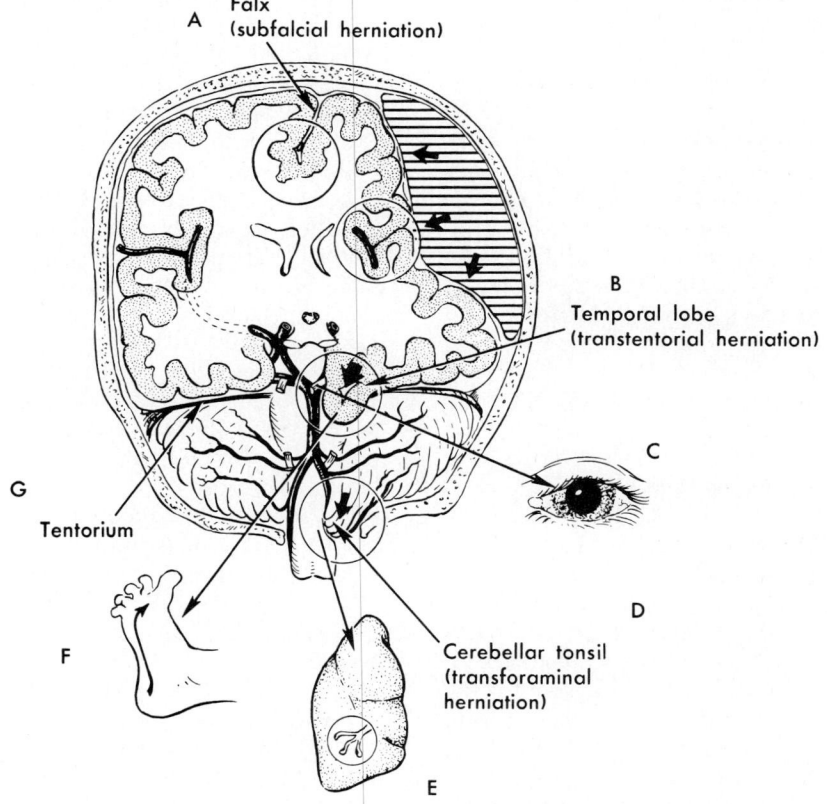

Fig. 20-10. Consequences of increased intracranial pressure. Expanding temporoparietal epidural hematoma with medial and downward pressure has produced subfalcial, transtentorial, and transforaminal internal herniations. Note distortion of falx, **A,** bulging of medial temporal lobe at tentorial edge, **B,** and herniation of cerebellar tonsil with descending pressure on brainstem, **D,** Also note how major blood vessels are collapsed in encircled areas. Some consequential effects of continuing and/or expanding pressure on neural structure with alterations in body functions are detailed: **C,** homolateral dilation and fixation of pupil with ptosis of eyelid; **E,** life-threatening respiratory arrest through indirect effects on respiratory centers in brainstem; **F,** contralateral Babinski sign showing extension of great toe and fanning of other toes on plantar stimulation (coronal view of head, ventral view of brainstem). (Modified from an original painting by Frank H. Netter, M.D.; from Clinical symposia. Copyright by Ciba Pharmaceutical Co., Division of Ciba-Geigy Corp., Summit, N.J. All rights reserved.)

Glasgow Coma Scale

	Stimuli	Score
Eyes open	Spontaneously	4
	To speech	3
	To pain	2
	None	1
Best verbal response	Oriented	5
	Confused	4
	Inappropriate	3
	words	2
	Incomprehensible	1
	None	
Best motor response	Obeys commands	5
	Localizes to pain	4
	Flexes to pain	2
	None	1

---

pressed by the herniating tissue, the pupilloconstrictor fibers in the top part of the nerve being the first affected. The ipsilateral pupil (when the lesion is in one hemisphere) remains dilated and is incapable of constricting. The pupil appears larger than that of the affected side and does not react to light. As cerebral pressure increases and both hemispheres are affected, there is bilateral pupil dilation and fixation—the pupil may respond to light slowly. Dilating pupils are a sign of impending tentorial herniation. When pupils dilate or change in ability to react, the physician should be notified immediately. A pupil that is fixed and dilated is sometimes referred to as a "blown pupil" and is an ominous sign.

Blood pressure and pulse

The effect of increased intracranial pressure on pulse and blood pressure is variable. Compensatory changes occur in the cerebral vasculature relative to hypoxia. Herniation, however, causes ischemia of the vasomotor center. This excites the vasoconstrictor fibers, causing the systolic blood pressure to rise. If the intracranial pressure continues to increase, blood pressure may fall, especially the diastolic blood pressure. An increased systolic blood pressure followed by a sharp drop in blood pressure is often seen as the patient's condition deteriorates.

Pressure in the vasomotor center also increases the transmission of parasympathetic impulses via the vagus nerve to the heart; as a result the pulse rate slows. Slowing of the pulse rate in conjunction with a rising systolic blood pressure is a significant observation that should be reported. For consistency, blood pressure and pulse should be taken in the same arm.

Respiration

Herniation produces respiratory dysrhythmias that are variable and related to the level of the brainstem compression or failure. The breathing pattern may be deep and stertorous or periodic (Cheyne-Stokes) respira-

tions. As intracranial pressure increases to fatal levels, respiratory paralysis occurs. The beginning of periods of apnea is significant. It is important to remember that the patient with a decreased level of consciousness will require assistance in keeping the airway clear. Persons with acute increased intracranial pressure require supplemental oxygen to prevent hypoxia, which can further increase intracranial pressure.

Temperature

Failure of the thermoregulatory center because of compression occurs later with increased intracranial pressure and gives rise to high, uncontrolled temperatures. Hyperthermia must be controlled, because it increases the metabolism of brain tissue.

Focal motor and sensory symptoms

Compression of the upper motor neuron pathway (corticospinal tract) interrupts transmission of impulses to the lower motor neuron, and progressive muscle weakness occurs. This often begins with the presence of drift and may progress to hemiparesis and hemiplegia. *Drift* is tested by asking the patient to close the eyes and extend the arms straight out in front for about 30 seconds. If one arm is weakened, it will drift downward without the patient being aware of it. Testing of the lower extremities includes the ability to push and pull against the tester, the ability to dorsiflex and plantar flex the feet, and the ability to do straight leg raises.

The presence of the *Babinski sign, hyperreflexia,* and *rigidity* are additional signs of decreased motor function. Seizures may occur. Herniation of the upper part of the brainstem produces *decerebrate rigidity* (fixed posture with arms, legs and trunk extended and with flexion of the palms and plantar joints) or decorticate rigidity (fixed posture with flexion of the arm, wrist, and fingers, with adduction of the arm and extensors and internal rotation of the legs). The worsening of existing motor defects is significant and should be reported to the physician.

Papilledema

The *blind spot* of the retina measures the size and shape of the optic papilla or optic disk. As intracranial pressure increases, the pressure is transmitted to the eyes through the cerebrospinal fluid and to the optic disk. Because the meninges of the brain reflect out around the eyeball, they permit the direct transmission of pressure along the spaces through the cerebrospinal fluid. As the optic disk swells, the retina is also compressed. The damaged retina cannot detect light rays. Visual acuity is lessened as the blind spot enlarges.

Vomiting

Projectile vomiting may be associated with increased intracranial pressure. The significance of vomiting and its frequency and character must be associated with other clinical signs.

Hiccuping

Compression of the vagus nerve (cranial nerve X) causes spasmodic contraction of the diaphragm. This compression occurs as brainstem herniation occurs. Hiccuping in a patient who is at risk for increased intracranial pressure or who has other symptoms should be reported to the physician immediately.

Diagnostic tests

The diagnosis of increased intracranial pressure can be made with the CT scan, which can show actual structural herniation as well as shifting of the brain. The displacement of the brain to the right or left occurs at a relatively late stage of increased intracranial pressure. Most of the time, however, acute increased intracranial pressure is a medical emergency, and there is little time for diagnostic tests. The diagnosis must be made on the basis of observation and neurologic testing. Although the frequency of "neuro checks" is often ordered by the physician, the nurse should use judgment to decide whether more frequent assessments and recordings are indicated. The presence of even subtle changes may be very significant.

In some postoperative or critically ill patients internal measuring devices are used to diagnose increased intracranial pressure. One of the most common requires the placement of a hollow screw through the skull into the subarachnoid space. The screw is attached to a Luer-Lok, which is connected to a transducer and oscilloscope for continuous monitoring. The transducer is fastened on level with the screw for accurate readings. A manometer may be attached for intermittent readings, or constant monitoring is available via the monitor.

It has become evident that the traditional clinical signs of increased intracranial pressure do not always correlate with the actual pressure changes as seen on the monitor. Many of the classic signs of increased pressure do not appear until the pressure has reached extremely high levels, and the chance to reverse the rising pressure and prevent permanent brain damage has already passed.

DATA ANALYSIS AND PLANNING

Nursing diagnoses

Possible nursing diagnoses for the patient with increased intracranial pressure include the following:
Airway clearing: ineffective
Alteration in comfort: pain
Breathing pattern: ineffective
Communication: impaired verbal
Mobility: impaired physical
Sensory perceptual alteration: visual
Thought process: alteration in
Tissue perfusion: alteration in cerebral

Expected patient outcomes

Because of the acute, emergent, and disabling nature of increased intracranial pressure, the outcomes are often the result of direct nursing and medical treatment. They include the following:
1. Cerebral edema is reduced.
2. Cerebral hypoxia is prevented or reduced by maintaining a clear airway and reducing cerebral pressure.

3. Activities that increase intracranial pressure are reduced.
4. Fluid intake is limited.
5. Intake and output are monitored.
6. Patient and family are supported and explanations given as appropriate.
7. Patient cooperates with therapeutic plan as much as possible.

IMPLEMENTATION

Assisting with implementation of therapeutic goals

The prevention of increased intracranial pressure may not be possible, but prevention of further rises in pressure and resulting damage to brain tissue is crucial. The detection of early signs is important to prevent irreversible effects.

The medical treatment of patients with increased intracranial pressure depends on the cause of the pressure. For example, if it is caused by an intracranial tumor, the tumor is removed surgically (p. 431). If surgery is not possible (or not indicated) efforts are made to reduce the pressure through drug therapy or direct physical measures.

Mechanical decompression

Rapidly rising intracranial pressure must be relieved directly by mechanical decompression. This may include the following:
1. Intracranial puncture with withdrawal of cerebrospinal fluid by needle or cannula
2. Continuous ventricular drainage via ventriculostomy tube
3. Removal of a piece of skull (craniotomy) to provide room for the cranial contents to expand
4. Burr holes made in the skull with or without evacuation of subdural hematoma if this is the cause of the pressure
5. Continuous drainage of subdural hematoma via subdural drain

Each of these measures requires careful monitoring by the nurse for signs of increased intracranial pressure and maintenance of asepsis at the entrance site into the skull.

MEDICATIONS

Medications are commonly ordered to promote rapid osmotic diuresis and to reduce intracranial pressure. Drugs commonly used include the following:
1. Intravenous urea (Urevert)
2. Intravenous mannitol
3. Hypertonic solutions of glucose (25% to 50%)
4. Corticosteroids such as dexamethasone (intravenously or intramuscularly)

All of these drugs cause dehydration and promote the movement of excess fluid from the brain tissues into the blood so that the fluid can be eliminated, lessening cerebral edema. Narcotics and other drugs that cause respiratory depression are avoided. Phenytoin sodium (Dilantin) may be given to prevent seizures.

CONSERVATIVE MEASURES

Conservative measures to reduce venous volume may be implemented. The head of the bed is elevated to 15 or 30 degrees, and the neck is kept in a neutral position. Positioning to avoid flexion of the hips, waist, and neck is important. Rotation of the head, especially to the right, has been found to increase intracranial pressure. Passive range of motion exercises do not increase intracranial pressure, unless they occur in association with multiple activities within a short period of time. Spacing of nursing activities is important in maintaining lower pressure levels.

Fluid intake may also be restricted. With the administration of osmotic diuretics, urine output must be carefully monitored. An indwelling catheter is often used. The Valsalva maneuver is eliminated to the extent it is possible because it causes increased intrathoracic pressure, which indirectly increases intracranial pressure. This includes not allowing the patient to become constipated or to strain during defecation. Suctioning should be performed only when necessary (and then with the patient well preoxygenated), because it causes coughing and gagging. Suctioning should not be performed at the same time as other procedures that cause increased intracranial pressure.

Oxygen therapy via mask or cannula is administered to improve brain oxygenation. Endotracheal intubation may be necessary. With the use of controlled ventilation, the P_{CO_2} can be lowered to below normal, which causes a slightly alkalotic pH. The decrease in the P_{CO_2} and the increase in the pH will decrease vasodilation and thereby decrease intracranial pressure.

EVALUATION

Evaluation of the patient with increased intracranial pressure includes frequent checks to evaluate neurologic status. Questions to ask include the following:
1. Is effective respiration occurring?
2. Are signs and symptoms of increased intracranial pressure decreased?
3. Is fluid intake limited and is careful measuring of intake and output occurring?
4. Are the patient and family being supported, and is the patient being kept as comfortable as possible?

Alterations in muscle tone and motor function

PATHOPHYSIOLOGY

Motor function disturbances are the most commonly encountered neurologic symptoms. Because the nervous system is designed primarily for the movement of the body in

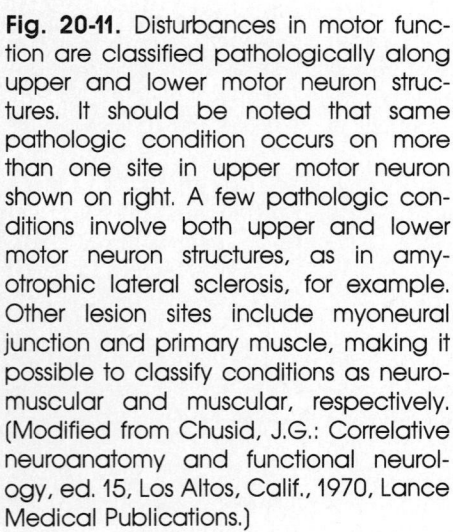
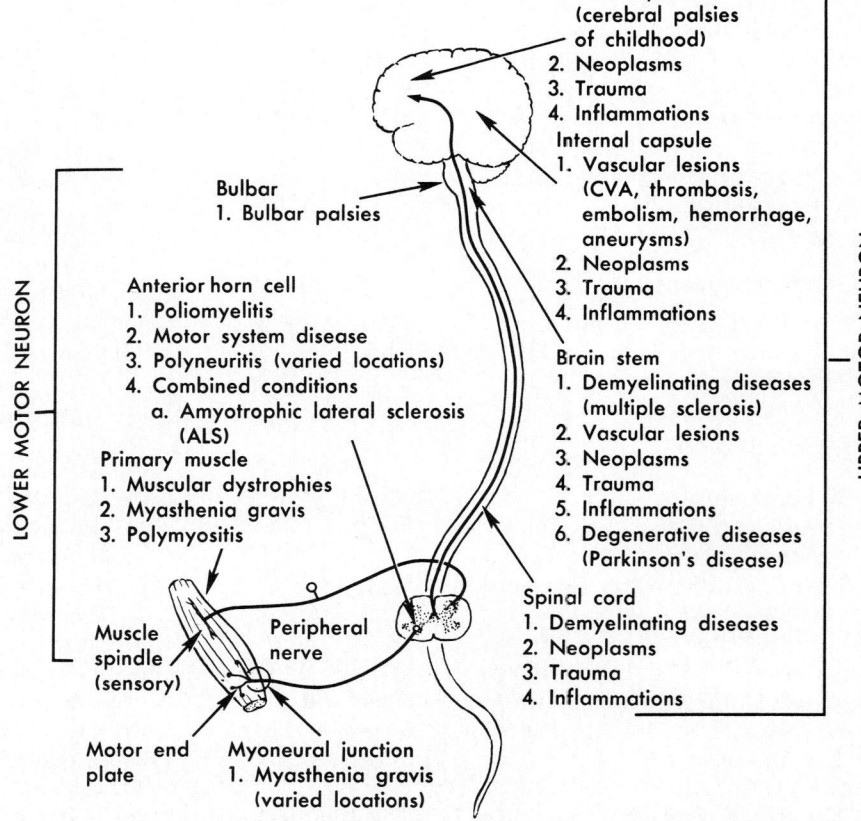

Fig. 20-11. Disturbances in motor function are classified pathologically along upper and lower motor neuron structures. It should be noted that same pathologic condition occurs on more than one site in upper motor neuron shown on right. A few pathologic conditions involve both upper and lower motor neuron structures, as in amyotrophic lateral sclerosis, for example. Other lesion sites include myoneural junction and primary muscle, making it possible to classify conditions as neuromuscular and muscular, respectively. (Modified from Chusid, J.G.: Correlative neuroanatomy and functional neurology, ed. 15, Los Altos, Calif., 1970, Lance Medical Publications.)

Motor cortex
1. Birth injuries (cerebral palsies of childhood)
2. Neoplasms
3. Trauma
4. Inflammations

Internal capsule
1. Vascular lesions (CVA, thrombosis, embolism, hemorrhage, aneurysms)
2. Neoplasms
3. Trauma
4. Inflammations

Brain stem
1. Demyelinating diseases (multiple sclerosis)
2. Vascular lesions
3. Neoplasms
4. Trauma
5. Inflammations
6. Degenerative diseases (Parkinson's disease)

Spinal cord
1. Demyelinating diseases
2. Neoplasms
3. Trauma
4. Inflammations

Bulbar
1. Bulbar palsies

Anterior horn cell
1. Poliomyelitis
2. Motor system disease
3. Polyneuritis (varied locations)
4. Combined conditions
   a. Amyotrophic lateral sclerosis (ALS)

Primary muscle
1. Muscular dystrophies
2. Myasthenia gravis
3. Polymyositis

Muscle spindle (sensory)

Peripheral nerve

Motor end plate

Myoneural junction
1. Myasthenia gravis (varied locations)

LOWER MOTOR NEURON

UPPER MOTOR NEURON

space and of the various parts in relation to each other, damage to it often causes serious problems in mobility. A loss of function, either motor or sensory, is called *paralysis.* A lesser degree of paralysis is called *paresis.* Damage to sensory pathways that are concerned with motor function may occur at the same time as the loss of motor function.

Injury or disease of motor neurons results in alterations of muscle strength, tone, and reflex activity. The specific clinical manifestations differ according to whether the lesion involves an upper motor neuron or a lower motor neuron (Fig. 20-11).

Lower motor neuron signs

The lower motor neurons (LMNs) consist of a large anterior horn cell located in the gray matter of the spinal cord (Fig. 20-12). They are also found in the motor cranial nuclei of the brainstem. This anterior horn cell, in conjunction with the anterior spinal nerve and the peripheral nerve involved, forms a motor unit that effects skeletal muscle activity (voluntary and reflex). When a lesion selectively involves some part of the lower motor neuron, it results in the following:

1. Flaccid muscle weakness or paralysis
2. Loss of reflex activity
3. Loss of muscle tone
4. Atrophy confined to the involved muscle or muscles
The degree of muscle weakness is directly related to the extent and severity of the lesion.

The involved muscles become *flaccid,* because the motor unit has been damaged and normal reflex activity has been interrupted. This flaccidity also is manifested in *hypotonia* and *hyporeflexia* and/or *areflexia* (reduced or absent muscle stretch reflexes). This interruption of the motor unit results in localized muscle atrophy or wasting. This atrophy also increases with nonuse of the muscle. In some LMN lesions, the affected muscle exhibits small localized, spontaneous and involuntary contractions called *fasciculations.*

Upper motor neuron signs

Upper motor neurons (UMNs) originate in the motor strip of the cerebral cortex and in multiple brainstem nuclei (Fig. 20-13). These axons then pass through the brainstem, deccusate (cross) in the medulla, and descend

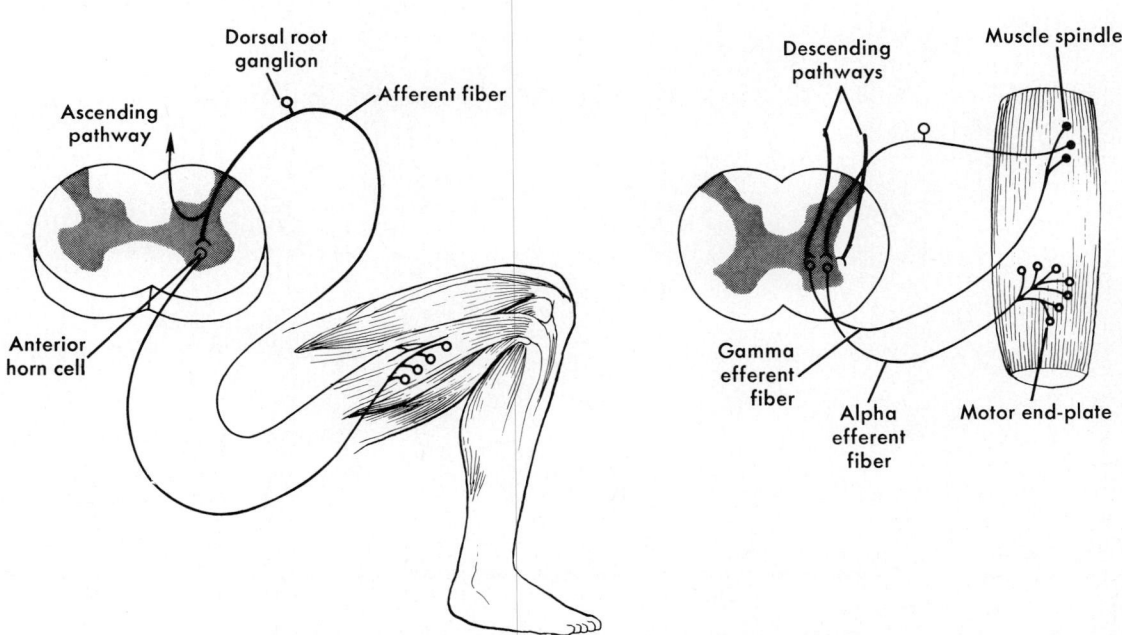

Fig. 20-12. Structures comprising lower motor neuron, including motor (efferent) and sensory (afferent) elements. Shown on right is anterior horn cell in anterior gray column of spinal cord and its axon terminating in motor end plate as it innervates extrafusal muscle fibers in quadriceps muscle. Detailed in enlargement on left are sensory and motor elements of gamma loop system. Gamma efferent fiber is shown innervating polar or end region of muscle spindle (sensory receptor of skeletal muscle). Contraction of muscle spindle fibers stretches central portion of spindle and causes afferent spindle fiber to transmit impulse centrally to cord. Muscle spindle afferent fibers, in turn, synapse on anterior horn cell and are transmitted via alpha efferent fibers to skeletal (extrafusal) muscle, causing it to contract. Muscle spindle discharge is interpreted by active contraction of extrafusal muscle fibers. (Adapted from Truex, R.C., and Carpenter, M.B.: Human neuroanatomy, ed. 6, Baltimore, 1969, The Williams & Wilkins Co.)

Fig. 20-13. Structures making up upper motor neuron, or pyramidal, system. Pyramidal system fibers are shown or originate primarily in cells in precentral gyrus of motor cortex; converge at internal capsule; descend to form central third of cerebral peduncle; descend further through pons, where small fibers are given off to cranial nerve motor nuclei along the way; form pyramids at medulla, where majority of fibers decussate; and then continue to descend in lateral column of white matter of spinal cord, where they synapse with anterior horn cells or all segments of cord. A few fibers descend without crossing at medulla level. (Adapted from original painting by Frank H. Netter, M.D. From Ciba Collection of Medical Illustrations. Copyright by Ciba Pharmaceutical Co., Division of Ciba-Geigy Corp. All rights reserved.)

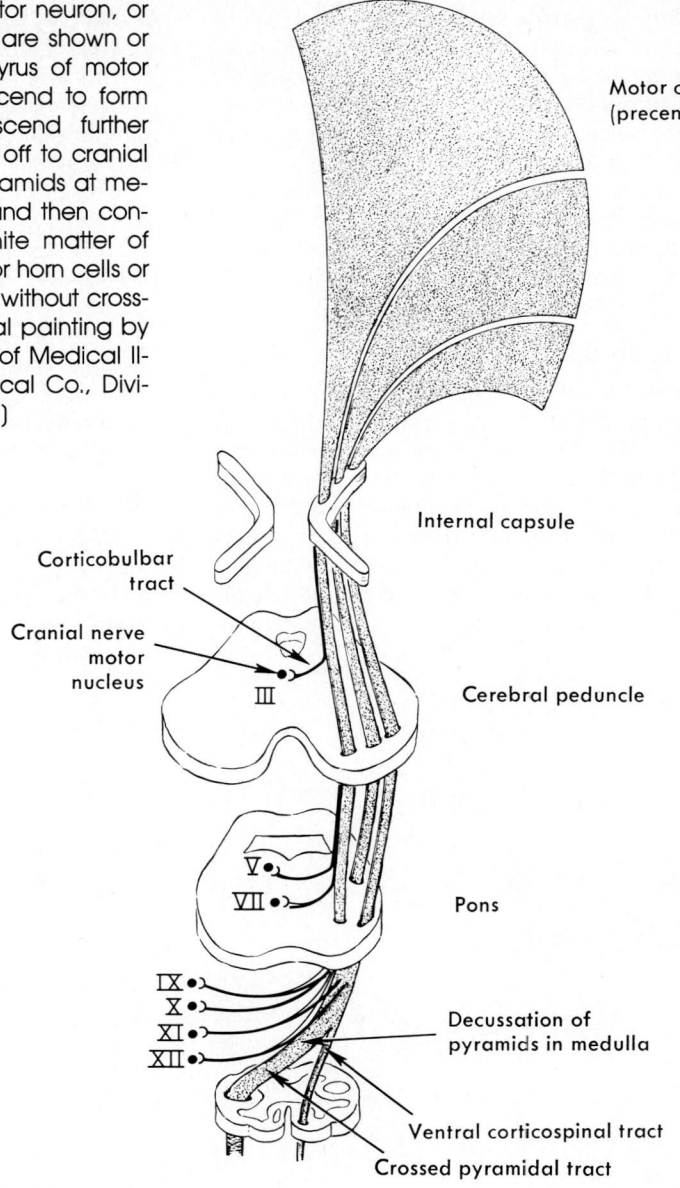

Clinical syndromes of UMN and LMN lesions

Motor component	UMN characteristics	LMN characteristics
Reflex	Hyperreflexia, extensor toe sign (Babinski's sign)	Hyporeflexia or areflexia
Muscle tonus	Hypertonia, clasp-knife spasticity, clonus	Hypotonia, flaccidity
Muscle movement	Paralysis or paresis of movements in hemiplegic distribution, etc.	Paralysis or paresis of individual muscles in peripheral nerve distribution
Muscle wasting	Late atrophy from disuse	Early atrophy or denervation
Muscle fasciculations	Not present	Present

in the spinal cord via the corticospinal tracts. These fibers synapse with LMNs in the spinal cord. The collective working of both the UMN and LMN is essential for fine, orderly, and smooth muscle movements.

When an UMN lesion is rostral to the medulla, as in a cerebrovascular accident, deficits will occur contralateral to the lesion and will result in *hemiplegia*. The distribution or degree of paralysis is not always equal or the same within the hemiplegic distribution. The following are upper motor neuron signs:

1. Paresis or paralysis of voluntary muscle tone and spasticity
2. Hyperreflexia
3. Late atrophy from disuse
4. Increased muscle tone

Initially, the muscles affected by an upper motor lesion are *flaccid (hypotonic)* and *hyporeflexic*. Gradually, and with variability, the reflex arcs become increasingly hyperreactive. Then paresis, or paralysis of voluntary muscle movement, occurs with increased tone and spasticity. The spasticity is characterized by *increased resistance to passive movement, hyperreflexia,* and *clonus*. (Clonus can be defined as a forced series of alternating contractions and partial relaxation of a muscle that occurs in some neurologic diseases.) An unilateral Babinski sign is present on the hemiparetic side.

Upper motor neuron lesions caudal to the medulla produce deficits ipsilateral to the lesion. Spinal cord injury is an example of this. If the cord is transected the lesion extends into both halves of the spinal cord; deficits will be demonstrated as quadriplegia or paraplegia, with loss of motor function, muscle tone, and reflex activity as well as somatic and visceral sensations below the level of injury.

ASSESSMENT

Both subjective and objective data are important in determining more about any abnormal muscle movements.

Subjective data

1. Patient's understanding of the problem and possible causes
2. Initial onset of problem
3. Measures that improve symptoms
4. Presence of clumsiness or incoordination
5. Presence of any abnormal sensation

If the lesion occurs suddenly, such as in spinal cord injury from trauma or a cerebrovascular accident, subjective symptoms of the muscle weakness may be minimal. Often, subjective symptoms occurring early in an illness involving abnormal muscle movements or sensations are ignored.

Objective data

1. Coordination
2. Muscle strength
3. Muscle tone

Electromyogram (EMG)

Purpose

To measure the contraction of a muscle in response to electrical stimulation.

Preparation of patient

1. No special preparation.
2. Patient teaching.
   a. Explain procedure.
   b. Time: approximately 45 minutes for one muscle study.
   c. Sensation: some discomfort when electrodes are inserted—persons with sensory neuropathies may experience more intense pain. Some discomfort when electrical current is used.
   d. Muscle may ache for a short time after the procedure.

Procedure

1. Electrodes are inserted into selected skeletal muscle.
2. Electrical current is passed through electrodes.
3. Machine graphs the variations of muscle potentials (voltage).

After procedure

1. Observe for signs of bleeding at site of electrode insertion
2. Plan rest period for patient
3. Medicate patient as needed for discomfort

4. Any atrophy of muscles
5. Presence of clones or fasciculations
6. Ability to move muscles, abnormal gait
7. Reflexes
8. Change in ability to carry on daily activities

Diagnostic testing

One of the most common diagnostic procedures to evaluate muscle dysfunction is electromyography. In motor disease, electrical activity of various types and abnormal patterns appear in resting muscle. An electromyogram (EMG) provides direct evidence of motor dysfunction and can be used to detect a dysfunction located in the motor neuron, the neuromuscular junction, or muscle fibers. It is particularly helpful in the diagnosis of lower motor neuron disease, primary muscle disease, and defects in the transmission of electrical impulses at the neuromuscular junction.

DATA ANALYSIS AND PLANNING

Nursing diagnosis

Possible nursing diagnoses for the patient with abnormal muscle movements include the following:
Bowel elimination, alteration in (constipation or incontinence)
Home maintenance management: impaired
Injury: potential for
Mobility, impaired physical
Self-care deficit: feeding, bathing/hygiene, dressing/grooming, toileting
Self-concept, disturbance in role performance
Sexual dysfunction
Skin integrity, impairment of (potential or actual)
Urinary elimination, alteration in patterns

Expected patient outcomes

Expected patient outcomes include the following:
1. Skin will remain intact and free of breakdown.
2. Joint deformities (that is, contractures) will not develop.
3. Patient can describe dosage, function, side effects, and toxic effects of medications to be taken at home.
4. Patient can demonstrate measures to prevent muscle or joint deformities.
5. Patient can describe measures to prevent skin breakdown.
6. Patient can describe and demonstrate range of motion.
7. Patient can list signs of skin breakdown that require professional assessment.
8. Patient can discuss plans for bowel and bladder care.
9. Patient can demonstrate activities of daily living that can be done alone and can describe methods of assistance for those functions which are dependent.
10. Patient does not have diarrhea or become constipated.
11. Patient can state plans for follow-up care.

IMPLEMENTATION

Successful nursing care of the patient with motor dysfunction includes those activities that prevent complications such as decubitus ulcers or joint contractures, as well as those that develop the person's optimal level of functioning.

Assisting with therapeutic goals
Safety needs

Patients with paralysis have significant safety needs. Protection of the patient from falling is a major one. When left alone, hemiplegic patients need to have the side rail raised on the side of the bed next to their affected side. A chair restraint may be helpful when the patient is up in a chair.

Also, the eye on the affected side of the body should be protected when the lid remains open and there is no blink reflex. If this is not done, damage to the cornea will occur, leading to corneal ulcers and blindness. Irrigation with a physiologic solution of sodium chloride, followed by artificial tear solution (methylcellulose) is sometimes used. An eye pad may be used to keep the eye closed. If a pad is used, it must be changed daily and the eye cleaned and carefully examined for signs of infection or drying of the cornea. Eye shields are preferable to pads, because there is no danger of lint entering the eye.

Skin care

Skin over bony prominences needs to be inspected regularly for signs of pressure. Paralyzed persons are at risk for decubitus formation. The following several factors account for this.
1. Muscles are not being used.
2. Interference with autonomic reflexes that monitor and maintain vasomotor tone may result in altered circulation to the paralyzed areas.
3. Accompanying sensory loss may prevent the individual from perceiving pain and pressure—the warning symptoms of tissue injury.

Persons who are physically capable of activity are taught to turn themselves in bed and to reposition themselves independently. Paraplegics are taught how to shift their weight in bed; for the quadraplegic patient these activities are done by the staff. If the person also has a loss of sensation, no external heat such as hot water bottles or heating pads should be used (the heat may not be felt and a burn could result). Paralyzed or weakened areas should be inspected daily for any signs of skin irritation; a mirror or other devices to assist in this assessment may be helpful.

Activity needs

The limbs of a person who has acute hemiplegia, as with the person who has paraplegia or quadriplegia, are often flaccid at first. Spasticity with a tendency to muscle contracture develops gradually. The joints then become flexed and fixed in useless positions with deformity unless preventive measures are taken by the nurse. There is a shortening of joint capsules and ligaments around the immobile joint, and the limb may be drawn into flexor or extensor contracture with or without muscle spasm.

Based on assessment of the joints that are vulnerable to contracture and deformity formation, the nurse should carefully place the limbs in a normal anatomic position to prevent deformity. Counterpositioning may be used. In hemiplegia, for example, the affected upper limb is pulled inward at the shoulder joint and the wrist drops; in the lower limb the knee flexes and the foot drops. In *counterpositioning* the nurse positions the patient so that the shoulder and upper arm are in abduction, the elbow is flexed, the wrist is dorsiflexed, the knee is in a neutral position, and the foot is dorsiflexed. If the person is supine, a pillow can be placed between the upper arm and body to hold the arm in abduction. Hand splints are often used to prevent hand deformity. Footboards may be used to prevent foot-drop, although some feel that these contribute to increased spasticity and should not be used routinely for patients with UMN lesions. High-topped tennis shoes can be effective to prevent foot deformity if initiated early enough. A sling may be useful for shoulder subluxation.

Positioning of the paralyzed person is extremely important. Knee flexion and foot-drop are serious complications that must be prevented. The development of a flexion contracture at the knee joint interferes with the person's ability to bear weight in an upright position and to transfer independently. As a result, the level of self-care and independence may be diminished. Subluxation of a shoulder joint in a person with hemiplegia, related to inadequate support of the joint when in an upright position, causes pain and limits therapy. Keeping the paralyzed person upright or semiupright for long periods of time results in hip deformities. Most joint deformities in a paralyzed person are preventable with early and continuing nursing interventions.

In addition to positioning, interventions for the person with paralysis include range of motion (ROM) exercises to all joints. These may be passive (carried out by the nurse) or active (carried out by the patient). Passive ROM is indicated at least three times daily for all joints that the person cannot voluntarily move.

Medications

Patients experiencing ongoing problems with spasticity may be given skeletal muscle relaxants to decrease tone and involuntary movements and to help relieve anxiety and tension. Common side effects include drowsiness and dizziness, which are potentiated when the medications are used in combination with alcohol, barbiturates, sedatives, hypnotics, or tranquilizers. Some commonly prescribed medications are the following:
1. Baclofen (Lioresal)—a derivative of GABA (an inhibitory neurotransmitter). Acts on the spinal cord.

2. Dantrolene sodium (Dantrium)—acts directly on skeletal muscle by impairing Ca^{++} release from the sacroplasmic reticulum. Can cause additional side effects of muscle weakness, slurred speech, drooling, and anuresis.
3. Diazepam (Valium)—centrally acting muscle relaxant and antianxiety agent.

Nutritional needs

Patience and persistence are necessary in giving food and fluids to the person with hemiplegia. So much difficulty may be encountered in swallowing food and fluids because of paralysis that the patient may believe that effort is not worthwhile. Important nursing measures are listed in box below.

Self-help devices for feeding are available. These include utensils with universal cuffs (Fig. 20-14), covered plastic cups, plate guards, and the Asepto syringe.

Elimination needs

The person with paralysis from an UMN or LMN lesion may experience problems with bowel and bladder control. This is discussed in Chapter 33.

Assisting with comfort and ADL
Activities of daily living

During the rehabilitative and acute phases, patients with paralysis are taught how to carry out ADL to the extent that they are able. A variety of self-help devices are available that assist with dressing with one hand, for example. The occupational therapist becomes involved in many of these activities, including homemaking. It is important to stress the concept of the rehabilitative team in managing these patients. Volunteers may also be included in helping the patient find meaningful diversional activities.

Nursing measures to improve nutrition

1. Make patients feel that problem is not overwhelming.
2. Give positive feedback to patient when any improvement is noted.
3. Turning the patient onto the back or unaffected side may help swallowing.
4. Avoid foods that cause choking, such as mashed potatoes.
5. Check affected side of mouth for accumulation of food and subsequent poor mouth hygiene—it may be helpful to irrigate mouth after eating.
6. Encourage patient to feed self as soon as possible.
7. Dentures should be used if at all possible.

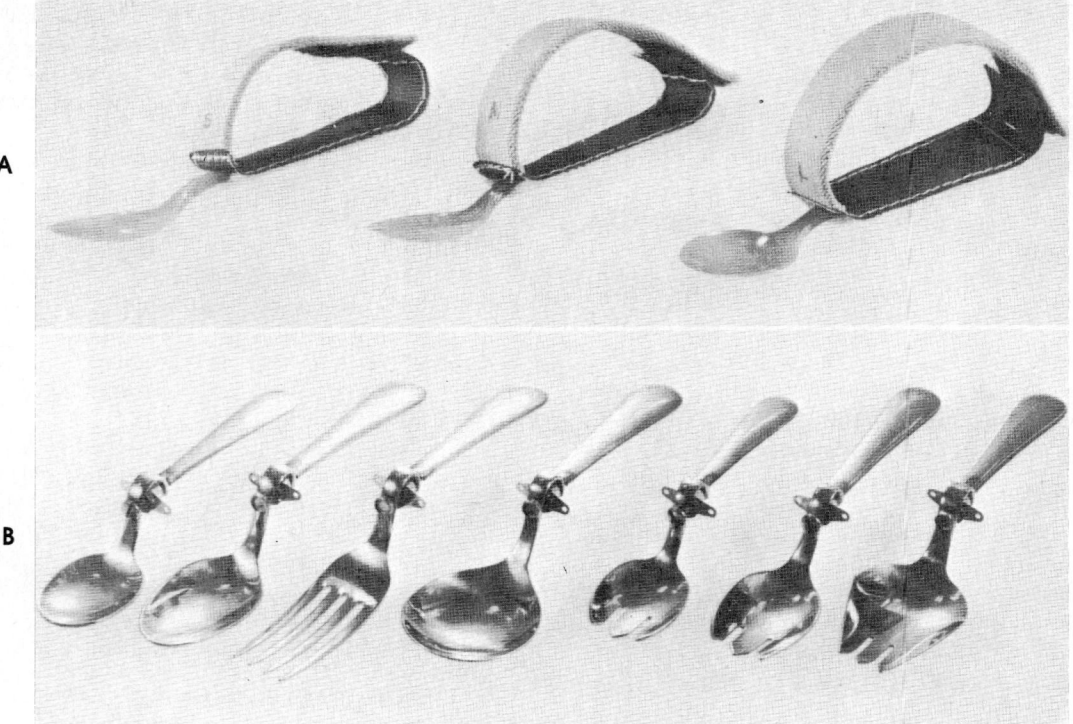

Fig. 20-14. Self-help devices for quadriplegic. **A,** Spoons with small, medium, and large universal cuff attachments that fit over hand. **B,** Swivel spoons, forks, and sporks (combination spoon and fork, last three on right), which are used with universal cuff. (Courtesy Fred Sammons, O.T.R., Chicago, Ill.)

Psychologic adjustment

The person with paralysis will need assistance in adjusting to the change in the body. The loss of the ability to function independently when paralyzed is traumatic. There also may be fears of rejection by loved ones, concerns about the future, and loss of self-esteem. A grief reaction similar to that described for the stages of death and dying may occur. At times, persons may relate to the paralyzed portion of the body as though it were not a part of them. Nursing interventions to help the patient cope with the loss of function and change in body image are essential.

Teaching

Teaching is an extremely important part of caring for the person with motor problems. Appropriate teaching activities are outlined in the box on p. 383.

EVALUATION

Evaluation of the patient experiencing motor dysfunction is made based on the perception of the patient as well as measurement against the defined patient outcomes. Questions to consider include the following:

1. Is the patient knowledgeable about range of motion?
2. Is the patient receiving adequate nutrition?
3. Is the patient as independent in ADL as possible?
4. Is the patient's fluid intake adequate?
5. Is the patient's skin intact?
6. Is the patient doing skin checks or asking staff to do them?
7. Are the joints freely moveable?
8. Does the patient have bowel and bladder control?
9. Can the patient state plans for follow-up care?
10. Does the patient verbalize knowledge of the medication regime?

Alterations in sensory function

PATHOPHYSIOLOGY

The presence of a lesion anywhere within the sensory system pathway, from the receptor to the sensory cortex, alters the transmission or perception of sensory information. The parietal lobe cortex is of major importance in interpretation of sensation with the exception of sight, hearing, smell, taste, and thermoregulation. Loss, decrease, or increase in sensation of pain, temperature, touch, and proprioception, singly or in combination, results in difficulty in daily living. Because these sensations normally help the person to be aware of alterations in the internal and external environments, any alteration in

Teaching for the patient with motor dysfunction

Safety needs

1. Always lock wheelchair when transferring patient
2. Check condition of affected eye frequently
3. Be aware of placement of affected extremities before movement
4. Protect paralyzed limbs from injury
5. Have patient wear shoes that fit well for ambulating

Skin care

1. Regular inspection of skin surfaces, using mirror or other device
2. Need to turn frequently
3. Weight shifts
4. No use of heating pads, hot water bottles, or excessively hot water for bathing

Activity needs

1. Range of motion
2. Proper positioning
3. Frequent changes in position

Medications

1. Use of medication, side effects, dosage, and timing
2. Reporting of side effects to physician
3. Importance of not combining medication with other mood-altering drugs or alcohol

Nutrition-diet

1. Foods that can be easily tolerated
2. Measures to decrease swallowing difficulty
3. Use of special appliances to assist with eating

ADL

1. Teaching techniques of bathing, grooming, dressing
2. Importance of having meaningful recreational activities
3. Bowel and bladder care

Other teaching

1. Importance of good fluid intake
2. Follow-up care—where to procure equipment, supplies
3. Methods for relieving feelings of frustration.

sensation lessens the ability to be completely and accurately protected.

One specific loss is that of *proprioception,* or the ability to know the position of the body and its parts without looking directly at the part. Lack of control of body temperature, or *hyperthermia,* is another dysfunction and occurs as a result of malfunction in the thermoregulatory center in the brain, such as that which occurs following brain surgery near the hypothalamus or from head injury.

Fig. 20-15 presents common patterns of sensory loss. A cerebral lesion results in various alterations in sensation contralateral to the lesion. This distribution results because all sensory fibers have decussated (crossed) before reaching the sensory cortex of the cerebrum. On the other hand, transection of the spinal cord results in total bilateral sensory loss distal to the lesion, because all pathways have been severed. The characteristic distribution of deficits with Brown-Sequard syndrome is ipsilateral (same side) loss of proprioception and vibratory sense and contralateral (opposite side) loss of pain, temperature, and crude touch sensation.

ASSESSMENT

The sensory examination is the most difficult part of the neurologic examination. Subjective data are collected as follows.

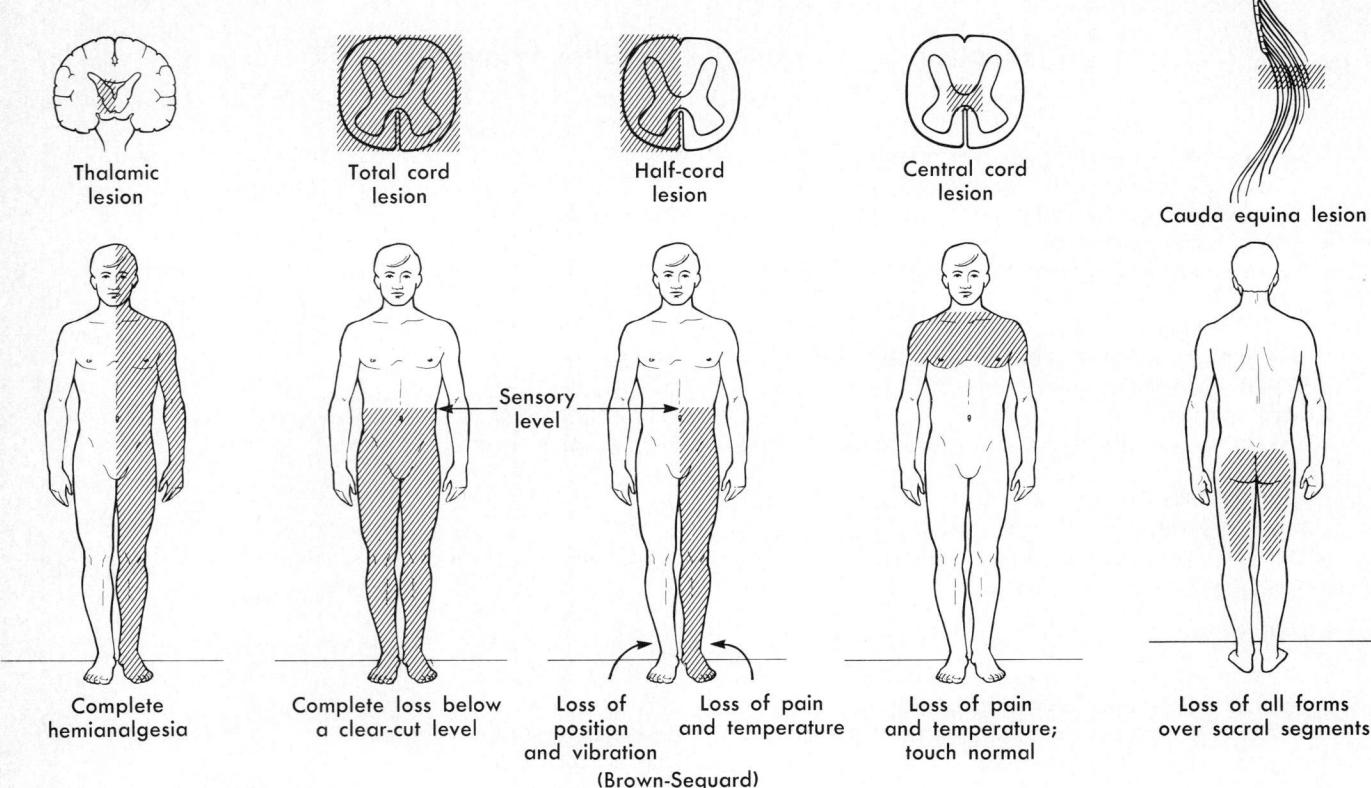

Fig. 20-15. Common patterns of sensory abnormality. Upper diagrams show site of lesion; lower diagrams show distribution of corresponding sensory loss. (Adapted from Bickerstaff, E.R.: Neurology for nurses, ed. 2, London, 1971, English Universities Press Ltd., and Hodder & Stoughton, Ltd.)

Subjective data

1. Patient's understanding of the sensory disturbance
2. Measures that relieve symptoms, including medications
3. Site of sensory abnormality
4. Onset of sensory problem
5. Presence of associated symptoms
6. Alteration in sensation
   a. Pain
   b. Touch
   c. Temperature
   d. Proprioception
   e. Stereognosis

DATA ANALYSIS AND PLANNING

Nursing diagnoses

Possible nursing diagnoses for the patient with sensory dysfunction include the following:
Anxiety
Comfort, alteration in: pain
Home maintenance management: impaired
Knowledge deficit
Mobility, impaired physical
Sensory perceptual alteration: kinesthetic and tactile
Skin integrity: impaired, potential

Expected patient outcomes

Expected patient outcomes for the patient with sensory dysfunction include the following:

1. Patient can demonstrate how to compensate for each sensory deficit or loss.
2. Patient can explain safety factors needed in activities of daily living to protect against injury.
3. Patient can demonstrate how to inspect the affected body parts for injury.
4. Patient can state signs and symptoms that would indicate worsening of the condition and the need to seek medical assistance.
5. Patient can state plans for follow-up care.

IMPLEMENTATION

Teaching

The most important nursing intervention for the patient with sensory dysfunction is teaching the person and family protective measures in relation to the sensory deficit or alteration. Teaching the person to use noninvolved senses to an increased extent helps to avoid injuries. For example, teaching the person with hypoesthesia (lessened touch) to visually inspect involved body parts regularly will help to prevent injuries.

EVALUATION

Evaluation of the patient with sensory dysfunction involves the patient and family. Questions to consider include the following:
1. Is the patient carrying out ADL in a safe manner?
2. Is the patient successfully compensating for sensory deficits?
3. Is the patient inspecting affected body parts for injury?
4. Is the patient following through with the prescribed follow-up care?
5. Can the patient state signs and symptoms that indicate the need to notify the physician?

Major health problems of the neurologic system

Functioning of the neurologic system can be interrupted for a variety of reasons. These include the following:
1. Interference with impulses because of conduction of impulses
2. Interference because of degenerative changes
3. Interference because of vascular problems
4. Interference because of infection
5. Interference because of trauma
6. Interference because of tumors
Some common neurologic disorders are listed in the box.

INTERFERENCE WITH FUNCTION BECAUSE OF PROBLEMS WITH CONDUCTION OF IMPULSES

Epilepsy or seizures

Epilepsy (convulsive disorder) is one of the oldest diseases known to humans. (For purposes of this text the terms *epilepsy, seizure disorder,* and *convulsive disorder* will be used interchangeably.) Seizures occur in all races, and affect males and females equally. There is no apparent geographic distribution. Epilepsy can begin at any age, but in many the onset is before the age of 20. The incidence is about 1 in every 200 to 300 persons.

There are numerous ways to classify seizures. One common way is the International Classification of Epileptic Seizures. In this classification, seizures are identified as partial (beginning locally), generalized (bilaterally symmetric and with no local onset), unilateral, or unclassified. Another way to classify seizures is based on the clinical features of the attack. The five groups in this type of classification are as follows:
1. Grand mal (major or generalized)
2. Petit mal
3. Psychomotor
4. Jacksonian and focal
5. Miscellaneous (myclonic, akinetic)
Table 20-3 shows the characteristics of each type of seizure.

PATHOPHYSIOLOGY

Epilepsy may be defined as a transitory disturbance in consciousness or in motor, sensory, or autonomic function with or without loss of consciousness. It is associated with sudden, excessive, and disorderly electrical discharges in the neurons of the brain. The patterns or forms of seizures vary and are dependent on the area of the brain from which the seizure arises. The pattern is

---

Health problems of the neurologic system

1. *Interference with function because of problems with conduction of impulses*
   a. Epilepsy or seizures
   b. Myasthenia gravis
2. *Interference with function because of degenerative diseases*
   a. Multiple sclerosis
   b. Parkinson's disease
   c. Amyotrophic lateral sclerosis (ALS)
   d. Alzheimer's disease
3. *Interference with function because of vascular conditions*
   a. Cerebrovascular accident (CVA)
   b. Intracerebral hemorrhage
4. *Interference with function because of infection/inflammation*
   a. Meningitis
   b. Encephalitis
   c. Brain abcess
   d. Poliomyelitis
   e. Guillain-Barré syndrome
   f. Neurosyphilis
5. *Interference with function because of trauma*
   a. Craniocerebral
   b. Spinal cord
   c. Peripheral nerve
6. *Interference with function because of tumors*
   a. Intracranial
   b. Intraspinal

Table 20-3. Characteristics of seizures

Type of seizure	Etiology	Characteristics	Clinical signs	Aura	Postictal period
Grand mal	Most common	Generalized, characterized by loss of consciousness for several minutes	Aura Cry Loss of consciousness The fall Tonic-clonic movements Incontinence	Yes Flashing lights Smells Spots before eyes Dizziness	Yes Need for sleep 1 to 2 hrs Headache common
Petit mal	Usually occur during childhood and adolescence Frequency decreases as child gets older	Sudden impairment in or loss of consciousness with little or no tonic-clonic movement Occurs without warning Has tendency to appear a few hours after arising or when person is quiet	Sudden vacant facial expression with eye focused straight ahead All motor activity ceases except perhaps for slight symmetric twitching about eyelids Possible loss of muscle tone Consciousness returns	No	No
Psychomotor	Occur at any age	Sudden change in awareness associated with complex distortion of feeling and thinking and partially coordinated motor activity Longer than petit mal	Behaves as if partially conscious Often appears intoxicated May do antisocial things such as exposing self or carrying out violent acts Autonomic complaints may occur Chest pain Respiratory distress Tachycardia Gastrointestinal distress Urinary incontinence	Yes Complex hallucinations or illusions	Yes Confusion Amnesia Need for sleep
Jacksonian-focal	Occur almost entirely in patients with structural brain disease	Dependent on site of focus May or may not be progressive	Commonly begin in hand, foot, or face May end in grand mal seizure	Yes Numbness Tingling Crawling feeling	Yes
Myoclonic	May antedate grand mal by months or years	May be very mild or may have rapid, forceful movements	Sudden involuntary contraction of muscle group, usually in extremities or trunk No loss of consciousness	No	No
Akinetic	Not common	Peculiar generalized tonelessness	Person falls in flaccid state Unconscious for minute or two	Rarely	No

stereotyped in the individual, although variations may occur with progression of cerebral lesions.

Seizures can involve essentially all parts of the brain at once, as in the generalized type, or only a minute focal spot. In the first type, the excessive neuronal discharges are thought to originate in the brainstem portion of the reticular activating system; these then spread throughout the CNS including the cortex and the deeper parts of the brain. The process may last from a few seconds to as long as 3 to 5 minutes, or it may stop immediately, as in a *petit mal seizure.* Stoppage of a seizure is thought to result from fatigue of the neurons involved in precipitating the seizure or by inhibition of certain structures within the brain. The excessive neuronal discharges may result in a *tonic convulsion,* with the contraction of all muscles at once, or a *clonic convulsion,* with alternate contraction and relaxation of opposing muscle groups. This gives the characteristic jerking movements of the body. Seizures are followed by inhibition of cerebral function with a variable length. This is called the *postictal period.*

When recurrent generalized seizure activity occurs at such frequency that full consciousness is not regained between seizures, it is called *status epilepticus.* This is a medical emergency and requires intensive medical and nursing care to prevent death from brain damage secondary to prolonged hypoxia and exhaustion.

Seizures occur in many childhood and adult illnesses. Causes include the following:

1. Cerebral anoxia
2. Hypoglycemia
3. Disturbance of calcium balance
4. Electrolyte imbalances
5. Disturbance in hydration
6. Injection of drugs and poisons with convulsive activity
7. Numerous metabolic disturbances and disorders
8. Infections that cause high temperature elevations
9. Generalized inflammatory processes
10. Degenerative tissue disorders
11. Hysteria

In many patients with epilepsy, a localized organic lesion serves as the focus for the abnormal neuronal discharges from the damaged brain tissue. These organic lesions include the following:

1. Neoplasms
2. Inflamed areas or abcesses
3. Sclerosis
4. Vascular formations or hematomas
5. Congenital malformations
6. Trauma
7. Other space-occupying lesions

ASSESSMENT

Both subjective and objective data are important to assess with the patient with seizures.

Subjective data

1. Patient's understanding of the seizure disorder and what might be causing it
2. Awareness of precipitating factors
3. Presence of an aura
4. Postictal feelings

An *aura* is defined as the set of symptoms that occurs before the seizure. An aura occurs in about 50% of all patients with *grand mal seizures* and usually includes a change in sensation or a change in affect. The exact character of the aura varies from person to person but may include numbness, flashing lights, dizziness, tingling of the arm, smells, or spots before the eyes. The patient may not be able to describe the aura precisely, but it gives conclusive evidence of the impending seizure and allows the patient to seek privacy and safety before it occurs.

During the postictal phase the individual is groggy and

Observations to be made about a person having a seizure

Aura	Presence or absence; nature if present; ability of patient to describe it (somatic, visceral, psychic)
Cry	Presence or absence
Onset	Site of initial body movements; deviation of head and eyes; chewing and salivation; posture of body; sensory changes
Tonic and clonic phases	Movements of body as to progression; skin color and airway; pupillary changes; incontinence; duration of each phase
Relaxation (sleep)	Duration and behavior
Postictal phase	Duration; general behavior; ability to remember anything about the seizure; orientation; pupillary changes; headache; injuries present
Duration of entire seizure	Length from aura to relaxation phase
Level of consciousness	Length of unconsciousness if present

Expected patient outcomes

Expected patient outcomes for the patient with myasthenia gravis include the following:

1. Patient can explain the action, side effects, and toxic effects of each anticholinesterase or cholinergic drug.
2. Patient can explain the reason for taking medication at the exact time.
3. Improved function occurs—patient has increased ability to carry out daily activities.
4. Patient can explain the need to monitor effects of medication on respiration, swallowing, and general muscle strength.
5. Patient can list drugs that act on the neuromuscular junction and are contraindicated.
6. Patient can demonstrate use of airway and ventilatory equipment.
7. Patient can explain need to avoid overexertion and emotional tension.
8. Patient can explain why it is better not to live alone.

IMPLEMENTATION

Assisting with the achievement of therapeutic goals
Medications

Two medications that are used in myasthenia gravis are neostigmine (Prostigmin) and pyridostigmine (Mestinon). These drugs block the action of cholinesterase at the myoneural junction and allow acetylcholine to act. Atropine or other anticholinergic agents that block the effects of acetylcholine can be used to treat the side effects of neostigmine and pyridostigmine. Treatment is planned so that the patient receives the drug in the amount tolerated without side effects and yet is able to carry out activities essential for normal living. Usually, the patient is allowed to adjust the dosage.

It is often difficult to distinguish between *myasthenic crisis* (too little drug) and *cholinergic crisis* (too much drug), because both conditions cause severe muscle weakness. Administering endramonium intravenously differentiates between the two conditions. A positive test (increase in strength) indicates underdosage of the drug. An increase in weakness is a sign of overdosage.

RESPIRATORY CARE

Respiratory complications are common for the patient with myasthenia gravis, and for this reason they are usually advised not to live alone. Upper respiratory infections are seen because patients may not have the energy needed to cough effectively and may develop pneumonia or airway obstruction. Aspiration is common. Many patients have airway equipment at home.

During acute episodes of the disease, the following are important:

1. Tracheostomy set at bedside, because respiratory status may change rapidly
2. Serial determinations of vital capacity, minute volumes, and tidal volumes
3. Suction as necessary
4. Nasogastric tube if swallowing is too dangerous (patient will not be able to cough to indicate if tube is in trachea, so careful assessment of the position of tube is important)

Assisting with comfort and ADL

Patients with severe symptoms of myasthenia gravis may be too weak to do anything for themselves. The nurse may have to turn and position the patient in addition to doing most of the other ADL. It is important to remember that the patient with myasthenia gravis will remain alert and will often be very frightened. Psychologic support and reassurance are essential.

Teaching for the patient with myasthenia gravis

1. Medications
   a. Importance of taking medication at time prescribed
   b. Dose individually determined and related to the activity of the person
   c. How to adjust dose to maintain muscle strength
   d. Side effects and how to monitor
   e. Medications to avoid
2. Respiratory care
   a. Avoid crowd during peak times for upper respiratory infections
   b. Eat only when sitting up
   c. Importance of seeking medical treatment at first sign of upper respiratory infecton
3. Pattern of activity
   a. Activities planned around time of day when fatigue is lessened
   b. Importance of frequent rest periods
   c. Plan so that minimum amount of energy is used in activities that are essential to remaining relatively self-sufficient, and conserve energy for other activities the patient wishes to take part in

Teaching

The patient with myasthenia gravis often has a great deal of control over his/her medication schedule and can do much to prevent respiratory problems. A well-informed patient is more likely to stay healthy.

Teaching should include the points listed in box on p. 392.

EVALUATION

Evaluation of the patient with myasthenia gravis is important. Involving the patient in this process is essential. Questions to consider are the following:

1. Is patient taking medication as ordered?
2. Can the patient explain the action, time element, and side effects of the medication?
3. Does the patient know what drugs to avoid?
4. Is the patient able to function in ADL?
5. Does the patient demonstrate knowledge of any necessary equipment?

INTERFERENCE WITH FUNCTION BECAUSE OF DEGENERATIVE DISEASES

The term *degenerative diseases* is used to refer to neurologic diseases in which there is a premature senescence of nerve cells, there is a known or suspected metabolic disturbance, or the cause of the disease is unknown. Included in this section are four such diseases. These are the following:

1. Multiple sclerosis
2. Parkinson's disease
3. Amyotrophic lateral sclerosis (ALS)
4. Alzheimer's disease

See Table 20-5 for a comparison of these four diseases.

Another degenerative disease is syringomyelia. This is a destruction of the gray and then white matter of the spinal cord that occurs as a result of the development of *syringes* (cysts filled with CSF). As a result there is destruction of nerve pathways in the spinal cord and interruption of the nerve impulses. This disease will not be discussed in further detail in below box, but it is one that the nurse should be aware of.

Drugs to be avoided by persons with myasthenia gravis

1. Muscle relaxants
2. Barbiturates
3. Morphine sulfate
4. Tranquilizers
5. Neomycin (potentiates muscle weakness because of effect on myoneural junction)

Table 20-5. Comparison of degenerative neurologic diseases

Disease	Pathologic signs	Effect	Medical treatment
Multiple sclerosis	Multiple foci (patches) of nerve degeneration throughout the brain and spinal cord	Demyelination causes nerve impulses to be interrupted (blocked) or distorted (slowed)	No specific treatment Symptomatic treatment Judicious use of ACTH or other corticosteroids
Amyotrophic lateral sclerosis	Destruction of myelin sheath of motor neurons of lateral tracts of spinal cord and brain	Demyelination causes nerve impulses to be interrupted (blocked) or distorted (slowed)	No specific treatment Symptomatic and supportive care
Parkinson's disease	Destruction of nerve cells of basal ganglia of brain	Decreased dopamine (neurotransmitter substance with anticholinergic effect)	Anticholinergic alkaloids Synthetic anticholinergic drugs Levodopa Carbidopa-levodopa Surgery in selected cases
Alzheimer's disease	Degeneration of neurofibrils and presence of plaque in brain	Destruction of neurons leading to impairments in intellectual functioning	No specific treatment Symptomatic and supportive care

Multiple sclerosis

Multiple sclerosis is a common degenerative neurologic disease. At least 500,000 persons suffer from it. The cause remains unknown despite research. Several hypotheses have been advanced as to the cause, including the following:

1. Mineral deficiency
2. Toxic substances
3. Disturbance of blood-clotting mechanism
4. Autoimmunity

The onset of symptoms usually occurs between the ages of 20 and 40. The course of the disease is estimated to be 12 to 25 years. Several studies have demonstrated an increased incidence of multiple sclerosis among siblings and even distant relatives. There has been no evidence to suggest a sexual mode of transmission.

PATHOPHYSIOLOGY

Multiple foci of demyelination are distributed randomly in the white matter of the brainstem, spinal cord, optic nerves, and cerebrum. During the demyelination process (primary degeneration) the myelin sheath and the sheath cells are destroyed, but there is early sparing of the axon cylinder. The outer myelin sheath destruction causes interruption or distortion of the impulse so that it is slowed or blocked. There is evidence of partial healing in areas of degeneration, which accounts for the transitory nature of early symptoms. In later stages the degeneration may extend to gray areas of the cord and limit healing.

Because of the wide distribution of areas of degeneration, there is a greater variety of signs and symptoms in multiple sclerosis than in other neurologic diseases. It is a chronic, remitting, and relapsing disease. The majority of persons recover from their early episodes, with remissions lasting for a year or more. Exacerbations may be aggravated or precipitated by fatigue, chilling, and emotional disturbances. In rare cases the disease may terminate in death within a few years of onset.

ASSESSMENT

Early symptoms of multiple sclerosis are usually transitory. Many persons may be considered neurotic because of the wide variety and temporary nature of symptoms and because of the emotional instability produced by the disease. Subjective symptoms are important in making the diagnosis.

Subjective data

1. Patient's understanding of disease
2. Presence of eye problems
   a. Diplopia
   b. Scotomas (spots before the eyes)
   c. Blindness
3. Presence of weakness or numbness of part of the body such as hand
4. Presence of unusual fatigue
5. Presence of tremor
6. Presence of emotional instability
7. Presence of bowel and bladder problems
8. Presence of impotence in men

Objective data

1. Documented abnormalities on neurologic testing
   a. Nystagmus
   b. Scanning speech
   c. Muscle weakness and spasms
   d. Changes in coordination
   e. Spastic ataxic gait
2. Behavior: presence of euphoria
3. Urinary incontinence, frequency or urgency
4. Difficulty in swallowing

It is suspected that the presence of euphoria is caused by patients' attempts to reassure themselves that their condition is not serious. Motor signs associated with multiple sclerosis have UMN characteristics. Pain is not a common symptom.

Diagnostic tests

There is no specific diagnostic test for multiple sclerosis. The determination of cerebrospinal fluid gamma globulin by chemical or electrophoretic methods or electroimmunodiffusion determination of cerebrospinal IgG is helpful. Testing of visual evoked potentials, which show evidence of early damage, has been closely linked with the early diagnosis of multiple sclerosis. Evoked potentials are electrical measurements of physiologic maturation of the human nervous system. They provide information about the primary sensory areas of the cortex.

DATA ANALYSIS AND PLANNING

Nursing diagnoses

Possible nursing diagnoses for the patient with multiple sclerosis include the following:

Anxiety
Bowel elimination, alteration in: constipation, incontinence
Comfort, alteration in pain
Communication
Home maintenance management; impaired
Knowledge deficit
Mobility, impaired physical
Self-care deficit: feeding, bathing/hygiene, dressing/grooming, toileting
Self-concept, disturbance in
Sensory perceptual alteration: visual
Sexual dysfunction
Skin integrity, impairment of: potential
Thought processes, alteration in
Urinary elimination, alteration in patterns

Expected patient outcomes

Expected patient outcomes for the patient with multiple sclerosis include the following:

1. Patient can explain how to prevent urinary bladder infection and discomfort.

2. Patient can explain the action, side effects, and toxic effects of medications to be taken at home.
3. Patient can state plan to balance rest and work activities.
4. Patient can explain plan for a balanced diet.
5. Patient can state the plan for inclusion of hobbies and other interests as related to mental health.
6. Patient can state importance of skin care and how to inspect skin.
7. Patient can explain safety measures necessitated by the disease.
8. Patient can explain exercise program to be followed, including frequent changes in position.
9. Patient can state how to secure community help.
10. Patient can state plans for follow-up care.
11. Patient can carry out daily activities for as long as possible.

IMPLEMENTATION

Assisting with the achievement of therapeutic goals
Medications

At present there is no specific treatment for multiple sclerosis. Favorable results seem to occur with the use of adrenocorticotrophic hormone (ACTH) and the corticosteroids. Their efficacy remains controversial. Some physicians prefer oral prednisone or intramuscular or oral dexamethasone (Decadron). ACTH may be given intramuscularly or intravenously. The effects of ACTH and the steroids on the demyelinating process is unknown. It is known from testing that (1) there is nothing to be gained from long-term treatment, and (2) there is possibly some gain from taking high doses of steroids at the start of an exacerbation, because the episode then seems to resolve more rapidly.

Elimination

Urinary frequency and urgency may respond to timed doses of propantheline bromide (Pro-Banthine). Prevention of urinary tract infection remains a problem, and such infections are a major cause of death. Cholinergic drugs such as bethanechol (Urecholine) may be helpful in the patient with atonic bladder. Oxybutynin chloride (Ditropan) is used to treat neurogenic bladder. It acts by exerting a direct antispasmodic effect on smooth muscles. Some patients are given prophylactic doses of medications such as trimethoprim and sulfamethoxazole (Bactrim, Septra) or nitrofurantoin (Macrodantin). Cystometric studies can be helpful in defining the specific bladder problem.

The patient should be encouraged to drink adequate fluids. Several glasses of cranberry juice a day may be helpful in decreasing urinary tract infection.

It may be necessary to have the patient take a stool softener such as docusate sodium (Colace) to prevent constipation.

Nutrition

A well-balanced diet with plenty of high-vitamin foods is important. Obesity should be avoided because it makes it more difficult for the patient to maneuver and to meet daily needs. High-fiber foods and prune juice may help reduce constipation.

Skin care

Many persons with multiple sclerosis have motor involvement that prevents them from moving about freely and changing position readily. Also, they may experience sensory disturbances that affect how they sense pressure. As a result, decubiti can easily develop. Patients must be taught the importance of turning at least every 2 to 3 hours. Other devices such as air mattresses may also be helpful.

Assisting with comfort and ADL
Activity and rest

Persons with multiple sclerosis should have a daily routine for rest and activity. They are usually advised to exercise regularly but never to the point of extreme fatigue. During an acute exacerbation, patients are often kept as quiet as possible, bed rest is maintained, and all activities are limited.

One side of the body is usually affected more than the other. The patient may learn to stabilize the gait by leaning toward the uninvolved side. Having the foot slap forward in taking a step may sometimes be overcome by putting the heel down in a pronounced fashion and rolling the weight forward on the side of the foot.

The judicious use of passive and active exercises, when the person is not in acute exacerbation, can be useful in maintaining function. The use of drugs such as diazepam (Valium) and dantrolene sodium (Dantrium) as well as baclofen (Lioresal) have been used to prevent spasticity.

Effort is made to maintain activity and work as long as possible. Patients can be helped to plan their activities so that they may continue to function even when the disease is well advanced.

Control of environment

Hot baths should be avoided, because the heat can increase weakness in the person with multiple sclerosis. Traveling in hot weather should be carefully planned to prevent travel during the warmest part of the day.

Persons with multiple sclerosis need a peaceful, relaxed environment. They may have slowness of speech and slowness in the ability to respond. Members of the family may need help in understanding this problem and meeting it calmly. The person may have sudden explosive emotional outbursts of crying or laughing. Reminding the patient of something sad may stop him/her from laughing, and holding the patient's mouth open may sometimes stop the crying.

Teaching

Teaching is important for both the patient with multiple sclerosis and his/her significant others. In late stages of the disease all functions of care usually have to be assumed by someone other than the patient. Teaching needs are listed in box on p. 396.

Teaching for the patient with multiple sclerosis

1. Use of medications, including side effects, dose, timing; importance of reporting side effects to physician
2. Importance of good fluid intake
3. Importance of spacing activities so that time is left for relaxation and fun activities
4. Range of motion exercises, as well as other exercises
5. Good, balanced diet
6. Emotional reactions of persons with multiple sclerosis
7. Safety factors to prevent injury
8. Positioning for prevention of decubiti
9. Importance of skin inspection
10. Importance of avoiding temperature extremes
11. Community resources and how to obtain them

EVALUATION

Evaluation should include the patient and care givers. Questions to consider include the following:
1. Is patient taking medication as ordered?
2. Can the patient explain the use of the medication?
3. Is an exercise program being followed?
4. Can daily functions be accomplished?
5. Is the patient infection free?
6. Is elimination occurring without difficulty?
7. Is the skin free of pressure sores?
8. Can the patient explain how community agencies may be of assistance?
9. Is patient reporting for follow-up care?

Parkinson's disease

Parkinson's disease is one of the more common diseases of the nervous system. It was first described in 1817 by James Parkinson. It affects both men and women in their middle and late years (50 to 60 years old). It affects all races and classes of persons.

PATHOPHYSIOLOGY

The pathologic process that occurs with Parkinson's disease is basically a *depigmentation* of the *substantia nigra* of the basal ganglia. The loss of neurons in the substantia is severe. Also, selective depletion of dopamine occurs and can be correlated with the degree of striatal degeneration. Without dopamine there is a loss of inhibitory influence and excitatory mechanisms are unopposed.

The cause of Parkinson's disease is not known, but the cluster of symptoms was found in many patients following the 1916-1917 epidemic of encephalitis. The characteristic symptoms are also sometimes found in arteriosclerotic patients, leading some to believe that arteriosclerosis may be a causative factor. Drug-induced parkinsonian syndromes are linked with the following drugs:
1. Reserpine (Serpasil)
2. Phenothiazines
3. Butyrophenones (e.g., haloperidol)

ASSESSMENT

Like many of the other neurologic diseases, Parkinson's disease starts with subtle symptoms and progresses slowly. The person may not be able to recall the onset of symptoms.

Subjective data

1. Patient's understanding of disease
2. Complaints of fatigue
3. Presence of incoordination
4. Defects in judgment and emotional instability
5. Heat insensitivity

Objective data

1. Presence of tremor (pill-rolling motion of the fingers or resting tremor)
2. Muscular response to movement (strength and rigidity)
3. Postural reflexes
4. Appearance of face, including skin
5. Presence of drooling
6. Gait
7. Sensory testing
8. Inability to carry out daily activities

The tremor is the outstanding sign of the disease. Two other frequent signs are muscular weakness with rigidity and loss of postural reflexes. It is essentially a problem of motion. Muscle rigidity prevents normal response and results in characteristic changes. These changes include a masklike appearance of the face and slowed, monotonous speech; drooling; shuffling gait that is propulsive and may not be able to be stopped until any obstruction is met; and moist and oily skin.

Diagnostic tests

There is no test that is diagnostic of Parkinson's disease. The clinical examination and history, along with the response of the patient to administration of medication used to treat Parkinson's disease, confirms the diagnosis.

Table 20-6. Medications used in Parkinson's Disease

Medication	Action/effects	Side effects	Comments
1. Anticholinergic alkaloids Scopolamine hydrochloride Hyoscyamine	Act against cholinergic excitatory effects More effective in lessening muscle rigidity than in controlling tremor	Central and peripheral cholinergic actions Blurring of vision Dryness of mouth and throat Constipation Urinary retention or urgency Ataxia Dysarthria Mental disturbances	Optimal results depend on dosage that provides compromise between improvement and development of side effects
2. Synthetic anticholinergic drugs Trihexphenidyl (Artane) Benztropine mesylate (Cogentin) Procyclidine (Kemadrin) Biperiden (Akineton)	Some degree of CNS anticholinergic action, but incapable of restoring striatal balance	Same as above	Same as above
3. Antihistamine drugs Diphenhydramine (Benadryl)	Exerts mild central anticholinergic properties	Sleepiness Dry mouth	Does not affect underlying process of Parkinson's disease
4. Levodopa	Assists in restoring striatal dopamine deficiency	Kidney, liver damage Nausea, vomiting Orthostatic hypotension Insomnia Agitation and mental confusion	Side effects common
5. Amantadine hydrochloride (Symmetrel)	Acts by blocking the reuptake and storage of catecholamines and allowing accumulation of dopamine in extracellular or synaptic sites	Mental confusion Visual disturbances Seizures	May not be effective for longer than 3 months
6. Carbidopalevodopa (Levodopa with inhibitor of the enzyme dopa decarboxylase)	Inhibitor limits metabolism of levodopa peripherally and provides more levodopa to brain	Same as levodopa	Fewer side effects than levodopa used alone

DATA ANALYSIS AND PLANNING

Nursing diagnoses

Except for "Sensory perceptual alteration: visual" (which is not a diagnosis for Parkinson's disease), the list of nursing diagnoses is the same as for multiple sclerosis (p. 394).

Expected patient outcomes

The expected patient outcomes for Parkinson's disease are the same as for multiple sclerosis (pp. 394-395).

IMPLEMENTATION

Assisting with the achievement of therapeutic goals
Medications

Treatment for Parkinson's disease is palliative and symptomatic and depends on pharmacologic manipulation of the disease. The severity of symptoms and the presence of associated disease processes determine the drugs to be used. Particular drugs and their characteristics can be found in Table 20-6.

After prolonged treatment with some of the drugs, there may be an increased appearance of side effects as well as a decrease in the effectiveness of the medication. It has been found helpful to admit some patients into the hospital for a *drug holiday*, during which all medications are withdrawn for a period of time. The medications are then restarted, and often much smaller doses are able to produce favorable results. This type of drug holiday must take place in the hospital. Complications such as aspiration pneumonia can occur, because immobility, rigidity, and other symptoms will return when the drugs are withdrawn.

Surgery

A surgical procedure has been used with some success in the treatment of selected patients with Parkinson's disease. It includes destroying portions of the globus pallidus (to relieve rigidity) or the thalamus (to relieve tremor) in the brain by stereotactic methods through the use of cautery, removal, or injection of alcohol. Operative techniques involving cooling or freezing with liquid nitrogen have been attempted with good results in selected cases. Medications used to control rigidity and tremor are discontinued several days preoperatively so that symptoms will be at their maximum during the surgery. Preoperative and postoperative care remain the same as for the patient undergoing cranial surgery and will be discussed later in this chapter. Many patients cannot be treated surgically. Results seem to be best in younger patients who have unilateral involvement following other diseases and who have marked tremor and rigidity.

Assisting with comfort and ADL

Activity

Special attention should be paid to posture. Lying on a firm bed without a pillow may help to prevent the spine from bending forward. Lying in the prone position also helps. Holding the hands folded behind the back when walking may help to keep the spine erect and prevent the arms from falling stiffly at the sides. The tremor is often less apparent when persons are sitting in an armchair, since they can grip the arms of the chair and partially control the tremor in their hands and arms.

Feeding

Feeding the patient becomes a real problem when the disease is far advanced, because of the danger of aspiration; aspiration pneumonia may be fatal. Unless the disease is well controlled by medication, drooling can be a problem and increases with general excitement. A bib can be used to protect the clothing during naps. When patients are dressed, garments with generous pockets for tissues will help them be less conspicuous and more comfortable.

Teaching

Teaching is important for the care giver and the patient with Parkinson's disease. The teaching is the same as that for the patient with multiple sclerosis (p. 396).

Evaluation

The evaluation of the care of the patient with Parkinson's disease is based on the expected patient outcomes and is the same as for the patient with multiple sclerosis (p. 396).

Amyotrophic lateral sclerosis

Amyotrophic lateral sclerosis (ALS) is a motor neuron disease that affects upper or lower motor neurons lying within the brain or spinal cord or a combination of the two. It is sometimes called Lou Gehrig's disease, because the famous New York Yankee baseball player died of ALS. It affects men more than women, and usually first appears in middle age, although it may occur in younger persons.

PATHOPHYSIOLOGY

In ALS the myelin sheaths are destroyed and replaced with scar tissue. There is direct involvement of the lateral tracts of the spinal cord with possible involvement of the medulla and the ventral tracts. The nerve impulses are distorted or blocked. Symptoms depend on which motor neurons are affected.

ASSESSMENT
Subjective data

1. Patient's understanding of disease
2. Presence of fatigue
3. Dysphagia
4. Difficulty with tasks involving fine finger movements

Objective data

1. Inability to carry out ADL
2. Muscle testing on neurologic examination
3. Evidence of involvement of brainstem and medulla
4. Weight loss

In ALS there is progressive muscle weakness, atrophy, and fasciculations. Spasticity of the flexor muscles is common. With involvement of the brainstem and medulla there is dysphagia, dysarthria, jaw clonus, tongue fasciculations, and respiratory difficulty. As the disease progresses, there is disability relative to both upper and lower limbs, and one side of the body becomes more involved. The person remains alert, and there is no sensory loss. Death usually occurs within 5 years of diagnosis, because of respiratory problems or bulbar paralysis.

Diagnostic tests

Initial testing may include an EMG (p. 379) to rule out other muscle diseases. There is no definitive test for ALS.

DATA ANALYSIS AND PLANNING

Nursing diagnoses

The nursing diagnoses for the patient with ALS are the same as that for the patient with multiple sclerosis with the addition of the following:

Airway clearance, ineffective
Communication, impaired verbal
Gas exchange, impaired
Nutrition, alteration in: less than body requirements

The diagnosis of "Sensory perceptual alteration: visual" is also not a diagnosis relevant to ALS.

Expected patient outcomes

The expected patient outcomes for ALS are the same as for multiple sclerosis (p. 394), with the addition that the patient is able to meet daily nutritional requirements.

IMPLEMENTATION

Assisting with the achievement of therapeutic goals

Treatment is directed toward relieving the symptoms of the disease. Prostheses are often supplied to support the weakened muscles. As the disease progresses, respirations are affected. At this time constant nursing attention is required. Providing adequate nutrition to the patient is a real challenge, and a nasogastric or gastrostomy tube may be necessary. Attention to prevention of skin breakdown and contractures is important.

Assisting with comfort and ADL

Nursing interventions include assistance with ADL as limb defects occur. Emotional support is extremely important. Patients and their families should be involved in making decisions about the types of interventions that will be used as the disease progresses. Some patients will decide to use ventilators at home as respiratory muscles become involved, whereas other patients will decide not to use any supportive devices. Because the patient remains alert until death, nurses should remember that they are dealing with someone who is probably very afraid.

EVALUATION

Because the outcomes in ALS are similar to those of multiple sclerosis, refer to that part of the chapter for the appropriate questions to ask (p. 396). An additional reference question is whether the patient is maintaining weight.

Alzheimer's disease

Alzheimer's disease is a degenerative disorder that affects the cells of the brain and causes impairment of intellectual functioning. It is recognized as the most common cause of dementia in the older adult. It affects men and women equally. Most newly diagnosed persons are in late middle age, but the disease has been documented in some persons as young as 40 years old.

PATHOPHYSIOLOGY

The changes in the brains of patients with Alzheimer's disease are visible in the cerebral cortex. The first change is the presence of microscopic "plaques" found in brain tissue. These plaques consist of a core surrounded by strands of fiberlike material. In addition, there is degeneration of some of the small fibers (neurofibrils) that run through the body of the nerve cells. These changes were first discovered in 1907 by the German neurologist Alzheimer.

ASSESSMENT

Subjective data

1. Patient's understanding of disease
2. Mental status part of neurologic examination
3. Onset of symptoms

Objective data

1. Inability to carry on ADL
2. Behavior: evidence of agitation, restlessness
3. Presence of incontinence

The patient with Alzheimer's disease goes through three rather distinct stages. These stages are described in box below.

The diagnosis of Alzheimer's disease is made after rul-

Clinical stages of Alzheimer's disease

Stage one
Mild mental impairment
Forgetfulness
Impairment in judgment
Lessening of initiative
Lack of spontaneity

Stage two
Confusion
Agitation
Irritability
Extreme restlessness
Incontinence of urine and stool
Need for constant supervision

Stage three
Total inability to care for self
Inability to communicate
Total incontinence

ing out other conditions in which there is memory loss. These include the following diseases:

1. Pernicious anemia
2. Drug reactions
3. Hormonal imbalances
4. Depression
5. Drug or alcohol abuse
6. Brain tumor
7. Chronic meningitis
8. Head trauma
9. Pick's disease
10. Parkinson's disease with dementia

The signs and symptoms of Alzheimer's disease occur progressively, but the rate at which they occur varies between individuals. In a few cases, there may be a very rapid decline, but in most cases there is gradual deterioration. Cause of death is often pneumonia or other infections.

Diagnostic tests

There is no diagnostic test that is specific for Alzheimer's disease. A CT scan is used to rule out other abnormalities. Often neuropsychologic testing can reveal characteristic changes in the ability to think.

DATA ANALYSIS AND PLANNING

Nursing diagnoses

The possible nursing diagnoses for the patient with Alzheimer's disease are the same as for the patient with multiple sclerosis (p. 394), with the following additions:

Injury: potential for
Sleep pattern disturbance
Violence, potential for

Expected patient outcomes

The expected outcomes for the patient with Alzheimer's disease are the same as those for the patient with multiple sclerosis, with several exceptions. The first is the addition of the outcome, "Safety is maintained." Another difference is that in many cases the person with Alzheimer's disease is mentally incompetent, so that the care giver needs to have major involvement in planning for the outcomes. The patient may not be able to have real input into them.

IMPLEMENTATION

Assisting with the achievement of therapeutic goals

There is no treatment that can cure, reverse, or stop the progression of Alzheimer's disease. Nursing care is directed toward maintaining nutrition, continence, hydration, and safety. Emotional support of both the patient and family is important. Appropriate drugs can sometimes be used to lessen anxiety, agitation, and unpredictable behavior.

Safety

One large area for intervention concerns safety. Because of forgetfulness, patients with this condition often do dangerous things. This includes walking outside without appropriate clothing, turning on burners, getting lost, and setting things on fire. The family must make plans to protect the patient from these hazards. This includes removing burner controls from the stove at night, double-locking all doors and windows, and keeping the person under supervision at all times. One very frustrating part of the illness is that many of the patients sleep for only short periods of time and are awake most of the night. This must be worked out if the caregiver is to get any rest.

EVALUATION

Evaluation of the patient with Alzheimer's disease focuses on the patient outcomes. Refer to the evaluation section for multiple sclerosis for appropriate questions to ask (p. 396). An additional question is whether the person is safely carrying out daily activities.

INTERFERENCE WITH FUNCTION BECAUSE OF VASCULAR CONDITIONS

Interference with function because of vascular conditions is common in neurologic nursing. In this section of the chapter the following two conditions will be discussed:

1. Cerebrovascular accident
   a. Thrombosis
   b. Embolus
   c. Hemorrhage
2. Intracerebral hemorrhage

Cerebrovascular accident

Cerebrovascular accident (CVA) is the most common disease of the nervous system and is one of the leading causes of death in the United States. In this section, the term *cerebrovascular accident* will be discussed as a general term. Most neurologists and neurosurgeons, however, refer more specifically to the cause of the CVA. These causes are as follows:

1. Thrombus
2. Embolus
3. Hemorrhage (this is discussed on p. 406)

The medical and nursing care may differ depending on the specific cause. *Stroke* is another term used when referring to CVA; clinically, stroke refers to the sudden and dramatic development of focal neurologic deficits.

Cerebrovascular accidents can be precipitated by many underlying factors and are frequently associated with other chronic diseases that cause vascular problems. These include heart disease, hypertension, kidney disease, peripheral vascular disease, and diabetes mellitus.

PATHOPHYSIOLOGY

The brain is very dependent on oxygen and has no reserve oxygen supply. When anoxia occurs, as in CVA,

---

Conditions causing CVA

Thrombus

Atherosclerosis in intracranial and extracranial arteries
Adjacency to intracerebral hemorrhage
Arteritis caused by collagen (autoimmune) disease or bacterial arteritis
Hypercoagulability such as in polycythemia
Cerebral venous thromboses

Emboli

Valves damaged by rheumatic heart disease (RHD)
Myocardial infarction
Atrial fibrillation (this arrhythmia causes variable emptying of left ventricle, blood pools and small clots form and
  then at times the ventricle will be emptied completely with release of small emboli)
Bacterial endocarditis and nonbacterial endocarditis causing clots to form on endocardium

Hemorrhage

Hypertensive intracerebral hemorrhage
Subarachnoid hemorrhage
Rupture of aneurysm
Arteriovenous malformation
Hypocoagulation (as in patients with blood dyscrasias)

Generalized hypoxia

Severe hypotension, cardiopulmonary arrest, or severe depression in cardiac output caused by arrhythmias

Localized hypoxia

Cerebral artery spasms associated with subarachnoid hemorrhage
Cerebral artery vasoconstriction associated with migraine headaches

---

cerebral metabolism is promptly altered, and cell death and permanent damage can occur within 3 to 10 minutes. Any condition that alters cerebral perfusion will cause hypoxia or anoxia. Hypoxia first leads to cerebral ischemia. Short-term ischemia (less than 10 to 15 minutes) causes temporary deficits but no permanent deficits. Long-term ischemia causes permanent cell death and results in cerebral infarction, with accompanying cerebral edema.

The type of permanent focal deficits will depend on the area of the brain that has been affected. The area of the brain affected depends on which cerebral vessels are involved. The vessel most commonly affected is the middle cerebral artery; the second most commonly affected is the internal carotid artery. Permanent focal deficits may be unknown when the patient is first seen because of generalized cerebral ischemia that may resolve.

Cerebral thrombosis

Thrombosis is the most common cause of a CVA, and the most common cause of cerebral thrombosis is atherosclerosis. CVA secondary to thrombosis is seen most often in the 60- to 90-year-old age group. Many of these persons have a history of hypertension or diabetes mellitus.

The onset of symptoms of CVA secondary to thrombosis tends to occur during sleep or soon after arising. This is thought to be related to the fact that elderly persons have decreased sympathetic activity, and recumbency causes a lowering of blood pressure, which can lead to brain ischemia. These persons often also have postural hypotension and poor reflex response to changes in position. Neurologic signs and symptoms very frequently worsen for the first 48 hours after thrombosis.

Cerebral embolism

Embolism is the second most common cause of CVA. Patients who have CVAs secondary to embolism are usually younger, and most commonly the emboli originate from a thrombus in the heart. The myocardial thrombus is most commonly caused by rheumatic heart disease with mitral stenosis and atrial fibrillation.

Transient ischemic attack

The term *transient ischemic attack* (TIA) refers to transient cerebral ischemia with temporary episodes of neurologic dysfunction. The neurologic dysfunction can be profound with complete loss of consciousness and loss of all sensory and motor function, or there may only be focal deficits. The most common deficit is contralateral weakness of lower face, hands, arms and legs, transient dysphasia, and some sensory impairment. Ischemic attacks may occur over days, weeks or months—between attacks the neurologic examination is normal. TIAs most commonly precede cerebral thrombotic attacks. They can be caused by any of the causes of CVA.

The major importance of TIAs is that they warn the patient and health care professional of the existence of an underlying pathologic condition. At least one third of patients who have TIAs will have a CVA in 2 to 5 years. TIAs need to be aggressively worked up to determine if preventative measures can be taken.

ASSESSMENT
Subjective data
1. Patient's understanding of disease or symptoms
2. Characteristics of onset of symptoms
3. Presence of headache—nature and location
4. Any sensory deficits
5. Visual ability—presence of diplopia, blurred vision
6. Ability to think clearly
7. Any other concomitant symptom

Objective data
1. Motor strength—paresis or plegia is common
2. Change in level of consciousness, including unconsciousness

---

Cerebral arteriogram (angiogram)

Purpose
To visualize the cerebral arterial system by injecting radiopaque material. Allows detection of arterial aneurysms, vessel anomalies, ruptured vessels, and displacement of vessels by mass lesions

Preparation of patient
1. Patient is given clear liquids morning of procedure.
2. Patient must be assessed for allergy to iodine.
3. If femoral approach is to be used, it is helpful to assess and mark the locations of the bilateral pedal pulses.
4. If the carotid artery is used, the neck circumference is measured as part of the baseline data.
5. Sedation may be given the night before and just before the procedure.
6. If the femoral approach is used, the groin site may be shaved the night before.
7. Immediately before the procedure, baseline vital signs, pulses, and neurologic checks should be done and recorded.
8. Patient teaching
   a. Explain procedure.
   b. Time: approximately 2 to 3 hours.
   c. Sensation: some discomfort in lying still for several hours. At the time of dye injection, most patients complain of feeling extremely hot and seeing flashes of light.

Procedure
1. Patient is positioned supine on the x-ray table.
2. Local anesthetic is used to anesthetize the area of puncture site.
3. Catheter is introduced percutaneously.
   a. In a four-vessel study, catheter is inserted into the femoral artery, innominate, carotid, and vertebral arteries.
   b. Each vessel is injected with the contrast dye as serial x-ray films are taken.
   c. Carotid or vertebral vessels may be used directly.
4. Catheter is withdrawn and pressure is applied to puncture site for at least 5 minutes.

After procedure
1. Patients usually kept in bed overnight.
2. Vital signs checked frequently (may be as often as every 15 minutes for a period of several hours), as well as neurologic checks with each vital sign check.
3. Site of puncture is assessed frequently for presence of hematoma.
   a. Femoral: check pulses distal to site for evidence of arterial occlusion.
   b. Carotid: check for difficulty breathing or swallowing; measure neck girth frequently.
4. Dye used in angiogram may raise intracranial pressure and cause decreased extremity strengths or change in level of consciousness.

3. Signs of increased intracranial pressure
4. Respiratory status
5. Ability to verbalize—presence of aphasia

The exact clinical picture varies depending on the area of the brain affected. The most common focal signs and symptoms are caused by disruption of flow through the midcerebral artery. These symptoms include the following:

1. Contralateral paralysis or paresis
2. Contralateral sensory loss
3. Sensory and motor loss most noticeable in face, neck, and upper extremities
4. Dysphasia or aphasia; occurs if dominant hemisphere is affected (left hemisphere in right-handed persons and most left-handed persons)
5. Spatial perceptual problems, changes in judgment and behavior, neglect of paralyzed side, and inability to recognize paralyzed extremity as own (*anosognosia*) if nondominant hemisphere is affected
6. Contralateral *homonymous hemianopsia*

Aphasia is a disorder of language caused by damage to the speech-controlling areas of the brain. It includes all areas of language, including speech, reading, writing, and understanding. These abnormalities can occur in a variety of ways as follows:

1. *Sensory aphasia*—inability to comprehend spoken word (also called receptive aphasia)
2. *Motor aphasia*—inability to use the symbols of speech (also called expressive aphasia)
3. *Global aphasia*—inability to understand the spoken word, as well as to speak

Diagnostic tests

A lumbar puncture (p. 363) is usually performed and may reveal increased spinal fluid pressure. If the CVA is caused by hemorrhage, there will be blood in the spinal fluid. A CT scan is also used to visualize affected areas; often it is done first to prevent herniation during the lumbar puncture if the pressure is extremely elevated.

Following TIAs, a cerebral angiogram may be done to discover blocked or occluded vessels. In some cases a digital subtraction angiogram (DSA) is done instead.

DATA ANALYSIS AND PLANNING

Nursing diagnoses

Possible nursing diagnoses for the patient with a CVA or TIA include the following:

Airway clearance, ineffective

Digital subtraction angiography (DSA)

Purpose

To identify abnormalities of the cerebrovascular system, using a process that removes overlying structures in an image, so that the clinically significant details can be displayed with enhanced visibility

Preparation of patient

1. Permit must be signed.
2. Food may be restricted before procedure.
3. Patient should be asked about allergy to iodine.
4. Patient teaching.
   a. Explain procedure.
   b. Time: approximately 45 to 60 minutes
   c. Sensation: some discomfort associated with the start of the IV. Injection of dye may be uncomfortable. Some patients may find need to lie still uncomfortable.

Procedure

1. Patient is positioned supine on the x-ray table.
2. Local anesthetic may be used to anesthetize the area of puncture site.
3. Catheter is introduced into vein, usually in the arm for cerebral studies.
4. Dye is injected as films are taken.
5. Catheter is withdrawn

After procedure

1. Vital signs are checked on return to floor.
2. Circulatory status of arm is assessed.
3. Injection site is checked for presence of hematoma.
4. Usually no activity restrictions—procedure can be done on an outpatient basis.
5. The computer performs the subtraction—a process that removes underlying structures in an image, so that the clinically significant details can be displayed with enhanced visibility.

from the immobility and dependency it causes and from

aneurysm and reduce the chances of hemorrhage. This is contingent on whether sufficient blood can be supplied from collateral vessels to preserve brain function. The procedure usually is performed in stages over several days. A clamp (Silverstone or Salibi) that has a detachable screw stem that can be tightened gradually is used. Usually the surgeon adjusts it each day, and the nurse assesses the patient closely and is instructed to release the clamp at once if there is evidence of inadequate blood supply, as shown by decreased neurologic status. Immediate removal of the clamps may prevent irreversible complications such as hemiplegia, aphasia, and loss of consciousness. If complete occlusion can be tolerated, the vessel may be permanently ligated. Serial embolizations of blood vessels that "feed" the aneurysm may also be done via the femoral or axillary route. The procedure is similar to a cerebral angiogram, and the postoperative care is the same. Thrombus formation with resultant cerebral embolism may complicate the patient's postoperative course following any surgery for a cerebral aneurysm.

Teaching

If the patient with an intracranial hemorrhage has neurologic deficits consistent with a CVA, the teaching is the same. Additionally, the points listed in the box below are important.

EVALUATION

In addition to those questions used to evaluate the patient who has had a CVA (p. 382), the following questions should be asked:
1. Is the patient's neurologic status stable?
2. Is the patient cooperating with the activity restrictions?
3. Is the patient relatively calm?
4. Does the patient verbalize understanding of the restrictions?
5. Does the patient verbalize understanding of surgery planned?

Teaching for a patient with intracranial hemorrhage

1. Importance of following activity restrictions.
2. Importance of keeping as free of stress as possible.
3. Very specific teaching about what activities are restricted.
4. Use of medication and what it does.
5. Information about preoperative and postoperative care will be useful.

INTERFERENCE WITH FUNCTION BECAUSE OF INFECTION/INFLAMMATION

Interference with function because of infection/inflammation is a fairly common occurrence. Specific conditions to discuss include the following:
1. Meningitis
2. Encephalitis
3. Brain abscess
4. Poliomyelitis
5. Guillain-Barré syndrome
6. Herpes zoster
7. Neurosyphilis

Because these conditions contain many common characteristics, they will be discussed together.

The nervous system may be attacked by a variety of organisms and viruses and may suffer from toxins of bacteria and viruses. These toxins reach the nervous system through a variety of routes. Untreated chronic otitis media and mastoiditis, chronic sinusitis, and fracture in any bone adjacent to the meninges may be the source of infection. Some organisms such as the tubercle bacillus reach the nervous system by means of the blood or lymphatic system. Meningitis can occur as a complication of an invasive procedure such as a lumbar puncture. The exact route of some other organisms is not known.

Meningitis
PATHOPHYSIOLOGY

Meningitis is an acute infection of the meninges. It is usually caused by one of the following organisms:
1. Pneumococci
2. Meningococci
3. Staphylococci
4. Streptococci
5. *Haemophilus influenzae*
6. Aseptic agents (usually viral)

Any other pathogenic organism, such as the tubercle bacillus, that gains access to the subarachnoid spaces can also cause meningitis. The incidence of bacterial meningitis is higher in fall and winter when upper respiratory tract infections are common. Children are more often affected than adults because of frequent colds and ear infections.

Once organisms reach the brain, the CSF in the subarachnoid spaces and in the pia arachnoid membrane becomes infected. The infection then spreads rapidly throughout the meninges and eventually invades the ventricles. Pathologic changes that occur include any or all of the following:
1. Hyperemia of the meningeal vessels
2. Edema of brain tissue
3. Increased ICP
4. Generalized inflammatory reaction with exudation of white blood cells into the subarachnoid spaces
5. Associated hydrocephalus caused by exudate blocking the small passage between the ventricles.

ASSESSMENT

Subjective and objective assessment are important in any patient with an infection of the nervous system. This assessment includes common characteristics to all infections/inflammations discussed in this section.

Subjective data

1. Patient's understanding of process and possible causes
2. Any history of infection such as upper respiratory infections
3. Measures that relieve symptoms
4. Presence of discomfort, including headache or stiff neck
5. Initial onset of symptoms
6. Presence of difficulty in thinking
7. Presence of muscle weakness, soreness, or incoordination

Objective data

1. Behavior: signs indicating discomfort or disorientation
2. Change in ability to carry out daily activities
3. Abnormalities on physical assessment part of neurologic examination
4. Temperature
5. Presence of vomiting
6. Pulse and blood pressure
7. Respirations

The onset of meningitis is usually sudden and characterized by severe headache, stiffness of the neck, irritability, malaise, and restlessness. Nausea, vomiting, delirium, and complete disorientation develop quickly. Temperature, pulse rate, and respirations are increased. Two pathologic signs that occur with meningitis are the following:

1. *Kernig's sign*—the inability of the patient to extend the legs completely without extreme pain
2. *Brudzinski's sign*—flexion of the hip and knee when the neck is flexed

Diagnostic tests

Most of the infections affecting the nervous system can be diagnosed by examining the cerebrospinal fluid. A CT scan and an EEG may also be used. These procedures were discussed earlier in this chapter.

DATA ANALYSIS AND PLANNING

Nursing diagnoses

Possible nursing diagnoses for the person with a neurologic infection include the following:
Airway clearance, ineffective
Anxiety
Bowel elimination, alteration in: incontinence
Breathing pattern, ineffective
Comfort, alteration in: pain
Communication, impaired verbal
Gas exchange, impaired
Home maintenance management: impaired
Knowledge deficit
Mobility, impaired physical
Self-care deficit: feeding, bathing/hygiene, dressing/grooming, toileting
Sexual dysfunction
Skin integrity, impairment of: potential
Thought processes, alteration in
Tissue perfusion, alteration in: cerebral
Urinary elimination, alteration in patterns

Not every diagnosis may apply to each infection/inflammation; much will depend on the severity of the deficit.

Expected patient outcomes

1. Patient can state the nature of the infection, infectious agent, and method of transmission.
2. Patient can explain how to prevent further infection.
3. Patient can state plans for follow-up care.
4. Patient can state and explain each medication—side effects, action, route, and dosage.
5. Patient remains neurologically intact.

Other patient outcomes are dependent on the nature of the disability. For instance, if the patient has motor deficits, the outcomes for the patient with motor dysfunction will be appropriate.

IMPLEMENTATION

Assisting with achievement of therapeutic goals

Treatment of meningitis consists of massive doses of the antibiotic or antibiotics specific for the causative organism. Treatment with multiple antibiotics is common. Culture and sensitivity studies demonstrate the most effective antibiotic. Usually a course of at least 10 days of parenteral administration is needed. The antibiotic may also be given directly into the spinal canal (intrathecally). The use of hyperosmolar agents or steroids may be necessary to decrease cerebral edema. Anticonvulsants may be given to prevent seizures.

Nursing care for the patient with meningitis includes the following:

1. General care given a critically ill patient
2. Darkened room, with noise kept to a minimum, because sensory stimulation can cause seizures
3. Careful neurologic checks at frequent intervals
4. Padded side rails
5. Observation for symptoms of inappropriate antidiuretic hormone (ADH), which is common in patients with meningitis

Residual damage from meningitis includes deafness, blindness, paralysis, and mental retardation. These complications are usually the result of chronic arachnoiditis. Hydrocephalus may also develop, requiring a shunting procedure.

Isolation of the patient depends on the causative organism. Check the infection control manual of your institution for specific guidelines.

EVALUATION

Evaluation of the patient with meningitis includes answers to the following questions:

1. Is the patient able to state the nature of his infection and how it occurred?
2. Can the patient explain how to prevent further infection?
3. Can the patient state plans for follow-up care?
4. Can the patient explain his medication regimen?
5. Does the patient remain neurologically intact?

If the patient has motor dysfunction, appropriate questions can be found on p. 382.

Encephalitis

PATHOPHYSIOLOGY

Encephalitis is inflammation of the brain tissues and its covering. Occasionally, the meninges of the spinal cord are also involved. It can have a variety of causes, including the following:

1. Syphilis
2. Exogenous poisoning such as that which follows the ingestion of lead or arsenic or inhalation of carbon monoxide
3. Reaction to toxins produced by infections such as typhoid fever, measles, and chickenpox
4. Reaction to vaccination
5. Various viruses, including arbovirus (those transferred by biting arthropod to humans)

Encephalitis caused by a virus and occurring in epidemic form was first described by von Economo in Austria, and the name *von Economo's disease* is still used to identify the widespread epidemic in the United States that followed the influenza epidemic in 1918. von Economo's disease was also called *sleeping sickness,* a term still used by lay persons. The demonstration that viruses can affect the central nervous system after a prolonged incubation period has resulted in considerable search for viral agents in many chronic neurologic diseases.

ASSESSMENT

The subjective and objective data for encephalitis are the same as for meningitis (p. 409). The onset of encephalitis is often abrupt, with a high fever, headache, meningeal signs, nuchal rigidity, and vomiting. Drowsiness or coma and focal or generalized convulsions usually develop within 24 to 48 hours after onset of symptoms. Focal neurologic signs develop, such as hemiplegia and cranial nerve palsies. There are typical findings in the CSF. Mortality may be as high as 60%.

DATA ANALYSIS AND PLANNING

The reader is referred to these headings in the discussion of meningitis. (p. 409).

IMPLEMENTATION

Nursing care consists of symptomatic or supportive care and careful observation. Any change in appearance or behavior should be reported, because the progress of this disease sometimes is extremely rapid. Bed rest is advocated. If disorientation is present, the patient must be attended constantly. During the time when temperature is increased, sponge baths or other hypothermia methods are used. There is no specific medical treatment for this disease. No isolation is necessary, because encephalitis is not transmitted from person to person. Prevention of arboviral infections includes destruction of larvae and elimination of breeding places. Control includes avoiding bites of the mosquito or tick vectors.

EVALUATION

Evaluation includes those questions defined under the evaluation section of meningitis (p. 410).

Brain abscess

A brain abscess is almost always secondary to a foci of infection somewhere else in the body. Common sites of the primary infection include the following:

1. Ear
2. Sinus or mastoid
3. Lung
4. Heart
5. Pelvic organs
6. Teeth
7. Skin

The three most common organisms involved are the streptococci, staphylococci, and pneumococci. Brain abscesses are most common in older children and young adults but may be seen at any age.

PATHOPHYSIOLOGY

In the first stage of brain abscess there is a localized inflammation of the brain with formation of exudate. Septic thromboses of some vessels occurs, and the surrounding brain tissue becomes necrotic and edematous. After a time (days to weeks) the inflammatory reaction decreases as the area is walled off. It is not uncommon for "satellite" abscesses to occur and for the abscesses to rupture into the ventricles. Brain abscesses are most commonly found in the temporal lobe and the cerebellum.

ASSESSMENT

The questions to ask in collecting data from the patient with a brain abscess are the same as for the patient with meningitis (p. 409). With a brain abscess, there may be a history of infection. The most common symptom is a constant or intermittent headache that is not relieved by medication and that is increased by straining.

The evolution of symptoms is variable. In some pa-

Symptoms of brain abscess

1. Constant and severe headache
2. Drowsiness
3. Confusion
4. Mental slowness
5. Focal or generalized seizures
6. Fever with bradycardia
7. Signs and symptoms of increased ICP

---

tients there may be a rapid progression of symptoms ending in death, whereas in others the course is more benign. Generally, however, the mortality is high with brain abscess, and residual disability often results.

Diagnostic tests

The diagnosis of brain abscess is made primarily on the basis of the history and examination of the CSF. EEG changes are present, and there will be areas of increased uptake on the CT scan.

DATA ANALYSIS AND PLANNING

The nursing diagnoses and the expected patient outcomes are the same for the patient with brain abscess as for the patient with meningitis (p. 409).

IMPLEMENTATION

Assisting with the achievement of therapeutic goals

Treatment consists of administering the appropriate antibiotics, often for extended periods of time. Combined antibiotics along with broad-spectrum antibiotics may be used. Agents to reduce ICP may be necessary. Ongoing assessment for signs and symptoms of increased ICP is important. These patients often must undergo long hospitalizations and periods of treatment; as a result, they may need a great deal of psychologic support.

Poliomyelitis

Poliomyelitis is an acute febrile disease caused by poliomyelitis virus types 1, 2, and 3. Paralysis is more common with type 1. With discovery of the Salk vaccine, its wide use since 1956, and the availability of the Sabin vaccine, this disease has become quite rare. At one time it was a serious crippler of children and young adults.

PATHOPHYSIOLOGY

The incubation period for poliomyelitis is from 7 to 21 days. The virus attacks the anterior horn cells of the spinal cord where the motor pathways are located and may cause motor paralysis. Sensory perception is not af-

fected, because posterior horn cells are not attacked. Poliomyelitis sometimes takes a somewhat different form and attacks primarily the medulla and basal structures of the brain, including the cranial nerves. This is called *bulbar paralysis*. If the medulla is involved, the patient may need respiratory assistance.

Guillain-Barré-Strohl syndrome (polyneuritis)

Guillian-Barré-Strohl syndrome is also known as acute inflammatory polyradiculoneuropathy and postinfectious polyneuritis. It is often serious because of the extent to which the nervous system is involved. The condition has become better known to the public since it was identified as a sequela of swine flu immunization. The disease is most common in persons aged 30 to 50 and is seen equally in men and woman. The cause is unknown, but it is thought to be either a viral agent or a result of an autoimmune reaction.

PATHOPHYSIOLOGY

With this disease there is patchy demyelination in peripheral nerves, nerve roots, root ganglia, and spinal cord. Axons are generally spared so recovery may occur early.

There may be variations in the pattern of onset of weakness as well as in the rate of progression of symptoms. The progression may stop at any point. If cranial nerves VII, IX, and X are involved, the patient may have difficulty in swallowing, speaking, and breathing. The vital centers in the medulla may be affected. Patients often recover fully, although a year or more may elapse before the patient is fully recovered.

ASSESSMENT

For appropriate subjective and objective data see the assessment of the patient with meningitis (p. 409). With Guillain-Barré syndrome there is symmetric muscle weakness and lower motor neuron paralysis (flaccidity). The paralysis usually starts in the lower extremities and ascends upward to include the thorax, upper extremities, and the face. Paresthesias may occur. Respiratory failure is possible as intercostal muscles are affected—without mechanical ventilation there is a 10% to 20% mortality. The bowel and bladder are rarely affected. Autonomic symptoms, such as fluctuating blood pressure, also occur.

DATA ANALYSIS AND PLANNING

See section on the patient with meningitis (p. 409).

IMPLEMENTATION

Assisting with achievement of therapeutic goals

A priority goal is the maintenance of respiratory function. Close observation of respiratory function is necessary. This should include serial measurements of the patient's vital capacity, tidal volume, and minute volume. Patients who develop respiratory failure require mechanical ventilation. Adrenocortical steroids are used at times to treat symptoms. Convalescence may require many months. Attention to the prevention of iatrogenic complications such as contracture, decubitus ulcers, muscle atrophy, and loss of range of motion is imperative to allow complete recovery.

Neurosyphilis
PATHOPHYSIOLOGY

In the late or chronic stage of syphilis, infection may involve the brain and spinal cord. The oculomotor nerves may be involved, causing inability of the pupil to react to light *(Argyll Robertson pupil)*. *Tabes dorsalis* is the name given to the involvement of the posterior columns of the spinal cord and the posterior nerve roots. Sensory symptoms predominate. The patient may have severe paroxysmal pain anywhere in the body, the most common location being in the stomach (gastric crisis). There may be areas of severe paresthesia. A common finding in tabes dorsalis is loss of position sense in the feet and legs. The patient is unable to sense where the feet are placed resulting in a highly characteristic slapping gait. There is increased difficulty walking in the dark, because the person relies on vision in placing the feet. Visual loss or blindness also can occur. Tabes dorsalis can cause trophic changes in the joints so that stability is lost *(Charcot's joint)*.

General paresis is the term used to designate another late manifestation of syphilis in which there is degeneration of the brain and deterioration of mental function, as well as evidence of other neurologic disease.

Herpes zoster

Herpes zoster, also known as shingles, is a common disease occurring at higher rates among the old and in patients with lymphomas, cancer, and Hodgkin's disease.

PATHOPHYSIOLOGY

The causative organism is the varicella virus, similar to the one that causes herpes simplex. It may occur as a result of a reactivation of the viral infection that lies dormant in the ganglion following a primary case of chickenpox. It is not communicable, except to persons who have not had chickenpox. There is an acute inflammatory reaction in the spinal or cranial sensory ganglions, the posterior gray matter of the cord, and the meninges.

ASSESSMENT

The subjective and objective data to be collected for a patient with herpes zoster is the same as for the patient with meningitis (p. 409). In addition, the objective data should include whether a rash is present.

The rash seen in herpes zoster consists of a vesicular, cutaneous eruption within a dermatome. It may be preceded by severe itching, pain in the area, fever, and malaise. There may be segmental weakness and atrophy in the same area as the sensory changes. A small percentage of patients present with ophthalmic herpes, with the rash and pain occurring along the distribution of the trigeminal nerve.

DATA ANALYSIS AND EXPECTED PATIENT OUTCOMES

The reader is referred to the sections under meningitis (p. 409).

IMPLEMENTATION

Assisting with the achievement of therapeutic goals

Treatment for herpes zoster consists mainly of supportive care with medication for control of pain. The pain may persist for some time after the rash disappears. Phenytoin (Dilantin) and carbamazerine (Tegretol) may be helpful for control of persistent pain. Steroid therapy started early in the disease course is believed to shorten the course but is not recommended for patients with suppressed immune responses. Special emphasis on rest, nutrition, and hydration during the acute period is important.

Control of environment

Isolation may be necessary for staff who have not had chickenpox. This is especially true for the pregnant employee. Also, patients with malignancies, lymphomas, or Hodgkin's disease who have not had chickenpox should be protected from exposure to the patient.

Because the virus is spread by direct contact and airborne routes, strict isolation is often necessary, at least until drainage from any lesions stop. The protective measures are listed in box below.

Isolation measures for herpes zoster

1. Private room with private toilet facilities
2. Gown, masks, and gloves required of care givers
3. Strict hand washing
4. Linen handled as isolation linen
5. Double-bagging of dressings
6. Disposable dishes if possible
7. Transport patients only as necessary
8. Isolation procedure for visitors

INTERFERENCE WITH FUNCTION BECAUSE OF TRAUMA

Interference with neurologic function can occur as a result of trauma. Parts of the nervous system commonly subjected to trauma include the craniocerebrum, the spinal cord, and the peripheral nerves. Traumatic lesions usually result from direct physical force or from sustained compression.

Craniocerebral trauma

Craniocerebral trauma, or head injury, causes death and serious disability in people of all ages. Head injury is the second most common cause of major neurologic deficits and the major cause of death between ages 1 and 35. Brain injury causes more deaths than does injury to any other organ. In some states the repeal of laws requiring motorcyclists to wear helmets has resulted in an estimated threefold increase in death and injury resulting from damage to the brain sustained in motorcyle accidents.

PATHOPHYSIOLOGY

Craniocerebral trauma may result in injury to the scalp, skull, and brain tissues, either singly or collectively. Some of the variables that may modify the extent of the injury to the head include the following:
1. Location and direction of the impact
2. Rate of the energy transfer
3. Surface area of the energy transfer
4. Status of the head at the time of the impact

Injuries vary from minor scalp wounds to concussions and open fractures of the skull with severe damage to the brain. The amount of obvious damage is not indicative of the seriousness of the trouble.

The skull indents and deforms when a physical impact occurs. Fractures commonly result, and they are classified as they are in other parts of the body.

Fractures can occur distal to the point of impact. The presence of a skull fracture does not necessarily indicate that brain injury has occurred, although *compound* and *depressed skull fractures* often cause serious complications. There is often a reverse correlation between skull damage and brain damage.

Fractures at the base of the skull are usually serious because of their location. When one is sustained, vital centers, cranial nerves, and nerve pathways may be permanently damaged. Trauma and the resulting edema may obstruct cerebrospinal fluid flow directly or indirectly, with resultant increased intracranial pressure. If the injury has caused a direct communication between the cranial cavity and the middle ear or the sinuses, meningitis or a brain abscess may develop. Bleeding from the nose and ears suggests a basal fracture. Serosanguineous drainage from these orifices may contain cerebrospinal fluid and should be noted.

The dura may remain intact in cerebral trauma and brain damage and is thought of as a closed head injury. If the dura is opened from a direct blow or from penetrating objects such as bone fragments, the injury is classified as an open head injury.

The effect of a blow on the cranium to the brain tissues within the skull is one of sudden movement. This effect can be likened to what happens as one stops suddenly when moving quickly with an open dish of fluid—some of the fluid spills. The only difference is that instead of spilling in the closed cavity, the brain tissue strikes the bony covering forcibly, causing a coup (at the site) or contrecoup (opposite the site) lesion.

Damage to the brain tissues may include concussion, contusion, or laceration. See the box below for a comparison of these injuries.

Lacerations of the scalp bleed profusely because of its

Damage of brain tissue caused by trauma

	Characteristics	Structural alteration	Effects
Concussion	Characterized by immediate and transitory impairment of neurologic function caused by mechanical force	No	May be loss of consciousness that is instant or delayed—usually reversible
Contusion	Likened to bruising with extravasation of blood cells	Yes	Injury may be at site of impact or at opposite site Often damage to cortex
Laceration	Tearing of tissues caused by sharp fragment or shearing force	Yes	Hemorrhage is serious complication

large blood supply. Hemorrhage resulting from craniocerebral trauma may occur at the following sites:

1. Scalp
2. Epidural
3. Subdural
4. Intracerebral
5. Intraventricular

Two of these, *epidural* and *subdural hematomas,* require careful and continuous observation by the nurse and pose special problems to the patient with a head injury. Epidural hematomas form as blood collects rapidly between the dura and skull. Bleeding in this area is commonly caused by laceration of the middle meningeal artery, which is capable of producing rapid clot formation. Common sites for bleeding include sites of basal and temporal skull fractures. If lethargy or unconsciousness develops after the patient regains consciousness, an epidural hematoma may be suspected. Bleeding needs to be controlled promptly and the blood evacuated.

A subdural hematoma forms as venous blood collects below the dural surface. Because the bleeding is under venous pressure, the hematoma formation is relatively slow. The clot formation will, however, cause pressure on the brain surface and may eventually displace brain tissue. If the expanding clot is not evacuated it can cause increased ICP with compression of vital areas. The focal neurologic signs of clot formation are related to the site of the clot. If a patient who has been conscious for several days to weeks after a head injury becomes unconscious or develops neurologic symptoms, a *subdural hematoma* should be suspected.

Most deaths from head injury are from cerebral edema caused by damage rather than the actual primary destruction of vital centers. Brain edema is a major cause of increased ICP. Along with the swelling, local and systemic disturbances in circulation occur with resulting anoxia. The brain damage may be severe and not related to the demonstrated structural damage.

ASSESSMENT
Subjective data

1. Patient's understanding of injury and resulting pathology—also patient's ability to understand
2. Information about nature of the injury—how it happened
3. Presence of headache, nausea, or vomiting
4. Presence of diplopia or other visual problems
5. Unusual sensations (paresthesias, ringing in ears)
6. History of bleeding from ear, nose, eye, or mouth
7. History of loss of consciousness

Objective data

1. Respiratory status (presence of patent airway, need for suctioning, need for intubation and mechanical ventilation)
2. Arterial blood gases
3. Level of consciousness and alertness
4. Pupils: size, equality, reactivity

5. Orientation
6. Motor status
7. Vital signs
8. Presence of bleeding
9. Presence of vomiting
10. Speech patterns—abnormalities

Because many persons with head injury, especially from motor vehicle accidents, have sustained other injuries, the intrathoracic and intraabdominal areas are checked carefully and the limbs are examined for fractures and injuries to nerves or arteries.

Diagnostic tests

Diagnostic tests performed for patients with head injury include skull x-ray films, CT scan, and possibly cerebral angiography. These procedures were described earlier in this chapter.

DATA ANALYSIS AND PLANNING
Nursing diagnoses

Possible nursing diagnoses for a patient with a head injury include the following:

Airway clearance: ineffective
Anxiety
Bowel elimination, alteration in: incontinence
Breathing pattern, ineffective
Comfort, alteration in: pain
Communication, impaired verbal
Gas exchange, impaired
Knowledge deficit
Mobility, impaired physical
Self-care deficit: feeding, bathing/hygiene, dressing/grooming, toileting
Sensory perceptual alteration: visual
Skin integrity, impairment of: potential
Thought processes, alteration in
Tissue perfusion, alteration in: cerebral
Urinary elimination, alteration in patterns

Expected patient outcomes

Expected patient outcomes for the patient with a head injury include the following:

1. ICP is kept within safe limits.
2. A patent airway and adequate gas exchange are maintained.
3. Patient makes progress toward independence in ADL.
4. Patient can safely compensate for visual field cuts and perceptual, motor, and sensory losses.
5. Patient can explain prescribed therapy to follow at home.
6. Patient can demonstrate exercises to maintain function.
7. Patient can demonstrate ability to comunicate within disease process restrictions.
8. Patient can explain homegoing medication regimen—side effects, desired effects, time, dose, and route.

9. Patient can explain how to obtain assistance from community agencies.
10. Patient can state plans for follow-up care.
11. Patient can explain importance of frequent position changes and demonstrate such positioning.
12. Skin remains clear.

IMPLEMENTATION

Assisting with the achievement of therapeutic goals

Immediate care is directed toward lifesaving measures and the maintenance of normal body function until the time when recovery is assured. The major aims of medical and nursing management are as follows:

1. To be constantly alert for changes in the patient's condition, especially changes that indicate any increase in ICP
2. To sustain the patient's vital functions until recovery allows the functions to resume
3. To manage complications that will be life threatening and interfere with full recovery

Respiratory care

It is extremely important to maintain a patent airway and ensure adequate oxygenation. Anoxia with a buildup of carbon dioxide can produce cerebral hypoxia and subsequent cerebral edema. It is important to assess the ability to clear the airway. Blood or mucus from injuries may block the airway, or the patient may have vomited and suctioning may be necessary. Inability to clear the airway can lead to airway obstruction as well as aspiration pneumonia. Oxygen should be given to the patient with a head injury, and if the patient cannot clear the airway an endotracheal tube should be used. Arterial blood gas levels are checked frequently to determine whether respiratory exchange is adequate. Suctioning should be done as necessary.

Rest and control of convulsions

The patient should be kept as quiet as possible. No vigorous effort should be made to "clean the patient up" during the first few hours after the accident. Side rails should always be on the bed, because restlessness may come on suddenly or convulsions may occur. The head of the bed is usually elevated 30 degrees. Restlessness may be caused by the need for a change of position, pain, or the need to empty the bladder. Codeine or other analgesics that do not depress the respiratory system are used for pain control. Anticonvulsants may be given to prevent seizures.

Vital signs and temperature control

The blood pressure, pulse, and respiratory rate are taken frequently until they have stabilized and remain within safe limits. A sudden sharp rise in temperature, which may go to 42° C or higher, and a sudden drop in blood pressure indicate that the regulatory mechanisms have lost control. The prognosis is poor. Measures are used to reduce temperature to normal, because hyper-

thermia causes increased brain metabolism. These measures include the following:

1. Administration of aspirin
2. Tepid sponge baths
3. Ice bags to the groin and axilla
4. Reduction of temperature in patient's room
5. Electrically controlled cooling mattress

Prevention of infection

The patient's ears and nose are checked carefully for signs of blood and serous drainage which would indicate that the meninges have been torn and that spinal fluid is escaping. No attempt should be made to clean out the orifices. Loose sterile cotton may be placed in the outer openings only. This procedure is performed with caution so that the cotton does not act as a plug to interfere with the free flow of fluid. The cotton should be changed whenever it becomes moist. If there is evidence of drainage of CSF from the nose, the patient should not cough, sneeze, or blow the nose. These activities may enable air to enter the cranial cavity where it may increase symptoms of increased ICP. If there is question about whether drainage from the nose is CSF a Tes-Tape will show a positive sugar reaction.

Meningitis is a possible complication when communication with the nose and ears occurs. With basal skull fracture, antibiotics are commonly used because of the high rate of infection following this type of fracture.

Medications

Medications are used to reduce cerebral edema and increased ICP, which are common problems in patients with head injuries. These medications include the following:

1. Osmotic diuretics that penetrate the brain slowly
   a. 30% solution of urea
   b. 20% mannitol
2. Dexamethasone

If the patient is receiving one of the diuretics and is not alert, a Foley catheter should be inserted to enable accurate accounting of output. Large amounts of urine can be anticipated.

Electrolyte balance

Careful monitoring of electrolytes is necessary. Several types of imbalance may occur with a head injury including the following:

1. Natriuresis (increased urinary excretion of sodium)
2. Inappropriate ADH syndrome (increased plasma levels of ADH, serum hyponatremia, and hypotonicity)
3. Hypernatremia
4. Cerebral sodium retention
5. Elevated plasma cortisol levels

Inappropriate ADH with large urinary output is usually treated with fluid restriction and sodium.

Elimination

The patient's intake and output should be carefully measured and recorded. The specific gravity of the urine is also measured and can yield clues to electrolyte imbalance. In acute situations these measurements are done hourly.

The urinary output should be approximately 0.6 to 1 ml/kg of body weight/hour. If osmotic diuretics have been given, this amount will be greater. An indwelling catheter may be necessary; appropriate measures should be used to prevent infection. The person with cranial trauma should also be assessed for symptoms of diabetes insipidus, a common occurrence.

Bowel function is not encouraged for several days following a head injury. Mild bulk laxatives, bisacodyl suppositories, or oil-retention enemas may be used. The patient is taught not to strain at stool. When the patient is receiving dexamethasone or other steroids it is important to check the stool for the presence of occult blood. This will also give a clue to the presence of stress ulcers, which are somewhat common after head injury. The ulcers are apparently caused by autonomic imbalances associated with the injury. Cimetidine (Tagamet) and antacids are routinely given if the patient with a closed head injury is receiving steroids.

Assisting with comfort and ADL
Emotional support

It is not uncommon that the patient with a head injury manifests loss of memory and loss of initiative. Behavioral problems associated with lack of judgment and restlessness may also occur. These patients need firm but gentle care, with specific guidelines for what behavior is allowed. The patient and family need to have gains in functioning pointed out, as it is easy to become frustrated and depressed when progress is slow.

Resumption of activities

The length of convalescence will depend on the amount of brain damage and how rapid the recovery has been. Patients are usually urged to resume normal activity as soon as possible. Headache and dizziness may be present for some time following a head injury. Some persons require intensive rehabilitation in a rehabilitation center. Recovery from head injury is most likely in those under age 20. Persons between the ages of 20 and 50 who remain in a coma longer than 2 weeks may not recover function.

Some patients are left with serious deficits that include hemiplegia. The nursing care of these patients is described in the section on patients who have had a stroke (p. 404).

Teaching

Patients with head injury may be seen in an emergency room but not admitted to the hospital. These patients need teaching about observations for complications. A sample set of instructions is found in the box below.

Teaching for the patient with a head injury who is left with deficits severe enough to require extended rehabilitation is similar to that for the patient with a motor problem. See p. 383 for a description of this teaching.

In addition, the following points are important:
1. Causes of increased ICP
2. Factors that can increase or decrease intracranial pressure
   a. No sneezing
   b. No heavy lifting, bending or straining
   c. No straining at stool
3. Signs and symptoms to report to the physician

EVALUATION

Evaluation of the patient with a head injury is based on the expected patient outcomes. Questions to ask include the following:
1. Are there symptoms of increased ICP?

Instructions for patient with a head injury

Patient should be awakened periodically through the first 24 hours to be sure he or she can wake up easily. Also, for the first 24 to 48 hours, the family should watch carefully for the following warning signs:
1. Vomiting—often with force behind it
2. Unusual sleepiness, dizziness, and loss of balance or falling
3. Complaint of seeing two of everything or blurry objects, jerking movement of the eyes.
4. Bleeding or discharge from nose or ears.
5. A slight headache may be expected; however, if it gets worse and the patient complains of feeling even worse when moving about, it should be reported
6. Convulsions (fits)—any twitching or movements of arms or legs that the patient is not able to stop
7. Any behavior or symptom that is not normal for the individual

Call a doctor at once if any of these signs are observed by the family
Call either your personal physician or the emergency services.

Courtesy Department of Nursing, University Hospital of Cleveland.

2. Is the patient able to carry on ADL as well as possible?
3. Does the patient carry on these activities safely?
4. Can the patient verbalize therapy program and demonstrate exercises?
5. Is the patient taking medication accurately?
6. Is the patient involved with community support as needed?
7. Is patient attending follow-up appointments?
8. Is skin intact?
9. Are joints freely mobile?

Because some patients with head injuries are mentally impaired, involvement of the family is important.

Spinal cord trauma

Spinal cord injury from accidents is a common and increasing cause of serious disability and death in the United States. Automobile, motorcycle, diving, surfing, and other athletic accidents and gunshot wounds are major causes of spinal cord injuries.

PATHOPHYSIOLOGY

The spinal cord may be damaged by lesions arising outside the cord or by intramedullary lesions. Intramedullary lesions are a less common cause and are usually the result of intramedullary tumors. Various types of lesions arising outside the cord eventually cause damage within it and compression of the cord (Fig. 20-16). (The word *lesion* here includes both disease and injury.) The anatomy and size of the spinal cord subject it to compression with even

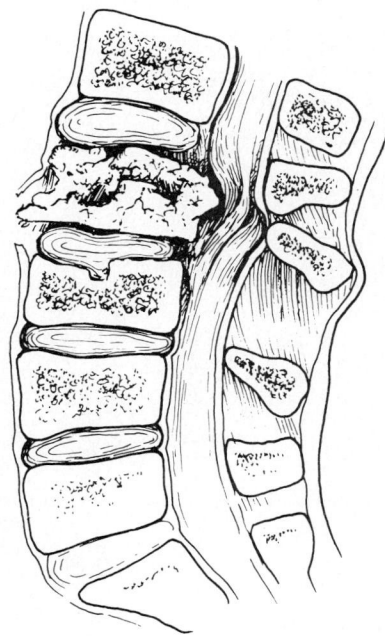

Fig. 20-16. Damage to spinal cord and distortion of adjacent structures that may occur in traumatic injuries to spine.

minimal inward encroachment. Edema then forms and contributes more to cord compression. With damage to any part of the vertebral column, the cord itself becomes more vulnerable to damage.

Severe traumatic lesions of the spinal cord may result in total transection of the spinal cord or a tearing of the cord from side to side at a particular level, with a complete loss of spinal cord functions. This total transection is also referred to as a "complete cord injury." With the complete injury there is loss of all voluntary movement below the level of the lesion. A partial transection or "incomplete injury" involves a partial transection or injury of the cord. The symptoms of incomplete injuries can vary depending on the nature of the injury and the resultant syndrome. Resultant syndromes can include the following:

1. Anterior cord syndrome
2. Central cord syndrome
3. Brown-Séquard syndrome
4. Conus medullaris syndrome
5. Cauda equina syndrome

See a neurologic text for further description of these syndromes.

Initially, in most spinal cord injuries there is a period of flaccid paralysis and a complete loss of reflexes. This is called spinal or neural shock, or areflexia, and it is a transitory event. During this period persons may require temporary respiratory assistance until recovery begins.

Within hours, days, or weeks the involved muscles gradually become spastic and hyperreflexic with the characteristic signs of an upper motor neuron lesion. These changes are thought to represent the release of the muscle stretch reflexes from the inhibitory influence of the damaged pyramidal tract, resulting in hyperactive responses.

The amount of disability that results from spinal cord injury is dependent on the level of injury. See the box on p. 418 below for specifics of muscle function following spinal cord injury.

Voiding

The center for micturition is located in the conus medullaris (S2-S4) and is linked to the detrusor muscle of the bladder by parasympathetic sensory and motor fibers that run in the pelvic nerves. Levels above the conus result in a bladder that is capable of emptying itself reflexly or involuntarily after the spinal shock phase. The bladder is hypertonic and it is variously known as an "upper motor neuron bladder" and "reflex neurogenic bladder." The emptying occurs spontaneously or automatically. The patient has no control over the act of micturition. Voiding may occur at intervals of 3 to 4 hours; there may be frequency, urgency, and incontinence. The reflex arc is intact in this type bladder. When the cord lesion is at or below the micturition center, there is destruction of the center or the sacral nerve roots; the reflex arc is no longer intact. This type of bladder condition is known as a "lower motor neuron bladder" or an "autonomous neurogenic bladder." Contractions of the bladder muscle

Muscle function after spinal cord injury

Spinal cord injury	Muscle function remaining	Muscle function lost
Cervical above C4	None	All, including respiration
C5	Neck	Arms
	Scapular elevation	Chest
		All below chest
C6-C7	Neck	Some arm, fingers
	Some chest movement	Some chest
	Some arm movement	All below chest
Thoracic	Neck	Trunk
	Arms (full)	All below chest
	Some chest	
Lumbosacral	Neck	Legs
	Arms	
	Chest	
	Trunk	

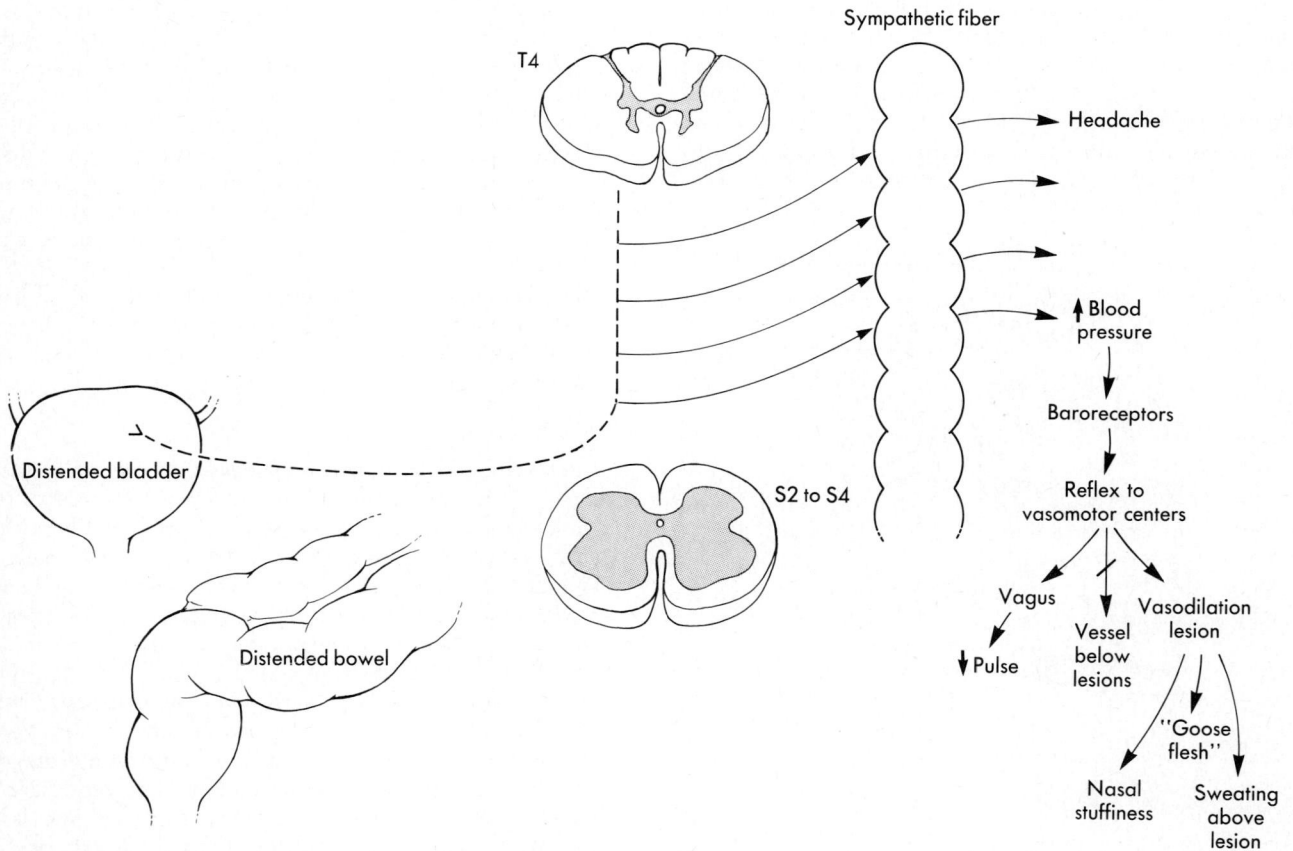

Fig. 20-17. Pictorial diagram of cause of automomic hyperflexia and results.

are the result of impulses transmitted through a mechanism within the bladder wall but are not of sufficient strength or duration to empty the bladder. Abdominal straining or manual compression is necessary for this to happen. Retention of urine and infection are common complications.

Autonomic dysreflexia

One complication of spinal cord injury that is extremely important to understand is autonomic dysreflexia. It occurs in patients with cord lesions above the sixth thoracic vertebra and most commonly in patients with cervical injuries (Fig. 20-17). The clinical signs include the following:

1. Bradycardia
2. Paroxysmal hypertension
3. Sweating
4. "Goose flesh"
5. Severe headache
6. Nasal stuffiness

Patients tend to develop individual symptoms of this condition and are soon able to recognize them.

The most common cause is visceral distention, which can include a distended bladder or impacted rectum. It is a medical emergency that requires immediate treatment, because it can lead to cerebrovascular accident, blindness or death. Treatment is discussed later in this chapter (p. 422).

Sexual function

In most cases, men experience impotence, decreased sensation, and difficulties with ejaculation. Impairment of fertility is common. The act of erection is under the control of sensory and parasympathetic fibers, while ejaculation requires sympathetic and parasympathetic innervation. Lesions above S2 leave the parasympathetic reflex arc intact; patients may be able to have an erection, but ejaculation is not usually possible. Lesions in the S2 to S4 area usually prevent erection and ejaculation. The higher the level of injury, the more likely a man with complete cord injury is able to perform sexually. The experience of orgasm is described as different than before the injury. Women with spinal cord injury are able to continue to perform sexually, although perception of sexual pleasure is usually altered.

ASSESSMENT

Assessment of the patient with spinal cord injury includes both subjective and objective data.

Subjective data

1. Patient's understanding of injury and resulting deficit
2. Information about nature of injury—how it happened
3. Presence of dyspnea
4. Unusual sensations (paresthesias, and so on)
5. History of loss of consciousness
6. Presence of pain
7. Absence of sensation—sensory level

Objective data

1. Respiratory status
2. Level of alertness and consciousness
3. Orientation
4. Pupil size, equality, and reactivity
5. Proper alignment of body in neutral alignment
6. Motor strength
7. Temperature, blood pressure, and pulse
8. Skin integrity
9. Bowel and bladder status and distention

As with the patient with a head injury, the patient with a spinal cord injury should be assessed carefully for the presence of other injuries, primarily fractures or head injury.

Diagnostic tests

It is most important to first detect if there has been any cervical vertebra fracture or displacement. X-ray films are always taken to detect any fracture-dislocations. These often occur before the patient is moved from the backboard or stretcher. Myelography may also be done to detect blockage. It can be carried out also without moving the patient if the dye is injected at the junction between the first cervical vertebra and the base of the skull. CT scanning may also be very helpful in ruling out spinal cord injury. These procedures were discussed earlier in this chapter.

DATA ANALYSIS AND PLANNING

Nursing diagnoses

Possible nursing diagnoses for the patient with spinal cord injury include the following:

Anxiety

Bowel elimination, alteration in: incontinence

Breathing pattern, ineffective

Comfort, alteration in: pain

Gas exchange, impaired

Home maintenance management, impaired

Knowledge deficit

Mobility, impaired physical

Self-care deficit: feeding, bathing/hygiene, dressing/grooming, toileting

Sensory perceptual alteration: tactile

Sexual dysfunction

Skin integrity, impairment of: actual or potential

Urinary elimination, alteration in patterns

Expected patient outcomes

The expected patient outcomes for a patient with spinal cord injury include the following:

1. Function is preserved to the extent possible—no increase in level of injury.
2. Vital functions such as respirations are compensated for until the spinal shock phase has passed.
3. Patient makes progress toward independence in ADL.
4. Patient can explain prescribed therapy to follow at home.

5. Patient and/or care giver can demonstrate exercises to maintain function.
6. Patient can explain medication regime—side effects, desired effects, time, dose, and route.
7. Patient can explain plans for follow-up care.
8. Patient can explain how to obtain community resources, including the Bureau of Vocational Rehabilitation.
9. Patient can explain importance of frequent position changes, including weight shifts.
10. Skin remains intact.
11. Patient can demonstrate inspection of skin.
12. Patient can explain need for assisted coughing and have care giver demonstrate.
13. Patient remains free of respiratory complications.
14. Patient can explain bladder program and demonstrate intermittent catheterization if appropriate.
15. Patient can explain bowel program and demonstrate digital stimulation if able.
16. Patient can explain autonomic dysreflexia and actions to be taken when it occurs.

IMPLEMENTATION

Assisting with achievement of therapeutic goals
Immediate stage

CERVICAL INJURIES. Immediate care after spinal cord injury is directed toward realignment of the cervial bony column in the presence of demonstrated fractures or dislocations. These measures include the following:
1. Simple immobilization
2. Skeletal traction
   a. Crutchfield tongs (Fig. 20-18).
   b. Vinke tongs
   c. Virginia tongs
   d. Stryker or Foster frame
3. Surgery for spinal decompression

Often surgical decompression is not performed until after a period of skeletal traction. This allows the patient's condition to stabilize and some initial swelling of the cord to subside. The beginning spontaneous healing of the fracture site provides more stability. With the introduction of the anterior surgical approach to the cervical spinal column, surgical intervention is safer and can be attempted earlier in the hospitalization. The primary advantage of the anterior surgical approach is that it provides immediate stabilization of the spinal cord by techniques of interbody cervical fusion and the direct removal of any extruded disk materials. See the box on p. 421 for care of the patient who has had surgical decompression.

Intubation and respiratory assistance may be required in the immediate stage following upper cervical cord injury. Any patient with a cord lesion at the C4 level probably will demand permanent ventilatory support. Careful monitoring of blood gas levels and regular pulmonary toilet are essential.

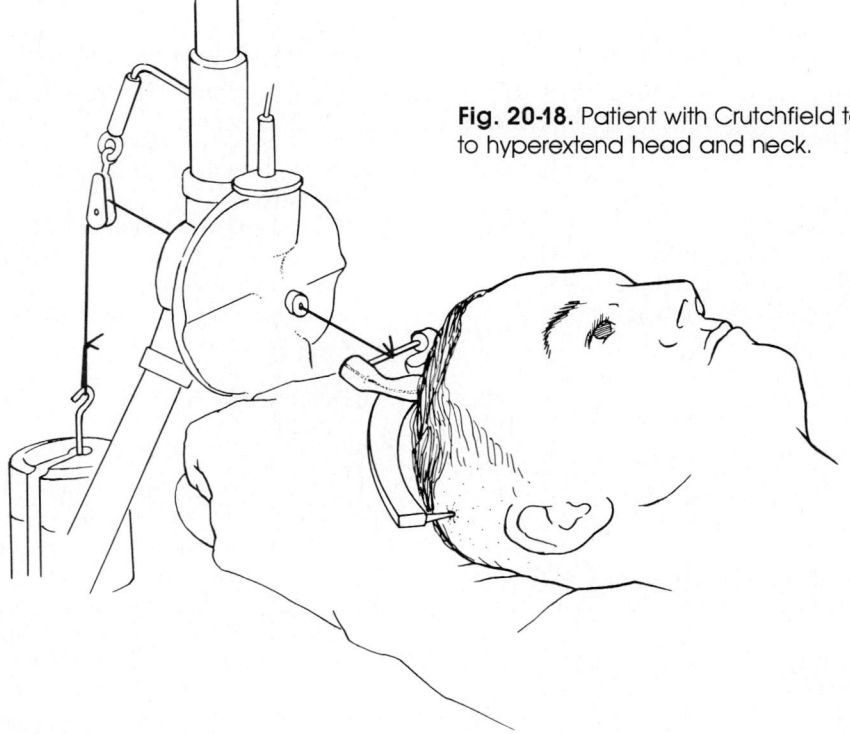

Fig. 20-18. Patient with Crutchfield tongs inserted into skull to hyperextend head and neck.

THORACIC AND LUMBAR INJURIES. Less immediate attention to thoracic and lumbar fracture immobilization is necessary for the patient with limited neurologic deficits. The patient is often treated with bed rest, hyperextension, and bracing. Stabilization of the spine may occur early in the recovery course or may be delayed until some healing has occurred.

MEDICATION

The use of adrenal corticosteroids for the prevention and alleviation of spinal cord edema is widespread. It is felt that the steroids assist in the reestablishment of membrane stability and in the control of central nervous tissue stability.

Intermediate stage

Throughout all stages of hospitalization of the patient with a spinal cord injury, nursing and medical interventions are directed toward restoration of structural or body integrity. All efforts are taken to ensure that the following occur:

1. Skin is intact.
2. Contractures do not develop.
3. Range of motion is maintained to the greatest degree possible.
4. Muscle tone is consistent with pathologic condition.
5. Bowel and bladder function are maintained.

The reader is referred to the section on care of the patient with a motor dysfunction (p. 380). Most of the care described there applies to the patient with a spinal cord injury. Additional care is described here.

POSITION AND MOVEMENT. In addition to frequent positioning, the patient with a spinal cord injury is usually placed on a bed with a firm surface or may even be placed on a Foster or Stryker frame. The physician should supervise moving of the patient and actually support the head and neck during the transfer. If at all possible, portable x-ray examinations and procedures should be done to minimize movement of the patient.

Care of the patient undergoing spinal decompression

Preoperative care

1. Clarify patient's knowledge of surgery and expected changes.
2. Explain expected postoperative measures (including positioning, bed rest).
3. Encourage patient and family to verbalize fears.
4. Baseline neurologic and physiologic data should be assessed and recorded.

Postoperative care

1. Monitoring
   a. Assess ability to move legs; ask patient to do straight leg raises, dorsiflexion, and plantar flexion. Assess ability to move arms and hands if cervical decompression has occurred.
   b. Assess degree and character of drainage.
      (1) Amount of drainage and bleeding should be minimal.
      (2) Initial dressing can be reinforced as needed.
   c. Assess ability of patient to swallow; observe for swelling of neck.
2. Promoting mobility
   a. Patient can be turned side to side and onto back.
   b. If decompression is in lumbar area, sitting is usually not permitted.
   c. If decompression is in thoracic area, patient should not use arms to pull or push; no trapeze on bed.
   d. Patient is encouraged to do active range of motion and leg exercises such as quadriceps setting.
3. Promoting psychologic comfort
   a. Patient is encouraged to verbalize fears and reactions once tissue diagnosis is in.
   b. Time should be spent with patient other than when giving direct care.
   c. Information about daily activities, tests, and procedures should be shared with patient.
   d. Medicate as needed for pain.
4. Preventing infection
   a. Incisional area kept clean and dry.
   b. Temperature checked frequently for first several days; report any elevation to physician.
   c. Report any redness, drainage, or hardness of wound.
   d. Incision often left open to air after first several days.

Care of the patient with autonomic dysreflexia

1. Place patient in sitting position to decrease blood pressure.
2. Check patency of catheter for kinking. If catheter is plugged, insert new catheter immediately.
3. Check rectum for impaction.
4. If it is necessary to remove impaction, dibucaine (Nupercaine ointment) should be instilled in the rectum for its anesthetic effect.
5. Send urine for culture if no other cause is found; urinary infection can lead to symptoms of autonomic dysreflexia.
6. Administer ganglionic blocking agent such as hexamethonium chloride or a vasodilator such as nitroprusside (Nipride) if conservative measures are not effective.

Early mobilization of the patient is important. When patients, especially quadriplegics, begin to sit up, it may be necessary to wrap their legs with Ace wraps to encourage venous return. Slowly increasing the angle of sitting is essential to prevent hypotension. For this reason a newly quadriplegic patient should use a recliner wheelchair until he or she is able to sit at a 90-degree angle for several hours.

Before the patient is permitted to be up following a spinal injury, a brace may be prescribed. All braces and corsets must be custom made; they are usually expensive, and the cost is dependent on the type of material used. The brace or corset should be applied before the patient gets out of bed. The patient should wear a thin, knitted undershirt next to the skin to keep the brace clean and to protect the skin. For some paraplegics, leg braces may permit them to stand and ambulate. Many find, however, that the effort to walk is not justified.

Urinary elimination

Since there is no sensation of needing to void in the patient with spinal cord injury, distention occurs easily. Usually a Foley catheter is inserted initially. Later, bladder training is started. Measures important in this training can be found in Chapter 33.

The presence of an indwelling catheter makes the patient highly susceptible to urinary infection. The best means of preventing infection is maintenance of fluid intake (3 to 4 liters a day) and meticulous aseptic technique. Drinking cranberry juice several times a day has been found helpful in preventing infection, along with prophylactic antibiotic therapy such as nitrofurantoin or sulfamethoxazole and trimethoprim (Septra, Bactrim).

Autonomic dysreflexia is one complication associated with urinary elimination in the patient with spinal cord injury. It is a medical emergency, and the nurse should be aware of the actions to take in preventing and alleviating the symptoms. The care required with the presence of symptoms is outlined above.

Bowel elimination

Patients are started on a bowel program early in the recovery period. At first, bisacodyl (Dulcolax) supposito- ries are given at regular intervals—usually every other night. This is followed by digital stimulation to further stimulate peristalsis. The goal is to eliminate the need for the suppositories. Other aids to bowel programs are the use of adequate fluids, stool softeners, and prune juice.

TEACHING

Teaching of the patient with spinal cord injury encompasses all of the points covered in teaching the patient with a motor dysfunction (p. 383) and sensory dysfunction (p. 384). In addition, the patient needs assistance in learning about the effects of their injury on sexual functioning. The important thought to keep in mind is that most patients with a cooperative partner are able to engage in a satisfying sexual relationship. The limitation depends on the site of the lesion and whether the cord injury is complete or incomplete. Generally, the higher the lesion, the more normal sexual function is likely to be. Patients with sacral lesions are the only patients with spinal cord injuries who are not able to have an erection and ejaculate. Education of the patient in terms of sexual function includes the points outlined here.

EVALUATION

The evaluation of the care of the patient with spinal cord injury is the same as that for the patient with a motor dysfunction (p. 382).

Peripheral nerve trauma

The peripheral nerves that lie outside the brain and spinal cord include the cranial nerves and spinal nerves and their branches and plexuses. The disorders involving the peripheral nerves are similar to those that affect the central nervous system and are the result of traumatic, degenerative, vascular, inflammatory, neoplastic, and metabolic causes. Important terms are found here.

Traumatic causes of peripheral nerve injuries include gunshot and knife wounds, fragmented fracture wounds, and surgical transections, as in denervation surgery and amputation. They result in stretching, laceration, and

---

Sexual functioning in patients with spinal cord injury

1. Reflexogenic erections occur not only as a result of stimulation of the genitalia, but also result from stimulation of "trigger points."
   a. Stroking the thigh
   b. Stimulating the rectum with a finger
   c. Manipulating the catheter
2. Male patients with catheters can either remove the catheter just before sexual activity or turn it back on the penis where it provides extra support.
3. Bowels should be emptied before intercourse to prevent incontinence.
4. Women patients who have a catheter can keep it in place if desired.
5. Women patients should realize that they maintain the ability to conceive—birth control should be practiced if pregnancy is not desired.

Common terminology with peripheral nerve trauma

Neuropathies	Noninflammatory disorders
Mononeuropathy	Disorder affecting one peripheral nerve
Polyneuropathy	Disorder involving multiple nerves
Neuritis	Inflammatory disorder
Neuralgia	Painful nerve disorder

compression of the peripheral nerve. The degree of injury is variable. Recovery is also variable—axons of peripheral nerves are capable of regeneration under favorable conditions.

PATHOPHYSIOLOGY

Following trauma (or disease) the axon undergoes secondary or *wallerian degeneration* distal to the lesion and for several segments proximal. The axon and myelin sheath degenerate and undergo fragmentation. The fragmented particles are completely ingested within several weeks; the axis cylinder remains. Schwann's cells and fibroblasts begin to proliferate, covering the degenerated fibers. During the regenerative phase, new axoplasm forms at the proximal edge of the injury and the regenerating fibers now grow distally and enter the empty neurolemmal sheath, which has in the meantime proliferated. Myelin then forms around the regenerated axon. When a nerve has been severely damaged and fibrous tissue is abundant, regeneration is interfered with by a tangled mass known as a traumatic neuroma; this may have to be removed surgically.

ASSESSMENT

Assessment includes both subjective and objective data.

Subjective data
1. Patient's understanding of condition
2. Alteration in sensation
   a. Pain
   b. Touch
   c. Temperature
   d. Proprioception
3. Site of sensory problem
4. Onset of problem
5. Presence of associated symptoms

Objective data
1. Presence of motor alterations

The clinical signs and symptoms resulting from peripheral nerve lesions depend on the exact location of the lesion and the specific function of the involved nerve or nerves. Because peripheral nerves contain both sensory and motor components, there may be deficits in both components distal to the site. There will be alteration in pain, touch, temperature, proprioception, and stereognosis. Motor alteration includes lower motor neuron signs such as flaccid paralysis and muscle wasting in the muscles innervated by the affected nerves.

DATA ANALYSIS AND PLANNING

The nursing diagnosis and expected patient outcomes are the same as those for the patient who has sensory (p. 384) or motor dysfunction (p. 380).

IMPLEMENTATION

Nursing care is specific to the areas of the body affected by the sensory and motor deficits. Plans for care include measures found in the section on motor dysfunction and sensory dysfunction. Promotion of good health habits in general assists in the creation of conditions favorable to nerve regeneration.

EVALUATION

The evaluation for the patient with peripheral nerve dysfunction is the same as for the patient with motor (p. 382) and sensory problems (p. 385).

Trigeminal neuralgia

Trigeminal neuralgia is one specific kind of peripheral nerve problem. It is also called *tic doloreaux*.

ASSESSMENT

Assessment is basically the same as for any patient with peripheral nerve trauma. Trigeminal neuralgia is characterized by excruciating, burning pain that radiates along one or more of the three divisions of the fifth cranial nerve (Fig. 20-19). The pain typically only extends to the midline of the face and head, because this is the extent of the tissue supplied by the offending nerve. There are areas along the course of the nerve known as trigger points and the slightest stimulation of these areas may initiate pain. Persons with trigeminal neuralgia try desperately to avoid triggering them.

IMPLEMENTATION

Assisting with the achievement of therapeutic goals
Medication

Carbamazapine (Tegretol) is the drug of choice for the treatment of trigeminal neuralgia pain. Drugs such as

nicotinic acid, thiamine chloride, analgesics, and even cobra venom have been tried with little success. Absolute alcohol may be injected into the peripheral branches of the trigeminal nerve. This provides relief for weeks to months.

Surgery

Permanent relief of pain is only obtained by surgery that consists of either inserting a fine needle through the

---

Postoperative concerns for the patient with trigeminal neuralgia

1. Preservation of eye function (if the upper branch is completely severed the corneal reflex is lost)
   a. Eye shield to prevent dust or lint from getting into the cornea
   b. Avoid contact with eye while bathing
   c. Eye baths with methylcellulose solution
   d. Inspect eye several times a day
2. Promoting mouth function (lower branch of fifth cranial nerve)
   a. Avoidance of hot food
   b. Food should be placed in unaffected side of mouth
   c. Mouth care after each meal
3. Safety concerns
   a. Electric razor should be used for shaving

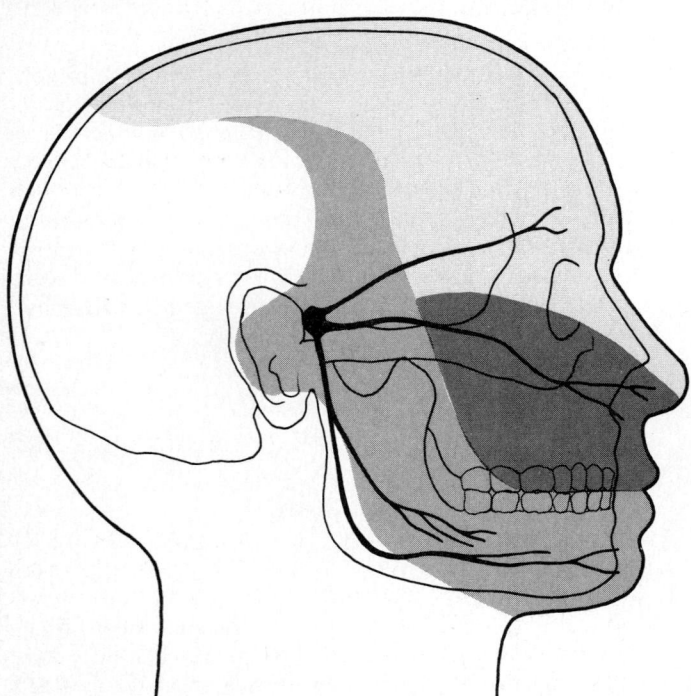

Fig. 20-19. Pathway of trigeminal nerve and facial area innervated by each of three main branches.

cheek or by surgical resection of the sensory root of the trigeminal nerve. This is not always successful. Preoperative care includes the following:

1. Measures of comfort
2. Allowing patient to voice questions or concerns
3. Education about procedure and what to expect

Postoperative care includes the measures listed in box on p. 424.

Within 24 hours after a fifth nerve resection, many patients develop herpes simplex (cold sores) about the lips. Usually the lesions heal in about a week.

Assisting with comfort and ADL

It is not uncommon for patients with trigeminal neuralgia not to have eaten properly for some time, since eating causes pain. They may be undernourished and dehydrated. They may not have washed or shaved or combed the hair for some time. Oral hygiene often has been neglected.

Measures to increase comfort preoperatively or of patients being treated nonsurgically are found in the following box.

Comfort measures for patients with tic doloreaux

1. Keep room free of drafts.
2. Avoid walking briskly to bedside of patient.
3. Place bed out of traffic area to prevent jarring of bed.
4. Avoid touching the patient's face.
5. Patients should not be urged to wash or shave the affected area nor to comb the hair.
6. Avoid hot or cold liquids that trigger pain.
7. Diet may have to be pureed and lukewarm and taken through straw.

Teaching for the patient with trigeminal neuralgia

1. Eye care—frequent inspection and washing with methylcellouse
2. Good oral hygiene
3. Avoidance of hot or cold food or liquids
4. Importance of seeing dentist at frequent intervals—dental caries will not cause pain.
5. Wearing of glasses outdoors to protect eye from dust or flying particles.

Teaching

Teaching of the patient with trigeminal neuralgia are found in the bottom box.

Bell's palsy (peripheral facial paralysis)

PATHOPHYSIOLOGY

Bell's palsy is thought to be caused by an inflammatory process involving the facial nerve (VII) anywhere from the nucleus in the brain to the periphery. Most patients recover spontaneously over a period of a few weeks, although recovery may be delayed or incomplete.

ASSESSMENT

Subjective and objective data are the same as for the patient with peripheral nerve trauma (p. 423). With Bell's palsy there is usually an abrupt onset of numbness or a feeling of stiffness of the face. Unilateral weakness of the facial muscles usually occurs, resulting in inability to wrinkle the forehead, close the eyelid, pucker the lips, or retract the mouth on that side. The face appears asymmetric with drooping of the mouth and cheek.

Other symptoms that may occur with Bell's palsy include the following:

1. Loss of taste
2. Reduction in saliva on affected side
3. Pain behind the ear
4. Ringing in ear or other hearing loss

DATA ANALYSIS AND PLANNING

See appropriate sections under the patient with peripheral nerve trauma.

IMPLEMENTATION

There is no specific therapy for Bell's palsy. Steroids given early in the course may speed recovery. Protection of the eyes when the eyelid does not close is important. Exercise and massage of the affected areas is sometimes recommended.

INTERFERENCE WITH FUNCTION BECAUSE OF TUMORS

Intracranial tumors

PATHOPHYSIOLOGY

Primary intracranial tumors, or neoplasms, arise from the intrinsic cells of brain tissues and the pituitary and pineal glands. Secondary or metastatic tumors are also a frequent contributing type of intracranial tumor. The prognosis for patients with an intracranial tumor is dependent on early diagnosis and treatment, because as the tumor grows it exerts pressure on vital centers and causes

Table 20-7. Type of brain tumor

Type	Incidence	Pathology
Astrocytoma (glioma)	Accounts for one half of brain tumors	Arises in any part of the brain connective tissue. Infiltrates primarily the cerebral hemisphere tissue. Not so well outlined as to be incised completely. Grows rapidly—most persons live months to years. Tumors assigned grade from 1 to 4, with 4 the most malignant. Different gliomas are as follows: 1. Astrocytomas 2. Oligodendrogliomas 3. Ependymomas 4. Medulloblastoma 5. Glioblastoma multiforme—most malignant
Meningioma	13% to 18% of all primary tumors in intracranial cavity	Arise from the meningeal coverings of the brain. They are usually benign but may undergo malignant changes. Usually encapsulated, and surgical cure is possible. Recurrence is possible.
Pituitary tumor	Occurs in all age groups, but more often in women	Arise from a varied number of tissues. Surgical approach is usually successful. Recurrence is possible.
Neuroma (schwannoma, neurofibroma)	Acoustic neuroma is most common.	Arises from Schwann's cells inside the auditory meatus on the vestibular portion of cranial nerve III. Usually benign, but may undergo cellular change and become malignant. Will regrow if not completely excised. Surgical resection is often difficult because of location.
Metastatic tumors	From 2% to 20% of all patients with cancer have metastasis to the brain.	Cancer cells spread to the brain via the circulatory system. Surgical resection is very difficult; even with treatment prognosis is very poor. Survival beyond a year or two is uncommon.

brain damage and death. Although approximately one half of all tumors are benign, they may also cause death by exerting pressure on vital centers.

Brain tumors are named for the tissues from which they arise. The more frequently encountered ones are described in Table 20-7. The brain, in addition, is also a frequent site for secondary tumors from other organs.

The symptoms of intracranial tumors result from both local and general effects of the tumor. Locally, the effects are from infiltration, invasion, and destruction of brain tissues at a particular site. There is also direct pressure on nerve structures, causing degeneration and interfer-

ence with local circulation. Local edema develops, and there is an increase in ICP. The increased ICP. is then transmitted throughout the brain and the ventricular system. Eventually, the ventricular system is distorted and displaced sufficiently to cause partial ventricular obstruction (Fig. 20-19). Papilledema results from the general effects of the increased ICP. Death is usually from brainstem compression resulting from herniation.

ASSESSMENT

It is important to assess both subjective and objective data in the patient with an intracranial tumor.

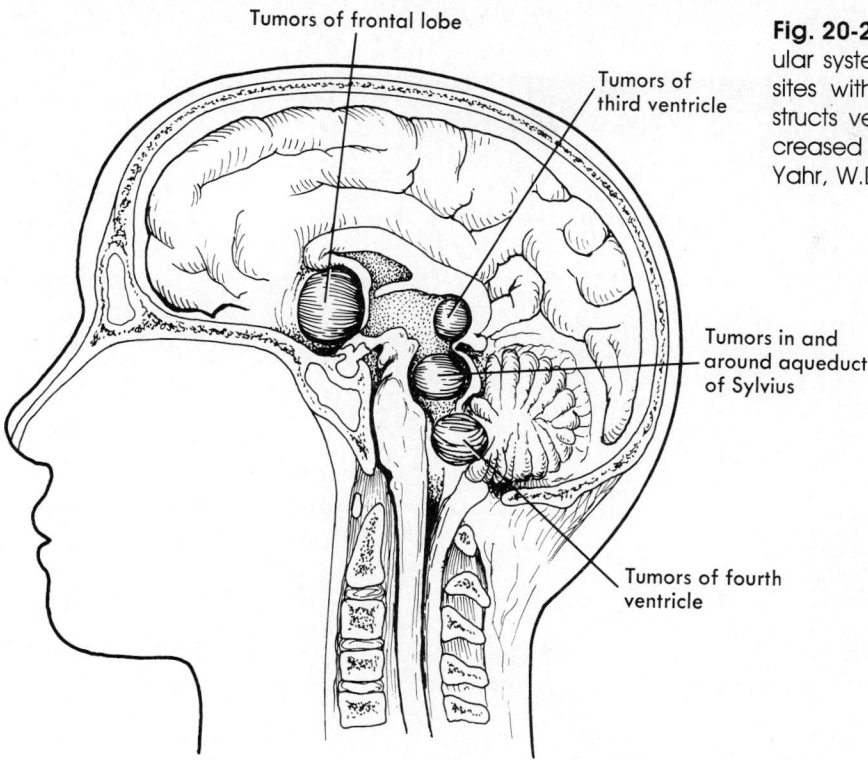

Tumors of frontal lobe

Tumors of third ventricle

Tumors in and around aqueduct of Sylvius

Tumors of fourth ventricle

Fig. 20-20. Sites of brain tumors adjacent to ventricular system. Note how developing tumor at varied sites with extension distorts, compresses, and obstructs ventricular system at some point so that increased intracranial pressure occurs early. (From Yahr, W.D.: Hosp. Med. **9:**8, 1973.)

Comparison of symptoms of tumors found in specific brain lobes

Area of the brain	Symptoms
Frontal lobe	Personality disturbances (range from subtle personality changes to frank psychotic behavior)
	Inappropriate affect
	Indifference of bodily functions
Precentral gyrus	Jacksonian seizures
Occipital lobe	Visual disturbances preceding convulsions
Temporal lobe	Olfactory, visual, or gustatory hallucinations
	Psychomotor seizures with automatic behavior
Parietal lobe	Inability to replicate pictures
	Loss of right-left discrimination

Subjective data

1. Patient's understanding of diagnosis
2. Changes in personality or judgment
3. Presence of abnormal sensations (paresthesia or anesthesia)
4. Visual problems—loss of visual acuity or diplopia
5. Complaints of unusual odors (often accompanies tumors of temporal lobe)
6. Presence of headache
7. Hearing loss
8. Inability to carry on daily activities

Objective data

1. Motor strengths
2. Gait
3. Level of alertness and consciousness
4. Orientation
5. Pupils: size, equality, and reactivity.
6. Vital signs
7. Funduscopic examination for evidence of papilledema
8. Presence of seizures
9. Speech abnormalities
10. Cranial nerve abnormalities
11. Symptoms of increased intracranial pressure

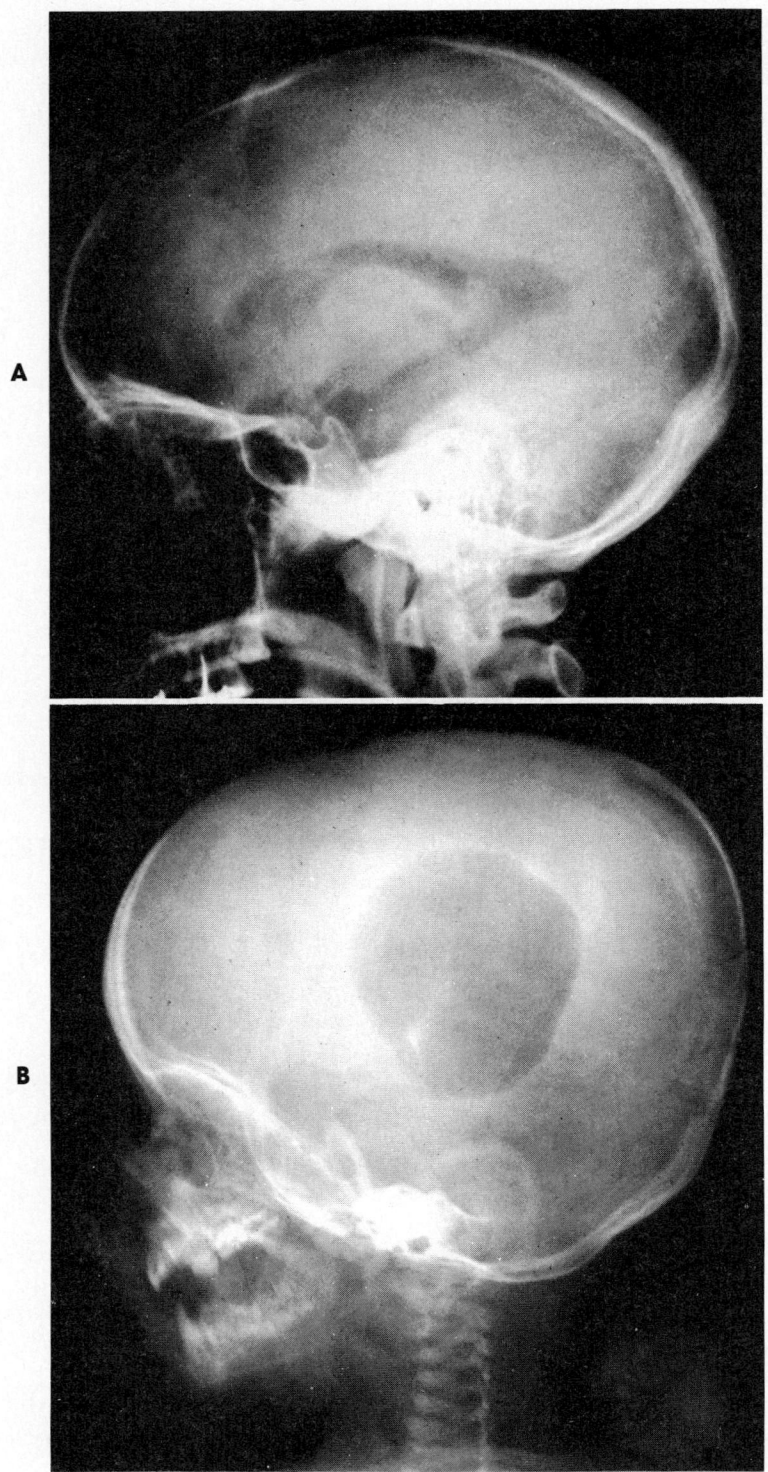

Fig. 20-21. Pneumoencephalogram. **A,** Lateral view showing outline of normal ventricle. **B,** Lateral view showing marked distention of ventricle with cerebrospinal fluid (caused by hydrocephalus).

Seizures occurring for the first time after middle age are very suggestive of a brain tumor in the cerebrum or its coverings. Intracranial tumors occuring within the cerebral lobes present disturbances that can be related to the function of the specific part of the brain.

Signs and symptoms of increased ICP resulting from intracranial tumors usually occur after localized signs and symptoms have been present for varying periods. See the previous discussion of increased ICP. Headache is at first transitory and later becomes constant; it increases in intensity with straining, coughing, stooping, and change of position. The headache is present in the morning and often awakens the person from sleep. Nausea and vomiting usually occur as the headache increases.

Diagnostic tests

No one procedure is entirely diagnostic of brain tumors, but the CT scan is often the basis of the diagnosis. Other tests that may be done include the brain scan and the EEG. These are discussed on p. 365 and p. 388. Another test that is used less frequently since the introduction of the CT scanner is the pneumoencephalogram (Fig. 20-20).

Other tests that may be helpful in locating the tumor are *arteriography* or *ventriculography*. Arteriography is described on p. 402. The ventriculogram is used when the suggested diagnosis is such that a spinal or lumbar puncture is contraindicated because of the presence of increased ICP.

Pneumoencephalogram

Purpose
To detect lesions of the ventricles and cisternal system using air as contrast

Preparation of patient
1. Prepare as if for surgery.
2. Permit must be signed.
3. Sedative may be given evening before procedure and just before test.
4. General anesthesia may be used.
5. Patient teaching:
   a. Explain procedure.
   b. Time: approximately 2 hours.
   c. Sensation: patient is usually very uncomfortable. Headache is usually severe during procedure; nausea and vomiting are common.

Procedure
1. Patient is positioned as for lumbar puncture (p. 363) or cisternal tap (p. 364).
2. After the tap is done and pressure measured the contrast medium (air or oxygen) is injected in amounts of 25 to 30 ml. Patient is watched carefully for headache, nausea, vomiting, or any change in vital signs or color.
3. Head of the table is gradually raised, and head may be rotated to assist air in filling ventricles.

After procedure
1. Patient is placed in bed with head flat. May be in bed 24 to 48 hours.
2. Constant attention with frequent vital signs and neurologic checks is needed until the patient is awake and alert.
3. Severe headache is common and may last for 48 hours.
4. Seizure precautions should be maintained if patient has history of seizures.
5. Tracheostomy set at bedside.
6. Reactions to procedure may be severe and include vomiting, shock, respiratory difficulty, and other signs of increased ICP.

Other
Pneumoencephalogram is not used as frequently because of the availability of the CT scanner. It is never done in the presence of increased ICP because of the danger of herniation.

Ventriculogram

Purpose

To detect pathology within the ventricular and cisternal system

Preparation of patient

1. Procedure is performed in the operating room.
2. Surgical permit must be signed.
3. Patient is prepared as if for surgery.
4. Top or back of head is partially shaved.
5. Intravenous or general anesthesia is commonly used.
6. Patient teaching
   a. Explain procedure.
   b. Time: variable. Often patient has craniotomy for tumor removal immediately after test.
   c. Sensation: none during procedure because of anesthesia.

Procedure

1. Patient is positioned, usually supine.
2. Trephine openings (burr holes) are made into the lateral ventricles.
3. Air is introduced directly via the ventricles.
4. X-ray films of the brain and ventricles are taken at intervals.

After procedure

1. Same as for pneumoencephalogram.
2. Observe site of burr hole for bleeding or drainage.
3. Observe for signs of neurologic deterioration that would indicate formation of intracerebral clot.

Another diagnostic test that has made significant recent advances in the detection of intracerebral tumors is the nuclear magnetic resonance scan (NMR), which is only available in major medical centers. One of the advantages of this test is that it requires no radiation.

DATA ANALYSIS AND PLANNING

Nursing diagnoses

Possible nursing diagnoses for the patient with an intracranial tumor include the:

Anxiety
Comfort, alteration in: pain
Communication, impaired verbal
Grieving, anticipatory
Knowledge deficit
Mobility, impaired physical
Sensory perceptual alteration: visual, auditory, kinesthetic, gustatory, tactile, olfactory
Thought processes, alteration in
Tissue perfusion, alteration in: cerebral

These diagnoses reflect the patient's initial diagnosis. Patient with tumors that have caused significant problems may present with nursing diagnoses indicative of increased ICP or motor dysfunction.

Expected patient outcomes

Expected patient outcomes for the patient with intracranial tumor in the early stages include the following:

1. Patient has ability to perform daily activities for as long as possible.
2. Patient can explain the specific therapy implemented and the desired outcome.
3. Patient can state signs and symptoms to report to physician.
4. Patient can explain medication regimen—dose, side effects, desired effects, route, and times.
5. Patient can explain care of the skin in relation to radiation therapy and the surgical incision.
6. Patient can explain plans for follow-up care.
7. Patient can explain and demonstrate any prescribed exercises.
8. Patient can explain how to obtain community support.
9. Patient is beginning to verbalize fears and concerns related to the diagnosis.

IMPLEMENTATION

Assisting with the achievement of therapeutic goals

The general methods of treatment for intracranial tumors include surgical removal when feasible, radiother-

---

Preoperative care of the patient having intracranial surgery

1. Baseline data of neurologic and physiologic status should be recorded.
2. Patient and family should be encouraged to verbalize fears.
3. Treatments and procedures are explained fully, even in unsure whether patient understands.
4. If head is shaved, it is usually done in the operating room.
5. Antiseptic shampoo may be ordered night before surgery and may be repeated in morning.
6. If hair is shaved, it is saved and given to patient or family.
7. Prepare family for appearance of patient following surgery.
   a. Head dressing
   b. Edema and ecchymosis of face common
   c. Temporary decreased mental status (possible)

---

apy, and chemotherapy. The choice of therapy is determined by the tumor type and site of the tumor. A combination of methods is often necessary.

When gliomas are located in areas that are not critical to vital functions, they are usually removed surgically. Most gliomas, however, infiltrate and are difficult to completely excise and treat. Surgery is often combined with radiotherapy and chemotherapy. When the tumor is located in a more critical area where removal would leave the patient with impaired function, a biopsy of the tumor is performed, it is "debrided" if possible, and the patient is treated with radiotherapy or chemotherapy.

Meningiomas are commonly treated by complete excision of the tumor (and overlying bone if infiltrated), because they are usually located in areas that permit removal. Meningiomas are often encapsulated, which aids in their removal.

Surgery

Intracranial surgery is commonly done for all types of pathologic conditions of the brain, including the relief of increased ICP and removal of tumors.

A surgical opening through the skull is known as *craniotomy*. It is a basic preparatory procedure for intracranial surgery. A series of burr holes is made first, and then the bone between the holes is cut with a Gigli saw to permit removal of the bone. Bone is then removed in such a way that it can be replaced if desired. Brain surgery may be done with the patient under hypothermia to lessen bleeding during the procedure. Drugs of hypotension may be used, such as norepinephrine bitartrate (Levophed). Patients may also be placed in a barbiturate coma during the surgery and for several days following it to lessen brain activity, metabolism, and oxygen needs. This may help to prevent worsening of deficits because of hypoxia.

When the brain lesion is in the supratentorium (above the tentorium or in the cerebrum), the incision is usually made behind the hairline. When the incision is into the infratentorium (below the tentorium or in the brainstem and cerebellum), it is made slightly above the nape of the neck.

Following craniotomy and removal of the bone, an incision is made into the meninges and the tumor is removed or other cranial surgery performed. The removed bone is carefully saved or preserved and may be replaced at the end of the surgery if there is not indication of infection or increased ICP. If it is not replaced, a bone prosthesis may later be placed over the deficit. The removal of part of the skull without replacement is called *craniectomy*. *Cranioplasty* is the repair of a cranial defect through use of a substitute bone material.

Tumors involving the pituitary gland that do not extend outside the sella turcica are usually removed using a transsphenoidal approach. After the surgery, packing is placed inside the nose and remains for 3 to 4 days. A muscle graft from the thigh is used to close the defect in the dura. With this type of surgery, recovery is relatively rapid and the patient has no loss of hair or external cranial incision.

Preoperative preparation of both the patient and family is important. They both are usually very threatened by the prospect of brain surgery. Specific fears may be related to those of a permanent change in appearance, dependency, or both. Preoperative care includes the points listed in above box.

During the postoperative period the patient is observed regularly for signs of increased ICP. The frequency of making and recording specific observations depends on the patient's condition. A device to measure ICP is often inserted during the surgery. Any change in the patient's vital signs, state of consciousness, pupillary response, or ability to move mucles is reported at once. Restlessness, often secondary to tissue hypoxia, may be the first warning of increased ICP. See p. 371 for specifics about ICP.

Specifics of postoperative care are dependent on the patient's condition. Most patients spend at least 1 or 2 nights in an intensive care unit, where arterial monitoring and close nursing observation is possible. Other details of postoperative care are found in the section on intracerebral hematomas (p. 406).

Hydrocephalus

Occasionally a catheter is placed in a ventricle of the brain to drain excess spinal fluid and to prevent hydrocephalus and increased ICP. The catheter is usually attached to a drainage system. The tubing and drainage receptacle should be sterile, and care must be taken to prevent kinking of the tubing. If drainage seems to have stopped, the neurosurgeon should be notified. At times, the nurse may adjust the level of the drainage device to facilitate drainage. This is only done with specific parameters for drainage and are ordered by the physician. For example the physician may order that the patient should drain 30 ml every 4 hours. The catheter is usually left in place for 24 to 48 hours and then is removed by the surgeon.

Hydrocephalus of a more permanent nature also occurs in the presence of intracranial tumors and is manifested by symptoms of increased ICP. Treatment consists of a shunting procedure. The different types of shunt procedures are named for their point of origin and termination and include the following:

1. Cyst to peritoneal
2. Lumbar-peritoneal
3. Ventricular-jugular
4. Ventricular-peritoneal

In this type of surgery excessive CSF is shunted away from the central nervous system and into either the peritoneal cavity (where it is absorbed) or into the jugular vein. At times a Ryckham reservoir is placed through a burr hole into the ventricle. This device can easily be palpated through the skin. Some of the shunts have an on-off valve, as well as a part that may be pumped to facilitate drainage. Valves that are inserted can be set for a pressure with some control over the amount of fluid drained.

Preoperative care is the same as for any patient having intracranial surgery. Key points of postoperative care are listed in box below.

Radiation therapy and chemotherapy

In some patients with intracranial tumors surgery may not be possible or indicated. In these cases radiation therapy and/or chemotherapy may be used. They are also used at times after intracranial surgery. See Chapter 14 for the care of the patient undergoing these treatments. One new and experimental chemotherapeutic treatment for brain tumors uses mannitol given via the arterial approach to open the blood-brain barrier. The chemotherapy is then given directly into the tumor area of the brain.

Assisting with comfort and ADL

Some patients who have had cranial surgery will have residual physical and mental limitations. The patient may have hemiplegia, aphasia, and personality changes. The rehabilitative care and planning are the same as for other patients with chronic and permanent neurologic disease

---

Postoperative care of the patient with a shunt

1. Monitoring
   a. Assess neurologic status frequently for any decrease in mental status.
   b. Observe for symptoms of subdural hematoma, one of the possible side effects of the surgery.
   c. Monitor for symptoms of overdrainage, as evidenced by headache, especially when patient is sitting upright or standing.
   d. Assess degree and character of drainage.
      1. Amount of drainage and bleeding should be minimal.
      2. Reinforce dressing as needed.
      3. Often incisional areas are left open to air after several days.
2. Maintain gastrointestinal status
   a. Check frequently for signs of paralytic ileus, because the manipulation of the bowel that occurs with the placement of the peritoneal part of the shunt can predispose the patient to this.
   b. Patient is usually kept NPO for first day, and then clear liquids are started.
   c. Regular diet is resumed as soon as good bowel sounds are present and patient tolerates liquids.
3. Maintaining comfort
   a. Patient may need more frequent pain medication because of involvement of abdominal area.
   b. Keep pressure off incisional sites.
4. Promoting mobility
   a. Turning to either side is permitted.
   b. Raise head of bed gradually when mobilizing patient.
   c. Patient is encouraged to ambulate as much as possible to encourage adaption to decreased ICP.

(see sections on the patient with motor dysfunction and the patient with a stroke). Regardless of the eventual prognosis and the diagnosis of the tumor, each patient should be helped to be as independent as possible for as long as possible.

EVALUATION

Evaluation of the patient with an intracranial tumor involves both the patient and the family. It is based on the expected patient outcomes. Pertinent questions to ask include the following:

1. Is the patient able to carry on ADL?
2. Can the patient explain their therapy and why it is occurring?
3. Can the patient state signs and symptoms to report to the physician?
4. Can the patient explain the medication regimen?
5. Is the patient taking medication as ordered?
6. Are any incisional areas healing?
7. Can the patient explain plans for follow-up care?
8. Can the patient explain how to obtain community support?
9. Is the patient carrying out prescribed exercises?
10. Is the patient verbalizing feelings and fears?

Intravertebral tumors

PATHOPHYSIOLOGY

Primary intravertebral tumors, or neoplasms, occur either extramedullary (involving tissues outside the cord) or intramedullary (involving tissue cells within the cord). Secondary or metastatic tumors may also involve the spinal cord, its coverings, and the vertebrae.

Extramedullary tumors of the intradural type may at first cause subjective nerve root pain. With tumor growth, this will include motor and sensory deficits relating to the level of the root and spinal cord involvement. As the tumor enlarges, it compresses the cord. Eventually, the patient loses all motor and sensory function below the level of the tumor.

An intramedullary tumor, beginning within the spinal cord, often presents as a central cord syndrome including segmental loss of pain and temperature function. In addition, there is often loss of anterior horn cell function, especially in the hands. Most of the central long tracts next to the gray matter become dysfunctional. There is gradual, progressive, and descending loss of pain and temperature sensations and motor weakness. Caudal motor and sensory functions are the last to be lost, including loss of bowel and bladder function.

ASSESSMENT

The subjective and objective data for the patient with an intravertebral tumor is the same as that for the patient with spinal cord injury (p. 419).

DATA ANALYSIS AND PLANNING

Nursing diagnoses and expected patient outcomes for the patient with a tumor of the spinal cord are the same as for the patient with a spinal cord injury (p. 419).

IMPLEMENTATION

Assisting with the achievement of therapeutic goals
Surgery

A spinal decompression is commonly done even when complete removal of the tumor is not considered possible. As much of the tumor as possible (and possibly bone) is removed to reduce the obstruction for a time. It can be done at any level of the vertebral column and may include several vertebrae. The operation is sometimes palliative. Care of the patient undergoing spinal decompression is found in the section on spinal cord injury (p. 421).

Assisting with comfort and ADL

Convalescent care and rehabilitation depend entirely on the type of tumor and whether it has been successfully removed. The decompression operation may give relief of symptoms for months and sometimes for years. If the tumor is a slow-growing one, radiation therapy may be given while the patient is in the hospital and continued after discharge.

EVALUATION

The evaluation of the care of the patient with an intravertebral tumor is the same as for the patient with a motor dysfunction (p. 382).

REFERENCES AND SUGGESTED READING

1. Allan, D.: Treating subarachnoid hemorrhage using carotid ligation, Nurs. Times **77:**1383-1385, 1977.
2. *Allwood, A., et al.: Cerebral artery bypass surgery, Am. J. Nurs. **80:**1284-1287, 1980.
3. Arnason, B.: Multiple sclerosis: current concepts and management, Hosp. Pract. **82:**81-89, 1982.
4. Bartel, M.: Dialogue with dementia: nonverbal communication in patients with Alzheimer's disease, J. Gerontol. Nurs. **5:**21-31, 1979.
5. Blount, M., et al.: Management of the patient with amyotrophic lateral sclerosis, Nurs. Clin. North Am. **14:**157-171, 1979.
6. Bowers, C., et al.: Severe head injury: current treatment and research, J. Neurosurg. Nurs. **14:**210-219, 1982.
7. Burnside, J.: Alzheimer's disease: an overview, J. Gerontol. Nurs. **5:**14-20, 1979.
8. *Cable, B., et al.: Test your neurologic nursing skills, Nurs. 80 **10:**40-43, 1980.
9. Carlson, C.: Psychological aspects of neurologic disability, Nurs. Clin. North Am. **15:**309-320, 1980.

*References preceded by an asterisk are particularly well suited for student reading.

10. Connolly, R., et al.: Update: head injury, J. Neurosurg. Nurs. **13**:195-201, 1981.

11. Conway-Rutkowski, B.: Carini and Owen's neurological and neurosurgical nursing, ed. 8, St. Louis, 1982, The C.V. Mosby Co.

12. Daly, B.: Intensive care nursing, Garden City, N.Y., 1980, Medical Exam Publishing Co.

13. Donahue, R.: Symposium on care of the patient with neuromuscular disease, Nurs. Clin. North Am. **14**:95-106, 1979.

14. Doolittle, N.: Arteriovenous malformation: the physiology, symptomatology, and nursing care, J. Neurosurg. Nurs. **11**:222-26, 1979.

15. Fedun, P.: Postoperative evaluation of patients undergoing microanastomosis for brain ischemia, J. Neurosurg. Nurs. **12**:46-53, 1980.

16. Felder, L.: Neurogenic bladder dysfunction, J. Neurosurg. Nurs. **11**:91-104, 1979.

17. Garrett, E.: Parkinsonionism: forgotten considerations in medical treatment and nursing care, J. Neurosurg. Nurs. **14**:13-18, 1982.

18. *Grinkel, J., et al.: Acute head injury: what to do, when and why, Nurs. '79 **9**:22-33, 1979.

19. Haberman, B.: Cognitive dysfunction and social rehabilitation in severely head-injured patients, J. Neurosurg. Nurs. **14**:220-224, 1982.

20. Hart, G.: Strokes causing left versus right hemiplegia: different effects and nursing implications, Geriatric Nurs. **4**:39-43, 1983.

21. Hollans, N., et al.: Overview of multiple sclerosis and nursing care of the multiple sclerosis patient, J. Neurosurg. Nurs. **13**:28-33, 1982.

22. Horvath, M.: Myasthenia gravis: a nursing approach, J. Neurosurg. Nurs. **14**:7-12, 1982.

23. *Howard, M., et al.: Psychological after effects of halo traction and a review of acute care, Am. J. Nurs. **12**:1839-1843, 1982.

24. *Johnson, L.: If your patient has increased intracranial pressure: your goal should be no surprises, Nurs. 83 **15**:58-64, 1983.

25. *Jones, S.: Glasgow Coma Scale, Am. J. Nurs. **79**:1551-1554, 1979.

26. *King, R.: Checking the patient's neuro status: the fine art of giving a physical, R.N. **45**:56-62, 1982.

27. King, R. et al.: Symposium on rehabilitative nursing: rehabilitation of the patient with spinal cord injury, Nurs. Clin. North Am. **15**:225-243, 1980.

28. Kirkland, J., et al.: Trigeminal neuralgia: approach to nursing care, J. Neurosurg. Nurs. **15**:149-153, 1983.

29. Levitt, R.: Understanding sexuality and spinal cord injury, J. Neurosurg. Nurs. **12**:88-89, 1980.

30. Martin, N., et al.: Comprehensive rehabilitation nursing, New York, 1981, McGraw-Hill Book Co.

31. Mauss-Clum, N.: Bringing the unconscious patient back safely: nursing makes the critical difference, J. Neurosurg. Nurs. **14**:32-43, 1982.

32. McClelland, P.: Behavioral problems after closed head injury, Top. Emerg. Med. **4**:42-50, 1983.

33. Mitchell, P.: Intracranial hypertension: implication of re-search for nursing care, J. Neurosurg. Nurs. **12**:145-154, 1980.

34. Mitchell, P., and Irvin, N.: Neurological examination: nursing assessment for nursing purposes, J. Neurosurg. Nurs. **9**:23-28, 1977.

35. Mitchell, P., and Maus, P.: Relating of patient's nursing activities to increased pressure variations: a pilot study, Nurs. Res. **27**:4-10, 1978.

36. Mitchell, P., et al.: Moving the patient in bed: effects of increased intracranial pressure, Nurs. Res. **30**:212-218, 1981.

37. Monson, R.: Autonomic dysreflexia: a nursing challenge, Rehabil. Nurs. **6**:18-19, 1981.

38. Nemeroff, D.: Transphenoidal hypophysectomy, J. Neurosurg. Nurs. **13**:303-312, 1981.

39. Nicholson, C.: Cranial bypass: a case study, J. Neurosurg. Nurs. **15**:165-168, 1983.

40. *Norman, E., et al.: Seizure disorders, Am. J. Nurs. **81**:983-1000, 1981.

41. *Norman, S.: The pupil check, Am. J. Nurs. **82**:588-591, 1982.

42. *Norman, S., and Baratz, R.: Understanding aphasia, Am. J. Nurs. **79**:2135-2138, 1979.

43. Norsworthy, E.: Nursing rehabilitation after severe head trauma, Am. J. Nurs. **74**:1319-1342, 1977.

44. O'Reilly, R.: Preparing the patient to computerized tomography, J. Neurosurg. Nurs. **11**:41-43, 1979.

45. *Pepper, G.: The person with spinal cord injury: psychological care, Am. J. Nurs. **77**:1330-1335, 1975.

46. Perdue, P.: Urgent priorities in severe trauma: life threatening head and spinal injuries, R.N. **44**:36-41, 1981. (Part 3.)

47. Plank, N.: Multiple sclerosis: an update and review, J. Neurosurg. Nurs. **11**:44-47, 1979.

48. Polhopek, M.: Stroke: an update on vascular disease, J. Neurosurg. Nurs. **12**:81-87, 1980.

49. *Reinisch, E.: Quick assessment for hemiplegic's functioning, Amer. J. Nurs. **81**:102-104, 1981.

50. Rhodes, M., et al.: Complications of posterior fossa craniotomy, J. Neurosurg. Nurs. **15**:19-21, 1983.

51. Ross, A., et al.: Neuromuscular diagnostic procedures, Nurs. Clin. North Am. **14**:107-121, 1979.

52. *Samond, R.: Guillain-Barre syndrome: helping the patient in the acute stage, Nurs. 80 **10**:34-41, 1980.

53. Shpritz, D.: Craniocerebral trauma, Crit. Care Nurs. **3**:49, 52, 55-56, 1983.

54. Smith, S.: Continuous intracranial monitoring: implications and applications for critical care, Crit. Care Nurse **3**:42-51, 1983.

55. Stevens, M.: Post concussive syndrome, J. Neurosurg. Nurs. **14**:239-244, 1982.

56. Taylor, J., and Bellinger, S.: Neurological dysfunction and nursing interventions, New York, 1980, McGraw Hill Book Co.

57. Terzian, M.: Neurosurgical intervention for the management of chronic intractable pain, Top. Clin. Nurs. **1**:75-88, 1980.

58. Wahlquist, G.: A great nursing challenge: recover and effective management of the patient with herpes simplex encephalitis, J. Neurosurg. Nurs. **13**:220-225, 1982.

59. *Wallech, C.: A neuro assessment procedure that won't make you nervous, Nurs. 82 **12:**50-58, 1982.
60. Webb, P.: Neurological deficit after carotid endarderectomies, Am. J. Nurs. **79:**654-658, 1979.
61. Wheeler, P.: Care of the patient with a cerebellar tumor, Am. J. Nurs. **77:**263-266, 1977.
62. Wilson, S.: Neuro nursing, New York, 1979, Springer Publishing Co.
63. Wing, S.: Cervical spine injuries: treatment and related nursing care, J. Neurosurg. Nurs. **9:**138-140, 1977.
64. Woods, N.F.: Human sexuality in health and illness, ed. 3, St. Louis, 1984, The C.V. Mosby Co.
65. Woodward, E.: The total patient: implications for nursing care of the epileptic, J. Neurosurg. Nurs. **14:**166-169, 1982.
66. *Young, M.: A bedside guide to understanding the signs of increased intracranial pressure, Nurs. 81 **11:**59-62, 1981.

Classic

67. Burnside, J.: Nursing and the aged, New York, 1976, The McGraw Hills Book Co.
68. Hurd, G.: Teaching the hemiplegic self care, Am. J. Nurs. **65:**64-68, 1965.
69. Mitchell, P., and Maus, N.: Intracranial pressure: fact and fancy, Nurs. 76 **6**(6):53-57, 1976.
70. *Olsen, E., et al.: The hazards of immobility, Am. J. Nurs. **67:**779-797, 1967.
71. Patient assessment: neurological assessment I, Am. J. Nurs. **75:**1511-1535, 1975.
72. Patient assessment: neurological assessment II, Am. J. Nurs. **75:**2037-2057, 1975.
73. Patient assessment: neurological assessment III, Am. J. Nurs. **76:**609-633, 1976.
74. Skelly, M.: Rethinking stroke: aphasic patients talk back, Am. J. Nurs. **75:**1140-1142, 1975.

21

The Patient with Eye Problems

BARBARA C. LONG

STUDY QUESTIONS

- Review anatomy and physiology of the eye. How does the aqueous humor differ from the vitreous humor? How does the aqueous humor enter and drain through the eye?

- Describe the effects on the eye of each of the following types of drugs: mydriatics, cycloplegics, miotics, adrenergic agents, osmotic agents.

- Consider bandaging your eyes for 1 day and carry out all your usual activities. What problems did you encounter? What did you find helpful?

- Describe how you would respond to a person who says, "I don't see as well as I used to. I don't need to go to an eye doctor; he'll only tell me I need glasses, and I already have a pair."

- In your community, what services and facilities are available to persons with limited vision? How are these financed?

ANATOMY AND PHYSIOLOGY

Anatomy of the eye

The eyeball is composed of three coats or layers of tissue, the sclera, the choroid, and the retina (Fig. 21-1). The tough outer coat, or *sclera,* is opaque (white) but becomes transparent anteriorly over the iris and pupil to form the *cornea.* The middle layer, the *choroid,* contains blood vessels and is modified anteriorly into the ciliary body, which is attached to the suspensory ligament and to the iris. The pupil is the space in the center of the doughnut-shaped iris. The inner coat, the *retina,* which does not have an anterior portion, contains the photoreceptors (rods and cones). These photoreceptors synapse in the retina with bipolar neurons and then with ganglion neurons, and these become the fibers of the optic nerve. The cones, which are less numerous than the rods, are found mostly near the center of the retina and are considered to be the receptors for bright daylight and color vision. The rods, found mostly in the periphery of the retina, are receptors for dim or night vision. Rods contain rhodopsin, a photosensitive protein that becomes rapidly depleted in bright light. The slow regeneration of rhodopsin, which is dependent on the presence of vitamin A, explains the time needed for the eyes to adjust from bright to dim light. Vitamin A deficiency affects night vision.

The interior of the eyeball is divided into two cavities, the anterior and the posterior. The *anterior cavity,* in front of the lens, is further subdivided into two *chambers,* an anterior chamber (between the cornea and the iris) and a posterior chamber (between the iris and the lens). The anterior cavity is filled with a clear liquid, the aqueous humor, which is produced in the ciliary body, drains into the posterior chamber, passes through the pupil into the anterior chamber, and drains out the canal of Schlemm at the junction of the iris and cornea (anterior

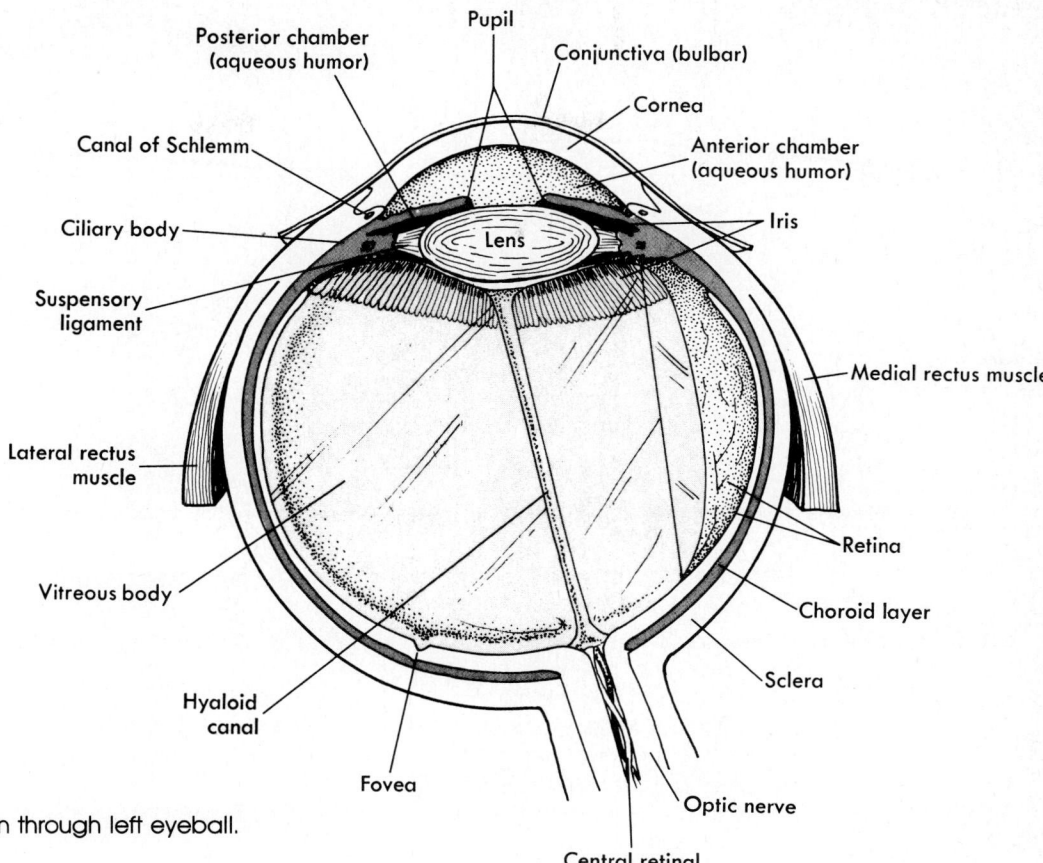

Fig. 21-1. Horizontal section through left eyeball.

Labels (clockwise from top): Pupil · Conjunctiva (bulbar) · Cornea · Anterior chamber (aqueous humor) · Iris · Medial rectus muscle · Retina · Choroid layer · Sclera · Optic nerve · Central retinal artery and vein · Fovea · Hyaloid canal · Vitreous body · Lateral rectus muscle · Suspensory ligament · Ciliary body · Canal of Schlemm · Posterior chamber (aqueous humor) · Lens

chamber angle). Obstruction of this drainage leads to glaucoma (p. 453). The *posterior cavity* of the eye is filled with a clear gelatinous substance, the vitreous humor, which helps maintain eye body. If vitreous humor is removed, the eye collapses.

Eye muscles are of two types, extrinsic and intrinsic. The extrinsic voluntary muscles outside the eyeball control extraocular movement. The intrinsic involuntary muscles within the eye are the ciliary body, which controls the shape of the lens, and the iris, which controls pupil size.

Physiology of vision

Light rays entering the eye bend (*refraction*) as they pass over the curved surfaces of the cornea and through various structures of the eye (cornea, aqueous humor, lens, vitreous humor), which have different densities, to focus on the retina.

The eyes adjust (*accommodation*) so as to see objects at various distances by flattening or thickening of the lens. Near vision requires contraction of the ciliary body, which decreases the distance between the edges of the ciliary body, thus relaxing the suspensory ligament attached to the lens. The lens then bulges to bend the light ray more acutely so that the rays focus on the retina.

Continual close vision may produce eye strain through constant contraction of the ciliary muscle; this can be relieved by frequent shifting of the eyes to distant objects. Accommodation is also facilitated by changing the size of the pupil. With near vision the iris constricts the pupil to force light rays to pass through the shortened but thicker lens. The pupils also constrict with bright lights to protect the retina from intense stimulation.

Light rays are absorbed by the photoreceptors on the retina and are changed to electrical activity in order to transmit the image to the cortex. The fibers of the optic nerve (cranial nerve II) divide at the optic chiasm, the medial portion of each nerve crosses to the opposite side, and the impulses are then transmitted to the visual cortex. Bilateral vision provides depth perception.

PREVENTION AND HEALTH EDUCATION

Vision is one of the most important senses. It orients us to the world around us. It provides pleasure through beautiful sights. It provides data to promote safety to our physical being and effective interaction with others. Vision also contributes to our self-concept and feeling of personal worth and well-being.

Because nurses have contacts with persons of all ages, they have opportunities to become involved in many activ-

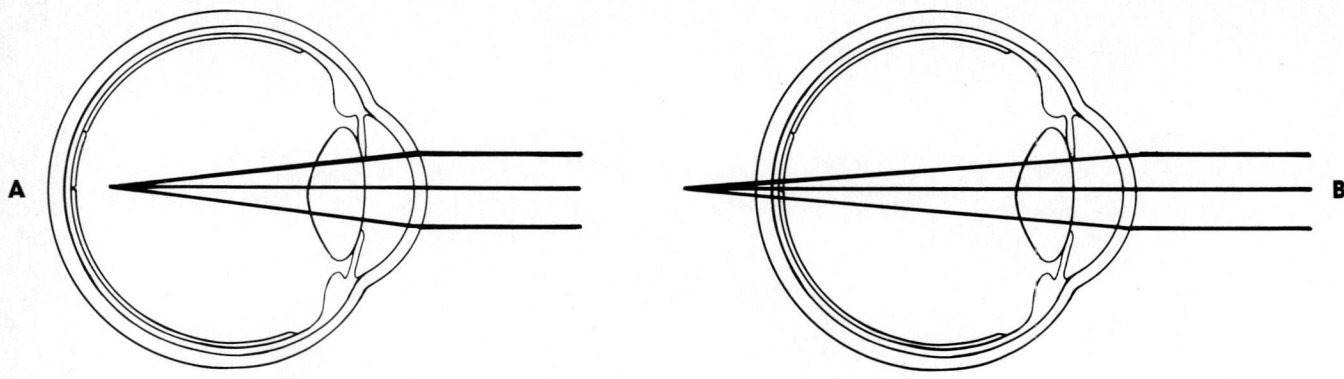

Fig. 21-2. A, Myopia (nearsightedness); image is focused in front of retina. **B,** Hyperopia (farsightedness); image is focused behind retina.

Persons who specialize in eye problems or corrective lenses

Ophthalmologist	Physician who specializes in diagnosis and treatment of eye diseases; may also prescribe lenses
Oculist	Same as ophthalmologist
Optometrist	Professional with special preparation in assessment of vision and in treatment of visual problems (e.g., prescribes lenses, visual training, or orthoptic exercises); is not a physician and does not treat eye disease
Optician	Person who grinds and fits lenses according to prescriptions written by ophthalmologist or optometrist

---

Terms describing visual acuity

Accommodation	Ability to adjust for far and near objects
Emmetropia	Normal eyesight; light rays focus on retina
Ametropia	Refractive error; light rays do not focus on retina
Myopia	Nearsightedness; light rays focus in front of retina (Fig. 21-2)
Hyperopia	Farsightedness; light rays focus behind retina
Presbyopia	Hyperopia from loss of lens elasticity because of age
Astigmatism	Irregular curvature of cornea; light rays do not focus at some point

---

ities that promote good vision and help to prevent injury or further impairment. This is accomplished by participation in promotion of visual acuity, promotion of safety measures, and detection of possible eye disorders.

Promotion of visual acuity

DETERMINATION OF VISUAL ACUITY

When light passes through the eye, the bending of the light rays and the location of the image depend on the shape and condition of ocular structures. The signs of presbyopia usually begin after age 40 years, and corrective lenses are commonly required, at least for reading. Persons with myopia, hyperopia, and astigmatism also frequently require corrective lenses.

MEASUREMENT OF VISUAL ACUITY

Distance vision is usually determined by use of a *Snellen chart* (Fig. 21-3). The person sits or stands 20 feet from the chart, covers one eye with a piece of stiff paper

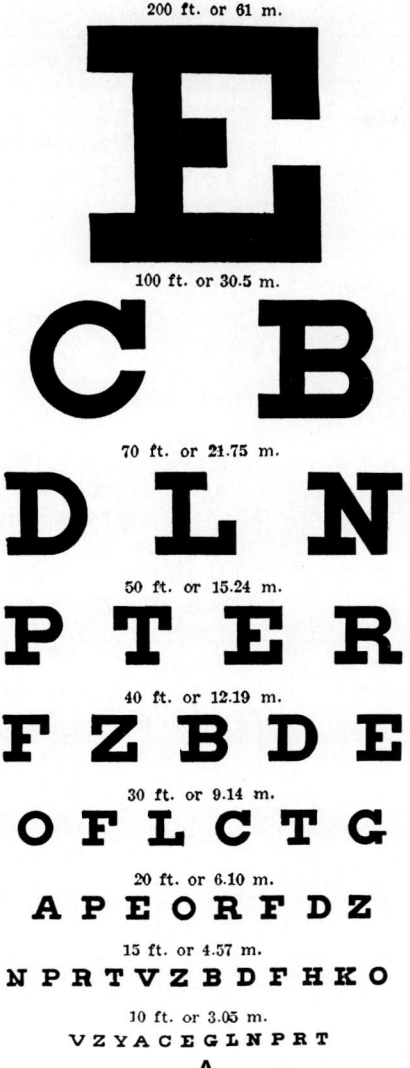

200 ft. or 61 m.

100 ft. or 30.5 m.

70 ft. or 21.75 m.

50 ft. or 15.24 m.

40 ft. or 12.19 m.

30 ft. or 9.14 m.

20 ft. or 6.10 m.

15 ft. or 4.57 m.

10 ft. or 3.05 m.

A

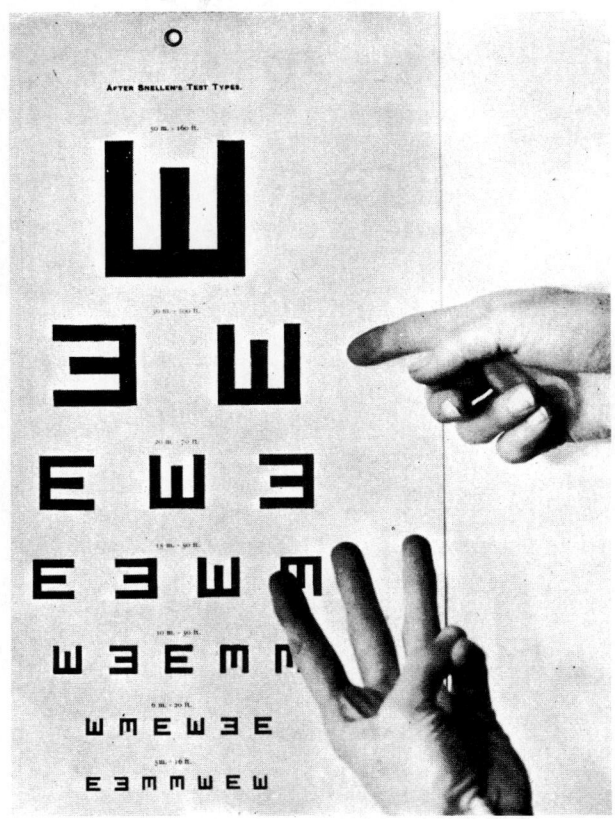

B

Fig. 21-3. Snellen chart used in testing vision. B, Modified Snellen chart, called "E" game, for testing vision of small children and persons unfamiliar with English alphabet.

or a plastic occluder, and reads the line as specified by the examiner. The eyes are tested with and without distance lenses.

Visual acuity is expressed as a fraction; a reading of 20/20 is considered normal. The upper figure refers to the distance at which the person can read the chart, and the lower figure indicates the distance at which a normal eye can read the line. For example, if an individual is able to read at 20 ft only the line that should be readable at 70 ft, he or she has 20/70 vision in the eye tested.

Near vision is tested by reading small print, such as newsprint, held 35 cm (14 in) from the eye. Any person with vision less than 20/30 in either eye is referred to an ophthalmologist or optometrist for further testing.

TYPES OF LENSES

Lenses may be worn as glasses or contact lenses (Table 21-1). Glasses may have one focus (for near or far vision),

bifocal (upper part for distance, lower part for near vision), or *trifocal* (for distance, intermediate, and near vision).

Contact lenses are usually chosen for cosmetic reasons or for sports activities because they do not fog or break easily. Persons who have lenses removed because of cataracts (but without lens implants) achieve better vision with contact lenses than with glasses. Some industrial occupations prohibit use of contact lenses because of irritation of the cornea by dirt or dust trapped under the lens.

Contact lenses are inserted after being cleaned thoroughly and immersed in a wetting agent such as methylcellulose. Conjunctival secretions provide the lubrication needed for the lenses to be worn in comfort. The lenses are held in place by capillary attraction and by the upper lid. If the person is injured or unconscious, the nurse removes the contact lenses. Lenses are stored separately in special containers, labeled left or right lens. Soft lenses are kept wet at all times with special solution or sterile saline solution.

Table 21-1. Types of corrective lenses

Lens	Characteristics	Benefits	Disadvantages
Glasses	Impact-resistant material (plastic or glass)	Plastic lenses are lighter in weight than glass	Plastic lenses are more expensive than glass and scratch easily
Contact lenses			
Hard	Hydrophobic, hard plastic Usually tinted Covers only the cornea	Least expensive Easy to clean Good optical quality	Easily lost Cannot be worn for long periods
Gas permeable	Hard plastic, permeable to oxygen and other gases Covers only cornea	Good optical quality Comfortable Can be worn longer than hard lenses	Expensive
Soft	Hydrophyllic, flexible plastic Covers cornea and part of sclera	Can be worn longer (up to 18 hours) Comfortable	Higher initial cost, need frequent replacement Must be kept wet to prevent damage More difficult to clean Absorb atmospheric pollutants
Extended wear	Same as soft lenses but contain more water	Can be worn continuously for several weeks	Expensive Require medical supervision Break easily

---

Removal of contact lenses

Hard lens

Method 1
  a. Place finger at outer canthus of eye.
  b. Pull skin obliquely upward, then straight down.
  c. Lens will appear on lower lashes as the upper lid moves downward.
  d. If lens moves off center, reposition it by gentle pressure on lid or lens itself.
Method 2
  a. Place finger or thumb of each hand at base of eyelashes (upper and lower).
  b. Bring eyelids together, trapping the lens (the lens will eject).
  c. If lens moves off center, reposition it by gentle pressure on lid or lens itself.
Method 3
  a. Using eye irrigation set, gently flush eye with sterile normal saline solution.
  b. Retrieve lens in curved basin.
Method 4
  a. Use small suction device shaped like a miniature "plumber's helper."
  b. Place over center of lens and pull lens off gently.

Soft lens

  a. Pull upper lid up with one thumb.
  b. Be sure lens is in place before attempting removal.
  c. Move lens over conjunctiva before grasping it, if possible. If lens does not move freely, put several drops of sterile saline solution in eye, close lid, and wait 1 minute before trying again.
  d. Grasp lens with thumb and forefinger or other hand and lift.

Promotion of eye safety

Everyone should know how to protect their eyes from injury. Many people keep unused eye medications and then use them for self-treatment at a later date. This is hazardous because it not only may lead to eye injury but may delay necessary treatment. Ophthalmic drugs may deteriorate, become more concentrated from evaporation of liquid, or become contaminated with bacteria or fungi.

Preventive goggles and break-resistant corrective lenses are available for persons who engage in very active physical activities such as sports and in selected occupations. Prompt and appropriate care of an injured eye may prevent serious vision impairment or loss of the eye (Table 21-2).

Secondary prevention

Early detection of eye disease is imperative for protection of vision. Inflammations of the eye are more easily detected than other eye disorders; the person usually complains of discomfort, and redness and discharge are easily observed. Glaucoma is the greatest threat to vision in older persons; the permanent vision loss it causes is preventable if the condition is identified early. Mass screening programs for glaucoma detection have been instituted in many communities, and everyone is urged to participate in these programs. All persons with symptoms suggestive of eye disease (Table 21-3) are urged to seek medical assistance.

Diseases of other parts of the body may also affect the

Eye safety measures

1. Avoid frequent rinsing of eyes with unprescribed solutions.
2. Discard any ophthalmic solution that is cloudy, discolored, has been open for ≥ 3 months, or contains particles.
3. Avoid self-treatment of an eye inflammation with a medication prescribed for a previous eye disorder.
4. To avoid eye strain:
   a. Use a good light for reading or doing work that requires careful visual focus.
   b. When reading or focusing eyes for long periods, look at distant objects for a few minutes at repeated intervals to rest eyes.
5. Avoid rubbing eyes.
6. Wash hands before touching eyes.
7. Wear safety glasses when engaging in activities that could injure the eyes.
8. Wear dark glasses for prolonged exposure to very bright light (such as sunlight on snow or water)
9. Flush eyes with copious amount of water when any irritating substances are accidentally introduced.
10. Do not attempt to remove foreign bodies from the cornea; cover eye and seek medical attention.
11. If a speck of dust blows in eye, pull upper lid over lower lid and let the tears wash the speck to the inner canthus or lower lid, where it may be safely removed.

Table 21-2. First aid for eye injuries

Injury	Interventions
Burns: chemical, flame	Flush eye immediately for 15 minutes with cool water or any available nontoxic liquid; seek medical assistance
Loose substance on conjunctiva: dirt, insects	Lift upper lid over lower lid to dislodge substance, produce tearing; irrigate eye with water if necessary; do not rub eye; obtain medical assistance if above interventions fail
Contact injury: contusion, ecchymosis, laceration	Apply cold compresses if no laceration present; cover eye if laceration present; seek medical assistance
Penetrating objects	Do not remove object; place protective shield over eye (e.g., paper cup); cover uninjured eye to prevent excess movement of injured eye; seek medical assistance

Table 21-3. Symptoms suggestive of eye disease

Symptom	Eye disease
Conjunctival redness	Conjunctivitis, blepharitis, sty
Crusting discharge	Conjunctivitis, blepharitis, sty
Ocular pain	Foreign body, sty, acute lid infection, glaucoma, keratitis, uveitis
Foreign body sensation	Foreign body, corneal erosion, blepharitis, chronic conjunctivitis
Blepharospasm	Keratitis, corneal ulcer
Multiple spots ("floaters")	Retinal detachment, intraocular hemorrhage, diabetic retinopathy
Photophobia	Uveitis, keratitis, glaucoma, corneal abrasions
Vision changes	
Blurred vision	Refractive error, cataract, glaucoma, uveitis, retinal detachment
Double vision	Strabismus
Halos around lights	Glaucoma
Blind spots	Hemorrhage, choroiditis
Sudden vision loss	Central retinal artery or vein occlusion

Table 21-4. Eye manifestations of systemic disorders

Disorder	Effect on eye
Diabetes mellitus	Senile cataracts occur earlier and progress more rapidly
	Diabetic retinopathy; retinal changes lead to decreased vision
	Vitreous hemorrhages
	Retinal detachment
Persistent systemic hypertension	Retinal hemorrhage, retinal edema, and retinal exudate lead to loss of sight
Cerebral vascular accident	Loss of sight in one half of visual field (hemianopia)
	Emboli may occlude retinal vessel
Demyelinating neurologic disorders (e.g., multiple sclerosis)	Nerve damage to eye
Increased intracranial pressure	Papilledema (swelling of optic disc)
Nutritional disorders	
Lack of vitamin A and B	Changes in conjunctiva, cornea, and retina
	Tears reduced
	Eyes and lids become reddened and inflamed
	Night blindness
Excess of vitamin A	Retinal damage

eye (Table 21-4). Early detection and treatment of these diseases can help to prevent loss of vision.

VISUALLY HANDICAPPED: BLIND

Vision is essential to most employment and necessary in countless experiences that make life enjoyable and meaningful. Yet in the United States there are an estimated 1 million legally blind persons. Approximately 1.5 million Americans are so visually handicapped that they cannot read ordinary newsprint even with the aid of corrective lenses. In underdeveloped countries there is a high incidence of blindness from preventable causes such as malnutrition and eye infections.

Although there has been a reduction of blindness in the United States from infections and certain diseases and injuries, blindness from diseases that occur most frequently among older persons, including diabetic retinopathy, glaucoma, cataract, and retinal degeneration, has increased. It is likely that the incidence of blindness will continue to increase because of the steady growth in the number of persons aged 65 and older.

Legal criteria of blindness

A person is considered legally blind when either of the following conditions exist:
1. Visual field no greater than 20 degrees
2. Central distance vision in better eye 20/200 or less with use of corrective lenses (eye can see at 20 ft what the normal eye can see at 200 ft).

Report of the National Advisory Eye Council, U.S. Department of Health, Education and Welfare, no. (NIH) 75-664, 1975.

Guidelines for communicating with blind persons

1. Talk in a normal tone of voice.
2. Do not try to avoid common phrases in speech, such as "See what I mean?"
3. Introduce yourself with each contact (unless well-known to the person).
4. Explain any activity occurring in the room.
5. Announce when you are leaving the room so the blind person is not put in the position of talking to someone who is no longer there.

Impaired vision

Vision impairment ranges from refractive errors correctable with lenses to total blindness, in which the person may not even be able to perceive light. For legal purposes blindness is defined very precisely in order to determine eligibility for assistance of various kinds. Although many nonseeing persons now prefer to be called *visually handicapped,* the term blindness is still in common usage.

Responses to loss of vision

IMPACT OF VISUAL LOSS

People who are born blind or develop blindness very early in life and who are raised as children who can see, neither overprotected or rejected, frequently are self-confident persons leading active productive lives.

Loss of vision may affect the self and the ability to interact with others and with the environment. The adult in whom blindness develops fairly rapidly usually has greater difficulty adjusting to the handicap. The impairment may cause a decrease in feelings of self-confidence and in the self-concept. Communication with others is affected, and a sense of isolation may develop. Familiar hobbies that require vision, such as reading, sewing, or crafts, may no longer be possible. Even listening to television creates problems when gaps in sound occur. Mobility or ability to carry out activities of daily living may be restricted or at least modified. Career options, job opportunities, and financial security may be affected. Blindness may influence the person's ability to remain independent, to feel socially adequate, or to feel that he or she is an esteemed contributing member of society.

COPING WITH VISUAL LOSS

After a person has been told that blindness will result, there is a normal reaction described as a period of mourning for the "dead" eyes. Grief and mourning over the loss of vision can cause emotional reactions such as denial, anger, guilt, resentment, hopelessness, helplessness, loneliness, and depression. These strong emotional feelings interfere with the blind person's ability to plan new ways of accomplishing tasks of living.

The ability to cope with the loss depends on the extent and duration of the handicap, the age at which it occurs, how the person has successfully coped in the past, and the presence of available support systems (family and friends).

Over time, persons with visual losses appear to be able to compensate for their deficit by an increase in sensitivity of the other senses. For example, some blind people compensate by increasing auditory acuity, tactile acuity, sense of smell, or kinesthetic awareness.

Nursing activities for the newly blind

COUNSELING

Newly blind persons who are trying to cope need an opportunity to talk about their feelings, concerns, and anxieties about the future. Once they have identified these feelings and concerns, they can be helped to identify their strengths and resources and to consider different approaches to dealing with tasks of everyday living. Alternate forms of recreation and pleasurable activities can also be explored. For example, the person who enjoyed reading may be interested in learning Braille or in using "talking books."

Some persons need assistance in developing a new self-image. It is not unusual for the person to reject initially any aids that officially identify them as "blind," such as the white cane. Patience is required; it sometimes takes a long time to change the self-image.

Persons who become blind do not develop impaired hearing or intelligence, yet some sighted persons insist on speaking loudly. Communication should be done naturally (see box, p. 444).

Facilitating independence in ADL for blind persons

1. Place clothing in specific locations in drawers or closets to facilitate clothing selection.
2. Keep furniture in specific places to facilitate mobility.
3. Encourage use of cane when walking in unfamiliar areas.
4. When assisting a blind person in walking, let the person take *your* arm (Fig. 21-4).
5. Provide descriptions of food on plate; describe location in terms of a clock face, for example, "The peas are at 7 o'clock."
6. Provide privacy while the newly blind person is learning to cope with eating.

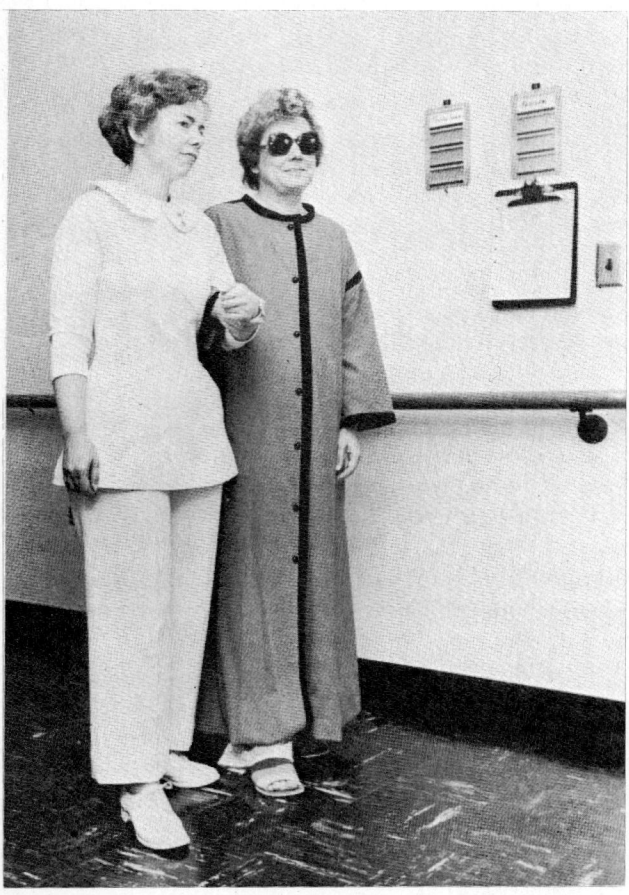

Fig. 21-4. Ambulation of patient who cannot see. Note that patient holds nurse's arm and is led without being held.

ASSISTANCE WITH ACTIVITIES OF DAILY LIVING

Given time, most blind persons develop ways of coping with activities of daily living (ADL) (see box above). One elderly blind lady was able to take her many medications accurately by devising a system using rubber bands and strings around the medication bottles to provide clues to when they were to be taken.

COMMUNITY SERVICES

Many federal, state, and local agencies provide services to persons with severe visual impairment. The health professional can refer these persons and their families to a social worker familiar with services and facilities available in their home area. Community health nurses often have this information readily available. Services to visually impaired persons include mobility training, personal counseling, vocational rehabilitation, relearning independent self-care, special education, and financial compensation in some instances. "Talking books" and tapes are available from public libraries as well as from organizations for the blind.

GOVERNMENT ASSISTANCE

Legal blindness entitles a person to certain federal assistance based on need. Blind persons are entitled to an extra personal deduction in reported income. Counseling and placement services are available through the Social and Rehabilitation Service (SRS) of the U.S. Department of Health and Human Services.

Major health problems of the eye

The most common disorders of the eye in adults include the following:

1. Inflammatory disorders of the eyelid, conjunctiva, cornea, choroid, ciliary body, and iris
2. Cataracts: opaqueness of the lens
3. Glaucoma: increased intraocular pressure
4. Retinal detachment

INFLAMMATORY EYE DISORDERS

Inflammations and infections may occur in any of the eye structures (Table 21-4), and account for more than half of eye disorders. Conjunctivitis is the most prevalent.

Table 21-4. Inflammatory disorders of the eye

Disorder	Description	Signs and symptoms	Medical therapy
Hordoleum (sty)	Staphylococcal infection of gland at eyelid margin	Localized abcess at base of eyelash, edema of lid, pain	Hot compresses to hasten pointing of abcess, topical antibiotic
Chalazion	Cyst from obstruction of sebaceous gland at eyelid margin	Initial edema and discomfort; later, painless mass in lid	Warm compresses and topical antibiotic initially; surgical removal if large and pressing on cornea
Blepharitis	Inflammation of lid margins, usually by staphylococci	Itching, redness, lid pain, lacrimation, photophobia; crusting ulceration; lids become glued together during sleep	Warm compresses followed by erythromycin or bacitracin eye ointment; steroid eye drops may be prescribed
Conjunctivitis (pink eye)	Inflammation of conjunctiva by viruses, bacteria (highly infectious), allergy, trauma (sunburn)	Redness of conjunctiva, lid edema, crusting discharge on lids and cornea of eye; itching with allergies	Cleansing of lids and lashes, warm compresses; topical antibiotics; steroid eye drops for allergies (contraindicated for herpes simplex virus); no eye patch
Keratitis	Inflammation of cornea by bacteria, herpes simplex virus, allergies, vitamin A deficiency	Severe eye pain, photophobia, tearing, blepharospasm, loss of vision if uncontrolled	Warm compresses; topical antibiotics for bacterial infections; atropine sulfate; idoxuridine for herpes simplex; eye patch, rest; corneal grafting if cornea injured
Corneal ulcer	Necrosis of corneal tissue from trauma, inflammation; may be superficial or may penetrate deeper tissue	Pain and blepharospasm may occur; ulcer may be outlined by fluorescein dye	Superficial ulcer: antibiotic eye drops, eye patch Deep ulcer: topical and systemic antibiotics, atropine sulfate, warm compresses, eye patch; cauterization; corneal transplant if necessary

PATHOPHYSIOLOGY

Most eye inflammations are caused by microorganisms, mechanical irritation, or sensitivity to some substance. Fortunately, a large percentage of inflammations are self-limiting, with no permanent scars. Severe corneal inflammation or ulceration can damage the cornea, causing visual impairment. Complications from uveitis can lead to formation of adhesions, secondary glaucoma, and loss of vision.

ASSESSMENT

Subjective data

Persons with inflammations of the eye may complain of itching, pain (mild to severe), lacrimation, sensitivity to light (photophobia), or spasms of the eyelids (blepharospasms).

Objective data

The external structures of the eye are routinely inspected during the physical examination (Chapter 3). Inflammations are identified by the presence of redness, edema of the lids, and pus or discharge. When considerable discharge is present, the lids may become glued together during sleep.

Corneal ulcers may be identified by instilling sterile fluorescein, a yellow-green harmless dye. Because fluorescein harbors the growth of microorganisms such as *pseudomonas,* only a new, unopened bottle should be used. Also available are single-use fluorescein-impregnated paper strips that are gently touched to the inside of the lower lid. The ulcer is then assessed by shining a penlight obliquely across the eye from the side. If pain and blepharospasm interfere with examination, a drop of anesthetic such as 0.5% proparacaine can be used.

Care of the person with an eye inflammation

1. Apply warm moist compresses as prescribed for healing and to decrease pain.
2. Irrigate eye, if prescribed, to remove discharge.
3. Administer prescribed eye medications.
4. Use eye pads only for inflammations without infection.
5. Dim bright lights if photophobia is present.
6. Give prescribed analgesics for pain.
7. Prevent spread of infection by:
   a. Using separate medication bottles or tubes for each eye if infection is present.
   b. Washing hands before touching eye.
   c. Using washcloths and towels only once if infection is present

---

Guidelines for application of warm moist eye compresses

1. Use sterile technique when infection or ulceration is present; clean technique may be used for allergic reactions.
2. Use separate equipment for bilateral eye infections.
3. Wash hands before treating each eye.
4. Temperature of compresses should not exceed 49° C (120° F).
5. Change compresses frequently over 10 to 20 minutes.
6. Do not exert pressure on eyeball.
7. Sterile petrolatum may be used on skin *around* eyes, if desired, to protect skin.
8. If sterility is not necessary, moist heat may be applied by means of a clean wash cloth.

DATA ANALYSIS AND PLANNING

Nursing diagnoses

Possible nursing diagnoses for persons with inflammations of the eye include the following:

Alteration in comfort: pain in eye

Potential for injury (spread of infection)

Expected patient outcomes

1. Patient states pain is decreased.
2. Infection does not spread to opposite eye.
3. If infection is present on discharge, the person can:
   a. State name, dosage, and frequency of eye medication to be taken and the need to destroy unused ophthalmic medications after therapy.
   b. Describe method and frequency of eye compresses to be used.
   c. Describe measures to prevent spread of infection to the uninvolved eye and to others in the household.
4. If corneal grafting has been performed, the person can:
   a. Describe the medication program.
   b. Describe activities and movements to be avoided.
   c. Describe the need for medical follow-up.

IMPLEMENTATION

Nursing interventions for the person with an eye inflammation consist primarily of giving eye treatments and medications to hasten healing and decrease pain, and helping prevent the spread of infection.

Assisting with achievement of therapeutic goals
Eye compresses

Warm moist compresses help relieve pain, promote healing, and help to cleanse the eye, which is normally cleansed by tears.

Cold moist saline compresses may be ordered to prevent or control edema and severe itching of the eyes and to help control bleeding immediately after eye injury. A small basin of sterile solution may be placed in a bowl of chipped ice at the bedside. Sterile forceps are used to wring out and apply the compress. If the compress does not need to be sterile, a washcloth or compress may be placed on pieces of ice in a basin. A rubber glove or small plastic bag packed with finely chipped ice may be applied to the eye and necessitates fewer compress changes.

Eye irrigation

Irrigation is used to remove secretions, discharge, foreign bodies, and chemical irritants from the eye. Physio-

Guidelines for eye irrigation

1. Place patient lying toward side to be irrigated to prevent fluid from flowing into other eye.
2. A plastic squeeze bottle is used unless very large amounts of fluid are needed.
3. Direct the irrigating fluid along the conjunctiva from the *inner* to the outer canthus (Fig. 21-5).
4. Avoid directing a forceful stream onto the eyeball.
5. Avoid touching any eye structures with irrigation equipment.
6. A piece of gauze may be wrapped around the index finger to raise upper lid for better cleaning if heavy discharge is present.
7. Place an emesis basin at side of face to collect irrigating fluid.

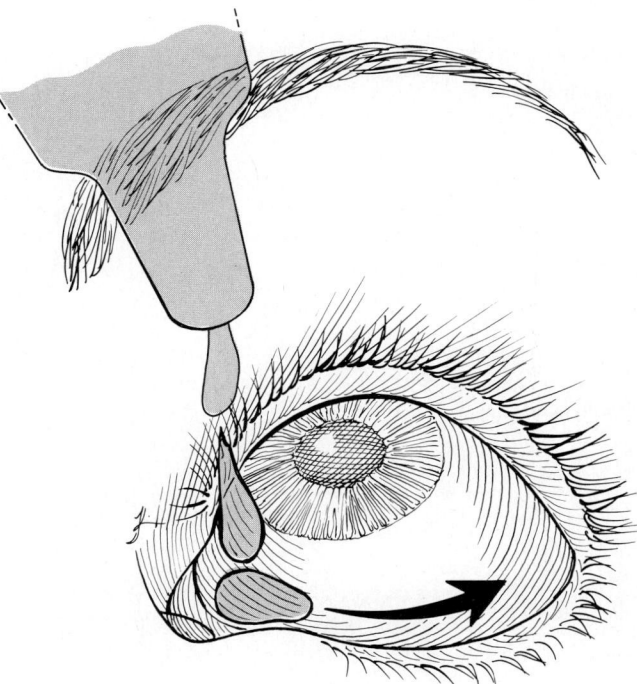

Fig. 21-5. Irrigating the eye. Fluid is directed along conjunctiva and over eyeball from inner to outer canthus.

Forms of eye medications

Ophthalmic solutions

1. Easily instilled
2. Do not interfere with vision
3. Cause few skin reactions
4. Do not interfere with mitosis of corneal epithelium
5. Disadvantage: do not remain in contact with eye for very long

Ophthalmic ointments

1. Remain in contact with eye for extended periods
2. Do not cause discomfort when instilled
3. Less absorption into lacrimal passageways
4. More stable than solutions
5. Disadvantages:
   a. Produce film across eye, which may interfere with vision
   b. May cause contact dermatitis
   c. May inhibit mitosis of corneal epithelium

logic saline solution or lactated Ringer's solution is commonly used because these isotonic solutions do not remove the electrolytes necessary for normal eye action. If only a small amount of fluid is needed, sterile cotton balls may be used to drip fluid into the eye.

Eye pads

Eye pads are contraindicated in general eye infections because they enhance bacterial growth. They may be used in photophobia when the inflammation is not caused by bacteria and to protect the eye when corneal ulceration is present. They are also used postoperatively to protect the eye from light and infection.

An eye pad is secured with two pieces of tape placed *diagonally* from cheek to forehead, one on each side of the pad. Plastic and paper tapes are used because they are easy to remove and do not cause allergic reactions.

Eye medications

Accuracy and safety in the administration of eye medications is essential to prevent irreparable damage to the eye. The correct eye to receive the medication must be identified. Labels must be checked carefully, and all medications with labels that are smeared or obliterated are discarded. Solutions that have changed color, are cloudy, contain sediment, or are outdated are also discarded. Elderly persons are particularly susceptible to side effects of medications.

Ophthalmic medications may be instilled as eyedrop solutions or ointment.

All patients should have their own bottles of eyedrops or tubes of ointment to prevent cross-infection. If an eye infection is being treated with an antibiotic and the same drug is being given prophylactically in the other eye, separate bottles or tubes are used.

Different types of drugs are used for treatment of eye diseases (Table 21-5). The most commonly used drugs for eye inflammations are antibiotic, steroid, and cycloplegic drugs (Tables 21-6 and 21-7).

Drugs applied topically to the eye can be absorbed and may cause systemic side effects. To avoid undesired systemic reactions, care should be taken with topically applied medications to give exactly what is ordered and no more.

Surgery

When the cornea is so damaged from corneal inflammation (keratitis) or from a corneal ulcer, corneal transplantation (keratoplasty) may be performed. Corneal grafts are taken from healthy donor eyes. Eye Banks for

---

Guidelines for instilling eye medications

Eyedrops

1. Wash hands before touching eyes.
2. Clean eyes before instilling eyedrops if crusting or discharge is present.
3. Ask patient to tilt head back and look up (Fig. 21-6).
4. Evert lower lid by pulling down gently on skin below eye.
5. Approach eye from side (not directly from front).
6. Place drops on *center* of conjunctival sac of lower lid.
7. Avoid touching eye with tip of dropper.
8. Ask patient not to squeeze eye shut (loss of medication down cheek).
9. Provide patient with a tissue.

Ointment

1. Follow steps 1 through 4 above.
2. Press the ointment from tube directly onto exposed conjunctival sac.
3. Avoid touching eye tissue with tube.

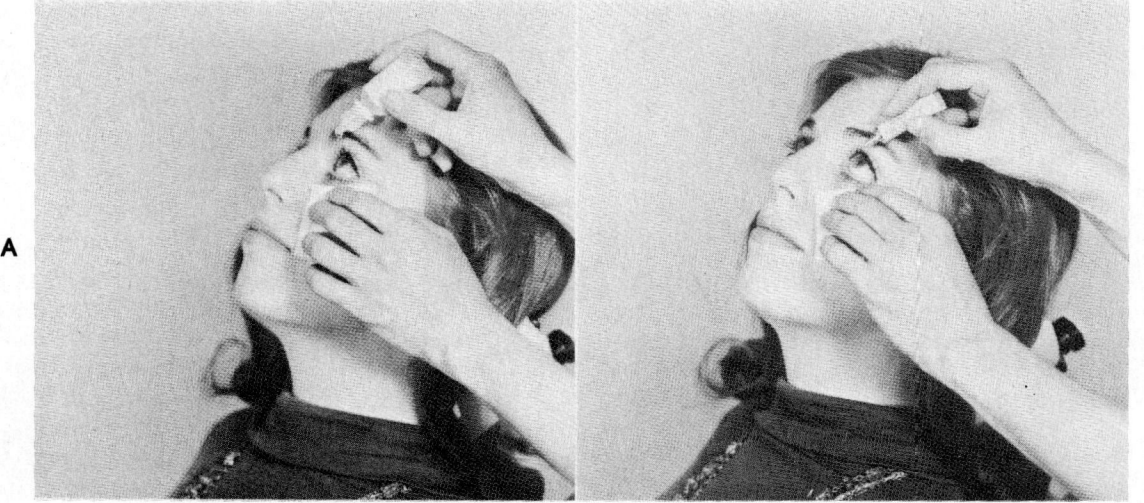

Fig. 21-6. To instill ophthalmic solution **(A)** or ointment **(B)** tilt patient's head backward supported by chair back or headrest. Use absorbent tissue pad under forefinger to depress lower lid to form conjunctival sac. Introduce medication into sac, never directly at or into eye. (Courtesy Eye and Ear Informary, University of Illinois Hospitals, Chicago, Ill.)

The patient with eye problems 449

Sight Restoration, Inc.,* a nonprofit organization, collects and distributes donated eyes throughout the United States.

Either total or partial replacement of the cornea may be performed (Fig. 21-7). The total penetrating graft is used most frequently, and although it is the more difficult of the grafts to establish, it is usually effective. A second transplant may be performed if the first is unsuccessful.

The surgery may be performed with local or general anesthesia. The new cornea is sutured in place, and an antibiotic is injected subconjunctivally. An eye shield is

*210 E. 64th St., New York, NY 10021.

applied, remains in place until the day after surgery, and is reapplied at night to prevent inadvertent injury during sleep. Glasses are worn during the day to protect the eye, and the patient can expect that some vision will be restored immediately. Vision improves over the following 6 to 12 months.

Corneal grafts heal very slowly because of the lack of blood vessels in the cornea. The patient is advised to avoid sudden, quick movement, jarring, bending, or lifting for 6 months. Sutures are not removed for 1 to 2 years.

The patient will need to use prescribed eyedrops after discharge and is instructed in their use. Topical antibiotics are usually given for 1 to 2 weeks, cycloplegics for 2

Table 21-5. Types of ophthalmic drugs

Type	Action	Uses
Mydriatic	Dilates pupil	Examination of interior of eye Prevents adhesions of iris with cornea in eye inflammations
Cycloplegic	Dilates pupil Paralyzes ciliary muscle and iris	Decreases pain and photophobia and provides rest in inflammations of iris and ciliary body and diseases of cornea Eye examinations
Miotic	Contracts pupil Permits better drainage of intraocular fluid	Glaucoma
Osmotic	Decreases intraocular pressure	Acute glaucoma Eye surgery
Secretory inhibitor	Decreases production of intraocular fluid	Glaucoma
Topical anesthetic	Decreases sensation (pain)	Surgery, treatments Eye inflammations
Topical antibiotic	Antiinfective	Eye inflammations
Steroid	Antiinflammatory	Eye inflammations and allergic reactions

Table 21-6. Mydriatic and cycloplegic drugs

Drug	Form and concentrations	Duration of effect
Mydriatric action		
Phenylephrine (Neo-synephrine)	Eyedrops, 1-10%	12 hr
Epinephrine (Epitrate)	Eyedrops, 1-2%	12 hr
Cycloplegic and mydriatic action		
Atropine sulfate (Atropisol, Isopto-Atropine)	Eyedrops, 0.5-1% Ointment, 1%	2-4 wk
Cyclopentolate (Cyclogyl)	Eyedrops, 0.5-2%	24 hr (cycloplegic) 2-3 days (mydriasis)
Homatropine (Isopto-Homatropine)	Eyedrops, 0.5-5%	1-2 days
Scopolamine hydrobromide	Eyedrops, 0.25-0.5%	1-2 days
Tropicamide (Mydriacyl)	Eyedrops, 0.5-1%	2-8 hr

Table 21-7. Other ophthalmic drugs

Drug	Form
Antibiotics and antiviral drugs	
Polymyxin B, bacitracin (Polysporin)	Ointment or eyedrops, 0.1-0.5%
Polymyxin B, neomycin, bacitracin (Neosporin)	Ointment
Bacitracin	Ointment, 500-1000 units/g
Idoxuridine (IDU)	Eyedrops, 0.1% solution
	Ointment, 0.5%
Gentamicin sulfate (Garamycin)	Eyedrops, 3% solution
Chloramphenicol (Chloromycetin, Chloroptic)	Oral, IV, subconjunctival
Steroids	
Prednisone	Topical, 0.25-0.5% suspension
	Oral, 5-15 mg
Prednisolone	Topical ointment, 0.1-0.25%
	Oral, 5-15 mg
Methylprednisolone (Depo-Medrol)	Subconjunctival, 0.5 mg
Triamcinolone (Aristocort)	Solution or ointment, 1%, subconjunctival
Dexamethasone (Decadron)	Solution, 0.1%
	Injection, 20 mg
Fluorometholone	Eyedrops, 0.1% solution
Anesthetics	
Proparacaine (Ophthaine, Ophthetic, Alcaine)	Eyedrops, 0.5% solution
Lidocaine (Xylocaine)	Local infiltration, 2-4% solution
Lubricants and tear substitutes	
Methylcellulose, gonioscopic	Eyedrops, 1% solution
Methylcellulose	Eyedrops, 0.1% solution

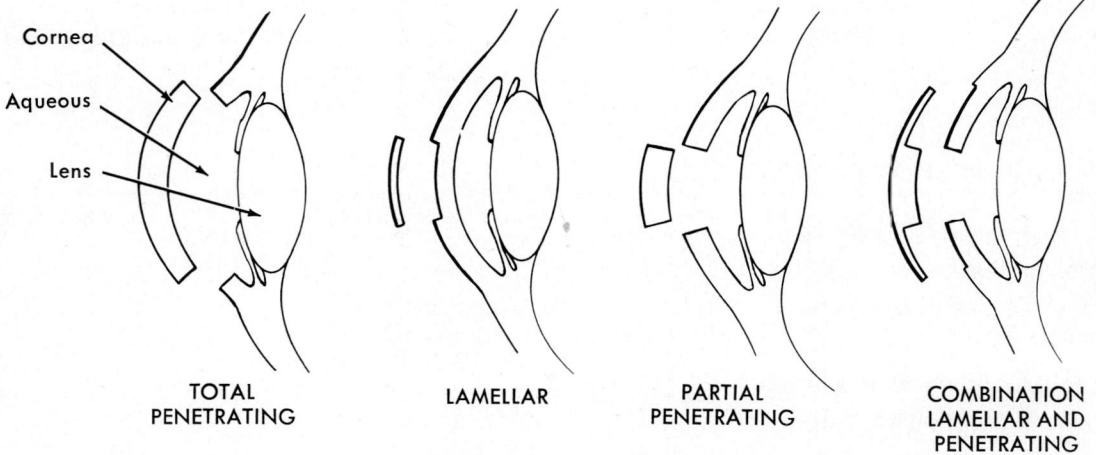

Fig. 21-7. Types of corneal grafts. Note that in lamellar graft, defect does not penetrate entire thickness of cornea.

to 4 weeks, and topical steroids in decreasing dosages for 6 to 8 months.[8]

Assisting with comfort

Pain from eye inflammations can be reduced by applying warm moist compresses several times each day and by instilling prescribed eyedrops (particularly the cycloplegic drugs, which put the iris and ciliary body at rest). If photophobia creates discomfort, bright lights can be dimmed. Mild analgesics such as aspirin or acetaminophen (Tylenol) usually suffice, but if pain is severe (as may occur with uveitis) a narcotic may be required.

Control of environment

When a highly infectious eye condition, such as acute bacterial conjunctivitis, is present, precautions need to be taken to prevent the spread of infection to others. Individual washcloths and towels should be used. Hands should be washed after any contact with the infected eye.

EVALUATION

When providing care for the patient with an eye inflammation or infection, consider the following:
1. Is the patient comfortable?
2. Is the uninvolved eye free of signs of infection?
3. Does the patient know how to carry out prescribed treatments after discharge?
4. If corneal surgery has been performed, does the patient know about activity limitations and need for continued medical follow-up?

Cataract

A cataract is a clouding or opacity of the lens that leads to gradual painless blurring of vision and eventual loss of sight (Fig. 21-8). The most common cause of cataract formation is aging (senile cataract); other causes include trauma, other eye diseases (for example, uveitis), systemic diseases (diabetes mellitus), or congenital defects (either hereditary or as a result of prenatal viral infections such as German measles).

PATHOPHYSIOLOGY

The lens of the eye is normally transparent, so that light rays can pass through. Biochemical changes may occur within the lens, or trauma may cause fiber changes that cause the lens to become cloudy and finally opaque, thus blocking the light rays from reaching the retina. A *mature cataract* is a developed cataract that separates easily from the lens capsule. It was previously thought that a cataract had to be mature ("ripe") before it could be extracted. Now cataracts are removed whenever the decreased vision interferes with activities of daily living. Cataracts may develop in both eyes, such as with senile cataracts, but usually at different rates.

ASSESSMENT

Acquired cataracts, either from aging or disease, usually develop gradually. Blurring of vision may occur immediately after trauma. The predominant symptom is progressive loss of vision; the degree of loss depends on the location and extent of the opacity. Persons with an opacity in the center portion of the lens can generally see better in dim light, when the pupil is dilated. The person with presbyopia may find that reading without glasses is possible in the early stages because of resulting myopia.

SURGERY

Surgery is the only method for treating cataracts, although only a small percentage of senile cataracts progress to the point where surgery is required. Patients of any age, even in their nineties, can be operated on with good results. The decision to remove the cataract depends on the degree of visual impairment, general health, and the use made of the eyes.

Because surgery is usually indicated only for advanced

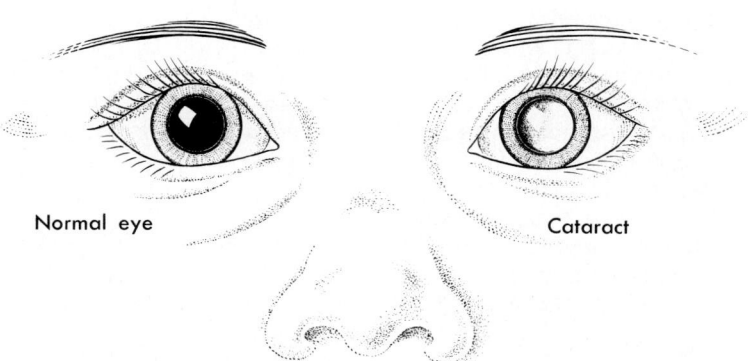

Normal eye   Cataract

Fig. 21-8. Cataract visible in left eye as white opacity of lens seen through pupil.

cataracts, elderly persons may believe they should wait until vision loss is far advanced before consulting an ophthalmologist. Delaying medical examination of the eye can lead to permanent vision loss if there is glaucoma, either alone or in combination with cataracts.

Surgical procedure

Cataracts usually are removed with the eye under local anesthesia. Removal has been simplified in many cases by the use of the enzyme alpha-chymotripsin, which weakens the zonular fibers that hold the lens in place. Cataracts may be removed within their capsule (intracapsular technique), or an opening may be made in the capsule and the lens lifted out without disturbing the membrane (extracapsular technique).

The most commonly used method of cataract removal is cryoextraction, using a supercooled metal probe that adheres to the wet surface of the cataract. Another method is phacoemulsification, which breaks up the lens and flushes it out in tiny pieces. A vibrating needle probe is used, and only one stitch is required to close the small incision. Healing is therefore quicker with phacoemulsification than with cryoextraction. The size and shape of the eye determine the most suitable method.

Preoperative care

The preparation of the eye on the day of surgery may include instillation of a combination of drugs into the eye at various intervals to dilate the pupil. The medications *must* be given at the prescribed times so that the eye is prepared at the time of surgery. If anesthetizing drops are instilled before the patient goes to the operating room, the patient is asked to close the eye and a pad is applied for protection. A sedative may also be prescribed preoperatively.

Postoperative care

Specific routines for care after eye surgery vary, and change rapidly as new techniques are developed. However, general goals of postoperative care are to *prevent* (1) increased intraocular pressure, (2) stress on the suture line, (3) hemorrhage into the anterior chamber, and (4) infection. Mydriatric and cycloplegic drugs may be prescribed before cataract surgery to keep the pupil dilated to prevent adhesions of the iris. Topical antibiotics may be given prophylactically.

Nursing interventions include the following:
1. Place patient on side not operated on or on back (to prevent pressure on affected eye).
2. Place bedside table at patient's side opposite that operated on to prevent turning to the affected side.
3. Apply metal eye shield at night to protect eye.
4. Assist with ambulation as necessary depending on extent of vision in unaffected eye.
5. Report complaints of severe pain or pressure within eye to physician (may suggest infection or hemorrhage).
6. Teach patient to avoid increasing intraocular pressure
   a. No bending or leaning over
   b. No straining (Valsalva manuever) or lifting.

Corrective lenses

Because the lens of the eye is removed, some form of auxiliary lens must be used, for example, cataract glasses, contact lenses (p. 439), or lens implants (Table 21-8).

More patients are now receiving lens implants at the time of surgery. The intraocular lens, which is made of polymethylmethacrylate, may be held in place either by suturing it to the iris (iris fixation) or by implanting it into the capsular sac. When the lens is implanted with-

Table 21-8. Corrective lenses after cataract surgery

Type	Advantages	Disadvantages
Lens implant	Cannot be lost or broken Better binocular vision No handling required	Possible complications: vitreous loss, inflammation
Contact lenses	Better visual correction than glasses Better cosmetic appearance Better binocular vision if only one lens removed	Awkward for some elderly persons to manage Easy to lose Difficult adjustment for some persons May cause irritation
Cataract glasses	More acceptable to some elderly persons No physical complications	Magnify objects by 25%; objects appear closer than they actually are Distort peripheral images and colors Heavy lenses May cause visual distortion if poorly positioned

out sutures, miotic agents (pilocarpine) are needed to prevent the iris from dilating too widely and causing the lens to slip.

GLAUCOMA

Glaucoma is eye disease characterized by increased intraocular pressure and associated with progressive loss of peripheral visual fields. It is responsible for about 15% of all blindness in the United States, and the incidence is increasing with the number of older persons in our population. Because early signs may be absent in some forms of glaucoma, many persons are unaware that they have glaucoma until loss of vision occurs. Early diagnosis and treatment are essential to prevent loss of vision.

PATHOPHYSIOLOGY

The anterior cavity of the eye in front of and to the sides of the lens is filled with aqueous humor, a free-flowing clear liquid similar to lymph. Aqueous humor is constantly being formed in the ciliary body located posterior to the iris, and it flows through the pupil into the anterior chamber (Fig. 21-9). The aqueous humor drains through Schlemm's canal, which encircles the eye and is located at the angle of the anterior chamber where the peripheral iris and cornea meet.

Normally there is a balance between the production and drainage of aqueous humor, permitting the intraocular pressure to remain relatively constant. The normal range of intraocular pressure is 10 to 21 mm Hg, with a mean value of 16 mm Hg. The pressure may vary up to 5 mm Hg as a result of diurnal changes.

Glaucoma results when the intraocular pressure is increased sufficiently to produce damage to the optic nerve. The increased pressure results from obstruction of drainage of the aqueous humor. The two major types of glaucoma are chronic open angle, which is most common, and acute angle closure, which is an ocular emergency (Table 21-9).

ASSESSMENT

Visual acuity testing is part of the routine physical assessment (Chapter 3). A more complete examination of visual acuity includes use of the Snellen chart (Fig. 21-3) and ocular refraction by an ophthalmologist or optometrist.

Visual *fields* (that which is visible during fixation of vision on one point) can be tested by various means. Gross measurement of peripheral vision can be accomplished as follows: Ask the person to focus steadily at a point directly ahead. Then place an object, such as a pencil or finger, peripherally beyond the line of vision. Advance it until the person states seeing it. Normally it should be seen at about 60 degrees laterally.

The ophthalmologist measures *intraocular pressure (IOP)* by means of a tonometer. There are various types of tonometers. The most common is the Schiøtz tonometer. The eye is anesthetized, and the tonometer is placed directly on the cornea (Fig. 21-11). Readings of > 24 mm Hg may suggest glaucoma. Temporary increases in IOP may occur from emotional stress. More elaborate tonometers, such as the air tonometer, which uses a jet of air to record the pressure, are frequently used by ophthalmologists and optometrists.

Nursing assessment consists of identifying any changes in vision as described by the patient and assessing degree of comfort.

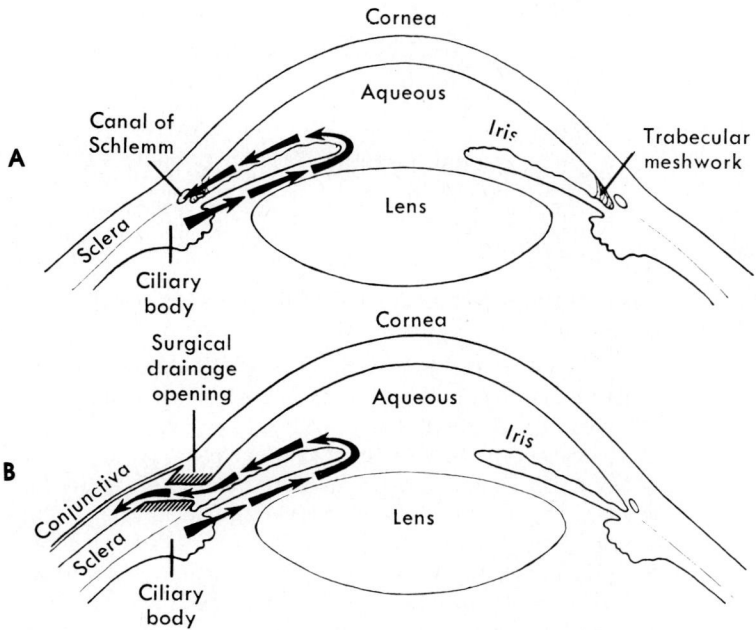

Fig. 21-9. A, Originating from ciliary processes, aqueous flows through pupil into anterior chamber and normally leaves eye by way of canal of Schlemm. **B,** In glaucoma, normal aqueous outflow is blocked. Purpose of glaucoma surgery is to create new channel through which aqueous can leave eye. (From Havener, W.J.: Synopsis of ophthalmology, ed. 5, St. Louis, 1979, The C.V. Mosby Co.)

Table 21-9. Types of glaucoma

Type	Characteristic	Signs and symptoms	Medical therapy
Chronic simple (open angle)	Most common type Results from degenerative changes	Slow loss of vision Early loss of peripheral vision (tunnel vision) (Fig. 21-10) Persistent dull eye pain Difficulty adjusting to darkness Failure to detect color changes Later: blurred vision, halos around lights, headaches, pain behind eyeball, nausea, vomiting	Eyedrops: miotics, carbonic anhydrase inhibitors, timolol maleate (Timoptic) Surgery: creation of permanent fistula to drain fluid
Acute (angle closure)	Ocular emergency Narrow angle of anterior chamber Blockage caused by pupil dilation from darkness, excitement, or a mydriatic drug	Severe eye pain radiating to head, blurring of vision, redness of eye, dilated pupil, colored halos seen around lights Marked increase in intraocular pressure for 24 to 48 hours leads to permanent blindness	Osmotic agents to lower intraocular pressure Miotics, carbonic anhydrase inhibitors Laser or surgical iridectomy or laser iridotomy
Absolute	Final stage of uncontrolled glaucoma	Eye is hard, sightless, and painful	Eye enucleation (removal)

DATA ANALYSIS AND PLANNING

Nursing diagnoses

Nursing diagnoses for the person with glaucoma may include the following:

Alteration in comfort: eye pain
Alteration in sensory perception: visual
Knowledge deficit

Expected patient outcomes

1. The patient states discomfort is decreased.
2. Vision is not decreased further.
3. When discharged the patient can:
   a. State recognition of lifetime need for eye medication
   b. State name, dosage, frequency, and side effects of prescribed eye medications
   c. Describe measures to prevent complications
   d. List signs indicating need to report immediately to ophthalmologist.

IMPLEMENTATION

Assisting with achievement of therapeutic goals
Medications

It is vital in the control of glaucoma that eye medications be given as prescribed. Drugs used in treatment of glaucoma are listed in Table 21-10. The purpose of pharmacologic therapy is to keep the pupil *constricted* to permit better drainage of the aqueous humor and to decrease the amount of aqueous humor produced. Pilocarpine is the miotic drug of choice in the treatment of chronic simple glaucoma. Mydriatic and cycloplegic agents are *contraindicated* in patients with glaucoma because they may further restrict drainage of aqueous humor. In severe acute conditions, osmotic agents are given to lower IOP by

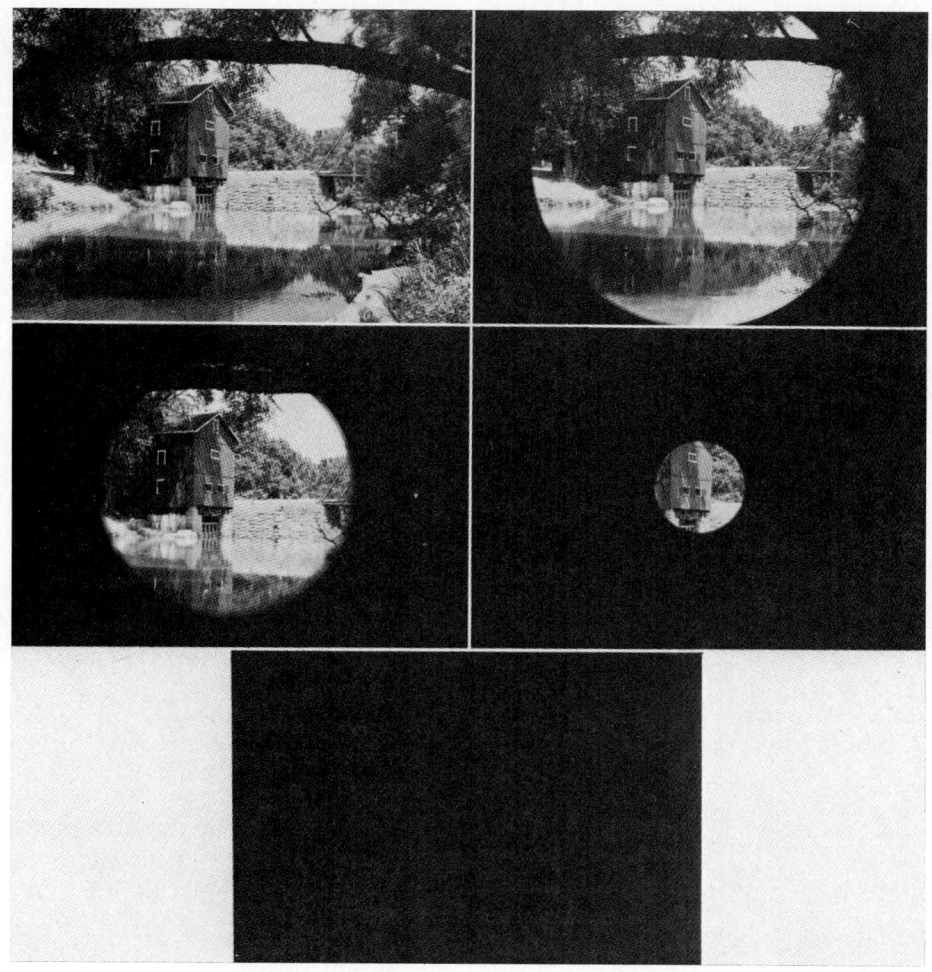

Fig. 21-10. Gradual loss of sight from glaucoma so insidiously destroys vision that person is unaware of impending blindness until extensive and irreversible damage is already present. (From Saunders, W.H., et al.: Nursing care in eye, ear, nose, and throat disorders, ed. 4, St. Louis, 1979, The C.V. Mosby Co.)

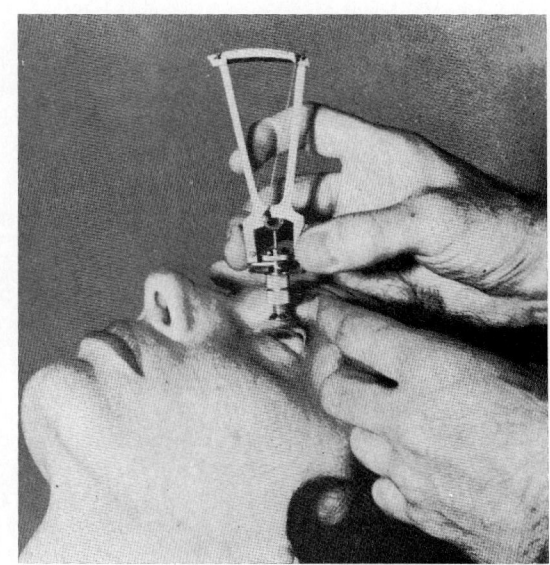

Fig. 21-11. Measurement of intraocular pressure with Schiøtz tonometer. (From Saunders, W.H., et al.: Nursing care in eye, ear, nose and throat disorders, ed. 4, St. Louis, 1979, The C.V. Mosby Co.)

Table 21-10. Drugs used in treatment of glaucoma

Drug	Form
Cholinergic drugs (miotics)	
Pilocarpine	0.5-3% solution (Ocusert)
Carbachol (Carbacel)	0.25-3% solution
Cholinesterase inhibitors (miotics)	
Physostigmine (Eserine)	0.25-1% solution or ointment
Isoflurophate (DFP) (Floropryl)	Ointment
Demecarium bromide (Humorsol)	0.125-0.25% solution
Echothiophate iodide (Phospholine iodide)	0.06-0.125% solution
Adrenergic agents	
Epinephryl borate (Eppy)	0.5-1% solution
Epinephrine hydrochloride (Glaucon)	0.5-2% solution
Epinephrine bitarrate (Epitrate)	2% solution
Carbonic anhydrase inhibitors	
Acetazolamide (Diamox)	125-250 mg tablets
	500 mg capsules, sequential
	500 mg vials for IM or IV use
Ethoxzolamide (Cardrase)	125-250 mg tablets
Dichlorphenamide (Daranide)	25-50 mg tablets
Methazolamide (Neptazane)	25-50 mg tablets
Osmotic agents	
Glycerin (glycerin, Osmoglyn, Ophthalgan)	Mix with equal amount of orange juice (oral)
Mannitol (Osmitrol)	10-20% solution for IV use
Urea (Ureaphil, Urevert)	30% solution for IV use
Beta-adrenergic blocker	
Timolol maleate (Timoptic)	0.25-0.5% solution

drawing fluid from the eye. Pain and blurred vision, commonly experienced at the beginning of treatment, disappear with prolonged use.

Surgery

Surgery may be performed in chronic simple glaucoma to produce a permanent filtration pathway for aqueous fluid. Filtering procedures, such as trabeculectomy, sclerotomy, iridencleisis, and trephining, provide a permanent fistula from the anterior chamber to the subconjunctival space. In selected cases, the production of aqueous fluid may be decreased by destroying part of the ciliary body. This may be accomplished by diathermy or cryosurgery. After surgery the patient usually is allowed out of bed at once, although one or both eyes may be bandaged for several days. Postoperative care is similar to that after cataract surgery (p. 452).

Surgery is usually performed in acute angle-closure glaucoma after initial vigorous pharmacologic therapy to decrease IOP. A portion of the peripheral iris is surgically excised (iridectomy) to maintain drainage.

Assisting with comfort

Pain usually decreases as the IOP decreases. Analgesics may be prescribed. Cold eye compresses may be helpful for painful eye spasms.

Teaching

Glaucoma is a chronic condition, and the patient with newly diagnosed glaucoma needs assistance in understanding and learning to live with the disease. Despite explanations from the physician, the person frequently hopes that an operation will provide a cure, that no further treatment will be necessary, and perhaps that the lost sight will be restored. It should be explained that *lost vision cannot be restored* but that further loss can usually be prevented and normal activities can be pursued if the person continues medical care. There usually is no restriction on the use of the eyes (see box, p. 457).

EVALUATION

Evaluation is based on the expected patient outcomes. Questions to ask include: Is the patient comfortable?

Teaching the patient with glaucoma

1. Medical supervision willl be required for the rest of life.
2. Eye drops *must* be continued as long as prescribed, even in the absence of symptoms
   a. Blurred vision decreases with prolonged use
   b. Avoid driving for 1 to 2 hours after administration of miotics.
3. To prevent complications:
   a. Have reserve bottle of eyedrops at home
   b. Carry eyedrops when away from home
   c. Carry card identifying glaucoma and the eyedrops solution prescribed.
4. Bright lights and darkness are not harmful.
5. There is no apparent relationship between vascular hypertension and ocular hypertension.
6. Report any reappearance of symptoms immediately to ophthalmologist.
7. If admitted to hospital for a different medical condition, alert the staff of continued need for prescribed eyedrops.
8. Avoid the use of mydriatic or cycloplegic drugs (for example, atropine) that dilate the pupils.

Does the patient know the chronic nature of the disease and treatment?

RETINAL DETACHMENT

PATHOPHYSIOLOGY

The retina is the part of the eye that perceives light; it coordinates and transmits impulses from receptor nerve cells to the optic nerve. It consists of two layers. Retinal detachment occurs when the two retinal layers separate as a result of accumulation of fluid or traction produced by contraction of the vitreous body (Fig. 21-12). As the detachment extends and becomes complete, blindness results. Myopic degeneration, trauma, and aphakia (absence of the crystalline lens) are the most frequent causes of retinal detachment. Detachment may follow sudden severe physical exertion, especially in persons who are debilitated. Most often, however, there is no apparent cause.

ASSESSMENT

Retinal detachment may occur suddenly or develop slowly. The person first notices flashes of light, followed by floating spots before the eye and progressive loss of vision. The floating spots are blood and retinal cells that are freed at the time of the tear and cast shadows on the retina as they seem to drift about the eye. The area of visual loss depends entirely on the location of the detachment. Usually there is a superior retinal detachment with inferior visual loss. When the detachment is extensive and occurs quickly, the patient may have the sensation that a curtain has been drawn before the eyes. The diagnosis is confirmed by ophthalmoscopic examination.

Ongoing nursing assessment includes the patient's subjective statements concerning changes in vision and observations related to signs of anxiety. The person with

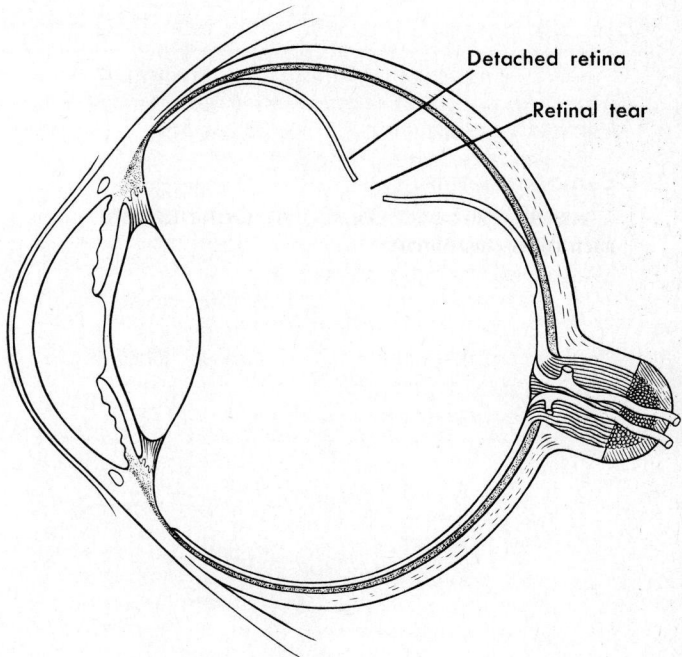

Fig. 21-12. Retinal detachment.

both eyes bandaged is assessed for ability to carry out activities of daily living.

DATA ANALYSIS AND PLANNING
Nursing diagnoses

Nursing diagnoses for the patient with retinal detachment may include the following:
Sensory perception alteration: visual
Anxiety
Potential for injury
Knowledge deficit

Patient teaching for retinal detachment

1. Report to ophthalmologist any signs of redetachment (flashes of light, increase in "floaters," blurred vision).
2. No reading for 3 weeks.
3. Check with physician concerning shampooing of hair.
4. Limited activity for 3 weeks.
5. No physical exertion for 6 weeks.
6. Check with physician concerning resumption of contact sports.
7. If eyedrops will be needed, teach appropriate technique.

Expected patient outcomes

1. No further vision loss occurs.
2. No injury occurs.
3. The patient can describe:
   a. Signs and symptoms indicating further retinal detachment
   b. Extent of limitations on activity.

IMPLEMENTATION

Assisting with achievement of therapeutic goals

Immediate care for the detachment of the retina includes keeping the patient quiet in bed with eyes covered to try to prevent further detachment. The head is positioned so the retinal hole is in the lowest part of the eye; that is, if the detachment is in the upper right, the patient is positioned flat on the right side. Activities are restricted.

Table 21-11. Surgical procedures for retinal detachment

Purpose	Procedure	Method
Removal of fluid from subretinal space	Drainage	Needle insertion
Sealing of retinal tear by creating inflammation to adhere retina to choroid	Cryosurgery	Supercooled probe applied to scleral surface over tear
	Diathermy	Application of diathermy (heat) to scleral surface over tear
	Photocoagulation	Strong light focused through pupil onto retinal tear
	Laser	Laser beam focused through pupil onto retinal tear
Splinting of choroid to retina until choroidal scar can seal tear	Scleral buckling	Tuck taken in sclera (to indent sclera and choroid) and sutured; buckle held in place with a piece of silicone held by a strap (Fig. 21-13)

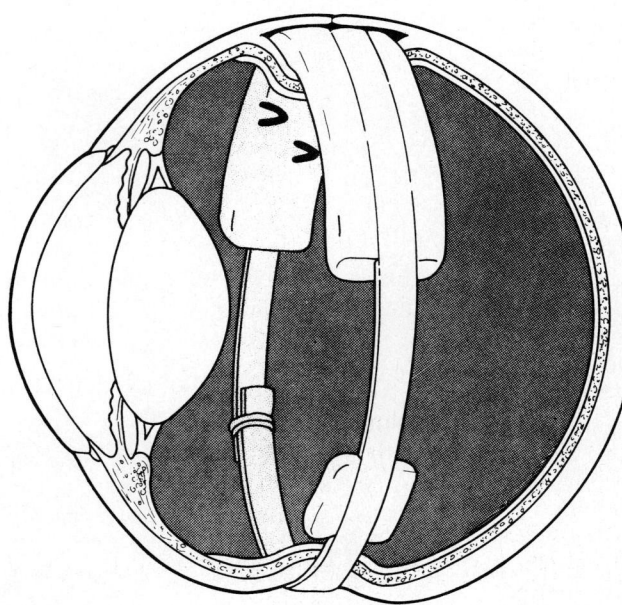

Fig. 21-13. Scleral buckle.

Promoting physical safety and comfort

Until treatment is instituted, both eyes are usually covered to decrease eye activity. Because the person cannot see, guidelines for communicating with blind persons (p. 443) are appropriate. Siderails are usually raised for safety precautions, and the call cord is always kept within easy reach.

Counseling

Anxiety frequently results from concern over possible loss of vision and feelings about having both eyes bandaged. Elderly persons may become confused when both eyes are covered and may need frequent orientation to place and time. Loss of orientation to time is not unusual for the person with both eyes bandaged. Radios are helpful for time orientation and for diversion.

Patients with retinal detachment may need opportunities to discuss their concerns if they so desire. Restoration of sight depends on the extent and duration of the retinal detachment and the degree of success of treatment. Therefore, reassurance to all patients that their sight will be restored cannot be made, although a large majority of persons do respond favorably with treatment.

Surgery

Early treatment is usually instituted because of the better prognosis with treatment. The procedures may be performed under local or general anesthesia. Different types of procedures may be carried out (Table 21-11).

Postoperative care

1. Position patient as instructed. This varies but usually includes the following:
   a. Position in bed with detached area *lowermost*
   b. Bedrest for 1 to 2 days.
2. Avoid jerking movements of the head, for example, combing hair, sneezing, coughing, vomiting.
   a. If nausea is present, give prescribed antiemetics.
   b. If cough is present, give prescribed cough medicine.
3. Assist with activities of daily living as necessary (e.g., wash back to prevent jerking of head).
4. Avoid reading if one eye is unbandaged (causes jerking of eyes). Television is permitted.
5. If eye discomfort is present (lid edema and conjunctival redness), apply prescribed warm compresses (p. 446).
6. Instill prescribed eyedrops (usually mydriatics).
7. Identify what patient knows about post-discharge activities and teach as necessary (see box, p. 458).

EVALUATION

Evaluation is based on expected patient outcomes. Questions to ask may include the following:
Is patient comfortable?
What is patient's reaction to restriction of activity and bandaging of eyes?
Does patient know expectations after discharge?

REFERENCES AND SELECTED READINGS*

1. American Foundation for the Blind: Directory of agencies serving the visually handicapped in the United States, New York, 1983, the William Byrd Press.
2. Boyd-Monk, H.: Examining the external eye, I. Nurs. 80 **10**(5):58-63, 1980. II. Nurs. 80 **10**(6):58-63, 1980.
3. *Boyd-Monk, H.: Helping the corneal transplant patient to see again, Nurs. 78 **8**(2):47-51, 1978.
4. *Boyd-Monk, H.: Screening for glaucoma, Nurs. 79 **9**(8):42-45, 1979.
5. Boyles, V.A.: Injection aids for blind diabetic patients, Am. J. Nurs. **77**:1456-1458, 1977.
6. Drugs in eye infections, Nurses Drug Alert **2**:100-103, 1978.
7. *Fernsberger, W.: Early diagnosis of acute angle-closure glaucoma, Am. J. Nurs. **75**:1154-1155, 1975.
8. *Gallagher, M.A.: Corneal transplantation, Am. J. Nurs. **81**:1845, 1981.
9. *Gould, H.: How to remove contact lenses from comatose patients, Am. J. Nurs. **76**:1483-1485, 1976.
10. *Jennings, B.: Intraocular lens for cataracts, AORN J **23**:664-672, 1976.
11. *Levenson, L., and Levenson, J.: Corneal transplantation, Am. J. Nurs. **77**:1160-1163, 1977.
12. *Neu, C.: Coping with newly diagnosed blindness, Am. J. Nurs. **76**:2161-2163, 1976.
13. *Resler, M.M., and Tumulty, G.: Glaucoma update, Am. J. Nurs. **83**:752-756, 1983.
14. *Reynolds, B.J.: Suddenly blind at 80, Nurs. 79 **9**(7):47-49, 1979.
15. Saunders, W.H., et al.: Nursing care in eye, ear, nose, and throat disorders, ed. 4, St. Louis, 1979, The C.V. Mosby Co.
16. *Shadick, M.H.: "I feel I'll be able to serve my patients more effectively because of my blindness," Occup. Health Nurs. **29**(2):16-18, 1981.
17. *Stern, E.J.: Helping the person with low vision, Am. J. Nurs. **80**:1788-1790, 1980.
18. *Wong, E.K., et al.: How ophthalmic drugs can fool you, RN **43**:36-44, 1980.

*References preceded by an asterisk are particularly well suited for student reading.

The Patient with Ear Problems

LINDA ANNE BROSEMAN

STUDY QUESTIONS

- Review the anatomy of the ear. What are the points of intersection between the external and middle ear? Between the middle and inner ear? Describe the pathway that sound takes to reach the brain.

- Walk around for 1 day with earphones on your head or earplugs in your ears. Describe your reactions. How do you think you would feel if you were told you would never hear well again?

- What agencies are available in your community that provide services for the hard-of-hearing or deaf persons?

ANATOMY AND PHYSIOLOGY

The ear and its structures will be discussed in three parts; the external ear, the middle ear and mastoid process, and the inner ear.

External ear

The external ear has two parts, the auricle (pinna) and the ear canal (Fig. 22-1). The *auricle* is generally made up of cartilage and skin, with little subcutaneous fat except for the lobule. The blood and lymphatic supply to the auricle are excellent. The nerve supply to the external ear is chiefly from cranial nerve V (trigeminal) and a branch of cranial nerve X (vagus) and from the cervical nerves.

The external ear and auditory *canal* provide a channel along which sound travels to the tympanic membrane. The outer third of the canal is lined with skin containing wax and sweat glands. The inner part of the canal is lined with squamous epithelium.

The external ear is separated from the middle ear by the *tympanic membrane (eardrum)*. It is a fairly tough membrane that serves to protect the middle ear and also vibrates with incoming sound waves for hearing.

Middle ear

The middle ear, which lies directly behind the eardrum, is a small air-filled space in the tympanic portion of the temporal bone. It contains three small bones, or ossicles: the *malleus, incus,* and *stapes.* The footplate of the stapes fits into the oval window, which is a small opening in the wall between the middle ear and the inner ear. The ossicles amplify sound waves received by the tympanic membrane and transmit them through the membrane in the oval window to the fluid in the inner ear.

Also communicating with the middle ear is the *eustachian tube,* a channel that extends into the nasopharynx. The eustachian tube allows air into the middle ear, thus equalizing pressure on both sides of the eardrum. The middle ear communicates posteriorly with mastoid air cells. Portions of the facial nerve (controlling movement of the face and supplying taste to the tongue) are located in the middle ear.

Inner ear

The inner ear, or *labyrinth,* contains both the organ of hearing (cochlea) and the organ of balance (vestibule and

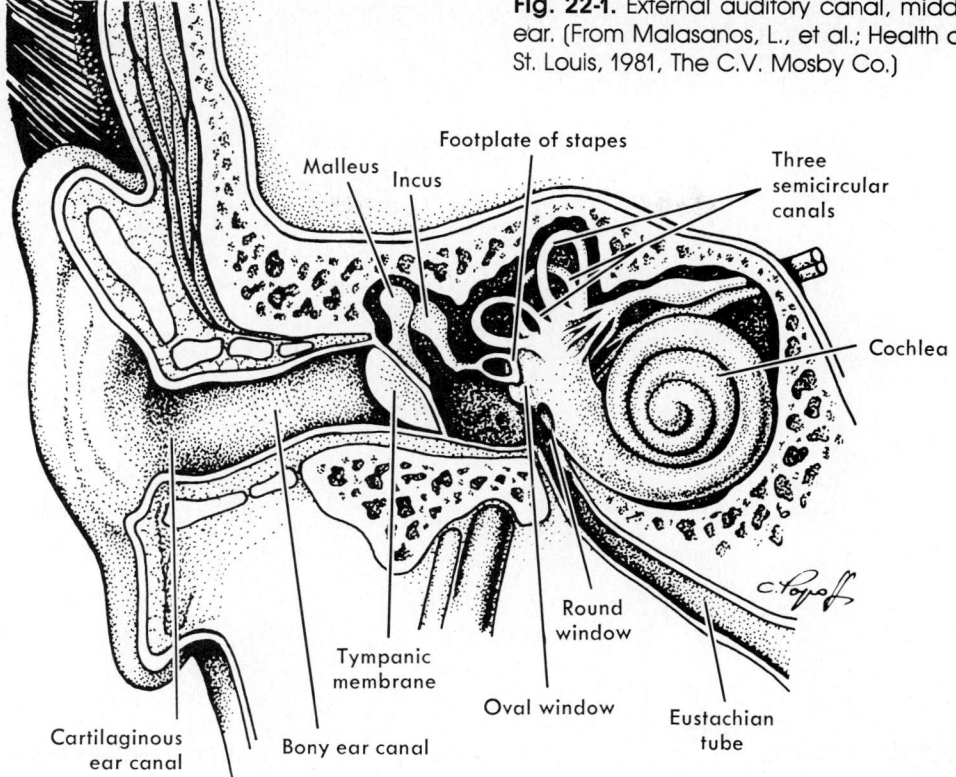

Fig. 22-1. External auditory canal, middle ear, and inner ear. (From Malasanos, L., et al.; Health assessment, ed. 2, St. Louis, 1981, The C.V. Mosby Co.)

Characteristics of sounds

Intensity	Pressure exerted by a sound, measured in decibels (db)
Loudness	Sensation of sound intensity experienced by a person
Frequency	Number of sound waves emanating from a source per second; expressed in hertz (Hz)
Pitch	Sensation of sound frequency experienced by a person

---

semicircular canals). The labyrinth, made up of delicate nerve tissue, will not recover if damaged. The inner ear is protected from damage by being situated deep in the head in the petrous bone.

Two separate fluids, the perilymph and the endolymph, are found in tiny channels in the labyrinth. The endolymph is contained in a membranous tube, which is then surrounded by the perilymph, which cushions the tube. The endolymph is in a contained closed system, while the perilymphatic spaces connect with the subarachnoid space and its cerebrospinal fluid.

The end organ of hearing, the organ of Corti, has thousands of tiny "hair cells" that project from its neuroepithelium. Sound waves enter the cochlea and mechanically bend the hair cells. At this time, sound, which had been a mechanical force, is converted into an electrochemical impulse. The impulse travels along the eighth cranial nerve (acoustic) to the temporal cortex of the brain, and is interpreted as meaningful sound. The hair cells are the most fragile elements in the ear and are crucial to hearing. In some instances persons with normal hair cells are unable to hear because of destruction of the acoustic nerve by a tumor.

Sound waves and hearing

Normal hearing depends on the ear's capacity to translate sound waves into meaningful sensations (Fig. 22-2). Sound is a form of energy generated by a vibrating source. Pure tones such as those generated by a tuning fork are simple sound waves. The human voice, however, produces more complex sound waves. Characteristics of sounds are described in box above.

Speech that is comfortably loud to a person with normal hearing ranges in intensity from approximately 40 to 65 db. Fig. 22-3 lists the decibel levels of various environmental sounds and situations.

A sound with a low frequency is perceived as a tone

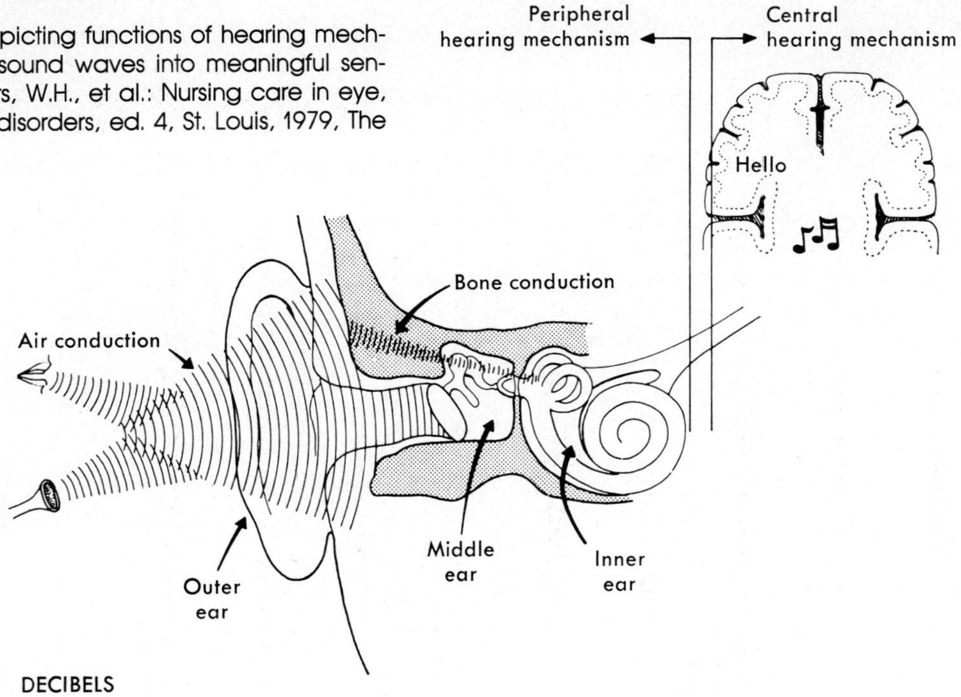

Fig. 22-2. Schema depicting functions of hearing mechanism as it translates sound waves into meaningful sensations. (From Saunders, W.H., et al.: Nursing care in eye, ear, nose, and throat disorders, ed. 4, St. Louis, 1979, The C.V. Mosby Co.)

Peripheral hearing mechanism ←→ Central hearing mechanism

Hello

Bone conduction

Air conduction

Middle ear

Inner ear

Outer ear

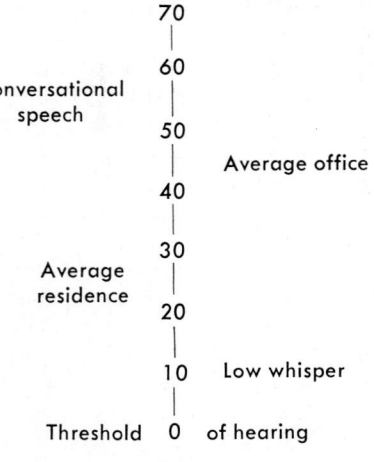

DECIBELS

140 — Jet engine
130
120
Thunder
110
100 — Rivet hammer
90
Air hammer
80
Heavy traffic
70
60
Conversational speech
50
Average office
40
30
Average residence
20
10 — Low whisper
Threshold 0 of hearing

DECIBELS

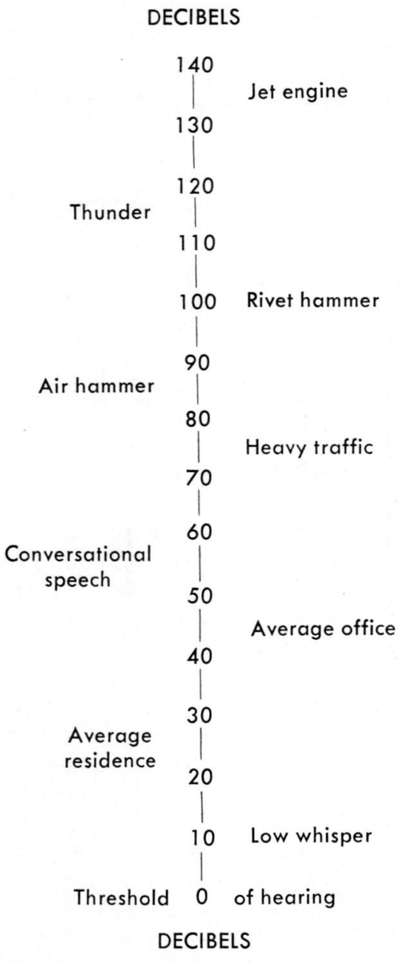

Fig. 22-3. Intensity range of human hearing. Intensity levels of various environmental sounds and situations. (From Saunders, W.H., et al.: Nursing care in eye, ear, nose, and throat disorders, ed. 4, St. Louis, 1979, The C.V. Mosby Co.)

low in pitch, whereas a sound with high frequency is perceived as a high-pitched tone. A child or young adult with normal hearing can often hear frequencies ranging from 20 to 20,000 Hz. Hearing is most sensitive for frequencies of 500 to 4000 Hz.

Sound reaches the inner ear by one of two ways: air conduction or bone conduction. Air conduction is the most sensitive. In *air conduction* sound waves pass through the ear canal to the ossicular chain to the inner ear (Fig. 22-2). In *bone conduction* hearing is caused by sound being transmitted through the bones of the skull to the inner ear. Sound energy is transformed in the inner ear into neural energy and is then "decoded" and interpreted by the brain as sound.

PREVENTION OF HEARING DIFFICULTIES

Hearing difficulties may begin at any age. Understanding the many causes of hearing loss is important for all health team members in all settings. Because nurses occupy a unique position in the health care system, they have the opportunity to be involved in many aspects of health care of the ear.

Care of healthy ears

A certain amount of cerumen (ear wax) in the ear canal is normal, and persons who have no wax have itching and scaling in the ear canal. Usually it is not necessary to clean the ears to remove wax. Occasionally, when the wax becomes impacted and causes pain or temporary deafness, it must be removed by the physician or person instructed in the procedure. Insertion of warm sweet oil (mineral oil or glycerin) or hydrogen peroxide in glyceryl

(Debrox) into the auditory canal for several days to soften the wax will facilitate removal.

All persons are taught not to insert anything into the ear beyond the extent of vision (including cotton swabs); wax or debris can be pushed further into the ear and cause pressure against the eardrum, or the eardrum itself can be damaged by the introduced article.

Prevention of ear infections

Before the advent of antibiotics, hearing loss was a frequent sequela of middle ear and mastoid process infections. Adequate treatment of upper respiratory tract and particularly of ear infections can prevent this loss. Persons need to be taught to blow the nose gently *with both nostrils open* to avoid contamination of the eustachian tubes with mucus, especially during an upper respiratory tract infection. Swimming in stagnant water or in water identified as being polluted may also lead to ear infection.

Individuals with upper respiratory infections should be encouraged to seek medical attention if they experience the following:

1. Increasing pain in the ear or increasing headache even after application of heat
2. Reddish fluid oozing from the ear (may indicate rupture of eardrum)
3. Temperature higher than 39° (102° F)
4. Convulsive twitching of facial muscles
5. Dizziness

Monitoring side effects of ototoxic drugs

Persons taking ototoxic drugs need to know the signs and symptoms of side effects of these drugs to prevent loss of hearing from developing. If symptoms of dizziness, decreased hearing acuity, or tinnitus (ringing in the ears) occur, the next dose of the drug is omitted and the physician is consulted. Audiometric testing may be necessary.

Monitoring noise pollution

A major cause of hearing loss is occupational hearing loss. Exposure to *industrial noise* levels greater than 85 to 90 db for months or years causes cochlear damage. Some 9 million workers are exposed daily to noise levels on the job that are potentially hazardous to hearing. Health team members in industry can help prevent deafness caused by noise of high intensity by teaching employees why they should wear earplugs. The nurse in industry faces a task that calls for special knowledge and training; courses are available to familiarize nurses with industrial hearing conservation requirements.

Concern with noise pollution as well as with other occupational hazards prompted the passage of the Williams-Steiger Occupational Safety and Health Act in 1970. *Unprotected* exposure to noise levels in excess of 90 db over an 8-hour day is considered excessive and should be avoided (Table 22-1).

Selected ototoxic drugs

The following drugs may affect the cochlea, vestibule or acoustic nerve:

Antibiotics

Streptomycin
Dihydrostreptomycin
Gentamicin (Garamycin)
Neomycin
Kanamycin
Vancomycin
Polymyxin B/Colistin
Chloramphenicol (Chloromycetin)
Capreomycin

Diuretics

Ethacrynic acid (Edecrin)
Furosemide (Lasix)
Acetazolamide (Diamox)

Salicylates

Acetylsalicylic acid (aspirin)

Other drugs

Quinine
Chloroquine
Nitrogen mustard
Bleomycin
Quinidine

Table 22-1. Permissible noise exposures

Duration per day (hr)	Sound level (dbA, slow)
8	90
6	92
4	95
3	97
2	100
1½	102
1	105
½	110
¼	115

From U.S. Department of Labor, Occupational Safety and Health Administration: Noise: the environmental problem, a guide to OSHA standards, Washington, D.C., 1979, U.S. Government Printing Office.

Other causes of noise-induced hearing loss include *firearms* and *high-intensity music*. With an M16 rifle or sport rifle, hearing loss tends to be greater in the ear opposite the dominant hand (that is, left-ear hearing loss in a right-handed person). With revolvers, hearing loss is equal in both ears. A person firing guns who notices tinnitus, sensation of fullness in the ear, or temporary hearing loss should stop firing guns or wear suitable ear protectors.

Sound in front of a rock band can reach up to 120 db, and hearing losses of up to 50 db have been measured in some members of rock bands. In the early stage, there is a loss of hearing *at* or *near* frequencies of 4000 Hz. Later the damage extends to both higher and lower tones, with the lower tones affected least.

If proximity to the high noise level cannot be avoided, *ear protectors or earplugs* should be worn. The earplugs are inserted into the external auditory canal and can reduce the noise reaching the middle ear by 10 to 30 db. Usually standard plugs are effective, but custom-made plugs molded to the person's ear canal may be obtained. If the noise level is extremely high (sound levels may reach 140 db or higher), individuals are not adequately protected with earplugs alone and must wear *ear muffs*. At times a *shield* must be worn over the entire head.

IMPAIRED HEARING: DEAFNESS
Implications of impaired hearing

More than 13 million people in the United States have some kind of hearing impairment. Of these persons, 6 million are seriously handicapped, and more than 1.7 million are totally deaf.

Hearing is as important as speech in our daily lives. Sound helps keep us *in touch with reality and our environment;* it adds esthetic pleasure as well as warnings of danger to our world. People with normal hearing perceive sound both consciously and unconsciously. One hears background noises, a clock ticking, or family conversations without concentrating on them; these sounds help us to be alert to our world. Other sounds, such as fire alarms or a child crying, signal us so that we consciously hear them and take action depending on our interpretation of the sound. This preconscious level of hearing is not perceived by persons who are hard of hearing. These persons perceive the world as being "dead" about them.

The sense of hearing is critical to *normal development and maintenance of speech.* Infants learn to speak by imitating sounds from others. They listen to the sounds they make in relationship to the sounds of others, a skill necessary in the formulation of adequate speaking skills. Congenitally deaf persons lack aural stimulation, which affects their development of speech and conceptual ability. This severe handicap can affect both personality development and responses on intelligence tests. People with lesser degrees of hearing loss who have learned speech normally also may have behavioral changes not necessarily proportional to the degree of hearing loss.

As hearing diminishes, the impact of not understanding others and not being understood may make people withdraw from social situations, and they may become anxious and insecure. Fear of inadequacy and inferiority may make them suspicious and depressed. When hearing is completely gone, they may find the silent world almost intolerable.

People who are hard of hearing or deaf are not easily recognized; they appear quite normal. When they fail to respond or respond inappropriately to oral communication, their actions are interpreted as slow or odd, and the speaker may withdraw. This withdrawal response of others may be perceived as rejection by the aurally handicapped person and may further increase isolation and withdrawal. The person who is hard of hearing or deaf may experience varying degrees of stress depending on personality, the extent and type of loss, the age of onset of loss, and the reaction of family and friends to the loss of hearing.

Early identification of hearing loss

The detection of persons with hearing impairment is an important nursing responsibility. Often the nurse is the first member of the health team to be approached by persons seeking help regarding problems. Behavioral clues useful in assessing hearing difficulties in adults are listed in box below.

Persons with faulty articulation in speech may be deaf. For persons to speak properly they must hear properly. This is not a simple hearing function but is tied to complex brain patterns. A congenitally deaf child will never be able to talk "normally," because there is no brain sequence of sound to speech. People who lose their hearing after normal speech has been learned will be able to talk normally for about 7 years after total deafness. Then, because of lack of auditory stimulus, the brain-speech patterns will deteriorate.

Persons who exhibit any of the behavioral clues of impaired hearing should have their ears examined by an oto-

---

Behavioral clues indicating difficult hearing

Any adult who
  Is irritable, hostile, hypersensitive in interpersonal relations
  Has difficulty in hearing upper frequency consonants
  Complains about people mumbling
  Turns up volume on television
  Asks for frequent repetition and answers questions inappropriately
  Loses sense of humor; becomes grim
  Leans forward to hear better; face serious and strained
  Shuns large- and small-group audience situations
  May appear aloof and "stuck-up"
  Complains of ringing in the ears
  Has an unusually soft or loud voice
  Repeatedly states, "What did you say?"

laryngologist, who will obtain a hearing test. In this way a complete evaluation of the hearing problem can be made to determine the extent of the loss, possibility of correction, and presence of more serious disease.

The nurse can help find and direct the person with a hearing loss, and the family to the appropriate agencies for assistance (p. 471). There may be ways of improving hearing through medical or surgical therapy. If the loss is irreversible, aural rehabilitation (p. 468) may make it possible for the person with a hearing loss to understand and communicate with others.

Classification of hearing loss

Hearing loss may be classified by severity (mild, moderate, or severe) or by type (conductive, sensorineural).

CONDUCTIVE HEARING LOSS

Any interference with conduction of sound impulses through the external auditory canal, the eardrum, or the middle ear produces a conductive hearing loss. The inner ear is not involved, and sound directed to it is heard clearly. *Amplifying sound* by use of hearing aids or raising the voice *may be useful* in permitting sound to reach the inner ear. Causes of conductive hearing loss are listed in box below. At present, the conductive type of hearing loss is more effectively treated by surgery than the sensorineural type.

SENSORINEURAL HEARING LOSS

Sensorineural hearing loss results from disease or trauma of the inner ear or its neural pathways. Treatment usually is not very effective for sensorineural hearing loss, because the damage has been done by the time

---

the individual sees the physician, and the process is irreversible. *Amplifying sounds by shouting causes distortion of sound* and may increase the hearing problem. Some surgical procedures have been developed to aid in restoring this type of loss. Cochlear implantation or cochlear stimulation are operations that attempt to replace part of the function of the cochlea, that of transducing the mechanical energy of sound vibrations to electrical energy which directly stimulates the auditory nerve.

Presbycusis

Presbycusis is the term used to describe hearing loss associated with the aging process. Some of the degenerative change is probably the result of atrophy of the ganglion cells in the cochlea. It is characterized by bilateral gradual loss of hearing beginning with a loss of high-frequency tones. Some relief is obtained from hearing aids and from cochlear implantation and stimulation.

Assessment of auditory acuity

The extent of assessment of auditory acuity by nurses depends on the nurse's preparation and focus of care. All nurses, however, should be prepared to carry out an inspection of the outer ear and at least a gross assessment of hearing ability for all persons entering a health care setting, regardless of the presenting problem (see Chapter 3). Gross assessment of hearing may be accomplished by evaluating the logical sequences of replies during the admission history. One method is to turn one's head away from the individual when asking a simple question that cannot be answered by a yes or no response.

A *complete* hearing assessment consists of *subjective data* from the history relating to the person's perceived difficulties with hearing or a family history of hearing loss. *Objective data* are obtained by inspection of the external structures of the ear and audiometric testing of hearing.

INSPECTION OF THE EARDRUM

An otoscope (Fig. 22-4) is necessary to examine the inner aspect of the ear canal and the eardrum. The largest speculum that the ear will accommodate is used. Care is needed when inserting the speculum so as not to push against the tympanic membrane or against the paper-thin skin adjacent to the tympanic membrane. The eardrum is important in physical assessment of the middle ear, because it serves as a translucent window through which disease processes in the middle ear may be inferred. The normal tympanic membrane has a wide range of colored hues, the most common being a pearly gray. Located in the membrane or seen through it are certain landmarks (Fig. 22-5).

AUDIOMETRIC TESTING

The inner ear cannot be examined visually. Functional examination is done by testing hearing by audiometry and by testing function of the semicircular canals by the caloric examination or by electronystagmography (p. 477).

Causes of specific types of hearing loss

Conductive hearing loss

Impacted cerumen
Foreign body in external auditory canal
Thickening, retraction, scarring or perforation of eardrum
Otosclerosis

Sensorineural hearing loss

Arteriosclerosis
Infectious diseases (mumps, measles, meningitis)
Ototoxic drugs
Neuromas of cranial nerve VIII
Blows to head or ears
Noise of high intensity
Old age (presbycusis)

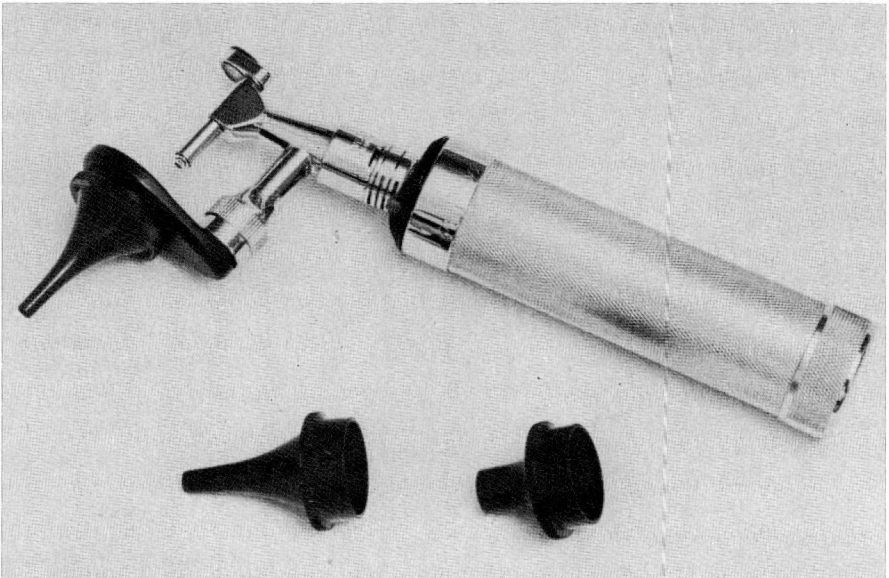

Fig. 22-4. Otoscope.

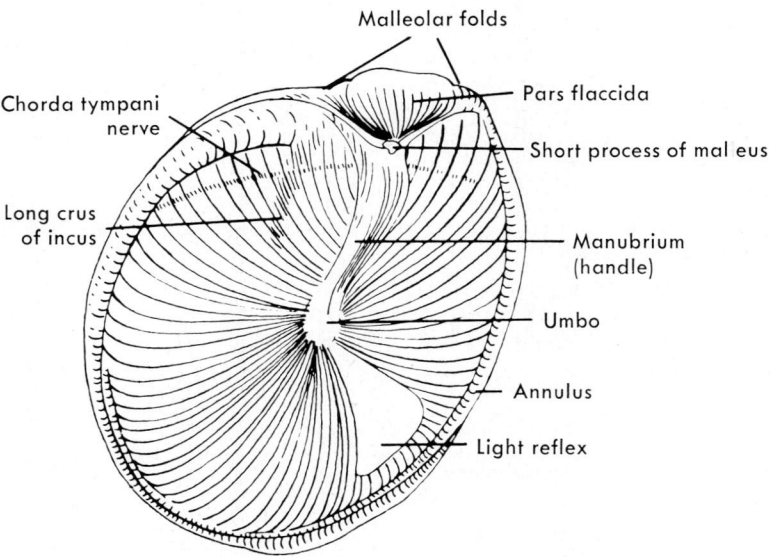

Malleolar folds

Chorda tympani
nerve

Pars flaccida

Short process of malleus

Long crus
of incus

Manubrium
(handle)

Umbo

Annulus

Light reflex

Fig. 22-5. Right tympanic membrane. (From Prior, J.A., and Silberstein, J.S.: Physical diagnosis: the history and examination of the patient, ed. 5, St. Louis, 1977, The C.V. Mosby Co.)

Functional examination for sensitivity (ability to hear sounds) and for speech discrimination (ability to distinguish different speech sounds) is done by audiometry. The graph of the hearing levels of both of these is called an audiogram (Fig. 22-6). *Hearing threshold* is defined as the lowest intensity of sound at which an auditory stimulus can be heard.

Audiologists (specialists in administering hearing tests) have developed audiometric tests to determine not only whether a hearing loss is present, but also the frequency of the loss, how well the person can understand speech,

and whether the problem site is in the middle ear (conductive loss) or inner ear or auditory nerve system (sensorineural loss) (Table 22-2).

Pure-tone audiometry must be performed in a specially constructed soundproof booth for best results. To test the sound intensity by air conduction, persons wear earphones and are instructed to signal (usually with a finger) when they first hear the tone and when they no longer hear it. The middle frequencies are tested first, and the operator alternately increases and decreases the intensity of the sound until the dial setting is found at which the

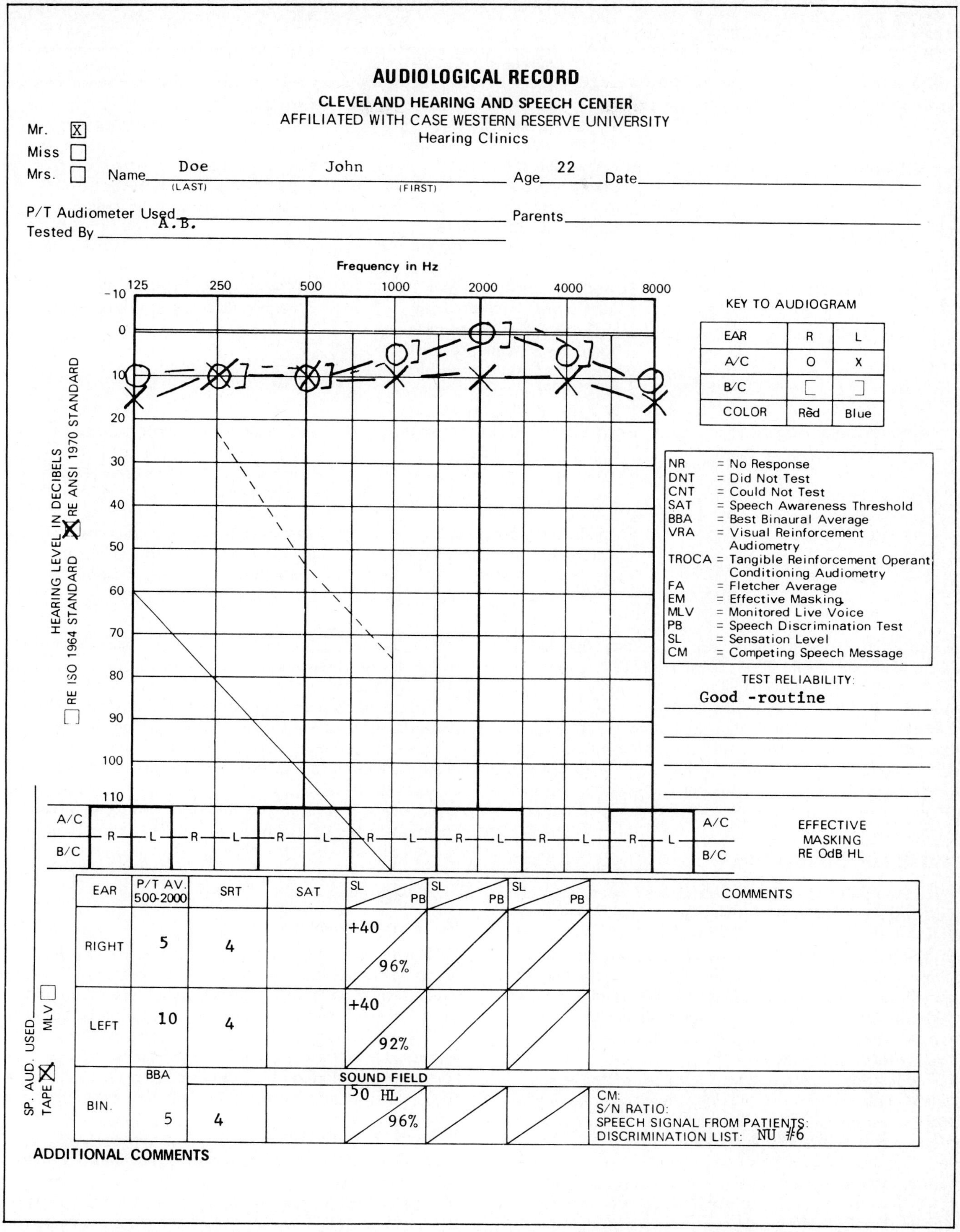

AUDIOLOGICAL RECORD

CLEVELAND HEARING AND SPEECH CENTER
AFFILIATED WITH CASE WESTERN RESERVE UNIVERSITY
Hearing Clinics

Mr. [X]
Miss [ ]
Mrs. [ ] Name Doe (LAST) John (FIRST) Age 22 Date_____

P/T Audiometer Used_____ Parents_____
Tested By A.B._____

Frequency in Hz

KEY TO AUDIOGRAM

EAR	R	L
A/C	O	X
B/C	[	]
COLOR	Rẽd	Blue

NR	= No Response
DNT	= Did Not Test
CNT	= Could Not Test
SAT	= Speech Awareness Threshold
BBA	= Best Binaural Average
VRA	= Visual Reinforcement Audiometry
TROCA	= Tangible Reinforcement Operant Conditioning Audiometry
FA	= Fletcher Average
EM	= Effective Masking
MLV	= Monitored Live Voice
PB	= Speech Discrimination Test
SL	= Sensation Level
CM	= Competing Speech Message

TEST RELIABILITY:

Good -routine

HEARING LEVEL IN DECIBELS
[X] RE ANSI 1970 STANDARD
[ ] RE ISO 1964 STANDARD

| A/C | R—L—R—L—R—L—R—L—R—L—R—L—R—L | A/C |
| B/C | | B/C |

EFFECTIVE MASKING RE OdB HL

EAR	P/T AV. 500-2000	SRT	SAT	SL / PB	SL / PB	SL / PB	COMMENTS
RIGHT	5	4		+40 / 96%			
LEFT	10	4		+40 / 92%			
	BBA			SOUND FIELD			
BIN.	5	4		50 HL / 96%			CM: S/N RATIO: SPEECH SIGNAL FROM PATIENTS: DISCRIMINATION LIST: NU #6

SP. AUD. USED
MLV [ ]
TAPE [X]

ADDITIONAL COMMENTS

Fig. 22-6. Normal audiogram. (Courtesy Cleveland Hearing and Speech Center, Cleveland, Ohio.)

Table 22-2. Types of audiometric testing

Test	Method	Use
Pure-tone audiometry	Person wears earphone; signals when sound is heard	General screening to identify persons requiring further testing
Impedance audiometry	Probe inserted in ear canal; measurements of middle ear pressure are obtained; does not require response from person	Assess presence or absence of abnormality of conductive mechanism of middle ear
Speech audiometry	Speech reception threshold: lowest intensity level in decibels at which person can correctly repeat selected bisyllabic words 50% of time; also a test of speech discrimination	Determine how well person can hear and understand speech
Electrocochleography; evoked-response audiometry	Response on EEG recording to clicks played to ear	Determine if central (brain) portion of hearing is intact or determine location of the lesion interfering with the transmission of sound
Tuning fork tests	Identification of sound made by tuning forks placed on head	Test hearing acuity and discriminate conductive vs sensorineural hearing losses

person being tested can just perceive sound (threshold). In audiometric testing the frequencies 125, 250, 500, 1000, 2000, 4000, and 8000 Hz are commonly employed to assess the hearing sensitivity of an individual.

Hearing loss is identified as the number of decibels reached before the person hears the sound for each specific frequency. Zero loudness is calibrated for that sound barely heard by a person with normal hearing. Up to a 20 db loss is considered to be within the normal range.

Aural rehabilitation

If hearing loss is irreversible and not amenable to surgical intervention, aural rehabilitation may make it possible for the individual to understand and communicate with others again. The purpose of aural rehabilitation is to maximize the hearing-impaired person's communication skills. Because the auditory sense is our primary mode of communication, it is imperative that hearing-impaired persons be given the opportunity to use their hearing for this purpose.

The hearing-impaired person must be helped to understand the implications of hearing loss for communication purposes (p. 464). This can be accomplished through discussions pertaining to daily communicative interactions at home, at work, or at play, often most helpful in determining how the individual's hearing impairment may have affected others. These insights are extremely important in planning appropriate rehabilitative strategies.

The person's acceptance of his/her hearing impairment, desire to seek help, and use of the facilities available, along with motivation, perseverance, and patience, contribute to the success of aural rehabilitation. Rehabilitation is affected by age and severity of impairment. For people who, although hard of hearing, have normally acquired communication skill, efforts are geared toward correcting, restoring, complementing, and maintaining those skills. For deaf persons who have not developed communication skills, efforts are made to teach language and speech skills by special methods.

HEARING AIDS

Nature of hearing aids

Hearing aids (Fig. 22-7) are commonly used by both hard-of-hearing individuals and deaf persons. Hearing aids are instruments through which sounds are amplified in a controlled manner. Generally a hearing aid consists of a *microphone* to receive and convert speech and other sounds into electric signals, an *amplifier* to increase the strength of the sound, a *receiver* to convert electric signals back to sound, and a *battery* to supply the electric power.

Benefits of hearing aids

Hearing aids are used to increase the intensity of the sound reaching the ear of the person with hearing loss. *Hearing aids do not improve the ability to hear, but they make the sound louder.* They are usually recommended when

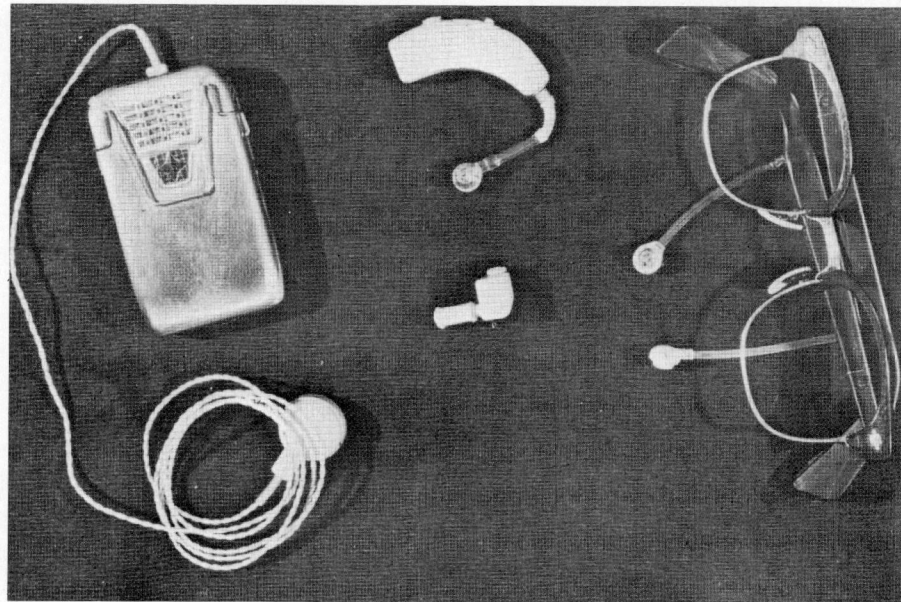

Fig. 22-7. Body and head borne hearing aids. *Left:* Body-type aid; button receiver is coupled to ear with insert, and component housing is either clipped to clothing or worn on body in harnessed cloth pouch. *Top center:* Behind-ear aid. *Center:* In-ear aid. *Right:* Eyeglass aid. (From Saunders, W.H., et al.: Nursing care in eye, ear, nose, and throat disorders, ed. 4, St. Louis, 1979, The C.V. Mosby Co.)

the person has difficulty understanding speech in everyday conversation.

When the person has difficulty with speech discrimination, benefits from an aid are more restricted. Persons with a *conductive* hearing loss *benefit most* from wearing a hearing aid, because their ability to understand speech is usually not impaired if the speech is loud enough.

Persons with *sensorineural* hearing losses often exhibit problems with amplification of sound. It should be noted, however, that this is the most common type of hearing loss and affects the majority of persons who are successfully wearing hearing aids. Appropriate aural rehabilitation will facilitate the adjustment to the amplification of sound in most instances. Elderly persons, who usually have sensorineural hearing loss, may lack the patience, concentration, or mental energy necessary to adjust to the hearing aid.

Obtaining a hearing aid

A person whose hearing problem indicates need for a hearing aid should be seen both by an otologist and an audiologist. The *otologist* determines the medical nature of the problem and decides whether there is any medical reason why a hearing aid cannot be worn. The *audiologist* can perform various tests and help determine if a hearing aid will benefit the person and what specific type of hearing aid will be best. Food and Drug Administration (FDA) regulations restrict the sale of hearing aids to those individuals who have received a medical evaluation, with the provision that any person over 18 years of age

can be permitted to waive the medical evaluation requirement provided certain criteria are met.

Over 1200 different models of hearing aids are available. They may be worn on the body, built into the temple bow of eyeglasses, or worn as individual units behind the ear (Fig. 22-8) or in the ear canal. Aids worn on the body are the most powerful and are generally fitted to persons with moderate to severe hearing losses. Aids worn in eyeglasses or behind the ear are generally equivalent in amplifying power. Implantation of hearing aids is under consideration, but as yet has not been shown to be superior to conventional aids.

Assisting the person with a hearing aid

Persons with hearing aids should know how to care for the aid and what to do if the aid fails to work. The aids have adjustable tone and volume controls, and several adjustments may have to be made before the aid is correctly set for the person's needs. Because a hearing aid is not selective when amplifying sounds, the amplified background sounds can often be annoying to the individual.

Persons who are reluctant to wear their hearing aids (often for cosmetic reasons) need counseling about the benefits of wearing the aid and the improvements in their ability to speak more distinctly. The aid may also serve to notify others to speak more distinctly. When a person with a hearing aid is hospitalized, it is important to encourage use of the aid during hospitalization and its safe storage when not in use.

OTHER TYPES OF AURAL REHABILITATION

Auditory training

Auditory training is used to encourage those who are hard of hearing to use their residual hearing more effectively. The training consists of helping the affected person to develop *listening skills.* It helps the hard of hearing person to do the following:

1. Establish attitudes of critical listening
2. Develop an awareness of the kinds of listening errors that are most likely to be made in view of the nature of the hearing impairment
3. Compensate for these errors by using other special clues that are still heard correctly
4. Improve listening habits and skills in general

Speech-reading

Speech-reading (commonly known as lipreading) is taught to *supplement the hearing function.* It includes the following:

Care of a hearing aid

1. Wash ear mold or plug frequently (daily is suggested) in mild soap and water using a pipe cleaner to cleanse the cannula
2. Dry ear mold or plug thoroughly before reconnecting it to the receiver
3. Avoid covering the hearing aid with heavy clothing. Men often wear the transmitter in their shirt pocket; women may fit it into a special pocket sewn on the outside of their underclothing
4. Arrange the microphone of the hearing aid so that it faces the speaker
5. Keep an extra battery and cord available at all times
6. Know what to do if the hearing aid fails to work:
   a. Check the on-off switch
   b. Inspect cleanliness of ear mold
   c. Examine battery for tightness or leaks
   d. Examine cord plug for tightness of insertion
   e. Examine cord plug for breaks
   f. Replace battery, cord, or both
   g. Take hearing aid to local service agency if these steps fail to correct the problem

---

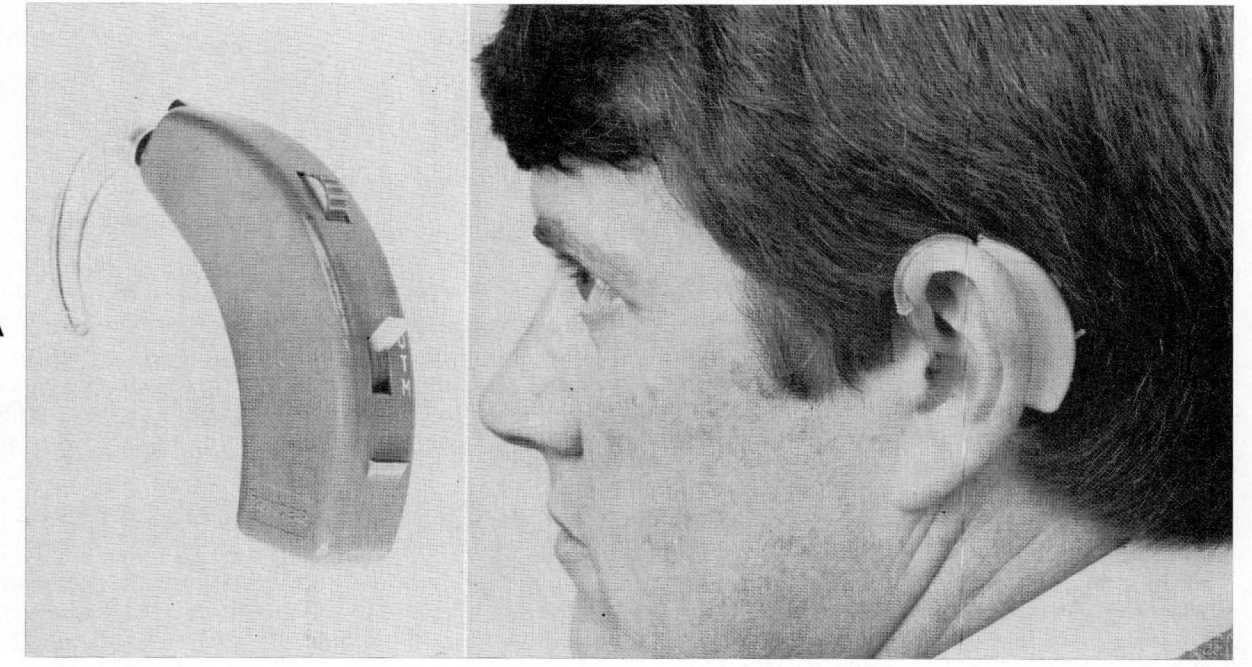

Fig. 22-8. A, Hearing aid. **B,** Hearing aid in place. (Courtesy HC Electronics, Inc. [Phonic Ear], Mill Valley, Calif.)

1. Lipreading
2. Study of facial expressions
3. Study of gestures and body movements used in speech
4. Use of environmental clues that facilitate hearing

Speech training

Speech training is given to *conserve, develop, or prevent deterioration of speech skills.* Clearness, pitch, quality, and rate of speech may deteriorate with loss of hearing and are the focus of speech training.

Agencies that provide assistance for the hearing impaired

American Annals of the Deaf, 5034 Wisconsin Ave., N.W., Washington, DC 20016. The April issue every year lists a directory of programs and services for the deaf available by state, including information about the type of facilities.

American Federation of the Physically Handicapped, Inc., 1370 National Press Building, Washington, DC 20004. Provides counseling and information.

American Speech and Hearing Association, 10801 Rockville Pike, Rockville, MD 20852. Membership is composed of professional persons who teach individuals who have hearing and speech problems.

Gallaudet College, 7th and Florida Ave., Washington, DC 20002. The only liberal arts college in the world for the deaf.

The John Tracy Clinic, 806 West Adams Blvd., Los Angeles, CA 90007. Provides information and correspondence classes for parents with deaf children.

National Association of Hearing and Speech Agencies, 919 18th St. N.W., Washington, DC 20006. Provides counseling and information.

State Office of Vocational Rehabilitation (in each state). Provides vocational training and placement services.

Veterans Administration. Provides audiology clinics and rehabilitative services for veterans.

Speech and hearing centers are found locally in many cities.

Facilitating communication for persons with impaired hearing

1. Get the person's attention by raising an arm·or hand.
2. Start with the light on your face; this will help the person speech read.
3. Talk directly to the person, facing him or her.
4. Speak clearly, but do not overaccentuate words.
5. Speak in a normal tone; do not shout. Shouting overemploys normal speaking movements and may cause distortion and be too loud for the person with sensorineural damage. If the person has conductive loss only, sometimes making the voice louder without shouting is helpful.
6. If the person does not seem to understand what is said, express it differently. Some words are difficult to "see" in speech reading, such as *white* and *red.*
7. Move closer to the person and toward the better ear if the person does not hear you.
8. Write out proper names or any statement that you are not sure was understood.
9. Do not smile, chew gum, or cover the mouth when talking to a person with limited hearing.
10. Inattention may indicate tiredness or lack of understanding.
11. Use phrases to convey meaning rather than one-word answers. State the major topic of the discussion first and then give details.
12. Do not show annoyance by careless facial expression. Persons who are hard of hearing depend more on visual clues for acceptance.
13. Encourage the use of a hearing aid if the person has one; allow him or her to adjust it before speaking.
14. If in a group, repeat important statements and avoid asides to others in the group.
15. Avoid the use of the intercommunication system as this may distort sound and cause poor communication.
16. Do not avoid conversation with a person who has hearing loss.

Adapted from Conover, M., and Cober, J.: Nurs. Clin. North Am. **5**:497, 1970.

COMMUNITY SERVICES

Selected agencies exist for helping the hearing-impaired person. The telephone company can provide information about special amplifiers or flashing lights that can be placed on doorbells or telephones. Services for persons with a hearing loss are offered by audiology clinics sponsored by universities, hospitals, community programs, local or state departments of health and education, or the Veterans Administration. National organizations are available to give information and counseling.

Communicating with the hearing-impaired person

Specific points to facilitate hearing or speech-reading for persons with impaired hearing are listed in the lower box on p. 471.

Hospital settings require identification of patients who have difficulty hearing. If a deaf or hard-of-hearing person is hospitalized, the new environment and unfamiliar faces may accentuate loneliness and isolation, and anxiety may reduce hearing even further.[11]

Persons who are hard of hearing depend on their other senses to provide information about changes in their environment. Patients are helped to use *visual cues* by placing them in a bed were they can observe activity and anticipate others approaching them. They will be easily startled if people suddenly enter the unit if the vision is obscured. Because hearing-impaired persons are often sensitive to light changes, they can easily be awakened by turning on a light. Many patients feel less isolated if the nurse *touches* them lightly on the arm to gain their attention and wakes them by touching them on the arm.

Special effort must be made to communicate information about the hospital routines to the deaf or hard-of-hearing patients, and to prepare them for special tests.

Table 22-3. Inflammations of the ear

Disorder	Description	Signs and symptoms	Medical therapy
External otitis	Inflammation of external ear; may be acute or chronic	Pain with movement of auricle, redness, scaling, itching, swelling, watery discharge, crusting of external ear	Application of astringents (Burow's solution), acidifiers (acetic acid), or antibiotics
Serous otitis media	Collection of sterile serum in middle ear; may be acute or chronic	Sense of fullness in ear, hearing loss, low-pitched tinnitus, ear-ache	Removal of eustachian obstruction by aspiration or insertion of tubes for drainage
Acute purulent otitis media	Infection of middle ear, usually by pneumococci, streptococci, staphylococci, or *Haemophilus influenzae*	Sense of fullness in ear, severe throbbing pain, hearing loss, tinnitus, fever	Antibiotics: If severe: bed rest, analgesics nasal vasoconstrictors Myringotomy if necessary
Acute mastoiditis	Acute infection of middle ear with extension to adjacent mastoid process	Pain in ear and over mastoid, fever, headache, profuse discharge from ear, vertigo	Hospitalization with high doses of IV antibiotics, mastoidectomy
Chronic otitis media	Chronic inflammation of middle ear; sequela of acute otitis media	Deafness, occasional pain, dizziness, chronic discharge from ear	Local debridement, topical and systemic antibiotics, mastoidectomy and tympanoplasty may be necessary
Labyrinthitis	Inflammation of inner ear	Severe and sudden vertigo, nausea and vomiting, nystagmus, photophobia, headache, ataxic gait	No specific treatment Antibiotics Dimenhydrinate for vertigo Parenteral fluids if nausea and vomiting persist

Major health problems of the ear

The most common health problems of the ear include the following:
1. Inflammations of the ear
   a. External otitis and furuncles
   b. Otitis media: serous, purulent (acute, chronic)
   c. Acute mastoiditis
   d. Labyrinthitis (inner ear)
2. Otosclerosis
3. Labyrinthine disorders

INFLAMMATIONS OF THE EAR

Inflammations may develop in the external ear, middle ear, or inner ear (Table 22-3).

PATHOPHYSIOLOGY

Inflammations of the *external* ear may be diffuse in the form of bacterial or fungal dermatitis or local in the form of furuncles (boils). If a furuncle develops in the external auditory meatus, pain may be severe because there is little expansile tissue, and pressure results.

Inflammations of the *middle* ear may be serous (sterile serum) or purulent (pus); development of these two forms differs (Fig. 22-9). Purulent otitis media may develop as an acute condition limited to the middle ear, it may spread into the mastoid area (mastoiditis), or it may become chronic.

Because the *inner* ear helps maintain balance as well as facilitate hearing, problems there disturb the function of the semicircular canals and loss of hearing. Severe suppurative labyrinthitis leads to permanent hearing loss. A special form of localized labyrinthitis tends to follow upper respiratory infections and involves the balance mechanism only.

ASSESSMENT

Persons with ear inflammations may be diagnosed and treated on an ambulatory basis. Because acute inflammations may become chronic, assessment of early signs of inflammation is important for early diagnosis and treatment.

Subjective symptoms of developing ear inflammations may include:
1. Pain in the ear or over the mastoid
2. Sense of fullness in the ear
3. Hearing loss
4. Tinnitus (ringing in the ears)
5. Vertigo (sensation of room spinning around)

Data to collect include onset, duration, and degree of involvement. Persons who are subject to ear infections are questioned about their knowledge of preventive measures and symptoms requiring medical attention.

Objective signs are seen mostly in external ear inflammations or with some middle ear infections. *Drainage* is described in terms of type (serous, purulent) and characteristic (watery, crusting). Inner ear inflammations may cause *nystagmus,* involuntary, rapid rhythmic movements of the eyes. Nystagmus and vertigo place the person at high risk for falls.

DATA ANALYSIS AND PLANNING

Nursing diagnoses are determined on the basis of collected data. Possible nursing diagnosis may include the following:

Knowledge deficit

Alteration in comfort: pain in ear

Potential for injury

Outcome criteria for the person with an ear inflammation include the following:
1. Discomfort in the ear is decreased.
2. The person can describe preventive measures and symptoms requiring medical attention.
3. No injury occurs.

IMPLEMENTATION

Assisting with achievement of therapeutic goals
Ear drops

Medications may be administered systemically, or locally in the form of ear drops or ointments.

Ear irrigation

The ear must sometimes be irrigated to remove wax, drainage, or debris. *Guidelines* for ear irrigations include the following:
1. Avoid ear irrigation:
   a. If eardrum is punctured (causes further inflammation)
   b. To remove a foreign body of vegetable origin (moisture will cause object to swell)
2. Use tap water or normal saline solution; hydrogen peroxide may be added to help dislodge wax
3. Warm solution to body temperature to prevent vestibular stimulation and consequent vertigo
4. Pull auricle up and back for adults to straighten canal

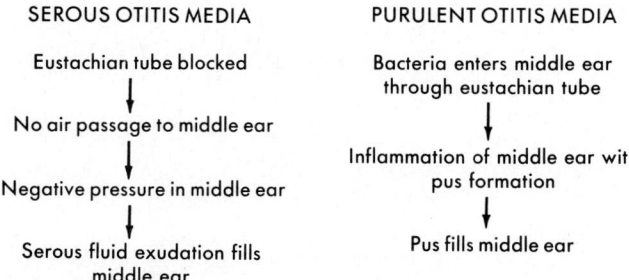

SEROUS OTITIS MEDIA	PURULENT OTITIS MEDIA
Eustachian tube blocked	Bacteria enters middle ear through eustachian tube
↓	↓
No air passage to middle ear	Inflammation of middle ear with pus formation
↓	↓
Negative pressure in middle ear	Pus fills middle ear
↓	
Serous fluid exudation fills middle ear	

Fig. 22-9. Pathogenesis of otitis media.

Instillation of eardrops

1. Warm solution to body temperature (no more than 38° C); vertigo may result from high or low temperatures (The bottle may be warmed by holding it in the hand for a few minutes.)
2. Have patient tilt head so ear is uppermost
3. Straighten ear canal by pulling up and back in adults (down and back in children)
4. Instill drops to run along canal wall to prevent air entrapment
5. Have patient hold head in position for 5 to 10 minutes
6. Gently insert piece of cotton moistened with eardrop solution into *external* auditory canal to keep drops from running out of ear
7. Dry external ear thoroughly to prevent skin irritation

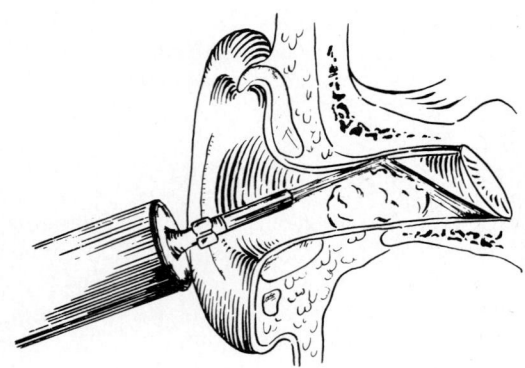

Fig. 22-10. Irrigation of external auditory canal with warm tap water. (From Saunders, W.H., et al.: Nursing care in eye, ear, nose, and throat disorders, ed. 4, St. Louis, 1979, The C.V. Mosby Co.)

5. Use a steady stream of solution against roof of auditory canal (Fig. 22-10) to prevent forcing material further into canal
6. Use *gentle* pressure
7. Do not obstruct canal with syringe or bulb; this may prevent outflow of solution and pressure against eardrum
8. Ask patient to lie on affected side or hold affected side down for several minutes to assure complete drainage of irrigating fluid
9. Dry external ear to prevent skin excoriation.

Surgery

MYRINGOTOMY. Myringotomy is an incision into the tympanic membrane (eardrum) to relieve pressure and facilitate drainage during acute otitis media. The myringotomy heals rapidly with only slight scarring and does not affect hearing. The procedure is usually performed on an ambulatory basis. The person is taught to protect the skin from ear drainage.

MASTOIDECTOMY. In a *simple* mastoidectomy, an incision is made in front of or behind the ear and the air cells of the mastoid bone are removed. A small rubber drain is inserted. Because the middle ear space, eardrum, and ear canal wall are left intact, hearing is not affected.

Radical mastoidectomy consists of a simple mastoidectomy plus removal of the ossicles, remnant of the eardrum, the bony ear canal wall, and all of the middle ear mucosa. Hearing is affected.

A *modified radical* mastoidectomy is a more commonly used procedure because it preserves as much of the eardrum and ossicles as possible. Hearing is better following the modified radical mastoidectomy than the radical surgery. For care of the person with ear surgery, see p. 476.

TYMPANOPLASTY. Tympanoplasty refers to a group of surgical procedures designed to restore hearing by plastic reconstruction of the bones of the middle ear. Continuity of the ossicles from the tympanic membrane to the oval window is reestablished. It is used for people who have perforation of the tympanic membrane or necrosis of one of the ossicles caused by a middle ear infection, stenosis, or trauma.

Assisting with comfort

Ear pain is often caused by buildup of fluid in the small encased ear spaces, causing pressure and thus discomfort. Pain usually decreases as the inflammation subsides or when the ear drains. Analgesics may be helpful.

Persons with vertigo usually prefer to keep the head motionless. Sudden movements or jarring are to be avoided. Support during walking is given the person with vertigo to prevent falls (pp. 477-478).

Teaching

Persons with ear inflammations need to know about (1) prevention of further infections, (2) care of the infected ear, and (3) signs indicating need for medical follow-up.

EVALUATION

Evaluation is based on expected patient outcomes. Questions to ask may include the following:

1. Is patient comfortable?
2. Can the patient describe care required at home?
3. Can the patient describe measures to prevent recurring infection?

Teaching the patient with ear infection

Prevention of further infection

1. Protection of ear canal during showers (cotton in *external* canal, use of shower cap over ears)
2. Avoidance of swimming during infection or following a perforated eardrum; avoidance of swimming in contaminated water when infection is healed
3. Adequate antibiotic therapy continued for prescribed number of days, even when symptoms disappear
4. Adequate and early treatment of upper respiratory infections and allergic conditions

Care of infected ear

1. Correct use of eardrops or ear irrigations (pp. 473-474) as necessary
2. Washing of hands before and after changing cotton plugs to prevent secondary infection
3. Protection of skin from ear drainage
   a. Place cotton *loosely* in outer ear to collect drainage
   b. Replace cotton plug when moist
   c. Keep external ear clean and dry

Signs requiring further medical attention

1. Fever
2. Return of ear pain
3. Headache
4. Behavioral changes (irritability, drowsiness, disorientation)

OTOSCLEROSIS

PATHOPHYSIOLOGY

Otosclerosis is a progressive condition in which the normal bone of the bony labyrinth is replaced by highly vascular spongy bone. The footplate of the stapes in the oval window becomes immobilized and ceases to vibrate effectively in response to sound pressure. The cause is unknown but appears to be hereditary. It is more common in women and appears between puberty and age 30.

ASSESSMENT

Subjective data include the presence of tinnitus and gradual hearing loss in both ears. The person is referred to an otologist for audiometric testing. Tuning fork tests will indicate that *bone conduction* is superior to air conduction.

SURGERY

The treatment for otosclerosis is primarily surgical, most commonly a *stapedectomy*. Surgery consists of removing the stapes and replacing it with some type of prosthesis (steel wire, polyethylene prosthesis, or Teflon piston). As soon as the new connection is made with the incus, the patient's hearing is improved. Hearing decreases temporarily during the early postoperative period as a result of drainage in the middle ear and ear canal,

postoperative edema, and inserted packing. Full effects cannot be evaluated until about 1 month postoperatively. Hearing improves permanently in the majority of cases. The care of the person experiencing ear surgery is summarized in the box on p. 476.

LABYRINTHINE DISORDERS

Common labyrinthine disorders include labyrinthitis (p. 472), Ménière's disease, and fluctuant hearing loss (Table 22-4).

PATHOPHYSIOLOGY

The membranous labyrinth of the inner ear is a closed system filled with endolymph. Disorders such as Ménière's disease or fluctuant hearing loss result from an overproduction or a decreased absorption of endolymph. The buildup of endolymph produces the symptoms. In Ménière's disease, vertigo (the sensation of rotation of the person or the room) is a predominant symptom; and the hearing loss is progressive. With fluctuant hearing loss, vertigo may or may not be present and the hearing loss fluctuates, although symptoms become worse with succeeding attacks.

Conditions that contribute to the occurrence of fluctuant hearing loss include poor circulation, diabetes mellitus, hyperlipoproteinemia, high salt intake, allergies, smoking, and syphilis.

Postoperative care of patients experiencing ear surgery

1. Position patient according to physician preference
   a. Operative ear uppermost prevents graft displacement
   b. Operative ear downward facilitates drainage
   c. Position of choice may prevent vertigo
2. Medicate for postoperative pain, nausea, or vertigo as necessary
3. Keep side rails up when patient is in bed; supervise walking if vertigo is present to prevent falls
4. Instruct patient to move slowly and avoid sudden movements to prevent vertigo
5. Give prescribed prophylactic antibiotics
6. Observe and report signs of complications
   a. Changes in hearing, tinnitus, or vertigo
   b. Bleeding
   c. Headache
   d. Signs of facial paralysis indicating injury to facial nerve (assymmetry when frowning, smiling, closing eyes, baring teeth, or blowing through lips)
7. Teach patient:
   a. Wear cotton in ear when outdoors for 1 week
   b. Avoid blowing nose or sneezing for 1 week; after healing is complete:
      (1) Blow nose with both nostrils open
      (2) Open mouth when sneezing
   c. Avoid getting ear wet
      (1) Avoid washing hair for 2 weeks
      (2) Wear shower cap over ears when bathing or showering
   d. Avoid exposure to persons with upper respiratory tract infections
   e. Avoid flying for 6 months

Table 22-4. Labyrinthine disorders

Disorder	Etiology	Signs and symptoms	Medical therapy
Ménière's disease	Cause unknown; stress may precipitate attacks	Recurrent episodes of vertigo; progressive deafness; tinnitus in the affected ear; attacks are irregular and sudden; nausea/vomiting with sudden motion of head during an attack	No treatment entirely successful Diuretics, low-salt diet, fluid restrictions During attack: anticholinergics (atropine), antihistimine, tranquilizers Between attacks: antivertiginous medication (meclizine [Antivert], dimenhydrinate [Dramamine]) desensitization with histamine Surgery: labyrinthectomy, endolymphatic sac depression
Fluctuant hearing loss	Cause unknown; thought to be more common than Ménière's disease	Fullness in the ear; roaring tinnitus; fluctuant hearing loss; vertigo may or may not be present	Diuretics, low-salt diet Antihistamines, tranquilizers (diazepam)

ASSESSMENT

Data to collect relate to *presence, extent,* and *duration* of the following symptoms during an attack episode. Additional data are collected about the person's knowledge of the condition to provide data for teaching.

Subjective data

1. Vertigo: usually described by the patient as a whirling sensation; a sitting or lying position is assumed to keep from falling; the vertigo may last for several hours or all day but is usually absent between attacks
2. Nausea: usually associated with vertigo
3. Tinnitus: ranges from buzzing sounds to painful, loud ringing sounds
4. Hearing loss: assess whether unilateral or bilateral (if bilateral, patient may not be able to answer questions or respond to directions during an attack)
5. Knowledge about disorder
   a. Circumstances precipitating attack
   b. Safety measures to be taken during attack
   c. Symptoms requiring medical intervention

Objective data

1. Vomiting: usually associated with vertigo
2. Diaphoresis: usually during severe attacks
3. Nystagmus: seen during attacks; note presence, whether in one or both eyes, and rapidity of eye movements

Diagnostic tests

Audiometric testing initially reveals low-tone sensorineural hearing loss. Neurologic consultation is usually obtained to rule out neurologic disease.

Specific diagnostic tests include *electronystagmography (ENG)* and a caloric test. ENG is a test used to measure nystagmus. It records the position and movement of the eyeball by recording the changes in the electrical field around the eye when there is a change in position of the eye. Electrodes are placed on the face around the eye; no discomfort is involved.

In the *caloric test,* cold water or air is irrigated in the external auditory canal. When labyrinthine function is normal, the person experiences vertigo and nystagmus. In labyrinthine disorders, the response is hyperactive or absent.

DATA ANALYSIS AND PLANNING

Nursing diagnoses that are identified based on patient data will depend on the extent of vertigo present and knowledge of the condition. Possible nursing diagnoses include the following:

Potential self-care deficit
Potential impairment of skin integrity
Potential for injury
Knowledge deficit

Expected patient outcomes include the following:

1. No injury or skin breakdown occur.
2. The patient can:
   a. Describe circumstances that may precipitate an attack and what to do when an attack occurs.
   b. State rationale for safety precautions.
   c. Describe symptoms requiring medical intervention.

IMPLEMENTATION

Assisting with achievement of therapeutic goals

About 10% of patients require surgery, such as labyrinthectomy, which destroys the membranous labyrinth and sacrifices the balance and hearing end organs. Relief from vertigo may not occur for several weeks in some cases. Ultrasonic labyrinthectomy is also used, especially for patients who have symptoms of vertigo but still have worthwhile hearing that should be preserved. A pencil-sized probe of the ultrasonic generator is applied directly to the bone through a mastoidectomy incision, and energy is directed into the labyrinth. Cryosurgical labyrinthectomy may also be used; it is performed similarly to ultrasonic surgery except that it is done through the ear canal. Care of the patient experiencing surgery is described on p. 476.

Promoting comfort and safety

Patients with vertigo and tinnitus are reluctant to move, because movement increases the symptoms. The immobility may lead to further discomforts and possible skin breakdown. Nursing care therefore centers on encouraging some movement while minimizing head movement when possible. Safety for the vertiginous patient takes high priority. specific nursing care activities include the following:

1. Assist patient with hygiene needs as necessary
2. Stand directly in front of patient when addressing him/her so patient's head does not have to turn
3. Encourage some movement in bed; assist patient to turn *slowly;* provide back care
4. Suggest patient try lying on *unaffected* side with eyes turned toward affected ear during an acute attack
5. Avoid bright, glaring lights
6. Encourage and facilitate eating; provide patient with desired foods and fluids (vertigo may cause anorexia)
7. Keep side rails raised when patient is in bed; provide support and assistance when patient walks
8. Teach patient
   a. Call nurse at first signs of an acute attack so medication can be given
   b. Do not walk alone when vertigo may occur
   c. Avoid reading when vertigo and tinnitus are present
   d. Avoid smoking with fluctuant hearing loss
   e. Nature of condition
      (1) Identification and avoidance of circumstances that precipitate an attack (for example, high salt or fluid intake, stress)
      (2) What to do when an attack occurs
         (a) If driving, pull over to curb and stop car
         (b) If standing, sit or lie down to prevent fall

484 Sensorimotor problems

PREVENTABLE FACTORS

Polio vaccine, screening of school-aged children for scoliosis, and screening tests for streptococcal infections with early treatment of the infection to prevent rheumatic fever are examples of preventive measures that can be employed on a community-wide basis in combating illnesses that cause musculoskeletal disability. Early attention to posture; good dietary habits; genetic counseling for individuals with sickle cell anemia and hemophilia; teaching of good body mechanics for individuals whose jobs entail lifting or carrying heavy objects; and concern and attention to the recommendations of the National Safety Council to help avoid accidents at home, on the job, and on the road are all examples of preventive measures that may be employed to decrease musculoskeletal disability within the general population.

PREVENTIVE HEALTH TEACHING

Promotion of safety

For those individuals who have limitations of motion or mobility, there are a variety of precautions and protective or safety devices that can be employed in the hospital or the home. Examples would be grab bars that can be mounted on a wall near a tub or toilet, safety arms that fit around a toilet, and rails that fasten onto the side of a bathtub. These devices provide the person with both a stable place to hold onto and a point of leverage for assuming a standing or sitting position. Throw rugs and obstacles should be removed from areas used by individuals with ambulatory difficulties, and floors should not be highly waxed. Wheelchairs should have adequate locking devices, and patients who must use wheelchairs should be taught how to lock and unlock the chair. Nurses should know where in the community needed equipment can be obtained.

PREVENTION OF MUSCLE AND JOINT COMPLICATIONS

Maintenance of joint mobility

For the individual with limited motion or mobility, range of motion exercises should be carried out to prevent joint stiffness or contracture from disuse. Whenever it is possible, except in conditions where there is acute joint inflammation, range of motion exercises should be performed several times a day. *Active range of motion* is most beneficial for the patient. Encouraging patients to do as much of their own care as they are able to do within the restrictions of their disability will often satisfy active range of motion requirements.

Several precautions should be mentioned. *Passive range of motion* exercises should not be performed past the point of the complaint of pain. Particularly in individuals with pathologic skeletal conditions (gross deformity, osteoporosis), fractures can result if a joint is forced through "normal" range of motion. Also, acutely inflamed, painful, or septic joints should be rested, since harm can be done by moving the joint before inflammation has subsided. The person who has pain is also likely to resist movement to avoid further pain.

Maintenance of posture

Although maintenance of good posture is important for all persons, it is especially important for the patient with chronic arthritic disease. Poor posture exerts further strain on already damaged joints and not only may cause pain and fatigue but predisposes to increased deformity.

The patient who must remain in bed for a long period of time in traction or in a cast should be in a bed with a firm mattress, and a bed board should be placed under the mattress. A firm bed lessens pain by preventing motion and consequent pull on painful joints and helps to keep the spine in good alignment. Boards should be long enough and wide enough to rest firmly on the main side and end rails of the bed, not on the bedsprings. The person with arthritis should either use no pillow or should use one small pillow that fits well down under the shoulders so that forward flexion of the cervical spine is not encouraged. Knees should not be flexed on pillows, and all patients who must be confined to bed most of the day should lie prone with a pillow under the abdomen for a part of each day to relieve supine pressure areas (inferior scapular areas, sacrum, coccyx, and ischial tuberosities) (Fig. 23-4).

Careful positioning with *trochanter rolls* (rolled towels or bath blankets to brace an extremity in the desired po-

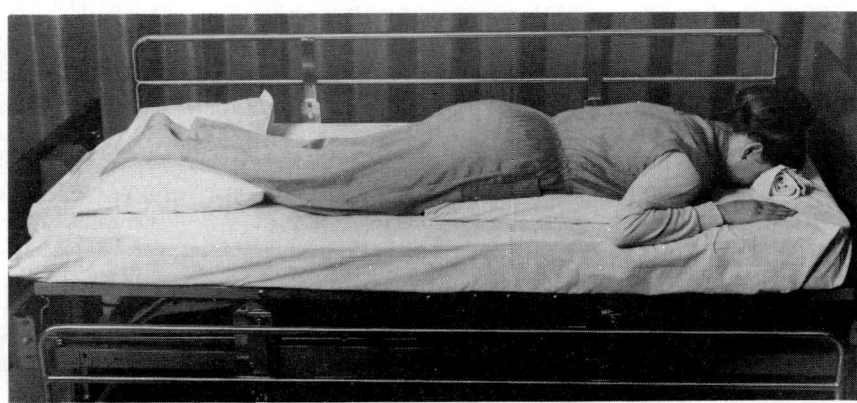

Fig. 23-4. Prone position. (From Rantz, M., and Courtial, D.: Lifting, moving, and transferring patients: a manual, ed. 2, St. Louis, 1981, The C.V. Mosby Co.)

sition), supportive pillows, attention to avoiding extreme flexion of joints, and care to avoid compressing nerves or arteries (the result of which can be neurologic or circulatory compromise) are all important considerations for both skin care and general maintenance of the patient.

The unaffected foot (or feet) should rest against a footboard at least part of the day. This helps to maintain the foot in a neutral position for a more normal walking position, prevents the weight of bedclothes from contributing to foot-drop, and provides a firm surface against which the person can do resistive foot exercises. Patients should be taught to check the position of their lower limbs when at rest. If their problem is nonneurologic, they should "toe in" to prevent external rotation contracture of the hip and pronation of the foot. These complications cause serious difficulty when walking is resumed.

For the general public, it should be remembered that poor posture throughout life may contribute to hypertrophic arthritis. Molding the pelvis correctly with a posterior pelvic tilt will help prevent increased curvature of the lower back with its resultant strain on muscles and joints. Holding the head up with the chin in takes a great deal of strain from the joints of the upper spine. It is surprising how many older persons can benefit from posture improvement even though damage may date from childhood. Nurses should teach patients good body mechanics to prevent muscle strain that could pull a joint out of alignment just enough for musculoskeletal changes to develop or to cause symptoms.

CONSERVATIVE MEASURES OF HEALTH TEACHING

The following are primarily for individuals with joint and muscle disorders. They can be restorative, preventive, or analgesic in nature.

Activity

Because many musculoskeletal disorders are problems of activity limitation, nursing care is directed toward improving activity. Absolute rest of a limb, joint, or part of the body may be ordered to prevent further tissue destruction and pain. As symptoms subside, activity will be gradually increased.

Clues such as pain, tiredness, and progressive loss of dexterity are helpful in recognizing the need for rest. The most frequent indicator that the patient has overused or misused a joint is an increase in pain or fatigue. Joint protection techniques that can be helpful, particularly for chronic inflammatory joint disorders, are as follows:

1. *Energy conservation techniques:* Examples are sliding rather than lifting objects and moving dishes, utensils, or equipment on a cart rather than carrying them.
2. *Avoiding positions of possible deformity:* Because flexor muscles are stronger than extensor muscles, joints tend to become deformed in a position of flexion. For example, avoid sitting for long periods, keeping the knees or elbows bent to avoid pain, and twisting motions to turn doorknobs or remove a jar lid.

3. *Learning to avoid holding muscles or joints in one position for a long time:*
   a. Activities need to be varied (as just mentioned).
   b. Active range of motion exercises are encouraged.
4. *Learning to use the strongest joints for activities:*
   a. Use good posture when sitting and standing.
   b. Work at a comfortable height.
   c. Use the knees and not the back when lifting objects.

Assistive, supportive, and safety devices

Although the occupational therapist may recommend specific assistive devices and teach the patient how to use them, the nurse needs to understand the need for them and encourage their use in self-care activities.

Supportive devices or ambulatory aids (walkers, canes, crutches) permit part of the person's weight to be transferred to the upper extremities. The physical therapist determines the specific device that is needed. Physical therapists generally select and teach the person how to use ambulatory devices. However, nurses may be called on to do this teaching. They must, in any case, know how to supervise the person who uses ambulatory aids. The most common gait patterns that may be used with a walker, cane, or crutches are the *three-point gait,* the *two-point gait,* and the *four-point gait.* These gait patterns are covered in Chapter 27.

Examples of *safety devices* used include the following:
1. Grab bars around toilets, tubs, and showers
2. Elevated toilet seats
3. Skid-proof mats or adhesive strips on tub floors
4. Hand rails along hallways and staircases
5. Nonskid wax applied to floors

Use of heat and cold

1. Moist heat is often used for relaxation of muscles and for sedative and analgesic effects.
2. Cold is often used to reduce or prevent swelling after trauma and to reduce pain and stiffness in some cases.
3. *Caution with heat or cold:*
   a. Apply with care to persons with decreased sensation.
   b. Check skin frequently for evidence of redness or burning.
   c. Moist compresses must be left on for 15 to 20 minutes to achieve maximal effectiveness.
   d. Dry heat must have a control device to regulate the heat at a low level.
   e. Do not use heat on joints that are or may be *infected.*
   f. Ice packs must be wrapped in toweling to protect the skin.

Splinting and bracing

Splints and braces (orthoses) are used to stabilize or support a joint to protect it from improper use or external trauma.
1. *Spring-loaded braces* are designed to oppose the action of unparalyzed muscles and to act as partial

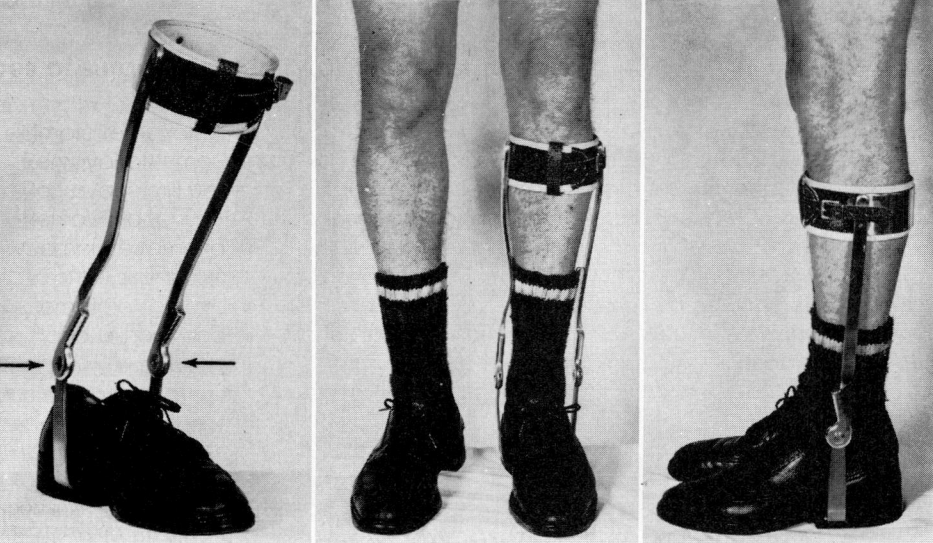

Fig. 23-5. Spring-loaded brace. (From Brashear, H., and Raney, R.: Shand's handbook of orthopaedic surgery, ed. 9, St. Louis, 1978, The C.V. Mosby Co.)

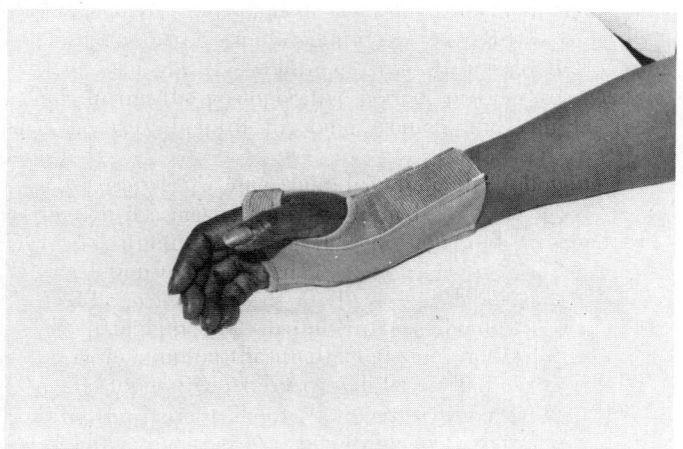

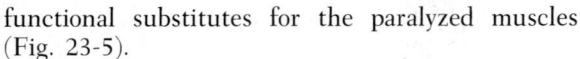

Fig. 23-6. Resting splints.

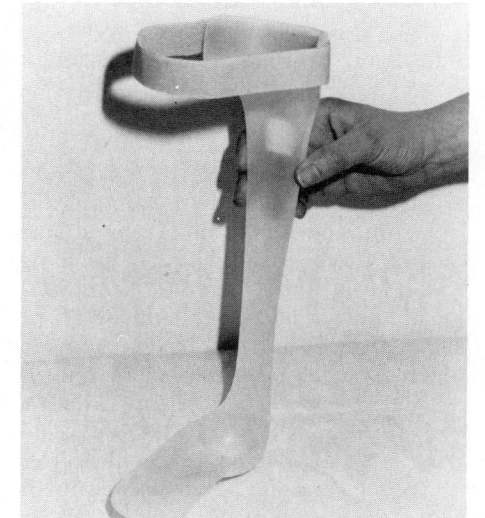

A

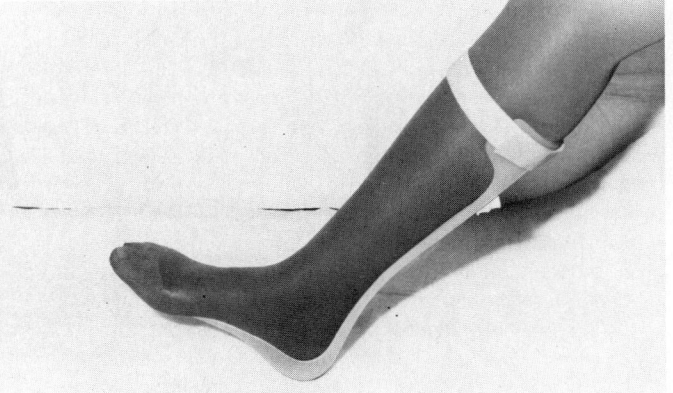

B

Fig. 23-7. Functional splints.

functional substitutes for the paralyzed muscles (Fig. 23-5).

2. *Resting splints* are designed to maintain a limb or joint in a functional position while permitting the muscles around the joint to relax (Fig. 23-6). They are used by the patient with rheumatoid arthritis to decrease muscle spasms that contribute to joint deformity.

3. *Functional splints* maintain the joint or limb in a usable position such as in the case of a drop wrist or foot-drop (Fig. 23-7).

Special considerations for splinting and bracing include the following:

1. Corrective shoes may be ordered for the feet to provide support and safety. These should be lacing shoes of an oxford type.

2. Observations of the patient's skin should be made

Guidelines for moving patient

1. If one side of the body is stronger than the other, *the patient should always be moved toward the strong side.* This guideline correlates with the principle that it is easier to move objects by pulling them than by pushing them. If the patient moves toward the strong side, the strong side is being used to pull the weak side through the required movement. The person assisting with the move should *support the strong side* to make it more effective.
2. If there is any question regarding the patient's ability to cooperate with the transfer, a second person should be standing by for assistance if needed.
3. If the person helping with the transfer has any doubt about his or her ability to accomplish the transfer safely, help should be obtained before attempting it.
4. The transfer should be accomplished using the strong muscles of the legs rather than the weak muscles of the back.
5. If lifting is required, there should be adequate help available. If adequate help is not available, the transfer should not be attempted at that time.
6. Whenever possible, pull sheets should be used to move the patent rather than trying to slide the patient (for example, from bed to cart).

---

after an orthosis has been worn, even for short periods, for areas of skin irritation. Adjustment may be needed by the *orthotist* (brace maker).

3. Patients must learn how to apply and remove braces or splints and how to care for them.
   a. Metal braces should be stored upright.
   b. Splints of molded materials should be stored away from sources of heat.
   c. Leather materials should be treated with Neatsfoot Compound or other leather preservative to prevent drying and cracking.
4. The brace should be adjusted if there is a change in weight (loss or gain).

Moving the patient

The student is referred to sources that are available regarding proper transfer techniques. A few basic guidelines are given in above box.

Major health problems of the musculoskeletal system

The disorders and injuries of the musculoskeletal system are vast in scope. They range from those that cause the patient minor discomfort and inconvenience to those that are life threatening. Listed here are some common musculoskeletal disorders that will be covered in this chapter:

1. Inflammatory disorders: rheumatoid arthritis, systemic lupus erythematosus, polymyositis (dermatomyositis), ankylosing spondylitis, gout, bacterial arthritis.
2. Nonarticular rheumatism: bursitis, carpal tunnel syndrome, Dupuytren's contracture.
3. Restrictive disorders: degenerative joint disorder, degenerative joint disorder of the spine, scoliosis.
4. Trauma: fractures of bone and soft tissue injuries.

INFLAMMATORY DISORDERS

The etiology, signs and symptoms, and medical therapy for the disorders to be covered are given in Table 23-1.

Rheumatoid arthritis

PATHOPHYSIOLOGY

Rheumatoid arthritis is a chronic, systemic, progressive inflammatory disorder that is more prevalent in women (3:1 over men) between 25 and 35 years of age. The inflammation begins in the synovial joints with edema, vascular congestion, fibrin exudate, and cellular infiltration. Continued inflammation leads to thickening of the synovium, particularly where it joins the articular cartilage. At these junctures, granulation tissue forms a *pannus,* or mantle, that covers the surface of the cartilage. The pannus also invades subchondral bone. As the amount of granulation tissue from inflammation increases, it interferes with normal nutrition of the articular cartilage. The cartilage becomes necrotic. The degree of erosion of the articular cartilage will determine the amount of articular disability. If large areas of cartilage are destroyed, adhesions form between the joint surfaces, and fibrous or bony union (ankylosis) develops between what were previously articulating surfaces. Destruction of cartilage and bone, in addition to some weakening of tendons and ligaments, may lead to subluxation or dislocation of joints. Invasion of the subchondral bone may cause eventual regional osteoporosis (increased bone porosity).

Text continued on p. 492.

Table 23-1. Rheumatic disorders

Disorder	Etiology	Signs and symptoms	Medical therapy
Inflammatory disorders			

Rheumatoid arthritis	Cause unknown
	Theories of causation:
	1. Immune mechanisms (antigen-antibody) such as interaction of the IgG class of immunoglobins with the rheumatoid factor (RF)
	2. Metabolic factors
	3. Infection with attention to viruses
	4. Genetic predisposition
		Local signs and symptoms:
		1. Generalized joint aching and stiffness and limitation in motion
		2. Gradual swelling, warmth, redness, and tenderness
		3. Changes in appearance of hands
		  a. Fusiform or spindle-shaped swelling of fingers
		  b. Swan-neck deformities of fingers
		  c. Ulnar deviation of the hands
		4. All joints can become involved: hips, knees, wrists, elbows, shoulders, and jaw
		Systemic signs and symptoms:
		Fatigue, malaise, fever, tachycardia, weakness, loss of weight, anemia; gradual bilateral, symmetric polyarthritis of small and large joints in all extremities
			Rest: complete bed rest during acute periods; otherwise 2 to 4 hr daily; rest for joints with splints
			Physical therapy:
			1. Active-assistive exercises to regular program of active exercises to preserve function
			2. Moist heat-packs or baths for muscle relaxing and relief of pain
			Medications: Table 23-2 lists medications prescribed in the treatment of the disorder.
			Reconstructive surgery may be necessary

Systemic lupus erythematosus (SLE)	Cause unknown Theories of causation: 1. Aberration of the immune system causes immune complexes containing antibodies to be deposited in tissue, thus damaging the tissue 2. Viral infections caused by or resulting from some immunologic abnormality 3. Genetic predisposition	General complaints: Moderate to severe—fever, weakness, fatigue, weight loss, sensitivity to sun, erythematous rash ("butterfly" pattern over bridge of nose and cheeks) Polyarthralgia and arthritis with pain and swelling Polyserositis (pleurisy and pericarditis) Anemia, thrombocytopenia, and renal, neurologic, and cardiac abnormalities Alopecia (hair loss) possible during periods of active systemic disease	No specific treatment; therapeutic program is ordered for the specific problems of the patient Medications (Table 23-2): adrenocorticosteroid therapy to control active manifestations of SLE; salicylates for joint pains; antimalariae drugs (Chloroquine) for cutaneous lesions

Polymyositis (dermatomyositis)	Cause unknown Theories of causation: 1. Reaction of the autoimmune system 2. Related to malignant tumors	Activities involving movement and lifting become difficult or impossible: 1. Climbing stairs 2. Arising from a chair 3. Combing the hair 4. Getting out of bathtub Weakness can lead to contractures and atrophy Difficulty with swallowing and presence of reflux esophagitis Decreased peristalsis Pulmonary function tests: may indicate impaired gas exchange, decreased vital and total lung capacity Muscle tenderness, transitory joint pain Dusky-red, patchy rash over elbows, dorsum of hands, knees, face, neck, shoulders (dermatomyositis) Weight loss	Symptomatic treatment Medications (Table 23-2): corticosteroids and mild analgesics Physical therapy to prevent contractures, preserve muscle strength Frequent small meals Antacids for reflux esophagitis May need complete bed rest with head of bed elevated Treatment of underlying malignancy if present

Ankylosing spondylitis	Unknown	Initial symptoms: mild with early morning stiffness and aching.
		Later: intermittent pain and restricted motion of the back.
		Extraspinal symptoms include:
		1. Pleuritic-like chest pain
		2. Achilles tendonitis
		3. Peripheral arthropathy (especially hips)
		4. Nonspecific symptoms:
		  a. Weight loss
		  b. Malaise
		  c. Fatigue
		  d. Mood change
		"Poker-back" deformity or kyphosis at the cervicodorsal junction
			Medications: salicylates to decrease inflammation; phenylbutazone (Butazolidin) or indomethacin (Indocin) for stronger antiinflammatory action
			Exercise program
			Hydrotherapy
			Surgery may be indicated

Continued.

Table 23-1. Rheumatic disorders—cont'd

Disorder	Etiology	Signs and symptoms	Medical therapy
Bursitis	Repeated trauma, strain, and overuse of joint	Deep-seated pain in area of bursa Pain on movement of involved extremity Passive and active range of motion limited in adjacent joint	Antiinflammatory agents are given (Table 23-2) Adrenocorticosteroids may be injected into bursa Rest of involved area Cold compresses during acute phase to help relieve discomfort
Degenerative joint disorder (DJD)	Cause of degeneration of articular cartilage is unknown Theories of causation: 1. Digestion of cartilage by enzymes and alteration of cartilage nutrition 2. Predisposition to excessive "wear and tear" of affected joints (chronic irritation) 3. Obesity and excessive weight on joints 4. Metabolic disturbances (for example, acromegaly) 5. Repeated joint hemorrhages 6. Trauma 7. Genetic predispositions 8. Congenital problems (for example, hip dislocations) 9. Stress on joints with aging process 10. Certain occupations such as coal mining and boxing	Pain in the movable joints, particularly on weight bearing Mild tenderness to aggravated pain on overuse of joint Joints become enlarged with loss of motion Crepitation Changes in alignment of affected part with flexion deformity Stiffness following periods of rest Changes in certain joints: 1. *Heberden's nodes*—bony protuberances on dorsal surface of distal interphalangeal joints of fingers 2. *Bouchard's nodes*—on proximal interphalangeal joints of fingers 3. *Coxarthrosis*—a degenerative change presenting with pain in hip with weight bearing; may progress to include groin and medial side of knee	Salicylates or nonsteroidal antiinflammatory drugs for relief of discomfort Weight reduction Physical therapy: 1. Exercise to preserve joint structure and function 2. Heat and massage for relief of pain and to relax muscles Drugs for analgesic and antiinflammatory effects: 1. Aspirin 2. Indomethacin (Indocin) 3. Naproxen (Naprosyn) Drugs as muscle relaxants 1. Methocarbamol (Robaxin) 2. Diazepam (Valium) 3. Meprobamate (Equanil) Intraarticular injections: corticosteroids Surgery
Restrictive disorders			

Degenerative joint disease of spine	Causes range from wide variety of disorders (see above)	1. Chief complaint: low back pain
		  a. Occasionally pain radiates to buttocks
		  b. There may be sciatic pain radiating down leg
		  c. Pain follows overactivity
			Same as for degenerative joint disease

Disorder	Etiology	Signs and symptoms	Treatment
		or periods of prolonged sitting, walking, or standing d. Difficulty in bending over or lifting objects Lateral deviation of spine away from midline (in thoracic spine region) One shoulder is higher than other Movement of chest is restricted on deep inspiration May complain of shortness of breath or difficulty in taking deep breath	
Scoliosis	Rickets Neuromuscular disorders Vertebral disorders Congenital Idiopathic (cause unknown)		Splints or braces or traction may be needed to place spine in functional position Therapeutic or corrective exercises Medications: salicylates Surgery may be necessary
Other disorders Gout	Metabolic disorder in synthesis of purines, or poor renal excretion of uric acid leading to hyperuricemia	Acute: rapid onset of severe pain in inflamed joints—most frequently large toe Presence of swelling and tenderness, malaise, headache, and high fever Chronic: always present in those who have familial tendency Acute exacerbations occur when not diagnosed or not treated Deposits of *tophi* (monosodium urate) in tissues, most noticeable in ears, on knuckles, and on great toe	Acute attack: reduce body pool of urates and serum uric acid via urinary excretion Long-term: Avoid acute attacks and avoid joint damage and renal failure Relief of pain during acute attack Rest of affected part Medications: 1. Colchicine (Col-Benemid) or allopurinol 2. Indomethacin (Indocin) 3. Phenylbutazone (Butazolidin) Increased fluid intake

Bacterial arthritis	1. Invasion of synovial membrane by microorganisms:
	  a. Gonococci
	  b. Meningococci
	  c. Staphylococci
	  d. Coliforms
	  e. Salmonella
	  f. *Haemophilus influenzae*
	2. Predisposition:
	  a. Susceptibility of the patient
	  b. Recent joint surgery or trauma
	  c. Intraarticular injections
	  d. Rheumatoid arthritis
		Pain
		Swelling
		Tenderness of joint
			Rest or immobilization
			Antibiotics specific for the organism
			Surgical drainage may be necessary

The course of rheumatoid arthritis varies greatly from person to person. It is marked by periods of exacerbation and remission. Some individuals have been known to recover from a first attack and never suffer a recurrence. For others, particularly those in whom the rheumatoid factor is found (seropositive rheumatoid disorder), the disorder tends to be chronically progressive. In a small number of individuals the disorder may be rapidly progressive, marked by unremitting joint destruction and diffuse vasculitis. Exacerbations can be triggered by physical or mental stress.

ASSESSMENT

Subjective data

The early manifestations of the disorder may lead the person to describe the location of aching and stiffness "in my arms," "in my hands," or "in my legs" as opposed to naming specific joints. This kind of discomfort may be present for some period of time before the person begins to see and feel the joint changes.

Objective data

1. Inspection and palpation: check same joints of *both sides of body* for symmetry, skin color, size and shape, tenderness, and swelling.
2. Evaluate passive range of motion of synovial joints.
   a. Note any deviation from normal (limited joint movement most important).
   b. Note presence of crepitation (*crepitus*), which is an audible grating sound made by movement of bony surfaces within the joint.
   c. Note pain with range of motion.
3. Inspect and palpate skeletal muscles bilaterally.
   a. Note atrophy, tone, and tenderness.
   b. Test muscle strength by resistive movements.

Diagnostic tests

1. Serologic tests
   a. Erythrocyte sedimentation rate: will be elevated
   b. Red and white blood cell count: will reveal anemia and leukocytosis
   c. Rheumatoid factor (RF): serum will show presence of large antibody-like protein molecules
2. Roentgenographic examinations
   a. Periarticular osteoporosis: joint surface erosion
   b. Later: narrowing of joint space, subluxation, and ankylosis
3. Joint aspiration: samples of synovial fluid from within the joint cavity will determine the presence of an aseptic inflammatory process; synovial fluid is cultured and examined microscopically.

DATA ANALYSIS AND PLANNING

Nursing diagnoses

Comfort, alteration in: pain in joints
Potential for injury due to loss of muscle strength and joint motion

Self-concept, disturbance in: body image
Self-care deficit: bathing/hygiene, dressing/grooming, toileting

Expected patient outcomes

1. Patient describes feeling more comfortable.
2. Patient has ability to move about with minimal limitations in range of motion.
3. Self-concept is more positive.
4. Patient is able to perform self-care activities.
5. Patient understands the disease and will continue with follow-up visits to clinics and physician's office.

IMPLEMENTATION

Assisting with achievement of therapeutic goals

1. Give prescribed medications on time and in prescribed doses (Table 23-2).
2. Assist with selection of foods; assist with feeding if necessary; encourage small, frequent meals.
3. Encourage and assist with range of motion exercises to increase mobility and muscle strength.

Assisting with comfort and ADL

1. Keep patient free of pain with prescribed medication.
2. Apply heat to joints as ordered by physician
3. Assist with self-care.

Counseling and teaching

1. Medications: importance of strict adherence to times and dosage; expected and side effects of prescribed drugs
2. Planning for rest periods and periods of activity
3. Planning gradual independence in ADL
4. Nutrition: food selections that meet daily requirements in all food groups
5. Instructions on the application, use, and care of splinting devices
6. Instructions on safety measures to prevent injury such as
   a. Using supportive shoes and avoiding of walking with slippers
   b. Avoiding use of scatter rugs or loose carpeting
   c. Avoiding use of wax on floors
   d. Using support devices on bathtub and in shower
7. Be wary of promises of a "cure" with gadgets, programs, and medicines; check with local chapter of the Arthritis Foundation for merit or lack or merit of community resources

EVALUATION OF CONSERVATIVE MEASURES

Based on expected patient outcomes the questions related to therapy would include the following:
1. Is the patient comfortable?
2. Is the potential for injury lessened?
3. Can the patient explain the need for follow-up care?
4. Can the patient explain the program of exercises?
5. Can the patient explain the importance of alternating rest and activity?

Table 23-2. Medications prescribed in the treatment of rheumatoid arthritis

Medication	Action	Side effects/ toxic effects	Precautions
Salicylates			
Examples: acetylsali-cyclic acid, choline salicylates	Analgesic, antipyretic, antiinflammatory	Gastric irritation, dose-related sali-cylism; skin rash; hypersensitivity	Take with food, milk, or antacid; space every 4-6 hr. to maintain an-tiinflammatory effect
Nonsteroidal antiinflammatory agents			
Indomethacin (Indo-cin)	Analgesic, antiinflam-matory	Headache; dizziness; insomnia; confu-sion; gastrointes-tinal irritation	Take with food, milk, or antacid; discontinue if central nervous sys-tem symptoms de-velop and notify phy-sician
Ibuprofen (Motrin)	Same as indomethacin	Same as indometha-cin but believed less irritating to gastrointestinal tract	Delayed absorption if taken with food
Tolmetin sodium (To-lectin)	Same as ibuprofen	Same as ibuprofen	Take with food or milk
Naproxen (Naprosyn)	Same as ibuprofen	Same as ibuprofen, also drowsines	Take with food, milk, or antacid; avoid driving until dosage effect es-tablished
Fenoprofen calcium (Nalfon)	Same as ibuprofen	Same os naproxen	Delayed absorption if taken with food; avoid driving until dosage effect estab-lished
Sulindac (Clinoril)	Same as ibuprofen	Same as ibuprofen; plus skin rash	Take with food, milk, or antacid; not to be used with acetylsali-cylic acid
Potent antiinflammatory agents			
Adrenocorticosteroids (for example, pred-nisone)	Interfere with body's normal inflammatory response	Fluid retention; so-dium retention; po-tassium depletion; hypertension; de-creased healing potential; in-creased suscepti-bility to infection; gastrointestinal irri-tation; hirsutism, os-teoporosis, fat de-posits; diabetes mellitus; myopathy; adrenal insuffi-ciency or adrenal crisis if abruptly withdrawn	Take with food, milk, or antacid; dosage not to be increased or decreased without physician's supervi-sion; take in morning if taken on once-a-day basis
Phenylbutazone (Bu-tazolidin)	Antiinflammatory; an-algesic at subcorti-cal site in brain	Gastrointestional irri-tation; hematologic toxicity; hyperten-sion, impaired renal function	Used for a short term (7-10 days); take with food or milk

Table 23-2. Medications prescribed in the treatment of rheumatoid arthritis—cont'd

Medication	Action	Side effects/ toxic effects	Precautions
Slow-acting antiinflammatory agents			
Antimalarials			
Hydroxychloroquine (Plaquenil)	Antiinflammatory (mechanism unknown); effect not expected to be noted for 6-12 mo after beginning therapy	Gastrointestinal disturbances; retinal edema that may result in blindness	Eye examination before beginning thearpy and every 6 mo thereafter
Chloroquine (Aralen)	Same as hydroxychloroquine	Same as hydroxychloroquine	Same as hydroxychloroquine
Quinacrine (Atabrine)	Same as hydroxychloroquine	Same as hydroxychloroquine but may be better tolerated; yellow discoloration of the skin	May be stopped periodically to prevent deepening of skin discoloration
Gold salts (Myochrysine, Solganol)	Antiinflammatory	Renal and hepatic damage; corneal deposits; dermatitis; ulcerations in mouth; hematologic changes	Urinalysis and complete blood count (CBC) before each injection; report dermatitis, metallic taste in mouth, or lesions in mouth to physician
Pencillamine (Cuprimine)	Antiinflammatory (mechanism unclear); effect not expected to be noted until several months after beginning treatment	Fever; rash; nephrotic syndrome; hematologic changes; gastrointestinal irritation; lupuslike syndromes; allergic reactions (33% probability if allergic to penicillin); retarded wound healing	Urinalysis, CBC, differential, hemoglobin, and platelet count at least weekly for 3 mo, then monthly; report skin rash, fever to physician; food interferes with absorption—take on empty stomach between meals

RECONSTRUCTIVE SURGERY

Orthopedic surgery may be necessary to correct ankylosed and deformed joints.

Replacement arthroplasty

Replacement arthroplasty is available for the shoulder, wrist, elbow, phalangeal joints of the fingers, hips (Fig. 23-8), knee (Fig. 23-9), and ankle. Since the hip and knee are the most commonly replaced, the discussion that follows will be limited to these two joints.

Rheumatoid arthritis, degenerative joint disease, and avascular necrosis are the major reasons for performing total joint or replacement arthroplasty. *Avascular necrosis* of the bone, or bone death, is caused by inadequate blood supply. It can be a complication of bone fractures, as well as corticosteroid treatment for rheumatoid arthritis and systemic lupus erythematosus. Pain (even at rest), restricted motion, and gait disturbances are characteristic. Surgery in the form of total joint replacement is performed to alleviate pain and increase motion.

The hip prosthesis consists of an acetabular portion (cup) and a femoral component. The designs of the various prostheses vary in size of the femoral head, shape and length of the femoral shaft, and design of the acetabular component. The care of the patient experiencing total hip or total knee replacement is outlined in boxes on pp. 496-497.

Expected patient outcomes following surgery

1. Patient continues with activities and weight-bearing restrictions for period recommended by surgeon.

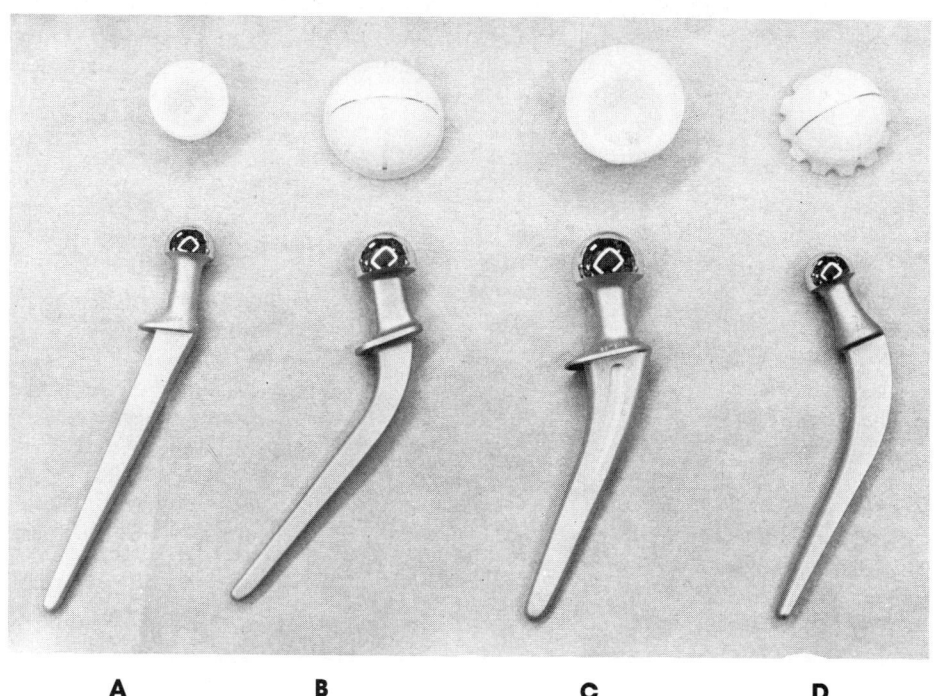

Fig. 23-8. Hip prostheses. **A,** Harris CDH (note offset cup). **B,** Trapezoidal-28. **C,** Aufranc-Turner (note offset cup). **D,** Charnley.

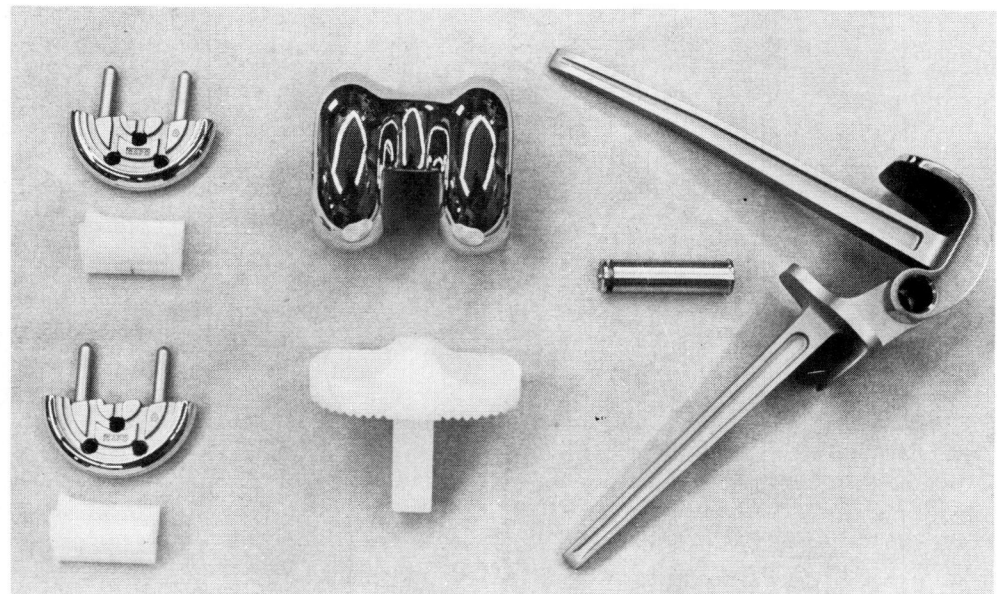

Fig. 23-9. Knee prostheses. *Left to right,* Polycentric knee, total condylar knee, and offset hinged knee with pin.

Types of surgical procedures for the patient with rheumatoid arthritis

Synovectomy: The early removal of synovial tissue to arrest the course of rheumatoid arthritis in a particular joint, and to maintain joint function and prevent recurrent inflammation. The knee and the wrist are the joints most often subjected to this procedure.

Arthrotomy: Opening into a joint. The procedure is done to
1. Explore the joint to determine the presence of a disease process.
2. Drain the joint.
3. Remove damaged tissue or foreign bodies within the joint.

Arthroplasty: Reconstruction of a joint that has been destroyed by injury or disease.
1. Purposes:
    a. Restore motion of the joint.
    b. Relieve pain.
    c. Correct deformity.
2. Types:
    a. Replacement of *part* of the joint with a *prosthesis* made of metal or other material such as the "cup" or "mold" arthroplasty of the hip joint.
    b. Surgical *reshaping* of the bones of the joint, which are then covered with *soft tissue* used as an interposition device.
    c. *Total joint replacement* where both sides of the joint are replaced by metal or polyethylene implants.

Total hip replacement

Preoperative care

1. Skin care:
    a. Preparation of the skin will follow the hospital's written procedure or the surgeon's written orders.
    b. The area must be kept free of contamination.
    c. The patient's environment must be as free as possible from potential sources of contamination.
2. Reassurance and education
    a. Patient needs to understand about the surgical procedure, postoperative care, and expectations after discharge.
    b. Patient is to sign the operative permit and have an understanding of its importance (informed consent).

Postoperative care

1. Positioning:
    a. Position will depend on the design of the prosthesis and the method of insertion.
    b. Generally the physician will order that the operated leg be kept in *abduction* with prescribed *limited flexion* of the hip.
2. Wound care: Drains are placed in the wound to prevent formation of a hematoma.
    a. Maintain constant suction through the self-contained vacuum of the Porto-Vac.
    b. Note amount and types of drainage.
    c. Keep area free of contamination. (Infection at the site of the prosthesis results in total failure of the surgery.)
3. Activity:
    a. Head of bed may be elevated about 60 degrees for short periods of time.
    b. Instruct patient on use of overbed trapeze and shifting weight using the unoperated leg and trapeze.
    c. Patient may be turned to the unoperated side with the operated leg in abduction.
    d. Encourage plantar flexion and dorsiflexion of the feet and quadriceps and gluteal-setting exercises to promote venous return, prevent thrombi, and maintain muscle tone.
    e. Ambulation will begin about the third or fourth postoperative day.
        (1) The patient is assisted to stand and cautioned not to flex the hip more than 60 degrees.
        (2) The amount of walking will vary with the patient's ability.
        (3) A walker is used for support. The amount of weight bearing will be ordered by the surgeon.

Total hip replacement—cont'd

Postoperative care—cont'd

4. Medications:
   a. Prophylactic anticoagulant drugs such as heparin may be given because of increased risk of thrombus formation. Many physicians prescribe aspirin for its anticoagulant effect.
   b. Narcotics are given for discomfort. Report excessive pain immediately.
5. Discharge:
   a. Patient must use crutches, avoid adduction, and limit hip flexion to 90 degrees for 2 months.
   b. A raised toilet seat extension must be used at home for at least 2 months to protect against extreme hip flexion.
   c. Patient will need a long-handled shoehorn and a reacher to pick up dropped items.
   d. Safety in the home must be reviewed with the patient (p. 484).

Total knee replacement

Preoperative care
Same as for total hip replacement.

Postoperative care

1. Plan of care same as for total hip replacement.
2. Activity:
   a. Patient is urged to do quadriceps-setting exercises and should begin to attempt straight-leg raising after drain is removed.
   b. *Active* flexion exercises are begun after removal of dressings.
   c. Ambulation with partial weight bearing using a walker or crutches will begin when the patient demonstrates quadriceps control and will continue for about 2 months.
   d. Patient must achieve active knee flexion to 70 degrees within the period determined by the surgeon; otherwise formed adhesions may need to be manipulated (flexed) under anesthesia.

---

2. Patient uses assistive devices as prescribed.
3. Incision heals without infection.

Systemic lupus erythematosus

PATHOPHYSIOLOGY

Systemic lupus erythematosus (SLE) is a chronic inflammatory disorder that affects women, particularly adolescent and young adults, four times more often than it affects men. The name of the disorder means "red wolf," after its characteristic rash, "likened to the damage wrought by a hungry wolf."

Once thought to be relatively rare and always fatal, the disorder has been found to be fairly common, and its course can be controlled by corticosteroids. Some patients may eventually die as a result of vascular lesions affecting the kidneys, central nervous system, or other vital organs; others may die of complicating secondary infections.

The pathologic manifestations of the disease include severe vasculitis with necrosis of the walls of the small arteries, renal involvement with thickening of the basement membrane of the glomerular tufts and necrosis of the glomerular capillaries, lymph node necrosis, synovitis, lesions of the nervous system, and the development of small white spots in the retina called *cytoid bodies*. The onset may be insidious or acute.

ASSESSMENT
Subjective data

1. Note that patients may express vague symptoms or simply say that they are "always tired."
2. Question patients about generalized weakness, loss of appetite, loss of weight, skin rashes, and specific joint discomfort (even at rest).
3. Identify the presence and extent of discomfort or stiffness of muscles or joints.
4. Identify the presence of sensitivity of eyes and skin to the sun.
5. Question patients regarding hair loss, which occurs during acute episodes.

Objective data

1. Observe for erythema over the cheeks and bridge of the nose, above the ears, on exposed part of the neck, and over other body areas.
2. Examine for loss of hair or partial loss at normal hairline.
3. Check for muscle strength and range of motion of joints.

Diagnostic tests

Depending on the organs involved, the patient may have findings of glomerulonephritis, pleuritis, pericarditis, peritonitis, neuritis, or anemia. Renal and neurologic manifestations are among the more serious manifestations of the disease.

Laboratory findings may be specific to the organs involved, as with proteinuria, abnormal cerebrospinal fluid, or roentgenographic evidence of pleural reactions. A positive lupus erythematosus (LE) cell reaction and immunofluorescent studies to identify the antibody responsible for LE cell reaction are helpful in making the diagnosis of the disease. Laboratory findings may also show the presence of anemia, thrombocytopenia, leukocytosis, or leukopenia. A *skin biopsy* is taken of the rash and studied for histopathologic evidence of the disorder.

DATA ANALYSIS AND PLANNING

Nursing diagnoses

Skin integrity, impairment of: actual
Nutrition, alteration in: less than body requirements
Activity intolerance
Comfort, alteration in: pain

Expected patient outcomes

1. Patient maintains skin integrity.
2. Patient has an appetite and maintains nutrition.
3. Patient has lessened fatigue and weakness and increased activity tolerance.
4. Patient is free of pain and discomfort.
5. Patient continues follow-up care by physician.

IMPLEMENTATION

Assisting with achievement of therapeutic goals

1. Medications: administer as prescribed—
   Corticosteroids
   Analgesics
   Antacids
2. Nutrition: encourage well-balanced diet consisting of all major food groups.
3. Activity: encourage planned program of exercises and joint range of motion.
4. Surgery: total joint replacement may be necessary, since avascular necrosis (p. 494) is also a complication of corticosteroid treatment of SLE.

Assisting with comfort and ADL

1. Administer medication for pain of joints and muscles.
2. Prevent skin lesions by protecting skin while in sunlight.
3. Help patient with gradual independence in ADL.

Counseling and teaching

1. Educate patient and family about the disorder.
2. Medications: have patient learn the use of those specifically prescribed.
3. Help the patient to plan periods of rest and exercise.
4. Explain how to avoid excessive exposure to sun.

EVALUATION

Based on expected patient outcomes, the questions related to therapy would include the following:
1. Has skin integrity been maintained?
2. Can the patient explain the need for rest periods alternating with periods of activity?
3. Can the patient explain the disorder and the need for continued follow-up care?

Polymyositis (dermatomyositis)

PATHOPHYSIOLOGY

Polymyositis (dermatomyositis) is a diffuse inflammatory disorder of the *striated* (voluntary) muscles. Females are affected twice as commonly as males. The disorder can occur at any age. The disorder usually runs a course of exacerbations and remissions and is first noted in the proximal muscles, in particular the pelvic and shoulder girdles. Other muscles, for example, neck flexors and muscles of swallowing, may become involved. There is primary degeneration of muscle fibers followed by degeneration or necrosis of parts or entire groups of muscle fibers. Lymphocytes and plasma cells may infiltrate blood vessel walls.

Involvement of the skin in the form of rash marks the disease as dermatomyositis. A reddish purple rash may be found chiefly in the sun-exposed areas (face, neck, shoulders, upper chest, and back). Increased evidence of malignant neoplasm has been found in persons over 40 years of age in the first 5 years of the illness.

ASSESSMENT

Subjective data

Polymyositis may vary in its mode of onset and in the rate of progression of symptoms, whether muscular, dermal, or articular. The clinical course may be one of spontaneous remissions and exacerbations.
1. Since muscular weakness is present in nearly all patients and particularly in the lower extremities, the patient is asked to describe the weakness and effect on ADL.
2. Questions are asked about joint and muscle pain, gastrointestinal problems, appetite, and weight loss.

Objective data

1. Weakness of myositis can lead to contractures and atrophy. Test strength of upper and lower extremities against resistance.
2. Observe patient for respiratory difficulty, since diaphragm may be affected by weakness.
3. Palpate muscles and joints for pain or tenderness.
4. Examine for dusky-red, patchy rash over elbows, dorsum of hands, knees, forehead, neck, shoulders, and chest (dermatomyositis).

Diagnostic tests

Manual muscle tests

Manual muscle tests are used to determine the degree of muscular weakness from the disorder. They are used also in cases of injury or muscle disuse. The physical therapist rates the strength of muscles in relation to gravity and applied resistance. Muscle testing is helpful in determining which muscle should be chosen for biopsy. When muscle-strengthening exercises are indicated, the test will indicate the group of muscles that requires the most therapy.

Muscle biopsy

Biopsy is performed to aid in the diagnosis of specific myopathic disorders. The muscle tissue may reveal degeneration, inflammatory reactions, or involvement of specific fibers.

A muscle biopsy is an operative procedure usually performed by a surgeon. A local or general anesthetic may be used. Following the procedure the patient will experience minor to moderate discomfort in the form of stiffness or pain at the operative site. The patient is encouraged to resume range of motion activity to avoid undue stiffness.

Electromyography

Electromyography measures the electrical activity of muscles; an *electromyogram* (EMG) is a recording of the electrical potential detected by a needle electrode inserted into skeletal muscle. The electrical activity can be heard over a loudspeaker and viewed on an oscilloscope and graph. Normal muscles at rest give off no electrical activity.

The EMG provides evidence of lower motor neuron disease, primary muscle disease, and defects in the transmission of electrical impulses at the neuromuscular junction, such as in myasthenia gravis. The test cannot be used to differentiate *specific* muscle disorders. There is no specific preparation of the patient, except to reassure the patient that the electrode needles will not cause electric shock and the procedure is not dangerous.

Serum enzyme tests

Serum glutamic-oxaloacetic transaminase (SGOT), creatine phosphokinase (CPK), and aldolase levels are elevated in the presence of active polymyositis or dermatomyositis.

DATA ANALYSIS AND PLANNING

Nursing diagnoses

Potential for impaired gas exchange
Potential for injury
Mobility, impaired physical
Nutrition, alteration in: less than body requirements
Self-care deficit: feeding, bathing/hygiene, dressing/grooming, toileting
Activity intolerance

Expected patient outcomes

1. Patient has increased energy for physical activities and self-care.
2. Patient maintains nutritional status.
3. Patient performs ADL without fatigue or discomfort.
4. Patient continues with physician's plan of treatment for remainder of life.

IMPLEMENTATION

Assisting with achievement of therapeutic goals

1. Muscular involvement may cause dysphagia or respiratory embarrassment. Oxygen and restoration of airway may be necessary.
2. Range of motion exercises must be done to prevent contractures and loss of function.
3. Assistance is needed with nutritional feedings. The patient may be taking small, frequent feedings.

Assisting with comfort and ADL

1. Assist patient with personal hygiene.
2. Analgesics may be prescribed for joint and muscle pain.

EVALUATION

Based on the expected patient outcomes the questions related to therapy would include the following:

1. Can the patient perform ADL with greater ease?
2. Is the patient maintaining nutritional status?
3. Is the patient able to describe the nature of the disorder and why there is a need for continued professional help?

Ankylosing spondylitis

PATHOPHYSIOLOGY

Ankylosing spondylitis is a chronic and usually progressive disorder of the sacroiliac and hip joints, the synovial joints of the spine, and the adjacent soft tissues leading to spinal fusion. Once considered a rare, predominantly male disorder, it is now recognized as affecting both sexes, with males being more severely affected. The onset is usually between ages 10 and 30. The progression of the disorder usually decreases after the age of 50, but limitation of movement of the spine persists. Fusion of the sacroiliac joints and spine up through the cervical vertebrae may occur over periods of 10 to 20 years (Fig. 23-10).

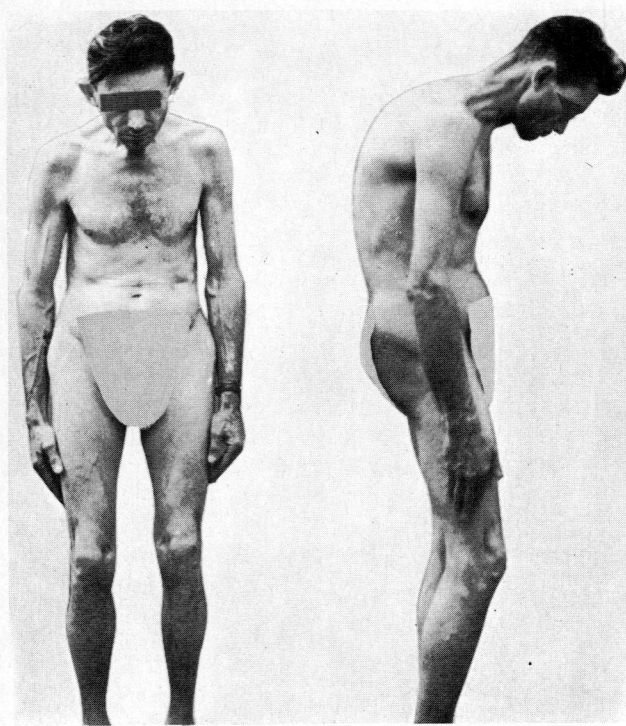

Fig. 23-10. Ankylosing spondylitis in 46-year-old man with ankylosis of entire spine in faulty position. (From Brashear, H., and Raney, R.: Shand's handbook of orthopaedic surgery, ed. 9, St. Louis, 1978, The C.V. Mosby Co.)

ASSESSMENT

Subjective data

Many persons with ankylosing spondylitis remain undiagnosed. The patient complains of low backache, stiffness, and alternating or bilateral "sciatica" that lasts for a few days at a time and subsides. Later the symptoms become more persistent and begin to include evidence of ankylosis of joints, particularly of the spine. The patient should be questioned about changes in body shape and any loss in height.

Objective data

1. Observe for pain on assuming or maintaining an erect position.
2. Examine patient's posture: patient appears bent forward at the waist, often compensating to achieve an erect position by flexing hips and knees.
3. Palpate for tenderness over the spine and sacroiliac region.
4. Note pain on motion and limitation in turning and bending upper body.

Diagnostic tests

Roentgenograms are most helpful in delineating the disorder. Changes in the sacroiliac joints are the earliest and most diagnostic. There is blurring of the bony mar-

gins, then sclerosis, and later ankylosis. Bony growths, called *syndesmophytes,* that bridge the adjacent vertebrae give the appearance of a "bamboo spine."

DATA ANALYSIS AND PLANNING

Nursing diagnoses

Impaired physical mobility
Comfort, alteration in: pain in joints and muscles; fatigue
Disturbance in self-concept: body image

Expected patient outcomes

1. Patient performs ADL without muscle or joint discomfort.
2. Patient has a positive self-concept.
3. There is no evidence of progressive spinal deformity.

IMPLEMENTATION

Assisting with achievement of therapeutic goals

1. Maintaining alignment of the spine
   a. Mattress should be firm.
   b. Bed board may be used.
   c. Patient should sleep flat without pillow.
   d. A back brace may be necessary for support.
2. Postural and breathing exercises
   a. Extension exercises should be performed to maintain erect posture and normal height and to strengthen paraspinal muscles.
   b. Abdominal lying should be done three to four times a day for 15 to 30 minutes.
   c. Breathing exercises will help increase breathing capacity.

Assisting with comfort

1. Apply heat to painful joints.
2. Apply hydrotherapy to entire body; this is best if done just before postural and deep breathing exercises.

EVALUATION

Based on expected patient outcomes the questions related to therapy would include the following:
1. Is the patient able to perform ADL with no discomfort?
2. Has progressive spinal deformity been prevented?

NONARTICULAR RHEUMATISM

Bursitis

PATHOPHYSIOLOGY

Bursitis is inflammation of a bursa, a small fluid-filled saclike cavity between two articular soft tissue layers. The bursa facilitates joint movements and acts like a pad to cushion joints. The joints most affected are the shoulders, elbows, hips, knees, and ankles. In some instances the inflammation of the bursa is preceded by tendonitis, that is, inflammation of a tendon, or by tenosynovitis, which is inflammation of a tendon and the tendon sheath.

ASSESSMENT

Subjective data

1. Ask patient to describe location and severity of pain and what preceded present shoulder pain.
2. Is patient being treated for inflammation of joints resulting from a known cause for the pain?
3. Does the patient have a history of rheumatoid arthritis?
4. Is the patient able to use the joint?

Objective data

1. Palpate the joint for tenderness and swelling of the soft tissues. The swelling will feel "boggy."
2. Observe degree of limited mobility of affected joint.

DATA ANALYSIS AND PLANNING

The *Nursing Diagnosis* is *Alteration in comfort: pain in joint bursa.* The *Expected Patient Outcomes* are that the patient will be free of pain and will be able to use the joint adjacent to the bursa in full range of motion.

IMPLEMENTATION

Assisting with achievement of therapeutic goals

1. Medications are given as prescribed for inflammation and discomfort.
2. Rest for the involved area may be necessary during the acute phase.
3. Modified joint and extremity exercises may be prescribed to prevent "frozen shoulder," for example.
4. *Cold* (not heat) is applied during acute phase; heat is avoided, as this increases the fluid exudate (additional fluid in the bursa). Heat may be used later.

SURGERY

Roentgenographic study may disclose a calcific mass in the subdeltoid area that may need to be removed.

EVALUATION

Based on expected patient outcomes the questions related to therapy include the following:
1. Is area free of pain?
2. Is full joint range of motion possible?

Carpal tunnel syndrome

PATHOPHYSIOLOGY

Carpal tunnel syndrome is caused by pressure being exerted on the median nerve at the wrist. The median nerve passes through a tunnel bounded by the carpal bones dorsally and the transverse carpal ligament volarly

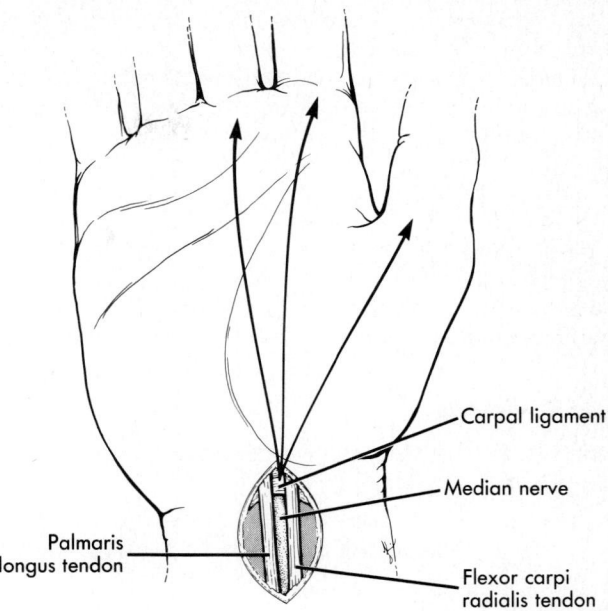

Fig. 23-11. Carpel tunnel syndrome. Volar aspect of wrist retracted to demonstrate position of median nerve. Distribution of median nerve is to thumb and first two fingers. (Adapted from Compare, E.L.: Orthopedic surgery, Chicago, 1974, Year Book Medical Publishers, Inc.)

(Fig. 23-11). Flexor tendons run through the tunnel parallel to the median nerve. The pressure on the nerve may derive from truama or from swelling of the tendon sheaths caused by other processes like rheumatoid arthritis. Generally the tenosynovitis is localized and not associated with any systemic disease. This condiiton is most common in middle-aged women.

ASSESSMENT

Subjective data

The symptoms that the patient describes are from the compression of the median nerve and include the following:
1. Episodes of burning pain or tingling in the hands that the patient says are relieved by vigorous shaking or exercising of the hand
2. Numbness (hypesthesia) affecting the thumb, index, and ring fingers, particularly after prolonged or forced flexion of the wrist, as in knitting or holding a book
3. Feeling of "swelling" in the affected hand
4. Complaint of difficulty grasping or holding onto small objects; "feels clumsy"

Objective data

1. There is no swelling in the hand, wrist, or fingers.
2. There is a wasting or depressed appearance of the soft tissue at the base of the thumb on the palmar surface (thenar eminence).

3. Symptoms can be elicited by tapping the median nerve at the wrist (Tinel's sign).
4. There is difficulty in abducting the thumb or opposing the thumb to the index finger (caused by weakness of the muscles of the thenar eminence).

DATA ANALYSIS AND PLANNING

The *Nursing Diagnosis* is *mobility, impaired ability to use hand and fingers.* The *Expected Patient Outcomes* are that the patient will have maximum function of hand, thumb, and fingers, and the incision will heal without infection.

IMPLEMENTATION

Assisting with achievement of therapeutic goals

1. Rest
2. Splinting of the wrist
3. Local injections of corticosteroids

SURGERY

Decompression by surgical release of the transverse carpal ligament and removal of tissues that may be compressing the median nerve.

EVALUATION

Based on expected patient outcome the questions related to therapy would include the following:
1. Has infection been avoided?
2. Is the patient able to use the hand and fingers with normal range of motion?

Dupuytren's contracture

PATHOPHYSIOLOGY

Dupuytren's contracture is a common problem particularly in men past middle age. The disorder is caused by a thickening and shortening of the palmar fascia on the ulnar side of one or both hands causing flexion of the ring finger and sometimes the small finger. There does not appear to be involvement of joints, muscles, tendons, or nervous or vascular tissue.

ASSESSMENT

Subjective data

The patient complains of a gradual decrease in the ability to extend the ring and small fingers.

Objective data

The most obvious appearance of the patient's hand is the flexed position of the ring finger and possibly the small finger. The skin of the palm is drawn down, forming tight puckers and nodules. The condition starts in one hand but often occurs in both hands. The patient cannot actively extend the fingers.

> ## Postoperative nursing care for patient having correction of Dupuytren's contracture
>
> 1. Hand is elevated to control swelling.
> 2. Ice packs may be ordered.
> 3. Fingers are checked for sensation, circulation, and finger movements.
> 4. Patient is encouraged to actively extend fingers.
> 5. In 2 to 3 days the patient begins use of hand in daily activities.

DATA ANALYSIS AND PLANNING

The *Nursing Diagnosis* is *mobility, impaired: inability to use flexed fingers.* The *Expected Patient Outcome* is that the patient will have full use of fingers and hand.

SURGERY

The major medical therapy is surgical removal of the involved palmar fascia. Postoperative care is listed in box above.

EVALUATION

Based on the expected patient outcome the question related to therapy would be: Does the patient have full use of hand and fingers?

RESTRICTIVE DISORDERS

Degenerative joint disease

PATHOPHYSIOLOGY

Degenerative joint disease, also known as *osteoarthritis, osteoarthrosis, hypertrophic arthritis,* or *senescent arthritis,* is the most common disorder of joint changes of persons past 40 years of age. Prevalence becomes almost universal in persons 65 years or older.

The disorder is characterized by progressive deterioration and loss of articular cartilage. It is thought to accompany aging but may develop secondary to other conditions (Fig. 23-12).

The articular cartilage, normally dense, white, translucent, and smooth, becomes yellow and opaque. Areas of the cartilage may become soft, and the surface becomes roughened, frayed, and cracked. Eventually this cartilage may be destroyed down to the bone. *Osteophytes,* or spurs of new bone that appear at the joint margins and at the sites of attachment of supporting structures, result in interference with joint function.

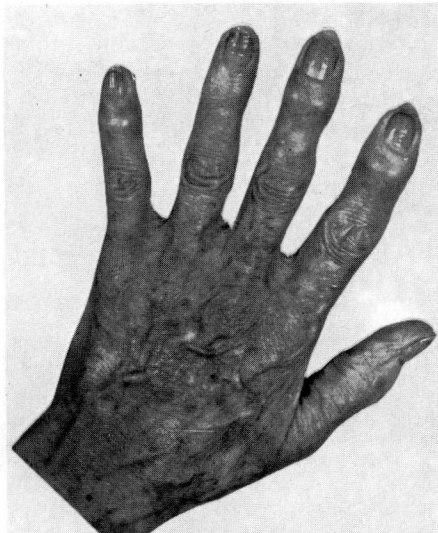

Fig. 23-12. Osteoarthritis of hand. Note enlargement of distal joints of index, middle, and little fingers (Heberden's nodes). (From Brashear, H., and Raney, R.: Shand's handbook of orthopaedic surgery, ed. 9, St. Louis, 1978, The C.V. Mosby Co.)

ASSESSMENT

Subjective data

The person with degenerative joint disorder is usually in good health. Questions that are asked include the following:
1. When does pain occur?
2. What measures give relief?
3. What joints are involved?

Objective data

Since signs and symptoms are usually local, inspection and palpation are the best evaluators.
1. Affected joints may appear normal.
   a. Check for tenderness, grating, and crepitus.
   b. Palpate for enlargement or irregularity in size of joint and flexion or lateral deformities.
2. Observe the person walking—is there a limp?
3. Evaluate range of motion of major joints.
4. Assess the vertebral column for limitation in cervical or lumbar areas.

Diagnostic tests

1. X-ray films may be normal if pathologic changes are mild.
2. Progressive changes include:
   a. Narrowing of joint spaces
   b. Marginal osteophyte formation
   c. *Eburnation* (sclerosis) of subchondral bone
3. Serologic and synovial fluid examinations will be essentially normal.

DATA ANALYSIS AND PLANNING

Nursing diagnoses

Comfort, alteration in: pain in affected joints
Potential impaired physical mobility
Activity intolerance
Self-care deficit in ADL: by pain and limited joint movement
Nutrition, alteration in: more than body requirements

Expected patient outcomes

1. Patient is free of pain.
2. Patient is able to be physically active.
3. Patient plans meals that are nutritious and that aid in maintenance of normal weight.
4. Patient plans to continue visits to the clinic or physician's office for follow-up care.

IMPLEMENTATION

Measures to relieve pain and discomfort and to promote mobility and increased ability to accomplish ADL are the same as for those of rheumatoid arthritis. The teaching plan would include the following:
1. Attention to posture
2. Prevention of weight gain
3. Use of ambulatory aids such as canes, crutches, or walkers to remove weight from painful joints
4. Alteration in ADL to avoid painful activities
5. Use of external measures such as local heat, prescribed exercises, and use of traction (if prescribed)

SURGERY

Specific procedures may be employed to
1. Relieve pain
2. Restore joint function
3. Prevent disability or further progression of the disease

These measures may include the following:
1. Osteotomy. Osteotomy is a procedure involving cutting a bone to change alignment, thereby correcting deformity in the bone or an adjacent joint. The procedure may be used to correct angulation or rotational deformities or to alter the weight-bearing surface in a diseased joint. The extremity is treated as in a fracture. Immobilization and care are similar to those for a patient with a fracture (p. 512).
2. Arthroplasty and total joint replacement. The surgery and care are the same as for rheumatoid arthritis (p. 496).
3. Arthrodesis (fusion). Arthrodesis is a form of surgery designed to cause the bones to grow firmly together. This procedure will be discussed under degenerative joint disease of the spine.

EVALUATION

Evaluation of progress can be made on the basis of expected patient outcomes.

Degenerative joint disease of the spine

PATHOPHYSIOLOGY

Degenerative joint disease of the spine is a common but difficult problem that merits special consideration. The spine has 23 intervertebral disk joints and 46 posterior facet joints, all of which are subjected to stresses and strains in holding the human body upright and moving it about. The vertebrae in the spinal column are articulated in a series of "couplets" that are able to move through an intervertebral disk joint and two posterior facet joints. The intervertebral disks are composed of an outer layer of cartilage called the *anulus fibrosus* and an inner layer of cartilage called the *nucleus pulposus*. The degeneration and dehydration of this cartilage results in a loss of elasticity.

The disk normally functions as a shock absorber. As it loses it resiliency, a strong force exerted across the disk can result in herniation of the nucleus through the anulus either posteriorly or laterally. This results in compression of a spinal nerve root and subsequent pain (Fig. 23-13). The facet joints that stabilize the spine are synovial joints, and their articular surfaces are covered with articular cartilage (Fig. 23-14). This means that these joints can be affected by rheumatoid arthritis as well as by degenerative joint disease. Osteophytes developing along the vertebral column can fuse and cause a limitation of motion, usually in the lumbodorsal region.

The intervertebral foramina in the cervical spine (C2-3 through C6-7) can become narrowed by spurs, thus creating pressure on the nerve roots in this area and resulting in neurologic symptoms.

ASSESSMENT

Subjective data

The patient seeks help because of pain and inability to walk or to carry on normal activities. Answers to the following questions should be sought:
1. Is low back pain relieved by recumbency?
2. Is pain aggravated by flexion of the trunk, coughing, or sneezing?
3. Is there a history of injury followed by back pain?

Objective data

1. Observe movements and walking.
   a. Patient appears to guard hips and back.
   b. Patient seeks frequent position changes.
2. Straight leg raising flexing the hip with the knee extended may produce sciatic pain.
3. Palpate for tender areas and spasm of the paravertebral muscles and posterior superior iliac spine.
4. Observe relief of discomfort when patient is supine with head elevated a few degrees and knees flexed.
5. Observe for muscle atrophy: If back problem has been longstanding, changes will be seen in affected leg.

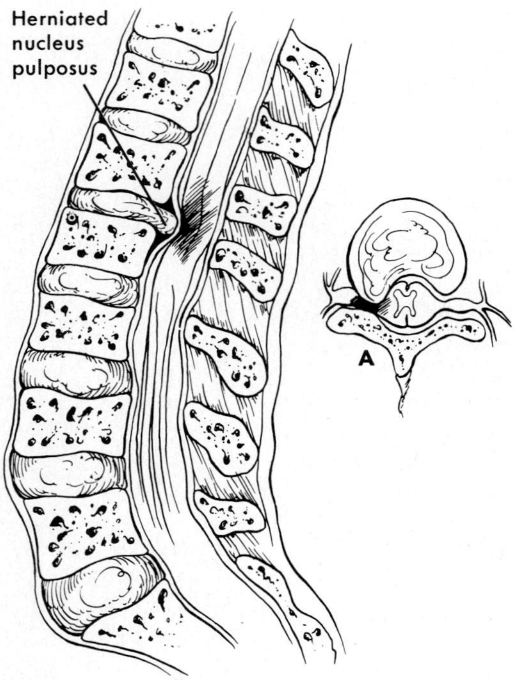

Fig. 23-13. Compression of spinal cord caused by herniation of nucleus pulposus into spinal cord. **A,** Pressure on nerves as they leave spinal canal.

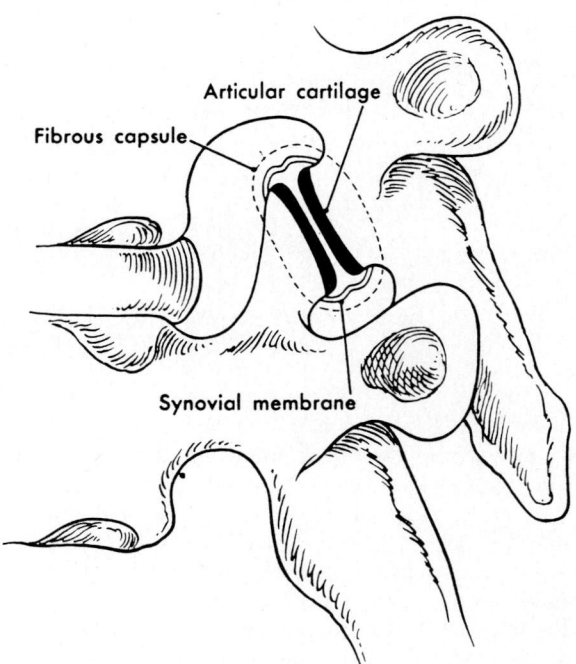

Fig. 23-14. Normal posterior facet joint.

Diagnostic tests
Neurologic examination

1. Neurologic signs and symptoms will help in determining the level of vertebrae involved. Sensory and motor changes depend on the nerve root involved.
2. Roentgenographic evaluation.
   a. For those patients whose symptoms are of short duration, the x-ray examination may fail to reveal any abnormality.
   b. For those patients with long-standing disorders, the x-ray examination may show significant narrowing of the disk space.
   c. Myelography, valuable in localizing the lesion, is reserved for confirmation of physical findings before surgery or to exclude conditions such as tumors.

DATA ANALYSIS AND PLANNING

Nursing diagnoses and expected patient outcomes are similar to those for degenerative joint disease.

IMPLEMENTATION

Assisting with achievement of therapeutic goals

Unless there is need for immediate surgery, the following are included in conservative management:
1. Provide a diet especially calculated for reduced caloric intake.
2. Prescribe bed rest with a firm mattress and bed boards.
3. Provide for position of comfort.
4. If there is loss of motor function, use a footboard or splint to prevent foot-drop and to keep bedclothes off the feet.
5. If there is sensory nerve loss, do not use hot water bottles or heating pads.
6. Patient should use a small bedpan with a small towel roll placed to support the lower back.
7. Traction may be ordered to relieve muscle spasm. This is usually accomplished by bilateral Buck's extension (p. 517).
8. Physical therapy may be used, specifically heat application and muscle relaxation techniques.

Counseling and teaching

1. Patients should learn to turn in bed in a logrolling fashion to maintain good spinal alignment: cross the arms over the chest, bend the uppermost knee to the side to which they wish to turn, and then roll over as a unit.
2. Constipation may be a problem.
   a. Urge patient to drink 3000 ml of fluids daily.
   b. Increase amount of roughage eaten; bran and fresh fruit are helpful.
   c. Give a mild laxative if necessary.
3. If brace or corset is ordered to provide external support for the spine, explain its need and application.

4. Teach principles of body mechanics.
   a. Avoid movements and positions that cause poor alignment of the spinal column and put strain on an injured nerve.
   b. Use a straight chair, not an overstuffed one.
   c. Avoid crossing the legs at the knees.
   d. Elevate the feet but flex the knees.
   e. During acute episodes, avoid stretching of the legs, such as driving a car or climbing stairs.
   f. In picking up items off the floor, bend the knees and keep the back straight.
5. When the acute episode subsides, the physician will order exercises designed to strengthen the back and abdominal muscles.

SURGERY

A laminectomy and/or spinal fusion may be performed. The nursing care is similar to that for a patient with a spinal fusion for scoliosis (p. 506).

EVALUATION

Evaluation is based on expected patient outcomes, which are the same as for degenerative joint disease (p. 503).

Scoliosis
PATHOPHYSIOLOGY

Scoliosis is a lateral deviation of the spine from the midline. It is an orthopedic problem that may show up during the school years, particularly during adolescence.

PREVENTION

Screening of school-aged children for scoliosis and early treatment exemplify a preventive measure that can be employed on a community-wide basis. Early attention to posture, good dietary habits, and teaching good body mechanics are valuable in preventing disability.

ASSESSMENT

Subjective data

1. Clothing does not fit correctly or hang well.
2. Patient is unable to breathe comfortably or take a deep breath (pain may not be a problem).

Objective data

Observation and palpation are most important. Observe the gait, posture, and ability to rise from a chair; compare heights of the shoulders. Palpate the spinal column with the patient in an upright position and bending forward. Palpate chest expansion on deep inspiration.

DATA ANALYSIS AND PLANNING

Nursing diagnoses

Potential alteration in comfort (back)
Potential activity intolerance

Expected patient outcomes

1. Patient avoids potential complications.
2. Patient maintains maximal functioning and independence.
3. Patient participates in long-range planning of care.

IMPLEMENTATION

Counseling and teaching

1. Splint or brace use (Milwaukee or Orthoplast braces are commonly used). Teach the patient to apply and remove the splint or brace and how to care for it (see pp. 486-487 for specific points).
2. Therapeutic exercises. Exercises are prescribed forms of activity designed to preserve joint mobility and to strengthen specific muscle group. These may include the following:
   a. Range of motion or isometric exercises
   b. Active resistive exercises (performed against resistance of another person or with weights)
3. Medications. Medications are rarely needed except for salicylates for antiinflammatory and analgesic effects.
4. Nutrition. A special diet is usually not prescribed except when the patient is overweight or laboratory studies indicate metabolic problems such as rickets. Assist the patient and family in planning meals that include fruits, and vegetables, proteins, and vitamins.

Nursing care of patient having spinal or scoliosis fusion

Postoperative care

1. The patient is kept absolutely flat for 1 to 14 days to avoid strain on the spine and dislodging the graft.
2. Position change is done by using a turning sheet and placing pillows between the legs to maintain proper alignment (Figs. 23-15 and 23-16).
3. Medication for pain is given, since pressure from edema at the operative site continues to cause pain.
4. Monitor vital signs, motor function, and sensation in the lower extremities.
5. Observe for sudden thromboembolic complications (p. 512) (pain in legs, chest pain).
6. Encourage the patient to move the legs and continue plantar flexion and dorsiflexion of feet.
7. Assess bowel and bladder function.
   a. A Foley catheter may be necessary for several days. Observe meticulous care to avoid infection.
   b. A stool softener may be ordered when the patient is able to take oral medications.
8. Inspect dressings for signs of bleeding or leakage of spinal fluid, and report drainage of spinal fluid at once.
9. Observe the condition of the dressing at the graft site.
10. Use care when turning the patient on the side of graft site if at the iliac crest.

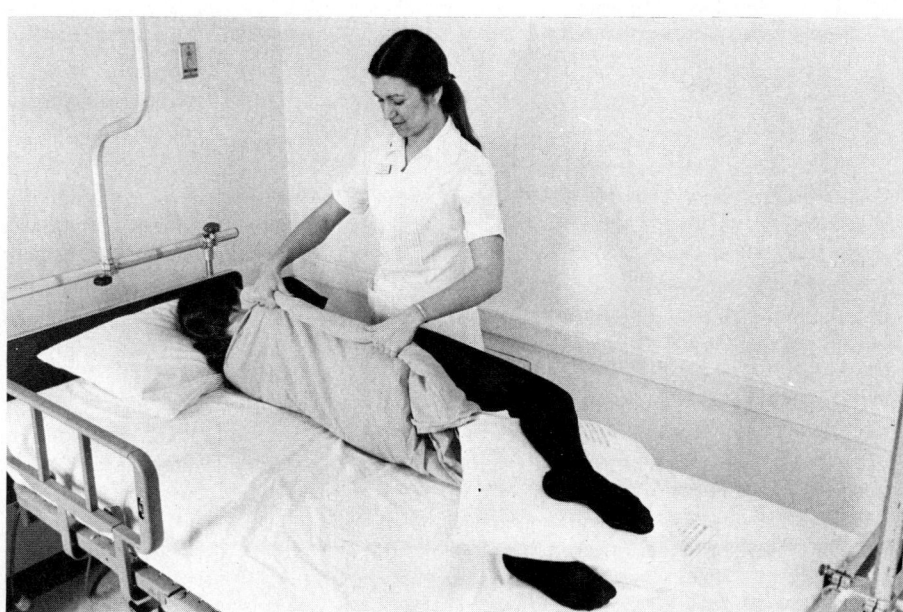

Fig. 23-15. Positioning a patient after back surgery by means of turning sheet extending from shoulders to thighs.

EVALUATION FOR CONSERVATIVE THERAPY

Based on expected patient outcomes the questions related to therapy would include the following:
1. Have spinal complications been avoided?
2. To what degree has the patient been able to function without back support?
3. Is the patient able to describe long-range plans of care?

SURGERY

Some forms of scoliosis are not amenable to treatment with bracing or body cast. An *arthrodesis* or *spinal fusion* may be performed to correct the scoliosis. Most commonly, lumbar fusion is performed through a posterior incision, with the bone for the graft being taken from the iliac crest. Scoliosis fusions involve internal devices such as Harrington rods or Dwyer screws and cables in conjunction with bone grafts.

Following surgery, the patient may be immobilized in a cast that extends from neck to pelvis. The cast remains on for 6 months. The care of the patient in a cast is covered on p. 515. The postoperative care for the patient having a posterior spinal approach with a bone graft from the iliac crest or a scoliosis fusion is described in box on p. 506.

EVALUATION FOR PATIENT WITH SPINAL FUSION

Based on the expected patient outcomes, the patient:
1. Can explain the nature of the surgery that has been performed.
2. Maintains maximum functioning (with brace if one is to be worn).
3. Is participating in physician's follow-up program.

OTHER RHEUMATIC DISORDERS
Gout
PATHOPHYSIOLOGY

Gout is an inflammatory type of arthritis caused by the deposits of sodium urate crystals in the joints and the connective tissues. The inflammatory process that results is extremely rapid, occurring over a few hours. Typically the great toe is involved, but other joints such as ankles, knees, or elbows may be affected. The disorder has a familial tendency; it affects males 20 times more frequently than females, and onset usually occurs after the age of 30.

ASSESSMENT
Subjective data

1. Acute episodes: chief complaint will be severe pain in great toe or other joints.
2. Question patient about previous episodes and what was done for relief.
3. Has there been weight gain?
4. Is there a history of gouty arthritis in the family?
5. Does the patient take medication for gout?

Objective data

1. Patient cannot tolerate touching the joint and will display guarding of the affected joint.
2. The joint is swollen and red (first metatarsal, tarsal joints, ankle, knee, or elbow) (Fig. 23-17).
3. There is a low-grade fever.
4. Nodular swelling may be visible in the subcutaneous tissues overlying the joints or in the cartilage of the helix of the ear.

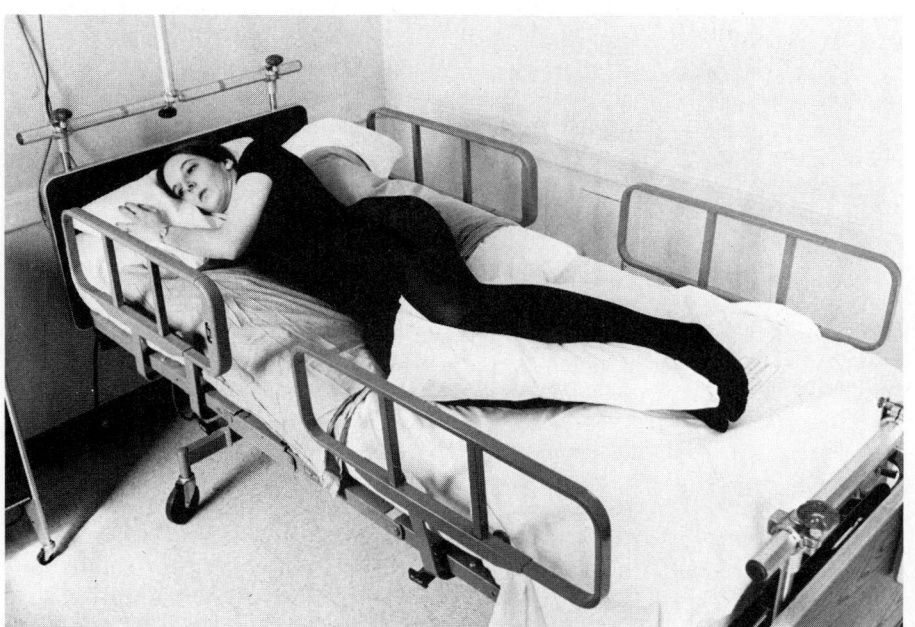

Fig. 23-16. Pillows behind the back provide support. Pillows between legs maintain anatomic alignment and decrease pull on lower back.

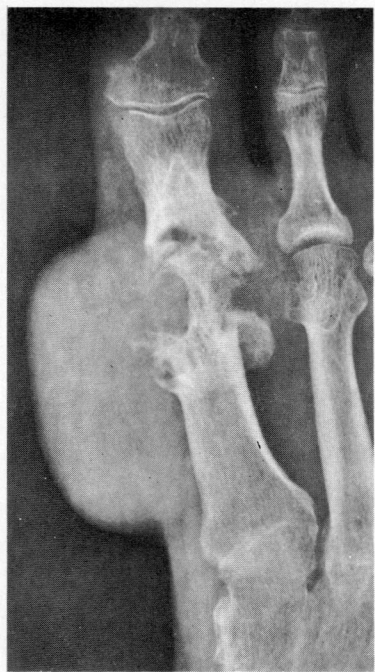

Fig. 23-17. Gout.

Medications for the patient with gout	
Colchicine	Given every hour until patient develops nausea, vomiting, diarrhea, or abdominal discomfort, or until joint pain is relieved
Probenecid (Benemid)	May be given on a regular, continuous basis to prevent acute attacks; facilitates excretion of uric acid by the proximal tubule of the kidney
Allopurinol (Zyloprim)	May be prescribed if probenecid is not tolerated; inhibits uric acid synthesis

Diagnostic tests

1. Serum uric acid level will be elevated (hyperuricemia).
2. The 24-hour urinary uric acid level may be elevated.
3. Synovial fluid from the joint shows presence of monosodium urate crystals.
4. Sedimentation rate will be elevated.
5. X-ray examination will reveal soft tissue swelling.

DATA ANALYSIS AND PLANNING

Nursing diagnoses

Comfort, alteration in: pain in affected joint
Potential injury to joints and kidneys

Expected patient outcomes

1. Patient is free of pain.
2. Patient avoids further episodes of gouty arthritis attacks.

IMPLEMENTATION

Assisting with achievement of therapeutic goals

1. Medications
   a. Colchicine for control of acute situation
   b. Specific uricosuric agents or uric acid inhibitors for interval (chronic) control

EVALUATION

Based on expected patient outcomes, the questions related to therapy include the following:

1. Is the patient free of joint pain?
2. Is the patient able to discuss medications and follow-up care to avoid attacks of gouty arthritis?

Bacterial arthritis
PATHOPHYSIOLOGY

Bacterial arthritis is inflammation of the synovial tissues caused by bacterial agents. The joint cavity may become involved and pus will be present in the synovial membrane and synovial fluid. If allowed to progress, the infection will cause abscesses in the synovium and subchondral bone and will destroy cartilage. Ankylosis of the joint will result.

ASSESSMENT

Subjective data

1. Ask patient to describe the onset of pain and changes noted in the joints.
2. Is patient being treated for another infection?
3. Is there a history of recent surgery or trauma?
4. Is there a history of recent sexual contact with a carrier of gonorrhea?

Objective data

1. Monitor the affected joint: it will be swollen and warm to touch.
2. Observe patient's resistance to movement.
3. Monitor body temperature; fever may be present.

4. Observe for contractures that may be present if infection is of long duration.

Diagnostic tests

1. Joint may be aspirated of synovial fluid to identify presence of organism.
2. Joint fluid white cell count will be elevated, and glucose content will be reduced.
3. Roentgenograms may show loss of joint space and lytic changes in bone.

DATA ANALYSIS AND PLANNING

Nursing diagnoses

Comfort, alteration in: pain in infected joints
Mobility, impaired physical

Expected patient outcomes

1. There is no evidence of infection.
2. Joint is free of pain.
3. Joint movements are free and within normal range of motion.

IMPLEMENTATION

Assisting with achievement of therapeutic goals

1. Antibiotics are given as prescribed; reactions to drugs are monitored.
2. Surgical drainage or system of irrigation and drainage may be employed. Drainage is monitored for amount and color.
3. As soon as infection subsides, encourage the patient to move the affected joint to prevent contracture.

Assisting with comfort and ADL

1. Give pain medication as prescribed.
2. During the acute stage, assist patient to rest and immobilize the joint to help control pain and prevent deformity.
3. Assist patient with self-care.

EVALUATION

Based on expected patient outcomes, the questions related to therapy include the following:
1. Has infection of the joint subsided?
2. Can patient demonstrate joint range of motion without discomfort?

TRAUMA

Fracture of bone and soft tissue injury

The etiology, signs and symptoms, and medical therapy are listed in Table 23-3.

PATHOPHYSIOLOGY AND BONE HEALING

A bone is said to be *fractured* or *broken* when there is an interruption in bone continuity. Commonly, a fracture is accompanied by *soft tissue* injury to surrounding tissues, that is, ligaments, muscle, tendons, blood vessels, and nerves.

A fracture may occur during normal activity or following a minimal injury when the bone is weakened by disease such as cancer or osteoporosis. This is called a *pathologic fracture* and causes collapse of the bone. A bone may fracture when the muscle is unable to absorb energy. This is called *fatigue fracture*.

The classification of fractures is given in box on p. 511.

Immobilization of a bone that is fractured is necessary for bone healing. Immobilization takes place by the following means
1. *Physiologic splintage.* This form of splintage will occur naturally, since guarding, avoidance of use, and muscle spasm will occur as a result of pain on movement.
2. *External orthopedic splintage.* This is accomplished with devices such as plaster casts and traction.
3. *Internal fixation.* In this method the opposing ends of the fracture are held in place by screws, plates, or rods.

Once immobilization is accomplished, new bone called *callus* begins to form by the following stages of growth:
1. *Hematoma formation.* Because blood vessels are injured, there is bleeding at the site of the fracture. The blood collects and fastens the broken ends together.
2. *Fibrin meshwork.* The hematoma becomes organized as fibroblasts invade the area, forming the fibrin meshwork. White blood cells wall off the area, localizing the inflammation.
3. *Invasion by osteoblasts.* The osteoblasts enter the fibrous area to help hold the union firm. Blood vessels develop, establishing a source of nutrients for building collagen. Collagen strands begin to incorporate calcium deposits.
4. *Callus formation* (Fig. 23-19).
   a. Osteoblasts continue to lay the network for bone buildup.
   b. Osteoclasts destroy dead bone and help to synthesize new bone.
   c. The collagen strengthens and continues to incorporate calcium deposits.
5. *Remodeling.* In this final step, excess callus is reabsorbed and trabecular bone is laid down along lines of stress.

Factors that impede or prevent callus formation include the following:
1. *Delayed healing or delayed union.* Delayed union occurs when the fracture does not heal within the usual time for healing.
   a. Reasons:
      (1) Callus is broken or torn apart by too much activity.
      (2) Edema at the fracture site impedes flow of nutrients to the area.
      (3) Immobilization is inefficient.
      (4) Infection is present at fracture site.

Table 23-3. Traumatic problems

Etiology	Signs and symptoms	Medical therapy

Fractures
1. Blow or injury (fall, accident)
2. Pathlogic fracture: weakened by disease such as cancer or *osteoporosis*
3. Fatigue facture: a bone fractures when muscles involved are unable to absorb energy, such as on long foot marches
	Complete fracture:
	1. Pain immediate and severe and aggravated by movement
	2. Loss of function of injured part
	3. Obvious gross deformity when compared to normal extremity
	4. Loss of rigidity of injured part
	5. Movement produces grating sound *(crepitus)* of bone fragments
	6. Localized swelling and discoloration (may not be apparent for several hours)
	7. Shock caused by severe injury and blood loss into damaged tissues
	NOTE: Symptoms may be absent in linear compacted fractures.
	1. There may be little or no swelling.
	2. Pain is present only when direct pressure is applied to fracture site or on use of limb or body part
		1. Immediate management:
		  a. Provide splint before moving patient or maintain support above and below fracture site until patient can be moved and immobilization applied with splints for transportation.
		  b. Elevate extremity to minimize edema.
		  c. Transport patient for emergency treatment.
		2. Observe injured part at frequent intervals for local changes in color, sensation, or temperature.
		3. Tetanus immunization is given if compound fracture is present.
		4. Cold applications are given to reduce hemorrhage and edema.
		5. Medication for pain (aspirin or narcotics) is given.
		6. Subsequent care of fractures: immobilization with reduction by closed reduction, open reduction, or internal fixation.

Fracture of the hip
1. Severe trauma or accident
2. Elderly people: bone breaks on turning or twisting the body because of
  a. Osteoporotic and degenerative changes (causing brittleness of the bones
  b. Fall caused by weakness of quadriceps
	Leg is shortened and externally rotated by the acute angle between shaft and neck of femur
	Impacted femoral neck fractures:
	1. Shortening and rotational changes possibly not obvious
	2. Only moderate discomfort even with movement
	3. Patient may bear weight on the extremity
		Same as above.

Classification of bone fractures

A. Classification as to types of fractures
1. *Complete* fracture: complete separation of the bone producing two fragments
2. *Incomplete* fracture: a partial break in the bone without separation of the bone
3. *Simple* or *closed* fracture: bone is broken; skin is intact
4. *Compound* or *open* fracture: the fracture parts extend through the skin
5. *Fracture without displacement:* bone is broken; bone fragments are in alignment in normal position
6. *Fracture with displacement:* bone fragments have separated at the point of fracture
7. *Comminuted fracture:* the bone has broken into several fragments
8. *Impacted ("telescoped")* fracture: one bone fragment is forcibly driven into another bone fragment
B. Classification as to line of fracture (Fig. 23-18)
1. *Greenstick:* splintering of one side of the bone (occurs most often in children with soft bones)
2. *Transverse:* break across the bone
3. *Oblique:* line of fracture at an oblique angle to the bone shaft
4. *Spiral:* line of fracture encircles the bone

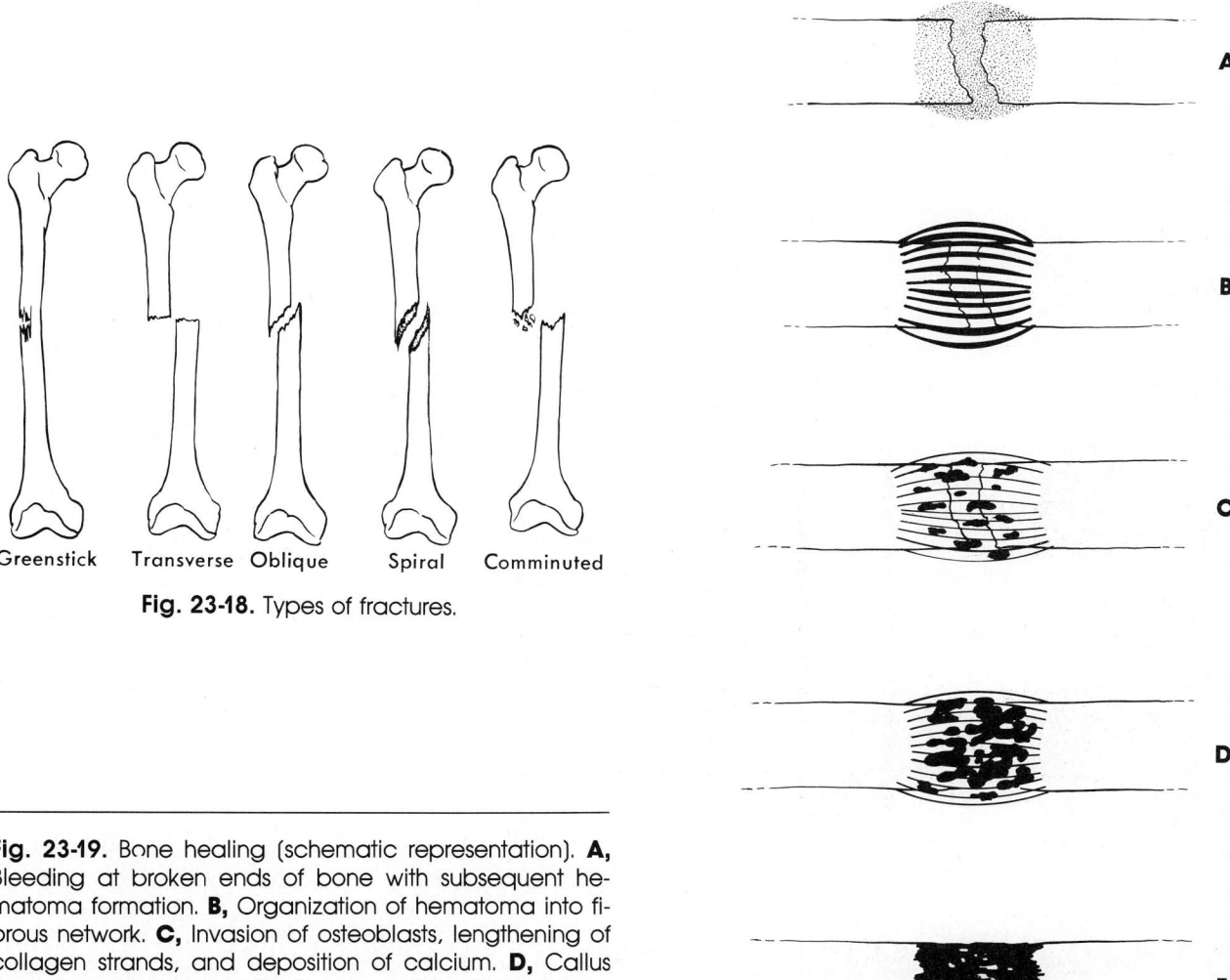

Greenstick Transverse Oblique Spiral Comminuted

Fig. 23-18. Types of fractures.

A

B

C

D

E

Fig. 23-19. Bone healing (schematic representation). **A,** Bleeding at broken ends of bone with subsequent hematoma formation. **B,** Organization of hematoma into fibrous network. **C,** Invasion of osteoblasts, lengthening of collagen strands, and deposition of calcium. **D,** Callus formation: new bone is built up as osteoclasts destroy dead bone. **E,** Remodeling is accomplished as excess callus is reabsorbed and trabecular bone is laid down.

(5) Patient is in poor nutritional state.
  b. Correction: More complete immobilization or open reduction for surgical measures.
2. *Nonunion.* Nonunion is the term used when healing does not occur even in a much longer period of time.
  a. Reasons:
    (1) Too much bone loss at time of injury to permit bridging of bone fragments.
    (2) Bone necrosis has occurred because of lack of blood supply.
    (3) Anemia, endocrine imbalance, or other systemic conditions are present.
  b. Correction:
    (1) Crutches may have to be used indefinitely.
    (2) A brace may be worn to support the limb.
    (3) Surgery may be performed to unite bone fragments with a bone graft.

• • •

The healing of bone fractures may be complicated by fat embolism and problems of immobilization.

FAT EMBOLISM

Pathophysiology

Fat embolism is the most serious complication of crushing injuries, multiple fractures, and fractures of long bones. The source of the emboli is thought to be the fat of the bone marrow. Pressure changes occurring within the fractured bones force molecules of fat from the marrow into the systemic circulation. Embolism to the pulmonary area may occur within the first 12 to 72 hours after injury or surgery on long bones.

Assessment

1. Observe for dyspnea, pallor, prostration, and collapse.
2. Observe for altered levels of consciousness and changes in the patient's behavior, or confusion. These are indicative of cerebral fat embolism.
3. Observe for petechial hemorrhages of the skin of the neck, shoulders, and axillary folds. (These usually appear about the second or third day after injury.)

Nursing care

1. Give respiratory support with oxygen; ventilator may be needed to decrease and inhibit further pulmonary edema.
2. Monitor vital signs. If heart failure occurs, the patient will be given digitalis.
3. Use measures to clear respiratory secretions as ordered by the physician.
4. Give medications as prescribed; these may include the following:
  (a) Rapid-acting diuretics
  (b) Bronchodilators
  (c) Antibiotics
  (d) Corticosteroids
5. Allay apprehension in both patient and family.

PROBLEMS OF IMMOBILIZATION

Cardiovascular system

Pathophysiology

The common problems associated with the cardiovascular system are as follows:
1. Increased incidence of deep vein thrombosis and pulmonary embolus
2. Increased work load on the heart

Failure of the vessels in the legs to assume or maintain vasoconstriction results in the pooling of venous blood, decreased venous return, and diminished cardiac output.

Assessment

1. Palpate peripheral pulses.
2. Monitor blood pressure and heart rate and force.
3. Observe for signs and symptoms of deep vein thrombosis (pain in leg) and pulmonary embolism (chest pain, cough).

Nursing care

1. Assist patient with active and passive range of motion and isometric exercises of extremities.
2. Reposition patient frequently within limitations as directed by physician's orders.

Respiratory system

Pathophysiology

Decreased movement, decreased stimulus to cough, and decreased depth of ventilation all contribute to the pooling of secretions in the bronchi and bronchioles.

Assessment

1. Observe for inability to cough.
2. Auscultate for sounds of moisture in the chest.

Nursing care

1. Reposition frequently within prescribed limitations.
2. Encourage active range of motion exercises of unaffected joints.
3. Prevent hypostatic pneumonia by having patient cough and deep breathe at regular intervals.

Skin integrity

Pathophysiology

Loss of skin integrity (abrasions, decubitus ulcers) is caused by friction, pressure, or tissue layers sliding on each other. The process of restricted circulation and tissue ischemia is intensified by infection, trauma, obesity, sweating, and poor nutritional state.

Assessment

1. Observe for areas of pressure and irritation, as may occur from the plaster cast or traction equipment or from pressure on the sacrum, elbows, and heels.
2. Monitor body temperature for elevation, which may indicate infection.

Nursing care

1. Prevent decubitus ulceration by keeping skin clean and dry, especially sacrum, elbows, and heels.

2. Turn the patient as physician permits to change points of pressure at frequent intervals. Some patients cannot be fully turned, for example, patients in traction. In this instance, other methods must be provided such as the following:
   a. Flotation pads that distribute pressure equally over large skin areas
   b. Air pressure mattresses that alternate pressures on the skin
   c. Sheepskin pads that decrease friction, distribute pressure, and reduce moisture
   d. Elbow and heel pads
3. Special beds may be necessary to turn the patient from supine to prone positions.
   a. The Stryker or Foster frame permits movement in a horizontal direction to two positions—supine and prone.
   b. The CircOlectric bed permits more position changes. Movement is vertical and can be stopped at any angle while good body alignment is maintained.
4. If decubitus ulcer results, follow hospital policy for special nursing measures.

Gastrointestinal system
Pathophysiology

Constipation is the most frequent complication of immobility. The change in normal dietary habits and fluid intake, lack of activity, and having to use a bedpan are contributing factors.

Assessment

1. Ask the patient about daily habits of evacuation.
2. Observe appetite and foods the patient selects.
3. Monitor the fluid intake.
4. Ask the patient what is normally taken for constipation.

Nursing care

1. Encourage the patient to be as active as possible within the limitations (turning, moving).
2. Encourage fluid intake to 2500 to 3000 ml/day unless contraindicated.
3. Assist the patient in selecting foods that have roughage or fiber content.
4. Give stool-softening agents and suppositories as prescribed.

Urinary system
Pathophysiology

Increased calcium from bone destruction, increased urinary pH (alkaline), increased citric acid (which causes the precipitation of calcium salts), stasis of urine in the bladder, and infection can all cause urinary problems.

Assessment

1. Observe quantity of fluid intake. Ask the patient about normal fluid intake.
2. Has the patient a history of urinary problems?
3. Ask the elderly male patient about urinary problems before admission. Some men will describe hesitancy and frequency because of an enlarged prostate gland.

Nursing care

1. Encourage fluid intake.
2. Limit calcium intake (milk) to dietary orders.
3. Monitor urinary output and report difficulties to the physician. (Potential is present for bladder infection and formation of renal stones.)

Musculoskeletal systems
Pathophysiology

Atrophy and weakness of the muscles will occur because of disuse. Bone growth (*osteoblastic*) and bone destruction (*osteoclastic*) activity is disrupted by immobility. The osteoclastic activity takes precedence, with the result that bone matrix is destroyed and calcium is released. The end result is *osteoporosis* and renal stones.

Nursing care

Encourage active and isometric exercises of unaffected limbs.

Fractures of the hip

The following is a review of the hip joint for a clearer understanding of what is involved in a fracture in this area. The hip joint is a ball-and-socket joint formed by the acetabulum, a deep round cavity in the innominate bone, and the rounded upper portion of the femur. The upper part of the femur is composed of a head, neck, greater and lesser trochanter, and shaft. The distal part of the femur ends in two condyles. The head of the femur fits into the acetabulum. The hip joint is surrounded by a fibrous capsule, ligaments, and muscles. The greater trochanter serves as a point of insertion for the abductor and short rotator muscles of the hip, whereas the lesser trochanter serves as a point of insertion for the iliopsoas muscle.

The blood supply to the femoral head is of paramount importance in fractures in or about the hip joint. The blood supply to the femoral head varies with age. The

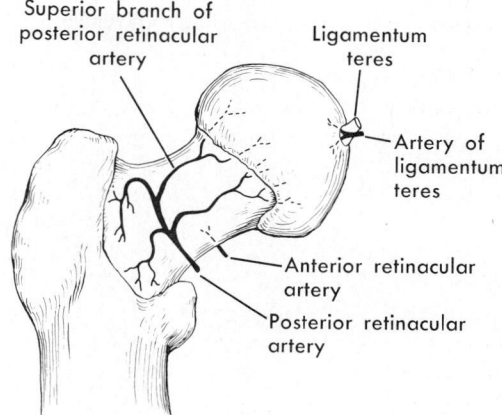

Fig. 23-20. Posterior view of the blood supply to head of femur.

chief source of blood supply to the femoral head in adults is the posterior retinacular artery (Fig. 23-20). The nutrient and periosteal vessels of the femoral shaft extend into the trochanteric region and lower part of the neck.

PATHOPHYSIOLOGY

Hip fractures occur more frequently in women than in men and more frequently in the elderly who have osteoporosis of the bone. There are two major types: *intracapsular fractures,* which occur within the hip joint and capsule and include subcapital, transcervical, and basal neck fractures (Fig. 23-21, A to C), and *extracapsular fractures,* which occur outside of the capsule and involve the trochanteric areas of the femur (Fig. 23-21, D).

REDUCTION OF THE HIP FRACTURE

Reduction is the term used for placing the bone fragments in their normal position for healing. Reduction is accomplished by closed manipulation (closed reduction), traction, or surgery (open reduction and internal fixation).

Closed manipulation (closed reduction)

When closed manipulation is used to reduce a fracture, the patient is often given a general anesthetic. The phy-

sician reduces the fracture by pulling on the distal fragment (manual traction) while countertraction is applied to the proximal fragment until the bone fragments engage or fall into their normal alignment. The physician may also apply direct pressure over the site of the fracture to correct angulation or lateral displacement of a fragment. Usually when this type of reduction is performed, a cast is applied to hold the fragments in the desired position while healing occurs.

An *intertrochanteric* fracture may be treated by closed reduction and the application of a hip spica cast. Russell traction may be used as a temporary measure.

The preoperative care of the patient includes the following:

1. Explain to patient what is to be expected: anesthesia, cleansing and preparation of the skin, immobilization of the body with a plaster cast, care following the surgery, and expectations after discharge.
2. Inspect skin to be covered by the cast for cuts, abrasions, and bruises and report to the physician. Skin lesions may need special care with disinfectant and dressing before a cast is applied.
3. For skin care, follow the hospital routine or prescribed orders.
4. Before plaster bandages are applied, all bony prominences are padded with sheet wadding or felt to pro-

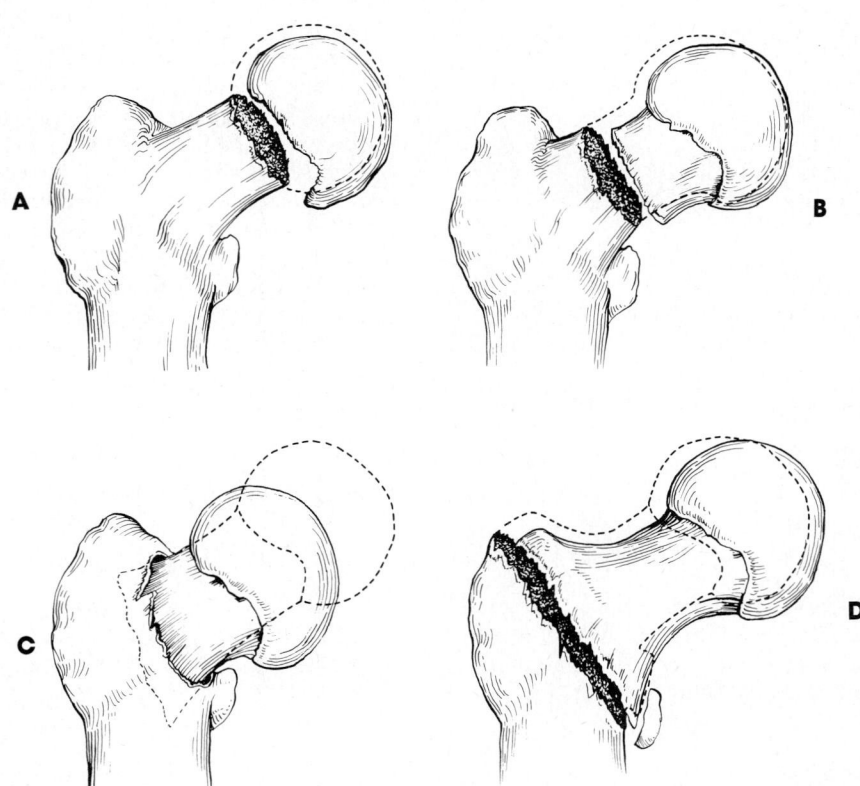

Fig. 23-21. Fractures of hip. **A,** Subcapital fracture. **B,** Transcervical fracture. **C,** Impacted fracture of base of neck. **D,** Intertrochanteric fracture.

tect them from pressure and resultant tissue ischemia. (This is done in the operating room.)
5. Have the patient sign the operative permit.
Postoperatively, care should follow the standard nursing format of assessment, analysis and planning, implementation, and evaluation.

Assessment
SUBJECTIVE DATA

1. Report tightness of the cast as evidenced by numbness or tingling of toes and loss of motor function of
the toes. Pressure pain may indicate nerve compression. Table 23-4 gives the signs and symptoms of
neurocirculatory impairment.
2. Report sudden pain and the expression of fright by
the patient, who may be experiencing pulmonary
embolism.
3. Report any complaint of inability to cough or
breathe comfortably; patient may be having pooling
of secretions in bronchi and bronchioles with beginning signs and symptoms of hypostatic pneumonia.

OBJECTIVE DATA

1. Observe for signs of delayed shock from excessive loss
of blood: faintness, dizziness, pallor, diaphoresis,
change in pulse rate, fall in blood pressure.
2. Observe for drainage from inside of cast; report bright
red drainage immediately.
3. Record urinary output.
4. Inspect skin distal to cast for edema, cyanosis, coldness, and delayed capillary refilling of toes.
5. Observe for inability or decreased ability to move body
part distal to site of fracture.

Data analysis and planning
NURSING DIAGNOSES

Potential for impairment of skin integrity
Mobility, impaired physical ability
Potential for deep vein thrombosis, pulmonary embolus
Potential for alteration of comfort with cast pressure
Potential for alteration in bowel elimination:constipation

EXPECTED PATIENT OUTCOMES

1. Skin is intact.
2. Range of motion is performed by extremities not in the
plaster cast.
3. Circulation has been maintained and deep vein thrombosis avoided.
4. Cast pressure has been avoided by careful handling.
5. Bowel elimination has been maintained.

Implementation
CAST CARE POSTOPERATIVELY

1. Support wet cast with flat of the hands.
   a. Cast can be cracked or broken by careless or inadequate support on moving patient.
   b. Support patient's head and extremities while
moving to bed.
   c. Cast may take several hours to days to dry, depending on cast thickness.
   d. Wrinkles or indentations caused by fingers will
cause pressure points on the body.
2. Place the patient in a cast on a firm mattress with
a bed board under the mattress; support the cast on
pillows to prevent flattening.
3. Provide for drying by evaporation by exposure to
circulating air.
   a. Hair dryer or cast dryer may be permitted to
provide *warm* moving air.
   b. Do not cover cast.
   c. Blankets may be used to protect body parts not
encased in plaster.
   d. Turn the patient every 2 hours to ensure drying
and prevent flattening pressure on the cast.
Turning to injured side will need the physician's
order.
4. Do not paint, varnish, or shellac cast; plaster of
paris is porous and allows circulation of air to the
skin.

ASSISTING WITH COMFORT AND ADL

1. Pain
   a. Give medication for discomfort as ordered.
   b. Continuous pain or pressure not relieved by

Table 23-4. Observations for signs and symptoms of neurocirculatory impairment

Observtion	Interpretation
Tissue color white	Decreased arterial blood supply
Tissue color blue	Venous stasis and poorly oxygenated tissue
Color slow to return to nail bed after appli-cation of moderate pressure	Decreased arterial blood supply
Edema	Fluid accumulating in tissues; poor venous return
Tissue cold or cool to touch	Decreased arterial blood supply
Patient unable to move parts distal to cast	Pressure on nerves innervating parts distal to cast
Patient complaint of heightened or de-creased sensation or paresthesia in part underlying or distal to cast	Pressure on nerves innervating parts underlying or distal to cast
Patient complaint of extreme pain unrelieved by elevation, analgesic, or repositioning	Pressure on nerve endings in parts underlying or distal to cast

NOTE: Comparison of tissue should be made with contralateral tissue to determine extent of deviation from normal.

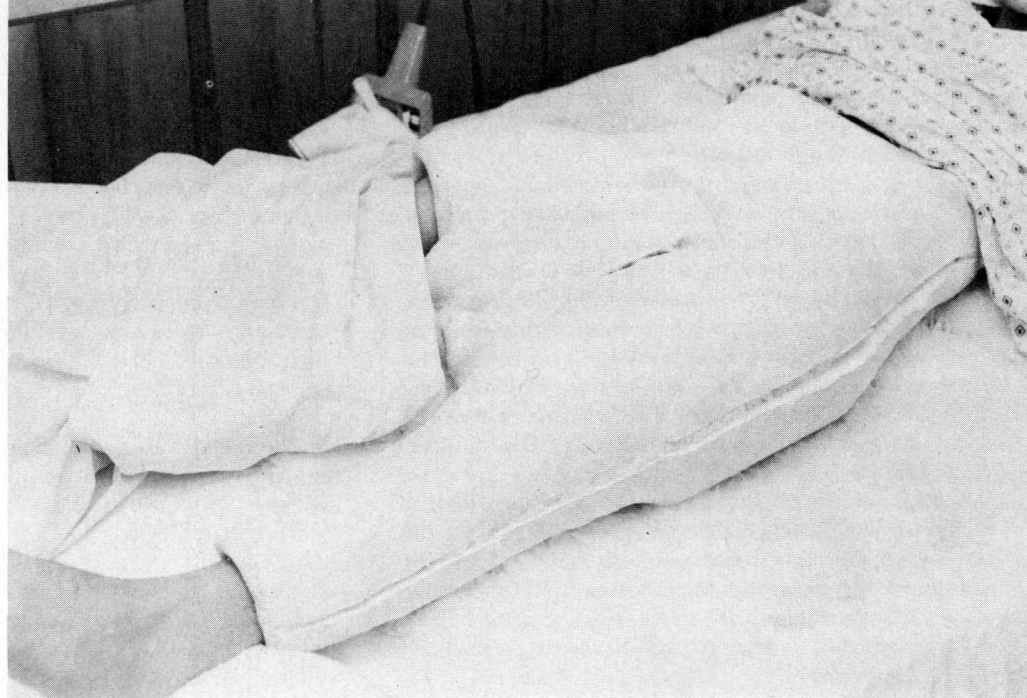

Fig. 23-22. Bivalved cast.

medication or change in position must be reported at once.

c. Continuous pressure on the peroneal nerve (located below the head of the fibula on the lateral aspect of the leg) may result in paralysis of the foot (foot-drop).

d. The cast may need to be bivalved (split in half lengthwise) to relieve pressure (Fig. 23-22).

2. Skin care

a. Assure patient that warmth from cast is normal and will be relieved.

b. Cleanse plaster off skin with warm water.

c. Use cream or lotion with care. These may cause the cast to stick to the skin.

d. Apply petal-shaped strips of adhesive tape or moleskin around rough edges of the cast.

e. Apply waterproof material around perineal area to prevent soiling of cast and potential irritation. If soiling occurs, remove surface stains with damp cloth and scouring powder. Allow to dry thoroughly.

3. Preventing deep vein thrombosis, pulmonary embolus, and hypostatic pneumonia

a. Provide orthopedic bed frame with a trapeze to assist the patient to move in bed.

b. Encourage active exercises of extremities not in the plaster cast.

c. Turn patient as directed by physician's orders.

d. Encourage deep breathing and coughing.

4. Toilet assistance

a. Use measures to prevent urine or stool from running back and under the cast. For a long leg cast or body cast, the physician may permit slight elevation of the head.

b. Use a fracture pan with support under the small of the back.

c. Encourage the patient to assist with self-care in bathing, oral hygiene, and grooming.

5. Abdominal discomfort

a. For abdominal distention a "window" or opening may be cut into the cast. Bladder distention can also be checked through the opening.

b. Constipation is a common complication of immobility. (A mild laxative may be necessary.)

6. Nutrition

a. Diet should include fruits, vegetables, proteins, and vitamins.

b. Even if patient has marked limitation of movement, encourage feeding self.

c. Do not increase calcium intake above patient's recommended dietary allowance. Decalcification and demineralization of bone take place during immobility regardless of quantity of calcium intake.

COUNSELING AND TEACHING. Many patients are discharged after the cast is dry and there is no evidence of neurocirculatory impairments. The patient and family or the care giver at home must be taught how to care for the cast and continue with care given in the hospital.

1. Never insert a sharp object (coat hanger, pencil) under the cast, since abrasions can become infected.

2. Weight bearing will not be permitted unless or-

dered by the physician. The amount of weight bearing will be prescribed.

3. The dietitian will assist the patient and family in planning nutritious menus. Caloric intake will be considered in the teaching plan to avoid weight gain.

4. Cast is removed when x-ray films show that union is sufficient to allow removal.
   a. The skin is usually dry and scaly.
   b. The skin is washed with mild soap and warm water, dried carefully, and lubricated with mineral oil.
   c. The patient begins to move the limb and perform prescribed exercises.
   d. The extremity must be elevated during sleep and at intervals during the day to control swelling.
   e. An elastic stocking may be ordered to help reduce dependent edema. The patient will need information about the elastic stocking (Chapter 27).

Evaluation

1. Is patient comfortable?
2. Does patient know how to care for the cast
3. Does patient know how to care for the limb after the cast is removed?

Reduction by traction

Traction is a steady pull on a part of the body is used to reduce and immobilize fractures, to overcome muscle spasm, to stretch adhesions, and to correct certain deformities. Traction is achieved by a system of ropes, pulleys, and weights connected to metal frame attached to bed.

When traction is used to treat a fracture, traction and counteraction are used to keep the bone fragments touching and in alignment. *Adjusting the traction and adding or subtracting weights are measures undertaken only by the physician.* X-ray films taken at intervals evaluate traction effectiveness.

Skin traction

Skin traction is achieved by applying wide bands of moleskin, adhesive, or other devices directly to the skin and attaching weights. The pull of the weights is transmitted indirectly to the involved bone. Buck's extension and Russell traction are the two most common forms of skin traction used for injury of the lower extremities in adults.

BUCK'S EXTENSION. Buck's extension is the simplest form of skin traction and provides for straight pull on the affected extremity (Fig. 23-23). It is often used to relieve muscle spasm and to immobilize a limb temporarily, such as the leg when a hip fracture has been sustained by an elderly person and internal fixation is to be performed within a short time. The skin of the leg is usually shaved, and tincture of benzoin is applied to protect it if adhesive substances are to be used. Adhesive tape or moleskin is placed on the lateral and medial aspects of the leg and

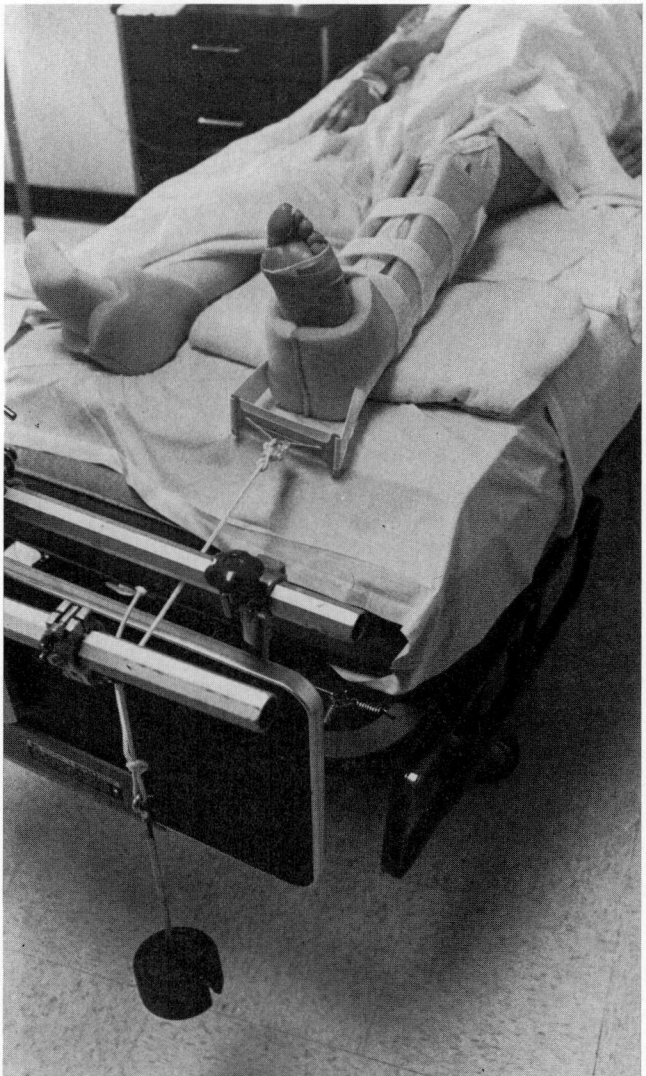

Fig. 23-23. Buck's extension.

secured with a circular gauze or elastic bandage. The tape should not cover the malleoli, since skin breakdown is certain to occur over these bony prominences. The tapes are attached to a spreader bar. The spreader bar should be sufficiently wide to pull the tapes away from the malleoli. Rope is attached to the spreader, passed through a pulley on a crossbar at the foot of the bed, and suspended with weights. The maximal weight that should be applied by skin traction is 3.6 kg (8 lb). Greater amounts of weight can cause skin damage. Commercial foam rubber Buck's traction boots are also in wide use. They are applied simply with Velcro straps.

RUSSELL TRACTION. *Russell traction* is sometimes used because it permits the patient to move about in bed somewhat freely and permits bending of the knee joint (Fig. 23-24). This is skin traction in which four pulleys are

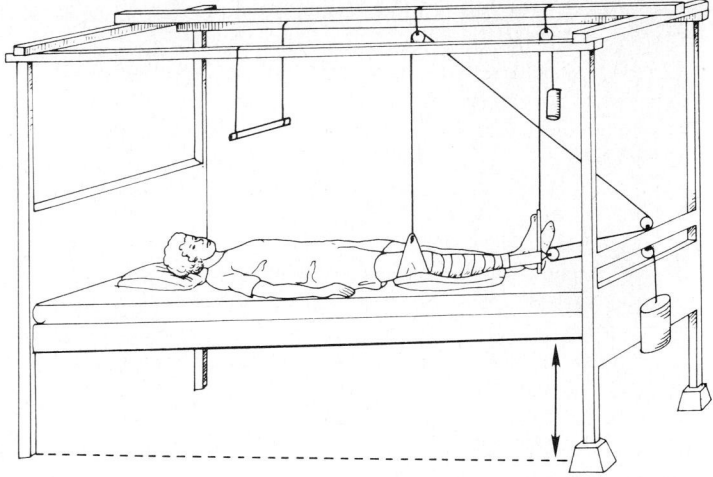

Fig. 23-24. Russell traction. Note that Balkan frame is attached to bed, leg is supported on pillows, and heel extends beyond pillow.

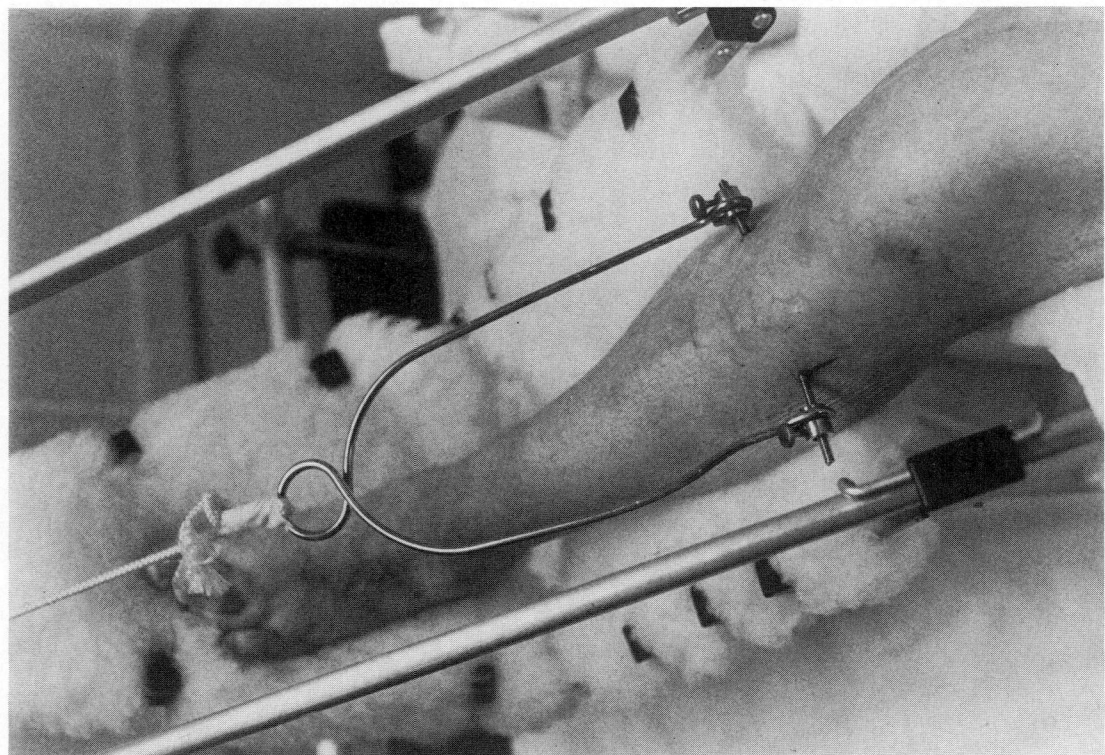

Fig. 23-25. Skeletal traction.

used. A Balkan frame must be attached to the bed before the procedure is started. Moleskin or adhesive is then applied to the leg as in Buck's extension. The knee is suspended in a hammock or sling to which a rope is attached. The rope is properly directed through a series of pulleys and finally suspended with weights to give a double pull from the crossbar to the footplate. Because of this double pull, the traction is equal to approximately double the weight used. A pillow may be placed under the thigh and under the leg. This traction results in slight flexion of the hip. The foot of the bed may be elevated to provide countertraction.

Russell traction is used in the treatment of intertrochanteric fracture of the femur when surgery is contrain-

dicated, especially in the aged. Bilateral Russell or Buck's traction may be used to treat back pain, since it immobilizes the patient and reduces muscles spasm.

Skeletal traction

Skeletal traction is traction applied directly to the bone. With the patient under general or local anesthesia a Kirschner wire or Steinmann pin is inserted distal to the fracture site (Fig. 23-25). The pin protrudes through the skin on both sides, and the ends may be covered with corks or metal protectors. Small sterile dressings are usually placed over the entry and exit sites of the pin. A metal U-shaped spreader or bow is attached to the pin. The rope for the traction is attached to the spreader.

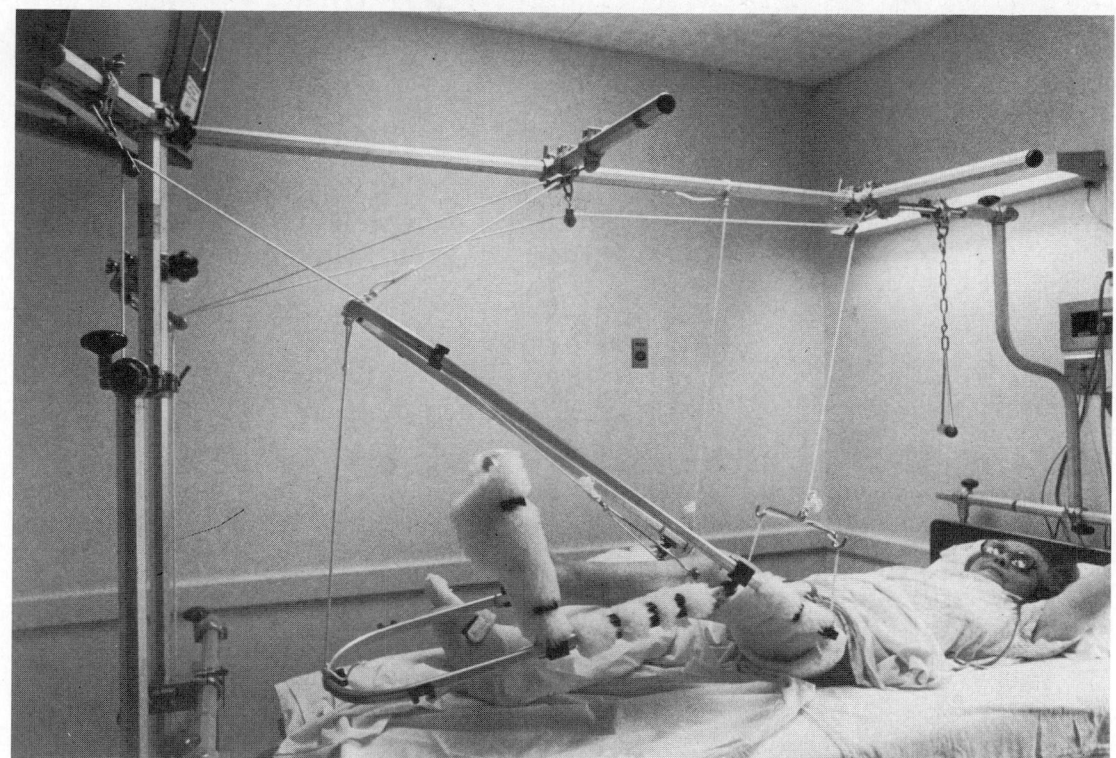

Fig. 23-26. Balance traction.

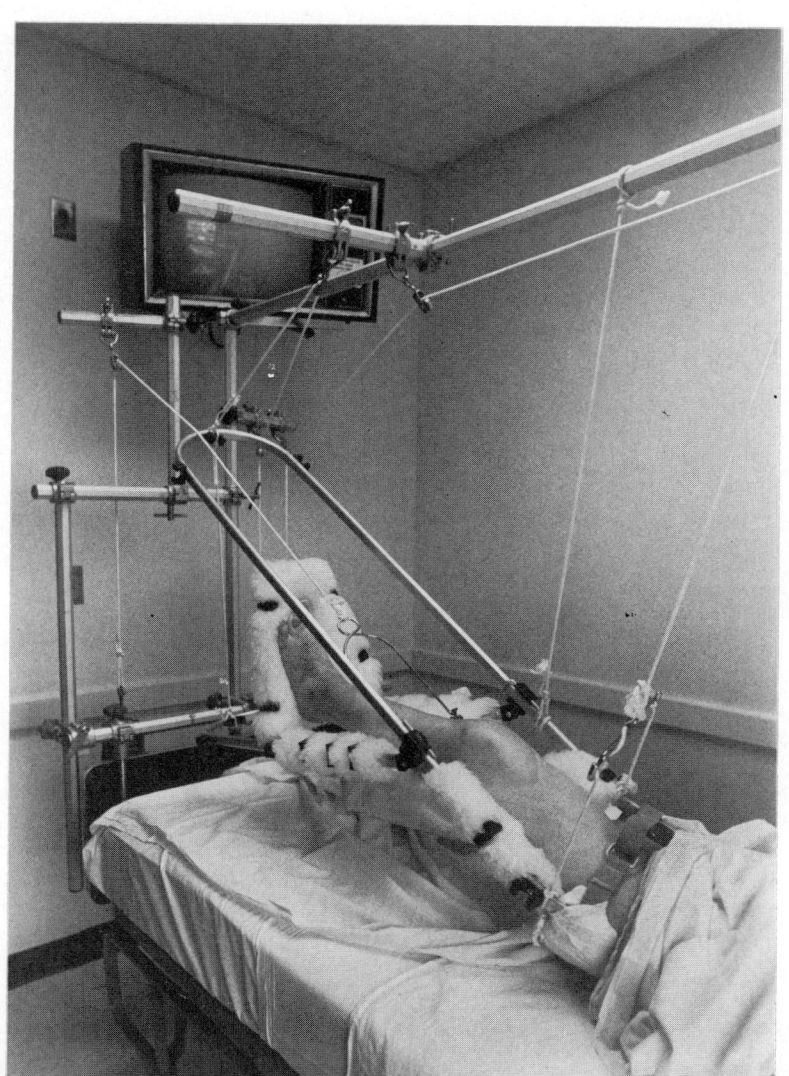

Fig. 23-27. Pearson attachment and Thomas splint.

Balanced suspension

Balanced suspension is used in conjunction with skin or skeletal traction (Fig. 23-26). Suspension of the affected extremity allows the patient more freedom to move about in bed without disturbing the line of traction. Nursing measures, such as bathing the patient, giving skin care, and placing the bedpan, are more easily accomplished. A full or half-ring *Thomas* or *Hodgen splint* may be used to suspend the leg. The areas under the popliteal space and heel are left open to prevent pressure. A *Pearson attachment* may be added to the Thomas splint if the knee is to be flexed or movement of the lower leg is permitted (Fig. 23-27). The patient may be turned toward the leg in the splint.

Assessment
SUBJECTIVE DATA

1. Complaints of pain or discomfort, burning or tingling are reported immediately, since patients in traction should have little or no pain or discomfort.

OBJECTIVE DATA

1. Examine the skin frequently for evidence of pressure or friction over bony prominences and in areas such as the groin (from Thomas splint) and the heel area.
2. Observe for signs and symptoms of thrombophlebitis that may develop from inactivity or from pressure on the popliteal vessels.
3. Observe for traction pull and body alignment as well as checking that there is no interference with traction weights.
4. Check peripheral pulses, color, and temperature of parts distal to traction.
5. Assess for altered sensation in extremity distal to site of injury, for example, inability to move the foot or wiggle the toes.
6. Inspect pin site of skeletal traction for sign of inflammation (infection).

Data analysis and planning
NURSING DIAGNOSES

Potential for alteration in bowel elimination: constipation

Mobility, impaired: physical

Potential for impairment of skin integrity

Knowledge deficit

EXPECTED PATIENT OUTCOMES

1. Bowel elimination has been maintained.
2. Traction and countertraction are maintained.
3. Patient is able to move about in bed within limitations of traction.
4. Patient discusses the purpose of traction and the expected bone healing process.

Implementation
ASSISTING WITH ACHIEVEMENT OF THERAPEUTIC GOALS

1. Maintaining traction and countertraction
   a. Patient needs explanation of traction in relation to fracture and physician's plan of therapy.

b. *Traction must not be released or altered.*
c. Amount of movement in bed will depend on the injury and the kind of traction used. The patient must understand the limitations of activity and the maintenance of correct body positioning.
d. *Traction weights must hang free.* The footplate must never push against the foot of the bed or the pulley (will negate traction) (Fig. 23-28). Ropes must run free in their pulleys.
2. Promoting nutrition
   a. Assist the patient with the selection of nutritional foods.
   b. Assist the patient with meals if the patient must lie flat or is unable to feed self.
3. Promoting elimination
   a. Use a small, flat bedpan (fracture pan), and support the back above the bedpan with a small pillow or a folded bath blanket.
   b. Offer a mild laxative at bedtime.
   c. Encourage fluids.
   d. Encourage intake of whole-grain cereals such as bran, fruits, and vegetables.
4. Maintaining integrity of skin
   a. Use the overhead attachment with trapeze bar to allow the patient to lift self and take some pressure off the back for short periods.
   b. The patient can lift up for skin care and change of bed linens with the help of the trapeze.
   c. Do not cover the Thomas ring; this will create dampness next to skin. Bathe the skin beneath the ring, dry it thoroughly, and powder the area lightly.
5. Promoting circulation and maintaining muscle strength
   a. Assist the patient in using the trapeze bar for lifting and turning to the degree permitted.
   b. Encourage exercise of the noninvolved extremities.

Evaluation

The questions related to therapy would include the following:
1. Does patient know the purpose of traction has been accomplished?
2. Is skin intact?
3. Have there been any problems with elimination?

Open reduction and internal fixation

Open reduction with internal fixation is used when other methods of reduction are not suitable. Although this method allows direct visualization of the injury, it also carries the risk of infection; consequently, surgery is performed under the most vigorous aseptic conditions.

Internal fixation is achieved by using a wide variety of metal devices. Pins, wires, intramedullary rods, compression plates, or nails may be tried. Each has its particular advantage and indication for use.

Following surgery the patient may be placed in a spica cast, in Buck's extension traction, or in Russell traction,

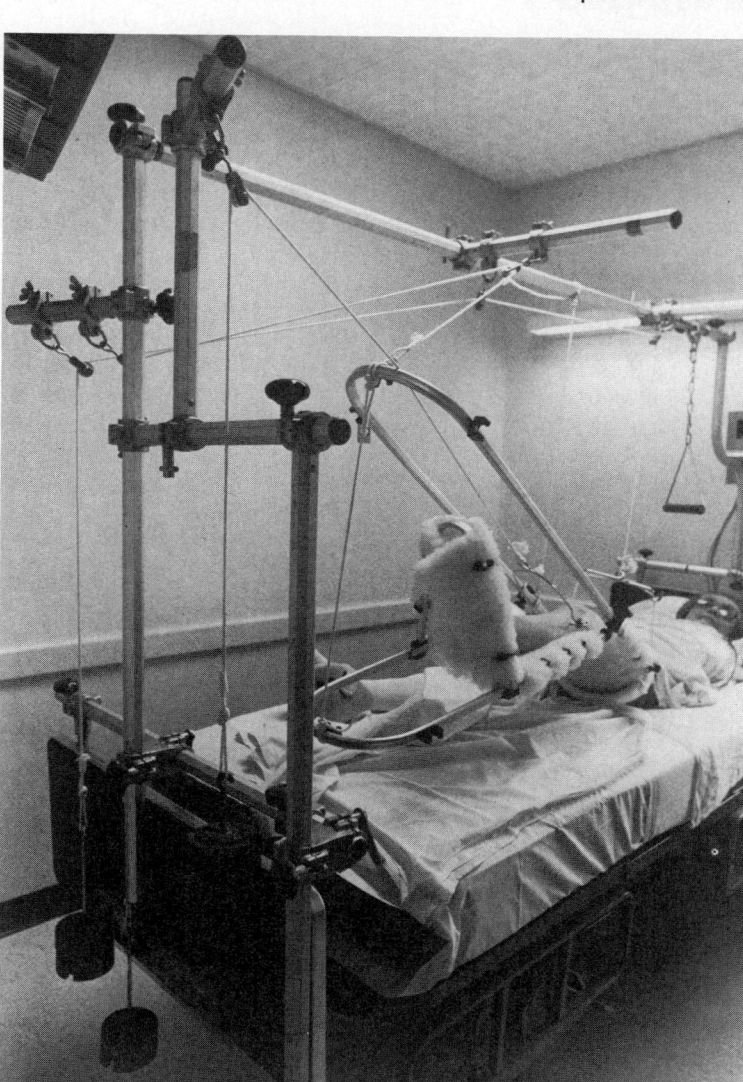

Fig. 23-28. Traction weights.

or the patient may be left free in bed. This last method permits early mobilization of the patient, thereby reducing systemic complications common in the elderly.

The preoperative care of the patient having internal fixation of the hip includes the following:

1. Relief of pain
   a. Medication is given for pain of the fracture and to reduce muscle spasms.
   b. Preoperative use of traction gives comfort and reduces muscle spasm. Mild analgesics can be very effective. Nursing measures that help in relief of discomfort include the following (discussed in traction section):
      (1) Good body alignment
      (2) Skin care
      (3) Assisting with position changes
      (4) Maintaining traction and countertraction
2. Coughing and deep breathing exercises are performed.

3. Explanation is provided of the surgical procedure and general nursing care after surgery.
4. Operative permit is signed by the patient.

Postoperatively, care should be as follows:

1. Traction. Buck's extension or a half-ring Thomas splint with a Pearson attachment may be used for a few days to overcome muscle spasms and allow soft-tissue healing (Figs. 23-23 and 23-26).
2. Preventing complications.
   a. Respiratory: encourage position changes, coughing and deep breathing, and adequate fluids.
   b. Circulatory:
      (1) Monitor vital signs at intervals for the first 24 to 48 hours.
      (2) Assess drainage on hip dressing.
      (3) Check peripheral pulses.
      (4) Observe for thrombophlebitis of lower extremity.
      (5) Encourage range of motion exercises.

c. Gastrointestinal: encourage good nutritional habits for elimination and for bone healing.
d. Wound infection:
(1) Monitor body temperature.
(2) Inspect dressing for drainage.
3. Positioning.
a. If traction was not used, check with the physician about turning the patient to either side.
b. Turn the patient every 2 hours initially; support the operative leg in abduction when Austin-Moore prosthesis is present or to promote patient comfort (Fig. 23-29). Place pillows under the fractured limb to place it at the same level as the trunk (Fig. 23-30).
c. Prevent external rotation of hip when patient is lying on back (use *trochanter roll*).
4. Early mobilization.
a. Mobilization may be started on the first postoperative day following internal fixation of an extracapsular fracture.
b. Partial weight bearing:
(1) Some fixation devices permit partial weight bearing on the operated leg; others, such as the Smith-Petersen nail, do not.
(2) Check on weight bearing status before getting the patient out of bed.

(3) Weight bearing may not be permitted for several months after some surgery.
c. Lift or assist the patient into a straight-back chair. Do not elevate the legs. Place the feet on the floor. If an Austin-Moore prosthesis is inserted, do not allow hip flexion beyond 60 degrees for 10 days.
d. Ambulation:
(1) During transfer, ambulation, and sitting remind the patient to maintain abduction of the operated hip to prevent dislocation of the prosthesis (if one has been inserted).
(2) A walker or crutches may be ordered when the patient is permitted partial weight-bearing ambulation.

Evaluation

The questions related to therapy would include the following:
1. Is patient comfortable?
2. Is healing occurring without infection?
3. Is patient transferring and ambulating according to prescribed weight-bearing restrictions?
4. Is patient able to engage in former activities?

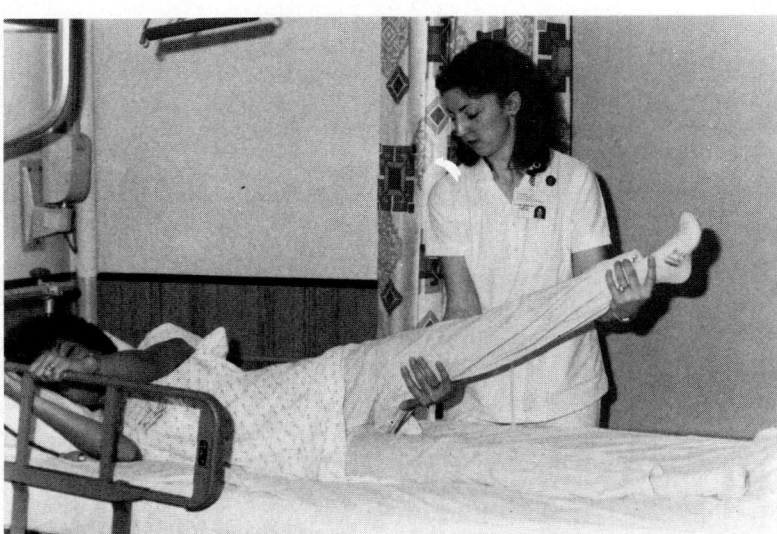

Fig. 23-29. Leg in abduction.

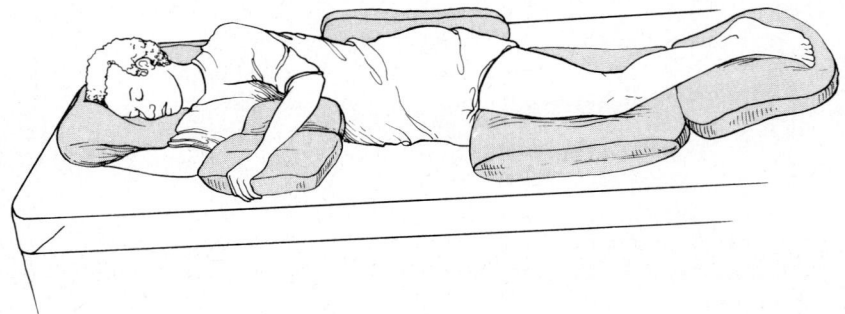

Fig. 23-30. Side-lying position.

REFERENCES AND SELECTED READINGS*

1. Adams, J.G.: Standard orthopaedic operations, ed. 2, Edinburgh, 1980, Churchill Livingstone.
2. Agee, B.L., and Herman, C.: Cervical logrolling on a standard hospital bed, Am. J. Nurs. **84:**315-318, 1984.
3. Anthony, C.P., and Thibodeau, G.A.: Textbook of anatomy and physiology, ed. 11, St. Louis, 1983, The C.V. Mosby Co.
4. *Berger, M.R., and Froimson, A.I.: Hands that hurt: carpal tunnel syndrome, Am. J. Nurs. **79:**264-265, 1979.
5. Brashear, H.R., Jr., and Raney, R.B., Sr.: Shands' handbook of orthopaedic surgery, ed. 9, St. Louis, 1978, The C.V. Mosby Co.
6. Brunner, N.A.: Orthopedic nursing: a programmed approach, ed. 4, St. Louis, 1983, The C.V. Mosby Co.
7. *Cohen, S., and Viellion, G.: Nursing care of a patient in traction, Am. J. Nurs. **79:**1771-1798, 1979.
8. *Darst, B.J.: I have a new hip, Am. J. Nurs. **78:**1489-1490, 1978.
9. *deToledo, C.H., et al.: The patient with scoliosis (four articles), Am. J. Nurs. **79:**1587-1612, 1979.
10. *Dickinson, G.R., and Gorman, T.K.: Adult arthritis: the assessment, Am J. Nurs. **83:**262-265, 1983.
11. Donahoo, C.A., and Dimon, J.H., III: Orthopedic nursing, Boston, 1977, Little, Brown & Co.
12. Donahoo, C.A., and Spickler, L., editors.: Core curriculum of orthopedic nursing, Atlanta, 1980, Orthopedic Nurses Association.
13. *Farrell, J.: Nursing care of the patient in a cast brace, Nurs. Clin. North Am. **13:**717-724, 1976.
14. Farrell, J.: Illustrated guide to orthopedic nursing, Philadelphia, 1977, J.B. Lippincott Co.
15. *Gallagher, L.: When your patient has a shoulder arthroplasty, here's how to help, Nurs. 80 **10:**46-49, 1980.
16. Hay, B.K., et al.: External fixation: option for fractures, AORN J.**34:**417-423, 1981.
17. Hilt, N., and Cogburn, S.: Manual of orthopedics, St. Louis, 1979, The C.V. Mosby Co.
18. Iveson, J.: Orthopaedic traction: you're pulling my leg! Nurs. Mirror **153:**44-45, Oct. 1981.
19. *Koerner, M.E., and Dickinson, G.R.: Adult arthritis: a look at some of its forms, Am. J. Nurs. **83:**255-262, 1983.
20. *Kryshyshen, P.L., and Fischer, D.A.: External fixation for complicated fractures, Am. J. Nurs. **80:**357-259, 1980.
21. Larson, C.B., and Gould, M.L.: Orthopedic nursing, ed. 9, St. Louis, 1978, The C.V. Mosby Co.
22. Lewis, R.C., Jr.: Handbook of traction casting and splinting techniques, Philadelphia, 1977, J.B. Lippincott Co.
23. McCarty, D.J., editor: Arthritis and allied conditions; a textbook of rheumatology, ed. 9, Philadelphia, 1979, Lea & Febiger.
24. Meyers, M.H., McNell, D.V., and Nelson, K.: Total hip replacement—a team effort, Am. J. Nurs. **78:**1485-1488, 1978.
25. Mitchell, G.: Orthopaedics: joint treatment . . . disorders of the hip, part 4, Nurs. Mirror **151:**26-28, Nov. 6, 1980.
26. Moskowitz, R.W.: Clinical rheumatology: a problem-oriented approach, ed. 2, Philadelphia, 1982, Lea & Febiger.
27. Mourad, L.: Nursing care of adults with orthopedic conditions, New York, 1980, John Wiley & Sons.
28. *Owen, B.D.: How to control that aching back, Am. J. Nurs. **80:**894-897, 1980.
29. *Porter, S.F., Dapper, M. J., and Foran, C.: Adult arthritis: hand splints, Am. J. Nurs. **83:**276-278, 1983.
30. Rantz, M.J., and Courtial, D.: Lifting, moving and transferring patients: a manual, St. Louis, 1977, The C.V. Mosby Co.
31. *Richards, M.: Osteoporosis . . . bane of the elderly, Geritr. Nurs. **3:**98-102, Mar. Apr. 1982.
32. *Schwaid, M.C.: Advice to arthritics: keep moving, Am. J. Nurs. **78:**1708-1709, 1978.
33. *Simpson, C.F.: Adult arthritis: heat, cold, or both? Am. J. Nurs. **83:**270-272, 1983.
34. *Simpson, C.F., and Dickson, G.R.: Adult arthritis: exercise, Am. J. Nurs. **83:**273-274, 1983.
35. *Strand, C.V., and Clark, S.R.: Adult arthritis: drugs and remedies, Am. J. Nurs. **83:**266-270, 1983.
36. Torbett, M.P., and Ervin, J.C.: The patient with systemic lupus erythematosus, Am. J. Nurs. **77:**1299-1302, 1977.
37. Turner, P.: Caring for emotional needs of orthopedic trauma patients, AORN J. **36:**566-570, 1982.
38. Volz, R.G., et al.: Upper extremity total joint replacement, AORN J. **28:**843-847, 1978.
39. *White, J.: Teaching patients to manage systemic lupus erythemtosus, Nurs. 78 **8:**26-35, 1978.

*References preceded by an asterick are particulary well suited for student reading.

UNIT VII
Gas Transport Problems

24 The Patient with Nose and Throat Problems
25 The Patient with Pulmonary Problems
26 The Patient with Cardiovascular Problems
27 The Patient with Peripheral Vascular Problems
28 The Patient with Hematologic Problems

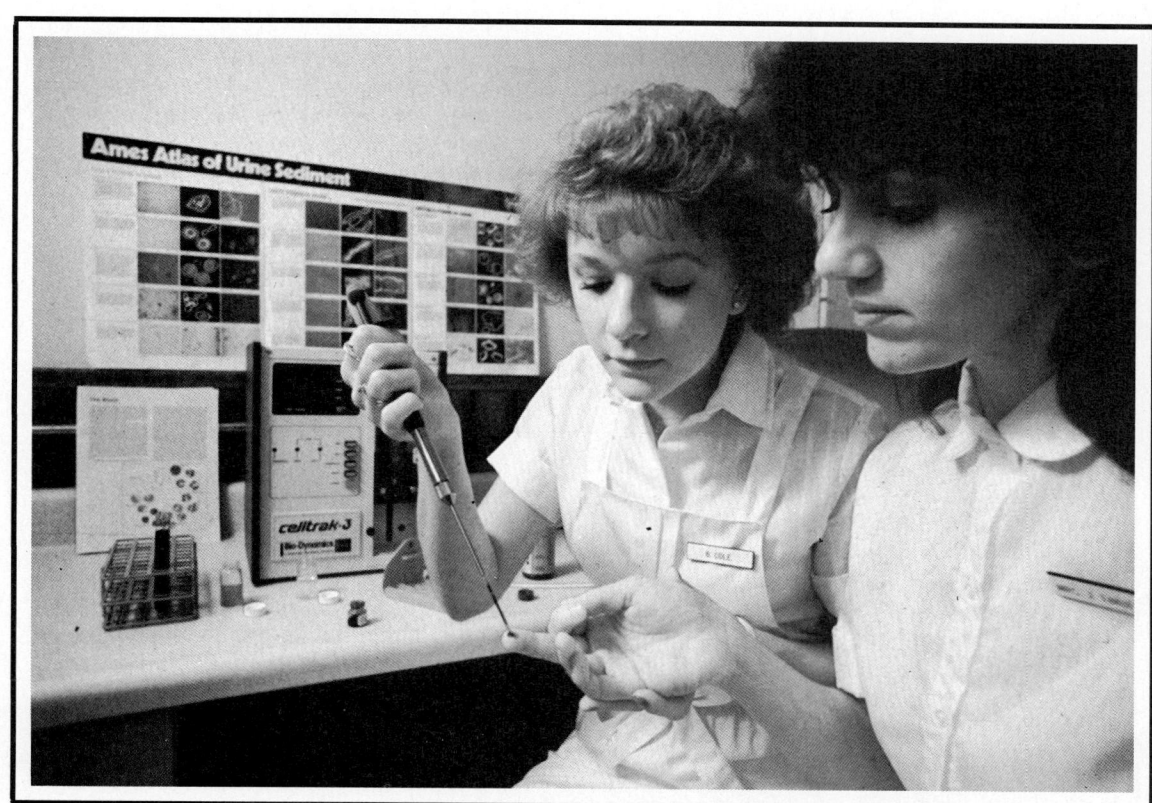

24

The Patient with Nose and Throat Problems

LINDA ANNE BROSEMAN

STUDY QUESTIONS

- Review the anatomy of the nose and throat.

- How do your mouth and throat feel when your nose is blocked and you are mouth breathing? What can you do to keep the mucous membranes moist?

- What actions can you take to prevent spreading a cold to others?

- What resources are available in your community to assist persons who have had a total laryngectomy?

Disorders of the nose and throat are very common, and nurses in particular are often asked to give advice about these problems. To be effective, nurses need a basic understanding of the structure and function of the organs of the upper airway, as well as knowledge of the medical and nursing regimens for problems affecting the upper airway.

ANATOMY AND PHYSIOLOGY

Nose and sinuses

The nose is supported by the nasal bones, the nasal processes of the maxillary bones, the cartilaginous and bony parts of the septum, and the upper and lower nasal cartilages. The septum, which divides the nares, is rarely straight in adults—usually at some time it has been injured.

The nasal cavities are located between the roof of the mouth and the frontal, ethmoid, and sphenoid bones. Three projections, which are lined with mucous membrane and called the *turbinate bones,* are located on the lateral walls of each nasal cavity (Fig. 24-1). Their pur-

pose is to increase the mucous membrane surface over which air passes as it travels to the nasopharynx, thus allowing for precipitation of inhaled particles and warming and moistening the inhaled air.

The mucous membrane posterior to the vestibule (anterior part) of the nose contains cilia that beat in a constant wavelike motion to carry mucus into the nasopharynx. Trapped in the mucus are bacteria, dust, and other foreign matter entering the nose. The olfactory epithelium is located in a small area superiorly and provides the end organ of smell.

There are four sets of paranasal sinuses located on either side of the head (Fig. 24-2). These sinuses are air-filled spaces in the skull that serve to lighten the head. They drain into the nasal cavities through openings behind the turbinates. The maxillary sinuses are the largest and most accessible. The sinuses are lined with mucous membrane continuous with that of the nose.

Upper throat: pharynx and tonsils

The pharynx is the space behind the oral cavity that extends from the base of the skull to the larynx. The

527

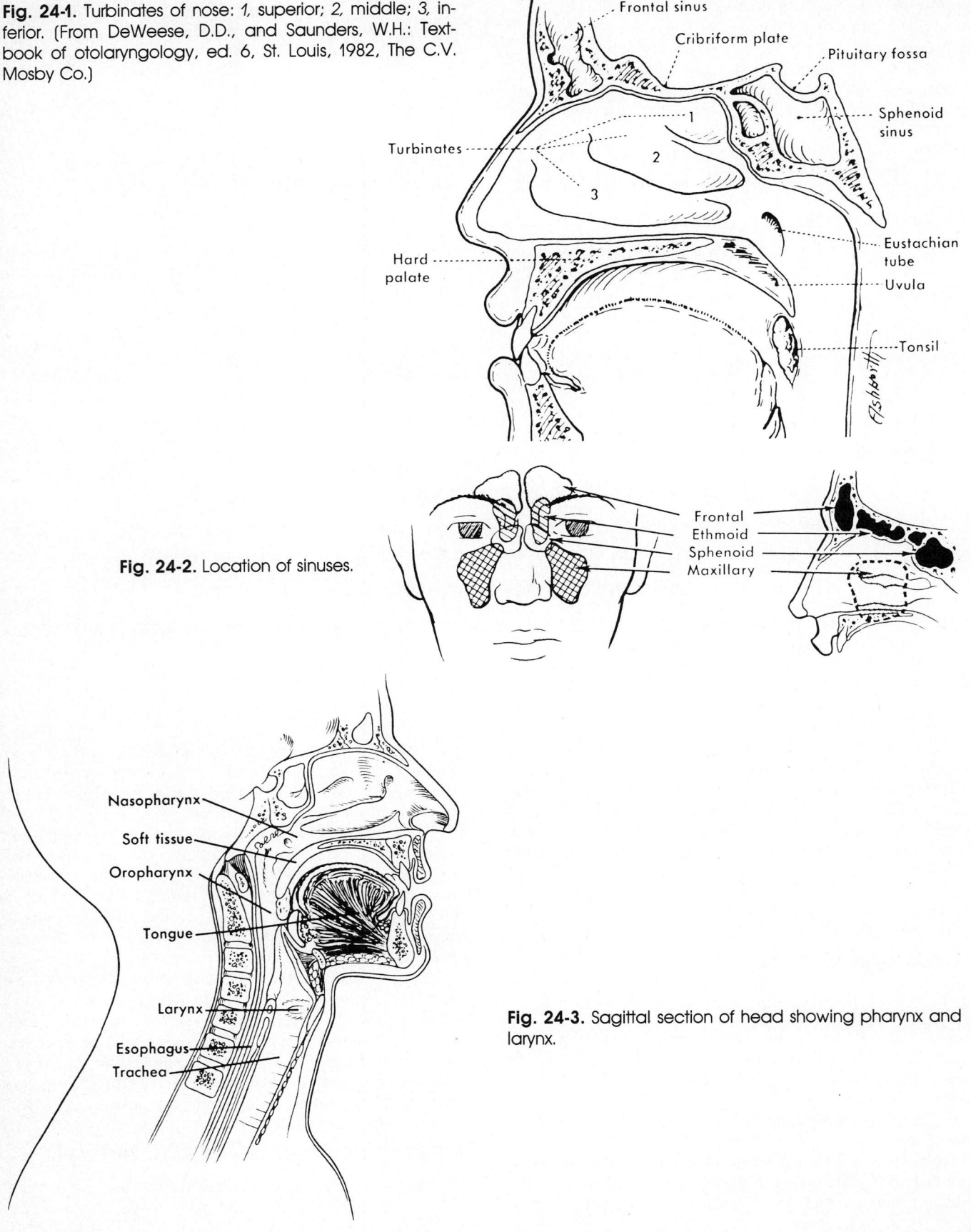

Fig. 24-1. Turbinates of nose: *1,* superior; *2,* middle; *3,* inferior. (From DeWeese, D.D., and Saunders, W.H.: Textbook of otolaryngology, ed. 6, St. Louis, 1982, The C.V. Mosby Co.)

Frontal sinus

Cribriform plate

Pituitary fossa

Sphenoid sinus

Turbinates

Eustachian tube

Hard palate

Uvula

Tonsil

1

2

3

Fig. 24-2. Location of sinuses.

Frontal
Ethmoid
Sphenoid
Maxillary

Nasopharynx

Soft tissue

Oropharynx

Tongue

Larynx

Esophagus

Trachea

Fig. 24-3. Sagittal section of head showing pharynx and larynx.

pharynx can be considered in three parts: the nasopharynx, the oropharynx, and the hypopharynx (Fig. 24-3). It is lined with mucous membrane.

The adenoids are located in the nasopharynx, the palatine tonsils anterior to the oropharynx, and the lingual tonsils in the hypopharynx. The adenoids and tonsils are lymphoid tissue and help to filter the circulating lymph of bacteria or other foreign matter that penetrate the body, especially by way of the nose or mouth.

Lower throat: larynx and hypopharynx

The larynx forms the upper extremity of the trachea. The framework of the larynx is made up of several cartilages held together by muscle and ligaments (Fig. 24-4). The cartilaginous framework protects the vocal cords and affords a stiffness that permits an airway. The thyroid cartilage, the "Adam's apple," is the largest cartilaginous element in the larynx and protects the inner structures. The hyoid bone forms an attachment for the larynx and tongue. The larynx is lined with mucosa continuous with that of the hypopharynx and trachea. The vagus nerve innervates the larynx.

The chief function of the larynx is to serve as an airway between the pharynx and trachea. A leaf-shaped lid of fibrocartilage (epiglottis) protects the glottis by covering the entrance to the larynx during swallowing to prevent aspiration of food or fluids. The closing of the glottis also allows for an increase of intrathoracic pressure, which is needed, for example, in coughing or lifting. This increased pressure increases the use of the muscles of the shoulder and thorax.

In addition, a most important function of the larynx is

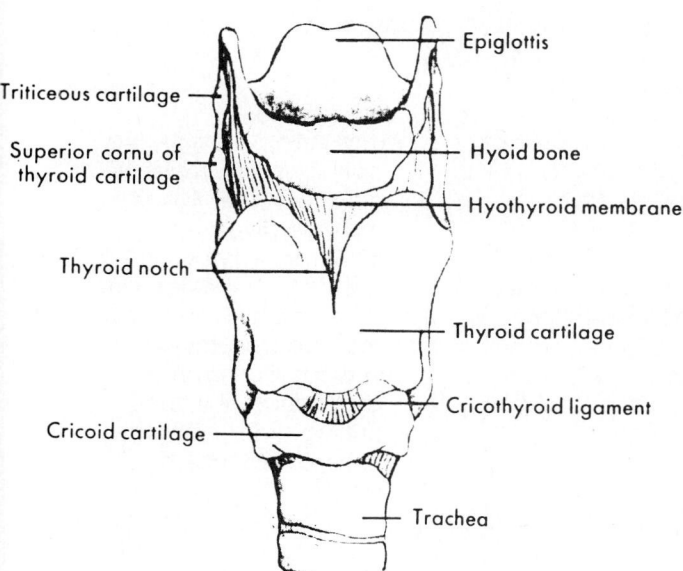

Fig. 24-4. Anterior aspect of larynx. (From Francis, C.C.: Introduction to human anatomy, ed. 6, St. Louis, 1975, The C.V. Mosby Co.)

phonation. The larynx creates sounds as a result of vocal cord vibrations that are formed into speech patterns by the movement of the pharynx, palate, tongue, teeth, and lips.

Major health problems of the nose and throat

Most disorders of the nose and throat may be categorized as inflammatory, obstructive, or malignant as follows:

1. Inflammatory disorders include rhinitis, sinusitis, pharyngitis, tonsillitis, peritonsillar abscess, and laryngitis.
2. Obstructive disorders include a deviated septum, hypertrophy of the turbinates, nasal polyps, foreign bodies, fractures (nasal, maxillary, zygomatic), and epistaxis.
3. Malignant disorders include carcinoma of the nasopharynx, of the maxillary and ethmoid sinuses, of the tonsil, and of the larynx.

INFLAMMATIONS OF THE NOSE AND THROAT

Inflammations may develop in the nose, sinuses, pharynx, tonsils, and larynx (Table 24-1).

PATHOPHYSIOLOGY

Inflammations of the upper airway structures may result from numerous viruses and bacteria. There are many filtrable viruses (such as the more than 30 identified rhinoviruses, adenovirus, echovirus, influenza and parainfluenza viruses, and coxsackie virus) that may serve as etiologic agents of inflammations. Bacteria include primarily streptococci, staphylococci, and pneumococci. A severe form of acute pharyngitis is often referred to as *strep throat* because of the frequency of streptococci as the causative organism. There is also increased evidence of gonococcal pharyngitis in both men and women caused by the gram-negative diplococcus *Neisseria gonorrhoeae*.

Inflammations of the upper respiratory tract, primarily in the nose and sinuses, may result as an allergic reaction to pollens of grasses and flowers, dust, animal dander, wool, and certain foods. Maxillary sinusitis may also occur as an extension of infection from abscessed teeth and tooth extraction, since the apices of many of the upper teeth roots are in close contact with the mucosal lining of the sinus.

The larynx is more susceptible to inflammation from irritants. Excessive use of the voice and excessive smoking are common causes. When the larynx becomes inflammed, laryngeal edema may cause respiratory obstruction.

Table 24-1. Inflammations of the nose and throat

Disorder	Etiology	Signs and symptoms	Medical therapy
Rhinitis (coryza, common cold)	Filterable virus	Initial: dryness of mucous membranes, chills, general malaise 12-24 hrs: profuse watery discharge, sneezing, tearing of eyes	Rest, fluids, moist inhalations, antihistamines and decongestants
Allergic rhinitis (hay fever)	Pollens or allergens	Sneezing, nasal obstruction, watery nasal discharge, frontal headache, itching of eyes and nose	Separation of person from sensitizing allergens, desensitization, antihistamines; submucous resection or polypectomy may be necessary
Chronic rhinitis	Follows repeated acute infections, allergy, or vasomotor rhinitis	Stuffiness and pressure in the nose; nasal discharge, which may be serous, mucopurulent or purulent; polyp formation; frontal headache; vertigo; sneezing	Antibiotics, removal of the offending allergens, antihistamines, polypectomy may be necessary
Sinusitis Acute	Streptococcus, staphylococcus, pneumococcus, *Haemophilus influenza*	Constant severe headache, pain over sinuses, orbital edema, nasal discharge, fever	Rest, analgesics, oral nasal decongestants, systemic antibiotics, local heat, topical nasal decongestants; antrum puncture may be necessary
Chronic	Same as above	Chronic purulent nasal discharge, dull sinus headache, loss of ability to smell	Surgery; sinus irrigations
Pharyngitis	Gram-positive bacteria or filtrable virus	Redness and soreness of throat, difficulty in swallowing, fever	Warm saline gargles, ice collar, aspirin, moist inhalations, antibiotics may be given
Tonsillitis	Usually streptococcus	Sudden onset of sore throat, dysphagia, fever, chills, malaise	Rest, fluids, warm saline gargles, antibiotics, analgesics, tonsillectomy may be performed
Laryngitis	Extension of inflammation from rhinitis, excessive use of voice, excessive smoking, irritating fumes, changes in temperature	From slight huskiness to total voice loss, sore throat, dry harsh cough	Symptomatic treatment, avoidance of further talking, steam inhalations, avoidance of smoking

Signs and symptoms seen with inflammations of the nose and throat result from the inflammatory process. Redness and edema of the mucous membrane occur early. Discharge from the nose and sinuses include fluid exudate from the inflammatory process (which may be serous or purulent if infection is present) as well as mucous secretions. General malaise and fever are part of the systemic response to inflammation. Fever is generally low in acute viral infections and higher with acute bacterial infections.

ASSESSMENT

Persons with inflammations of the nose and throat may be diagnosed and treated on an ambulatory basis. Since acute inflammations may become chronic, assessment of early signs of inflammation is important for early diagnosis and treatment.

Subjective symptoms may include the following:
1. Dryness of the nose, eyes, throat
2. General malaise
3. Headache
4. Sore throat
5. Watery nasal discharge
6. Nasal obstruction

Subjective data should also include the person's knowledge of preventive measures and symptoms requiring medical intervention.

Objective data include fever and drainage (serous, mucopurulent, purulent). Polyps (pale, soft, edematous outpouchings of nasal or sinal mucosa) may be present and are usually bilateral in inflammation of the nose or sinus. Causative organisms may be determined by culture.

DATA ANALYSIS AND PLANNING

Nursing diagnoses

Nursing diagnoses are determined on the basis of collected data and may include the following:
Knowledge deficit
Alteration in comfort: pain (headache, throat, sinus)

Expected patient outcomes

The patient can describe the following:
1. Ways to prevent future attacks
2. Measures for relief of discomfort
3. Plans for increased fluid intake
4. Medication program and dangers of using over-the-counter preparations

IMPLEMENTATION

Most persons with acute upper respiratory infections are ambulatory, therefore, the major thrust of nursing care is on teaching the person about the condition and proper self-care (see lower box on p. 533). With chronic infections, surgery may be indicated.

Surgery

Various types of surgery may be performed depending on the location and the type of infection (Table 24-2).

Nasal surgery

Most nasal surgery on adults is done under local anesthesia. The nose is usually packed with ½-inch gauze at the conclusion of the operation. Commonly used packs are petrolatum-impregnated gauze, Adaptic gauze, iodoform gauze with bacitracin, and Cortisporin-impregnated

Table 24-2. Surgeries for inflammations of nose and throat

Surgery	Procedure	Use
Antrum puncture	Perforation and irrigation with saline of maxillary sinus (antrum) with a trocar and canula	Acute sinus infection not relieved by conservative measures
Caldwell-Luc	Cleaning out of maxillary sinus through incision under upper lip	Chronic maxillary sinusitis
Ethmoidotomy, sphenoido-tomy	Incision into ethmoid or sphenoid sinus for drainage; incision is intranasal or externally through an eyebrow incision	Chronic sinusitis of ethmoid or spenoid sinus
Osteopathic flap	Complete removal of diseased mucosa of frontal sinus with obliteration of sinus; space is packed with subcutaneous fat obtained from abdomen	Chronic frontal sinusitis
Tonsillectomy and adenoid-ectomy	Removal of tonsils and adenoids	Repeated occurrences of acute tonsillitis (five episodes in 1 year), peritonsillary abscess, enlarged tonsils causing obstruction

gauze. The latter is particularly effective in reducing the odor of the nasal pack. If the packing should slip back into the throat, the surgeon is notified immediately. The pack is usually removed and replaced as necessary. In some persons, packing may remain in the nares as long as 1 week, while in others it is removed in 48 hours.

Following nasal surgery, there is danger of hemorrhage, and the patient is monitored for signs of bright red bleeding. If bleeding is pronounced, the surgeon may repack the nose.

Frequent mouth care and oral fluid intake are necessary since the person may be mouth breathing. Packing blocks the passage of air through the nose, creating a partial vacuum during swallowing, and the patient may complain of a sucking action when attempting to drink. Postnasal drainage, the presence of old blood in the mouth, and the loss of the ability to smell lessen the person's appetite. Because it is difficult to eat while the nose is packed, most persons prefer a liquid diet until the packing is removed, but they can have whatever food is tolerated.

Sinus surgery

If the person has recurrent attacks of sinusitis, it may be necessary to provide better drainage by permanently enlarging the sinus openings or by making a new opening and removing the diseased mucous membrane.[9] Surgery usually is performed during the subacute stage of infection. Surgery on the sinuses is done under general as well as under local anesthesia.

The care of the patient experiencing sinus surgery is similar to that of nasal surgery. A gross check of the person's visual acuity is advisable after sinus surgery to be sure that there is no damage to the optic nerve. A check for diplopia is advisable to determine damage to the nerves of muscles at the globe of the eye.

Tonsillectomy

Tonsillectomy for the adult may be performed under local or general anesthesia. Hemorrhage may occur postoperatively. The physician may be able to control minor postoperative bleeding by applying a sponge soaked in a solution of epinephrine to the site. The person who is bleeding excessively often is returned to the operating room for surgical treatment to stop the hemorrhage. This may be done by ligating or by cauterizing the bleeding vessel. If sutures must be used, the person will have more pain and discomfort than following a simple tonsillectomy. The patient may not be able to take solid food for several days. Some surgeons no longer prescribe aspirin for pain after tonsillectomy, as it increases the tendency to bleed. Acetaminophen or another aspirin substitute is usually ordered.

A tough, yellow, fibrous membrane that forms over the operative site begins to break away between the fourth and eighth postoperative days, and hemorrhage may oc-

---

Care of the patient experiencing nasal or sinus surgery

Preoperative care
1. Inform patient that discoloration about eyes may occur postoperatively
2. Give nothing by mouth for 6 hours before surgery
3. Give prescribed sedative and narcotic

Postoperative care
1. Monitor for and report signs of bleeding
   a. External dressing
   b. Expectoration or vomiting of bright red blood
   c. Back of throat
2. Check patient's visual acuity after sinus surgery
3. Change dressing *under* nose, if soiled
4. Give mouth care
5. Encourage oral fluid intake
6. To decrease local edema around nose and eyes
   a. Keep patient in mid-Fowler's position
   b. Apply ice compresses, if desired, over nose for 24 hours (patient may do this for self)
7. Teach patient in regard to following:
   a. After packing is removed, avoid blowing nose for 48 hours
   b. Report fever to surgeon (sign of infection)
   c. Expect stools to be tarry (from swallowed blood) for several days
   d. Avoid constipation (Valsalva's maneuver can initiate bleeding)

Postoperative care for tonsillectomy

1. Side-lying position until awake, then mid-Fowler's
2. Monitor for signs of hemorrhage
   a. Repeated swallowing
   b. Vomiting of bright red blood
   c. Increased pulse rate while sleeping
3. Diet
   a. Offer fluids when vomiting has ceased
      1. Encourage patient to take large swallows (more comfortable than small sips)
      2. Avoid using a straw (suction may cause bleeding)
      3. Ice-cold fluids better tolerated
   b. Offer bland nourishment
      1. Ice-cream, cold custards, cream soups, and bland juices (for example, pear) offered initially
      2. Refined cereal and soft-cooked egg usually better tolerated morning after surgery
      3. Avoid citrus juices, hot fluids, rough or highly seasoned foods for one week
   c. Relieve throat discomfort
      1. Apply ice collar if desired
      2. Give prescribed analgesic (avoid aspirin)
   d. Teach patient as to the following:
      1. Avoid vigorous exercise, coughing, sneezing, clearing throat, and vigorous nose blowing for 1 to 2 weeks
      2. Report signs of bleeding immediately to physician
      3. Drink fluids (2 to 3 L/day) until mouth odor disappears
      4. Stools may be tarry for several days from swallowed blood
      5. Throat discomfort may increase slightly between fourth and eighth postoperative day (membrane separation)

Teaching the patient with an inflammation of the nose or throat

1. Get additional rest (hastens recovery)
2. Drink at least 2 to 3 L of fluid every day
3. Medications
   a. Antihistamines are effective primarily during the initial period only; care should be taken when driving or working with heavy machinery when taking antihistamines
   b. Take any prescribed antibiotics for bacterial infections for the prescribed period of time
   c. If using nose drops
      1. Place no more than 3 drops of solution in each nostril at one time (unless otherwise prescribed)
      2. Keep head tilted back for about 5 minutes to permit solution to reach posterior nares
      3. Insert 1 to 2 additional drops after 10 minutes if marked congestion is still present
   d. If using atomizer:
      1. Occlude opposite nostril with finger pressure to prevent entrance of air
      2. Administer no more than 3 sprays of solution in each nostril at one time
4. Promote throat comfort through use of the following:
   a. Warm saline gargles
   b. Ice collar
   c. Aspirin lozenges
   d. Moist inhalators
5. Avoid further upper respiratory infections
   a. Avoid direct exposure to others with respiratory infections, if possible
   b. Teach all persons to cover mouth when coughing or sneezing
   c. Wash hands after disposing of waste products

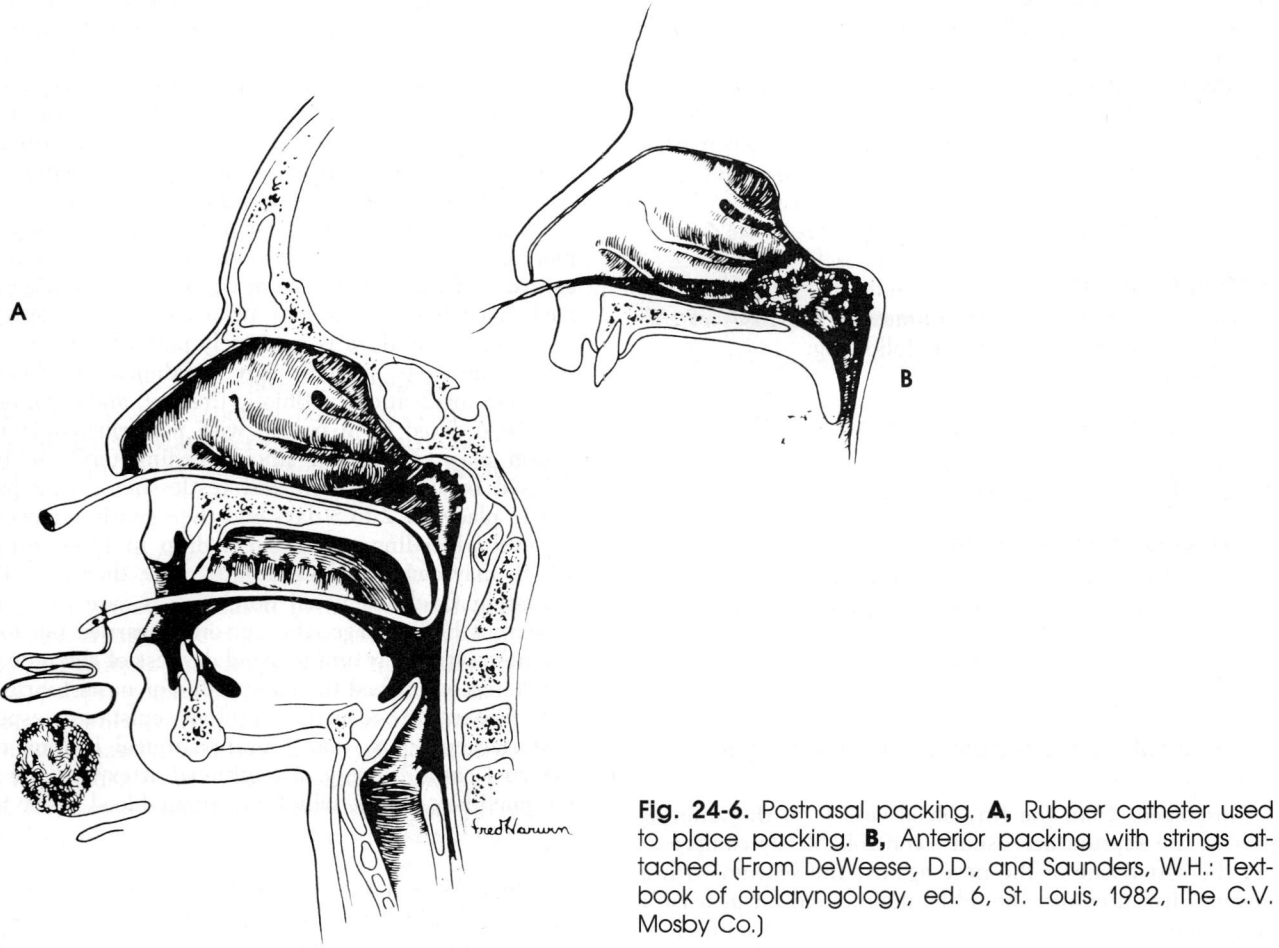

Fig. 24-6. Postnasal packing. **A,** Rubber catheter used to place packing. **B,** Anterior packing with strings attached. (From DeWeese, D.D., and Saunders, W.H.: Textbook of otolaryngology, ed. 6, St. Louis, 1982, The C.V. Mosby Co.)

Table 24-4. Surgeries to relieve nasal obstruction or trauma

Surgery	Description	Comments
Nasal polypec-tomy	Removal of polyps from nose	Local anesthesia given; nasal packing for 24 hours
Submucous re-section	Removal of obstructive parts of cartilage and bone from nasal sep-tum	Local anesthesia given; both nostrils packed to provide splinting
Nasosepto-plasty	Reconstruction of nasal septum	Same as for submucous resec-tion
Rhinoplasty	Reconstruction of external nose following trauma or for cosmetic reasons	Often combined with septoplasty following nasal trauma; nose is splinted after surgery; nasal packing

EVALUATION

Evaluation is based on expected patient outcomes. Questions to ask may include the following:

1. Is the patient comfortable?
2. Can the patient describe care required at home following surgery?
3. Can the patient describe ways to prevent nosebleeds?
4. Can the patient describe the expected time frame for positive cosmetic effects following rhinoplasty?

MALIGNANCIES OF THE NOSE AND THROAT

Malignancies may develop in the nasopharynx, sinuses, tonsils, and larynx (Table 24-5).

PATHOPHYSIOLOGY

Nasopharyngeal carcinomas obstruct the nose; they metastasize early to the neck. Carcinomas of the maxillary and ethmoid sinuses may erode the adjacent nasal walls and bleed easily. Carcinoma of the maxillary sinus cause dental problems initially; other effects may include nasal obstruction, nosebleeds, and displacement of the eye. Carcinoma of the ethmoid sinus causes outward displacement of the eye, disturbance of the sense of smell, and nosebleeds. The prognosis is grave.

Malignancy of the tonsils is second only to malignancy of the larynx in malignancies of the upper respiratory tract.[2] The malignancy can be one of three types: carcinoma, lymphoepithelioma, or lymphosarcoma. Carcinomas are more common in men, possibly related to the increased incidence of smoking among men. The carcinomas spread upward into the soft palate and usually metastasize early to the neck.

Squamous cell carcinoma of the *larynx* is increasing in frequency. It is estimated that in the United States there are over 10,000 new cases every year.[2] Cancer of the larynx limited to the true vocal cords grows slowly because of the limited lymphatic supply. Elsewhere in the larynx (for example, the epiglottis, false vocal cords), lymph vessels are abundant; and cancer of these tissues often spreads rapidly and metastasizes early to the deep lymph nodes of the neck.

Cancer of the larynx is eight times more common in men than in women, and it occurs most often in persons over 60 years of age. There appears to be some relationship between cancer of the larynx and heavy smoking, alcohol abuse, chronic laryngitis, vocal abuse, and family predisposition to cancer. Because of the increase in the number of women who are heavy smokers, the incidence of carcinoma of the larynx among this group is increasing.

ASSESSMENT

Persons with carcinomas of the nose, sinuses, tonsils, or larynx can have a variety of symptoms.

1. Nasal obstruction, either unilateral or bilateral
2. Bleeding from the nose
3. Dental problems, for example, loosening of the upper teeth, or poorly fitting dentures
4. Disturbance of the sense of smell
5. Eye problems: displacement, tearing, diplopia
6. Local ulceration of the tonsil with or without pain
7. Hoarseness

Hoarseness is an early symptom of cancer of the vocal cords. If treatment is given when hoarseness appears (caused by the tumor's preventing the complete approximation of the vocal cord), a cure usually is possible.

Diagnostic tests

The nose may be examined by the physician by direct inspection using a nasal speculum. A laryngeal mirror is

Table 24-5. Malignant disorders of nose and throat

Disorder	Description	Signs and symtoms	Medical therapy
Nasopharyngeal carcinomas	Carcinomas that obstruct nose first on one side then the other	Nasal obstruction, early metastasis to neck, bleeding	Surgery, radiation therapy
Carcinoma of maxillary and ethmoid sinuses	Relatively uncommon	Loosening of upper teeth; nasal obstruction, nosebleeds, displacement of eye, anosmia, tearing and diplopia	Surgery that removes entire upper jaw (maxillectomy) and one eye (orbital exenteration); radiation therapy
Cancer of tonsil	May be carcinoma, lymphoepithelioma, or lymphosarcoma	Local ulceration, enlarged tonsil, pain	Surgery, irradiation
Carcinoma of larynx	Squamous cell carcinoma of vocal cords and surrounding tissue	Progressive hoarseness that lasts longer than 2 weeks	Partial or total laryngectomy

used to visualize the larynx. Roentgenograms of the sinuses may help to establish the diagnosis.

Direct laryngoscopy

A direct laryngoscopy is performed on all persons with suspicious lesions of the larynx.[9] It is usually performed under local anesthesia with 10% cocaine or under general anesthesia. A sedative (for example, secobarbital, meperidine, or other narcotic) and atropine sulfate (to decrease secretions) are given 1 hour before the examination. The person is placed in a reclining position with the head in a head holder or with the head extended over the edge of the table and manually supported by a physician or nurse. The laryngoscope is inserted through the mouth and hypopharynx, making the interior of the larynx easily visible. Minor surgical procedures, such as a biopsy, may be performed through the laryngoscope.

If local anesthesia has been given, the patient should not eat or drink anything until the gag reflex returns, usually within 2 hours. The gag reflex can be tested by touching the back of the throat with a tongue blade or applicator. After the gag reflex returns, the patient should first try to drink water, since if it is accidentally aspirated into the trachea or lungs, it is the fluid least likely to cause aspiration pneumonia.

Surgery

The treatment for metastatic disease of the nose and throat is primarily surgical. Radiation therapy may also be indicated.

MAXILLECTOMY AND ORBITAL EXENTERATION

Surgery for malignancies of the sinuses often consists of removal of the entire upper jaw (maxillectomy) and one eye (orbital exenteration). Split-thickness skin grafts (see Chapter 37) are usually applied to the operative area. Postoperatively, the deformity of the jaw is managed with a dental prosthesis, which closes off the defect in the mouth. Several different prostheses may be needed before a final one fits because of shrinking of the cavity as healing progresses. Radical surgery is required because of the danger of recurrence.

Postoperative care includes the following:
1. Monitor for signs of meningitis (fever, headache, neck rigidity)
2. Provide care related to nasogastric intubation (see Chapter 32)
3. Provide tracheostomy care, if indicated (see Chapter 25)
4. Provide mouth care
   a. Use a gentle spray or oral irrigation
   b. Use saline with hydrogen peroxide, weak sodium bicarbonate, or prescribed antibiotic solution
   c. Aspiration of drainage may be necessary (care is taken to prevent trauma from suction tip)
5. Provide pain medication as needed
6. Give prescribed prophylactic antibiotics
7. Encourage early ambulation
8. Provide emotional support

Persons who undergo radical surgery of this type have a number of emotional adjustments to make.[37,48] The alteration in their physical appearance is readily visible; the person feels conspicuous and different. In addition to disfigurement, the person has all the normal fears of surgery and of cancer. Fear, anger, and grief are normal reactions to the situation. Fear is focused on concerns about the future, the ability to live normally, and also of being rejected. Anger and grief are common responses to the loss and the helplessness to control the loss. Oral communication also may be a problem immediately following surgery, and every effort is made to allow the person to express needs and feelings by writing if necessary. Conveying compassion and concern to the person is important.

LARYNGECTOMY

Partial laryngectomy

If a tumor is limited to portions of the vocal cords or areas just above them, a *partial laryngectomy* may affect a cure. Patients suitable for partial laryngectomy have only one diseased vocal cord, and there is complete mobility of both cords.[9]

The most common technique for partial laryngectomy is a *laryngofissure,* an opening into the larynx through the thyroid cartilage and removal of the involved cord and tumor. As healing takes place, scar tissue fills the defect where the diseased cord was removed and becomes a vibrating surface within the larynx. This tissue permits husky but acceptable speech.

A *hemilaryngectomy* is sometimes performed through the same operative approach as a laryngofissure. One side of the thyroid cartilage behind the true and false vocal cords is also removed. A *supraglottic partial laryngectomy* is performed for carcinoma of the epiglottis and adjacent structures above the level of the true vocal cords. The vocal cords are left intact. The postoperative rehabilitation of persons with these two procedures is more arduous than those with a laryngofissure.

Total laryngectomy

When cancer of the larynx is advanced, total laryngectomy may be performed. This includes removal of the epiglottis, thyroid cartilage, hyoid bone, cricoid cartilage, and three or four rings of the trachea. The pharyngeal opening to the trachea is closed, the anterior wall of the hypopharynx is closed, and the remaining trachea is brought out to the neck wound and sutured to the skin. It forms an opening (permanent tracheostomy) through which the patient breathes (Fig. 24-7).

Preoperative care

The person who is to have a laryngectomy is told by the physician that breathing will occur through a special opening made in the neck and that normal speech will

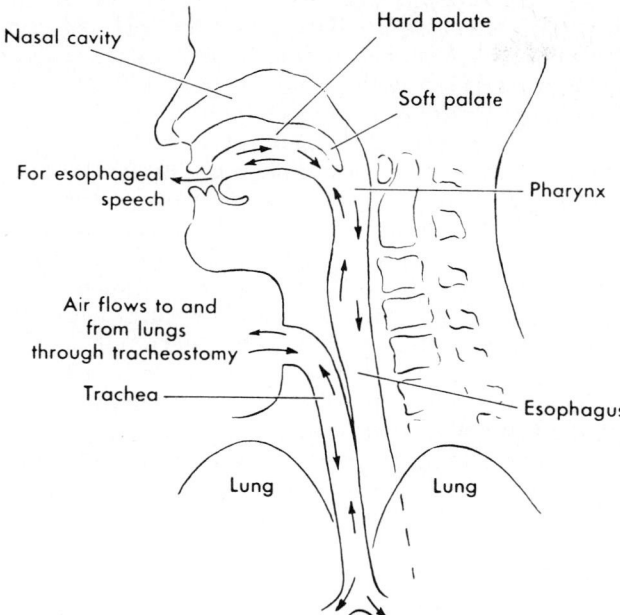

Fig. 24-7. Permanent opening in trachea following total laryngectomy. Note that nose is not used for breathing and that all air enters through tracheostomy opening. Air swallowed through mouth is used to produce laryngeal speech. (Redrawn from Saunders, W.H., et al: Nursing care in eye, ear, nose, and throat disorders, ed. 4, St. Louis, 1979, The C.V. Mosby Co.)

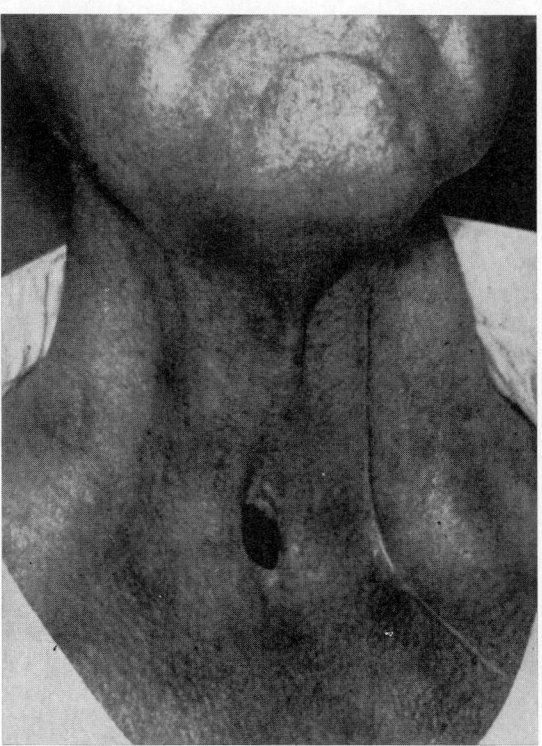

Fig. 24-8. After laryngectomy. Note scars of bilateral radical neck dissections. (From DeWeese, D.D., and Saunders, W.H.: Textbook of otolaryngology, ed. 6, St. Louis, 1982, The C.V. Mosby Co.)

not be possible. This is often depressing to the patient, because it threatens economic status as well as life. In some instances, it is helpful to receive a visit from another person who has made a good recovery from laryngectomy and who has undergone rehabilitation successfully. In other instances, this visit may depress the patient further. Careful assessment must be made to determine if the person will benefit from such a visit and whether the visit should be made preoperatively, immediately after surgery, or later in the recovery period.

Often no one else can give a person the reassurance that speech can be regained as well as a fellow patient. Many large cities have a "Lost Chord Club" or a "New Voice Club," and the members are willing to visit hospitalized patients. Information regarding these clubs may be obtained by writing to the International Association of Laryngectomees.* Local speech rehabilitation centers may supply instructive films and other resources. The local chapter of the American Cancer Society and the local health department also have information available. If possible, the family also should learn about the method of esophageal speech that the person will learn to use.

Postoperative care

Postoperative care of the person is essentially the same as that described for tracheostomy (Chapter 25) except

*American Cancer Society, 777 Third Ave., New York, NY 10017.

that these persons will have a *laryngectomy tube* in place, a tube that is shorter and wider in diameter than a tracheostomy tube. Some patients may not have a tube in the stoma after the operation because the stoma is a permanent one kept open initially by the sutures and because their surgeon believes that there is less tissue reaction and a better stoma if no tube is used. If a laryngectomy tube is used, it will remain until the wound is healed and a permanent fistula has formed, usually in 2 to 3 weeks (Fig. 24-8). Frequent suctioning is necessary in the early postoperative period to keep the trachea free of secretions.

A *nasogastric tube* is usually inserted during the surgical procedure for the instillation of food and fluids at regular intervals postoperatively for about 10 days (Fig. 24-9). The use of the tube to give food is thought to minimize contamination of the pharyngeal and esophageal suture lines and to prevent fluid from leaking through the wound into the trachea before healing occurs. The nasogastric tube is removed as soon as the person can safely swallow. The person then needs careful attention in the first attempts to swallow. There may be the sensation of choking as well as severe coughing that is frightening and painful. Aspiration cannot occur because the trachea no longer communicates with the esophagus.

The sense of smell is affected after laryngectomy because breathing through the nose is impossible, therefore, the patient does not receive olfactory sensations.

Speech rehabilitation

Speech rehabilitation may be started as soon as the esophageal suture line is healed. In addition to the Inter-

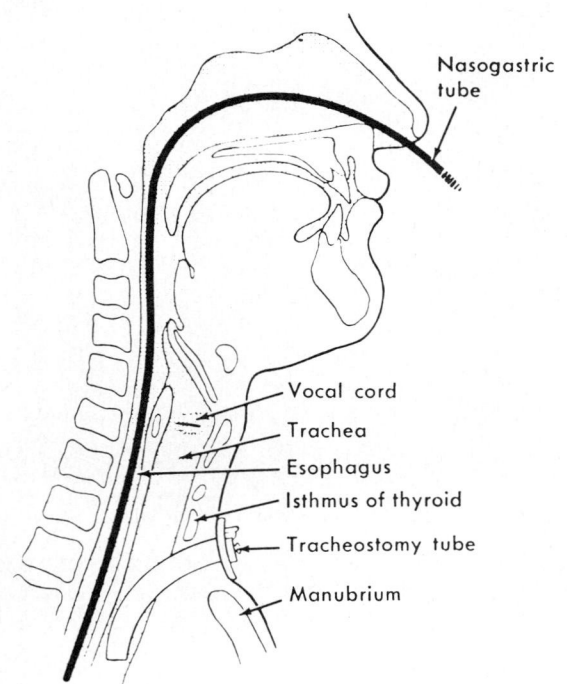

Fig. 24-9. Position of tracheostomy tube and nasogastric tube if both are used.

national Association of Laryngectomees and the local chapter of the American Cancer Society, information on laryngeal speech can be obtained from the American Speech and Hearing Association.*

Most persons learn esophageal speech best at a special clinic. Although some persons may need to go to a nearby city for this instruction, they usually must remain away from home for only 1 to 2 weeks. Motivation and persistent effort are essential in learning this kind of speech; encouragement and support from the professional staff and the person's family and friends are important to the person's morale. About 75% of all persons who have their larynx removed master some sort of speech, and the average person can return to work 1 to 2 months after leaving the hospital.

To learn esophageal speech, the person must first practice burping. This provides the moving column of air needed for sound, while folds of tissue at the opening of the esophagus act as the vibrating surface. The person must learn to coordinate articulation with esophageal vocalization made possible by aspirating air into the esophagus. The new voice sounds are natural although somewhat hoarse. The qualities of speech provided by the use of the nasopharynx are still present, however. The person may have digestive difficulty during the learning period, caused by swallowing air during practice, by unusual strain on abdominal muscles, and by nervous tension. The person can be told that digestive difficulty may occur but that it abates with proficiency in speaking.

If the person is unable to learn esophageal speech in 60 to 90 days after surgery, a speech aid such as a vibra-

---

*American Speech and Hearing Association, 10801 Rockville Pike, Rockville, MD 20852.

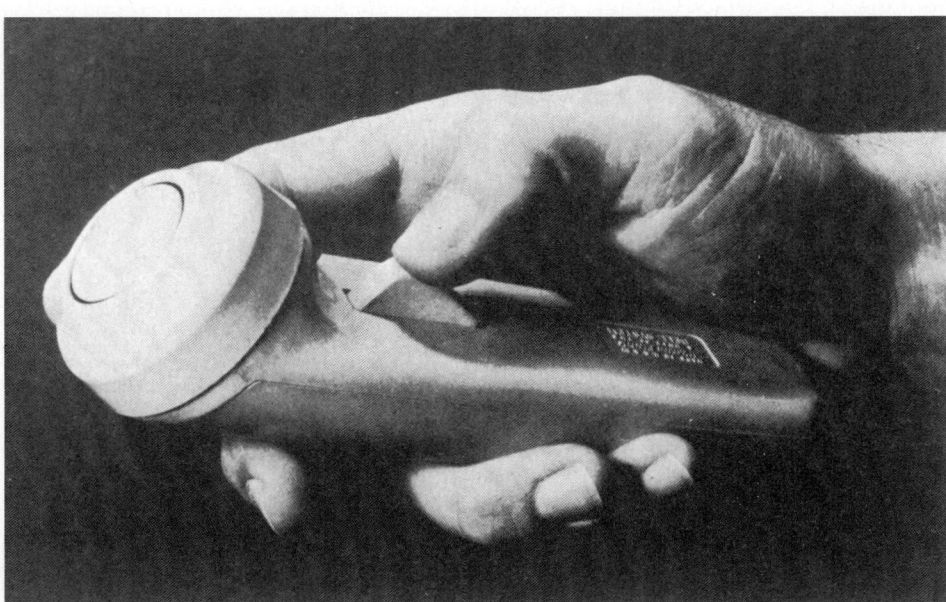

Fig. 24-10. Battery-powered electronic artificial larynx for patient who has total laryngectomy and cannot learn esophageal speech. (Courtesy Illinois Bell Telephone Co.)

tor or an electronic artificial larynx (Fig. 24-10) may be prescribed. Various mechanical devices are available, and the new ones permit a natural type of speech, providing pitch inflections and volume control. The local chapter of the American Cancer Society or the local telephone company can provide information about the purchase of these devices.

Discharge teaching

Persons with laryngectomies must take some special precautions as follows:

1. Care must be taken while bathing or taking a shower that water is not aspirated through the opening into the lungs.
2. Swimming or boat trips may be permitted with precautions; a snorkle device to fit over the stoma is available to laryngectomees so that swimming can be permitted.
3. Persons with laryngectomies are advised to wear a scarf or a shirt with a closed collar that covers the opening, yet is of porous material to warm the air and screen for dust.

Usually by the time of discharge, persons with laryngectomies do not need to be suctioned but can cough up secretions. If suctioning is deemed necessary, the person or family are taught how to provide the care and where to obtain the supplies. Suction equipment can be rented for home use or obtained in many communities through the local chapter of the American Cancer Society.

RADICAL NECK DISSECTION

Radical neck dissection often accompanies total laryngectomy because of the possibility of metastases to the neck from carcinoma of the larynx. It is always indicated when cervical nodes are palpable at the time of surgery. The surgery is aimed primarily at removing the cervical lymph nodes. To do that, the sternocleidomastoid muscle, the internal jugular vein, and spinal accessory nerve have to be sacrificed. These resections cause atrophy of the trapezius muscle, and the shoulder drops on one side.

Persons can be taught to do exercises to gradually replace the function of the lost muscles with other muscles. A person may have some difficulty lifting the head; this can be facilitated by placing the hands behind the head. A mid-Fowler's position can facilitate breathing.

Pressure dressings are best avoided in radical neck dissection because they compromise the blood supply to the skin flaps protecting the vital neck structures. Low suction, such as by a Hemovac, is used to drain fluid and thus prevent pressure on the flaps.

There is some readily visible alteration of appearance that may cause the person to feel somewhat conspicuous. Anger, grief, or denial may be part of the person's normal response to the change in body image.

Radical neck dissection can be performed without laryngectomy for persons whose primary malignant lesion is in the tongue, tonsil, lip, nasopharynx, or thyroid. Often the procedure is termed a *composite resection*. Composite resections may include a radical neck dissection in addition to either the removal of the mandible; removal of the mandible and resection of the floor of the mouth; or removal of the mandible, floor of the mouth, and the tongue. The nursing care for these patients is similar to the care given for maxillectomy and orbital exenteration. Emotional reactions to this type of radical surgery may be profound. Disfigurement is readily visible, and reactions to the change in body are marked.

REFERENCES AND SELECTED READINGS*

1. Argawal, M.K., and others:Fibrosarcoma of nose and paranasal sinuses, J. Surg. Oncol. **15:**53-57, 1980.
2. American Cancer Society: 1984 cancer facts and figures, New York, 1984, The American Cancer Society.
3. *Blues, K.: A framework for nurses providing care to laryngectomy patients, Ca. Nurs. **1:**441-446, 1978.
4. Brown, M.H.: Cancer audit, nursing patient care outcome, audit criteria: laryngectomy with radical neck dissection, Ca. Nurs. **1:**331-334, 1978.
5. Cachin, Y., and others: Nodal metastasis from carcinomas of the oropharynx, Otolaryngol. Clin. North Am. **12:**145-154, 1979.
6. Carpenter, R.J., DeSanto, L.W., and Devine, K.D.: Reconstruction after total laryngopharyngectomy, Arch. Otolaryngol. **105:**417-422, 1979.
7. Conservation surgery of the larynx (clinical conference), Clin. Bull. **10:**70-75, 1980.
8. *Daly, K.M.: Oral cancer, everyday concerns, Am. J. Nurs. **79:**1415-1417, 1979.
9. DeWeese, D.D., and Saunders, W.H.: Textbook of otolaryngology, ed. 6, St. Louis, 1982, The C.V. Mosby Co.
10. *Dropkin, M.J.: Compliant behavior and changed body image, Am. J. Nurs. **79:**1294, 1979.
11. *Dupont, J.: Ambulatory nursing, EENT emergencies, Nurs. 79 **9**(11):65-70, 1979.
12. Elman, A.J., and others: In situ carcinoma of the vocal cords, Cancer **43:**2422-2428, 1979.
13. *Ewing, D.: Electronic larynx for aphonic patients, Am. J. Nurs. **75:**2153-2157, 1975.
14. Fiumara, N.J.: Pharyngeal infection with Neisseria gonorrhoeae, Sex. Transm. Dis. **6:**264-266, 1979.
15. *Gannon, E.P.: Giving your patient meticulous mouth care, Nurs. 80 **10**(3):70-75, 1980.
16. *Gardner, M.E.: Notes from a waiting room, Am. J. Nurs. **80:**86-89, 1980.
17. Glazer, D.C.: Audiologic management of head and neck carcinoma patients, J. Speech Hear. Disord. **45:**216-222, 1980.
18. *Honeysett, J.: Epistaxis, Nurs. Times **78**(14):578-581, 1982.
19. Howard, J.C., and others: Effectiveness of antihistamines in the symptomatic management of the common cold, JAMA **242:**2414-2417, 1979.
20. *Hutchinson, R.: The common cold primer, Nurs. 79 **9**(3):57-61, 1979.

---

*References preceded by an asterisk are particularly well suited for student reading.

21. Hybels, R.L.: Selected new techniques of laryngeal surgery, Sur. Clin. North Am. **60:**637-647, 1980.

22. Johnson, J.T., Newman, R.K., and Olson, J.E.: Persistent hoarseness: an aggressive approach for early detection of laryngeal cancer, Postgrad. Med. **67:**122-126, 1980.

23. *Kaur, H.: Nursing care study: a lump in his throat, Nurs. Mirror **154**(25):36-38, 1982.

24. Keeling, B.: Giving and getting the courage to face death, Nurs. 78 **8**(11):38-41, 1978.

25. *Kerth, C.C.: Wound management following head and neck surgery, Nurs. Clin. North Am. **14:**761-778, 1979.

26. Key, G.: Stopping nosebleeds in the elderly: pressure, cautery, or packing? Geriatrics **36:**74-80, 1981.

27. Kraus, S.J.: Incidence and therapy of gonococcal pharyngitis, Sex. Transm. Dis. **6:**143-147, 1979.

28. *Larsen, G.L.: Rehabilitation for the patient with head and neck cancer, Am. J. Nurs. **82:**119-120, 1982.

29. Liston, S.L., and Siegel, L.G.: Nasal and sinus disorders in the elderly: which ones are life-threatening? Geriatrics **36:**91-102, 1981.

30. *Masterson, A.: Larynx reconstruction, Nurs. 79 **9**(3):78-80, 1979.

31. *McConnell, E.A.: How to truly help the patient with radical neck dissection, Nurs. 76 **6:**58-65, 1976.

32. *McCormick, G.P., and others: Artificial speech devices, Am. J. Nurs. **82:**121-122, 1982.

33. Moore, J.C.: Establishment of an outpatient ENT clinic, AORN J. **31:**620-626, 1980.

34. *Newman, M.: Nursing care study: carcinoma of the lateral wall of the nose, Nurs. Mirror **147**(18):24-26, 1978.

35. Newmann, R.K., and Johnson, J.T.: Nasal airway obstruction: approach to diagnosis and treatment, Postgrad. Med. **68:**184-190, 1980.

36. *Nicholson, E.: Personal notes of a laryngectomee, Am. J. Nurs. **75:**2157-2158, 1975.

37. *Oser, J.: Oral cancer; coping with the changes, Am. J. Nurs. **79:**1418-1419, 1979.

38. Streptococcal pharyngitis, Compr. Ther. **5:**51-58, 1979.

39. *Price J.: Oral health for the geriatric patient, J. Geriatr. Nurs. **5**(2):25-29, 1979.

40. Russ, J.E.: Management of osteosarcoma of maxilla and mandible, Am. J. Surg. **14:**572-576, 1980.

41. Schwartz, S.L.: Carotid catastrophe, Am. J. Nurs. **79:**1566-1567, 1979.

42. *Schweiger, J.L.: Oral assessment, Am. J. Nurs. **80:**654-657, 1980.

43. Sheehan, M.: Reflections of a cancer nurse, Ca. Nurs. **1:**309-311, 1978.

44. Steiner, W.: Techniques of diagnostic and operative endoscopy of the head and neck, Endoscopy **11:**51-59, 1979.

45. Stone, J.W.: External rhinoplasty, Laryngoscope **90:**1626-1630, 1980.

46. *Stuart, M.: Skin flaps and grafts after head and neck surgery, Am. J. Nurs. **78:**1368-1375, 1978.

47. Symposium on reconstruction of the larynx and trachea, Otolaryngol. Clin. North Am. **12:**735-917, 1979.

48. *Tierney, E.: Accepting disfigurement when death is the alternative, Am. J. Nurs. **75:**2149-2150, 1975.

49. *Trowbridge, J., and Williams, C.: Oral care of the patient having head and neck irradiation, Am. J. Nurs. **75:**2146-2149, 1975.

50. *Wegmann, J.A., and Ogrinc, M.: Oncology nursing conflict: a case presentation of holistic care and the family in crisis, Ca. Nurs. **4**(1):43-48, 1981.

51. *Wong, R.: Sore throat, Am. J. Nurs. **77:**1796-1798, 1977.

52. Yarington, C.T., Jr.: Sinusitis as an emergency, Otolaryngol. Clin. North Am. **12:**447-454, 1979.

53. Zapka, J., and Averill, B.W.: Self-care for colds: a cost-effective alternative to upper respiratory infection management, Am. J. Public Health **69:**814-816, 1979.

PATIENT INFORMATION

Helping words for the laryngectomee (Brochure, 26 pages, free), International Association of Laryngectomees, 777 Third Ave. New York, NY 10017.

Looking forward: a guidebook for the laryngectomee, (Brochure, 56 pages, small charge) Schmidt Printing Inc., 1416 Valley High Dr., Rochester, MN 55901.

25

The Patient with Pulmonary Problems

WILMA J. PHIPPS

STUDY QUESTIONS

- What is the quality of air in the community in which you reside? if air pollution is a problem, what are the major contributing factors (industries, automobile exhaust, and so on)? Are there community groups working to improve the problem? If so, what activities are they involved in and how might a nurse be helpful to their efforts?

- Where is the branch of the American Cancer Society and the American Lung Association nearest your community? What services do they provide for health professionals and for patients?

- What is the tuberculosis case rate in the area in which you live? Is this higher or lower than the national rate of 11/100,000 population? List the factors that contribute to a higher or lower case rate in your community.

- List the services available in your community to assist persons who wish to stop smoking and to which you could refer patients or friends.

- Design a teaching plan or project that you believe would help convince teenagers they should not smoke. Would you use a different approach for females than for males?

- Plan a 3,000-calorie, high-protein diet for a 60-year-old man with pulmonary emphysema who is very short of breath and finds eating to be a chore.

ANATOMY AND PHYSIOLOGY OF THE RESPIRATORY TRACT

The main purpose of respiration is to provide oxygen to body cells and to remove excess carbon dioxide from them. For respiration to take place there must be a way to deliver oxygen (O_2) to the body and a circulatory system to carry it to the cells and to remove carbon dioxide (CO_2) from them. The transport of O_2 is accomplished through the upper and lower airway.

The upper airway consists of the nose and nasopharynx, mouth and oropharynx, and the larynx. The lower airway is made up of the trachea, mainstem bronchi, bronchioles, and alveolar ducts, which lead to the alveoli themselves. The airway, in addition to providing a passageway for air, serves three functions: *filtering, warming,* and *humidifying* air.

Air inspired through an intact respiratory tree is cleansed of all particles larger than $2\mu m$ in diameter before reaching the alveolus. The removal of this particulate matter, such a dust and bacteria, preserves the sterility of the alveolus. Foreign material is filtered through several mechanisms. *Goblet cells* in the epithelial layer of the airway secrete copious amounts of a thick mucopolysaccharide substance, mucus, which coats the airways and entraps particles. *Cilia,* which are found as far into the respiratory tree as the bronchi, then propel the mucus and foreign material up into the pharynx where it can be expelled by coughing or sneezing.

The *warming* and *humidifying* functions are made possible by the rich capillary blood supply in the submucosal layer of the airways. During inspiration, air is heated to body temperature, and up to 1000 ml of water is used per day to raise the humidity of the inspired air to at least 80%. On expiration some of this water is reabsorbed, thus conserving fluid; an average of 300 ml per day is lost in normal respiration.

The basic gas exchange unit of the respiratory system is the alveolus. Alveoli, which number over 300 million in the healthy adult, are minute sacs that arise from alveolar ducts. The ducts are composed of smooth muscle that is capable of expanding and contracting; the alveolus itself is composed of a single layer of squamous epithelium and an elastic basement membrane. These two layers, in addition to the endothelial and basement layers of the adjacent capillary, form the *alveolar-capillary membrane* or *interface.* It is across this membrane, a distance of less than $1\mu m$, that gas exchange takes place.

The lungs themselves are subdivided into lobes (Fig. 25-1). The right lung has three lobes: upper, middle, and lower. The left lung has two lobes: upper and lower. Air is conducted to each lobe through lobar bronchi that branch off the mainstem bronchus. An important difference between the right and left lungs is the size of the airways leading to them. The right bronchus is significantly wider and shorter and extends at a straighter angle from the trachea, making it the more likely lodging point for aspirated material. The left bronchus is narrower and extends at more of a right angle off the trachea, making

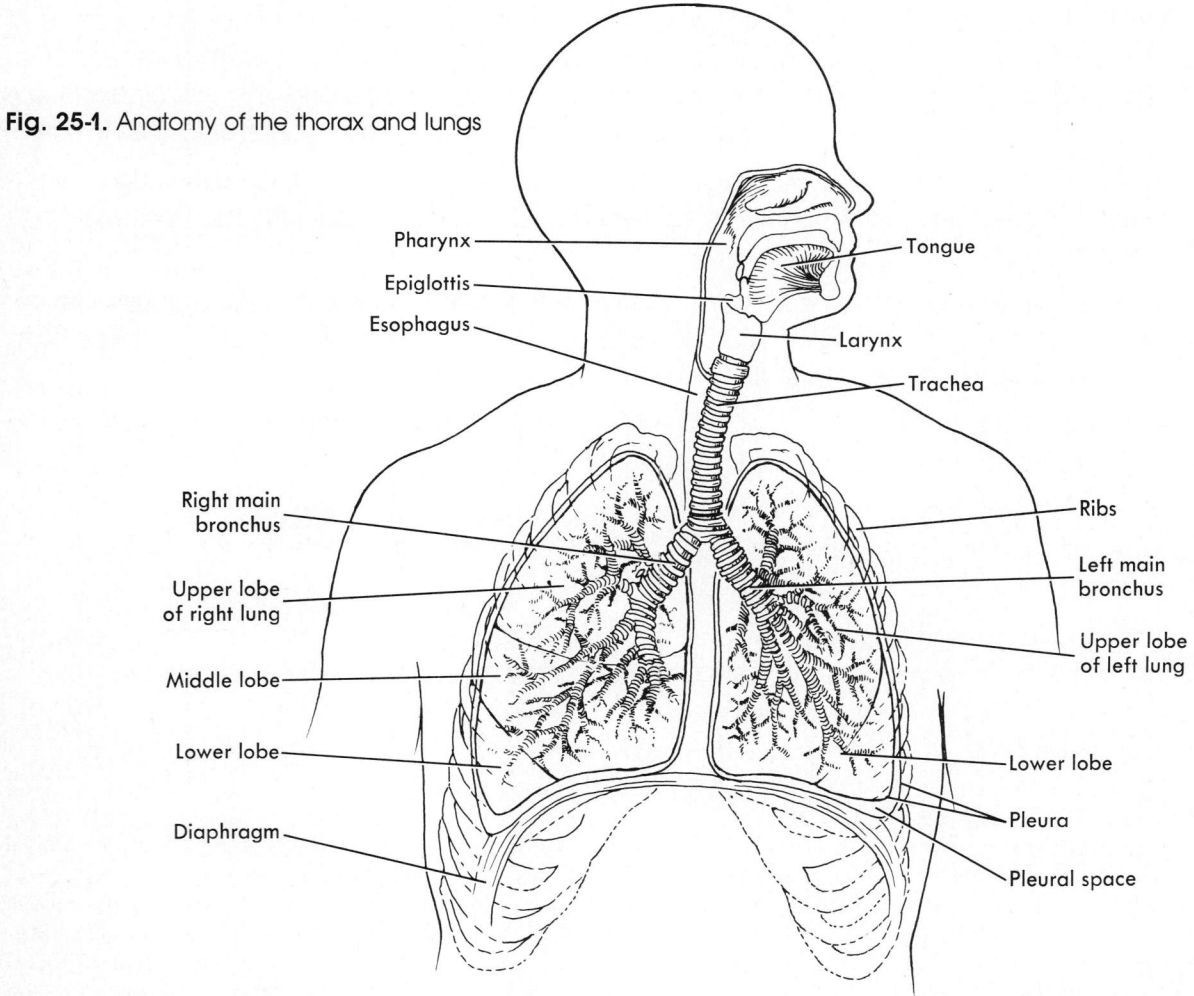

Fig. 25-1. Anatomy of the thorax and lungs

it more difficult to suction secretions from the left lung.

The lungs lie in and are protected by the thoracic cavity. This bony cage is composed of the sternum and ribs anteriorly and the ribs, scapulae, and vertebral column posteriorly. On the anterior surface, the apices of the lungs lie just above the clavicle and extend posteriorly to the eleventh or twelfth rib.

The thoracic cavity is lined with pleurae. The pleura is a continuous *serous* membrane, one surface of which lines the inside of the rib cage (parietal pleura) while the other surface (visceral pleura) covers the lungs. The space between the two surfaces is known as a *potential space*. It normally contains a few milliliters of serous fluid that prevents friction rub when the two surfaces come together.

There are three processes involved in respiration. These are ventilation, perfusion, and diffusion. *Ventilation* involves the movement of air in and out of the tracheobroncheal tree, thereby delivering oxygen to the alveoli and removing carbon dioxide. *Perfusion* refers to the blood flow in the capillary bed in the lung. Fear or an injection of adrenalin increases perfusion while vagal stimulation or acetylcholine decreases it. During *diffusion* there is movement of gases (O_2 and CO_2) across the alveolarcapillary membrane, with the flow being from the area of greater concentration to that of lesser concentration, resulting in alveocapillary equilibrium.

Pulmonary ventilation

Air moves in and out of the lungs as a result of the principle of fluid flow; that is, movement is from an area of greater pressure to an area of lower pressure. At the start of inspiration the atmospheric air pressure is greater than alveolar pressure; therefore air moves through the respiratory passageway into the alveoli. When the alveolar pressure exceeds atmospheric pressure, expiration occurs, and air moves out of the lungs into the atmosphere.

The pressure gradient between the alveoli and the atmosphere is established by changes in the size of the thoracic cavity. As the size of the thorax increases, pressure decreases, and air flows into the lung. Thoracic size is increased by contraction of the diaphragm and the external intercostal muscles. The diaphragm descends as it contracts and flattens, increasing the longitudinal diameter of the thorax. The external intercostal muscles pull the ribs up and out, elevating the sternum and increasing both the anteroposterior and lateral diameters of the chest. The accessory muscles (scalene, sternocleidomastoid, trapezius, and pectoralis) are active only in labored respiration.

As the thorax expands, it pulls the lungs with it because of cohesion between the moist surfaces of the lungs and chest wall. Expiration is normally a passive process that results from the elastic recoil of the lungs and thoracic muscles. Any condition that interferes with contraction of the diaphragm or intercostal muscles will decrease pulmonary ventilation.

Control of respiration

Breathing is an automatic process but it may also be controlled voluntarily; that is, humans do not have to think about breathing but can breathe slower or faster at will. Voluntary control of respiration is centered in the cerebral cortex, from which impulses are sent to innervate the muscles of respiration.

Automatic control of respiration is centered in the medulla and pons. The pons is responsible for maintaining rhythmicity of respirations. The respiratory center that is located in the medulla is controlled primarily by the carbon dioxide tension (PCO_2), oxygen tension (PO_2), and acidity (pH) of arterial blood (p. 599). Chemoreceptors in the carotid bodies (near the carotid bifurcation) and aortic bodies (near the arch of the aorta) are stimulated by a rise in PCO_2 or by a fall in PO_2 or pH of arterial blood (more acid), leading to an increase in respiratory rate. Additional chemoreceptors near the medulla are sensitive to small changes in PCO_2. Other factors that influence respirations include emotions, pain, stretching of the anal sphincter, and stimulation of the pharynx or larynx.

Gas exchange in the lung

In the alveoli, oxygen diffuses across the alveolarcapillary membrane from the alveoli into the blood because the partial pressure of oxygen (oxygen tension, PO_2) of *alveolar air* (100 mm Hg) is greater than the PO_2 of venous blood (40 mm Hg). Carbon dioxide diffuses in the opposite direction because the PCO_2 of *venous blood* (46 mm Hg) is greater than the PCO_2 of alveolar air (40 mm Hg). The pulmonary diffusion capacity for carbon dioxide is much greater than the capacity for oxygen, and thus carbon dioxide diffuses more easily. Diffusion capacity of oxygen is decreased by the lower PO_2 of atmospheric air (high altitudes), by decreased surface area in the alveoli, or by decreased alveolar ventilation volumes (amount of oxygen reaching the alveoli).

Oxygen—carbon dioxide exchange

For breathing to take place normally, several factors are necessary: (1) an adequate supply of oxygen in the environment, (2) a patent airway, (3) a normally functioning bellows motion of the chest wall and diaphragm, (4) an adequate number of functioning alveoli and capillaries that together form a terminal respiratory unit (TRU), (5) an adequate amount of hemoglobin to carry oxygen to the cells, (6) an intact circulatory system and an effective heart pump, and (7) a functioning respiratory center. Problems in one or more of these can result in inadequate exchange of oxygen and carbon dioxide and, if severe enough, can cause death. Table 25-1 lists some of the conditions than can lead to inadequate oxygencarbon dioxide exchange. Each of these factors is discussed here.

Table 25-1. Factors interfering with oxygenation and normal oxygen–carbon dioxide exchange

Necessary component	Interference
Adequate supply of oxygen	Inhalation of air containing oxygen at subnormal pressure caused by: Smoke inhalation Carbon monoxide poisoning High altitudes Dilution of inspired air with inert gases (nitrogen, helium, hydrogen, methane, or anesthetic gases such as nitrous oxide)
Patent airway	Interference with the passage of oxygen from air through tracheobronchial tree to alveolar-capillary membrane caused by mechanical obstruction such as drowning, foreign bodies in tracheobronchial tree: Children (aspiration of objects such as pennies, pins, jacks) Unconscious adults (tongue obstructing airway, aspirated vomitus, loose dentures) Mucus plug resulting in atelectasis Allergic reactions resulting in bronchoconstriction, increased mucus secretions, and increased capillary permeability
Normally functioning bellows	Trauma to chest wall with possible sequelae of paradoxical breathing, pneumothorax, mediastinal shift Muscle or nerve trauma or impairment (quadriplegia, paraplegia, poliomyelitis, myasthenia gravis, Guillain-Barré-Strohl syndrome, Landry ascending paralysis, muscular dystrophy)
Adequate functioning alveoli and capillaries (TRU)	Pulmonary edema Adult respiratory disease syndrome (interstitial edema) Physiologic shunts Damage to alveolar-capillary membrane secondary to conditions such as pulmonary emphysema
Adequate amount of hemoglobin	Severe anemia Carbon monoxide poisoning Methemoglobinemia
Intact circulatory system and pump	Congestive heart failure Hemorrhage
Functioning respiratory center	Depression of respiratory center by drugs (heroin, morphine, barbiturates, alcohol, or a combination of alcohol with a tranquilizer or barbiturates) Increased intracranial pressure (head injury or disease such as meningitis)

MAINTAINING AN ADEQUATE SUPPLY OF OXYGEN IN THE ENVIRONMENT

High altitudes do not change the composition of the air, but the oxygen pressure (PO_2) decreases.[54] Persons exposed to high altitudes, such as pilots, astronauts, mountain climbers, and those moving to high altitudes, will have various reactions depending on the rate at which hypoxia develops, the degree of oxygen requirements as determined by physical exertion, and the duration of exposure.[54]

The initial reaction to high altitudes results in the same signs and symptoms seen in anyone experiencing oxygen lack. Headache, dizziness, breathlessness, weakness, nausea, sweating, palpitation, dimness of vision, partial deafness, and sleeplessness occur with moderate hypoxia.[54] With exertion, dyspnea and other symptoms worsen. These signs and symptoms have been referred to as *mountain sickness* since they are evident as persons drive or take a train through higher altitudes than they have been accustomed to.

These symptoms gradually disappear over days or weeks depending on the altitude, and the person will be able to carry out more activities without becoming short of breath. This is known as *acclimatization* and is caused in part by an increased capacity for supplying oxygen to the tissues and in part by overcoming the consequences of hypocapnia produced by excessive breathing.[54]

The factors involved in acclimatization include (1) a sustained increase in alveolar ventilation, (2) adjustment in the acid-base composition of the blood and other body fluids, (3) an increase in oxygen-carrying capacity, and (4) an increase in cardiac output.[54]

Persons moving to higher climates, such as mountain climbers, are advised to allow time for their bodies to adjust to changes in various altitudes. Trained climbers, especially those ascending to very high altitudes, allow themselves weeks or even months at base camps at various altitudes in preparation for their ascent.[54]

MAINTAINING A PATENT AIRWAY

Several measures may be used to ensure a patent airway. The most basic measure involves simply positioning the person in such a way as to prevent obstruction of the airway. This is most relevant in resuscitation or in caring for an unconscious person. The position of choice is supine or side-lying with neck hyperextended. Persons who are unconscious or very lethargic may suffer airway obstruction if the tongue is allowed to fall back and cover the glottis; the side-lying position prevents this from happening (see Fig. 19-14).

When a person has a mechanical obstruction of the airway and is expected to be unconscious for some time, it may be necessary to use an artificial airway (p. 613).

MAINTAINING BELLOWS FUNCTION OF THE CHEST WALL AND DIAPHRAGM

Whenever there is interference with the bellows function of the chest wall, there will be changes in the breathing pattern. The major cause of disruption of the bellows function is trauma to the chest involving fractures of the ribs or penetrating chest wounds (p. 592). These conditions and their sequelae of paradoxic breathing and pneumothorax are discussed on p. 593.

MAINTAINING AN ADEQUATE NUMBER OF TERMINAL RESPIRATORY UNITS

The individual with pulmonary disease may have impaired ability to aerate alveoli. The impairment may be related to several factors. These include (1) inability to move adequate amounts of air in and out of the lungs, (2) interference with alveolar expansion secondary to an accumulation of secretions resulting in collapse of portions of the lungs (*atelectasis*), and (3) restriction of lung expansion by mechanical factors such as air in the pleural space (*pneumothorax*) or fluid or blood in the pleural space (*pleural effusion* or *hemothorax*). An increase in respiratory rate and pulse rate indicates that the body is trying to compensate for hypoxia. Patients who must make a conscious effort to breathe become very tired. They also become very anxious because of shortness of breath and hypoxia.

MAINTAINING TRANSPORTATION OF OXYGEN AND ADEQUATE OXYGENATION OF TISSUES

For oxygen to be supplied to the cells there must be (1) an adequate amount of hemoglobin available to transport oxygen and (2) an effective heart pump and circulatory system to deliver the oxygen to the tissues. The amount of oxygen delivered to body tissues each minute equals the cardiac output in liters per minute times the number of milliliters of oxygen contained in 1 L of arterial blood. In the resting state this is about 5×200, or 1000 ml O_2/min. About one fourth of this is used by the tissues, and three fourths returns to the heart in mixed venous blood. During exercise the amount of oxygen contained in 1 L of arterial blood does not increase, but the cardiac output does increase. With a cardiac output of 24 L/min, the oxygen delivered would be 24×200, or 4800 ml/min. The tissues would use three fourths of this amount, and only one fourth would be returned to the heart in mixed venous blood.[110]

An inadequate amount of hemoglobin, such as occurs in anemia, or an inadequate heart pump, or a problem with the circulatory system can each have a deleterious effect on the delivery of oxygen. In these situations the basic problem is treated in an attempt to increase the amount of available hemoglobin, to strengthen the heart pump and thus increase the cardiac output, or to improve the circulatory system. As can be seen in Table 25-1, severe anemia, carbon monoxide poisoning, methemoglobinemia, congestive heart failure, and hemorrhage are possible interferences that will need to be corrected before an optimal amount of oxygen will be available to the tissues.

If hypotension is present secondary to hemorrhage or a failing heart pump there may be several sequelae. These include (1) anginal pain, since the coronary vessels that normally extract almost the maximal amount of oxygen from the blood cannot significantly increase oxygen uptake to meet their needs and (2) changes in sensorium and behavior secondary to cerebral anoxia. If this situation continues and there is inadequate oxygenation of tissues, respiratory or cardiac arrest may result. If an arrest occurs, cardiopulmonary resuscitation (CPR) must be instituted. CPR is discussed in detail in Chapter 26, and the reader is referred there for details.

MAINTAINING A FUNCTIONING RESPIRATORY CENTER

Hypoventilation or apnea can occur if there is depression of the respiratory center by general anesthesia, morphine, heroin, barbiturates, or alcohol. Diseases of the central nervous system, such as bulbar poliomyelitis or meningitis, also will depress the respiratory center, as will an increase in intracranial pressure. In these situations the patient's respirations will have to be assisted until the patient is able to maintain his/her own breathing. Intubation with an endotracheal tube, supplemental oxygen, and artificial respiration with a ventilator may all be required. The conditions causing depression of the respiratory center will need to be identified and treated while the person's ventilation is being maintained. Details of management of patients in respiratory failure are discussed on p. 612.

PHYSIOLOGIC CHANGES WITH AGING

Several changes occur in the lungs and other parts of the respiratory tract with aging.

Structural alterations in the thorax may limit lung expansion. Ribs do not move as freely because of cartilage calcification and partial contraction of respiratory muscles.[25] Kyphosis (hunchback) decreases the transverse measurement of the thorax.

The lungs become more rigid and less elastic. There is an increase in residual capacity and a decrease in vital capacity secondary to a decrease in the strength of the inspiratory and expiratory muscles. The result is incomplete lung expansion and basilar lung collapse. These changes may *not* cause an obvious decrease in lung performance unless there is an increase in activity or stress when dyspnea and other symptoms occur.[25]

As a result of these changes the aged are very vulnerable if they develop a pulmonary infection or other illness that places stress on their already compromised respiratory system.

Because of the changes in the thorax and altered muscle strength there is less ability to clear the airway and cough effectively.

PREVENTION AND HEALTH EDUCATION

Disorders of the respiratory tract are probably the most common health problems for most persons in the Western world.

The objectives of health education in relation to pulmonary diseases are the same as for other diseases. Prevention, early diagnosis, prompt and often continued treatment, limitation of disability, and rehabilitation should be emphasized for all persons. Early symptoms of respiratory diseases are probably those most often ignored by the general population. Perhaps this is because, with the exception of influenza and some types of pneumonia, respiratory diseases often develop slowly and progress without the individual's awareness.

Because of the deleterious effects of cigarette smoking on the cardiopulmonary systems, a concerted effort is indicated to teach persons about the hazards of smoking. In recent years many organizations, but most notably the American Lung Association (ALA), the American Cancer Society (ACS), the American Heart Association (AHA), and the federal government have launched campaigns to reduce cigarette smoking in the United States. A major emphasis has been on preventing children and teenagers from beginning to smoke. These campaigns have been somewhat successful, and it is now estimated that only one third of the adult population in the United States smokes. However, the number of women smokers has increased, and this is reflected in the ever-rising increase in morbidity and mortality from lung disease, especially cancer of the lung and chronic obstructive pulmonary diseases, among women.

Primary prevention: prevention of disease

Since the cause of many respiratory disorders is known, prevention is possible. The major emphasis is on

---

Prevention of respiratory infections

Preventing spread of infection

1. Isolate the infected person
2. Teach the infected person to cover nose and mouth when coughing or sneezing so that droplet nuclei are not released into the air

Maintaining resistance to infection

1. Eat a balanced diet
2. Get adequate rest and sleep
3. Avoid crowds during periods of prevalent respiratory infections
4. Receive annual influenza immunization if over age 65 or if younger with chronic heart, lung, or renal disease

---

Early detection of major pulmonary disorders

1. Signs or symptoms requiring immediate medical follow-up
   a. Chronic cough
   b. Sputum
   c. Dyspnea (shortness of breath)
2. American Cancer Society recommendations for screening for cancer of the lung
   a. Yearly chest x-ray examination for men over age 40
   b. Yearly examination for heavy cigarette smokers over age 50, for persons who started smoking at age of 15 or less, and for smokers working in or near asbestos

avoiding respiratory infections and educating the public about the risks of cigarette smoking. Health practices helpful in preventing infection are outlined in upper box on p. 548.

Secondary prevention: early detection

Medical attention should be sought for respiratory symptoms that do not subside within 2 weeks. Guidelines for early detection are listed in lower box on p. 548.

Major health problems of the respiratory system

There are several ways to classify disorders affecting the lung and respiration but one of the most useful and commonly used is to divide them into restrictive and obstructive diseases.

In *restrictive lung disease* there is a restriction in lung volume and a reduction in lung compliance. As a result there is a reduction in total lung capacity (TLC) and a decrease in vital capacity (VC) to less than predicted normal.

In contrast, in *obstructive lung disease* there is an increase in airway resistance resulting in prolonged exhalation. This results in an increase in residual volume (RV) while TLC may be normal or increased. Thus pulmonary function tests are necessary to establish the diagnosis. A comparison of the characteristic changes in pulmonary function tests for restrictive and obstructive disease is shown Table 25-2.

There are several conditions that can cause restrictive pulmonary disease and not all of these will be discussed here. Some of the conditions that will *not* be discussed include atelectasis; fluid or air in the pleural space;

Table 25-2. Comparison of pulmonary function test results in restrictive and obstructive disease

Test	Restrictive	Obstructive
FVC	Decreased	Decreased or normal
RV	Decreased	Increased
TLC	Decreased	Normal or increased
RV/TLC	Normal or increased	Significantly increased
$FEV_{1.0}$/FVC	Normal or increased	Decreased
$FEV_{3.0}$/FVC	Normal or increased	Decreased

From Morrissey, W: Respiratory diseases. In Kaye, D., and Rose, L.F., eds.: Fundamentals of internal medicine, St. Louis, 1983, The C.V. Mosby Co.

changes in the bony thorax, such as kyphoscoliosis, limitation of thoracic mobility from abdominal tumors, ascites, or paralytic ileus; neuromuscular depression from disease or drugs, that is, Guillian-Barré syndrome, poliomyelitis, myasthenia gravis, and CNS depression from heroin or morphine.

Conditions that result in restrictive or obstructive pulmonary disease that will be discussed in this chapter are the following.

I. Restrictive pulmonary disorders
  A. Infectious diseases of the pulmonary tract
    1. Viral: acute bronchitis
    2. Bacterial: pneumonia, tuberculosis
    3. Fungal: histoplasmosis, coccidiomycosis, blastomycosis
  B. Occupational lung disease
    1. Inhalation of inorganic dust: silicosis
    2. Inhalation of organic dust: allergic alveolitis (farmer's lung)
  C. Adult respiratory distress syndrome (ARDS)
  D. Carcinoma of the lung
II. Obstructive pulmonary disorders
  A. Chronic bronchitis
  B. Pulmonary emphysema
  C. Asthma

RESTRICTIVE PULMONARY DISORDERS

Infectious diseases of the pulmonary tract

For an infection of the lung to occur, pathogens must be able to enter the lower respiratory tract. This means that the defense mechanisms of the lung must be overcome in some manner. There are many lung defense mechanisms including upper airway defenses, lower respiratory tract clearance mechanisms, and intrapulmonary detoxification mechanisms. These mechanisms are outlined on pp. 550-551.

VIRAL INFECTIONS

Many respiratory diseases are probably caused by viral infections. Presently, over 30 diseases have been found to be directly related to viral infections, and there are probably many more. Some diseases may be caused by one virus, or different viruses may cause the same symptoms.

If specific signs are not evident, the clinical illness is termed a common cold, viral infection, fever of unknown origin (FUO), or acute respiratory illness. The most common specific respiratory diseases caused by the various viruses are epidemic pleurodynia (Bornholm's disease), acute laryngotracheobronchitis, viral pneumonia, and influenza. Most adults have developed antibodies for the more common viruses, and most viral infections are relatively mild. However, they are frequently complicated by secondary bacterial infections. When new strains of the influenza virus develop, severe epidemics may ensue, and many people may die from secondary infections such as pneumonia.

Lung defense mechanisms

I. Upper airway defenses against pulmonary infection
  A. Removing particulate matter from inspired air
    1. Particles greater than 20 μm settle back on surfaces
    2. Particles 5-10 μm deposited in nose
    3. Particles 0.1-10 μm remain suspended in air for long periods and are then inhaled
    4. Particles 1-5 μm deposited in tracheobronchial tree
      a. Droplet nuclei 2-4 μm (dried particles from sneezing, coughing, talking)
      b. May contain viruses or bacteria
      c. Spread organisms from person to person
  B. Minimizing the microbial population on membranes of upper respiratory tract
    1. Mucociliary transport
      a. Posterior two thirds of nasal cavity, sinuses, and nasopharynx lined by *ciliated epithelium* covered with thin layer of mucus
      b. Dense concentration of small blood vessels present beneath ciliated epithelium and mucous layers
      c. Mucus and fluid produced = 1000 ml/24 hr in normal persons
      d. Mucus and fluid carried at rate of 5-10 mm/min back into hypopharynx by beating action of cilia
      e. Substances in secretions inhibit microbial growth and prevent organisms from sticking to mucous membranes
        (1) Immunoglobulins (secretory IgA)
        (2) Lysozyme
        (3) Complement
  C. Minimizing possibility of aspiration
    1. Motor function of upper airway
      a. Laryngeal mechanism—closes glottis when swallowing to protect larynx
        (1) Gag reflex also closes glottis
        (2) Clearing throat, spitting, clear upper airway
    2. Contamination of lower respiratory tract
      a. Impaired clearance of particles in upper airway = spread of bacteria
      b. Accumulation of debris and microbes → penetration of tissues = sinusitis, otitis media
      c. Accumulation of debris and microbes → aspiration into trachea; lung abscess caused by anaerobic bacteria secondary to severe gingival disease
      d. Intoxication or distraction → aspiration
      e. Normal sleep → minor aspiration
      f. Aspiration of pharyngeal contents → lung → bacterial pneumonia
II. Lower respiratory tract clearance mechanisms
  A. Pulmonary reflex
    1. Cough—an involuntary reflex elicited by stimulation of irritant receptors in subepithelium of hypopharynx, larynx, and tracheobronchial tree: mediated by vagus nerve
      a. Facilitator of mucociliary clearance
      b. Aids in dealing with gross contamination from above larynx
    2. Bronchoconstriction—reflex response to airway irritants
      a. Decreased size of bronchus and forced expiration and cough propel debris toward mouth
      b. Excessive bronchoconstriction (asthma) = decreased expiratory airflow, air trapped in lung, effective cough difficult
  B. Mucociliary clearance
    1. Mucus secreted by epithelial goblet cells from submucosal glands 0.10-100 ml passes up trachea into hypopharynx and is swallowed; amount and nature of mucus secreted are controlled, in part, by parasympathetic nervous system affected by neurohumoral stimulation (adrenergic or cholinergic), and by direct mucosal irritation
    2. Cilia (200 cilia/each cell surface) beat rhythmically 1200 beats/min mouthward beginning at terminal bronchioles → larynx; beating of cilia → overlying mucous layer → mouthward at rate of 0.5 mm/min in small airways to about 10 mm/min in major bronchi
    3. Clearance increased by:
    a. Bronchodilator drugs
      (1) β-Adrenergic agents (ephedrine) stimulate transport of water and salt into mucus = ↓ viscosity of mucous
      (2) Methylxanthines (aminophylline)— ↑ mucous production and ciliary activity

Adapted from Light, B.: Respiratory infections. In Kryger, M.H., editor: Pathophysiology of respiration, New York, 1981, John Wiley & Sons, Inc.

4. Ciliary function depressed by:
   a. Chronic exposure to airway irritants—cigarette smoke and other irritants
   b. Pharmacologic agents—100% O_2, anticholinergic agents, alcohol
   c. Infection such as viral bronchitis
5. Mucous production increased by:
   a. Chronic irritation of respiratory tract → increase in number of mucus-secreting gobler cells = ↑ mucus
   b. Inflammatory response to irritation → ↑ numbers of phagocytic cells and amount of cellular debris in mucus (especially DNA) = ↑ viscosity of mucus, which is less readily moved along by ciliary action
6. Immotile cilia—congenital impairment
   a. *Kartagener's syndrome*—sinusitis, recurrent lung infection and sinusitis
   b. *Cystic fibrosis*—infection, chronic inflammatory increases in respiratory mucous volume and viscosity = impaired lung clearance and progressive lung damage
III. Intrapulmonary detoxification mechanism
   A. Phagocytes
      1. Alveolar macrophage
         a. Phagocytosis of particles—inhaled particulate debris, bacteria, or cell constituents
         b. Kills most microbes
      2. Polymorphonuclear neutrophil present in blood (normally only small number in lung)
         a. Avid phagocyte—kills microbes
         b. Defends against established infectious processes
         c. Infection—products of inflammation attract neutrophils to site of infection (chemotaxis)
      3. Factors interfering with phagocytosis
         a. Inhibition of alveolar macrophage function
            (1) Cigarette smoke
            (2) Other inhaled pollutants—ozone, nitrogen dioxide, oxygen
            (3) Drugs—corticosteroids, antineoplastic and antiinflammatory cytoxic agents, and ethanol (alcohol)
            (4) Metabolic derangements—uremia, hyperglycemia of diabetes mellitus
            (5) Acquired granulocytopenia—bone marrow depression from cytotoxic drugs
   B. Immunoglobulins
      1. IgG and IgA—most important for lung defense; present in secretions of respiratory tract as well as in blood
         a. IgA antibodies—specific for viral antigens; neutralize viruses and prevent infection
         b. IgG predominates in terminal lung units; antigen-specific IgG contributes to local defense against bacterial infections (important in neutralizing highly pathogenic encapsulated bacteria [especially *Streptococcus pneumoniae* and *Hemophilus influenzae*], which are resistant to phagocytosis)
   C. Cell-mediated immunity (CMI)
      1. One half of lymphocytes in and around airways are rhymus-derived lymphocytes, or *T cells*
         a. Found in lymphoid aggregates adjacent to bronchi (bronchus-associated lymphoid tissues, or BALT)
         b. T cells important in:
            (1) Resistance to some viral infections
            (2) Resistance to most fungal infections
            (3) Infections by organisms that survive and multiply inside host cells: *Mycobacterium* tuberculosis, *Brucella, Listeria monocytogenes,* and *Pneumocystis carinii*
      2. Impaired CMI = ↑ susceptibility to infection
         a. Deficient T cell function (anergy) associated with:
            (1) Neoplasms—lymphoma
            (2) Cytotoxic or corticosteroid therapy
            (3) Systemic diseases—sarcoidosis, malnutrition
         b. Some lung infections occur almost exclusively in severely impaired CMI—pneumonia caused by cytomegalovirus, herpes zoster, Aspergillus species, or Pneumocystis carinii

Table 25-3. Signs and symptoms and medical therapy for acute bronchitis

Etiology	Signs and symptoms	Medical therapy
Any of 30 different viruses	Chills, malaise muscular aches, headache, dry scratchy throat, hoarseness, cough, tightness and soreness in chest after coughing	No specific therapy. Therapy directed to relief of symptoms, i.e., cough medicine, vaporizer. Fluid intake 3-4 L/day. Bland diet Antibiotics for elevation in temperature Rest Avoiding exposure to further infection

Acute bronchitis

Pathophysiology

Bronchitis can be acute or chronic. Acute bronchitis is an inflammation of the bronchi and sometimes the trachea (tracheobronchitis). It is often caused by an extension of an upper respiratory tract infection such as the common cold and is therefore communicable. It also may be caused by physical or chemical agents such as dust, smoke, or volatile fumes. As air pollution increases, the incidence of acute bronchitis increases.

Assessment

SUBJECTIVE DATA
1. Onset and duration of symptoms (see Table 25-3)
2. What taken for cough and its effectiveness

OBJECTIVE DATA
1. Vital signs—temperature may be elevated; tachypnea frequent with severe bronchitis
2. Rasping cough with mucoid sputum
3. Chest percussion—normal.
4. Auscultation—vesicular breath sounds, vocal fremitus normal, adventitious sounds—localized rales and sibilant rhonchi

Data analysis and planning

NURSING DIAGNOSIS. Possible nursing diagnoses for a patient with acute bronchitis include the following:
Ineffective airway clearance
Ineffective breathing pattern
Impaired gas exchange

EXPECTED PATIENT OUTCOMES. The patient's symptoms are improved in the following ways:
1. Temperature returns to normal.
2. Cough and sputum are decreased.
3. Headache and muscle aches are absent.

Implementation

1. Assisting with achievement of therapeutic goals
    a. Assist patient to cough effectively
Coughing is normally a mechanism that aids in the removal of inhaled foreign materials. When an infection is present the throat becomes dry and irritated and there is an increase in mucus production as part of the lung defense mechanisms.

Receptors for the cough reflex are located in the tracheal and bronchial mucosa with the largest concentration of them being found in the larynx, carina, and bifurcations of the large and medium-sized bronchi. When these receptors are stimulated, impulses are transmitted primarily via the afferent vagus nerve to the medulla and then are passed via efferent nervous pathways (vagus, phrenic, and spinal motor nerves) to expiratory musculature (larynx, tracheobronchial tree, diaphragm, and abdominal wall).[37]

To produce an effective cough there must be a deep inspiration followed by maximum expiratory effort against a closed glottis. This results in a tremendous increase in intrathoracic pressure. As the glottis opens, mucus and inhaled particles are forced out of the airways at high velocity.[73]

Persistent coughing can be very annoying and tiring to the patient and those around her/him. Complications of persistent coughing include insomnia, exhaustion, vomiting, urinary incontinence, rib or muscle trauma, pneumothorax, or fainting.

If cough is present, give prescribed medication. Table 25-4 lists commonly used medications and their desired effects.

Assist with coughing as necessary by supporting chest (front and back) as patient coughs. Teach patient to cough effectively to maintain a clear airway and collect required specimens. Take a deep breath, force it out down to residual volume, contract the diaphragm and exhale forcefully.
    b. Provide for good drainage of tracheobronchial secretion
    c. If antibiotics are prescribed, give on time to maintain therapeutic blood levels
    d. If steam vaporization is prescribed, administer it using precautions described on p. 557.
2. Assisting with comfort
    a. Place patient in position of comfort; semi-Fowler's or high-Fowler's position may be helpful
    b. Assist with ADL as necessary during acute phase of illness
3. Teaching
The patient should be taught to avoid persons with upper respiratory infections. If respiratory infection does occur, the patient should seek medical attention.

If the patient smokes cigarettes, he/she should be encouraged to quit smoking. Group programs are helpful to some persons and the local branches of the American Lung Association or American Heart Association can sup-

Table 25-4. Medications used to treat cough

Desired effect	Medications prescribed
↑ Secretions	Expectorants
	Ammonium chloride
	Ammonium carbonate
	Sodium iodide
	Potassium iodide (saturated solution; SSKI)
	Ipecac
	Terpin hydrate
↓ Secretions	Anticholinergic agents
	Atropine
Thin secretions	Mucolytic agents
	Acetylcysteine (Mucomyst)
	Desoxyribonuclease (Domavac)
Depress cough reflex	Antitussives
	Narcotic
	Codeine
	Nonnarcotic agents
	Benzonatate (Tessalon)
	Noscapine (Nectadon)
	Dextromethorphan hydrobromide (Romilar)
	Carbetapentane citrate (Toclase)
	Levopropoxyphene napsylate (Novrad)
	Chlophedianol hydrochloride (Ulo)

Organisms causing infectious pneumonia in adults

I. Typical or classic pneumonia syndrome
  A. Bacterial pneumonia
    1. Common
      a. *Streptococcus pneumoniae*
    2. Uncommon
      a. *Haemophilus influenzae*
      b. *Staphylococcus aureus*
II. Atypical pneumonia syndrome
  A. Common
    1. *Mycoplasma pneumoniae*
  B. Uncommon
    1. *Legionella pneumophila*
III. Aspiration pneumonia syndrome
  A. Hospitalized, debilitated, or antibiotic-treated patients
    1. Mixed anaerobic/aerobic pharyngeal flora
    2. *Staphylococcus aureus*
    3. *Klebsiella pneumoniae*
    4. *Pseudomonas aeruginosa*
    5. *Serratia marcescens*
    6. *Acinetobacter* species
    7. Enteric gram-negative aerobes *(Eschercichia coli, Enterobacter, Proteus)*
  B. Outpatients with normal pharyngeal flora
    1. Mixed anaerobic/aerobic pharyngeal flora
IV. Hematogenous pneumonia syndromes
  A. *Staphylococcus aureus*
  B. *Escherichia coli*
  C. Enteric/pelvic anaerobes

From Frame, P.T.: Basics RD **10:**1-8, 1982.

---

ply the names of local programs to assist persons to stop smoking.

BACTERIAL INFECTIONS

Pneumonia

Pathophysiology

Pneumonia is an inflammatory process in which there is consolidation caused by exudate filling the alveolar spaces. Gas exchange cannot take place in consolidated areas, and blood is shunted around the nonfunctioning alveloi. *Hypoxemia* may occur depending on how much lung tissue is involved.

About 60% of patients with pneumococcal pneumonia have some degree of pleural effusion. Empyema may also occur in some patients with pneumonia.[32]

Acute pneumonias are responsible for 10% of hospital admissions in the United States. Pneumonia can occur in any season but is most common during winter and early spring. Persons of any age are susceptible, but pneumonia is more common among infants and the elderly. Pneumonia is often caused by aspiration of infected materials into the distal bronchioles and alveoli. Certain individuals are especially susceptible. This includes persons whose normal respiratory defense mechanisms are damaged or altered (those with chronic obstructive pulmonary disease, influenza, and tracheostomy, and those who have recently had anesthesia); persons who have a disease affecting antibody response (those with multiple myeloma, hypogammaglobulinemia, and so on); and alcoholics in whom there is increased danger of aspiration and persons with delayed white blood cell response to infection. Increasingly, nosocomial pneumonia (acquired in the hospital) is a cause of morbidity and mortality. This is the direct result of an increase in the number of patients with impaired defenses resulting from certain types of therapy and of an increase in the number of patients whose lives are being prolonged with life support therapy.

Pneumonia is a communicable disease; the mode of transmission is dependent on the infecting organism. Pneumonia is classified according to the offending organism rather than the anatomic location (lobar or bronchial) as was the practice in the past. A recent classification of pneumonia in adults is presented in box above.

Typical or classic pneumonia

Typical or classic pneumonia occurs in both males and females of any age. It is found both in persons without underlying disease and in those with diminished defense mechanisms. Commonly, there is a history of alcoholism, recent respiratory tract infection, or viral influenza.

Assessment

SUBJECTIVE DATA

1. Onset and duration of cough, fever, and shaking chills
2. Color and consistency of sputum
3. Therapy used since onset of infection
4. See Table 25-5 for common signs and symptoms of pneumonia

SPUTUM

Material that is coughed up and expectorated from the bronchial tree is called sputum. It consists of secretions from the mucus glands and the goblet cells present in the airways.[73]

Microscopic examination of sputum can help establish a diagnosis. Constituents indicative of infection include polymorphonuclear neutrophils (pus cells) and ciliated bronchial esbithelial cells, which are an index of damage to bronchial epithelium.

Color of sputum is not always an accurate diagnostic tool. Microscopic examination is essential to distinguish between allergic and infected sputum. Allergic sputum (asthma) usually contains an increased number of eosinophils. Consistency of sputum is described as being thick, thin, or tenacious.

OBJECTIVE DATA

1. Tachypnea
2. Guarding and restricted motion of the chest on the affected side
3. Palpation of chest to check for limited expansion and increased tactile fremitus on the affected side
4. Percussion of chest to check for dull to flat sounds
5. Auscultation to check for
   a. Breath sounds increased in intensity; bronchovesicular or bronchial breath sounds over affected area

---

Sputum color analysis

1. Colorless or clear mucoid: noninfectious process
2. Creamy yellow: staphylococcal pneumonia
3. Green: *Pseudomonas* pneumonia
4. "Currant jelly": *Klebsiella* pneumonia
5. Rusty: pneumococcal pneumonia

---

   b. Vocal fremitus—increased bronchophony, egophony, and presence of whisper pectoriloquy
   c. Adventitious sounds—inspiratory rales, terminal third of inspiration

DIAGNOSTIC TESTS. The diagnosis of bacterial pneumonia is made from the patient's history, parenchymal infiltrates on the chest film, leukocytosis (increase in number of neutrophils), and sputum culture. Hypoxemia and hypocapnia may also be present.

A chest roentgenogram showing lobar consolidation is most common with pneumococcal or *Klebsiella* infections. Multiple infiltrates are more common with *Staphylococcal* and *Haemophilus* infections.[32]

Sputum specimens are collected for microscopic examination and for culture and sensitivity. The best sputum specimens are obtained from a deep, spontaneous cough. The sputum specimens are removed as soon as possible, labeled, and sent to the laboratory. Oral hygiene is provided after a patient has expectorated sputum.

Data analysis and planning

NURSING DIAGNOSES. Possible nursing diagnoses for a patient with bacterial pneumonia include the following:
Ineffective airway clearance
Ineffective breathing pattern
Impaired gas exchange
Alteration in tissue perfusion: cardiopulmonary
Alteration in comfort: pleuritic chest pain

EXPECTED PATIENT OUTCOMES. The patient's signs and symptoms are improved in the following ways:
1. Temperature returns to normal.
2. Cough and sputum are reduced.
3. Breath sounds return to normal.
4. Pain is relieved.

Implementation

ASSISTING WITH ACHIEVEMENT OF THERAPEUTIC GOALS
MEDICATIONS

1. Before beginning administration of prescribed antibiotic sputum is collected for culture. If blood culture is ordered blood is also drawn before therapy is begun.
2. Antibiotic blood levels are monitored by giving antibiotics at scheduled times. (Table 25-5 lists the antibiotic therapy currently employed in treating pneumonia.)
3. Give medication prescribed to relieve pain. Codeine may be prescribed to relieve pain since it is less likely to inhibit the cough reflex than more potent narcotics.

OXYGEN THERAPY

Oxygen by mask or cannula (Figs. 25-2 and 25-3) is usually ordered when PO_2 is less than 60 mm Hg.[32] When supplemental oxygen is necessary it may be administered by nasal prongs or by mask. The method used will depend on the patient's condition and the concentration of oxygen required. The nurse should be familiar with the various devices used to administer oxygen, and when oxygen is in use the nurse should check the equipment frequently to be sure that it is working properly.

When the patient is having difficulty exchanging oxygen and carbon dioxide, such as occurs in pulmonary edema, oxygen may be given under positive pressure. In some situations, such as chronic obstructive pulmonary disease, low-flow rates of oxygen are indicated. The use of low-flow oxygen is discussed on p. 613. In all situations, the nurse should remember that a patient suffering from hypoxemia may not be breathless or cyanotic, since cyanosis does not occur until there is 5 g or more of deoxygenated hemoglobin. In a person with anemia all the available heme is completely saturated with oxygen and thus these patients are never cyanotic even though they may be hypoxemic. For this reason an increase in

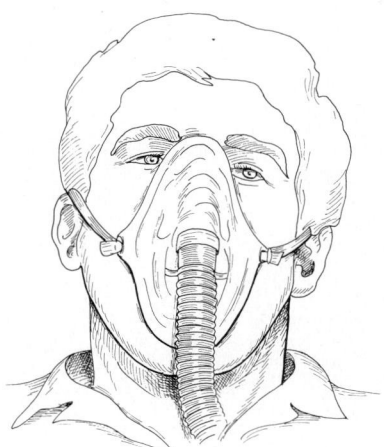

Fig. 25-2. Simple face mask. (From Abels, L.F.: Mosby's Manual of Critical Care, St. Louis, 1979, The C.V. Mosby Co.)

the pulse rate may be the first indication that the patient is experiencing hypoxemia. When patients are receiving oxygen therapy they will be monitored by arterial blood gas studies. These studies are explained on p. 596.

FACILITATING BREATHING

Assist patient to breathe deeply and expand chest to increase ventilation.

1. Place patient in position to facilitate breathing—usually upright or semiupright position (Fig. 25-4).
2. A pillow may be placed lengthwise at patient's back to provide support and thrust thorax slightly forward, allowing freer use of the diaphragm.
3. The patient who must be upright to breathe may find it restful to rest head and arms on a pillow placed on an overbed table (Fig. 25-5).
4. For the patient with severe hypoxemia, safety side rails should be in place. Patient can use them to assist in moving about in bed.
5. Some patients may breathe best when sitting up in a large armchair while leaning on a smaller chair placed in front of them. This chair is blocked to prevent it from slipping.

PROVIDING VENTILATION, HUMIDITY AND TEMPERATURE OF COMFORT

1. Most patients are most comfortable if air is cool and not too humid. An air-conditioned room may make the patient more comfortable.
2. If patient has nose, throat or bronchial irritation, warm, moist air from a *humidifier* or *vaporizer* may be helpful.
3. Because of concern about cross-infection from room humidifers, the precautions listed here are recommended by the Centers for Disease Control (CDC).

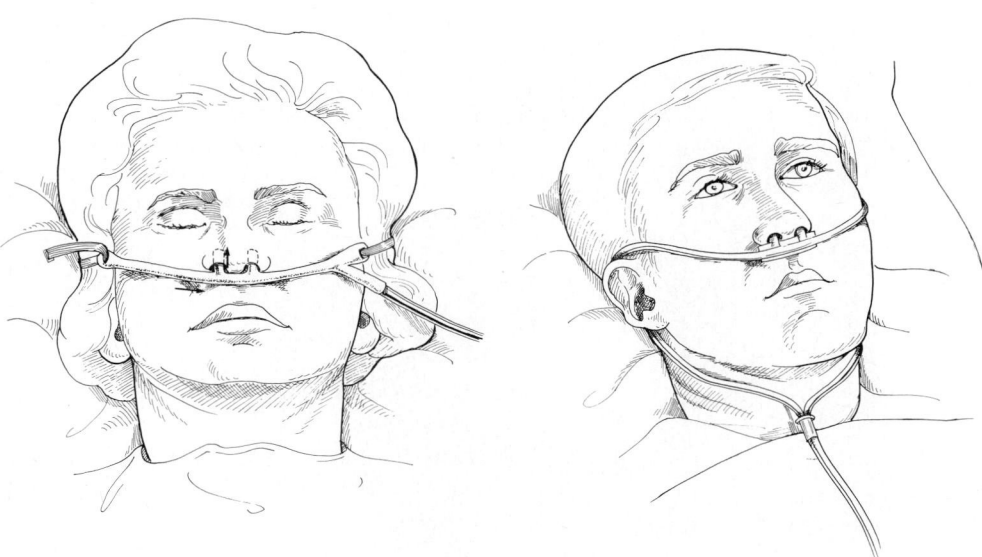

Fig. 25-3. Two types of nasal cannulas. (From Abels, L.F.: Mosby's Manual of critical care, St. Louis, 1979, The C.V. Mosby Co.)

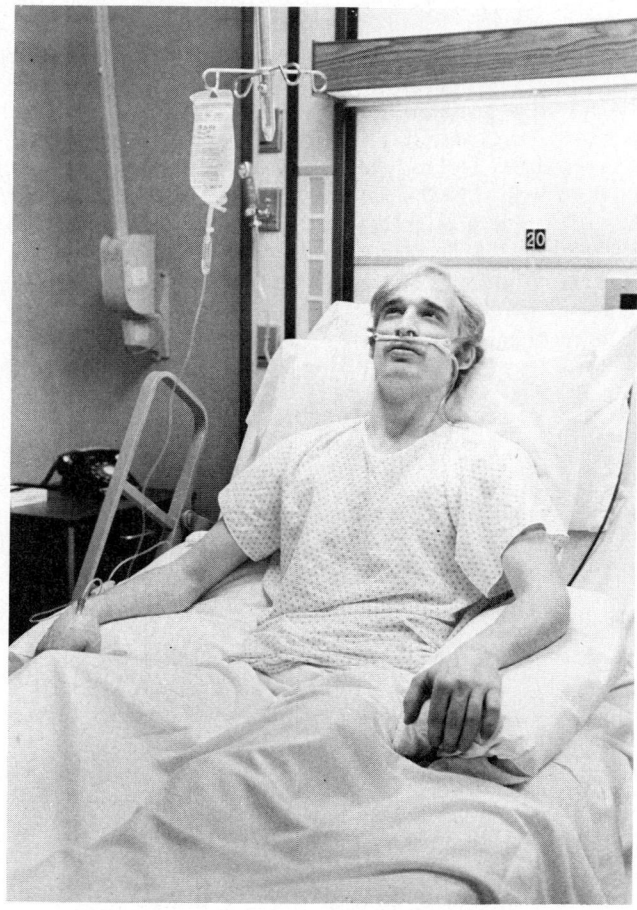

Fig. 25-4. Patient sitting upright with pillows under head and each arm to promote chest expansion and comfort.

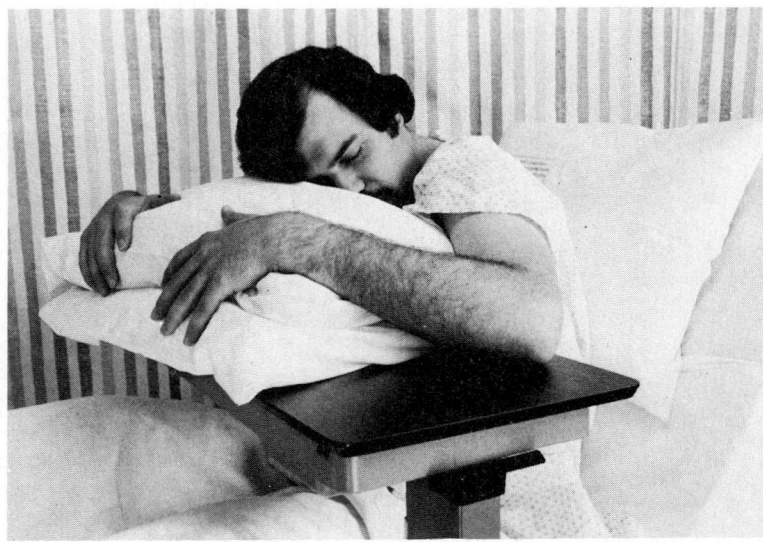

Fig. 25-5. Pillows placed on over-bed table provide comfortable support for the patient who must sleep in a sitting position.

Precautions when using humidifier

1. Use only a direct *heated* humidifier or nebulizer with a bacterial filter. Cold vapor or cool mist humidifiers are not recommended because they cannot withstand daily sterilization.
2. Use only sterile water in the humidifier and drain remaining water each time the humidifier is refilled, or at least every 24 hours. Tap water is not safe to use because it is frequently contaminated with *Pseudomonas, Flavobacterium, Acinetobacter,* or other organisms.
3. Establish a routine maintenance schedule.
4. Set medical guidelines to determine which patients should receive humidification and which should not. It may not be advisable to use humidifiers for immunosuppressed patient.
5. Do not send humidifying unit home with patients because of the concern about transporting highly resistant hospital organisms into the community.

VAPORIZERS

Small electric vaporizers can be purchased at most local drugstores. However, when the person cannot afford to purchase one, the nurse can assist in improvising equipment for inhalation and for proper humidity. An empty coffee can or a shallow pie tin can be filled with water and placed on an electric plate in the person's room to increase humidity. If the inhalation is to be directed, an ordinary steam kettle or a tea kettle with a longer improvised paper spout may be used. The paper should be changed frequently. A few drops of menthol or oil of eucalyptus can be put into the water. Benzoin will cause corrosion in the kettle, which is exceedingly difficult to remove. The kettle and electric plate should be placed a safe distance from the face so the medicated steam can be breathed freely, and yet the person will not be burned by accidentally tipping the kettle or by touching the hot plate. After the 25- to 30-minute treatment, equipment should be removed from the bedside.

HYDRATION

Dehydration will result in thick, tenacious secretions. The best liquefying agent is water, and it is preferable to adequately hydrate the patient rather than attempt to loosen secretions with mist therapy. If the patient does not have cardiovascular disease requiring fluid restriction, a fluid intake of 3 to 4 L/day should be provided.

ASSISTING WITH COMFORT AND ADL

1. Place patient in position of comfort—patients are usually most comfortable with head of bed elevated 45 to 90 degrees
2. Support the patient's chest during coughing

CONTROL OF ENVIRONMENT

1. Respiratory isolation is required for patients with staphylococcal pneumonia. Other forms of pneumonia do not require isolation.
2. Hand washing is the most important way to prevent spread of pneumonia from one patient to another via the hands of hospital personnel.

COUNSELING AND TEACHING

The major emphasis is on prevention.
1. Two vaccines are now available to prevent respiratory infections: influenza vaccine and pneumococcal vaccine.
2. Persons at high risk for developing complication of influenza (pneumonia) should be immunized unless they are allergic to eggs or egg products or had a previous reaction to vaccine.
   a. Influenza vaccine given yearly.
   b. *Pneumonia polysaccharide* vaccine given only every 3 to 5 years.[32]
3. Attention needs to be paid to reducing the likelihood of gram-negative colonization of patients. For this reason many hospitals have instituted tighter control policies on the use of antibiotics except in situations where a review panel of physicians approves their use. A reduction in use of antibiotics also reduces the incidence of antibiotic-resistant hospital flora, which are the source of many nosocomial infections. (See Chapter 13.)

Complications of pneumonia

With the advent of antibiotics and better diagnostic measures such as x-ray procedures, complications during or following pneumonia are rare in otherwise healthy persons. Atelectasis, delayed resolution, lung abscess, pleural effusion, empyema, pericarditis, meningitis, and relapse are complications that were common in the past. The fact that pneumonia and influenza rank fifth as a cause of death in the United States is an impressive reason for strict adherence to the prescribed medical treatment. Careful and accurate observation as well as sufficient time for convalescence will also help to ensure the average patient a smooth recovery. Aged persons and those with a chronic illness are likely to have a relatively long course of convalescence from pneumonia, and there is a greater possibility of their developing complications. There has been an increase in the incidence of staphylococcal pneumonia subsequent to influenza. Consolidation of lung tissue, pleural effusion, and empyema frequently occur soon after onset of this type of pneumonia and may cause death.

Evaluation

1. Are the patients signs and symptoms improved?
2. Can the patient state when influenza of pneumonia vaccine should be taken?

Atypical pneumonia
Epidemiology

The most common form of atypical pneumonia in adults is caused by *Mycoplasma pneumoniae*. *Legionella pneumophila* is an uncommon cause of atypical pneumonia. It occurs more commonly in older adults and in persons who smoke or have abnormal pulmonary defenses.[32] *Legionella pneumophila* is the agent causing Legionnaires' disease (legionellosis). It is three times more common in men than in women. A number of conditions are felt to predispose one to legionellosis. These include chronic renal disease, chronic bronchitis or emphysema, diabetes, cancer, immunosuppressive medications, and smoking. It is estimated that about 25,000 cases of Legionnaires' disease occur each year.[87]

Both epidemics and sporadic cases of Legionnaires' disease occur. Epidemics have been associated with common source exposures such as air conditioning, water-cooling towers, and excavation sites. *Legionella pneumophila* has been isolated from soil and fresh water and from shower heads in hospitals.

Fine inspiratory rales may be present, but there is no evidence of consolidation. A roentgenogram of the chest shows patchy segmental infiltrates, which may progress from unilateral to bilateral. Pleural effusion is uncommon. Patients with legionellosis may have renal failure, hyponatremia, hypophosphatemia, and an elevation of creatine phosphokinase.

Medical therapy

The usual treatment for both *Mycoplasma pneumoniae* and *Legionella pneumophila* pneumonia is erythromycin (Table 25-5). If a patient is seriously ill with Legionnaires' disease, rifampin may be added to the treatment with erythromycin. Rifampin should never be used alone because of the high likelihood of resistant organisms developing during monotherapy. Because relapses have occurred within 1 to 2 weeks of therapy, it is recommended that treatment for Legionnaires' disease be continued for 3 weeks.

The overall mortality of Legionnaires' disease is almost 15%. Most of this is attributed to respiratory failure.

When *Myoplasma* pneumonia is untreated, the fever and malaise generally resolve in 1 to 2 weeks. Serious systemic complications are quite rare, although hemolytic anemia, disseminated intravascular coaglation (DIC), thrombocytopenic purpura and renal failure, myocarditis and pericarditis, meninogencephalitis and other neurologic syndromes, arthritis, and hepatitis have been reported.[58] The mortality for *Mycoplasma* pneumonia is less than 1%.[32]

Aspiration pneumonia

The common factor in all forms of aspiration pneumonia is the aspiration of material into the airways. Aspiration pneumonia may occur while the patient is in the hospital and diligent nursing care may prevent it. The types of aspiration pneumonia are listed in box below.

Hematogenous pneumonia

Bacterial infections of the lung can also occur when pathogenic organisms are spread to the lungs through the blood stream. See Table 25-5 for etiology, signs and symptoms, and medical therapy of this type of pneumonia.

Types of aspiration pneumonia

Noninfectious aspiration pneumonia

1. Aspiration of gastric acid
   a. Only a small quantity of aspirated gastric acid will cause severe respiratory distress within a few seconds.
   b. Bacterial superinfection, if it does occur, does not become evident for 48 to 72 hours.
2. Aspiration of large quantities of inert substances.
   a. Common subtances include water, barium, tube-feeding liquids, and nonacid gastric contents.
   b. Aspirated substances obstruct airways, causing respiratory distress.
   c. Secondary bacterial infection may occur in lung segments that have obstructed airways.
3. Noninfectious aspiration syndrome is witnessed or identified from suctioning of foreign material from lungs.

Bacterial aspiration pneumonia

1. High-risk persons
   a. Persons with disorders of consciousness (for example, anesthesia, coma, seizures, alcoholism).[32]
   b. Persons with poor cough mechanisms (for example, laryngeal dysfunction, respiratory muscle paralysis).
2. Mixed anerobic and aerobic flora of the upper respiratory tract is most common cause.

Table 25-5. Signs and symptoms and medical therapy for pneumonia

Pneumonia	Etiology	Signs and symptoms	Medical therapy
Classic syndrome	Common cause *Streptoccus pneumoniae;* uncomplicated	Sudden onset with shaking chill Fever (39° to 40° C), pleuritic chest pain, productive cough Sputum—green and purulent and may be blood tinged; "rusty" Respirations—rapid and shallow with "grunting" at end of each breath Nasal flaring, intercostal rib retraction, use of accessory muscles, and cyanosis may be present	*Drugs of choice* Penicillin G procaine, IM Aqueous crystalline penicillin G, IV Penicillin V *Other effective drugs* Erythromycin, clindamycin, cephalosporins, other penicillins, trimethoprim with sulfamethoxazole
	Streptococcus pneumoniae; complicated (empyema, metastatic infection) *Haemophilus influenzae*		Penicillin G Ampicillin *Other effective drugs* Chloramphenicol, cefamandole, trimethoprim with sulfamethoxozole
	Staphyloccus aureus		Nafcillin *Other effective drugs* Methicillin, oxacillin, cefazolin, cephalothin, vancomycin, clindamycin
	Staphyloccus aureus (methicillin resistant) *Klebsiella pneumoniae*		Vancomycin, IV Cefazolin, IV, plus gentamicin or tobramycin
Atypical syndrome	Common cause *Mycoplasma pneumoniae*	Onset gradual over 3-4 days Malaise, headache, sore throat, dry cough May have chest wall soreness from coughing	*Drug of choice* Erythromycin *Other effective drugs* Tetracycline
	Uncommon cause *Legionella pneumophila*	Above plus abdominal pain and diarrhea Temperature 40° C or greater Shaking chills Respiratory distress Renal failure, hyponatremia, hypophosphatemia, elevated creatine phosphokinase	*Drug of choice* Erythromycin *Other effective drugs* Rifampin, gentamicin

Continued.

Table 25-5. Signs and symptoms and medical therapy for pneumonia—cont'd

Pneumonia	Etiology	Signs and symptoms	Medical therapy
Aspiration pneumonia	Common factor in all forms of aspiration pneumonia is aspiration of material into airways	Mixed anaerobic aspiration pneumonia: the clinical course is mild and gradual in the early stages. There is cough and low-grade fever over several days or weeks, slowly progressing to expectoration of large amounts of foul-smelling sputum.[11] The chest film reveals pneumonitis in dependent portions of the lung. The lateral segments of the upper lobes are dependent in the lateral decubitus position, and the superior segments of the lower lobes are dependent in the supine position. Later, abscess formation occurs in these segments of the lung and empyema is not uncommon.[32] When aspiration pneumonia is acquired in the hospital it may be insidious in onset, and the only early symptoms may be an unexplained fever and mild tachypnea. If the involved organisms are staphylococcal or gram-negative pathogens, the patient's condition can take a rapid downhill course accompanied by bacteremia and septic shock.[32]	Symptomatic bacterial infection present—antibiotics specific to that organism will be used.
Hematogenous	Occurs when pathogenic organisms are spread to the lungs via the bloodstream. *Staphylococcus aureus* and *Escherichia coli* are the most commonly involved agents. Most often the patient has an endovascular focus of infection (infected intravascular catheter, endocarditis, or intravenous drug abuse) *Escherichia coli* pneumonia is seen in patients with deep-seated *Escherichia coli* infections, such as intraabdominal abscess, pyonephrosis, or empyema of the gallbladder.	Pulmonary symptoms minimal compared with the symptoms of septicemia Nonproductive cough and pleuritic chest pain similar to that seen in pulmonary embolism are most common complaints	*Drugs of choice* Nafcillin, IV, ampicillin, IV, plus gentamicin or tobramycin Clindamycin, IV, plus gentamicin or tobramycin

TUBERCULOSIS

In the past few years the greatest numbers of tuberculosis cases have been found in the counties with the largest populations, especially when the county encompasses a major city, and the rates are highest in the largest metropolitan areas. Other regions in which the case rates are higher than the average are counties close to the Mexican border and a few areas in which there is a large population of American Indians. Tuberculosis rates are also higher than the average in areas of the United States where there are large numbers of immigrants from countries in which tuberculosis is far more prevalent than in the United States. For example, Southeast Asian refugees accounted for approximately 7.8% of the reported cases for 1980.[18] Canadian reports have shown similar findings. These figures point out that with a few exceptions most countries of the world have much higher tuberculosis morbidity and mortality than has the United States. In general, Latin America, Africa, Asia, and Oceania have considerably higher case rates than do the United States and the English-speaking and Western European countries. Thus Americans residing for prolonged periods of time in countries where the tuberculosis rates are very high run an increased risk of becoming infected with tubercle bacilli.

As has been true for several years, the new active case rate for men is double that for women (Fig. 25-6). In both white men and white women the greatest number of cases are found in those age 65 and over. In other races the greatest number of cases also occur in men age 65 and over and in women between age 25 and 44 and over age 65. The case rates for children under age 5 and those age 5 to 14 have shown a decline every year since 1964.

There has been a steady decrease in the number of cases of tuberculosis since the introduction of effective chemotherapeutic agents (Fig. 25-7). As could be expected, the death rate has also decreased. Today the case rate is 11/100,000 population, and the death rate is around 2/100,000 population. However, the tuberculosis death rate for males is more than double that for females, and the death rate for nonwhites is three times that for the white population.

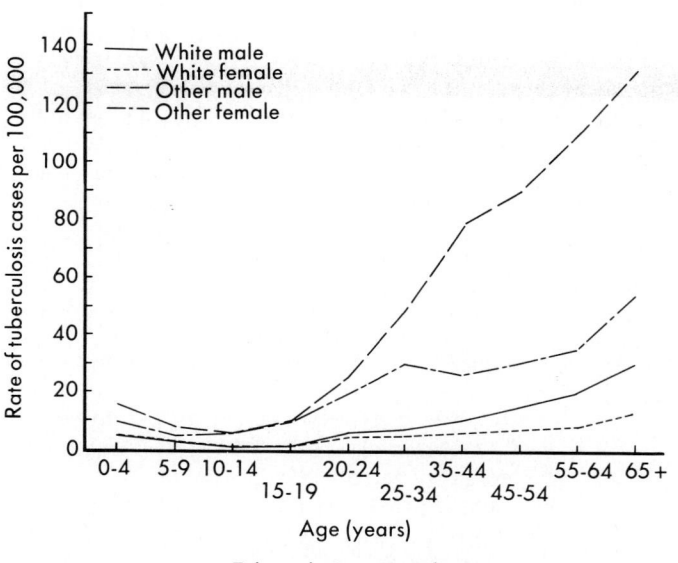

Fig. 25-6. Tuberculosis case rates by race and sex in the United States 1982. (From Centers for Disease Control: Annual Summary 1982: reported Morbidity and Mortality in the United States, Morbid. Mortal. Weekly Rep. 31:54, 1982.)

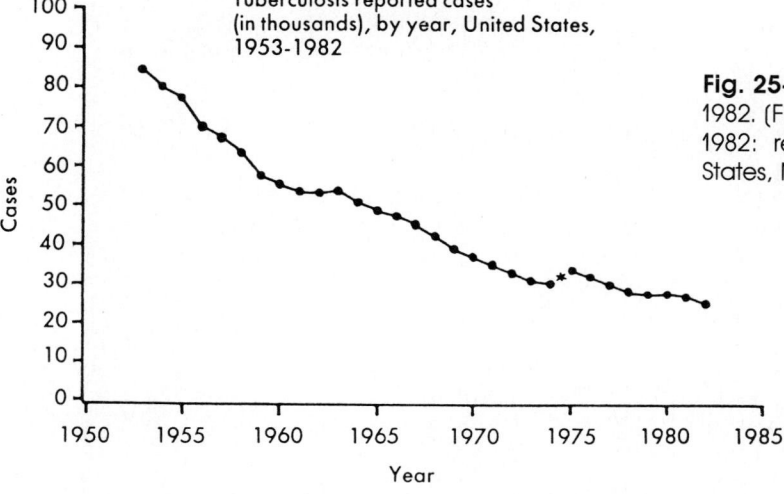

Fig. 25-7. Tuberculosis cases in the United States, 1953 to 1982. (From Centers for Disease Control: Annual Summary 1982: reported Morbidity and Mortality in The United States, Morbid. Mortal. Weekly Rep. 31:54, 1982.)

In an attempt to eliminate tuberculosis from the United States, concerted efforts must be made to prevent persons from becoming infected with the tubercle bacillus. Measures to do this are discussed under prevention on p. 563.

Pathophysiology

When an individual with no previous exposure to tuberculosis (negative tuberculin reactor) inhales a sufficient number of tubercle bacilli into the alveoli, tuberculosis *infection* occurs. The body's reaction to the tubercle bacilli depends on the susceptibility of the individual, the size of the dose, and the virulence of the organisms. Inflammation occurs within the alveoli (parenchyma) of the lungs, and natural body defenses attempt to counteract the infection. Lymph nodes in the hilar region of the lung may be involved as they filter drainage from the infected site. The inflammatory process and cellular reaction produce a small, firm, white nodule called the *primary tubercle*. The center of the nodule contains tubercle bacilli. Cells gather around the center, and usually the outer portion becomes fibrosed. Thus blood vessels are compressed, nutrition of the tubercle is interfered with, and necrosis occurs at the center. The area becomes walled off by fibrotic tissue around the outside, and the center gradually becomes soft and cheesy in consistency. This latter process is known as *caseation*. This material may become calcified (calcium deposits), or it may liquefy and is known as *liquefaction necrosis*. The liquefied material may be coughed up, leaving a *cavity* or hole in the parenchyma of the lung. The cavity or cavities are visible on chest x-ray films and result in the diagnosis of *cavitary* disease. Most individuals who are exposed to tuberculosis and develop a tuberculosis infection (confirmed by a positive tuberculin test) do not develop an active case of tuberculosis. The only x-ray evidence of their tuberculosis infection is a calcified nodule known as the *Ghon tubercle*. The evidence on x-ray film of enlarged hilar lymph nodes and a Ghon tubercle is sometimes referred to as the *primary complex*.

Persons who have been exposed to the tubercle bacillus become sensitized to it, and this is confirmed by a positive tuberculin test. Sensitization, once developed, usually remains throughout life unless something interferes with the immune response. Recent evidence suggests that about 50% of tuberculin reactors who take isoniazid for 1 year convert back to negative test results. A positive tuberculin test does not mean that one has tuberculosis, however, and nurses should explain this fact to persons who are having the test.

Tuberculosis infection is unlike other infections. Usually, other infections disappear completely when overcome by the body's defenses and leave no living organisms and generally no signs of infection. However, a person who has been infected with tubercle bacilli harbors the organism for the remainder of his/her life. Tubercle bacilli remain in the lungs in a dormant, walled-off, or so-called resting, state. When a person is under physical or emotional stress, these bacilli may become active and be-

Table 25-6. Classification of tuberculosis

Class	Description	Therapy
0	No TB exposure, not infected	None
1	TB exposure, no evidence of infection	Preventive chemotherapy may be given for persons converting their tuberculin test from negative to positive
2	TB infection, no disease	Isoniazid (INH) for 1 year (preventive chemotherapy) for *positive reactors* under age 35
3	TB: current disease (Persons with completed diagnostic evidence of TB: both a significant reaction to tuberculin skin test and clinical and/or x-ray evidence of TB)	Antituberculosis drugs: at least 2 of the first-line drugs (INH, ethambutol, rifampin, streptomycin)
4	TB: no current disease (persons with previous history of TB or with abnormal x-ray films but no significant tuberculin skin test reaction or clinical evidence)	No new therapy (persons may still be receiving chemotherapy)
5	TB: suspect (diagnosis pending) (Used during diagnostic testing of suspect persons, for no longer that a 3-month period)	Preventive chemotherapy may be instituted

gin to multiply. If body defenses are low, active tuberculosis may develop. Most persons who have active tuberculosis developed it in this manner. However, it is generally accepted that only 1 out of 20 persons with a positive tuberculin test will ever develop active tuberculosis, and the incidence is expected to be much lower among those who receive preventive therapy with isoniazid.

Classification

The classification used by states and territories of the United States when reporting morbidity statistics to the CDC of the Public Health Service is outlined in Table 25-6. The six basic classifications cover the total child and adult population, those unexposed to tuberculosis, those uninfected even though exposed, those with evidence of tuberculosis infection without disease, those with current disease, those with evidence of tuberculosis without current disease, and those in whom tuberculosis is suspected (diagnosis pending).

Prevention

To eliminate tuberculosis, the organism must be prevented from being transmitted from one person to another. Preventive measures are directed toward the recommendations described under classification. Preventive therapy emphasis is on (1) finding all persons who have tuberculosis and getting them under adequate treatment, (2) identifying persons who should be on preventive chemotherapy and getting them under treatment, and (3) locating persons who had tuberculosis in the past who did not receive adequate treatment with chemotherapy and treating them.

Persons over 35 years of age without the risk factors listed here are not given preventive chemotherapy because of the risk of isoniazid-associated hepatitis. Although the risk is small, it is age related and increases from less than 0.2% in those under age 20 to up to 2.3% in those 50 to 64 years of age.

If isoniazid-associated hepatitis occurs, the symptoms are quite mild and nonspecific and resemble those of any viral illness. (See Chapter 31 for a discussion of viral hepatitis.)

Contraindications to the use of isoniazid preventive therapy are (1) previous isoniazid-associated liver disease; (2) severe adverse reactions to isoniazed, including fever, chills, rash, and arthritis; and (3) *acute* liver disease of any cause.

Persons receiving isoniazid preventive chemotherapy should be seen monthly by a health care provider for the purpose of reinforcing the necessity of taking the chemotherapy regularly and to monitor the patient for any serious side effects.

Vaccination

Efforts continue in search of a more satisfactory tuberculosis vaccine. Presently, BCG (bacillus Calmette-Guérin) vaccine is in use in many countries throughout the world. This vaccine contains attenuated tubercle bacilli that have lost their ability to produce disease. It is administered only to persons who have a negative reaction to the tuberculin test. It is not widely used in the United States because of disagreements among physicians as to its safety and effectiveness. Also, vaccination with BCG induces hypersensitivity to tuberculin in vaccinated persons. Thus the tuberculin test loses its value as a diagnostic tool for these persons, and this is one of the major objections to its use in the United States.

The vaccine should be given only be persons who have had careful instruction in the proper technique. A multiple-puncture disk is used. When there is a positive reaction to skin testing with tuberculin, when acute infectious disease is present, or when there is any skin disease, BCG vaccine is not given. Possible complications

---

Persons who should be considered for preventive chemotherapy

1. Persons known to be exposed to tuberculosis who may be in the process of converting their tuberculin test (recent converters under 35 years of age)
2. Household contacts of persons diagnosed as having tuberculosis, especially children under age 5
3. Positive reactors to the tuberculin test under age 35
4. Tuberculin reactors over age 35 who are at special risk:
   a. Those receiving corticosteroid therapy
   b. Those receiving immunosuppressive therapy
   c. Those having a disease that impairs the immune response
5. Persons with;
   a. Leukemia or lymphoma
   b. Silicosis
   c. Diabetes difficult to control
   d. Gastrectomy

following vaccination are local ulcers, which occur in a relatively high percentage of persons vaccinated, and abscesses or suppuration of lymph nodes, which occur in a small percentage.

In countries where living conditions are such that transmission of the disease is to be expected, BCG vaccine is given early in life and then repeated after 12 to 15 years. The intradermal method is used to administer the vaccine so that a uniform controlled dose can be given. BCG vaccine is not generally recommended for use in the United States, although some highly susceptible groups such as migrant workers may be immunized.

Assessment
Subjective data

It is important to determine whether the patient was exposed to a person with active tuberculosis. Often the cause of the infection is unknown and may never be determined. At the same time close contacts of the patient need to be identified so that they may have follow-up to determine if they have active disease or have a positive tuberculin test.

Objective data

1. Presence of cough
2. Afternoon temperature elevation
3. Night sweats

TUBERCULIN SKIN TESTING. Tuberculin skin testing provides evidence of whether the individual tested has been infected by tubercle bacilli. It is based on the fact that a hypersensitivity reaction develops to certain products of *Mycobacterium tuberculosis.* This cell-mediated or delayed hypersensitivity reaction is manifested by induration caused by cellular infiltration at the site of the injection in persons who have been sensitized to the tubercle bacillus. Such persons are called "reactors." In the past the terms *negative* and *positive* were used to describe the results of tuberculin testing. In 1981 the American Thoracic Society (ATS), the medical section of the American Lung Association, suggested that the terms positive and negative are not the most accurate way to describe the results of tuberculin skin testing.[8] They recommend that the number of millimeters of induration be recorded and then interpreted appropriately.

Two substances may be used for tuberculin skin testing: OT (old tuberculin), which is prepared from dead tubercle bacilli and contains their related impurities; and PPD (purified protein derivative), which is a highly purified product containing protein from the tubercle bacilli.

The tuberculin test that gives the most accurate results is the *Mantoux test,* or intracutaneous injection of either PPD or OT. A tuberculin syringe and a short (½-inch), sharp, 24- to 26-gauge needle are used. With the skin (usually the inner forearm is used) held taut, the injection of 0.1 ml of PPD or OT is made into the superficial layers, and it produces a sharply raised white wheal. Weak dilutions are used first. If there is no reaction, stronger dilutions are used. This precaution prevents severe local reactions that might occur in highly sensitive

individuals if the higher dilutions were used initially. The most frequently used strength of PPD is an intermediate strength of 0.0001 mg/dose, or 5 tuberculin units (5 Tu). PPD is also available in first- and second-strength dilutions. For broad-screening and case-finding purposes, a single test of intermediate strength is recommended. Interpretations of the test are made after 48 hours. A tuberculin reaction may begin after 12 to 24 hours with an area of redness and a central area of induration, but it reaches its peak in 48 hours. The area of induration (not the erythema) indicates how positive the test is. Induration should be examined in a good light and palpated gently. Tuberculin reactions should always be measured and recorded in millimeters at the largest diameter of the induration. When successive dilutions are being used, it is advisable to have tests read by the same person so that individal variation in interpretation can be prevented. If the test is negative, there may be no visible reaction or there may be only slight redness with no induration.

One of the most important steps in tuberculin testing is the accurate measurement of reaction. A reaction is considered to be significant when it is 10 mm or more in diameter. Reactions between 5 and 9 mm are considered to be doubtful reactions and are more likely to indicate infection with atypical acid-fast bacilli than with *Mycobacterium tuberculosis,* except in persons who are suspects or close contacts of persons with tuberculosis. In this instance a reaction of 5 mm or more is considered significant.[8]

ROENTGENOGRAPHIC EXAMINATIONS. Persons with positive tuberculin tests will have chest x-ray examinations to determine if there is evidence of active tuberculosis. Standard posteroanterior and lateral chest films are usually ordered. Body-section roentgenograms (planography, tomography) also may be ordered. These views are helpful in defining nodules, cavities, cysts, calcification and vascular details in the parenchyma of the lung.

Tuberculous lesions usually occur in the apical and posterior segments of the upper lobe or in the superior segment of the lower lobe.

Pleural effusion may be the only x-ray finding evident with pleural tuberculosis.

SPUTUM EXAMINATION. For the diagnosis of tuberculosis to be made there must be growth of *M. tuberculosis.*

Tests to be done on sputum are explained to the patient so that a suitable specimen will be obtained. The patient is instructed to collect only sputum that has come from deep in the lungs. When instructed inadequately, patients often expectorate saliva rather than sputum. They are likely to exhaust themselves unnecessarily by shallow, frequent coughing that yields no sputum suitable for study and that affords them little relief from discomfort. *The first sputum raised in the morning is usually the most productive of organisms.* During the night, secretions accumulate in the bronchi, and just a few deep coughs will bring them to the back of the throat. If patients do not know this fact, on awakening they may almost unconsciously cough, clear their throats, and swallow or expectorate before attempting to produce the specimen.

The patient should be supplied with a wide-mouthed container and instructed to expectorate directly into it. Because the outside of the container may be contaminated, the container is placed in a disposable water-tight bag before being sent to the laboratory. Usually 4 ml of sputum is sufficient for testing. It is recommended that early morning specimens be collected on three consecutive days.

SPUTUM COLLECTIONS USING SALINE INHALATION

Inhalation of a heated saline solution is used to help some persons raise sputum for specimens. A 10% solution of saline in distilled water is placed in a heated nebulizer, and a fine spray is produced by attaching the nebulizer to compressed air or oxygen. When inhaled, the heated vapor condenses on the surface of the tracheobronchial mucosa and stimulates production of secretions.

Patients who have difficulty raising sputum for specimens can learn this procedure readily. The patient is taught how to deep breathe and cough before the procedure. The mouth is placed over, but not sealed around, the nebulizer before inhaling. Inhalation of the vapor is repeated for a few minutes or until coughing is stimulated. Some patients begin to cough after the first inhalation. The patient should have a supply of tissues to cover the cough and should expectorate sputum into the collection container.

It is important to encourage patients to rest for a few seconds between periods of inhaling and coughing so that they do not become overtired. If the patient complains of light-headedness or dizziness caused by hyperventilation, sitting quietly and breathing slowly for a few minutes will normally bring relief. If nausea occurs, the inhalations should be discontinued. The patient usually feels nauseated for only a few minutes, and it may be associated with factors other than inhalation. The advantage of this method of raising sputum is that the patient can do the procedure at any time of the day and needs no special preparation.

If the patient is suspected of having tuberculosis and specimens are being collected for screening purposes, the hospital or outpatient personnel should use appropriate precautions. The room should be well ventilated so that there are frequent changes of air. If the patient is known to have sputum positive for tubercle bacilli, the extra precaution of wearing a high-filtration mask may be taken. Special ultraviolet lights may be installed to rid the rising circulating air of infectious droplets. They are intalled high enough to protect the patient and the personnel from direct exposure to the light.

GASTRIC WASHINGS

Gastric aspiration is occasionally used to collect gastric contents, which may contain swallowed sputum. It is usually done when the diagnosis or suspected diagnosis is tuberculosis. Since most patients swallow sputum when coughing in the morning and during sleep, and examination of gastric contents may reveal causative organisms. Breakfast is withheld for gastric aspiration. (The procedure for passing the nasogastric tube is the same as that discussed in Chapter 32.) Once the tube is passed, a large syringe is attached to the end, and by gentle suction a specimen of stomach contents is withdrawn. The specimen is placed in a covered bottle, and the tube is withdrawn. The specimen is examined microscopically on slides, and culture media are inoculated as is done with other sputum samples. For the patient the disadvantages of this method of sputum collection are the discomforts of going without food and the passage of the nasogastric tube.

• • •

Results of roentgenograms and sputum examinations will either rule out the possibility or confirm a diagnosis of tuberculosis. Bacteriologic confirmation of the presence of *M. tuberculosis* is necessary to establish the diagnosis of tuberculosis. Because it is impossible to differentiate between typical and atypical acid-fast bacilli by a sputum smear, cultures are obtained on all persons. Cultures are also used for antimicrobial susceptibility (sensitivity) studies. *Despite the introduction of improved culture media, the tubercle bacillus grows slowly on artificial media, and culture reports will not be available for 3 to 6 weeks.*

Blood-streaked sputum in the absence of pronounced coughing may be the first indication to the person that anything is wrong. Pathologic changes may have occurred in the lungs, but sputum examination may not show tubercle bacilli. However, if the nodules produced in the parenchyma of the lung become soft in the center and then caseated and liquefied, the liquefied material may break through and empty into the bronchi and be raised as sputum. Cavities in the lung may appear on x-ray film and may be present in more than one lobe of the lung.

Data analysis and planning

Possible nursing diagnoses for the person with tuberculosis include the following:

Alteration in tissue perfusion: cardiopulmonary
Ineffective airway clearance
Knowledge deficit

Expected patient outcomes include the following. The person or significant other can:

1. Explain how tuberculosis is spread and those measures necessary to prevent spread (keep taking chemotherapy, cover mouth and nose when coughing or sneezing).
2. State name, dosage, actions, and side effects of prescribed medications.
3. State why at least two chemotherapy agents must be taken uninterruptedly.
   a. Explain drug-resistant organisms and relate this to the need to take chemotherapy uninterruptedly.
   b. Explain why the health care provider should be notified immediately if for any reason (for example, side effects) chemotherapy cannot be taken.
4. State where to receive new supply of chemotherapy and date it is to be obtained.

5. State plans for follow-up care.
   a. List signs and symptoms that indicate need for immediate medical care (increased cough, hemoptysis, unexplained weight loss, fever, night sweats).
   b. State when next sputum test or roentgenogram is to be taken and where.
   c. State plans for ongoing follow-up care.

Implementation
Assisting with achievement of therapeutic goals

MEDICATIONS. Treatment with at least two of the first-line or primary drugs (isoniazid, ethambutol, rifampin, or streptomycin) is instituted (Table 25-7). The most commonly prescribed drugs are isoniazid, 300 mg/kg, and ethambutol (EMB), 15 mg/kg, given once a day for 18 to 24 months.

If the person's organisms are resistant to the first-line drugs, second-line drugs are prescribed (Table 25-7). A person may be infected with drug-resistant bacilli inhaled from a person with drug-resistant tuberculosis. Drug resistance is more common in persons of Hispanic or Asian origin and in Americans who were infected while in Asia.[104] Primary drug resistance rates vary widely in the United States and Canada, and nurses need to know the local resistance rates for the area in which they are working. It can be postulated that resistance rates will be higher in those areas where large numbers of Hispanics and Asians live. Resistance to isoniazed is more common than resistance to other antituberculosis drugs.

At least two drugs and preferably three are prescribed when resistant organisms are present. The ones used will depend on the findings of sensitivity studies. All these drugs are more toxic than the first-line drugs, and viomycin, capreomycin, kanamycin, and streptomycin are usually not given together because of their toxic effect on the eighth cranial nerve and the kidneys. Some persons with resistant organisms may require more than 18 months of therapy. The most commonly prescribed drugs used to treat tuberculosis caused by resistant organisms are rifampin (RIF) and ethambutol.

Controlling the environment to prevent contamination of air with droplet nuclei of M. tuberculosis

Preventing contamination of air with tubercle bacilli is accomplished by: (1) treating the patient with antituberculosis drugs, and (2) preventing contamination of air with tubercle bacilli. The most effective way to achieve both of the above is by patient teaching (see box).

Evaluation

1. Does patient cover nose and mouth when coughing, sneezing or laughing?
2. Are the patient's sputum cultures negative, indicating that antituberculosis drugs are effective and are being taken as prescribed?

Table 25-7. Drugs used to treat tuberculosis

Drugs	Most common side effects	Tests for side effects
First-line drugs		
Isoniazid (INH)	Peripheral neuritis, hepatitis, hypersensitivity, convulsions	SGOT/SGPT (not as a routine)
Ethambutol (EMB)	Optic neuritis (reversible with discontinuation of drug; very rare at 15 mg/kg), skin rash	Red-green color discrimination and visual acuity
Rifampin	Hepatitis, febrile reaction, purpura (rare)	SGOT/SGPT (not as a routine)
Streptomycin (SM)	Eighth cranial nerve damage, nephrotoxicity (rare)	Vestibular function, audiograms; BUN and creatinine
Second-line drugs		
Viomycin	Auditory toxicity, nephrotoxicity, vestibular toxicity (rare)	Vestibular function, audiograms; BUN and creatinine
Capreomycin	Eighth cranial nerve damage, nephrotoxicity	Vestibular function, audiograms; BUN and creatinine
Kanamycin	Auditory toxicity, nephrotoxicity, vestibular toxicity (rare)	Vestibular function, audiograms, BUN and creatinine
Ethionamide	Gastrointestinal disturbance, hepatotoxicity, hypersensitivity	SGOT/SGPT
Pyrazinamide (PZA)	Hyperuricemia, hepatotoxicity	Uric acid, SGOT/SGPT
Para-aminosalicyclic acid (aminosalicylic acid; PAS)	Gastrointestinal disturbance, hypersensitivity, hepatotoxicity, sodium load	SGOT/SGPT
Cycloserine	Psychosis, personality changes, convulsions, rash	Psychologic testing

---

Patient teaching to prevent transmission of tuberculosis

1. Patient must take antituberculosis drugs as prescribed.
   a. Drugs are always taken in combination of two or three drugs.
   b. Drugs must be taken uninterruptedly.
   c. Both of the above are necessary to prevent development of resistant strains of *M. tuberculosis.*
2. Preventing contamination of air with *M. tuberculosis.*
   a. Cover nose and mouth with disposable tissues when coughing, sneezing, or laughing.
   b. Place used tissues in paper bag which will be burned.

Table 25-8. Incidence and prevention of fungal infections

Type of infection and source	Incidence	Prevention
Histoplasmosis		
Soil contaminated with fowl excreta. Bats may be infected and areas they inhabit (caves, attics, hollow trees) can be extremely infectious.	Quite high in United States. Endemic areas in Missouri, Kentucky, Tennessee, Southern Illinois, Indiana, and Ohio.	Locate areas where soil is infected with fowl excreta. Teach public to avoid inhalation of dust from infected soil. Infants and the elderly are especially susceptible.
Coccidioidomycosis		
Soil contaminated with spores. Heavy rainfall in the desert enhances growth of the fungus—sunlight inhibits it. Liberation of dust in the spring disperses anthrospores, which are inhaled.	Endemic to well-defined areas in southwestern United States, Mexico, and South America. In United States, endemic in San Joaquin Valley, Southern Arizona, New Mexico, and Southwestern Texas.	Wearing of masks by persons working in desert dust, archeologists, construction workers.
Blastomycosis		
Soil contaminated with spores that are carried on air currents and inhaled by humans and animals. Dogs can acquire the disease. Not believed to be spread from animals to man. Believed that both humans and animals infected by inhaling spores.	Most prevalent in the United States and Canadian valley areas surrounding the Mississippi, Missouri, Ohio, and St. Lawrence rivers. Also present in Africa, South America, and Mexico.	Avoid inhalation of spores in areas where cases have been identified.

FUNGAL INFECTIONS

There are three major fungal infections of the lungs: *histoplasmosis, coccidioidomycosis,* and *blastomycosis.* They are classified as deep mycoses because there is involvement by the parasite of deeper tissues and internal organs.[109] The incidence and prevention of these fungal (mycotic) infections are discussed in Table 25-8.

Histoplasmosis
Pathophysiology

The spores are inhaled and phagocytized by alveolar macrophages within which they germinate. They form yeast cells, and multiply by budding. In persons previously uninfected there is a primary or initial infection that resembles the infection in primary tuberculosis with involvement of regional lymphatics and early dissemination via lymphatics and blood to other organs. Yeast cells spread hematogenously and are phagocytized by reticuloendothelial cells in the liver, spleen, and bone marrow. The process in the lung is similar to that seen in tuberculosis with necrosis and healing by fibrosis encapsulation. Eventually, the areas show calcification in the original parenchymal foci in the lung and in the hilar lymph nodes. Usually the initial infection is self-limiting and does not require antifungal chemotherapy. However, some persons, such as infants and adults with immmunologic incompetence (lymphoma), may develop a rapidly progressive primary infection that will be fatal without antifungal therapy.

Reinfection histoplasmosis and *progressive histoplasmosis* can also occur. Reinfection with *histoplasma* causes an illness resembling the initial infection. Since some degree of immunity to histoplasmosis is conferred by the initial infection, the extent of disease will be modified by the degree of fungal immunity.[3] Heavy inoculation may cause *pneumonitis,* which is usually self-limiting over days to weeks. The onset is acute with nonproductive cough, fever, malaise, and dyspnea. Some persons who are fully immune may develop a hypersensitivity-like pneumonitis with small, discrete granulomatous foci that may give a *miliary* appearance on x-ray examination. This means that the infection is spread throughout the lung, giving the appearance of the presence of small millet seeds throughout the lung.

Progressive histoplasmosis is usually chronic; chronic pulmonary histoplasmosis is the most frequently encountered symptomatic form of the disease. It develops almost exclusively in middle-aged white men who have chronic obstructive pulmonary disease. There are recurrent episodes of necrotizing segmental or lobar granulomatous pneumonitis, which have a tendency to cavity formation, contraction, fibrosis, and compensatory emphysema.

Progressive disseminated histoplasmosis usually occurs as a consequence of the initial infection in persons with very low resistance to the infection (infants, persons with immunologic incompetence). Rarely, it can occur in adults of both sexes and all ages with no known immune disorder. These persons have fever, weakness, weight loss, hepatosplenomegaly, leukopenia, and mucous membrane ulceration involving the oropharynx, tongue, or larynx.

Adrenal insufficiency occurs in about 50% of these persons.[3]

Coccidiodomycosis
Pathophysiology

The process following inhalation of spores is believed to be very similar to that described under histoplasmosis. The arthrospores reach the alveoli, where they are phagocytized. If the disease becomes disseminated there is marked hilar adenopathy, and fungi can be isolated from lymph nodes. A pneumonic disease with necrosis and cavitation may occur after development of delayed hypersensitivity.[109] The disease process is controlled and resolved in most persons as the result of cell immunity to infection. Thus progressive disseminated coccidioidomycosis or progressive pulmonary disease is found only in those persons whose ability to resist infection or develop immunity has been compromised in some way. Susceptibility to infection is in part genetically determined. Coccidioidomycosis is 50 times more common in Filipino men and 10 times more common in black men than it is in white men.[109] This increased susceptibility to progressive disease in these groups of men parallels their susceptibility to tuberculosis. The increased susceptibility of some races to diseases such as coccidiodomycosis and tuberculosis is believed to be the result of a genetically determined impairment of their capacity to develop cellular immunity to infection.[109]

Skin testing with coccidioidin, 1:10 or 1:100, is available to test for the disease. The test is read in 48 hours. It takes 3 to 6 weeks after exposure for the test to become positive. In severe disseminated disease the test may be negative, indicating that the patient's immune system is no longer able to respond.

Roentgenograms of the chest may exhibit pneumonic infiltrate, hilar adenopathy, pleural effusion, or a cavitary lesion.[53] About 5% of persons with primary pulmonary involvement will have residual lung lesions such as cavities or nodules. Only about 0.5% of infected individuals go on to develop a severe, progressive mycosis.

Extrapulmonary dissemination of coccidioidomycosis can occur. One of the most frequent sites of dissemination is the meningeal surfaces of the brain. If there is any indication of involvement of the central nervous system, a lumbar puncture is performed. A positive complement fixation titer in the spinal fluid is diagnostic of meningitis.[53]

Dissemination can also occur to skin, soft tissue, and bones, and the patient is monitored by physical examination of the skin, gallium scanning of soft tissues, and bone scans. A bone scan should be performed before starting amphotericin B therapy.

Surgical intervention for localized lesions may involve either excision or drainage to facilitate healing.

Blastomycosis
Pathophysiology

Although skin lesions are the first evidence of blastomycosis, it is believed that the initial site of infection is in the lung. It is assumed that spores are inhaled and phagocytized in the alveoli as part of the primary infection. Thus the pathogenesis of blastomycosis is similar to that of tuberculosis, histoplasmosis, and coccidiodmycosis. The infection is spread by the lymphatics and spread throughout the body. The skin lesions represent metastatic infection from the primary pulmonary disease.[109]

Acute pulmonary blastomycosis in the form of a self-limited pneumonia can occur. Otherwise, blastomycosis is a chronic progressive disease with a mortality of about 90% when untreated. For this reason it is recommended that every person in whom the diagnosis is established be treated.[75]

Assessment of the patient with fungal infection

SUBJECTIVE DATA
1. Onset and duration of signs and symptoms. (See Table 25-9 for common signs and symptoms.)
2. History of exposure to soil contaminated with spores

OBJECTIVE DATA
1. Palpation of chest to check for limited expansion
2. Percussion of chest to check for dull to flat sounds
3. Auscultation to check for type of breath sounds or adventitious sounds

DIAGNOSTIC TESTS
1. Direct demonstration of intracellular yeasts in smears of bone marrow and biopsy of lumph nodes, liver and spleen. Cultures of bone marrow, blood or sputum.
2. Serologic tests. Aggulutination, precipitation and complement-fixation tests are used to help establish diagnosis of histoplasmosis and coccidioidomycosis. Serology tests become positive about 1 month after the primary infection. Titers of serial tests are used to determine activity of the infection.
3. Skin testing. Skin test for histoplasmosis is only used for screening purposes. In endemic areas between 90% and 95% of young adults have positive test results. The person should be tested with histoplasmin, tuberculin, blastomycin, and coccidiodin because of the likelihood of cross-reaction. The strongest reaction indicates the likely cause of the infection.
4. In histoplasmosis and coccidioidomycosis, chest films demonstrate a nodular infiltrate similar in appearance to tuberculosis. In blastomycosis, chest films may be nonspecific.
5. White blood cell count is usually normal. In acute causes may increase to 13,000 mm^2.
6. Leukopenia and anemia may be present in persons with disseminated disease.

Data analysis and planning

NURSING DIAGNOSES. Possible nursing diagnoses for a person with severe mycotic infection include:
Ineffective breathing pattern
Ineffective airway clearance
Impaired gas exchange
Alteration in comfort: chest pain
Knowledge deficit

Table 25-9. Signs and symptoms and medical therapy for fungal infections

Type of infections	Etiology	Signs and symptoms	Medical therapy
Histoplasmosis	Inhalation of spores of *Histoplasma capsulatuum*	*Severe infections* Acute onset with fever, chest pain, dyspnea, prostration, weight loss, widespread pulmonary infiltrates, hepatomegaly, and splenomegaly. Some persons show no symptoms, others have benign acute pneumonitis	*Drug(s) of choice* Amphotericin B (Fungizone intravenous) *Newer drug* Ketoconazole (Nizoral)
Coccidioidomycosis (Valley fever, San Joaquin Valley fever)	Inhalation of spores of *Coccidioidoides immitis*	Asymptomatic upper respiratory tract infection in about 60% of those who inhaled spores, 40% have symptoms ranging from flulike illness to frank pneumonia	Amphotericin B IV Therapy required for only 10% of those with symptoms, remainder have spontaneous remission
Blastomycosis	Believed to be inhalation of *Blastomyces dermatitidis*	Skin lesions that appear as small papular or pustular lesions on exposed parts of the body such as hands and face Lesions develop peripherally, may become raised and *do not* itch	Amphotericin B IV

EXPECTED PATIENT OUTCOMES
1. Temperature returns to normal.
2. Chest pain is reduced.
3. Patient knows source of infection and can teach others to avoid infected areas (Table 25-9).

Implementation

ASSISTING WITH ACHIEVEMENT OF THERAPEUTIC GOALS
1. Place patient in position to faciliate breathing.
2. Administer medications as prescribed and monitor patient for side effects.
   a. Amphotericin B (Fungizone Intravenous) is the standard therapy for mycotic infection. The dose and length of therapy are determined by the difficulty in eradicating the infection and the likelihood of replapse.[3] The therapy may last 2 to 3 weeks or 2 to 3 months.
   b. Amphotericin B must be given intravenously and has many toxic properties including local phlebitis, systemic reactions, renal toxicity, hypokalemia, and anemia. In rare instances anaphylaxis, bone marrow suppression, and cardiovascular and hepatic toxicity develop.
   c. Systemic toxicity (chills, fever, aching, nausea, and vomiting) can be lessened by premedication with 600 mg of aspirin along with 25 to 50 mg of diphenhydramine (Benadryl) or promethazine (Phenergan) or 10 mg of prochlorperazine (Compazine) orally.[3] Heparin and hydrocotisone succinate (Solu-Cortef) are sometimes added to the infusions to minimize phlebitis.
   d. A reversible azotemia occurs regularly when amphotericin B is administered. The level of azotemia is monitored by biweekly BUN or serum creatinine determinations. A BUN of greater than 40 or a creatinine nearing 3.0 indicates a need to temporarily reduce or stop the drug. Therapy is not continued until the axotemia is improved.[3] Serum potassium levels are checked biweekly, and hypokalemia is treated with oral potassium. Anemia is common, and the hematocrit usually stabilizes at 25% to 35%.[3]
   e. Ketocoanzole (Nizoral) is a newer drug, administered orally, that is effective in the treatment of systemic mycotic infections. It is given daily for a minimum of 6 months. Toxicity appears to be minimal; pruritus, minor gastrointestinal intolerance, and liver function abnormalities have been reported. It is not known whether late relapses of histoplasmosis will occur in persons treated with ketoconazole, since the drug has been in use for only a short time.
   f. Resectional pulmonary surgery is seldom required, and it is reserved for patients with adequate pulmonary reserve and residual cavities who are not able to tolerate amphotericin B.[3]
3. Assisting with comfort and ADL
   a. Take measures to reduce fever (if present) by cool sponge baths, and so on.
   b. Maintain room temperature desired by patient.
4. Counseling and teaching
   a. Review precautions to take in preventing reinfection (avoid infected areas).
   b. Assist patient with plans for recuperation after leaving hospital.

Evaluation
1. Is patient comfortable?
2. Are the patient's signs and symptoms improved?
3. Is the amphotericin infection site free of complications?

Occupational lung diseases

EPIDEMIOLOGY AND ETIOLOGY

There are many pulmonary diseases that are believed to be caused by substances inhaled in the work place. They are more common (1) in blue-collar workers than in white-collar workers, (2) in industrialized areas than in rural areas, and (3) in small and medium-sized businesses than in larger industrial plants.

In some instances it is debatable whether a person's lung disease is clearly occupation specific. This is especially so in cases of bronchitis, asthma, emphysema, or cancer since all of these conditions can be caused or aggravated by several factors found in many different occupations and by nonoccupational factors such as smoking and pollution of the atmosphere.[9]

Millions of Americans are believed to be suffering from job-related diseases. Since these diseases are not reportable, exact statistics do not exist. The Department of Health and Human Services has estimated that 400,000 persons develop job-related diseases each year. They also estimate that there are 100,000 deaths each year from occupational diseases. The National Heart, Lung, and Blood Institute stated in a 1977 report that lung diseases cause more than half of these deaths.[9] Over $5 billion a year is paid out in workers' compensation for job-related illnesses and injuries.[9]

PREVENTION

Occupational lung diseases are preventable. However, there must be a concerted effort by the public, governmental agencies, and industry if these diseases are to be prevented.

Governmental action has been slow and has only occurred, in some instances, in response to public interest groups that have lobbied for stricter regulation of harmful substances. However, countervailing political pressures have sometimes prevented laws from being passed or have resulted in less strict laws being passed because of the costs involved in meeting the strict standards required to control certain hazards.

The American Lung Association believes that several things need to be done to reduce the incidence of occupational-related lung diseases: (1) education of the public about the relationship between polluted air in the work place and lung diseases; (2) general commitment to reducing, eliminating, or avoiding air pollution of the work place; and (3) elimination of the most prevalent and notorious lung hazard: cigarette smoke.[9]

Education of the public includes not only employers and employees but also engineers and planners who design operations; buyers and purchasers who select ingredients, cleaning agents, and equipment; and physicians who see persons with occupational-related diseases. Many times workers who are instructed about the hazards involved in certain occupations and work places are helpful in deciding what preventive measures need to be taken to combat or minimize the effects of hazards. The commitment to reduce, eliminate, or avoid pollution of work place air requires full consideration of possible health effects whenever operations are planned and improvement of conditions whenever possible.

It is well documented that smokers get occupational lung diseases more often than nonsmokers and that smokers' lungs are more vulnerable to the effects of these diseases than are nonsmokers' lungs. The combined effects of cigarette smoke and industrial pollutants are very great. The risk of developing chronic bronchitis, emphysema, lung cancer, and heart disease is much increased when the worker smokes.[9] Some of these risks, such as lung cancer in asbestos workers who also smoke, are becoming more commonly known.

Occupational lung diseases can be divided into several categories. The major ones are (1) the pneumoconioses, including silicosis and coal miner's pneumoconiosis (black lung disease); (2) asbestos-related lung disease; and (3) hypersensitivity diseases, including occupational asthma, allergic alveolitis (farmer's lung), and byssinosis (brown lung disease). The etiology, pathophysiology, signs and symptoms and prevention of these diseases are listed in Table 25-10.

The medical therapy and nursing care of these patients is dependent on the patient's signs and symptoms and complications. The reader is referred to other sections of this chapter for discussion of these topics.

The major role of nurses is to be knowledgeable about the etiology and prevention of these diseases so that appropriate information and teaching can be presented to the public.

Table 25-10. Major occupational lung diseases

Type	Etiology and epidemiology	Pathophysiology	Signs and symptoms
Pneumoconioses*	1 million people in United States run risk of developing silicosis		
Chronic silicosis	Inhaled silica dust; commonest form seen in miners, foundry workers, and others who inhaled relatively low concentrations of dust for 10-20 yr	Dust accumulated in tissue → tissue reaction with whorl-shaped nodules throughout lungs	Breathlessness with exercise
Coal worker's pneumoconiosis (CWP; "black lung disease")	150,000 coal miners in the United States at risk; amount, size, and nature of dust in air vary according to type of coal, machinery, and technique used, efficiency of ventilation, and other dust control measures; 10-30% of all coal miners develop simple form of the disease; more prevalent in miners of anthracite, or hard coal; other minerals found in miner's lung (silica, kaolin, mica, beryllium, copper, cobalt, and others); unknown whether these minerals contribute to development or progression of CWP	Simple CWP: dust accumulation in lungs visible on x-ray film; over years dust piles up and respiratory bronchioles are dilated (called focal emphysema)	Simple CWP: no symptoms, no respiratory difficulty

From American Lung Association: Occupational lung diseases: an introduction, New York, 1979, The Association.
*Also known as "dust in the lungs."

Continued.

Table 25-10. Major occupational lung diseases—cont'd

Type	Etiology and epidemiology	Pathophysiology	Signs and symptoms
Pneumoconioses*—cont'd			
Complicated CWP or progressive massive fibrosis (PMF)	3% of persons with simple CWP develop complicated form; more often occurs in miners with heavy deposits of coal dust in lungs; may appear suddenly years after miner has left the mines; can stop suddenly for no discernible reason; smoking seems to have no affect on development of CWP, but smoking has adverse effect on miners' health; miners who smoke have 5-6 times more lung obstruction than non-smoking miners; cigarette smoking causes chronic bronchitis and emphysema as in nonminers	Fibrosis develops in some of dust-laden areas; fibrosis spreads and fibrotic areas coalesce, eventually most of lung is stiffened and useless; silica plays some role in fibrosis but despite international research, role of silica in CWP is not understood	PMF shortens life span; may die from respiratory failure, cor pulmonale, or superimposed infection. Prevention: dust control; reduced levels of coal dust can lower simple CWP and reduce number of miners who develop complicated CWP
Asbestos-related lung disease†	Asbestos is one of the most dangerous occupational hazards; can cause both fibrosis and cancer in asbestos workers; also a general environmental hazard because of its extensive use before health hazards were recognized; most dangerous to those who mine the ores and process the crude material into pure form; no asbestos mines in United States, but it is processed and used in United States; federal agencies and state governments moving to tighten controls on use of asbestos; lung cancer associated with all types of asbestos; 20-25% of deaths of workers with heavy exposure are from lung cancer; cancer is related to degree of asbestosis and to cigarette smoking, which enhances carcinogenic properties of asbestos; asbestos worker who smokes is 90 times as likely to get lung cancer as smoker who never worked with asbestos	Asbestos occurs in several different forms or ores; commercially important ores are chrysolite, crocidolite, and amosite; most hazardous medically are crocidolite and amosite; fibrosis caused by asbestos is called *asbestosis;* asbestos fibers accumulate around terminal bronchioles; body surrounds fibers with iron-rich tissue = asbestos body with characteristic picture on x-ray film; more asbestos bodies as more fibers are inhaled; after 20-30 yr of exposure, fibrosis begins in lungs; if heavy exposure, fibrosis appears in 4-5 yr	After fibrosis begins, cough, sputum, weight loss, increasing breathlessness; most die within 15 yr of first symptoms

†Asbestos is a fire-proofing and insulating agent.

Table 25-10. Major occupational lung diseases—cont'd

Type	Etiology and epidemiology	Pathophysiology	Signs and symptoms
Asbestos-related lung disease†—cont'd			
	Mesothelioma (cancer of the pleura) accounts for 7-10% of deaths of asbestos workers; inoperable and always fatal; can occur after very little exposure to crocidolite; has been reported in wives of asbestos workers and in persons living near asbestos plants; cigarette smoking not a contributing factor; only a few fine, straight crocidolite fibers are necessary; asbestos workers have a higher incidence of other cancers (esophagus, stomach, and intestines); swallowing of asbestos-contaminated sputum responsible for these cancers	Occurs in persons exposed to crocidolite fibers of a certain size; a few cases involve amosite fibers; needlelike shape of crocidolite fibers enables them to pass through lung tissue to pleura	Prevention: number of asbestos-related diseases has been increasing despite recognition of hazards and dust-control measures; much tighter controls are needed; some countries have taken such steps; there is need for massive efforts to educate general public of danger of asbestos
Hypersensitivity diseases	Hypersensitivity diseases fall into occupational category when antigen is found primarily in work place; lung hypersensitivity can occur in bronchi, bronchioles, or alveoli; coarse dust causes bronchial reactions; fine dust provokes small airway and alveolar reations		
Occupational asthma	More common in the 10% of the population who are atopic (genetic tendency to develop an allergy); nonatopic persons can also become sensitized; substances with antigenic properties include detergent enzymes, plantinum salts, cereals and grains, certain wood dusts, isocyanate chemicals used in polyurethane paints and other products, agents used in printing and some pesticides.	Hypersensitivity reaction mediated by histamine → bronchoconstriction and ↑ mucous production; repeated attacks if cause unrecognized and asthma is untreated may lead to permanent obstructive lung disease; asthmatic response that is well established can be provoked by other factors (house dust, cigarette smoke) and by fatigue, breathing cold air, and coughing	Wheezing is major symptom Prevention: total elimination of antigen, desensitization not successful

Continued.

Table 25-10. Major occupational lung diseases—cont'd

Type	Etiology and epidemiology	Pathophysiology	Signs and symptoms
Hypersensitivity diseases—cont'd			
Allergic alveolitis (farmer's lung)	Hypersensitivity disease caused by fine organic dust inhaled into smallest airways: cause of farmer's lung is moldy hay; other dusts can cause allergic alveolitis: these include moldy sugar cane and barley, maple bark, cork, animal hair, bird feathers and droppings, mushroom compost, coffee beans, and paprika; often disease is named for cause (mushroom worker's lung, etc); fungus spores growing in the apparent antigen are thought in many cases to be real cause of the disease	Alveoli are inflamed, inundated by WBCs, sometimes filled with fluid if exposure infrequent or level of dust low, symptoms are mild, and treatment not sought, chronic form develops over times; eventually, fibrosis occurs, and fibrosis may be so well established that it cannot be arrested	Symptoms begin some hours after exposure to offending dust and include fatigue, shortness of breath, dry cough, fever, and chills; symptoms may be severe enough to require emergency treatment and hospitalization; acute attacks treated with steroids; recovery may take 6 wk and patient may suffer residual lung damage; real cure is permanent separation of patient and antigen. Prevention: Properly dried and stored farm products (hay, straw, sugar cane) do not cause allergic alveolitis; presumably fungi only grow in moist conditions.
Byssinosis (brown lung)	Occupational disease occurs in textile workers; mainly in cotton workers but also afflicts workers in flax and hemp industries; cause is found in bales of raw cotton that contain not only cotton fibers but fragments of cotton plant; something in plant matter, rather than pure cotton is cause	Chronic bronchitis and emphysema develop in time; constriction of bronchioles in response to something in crude cotton; symptoms of asthma and allergy persist as long as there is exposure to cotton antigen	Tightness in chest on returning to work after a weekend away (Monday fever); strong relationship between amount of dust inhaled and symptoms; persistent productive tight chest with chronic bronchitis and emphysema; person leaves industry as respiratory cripple. Prevention: dust control measures; pretreating bales of cotton by washing with steam and other agents may inactivate causative agent; try to detect persons who are likely to become sensitized to cotton dust and keep them out of high-risk areas

Adult respiratory distress syndrome

Adult respiratory distress syndrome (ARDS) was first described by T.L. Petty in 1967. ARDS is often fatal and is characterized by severe dyspnea, hypoxemia, and diffuse bilateral pulmonary infiltrations following lung injury in previously healthy persons. Before 1967, what is now known as ARDS was known by several other names including pump lung, traumatic wet lung, shock lung, progressive pulmonary congestion, and Da Nang lung.

The etiology, signs and symtpoms and medical therapy for ARDS are summarized in Table 25-11.

PATHOPHYSIOLOGY

Several changes occur in ARDS. First, there is damage to the alveolar-capillary membrane. The damage can be on either the alveolar or capillary side of the membrane. Second, as a result of damage to the alveolar-capillary membrane, there is an increase in vascular permeability, and fluid may leak into the interstitial space and into the alveoli, causing pulmonary edema. Fluid and red blood cells can be found in the interstitial space and in the alveoli. Later, hyaline membranes (made up of proteins, mainly fibrinogen) that have leaked into the alveoli are seen.[79] The alveolar-capillary damage and the presence of interstitial and pulmonary edema impair gas exchange between the alveoli and the capillaries, and ventilation-perfusion abnormalities result (p. 583). Third, surfactant is inactivated resulting in an increase in surface tension and collapse of alveoli, especially smaller ones that are more dependent on surfactant to reduce their surface tension and keep them open. As areas of the lung become atelectatic, it is more difficult to inflate them with each breath, compliance decreases, and the work of breathing increases. The atelectasis also further increases the ventilation-perfusion disparity. The end result of these processes is severe hypoxemia, which is resistant to oxygen therapy. These changes are summarized in Fig. 25-8.

There are many similarities between infantile respiratory distress syndrome (IRDS) and ARDS. For example, deficient surfactant plays a major role in IRDS. In both ARDS and IRDS there is congestive atelectasis, alveolar debris, and hyaline membrane formation. The approach to treatment is comparable in IRDS and ARDS.[79]

The chest x-ray film shows diffuse, bilateral, and usually symmetric interstitial and alveolar infiltrations. These x-ray findings are commonly described as a "wet snowstorm."

Nursing care of patients with ARDS depends on the patient's signs and symptoms. The patient is critically ill

Table 25-11. Etiology, signs and symptoms, and medical therapy of ARDS

Etiology	Signs and symptoms	Medical therapy
Shock, trauma, infection, drug overdoses, and pulmonary infections See box on p. 576 for summary of clinical conditions associated with ARDS	Latent period of 18 to 24 hours after time of lung injury until symptoms develop Tachypnea, labored breathing, air hunger, and cyanosis	Mechanical ventilator support with volume-cycled ventilator attached to endotracheal or tracheostomy tube PEEP (p. 621) Drug therapy to treat specific symptoms such as shock and infection

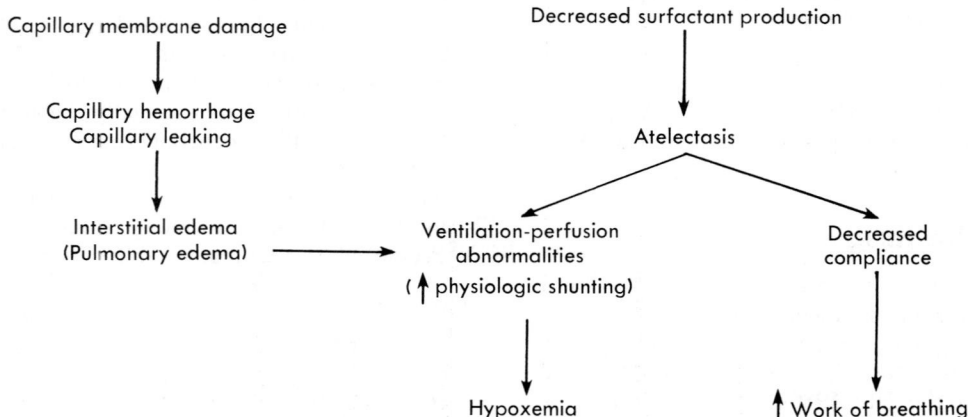

Fig. 25-8. Pathophysiologic events in adult respiratory distress syndrome.

588 Gas transport problems

ever, gentle squeezing of the tube is usually sufficient to move the bloody drainage along in the tubing. Special caution should be used in stripping tubes of patients with a known history of fragile tissue, such as occurs in emphysema.[24] The nursing measures necessary in maintaining chest tubes and closed drainage are listed in box below.

SUCTION

Suction is usually used to speed reexpansion of the lung after surgery, using either wall suction or an Emerson suction machine (Fig. 25-16, B). Commonly −10 to −30 cm of suction is applied, according to the surgeon's preference. When it is particularly important to regulate the exact amount of suction used, a control or "breaker" bottle is added to the system between the suction source and the patient's drainage bottle. The use of a control or "breaker" bottle controls the amount of suction that is applied to the water sealed bottle and thus to the patient's pleural space. The stopper in the control bottle has three openings. One is connected to the water-seal bottle, one is connected to the suction source, and the third contains

a glass rod that is under water and open to the outside (Fig. 25-17). The amount of suction produced will be determined by the distance between the surface of the water and the tip of this tube. When the suction source is turned on, the level of water in the open tube will sink in proportion to the amount of negative pressure in the system. Thus if there is 15 cm of water between the surface of the water and the tip of the tube, the amount of negative pressure in the system will be 15 cm of water pressure. Since the water will be at the bottom of the tube when this amount of pressure is reached, any increase in negative pressure will cause air to be drawn in from the outside, *breaking* the suction at this level. Therefore it can be expected that the water in the control bottle will bubble almost continuosly. If it fails to bubble at all, the desired level of suction is not being attained. When the water in the control bottle is not bubbling, the tubing should be checked for air leaks. If there are no leaks and bubbling still does not occur, the surgeon should be notified at once since the air leak in the pleura may be so great that the amont of negative pressure is not sufficient to overcome it. In this instance water may be added

---

Maintaining chest tubes and closed chest drainage

1. Mark water level in bottle with strip of adhesive tape so that amount of drainage can easily be determined. Write date and hour on tape.
2. Fasten tubing to the bed so that there are no dependent loops between the bottles and the bed (Fig. 25-16). Dependent loops allow fluid to collect in tubing and impede removal of air and fluid from pleural space.
3. Be sure that tip of chest tube is 1 to 2 cm under water so that if the bottle accidently tips over, the tube will remain under water.
4. Check the tubes for fluctuation fequently. If the column of water is not fluctuating:
   a. Be sure patient is not lying on tubes.
   b. Check connections to be sure chest tube system is intact.
   c. Ask patient to cough or change position to see if fluctuation is restored.
   d. Fluctuation will stop when lung is reexpanded.
5. Milk or strip chest tubes as ordered (sometimes every hour). This is accomplished by gently exerting pressure along the chest tube with the right hand while holding the chest tube firmly with the left hand. Holding the tube with the left hand prevents tugging on it while the tube is being milked or stripped. See p. 586 for precautions about milking tubes.
6. Keep two hemostats at the bedside so that the chest tube can be clamped if a bottle is accidentally broken. When a bottle is broken, the chest catheter should be clamped and then reconnected to a sterile setup as soon as possible. Sterile water should be used in the bottle. As soon as the system is reconnected with the tip of the tube under water, the clamp should be removed. Except in case of an emergency, such as a broken bottle, most thoracic surgeons prefer that tubes not be clamped, and a specific order is written if clamping is desired.
7. Never clamp chest tubes unless a bottle breaks (a rare occurrence) or without a written order. When chest tubes are clamped, air (positive pressure) may be trapped in the pleural space and further collapse the lung. If a patient is being transported from one place to another such as to the x-ray department, tubes should not be clamped unless for only a few minutes.
8. Never lift chest tube bottles above the level of the patient's chest, since this would allow fluid to be pulled into the pleural space.
9. The water-seal bottles should be placed on the floor so that they will not be broken by a lowered side-rail. When a Hi-Lo bed is being used, care is taken not to lower the bed onto the bottles.

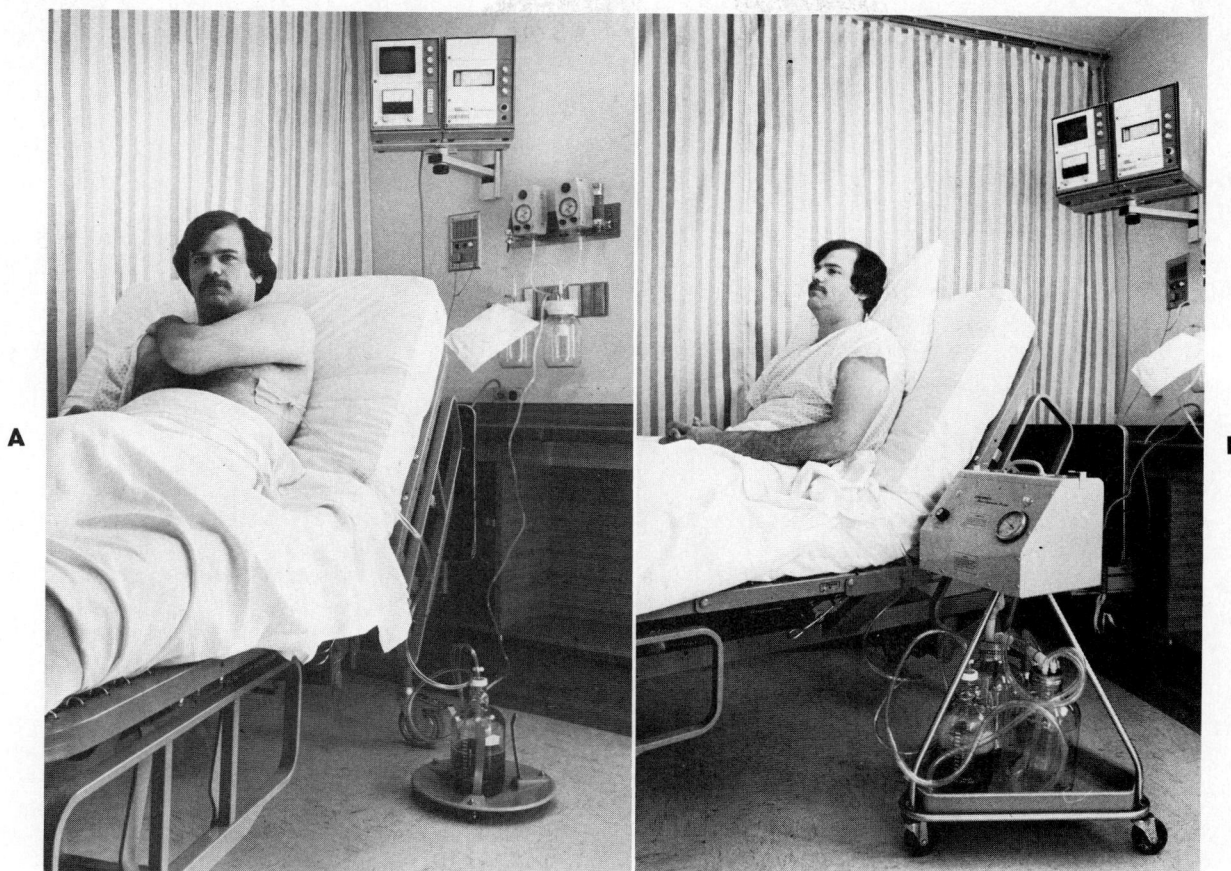

Fig. 25-16. Chest tube with water-seal suction. **A,** Wall outlet provides source of suction. Note holder used to secure bottle in upright position. **B,** Emerson suction machine as source of vacuum.

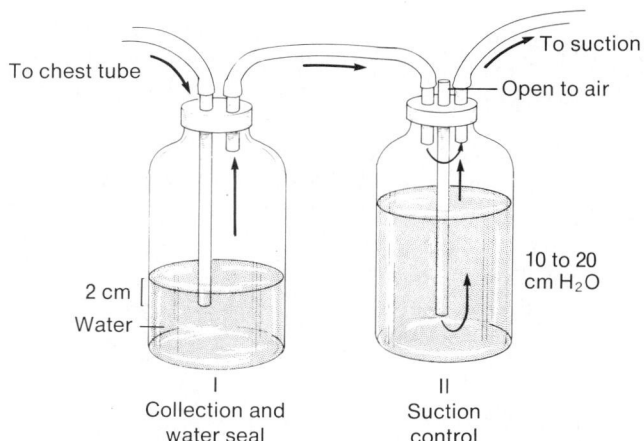

Fig. 25-17. Two bottle drainage system showing water-seal bottle connected to suction control ("breaker") bottle. Note that glass rod in suction control bottle is open to the air. This bottle regulates the amount of suction exerted on the pleural space. (From Abels, L.F.: Mosby's manual of critical care, St. Louis, 1979, The C.V. Mosby Co.)

to the control bottle to increase the distance between the surface of the water and the tip of the tube, thereby increasing the amount of negative pressure being exerted on the pleural space.

The distance the tube is placed under water in the control bottle is determined by the surgeon. A bottle and suction may be attached to one or both tubes. Most commonly it is attached to the upper tube, since this is where air is most likely to be leaking from the pleural surface. A small empty trap bottle is usually attached by tubing between the control bottle and the suction source. The purpose of this bottle is to protect the suction motor from becoming wet should the control bottle overflow.

AMBULATION

There is no contraindication to ambulating with a chest tube in place. As long as the water-seal bottle remains below the level of the chest, the patient may assume any position of comfort in bed or may be out of bed in a chair.

REMOVAL OF THE CHEST TUBE

Chest tubes are removed when there is no fluctuation of fluid in the tubing, and when roentgenograms confirm the full reexpansion of the lung. The patient should receive medication for pain 30 minutes before removal of the tube. Physicians vary in the exact procedure used to remove the tube, but generally a sterile scissors, 4-inch × 4-inch gauze squares, and adhesive tape are the materials required. The suture holding the tube in place is cut, the patient is asked to exhale deeply, and the tube is removed. Some physicians cover the site with a Telfa dressing instead of gauze squares to ensure an airtight dressing. The dressing is covered securely by three strips of 2-inch adhesive tape. If a purse-string suture was used, it is retied and a dry sterile dressing is placed over the site.

PROMOTING ARM EXERCISES. Passive arm exercises are usually started the evening of surgery. The purpose in putting the patient's arm through range of motion is to prevent restriction of function. Most patients are reluctant to move the arm on the operative side, but with proper preoperative instruction and postoperative follow-through they do so readily. It is important for both the patient and nurse to understand that the longer the arm is unexercised, the stiffer it will become. The patient should put both arms through active range of motion two or three times a day within a few days. The recommended exercises are similar to those done following mastectomy (Chapter 36). The exercises are best done when the patient is upright or lying on the abdomen. Exercises such as elevating the scapula and clavicle, "hunching the shoulders," bringing the scapulae as close together as possible, and hyperextending the arm can only be done in these positions. Since lying on the abdomen may not be possible at first, these exercises are done with the patient sitting on the edge of the bed or standing.

PROMOTING NUTRITION. The patient is encouraged to take fluids postoperatively and to progress to a general diet as soon as it is tolerated. Forcing fluids helps to liquefy secretions and makes them easier to expectorate. A diet adequate in protein and vitamins (especially vitamin C) facilitates wound healing.

Care following pneumonectomy

The postoperative care discussed above applies to all patients with resectional surgery except those having a pneumonectomy. The special care required following pneumonectomy is outlined on p. 591.

Thoracoplasty

A thoracoplasty is an extrapleural procedure involving the removal of ribs. By removing ribs it is possible to reduce the size of the chest cavity. Before the widespread use of resectional surgery, thoracoplasty was the basic surgical treatment for tuberculosis. Today thoracoplasty is used (infrequently) primarily to prevent or treat the complications of resectional surgery. When it is felt that a patient's lung may not be able to expand sufficiently after a resection to fill the space, a thoracoplasty is done 2 or 3 weeks before the resection. It also may be done before pneumonectomy, since this will reduce the chance of mediastinal shift after surgery. This type of thoracoplasty is often called a *preresection* or *tailoring* thoracoplasty; that is, the chest wall is tailored to reduce its size.

If the remaining portions of the lung fail to reexpand sufficiently after resection or if another complication such as empyema occurs, a thoracoplasty is performed. In general, it is employed when there is a space in the chest that cannot be obliterated by other means. Usually no more than three ribs are removed, and therefore paradoxical motion following thoracoplasty is seldom seen anymore. Paradoxical motion is discussed under chest injuries (p. 593).

Complications of chest surgery

There are two major complications that are specific to chest surgery, empyema and bronchopleural fistula. The patient may have empyema with or without bronchopleural fistual. The signs and symptoms and treatment of these complications are outlined in Table 25-15.

Evaluation for the patient having resectional surgery

1. Is the patient able to be up and about independently?
2. Does the patient have full use of the arm and the operative side?
3. Is the surgical wound free of infection?
4. Does the patient understand prescribed follow-up therapy such as radiation or chemotherapy?
5. Is the patient able to express concerns regarding diagnosis of cancer and his/her future?
6. Does the patient know signs and symptoms that indicate the need for immediate medical follow-up?

Special care following pneumonectomy

1. Chest tubes are not necessary since there is no lung left to reexpand on the operative side.
2. Patient may lie on back or *operated side only.* Patient is not allowed to lie with operative side uppermost because of fear that the sutured bronchial stump may open, allowing fluid to drain into the unoperated side and drown the patient.
3. Pressure in the operative side will be checked in the operating room after the chest is closed. A pneumothorax apparatus (which can instill or remove air) will be used to check the pressure in the operative space, and air will be removed or instilled as necessary to bring the pressure to slightly negative (slightly less than 760 mm Hg).
4. The surgeon will palpate the patient's trachea at least daily to determine if it is in midline. Deviation of the trachea toward either the operated or unoperated side is a sign of *mediastinal shift.* If pressure builds up in the operated side, the trachea will deviate toward the unoperated side. The treatment is to remove air (positive pressure) with a pneumothorax aparatus. Mediastinal shift toward the "good" lung can seriously comprise ventilation and needs to be treated promptly. Deviation of the trachea toward the operated side indicates that more pressure (air) needs to be instilled into the empty space.
5. The patient with a mediastinal shift resembles the patient in congestive heart failure. Neck veins are distended, the trachea is displaced to one side, pulse and respirations are increased, and dyspnea is present.
6. Serous drainage will collect in the operated space and over time will congeal to the consistency of axle grease. This is often sufficient to keep the mediastinum from shifting toward the operative side. Persistent mediastinal shift toward the operative side may have to be treated with *thoracoplasty* (removal of ribs) to reduce the size of the remaining space and assist in maintaining the mediastinum in midline. Thoracoplasty is described on p. 590.
7. It usually takes 2 to 4 days for the remaining lung to adjust to the increase in blood flow. For this reason the amount of fluids and blood given intravenously is monitored closely to prevent fluid overload. CVP monitoring is common. Rales are commonly heard over the base of the remaining lung and vascular markings will be more prominent on x-ray films. Any increase in rales, in pulse or blood pressure, and in dyspnea may indicate circulatory overload and should be reported immediately. Treatment may include diuretics and/or digitalization along with discontinuing intravenous fluids.
8. Deep breathing, coughing and arm exercises are the same as described earilier (p. 585).
9. Patients who have had a lung removed may have a lowered vital capacity, and exercise and activity should be limited to that which can be done without dyspnea. Since the body must be given time to adjust to having only one lung, the patient's return to work may be delayed.
10. If the diagnosis is cancer, radiation therapy is usually given, and it may be started before the patient leaves the hospital. (See Chapter 14 for further discussion of nursing care for patients receiving radiation therapy.)
11. The patient who has had a pneumonectomy for cancer is urged to report to the physician at once if hoarseness, dyspnea, pain on swallowing, or localized chest pain develop, since these difficulties may be signs of complications.

Table 25-15. Empyema and bronchopleural fistula

Complications	Signs and symptoms	Treatment
Empyema		
Pus in the pleural space is a dreaded complication of thoracic surgery. Pus may drain from chest tube(s) or if chest tubes are already removed can be obtained on thoracentesis (insertion of a needle attached to a syringe with a three-way stopcock used to remove fluid, blood, or pus from pleural space).	Unexplained elevation in temperature Evidence of pleural exudate on x-ray film	*Dependent drainage* by thoracentesis, intercostal chest tube, open drainage with rib resection. Chest tube may be connected to water-seal bottle or cut off and allowed to drain into chest dressings. Water-seal no longer necessary if empyema space has a thick wall and there is no danger of lung collapse. Over time as empyema drains out tube the space becomes smaller and fills in with granulation tissue. If space persists a thoracoplasty will be necessary.
Bronchopleural fistula		
Opening in the sutured bronchus that permits communication with pleural space. Space usually becomes infected and empyema develops.	Fever, leukocytosis, anorexia, expectoration of purulent sputum, and evidence of pleural exudate on x-ray film	Chest tubes connected to water-seal since there is a direct communication between bronchus (positive pressure being inspired) and the pleural space. A persistent bronchopleural fistula is treated by thoracoplasty and a muscle implant to seal off the bronchus.

CHEST TRAUMA

Trauma to the chest is a major problem most often seen first in the emergency department. The injuries to the chest range from a few fractured ribs to major trauma to the chest wall, sternum, lungs, heart, and major blood vessels. Injuries to the chest are broadly classified into two groups—blunt and penetrating. *Blunt* or nonpenetrating injuries include fractures of the ribs in which there is no damage to the pleura and lung. These injuries occur most commonly as the result of automobile accidents, falls, or blast injuries. Automobile accidents in the United States kill approximately 45,000 persons each year. Of this number, 40% have a major thoracic injury.[57] The injury is most often sustained when striking the steering wheel or being hurled from the car.

Fractures of the ribs

PATHOPHYSIOLOGY

The fourth, fifth, sixth, seventh, and eighth ribs are most commonly fractured. Fractures of the ribs are caused by blows, crushing injuries, or strain caused by severe coughing or sneezing spells. If the rib is splintered or the fracture displaced, sharp fragments may penetrate the pleura and the lung. Persons with possible rib fractures should have an x-ray examination of the chest and should be observed carefully for signs of pneumothorax or hemothorax.

ASSESSMENT

Subjective data

Subjective data to collect include the nature of the injury and when it occurred. If patient is too badly injured to answer questions, data is obtained from those accompanying the patient.

Objective data

1. Pain at site of injury that increases on inspiration
2. Area tender to the touch
3. Patient splints chests and takes shallow breaths

IMPLEMENTATION

Assisting with achievement of therapeutic goals
Initial care for fractured ribs

If ribs are fractured and the rib has not penetrated the pleura, the chest is strapped with adhesive tape, or an Ace bandage or chest binder is applied.

1. Check strapping to be sure it is secure.
2. Give analgesics as ordered.

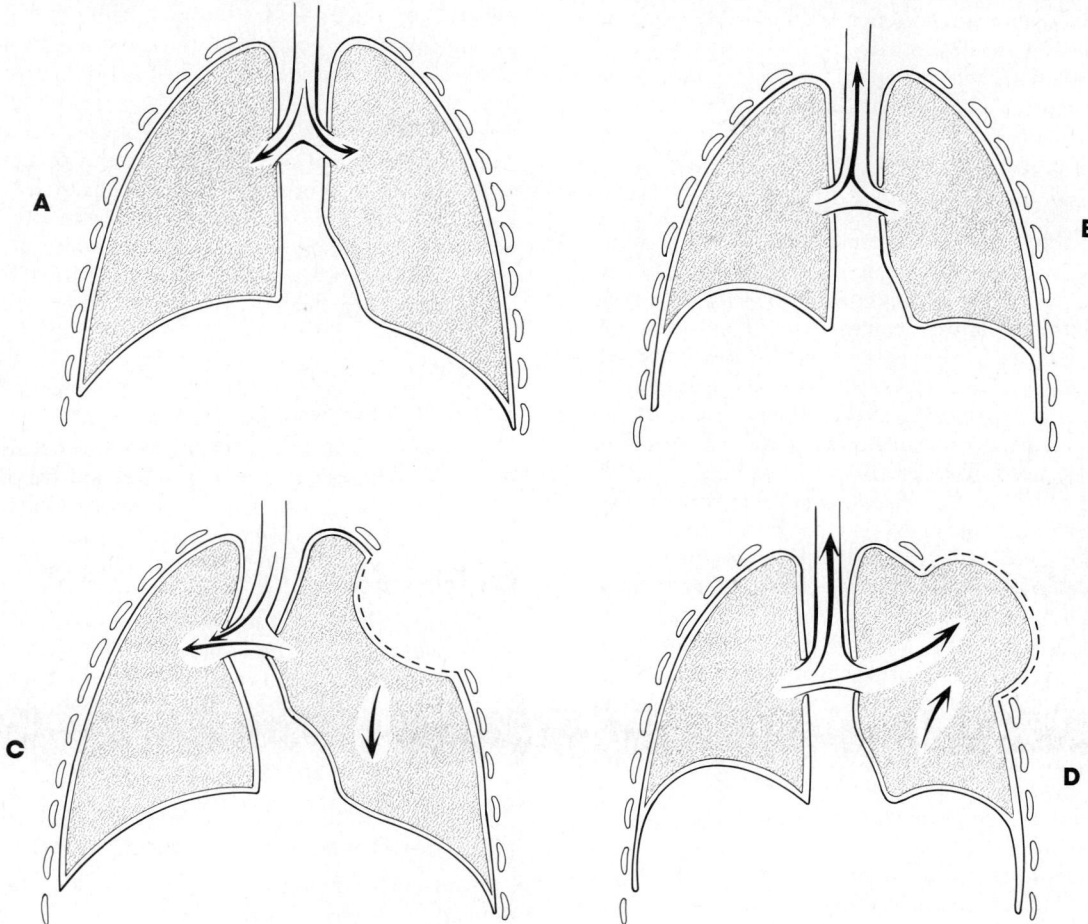

Fig. 25-18. Normal respiration. **A,** inspiration **B,** expiration. *Paradoxical motion* **C,** inspiration, area of lung underlying unstable chest wall sucks in on inspiration. **D,** same area balloons out on expiration. Note movement of mediastinum toward opposite lung on inspiration.

Assisting with comfort

1. Place patient in position of comfort. May be able to breathe easier in Fowler's or semi-Fowler's position.
2. If pain persists despite analgesics, notify the physician, who may infiltrate the intercostal spaces above and below the fractured rib(s) with 1% procaine.

Paradoxical breathing

PATHOPHYSIOLOGY

When several ribs are fractured, the chest wall on the injured side becomes unstable and the result is a *flail chest*. The chest wall no longer provides the rigid bony support that is necessary to maintain the bellows function required for normal ventilation. This causes paradoxical breathing. In *paradoxical breathing* the portion of the lung underlying the unstable chest wall moves opposite to the remainder of the lung (Fig. 25-18). On inspiration that portion of the lung sucks in while the remaining lung expands. On expiration it balloons out as the remaining lung contracts. This results in a vicious cycle of events leading to *hypoxia*.

ASSESSMENT

Subjective data

Subjective data to collect include the nature of the injury and when it occurred. Often the patient is too badly injury to answer questions, and data are obtained from those accompanying patient.

Objective data

1. Pain is severe and increases with each respiratory movement.
2. Mediastinum oscillates or "flutters" with each respiration.

3. If there is severe interference with cardiac function, neck veins will be distended.
4. Vital signs: increased pulse and respiratory rate. Blood pressure will fall if paradoxical motion is not relieved.

IMPLEMENTATION

Initial care for paradoxical breathing

Internal stabilization is the treatment of choice and is best obtained by use of a volume-controlled ventilator attached to a cuffed tracheostomy tube (p. 614). The ventilator is set to automatically control the patient's respirations. The patient who is breathing against the ventilator will need to be sedated. Narcotics, sedatives, and even muscle relaxants may have to be given. When the patient also has a head injury, narcotics are contraindicated, and muscle relaxants will be used until ventilatory control is achieved. Once the person is quiet and is no longer resisting the ventilator, hyperventilation can be used to depress the respiratory center so that ventilatory control is maintained.[57] The patient will require meticulous tracheostomy care to maintain a clear airway and to prevent infection. It takes 2 to 3 weeks for the chest wall to stabilize and the patient to be weaned for the ventilator. During this time the attention of experienced respiratory therapists, frequent blood gas studies, and constant care by skilled nursing personnel will be required. Culture and sensitivity studies of tracheal aspirations should be repeated at least every 4 to 5 days. These can be obtained by collecting the tracheal aspirate in a Luken's tube.

External stabilization was widely used before the development of modern mechanical ventilators and still may be used occasionally. Under local anesthesia a small incision is made, and stainless steel wire is attached to the ribs or sternum to pull the chest wall outward. The wire is connected to a rope and pulley with about 2.25 kg (5 pounds) of weight. Usually in 14 to 21 days the chest wall becomes rigid enough to permit removal of the traction.

Penetrating chest wounds

PATHOPHYSIOLOGY

When a knife, bullet, or other flying missile enters the chest, a penetrating wound occurs. The major problem in penetrating injury is not injury to the chest wall but injury to the structures within the chest cavity. Penetration of the lung is associated with leakage of air from the lung into the pleural cavity (pneumothorax) (Fig. 25-19, *B*). Blood may also leak into the pleural cavity (hemothorax). As the air or fluid accumulates in the pleural cavity, it builds up positive pressure, which causes the lung to collapse and may even cause a mediastinal shift. This compresses the opposite lung and interferes with cardiac action. The person then has serious difficulty in breathing and may go into shock.

ASSESSMENT

Subjective data

Subjective data to collect include the nature of the injury and when it occurred. If the patient is too badly injured to answer questions, data is obtained from those accompanying the patient.

Objective data

1. Signs of shock—weak and thready pulse, falling blood pressure, and cold and clammy skin.
2. Severe shortness of breath.
3. Check for mediastinal shift—trachea deviated from midline.

IMPLEMENTATION

Initial care for penetrating chest wounds

If an open sucking wound of the chest has been sustained, it should be covered immediately to prevent air from entering the pleural cavity and causing a pneumothorax. Several thicknesses of nonporous material such as plastic food wrap may be used, and these are anchored with wide adhesive tape, or the wound edges may be taped tightly together. If an object such as a knife is still in the wound, it must never be removed until a physician arrives. Its presence may prevent the entry of air into the pleural cavity, and its removal may cause further damage. The person who has sustained a penetrating wound of the chest should be placed in an upright position and taken to the nearest emergency room.

Emergency treatment is directed toward sustaining

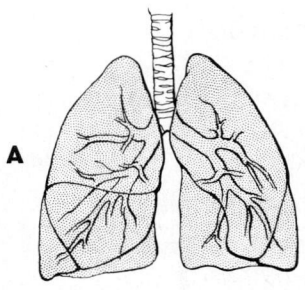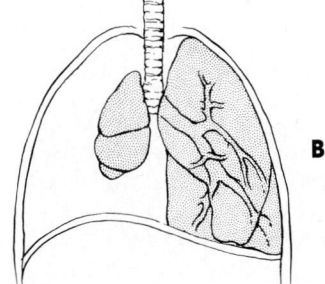

Fig. 25-19. A, Normal expanded lungs **B,** Complete collapse of right lung caused by air in pleural cavity (pneumothorax).

oxygen exchange and correcting circulatory failure. Usually the patient is intubated with an endotracheal tube and then is checked for air or blood in the pleural cavity. An emergency thoracentesis is done, and air and fluid are removed by syringe. Usually a catheter is inserted into the pleural space and connected to water-seal drainage (p. 586). If the lung fails to reexpand with this treatment or there is evidence of internal bleeding, surgical exploration may be necessary and will be done as soon as shock and other complications are under control.

To monitor the patient for hypovolemia a central venous pressure (CVP) line is inserted. This line can also be used to administer intravenous fluids and blood as necessary. The CVP is a very effective way to monitor for cardiac tamponade. A pressure above 15 cm of water or a rising CVP in a patient in shock with penetrating trauma in the region of the heart often indicates cardiac tamponade.[57] It is suspected that cardiac injury and tamponade may be present, a *pericardiocentesis* will be done.

Pneumothorax

PATHOPHYSIOLOGY

Pneumothorax is a condition in which there is air in the pleural space between the lung and the chest wall (Fig. 25-19, *B*). It usually results from the rupture of an emphysematous bleb on the surface of the lung, but it may also follow severe bouts of coughing in persons with a chronic pulmonary disease such as asthma. It also occurs when wounds have penetrated the chest wall and perforated the pleura. As atmospheric pressure builds up in the pleural space, the lung on the affected side collapses; and the heart and mediastinum shift toward the unaffected lung. If untreated, the person may die. If the cause of the condition is trauma, the immediate treatment is to seal the chest wound surgically and then to aspirate air from the pleural space.

A *spontaneous pneumothorax* occurs without warning. Roentgenograms are always ordered to determine the amount of collapse of the lung as well as the degree of mediastinal shift. When roentgenograms are taken, the patient needs help to prevent overexertion.

ASSESSMENT

Subjective data to collect include the nature of the injury and when it occurred. Objective data to collect include assessment of the following:
1. Sudden, sharp pain in chest
2. Dyspnea, anxiety, diaphoresis, weak and rapid pulse
3. Cessation of normal chest movements on affected side
4. Trachea deviation toward unaffected side
5. Hyperresonance on percussion
6. Breath sounds decreased or absent
7. Vocal fremitus depressed or absent
8. No adventitious sounds

IMPLEMENTATION

Assisting with achievement of therapeutic goals
Initial care for spontaneous pneumothorax

When a spontaneous pneumothorax is suspected, a physician should be summoned immediately. The patient should not be left alone, should be reassured, and should be urged to be still and not move about. Oxygen and equipment for a thoracentesis should be prepared. Air is immediately aspirated from the affected pleural space, and the intrapleural pressure is brought to normal if possible. If air continues to flow into the pleural space, a chest tube will be inserted and connected to water-seal drainage (p. 586).

Vital signs are monitored every 15 minutes until stabilized and then every hour for the first 24 hours.

Assisting with comfort
1. Place patient in upright position to facilitate breathing and comfort
2. Assist patient to keep physical activity at minimum for 24 hours
   a. Place call light and so on within easy reach of patient.
   b. Caution patient not to stretch, reach, or move suddenly

Follow-up care for spontaneous pneumothorax

When air no longer is expelled from the pleural space through the underwater drainage system and a roentgenogram reveals that the lung has completely reexpanded, the chest tube is removed and the person is allowed out of bed. Stenuous exertion, which increases rate and depth of respirations, should be avoided, but relatively normal activity may be resumed rather quickly. If there are frequent recurring episodes, some physicians instill silver nitrate into the pleural space to cause adhesions between the visceral and parietal pleurae. If this procedure is unsuccessful, the portion of the lung containing the defect may be resected and the parietal pleura abraded so that it will adhere to the visceral pleura and obliterate the pleural space.

OBSTRUCTIVE LUNG DISEASES

Chronic obstructive pulmonary disease

As mentioned on p. 549, *chronic obstructive pulmonary disease (COPD)* refers to diseases that produce obstruction of airflow and includes *asthma, chronic bronchitis,* and *pulmonary emphysema.* The disease spectrum associated with this diagnosis ranges from pure obstructive airway disease with the presence of bronchitis but no emphysema, through various combinations, to severe emphysema without bronchitis. The pathophysiologic processes that cause these changes are neither static nor are they necessarily progressive. Thus all stages are possible, from reversible abnormalities to relentlessly progressive cardiopulmonary insufficiency. There has been much confusion concerning the clinical use of the terms *chronic bronchitis, emphysema,* and *asthma;* therefore the term *chronic obstructive pulmonary disease* is now frequently used rather than a designation of the specific disease. Frequently by the time medical attention is sought, pathologic changes have occurred and symptoms are often moderately severe.

The incidence of COPD has increased spectacularly in recent years. Both the prevalence of COPD and the death rate attributed to it have reached epidemic proportions according to the American Lung Association.[7] During the 1970s, there was a sevenfold increase in the mortality attributed to COPD, and in 1980 COPD was the sixth leading cause of death following heart disease, neoplasms, strokes, accidents, and influenza-pneumonia.[7]

This increase in death rate from COPD is believed to be related to (1) the growing tendency of physicians to list it as a primary cause of death, (2) the greater use of pulmonary function testing, and (3) more emphasis in medical literature on the importance of this syndrome.[7] Despite these facts, it is believed that the mortality is even higher than reported since many persons who were reported to have died from pneumonia, asthma, or congestive heart failure probably had COPD. The major factors in this increase in mortality, in addition to improved reporting and the increased aging of the population, is a history of cigarette smoking.[7] These diseases are more prevalent among men than women, but death rates are now showing a higher percentage rate of increase in women than in men. This is believed to be directly related to the increase in smoking among women.

CHRONIC BRONCHITIS

Chronic bronchitis is defined *symptomatically* by hypersecretion of mucus and recurrent or chronic productive cough for a minimum of 3 months per year for at least 2 consecutive years in patients in whom other causes have been excluded. It is characterized *physiologically* by hypertrophy and hypersecretion of bronchial mucous glands. The etiology, signs and symptoms, and medical therapy are outlined in Table 25-16.

Pathophysiology

Persons with chronic bronchitis are susceptible to infection because of their inability to clear their bronchial tree of excess mucus. Bacteria proliferate in the mucous secretions in lumen of the bronchi. The most common infectious agents are *Streptococcus pneumoniae* and *Haemophilus influenzae.* As bacteria multiply, they exert a neutrophilic chemotaxis, and pus cells migrate from between bronchial epithelial cells to produce a mucopurulent exudate in the lumen, or it may progress to ulceration and destruction of the bronchial wall. When this occurs, granulation and fibrotic tissue replace the normal ciliated epithelium with flattened squamous epithelium.[41] The scarring in the airways leads to stenosis and airway obstruction. Small airways may be completely obliterated and others may become dilated. This chain of events further traps secretions and promotes multiplication of bacteria. Airway obstruction will occur first in airways that

are less than 2 mm in diameter.[41] Small airway obstruction can be detected only by pulmonary function tests, and this is why symptoms alone are not sufficient to establish the diagnosis.

Cor pulmonale (right ventricular hypertrophy, which develops as the result of increased pulmonary vascular resistance in response to hypoxemia and hypercapnia), right-sided heart failure, and respiratory failure are frequent complications of chronic bronchitis.

Assessment
Subjective data

1. When productive cough first noticed
2. Smoking history
3. Measures followed at home to improve breathing
4. Medications taken and their effectiveness in relieving symptoms

Objective data

1. Edema of ankles and degree
2. Auscultation—bronchovesicular rhonchi, rales
3. Cough with copious production of yellow or green sputum
4. Epigastric fullness
5. Distended neck veins
6. Appears overweight
7. Appears slightly cyanotic

Diagnostic tests

Diagnostic tests used in establishing a diagnosis of chronic bronchitis include sputum analysis, pulmonary function tests, and arterial blood gas levels.

SPUTUM ANALYSIS. Sputum collection is discussed on p. 564. The type of cells present in the sputum helps to differentiate between allergic inflammation of the airways, as seen in bronchial asthma, and nonspecific inflammation, as seen in chronic bronchitis.[41] In chronic bronchitis polymorphonuclear leukocytes (neutrophils) are found. The sputum often changes color to green or yellow not from infection but from the action of the enzyme myeloperoxidase, which is associated with cellular breakdown under stasis from retained secretions.

The sputum specimen must be fresh and transported to the laboratory immediately for bacteriologic examination.

PULMONARY FUNCTION TESTS. Pulmonary function tests are explained on p. 583. The findings that are common in patients with chronic bronchitis can be found in Table 25-17. Pulmonary function tests results may improve slightly after the administration of bronchodilators.

ARTERIAL BLOOD GAS LEVELS. Arterial blood gas studies have become a common tool to aid in physiologic diagnosis and therapeutic management of patients. These studies determine blood pH, carbon dioxide tension (P_{CO_2}), oxygen tension (P_{O_2}), and percent of oxyhemoglobin saturation (S_{aO_2}). Blood gas studies are obtained to assess the adequacy of oxygenation and ventilation and to assess acid-base status. The blood sample is obtained from the radial, brachial, or femoral artery using a preheparinized

Table 25-16. Etiology, signs and symptoms, and medical therapy for chronic bronchitis and pulmonary emphysema

Bronchitis	Pulmonary emphysema
Etiology	
Inhalation of physical or chemical irritants or viral or bacterial infections.	Not known. Believed that some change in the enzyme-inhibitor balance occurs allowing proteolytic enzymes to attack lung tissue.
Most common inhaled irritant is cigarette smoke.	Not known why some smokers develop bronchitis and others develop emphysema. A_1-antitrypsin deficiency occurs in some persons who develop severe, disabling emphysema early in life. There is a familial tendency for this type of emphysema.
Signs and symptoms	
Early symptoms	Dyspnea on exertion may be in acute respiratory distress.
Productive cough on awakening. Often ignored by cigarette smokers who refer to it as their "cigarette cough."	Using accessory muscles to breathe. Ruddy color.
Later symptoms	Thin with a "barrel chest."
Significant physical incapacity. Breathlessness even when walking on a flat surface. Noticeable shortness of breath (SOB) and use of accessory muscles to breathe. Cyanosis is common. Ankle edema, bloated appearance, distended neck veins. Sometimes referred to as "blue bloater."	Usually able to maintain resting P_{O_2}
	Cyanosis uncommon
	Sometimes referred to as "pink puffer."
	Late in disease
	P_{CO_2} ↑
Late in disease	Cor pulmonale and respiratory failure may arise as complications.
Cor pulmonale (right ventricular hypertrophy), right-sided heart failure, and respiratory failure are frequent complications	
Pulmonary function test findings	
↓ Expiratory flow rates	↓ Expiratory flow rates, especially forced expiratory volume and maximal midexpiratory flow.
↓ Vital capacity	↑ Total lung capacity
↑ Residual volume	↑ Residual volume
Total lung capacity is usually within normal limits.	Vital capacity may be normal or slightly reduced until late stages of disease. FEV_1/VC ratio is changed.
Arterial blood gas findings	
Low resting P_{O_2}	P_{O_2} normal or slightly reduced at *rest* but falls during exercise.
Elevated P_{CO_2} (if obstruction severe)	Normal P_{CO_2}.
During exercise P_{CO_2} ↑ and P_{O_2} may also ↑	Late in disease P_{CO_2} is elevated.

Continued.

Table 25-16. Etiology, signs and symptoms, and medical therapy for chronic bronchitis and pulmonary emphysema—cont'd

Bronchitis	Pulmonary emphysema

Medical therapy

Medical therapy for chronic bronchitis and pulmonary emphysema is similar and is dependent on symptoms, pulmonary function test results and blood gas findings. Therapy may include all or some of the modalities outlined here.

Supportive measures

Education of patient and family about:
    Avoidance of cigarette smoke
    Avoidance of other inhaled irritants
    Avoidance of persons with upper respiratory infections
    Control of environmental temperature and humidity
    Proper nutrition
    Adequate hydration

Specific therapy

Medications
    Bronchodilators (Table 25-18)
    Antimicrobials
        Tetracycline or ampicillin usually prescribed to treat respiratory tract infections.
    Corticosteroids
        May be prescribed to alleviate acute symptoms. Prednisone most often used.
    Digitalis
        May be prescribed to treat left ventricular failure.

Respiratory therapy

Aerosol therapy
    Used to deliver bronchodilators through metered cartridge devices or hand-bulb nebulizers.
Oxygen therapy
    Required for patients who are unable to maintain a Po_2 of 50 mm Hg or more at rest or who cannot carry out ADL without becoming short of breath. 1 to 2 L of O_2 given by nasal prongs (p. 554).

Physical conditioning

Relaxation exercises
    Progressive relaxation exercises are encouraged. Best practiced before meals or 2 hours or more after eating, since digestion seems to interfere with ability to relax.
Meditation
    Meditation is becoming more widely used to assist patients to relax.
Breathing retraining
    Pursed-lip breathing
    Leaning forward position for exhalation
    Abdominal breathing
    Inhalation-exhalation exercises
    Exhalation with exertion
Rehabilitation
    Muscle reconditioning programs specific for the patient

syringe to prevent clotting. The syringe is capped after obtaining the blood sample to prevent contact with air and is placed in a container of ice water until analyzed. Pressure is maintained over the puncture site for at least 2 minutes after needle withdrawal to prevent bleeding.

Gas tensions refer to partial pressure, or that part of the total pressure exerted by a specific gas. For example, pressure exerted by the atmosphere at sea level is 760 mm Hg. The amount of oxygen in air at sea level is 21%; that is, 21% of the total pressure is exerted by oxygen. Since 21% of 760 is approximately 159, the Po_2 of air at sea level is 159 mm Hg. Definitions of gas exchange functions and their normal values are given in the box below.

The measurement of oxygen values includes both the

P_{O_2} and Sa_{O_2}. The P_{O_2} measures oxygen dissolved in the blood; however, the amount of oxygen carried in the blood in this form is small, since most oxygen is transported in chemical combination with hemoglobin. Oxyhemoglobin saturation refers to that percentage of the hemoglobin that is combined with oxygen. More than 90% of the oxygen-carrying capacity of blood is accounted for by oxyhemoglobin, with the partial pressure of oxygen acting as the driving force for this chemical combination. Therefore both P_{O_2} and Sa_{O_2} levels must be examined to determine the adequacy of oxygenation of the tissues.

It is particularly important to understand the relationship of the P_{O_2} to oxyhemoglobin saturation in order to assess adequacy of tissue oxygenation. This relationship is not directly linear; many factors affect the affinity of the heme molecule for oxygen. A sigmoid curve (Fig 25-20) represents the saturation percentages that occur at various P_{O_2} levels. Most significant of the factors that affect the ability of the blood to carry oxygen is the partial pressure of the oxygen itself in the blood. As can be seen in the oxyhemoglobin dissociation curve, in the upper portion of the curve, hemoglobin has an increased affinity for oxygen, so that large changes in P_{O_2} levels can be tolerated without significantly changing the saturation. For example, at a P_{O_2} of 100 mm Hg, hemoglobin saturation is almost total, 97%; even if the P_{O_2} should fall to 70 mm Hg, the saturation would only decrease to 94%. This serves as a protective mechanism that ensures adequate tissue oxygenation even when there is mild hypoxemia. It should be noted, however, that once the P_{O_2} level falls below 60 mm Hg, saturation begins to decrease sharply, thus reducing the ability of the hemoglobin to transport oxygen.

Other factors that influence the oxygen affinity of hemoglobin are temperature, pH, and P_{CO_2}. At higher temperatures, increased levels of P_{CO_2} (hypercapnia), and acidosis, the curve shifts to the right. This means that at any given P_{O_2} the hemoglobin has less affinity for oxygen and lower saturations will result. The converse of this is also true; with decreased temperature, decreased P_{CO_2}, and alkalosis, higher saturations occur with any given P_{O_2}.

The P_{CO_2} is used as a measurement to determine the adequacy of ventilation and is dependent on the amount of carbon dioxide produced by the body and the ability of the lungs to eliminate it. *Hypoventilation* therefore is shown by an elevated P_{CO_2}, while *hyperventilation* is indicated by a decrease in P_{CO_2} below nromal levels.

The pH refers to the acidity of the blood and is an expression of the hydrogen ion concentration. Because pH is expressed as a negative logarithm, as hydrogen ion concentration increases and blood becomes more acid, the pH value falls. When hydrogen ion concentration decreases, the blood becomes more alkaline and the pH value rises.

The P_{CO_2} is related to the pH because of the chemical reaction of carbon dioxide and water in the blood, which results in the formation of carbonic acid. Carbonic acid,

---

Definitions and normal values of gas exchange functions

pH	Acidity of blood	7.35 to 7.45
P_{CO_2}	Partial pressure of carbon dioxide in blood	38 to 42 mm Hg
P_{O_2}	Partial pressure of oxygen in blood	80 to 100 mm Hg
Sa_{O_2}	Percentage of available hemoglobin saturated with oxygen	95% to 98%

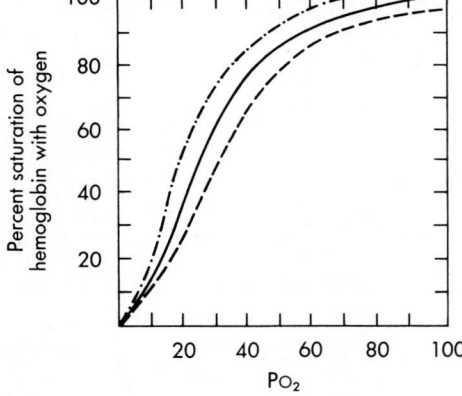

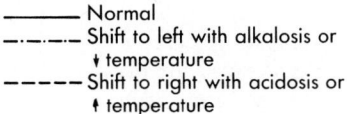

— Normal
—·—·—· Shift to left with alkalosis or ↓ temperature
– – – – Shift to right with acidosis or ↑ temperature

Fig. 25-20. Oxyhemoglobin dissociation curve. (Reproduced with permission from Comroe, J.H., Jr.: Physiology of respiration, ed. 2, Copyright, 1974, by Year Book Medical Publishers, Inc. Chicago.)

in turn, dissociates to form hydrogen and bicarbonate ions, as illustrated in the following equation:

$$CO_2 + H_2O \rightleftharpoons H_2CO_3 \rightleftharpoons HCO_3^- + H^+$$

The maintenance of a normal pH is dependent on a ratio of 20 bicarbonate ions to 1 hydrogen ion. It can be seen from the equation that the presence of an elevated PCO_2 will result in an excess of hydrogen ions. When this occurs, the pH falls and the patient is said to be in *respiratory acidosis*. Conversely, when PCO_2 is decreased, the pH increases and the result is termed *respiratory alkalosis*.

Data analysis and planning
Nursing diagnoses

Possible nursing diagnoses for a patient with chronic bronchitis include the following:
Ineffective airway clearance
Ineffective breathing pattern
Impaired gas exchange
Alteration in tissue perfusion: cardiopulmonary
Alteration in fluid volume: excess
Alteration in nutrition: potential for more than body requirements
Anxiety
Sleep pattern disturbances
Self-care deficit
Knowledge deficit

Expected patient outcomes

Because it is often impossible clinically to determine if the patient has chronic bronchitis or pulmonary emphysema, and the patient often has some degree of both, the outcome criteria for COPD will be presented after the discussion of pulmonary emphysema.

In general the goals of treatment for the patient with chronic bronchitis are to (1) improve the patient's symptoms, (2) improve the ability to carry out ADL, and (3) reduce the progression of the disease when the disease is detected early.[41] Specifics of therapy are presented after the discussion of emphysema, since the treatment for both of these diseases is similar.

EMPHYSEMA

Emphysema is defined *pathologically* by destructive changes in alveolar walls and enlargement of air spaces distal to the terminal nonrespiratory bronchioles. It is characterized *physiologically* by increased lung compliance, decreased diffusing capacity, and increased airway resistance. The etiology, signs and symptoms, and medical therapy are outlined in Table 25-16.

Pathophysiology

The diagnosis of emphysema is inferred from pulmonary function tests that show a decrease in airflow. The type of emphysema can be determined only by descriptive morphology. There are two principal types of emphysema morphologically—*centrilobular* emphysema (CLE) and *panlobular* emphysema (PLE). In CLE, there is distention

and damage of the respiratory bronchioles selectively. Openings develop in the walls of the bronchioles; they become enlarged and confluent and tend to form a single space as the walls enlarge. The disease tends to be unevenly distributed throughout the lung but usually is more severe in the upper portions.

In PLE, there is a more uniform enlargement and destruction of the alveoli in the pulmonary acinus. PLE is usually more diffuse and is more severe in the lower lung. It is found in elderly persons who have no evidence of chronic bronchitis or impairment of lung function.[7] It occurs just as commonly in women as in men, but PLE is less frequent than CLE. PLE is a characteristic finding in persons with homozygous alpha$_1$-antitrypsin deficiency.[7]

Because of destruction of tissue, there is physiologic obstruction by collapse of airways on expiration. As a result, full exhalation is difficult, air trapping ensues, and the diaphragm becomes fixed in a flattened position.

Assessment
Subjective data

1. Onset and duration of symptom
2. Measures followed at home to improve breathing
3. Use of supplemental oxygen at home during the day or during sleep
4. Medications taken and their effectiveness in relieving symptoms
5. Smoking history

Objective data

1. Rapid respirations
2. Activities that cause patient to become dyspneic
3. Barrel chest
4. Palpation
   a. Diminished chest expansion
   b. Decrease in tactile fremitus
5. Percussion
   a. Resonant to hyperresonant
   b. Diaphragm moves very little
6. Auscultation
   a. Breath sounds exhibit decreased intensity, usually prolonged expiration
   b. Vocal fremitus is normal or decreased
   c. Adventititious sounds reveal occasional sonorous and/or sibilant rhonchi, fine rales in late inspiration

Diagnostic tests

Because patients with emphysema are very vulnerable to lung infections, sputum tests for culture and sensitivity are frequently ordered. Pulmonary function tests and arterial blood gas findings will be necessary to determine degree of impairment and therapy.

Data analysis and planning
Nursing diagnosis

Possible nursing diagnoses for a patient with pulmonary emphyema include the following:

Ineffective breathing pattern
Impaired gas exchange
Alteration in tissue perfusion: cardiopulmonary
Ineffective airway clearance
Alteration in nutrition: less than body requirements
Anxiety
Activity intolerance
Sleep pattern disturbance
Self-care deficit
Disturbance in self-concept

Expected patient outcomes for the person with COPD

The person or significant others can:

1. Explain dietary changes required after discharge.
   a. Explain food and fluid requirements and plan for meeting them.
   b. List specific foods to be avoided.
   c. Explain plan for frequent, small feedings of soft foods that do not require much chewing, and the need for increased time for eating if indicated.
2. Explain any home medication or treatment program.
   a. State name, dosage, action, and side effects of each home medication.
   b. Explain how and when to use medications ordered on a prn basis (for example, bronchodilators, antibiotics, steroids, antacids).
   c. Demonstrate techniques necessary for follow-up care (for example, segemental postural drainage, clapping and vibrating, inhalation therapy treatments [IPPB]).
3. Explain exercise program to be followed at home.
   a. Demonstrate effective methods of coughing.
   b. Demonstrate efficient breathing patterns with emphasis on increasing time of exhalation in relation to inhalation (for example, use of diaphragm, expansion of lower thoracic cage, use of abdominal muscles, use of pursed-lip breathing).
4. Explain health maintenance or therapeutic follow-up program.
   a. Explain basic pathologic condition and overall treatment for medical problem in own words.
   b. Explain need to avoid respiratory irritants and infectious agents and identify sources of these in environment (for example, tobacco smoke, industrial pollutants, allergens, persons with upper respiratory tract infections).
   c. List signs or symptoms requiring institution of specific therapy or contact with physician (for example, change in amount, color, consistency of sputum; increased cough, hemoptysis, drowsiness, changes in behavior, increasing fatigue, weight gain, increase in peripheral edema, change in color of stool).
5. Explain how to obtain professional and community resources necessary to structure a satisfactory environment at home.
   a. State how to contact other agencies (for example, vocational counselor, Visiting Nurses Association).
   b. Describe how to obtain and maintain any needed equipment or supplies (for example, oxygen, nebulizers, humidifiers, mistometers, IPPB, syringes, medications).
6. State plans for ongoing follow-up care.

Implementation
Facilitating breathing

1. Teach patient to slow respiratory frequency and to breathe slowly and rhythmically.
2. Discourage patient from taking big gulps of air.
3. Teach patient to increase inspiratory: expiratory ratio so that expiration takes twice as long as inhalation.
   a. Teach patient to count in seconds and to concentrate on increasing time taken to exhale.
   b. Count to 5 on inhalation and to 10 on exhalation.

Teach pursed-lip breathing if the patient is not already using it. Teach the forward-leaning position for exhalation. Using a forward-leaning position of 30 to 40 degrees with the head tilted at a 16- to 18-degree angle is a very effective way to improve exhalation. As mentioned earlier, patients with emphysema have increased TLC and residual volume (RV) with the diaphragm in a fixed flattened position. For this reason, the diaphragm cannot assist in exhalation as it does normally. Leaning forward allows more air to be removed from the lungs on exhalation. The leaning-forward position can be achieved in either a sitting or standing position. For example, (1) the patient can sit on the edge of the bed or a chair and lean forward on two or three pillows placed on a table or overbed stand; (2) the patient can sit in a chair with the legs spread apart shoulder width (or wider, if obese) with the elbows on the knees and the arms and hands relaxed; or (3) the patient can stand with the back and hips against the wall with the feet spread apart and about 12 inches. (30 cm) from the wall. The patient then relaxes and leans forward.[84] In these positions, the patient cannot use the accessory muscles of respiration, and the upward action of the diaphragm is improved.

ABDOMINAL BREATHING AND EXERCISES. Teach abdominal breathing, leg raising exercises, inhalation-exhalation exercises, and muscle reconditioning exercises.

Abdominal breathing improves the breathing efficiency of persons with COPD, because it assists the patient to elevate the diaphragm. Abdominal breathing can be taught in the sitting or lying position. In the sitting position, the patient sits on the side of the bed or in a chair and holds a small pillow or a book against the abdomen. The patient then exhales slowly while leaning forward and pressing the pillow or book against the abdomen. In the lying position, a small pillow or a book is placed on the abdomen and the patient is asked to "puff out" the abdomen and raise the pillow or book as high as possible. The patient then exhales slowly through pursed lips while pulling in on the abdominal muscles. Manual pressure on the upper abdomen during expiration facilitates

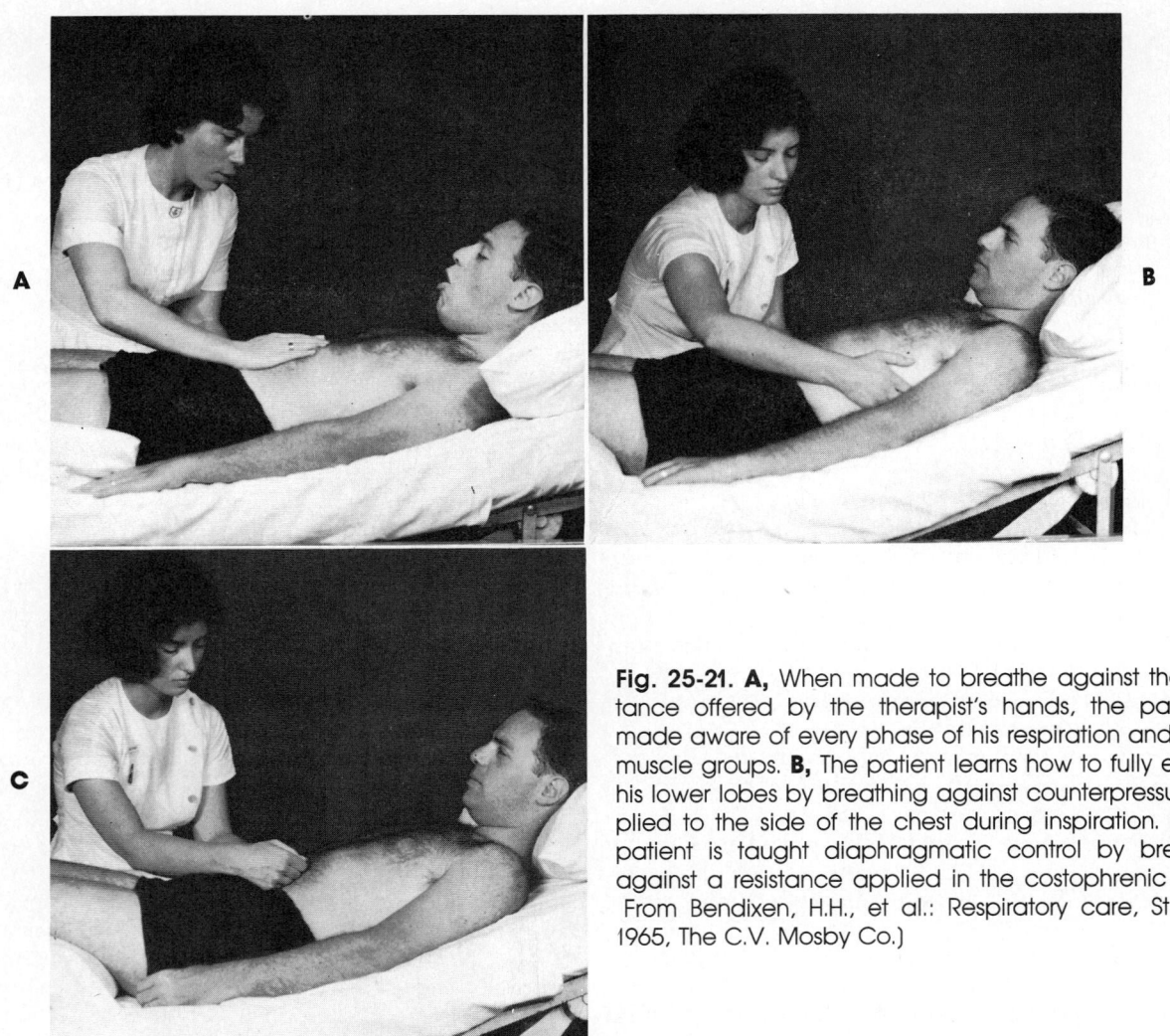

Fig. 25-21. A, When made to breathe against the resistance offered by the therapist's hands, the patient is made aware of every phase of his respiration and use of muscle groups. **B,** The patient learns how to fully expand his lower lobes by breathing against counterpressure applied to the side of the chest during inspiration. **C,** The patient is taught diaphragmatic control by breathing against a resistance applied in the costophrenic angle. From Bendixen, H.H., et al.: Respiratory care, St. Louis, 1965, The C.V. Mosby Co.)

this maneuver (Fig. 25-21). In addition to abdominal breathing, exercises to strengthen the abdominal muscles will assist patients to use their abdominal muscles more effectively in emptying their lungs.

This "controlled" breathing pattern is to be used while performing various activities of daily living—from sitting, standing, walking, and climbing stairs to more complex activities. As this pattern becomes natural, it will be used automatically during periods of increased shortness of breath. Persons who do not know how to use controlled breathing tend to increase their respiratory rate and their work of breathing when they are short of breath. As a result, physiologic obstruction increases, oxygen requirements increase, and effective ventilation decreases. Changing a person's respiratory pattern requires a great deal of effort by both the individual and those providing care.

This same method of teaching augmented abdominal (diaphragmatic) breathing can be used to teach the patient to cough. The difference is that expiration is forced down to residual volume. This maneuver often stimulates the cough reflex. If it does not, the person is taught to actively cough at the end of full expiration. Physiologically, forced expiration simulates the effects of a cough and is therefore more effective than telling the patient to take a deep breath and then cough.

Leg-raising exercises, with each leg being raised alternately as the patient exhales, is one way to strengthen abdominal muscles. Another way is to have the patient raise the head and shoulders from the bed while he or she exhales. Not all patients can do all exercises, but most can do some of them on a daily or twice daily basis. With practice and encouragement the patient can do the exercises 10 times each morning and evening after clearing the lungs as completely as possible of secretions.

Inhalation-exhalation exercises emphasize the need to prolong exhalation about four to five times longer than inhalation. Patients who are up walking can be taught to count in seconds and to concentrate on exhaling slowly and fully. While learning to *exhale with exertion,* the pa-

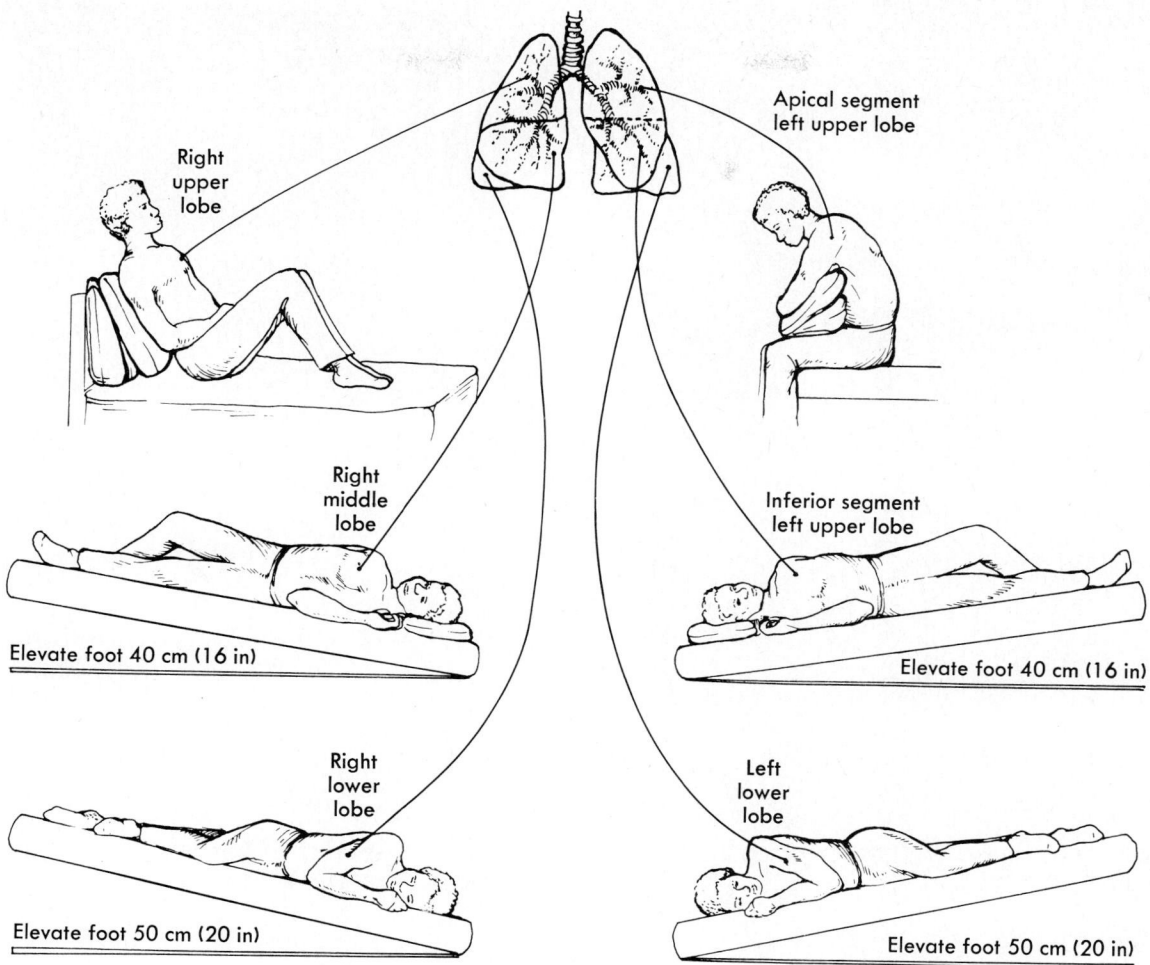

Fig. 25-22. Postural drainage requires that the patient assume various positions to facilitate the flow of secretions from various portions of the lung into the bronchi, trachea, and throat so that they can be raised and expectorated more easily. Drawing shows the correct position to drain various portions of the lung.

tient exhales during an activity such as bending over or sitting down.[84]

Muscle reconditioning refers to a variety of exercises that will tone muscles. For patients who are able to be up and about, walking, using a treadmill, or riding a stationary bicycle is helpful. The exercise period is started slowly with 10 minutes twice daily three times a week, increasing to 20 minutes twice daily three times a week. The patient needs to be assessed for his or her ability to carry out such an exercise program, and a staff member should be present during the exercise period.

PULMONARY PHYSIOTHERAPY. The person who has difficulty in breathing may be taught how to increase the efficiency of his/her breathing pattern. Breathing exercises are usually a part of pulmonary physiotherapy, which may also include *segmental postural drainage, clapping,* and *vibrating.* Although pulmonary physiotherapy activities may be performed by a physical therapist, they are often part of a nurse's responsibility. Regardless of where the pri-

mary responsibility lies, nurses must be familiar with the techniques so that they can demonstrate and reinforce them and be sure that the individual is doing them correctly. Also, the need for pulmonary physiotherapy may occur at a time when the physical therapist is not available to the patient.

SEGMENTAL POSTURAL DRAINAGE

Segmental postural drainage with clapping and vibration is a technique used to combine the force of gravity with the natural ciliary activity of the small bronchial airways to move secretions upward toward the main bronchi and the trachea. From this point the patient can cough them up, or they can be suctioned. In the treatment of chronic obstructive pulmonary disease, drainage of all segments is usually accomplished by placing patients in various postural drainage positions (Fig. 25-22). Treatment may also be directed at draining specific areas of the lung. While the patient is in each position, *clapping* with

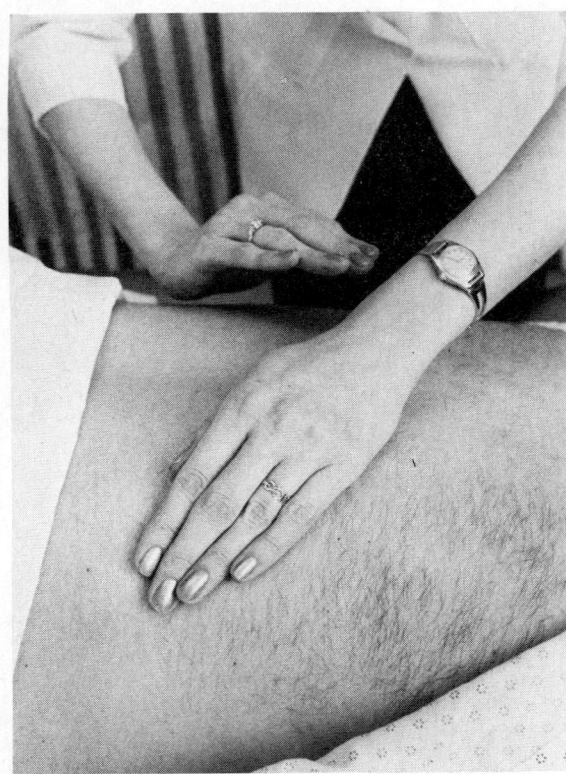

Fig. 25-23. Position of the hands for clapping the chest to loosen secretions.

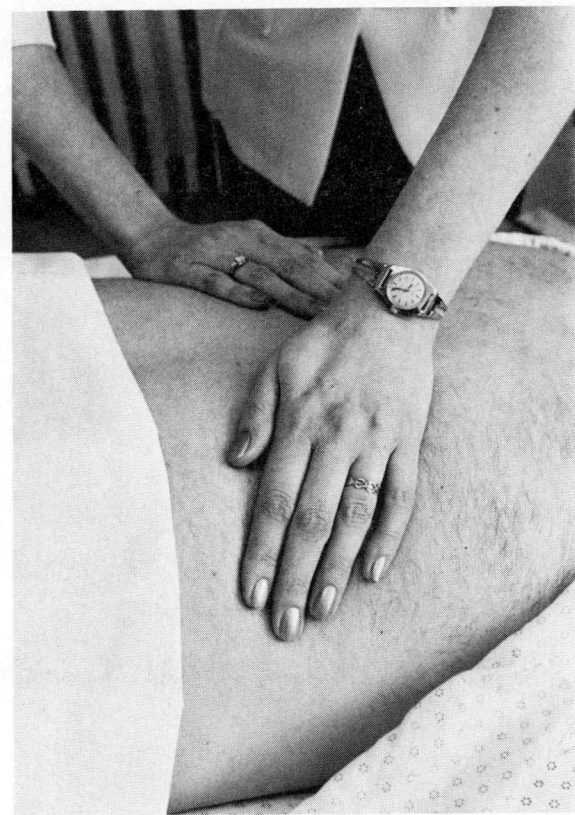

Fig. 25-24. Position of the hands for vibrating the chest at the end of prolonged expiration.

a cupped hand is done over the area being drained. This maneuver helps to loosen secretions and stimulate coughing (Fig. 25-23). After clapping of the area for approximately 1 minute, the patient is instructed to breathe deeply. *Vibrating* (pressure applied with a vibrating movement of the hand on the chest) is performed during expiratory phase of the deep breath (Fig. 25-24). This assists the patient to exhale more fully. The procedure is repeated as necessary. When the patient cannot tolerate a head-down position, a modified position is used.

Positions that provide gravity drainage of the lungs can be achieved in several ways, and the procedure selected usually depends on the age and general condition of the person as well as the lobe or lobes of the lungs where secretions have accumulated. A young person usually can tolerate greater lowering of the head than an elderly person whose vascular system adapts less quickly to change of position. A severely debilitated patient may only be able to tolerate slight changes in position.

Postural drainage can be achieved in several ways. Electric hospital beds can be tilted into a head-down position with little difficulty. If an electric bed is not available (for example, in the home), blocks can be placed under the casters at the foot of the bed or a hydraulic lift can be used under the foot of the bed. If these are not available, the foot of the

bed can be supported on the seat of a firm chair to provide a position in which the head is lowered.

The nurse needs to know the part of the lung affected and how to position the patient to drain that portion of the lung. For example, if the right middle lobe of the lung is affected, drainage will be accomplished best by way of the right middle bronchus. The patient should lie supine with the body turned at approximately a 45-degree angle. The angle can be maintained by pillow supports placed under the right side from the shoulders to the hips. The foot of the bed is raised about 30 cm (12 inches). This position can be maintained fairly comfortably by most patients for half an hour at a time. On the other hand, if the lower posterior area of the lung if affected, the foot of the bed can be raised 45 to 50 cm (18 to 20 inches) with the patient assuming a prone position for drainage. A summary of the positions for segmental postural drainage is given in Table 25-17.

Postural drainage and percussion should be planned so as to achieve maximal benefit. The best time is generally in the morning soon after arising and at night before retiring. Frequency of treatments will depend on each person's needs, but care should be taken to avoid exhaustion, which will result in shallow ventilation and negate the positive effects of the treatment.

Table 25-17. Positions for segmental postural drainage, clapping, and vibrating

Area of lung	Position of patient	Area to be clapped or vibrated
Upper lobe		
Apical bronchus	Semi-Fowler's position, leaning to right, then left, then forward	Over area of shoulder blades with fingers extending over clavicles
Posterior bronchus	Upright at 45-degree angle, rolled forward against a pillow at 45 degrees on left and then right side	Over shoulder blade on each side
Anterior bronchus	Supine with pillow under knees	Over anterior chest just below clavicles
Middle lobe (lateral and medial bronchus)	Trendelenburg's position at 30-degree angle or with foot of bed elevated 35-40 cm (14-16 inches), turned slightly to left	Anterior and lateral right chest from axillary fold to midanterior chest
Lingula (superior and inferior bronchus)	Trendelenburg's position at 30-degree angle or with foot of bed elevated 35-40 cm (14-16 inches), turned slightly to right	Left axillary fold to midanterior chest
Apical bronchus	Prone with pillow under hips	Lower third of posterior rib cage on both sides
Medial bronchus	Trendelenburg's position at 45-degree angle or with foot of bed raised 45-50 cm (18-20 inches) on right side	Lower third on left posterior rib cage
Lateral bronchus	Trendelenburg's position at 45-degree angle or with foot of bed raised 45-50 cm (18-20 inches) on left side	Lower third of right posterior rib cage
Posterior bronchus	Prone Trendelenburg's position at 45-degree angle with pillow under hips	Lower third of posterior rib cage on both sides

Patients having postural drainage of any kind are encouraged to breathe deeply and to cough forcefully to help dislodge thick sputum and exudate that is pooled in distended bronchioles, particularly after inactivity. Humidity, bronchodilators, or liquefying agents often are given 15 to 20 minutes before postural drainage is started, since they facilitate the removal of secretions. The patient may find that sputum can best be raised on resuming an upright position even though no drainage appeared while lying down with the head and chest lowered.

Since some patients complain of dizziness when assuming positions for postural drainage, the nurse stays with the patient during the first few times and reports any persistent dizziness or unusual discomfort to the physician.

Postural drainage may be contraindicated in some persons because of heart disease, hypertension, increased intracranial pressure, extreme dyspnea, or advanced age. However, most people can be taught to assume the positions for postural drainage and can proceed without help after being supervised once or twice.

Chest percussion (clapping) is contraindicated in the case of pulmonary emboli, hemorrhage, exacerbation of bronchospasms, severe pain, and over areas of resectable carcinoma. Often patients with a chronic pulmonary problem need to be taught to do postural drainage independently so that they can continue at home. The position usually is maintained for 10 minutes at first, and the period of time is gradually lengthened to 15 to 20 or even 30 minutes as the patient becomes accustomed to the position. At first, elderly persons usually are able to tolerate these positions only for a few minutes. They need more assistance than most other patients during the procedure and immediately thereafter. They should be assisted to a normal position in bed and requested to lie flat for a few minutes before sitting up or getting out of bed. This helps to prevent dizziness and reduces the danger of accidents.

The patient may feel nauseated because of the odor and taste of sputum. Therefore the procedure should be timed so that it comes at least 1 hour before meals. A short rest period following the treatment often improves postural drainage. Aromatic mouth washes should be available for frequent use by any patient who is expectorating sputum freely.

OXYGEN THERAPY. Oxygen therapy is required for patients with COPD who are unable to maintain a PO_2 of 50 mm Hg or more at rest and for those who cannot carry out ADL (bathing, eating, dressing, toileting) without be-

Table 25-18. Bronchodilators commonly used to treat COPD

Name	Mode of action
Methylxanthines	
Aminophylline	Block action of phosphodiesterase and interfere with degradation
Theophylline	of cyclic AMP, resulting in bronchodilation
Dyphylline	
Sympathomimetics*	
Beta$_1$-receptor sites	Activate adenylcyclase leading to increased production of
Epinephrine (adrenaline HCl)	cyclic AMP, resulting in relaxation of smooth muscle of airway;
Isoproterenol (Isuprel)	increase in cyclic AMP also inhibits release of chemical me-
Beta$_2$-receptor sites	diators that cause bronchospasm (histamine and SRS-A).
Terbutaline (Brethine)	
Metaproterenol (Alupent)	
Isoetharine (Bronkosol)	

*Beta-adrenergic drugs.

coming very short of breath. In these instances, 1 to 2 L of oxygen is usually given via nasal prongs. In addition, some patients only require supplemental oxygen during sleep. Patients who complain of restlessness, insomnia, or headaches may be helped to sleep more comfortably if they receive low flow oxygen during the night. Because many patients with COPD have chronic carbon dioxide retention, they need to understand that the risk of high flow rates of oxygen tension to greater than 60 to 70 mm Hg may remove the hypoxic drive and put them into respiratory failure. (See section on respiratory failure later in this chapter.)

Portable oxygen units are available that allow the patient to be up and about while receiving oxygen.

Medications

The types of medications that may be prescribed for persons with COPD include bronchodilators, expectorants, antimicrobials, corticosteroids, digitalis, diuretics, and psychopharmacologic agents.

BRONCHODILATORS. There are two basic categories of *bronchodilators*— sympathomimetic (adrenergic) agents and xanthine compounds. These bronchodilators act at different sites and appear to work synergistically when used together.[7] Table 25-18 lists the commonly used bronchodilators and their mode of action. Adrenergic agents that work at beta$_2$ sites located in smooth muscles of the airways have fewer cardiac side effects than do beta$_1$-agents whose receptor sites are in the myocardium. For this reason, isoetharine, metaproterenol sulfate, and terbutaline sulfate may be prescribed for patients with hypertension and those who have excessive palpitations or tachycardia from beta$_1$-agents.

AEROSOL THERAPY

Aerosol therapy is one of the most effective ways to deliver bronchodilators. There are several ways in which aerosolization of medications can be achieved. The in-

clude a Freon-propelled, metered-dosage cartridge inhalator; hand-bulb nebulizer; compressor pump; or IPPB machine.[41] In general, metered-dosage cartridge inhalators and hand-bulb nebulizers are used more commonly than IPPB (see box, p. 607). However, IPPB is still used to deliver aerosols to persons who cannot inhale repetitively to near TLC or in those persons who are unable to use a hand-bulb nebulizer because of lack of coordination or fatigue. When administering bronchodilators, the solution should be diluted with either water or saline. Some experts recommend that the diluent be water, since saline solutions already contain a solute (NaCl) in water.[41] All bronchodilator solutions are high-molecular weight concentrated solutions and have a high solute content. When they are diluted with water, there is a maximal decrease in solute concentration; thus smaller particle size and deeper depositon of the aerosol result.[41]

Aerosol devices are excellent sites for bacterial growth, and patients using such equipment at home should be advised how to clean them appropriately.

EXPECTORANTS. Although expectorants are sometimes prescribed, some experts believe they do more harm than good.[41] Water is still considered to be the best expectorant, and adequate hydration without fluid overload should be encouraged. Usually 2.0 to 2.5 L of fluids daily are recommended unless the patient has *cor pulmonale* and is on fluid restriction.

ANTIMICROBIALS. Antimicrobials are prescribed to treat respiratory tract infections in persons with COPD. The most commonly used ones are *tetracycline* and *ampicillin*, 1 to 2 g/day for 7 to 10 days. Some patients have a prescription on hand and self-administer the antimicrobial after telephone consultation with their physician. Antimicrobials should be started within 24 hours of the first sign of a respiratory infection (increased sputum production and purulence).[41] Patients who are febrile or have other signs and symptoms of infection that do not respond to the prescribed therapy should have a Gram stain and

---

Teaching patient to use hand nebulizer

The steps to be followed in teaching a person to use a hand nebulizer:
1. Exhale fully.
2. Position nebulizer in mouth *without* sealing lips around it.
3. Take a deep breath through mouth while squeezing the bulb of the nebulizer *once.*
4. Hold breath for 3 to 4 seconds at full inspiration.
5. Exhale slowly through pursed lips.

Usually one inhalation is sufficient. Several inhalations of a bronchodilator may cause medication overdosage and result in side effects (tachycardia, palpitation, nervousness).

Foods to increase protein and caloric intake

1. Offer frequent small feedings of foods high in protein and calories, for example:
   a. Milk shakes
   b. Flavored gelatin or pudding with whipped cream
   c. Cream soups made with half and half
   d. Peanut butter spread on crackers, bananas, pears, or apples
   e. Crackers and cheese, nuts, dried fruits, and ice cream readily available for snacks
2. Avoid foods that are difficult to chew or to digest; patient usually will indicate desires in this regard

---

culture and sensitivity studies. When antibiotics are used inappropriately, especially in patients who are not adequately clearing their lungs of secretions, superinfection with bacteria or fungi may occur.[41]

CORTICOSTEROIDS. Corticosteroids may be prescribed for patients with intermittent bronchial obstruction and blood or sputum eosinophilia whose condition is not controlled by bronchodilators.[41] Usually a short course of corticosteroids is prescribed to alleviate acute symptoms. Prednisone is often prescribed for a total of 7 to 10 days. In some patients with asthma, a longer course of prednisone may be prescribed and some patients will be on low-maintenance doses (5 to 10 mg/day) for several months or even years. Long-term corticosteroid therapy is usually not recommended for patients with chronic bronchitis or emphysema unless their disease is rapidly progressing.[41]

Persons who are on long-term steroid therapy should have a tuberculin test before initiation of therapy. Those with tuberculin reaction of 10 mm induration or more are candidates for isoniazid therapy (p. 566). The purpose of isoniazid therapy is to prevent reactivation of tuberculosis that can occur in persons receiving prolonged steroid therapy.

DIGITALIS. Digitalis may be prescribed for patients with COPD and left ventricular failure. The patient receiving a digitalis preparation should be carefully monitored for side effects (Chapter 26).

Patients with increased dyspnea secondary to pulmonary edema, or with right ventricular failure, or corticosteroid-induced fluid retention may benefit from *diuretics.*

When diuretics are given, the patient should be carefully monitored for side effects. Those on thiazide diuretics will need to be taught about eating foods high in potassium such as bananas, oranges, prunes, and raisins.

PSYCHOPHARMACOLOGIC AGENTS. Psychopharmacologic agents may need to be prescribed for some patients with severe emotional disturbances. The type of agent and size of dose are individually determined; but in general, the older the patient, the smaller the dose. When these agents are prescribed, a pharmacology book should be referred to for information about the side effects and precautions to be used in administering these agents.

Maintaining adequate nutrition and fluid intake

Persons with COPD may be very short of breath, and eating can become a real problem to the person who is breathless. The patient may be overweight early in the disease and will be urged to lose weight and keep it at normal or slightly below normal levels.

In later stages of COPD patients are often malnourished because of dyspnea and reduced energy levels. Suggestions to increase protein and caloric intake are listed in lower box above.

Assisting with comfort and ADL

1. Place patient in position of comfort, usually Fowler's or high Fowler's
2. Assist patient with progressive relaxation exercises and meditation (see boxes, p. 608)

tively. When an endotracheal tube is removed, the normal airway is restored and the patient is usually able to cough without difficulty. However, when a tracheostomy tube is removed, there is an air leak at the incision site. This air leak prevents the buildup of intrathoracic pressures high enough to produce an effective cough until the incision is healed. The patient can be taught to place two or three fingers firmly over the dressing that covers the tracheostomy site to reduce the air leak. If this is not successful in helping to generate a cough that clears the airway, the stoma can be suctioned. Frequent use of the stoma for suctioning, however, can delay closure and healing of the tracheostomy incision.

MECHANICAL VENTILATION

If the patient is unable to maintain ventilation (as indicated by a rising arterial P_{CO_2}) mechanical ventilation is necessary.

Many different kinds of respirators are available. In general, there are two kinds, pressure cycled and volume cycled. The Bird and Bennett (PR series) (Fig. 25-30) are pressure-limited ventilators, whereas the Möerch, Emerson, Engstrom, Air Shields, Bennett MA-1, Siemen's Servo, and Ohio 560 are volume-limited machines (Fig. 25-31). Both types of machines can be used intermittently or continuously to assist or to control respiration.

When a *pressure-cycled* ventilator is used, the machine is set to deliver a predetermined amount of pressure (usually 15 to 25 cm of water) with each breath. When this pressure is reached, the machine turns off and normal exhalation begins. The volume of gas delivered to the patient is not necessarily constant because it depends on the resistance of the entire system, including the patient's lungs. For this reason the expired tidal volume must be monitored frequently and adjustments made in the respirator controls as needed.

With a *volume-controlled* machine a *constant volume* of air is delivered with each breath. The volume is preset and is delivered to the patient at whatever pressure is necessary to attain that volume. A volume-cycled machine should have a pressure cutoff valve. Such a mechanism allows a pressure limit to be set. If the pressure required to deliver the set volume exceeds the pressure limit, the machine will turn off before the entire volume is delivered. The pressure limit on a volume-cycled machine usually has an audible alarm. The nurse can set the limit slightly above (approximately 5 cm of water) the pressure required to ventilate the patient. The alarm will then go off if the patient coughs, accumulates secretion, or starts to resist the machine.

Regardless of which type of ventilator is used, mechanisms for various regulations are necessary if the machine is to be adjusted to each patient. It is preferable to have a respirator that can be used to assist or control the patient's breathing. "Assist" means that the patient's own inspiratory effort triggers (turns on) the machine. Most respirators have a *sensitivity control knob* that can be adjusted to respond to weak inspiratory efforts. "Control"

implies the use of automatic cycling. The patient may be apneic and the machine set at the desired rate; the patient's own respiratory rate may be too slow, and the automatic cycling can be used to force an increase in the rate; or the patient's own respiratory efforts can be ignored and an automatic rate used to ventilate the patient. (Some machines with automatic cycling do not allow for the latter adjustment.) It is also helpful to be able to regulate the flow rates at which the gas is delivered to the patient. For example, patients breathing at rapid rates and high volumes need faster flow rates than those breathing slowly and at moderate volumes. A final necessity is the ability to regulate the inspired concentration of oxygen from 20% (room air) to 100%.

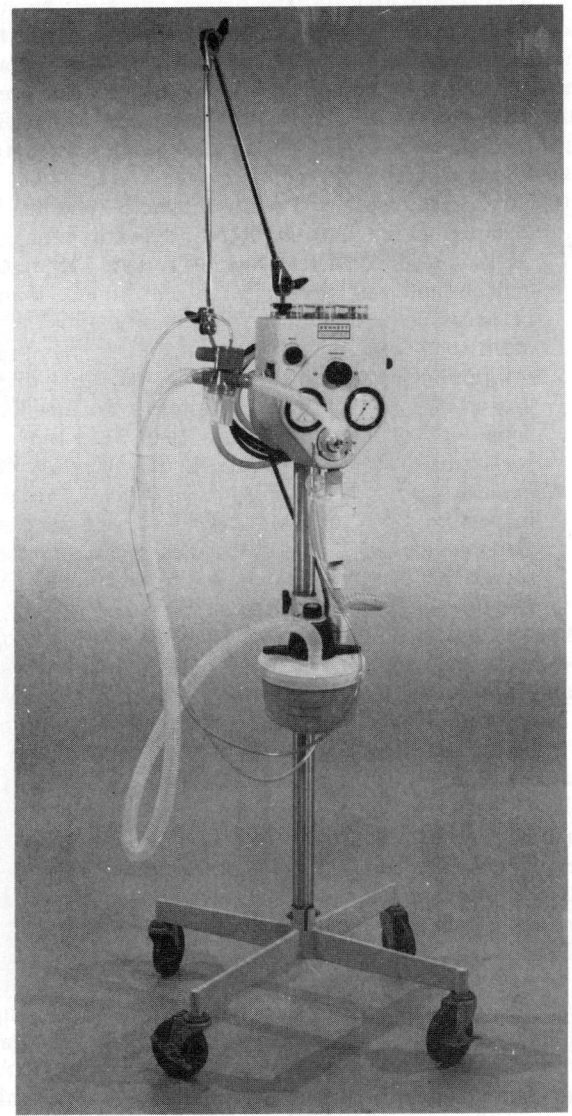

Fig. 25-30. Pressure-cycled ventilator, Bennett, PR-1. (From Abels, L.F.: Mosby's manual of critical care, St. Louis, 1979, The C.V. Mosby Co.)

All respirators used for mechanical ventilation must do the following:

1. Provide for the heating and humidifcation of inspired air
2. Provide a means for measurement of expired volumes
3. Be dependable for long periods of use
4. Be easily cleaned

Any patient on continuous mechanical ventilation should be "sighed" (given a deep breath) several times an hour. Some respirators automatically "sigh" the patient, while with others the patient is "sighed" manually using a self-inflating (Ambu) or anesthesia bag. This periodic deep breathing is necessary to prevent alveolar collapse and resultant atelectasis.

Positive-end expiratory pressure

Positive end-expiratory pressure (PEEP) is ventilator mode that has been shown to increase the effectiveness of mechanical ventilation in certain patients. PEEP involves the maintenance of positive pressure, at the end of expiration, rather than allowing airway pressure to return to normal (atmospheric) as usually occurs. By maintaining positive pressure, alveoli that would otherwise collapse on expiration are held open, thus increasing the opportunity for gas exchange across the alveolar-capillary membrane. This is accomplished by the increase in functional residual capacity. The result is a decrease in physiologic shunting and the ability to achieve a higher level of PO_2 with lower concentrations of delivered oxygen (FIO_2). PEEP has its greatest use in the treatment of

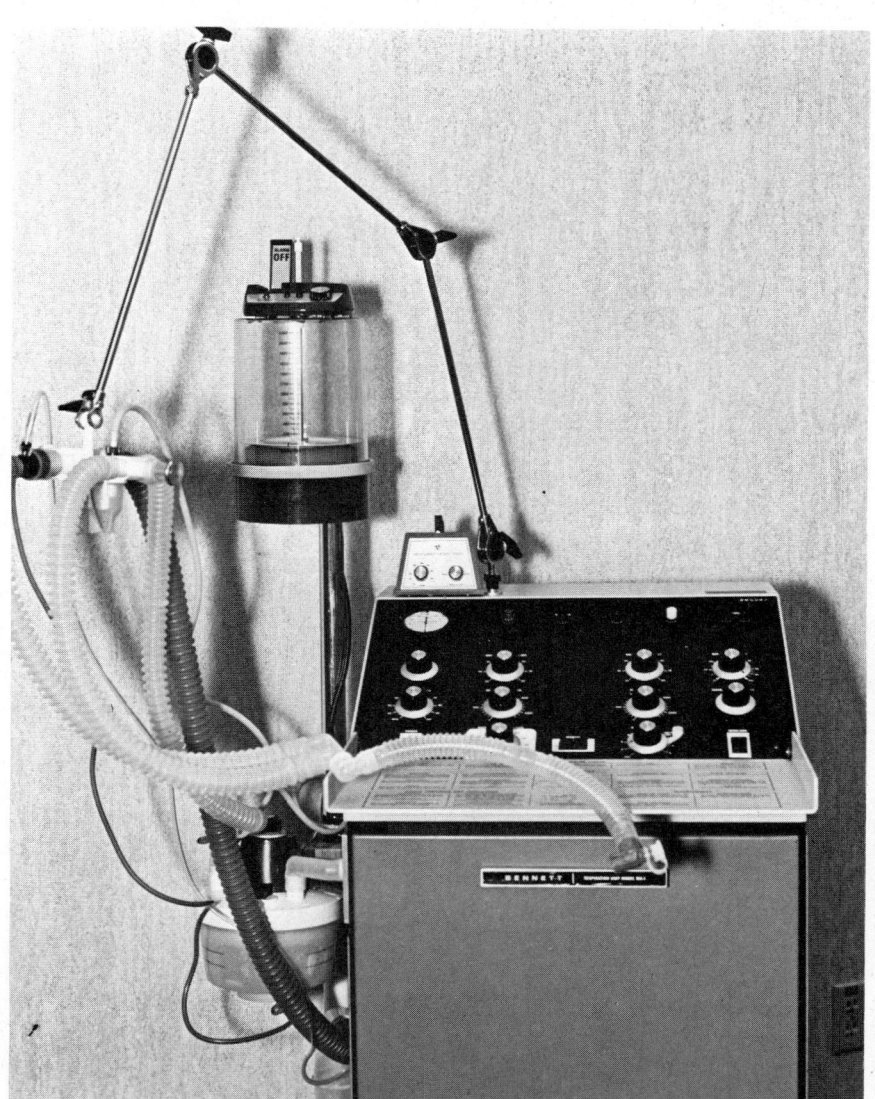

Fig. 25-31. Volume cycled ventilator, Bennett, MA-1. (From Abels, L.F.: Mosby's manual of critical care, St. Louis, 1979, The C.V. Mosby Co.)

ARDS, but is also used in treating any patient who would otherwise require unacceptably high concentrations of oxygen.

The hazards of PEEP are related to the increase in intrathoracic pressure. Most serious of the dangers related to this technique is the increased incidence of pneumothorax, particularly in those with friable lung tissue, as seen in persons with emphysema or lung cancer. The sudden disappearance of breath sounds on one side, in conjunction with signs of respiratory distress, in the patient being ventilated with PEEP *must be taken as an indication of a pneumothorax.* This can develop into a life-threatening episode if the pneumothorax is large, and the physician must be called immediately. Another less serious consequence of PEEP may be a reduction in venous return, which is impeded by the increased intrathoracic pressure, and a subsequent fall in cardiac output. This effect seems to be particularly common in patients who are relatively dehydrated and can sometimes be avoided by careful fluid administration.

Weaning from the ventilator

The nurse plays an important role in weaning the patient from the ventilator. Both physiologic studies (blood gases, tidal volume) and clinical status determine the patient's readiness to breathe without mechanical assistance. Before weaning, the patient should have been taught breathing exercises. When the patient is taken off the respirator, a nurse in whom the patient has confidence should be present. It is also helpful if the environment around the patient is calm. Much of the success of weaning is dependent on the interrelationship between the patient's physiologic and psychologic responses. If the patient becomes very anxious and takes rapid, shallow breaths, being off the respirator will be poorly tolerated. If a pattern of controlled breathing can be maintained, success is more likely. Weaning is usually begun with short periods off the respirator. The amount of time off the respirator is increased according to the patient's tolerance. The nurse must carefully assess the adequacy of the patient's ventilation during the time off the respirator. If, in the nurse's judgment, the patient cannot tolerate breathing on his or her own because of inadequate tidal volume, cyanosis, tachycardia, diaphoresis, or restlessness, mechanical assistance should be reinstituted.

A more recent technique of weaning is the use of *intermittent mandatory ventilation* (IMV). This involves the addition of an oxygen reservoir with a one-way valve to the respirator circuit. The rate on the ventilator is reduced below the patient's normal rate. The ventilator then delivers the set minimum, and the patient spontaneously breathes several breaths in addition to this from the oxygen reservoir. For example, if the patient's natural respiratory rate is 16, the ventilator might be set to deliver 10 breaths per minute. The patient will then take an additional six breaths independently. In this way, the pa-

tient can gradually build up strength and gain respiratory independence without having to be taken completely off the ventilator for periods of time.

Throughout the treatment of the patient in respiratory failure, ventilation should be carefully monitored by blood gas studies and simple spirometry (tidal volume, vital capacity). Alert nursing observation of the patient can determine the adequacy of ventilation. Meticulous attention is given to maintaining a patent airway, which is the prime nursing responsibility. (See specialized material for further detail.[56,81,100,103]

REST

The patient who is subjected to many treatments can become excessively fatigued, further compromising ventilatory capacity. Frequent rest periods must be interspersed with treatments, and it is the nurse's responsibility to see that the patient is provided with a quiet environment and is not disturbed by unnecessary interruptions at rest times. Unfortunately, persons who have severe insufficiency must have frequent treatments and interventions; it is *not* appropriate, although the person may be quite tired, to allow the patient to sleep through the night and omit treatments. This will inevitably lead to a worsened status.

Although persons with respiratory insufficiency are often anxious and frightened, sedation is contraindicated because it depresses respirations. Therefore it is especially important that the nurse be supportive of the patient and be skillful in assisting the patient to breathe effectively. The patient can be extremely demanding, and the nurse must understand the fear and anxiety that is often the basis for the patient's behavior.

MONITORING

Aggressive, constant nursing care is essential for these patients. The nurse must be continually alert to clinical changes that represent changes in the patient's ventilation. Increasing confusion and behavioral changes often indicate an elevated P_{CO_2}. The behavioral changes may range from pugnacious, combative behavior to lethargy. Other clinical signs of *hypercapnia* are flushed skin color caused by reflex vasodilation, muscle twitching, and headache. Signs commonly seen in *hypoxia* include tachycardia, increased pulse rate, cyanosis, changes in blood pressure, and changes in behavior. In *early* stages of hypoxia, the blood pressure is elevated as a result of vasoconstriction and increased peripheral resistance. In *later* stages the blood pressure falls to hypotensive levels, and circulatory arrest can occur. It is important to point out that cyanosis is not an early sign of hypoxia, since it does not occur until arterial oxygen saturation is less than 85%; thus the nurse needs to be alert to earlier signs of hypoxia mentioned previously.

REFERENCES AND SELECTED READINGS*

1. Agle, D.P., and Baum, G.L.: Psychological aspects of chronic obstructive pulmonary disease, Med. Clin. North Am. **61:**749-758, 1977.
2. Albanese, A., and Toplitz, A.: A hassle-free guide to suctioning a tracheostomy, RN **45:**24-30, 1982.
3. Alford, R.H.: Histoplasmosis. In Conn, H.F.: Current therapy 1982, Philadelphia, 1982, W.B. Saunders Co.
4. American Academy of Pediatrics: Report of the Committee on Infectious Diseases, ed. 19, Evanston, Ill., 1982, The Academy.
5. American Cancer Society: Cancer facts and figures 1984, New York, 1983, The Society.
6. American College of Chest Physicians: A report of the Committee on Emphysema: recommendations for continuous oxygen therapy in chronic obstructive lung disease, Chest **64:**505-507, 1973.
7. *American Lung Association: Chronic obstructive pulmonary disease, New York, 1981, The Association.
8. American Lung Association: Diagnostic standards and classification of tuberculosis, New York, 1981, The Association.
9. *American Lung Association: Occupational lung disease: an introduction, New York, 1979, The Association.
10. American Thoracic Society: Treatment of myobacterial disease, Am. Rev. Respir. Dis. **115:**185-187, 1977.
11. Bartlett, J.G., and Garbach, S.L.: The triple threat of aspiration pneumonia, Chest **68:**550-556, 1980.
12. Brenner, D.J., et al.: Classification of the legionnaires' disease bacterium: an interim report, Curr. Microbiol. **1:**71-75, 1978.
13. *Bricker, P.L.: Chest tubes. The crucial points you mustn't forget, RN **43:**21-26, 1980.
14. *Callahan, M.: C.O.P.D. makes a bad first impression, but you'll find wonderful people underneath, Nurs. 82 **12:**67-72, 1982.
15. *Cameron, T.J.: Fiberoptic bronchoscopy, Am. J. Nurs. **81:**1462-1465, 1981.
16. *Cardin, S.: Acid-base balance in the patient with respiratory disease, Nurs. Clin. North Am. **15:**593-601, 1980.
17. Carr, D.T., and Rosenow, E.C.: Bronchogenic carcinoma, Basics RD **5:**1-6, 1977.
18. Center for Disease Control: Annual summary 1982: reported morbidity and mortality in the United States, Morbid. Mortal. Weekly Rep. **31:**54, 1983.
19. *Cimprich, B., Gaydos, D., and Langan, R.: A preoperative teaching program for the thoracotomy patient, Ca. Nurs. **1:**35-39, 1978.
20. *Cohen, S.: Pulmonary function tests in patient care: programmed instruction, Am. J. Nurs. **80:**1135-1161, 1980.
21. *D'Agostino, J.S.: Teaching tips for living with C.O.P.D. at home, Nurs. 84 **14:**57, 1984.
22. *D'Agostino, J.S.: You can breathe new life into your COPD patients, Nurs. 83 **13:**72, 74-77, 1983.
23. Daly, B.: Intensive care nursing, New York, 1980, Medical Examination Publishing Co.
24. *Duncan, C., and Erichson, R.: Pressures associated with chest tube stripping, Heart Lung **11:**166-171, 1982.
25. Ebersole, P., and Hess, P.: Toward healthy aging, St. Louis 1981, The C.V. Mosby Co.
26. Eickhoff, T.C.: The current status of BCG immunization against tuberculosis, Ann. Rev. Med. **28:**411-423, 1979.
27. *Einstein, H.E.: Coccidioidomycosis, Basics RD **9:**1-6, 1980.
28. *Elpern, E.H.: Asthma update: Pathophysiology and treatment, Heart Lung **9:**665-670, 1980.
29. *Erickson, R.: Chest tubes. They're really not that complicated, Nurs. 81 **11:**34-43, 1981.
30. *Erickson, R.: Solving chest tube problems, Nurs. 81 **11:**62-68, 1981.
31. Erickson, R.: To cough or not to cough, Nurs. 82 **12:**124-126, 1982.
32. *Frame, P.T.: Acute infectious pneumonia in the adult, Basics RD **10:**3, 1982.
33. Fromm, C.: Using basic laboratory data to evaluate patients with acute respiratory failure, Crit. Care Q. **1:**43-52, 1979.
34. *Fuchs, P.L.: A.R.D.S.: physiology, signs, and symptoms, Nurs. 83 **13:**52-53, 1983.
35. *Fuchs, P.L.: Asthma, signs, and symptoms, Nurs. 83 **13:**36-37, 1983.
36. *Fuchs, P.L.: Before and after surgery: stay right on respiratory care, Nurs. 83 **13:**47-50, 1983.
37. Gong, H.: Evaluation and management of patients with cough, sputum, or hemoptysis. In Selecky, P., editor: Pulmonary disease, New York, 1982, John Wiley & Sons, Inc.
38. *Greenwood, B.S.: The before and after of good postop pulmonary care, Nurs. 82 **12:**68-69, 1982.
39. Hanson, E.I.: Effects of chronic lung disease on life in general and on sexuality: perception of adult patients, Heart Lung **11:**435-441, 1982.
40. *Hanson, R.R., and Kasik, J.E.: The pneumoconioses, Heart Lung **6:**645-652, 1977.
41. *Hodgkin, J.E.: Chronic obstructive pulmonary disease, Park Ridge, Ill., 1979. American College of Chest Physicians.
42. Hudgel, D.M., and Madsen, L.A.: Acute and chronic asthma: a guide to intervention, Am. J. Nurs. **80:**1791-1795, 1980.
43. *Hughes, J.M.: Postoperative pulmonary care: past, present, and future, Crit. Care Q. **6:**67, 1983.
44. Humidifiers: tips given on trimming infection hazards, Hosp. Infect. Control **8:**24-26, 1979.
45. *Hunter, P.M.: Bedside monitoring of respiratory function, Nurs. Clin. North Am. **16:**211-224, 1981.
46. Jones, R.W., and Weill, H.: Occupational lung disease, Basics RD **6:**1-6, 1978.
47. Kamholz, S.L., and Pinsker, K.L.: Bacterial pneumonia. In Conn, H.F.: Current therapy 1982, Philadelphia, 1982, W.B. Saunders Co.
48. Karetzky, M.S., and Khan, A.U.: Review of current concepts in aspiration pneumonia, Heart Lung **6:**321-326, 1977.
49. Keyes, J.L.: Blood gas analysis and the assessment of acid-base status, Heart Lung **5:**247-255, 1976.

*References preceded by an asterisk are particularly well suited for student reading.

50. *Kirilloff, L.H., and Tibbals, S.C.: Drugs for asthma. A complete guide, Am. J. Nurs. **83:**55-61, 1983.

51. *Kirkis, E.J.: Infection consult: common error can cause pneumonia, RN **45:**97-98, 1982.

52. *Koss, J.A., and Christoph, C.: Oxygen therapy and other respiratory therapy in acute respiratory failure, Crit. Care Q. **1:**53-63, 1979.

53. Kravetz, H.M.: Coccidioidomycosis. In Conn, H.F.: Current therapy 1982, Philadelphia, 1982, W.B. Saunders Co.

54. Kryger, M., editor: Pathophysiology of respiration, New York, 1981, John Wiley & Sons, Inc.

55. *Landis, K., and Smith, S.: The mechanically ventilated patient: a comprehensive nursing care plan, Crit. Care Q. **6:**43, 1983.

56. Langston, H.T., and Barker, W.S.: The adult thoracic surgical patient. In Neville, W.E., editor: Intensive care of the surgical cardiopulmonary patient, ed. 2, Chicago, 1983, Year Book Medical Publishers, Inc.

57. Leininger, B.J.: Thoracic trauma, In Neville, W.E.: Intensive care of the surgical cardiopulmonary patient, ed. 2, Chicago, 1983, Year Book Medical Publishers, Inc.

58. Levine, D.P., and Lerner, M.: The clinical spectrum of *Mycoplasma pneumoniae* infections, Med. Clin. North Am. **62:**961-978, 1978.

59. *Linn, L.J.: Psychosocial needs of patients with acute respiratory failure, Crit. Care Q. **1:**65-74, 1979.

60. Malasanos, L., et al.: Health assessment, ed. 2, St. Louis, 1981, The C.V. Mosby Co.

61. *Martini, N.: Lung cancer—an overview, Ca. Nurs. **1:**31-33, 1978.

62. McCauley, K., and Weaver, T.E.: Cardiac and pulmonary diseases: nutritional implications, Nurs. Clin. North Am. **18:**81-96, 1983.

63. Mennies, J.H.: Smoking: the physiologic effects, Am. J. Nurs. **83:**1143, 1983.

64. Miller, W.C.: Chronic bronchitis, bronchiectasis, and emphysema. In Conn, H.F.: Current therapy 1982, Philadelphia, 1982, W.B. Saunders Co.

65. Mizuki, J.: There's no place like home, Am. J. Nurs. **84:**647, 1984.

66. Moorthy, S.S., LoSasso, A.M., and Gibbs, P.S.: Respiratory failure in patients following surgery and trauma, Crit. Care Q. **1:**15-25, 1979.

67. Mountain, C.F.: Primary lung cancer. In Conn, H.F.: current therapy 1982, Philadelphia, 1982, W.B. Saunders Co.

68. Nielsen, L.: Mechanical ventilation: patient assessment and nursing care, Am. J. Nurs. **80:**2191-2217, 1980.

69. Nursing Grand Rounds: Adult respiratory distress syndromes: a true test of nursing skills, Nurs. 80 **10:**51-56, 1980.

70. Nursing Grand Rounds: Fighting the frustrations of status asthmaticus, Nurs. 82 **12:**58-63, 1982.

71. *Nursing Grand Rounds: Teaming up to send the end-stage COPD patient home, Nurs. 84 **14:**65-68, 1984.

72. Oermann, M., et al.: Patient sensations following a tracheostomy: a discussion, Crit. Care Q. **6:**53, 1983.

73. Ostrow, D.: Symptoms and signs. In Kryger, M., editor: Pathophysiology of respiration, New York, 1981, John Wiley & Sons, Inc.

74. Pare, J.A., and Fraser, R.G.: Synopsis of diseases of the chest, Philadelphia, 1983, W.B. Saunders Co.

75. Penn, R.L.: Blastomycosis. In Conn, H.F.: Current therapy 1982, Philadelphia, 1982, W.B. Saunders Co.

76. Pennoyer, D., and Sheffer, A.L.: Asthma in adults. In Conn, H.F.: Current therapy 1982, Philadelphia, 1982, W.B. Saunders Co.

77. Perdue, P.: Urgent priorities in severe trauma: life-threatening respiratory injuries, RN **44:**27-33, 1981.

78. *Petersen, G.M.: Application of oxygen therapy devices, Nurs. Clin. North Am. **16:**241-257, 1981.

79. Petty, T.L.: Adult respiratory distress syndrome. In Kryger, M.H., editor: Pathology of respiration, New York, 1981, John Wiley & Sons, Inc.

80. Pfister, S.: Respiratory arrest: are you prepared? Nurs. 82 **12:**34-41, 1982.

81. *Phipps, W.J., Barker, W.L., and Daly, B.J.: Respiratory insufficiency and failure. In Meltzer, L.E., Abdellah, R.G., and Kitchell, J.F.: Concepts and practices of intensive care for nurse specialists, ed. 2, Bowie, Md., 1976, The Charles Press.

82. *Rhodes, M.K.: Recognizing and caring for the patient with Legionnaire's disease, Nurs. 80 **10:**104E, 1980.

83. *Rhodes, M.: Update on chest traums, Crit. Care Q. **6:**59, 1983.

84. Rifas, E.M.: How you and your patient can manage dyspnea, Nurs. 80 **10:**34-41, 1980.

85. Rifas, E.M.: Teaching patients to manage acute asthma. The future is now, Nurs. 83 **13:**77-80, 1983.

86. *Risser, N.L.: Preoperative and postoperative care to prevent pulmonary complications, Heart Lung **9:**57-67, 1980.

87. Rogers, B.H., et al.: Opportunistic pneumonia: a clinicopathological study of five cases caused by an unidentified acid-fast bacterium, New Engl. J. Med. **301:**959-961, 1979.

88. *Rokosky, J.S.: Assessment of the individual with altered respiratory function, Nurs. Clin. North Am. **16:**195-209, 1981.

89. Selecky, P.A.: Pulmonary disease, New York, 1982, John Wiley & Sons, Inc.

90. Shapiro, B.A., Harrison, R.A., and Trout, C.A.: Clinical application of respiratory care, ed. 2, Bowie, Md., 1979, The Charles Press.

91. *Sjobers, E.L.: Nursing diagnoses and the COPD patient, Am. J. Nurs. **83:**245-248, 1983.

92. Slonim, N.B., and Hamilton, L.H.: Respiratory physiology, ed. 4, St. Louis, 1981, The C.V. Mosby Co.

93. Spires, R.: Tuberculosis today. The siege isn't over yet, RN **43:**43-47, 1980.

94. Stevens, P.M.: Positive and expiratory pressure breathing, Basics RD **5:**1-6, 1977.

95. *Stewart, E.: To lessen pain: relaxation and rhythmic breathing, Am. J. Nurs. **76:**958-959, 1976.

96. Straus, M.J.: Lung cancer: clinical diagnosis and treatment, ed. 2, New York 1982, Grune & Stratton, Inc.

97. *Sumner, S.M., and Lewandowski, V.: Guidelines for using artificial breathing devices, Nurs. 83 **13:**54-57, 1983.

98. Symposium on respiratory care, Nurs. Clin. North Am. **16:**193-297, 1981.

99. Thomson, P.S., and Willis, J.C.: Compliance challenges in a Black Lung Clinic, Nurs. Clin. North Am. **17:**513-521, 1982.

100. Traver, G.A.: Respiratory nursing: the science and the art, New York, 1982, John Wiley & Sons, Inc.

101. U.S. Center for Disease Control, Tuberculosis branch: Tuberculosis statistics: cities and states—1976, Atlanta, 1977, The Center.

102. U.S. Department of Health and Human Services/Public Health Service, Center for Disease Control: Morbid. Mortal. Weekly Rep. **31:**10, March 19, 1982.

103. Wade, J.: Comprehensive repiratory care; physiology and technique, ed. 3, St. Louis, 1982, The C.V. Mosby Co.

104. *Weg, J.G.: Tuberculosis and other mycobacterial disease. In Conn., H.F.: Current therapy 1982, Philadelphia, 1982, W.B.Saunders Co.

105. West, J.B.: Ventilation/blood flow and gas exchange, ed. 3, Oxford, England, 1980, Blackwell Scientific Publications.

106. Woodin, L.M.: Your patient with pneumothorax: a patient in distress, Nurs. 82 **12:**50-56, 1982.

107. Worthington, L.: Hypoxemia: why giving oxygen isn't enough, RN **43:**49-53, 1980.

108. Wyngaarden, J., and Smith, L.: Cecil textbook of medicine, ed. 16, Philadelphia, 1982, W.B. Saunders Co.

109. Youmans, G.P., Patterson, P.Y., and Sommers, H.M.: The biologic and clinical basis of infectious diseases, Philadelphia, 1976, W.B. Saunders Co.

Classic

110. Comroe, J.H.: Physiology of respiration, ed. 2, Chicago, 1974, Year Book Medical Publishers, Inc.

111. *Hunt, W.J., and Bespalec, D.A.: An evaluation of current methods of modifying smoking behavior, J. Clin. Psychol. **30:**431-438, 1974.

112. *Jacquette, G.; To reduce hazards of tracheal suctioning, Am. J. Nurs. **71:**2362-2364, 1971.

113. *Nett, L., and Petty, T.L.: Oxygen toxicity, Am. J. Nurs. **73:**1556-1558, 1973.

114. *Petty, T.L.: A chest physician's perspective on asthma, Heart Lung **1:**611-620, 1972.

115. *Wagner, M.M.: Assessment of patients with multiple injures, Am. J. Nurs. **72:**1822-1827, 1972.

116. Ziskind, M.M.: The acute bacterial pneumonias in the adult. In American Thoracic Society: Basics of RD, New York, 1974, The Society.

26

The Patient with Cardiovascular Problems

EILEEN WALSH-ESSIG, H. FRED FARLEY, and MARY A. (SANDY) WYPER

STUDY QUESTIONS

- Review the developmental anatomy of the heart, specifically as it pertains to the pericardium, myocardium, and endocardium.

- Review the electrophysiology of the heart.

- Review the guidelines for oxygen therapy in your fundamentals nursing text or nursing skills book.

- Review the process of wound healing (see Chapter 19). How can this process be applied to a myocardial infarction?

- Examine the chart of a patient who has had a myocardial infarction. What changes can be noted in the serum enzyme levels? What nursing diagnoses were identified?

- What drugs improve, regulate, and/or stimulate the action of the heart?

- What is the rationale for the use of diuretic therapy in the treatment of heart failure?

- Examine the chart of a patient with congestive heart failure. Compare and contrast the patient's symptoms with the usual symptoms of CHF. From the description of the patient's symptoms, does the patient have left- or right-sided heart failure or both? What nursing diagnoses were identified?

Heart disease remains the leading cause of death in the industrialized nations. In the United States alone, cardiovascular disease (CVD) is responsible for approximately 1 million deaths every year. Fortunately, during the past 2 decades cardiovascular research has significantly increased our understanding of the structure and function of the cardiovascular system in health and disease, and during the last 15 years there has been a steady decline in mortality from cardiovascular disorders. It is hoped that effective application of the increased knowledge of CVD and its risk factors will enable health care professionals to assist persons more effectively in achieving and maintaining optimal health.

ANATOMY AND PHYSIOLOGY
Basic structure of the heart

The heart is a small organ (about the size of a fist) located in the middle and slightly to the left of the mediastinum, where it is partially overlapped by the lungs. The lower border, which forms a blunt tip (apex) to the left, rests on the diaphragm.

The heart is enclosed by a loose, inelastic sac (*pericardium*) that consists of two layers: the inner layer (visceral pericardium) and the outer layer (parietal pericardium). The two pericardial surfaces are separated by a pericardial space that normally contains approximately 10 to 20 ml of thin, clear pericardial fluid. This lubricating fluid moistens the contacting surfaces of the pericardial layers and serves to reduce the friction produced by the pumping action of the heart. If too much fluid collects in the pericardial space (pericardial effusion), pressure is exerted on the heart muscle, leading to decreased pumping efficiency.

There are three layers of cardiac tissue:

Epicardium: Outer layer of the heart
   Same structure as the visceral pericardium

Myocardium: Middle layer of the heart
   Composed of striated muscle fibers
   Responsible for the heart's contractile force

Endocardium: Inner layer of the heart
   Consists of endothelial tissue
   Lines the inside of the chambers and covers the heart valves

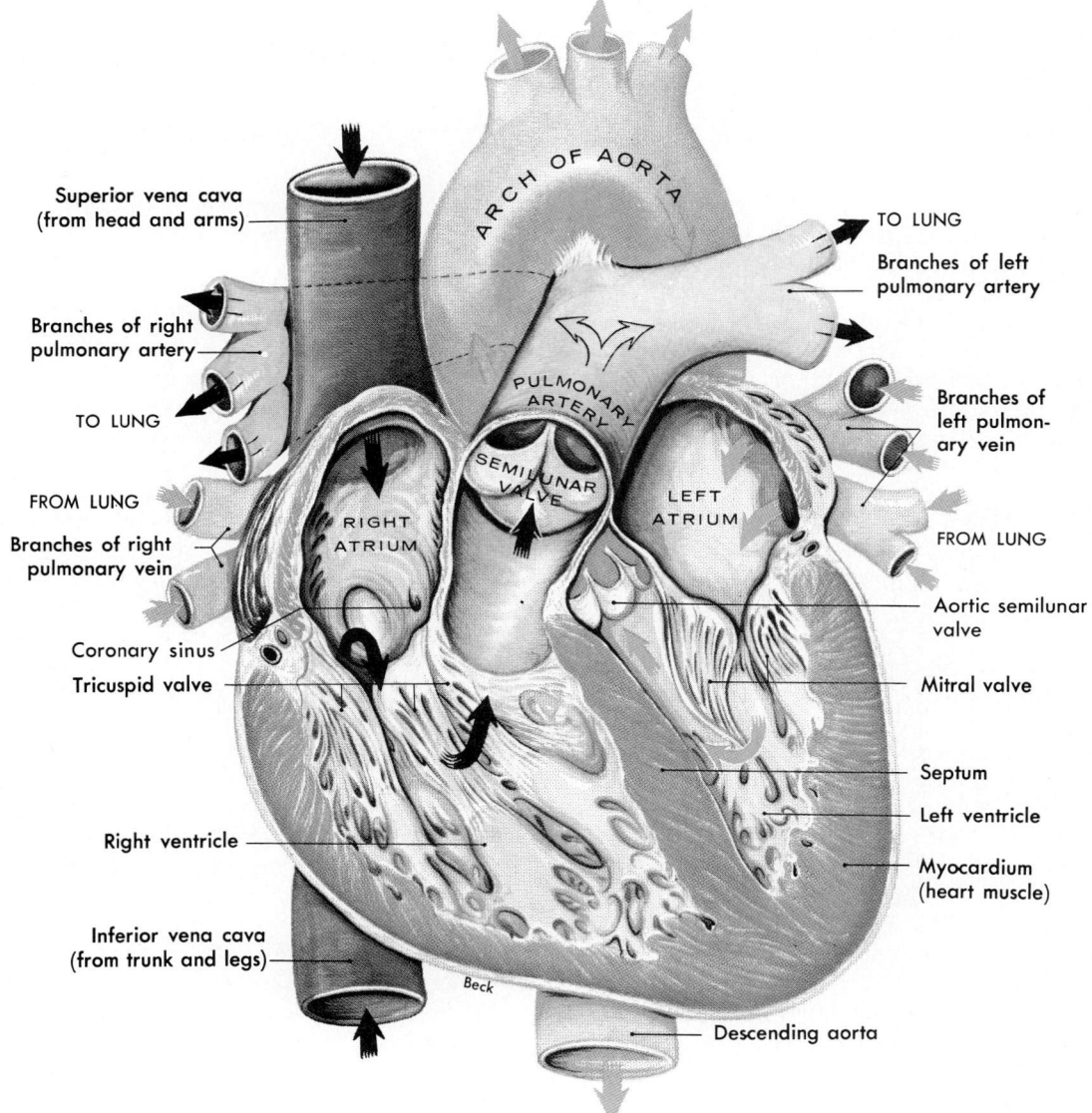

Fig. 26-1. Frontal section of heart showing four chambers, valves, openings, and major vessels. Arrows indicate direction of blood flow. Black arrows represent unoxygenated blood; gray arrows represent oxygenated blood. Two branches of right pulmonary vein extend from right lung behind heart to enter left atrium. (From Anthony, C.P., and Thibodeau, G.A.: Textbook of anatomy and physiology, ed. 11, St. Louis, 1983, The C.V. Mosby Co.)

CHAMBERS

The heart is divided into two halves by a muscular wall (septum) (Fig. 26-1). Each half has an upper collecting chamber (atrium) and a lower pumping chamber (ventricle). Oxygen-poor venous blood enters the right atrium, flows from the right atrium to the right ventricle (mainly by gravity) when the tricuspid valve is opened, and is pumped into the pulmonary artery to the lungs. Oxygen-rich blood returns from the lungs to the left atrium, enters the left ventricle when the mitral valve is opened, and is ejected into the aorta for distribution to the peripheral tissues.

The overall workload of the right ventricle is much lighter than that of the left ventricle, because the pulmonary system is a low-pressure system. The left ventricle has thick walls, because it must contract against a high-pressure systemic circulation to deliver blood to the peripheral tissue.

VALVES

The four cardiac valves are flaplike structures that function to maintain unidirectional (forward) blood flow through the heart chambers. These valves open and close in response to pressure and volume changes within the cardiac chambers. The cardiac valves can be classified into two types: the atrioventricular (AV) valves, which separate the atria from the ventricles, and the semilunar valves, which separate the pulmonary artery and the aorta from their respective ventricles.

Atrioventricular valves

The AV valves are the *tricuspid* valve, located between the right atrium and the right ventricle, and the bicuspid *(mitral)* valve, located between the left atrium and left ventricle. The tricuspid valve contains three leaflets held in place by fibrous cords called the *chordae tendineae,* which in turn are anchored to the ventricular wall by the papillary muscles. The mitral valve on the left side of the heart has two valve cusps or leaflets. It is attached in the same manner as the tricuspid valve. The chordae tendineae are important, because they support the AV valves during ventricular systole to prevent valvular prolapse into the atrium. There is a degree of leaflet overlapping during closure of the AV valves that helps to prevent the backward flow of blood. Damage to the chordae tendineae or to the papillary muscles would permit valvular regurgitation of blood back into the atrium during ventricular systole. The AV valves are *closed during ventricular systole (contraction) and open during diastole (relaxation).*

Semilunar valves

The semilunar valves include the *aortic* and *pulmonic* valves. The structural design of the semilunar valves is quite different from the AV valves; each consists of three cuplike cusps. They lie between each ventricle and the great vessel into which it empties. These valves are *open during ventricular systole* to permit blood flow into the aorta and pulmonary arteries and *closed during diastole* to pre-

vent retrograde flow from the aorta and pulmonary artery back into the ventricle when it is relaxed.

CORONARY ARTERIES

The coronary arteries arise at the beginning of the aorta right behind the aortic valve (Fig. 26-2). The function of the coronary artery system is to provide an adequate blood supply to the myocardium.

There are two main coronary arteries, the left and the right. The left coronary artery, which supplies the left side of the heart, divides into two main branches, the *left anterior descending* (LAD) and the *circumflex coronary* arteries (CCA). The right coronary artery (RCA) supplies the right side of the heart. There are very few connections (anastomoses) between the main coronary arteries; therefore blockage of a coronary artery or one of its branches will cause diminished blood flow (ischemia) to the portion of cardiac muscle supplied by that vessel and may result in angina pectoris or a myocardial infarction. Such blockages may be caused by clots or, more commonly, by fatty deposits in the walls of the arteries (coronary atherosclerosis).

Conduction system

The mechanical contraction of the heart is the product of a stimulus-response process. The resting myocardial cell has a membrane potential (that is, an electrical charge) as a result of the relative distribution of extracellular and intracellular sodium and potassium ions. Whenever the cell is stimulated, the membrane potential undergoes a change. A graphic record of this change forms the basis for an electrocardiogram (ECG). The change in electrical potential in response to a stimulus is known as the action potential. The two components of the action potential are *depolarization* (generation of the impulse) and *repolarization* (return of cell to resting state). The electrical current stimulates the release of calcium ions, which catalyze the reaction of myocardial contraction.

The primary structures of the conduction system are listed in box on p. 629 and illustrated in Fig. 26-3.

The sequence of cardiac activation is as follows:
1. Depolarization is initiated by an impulse from the SA node.
2. The impulse spreads through both atria.
3. The impulse reaches the AV node, which delays the impulse about 0.1 second.
4. The impulse is transmitted along the branches of the bundle of His to the Purkinje fibers, activating both ventricles almost simultaneously.
5. Activation of ventricular muscle proceeds from apex toward base of heart.

Cardiac cycle

The cardiac cycle has two phases, diastole and systole. Relaxation and filling of the chambers take place during diastole. Contraction and emptying occur during systole.

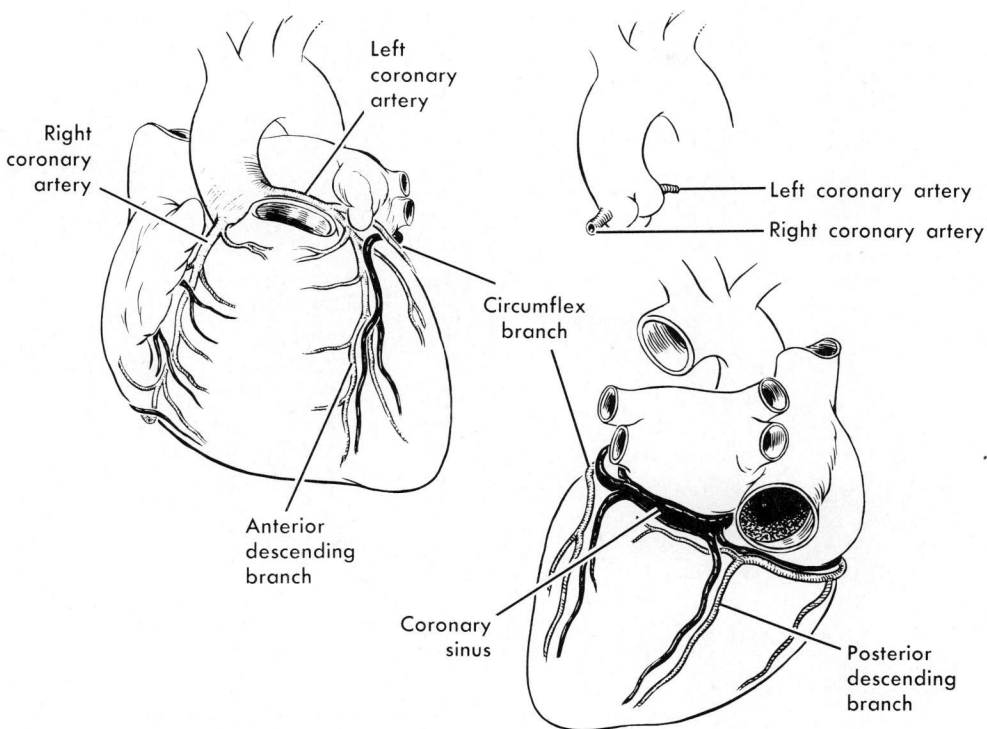

Fig. 26-2. Coronary blood vessels. (From King, O.M.: Care of the cardiac surgical patient, St. Louis, 1975, The C.V. Mosby Co.)

Structure of the conduction system of the heart

Sinoatrial (SA) node	Pacemaker node located in right atrium near opening of superior vena cava
Internodal tracts	Connect SA and AV nodes
Atrioventricular node (AV)	Located on right side of interatrial septum
Bundle of His	Thick cable of fibers starting at the AV node, bifurcating into left and right bundle branches (LBB and RBB) down the two sides of the interventricular septum; the LBB bifurcates into anterior and posterior divisions
Purkinje fibers	Network of fibers at end of Bundle of His that transmits impulse to both ventricular walls

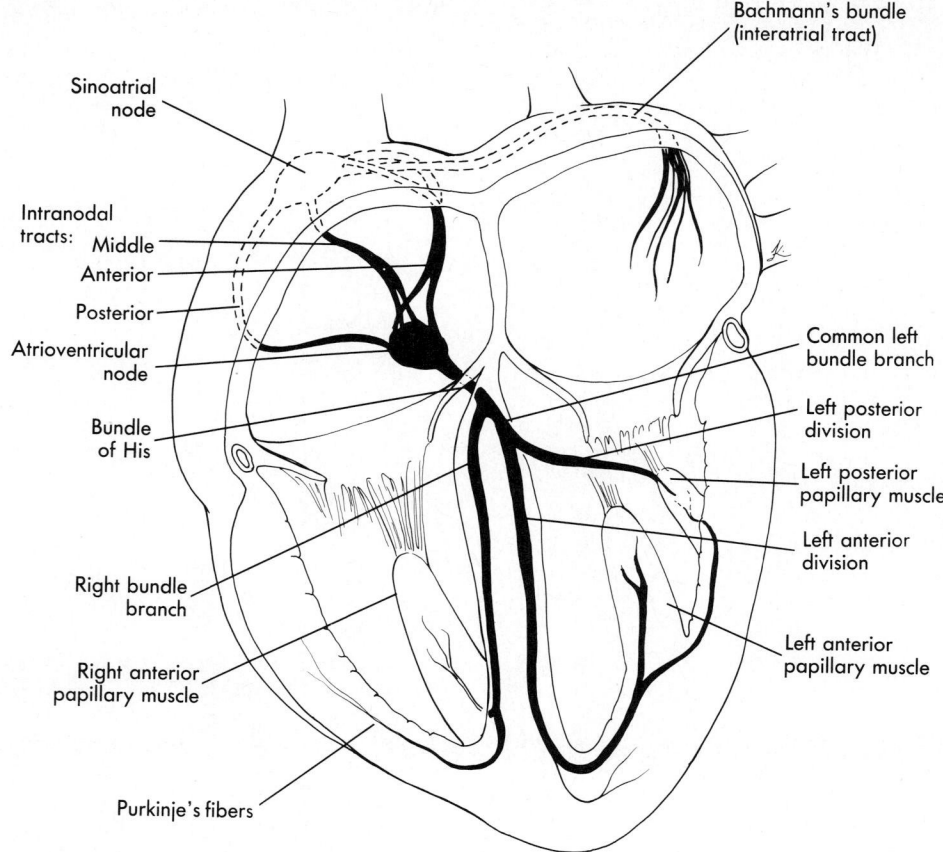

Fig. 26-3. Schematic diagram of heart illustrating conduction system.

DIASTOLE

It is useful to envision the cardiac cycle starting at a point immediately after ventricular systole. At this time the AV valves are closed, and the atria are rapidly filling with blood (atrial diastole). Ventricular diastole is conceptualized in three phases:

1. *Isovolumetric ventricular relaxation:* ventricular muscle relaxed but not yet filling
2. *Rapid ventricular filling:* passive gravity flow of blood from atria to ventricles; starts when atrial pressure exceeds ventricular pressure and AV valves open
3. *Slow ventricular filling:* occurs as increasing blood volume causes ventricular pressure to rise, which slows further filling

SYSTOLE

Electrical activation (depolarization) precedes mechanical contraction of both the atria and the ventricles. Atrial systole occurs immediately after depolarization of the atria while the electrical impulse is delayed by the AV node. At this time the remaining blood in the atria is propelled into the ventricles. The ventricles are then depolarized, and ventricular systole begins. This process also has three phases:

1. *Isovolumetric ventricular contraction:* increase in myocardial tension and intraventricular pressure without change in blood volume; AV valves close
2. *Maximal ventricular ejection:* greater pressure in ventricles than in aorta or pulmonary artery forces open semilunar valves, and blood is pumped into pulmonary and systemic circulation
3. *Reduced ventricular ejection:* ventricles remain contracted and small quantity of blood is ejected from momentum built up by contraction; higher pressure in aorta and pulmonary artery than in ventricles causes closure of semilunar valves, the end of ventricular systole

The familiar "lub-dub" heard when listening to the heart corresponds with the closure of the valves. The first sound results from closure of the atrioventricular valves at the beginning of ventricular systole. The second sound results from closing of the semilunar valves at the end of ventricular systole. (See Chapter 3 for auscultation of heart sounds.)

Cardiac output

The amount of blood ejected from the left ventricle into the aorta per minute is called *cardiac output (CO).*

CO is equivalent to *stroke volume (SV)* (volume of blood ejected from the left ventricle with each contraction) multiplied by *heart rate (HR)* (number of heart beats per minute:

$$CO = SV \times HR$$

The average adult CO is 5.6 L/min. However, during periods of strenuous exercise the CO may reach 20 to 25 L/min.

CO is therefore dependent on the relationship between the stroke volume and the heart rate. Despite fluctuations in one of these two variables, CO can be maintained at relatively constant levels by compensatory adjustments made in the other variable. For example, if the heart rate slows, the time for ventricular filling (diastole) is lengthened. This allows for an increase in preload and a subsequent increase in stroke volume. Conversely, if the stroke volume fails, the heart rate can increase to compensate temporarily and to maintain cardiac output. Therefore the actual determinants of cardiac output are the mechanisms regulating stroke volume and the heart rate.

CONTROL OF STROKE VOLUME

Three significant factors affecting stroke volume and thus cardiac output are preload, contractility, and afterload.

Preload

Starling's law of the heart states that myocardial fiber responds with a more forceful contraction when it is stretched. An example of this phenomenon is that of increasing the stretch of a rubber band to obtain a more forceful recoil when the rubber band is released. Myocardial fibers can be stretched by increasing the volume of blood delivered to the ventricles during diastole. The degree of myocardial stretch before contraction is expressed in terms of preload. *Preload is related to the volume of blood distending the ventricles at the end of diastole.* It is determined by the amount of venous return and the ejection fraction, which determines the amount of blood left in the ventricle at the end of systole.

Contractility

Contractility refers to a change in the inotropic state (force of contraction) of the muscle without a change in myocardial fiber length or preload. Contractility can be increased by sympathetic stimulation or by the administration of substances such as calcium or epinephrine. Increased contractility improves ventricular emptying during systole, thereby increasing the stroke volume.

Afterload

Afterload is defined as *the amount of tension the ventricle must develop during contraction* to eject blood from the left ventricle into the aorta. The major impedance against which the left ventricle must pump is primarily determined by *peripheral vascular resistance.* Increase in pressure resulting from hypertension or vasoconstriction pro-

---

Factors affecting heart rate

Increase heart rate

Emotions (fear, anger)
Pain
Decreased blood pressure
Increased body temperature
Exercise
Epinephrine

Decrease heart rate

Stimulation of baroreceptors in carotid sinus or aortic arch
Decreased body temperature
Sudden intense visceral pain

---

duces an increased resistance to pumping and will require an increase in ventricular tension to eject blood.

Dilation of the ventricles also affects afterload by increasing ventricular volume and thus increasing the work load of the heart to eject the blood. Excessive elevation of the afterload may impair ventricular emptying. thereby reducing stroke volume and cardiac output.

CONTROL OF HEART RATE

Under normal circumstances, heart rate is regulated by the activity of the sinoatrial (SA) node. The number of electrical impulses initiated per minute by this pacemaker is primarily the result of its innervation by fibers from both the sympathetic and the parasympathetic branches of the autonomic nervous system (ANS). Impulses from the sympathetic branch have a positive chronotropic effect (increase heart rate), and those from the parasympathetic branch have a negative chronotropic effect. Parasympathetic innervation occurs by way of the vagus nerve and is commonly thought to act as a "brake" that maintains resting heart rate at 65 to 75 beats/min. Some of the common conditions associated with increased or decreased impulse initiation by the SA node are listed in the box above. In addition to factors that influence the SA node, disturbances in the heart's conduction system and excitation of other pacemaker cells can affect heart rate. These will be discussed in more detail in the next section on cardiac arrhythmias (p. 632).

In summary, ventricular function and therefore CO are influenced by heart rate and stroke volume. Heart rate is primarily controlled by the ANS, and stroke volume is dependent on the three distinct variables of preload, contractility, and afterload.

Physiologic changes with aging

Unless there are cardiac conditions present, such as congestive heart failure or hypertension, most elderly persons have a slightly smaller heart than younger persons as a result of atrophy of muscle cells. However, the following changes occur in the elderly:

1. Decreased cardiac output
2. Decreased contractile strength
3. Reduced enzymatic stimulation.[26]

Because the basal metabolic rate and body size have decreased, the decreased CO is usually sufficient for maintaining usual activities. Problems may occur when an increase in CO is required, such as during increased activity and illness or some other stressful event.

The heart may respond to increased circulatory needs by a pulse rate that does not increase as rapidly as in younger persons and that takes an increased time to return to normal

Early signs of decreased cardiac function may be blurred in the elderly. Confusion or decreased mental function may be the early signs of a significant decrease in CO and may lead to lack of identification of other pertinent symptoms, such as fatigue or dyspnea. Anginal pain may also go unreported during early stages of myocardial ischemia because of decreased sensitivity to pain.

CARDIAC ARRHYTHMIAS

Cardiac arrhythmias (abnormalities of heart rate or rhythm) are the result of disturbances in the initiation or conduction of electrical impulses within the heart. Some arrhythmias represent disturbances in both impulse initiation and impulse conduction.

The hemodynamic consequences of arrhythmias are extremely variable. Some cause no significant alteration in CO, although they may produce annoying symptoms such as a "fluttering" feeling in the chest or the sensation that the heart has "flipped over." Other arrhythmias cause reductions in CO that result in symptoms of decreased perfusion. This is particularly likely if the arrhythmia is associated with a very fast or very slow heart rate. Two arrhythmias, ventricular fibrillation and ventricular standstill, cause death if not promptly treated, because they result in *no* CO. There are many causes of arrhythmias, some of which are not primarily related to a cardiovascular disease.

Accurate assessment of heart rate and rhythm and comparison of findings with baseline data will allow the nurse to detect some changes in the heart's electrical activity, but not all arrhythmias are easily noted by physical assessment. A visual display of cardiac electrical activity on the oscilloscope of a cardiac monitor or a graphic record such as an ECG is always required for definitive identification of cardiac arrhythmias.

Electrocardiogram (ECG)

An ECG is a graphic record of the electrical activity of the heart muscle. The recording is made at a standard speed on a grid that allows measurement of both the intensity of electrical events (voltage) and their duration. Intensity is measured on the vertical axis in millivolts (mV), and time is measured on the horizontal axis in seconds. Each small square on the grid is equivalent to a known unit of time (0.04 sec) and voltage (0.1 mV) that allows rapid calculation of both these parameters (Fig. 26-4).

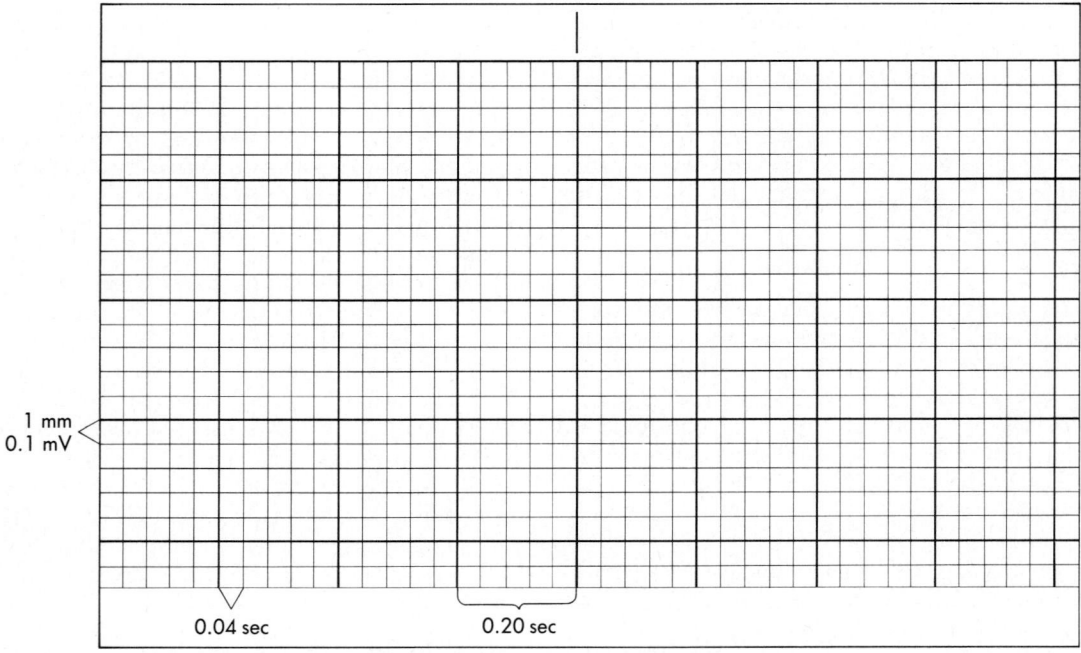

Fig. 26-4. Components of ECG paper.

The ECG may be recorded by a special technician or by health care professionals who have been trained in the procedure. It is essential that the patient be relaxed and cooperative, so the nurse must be able to explain both the purpose of this test and the procedure itself. An important point to emphasize is the fact that the ECG machine is merely *recording* electrical energy produced by the body and is not delivering any electrical current to the body. The patient's comfort and safety are maintained by preventing unnecessary exposure and by ensuring adequate grounding of the ECG machine.

In brief, recording electrodes are placed on the patient's four extremities and on the anterior thorax. A conductive substance (jelly, paste, or a specially prepared disposable pad) is placed between the skin and the electrodes to facilitate achievement of a high-quality recording. The patient must sit or lie still during the procedure, which is not painful and takes less than 5 minutes. The operator controls the ECG machine, which is designed to record electrical activity in several different planes.

Typically, 12 different views are recorded, hence the term *12-lead ECG* (Fig 26-5). The twelve typical views of the heart's electrical activity actually represent three different methods of recording and provide information about activation on both the frontal (vertical) and horizontal planes. The subdivisions of the 12-lead ECG and the names of the leads are described in box on p. 634.

Normal cardiac electrical activity as described earlier in the chapter, and the resultant electrocardiographic findings are found in Table 26-1. When cardiac electrical activity occurs in a normal manner, a *cardiac complex* such as the one schematically depicted in Fig. 26-6 is produced. The voltage and major deflection (above or below the isoelectric baseline) of each component of the cardiac complex vary with the specific lead being re-

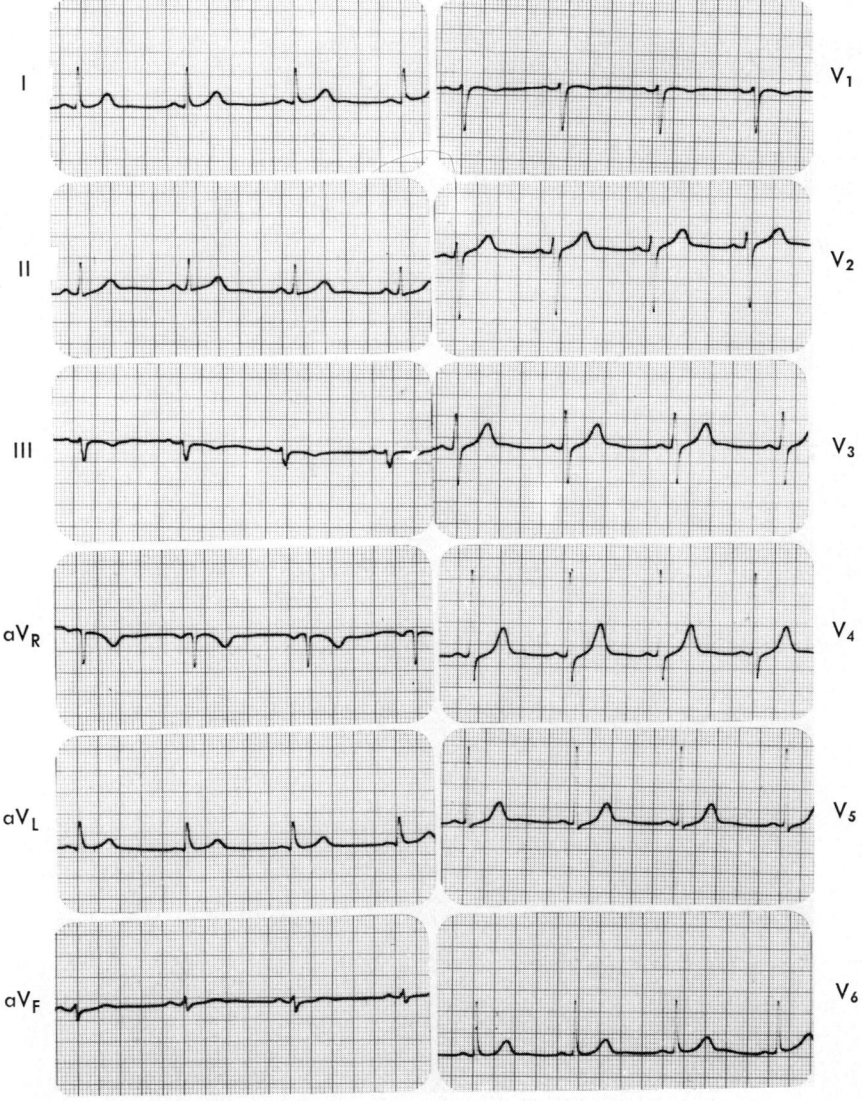

Fig. 26-5. Twelve-lead ECG showing normal sinus rhythm. (From Andreoli, K.G., et al.: Comprehensive cardiac care: a text for nurses, physicians, and other health practitioners, ed. 5, St. Louis, 1983, The C.V. Mosby Co.)

Components of the 12-lead electrocardiogram

Standard (bipolar) limb leads	Lead I, II, III
Augmented (unipolar) limb leads	aVR, aVL, aVF
Chest leads	V_1 through V_6

Table 26-1. Normal cardiac electrical activity and resultant electrocardiographic findings

Cardiac electrical event	Electrocardio-graphic finding
Firing of S-A node	Not recorded
Spread of impulse through the atria (atrial depolarization)	P wave
A-V node delay	Isoelectric baseline between P and QRS
Atrial repolarization	Not recorded
Spread of impulse through the ventricles (ventricular depolarization)	QRS complex
Ventricular repolarization	T wave

corded. A chest lead is compared with one of the standard leads shown in Fig. 26-7.

The nature of cardiac arrhythmias can be inferred by observing the presence, rate, and regularity of the various components of the cardiac complex and the relationship between the component parts. Ischemia, injury, or infarction of the myocardium as well as an assortment of other conditions (some of which do *not* represent cardiac pathology) may alter the size, shape, or configuration of various components of the cardiac complex.

In summary, the ECG shows only the electrical activity of the heart, which may or may not be disturbed by a pathologic process. It does not show the actual physical state of the heart or indicate its ability to function as a pump. Its most important diagnostic uses are the interpretation of abnormal cardiac rhythms and the identification of coronary atherosclerotic heart disease.

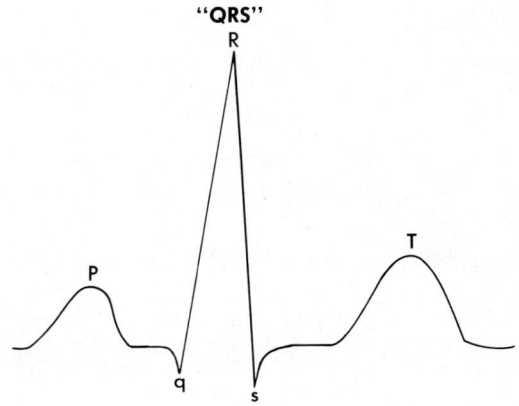

Fig. 26-6. Normal cardiac complex as seen in lead II.

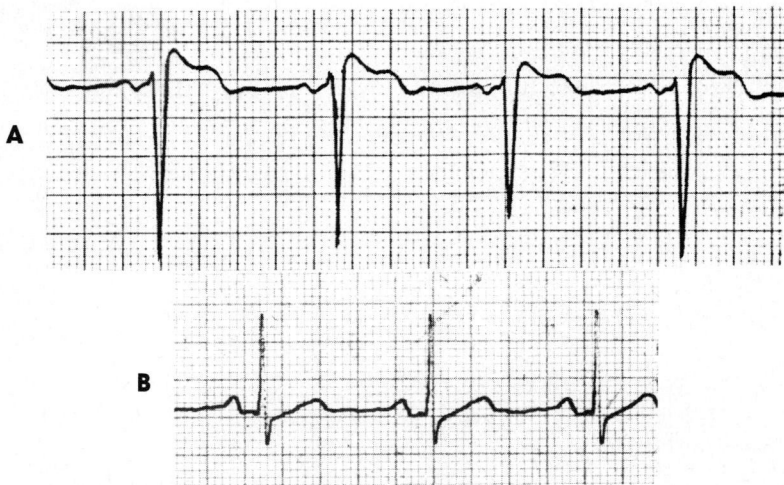

Fig. 26-7. A, Normal ECG in lead V_1. **B,** Normal ECG in lead II.

Cardiac monitors

It is common practice to assess on a continuing basis the cardiac electrical activity of persons who are known or suspected to have arrhythmias or who are prone to develop arrhythmias. This assessment is carried out through the use of a cardiac monitor that displays information from *one* electrocardiographic lead on an oscilloscope. The lead chosen for display varies with the condition of the patient, but standard lead II or MCL$_1$ (a close facsimile of V$_1$) is frequently used. Fig. 26-8 shows

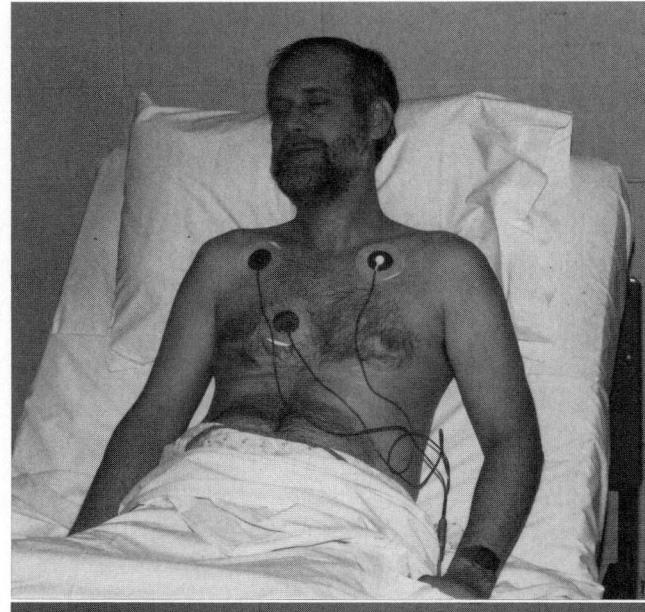

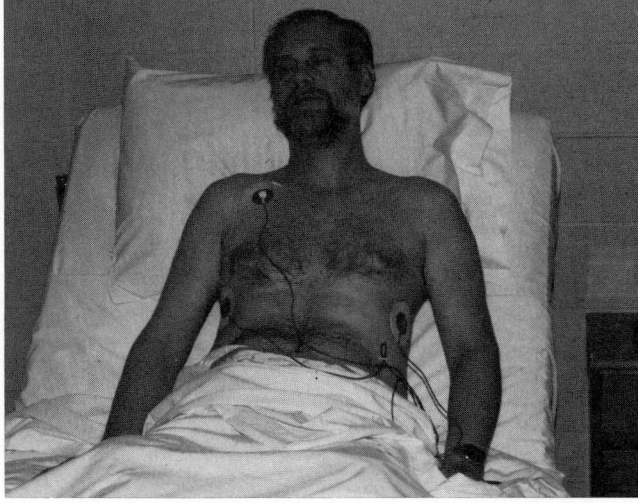

Fig. 26-8. A, Placement of ECG electrodes on anterior chest wall for lead V$_1$. Grounding electrode is on upper right chest, negative electrode on upper left chest, and positive electrode on right fourth intercostal space (along sternal border). **B,** Placement of ECG electrodes on anterior chest wall for lead II. Grounding electrode is on lower right chest, positive electrode on lower left chest, and negative electrode on upper right chest.

the placement of electrodes on the chest for these two leads.

Most monitors provide a visual display of both cardiac electrical activity and the current heart rate. Preset alarms warn of heart rates that exceed or drop below limits considered acceptable for each specific patient. More sophisticated monitors are designed to detect and tentatively interpret arrhythmias through the use of a computer. Other physiologic parameters such as body temperature, systemic arterial pressure, and pulmonary artery pressures can also be monitored on a continual basis.

Acutely ill persons are monitored in intensive care settings, but the increased use of battery-powered ECG transmitters that do not require direct connection of the patient to the oscilloscope (*telemetry monitoring equipment*) has expanded the use of such equipment to other patients as well. This development has resulted in the need for nurses working on general medical-surgical units to become familiar with monitoring equipment and to acquire some basic skills in rhythm interpretation.

Attachment to a cardiac monitor does not significantly alter a person's need for nursing care. Placement of the monitoring electrodes on the anterior thorax rather than the extremities leaves the patient relatively free to carry on usual activities. Special attention should be paid to the electrode sites to ensure a constant tight seal between the electrode and the skin and to note the development of any skin irritation. If a rash appears, the electrodes must be switched to alternate sites. Instructions supplied by individual electrode manufacturers guide the nurse in the application procedure and in necessary routine maintenance. Periodic checking of the monitoring system to ensure proper grounding and secure connection of all component parts is another general nursing responsibility.

Format for rhythm interpretation

A permanent graphic record of the heart's electrical activity can be obtained by either a standard ECG machine or a "write-out" component of a cardiac monitor. The monitor "write-out" is usually activated automatically when the monitor alarm sounds and can also be activated manually whenever a written record is desired for analysis. The record produced is commonly called a *rhythm strip* and should be at least 6 seconds long for proper interpretation. A longer strip may be required if the heart rhythm is irregular.

Interpretation of a rhythm strip involves knowledge of normal electrophysiology and a measure of deductive reasoning. Systematic collection and analysis of the data listed in the box on p. 636 is required. (The important segments and intervals of a single cardiac complex are schematically depicted in Fig. 26-9.)

NORMAL SINUS RHYTHM

The term *normal sinus rhythm* implies that cardiac electrical activity is within normal limits as indicated by the following criteria (see Fig. 26-10).

Rhythm strip analysis

1. **Heart rhythm.** Does this produce a pulse that is regular or irregular? Assess by noting whether the distance between QRS complexes (R-R) interval is consistently the same.
2. **Heart rate.** Number of ventricular contractions/min. Calculate by counting QRS complexes in 6 seconds and multiplying by 10 or by dividing number of small squares between two consecutive QRS complexes into 1500 (1500 × 0.04 sec = 60 sec). The latter method can be employed only if the rhythm is regular.
3. **Presence of P wave.** Indicates atrial depolarization.
   a. Do P waves occur regularly? The sinus node normally fires in a rhythmic fashion. Assess by noting whether P-P interval is consistent.
   b. Atrial rate: number of atrial contractions per minute. Calculate as with heart rate but use P waves.
   c. Is each wave followed by a QRS complex? If so, this verifies conduction of impulse from atria into ventricles; if not, a conduction defect is present.
4. **P-R interval.** Time from onset of atrial depolarization to onset of ventricular depolarization. It includes passage of impulse through the AV node.
   a. Length of P-R interval. Measure from beginning of P to beginning of QRS. Normal duration is 0.12 to 0.20 sec. Longer than 0.20 sec indicates a conduction delay in AV node.
   b. Is length of P-R interval consistent? If not, it may indicate lack of association between P and QRS.
5. **QRS duration.** Time needed for ventricular depolarization. Normal duration is 0.06 to 0.10 sec. Longer than 0.10 sec indicates abnormal ventricular depolarization.
6. **S-T segment and Q-T interval.** Assessment of these portions of the cardiac complex provides additional diagnostic information but is not required for rhythm interpretation.

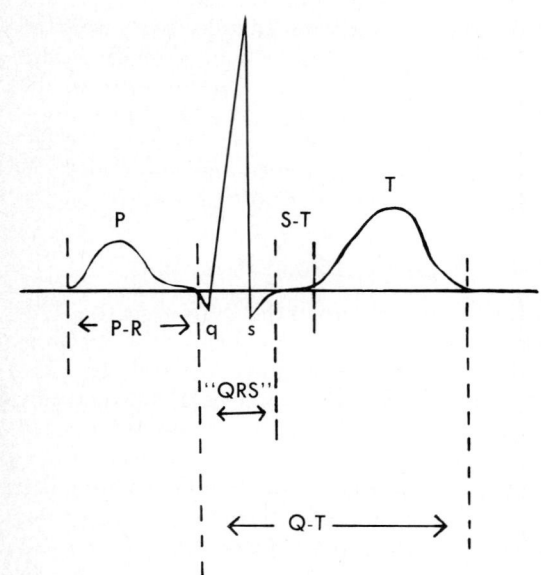

Fig. 26-9. Normal cardiac complex showing segments and intervals.

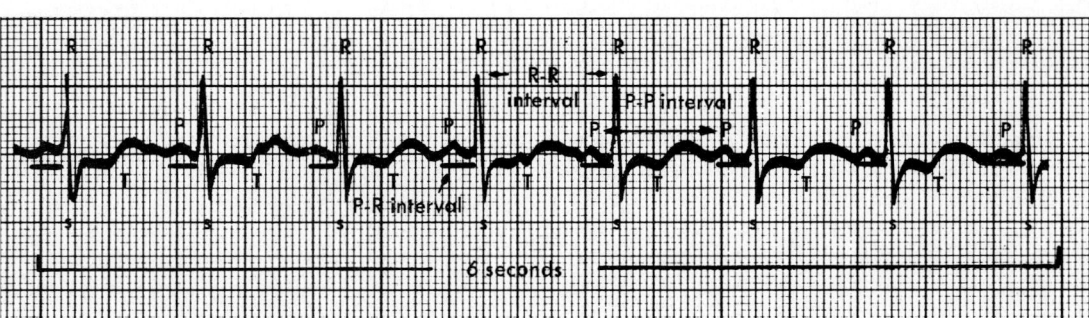

Fig. 26-10. Normal sinus rhythm showing R-R, P-P, and P-R intervals.

Table 26-2. Summary of selected cardiac arrhythmias

Arrhythmia category/name	Predisposing factors	ECG appearance	Significance/hemodynamic effects
Disturbances of impulse initiation			
Arrhythmias of the sinus node			
Sinus tachycardia	Increased metabolic demands: fever, exercise, excitement Compensatory response to blood loss, anemia, heart failure	Same as normal sinus rhythm except atrial and ventricular rates 100 to 150 beats/min	Increases cardiac output initially; prolonged episodes may lead to ↓ stroke volume
Sinus bradycardia	Peak cardiac efficiency (athletes) Parasympathetic stimulation, increased intracranial pressure, ↓ O_2 in sinus node	Same as normal sinus rhythm except atrial and ventricular rates 40 to 60 beats/min	Decreases cardiac output if not compensated by ↑ stroke volume
Sinus arrhythmia	Respiratory variation in impulse initiation by sinus node	Same as normal sinus rhythm except phasic shortening then lengthening of P-P (and consequently R-R) interval	Usually none
Ectopic arrhythmias			
Premature beats	Sympathetic stimulation, electrolyte imbalance, myocardial ischemia, chemical stimuli (caffeine, nicotine), distension of cardiac chambers, mechanical irritation (pacemaker catheter)	Cardiac complex comes "early" compared to normal rhythm *Atrial:* complex has P wave and normal QRS *Ventricular:* complex has no P and wide, bizzare QRS	Serves as a warning of cardiac irritability; ventricular more serious than atrial Do not usually cause ↓ in CO unless very frequent
Ectopic tachycardias	Same as for premature beats; drug toxicity may also be a factor (especially digitalis and some antiarrhythmic agents)	Rapid heart rate—usually >150 beats/min Rhythm often regular *Atrial:* P wave present (may merge into previous T wave); QRS usually normal *Ventricular:* no P wave before QRS; QRS wide and bizarre	May cause palpitations, dizziness Seldom seen in clients without heart disease; A serious arrhythmia CO ↓
Fibrillation			
Atrial	Same as for other ectopic rhythms; often associated with heart disease	Rhythm "irregularly irregular" No normal P waves seen QRS usually normal Heart rate variable	Loss of atrial contraction causes some ↓ in CO; situation worse if heart rate is rapid May persist as a chronic arrhythmia
Ventricular	Same as for other ectopic rhythms; often associated with acute myocardial infarction, electrocution	No recognizable QRS; pattern totally chaotic	Death-producing arrhythmia; no cardiac output Requires immediate termination

Continued.

Table 26-2. Summary of selected cardiac arrhythmias—cont'd

Arrhythmia category/name	Predisposing factors	ECG appearance	Significance/hemodynamic effects
Disturbances of impulse conduction *Delays in impulse conduction*			
First-degree AV block	↓ O_2 in AV node Infections Drug effects (especially digitalis)	Same as NSR except P-R interval >0.20	Warns of impaired conduction
Bundle branch block	Degeneration or ischemia in conduction system; congenital anomalies; drug effects	Same as NSR except QRS duration >0.10	Same as first-degree block
Nonconduction of some impulses			
Second-degree heart blocks	Same as for first-degree or bundle branch blocks Often associated with myocardial infarction	P waves usually occur regularly at rates consistent with sinus node initiation Not all P waves followed by QRS; P-R interval may lengthen before nonconducted P wave or may be consistent QRS may be normal or prolonged	Hemodynamic effects depend on frequency of nonconduction and underlying sinus rate; significant ↓ in heart rate will cause ↓ in CO A serious arrhythmia
Nonconduction of all impulses			
Complete heart block (third-degree)	Same as for second-degree blocks	Ventricles controlled by subsidiary pacemaker; heart rate usually <70 beats/min; may be as low as 30 to 40 beats/min No relationship of P waves to QRS (P-R interval constantly varies) QRS often wide and bizzare	Usually associated with ↓ CO and requires prompt intervention
Ventricular standstill	Same as for second-degree blocks	Failure of even subsidiary pacemakers P waves often present No QRS complex	Death-producing arrhythmia Requires immediate intervention (cardiopulmonary resuscitation and other therapies)

1. P waves present and regular. If the SA node is initiating electrical activity in a rhythmic manner, atrial depolarization should occur in a rhythmic manner.
2. Atrial rate (P waves) between 60 and 100 beats/min. This represents the range of normal rates for SA node
3. Each P wave is followed by a QRS complex. This verifies conduction of the impulse initiated by the SA node into the ventricles and implies that the heart rhythm is regular and the heart rate is also between 60 and 100 beats/min.
4. In addition, a normal P-R interval and QRS duration indicate normal functioning of all components of the conduction system.

Common arrhythmias

This discussion is intended as a brief introduction to the more common arrhythmias. Because of the complexity of this topic, some of the information is somewhat oversimplified. Nurses who are responsible for arrhythmia interpretation must undertake an in-depth study of electrophysiology and electrocardiography. Many continuing-education courses have been designed to enable the nurse to gain the specialized knowledge and skills required for this activity.

The arrhythmias will be discussed according to the two basic arrhythmia mechanisms: disturbances of impulse initiation and disturbances of impulse conduction. In addition to the description that follows, Table 26-2 summarizes the important features of each arrhythmia. Common treatment modalities are outlined in Table 26-3.

DISTURBANCES OF IMPULSE INITIATION

Most arrhythmias represent disturbances in impulse initiation. The disturbance may occur within the SA node or elsewhere in the heart (ectopic site).

Arrhythmias of the sinus node
Sinus tachycardia

Sinus tachycardia is the result of the SA node firing at a faster than normal rate (that is, greater than 100 beats/min). Any condition that increases the body's demand for oxygen may cause this arrhythmia, which is a normal response to exercise, excitement, and fever. Sinus tachycardia may also be a compensatory response to anemia, heart failure, and hemorrhage. The ECG appearance (Fig. 26-11) is the same as with normal sinus rhythm except for the faster atrial and ventricular rates (usually 100 to 150 beats/min). The general result of sinus tachycardia is an increased CO, although a prolonged episode may precipitate ventricular failure. When the underlying

Table 26-3. Summary of general treatment modalities for cardiac arrhythmias

Therapeutic aim/treatment	Indications for use
Increase heart rate	
Atropine	Sinus bradycardia (very slow rates)
Epinephrine, isoproterenol	Second- and third-degree heart blocks
Artificial pacemaker	Second- and third-degree heart blocks
	"Overdrive" of ectopic rhythms refractory to more usual therapy
Decrease heart rate	
Reduction of metabolic demands	Sinus tachycardia
Treatment of underlying cause of decreased stroke volume	Sinus tachycardia
	Ectopic tachycardias
Antiarrhythmic agents	Ectopic tachycardias
Verapamil	
Propranalol (Inderal)	
Suppression of ectopic impulse formation	
Antiarrhythmic agents	Premature beats
Bretylium tosylate (Bretylol)	Ectopic tachycardias and fibrillation
Disopyramide (Norpace)	
Lidocaine	
Quinidine	
Procainamide (Pronestyl)	
Verapamil	
Cardioversion	Ectopic tachycardias and atrial fibrillation
Defibrillation	Ventricular fibrillation

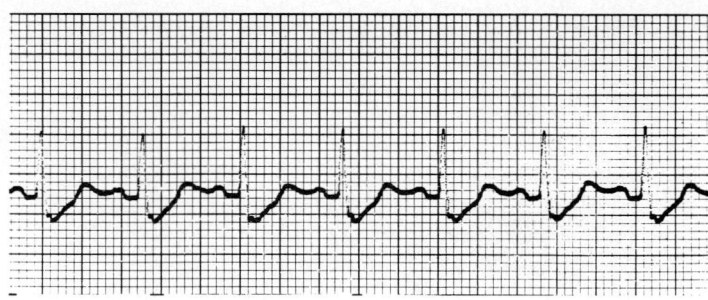

Fig. 26-11. Sinus tachycardia. Lead II showing heart rate of 115, regular rhythm, normal PR interval, and normal QRS duration.

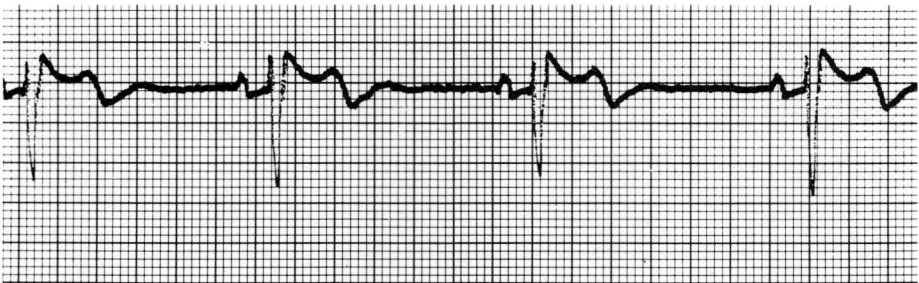

Fig. 26-12. Sinus bradycardia (lead V_1). P waves are present and regular. Atrial and ventricular rates are 44. Each P is followed by a QRS.

cause has been treated, the SA node returns to a normal rate.

Sinus bradycardia

Sinus bradycardia is the result of the SA node firing at a slower than normal rate (that is, less than 60 beats/min). This arrhythmia may be a normal finding in athletes or others whose heart muscles contract at peak efficiency. It may also be the result of stimulation of the parasympathetic nervous system, increased intracranial pressure, or lack of blood and oxygen in the SA node. The ECG appearance (Fig. 26-12) is the same as for normal sinus rhythm except for the slower atrial and ventricular rates (usually 40 to 60 beats/min). The general result of sinus bradycardia is a decreased CO, although the heart may compensate for the decreased rate by increasing stroke volume. If the person with sinus bradycardia shows clinical signs of decreased perfusion, atropine may be used to speed up the action of the SA node. On a long-term basis, a pacemaker may be required.

Sinus arrhythmia

Sinus arrhythmia is the term applied to irregularities in the rate of firing of the SA node that occur in a phasic, predictable manner. The rate alternately speeds up for a few beats and then slows down for a few beats. Assessment of the person's respiratory pattern reveals that the heart rate speeds up during inspiration and slows down during expiration. Except for the irregular P-P (and therefore R-R) intervals, this meets the other criteria for normal sinus rhythm. Sinus arrhythmia is a benign condition and does not require treatment.

Ectopic arrhythmias

Arrhythmias resulting from electrical impulse formation in ectopic sites can be classified according to the frequency with which the ectopic impulses occur. The frequency varies from occasional (premature beats) to one that exceeds the frequency of impulse initiation by the SA node (ectopic tachycardias and fibrillation).

Premature beats

Premature beats may arise in the atria, the AV junctional region, or the ventricles. This arrhythmia causes the heart rhythm to be irregular because of the periodic early occurrence of an abnormal cardiac complex. In this instance, "early" means resulting in an R-R interval that is shorter than that between two consecutive normal cardiac complexes. The specific characteristics of the abnormal cardiac complex allow the interpreter to infer the location of the ectopic focus; for example, atrial premature beats have a P wave and normal QRS, whereas ventricular premature beats have no P wave and a bizarre, widened QRS (Fig. 26-13).

Premature beats represent the occasional firing of an ectopic focus that has been made irritable by the presence of a stimulus such as increased activity of the sympathetic nervous system, hypoxia, caffeine and nicotine ingestion, electrolyte imbalances, and distention of a group of cells by abnormally large blood volumes. This is not an all-

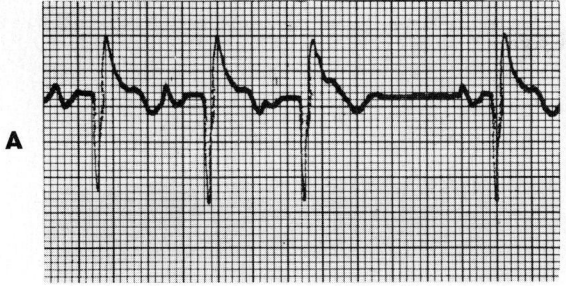

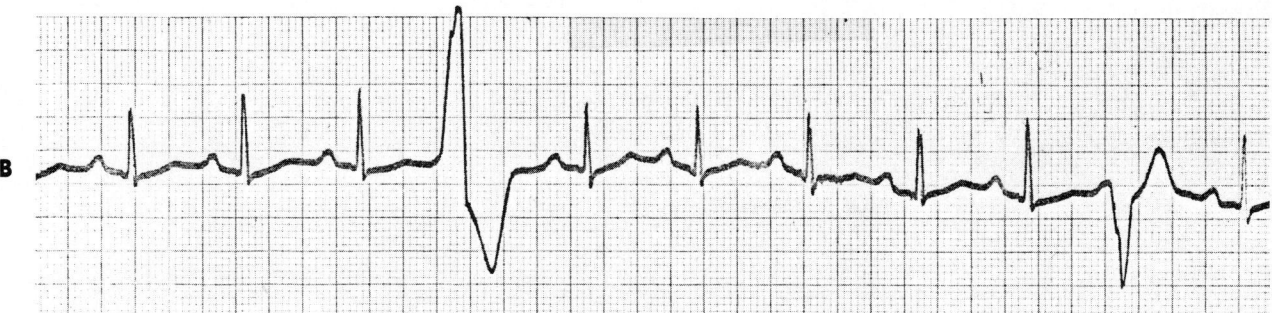

Fig. 26-13. A, Premature atrial beat (lead V₁). Third beat is premature atrial beat with abnormal early P wave followed by normal QRS complex. **B,** Premature ventricular beats (lead II). Fourth and tenth beats are premature with no P wave and wide, bizarre QRS. Different shapes of PVBs indicate two different ectopic sites in ventricles.

inclusive list of potential stimuli but is intended to demonstrate the wide variety of possibilities. Ventricular premature beats are considered more serious than those arising above the ventricle, but as a group, premature beats do not generally cause significant alterations in CO. They may be completely unnoticed by the person but may also be a cause of "palpitations."

Treatment of premature beats depends on the location of the ectopic focus, the frequency of occurrence, and the clinical condition of the patient. Frequent premature beats warn of increasing irritability of the ectopic focus, and treatment is aimed at preventing the development of more serious arrhythmias.

Ectopic tachycardias

Ectopic tachycardias arise from the same assortment of ectopic foci as premature beats but indicate much more severe irritability. These arrhythmias frequently start and end abruptly; therefore the term *paroxysmal* is often included in the name, for example, *paroxysmal atrial tachycardia* (*PAT*) or *paroxysmal ventricular tachycardia*. An ectopic tachycardia may last a few seconds or as long as several hours, but regardless of its duration, it represents loss of control of the usual pacemaking function of the SA node. Initiation of cardiac electrical activity is regulated by the ectopic focus until the arrhythmia can be terminated.

General ECG characteristics of ectopic tachycardias include a rapid heart rate (often 150 beats/min or greater) and a regular rhythm. Those arising above the ventricles have normal cardiac complexes (that is, P waves preceding normal QRS complexes), whereas those initiated in the ventricles have wide, bizarre QRS complexes not preceded by P waves.

Paroxysmal atrial tachycardia can be precipitated by stress, excessive caffeine or alcohol intake, and distention of the atria related to heart failure or malfunction of one of the AV valves. An episode may be so brief as to make treatment unnecessary, but prolonged bouts may result in decreased CO because of decreased ventricular filling time. Stimulation of the parasympathetic nervous system by induced vomiting or pressure applied to the carotid sinus region by a physician frequently terminates this arrhythmia. Rapid-acting forms of digitalis or cardioversion (p. 648) may also be employed.

Paroxysmal ventricular tachycardia is a serious problem not commonly seen in persons who do not have heart disease of some type. It is a frequent complication of acute myocardial infarction. Because electrical activity is initiated in the ventricles and does not proceed in an orderly sequence, coordination of atrial and ventricular contraction is lost. CO is therefore almost always significantly decreased. Prompt treatment is essential and may take the form of intravenous lidocaine or procainamide. If the patient loses consciousness, immediate cardioversion is required.

Fibrillation

Fibrillation is the result of extremely rapid, chaotic firing of an ectopic focus. The hemodynamic consequences of this arrhythmia mechanism vary so drastically, depending on the site of the ectopic focus, that atrial and ventricular mechanisms must be discussed separately.

ATRIAL FIBRILLATION. Atrial fibrillation is a common arrhythmia. It is usually associated with organic heart diseases such as mitral stenosis or chronic heart failure, but it may also follow the injudicious use of alcohol, excessive

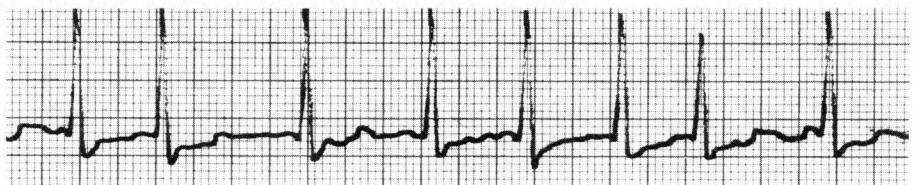

Fig. 26-14. Atrial fibrillation (lead II). Atrial rate is rapid with varying conduction to ventricles, rhythm is irregular, QRS complex is normal, no definite P waves are visible.

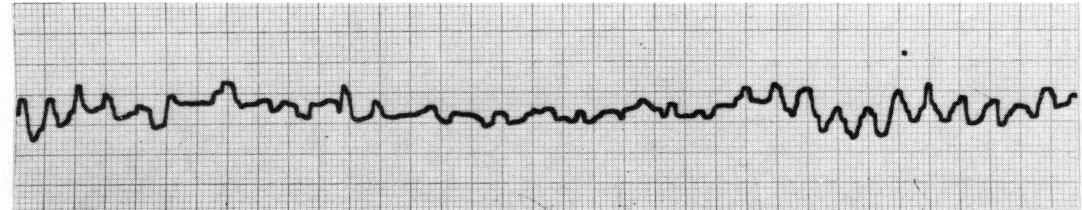

Fig. 26-15. Ventricular fibrillation (lead II). Tracing shows electrical chaos in myocardium. There are no QRS complexes and no definite P waves visible.

smoking, or large meals. The atrial ectopic focus fires 350 to 600 times a minute, which again results in the SA node losing control of impulse initiation. Electrical impulses move through the atria so quickly that they are not depolarized as a unit (therefore there are no normal P waves on the ECG), and they do not contract as a unit. Rather, individual muscle fibers contract and relax, giving an overall "twitching" effect. Loss of atrial contraction means that about 20% of the CO is never propelled into the ventricles. The other 80% falls into the ventricles because of the force of gravity and pressure changes within the chambers.

The AV node is incapable of conducting 350 or more impulses per minute into the ventricles, so ventricular depolarization occurs in a more or less random fashion. The QRS complexes are normal, since the stimulus goes through the ventricular conduction system in the usual manner, but the rhythm is "irregularly irregular," that is, has no discernible pattern (Fig. 26-14). The irregular pattern of ventricular contraction results in varying amounts of blood being ejected with each beat. Some contractions are associated with so little output that no peripheral pulsations are produced. This creates an apical-radial pulse deficit. The heart rate of a person in atrial fibrillation should always be calculated from an apical pulse or from an ECG rhythm strip.

The hemodynamic consequences of atrial fibrillation depend largely on the heart rate of each specific episode. With more rapid heart rates (that is, 150 beats/min or greater), signs of decreased perfusion are likely to occur. Digitalis preparations are frequently employed to slow the ventricular rate. This occurs because of the delaying ac-

tion of digitalis on conduction through the AV node. Once the heart rate has been controlled, quinidine is usually given to suppress the irritability of the atrial ectopic focus. When treatment with quinidine is initiated, the patient is watched closely, since many persons are allergic to this drug. Flushing, ringing in the ears, syncope, or an increase in pulse rate are brought to the physician's immediate attention. Diarrhea is a common side effect of quinidine therapy and can usually be treated symptomatically for a day or so until the gastrointestinal system adjusts to the drug.

Atrial fibrillation of recent onset may also be terminated electrically by cardioversion. If the underlying cause of this arrhythmia cannot be reversed, it may persist for months or years with little consequence to the person as long as the heart rate is not rapid. Long-standing atrial fibrillation is not likely to respond to cardioversion, since the SA node is not apt to resume its pacemaking role after a long period of dormancy.

VENTRICULAR FIBRILLATION. *Ventricular fibrillation* is the term given to rapid, chaotic electrical activity initiated by a ventricular ectopic focus. This death-producing arrhythmia may result from ischemia in the ventricles, electrocution, drowning, electrolyte imbalances, and toxic doses of digitalis or quinidine. As is the case in atrial fibrillation, extremely rapid firing of the ectopic focus causes the loss of coordinated depolarization and contraction. The important difference between atrial and ventricular depolarization, however, is that the ventricles contract normally in atrial depolarization, whereas in ventricular depolarization the ventricles do not contract at all. On the monitor, ventricular fibrillation is characterized by the absence of recognizable QRS complexes (Fig. 26-15).

The person with ventricular fibrillation has neither a palpable pulse nor detectable heart sounds and quickly loses consciousness. The definitive treatment for this arrhythmia is defibrillation (p. 648) performed by either a physician or a specially trained nurse. If a defibrillator is not immediately available, cardiopulmonary resuscitation (CPR) should be instituted to ensure perfusion of the brain, but this intervention does not reverse the arrhythmia.

DISTURBANCES OF IMPULSE CONDUCTION

Disturbances of impulse conduction may occur at the AV node or within the intraventricular conduction system (the right and left bundle branches). The most serious result of this type of arrhythmia is the failure of some or all of the impulses initiated by the SA node to reach the ventricles. Ventricular depolarization then occurs less frequently than it would if conduction were normal; heart rate decreases, and CO is likely to be diminished.

Delays in impulse conduction

Conduction defects can be viewed as existing along a continuum. The less serious problems, first-degree AV block and bundle branch block, represent only delays in impulse conduction. In spite of the names applied to these conditions, no impulses are actually blocked from reaching the ventricles.

First-degree AV block

First-degree AV block is the result of delayed impulse conduction through the AV node. It is manifested on the ECG by a prolonged P-R interval (greater than 0.20 sec). Decreased circulation of blood and oxygen to the AV node, infectious processes, and suppression of conduction by various drugs such as digitalis preparations are some of the common causes of first-degree AV block. Since this arrhythmia has no effect on heart rate, it has no hemodynamic consequences and is significant only as a warning of impaired conduction. There is usually no treatment.

Bundle branch block

Bundle branch block is the result of a failure of impulse conduction in one division of the intraventricular conduction system. As long as only one major component is involved (the right or the left bundle branch), impulses continue to reach the ventricles and achieve depolarization, although by an abnormal route. This conduction abnormality is manifested on the ECG by QRS complexes whose duration exceeds the 0.10 sec upper limit of normal. The exact configuration of the QRS complex in selected leads of a 12-lead ECG determines the diagnosis of right or left bundle branch block.

Inadequate circulation to the intraventricular conduction system, congenital anomalies, degenerative diseases of the conduction system, and drug effects are some of the causes of bundle branch block. Although bundle branch blocks also have no hemodynamic consequences, they are considered a more serious problem than first-degree AV block because of their propensity to progress to more significant conduction disturbances.

Nonconduction of some impulses (second-degree heart blocks)

Second-degree heart blocks are a group of conduction disturbances that result from the failure of some, but not all, of the impulses initiated by the sinus node to reach the ventricles. The site of the conduction disturbance may be either the AV node or the intraventricular conduction system, and the frequency of nonconduction episodes may be only periodic or as often as every other cardiac cycle. The specific names given to second-degree heart blocks reflect both the frequency of nonconduction and the site of the pathologic condition. For example, a Mobitz I second-degree block indicates periodic nonconduction in the AV node. (The reader is referred to more specialized texts for an in-depth discussion of this topic.)

The absence of QRS complexes after some of the P waves initiated by the sinus node is the primary ECG characteristic of second-degree heart blocks. Unless there is also a disturbance in the sinus node, the P waves should occur regularly at a rate between 60 and 100 beats/min. The obvious result of this phenomenon is a heart (ventricular) rate that is *less than* the atrial rate. Whether or not the second-degree block creates a condition of decreased cardiac output depends on the following;

1. The rate at which the sinus node is firing (The more P waves there are, the less serious the consequences of occasional nonconduction.)
2. The frequency with which nonconduction occurs
3. The ability of the ventricles to regulate stroke volume

Many episodes of second-degree heart block require therapeutic intervention to increase the heart rate. Atropine is used at times to improve conduction through the AV node, but the most dependably effective intervention is the installation of an artificial pacemaker (p. 645). It should be noted that interventions for conduction disturbances do not generally remove the underlying cause but merely serve to maintain an adequate heart rate.

Nonconduction of all impulses (complete heart block)

Complete heart block, sometimes called *third-degree block* occurs when no impulses initiated by the sinus node are conducted into the ventricles. The same causes discussed in relation to first- and second-degree blocks apply to this serious conduction defect. In the absence of stimulation from the sinus node, subsidiary pacemaking cells in the ventricles take over control of the electrical activity for this region of the heart. In effect, complete heart block repesents activity of two independent pacemakers. The SA node controls electrical activity in the atria, and a slower, less dependable pacemaker controls the ventricles.

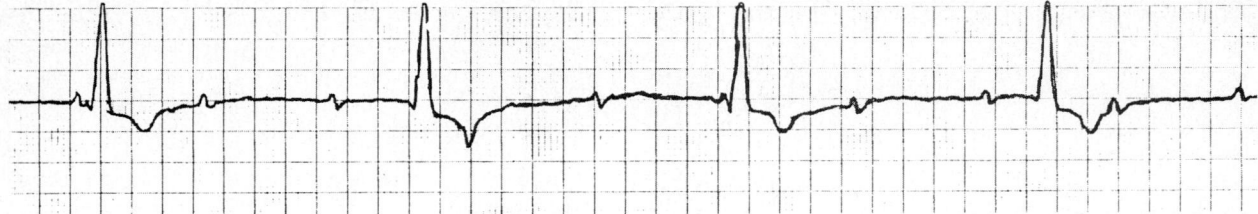

Fig. 26-16. Complete heart block (lead II). Atrial rate is 75; ventricular rate is less than 30. P waves have no consistent relationship to QRS complex.

On the ECG, this is manifested by P waves occurring at one rate and QRS complexes occurring at a different, slower rate (usually 20 to 40 beats/min) (Fig. 26-16). Since the stimulus for ventricular depolarization arises in the ventricles and travels through the ventricles in a delayed, abnormal manner, the QRS complexes are likely to have a wide, bizarre contour. The lack of association between the P waves and the QRS complexes is shown by the lack of a consistent P-R interval.

Complete heart block is associated with both acute and chronic cardiovascular diseases. The slow heart rate that results almost always requires therapeutic intervention. Some persons with chronic degenerative diseases of the conduction system have periodic, transient episodes of complete heart block that produce symptoms known as *Stokes-Adams syndrome.* This condition is characterized by dizziness, fainting, and possible loss of consciousness resulting from a *sudden* decrease in heart rate and CO. Stokes-Adams attacks occur most often in elderly individuals and are of great concern, since they may lead to serious physical injury or death. Once the presence of Stokes-Adams syndrome has been detected, therapy in the form of a permanent pacemaker greatly improves the prognosis of these individuals. Temporary pacemakers are used in acute care settings to maintain the heart rate of persons with complete heart block until the condition either resolves or gives indication of requiring permanent therapy.

Ventricular standstill

Failure of the ventricles to initiate their own electrical activity in the absence of stimulation from the SA node or any other supraventricular pacemaker is called ventricular standstill. This death-producing condition is characterized by no evidence of ventricular depolarization on the ECG, that is, no QRS complexes. P waves may be present, or the tracing may have a "straight-line" appearance.

The person with ventricular standstill has no peripheral pulse and no detectable heart sounds and loses consciousness. These signs are the *same* as those occurring with ventricular fibrillation; these two arrhythmias cannot be distinguished by clinical evidence. An ECG tracing is essential in making a definitive diagnosis. CPR should be instituted at once for ventricular standstill, and

---

> ## Therapies to relieve underlying cause of arrhythmias
>
> Oxygen to relieve hypoxia
> Provision of depleted serum electrolytes (especially potassium)
> Treatment of heart failure
> Relief of anxiety
> Removal of noxious stimuli (for example, caffeine)

cardiac stimulants such as epinephrine (Adrenalin) are administered intravenously or directly into the myocardium. Again, installation of a temporary pacemaker is often the only treatment that is effective over the long term. Prophylactic placement of temporary pacemakers has become common practice for individuals displaying evidence of progressive deterioration in cardiac conduction. The aim is to prevent the occurrence of ventricular standstill.

Treatment modalities

There are three major treatment modalities employed for cardiac arrhythmias:

1. Therapy aimed at relieving the underlying cause of the arrhythmia (see box)
2. Drug therapy aimed at suppression of impulse formation by ectopic sites or enhancement of impulse formation by the SA node
3. The use of electrical stimuli to suppress ectopic impulse formation or to initiate impulse formation in a regulated manner

The list of *antiarrhythmic drugs* in current use appears to grow almost daily. The development of drugs that are effective and free of dangerous or annoying side effects has been a challenge to the pharmaceutical industry. The more common drugs are listed in Table 26-3; the reader is referred to pharmacology texts for specific information regarding antiarrhythmic agents.

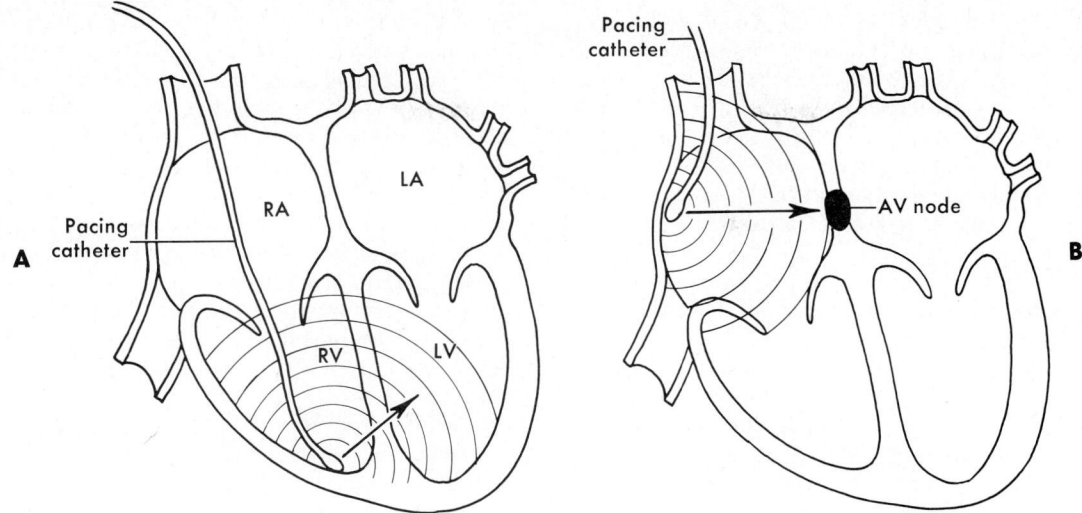

Fig. 26-17. A, Ventricular pacing. Impulses are initiated in ventricle. **B,** Atrial pacing. Impulses are initiated in atrium and travel to ventricles by normal conduction system.

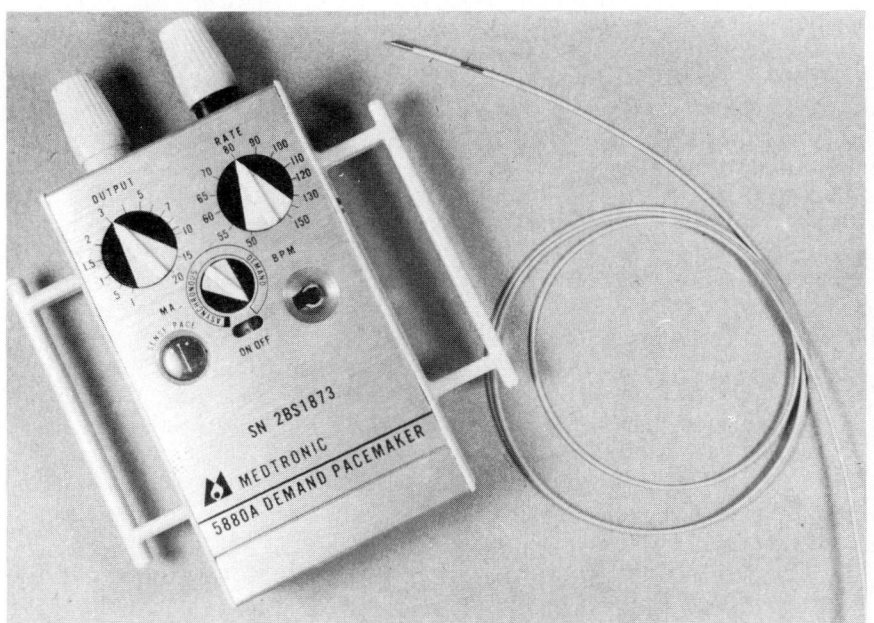

Fig. 26-18. Temporary (external) pacemaker. Pulse generator is battery powered. Electrode is passed into heart before being attached to pulse generator.

The use of various forms of electrical stimuli in the treatment of cardiac arrhythmias has a number of nursing implications; therefore these modalities wil be discussed in some detail.

PACEMAKERS

An artificial pacemaker is a mechanical device that electronically stimulates impulse initiation within the heart. The pacemaker system is composed of a battery-powered energy source (technically called a *pulse generator* but more commonly called a *pacemaker*) and a wire or catheter that delivers the electronic stimulus to a point of contact in the atrial or ventricular myocardium. The purpose of artificial pacing is control of heart rate.

Pacemakers are primarily used in the treatment of conduction defects, in which case the catheter is placed in the ventricle to ensure adequate depolarization beyond the site of impulse blockage (Fig. 26-17, A). These devices are also employed to remedy inadequate impulse initiation by the SA node and to suppress myocardial irritability that does not respond to antiarrhythmic therapy. In these instances the catheter may be placed in the atrium, since the underlying problem does not involve failure of the conduction system (Fig. 26-17, *B*). Atrial pacing has been technically difficult to achieve, although continual advances in catheter design will undoubtedly lead to increased use of this pacing mode in the future. Ventricular pacing is "nonphysiologic," since it does not result in coordination between atrial and ventricular mechanical activity. The CO thus achieved, however, is adequate for the great majority of persons requiring pacemakers.

Pulse generators

The pulse generator has a number of controls that can be easily manipulated in a temporary system (Fig. 26-18) and that are more easily manipulated than has previously been the case in permanent systems because of improvements in technology. These controls include energy output, heart rate, and pacing mode (asynchronous or demand).

Energy output refers to the intensity of the electronic stimulus delivered to the myocardium. Output is measured in milliamperes (mA), and relatively low levels of energy (approximately 1.5 mA) are usually sufficient to cause depolarization if the catheter is in proper contact with the myocardium. Energy output is set by the physician at the time of pacemaker insertion after determination of the "threshold level" of stimulation, that is, the lowest output that will achieve depolarization. Because of continuous minor fluctuations in the threshold, energy output is usually set at twice the initial level.

Heart rate is set according to the clinical condition of the patient and the desired therapeutic aim. With rare exceptions, the rate is set between 70 and 80 beats/min when the aim is simple maintenance of adequate cardiac output. If the purpose of pacing is the suppression of myocardial irritability, the rate is set higher, often as high as 100 to 120. The heart rate setting reflects the *lowest* anticipated heart rate in a properly functioning pacemaker system.

There has been a considerable evolution in *pacing modes* since the original introduction of artificial pacemakers (see box). *Fixed-rate pacing* is the oldest mode and is characterized by the constant stimulation of the myocardium at a preset rate. The danger with fixed-rate pacing is the possibility of competition between the pacemaker and naturally occurring electrical activity which, in the worst case, could result in ventricular fibrillation.

Because of this hazard and the development of safer approaches to pacing, fixed-rate pacing is rarely used today.

Demand pacing is the most frequently used mode and is characterized by stimulation of the myocardium *only* when the person's natural heart rate falls below the preset limit. This requires that the pulse generator perform two different functions. It must recognize the absence of natural electrical activity and stimulate the heart accordingly. In addition, the pulse generator must "sense" the presence of natural electrical activity that maintains the desired heart rate and withhold the pacing stimulus under those circumstances. These two functions are independent and must be assessed separately.

Temporary pacemakers

Temporary pacemakers are used in the following situations:

1. Emergency treatment of ventricular standstill
2. Short-term treatment of conduction defects causing decreased CO
3. Prophylactic management of persons who are prone to the sudden development of complete heart block.

A temporary pacing system is characterized by an *external* pulse generator attached to the distal end of the pacing catheter. The catheter may be advanced through the venous system to make contact with the endocardial surface of the heart, or it may be sutured directly to the epicardial surface. The transvenous approach can be employed at the bedside under ECG guidance or in a special procedure room under fluoroscopy. Direct suturing of the catheter to the epicardium is performed during cardiac or thoracic surgery.

If the patient is connected to a cardiac monitor, the presence of the pacing stimulus (a small vertical spike that indicates that the pulse generator has sent a stimulus to the heart) and evidence that the stimulus actually causes depolarization (either a P wave or a QRS complex immediately following the stimulus, depending on where the catheter has been placed) will be noted (Fig. 26-19).

The pulse generator may be secured to an arm if the antecubital fossa is the insertion site of the pacing catheter. If a subclavian site is used (an approach that has become more common because it leads to greater catheter stability), the pulse generator may be taped to the chest or placed in a chest pocket on specially prepared hospital

---

Types of pacing modes

1. Stimulation of ventricles only
   a. QRS inhibited (demand) pacing
   b. P-wave triggered ventricular pacing (SA node still determines heart rate, and atrial kick is maintained)
2. Stimulation of atria only (requires the presence of a normal conduction system below the atria)
3. Stimulation of both atria and ventricles (simulates the normal impulse formation and conduction; has artificial P-R interval to maintain synchronous contraction of the cardiac chambers)

gowns. Nursing care of patients with temporary pacemakers is summarized in the box below.

Permanent pacemakers

Permanent pacemakers are used in the long-term treatment of persistent arrhythmias that are amenable to this type of therapy. The pacing system is totally implanted with the pulse generator generally placed in a subcutaneous "pocket" beneath the clavicle (Fig. 26-20). As with temporary pacing systems, the catheter may be placed in contact with the heart by either the transvenous or epicardial approach.

Permanent pacemakers (Fig. 26-21) are inserted in the operating room or in a special procedure room. The

---

Nursing care of the person with a temporary pacemaker

1. Assessment of pacemaker function
   a. Monitor heart rate to verify that it has not dropped below the preset level
   b. If patient is connected to cardiac monitor, monitor presence of pacing stimulus and that a P wave or a QRS complex immediately follows the stimulus
2. Maintenance of system integrity
   a. Ensure that catheter terminals are securely connected to pulse generator
   b. Ensure that pulse generator is attached to person in such a way that accidental dislodgement of the system does not occur
3. Maintenance of patient safety and comfort
   a. Monitor for signs of infection at catheter insertion site
   b. Encourage range of motion in extremity to which pulse generator is attached, as permitted
   c. Ensure that patient avoids contact with any electrical machinery that is not properly grounded
   d. Give simple explanations concerning the purpose of the pacing system and any needed restrictions on activities to prevent anxiety.

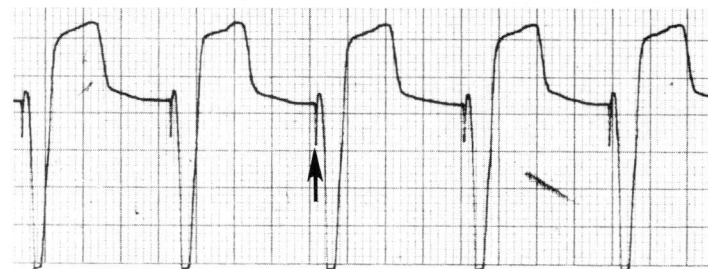

Fig. 26-19. Pacemaker ECG (lead V_1). Rate is 78, rhythm is regular. Pacing stimulus (arrow) followed by QRS. Pacing wire is in ventricle. QRS is wide and bizarre.

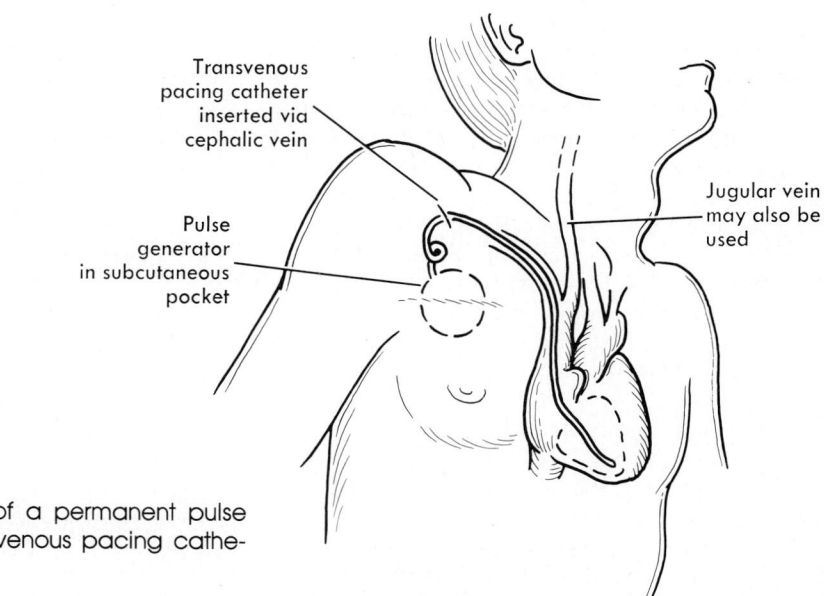

Transvenous pacing catheter inserted via cephalic vein

Pulse generator in subcutaneous pocket

Jugular vein may also be used

Fig. 26-20. Thoracic placement of a permanent pulse generator (pacemaker) and transvenous pacing catheter.

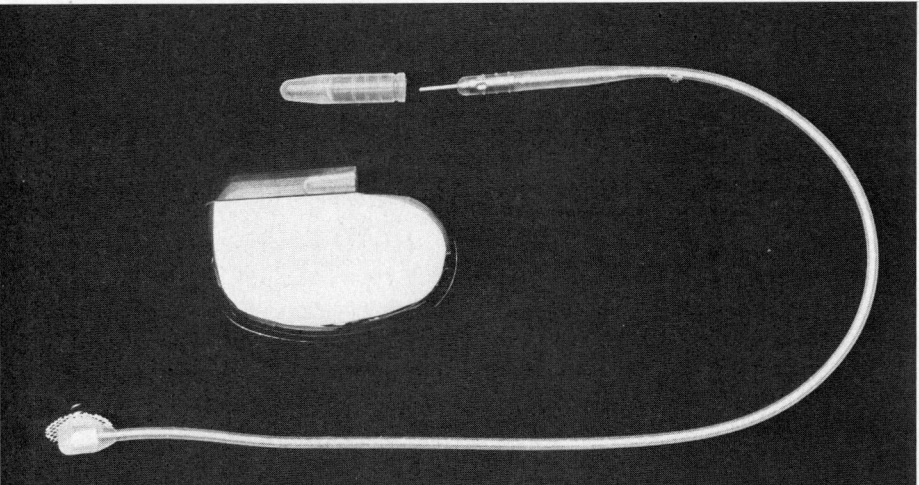

Fig. 26-21. One type of implantable pacemaker (pulse generator) usually implanted subcutaneously in right anterior chest below clavicle.

Teaching the person with a permanent pacemaker

1. Rationale for pacemaker insertion
2. Expected outcomes of treatment
3. Monitor pulse daily and report unusual changes to physician
4. Carry out usual physical activity (with avoidance of contact sports)
5. Use only electrical equipment that is in good working order
6. Show pacemaker identification to security officers at airport detector stations; request hand scanner to avoid false activation of metal detector
7. Carry identification card that states:
   a. Type of pacemaker and model number
   b. Heart rate and energy output settings
   c. Manufacturer's name and address
   d. Physician's name and phone number
8. Plan for regular medical follow-up.

---

transvenous approach to insertion does not require general anesthesia, a fact that decreases the risk of this procedure. The generator is powered by a battery that has an expected life of 4 to 6 years. Research is directed toward power sources that may function for 10 or more years.

Manipulation of heart rate and energy output has been difficult at best once the permanent unit was implanted; however, recent technologic advances have resulted in programmable pulse generators that allow variation in both the preset heart rate and the energy output. The latter manipulation has proved useful in reducing battery drain.

Immediate postinsertion care of a person with a permanent pacemaker includes relief of incisional discomfort, monitoring for infection, and assessment of the system's functioning. Attachment of the person to a cardiac monitor for 24 to 48 hours following insertion is the usual practice. Long-term follow-up of these persons is essential and is especially important within the last year of anticipated battery life. Pacemaker clinics have been established to facilitate follow-up, and in some instances, telecommunications systems allow telephone assessment of functioning. Literature published by pacemaker manufacturers and by the American Heart Association can be incorporated into teaching plans for persons with permanent pacemakers.

DEFIBRILLATION AND CARDIOVERSION

Defibrillation

Defibrillation operates on two electrophysiologic principles. The first is that electricity is a stimulus that can initiate depolarization. The second is that premature discharge of either a normal pacemaker or an ectopic focus can upset its rhythmicity and momentarily suppress its activity. The application of a large amount of electrical energy (400 joules) to the chest wall of a person in ven-

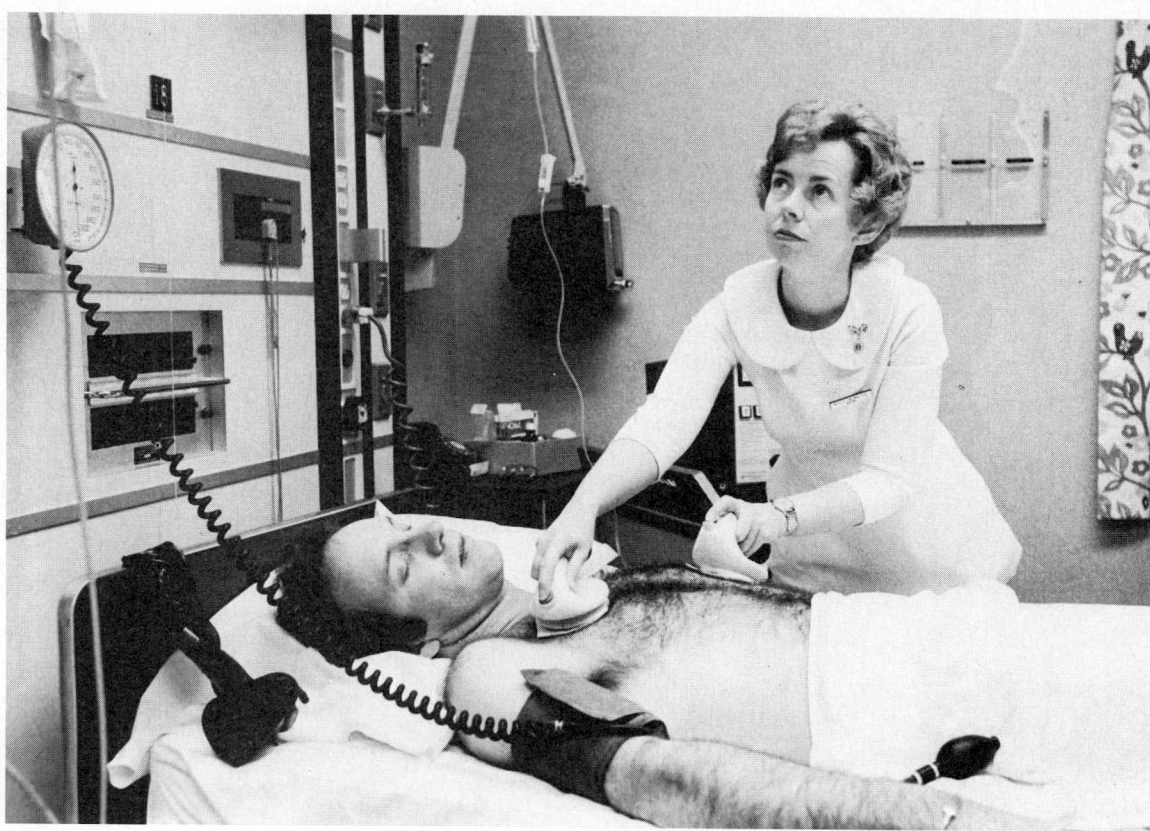

Fig. 26-22. Nurse defibrillating patient.

tricular fibrillation allows enough current to reach the heart to cause depolarization of all the cells simultaneously. This serves to suppress the ectopic focus and, it is hoped, allows the SA node to regain control of cardiac electrical activity.

Defibrillation is achieved by placing the paddles from the defibrillator close to the sternum on the upper right chest and just below and lateral to the nipple line on the lower left chest along the "long axis" of the heart) (Fig. 26-22). Either conducting gel or saline-soaked pads (as pictured) must be applied between the paddles and the skin to ensure conductance of the electrical energy. The machine is triggered in such a way that the electrical energy is discharged simultaneously through both paddles.

Failure of defibrillation to achieve the desired results may be caused by profound myocardial ischemia, acidosis, or inadequate functioning of the SA node. Usual practice is to administer a second shock immediately and then proceed with adjunctive therapy if needed. An endotracheal tube is inserted so that adequate oxygenation can be achieved. Sodium bicarbonate is administered intravenously to reverse acidosis, and epinephrine may be used to stimulate the SA node. The American Heart Association Standards for Advanced Life Support serve as a guide for training health professionals to deal with life-threatening arrhythmias such as ventricular fibrillation and as criteria for evaluating their performance.

Cardioversion

Cardioversion differs from defibrillation in only one substantial respect. It is a synchronized procedure designed to deliver the electrical energy to the heart at a set time during the cardiac cycle. In brief, once the machine has been discharged, the shock is withheld until the next QRS complex occurs. The purpose of synchronization is to prevent ventricular fibrillation from occurring as the result of an improperly timed electrical stimulus. It is clear that cardioversion is *never* used to terminate ventricular fibrillation, since there are no QRS complexes to trigger the release of the electrical energy.

Cardioversion is largely an elective procedure that requires the person's consent. Exceptions would be made if the patient's clinical condition were deteriorating too rapidly to obtain consent. Premedication is given to allay the anxiety that naturally accompanies the thought of enduring an "electric shock." Valium is frequently administered intravenously for this purpose because of its muscle relaxant and amnesic properties. An oral airway, oxygen, and emergency drugs should be available during this procedure.

Major health problems of the heart

Alterations in cardiac functioning or structural defects of the aorta affect circulation and may therefore be life threatening. The following common cardiac and aortic disorders are discussed in this chapter:

1. Interference with coronary blood flow: coronary artery disease (angina pectoris, myocardial infarction)
2. Pump incompetence or failure: congestive heart failure
3. Inflammations of the heart: pericarditis, myocarditis, endocarditis, rheumatic heart disease, cardiovascular syphilis, alcoholic cardiomyopathy
4. Inadequate valve functioning: stenosis or insufficiency of the heart valves (mitral, aortic, tricuspid)
5. Weakening of aortic wall: aortic aneurysms

CORONARY ARTERY DISEASE

Pathophysiology

Coronary artery disease (CAD) refers to a variety of pathologic conditions that obstruct blood flow through the arteries that supply the heart. Atherosclerosis is the most common etiologic factor.

Atherosclerosis, the predominant type of arteriosclerosis in humans, is characterized by the accumulation of fatty materials (lipids) and fibrous tissue within the arterial walls. As these atherosclerotic changes progress, the lumen of the vessel becomes narrowed and blood flow is obstructed to those areas of the myocardium supplied by the artery. Since this is a form of arteriosclerosis, the arterial wall also loses its elasticity and becomes less responsive to changes in blood volume and pressure.

Although several theories have been postulated to explain the pathogenesis of atherosclerosis, the etiology of this condition remains unclear. Atherosclerotic lesions usually develop near the origin and bifurcation of the main coronary arteries (see Fig. 26-2). The left coronary artery is more often affected than the right coronary artery. The disease process is initially localized but then becomes diffuse with advancing coronary atherosclerosis.

The first lesion to form within the coronary arterial wall is called a fatty streak (Fig. 26-23). This lesion begins to appear in coronary vessels as early as 15 years of age. Lipid-filled cells or "foam cells" invade the intimal wall and produce a fatty streak. As the disease progresses, raised thick fibrous plaques form and with increasing size limit the luminal capacity of the vessel. These lesions are typically characteristic of advancing atherosclerosis.

An even more advanced stage of atherosclerosis is represented by a calcified fibrous plaque or complicated lesion. This calcified deposit can rupture and hence greatly increase the risk of spasm, thrombus formation, and embolization. It is this final type of atherosclerotic lesion that gives rise to the symptoms of CAD. The arterial lumen becomes so narrowed that there is a great imbalance between myocardial oxygen supply and myocardial oxygen demand. When the artery becomes occluded more than 70%, manifestations of myocardial ischemia can occur.

Conditions that obstruct coronary blood supply

Atherosclerosis
Arteriosclerosis
Arteritis
Coronary artery spasms
Coronary thrombosis
Embolism
Infectious disease

Manifestations of myocardial ischemia

Angina pectoris
Myocardial infarction
Sudden death

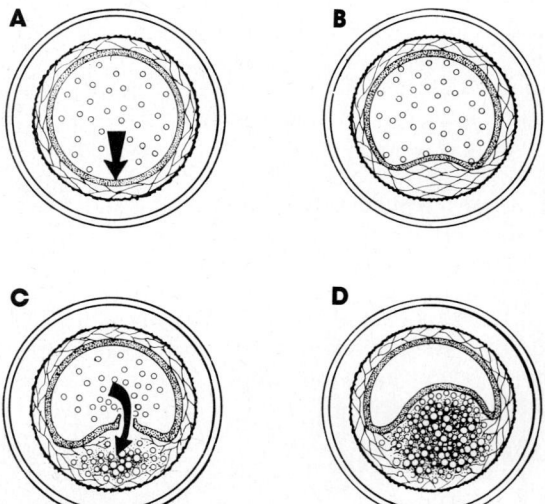

Fig. 26-23. Progressive development of coronary atherosclerosis. **A,** Injury to intimal wall. **B,** Lipoprotein invasion of smooth muscle cells. **C,** Development of fatty streak and fibrous plaque. **D,** Development of complicated lesion.

RISK FACTORS

The result of extensive clinical research has led to the identification of several contributing factors that place an individual at risk for the development of coronary artery disease. The cummulative effect of these risk factors accelerates the atherosclerotic process. Risk factors are grouped into two basic categories: those which cannot be altered by the individual (nonmodifiable) and those which the individual has the capacity to change (modifiable).

Nonmodifiable risk factors

Age

1. Morbidity and mortality of coronary artery disease increase with age.
2. Nearly one of four deaths from myocardial infarctions occur before age 65.[1]
3. Clinical symptomatology may be seen in persons in their teens and 20s.
4. The incidence of CAD steadily rises in the 30- to 50-year age group.

Sex

Men are at a greater risk for the development of CAD. Women are usually not affected by this disease until after menopause. The postmenopausal increase has been attributed to decreased levels of estrogens and rising blood lipids.

Race

There is a higher mortality rate from CAD in nonwhites who are less than 65 years of age. An associative factor that may contribute to this finding is that black Americans have a 45% greater chance of developing hypertension.[1]

Risk factors for coronary artery disease

Nonmodifiable risk factors
Age
Sex
Race
Family history

Modifiable risk factors
Cigarette smoking
Hyperlipidemia
Diabetes mellitus
Hypertension
Obesity
Lack of exercise
Stress
Oral contraceptives

Family history

A familial tendency toward the development of CAD has been demonstrated. The presence of coronary atherosclerosis in a parent or sibling under 50 years old is associated with the same finding in another family member. The extent to which genetic and environmental factors contribute to this disorder, however, is still not known.

Modifiable risk factors

Cigarette smoking

Cigarette smoking is a major contributing factor of CAD. Cigarette smokers have a two to three times greater risk of death from CAD than nonsmokers. This risk is related to the number of cigarettes smoked per day; the more cigarettes smoked, the greater the risk. Individuals who quit smoking are at a lesser risk than smokers.

Although the exact relationship between cigarette smoking and coronary atherosclerosis is unclear, it is thought to be associated with the effects of nicotine and the higher content of carbon monoxide produced by the smoker. Nicotine increases myocardial workload and subsequent oxygen demand. Carbon monoxide interferes with oxygen transport. The combination of these two factors may place an inordinate demand on a diseased heart.

Hyperlipidemia

Hyperlipidemia refers to the elevation of cholesterol and triglyceride levels within the blood. Cholesterol can be obtained directly from dietary sources or manufactured by the liver and intestine. Triglycerides are derived from fatty acids found in adipose tissue or the diet. Cholesterol and triglycerides are involved in the transportation, digestion, and absorption of fats.

Individuals with cholesterol levels in excess of 300 ml/dl have four times the risk of CAD of those with levels less than 200 mg/dl. There is also clinical evidence that high levels of a specific type of lipid-protein complex, the *low-density lipoproteins*, are indicative of CAD. These lipoproteins transport plasma lipids and contain approximately 50% cholesterol. In contrast, the high-density lipoproteins are thought to have an antiatherogenic effect.

Diabetes mellitus

Individuals with diabetes mellitus are at much greater risk for CAD. Coronary atherosclerosis has been found to be two to three times more prevalent in persons with diabetes, regardless of blood lipid levels. Despite this, it is difficult to isolate diabetes as a single causative factor since it is also associated with hypertension and obesity.

Hypertension

The relationship between high blood pressure and CAD has been attributed to the effects of hypertension on the coronary vessels. Consistent elevation in systolic or diastolic blood pressure is associated with coronary atherosclerosis.

Obesity

Obesity or excess body weight in relation to height increases the workload and hence the oxygen demand of the heart. Its effect as a risk factor is questionable, although obesity highly correlates with hypertension, hyperlipidemia, and diabetes. Specifically, obesity tends to be associated with increased caloric intake and elevated levels of low-density lipoproteins.

Lack of exercise

The lack of exercise has not been clearly linked to CAD. It has been demonstrated, however, that exercise can improve the efficiency of the heart by the reduction of heart rate and blood pressure. Other physiologic effects of regular exercise, such as decreased levels of low-density lipoproteins, lowered blood glucose levels, and improved cardiac output, have been associated with a lesser chance of CAD.[16] The psychologic benefits of exercise, reduced anxiety and depression, may also be of significance.

Stress

The effect of stress on the pathogenesis of CAD is controversial. Stress stimulates the cardiovascular system by the release of catecholamines, which in turn increase the heart rate and produce vasoconstriction. Stress also plays a major role in those individuals characterized by type A behavior. Behaviors including ambitiousness, aggressiveness, competitiveness, impatience, muscle tenseness, vigorous speech, and rapid pace in all activities are indicative of the type A behavior pattern.[17] These individuals are by virtue of their stressful life-style more likely to develop CAD.

Oral contraceptives

The use of oral contraceptives or birth control pills has been associated with an increased risk of CAD. Oral contraceptives cause changes in blood pressure and predispose to thrombus formation and emboli.

Angina pectoris

PATHOPHYSIOLOGY

Angina pectoris or chest pain is a clinical syndrome produced by insufficient coronary blood flow. There is imbalance between myocardial oxygen supply and myocardial oxygen demand, which creates transient myocardial ischemia. The underlying mechanism to account for the experience of pain is probably related to the change from aerobic to anaerobic metabolism. By-products from anaerobic metabolism, specifically lactic acid, may initiate sensory receptors and cause pain. The release of other substances from the ischemic cells may also produce pain in this manner. Since the basic problem in angina is an imbalance between oxygen supply and demand, the primary goals of therapy are directed to the restoration of this balance (Table 26-4).

Two subcategories of angina should be distinguished from the classic condition. These are unstable angina and variant angina. A brief description of these forms of angina is presented here. For further information, consult a cardiology text.

Table 26-4. Coronary artery disorders

Disorder	Etiology	Signs and symptoms	Medical therapy
Angina pectoris	Atherosclerosis Hypertension Diabetes mellitus Thromboangiitis obliterans Severe anemia Arteritis Aortic insufficiency	Substernal chest pain, retrosternal chest pain, pain radiating to neck, jaw, back and arms; dyspnea, diaphoresis, nausea, apprehension	Avoidance of precipitating factors Reduction of modifiable risk factors Medication: nitrates, beta adrenergic blocking agents, calcium channel blockers Oxygen therapy ECG monitoring

Myocardial infarction	Atherosclerotic progression associated with hypertension or diabetes
	Coronary thrombosis
	Prolonged constriction of coronary arteries
		Substernal chest pain; pain radiating to neck, jaw, back and arms; dyspnea, diaphoresis, nausea and vomiting, marked anxiety and apprehension	Medications: analgesics, antiarrhythmics, anticoagulants, stool softener, sleeping pill
			Oxygen therapy
			ECG monitoring
			Dietary restrictions
			  Low cholesterol,
			  No added salt (NAS)
			  No caffeine
			  Fluid restriction
			Activity restrictions

Unstable angina

Unstable angina frequently refers to preinfarction angina, crescendo angina, or intermittent coronary syndrome. This type of angina is characterized by an increase in the severity, frequency, or duration of symptoms without infarction.

Variant angina

Variant angina or Prinzmetal's angina is thought to develop from intermittent coronary artery spasm with or without atherosclerotic heart disease. This type of anginal pain can occur during normal activities and is not necessarily precipitated by exercise or stress. Anginal pain in this condition develops at the same time of day or night, demonstrating a cyclic pattern.

ASSESSMENT

Subjective data

Data is collected concerning the patient's perception of the anginal pain.
1. Location and radiation to other sites (Fig. 26-24)
2. Quality of pain
   a. Tightness or heaviness in chest
   b. Pressure or squeezing sensation
3. Onset and duration of pain
4. Associated factors: exertion, exposure to cold, exposure to hot, humid conditions, stress, heavy meal
5. Relieving factors: rest, nitroglycerin

Objective data

1. Patient behavior: apprehensive, gripping sternum with hands

2. Change in vital signs: increase in heart rate, respiratory rate, and blood pressure
3. Change in location, frequency, and severity of anginal pain (An individual usually experiences anginal pain in the same location and at the same frequency; over a period of years, the frequency and severity increase; less exertion may cause pain.)
4. Change in cardiac rhythm
5. Presence of risk factors

Diagnostic tests

The diagnosis of ischemic heart disease is frequently made on the basis of the patient's history. Diagnosis of angina may also be facilitated by electrocardiogram (ECG) (p. 632), Holter monitor, chest x-ray film, and stress testing.

Electrocardiogram

Characteristic findings of ischemia, S-T segment depression, and T wave inversion may be seen during chest pain. The absence of ECG changes does not exclude the diagnosis of ischemia.

Holter monitor

A Holter monitor is a small portable ECG monitor about the size of a large transistor radio. In nonacute situations, a patient can be connected to this monitor to evaluate chest pain during performance of daily activities. Two wires are attached to the patient's chest and connected to the monitor. The monitor is then worn for 24 hours, during which time the patient maintains a log of daily activities, medications, and unusual sensations.

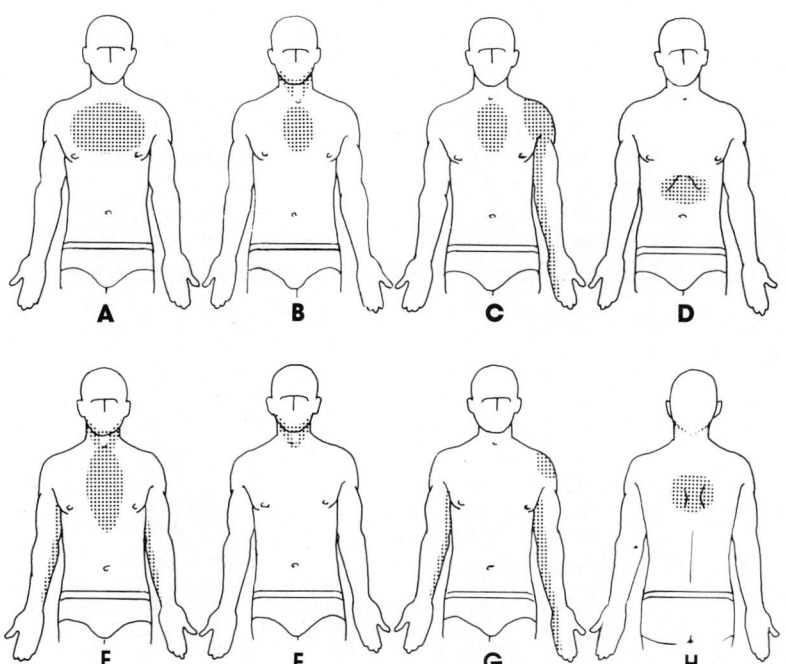

Fig. 26-24. Sites where ischemic myocardial pain may be referred. **A,** Upper chest. **B,** Beneath sternum radiating to neck and jaw. **C,** Beneath sternum radiating down left arm. **D,** Epigastric. **E,** Epigastric radiating to neck, jaw, and arms. **F,** Neck and jaw. **G,** Left shoulder, inner aspect of both arms. **H,** Intrascapular.

Chest x-ray film

A chest x-ray film may aid in the diagnosis of ischemic heart disease if there is calcification of the coronary arteries. An enlarged heart may reflect the presence of ischemia.

Stress testing

Stress testing or exercise electrocardiography is a noninvasive test used to evaluate cardiovascular response to controlled physical work loads. The indications for performing a stress test are identified here.

During stress testing, the patient pedals a stationary bicycle or walks on a treadmill. Throughout the testing, the patient's blood pressure and ECG are recorded. Conditions that require termination of the testing are listed in the box below. The risk of developing a myocardial infarction is less than 1 in 500; the risk of death is less than 1 in 10,000.[51]

Indications for stress testing

Evaluate symptoms of CAD

Determine physical work capacity and aerobic capacity

Determine functional capacity following a myocardial infarction

Determine limitations for exercise programming

Evaluate arrhythmias that develop during exercise

Screen patients over age 40 and at risk for CAD

Evaluate effect of pharmacologic agents on arrhythmias and angina

---

Conditions requiring termination of stress testing

Ventricular tachycardia

Marked decrease in peak systolic blood pressure

Marked decrease in heart rate

Vertigo

Frequent premature ventricular beats

Anginal pain

Severe dyspnea

Severe anxiety

Diagnostic ST segment depression on ECG

Adequate patient preparation is extremely important. The patient should do the following:

1. Get adequate rest the night before the test
2. Avoid coffee, tea, and alcohol the day of the test
3. Avoid smoking and taking nitroglycerin during the 2-hour period immediately before the test
4. Eat a light breakfast or lunch at least 2 hours before the test
5. Wear comfortable, loose-fitting clothes; women need to wear a bra for support
6. Wear sturdy, comfortable walking shoes
7. Consult with the physician regarding the taking of medications before the test (Digoxin, propranolol, and vasodilators may affect the results of the stress test.)
8. Inform the physician if any unusual sensations develop during the test (for example, chest pain, dizziness)
9. Rest after the test; do *not* take a hot shower; a warm bath 1 to 2 hours after the test is permitted.

DATA ANALYSIS AND PLANNING

Nursing diagnoses

Possible nursing diagnoses for the patient with angina include the following:

Comfort, alteration in: chest pain

Activity intolerance

Tissue perfusion, alteration in: cardiopulmonary

Knowledge deficit

Expected patient outcomes

The patient can do the following:

1. Describe the medication regimen.
2. Describe events that may precipitate anginal attacks and plans for avoidance of such events.
3. Describe activity plans to balance myocardial oxygen demands with supply.
4. Describe the purpose, rationale; and preparation for diagnostic testing.
5. Indicate plans for medical follow-up.

IMPLEMENTATION

Assisting with achievement of therapeutic goals

1. Administer medications as prescribed. If angina is present, give nitroglycerin sublingually. Repeat dosage in 5 minutes if pain does not subside. Repeat two or three times at 5-minute intervals.
2. Monitor for arrhythmias.
3. Administer oxygen per nasal cannula as prescribed.
4. Monitor effects of daily activities on cardiac status; occurrence of arrhythmias and need for oxygen.

Assisting with comfort

1. Provide a calm environment to decrease stress and anxiety

2. Relieve pain
3. Provide rest periods if fatigue present during daily activities

Teaching

A major nursing intervention is teaching the patient about the following:
1. Prescribed medications
2. Measures to minimize precipitating events (exertion, stress, overeating, exposure to cold or hot, humid conditions)
3. Effects of exercise on reduction of myocardial oxygen needs

Specific points to include in the teaching are described here.

Effect of medications

Nitrates (nitroglycerin [Nitro-bid, Transderm], isosorbide) are given to dilate coronary arteries and collateral vessels of the heart and to dilate peripheral vessels, especially the veins. Specific patient instructions for taking nitrates are listed in the box below.

Beta (β) adrenergic blocking agents (propranolol, nadolol) lower oxygen demands during exercise and improve the oxygen supply/demand balance. They lower heart rate and blood pressure. Beta blockers should be withdrawn gradually.

Calcium channel blockers (nifedipine, diltiazem, verapamil) decrease the work load of the heart. They decrease heart rate and improve oxygen supply by dilating coronary arteries.

EVALUATION

Evaluation will be based on expected patient outcomes. Questions to ask may include the following:
1. Is patient able to control pain by use of prescribed medication?
2. Does the patient know action, usage, and side effects of prescribed medications?
3. Can patient describe ways to minimize events that may precipitate anginal pain?
4. Is patient engaged or planning to engage in a regular exercise program?

Teaching the patient with angina pectoris

1. Use of nitrate medications
   a. Use nitroglycerin prophylactically to avoid pain known to occur with certain activities
   b. Burning sensation on tongue indicates nitroglycerin is activated
   c. Throbbing sensation in head and flushing may be felt
   d. Sit and stand slowly after taking nitroglycerin
   e. Place nitroglycerin tablets under the tongue at the onset of anginal pain; second tablet can be taken after 5 min and third tablet after another 5 min if pain is unrelieved
   f. Call physician if pain does not subside after third nitroglycerin tablet; go to nearest emergency department; do not drive yourself
   g. Always carry nitroglycerin
   h. Store nitroglycerin in dark bottle and keep in dry place
   i. Replenish nitroglycerin supply every 6 months or before expiration date
   j. Remove all old nitrate ointment just before application of new cream.
2. Ways to minimize precipitating events
   a. Avoid overexertion
   b. Try to reduce stress and anxiety, which cause blood vessels to constrict
   c. Avoid overeating, as it places an increased work load on the heart
   d. Avoid cold weather (constricts coronary vessels to conserve body heat, hence anginal pain can develop more easily)
   e. Dress warmly in cold weather
   f. Avoid hot, humid conditions (increases work load of heart)
   g. Walk downhill and with wind since walking uphill and against wind increase work load of heart.
3. Effects of exercise program in reduction of myocardial oxygen needs
   a. Engage in regular exercise program
   b. Exercise conditions heart muscle and can decrease oxygen demand during exercise
   c. Space exercise period with rest periods
   d. Take nitroglycerin before exertion
4. Need for regular medical follow-up

Myocardial infarction

PATHOPHYSIOLOGY

Myocardial infarction is a sudden complete blockage within a major coronary artery or one of its branches. The extent of myocardial damage is variable. It can cause necrosis with subsequent scar formation or fibrosis, or it can cause sudden death.

Prolonged ischemia lasting more than 35 to 45 minutes produces irreversible cellular damage and necrosis. The contractile properties of cardiac muscle within the necrotic areas become permanently impaired (Fig. 26-25). The final extent of the infarct is dependent on the ability of the surrounding ischemic tissues to recruit collateral circulation. Collateral circulation is the inherent development of new vessels within the heart to compensate for the damaged artery.

The clinical features of a myocardial infarct are determined by the site and extent of the disease process. An occlusion in the *left* anterior descending artery is referred to as an *anterior wall infarct*. Since this arterial branch supplies the left ventricle, it is often associated with a substantial loss of ventricular muscle mass, which causes severe hemodynamic consequences. A blockage in the *right* coronary artery (RCA) results in an *inferior wall infarct*. Because of the close proximity of the RCA to the conduction system, serious arrhythmias may develop. Occlusion of the *circumflex* artery produces a *lateral wall infarct*. Symptoms of hemodynamic instability develop when a large area of the heart is affected. The etiology, signs and symptoms, and medical therapies to correct this life-threatening emergency are outlined in Table 26-4.

ASSESSMENT

Subjective data

1. Patient's perception of the pain
   a. Location and radiation to other sites (Fig. 26-24)
   b. Quality of the pain
      1. Crushing or viselike sensation
      2. Abdominal pain
      3. Indigestion
   c. Onset and duration of pain
      1. Sudden onset
      2. More severe and prolonged than anginal pain
   d. Associated factors: exertion, stress, at rest
   e. Relieving factors: not relieved by rest or nitroglycerin
2. Feeling of uneasiness or impending doom.
3. Associated symptoms: dyspnea, nausea, dizziness, weakness
4. History of cardiac disease

Objective data

1. Behavior: apprehensive
2. Changes in vital signs: increased pulse rate, decreased blood pressure
3. Associated signs: diaphoresis, vomiting, sudden arrhythmias
4. Breath sounds: presence of rales, rhonchi
5. Change in cardiac rhythm
6. Presence of risk factors
7. Serum enzyme levels (see p. 657).

Diagnostic tests

Several diagnostic tests are used to detect a myocardial infarction. These include blood tests, ECG, and serum enzymes. Other diagnostic procedures, such as nuclear studies and pulmonary artery catheterization, are also of medical importance.

Blood tests

A nonspecific reaction to myocardial injury is an elevation in white blood cell count (12,000 to 15,000/mm^3). This increase begins a few hours after the onset of pain and lasts for 3 to 7 days. In general, high white blood cell

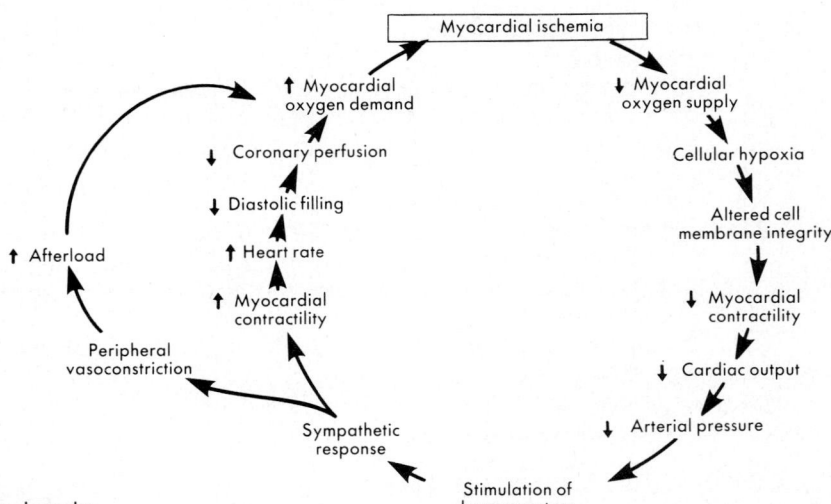

Fig. 26-25. Effects of prolonged myocardial ischemia.

counts are associated with larger infarcts. Also, the erythrocyte sedimentation rate (ESR) rises during the first week after the infarction and remains elevated for several weeks.

SERUM ENZYMES. As infarcted cardiac muscle cells die, cellular components are released into the vascular system. Some of these components are enzymes that can be evaluated by blood levels. Creatine phosphokinase (CPK), serum glutamic-oxaloacetic transaminase (SGOT) and lactic dehydrogenase (LDH) are found to be elevated at varying times following a myocardial infarction (Fig. 26-26).

Since these enzymes are not exclusively found in the heart, measurements of enzyme fractions or *isoenzymes* are more diagnostic of myocardial insult. Isoenzymes levels of CPK are the most reliable indicators of cardiac damage. The CPK isoenzyme that contains the MB subunits, $CPK(MB)_1$, is elevated for 48 hours after a transmural infarction. LDH can be fractionated into five distinct isoenzymes. Of these, LDH_1 and LDH_2 are most important. LDH_2 is more abundantly found in serum, whereas heart muscle in rich in LDH_1. An elevation in serum LDH_1, therefore, is confirmation of a myocardial infarction.

Radionuclide imaging

Radionuclide imaging is a noninvasive procedure that aids in evaluating the myocardium and coronary arteries. The two most commonly used techniques are pyrophosphate scanning and thallium scanning. Even though these scans involve radioactive materials, they are safe for both patients and hospital personnel.

PYROPHOSPHATE SCANNING. A radionuclide, technetium-99m pyrophosphate, is injected intravenously. The patient is scanned after 2 to 3 hours. This radionuclide is actively taken up by damaged myocardial tissue, producing a "hot spot" image. The scan takes 15 minutes to complete and is not painful. The scan will be negative during the first 12 hours after an infarction. Peak activity is evidenced at 36 hours.

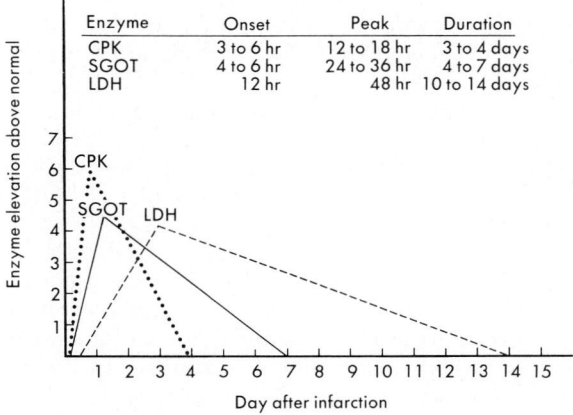

Fig. 26-26. Patterns of serum enzyme levels following myocardial infarction.

THALLIUM SCANNING. Thallium-201 is an intracellular ion that is actively transported into normal cells. If the cell is ischemic or infarcted, the thallium will not be picked up and a "cold spot" image is produced. This radioisotope is injected intravenously with the patient at rest or during stress testing.

Gated pool imaging

This particular type of imaging involves the intravenous injection of technetium-99m. After 3 to 5 minutes, the patient is placed in a supine position, and computer outlines of the left heart during all cardiac cycles are obtained. This procedure is used to evaluate left ventricular function and specifically to calculate the ejection fraction.

Pulmonary artery catheterization

Pulmonary artery catheterization has the following uses:
1. Assess the function of the right and left ventricles
2. Monitor for complications of myocardial infarction (cardiogenic shock, pulmonary edema)
3. Monitor effects of cardiovascular drugs
4. Determine preoperative hemodynamic status
5. Monitor postoperative cardiac function.

The entire procedure usually lasts about 30 to 45 minutes. A flexible multilumen catheter (Table 26-5) is inserted into the anticubital vein by means of a cutdown. The catheter is threaded through the superior vena cava, the right atrium, right ventricle, pulmonary artery, and lastly into a small branch of this artery (Fig. 26-27). Throughout the insertion, representative waveforms are viewed on an oscilloscope and pressure readings are obtained (p. 684).

DATA ANALYSIS AND PLANNING

Nursing diagnoses

Nursing diagnoses for the patient with myocardial infarction may include the following:
Comfort, alteration in: chest pain
Tissue perfusion, alteration in: cardiopulmonary
Activity intolerance
Anxiety
Knowledge deficit

Expected patient outcomes

1. Patient states he/she is feeling more comfortable.
2. Patient is participating in a program of progressive activity.
3. Patient can:
   a. Explain the nature of myocardial infarction and how the healing process relates to the treatment regimen.
   b. Describe risk factors that can be modified and plans to alter life-style.
   c. Describe prescribed medication regimen.
   d. Describe any dietary restrictions.

Table 26-5. Pulmonary artery catheter lumens

Type of lumen	Location	Purpose
Proximal	Right atrium	Administer intravenous fluids Obtain CVP readings
Distal	Pulmonary artery	Measure pulmonary artery pressure Measure pulmonary capillary wedge pressure (PCWP)
Balloon	Branch of pulmonary artery	Inflate balloon to obtain PCWP
Thermistor	Pulmonary artery	Measure CO

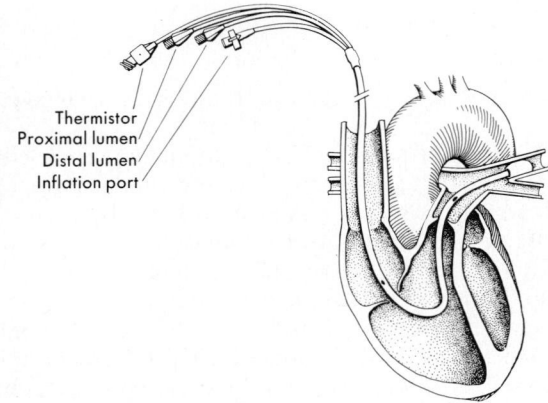

Thermistor
Proximal lumen
Distal lumen
Inflation port

Fig. 26-27. Placement of Swan-Ganz catheter.

e. Describe plans to continue progressive activity and resumption of sexual activity (if appropriate).
f. State the purpose and rationale of diagnostic testing.
g. Describe the rationale for and type of surgery to be performed, when indicated.
h. State plans for ongoing medical care.

IMPLEMENTATION

Assisting with achievement of therapeutic goals

1. Administer medications as prescribed
   a. Intravenous lidocaine is usually given prophylactically to prevent ventricular fibrillation
   b. Anticoagulants (heparin or coumadin) may be prescribed to decrease incidence of thrombophlebitis and pulmonary embolism
   c. *Avoid giving intramuscular injections* since these alter serum enzyme levels
2. Administer oxygen via nasal cannula to correct ventilation-perfusion abnormalities during the initial 24 to 48 hours; maintain oxygen therapy with persistent pain, hypotension, dyspnea, or arrhythmias
3. Monitor for cardiac arrhythmias (for example, premature ventricular beats, ventricular fibrillation)
4. Monitor vital signs for signs of cardiogenic shock (decreased blood pressure, tachycardia, cold clammy skin, mental confusion)

5. Maintain patient on prescribed low cholesterol, low-salt diet without caffeine-containing beverages
6. Administer stool softener to prevent constipation effects of opiates and decreased mobility and to prevent Valsalva maneuver (see Chapter 32) when straining at stool
7. Maintain patient on prescribed bedrest for 24 to 48 hours; encourage progressive ambulation when permitted

Assisting with comfort

1. Administer morphine intravenously to relieve pain and apprehension and to produce vasodilation
2. Administer prescribed tranquilizer (for example, diazepam [Valium]) to decrease anxiety and restlessness
3. Administer prescribed sleeping pill to promote sleep
4. Provide a calm environment
5. Answer patient's and family member's questions
6. Provide explanations for necessary monitoring and diagnostic tests
7. Plan patient care activities to minimize interruptions in rest

Counseling and teaching

Education of the patient and family enables them to assume a more active role in the patient's health care. A great deal of anxiety and apprehension can be allayed by providing information about the cardiac condition and its management. Major points for teaching are outlined in the box on p. 659.

During the hospitalization, many patients experience denial, depression, and anxiety. Generally, patients tend to become more anxious on the second day of hospitalization after the immediate threat of death from infarction has passed. Depression may occur several days later and may continue after the patient is discharged. Most persons who experience a myocardial infarction, however, adjust extremely well. Over 85% of all patients with uncomplicated myocardial infarctions are able to return to work. This, along with resuming normal sexual functioning, aids tremendously in the adjustment process.

The patients and their partners may need teaching and reassurance regarding resuming *sexual activities*. Many feel that their sex life is over after a myocardial infarction. Education should aim at supplying information and

---

Teaching the person with a myocardial infarction

1. Effect of myocardial infarction, the healing process, and treatment regimen
2. Effect of medications in the treatment of myocardial infarction
3. Association between risk factors and coronary artery disease
   a. Identify nonmodifiable risk factors
   b. Identify modifiable risk factors (especially cigarette smoking)
4. Effect of dietary restrictions on CAD: low salt, low cholesterol, no caffeine, fluid restrictions
5. Effect of activity on heart and need to participate in a progressive activity plan
6. Resumption of sexual activity (if appropriate)
   a. Abstention of sexual intercourse as directed, usually for 4 to 6 weeks (sexual closeness, for example, cuddling, may be started earlier as desired)
   b. Reporting to physician the following symptoms occurring during or following intercourse
      1. Dyspnea or increased heart rate continuing for more than 15 min after intercourse
      2. Extreme fatigue
      3. Chest pain during intercourse
      4. Palpitations for more than 15 min after intercourse
      5. Insomnia after intercourse

---

dispelling misinformation. Once patients with an uncomplicated myocardial infarction are capable of walking two flights of stairs without difficulty, they are generally able to perform sexual intercourse safely. Approximately 80% of all postcoronary patients will be able to resume sexual activity without serious risk. The other 20% need not totally abstain, but their sexual activity should be limited according to their cardiac capacity.

EVALUATION

Evaluation will be based on the expected patient outcomes. Some questions to ask may include the following:
1. Was chest pain decreased?
2. Was need for additional oxygen decreased?
3. Is activity tolerance increasing as evidenced by absence of fatigue, dyspnea, or discomfort with increasing activity?
4. Does the patient know the nature of the disorder, ways to decrease possibility of further ischemic attacks, activity prescription?
5. Has the patient made plans for follow-up medical care?

Cardiac surgery for myocardial ischemia

Surgical intervention is often necessary for patients with severe myocardial ischemia that is uncontrolled by medical therapy. Recommendation for surgery is based on the assessment of the expected benefits of the procedure and the inherent surgical risks. Patients with cardiomegaly, severe congestive heart failure, recent myocardial infarction, high left ventricular end-diastolic pressure, and an inadequate ejection fraction are at higher risk.

CORONARY ARTERY BYPASS GRAFT

Correction of myocardial ischemia is usually done through a bypass procedure in which a graft is sutured above and below the area of blockage in the coronary artery. Any number of bypasses can be performed depending on the location and extent of the blockages. Blood flow to the ischemic areas of the heart is then conducted through the new grafts, thus "bypassing" the obstruction.

Bypass grafts are obtained from sections of the saphenous vein or the internal mammary artery. The saphenous vein is harvested from the inner thigh and sectioned. Removal of this vein does not compromise circulation in the leg, since there are numerous other vessels to assist in this function.

The heart is exposed through a median sternotomy or anterolateral thoracotomy; retractors are used to spread the chest wall. Saphenous vein sections are grafted from the aorta to the point beyond the blockage. The internal mammary artery remains attached proximally to the subclavian and distally to the coronary artery beyond the occlusion (Fig. 26-28). Cardiopulmonary perfusion is used during bypass grafting to allow the ·surgeons access to the operative site and to maintain blood flow to vital organs.

Cardiopulmonary bypass

Most heart surgeries require partial or total cardiopulmonary bypass (Fig. 26-29). In *partial* bypass, pulmonary circulation is not interrupted. Oxygenated blood is drained from the left side of the heart, passed through a pulsatile pump, and returned through the descending aorta or common femoral artery. *Total* cardiopulmonary bypass involves both circulation and oxygenation of the extracted blood. Cannulas are placed in the right atrium to drain venous blood. The machine oxygenates this blood

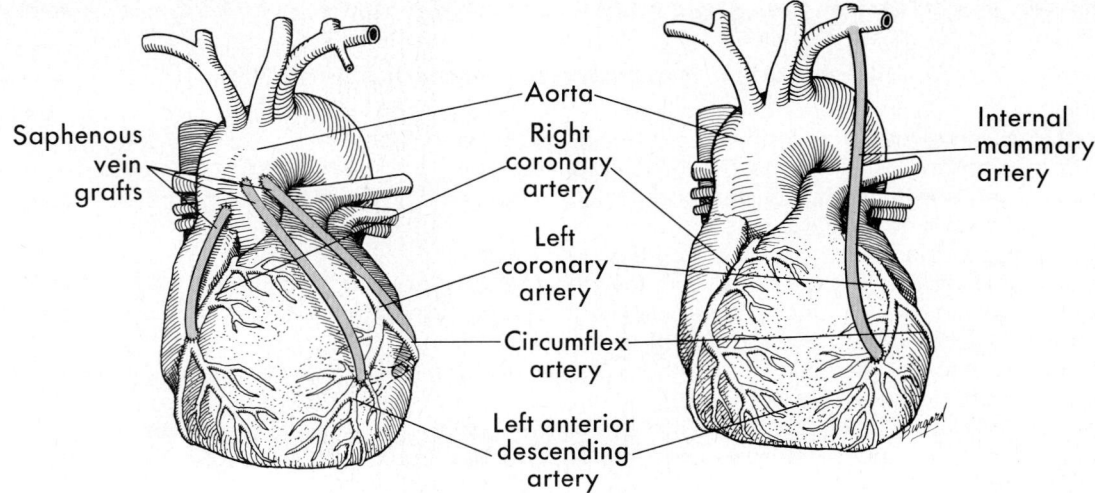

Fig. 26-28. Coronary artery bypass grafts.

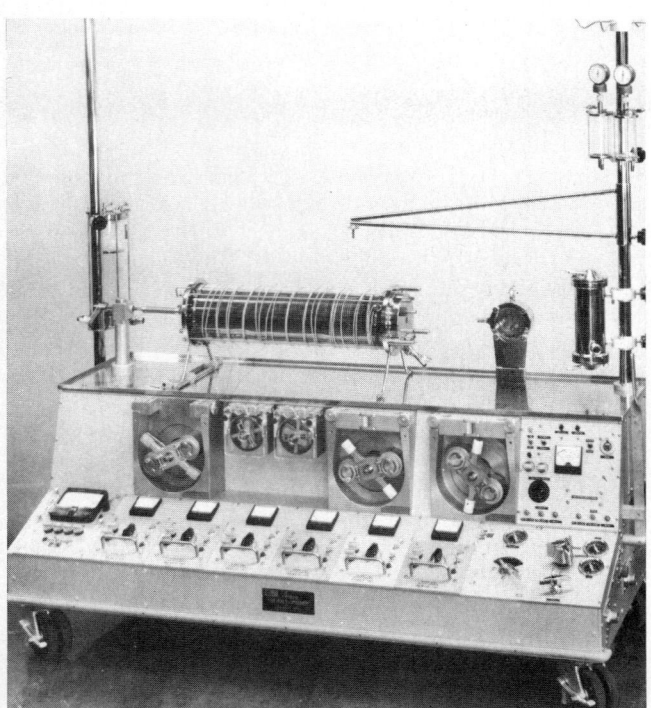

Fig. 26-29. Cardiopulmonary bypass machine used during heart surgery. (Courtesy, PEMCO, Inc., Cleveland, Ohio.)

Types of equipment

Many different types of equipment are used during cardiac surgery. Some of these and their uses are described in the following list:

1. Endotracheal tube, ventilator: to maintain open airway, ventilation, and access to secretions
2. Cardiac monitor: to identify arrhythmias
3. Intravenous line: to replace fluids, monitor central venous pressure, administer medications
4. Arterial line: to monitor blood pressure, obtain arterial blood samples
5. Pulmonary artery catheter (Swan-Ganz): to monitor pulmonary artery pressure, capillary wedge pressure, and cardiac output
6. Chest tube: to drain blood and air from chest
7. Epicardial pacing wires: to facilitate temporary cardiac pacing, if necessary
8. Urinary catheter; to monitor fluid status

Preoperative care

Preoperative care consists of (1) altering medications, (2) preparing the operative site, and (3) providing patient teaching. Digitalis preparations are discontinued on the day of surgery. Diuretics are also withheld so that the patient is adequately hydrated. Anticoagulants (couma-

and pumps it back into the ascending aorta or femoral artery.

Besides the capability of the heart-lung machine to provide extracorporeal circulation, it also serves as a direct route for medication administration and systemic hypothermia. Cooling of the machine solutions and subsequent body cooling lowers oxygen consumption by decreasing cellular metabolism.

Preoperative teaching for the patient experiencing coronary artery bypass surgery

1. Simple explanation of anatomy of heart, function of coronary arteries, and effect of CAD (use of heart drawings and models is helpful)
2. Explanation of surgery
   a. Removal of saphenous vein
   b. Use of internal mammary artery
   c. Effect on cardiac function
3. Definition of terms: *bypass, graft*
4. Explanation of events on day of surgery
   a. Preoperative medications
   b. Length of time in surgery (2 to 4 hours)
   c. Length of time until able to see family (1 ½ to 2 hours after surgery)
5. Explanation of the intensive care unit
   a. One large room, very busy, and noisy 24 hours a day; difficult to obtain sleep
   b. Nurse will be available at all times
   c. Visiting hours for family
   d. Length of stay in unit (2 to 3 days)
6. Explanation of monitors
   a. Round patches on chest connected to cardiac monitor
   b. Monitor makes beeping sound at all times
7. Explanation of lines
   a. Intravenous routes for fluid and medications
   b. Central venous line in chest or groin to monitor fluid status
   c. Faucetlike line to obtain blood samples without a needle prick
8. Explanation of drainage tubes
   a. Catheter draining urine from bladder
   b. Chest tube draining bloody fluid from incision (usually removed day after surgery)
9. Explanation of breathing tube
   a. Tube in windpipe connected to machine called ventilator
   b. Unable to speak with tube (can mouth words or write notes to communicate)
   c. Tube removed when patient is fully awake and stable
   d. Secretions in lungs or tube removed by nurse
10. Explanation and demonstration of activity and exercises
    a. Purpose of activity and exercises is to promote circulation, keep lungs clear, and prevent infection
    b. Activity will include:
       1. Turning from side to side in bed
       2. Sitting on edge of bed on night of surgery
       3. Sitting in chair day after surgery
    c. Range of motion exercises to arms and legs
    d. Effective deep breathing (use of sustained maximal inspiration, holding breath for 3 to 5 sec at end of deep inspiration)
    e. Effective coughing (coughing twice in succession with pillow splinting chest)
    f. Use of incentive spirometer (similar technique used to take deep breath)
11. Explanation of pain medication
    a. Pain will be present at chest incision and leg incision
    b. Medication reduces pain and makes activity and exercises easier
    c. Encourage use of pain medication
12. Explanation of diet
    a. After removal of breathing tube, will be given ice chips and water
    b. Clear liquids with gradual progression to regular diet

din, heparin) and other medications with anticoagulant effects (aspirin) are discontinued 48 hours before surgery.

In preparing the operative site, the patient showers with a special antimicrobial soap on the night before surgery. The chest and abdomen are shaved from neck to groin and from the left to the right midaxillary lines. If saphenous veins are needed for grafting, the inner aspects of the legs are also shaved.

Preoperative teaching is essential for a patient undergoing cardiac surgery. Involvement of the patient's family or significant others is also of importance in preparing the patient for surgery. Preoperative teaching for the patient experiencing coronary artery bypass surgery is summarized in box on p. 661. Adequate time should be provided for patient questions and concerns.

Postoperative care

Postoperative care centers around promoting oxygenation, maintaining fluid and electrolyte balance, promoting comfort, and preventing complications (thrombophlebitis, pulmonary embolism, cardiac tamponade, cardiac arrhythmias, and cardiac failure).

Promoting oxygenation

1. Ventilate with supplemental oxygen
2. Turn from side to side
3. Keep head of bed elevated at least 10 to 20 degrees
4. Assess quality of breath sounds
5. Monitor arterial blood gases
6. Encourage performance of range of motion exercises
7. Encourage progressive activity level
8. Daily chest x-ray films will be obtained
9. Monitor patency and drainage from chest tube
10. Assist with deep breathing, coughing, and use of incentive spirometer

Maintaining fluid and electrolyte balance

Crystalloid fluids are given intravenously to maintain adequate circulating blood volume. Colloids (whole blood, packed cells, plasma, or plasma expanders) are given depending on the hemoglobin and total protein concentrations. Potassium is frequently required after heart surgery, and the patient is monitored for signs of hypokalemia. Nursing activities include the following:

1. Maintain prescribed flow rate of parenteral fluids
2. Maintain patency of chest tube and urinary catheter
3. Record amount of drainage accurately
4. Assess for signs of fluid loss (dry skin, dry mucous membranes, decreased skin turgor) and fluid overload (peripheral edema, neck vein distention, moist respirations)
5. Monitor central venous pressure (CVP) readings
6. Monitor daily weight
7. Assess serum electrolytes (especially potassium) and hematocrit
8. Monitor Swan-Ganz parameters: pulmonary artery pressure, pulmonary capillary wedge pressure

Promoting comfort

1. Administer narcotic analgesics (morphine sulfate or meperidine) on a fairly regular basis during first 48 to 72 hours to relieve severe pain
2. Provide frequent oral hygiene until patient is taking fluids regularly
3. Eliminate unnecessary environmental stimuli (noise, lights) that impair ability to rest/sleep
4. Change linens if profuse nights sweats occur; assure patient that this commonly occurs
5. Group daily activities to allow for periods of uninterrupted rest/sleep
6. Encourage use of splinting devices (pillow, blanket) during coughing
7. Provide explanations for activities, as necessary
8. Monitor patient for changes in behavior and encourage patient to express concerns

Preventing complications

1. Thrombophlebitis/pulmonary embolism
   a. Encourage leg exercises until patient is ambulatory
   b. Encourage use of elastic stockings
   c. Encourage ambulation when permitted
2. Tamponade (compression of heart from accumulation of blood or fluid under pericardium)
   a. Monitor color and amount of chest tube drainage (change in color to bright red, sustained bleeding, or sudden cessation of drainage)
   b. Assess for increase in bleeding from midsternal incision
   c. Assess for other signs (restlessness, diaphoresis, hypotension, increased CVP, decreased urinary output)
3. Cardiac arrhythmias
   a. Maintain continuous ECG monitoring
   b. Assess cardiac rhythm
   c. Monitor daily electrolyte values (especially potassium)
   d. Medicate with antiarrhythmic drugs as prescribed
   e. Assist in treatment of other underlying causes of arrhythmias (decreased oxygenation)
4. Cardiac failure
   a. Monitor for signs of low cardiac output (hypotension, increased heart rate, restlessness, lethargy)
   b. Monitor CVP readings
   c. Monitor hourly urine output during initial period
   d. Monitor Swan-Ganz parameters
   e. Administer blood products and volume expanders as prescribed

Discharge planning

The usual hospital stay is 7 to 10 days after surgery, barring any complications. The patient and family need to know that it takes at least 3 to 6 months to experience significant improvements in preoperative symptoms such as dyspnea or pain.

Before discharge, the patient and family need specific guidelines for physical activity level. Activities are encouraged at a slow progressive pace unless overexertion occurs. Daily walking with a gradual increasing weekly distance is highly recommended. Patients are cautioned to avoid heavy lifting (greater than 30 pounds) and activities that require repetitive arm movements, such as vacuuming and playing golf. Patients are instructed not to drive a car or perform heavy labor until permitted by the physician.

Sexual intercourse can be resumed within the third or fourth postoperative week. Couples are cautioned to avoid sexual positions in which the patient would be supporting weight. Large meals or the consumption of alcohol should be avoided before sexual activity.

In summary, the following patient outcomes are expected:
1. Describe extent of permissible activity
   a. Describe plans for progressive return to physical activity as recommended by physician
   b. State awareness of when sexual activity may be resumed
   c. Describe criteria to use as a guide in determining if overexertion occurs (fatigue, dyspnea, pain)
   d. Describe plans to return to work if employed
2. Plan meals incorporating a balanced diet with any prescribed modifications
3. Describe any medication regimen
4. Describe plans for follow-up care
   a. Explain basis of any symptoms that may persist (dyspnea, pain, night sweats)
   b. Describe signs or symptoms requiring immediate medical attention (fever, increasing dyspnea, chest pain with minimal exertion)
   c. State plans for ongoing medical care

PERCUTANEOUS TRANSLUMINAL CORONARY ANGIOPLASTY

An alternative approach to coronary bypass surgery for selected patients with myocardial ischemia is percutaneous transluminal coronary angioplasty (PTCA). The procedure consists of mechanically dilating the coronary vessel wall by compressing the atheromatous plaque.

During PTCA, a specially designed catheter is inserted under fluoroscopy (similar to cardiac catheterization) and advanced to the site of the coronary obstruction. Once in position, a balloon on the catheter is inflated to provide compression and rupture the atheromatous plaque.

About 5% to 10% of patients undergoing PTCA require emergency coronary bypass surgery because of coronary occlusion,[74] therefore preparation is similar to preoperative preparation for coronary bypass surgery.

Following a successful PTCA, the patient may return either to the general cardiology unit or to an intensive care unit. Thrombosis may occur after treatment, therefore anticoagulants are usually given prophylactically. ECG monitoring is maintained the first day to monitor for arrhythmias indicating myocardial ischemia. The pa-

tient with an uncomplicated recovery may be discharged in 2 to 4 days after PTCA.

CARDIOGENIC SHOCK

Cardiogenic shock is a shock state of primary cardiac origin. It is most frequently caused by myocardial infarction but may also result from other cardiac disorders that lead to low cardiac output.

PATHOPHYSIOLOGY

Cardiogenic shock occurs when cardiac function is severely impaired and cardiac output is low. As the shock progresses, there is decreased coronary artery perfusion leading to development of cardiac muscle ischemia that leads to further decreased function (Fig. 26-30). Mortality is high.

MEDICAL THERAPY

Cardiogenic shock is a medical emergency that requires immediate intervention and constant attention to prevent irreversible cell damage and death. Therapy is aimed at correcting factors that contribute to decreased tissue perfusion, such as cardiac arrhythmias, hypoxemia, and pain.

Invasive monitoring lines that are usually placed include catheters in the pulmonary artery, systemic artery, and urinary bladder. The left ventricular end-diastolic

---

Causes of cardiogenic shock

Myocardial infarction
Critical aortic stenosis
Intractable arrhythmias
Ruptured aortic aneurysm
Severe congestive heart failure
Massive pulmonary embolism
Cardiac tamponade

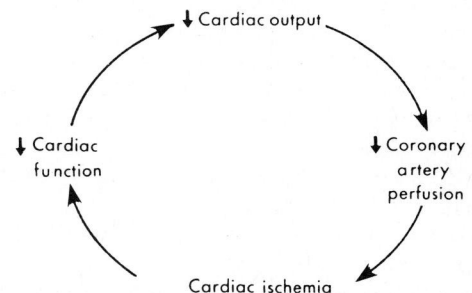

Fig. 26-30. Sequence of events in cardiogenic shock.

pressure (LVEDP) is reflected in the pulmonary capillary wedge pressure, which is used as a guide to fluid therapy.

The following therapy may be initiated:

1. Vasopressors and cardiotonic agents (for example, dopamine, norepinephrine) to raise systemic arterial pressure without increasing cardiac work load; vasopressors are titrated to maintain systolic pressure, preferably above 90 mm Hg.
2. Hyperventilation and buffering agents (for example, sodium bicarbonate) to counteract lactic acidosis
3. Intravenous fluids if hypovolemia is present: care must be taken to prevent fluid overload with resulting pulmonary edema
4. Use of intraaortic balloon counterpulsation, if necessary (see below)

General care of the patient experiencing shock is described in Chapter 11.

Intraaortic balloon counterpulsation

A counterpulsation device facilitates blood circulation by decreasing aortic pressure during systole and increasing it during diastole. The overall effects include the following:

1. Increase in coronary artery perfusion
2. Decrease in preload (degree to which the myocardium is stretched before contracting)
3. Decrease in afterload (resistance against which blood is expelled).

In addition to the situations producing cardiogenic shock, the intraaortic balloon pump may be used in unstable cardiac patients before and during open heart surgery and in assistance when removing these patients from cardiopulmonary bypass postoperatively.

Technique

The intraaortic balloon is inserted percutaneously or by cutdown into the right or left femoral artery. It is advanced into the thoracic aorta and sutured into place at the insertion site after the balloon tip has been correctly positioned just distal to the left subclavian artery (Fig. 26-31). The end of the balloon catheter is attached to a pump console, which alternately inflates and deflates the balloon using either helium or carbon dioxide gas.

The timing of the inflation-deflation sequence is of the utmost importance in obtaining maximal counterpulsation effect. Using the ECG to trigger the pumping mechanism and the arterial waveform to determine effectiveness of the counterpulsation, the balloon is timed to inflate just at the beginning of ventricular diastole, immediately after closure of the aortic valve. The balloon remains inflated during diastole and is then timed to deflate immediately before the next ventricular systolic ejection or just before the aortic valve reopens. Improper balloon timing not only defeats the purpose of counterpulsation, but also could be directly damaging to the myocardium. This is particularly true in early inflation or late deflation, in which the heart would be ejecting blood against a partially inflated balloon.

Nursing management

1. Monitor vital signs and indices of cardiac function at frequent intervals as specified
2. Position patient:
   a. Head of bed elevated no more than 30 degrees to prevent balloon migration upward in aorta
   b. Reposition patient every 2 hours on alternate sides to prevent skin breakdown and other consequences of immobility
   c. Avoid hip flexion on catheterized side; restrain leg if necessary
3. Monitor circulation of both legs before catheter insertion and hourly thereafter until balloon is removed
4. Keep dressing on balloon insertion site clean and dry; change every 24 to 48 hours using sterile technique
5. Administer prescribed heparin or low molecular weight dextran to prevent blood clotting or emboli

Considerable psychologic support is necessary for the patient and family during such critical therapy. Not only is the physical size and noise of the pump console very intimidating, but its presence only reinforces everyone's awareness of the frailty of the patient's heart and uncertainty about the future. Careful but simple explanations of the pump's action are necessary for patients who are alert enough to understand; it is important that they not get the mistaken idea that the pump is working instead of their heart. Some patients with this type of misunderstanding fear that they will die if the pump stops even momentarily. Such terrific fear makes them anxious and restless and further increases the body's demand for oxygen. Continuous reassurance and repeated simple expla-

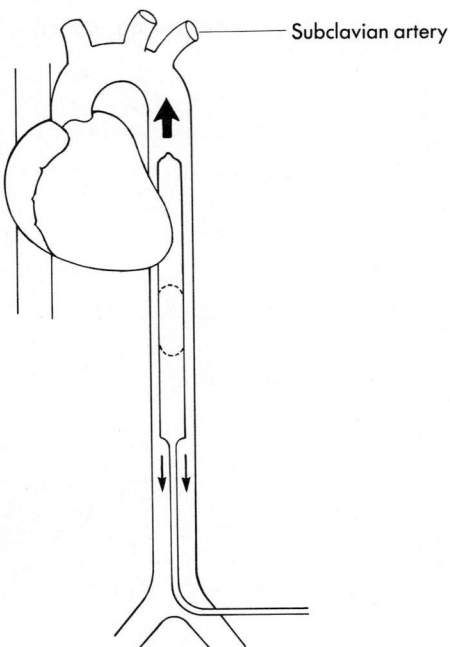

Subclavian artery

Fig. 26-31. Representation of triple-segmented intraaortic balloon positioned just distal to left subclavian artery.

nations are essential. Some patients may benefit from mild sedation.

CONGESTIVE HEART FAILURE

Heart failure (also known as congestive heart failure, cardiac decompensation, cardiac insufficiency, and cardiac incompetence) is a state in which the heart no longer is able to pump an adequate supply of blood to meet the demands of the body. It can be classified as acute or chronic. *Acute* heart failure develops quickly and often without warning. The clinical picture may include shock, cardiac arrest, or sudden death as a result of the myocardium failing to function adequately. Acute heart failure may result from decreased effectiveness of the heart after myocardial infarction. *Chronic* heart failure develops gradually, and the patient is seen initially with milder symptoms. The heart has the capability to compensate for the decreased performance, thus lessening the severity of symptoms.

ETIOLOGY

The causes of heart failure can be divided into three groups (see box). *Preload* is the ventricular blood volume at end diastole, the maximal ventricular blood volume for that beat of the heart. According to Starling's law, once the preload has reached a given limit, the effectiveness of the contraction diminishes, resulting in heart failure. *Afterload* is the force that the ventricle must develop to eject blood into the circulatory system. This is the pressure against which the heart must work.

PATHOPHYSIOLOGY

Inadequate cardiac output triggers a number of compensatory responses in an effort to maintain the heart's functions. If cardiac output continues to fall despite the cardiac compensatory mechanisms, renal perfusion is affected. The kidney then compensates by increasing sodium reabsorption which increases water absorption. The result is fluid overload and edema (Fig. 26-32).

Initially, one side of the heart fails. Since the left ventricle is most often affected by coronary atherosclerosis and hypertension, heart failure usually begins there. However, since both ventricles are part of the same system, the right ventricle usually becomes impaired as well.

The symptoms of heart failure are the result of excessive fluid retention by the body. The congestion that results can involve either the venous system or the pulmonary system or both. As the effectiveness of the heart decreases, venous stasis occurs and venous pressure increases. The result is further fluid retention by the kidneys. Symptoms are summarized in the box on p. 666.

Causes of heart failure

1. Direct damage to the heart: myocardial infarction, myocarditis, myocardial fibrosis, ventricular aneurysm
2. Ventricular overload
   a. Preload: mitral or aortic regurgitation, atrial or ventricular septal defects, rapid infusion of intravenous solutions
   b. Afterload: aortic or pulmonary valve stenosis, systemic or pulmonary hypertension
3. Constriction of ventricle: cardiac tamponade, constrictive cardiomyopathies, pericarditis

---

Compensatory responses to inadequate cardiac output

Response	Effect
Stimulation of sympathetic nervous system	Increased rate and force of myocardial contraction
Ventricular dilation	Stretching of fibers allows for more forceful contraction thus increasing stroke volume
Hypertrophy of myocardium	More effective contraction of heart, thus increasing cardiac output
Kidneys: sodium and water retention	Expands blood volume, increases cardiac output

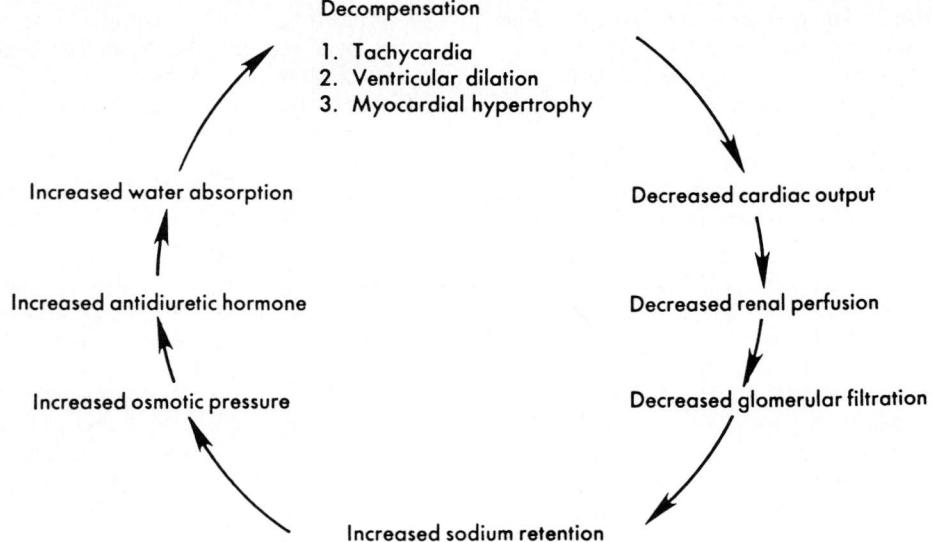

Decompensation

1. Tachycardia
2. Ventricular dilation
3. Myocardial hypertrophy

Increased water absorption

Decreased cardiac output

Increased antidiuretic hormone

Decreased renal perfusion

Increased osmotic pressure

Decreased glomerular filtration

Increased sodium retention

Fig. 26-32. Sequence of events compounding decompensation in chronic heart failure.

> ## Signs and symptoms of congestive heart failure
>
> ### Left ventricular failure
> Dyspnea
> Orthopnea
> Cheyne-Stokes respirations
> Cough
>
> ### Right ventricular failure
> Peripheral edema
> Liver engorgement
> Distended neck veins
>
> ### General symptoms
> Fatigue
> Angina pectoris
> Anxiety

Left ventricular failure

In left ventricular failure, the left ventricle cannot pump oxygenated blood coming from the lungs at a volume necessary to meet the demands of the body. Symptoms are the result of congestion of the lungs with fluid that is forced from the pulmonary circulation into the pulmonary tissues, causing pulmonary edema (p. 673) and pleural effusion.[20,94] Fluid may be present in the interstitial tissues, alveoli, bronchioles, or pleural space.

Dyspnea

Dyspnea, or labored breathing, is an early symptom of left ventricular failure. It is caused by interference with gas exchange as a result of the fluid in the alveoli. It may occur or become worse only on physical exertion, such as climbing stairs, walking up an incline, or walking against the wind, since these activities require increased amounts of oxygen.

Orthopnea

Difficulty in breathing when lying flat may be present, and persons often must sleep propped up in bed or in a chair. When the person is lying flat, there is decreased ventilation and the blood volume in the pulmonary vessels is increased. The orthopnea is often described by the number of pillows required for the patient to rest comfortably when in bed, for example, "three-pillow orthopnea."

Although orthopnea may occur immediately after lying down, it often does not occur for several hours. At that time, it causes the person to wake with severe dyspnea and coughing. This condition is known as *paroxysmal nocturnal dyspnea* and results from the accumulation of fluid in the lungs as the person is lying in bed. The patient usually experiences a feeling of suffocation and often awakens in panic.

Apnea and hyperpnea (Cheyne-Stokes)

In heart failure, the patient may experience alternating periods of apnea and hyperpnea. Often because of respiratory insufficiency, an inadequate amount of oxygen makes the respiratory center in the brain insensitive to the amounts of carbon dioxide in the arterial blood, and respirations cease (apnea). When the carbon dioxide content in the arterial blood increases enough to stimulate the respiratory center or when the oxygen level in the blood drops to a level that is low enough to stimulate the respiratory center, hyperpnea results. These periods of overbreathing result in greater than normal decreases in carbon dioxide content of arterial blood, producing another period of apnea. Periodic overbreathing often begins as the patient goes to sleep and decreases as sleep deepens and ventilation decreases.

Cough

A persistent hacking cough is often a symptom of left-sided heart failure. It results from congestion of trapped fluid, which is irritating to the mucosal lining of the lungs and bronchi. The cough is usually productive of large quantities of frothy sputum which is occasionally blood tinged. On auscultation *rales* may be heard. Rales are the moist popping and crackling sounds heard most often at the end of inspiration.

Right ventricular failure

In right ventricular failure the right ventricle compensates in response to an increase in pulmonary artery pressure. The heart becomes less effective and is unable to maintain adequate output against the increased resistance. This results in blood damming back into the systemic circulation, leading to *peripheral edema.* This edema is of the pitting type, is nontender, and occurs in dependent parts (legs or sacrum). As the edema becomes more pronounced, it progresses up the legs into the thighs, external genitalia, and lower trunk. As the tissue becomes extremely engorged, the skin cracks, and fluid may "weep" from the tissues.

The *liver* may also become engorged with intravascular fluid, resulting in enlargement and tenderness in the right upper abdominal quadrant. As venous stasis increases, pressure within the portal system becomes so great that fluid is forced through the blood vessels into the abdominal cavity (ascites). The ascitic fluid can reach volumes of more than 10 L, displacing the diaphragm and resulting in severe respiratory distress. A paracentesis (see Chapter 31) may be required to relieve the pressure on the diaphragm. *Distended neck veins* are a result of the increased systemic venous pressure and are usually observed when the patient is in a sitting position (see Fig. 11-2).

General symptoms of heart failure

Fatigue

Persons with heart failure commonly note fatigue following activities that ordinarily are not tiring. The fatigue results from impaired blood circulation to tissues as a result of the decreased CO. The reduction in tissue oxygen decreases the production of adenosine triphosphate (ATP), the immediate energy source for muscle contractions. In addition, the impaired circulation causes a decrease in the removal of metabolic waste products, and the result of this is further decreased muscle function.

Anginal pain

Cardiac pain is *not* a typical symptom of heart failure; however, angina pectoris can occur from the decrease in CO. It is most likely to occur in patients with CAD, which increases the patient's sensitivity to a deficiency in the oxygen content in the circulating blood. As heart failure develops, the blood is less effectively oxygenated and angina occurs. As the fluid overload state is corrected, the chest pain resolves.

Anxiety

Most persons are aware of the importance of an effective functioning heart to maintain life, and they are acquainted with the symptoms that indicate a failing heart. Therefore anxiety usually occurs when symptoms of heart failure are present. Anxiety can cause increased breathlessness, which is interpreted by the patient as a increase in the severity of the heart failure, and this in turn increases the anxiety.

ASSESSMENT

Subjective data

1. Shortness of breath: occurrence, extent
2. Orthopnea: degree
3. Recent weight gain
4. Pedal edema (that is, are shoes usually tight?)
5. Ability to perform daily activities; degree of fatigue
6. Discomfort: anginal or abdominal pain
7. Concerns, anxious feelings
8. Usual coping skills
9. Knowledge of condition

Objective data

1. Neck vein distention: presence, degree
2. Edema: site, degree of pitting
3. Abdominal distention
4. Daily weights: weigh on litter scale if severe heart failure present; weigh at same time of day (usually in morning after emptying bladder, before breakfast) and with same amount of clothing
5. Adventitious breath sounds
6. Gallop rhythm of heart on auscultation
7. Level of consciousness
8. Pulse changes and respiratory effort with activity

DIAGNOSTIC TESTS

The more common diagnostic tests for patients with congestive failure are ECG, echocardiogram (p. 632), chest x-ray films, and cardiac catheterization (p. 684).

DATA ANALYSIS AND PLANNING

Nursing diagnoses

Possible nursing diagnoses for the patient with congestive heart failure may include the following:

Anxiety
Activity intolerance

Breathing pattern, ineffective
Cardiac output, alteration in: decreased
Comfort, alteration in: pain
Fear
Gas exchange, impaired
Sleep pattern disturbance
Thought process, alterations in
Tissue perfusion, alteration in: cerebral, cardiopulmonary, renal, gastrointestinal, peripheral

Expected patient outcomes

1. Breathing is easier
2. Edema is reduced
3. Normal respiratory rate is achieved without the use of supplemental oxygen
4. Fatigue is decreased
5. The patient can:
   a. Describe a plan for activity that will avoid fatigue or dyspnea
   b. Plan a diet incorporating any prescribed sodium or fluid restrictions
   c. Describe the medication therapy
   d. Describe signs and symptoms requiring health care follow-up
   d. State plans for follow-up care.
6. If the patient will be on oxygen therapy at home, the patient can describe usage and precautions

IMPLEMENTATION

Assisting with achievement of therapeutic goals

The primary goals of the treatment of congestive heart failure are to restore a balance between the supply and demand for blood by body tissues and to remove excessive fluid from the circulating blood volume.[20] The desired outcome of medical therapy is improvement in signs and symptoms. These objectives are accomplished by optimizing cardiac output and by reducing the requirements of the body for oxygen. Fig. 26-33 shows the effects of medications that may be used.

At many acute care hospitals, patients with acute

Medical therapy for congestive heart failure

1. Reducing oxygen requirements of body
   a. Oxygen therapy
   b. Positioning of patient to facilitate breathing
   c. Rest
2. Optimizing cardiac output
   a. Digitalis therapy
   b. Diuretic therapy
   c. Sodium-restricted diet

---

congestive heart failure are admitted to medical or cardiac intensive care units. Occasionally, the physician may elect to place the patient in the usual room accomodations, where the environment is less stressful and where family members can visit more routinely.

Providing oxygenation

In heart failure, the oxygen content of the bloodstream may be markedly reduced because of the less effective oxygenation of the blood as it passes through the congested lungs. The patient may be more comfortable and better able to rest when receiving oxygen, since it helps in reducing dyspnea and fatigue. Oxygen is usually administered by nasal cannula at 2 to 6 L/min. Baseline arterial blood gases are obtained at initiation of oxygen therapy and intermittently during therapy to assess effectiveness of the treatment.

Breathing is often made easier by maintaining the patient in semi-Fowler's or high Fowler's position. These positions maximize oxygenation by permitting greater lung expansion. The patient is often orthopneic and tends to breathe more easily sitting than lying in bed. If the patient is sitting in a chair, the feet are elevated to reduce pooling of fluid in the dependent limbs. When the patient is in high Fowler's position in bed, a pillow may be placed lengthwise behind the shoulders and back in such a manner that full expansion of the rib cage is possible. The arms may be supported on pillows to reduce the pull on the shoulder muscles (Fig. 26-34). An over-the-bed table may be placed close to the patient to allow resting of the head and arms.

Promoting rest and activity

Reducing the requirement for oxygen can best be effected by providing the patient with the degree of activity that does not compromise myocardial function, as demonstrated by the presence of symptoms. For mild heart failure, the patient may be treated on an ambulatory basis with only a regimen of less strenuous activity and more rest than usual.

For severe heart failure, a program of bed rest or limited activity may be necessary until symptoms abate. Permissible activity will be based on symptoms such as dyspnea and fatigue. A careful assessment must be made each day to determine the amount of rest required. If the patient has difficulty relaxing because of apprehension or anxiety, a tranquilizer may be prescribed.

Ambulation is started slowly to avoid overloading the heart. The regimen varies depending on individual patient response. When a patient has been on restricted bed rest, activities progress slowly from dangling, to sitting, to walking increased distances under close supervision. If signs of dyspnea, fatigue, or increased pulse rate that does not stabilize readily occur, the patient is returned to bed. Oxygen is given for dyspnea, and the physician is notified.

The plan for increased activity is explained to the patient and family. They should understand that if activity tires the person excessively, it may be curtailed. Overac-

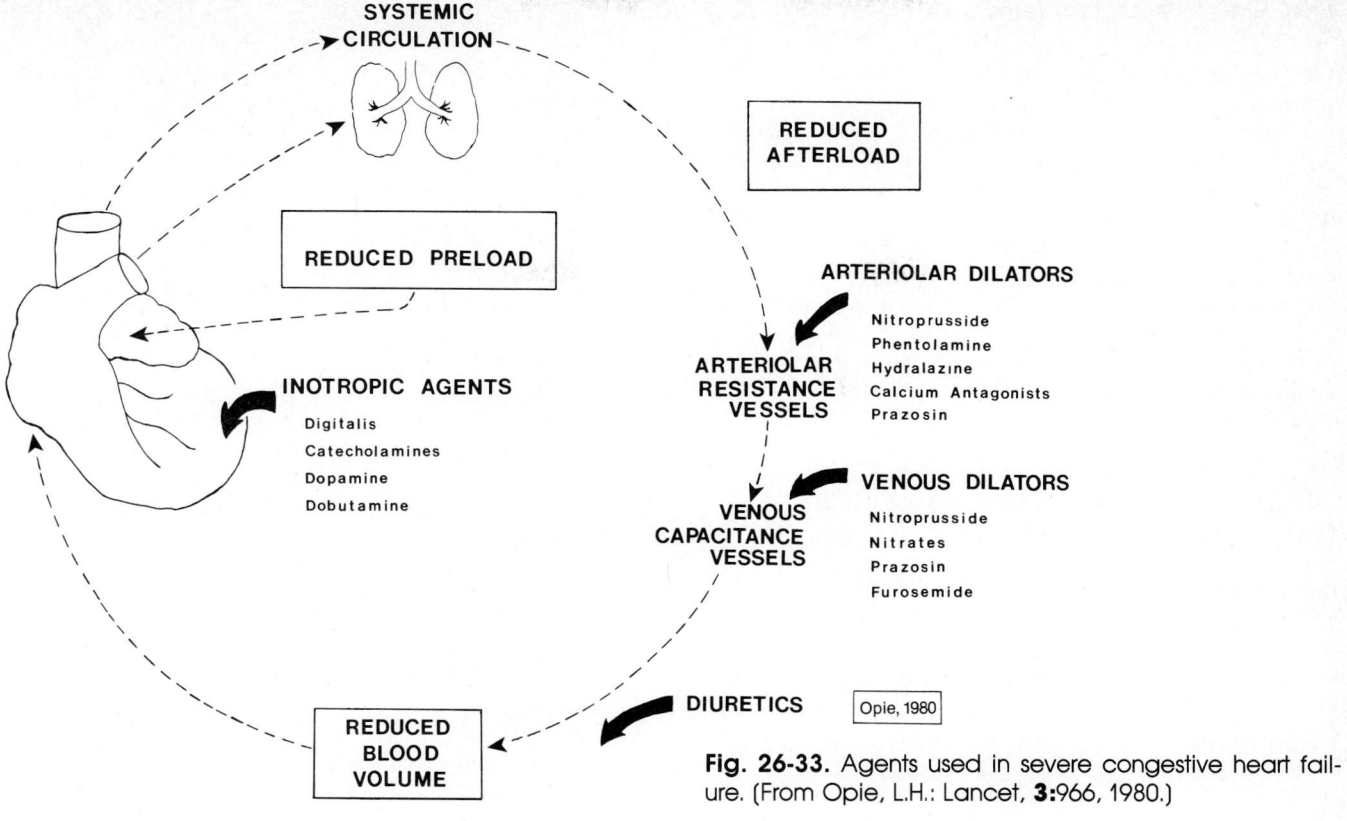

SYSTEMIC
CIRCULATION

REDUCED
AFTERLOAD

REDUCED PRELOAD

ARTERIOLAR DILATORS

Nitroprusside
Phentolamine
Hydralazine
Calcium Antagonists
Prazosin

ARTERIOLAR
RESISTANCE
VESSELS

INOTROPIC AGENTS

Digitalis
Catecholamines
Dopamine
Dobutamine

VENOUS DILATORS

Nitroprusside
Nitrates
Prazosin
Furosemide

VENOUS
CAPACITANCE
VESSELS

DIURETICS   Opie, 1980

REDUCED
BLOOD
VOLUME

Fig. 26-33. Agents used in severe congestive heart failure. (From Opie, L.H.: Lancet, **3:**966, 1980.)

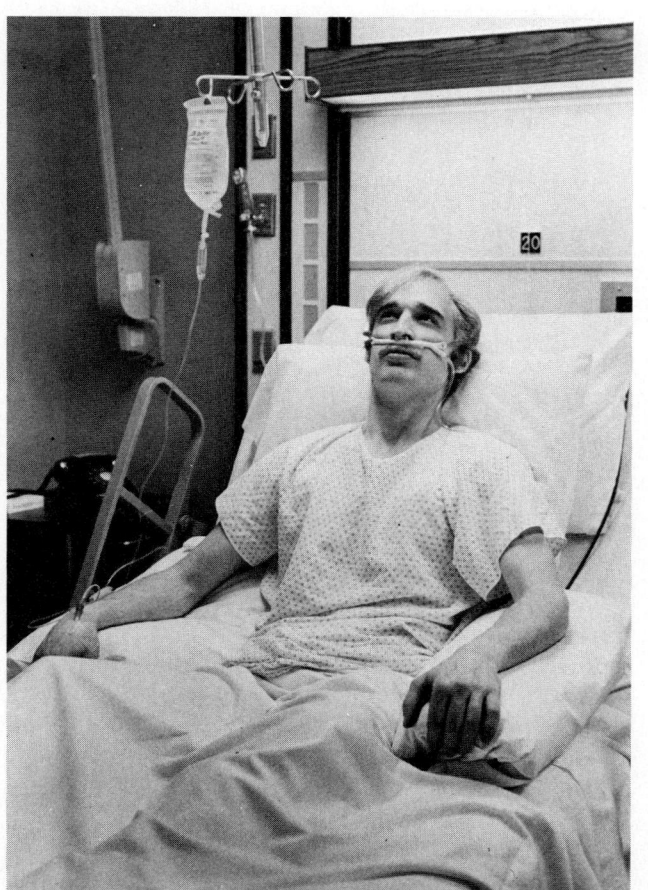

Fig. 26-34. Patient sitting upright with pillows under head and each arm to promote chest expansion and comfort.

tivity can produce physical and mental setbacks that delay ultimate recovery.

Rest to the heart is also promoted by preventing constipation, since straining at defecation places an extra burden on the heart. During straining against a closed glottis (Valsalva maneuver), venous return to the heart is decreased as a result of increased intrathoracic pressure. When this pressure is released after straining, a large amount of venous return creates an increased work load on the heart. The feces can be kept soft by stool softeners or bulk-forming laxatives. If an enema is necessary, it should be of low volume and given with a small rectal tube inserted only 3 to 4 inches.

Digitalis therapy

Digitalis is the major therapeutic approach in the treatment of congestive heart failure. Digitalis and its deriva-

tives usually are effective in improving myocardial function in persons with congestive heart failure. The positive inotropic action of digitalis preparations enhances mechanical performance by strengthening the force of myocardial contraction. This leads to increased CO and in-

---

Factors predisposing to digitalis toxicity

Hypokalemia: potentiates the effects of digitalis
Severe liver and kidney disease: the liver inactivates digitalis; the kidney excretes it
Primary myocardial disease: myocardium is more sensitive to the drug
Elderly persons: decreased tolerance from decreased metabolism

---

Signs and symptoms of digitalis toxicity

Cardiovascular effects

Bradycardia
Tachycardia
Bigeminy (double beats)
Ectopic beats
Pulse deficit (difference between apical and radial pulse)

Gastrointestinal effects

Anorexia
Nausea and vomiting
Abdominal pain
Diarrhea

Neurologic effects

Headache
Double, blurred, or colored vision
Drowsiness, confusion
Restlessness, irritability
Muscle weakness

Table 26-6. Digitalis preparations

Generic name	Trade name	Route	Onset	Duration
Purple foxglove				
(Digitalis purpurea)				
Powdered digitalis	Digifortis	Oral	Slow	Long
	Digiglusin			
Digitoxin	Crystodigin	IV	Slow	Long
	Purodigin	Oral		
	Digitaline Nativelle			
	Unidigin			
Gitalin	Gitaligin	Oral	Fast	Moderate
White foxglove				
(Digitalis lanata)				
Digoxin		Oral	Fast	Moderate
	Lanoxin	IV		
		IM		
Deslanoside	Cedilanid-D	IV	Fast	Short
		IM		
Lanatoside C	Cedilanid	Oral	Variable	Short
Acetyldigitoxin	Acylanid	Oral	Moderate	Short
Strophanthus gratus				
Ouabain		IV	Fast	Short

creased blood flow to the kidneys. Digitalis preparations also decrease heart rate (automaticity) and cardiac conduction velocity, which permits the ventricles to relax more to allow time for better filling of the ventricles with blood.

DIGITALIZATION. When acute congestive heart failure occurs, the physician usually orders an optimal therapeutic dose of a digitalis preparation to slow the ventricular rate and decrease symptoms. This larger dose given over a short period of time, usually 24 to 48 hours, is called a *loading* or *digitalizing* dose. In some instances the dose may approach the toxic level. After the optimal therapeutic dose has been determined, the person is given a daily maintenance dose.

Numerous types of digitalis preparations may be used (Table 26-6). For rapid digitalization in emergency situations, deslanoside (Cedilanid-D), or ouabain is usually selected. Digoxin or digitoxin is most commonly used for maintenance drug therapy. Digoxin has a more rapid effect than digitoxin, yet it has sufficient duration for adequate maintenance therapy. Response to a digitalis preparation is evaluated on the basis of relief of symptoms.

NURSING IMPLICATIONS
1. Take apical pulse before administering digitalis preparations; withhold medication and notify physician if pulse is below 60
2. If giving digoxin intramuscularly, inject it deeply and massage area well, since drug is a tissue irritant
3. Observe for signs of digitalis toxicity
4. Monitor serum potassium blood levels (hypokalemia is the most common cause of digitalis toxicity)
5. Give potassium supplements (if prescribed)

Diuretic therapy

Diuretic therapy is not a substitute for digitalis therapy. The purpose of diuretic therapy is to decrease cardiac work load by reducing circulating volume, and thus decrease symptoms. Diuretics are potentially dangerous medications, and their use is instituted only after symptoms of heart failure persist following digitalization and sodium restriction.

Essential to proper initiation of diuretic therapy is determining how much fluid should be removed from the patient by establishing a "dry weight" or edema-free weight. This is accomplished by gradually removing fluid by use of diuretics and assessing the patient's blood pressure. When the patient becomes hypotensive, particularly orthostatic, this signals the physician that too much fluid has been removed. The patient is then permitted to reaccumulate a small amount of fluid until hypotension no longer occurs. This weight is then considered the patient's dry weight.

Types of common diuretic drugs are listed in Table 26-7. Currently the *thiazides* are the diuretics of choice in the treatment of heart failure. The thiazides are inexpensive, easy to take, and effective when taken over a long time. Because these potent drugs can lead to electrolyte imbalance, serum chemistry levels are observed closely, particularly at the onset of therapy. The major complication is hypokalemia, which may produce ECG changes and cause digitalis toxicity. Foods high in potassium are encouraged, and potassium supplements may be prescribed.

If thiazides are ineffective, an oral aldosterone antagonist, such as spironolactone (Aldactone) or triamterene (Dyrenium), may be given with the thiazide. These drugs work by competitive inhibition of aldosterone, resulting in retention of potassium and excretion of sodium and water.

The most potent duretics currently available are furosemide (Lasix) and ethacrynic acid (Edecrin). These medications are reserved for severe congestive heart failure or when other forms of treatment are ineffective in

Table 26-7. Diuretics used in the treatment of heart failure

Type	Example	Onset/peak/duration	Side effects
Thiazide	Chlorothiazide (Diuril)	2 hr/4 hr/6-12 hr	Gastrointestinal upsets (can be minimized by taking medication with meals); hypokalemia; hyperglycemia
	Hydrochlorothiazide (Esidrix, Hydrodiuril)	2 hr/4 hr/6-12 hr	
Loop	Furosemide (Lasix)	1 hr/1-2 hr/6-8 hr	Similar to thiazide diurectics; also ototoxicity and blood dyscrasias
	Ethacrynic acid (Edecrin)	30 min/2 hr/6 hr	
Potassium-sparing	Spironolactone (Aldactone)	Gradual/3 days/2-3 days after therapy discontinued	Gastrointestinal irritation; hyperkalemia
	Triamterene (Dyrenium)	Rapid/7-9 hr/12-16 hr	

relieving symptoms. These agents also increase renal blood flow and therefore may prove effective in treating heart failure when renal function is also impaired. Therapy is best initiated in the hospital setting so that electrolyte and acid-base balance may be monitored.

Sodium-restricted diet

Edema is often effectively controlled in patients with heart failure by restriction of sodium intake. The degree of restriction depends on the severity of the failure and the extent of diuretic therapy. The severely restricted sodium diet is rarely prescribed, because this diet is unpalatable and expensive, which results in poor patient compliance.

The amount of sodium in the normal diet is 3 to 10 g/day. Sodium restriction in persons receiving diuretics may not be dropped below 3 to 5 g/day because of the dangers of hyponatremia. In mild cardiac failure, sodium may be restricted to 1 to 2 g/day; this is known as a no-added salt (NAS) diet. It is essentially a normal diet, except that no extra salt is added to prepared foods and obviously salted foods such as potato chips are omitted. For moderate or

---

Care of the patient with congestive heart failure

Assisting with achievement of therapeutic goals

1. Reinforce importance of conservation of energy and planning of activities to avoid fatigue
2. Provide diversional activity that will assist in conserving energy
3. Assist in maintaining an adequate nutritional intake while observing prescribed dietary prescriptions (sodium restrictions)
4. Monitor signs of fluid and electrolyte imbalance
5. Medicate patient as prescribed
   a. Careful and timely administration of diuretics
   b. Assess apical heart rate before administering digitalis preparations
   c. Observe patient for signs of digitalis toxicity (p. 670)
   d. Give pain medication or tranquilizer as indicated
6. Assess and record weight daily
7 Administer oxygen therapy as prescribed.

Assisting with comfort and ADL

1. Assist with ADL as necessary
2. Encourage independence within the patient's limitations
3. Position patient carefully to promote comfort, ease of respirations, and venous return
4. Give meticulous skin care in patients with edema
   a. Careful washing of skin
   b. Frequent application of skin lotion
   c. Frequent repositioning
   d. Use of flotation mattress or waterbeds for severe edema
   e. Massage
5. Provide patient and family with opportunities to explore their concerns

Teaching

1. Need to monitor for signs and symptoms of congestive heart failure including daily weights, pedal edema, change in respiratory status
2. Need to avoid fatigue and plan for rest periods
3. Instructions for home oxygen therapy, if appropriate
4. Name, purpose, dosage, frequency, and side effects of prescribed medications (digitalis preparation, diuretic)
5. Dietary planning
   a. Rationale for sodium or fluid restrictions, as appropriate
   b. Foods to be avoided depending on diet prescription
   c. Small frequent feedings to decrease exertion and decrease GI blood requirements, which can tax the failing heart
6. Need for medical follow-up.

severe heart failure, the amount of sodium permitted is specifically prescribed. Vitamin supplements are usually required when severely restricted sodium diets are prescribed.

Low-sodium diets can be made more appealing by adding salt substitutes to food in place of table salt. Since many salt substitutes contain potassium, the patient's need for potassium must be assessed. Often the increased potassium is beneficial when the patient is on diuretic therapy. The use of herbs often makes the food more appetizing.

Fluid restriction is less commonly instituted than in the past as long as the person is on a sodium-controlled diet and is receiving diuretics or digitalis. If fluids are restricted, the amount of fluid permitted is prescribed by the physician and a plan is made, in conjunction with the patient if possible, to space the fluids over the day.

Assisting with comfort and ADL

A careful assessment must be made each day to determine the extent to which the person can perform ADL such as eating and bathing. Most patients prefer to maximize their independence, and this is encouraged within the limitations of their symptoms.

Edematous skin is poorly nourished and very susceptible to breakdown. Edema of the sacrum is prevalent in patients with heart failure who are restricted to bed rest, and decubiti can develop quickly. Measures to prevent skin breakdown are instituted early.

Counseling and teaching

Since anxiety increases the symptoms of heart failure, measures are taken to help the person decrease anxiety. These measures include the following:
1. Identifying the feelings and the content related to these feelings
2. Identifying strengths that can be used for coping
3. Learning what can be done to decrease the anxiety, (for example, learning about measures to control heart failure and measures to reduce stress (see Chapters 8 and 9).

Working with family members in the same manner is also helpful to decrease their anxiety so they can be of greater support to the patient.

Patients who will be receiving oxygen therapy at home need to know how to manage the therapy. Instructions should include the following:
1. Indication for initiating oxygen therapy
2. How to initiate oxygen therapy
3. Mechanism for reordering oxygen supply
4. Precautions necessary when oxygen therapy is being used[28]

Teaching patients about their dietary restrictions, need for rest, and dietary regimen needs to be started early in the patient's hospitalization to permit time for learning and asking questions. The patient may need frequent interactions with the dietitian and nurse before being able to follow a prescribed sodium diet.

EVALUATION

Evaluation will be based on the expected patient outcomes. Questions to ask may include the following:
1. Is patient breathing easier?
2. Is patient comfortable?
3. Does the patient know how to monitor activity to prevent fatigue?
4. Is the patient free of skin breakdown.
5. Can the patient describe dietary restrictions?
6. Can the patient describe the medication regimen?

Pulmonary edema

Acute pulmonary edema is the rapid effusion of serous fluid from plasma into the pulmonary interstitial tissue and alveoli. It is a medical emergency that requires immediate care. The causes of pulmonary edema include the following:
1. Severe left ventricular failure
2. Inhalation of irritating gases
3. Rapid administration of intravenous fluids (whole blood, plasma, crystalloid fluids)
4. Barbiturate or opiate overdose

The signs and symptoms of pulmonary edema are listed in box below.

MEDICAL THERAPY

1. High Fowler's position
2. Morphine sulfate, 10 to 15 mg intravenously (decreases anxiety, slows respirations, reduces venous return
3. Oxygen at 40% to 70% by face mask
4. Intubation may be necessary for a short period to deliver adequate tidal volume and oxygen concentration and to remove secretions
5. Aminophylline may be given IV to dilate bronchi, increase urinary output, and increase CO
6. Treatment for congestive heart failure may be instituted (rapid digitalization, diuretic therapy with furosemide)

Signs and symptoms of pulmonary edema

Restlessness
Vague uneasiness
Dyspnea
Tachycardia
Pallor or cyanosis
Cough productive of large quantities of blood-tinged frothy sputum
Audible wheezing

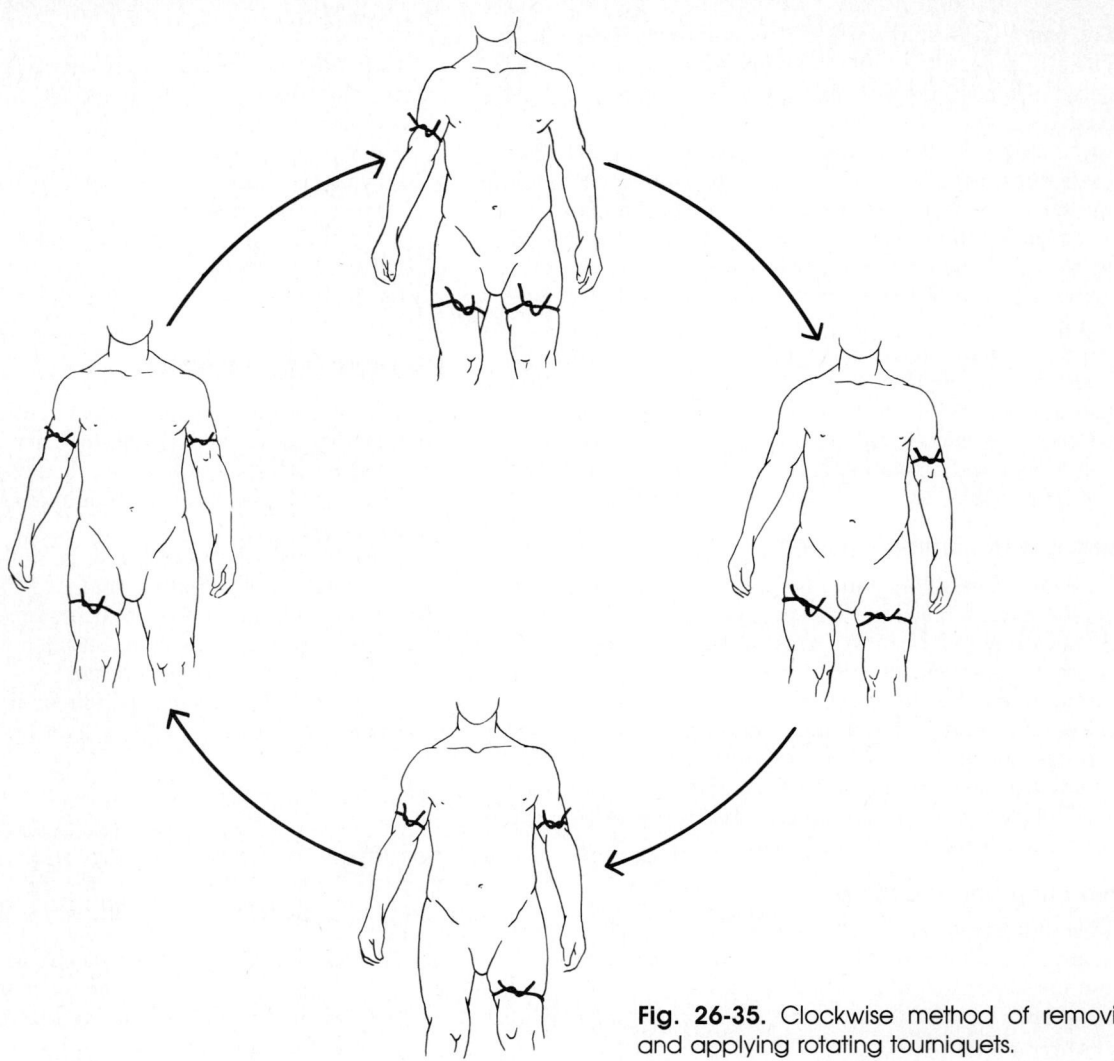

Fig. 26-35. Clockwise method of removing and applying rotating tourniquets.

7. Monitoring of serum potassium level (potassium loss through large diuresis)

Two more radical treatments that may be used when the preceding regimens fail include phlebotomy and rotating tourniquets. The purpose of phlebotomy is to decrease the amount of circulating blood to decrease pulmonary engorgement; however, this removes hemoglobin that may further contribute to hypoxemia.

The purpose of rotating tourniquets is to pool blood in the extremities, thus reducing cardiac overload. As much as 1 L of blood may be trapped in the extremities when tourniquets are used. The tourniquets are placed on three extremities at one time (Fig. 26-35). Every 15 minutes, in clockwise or counter-clockwise motion, one tourniquet is removed and another reapplied. Thus each extremity is occluded for 45 minutes. A rotating tourniquet machine uses blood pressure cuffs as tourniquets and automatically pumps and deflates the cuffs to obtain the desired effect. Since the purpose of this therapy is to occlude venous blood, the tourniquets should not obliterate arterial pulses in the extremity. If an extremity does not return readily to normal color on release of a tourniquet, the physician is informed. When the procedure is terminated, the tourniquets are released, one every 15 minutes to prevent a sudden increase in venous return and recurrence of pulmonary edema.

INFLAMMATORY HEART DISORDERS
PATHOPHYSIOLOGY

Inflammation has been defined as a complex of sequential changes in tissues in response to injury.[41] Bacterial invasion, trauma, chemicals, radiation, or heat can all initiate the inflammatory response (see Chapter 6).

The many tissues of the heart are susceptible to inflammation. Local changes in the affected tissues will produce signs and symptoms as the process of inflammation progresses. Humoral substances released by damaged tissues will leak into surrounding fluids, causing edema.

Table 26-8. Inflammatory heart disorders

Disorder	Etiology	Signs and symptoms	Medical therapy
Pericarditis	Infection (virus, bacteria), complication of systemic disease, trauma, neoplasm	*Acute:* Severe precordial chest pain referred to neck, shoulder, left arm; intensified when lying supine, coughing or breathing deeply or swallowing Pericardial friction rub Fever, leukocytosis, ECG changes Cardiac tamponade *Chronic:* Dyspnea, fatigue, congestive heart failure	*Acute:* Treatment of underlying condition Supportive care: salicylates, indomethacin, corticosteroids Pericardiocentesis for injection of antibiotic or sclerosing agent Pericardial fenestration *Chronic:* Digitalization, diuretics Low-sodium diet Pericardiectomy for severe cases
Myocarditis	Infection, drugs, chemicals, radiation, metabolic disorders	May be asymptomatic Nonspecific complaints of dyspnea on exertion, palpitations, precordial chest pain, fever, tachycardia	Antibiotics Corticosteroids for severe cases Antiarrhythmic drugs for arrhythmias
Endocarditis	*Streptococcus viridans,* staphylococci, enterococci; associated with rheumatic valvular disease and intrusive procedures, drug addition	Gradual onset: malaise, achiness, fever Splenomegaly, clubbing of fingers, Osler's nodes on fingers, petechiae in conjunctiva and mouth, cardiac murmur, anemia	Bed rest Antibiotics (IV) Prolonged antibiotic therapy Incision and drainage of abscesses Valve replacement
Rheumatic fever	Unknown; seen in conjunction with group A beta-hemolytic streptococcal pharyngeal infections	Symptoms follow pharangeal infection in 1 to 4 weeks Joint pain—recurrent Heart murmur, friction rub, cardiac arrhythmias, congestive heart failure	Antibiotics Antiinflammatory drugs (salicylates, corticosteroids) Early ambulation
Cardiovascular syphilis	Result of early syphilitic infection	Signs of aortic aneurysms, aortitis, aortic valve insufficiency, congestive heart failure	Penicillin Surgery for aneurysm or aortic valve insufficiency, if feasible Treatment of congestive heart failure, if develops
Alcoholic cardiomyopathy	Chronic alcoholism	Gradual onset: fatigue, dyspnea on exertion Pulmonary rales, cardiac murmur, edema, hypertension, increased central venous pressure, congestive heart failure, thromboemboli	Symptomatic Treatment of congestive heart failure Vasodilators and prolonged bed rest to decrease size of enlarged heart

In the heart, this process can rapidly progress to heart failure and result in systemic problems. Inflammation may occur in the pericardium (pericarditis), myocardium (myocarditis, cardiomyopathy), or endocardium (endocarditis, rheumatic heart disease, cardiovascular syphilis) (Table 26-8).

Pericarditis

Pericarditis is an inflammatory process of the visceral or parietal pericardium. It may result from various factors.

Pericarditis may be acute or chronic and may spread from or to the myocardium. *Acute pericarditis* is further classified as fibrinous or exudative. The exudate accompanying acute pericarditis may be serous, purulent, or hemorrhagic. When fluid accumulates in the pericardial sac, *cardiac tamponade* (compression of heart from blood or fluid) may occur with impairment of ventricular filling and emptying. If not diagnosed and treated promptly, the severe reduction in CO can result in shock and death.

Chronic pericarditis is referred to as chronic constrictive or adhesive pericarditis. It is three times more prevalent in men than women. It may result from fibrosing of the pericardial sac secondary to trauma or neoplastic disease. In the majority of cases, no specific pathogen can be identified as the causative agent. Chronic pericarditis is often associated with other disease processes. If the pericardium becomes a constrictive band surrounding the heart, it will prevent adequate filling and emptying of the ventricles, thus decreasing CO and ultimately producing cardiac failure.

Myocarditis

Myocarditis is an inflammatory disease of the myocardium. It may be classified as acute or chronic and can be either focal or diffuse in nature. Frequently, the inflammatory process develops secondary to acute endocarditis or pericarditis.

Infection may result in different ways:
1. Invasion by organisms of the myocardial tissue
2. Production of toxins (diphtheria)
3. Autoimmune reaction (rheumatic fever, systemic lupus erythematosus)

Worldwide, the more frequent infectious agents are rickettsiae, bacteria, protozoans, and metazoans. In North America, viral causes predominate, including Coxsackievirus, echovirus, and viral encephalitis, rabies, and herpes simplex.

Endocarditis

Endocarditis is an infection of the endocardium and most often of the heart valves. The more recent method of classification of infective endocarditis is on the basis of the causative organism, for example, enterococcal endocarditis or streptococcal endocarditis. It may occur in acute or subacute forms. Acute endocarditis occurs rapidly, often on normal heart valves, and if untreated may cause death within days or weeks. The subacute form

---

Causes of pericarditis

Infection: viral, bacterial, fungal
Complications of systemic disease
    Rheumatoid arthritis
    Systemic lupus erythematosus
    Scleroderma
    Uremia
Trauma
    Closed chest trauma (for example, automobile accident)
    Myocardial infarction
Neoplasm: neoplastic infiltration, myxoma

Symptoms of cardiac tamponade

Diminished or absent point of maximal impulse (PMI)
Diminished peripheral pulses
Distended neck veins (secondary to increased CVP)
Decreased blood pressure (secondary to ineffective pumping action)
Narrowing pulse pressure (difference between systolic and diastolic blood pressure)
Paradoxical pulse (decrease in pulse strength during inspiration)
Diminished heart sounds

Disorders associated with chronic pericarditis

Rheumatic heart disease
Congenital heart disease
Hypertensive heart disease
Systemic lupus erythematosus
Rheumatoid arthritis
Scleroderma
Myxedema
Renal failure

develops more gradually, usually on previously damaged heart valves, and responds well to treatment.

The infecting organisms are carried by a turbulent blood flow and deposited on the heart valves or elsewhere on the endocardium. The turbulent blood flow occurs in areas of myocardial anomalies, such as prolapsed mitral valves or ventricular septal defects. The organisms bombard the heart valves, become embedded in the valve matrix, and result in vegetative growths that may scar and perforate the leaflets. Further risk results if the vegetative growths break free of the valves, enter the bloodstream, and cause emboli. If the vegetative emboli enter organs such as the spleen or kidney, abscesses may form.

Rheumatic heart disease

Rheumatic fever is an acute inflammatory reaction. It is important in the discussion of inflammatory heart disease, as it has tremendous potential for causing chronic heart problems. In the United States today approximately 1,750,000 adults and 100,000 children have rheumatic heart disease.[1] Symptoms of cardiac involvement usually follow a group A beta-hemolytic streptococcus pharyngeal infection. Ninety percent of the victims are between the age of 5 and 15.

Rheumatic fever may progress with mild symptoms and go undiagnosed, or the disease may be subclinical with no symptoms. The patient develops cardiac manifestations years later. On careful history taking, a recollection of a childhood illness confirming the likelihood of rheumatic fever is usually found.

The pathophysiology of rheumatic heart disease remains unclear. The pericardium, myocardium, or endocardium can be involved. The affected tissue develops small areas of necrosis (Aschoff bodies), which heal, leaving scar tissue. Myocardial changes are usually reversible. In the pericardium and endocardium, however, the disease process is usually not reversible and produces the disabling effects of rheumatic heart disease. The valves are typically most affected and become fibrous and incompetent. The leaflets of a valve may fuse during the healing phase.

Cardiovascular syphilis

Cardiovascular syphilis usually occurs from 10 to 30 years after the primary syphilitic infection. Since the highest incidence of primary syphilis is among persons in their early twenties, persons with symptoms of cardiovascular syphilis are usually over 30 years of age.

Cardiovascular syphilis is an extremely dangerous complication of primary syphilis. The spirochetes attack the aorta, the aortic valve, and the myocardium. The ascending aorta is often affected. The wall of the aorta becomes weakened and an aneurysm (p. 686) develops. As the aneurysm grows, it may press on neighboring structures, such as the intercostal nerves, resulting in chest pain. An aneurysm may be present without symptoms. It may rupture as it increases in size. Because of this, the patient is encouraged to avoid strenuous activities that might cause a sudden increase in blood pressure.

Spirochetes may also attack the aorta more diffusely, causing *aortitis*. The aorta becomes dilated, and calcium plaques are laid down. The junction of the aorta with the coronary arteries becomes constricted, resulting in angina (p. 652). Thrombi may also develop in the aorta, leading to the development of emboli and resulting in myocardial infarction or cerebral emboli.

Spirochetes may also attack the aortic valve, resulting in scarring. Aortic insufficiency may develop. This is often complicated by heart failure.

Alcoholic cardiomyopathy

When any form of ethanol (the chief substance in alcoholic beverages) is consumed in large quantities over a period greater than 5 years, it has a direct toxic effect on cardiac tissue. Additives in alcoholic beverages may also create their own toxic effects. Persons with alcoholic cardiomyopathy are usually well-nourished individuals; only 15% of these patients have thiamin deficiency as is seen in many alcoholics.

Alcohol cannot function as an adequate source of calories. The oxidation rate of alcohol cannot be accelerated to meet demands for increases in energy. In chronic alcoholism, these metabolic disturbances result in visceral fatty degeneration of heart tissue. In the early stages, the disease process may be totally reversed by abstinence from alcohol.

ASSESSMENT

Subjective data

1. Presence, duration and extent of symptoms: malaise, achiness, lassitude, chills and fever, chest pain, anorexia
2. Energy levels, rest/sleep patterns
3. Weight loss
4. Knowledge of preventive measures, if appropriate (infective endocarditis, rheumatic fever, alcoholic cardiomyopathy)
5. Possible causative agent (drugs, recent infections)

Objective data

Objective data should include an assessment for heart failure (p. 667). Both fluid status and cardiac status are assessed.

1. Fluid status
   a. Peripheral edema, distended neck veins
   b. Auscultation of breath sounds
   c. Skin turgor
   d. Daily weights
2. Cardiac status
   a. Heart sounds: presence of murmurs, friction rubs
   b. Pulse rate, rhythm, presence of paradoxical pulse (decreased intensity during inspiration) seen with pericarditis

Diagnostic tests

The most frequently used diagnostic tests include the following:

1. Chest x-ray film
2. ECG
3. Echocardiogram (p. 682)
4. Cardiac catheterization with angiographic studies (p. 684)
5. Cardiac biopsy may be required for a definitive diagnosis

Pericardiocentesis

When fluid collects in the pericardial sac, the physician may perform a pericardiocentesis (surgical puncture of the pericardial cavity for aspiration of fluid). Laboratory analysis and culture and antibiotic sensitivity will be performed on the aspirated fluid to determine the causative agent. A pericardiocentesis may also be performed as a treatment modality when there is a large amount of pericardial fluid. Occasionally, after removal of the fluid, the physician may instill antibiotics directly into the pericardial sac.

DATA ANALYSIS AND PLANNING

Nursing diagnoses

Possible nursing diagnoses for the patient with inflammatory heart disease include the following, depending on extent of inflammation and presence of congestive heart failure:

Breathing pattern, ineffective
Cardiac ouptut, alteration in: decreased
Comfort, alteration in: pain
Coping, ineffective individual
Fluid volume, alteration in: excess
Activity intolerance
Gas exchange, impaired
Knowledge deficit
Nutrition, alterations in: less than body requirements
Tissue perfusion, alteration in: cerebral, cardiopulmonary, renal, gastrointestinal, peripheral

Expected patient outcomes

1. Patient states he/she is feeling more comfortable.
2. Patient breathes with relative ease.
3. Patient can:
   a. Describe the rationale for the degree of rest and activity prescribed and plan activities within the established prescription.
   b. Demonstrate ways to carry out ADL to conserve energy.
   c. Plan a diet to include adequate nutrients and fluids and avoidance of sodium, if so prescribed.
   d. Describe the medication program.
   e. Describe activities that require prophylactic antibiotics.
   f. State plans for regular medical follow up.

IMPLEMENTATION

Assisting with achievement of therapeutic goals

1. Reinforce importance of bed rest during acute phase
2. Provide diversional activities for patient particularly, when on bed rest and during extended hospitalizations
3. Assist in maintaining adequate nutritional intake while observing prescribed dietary restrictions (fluids or salt may be restricted)
4. Monitor for signs of fluid overload and electrolyte imbalance
5. Medicate patient as prescribed
   a. Careful and timely administration of antibiotics
   b. Assessment of heart rate before administering digitalis preparations
   c. Documentation of rate and rhythm of patient's pulse, particularly if patient is receiving antiarrhythmic medications

Assisting with comfort and ADL

The patient on bed rest will require assistance with ADL. The patient is encouraged to be as independent as possible but should not be allowed to overdo. Rest periods need to be spaced with activities. As the patient begins to progress and can tolerate being out of bed, particular care is taken to assist the patient with ADL while at the same time continuing to encourage independence.

The patient with congestive heart failure will frequently experience peripheral edema. As edema increases, the patient becomes increasingly uncomfortable. Careful positioning and frequent changes in position may increase comfort while also protecting the skin from breakdown.

Pain management can be a significant problem in the patient with inflammatory heart disease. Pain severity and characteristics are assessed and pain medications given as indicated. It is important to document pain characteristics and responses to pain medications. A change in the character of the pain could indicate complications, such as myocardial infarction or cardiac tamponade (with pericarditis).

Teaching

The patient with infective endocarditis needs to learn methods of prevention. Good oral hygiene is imperative, and all intrusive approaches, such as catheterization, are avoided if possible. Prophylactic antibiotic therapy should be taken before any intrusive procedures, such as dental procedures, genitourinary or gastrointestinal procedures, or surgeries are performed.

Persons with a history of rheumatic fever are often given prophylactic penicillin until about age 25. Adults who experience rheumatic fever are given prophylactic penicillin for about 5 years after an attack. Persons need to know the importance of receiving the antibiotic for the prescribed time period even when they are feeling well.

Teaching the patient with an inflammatory heart disorder includes the following:

1. Need for continued antibiotic therapy after symptoms subside
2. Need to monitor for signs of congestive heart failure
   a. Daily weight for sudden increase
   b. Pedal edema
   c. Changes in respiratory status
3. Rationale and side effects of prescribed medications
4. Rationale for any dietary restrictions
5. Need for ongoing medical care

EVALUATION

The evaluation is based on the expected patient outcomes. Questions to ask may include the following:
1. Is the patient free of pain?
2. Is the patient breathing with ease?
3. Does the patient know the rationale for prescribed therapies and medication regimen?
4. Does the patient have a plan for rest periods if fatigue is a problem?
5. Has the patient made plans for follow-up care?

VALVULAR HEART DISEASE

PATHOPHYSIOLOGY

Valvular heart disease is a general term that refers to any one of a variety of conditions that affect the valves within the heart. Normal valves function to maintain a unidirectional flow of blood through the cardiac chambers by passively opening and closing in response to variant pressure gradients. The mitral and tricupsid valves (atrioventricular valves) prevent the backflow of blood from the ventricles into the atria during systole. Movement of these atrioventricular valves is facilitated by the chordae tendinae and papillary muscles (Fig. 26-1). Similarly, the aortic and pulmonic valves (semilunar valves) prevent the backflow of blood from the aorta and pulmonary artery into their respective ventricles during diastole.

The two basic problems that compromise the normal function of the valves are stenosis and insufficiency. *Stenosis* is a thickening of the valvular tissue, which causes a narrowing of the valvular orifice. *Insufficiency* refers to the inability of the valve to close completely. An insufficient or incompetent valve allows blood to flow in a retrograde or regurgitant manner.

The predominant etiological factor in the development of a stenosed or insufficient valve is rheumatic fever. Throughout the course of this disease, large hemorrhagic and fibrinous lesions vegetate along the inflamed edges of the valves.[41] These lesions frequently develop on adjacent valve leaflets so that the edges adhere together. As the disease process progresses, the leaflets become so scarred there is permanent leaflet fusion and limited valvular movement of the normally free-flapping edges.

Since these underlying pathologic changes occur over a period of time, the clinical signs and symptoms of a stenosed or insufficient valve do not usually manifest until 10 to 40 years after the onset of rheumatic fever. Furthermore, the extent of valvular damage is largely dependent upon its normal degree of motion. Since the pressures and consequent valvular movement on the left side of the heart are greater than those on the right, the mitral and aortic valves are more susceptible. The tricupsid and pulmonic valves are much less frequently affected by rheumatic fever.

The etiology, signs and symptoms, and medical therapy of valvular heart disorders are outlined in Table 26-9 for each type of disorder. Additional information about specific valvular disorders is provided in the sections that follow.

Mitral stenosis

Mitral stenosis is more often found in women than men. As rheumatic fever is the primary factor in its development, the progressive destruction of the valve occurs over a 20-year period. Mitral commissures (junctions between adjacent cusps) fuse and the valvular leaflets or cusps thicken and calcify. The chordae tendinae also become short and thick. These underlying changes result in a narrowed mitral valve that impedes the normal flow of blood.

To accommodate the increased work load required to move blood through this narrowed orifice, the left atrium hypertrophies. The resultant left atrial pressure exerts further pressure onto the pulmonary vasculature, causing pulmonary hypertension and pulmonary congestion. Eventually these conditions result in right ventricular failure and right-sided heart failure.

Another common complication of mitral stenosis is atrial fibrillation. Structural changes in the atrial wall from the increased pressure predispose to this arrhythmia. The coupling of atrial fibrillation and pooling of blood in the atria increases the likelihood of thrombus formation and arterial embolization.

Mitral insufficiency

In contrast to mitral stenosis, mitral insufficiency is more commonly seen in men than women. Although the same pathological processes occur as a result of rheumatic fever, several other acquired and congenital conditions can contribute to its development. The end result is that the mitral valve leaflets fail to close fully. Consequently, a variable amount of blood leaks back through the valve from the left ventricle into the atrium.

The left atrium dilates and hypertrophies to compensate for the increased atrial pressure. The left ventricle also hypertrophies to respond to the increased preload that results from the blood passing through the incompetent valve during diastole. In time, ventricular function becomes so compromised that there is a decrease in CO.

Aortic stenosis

Aortic stenosis constitutes 25% of all valvular heart diseases. Diseases of the aortic valve do not usually occur as a single entity; most often there is involvement of the

Table 26-9. Valvular heart disorders

	Etiology	Signs and symptoms	Medical therapy
Mitral insufficiency	Rheumatic fever Papillary muscle dysfunction (for example, myocardial infarction, ventricular aneurysm) Ruptured chordae tendinae Floppy valve syndrome: prolapsed mitral valve Bacterial endocarditis Congenital abnormalities	Excessive fatigue, weakness, exhaustion Weight loss Exertional dyspnea, orthopnea, paroxysmal nocturnal dyspnea, rales Late stages: pulmonary edema, right-sided heart failure *Auscultation:* Palpable thrill at apex S_1 absent, soft, or buried in murmur Murmur: high pitched, blowing, swishing, throughout systole (at apex) S_3, low pitched	Activity limitations Sodium-restricted diet Diuretics Digoxin Treatment of atrial arrhythmias Surgery: valvuloplasty, valvular replacement, annuloplasty
Mitral stenosis	Rheumatic fever May be associated with congenital anomalies "Parachute" mitral valve	Excessive fatigue, weakness Dyspnea, exertional dyspnea, orthopnea, paroxysmal nocturnal dyspnea Dry cough, bronchitis, rales Pulmonary edema Recurrent pulmonary emboli Hemoptysis Right-sided heart failure *Auscultation:* Palpable thrill at apex S_1 snapping, increased, loud Murmur: soft, low pitched, rumbling, diastolic (at apex)	Sodium-restricted diet Diuretics Activity limitations Oxygen therapy Anticoagulant therapy Surgery: valvulotomy, valve replacement
Aortic insufficiency	Rheumatic fever Severe hypertension Bacterial endocarditis Syphilis Dissecting aortic aneurysm Traumatic valve rupture Marfan's syndrome Congenital anomalies	Palpitations, sinus tachycardia Exertional dyspnea, orthopnea, paroxysmal nocturnal dyspnea Excessive diaphoresis Angina Late stages: left and right sided heart failure *Auscultation:* Murmur: high pitched, blowing, diastolic (third intercostal space) Systolic ejection murmur at base	Digoxin Sodium-restricted diet Diuretics Nitroglycerin (angina) Penicillin therapy (if syphilis a cause) Surgery: valve replacement, valvuloplasty

Table 26-9. Valvular heart disorders—cont'd

	Etiology	Signs and symptoms	Medical therapy

Aortic stenosis	Congenital anomalies
	Acquired:
	  Rheumatic fever
	  Arteriosclerosis
	  Idiopathic hyper-
	  tropic subaortic
	  stenosis
	  Calcification of
	  leaflets
		Angina
		Syncope
		Fatigue, weakness
		Exertional dyspnea, orthopnea, paroxysmal nocturnal dyspnea
		Pulmonary edema, rales
		Late stages: right-sided heart failure
		Auscultation:
		Murmur: low pitched, rough, rasping, systolic (at base or carotids)
		Systolic thrill at base of heart
			Activity limitations
			Sodium-restricted diet
			Diuretics
			Digoxin
			Nitroglycerin (angina)
			Surgery: valve replacement

Tricuspid stenosis	Rheumatic fever Carcinoid heart disease Fibroelastosis Endomyocardial fibrosis	Pulmonary congestion, dyspnea Right-sided heart failure Decreased CO: weakness, fatigue, weight loss, hypotension Late stages: cirrhosis, jaundice, malnutrition	Sodium-restricted diet Digoxin Diuretics Surgery: valvuloplasty, valve replacement
Tricuspid insufficiency	Rheumatic fever Bacterial endocarditis Trauma Carcinoid heart disease Endomyocardial fibrosis Infarction of right ventricular papillary muscle Congenital anomalies	Right-sided heart failure Decreased CO: weakness, fatigue, weight loss, hypotension *Auscultation:* Murmur: blowing, throughout systole (left sternal border, increases with inspiration)	Sodium-restricted diet Digoxin Diuretics Surgery: narrowing of annulus, valve replacement

mitral valve. Aortic stenosis develops as a congenital or acquired condition. Clinical symptoms of aortic stenosis are not manifested until the valve is one third its normal size, which is some 10 to 30 years beyond the inception of the disease process. The asymptomatic nature of this disease is largely caused by the tremendous compensatory abilities of the left ventricle.

With an increase in ventricular volume, a greater pressure is needed to eject blood through the narrowed aortic orifice during systole. This added pressure produces ventricular hypertrophy with a concomitant increase in myocardial oxygen demand. The oxygen demand exceeds the supply because of inadequate coronary artery perfusion. These underlying changes give rise to the classic symptom of angina.

The progressive stenosis accompanied by ventricular hypertrophy in the presence of mitral valve disease causes a decrease in CO. Symptoms of pulmonary congestion and eventually right-sided heart failure ensue.

Aortic insufficiency

Rheumatic fever accounts for approximately 80% of all cases of aortic insufficiency. In this instance the valve fails to close completely and this results in a retrograde blood flow from the aorta into the left ventricle during diastole. The ventricle hypertrophies to hold all the regurgitant blood. Over time, the left ventricle cannot withstand the added work load, leading to the development of decreased CO, left ventricular failure, and right-sided heart failure.

Tricuspid stenosis

Tricuspid stenosis is a relatively uncommon valvular lesion that usually coexists with stenosis of the mitral or aortic valves. The major cause of this disease is rheumatic fever. The leaflets become thick and fuse together, and the chordae tendinae also become short and thick. Hence during diastole there is a reduction in blood flow through the compromised valve. This blockage further causes a backflow of blood in the systemic circulation. Engorgement of the superior and inferior vena cava precede the development of right-sided heart failure.

Tricuspid insufficiency

Tricuspid insufficiency is a very rare disorder that is more prevalent in children than adults. The disease usually develops secondary to marked dilation of the right ventricle and the tricuspid valve ring.[47] The valve itself widens and the leaflets are unable to close properly. Therefore there is regurgitant blood flow to the right atrium during systole. The right atrium hypertrophies to accommodate the increased volume, but invariably the CO decreases with the concomitant decreased blood flow to the left side of the heart. Eventually the excess volume in the atrium causes right-sided heart failure.

Pulmonic valve disease

Lesions of the pulmonic valve are extremely rare in adults. This valve is less likely to be affected by rheumatic fever and bacterial endocarditis. For a more detailed discussion of congenital pulmonic stenosis, refer to a standard pediatric text.

ASSESSMENT

Assessment data that the nurse obtains are essentially the same for any patient with valvular heart disease. Many of the symptoms are related to decreased CO.

Subjective data

1. Fatigue and weakness: extent, ability to carry out ADL
   These symptoms result from inadequate CO with subsequent impairment in cellular oxygenation
2. Shortness of breath: occurrence, type
   The patient may have dyspnea on exertion (DOE), orthopnea, or paroxysmal nocturnal dyspnea (p. 666) depending on the degree of heart failure
3. Pain in chest (angina): occurrence, measures used to relieve pain
4. Palpitations: occurrence
   Palpitations are a sensation in the chest described as a bounding or pounding of the heart
5. Syncope: occurrence
   A patient may verbalize feelings of light-headedness, dizzy spells, or fainting; these symptoms can be associated with a decrease in CO
6. Peripheral edema: site, extent, time of day
   Swelling of legs during the day with decreased swelling at night when legs are elevated is usually reported

Objective data

1. History of rheumatic fever
2. Observation/inspection
   a. Position and comfort level of patient
   b. Character and rate of breathing
   c. Use of supplemental oxygen
   d. Skin color and temperature
   e. Nailbed color and blanching (capillary filling)
   f. Diaphoresis
3. Auscultation
   a. Cardiac rate and rhythm
   b. Presence or change in heart sounds (murmurs, S_3, S_4, friction rub)
   c. Character of heart sounds at all auscultatory sites (aortic, pulmonic, tricuspid, mitral)
   d. Presence of adventitious breath sounds (rales, rhonchi)
   e. Difference between right and left lung fields
4. Palpation
   a. Warmth of extremities
   b. Equality and symmetry of pulses
   c. Presence of edema
   d. Signs of phlebitis (increased calf diameter, positive Homans' sign)
5. Change in body weight
6. Adherence to diet and medications

Diagnostic tests

There are four major diagnostic tests used to determine the presence of valvular heart disease: chest radiograph, ECG, echocardiogram, and cardiac catheterization. Table 26-10 summarizes the findings that are indicative of each specific type of valvular disease.

Chest radiograph

A chest radiograph demonstrates the overall size and configuration of the heart and its chambers. Calcification in the pericardium, myocardium, valves, or large blood vessels is also evident on the film. Most cardiac abnormalities are detected with a standard anterior-posterior and lateral view of the chest.

Electrocardiogram

An ECG (p. 632) is helpful in the diagnosis of valvular heart disease. Hypertrophy of either chamber as well as specific arrhythmias can be detected.

Echocardiography

Echocardiography is most useful in the detection of abnormalities in the mitral and aortic valves. It is some benefit in the diagnosis of tricuspid valve disease.

Echocardiography is a noninvasive technique that uses ultrasound to assess both the structures and motions within the heart. A small transducer is placed on the patient's anterior left chest and moved in various directions to visualize specific cardiac areas. This small transducer functions as a transmitter and receiver. It transmits high-frequency sound waves to the heart and then receives back the reflected or echoed ultrasonic beams from the patient's heart. The ultrasonic beam is converted into electrical energy so that lines and spaces are displayed on the oscilloscope. These lines and spaces represent bone, cardiac chambers, valves, the septum, and muscle. A representative copy of the echocardiogram is obtained on paper to become a permanent record of the findings.

Since echocardiography is a noninvasive procedure, it

Table 26-10. Findings in valvular heart disorders

Disorder	Chest radiograph	ECG	Echocardiogram	Cardiac catheterization
Mitral stenosis	Left atrial enlargement Mitral valve calcification Right ventricular enlargement Prominence of pulmonary artery	Left atrial hypertrophy Right ventricular hypertrophy Atrial fibrillation	Thickened mitral valve Left atrial enlargement	Increased pressure gradient across valve Increased left atrial pressure Increased PCWP Increased right heart pressures Decreased CO
Mitral insufficiency	Left atrial enlargement Left ventricular enlargement	Left atrial hypertrophy Left ventricular hypertrophy Atrial fibrillation Sinus tachycardia	Abnormal mitral valve movement Left atrial enlargement	Mitral regurgitation Increased atrial pressure Increased LVEDP* Increased PCWP Decreased cardiac output
Aortic stenosis	Left ventricular enlargement Aortic valve calcification May have enlargement of left atrium, pulmonary artery, right ventricle, right atrium	Left ventricular hypertrophy	Thickened aortic valve Thickened ventricular wall Abnormal movement of aortic leaflets	Increased pressure gradient across valve Increased LVEDP*
Aortic insufficiency	Left ventricular enlargement	Left ventricular hypertrophy Tall R waves Sinus tachycardia	Left ventricular enlargement Abnormal mitral valve movement Increased movement of ventricular wall	Aortic regurgitation Increased LVEDP* Decreased arterial diastolic pressure
Tricuspid stenosis	Right atrial enlargement Prominence of superior vena cava	Right atrial hypertrophy Tall peaked P waves Atrial fibrillation	Abnormal valvular leaflets Right atrial enlargement	Increased pressure gradient across valve Increased right atrial pressure Decreased CO
Tricuspid insufficiency	Right atrial enlargement Right ventricular enlargement	Right ventricular hypertrophy Atrial fibrillation	Prolapse of tricuspid valve Right atrial enlargement	Increased atrial pressure Tricuspid regurgitation Decreased CO

*Left ventricular end-diastolic pressure.

Cardiac catheterization

Right side	Left side
Purpose	
Confirm suspected valvular heart disease—congenital or acquired	Evaluate pressures on left side of heart
	Assess competency of valves
	Assess left ventricular function
Procedure	
Cutdown made in large vein in patient's arm	Cutdown made in large artery in patient's arm or groin
Catheter threaded via fluoroscopy through superior vena cava, right atrium, right ventricle, pulmonary artery and pulmonary capillaries	Catheter threaded via fluoroscopy through aorta, aortic arch, descending aorta, aortic valve, and left ventricle
Blood sample obtained to determine oxygen content and saturation	Blood sample obtained to determine oxygen content and saturation
Pressures recorded for each chamber/vessel	Pressures recorded for each chamber/vessel
	Pressure gradient measurement across valves obtained

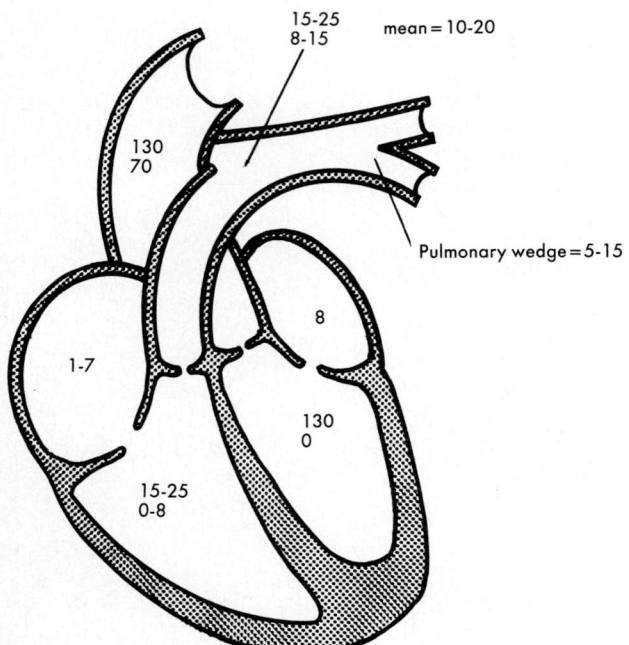

15-25
8-15

mean = 10-20

130
70

Pulmonary wedge = 5-15

8

1-7

130
0

15-25
0-8

Fig. 26-36. Pressure readings in mm Hg in chambers of heart and major blood vessels.

is safer than cardiac catheterization. Hence, whenever possible, it precedes the cardiac catheterization. There is no special preparation required for the test. The patient can eat and take medications as usual. Most importantly, the patient should be told about the purpose and procedure of this test. The patient must be aware of the importance of lying still for approximately 30 to 60 minutes. After the test the patient may resume normal activities, since there are no adverse effects from this test.

Cardiac catheterization

Cardiac catheterization is an extremely valuable diagnostic procedure that provides information about the structure and function of the cardiac chambers, valves, and vessels. Since this is an invasive procedure, it is usually performed after several other diagnostic tests. A catheterization is performed on either the right or left side of the heart depending on the suspected valvular dysfunction. The purpose and procedure of each type are outlined in box above.

Normal pressure readings and oxygen concentrations for the chambers and great vessels are listed in Fig. 26-36. The right side of the heart is a low-pressure system with less oxygen saturation, since the blood there is going to the lungs. In contrast, the left side of the heart is a relatively high-pressure system with full oxygen saturation, as the blood there is returning from the lungs. Any changes in normal pressures and oxygen saturation are significant. Abnormalities in pressure gradients across valve are also indicative of valvular heart disease.

Types of valve repair

Valvuloplasty	Repair of valve, suturing of torn leaflets
Annuloplasty	Repair of ring or annulus of incompetent valve, tightening and suturing of annulus
Valvulotomy/commissurotomy	Repair of a leaflet or commissure, fibrous band, or ring

---

DATA ANALYSIS AND PLANNING

Nursing diagnoses

Potential nursing diagnoses for the patient with valvular heart disease include the following:

Activity intolerance
Cardiac output, alteration in
Knowledge deficit

Expected patient outcomes

The patient can do the following:

1. Explain required dietary changes including any sodium or fluid restrictions.
2. Describe any medication therapy.
3. Describe a work, rest, and activity program to conserve energy.
4. State the purpose and procedure for diagnostic tests.
5. Describe the rationale for and type of surgery to be performed, if surgery is indicated.
6. State plans for medical follow-up, including ongoing laboratory tests, if required.

IMPLEMENTATION

Assisting with achievement of therapeutic goals

1. Administration of medications, as prescribed (diuretics, digoxin, antiarrhythmics)
2. Continued monitoring
   a. Daily intake and output
   b. Daily weights
   c. Respiratory rate and rhythm
   d. Auscultation of breath sounds and heart sounds every 4 hours of every shift
   e. Condition of skin and mucous membranes
   f. Capillary perfusion
   g. Equality and strength of peripheral pulses
   h. Presence and extent of edema
   i. Blood pressure

Assisting with comfort and ADL

1. Identify those activities of daily living which are fatiguing and for which patient may need some assistance
2. Design with patient a plan that will allow for completion of daily activities
3. Incorporate rest periods between activities

4. Maintain use of supportive oxygen therapy during activities, as necessary

Teaching

1. Effect of a sodium-restricted or fluid-restricted diet on cardiac function, as appropriate
2. Effects of medications: diuretics, cardiac glycosides, anticoagulants
3. Prophlactic use of antibiotics before and after dental work
4. How to check for buildup of fluid in legs
5. Purpose and procedure for diagnostic tests (echocardiogram, cardiac catheterization)
6. Purpose and nature of surgical intervention, if appropriate

Surgery

Surgical intervention is indicated for a patient whose life-style is severely compromised by valvular heart disease. If a patient experiences hemodynamically debilitating symptoms that are unsuccessfully managed by conventional medical therapies, surgery is then the recommended treatment modality. There are two basic surgical procedures: repair of the valve problem or replacement of the valve.

Repair of valve

Several terms are used to describe the specific anatomical structure undergoing repair. Valvulotomy or commissurotomy can be done as a closed or open procedure. A closed approach involves the removal of a rib with a small incision into the left atrium. A dilator is then used to widen the narrowed valve and free the stenosed leaflet. The atrium is also palpated for thrombi. In the open technique, used also for valvuloplasty and annuloplasty, the thorax is incised and the heart completely exposed.

Replacement of valve

There are many types of valves that can be used for replacement. A valve is selected on the basis of location of the incompetent valve, the underlying pathologic changes, and the age of the patient. The size of the prosthetic valve is of major importance. Valves are grouped according to their design and function: caged-ball valves, tilting-disc valves, and biological valves (Fig. 26-37).

A   **B**   **C**

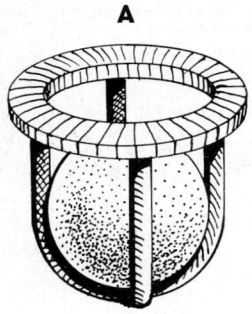
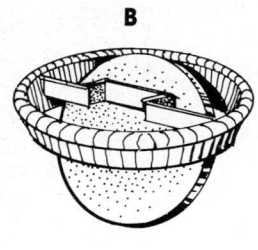
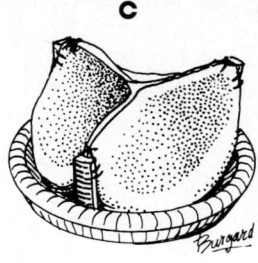

Fig. 26-37. Heart valve replacements. **A,** Caged-ball valve. **B,** Tilting-disc valve. **C,** Biological valve.

Specific nursing care for the patient with valvular surgery

Preoperative care
1. Discontinue administration of digoxin and diuretics at least 2 days before surgery (to avoid digitoxic arrhythmias precipitated by cardiopulmonary bypass)
2. Administer vitamin K preoperatively to return prothrombin time to normal
3. Give antibiotics as ordered to decrease incidence of postoperative endocarditis
4. Prepare patient for surgery, providing explanation of procedure.

Postoperative care
1. Administer anticoagulant therapy 5 to 7 days after valve replacement to prevent thrombus formation
2. Assess apical heartbeat: a "click" sound is usually heard; reassure patient that this sound is normal; assess for development of murmur
3. Explain medication regimen to patient
    a. Need for antibiotics for approximately 1 month following valve replacement
    b. Need for cardiac glycosides to improve cardiac function and control arrhythmias for prescribed time (usually 3 to 6 months after surgery)

Caged-ball valves are the most durable. Their use, however, is restricted to patients with a large enough annulus and chamber to accommodate the cage itself. It is never used for tricuspid valve replacement because of the limited capacity of the right ventricle.

Tilting-disc valves require less space than caged-ball valves. The valve tilts when open and returns to flat position when closed. Similar to the caged-ball valve, the tilting-disc valve has a great potential for clot formation around the valve.

Biological valves are derived from animal cardiac tissue or human cadaver donors. These valves carry less risk for thromboembolism; however, they tend to degenerate over time.

Preoperative and postoperative care

Nursing care for the patient undergoing valvular heart surgery is essentially the same as that for patients undergoing coronary bypass surgery (p. 661). Specific nursing care related to valvular surgery is listed in box above.

EVALUATION

Evaluation will be based on expected patient outcomes. Some questions to ask may include the following:
1. Can patient describe the nature of the valvular disorder?
2. Is patient able to describe a work, rest, and activity program to conserve energy?
3. Is patient able to explain any required dietary changes?
4. Can patient explain medication regimen?
5. Has patient made plans for continued medical follow-up?

ANEURYSMS
PATHOPHYSIOLOGY

An aneurysm is a local or diffuse dilation of an artery. It occurs secondary to a variety of disease processes, although arteriosclerosis is the predominant etiological factor (see Table 26-11). Regardless of the pathogenesis, the

Table 26-11. Aneurysms

Type	Etiology	Signs and symptoms	Medical therapy
Abdominal aortic	Arteriosclerosis Hypertension Cystic medial necrosis Trauma Syphilis Other infections	Pulsating mass in mid-upper abdomen Systolic bruit over aorta Pain in mid-upper abdomen or in lower back or groin Long-standing cramps in buttocks, thighs, calves	Antihypertensive medications Pain medications Inotropic agents (for example, propranolol [Inderal]) Surgery: resection of aneurysm with graft replacement
Thoracic aortic	Arteriosclerosis Infection Congenital disorders causing cystic medial necrosis Trauma Syphilis Hypertension	*Ascending aorta:* Chest pain: deep, diffuse, aching *Transverse aorta:* Dyspnea, cough, hoarseness *Dissecting aneurysm:* Tearing sensation in chest, pain radiating to neck, shoulders, lower back, abdomen	Antihypertensive medications Negative inotropic agents (for example, propranolol [Inderal]) Surgery: Resection of aneurysm with graft replacement Aortic valve replacement (if aortic insufficiency)

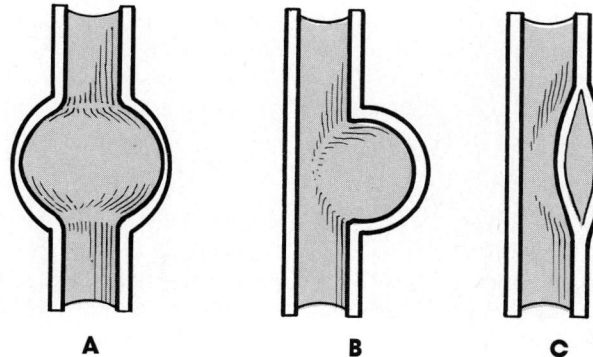

Fig. 26-38. Types of aneurysms. **A,** Fusiform. **B,** Saccular. **C,** Dissecting.

musculoelastic middle (media) layer of the artery becomes weakened, and it produces stretching of the inner (intima) and outer (adventitia) layers. Blood pressure within the vessel continues to weaken its walls and to enlarge the aneurysm.

The extent of arterial damage and clinical symptomatology vary greatly according to the type, size, and location of the aneurysm. An aneurysm is classified on the basis of its shape and subsequent damage to the affected artery (Fig. 26-38). The *fusiform aneurysm,* the most common type, assumes a spindle shape around the entire circumference of the vessel. In contrast, a *saccular aneurysm* affects only a part of the arterial circumference. This type of aneurysm appears as a unilateral sac or outpouching on the side of the artery. Also, a saccular aneurysm is more likely to rupture. A *dissecting aneurysm* develops from a split or tear in the intimal wall overlying a diseased media. This relatively uncommon occurrence leads to the accumulation of blood in a newly formed cavity between the vessel layers.

Although these types of aneurysms can develop in any artery, the major site for aneurysm formation is the aorta. Since the aorta has such a large diameter and is subject to great pressures, it is often the location for underlying disease processes. Aortic aneurysms are found in the thoracic segment and, more commonly, in the abdominal portions (Fig. 26-39). Since there is some difference between aneurysms in these locations, they are discussed as separate entities.

Thoracic aortic aneurysms

Aneurysms within the thoracic area can develop in the descending, ascending, or transverse section of the aorta. Hypertensive men between 50 and 70 years of age are typically subject to this disease.

Aneurysms in the *descending aorta* are usually fusiform and originate just distal to the left subclavian artery. A

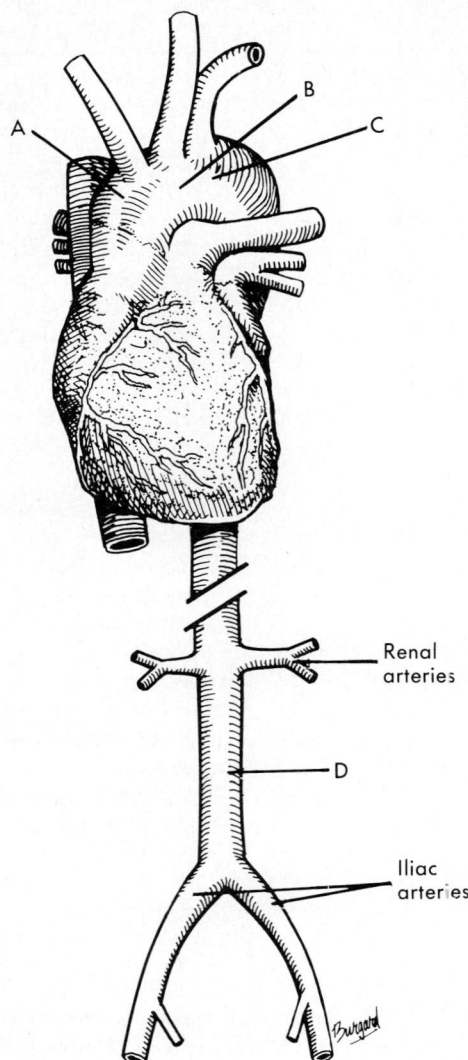

Fig. 26-39. Common sites of aortic aneurysms. *A,* Ascending aorta. *B,* Transverse aorta. *C,* Descending aorta. *D,* Abdominal aorta.

patient with this form of aneurysm is asymptomatic. Symptoms of chest pain are associated with aneurysms of the *ascending aorta.* Less frequent are aneurysms of the *transverse aorta* or aortic arch. Symptoms of this type directly relate to the aneurysms's compression on surrounding structures, such as the lungs, trachea, and larynx.

Abdominal aortic aneurysms

Aneurysms of the abdominal aorta are more prevalent in hypertensive men over 60 years of age. The vast majority of these aneurysms develop just below the renal arteries but above the iliac bifurcation. An abdominal aneurysm grows slowly, hence the patient is usually asymptomatic. It can leak into the retroperitoneal or pelvic cavity, or dissect into the duodenum. As the aorta exceeds its normal 3 to 4 cm diameter at this point, there is an increased probability of rupture.

The prognosis for a patient with an abdominal aortic aneurysm depends not only on the size of the defect but, more importantly, on the extent of arteriosclerotic heart disease. More than half of those with untreated abdominal aneurysm die within 2 years of diagnosis; over 85% die within 5 years.

DIAGNOSTIC TESTS

Radiography

An aneurysm is most often detected accidentally by routine chest or abdominal radiograms; since symptoms are rarely manifested. Radiographic findings show widening of the aorta with a ring of calcification outlining the aneurysm and displacement of surrounding structures.

Angiography

An aortogram reveals the size and location of an aneurysm. This test determines whether an aneurysm is leaking, expanding, or dissecting. An aortogram is performed by insertion of a catheter into the femoral, brachial, or axillary artery. The patient may experience a burning sensation when the contrast dye is injected. Following injection of the contrast material, a series of radiograms are taken at intervals to determine an accurate flow study.

After the procedure, the patient must remain on strict bed rest for 6 to 12 hours with only minimal flexion of the cannulated joint. Vital signs are monitored every 15 minutes for 2 hours. Assessment of pulses, skin color, temperature, movement, and numbness distal to the site is also important. The injection site is inspected whenever vital signs are taken for the presence of bleeding, swelling, or hematoma.

Sonography

Ultrasound is also helpful in determining the shape and location of the aneurysm. Special conducting gel is applied to the skin. The Doppler probe head is placed over the gel to intensify sounds of pulse vibration. Blood flow and presence of bruit are detected. Since this is a noninvasive procedure, there are no special precautions or posttest care.

SURGERY

Surgery is the treatment of choice for patients with large or dissecting aneurysms or with those aneurysms that produce symptoms with a significant risk of rupture. Elective resection at the time of the first symptoms is often advised, since emergency surgery increases surgical risks. Complications of surgery include massive hemorrhage, injury to adjacent structures (duodenum, ureters, kidneys), myocardial infarction, renal failure, stroke, or graft infection.

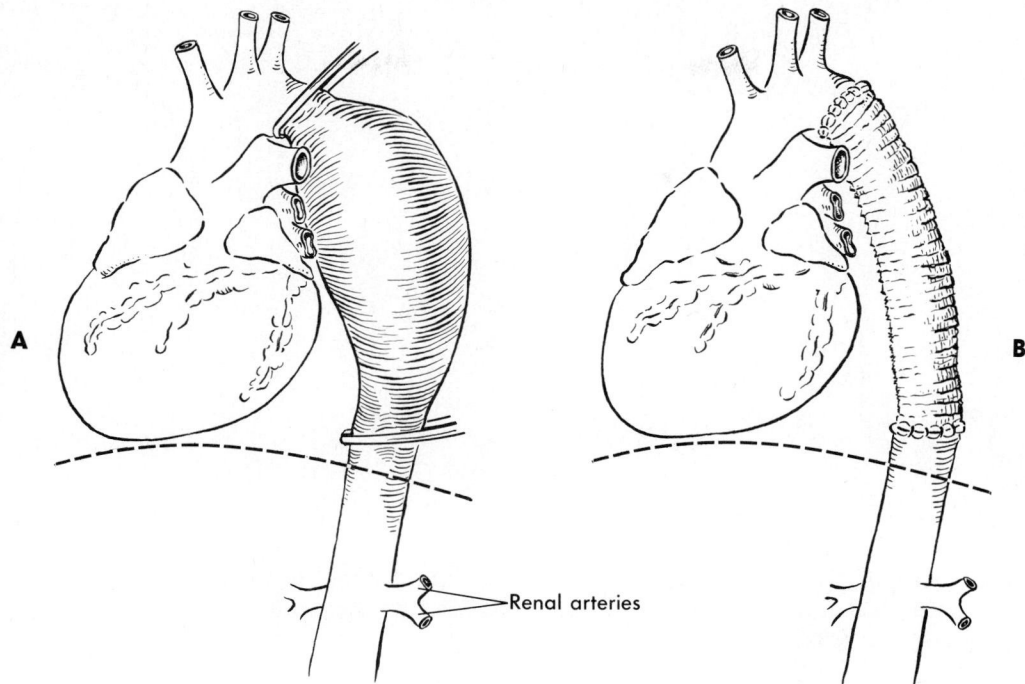

A

B

Renal arteries

Fig. 26-40. Aneurysm of descending thoracic artery. **A,** Resection of thoracic aorta with cardiovascular clamps in place. **B,** Permanent replacement graft after resection of aneurysm. (Redrawn from Bloodwell, R.D., et al.: Surg. Clin. North Am., **46:**901-911, 1966.)

Procedures

Thoracic aorta

Surgical intervention for the patient with an aneurysm of the thoracic aorta is comparable to open heart surgery. A midline thoracic incision is made, and the aneurysm is exposed. Cardiopulmonary bypass (p. 659) is used to maintain tissue oxygenation during clamping of the aorta. Hypothermia may also be indicated to decrease the metabolic requirements of the tissues. While the aneurysm itself is being resected, cross-clamps are placed above and below the aorta to prevent blood flow into the operative area (Fig. 26-40). An artificial patch or tube (Teflon or Dacron) is grafted on the area.

Abdominal aorta

Surgical intervention for the removal of an abdominal aortic aneurysm is performed without use of heart and lung bypass, since arterial blood flow to lower extremities can safely be interrupted during the operative procedure. An abdominal incision is made, the aneurysm is opened, and any clots and debris are removed. A synthetic graft in the form of a patch or tube is sutured onto the tissues. Once the graft is replaced, the remaining arterial wall is sutured over the graft (Fig. 26-41).

Preoperative preparation

The physician explains the surgical risks in obtaining informed consent for the surgery. The nurse provides

support for the patient during the decision-making process, since the surgery is associated with some mortality and morbidity.

The preparation and postoperative care for resection of a thoracic aortic aneurysm are similar to that for cardiac surgery (p. 661). Resection of an abdominal aortic aneurysm is similar to other abdominal surgery. Some surgeons additionally require a bowel preparation for optimum preparation, should bowel surgery be necessary. Heparin is usually given during surgery, before clamping of the artery.

Postoperative care (abdominal aortic aneurysm)

1. Monitor the following parameters:
   a. Vital signs until stable
   b. Central venous pressure (CVP) to assess fluid status
   c. Hourly circulation checks with assessment of all pulses distal to graft site (femoral, posterior tibial, posterior tibialis, dorsalis pedis)
      (1) Absent pulses more than 6 to 12 hours indicate arterial occlusion
      (2) Poor peripheral occlusion: marked decrease in blood pressure, weak thready pulses, cool skin temperature, diaphoresis
      (3) Advanced occlusion: pain, cramping, numbness in extremities; legs may be white or blue, and cool to cold

A   B   C

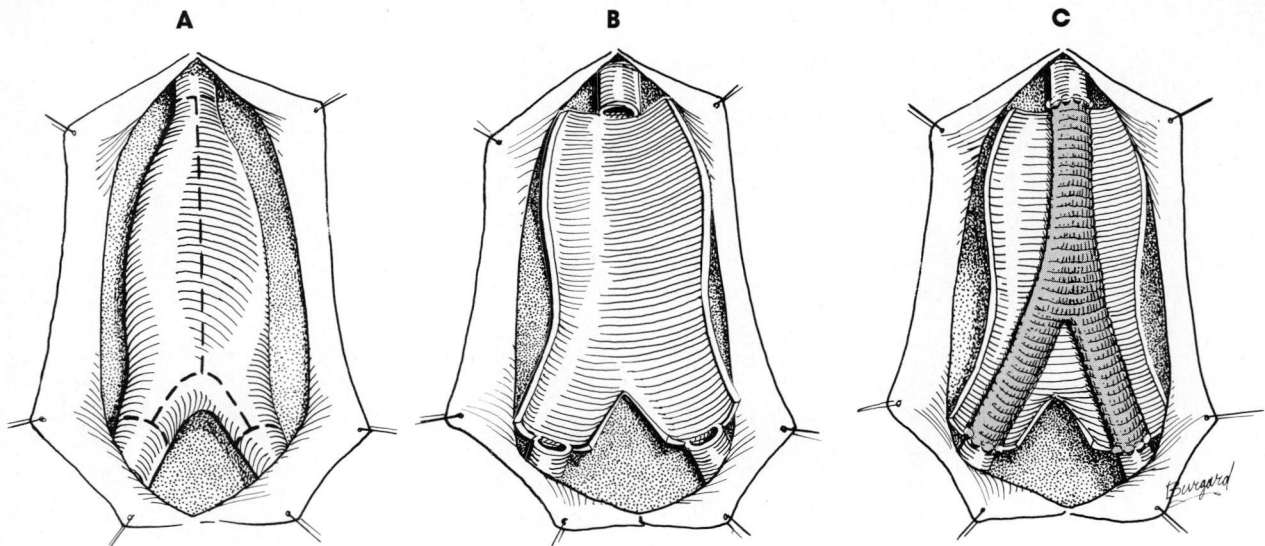

Fig. 26-41. Abdominal aneurysm. **A,** Aneurysm of aorta and iliac arteries. **B,** Bifurcation graft used to replace excised aneurysm. **C,** Closure of posterior peritoneum over graft and suture line.

   d. Renal function (since aorta was clamped during surgery, preventing blood flow to kidneys)
      (1) Hourly urine flow greater than 25 to 30 ml through indwelling catheter
      (2) Urine color (hematuria may occur with renal damage)
      (3) Daily blood urea nitrogen (BUN)
   e. Presence of back pain (indicative of retroperitoneal hemorrhage or thrombus at graft site)
2. Keep patient flat in bed without sharp flexion of hip and of knee to avoid pressure on femoral and popliteal arteries
3. Medicate for pain
4. Institute pulmonary ventilatory measures (deep breathing and coughing, and so on); use firm abdominal support to incision during coughing
5. Monitor for postoperative ileus and distention (patient may have an indwelling nasogastric tube)
6. Prevent postoperative thrombophlebitis
   a. Check for pain or cramps in calf, tenderness in specific areas of leg, redness along course of vein
   b. Encourage dorsiflexion and plantar flexion of feet
   c. Use elastic stockings

REFERENCES AND SUGGESTED READINGS*

1. American Heart Association: Heart facts, Dallas, 1984, The Association.
2. American Heart Association: Living with your pacemaker, 1979, The Association.
3. Andreoli, K.G., et al.: Comprehensive cardiac care: a text for nurses, physicians, and other health practitioners, ed. 5, St. Louis, 1983, The C.V. Mosby Co.
4. Angina pectoris: guidelines for treatment and prevention, Atlanta, 1979, Pritchett and Hull Associates, Inc.
5. Barbarowicz, P.: An active partnership for the health of your heart (after your coronary bypass surgery), Stanford, Calif., 1976, American Heart Association.
6. Barboriak, J.J., and Menahan, L.A.: Alcohol, lipoproteins, and coronary heart disease, Heart Lung **8:**736-740, 1979.
7. *Baum, P.L.: Abdominal aortic aneurysm? The patient takes AAA care, Nurs. 82 **12**(12):34-41, 1982.
8. Berne, R.M., and Levy, M.N.: Cardiovascular physiology, ed. 4, St. Louis, 1981, The C.V. Mosby Co.
9. *Bitran, D., et al.: Intra-aortic balloon counterpulsation in acute myocardial infarction, Heart Lung **10:**1021-1027, 1981.
10. Blowers, M.G., and Smith, R.J.: How to read an ECG: basic interpretation for nurses and other health workers, Oradell, N.J., 1977, Medical Economics Co.
11. *Boggs, B., Malone, D., and McCulloch, C.: A coronary teaching program in a community hospital, Nurs. Clin. North Am. **13:**457-497, 1978.
12. Brzenski, T.S.: Pacemakers: pulse of life, A.O.R.N. J. **32:**967-976, 1980.

*References preceded by an asterisk are particularly well suited for student reading.

13. *Burden, L.L., and Atwell, K.: The treacherous waters of unstable angina pectoris, Nurs. 83 **13**(12):50-55, 1983.

14. *Cain, R.S., Ferguson, R.M., and Tillisch, P.: Variant angina: a nursing approach, Heart Lung **8**:1122-1126, 1979.

15. Campuzano, M.: Self-care following coronary artery bypass surgery, Focus Crit. Care **9**:55-56, 1982.

16. *Cantwell, J.D.: Exercise and coronary heart disease: role in primary prevention, Heart Lung **13**:6-13, 1984.

17. Chesney, M.A., and Rosenman, R.H.: Type A behavior: observations on the past decade, Heart Lung **11**:12-18, 1982.

18. Child, J.S.: Aortic valvular stenosis, Hosp. Med. **18**:325-32II, Nov. 1982.

19. *Cohen, S.: New concepts in understanding congestive heart failure. I. How the clinical features arise, Am. J. Nurs. **81**:119-142, 1981.

20. *Cohen, S.: New concepts in understanding congestive heart failure. II. How the therapeutic approaches work, Am. J. Nurs. **81**:357-380, 1981.

21. *Connors, J.P., and Avioli, L.V.: An update on cardiac surgery, Heart Lung **10**:323-328, 1981.

22. Conover, M.B.: Cardiac arrhythmias: exercises in pattern interpretation, ed. 2, St. Louis, 1978, The C.V. Mosby Co.

23. Conover, M.B.: Understanding electrocardiography, ed. 4, St. Louis, 1984, The C.V. Mosby Co.

24. *Cromwell, V., et al.: Understanding the needs of your coronary bypass patients, Nurs. 80 **10**(8):34-45, 1980.

25. Crumlisch, C.M.: Cardiogenic shock: catch it early! Nurs. 81 **11**(8):34-41, 1981.

26. Ebersole, P., and Hess, P.: Toward healthy aging, St. Louis, 1981, The C.V. Mosby Co.

27. *Edwards M., and Payton, V.: Cardiac catheterization: technique and teaching, Nurs. Clin. North Am. **11**:271-281, 1976.

28. *Ellmyer, P., and Thomas, N.: A guide to your patient's safe home use of oxygen, Nurs. 82 **12**(1):55-57, 1982.

29. Fletcher, G.F.: Exercise and coronary risk factor modification in the management of atherosclerosis, Heart Lung **10**:811-813, 1981.

30. Fletcher, G.F.: Exercise and exercise testing: current state of the art, Heart Lung **13**:5-6, 1984.

31. Fletcher, G.F.: Long-term exercise in coronary artery disease and other chronic disease states, Heart Lung **13**:28-46, 1984.

32. Foster, S.B., and Canty, K.A.: Pump failure following myocardial infarction, Heart Lung **9**:293-298, 1980.

33. Fuhs, M.F.: Smoking and the heart patient, Nurs. Clin. North Am. **11**:361-369, 1976.

34. *Furman, S.: Recent developments in cardiac pacing, Heart Lung **7**:813-826, 1978.

35. Galen, R.S.: Enzymes in the diagnosis of myocardial infarction, Heart Lung **10**:484-485, 1981.

36. Gilbert, C.J., and Akhtar, M.: Right heart catheterization for intracardiac electrophysiologic studies: implications for the primary care nurse, Heart Lung **9**:85-92, 1980.

37. *Giving cardiac care. Nursing Photobook Series, Springhouse, Pa., 1981, Intermed Communications, Inc.

38. Glancy, D.L.: Medical management of adults and older children undergoing cardiac operations, Heart Lung **9**:277-283, 1980.

39. Goldman, M.J.: Principles of clinical electrocardiography, ed. 11, Los Altos, Calif., 1982, Lange Medical Publications.

40. Graboys, T.B.: Clinical pharmacology of antiarrhythmic agents, Heart Lung **8**:706-710, 1979.

41. Guyton, A.C., et al.: Textbook of medical physiology, ed. 6, Philadelphia, 1981, W.B. Saunders Co.

42. *Hammond, C.E.: Protecting patients with temporary transvenous pacemakers, Nurs. 78 **8**(11):82-86, 1978.

43. Hansen, M.S., Woods, S.L., and Wills, R.E.: Relative effectiveness of nitroglycerin ointment according to site of application, Heart Lung **8**:716-720, 1979.

44. Heger, J.J., et al.: New drugs for the treatment of ventricular arrhythmias, Heart Lung **10**:475-483, 1981.

45. *Houser, D.: What to do first when a patient complains of chest pain, Nurs. 76 **6**(11):54-56, 1976.

46. Iskandrain, A.S., Hakki, A., and Segal, B.L.: Acquired stenosis, Hosp. Med. **19**(1):55-66, 1983.

47. Isselbacher, K., et al.: Harrison's principles of internal medicine, ed. 9, New York, 1980, McGraw-Hill Book Co.

48. *Janz, N., and Lampman, R.M.: Coaching your cardiac patient along the path to recovery, Nurs. 81 **11**(12):36-41, 1981.

49. *Jasinkowski, N.: Aortic bypass: trimming the postop risks, RN **46**:41-45, 1982.

50. Johnson, G.P., and Johanson, B.C.: β-blockers: an expert's guide to what's on the market, Am. J. Nurs. **83**:1034-1043, 1983.

51. *Johnson, P., et al.: Cardiovascular system. In Diagnostics: nurse's reference library, Springfield, Pa, 1981, Intermed Communications, Inc.

52. Johnston, B.L.: Exercise testing for patients after myocardial and coronary bypass surgery: emphasis on predischarge phase, Heart Lung **13**:18-27, 1984.

53. Kaltenbach, M., et al.: Cardiomyopathy and myocardial biopsy, New York, 1978, Springer-Verlag New York, Inc.

54. Kannel, W.B., and Dawber, T.R.: Contributors to coronary risk: ten years later, Heart Lung **11**:60-64, 1982.

55. *Kern, L.S., and Gawlinski, A.: Stage-managing coronary artery disease, Nurs. 83 **13**:34-40, 1983.

56. *Klein, D.M.: Angina: physiology, signs and symptoms, Nurs. 84 **14**:44-46, 1984.

57. Kloosterman, N.D.: Prevention of ICU psychosis, Focus Crit. Care **10**:59-61, 1983.

58. *Kluge, R.M.: Infections of prosthetic cardiac valves and arterial grafts, Heart Lung **11**:146-151, 1982.

59. *Kovalesky, A.: Mitral valve prolapse, Nurs. 81 **11**(4):58-61, 1981.

60. Kroncke, G., and Boake, W.: Practical advice for your pacemaker patients, Fam. Pract. recertification **1**:75-76, 1979.

61. *Kroncke, G., et al.: What to do when your patient's pacemaker stops working, Nurs. 81 **11**(10):74-78, 1981.

62. Kumpuris, A.G., Paizner, A.E., and Luchi, R.J.: The role of serum digitalis levels in clinical practice, Heart Lung **8**:711-715, 1979.

63. Lakier, J.B.: Myocardial infarction management: the first 24 hours, Hosp. Med. **19**:66D-66Q, 1983.

64. Leibrandt, T., et al.: Cardiovascular disorders. In Disease: nurse's reference library, Springhouse, Pa., 1982, Intermed Communications, Inc.

65. Levy, R.I.: Medicine for the layman: heart attacks, Washington, D.C., 1980, U.S. Department of Health and Human Services.

66. *Lovvorn, J.: Coronary artery bypass surgery: helping patients cope with postop problems, Am. J. Nurs. **82:**1073-1075, 1982.

67. *Mallison, M.: Updating the cholesterol controversy: verdict, diet does count, Am. J. Nurs. **78:**1681, 1978.

68. *Manwarning, M.: What patients need to know about pacemakers, Am. J. Nurs. **77:**825-830, 1977.

69. *Marinelli-Miller, D.: What your patient wants to know about angiography, but may not ask, RN **46:**52-54, 1983.

70. Marriott, H.J.L.: Practical electrocardiography, ed. 7, Baltimore, 1983, Williams & Wilkins Co.

71. *McCauley, K.: Probing the in's and out's of congestive heart failure, Nurs. 82 **12**(11):60-65, 1982.

72. Michaelson, C.: Congestive heart failure, St. Louis, 1983, The C.V. Mosby Co.

73. Pantaleo, N., et al.: Thallium myocardial scintigraphy and its use in the assessment of coronary artery disease, Heart Lung **10:**61-71, 1981.

74. *Purcell, J.A., and Giffen, P.: Percutaneous transluminal coronary angioplasty, Am. J. Nurs. **81:**1620-1626, 1981.

75. Riedinger, M.S., Shellock, F.G., and Swan, H.J.C.: Reading pulmonary artery and pulmonary capillary wedge pressure waveforms with respiratory variations, Heart Lung **10:**675-678, 1981.

76. Roberts, R.: Diagnostic assessment of myocardial infarction based on lactate dehydrogenase and creatine kinase isoenzymes, Heart Lung **10:**486-506, 1981.

77. *Rossel, C.L., and Alyn, I.B.: Living with a permanent cardiac pacemaker, Heart Lung **6:**273-279, 1977.

78. *Rossi, L.P., and Antman, E.M.: Calcium channel blockers: new treatment for cardiovascular disease, Am. J. Nurs. **83:**382-388, 1983.

79. Sadler, P.D.: Incidence, degree, and duration of postcardiotomy delirium, Heart Lung **10:**1084-1092, 1981.

80. Sadler, P.D.: Nursing assessment of postcardiotomy delirium, Heart Lung **8:**745-750, 1979.

81. Sanderson, R.G., and Kurth, C.L.: The cardiac patient: a comprehensive approach, ed. 2, Philadelphia, 1983, W.B. Saunders Co.

82. *Saul, L.: Heart sounds and common murmurs, Am. J. Nurs. **83:**1679-1689, 1983.

83. Schlesinger, Z., and Barilay, J.: Prolonged rehabilitation of patients after acute myocardial infarction and its effects on a complex of physiological variables, Heart Lung **9**1038-1043, 1980.

84. *Scordo, K.A.: Taming the cardiac monitor. I, Nurs. 82 **12**(8):58-64.

85. *Scordo, K.A.: Taming the cardiac monitor. II, Nurs. 82 **12**(9):60-69, 1982.

86. *Scordo, K.A.: This procedure called PTCA: your patient's CABG substitute? Nurs. 82 **12**(2):50-55, 1982.

87. *Sears, M.F., and Heise, C.: Troubleshooting the Swan-Ganz catheter, Heart Lung **9:**303-305, 1980.

88. Seger, U., and Schlesinger, Z.: Rehabilitation of patients after acute myocardial infarction: an interdisciplinary family-oriented program, Heart Lung **10:**841-847, 1981.

89. *Stanford, J.F., et al.: Antiarrhythmic drug therapy, Am. J. Nurs. **80:**1288-1295, 1980.

90. Swartz, M.H., and Dack, S.: Mitral valve prolapse syndrome, Hosp. Med. **18**(12):49-64, 1982.

91. *Sweetwood, H.: patients with pacemakers, Nurs. 77 **7**(3):44-51, 1977.

92. *Tannenbaum, R., et al.: The pain of angina pectoris: how to recognize it, how to manage it, Nurs. 81 **11**(9):44-45, 1981.

93. *Tanner, G.: Heart failure in the MI patient, Am. J. Nurs. **77:**230-234, 1977.

94. *Taylor, D.: Congestive heart failure, Nurs. 83 **13**(9):44-45, 1983.

95. Tirrell, B.E., and Hart, L.K.: The relationship of health beliefs and knowledge to exercise compliance in patients after coronary bypass, Heart Lung **9:**487-493, 1980.

96. *VanMeter, M.: Balloon flotation catheters today: what they tell you, why they're vital, RN **46:**36-41, 1983.

97. *Viebrock, R., and Barth, R.: The pacemaker patient: how you can spare him needless alarm, RN **43:**38-42, 1980.

98. *Visalli, F.: The Swan-Ganz catheter, Nurs. 81 **11**(1):42-47, 1981.

99. *Waggoner, P.C.: Postoperative care of the patient undergoing cardiac valve replacement: a nursing perspective, Crit. Care Q. **4:**57-65, Dec. 1981.

100. Walsh-Essig, M.E.: A restudy of structured repetitive preoperative teaching to coronary artery bypass patients, master's thesis, Cleveland, 1982, Case Western Reserve University.

101. Way, L.W.: Current surgical diagnosis and treatment, ed. 6, Los Altos, Calif., 1983, Lange Medical Publications.

102. Weiland, A.P.: A review of cardiac valve prostheses and their selection, Heart Lung **12:**498-504, 1983.

103. Wenger, N.K.: Early ambulation physical activity: myocardial infarction and coronary artery bypass surgery, Heart Lung **13:**14-18, 1984.

104. Wenger, N.K., Hurst, J.W., and McIntyre, M.C.: Cardiology for nurses, New York, 1980. McGraw-Hill Book Co.

105. Westfall, V.E.: Electrical and mechanical events in the cardiac cycle, Am. J. Nurs. **76:**234-235, 1976.

106. Winslow, E.H., and Mac Vaugh H.: Coronary artery surgery: operative technique and patient education, Nurs. Clin. North Am. **11:**371-383, 1976.

107. Wyngaarden, J.B., and Smith, L.H.: Textbook of medicine, ed. 16, Phiadelphia, 1982, W.B. Saunders Co.

108. Wyper, M.A., and Daly, B.J.: Care of the patient with cardiovascular disease. In Daly, B.J.: Intensive care nursing, ed. 2, Garden City, N.Y., 1980, Medical Examination Publishing Co.

109. Yalof, I.: The multidisciplinary team: an effective approach to management of the cardiac surgery patient, Heart Lung **8:**699-705, 1979.

110. Young, L.E.: Nursing interventions with obese cardiac patients, Nurs. Clin. North Am. **13:**449-456, 1978.

111. Zeluff, G.W., Cashion, W.R., and Jackson, D.: Evaluation of the coronary arteries and myocardium by radionuclide imaging, Heart Lung **9:**344-349, 1980.

27

Peripheral Vascular Diseases

GRACE McCARTHY HARLAN and BARBARA J. DALY

STUDY QUESTIONS

- Review the anatomic structure of the artery and the vein and their specific function in maintaining circulation to the peripheral tissues.

- Describe the relationship of the arteries and veins to the lymphatic system.

- List risk factors that influence the development of arteriosclerosis and atherosclerosis, and the major complications that follow vascular changes.

- List self-care measures you would include in a teaching plan that would help persons with peripheral vascular disease of an extremity.

The term *peripheral vascular disease* refers to a number of diseases of the blood vessels that affect any part of the vascular sytem. Diseases of the heart and coronary arteries are excluded from this classification. This chapter will therefore concentrate on arterial and venous diseases of the lower extremities. Since the lymphatic system complements the function of the vascular system, the interruption of the transport of lymph and tissue fluids from the interstitial space to the veins will also be covered in this chapter.

ANATOMY AND PHYSIOLOGY

All the cells of the body are directly dependent on an intact and functioning vascular system. This vascular system is a closed circuit consisting of the systemic circulation and the pulmonary circulation connected to the right and left sides of the heart. Blood is conveyed from the left side of the heart to the tissues and back to the right side of the heart.

Arteries conveying blood via the aorta away from the heart supply nutrients, oxygen, and regulatory substances to the body tissues (Fig. 27-1). The veins carry back the waste products. As the arteries approach the tissues they branch into smaller vessels called *arterioles*, which connect with the capillary vessels. These vessels are located within the tissues and allow for the movement of nutrients, oxygen, and regulatory substances into the cells and the removal of cellular secretions, waste products, and carbon dioxide out of the cells back into the blood. The movement out of the cells is into small veins called *venules* and into large veins that carry the blood back to the heart (Fig. 27-2).

Arteries

Arteries are composed of three coats: an inner coat (*tunica intima*), a middle coat (*tunica media*), and an outer coat (*tunica adventitia*). These coats give the artery its elasticity, muscularity, and its wall thickness. These characteristics and the diameter of the artery enable the arteries to receive blood under very high pressure with each contraction of the heart and to move blood through them rather rapidly to the arterioles and the capillaries.

Capillaries

The capillaries are minute, thin-walled vessels that connect the smallest arteries, the *arterioles*, with the smallest veins, *venules*. It is through the capillaries that the cellular exchange essential to life takes place.

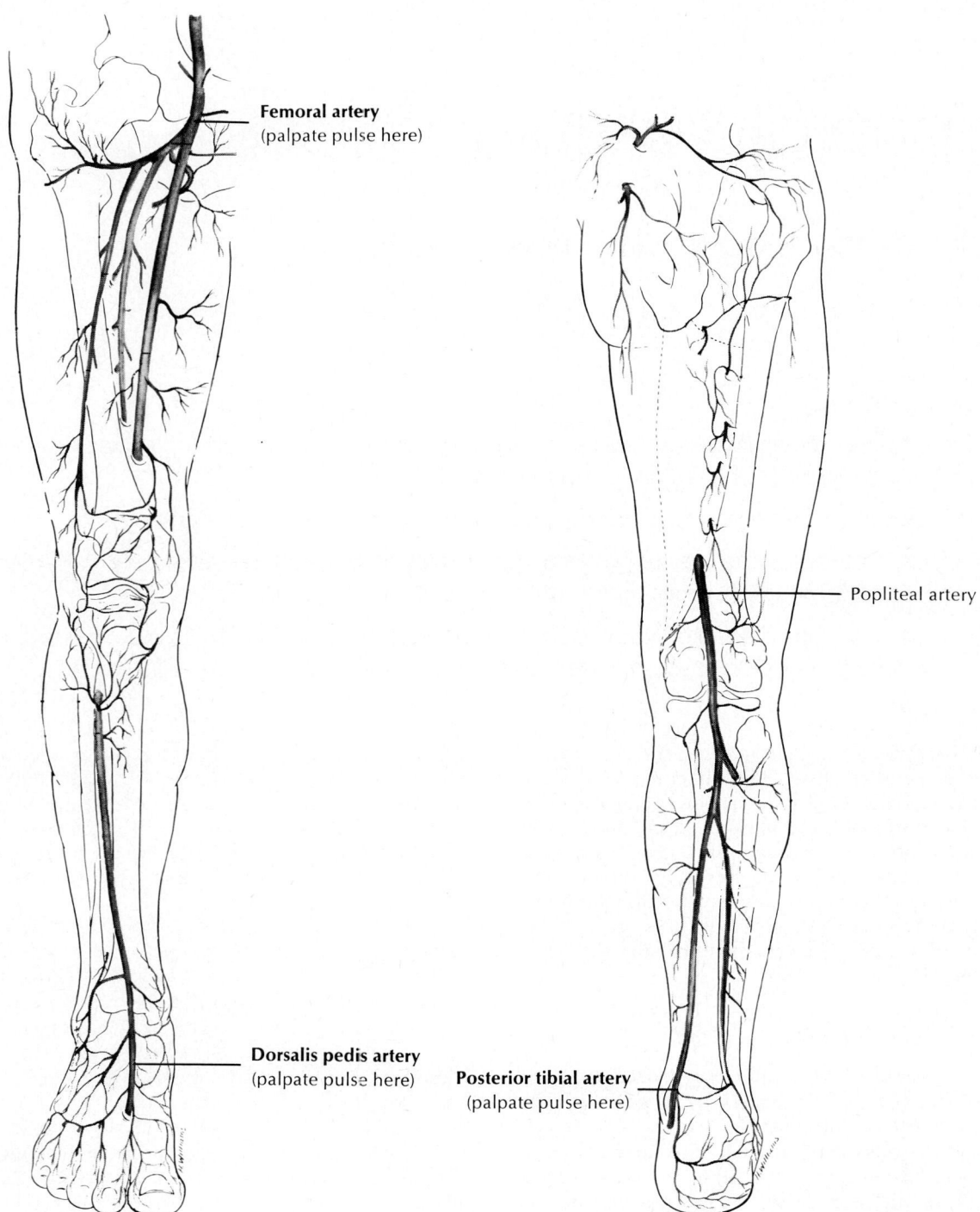

Fig. 27-1. Arteries of the lower extremity (Adapted from Francis, C.C., and Martin, A.H.: Introduction to human anatomy, ed. 7, St. Louis, 1975, The C.V. Mosby Co.)

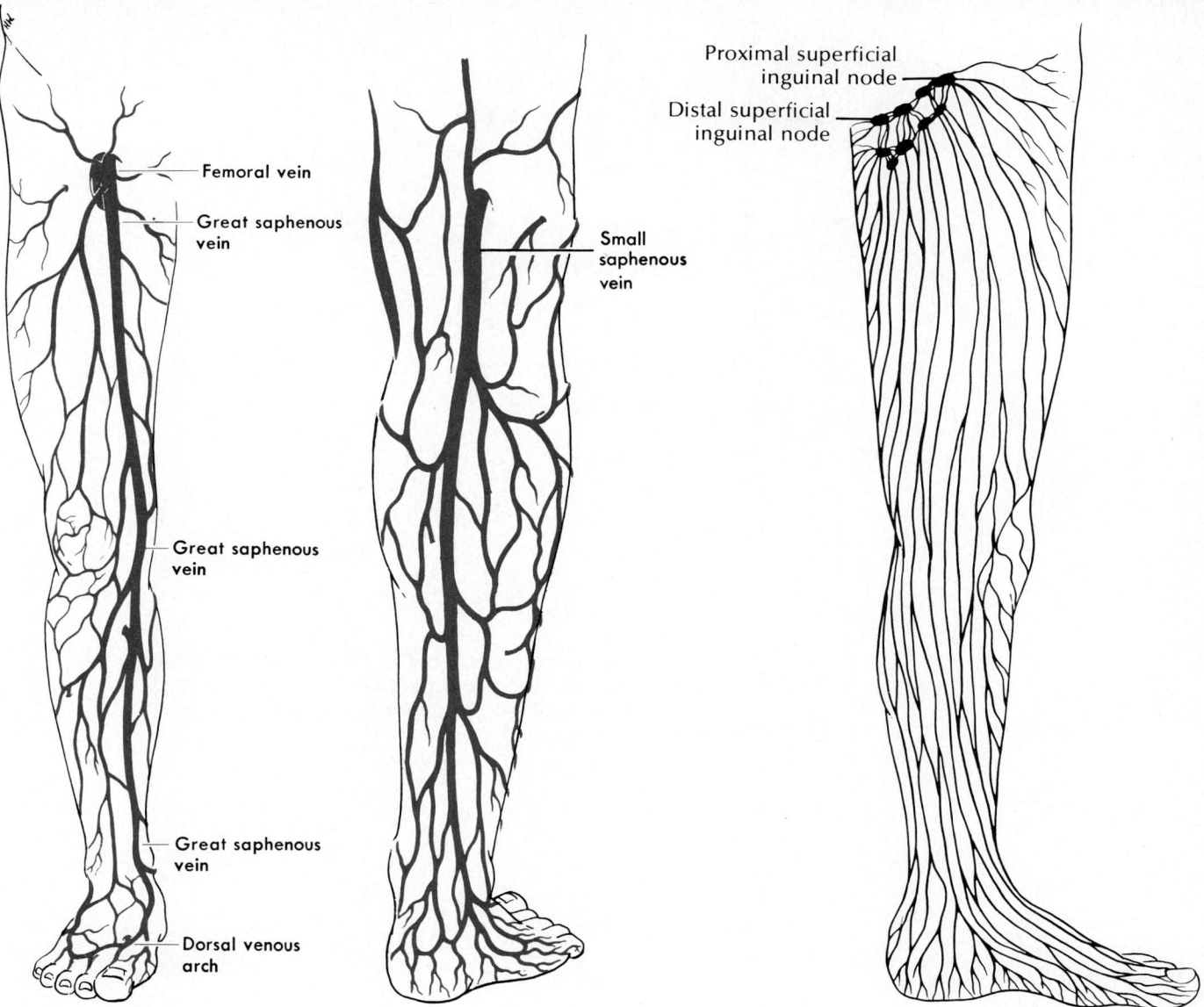

Fig. 27-2. Superficial veins of leg and foot. (From Anthony, C.J., and Thibodeau, G.A.: Textbook of anatomy and physiology, ed. 11, St. Louis, 1983, The C.V. Mosby Co.)

Fig. 27-3. Superficial lymphatics of medial aspect of lower extremity (after Sappey). (From Francis C.C., and Martin, A.H.: Introduction to human anatomy, ed. 7, St. Louis, 1975, The C.V. Mosby Co.)

Veins

The capillaries join with the venules, which in turn become veins that return the blood to the right side of the heart. The structural elements of the veins are the same as those of the arteries. They also are composed of three coats. The main differences between the veins and the arteries are as follows:

1. Veins are less elastic.
2. Many veins have valves.
3. The walls in veins are thinner, which causes them to collapse more readily.

Lymphatic system

The lymphatic system is made up of small, thin, vein-like vessels that are found throughout most of the body. These lymphatic vessels tend to lie near the veins (Fig. 27-3). These tiny vessels begin as lymph capillaries that drain the tissue spaces of *lymph,* a fluid similar to plasma

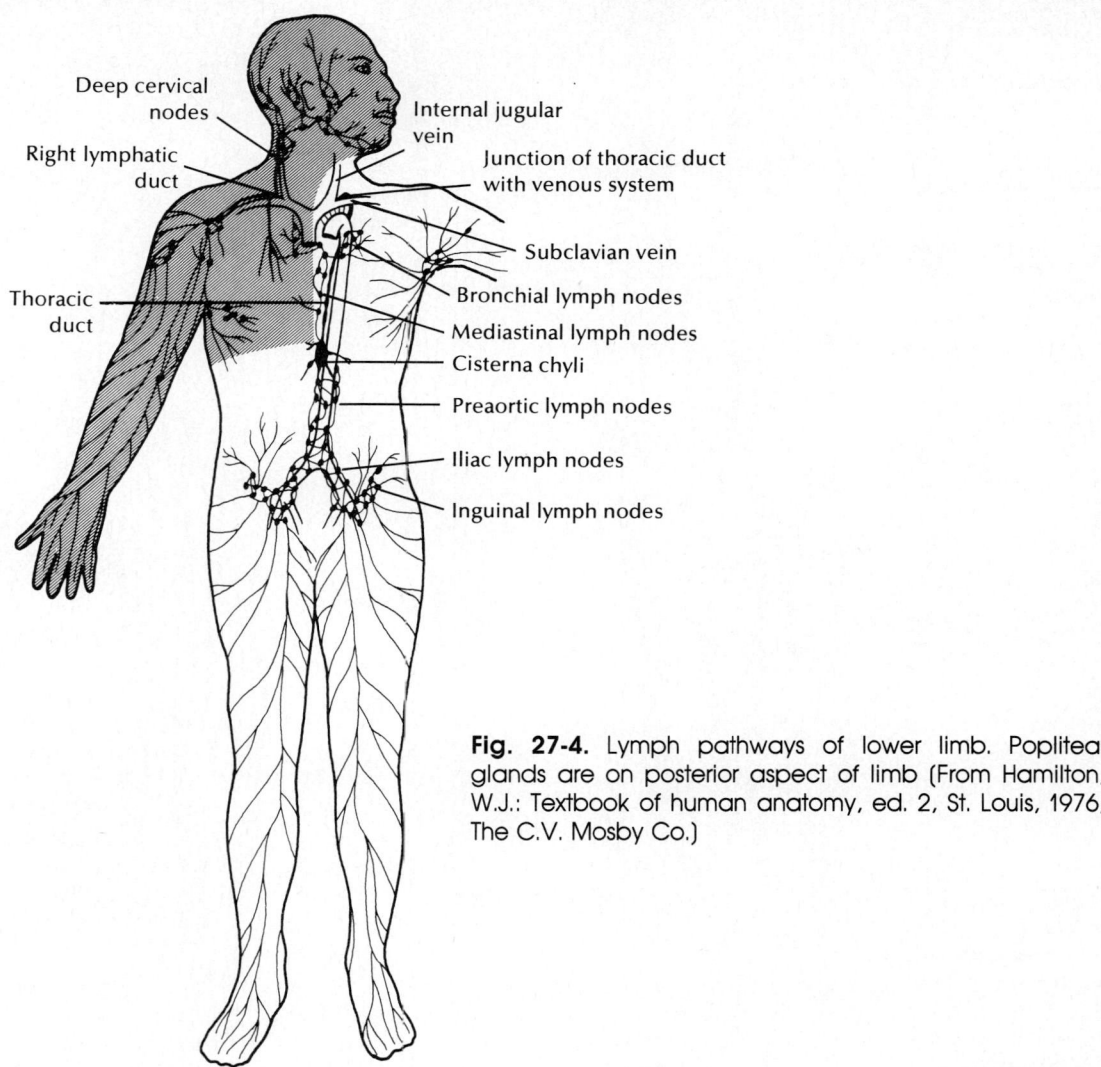

Deep cervical nodes

Right lymphatic duct

Thoracic duct

Internal jugular vein

Junction of thoracic duct with venous system

Subclavian vein

Bronchial lymph nodes

Mediastinal lymph nodes

Cisterna chyli

Preaortic lymph nodes

Iliac lymph nodes

Inguinal lymph nodes

Fig. 27-4. Lymph pathways of lower limb. Popliteal glands are on posterior aspect of limb (From Hamilton, W.J.: Textbook of human anatomy, ed. 2, St. Louis, 1976, The C.V. Mosby Co.)

and tissue fluid. The lymph flows through small, oval bodies called lymph nodes before entering the bloodstream. From the lymph nodes, the flow finally empties into the large thoracic duct that joins the jugular veins in the neck (Fig. 27-4).

Physiologic changes with aging

With advancing age, changes occur in the vascular system. Major changes appear to occur in the vessel walls. There are gradual changes that occur especially in the intimal connective tissue, in the elastic media; and in the collagen fibrils. As these changes occur, the blood vessels become less resilient and less able to accommodate the volume of blood flow.

As the blood vessels lose their elasticity and flexibility, they tend to dilate and become tortuous, causing an increase in resistance to blood flow termed *peripheral vascular resistance*. Blood flow through the vessels is diminished, resulting in decreased supplies of oxygen and

nutrients to the capillaries and the tissue cells and an excess accumulation of carbon dioxide and acid metabolites in the tissues.

Superimposed on these age-related vascular changes is the development of *arteriosclerosis* (commonly referred to as "hardening of the arteries"). This process of vascular change is thought to begin within the first year of life and continue throughout life. Changes in blood vessels can be local or generalized systemically. Atherosclerosis, for example, causes generalized effects.

As the life span of the population increases, peripheral vascular diseases and their complications are seen more often in care facilities that provide medical, surgical, and nursing care.

PREVENTION AND HEALTH EDUCATION

Health teaching about the factors influencing peripheral vascular disease should be done by the nurse working in any clinical setting. All individuals will benefit from

---

**Risk factors for peripheral
vascular disease**

Cigarette smoking
Elevated blood serum cholesterol and triglycerides
Nutritional excesses: calories, fats, carbohydrates, salt
Obesity
Physical inactivity
Emotional stress

---

education about changes that occur in the vascular system with advancing age. The person with peripheral vascular disease has a chronic, potentially disabling disease and is subject to periods of exacerbation and complications such as infection, thrombosis, or even amputation.

The person must learn about the disease as it affects and is affected by life-style and daily habits. The single most important factor in health education is prevention.

Risk factors

The risk factors predisposing to the development of vascular changes and potential health problems are listed in the above box.

Counseling and teaching

Because of the upright posture of humans, the danger of peripheral vascular disease in the lower extremities is always present. The activity and exercise habits of the individual may need particular attention. Other areas for counseling and teaching are as follows:

1. Promoting activity. Exercise by walking and moving about to:
    a. Promote muscle contraction and relaxation.
    b. Improve return of venous blood from the extremities to the heart and aid in the development of collateral circulation.
        (1) Avoid standing or sitting for long periods.
        (2) Avoid crossing the legs at the knees and thus placing pressure on the popliteal vessels.
        (3) Develop the habit of rotating the foot at the ankle, bending the foot up and down, and straightening the knees at intervals.
2. Preventing compromise of circulation
    a. Persons with peripheral vascular disease must not wear anything that constricts and further impedes circulation.
        (1) Avoid rolled garters, socks with tight bands, girdles, or pantyhose.

(2) Avoid tight waistbands; suspenders may be preferred to belts for men.
(3) Loosen and relace shoe laces several times a day to prevent edema of the feet at the end of the day.
(4) Sleep on a firm mattress; soft mattress may allow flexion of the trunk at the hips, which will impede circulation to the lower extremities.
    b. Persons with peripheral vascular disease must avoid vasoconstriction with lessening of circulation in the extremities.
        (1) Avoid exposure to cold and chilling.
        (2) In cold weather, wear warm covering on all parts of the body.
        (3) Maintain a warm environment of about 70° F (21° C).
3. Counseling for proper nutrition
    a. Avoid obesity and control weight.
        (1) Obesity places an added burden on the heart and blood vessels to circulate blood effectively, and excess fat tissue tends to compromise vessels and increase venous congestion.
        (2) Change eating habits and caloric intake.
        (3) Match caloric intake with metabolic needs.
    b. Avoid or control the development of atherogenic disease and its sequelae such as stroke and myocardial infarction (Chapter 26); doing so can reduce or control the extent of disease.
        (1) Reduce or eliminate saturated fats.
        (2) Reduce carbohydrates and thus serum triglycerides.
        (3) Plan meals that are within caloric restrictions.
        (4) Include foods high in B-complex vitamins to maintain tonicity of smooth muscle of blood vessels.
        (5) Include foods high in vitamin C, essential to healing and prevention of both internal and external hemorrhage.
4. Teaching effects of smoking. Smoking is one of the greatest risk factors in the development of peripheral vascular disease. Smoking exerts an influence on circulation.
    a. Nicotine causes vasoconstriction and spasms of the arteries.
    b. Nicotine increases the heart rate, causing greater strain on the circulatory system.
    c. The inhaled carbon monoxide in cigarette smoke raises the carboxyhemoglobin level and reduces the oxygen-carrying capacity of the blood to the tissues.
5. Preventing skin breakdown. Resistance to infection is low when tissues are inadequately nourished and oxygenated.
    a. Keeping extremities warm:
        (1) Aids in vasodilation and improved circulation to affected part.

(2) In the presence of peripheral vascular disease and peripheral nerve degeneration and decreased sensitivity to heat:
    (a) Avoid hot water bottles, heating pads, or other forms of local heat to the legs or feet.
    (b) Avoid soaking feet in hot or even very warm water. Water should be 90° F (32° C).
    (c) Use warm bath to warm entire body.
    (d) Wear loose woolen bed socks at night.

b. Teaching care of feet.
    (1) Daily bath is recommended except for the elderly, for whom two or three baths a week are sufficient.
    (2) Dry skin by gentle patting.
    (3) Check skin for changes on legs and feet
        (a) Dry skin and scaling: fewer baths may be indicated; lubricate skin with lanolin or a moisturizing agent after bathing and between baths.
        (b) Swelling around varicosities, and hard, reddened or painful areas may indicate phlebitis. Report to physician at once.
        (c) Report changes in toenails.
    (4) Wash feet daily in tepid water, dry thoroughly. Pay special attention to areas between the toes and inspect for calluses and blisters. Massage skin and nails gently with lubricant.
    (5) Do not use alcohol: has drying effect.
    (6) Powder may be used: remove excess.
    (7) Change socks at least once daily.
    (8) Do not use over-the-counter foot preparations; they are too strong for feet with impaired circulation.
    (9) Prevent ingrown toenails.
        (a) Soak feet in tepid water.
        (b) With nail clippers, cut nails straight across and round slightly at edges with a file.
        (c) Do not use pocket knife, razor blade, or scissors.
        (d) Elderly persons with poor eyesight should see a podiatrist.
        (e) Thickened or deformed nails should be treated by a podiatrist or a physician.
    (10) Medical care should be sought for blisters, corns and calluses, and areas of thickened skin.

c. Preventing trauma and pressure.
    (1) Do not walk barefoot.
    (2) Do not scratch skin lesions or mosquito or insect bites.
    (3) Use calamine lotion for itching (pruritus).
    (4) Alternate shoes daily to allow for airing.
    (5) Dry wet shoes on shoe trees to preserve their shape.
    (6) Shoes should be comfortable, give good support to the feet, and be safe to walk in. Rubber-soled shoes are not advised: they retard evaporation and may contribute to the development of fungal infection.
    (7) Avoid pressure of bed covers on the toes and feet. Improvise a board at the foot of the bed to keep the weight of covers off the feet.

d. Treating ulceration. Preventing infection is one of the most difficult problems in caring for persons with ulcers. Despite precautions, some persons with peripheral vascular disease develop areas of ulceration because of trauma or pressure. The ball of the foot, the ankle, and the lower calf are the most commonly involved areas.
    (1) Wet-to-dry dressings are often used for debridement (removal of necrotic and sloughed tissue that adheres to the dried dressing).
    (2) Complete bed rest may not be ordered. Most physicians feel the arterial circulation and healing are improved by a moderate amount of moving about some part of the day.
    (3) Keep extremity warm, but avoid direct pressure on ulcerated areas. A bed cradle with a 25-watt bulb will provide warmth and will improve ulcer healing. The physician will order length of time and distance of bulb from limb.
    (4) Apply topical ointment as ordered by the physician. A wide variety of antibiotic and antibacterial topical agents are used, such as penicillin, nitrofurazone (Furacin), bacitracin, and neomycin. Streptokinase-streptodornase (Varidase) may be ordered to be applied locally.

Major health problems of the peripheral vascular system

Changes in the peripheral vascular system may cause local arterial or venous disorders or may result in a systemic effect (for example, hypertension). Major peripheral vascular disorders that will be discussed in this chapter are listed here.

1. Arterial disorders
    a. Atherosclerosis
    b. Atherosclerosis obliterans
    c. Thromboangiitis obliterans (Buerger's disease)
    d. Raynaud's phenomenon
    e. Arterial embolism
    f. Aneurysms of the extremity and arteriovenous fistula

2. Venous and lymph disorders
   a. Thrombophlebitis
   b. Varicose veins
   c. Lymphedema
3. Hypertension

ARTERIAL DISORDERS

Since the function of the arteries is to transport blood from the heart to the tissues, any disturbance in the structure of the arteries interferes with this function. The result is diminished blood and decreased oxygen supply to the tissues. The symptoms of arterial disease are not caused by the degree of obstruction or narrowing but by the degree to which the involved body part is deprived of circulation. This in turn is affected by such factors as blood pressure and presence or absence of collateral circulation. For example, 50% occlusion of one artery may cause severe symptoms, while 50% occlusion of another artery will cause no symptoms if collateral circulation is sufficient to provide oxygenation. The etiology, signs and symptoms, and medical therapy for the different arterial disorders are listed in Table 27-1.

PATHOPHYSIOLOGY

Atherosclerosis

Atherosclerosis is generally viewed as a type of arteriosclerosis or as a part of the aging process. This disease involves the development of lesions on the intimal wall.

Three types of lesions have been identified: (1) fatty streaks, which consist of smooth-muscle cells and lipid depositions that are present in the aorta of all individuals by age 10 years, but which do not necessarily progress to produce disease; (2) fibrous plaques, which involve a thickening of the intima and are surrounded by lipids,

Table 27-1. Arterial disorders

Disease	Etiology	Signs and symptoms	Medical therapy

Atherosclerosis	The aging process
	Risk factors (p. 696)
	  Hypercholesteremia
	  Plasma triglycerides
	  Obesity
	  Stress
	  Cigarette smoking
	Poor dietary habits
	Inborn errors of carbohydrate metabolism
	Other variables
	  Diabetes and elevated blood sugar
	  Hypertension
	  Hypothyroidism
		May not appear for 20 to 40 years
		Pain in lower limbs brought on by walking and exercise *(intermittent claudication)*
			Place on exercise program to improve collateral circulation
			Teaching program on care of feet (p. 698)
			Drug therapy with vasodilators (p. 704)
			Changes in dietary habits
			Stop smoking

Atherosclerosis obliterans	Late stage of atherosclerosis Risk factors same as for atherosclerosis	Early Tingling and numbness in the toes Extremity "feels" cold—"can't keep feet warm" Extremity muscles become tired and "achy" on exercise or walking Later Increased pain in feet and calves on walking or exercises *(intermittent claudication)* most common symptom Absence of palpable pulses is most reliable sign Skin: cold and white Ischemic rest pain caused by lack of oxygen to tissues	Surgical intervention may be the only alternative in the presence of an arterial occlusion

Continued.

Table 27-1. Arterial disorders—cont'd

Disease	Etiology	Signs and symptoms	Medical therapy

Thromboangiitis obliterans	Secondary to atherosclerosis
	Secondary to thrombosis and spasms
	Tobacco plays primary role
	Hypercoagulability plays a role
		Intermittent claudication is first symptom noticed
		Coldness or sensitivity to cold is an early symptom
		Burning pain is *intensified* by smoking or chilling
		Pulsations are impaired or absent
		Later
		  Redness or cyanosis in extremity of one or more digits
		  Ulceration and gangrene occur spontaneously or with trauma
		  Changes occur in skin and nails
			The same as for atherosclerosis
			Treat ulcers
			Sympathectomy
			In the presence of gangrene, amputation may be choice of treatment for the part or all of extremity involved

Raynaud's phenomenon	Emotional or thermal (cold) stimuli
	Trauma of high-speed vibratory tools under conditions of cold
	Result of occupational hazards as above and repeated percussive forces, as with operators of chain saws and typists
	Secondary to
	  Scleroderma
	  Occlusive arterial disease
	  Rheumatoid arthritis (Chapter 23)
		Chief complaint: cold, numbness or tingling in one or more digits (generally unilateral)
		Intermittent attacks of pallor or cyanosis followed by redness on abatement of spasms
		Symptoms intensify on exposure to cold and with emotional reactions
		Advanced cases: small ulcerated areas and gangrene appear at the tips of the digits (caused by trauma to severely ischemic tissues).
			Main objective is to arrest progress of the disease
			Stop smoking
			Keep body warm, prevent injury to feet and hands
			Vasodilator drugs (p. 704)
			Sympathectomy may be physician's choice (p. 704)
			Amputation may be necessary to treat progressive gangrene

Arterial embolism	Advanced aortic atherosclerosis
	Released thrombi from chambers of the heart as result of
	  Atrial fibrillation
	  Myocardial infarction
	  Congestive heart failure
	Vascular disease such as damaged vessel
	Fragmentation of embolus to more distal vessels
	Immobility
	Anemia
	Dehydration
	Postsurgical release of embolus
		Depends on size of embolus, organ involved, and state of collateral vessels
		Numbness or tingling of extremity
		Weight bearing may suddenly become difficult
		Sense of coldness in extremity
		Sudden occlusion
		  Acute, severe pain at site of thrombus formation
		  Burning or aching pain in the tissues distal to the occlusion
		  Arterial pulses absent distal to site of occlusion
		  Loss of sensory and motor function
		  Extremity becomes pale, mottled, and numb
			Vasodilators (p. 704) to improve collateral circulation
			Sympathetic block of lumbar ganglia may be performed to dilate other vessels
			Oxygen to alleviate hypoxemia and dyspnea
			Heparin and coumadin given to prevent further emboli (p. 704)
			Thrombolytic agents Streptokinase and urokinase may be used to attempt embolic lysis (p. 704)

Table 27-1. Arterial disorders—cont'd

Disease	Etiology	Signs and symptoms	Medical therapy
Arterial embolism—cont'd		Cyanosis and gangrene may occur if blood supply is completely cut off from the tissues Fainting, nausea, vomiting, and signs of pronounced shock may appear	
Aneurysm of extremity and arteriovenous fistula	Weakening of the vessel wall secondary to Trauma Congenital vascular disease Infection Atherosclerosis	May be asymptomatic Presence of large pulsating mass is felt in area of artery Presence of a *bruit,* or soft blowing sound, heard with the stethoscope At other times there may be pain, coldness, numbness distal to aneurysm Associated with arteriovenous fistulas are signs of venous insufficiency, such as mottled, darkened skin, edema of the extremity, increased skin temperature when compared with normal extremity Both conditions: in time atrophy, cyanosis, trophic changes, and gangrene may occur	Choice of treatment is Closure of the fistula Removal of portion of the aneursym Antihypertensive medicines in the presence of hypertension (p. 723)

collagen, and elastic fibers; and (3) the complicated lesion associated with disease, which is a large mass consisting of lipids and extracellular and intracellular debris.

The result of atherosclerosis is narrowing of the artery with progression to obstruction, thrombosis, aneurysm development, and rupture. Other consequences can be reduction of nutrients and oxygen to the tissues, resulting in ischemic necrosis of the tissue cells.

Atherosclerosis obliterans

Atherosclerosis obliterans is the most common form of obstructive disease of the aorta and large and medium-sized arteries. It is caused by atherosclerosis of the intima with medial arteriosclerosis. The femoral artery is the most commonly involved. The disease can occur as early as 30 years of age, but its greatest incidence is between 50 and 70 years of age.

If the obstruction progresses slowly, preexisting collateral channels can convey blood around the obstruction. Under increased pressure caused by the arterial obstruction, the collateral vessels will dilate and carry increased arterial flow. Appearance of symptoms will depend on the size of the obstructed artery, how fast the obstruction has

occurred, and the development of effective collateral circulation.

Thromboangiitis obliterans (Buerger's disease)

Thromboangiitis obliterans, commonly referred to as *Buerger's disease,* is an obstructive, idiopathic disease affecting small- and medium-sized arteries and veins. The primary pathophysiologic event is an inflammatory process associated with thrombosis and spasm. It occurs as a focal rather than a diffuse process, affecting the lower extremities more often than the upper extremities. The disease is most common in men between 25 and 40 years of age and has been reported in all races and many areas of the world.

Raynaud's phenomenon

Raynaud's phenomenon is the term used to describe the intermittent episodes of arterial spasms of the extremities that result in coldness, pain, pallor, and cyanosis, most often in the hands. Symptoms are most likely to occur at an early age, often in the teens. Of those diagnosed, 80% are women.

Little is known about the actual pathophysiologic

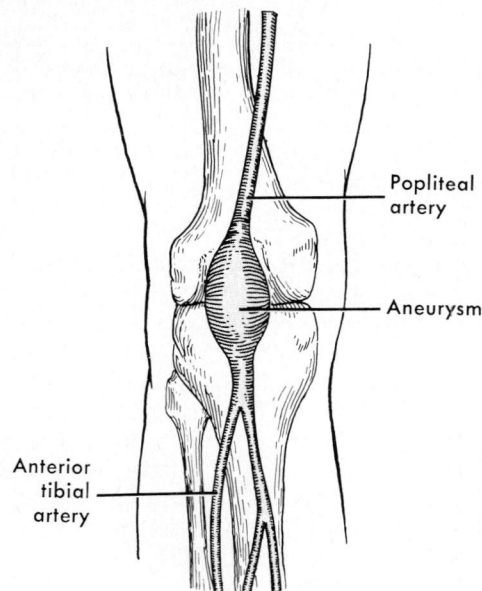

Fig. 27-5. Posterior view of knee with aneurysm of popliteal artery.

changes that occur in the blood vessels, except that intimal thickening occurs over time, causing reduction of blood flow to the extremity.

Generally the condition is unilateral and may affect only one or two digits.

Arterial embolism

Arterial emboli are blood clots floating in the circulating blood. These clots most commonly originate in the heart as a result of atrial fibrillation, myocardial infarction, congestive heart failure, or a vascular disease. The clot may be a fragment of an arteriosclerotic plaque loosened from the aorta. An embolus is carried into the arterial system, where it plugs an artery that is too small to allow it to pass. The embolus may lodge at a bifurcation, or division, of arteries. An embolus lodging at the bifurcation of any artery is called a *saddle embolus*. Over half of the emboli to the lower extremity will lodge in the femoral or the popliteal artery.

Aneurysm of the extremity and arteriovenous fistula

An *aneurysm* is an enlarged, dilated portion of an artery. Although it may follow trauma, such as an automobile accident, it is most commonly associated with atherosclerosis. The destruction of the medial layer leads to weakening of the wall of the artery and to the eventual formation of an aneurysm. Aneurysms of the arteries of the lower extremities, particularly in the popliteal area, are common in persons over 60 years of age who have pronounced arteriosclerosis (Fig. 27-5). Thrombi form at the site of the aneurysm, and emboli may travel to obstruct more distal portions of the artery.

An *arteriovenous fistula* is an abnormal communication between an artery and a vein caused by congenital anomaly or by trauma. In an arteriovenous fistula the blood in the artery bypasses the capillary bed, which has a strong resistance to blood flow, and flows instead directly into the vein. Persistance of this high-pressure flow in the vein eventually results in venous dilation and may be associated with aneurysm formation.

ASSESSMENT

Subjective data

1. Onset of symptoms: slow and progressive or sudden
2. Changes noted in skin color and temperatue of extremities
3. Discomfort in legs with walking or at rest
4. Effect of cold temperatures on extremities
5. Smoking habits
6. Relief measures used for discomfort in extremities
7. Changes noted in general appearance of either extremity, for example, "swelling"

Objective data

1. General appearance, for example; thin, emaciated, dehydrated, comatose
2. Color and temperature of extremities
3. Palpation of peripheral pulses (Fig. 27-6)
4. Assessment of sensation of extremities
5. Assessment traumatized areas not healing
6. Compare both extremities on points 2 to 5

Diagnostic tests

One or more of the following tests are used as part of the clinical examination to help in diagnosis of vascular disease and determine the treatment that will follow.

Angiography (arteriography)

Angiography is an x-ray procedure that permits visualization of the vascular tree through the intravascular injection of radiopaque contrast medium such as Hypaque or Renografin. The collateral vessels will fill with the contrast dye, thus permitting visualization of vessels distal to an obstruction if one is present. Calcified atherosclerotic plaques at the site of the occlusion may be visualized, and calcification can sometimes be traced the length of the artery.

The patient is watched closely for allergic reaction to the dye, such as dyspnea, nausea, vomiting, numbness of the extremities, diaphoresis, and tachycardia. The site of the injection must be monitored for signs of irritation and thrombosis. Antihistaminic drugs, epinephrine, and oxygen are used to treat hypersensitivity reactions to the dye. Warm moist packs may be ordered to the inflamed site of the injection.

Peripheral pulses distal to the injection site are checked every hour for 4 to 8 hours after the test.

Intermittent claudication test

Some physicians believe that the *intermittent claudication test* is the hallmark and specific symptom of ather-

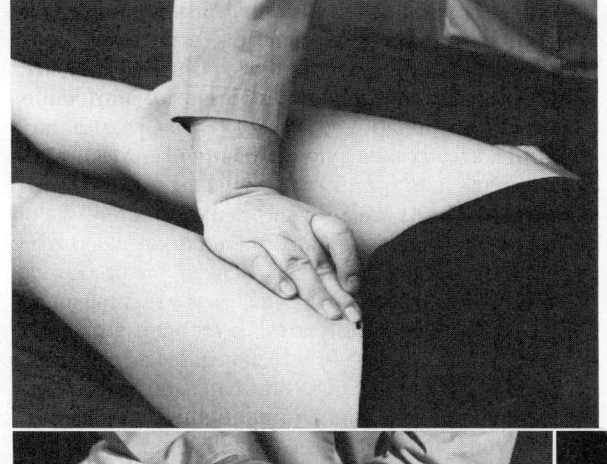

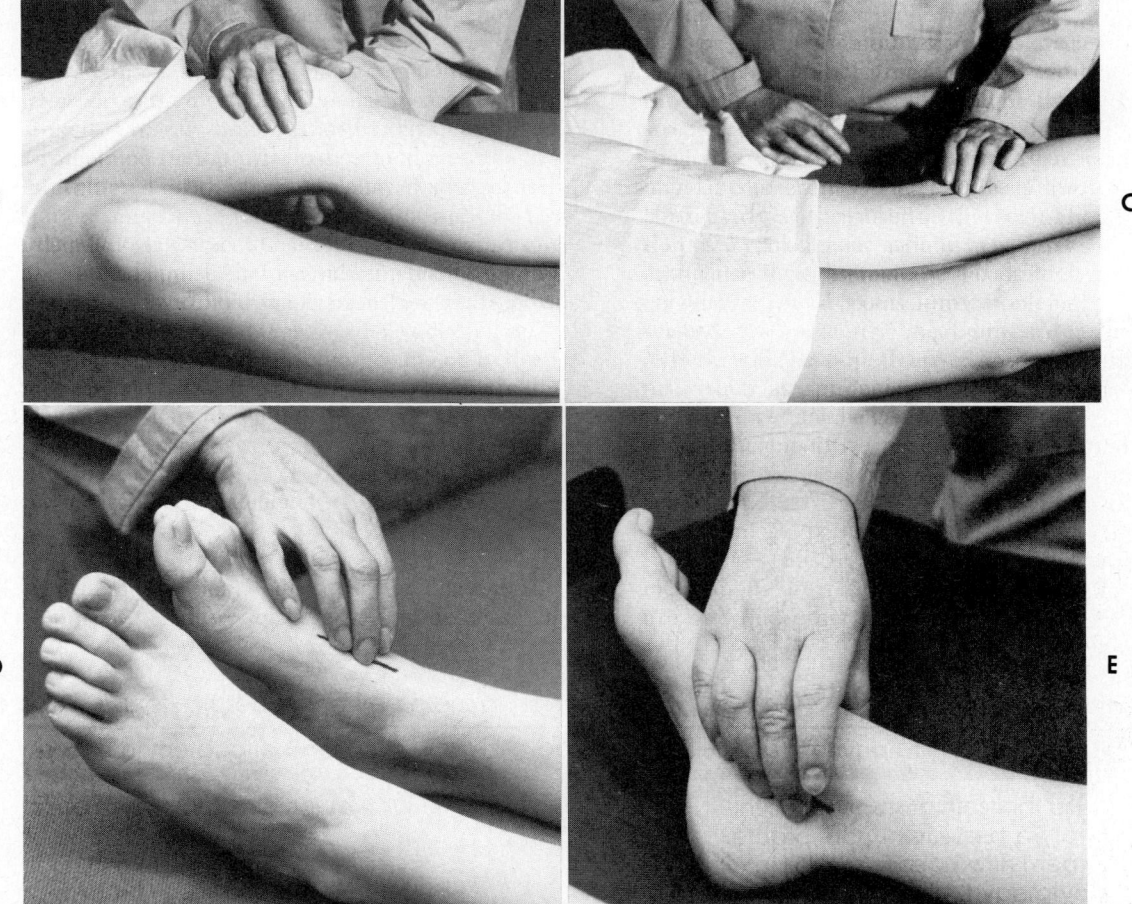

Fig. 27-6. A, Palpation of femoral pulse. **B,** Palpation of popliteal pulse with client in dorsal recumbent position. **C,** Palpation of popliteal pulse with client in the prone position. **D,** Palpation of dorsal pedal pulse. **E,** Palpation of posterior tibial pulse. (From Malasanos, L., et al.: Health assessment, ed. 2, St. Louis, 1981, The C.V. Mosby Co.)

osclerosis. The patient walks or exercises until pain occurs in the extremity. The time is recorded for the onset of pain and the relief of pain following a timed period of rest.

The pain in the muscles is caused by the peripheral vascular arterial insufficiency to the mucles and the accumulation of toxic wastes in the ischemic tissues.

Plethysmography

Plethysmography measures variations in the electrical resistance associated with changes in blood volume. Venous flow is occluded with a cuff, and, as blood pools in the extremity, changes in resistance are measured via electrodes that are connected to a recorder from the extremity. It is a common tool used for assessing arterial flow to the hands, feet, and calves. It is sometimes used in combination with exercise to gain more information about functional capacity during exercise.

Lumbar sympathetic block

The *lumbar sympathetic block* is used to evaluate peripheral circulation. A local anesthetic is injected into the lumbar epidural space to block the sympathetic nerves that go to the legs. Blocking these nerves to the muscles of the blood vessels produces vasodilation and a definite warming and drying of the skin on the same side as the injection. In the presence of atherosclerosis the blood vessels fail to dilate, and the change in the skin may be minimal or absent.

Oscillometry

Oscillometric readings help determine the effectiveness of the larger arteries by measuring their pulsations. A pneumatic cuff is placed around the extremity at desired levels and is connected to a delicate diaphragm that transmits arterial pressure to a needle attached to a dial. The reading is measured in units called the *oscillometric readings*.

DATA ANALYSIS AND PLANNING

Nursing diagnoses

Possible nursing diagnoses for the person with arterial disorders may include the following:

Comfort, alteration in: pain in legs

Injury, potential for

Mobility, impaired physical

Tissue perfusion, alteration in: peripheral

Anxiety

Knowledge deficit

Expected patient outcomes

Expected patient outcomes are related to the nursing diagnoses and include the following:

1. Patient will have relief of pain
2. No injuries will occur
3. Anxiety will be relieved
4. Ambulation is increased
5. The patient can
   a. Describe the nature of the disorder
   b. Describe factors that precipitate exacerbation of symptoms
   c. Describe the treatment regimen
   d. Describe plans for follow-up care

IMPLEMENTATION

Assisting with achievement of therapeutic goals
Medications

Vasodilators may be used in elected instances, that is, for atherosclerosis, Raynaud's phenomenon, and arterial embolism. They may be tried but generally are not prescribed for thromboangiitis obliterans, because dilation of all blood vessels may divert blood flow away from the partially occluded vessels.

Patients being treated with medications for peripheral vascular disease must understand the purpose of the medication and the way in which it is to be taken.

ANTICOAGULANTS. Anticoagulants commonly used in the treatment of venous and arterial thrombosis are as follows:

Heparin

Coumadin

Ethyl biscoumacetate (Tromexan)

Dicumarol

Prothrombin

They act by doing the following:

1. Prolonging the clotting time of blood
2. Preventing thrombus formation when used with threatened thrombosis or thrombophlebitis
3. Preventing further extension of a clot and formation of new clots

Patient teaching is as follows:

1. Prothrombin time may be done two or three times a week, eventually every 1 to 4 weeks.
2. Dosage may change with each blood test.
3. Recognize signs of bleeding from any site and report them immediately. Bleeding from the gums while brushing the teeth may be an early sign.
4. Carry identification card or wear Medic-Alert bracelet with drug name and name and number of physician.
5. Do not take any other medications, especially aspirin, without consulting the physician.

VASODILATORS. Vasodilators commonly used in the treatment of peripheral vascular diseases are as follows:

Papaverine

Phenoxyhenamine (Dibenzyline)

Azapetine (Ilidar)

Tolazoline (Priscoline)

Isoxsuprine (Vasodilan)

Cyclandelate (Cyclospasmol)

Dibenzylchlorethamine (Dibenamine)

Nylidrin (Arlidin)

Nicotinyl alcohol (Roniacol)

They act by lessening vasospasm in the arterioles of the lower extremities when:

1. Arteriosclerosis has caused narrowing of the blood vessels
2. A thrombus has formed and caused partial or total obstruction

Patient teaching is as follows:

1. Toxic reactions to medications must be reported at once.
2. Toxic signs include palpitation, tachycardia, nausea and vomiting, pruritus and abnormal skin sensations, and drop in blood pressure causing dizziness.

FIBRINOLYTICS. Fibrinolytics commonly used topically or systemically are as follows:

Streptodornase-streptokinase (Varidase)

Trypsin (Tryptar)

Fibrinolysin (Elase)

There are ointment forms that do the following:

1. Dissolve fibrinous material and purulent accumulations

2. Remove necrotic tissue in debridement procedure
Patient teaching is as follows:
1. These topical medications are ordered in treatment of leg ulcers.
2. Patient may be applying antibiotics in conjunction with the enzymes to promote more rapid healing.
3. Medications are usually applied topically in the form of wet dressings.

MEDICATIONS FOR SYSTEMIC USE

Streptokinase and urokinase are more recent fibrinolytic agents used in treating thrombosis. Both are given intravenously or intraarterially. Their disadvantages are that streptokinase has a high incidence of allergic reactions, and the high cost of urokinase prevents its wide use.

Surgery

Surgery may be necessary for several of the vascular disorders.

ARTERIAL BYPASS SURGERY AND RECONSTRUCTION. If *atherosclerosis obliterans* is rapidly progressing and intermittent claudication has become gravely disabling, surgery to correct the obstruction is indicated. The most common procedure is a bypass of the obstructed arterial segment, using prosthetic material such as Teflon or Dacron or autogenous (the patient's own) artery or vein, such as the saphenous vein. The bypass may involve the aorta itself, as with an aortofemoral bypass, or more distal vessels such as the femoral-popliteal (Fig. 27-7). Procedures that may be performed either in conjunction with a bypass or by themselves include *patch grafting* (replacing a damaged segment of the arterial wall with a vein patch), *profundo-*

Surgical procedure for arterial disorders

Atherosclerosis obliterans	Arterial bypass and reconstruction or amputation of limb
Raynaud's phenomenon	Sympathectomy
Arterial emboli	Embolectomy or endarterectomy
Aneurysm	Surgical removal of aneurysm
Arteriovenous fistula	Surgical closure of fistula

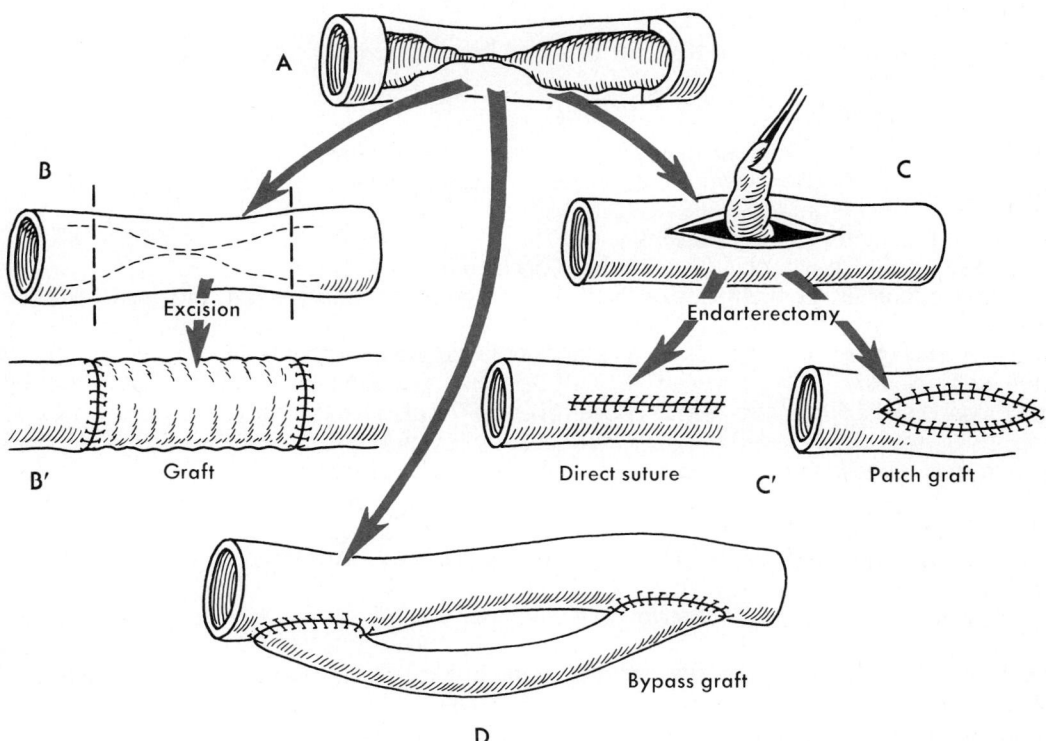

Fig. 27-7. A, Obstructed artery. Methods of restoring arterial blood flow include **B,** excision, **B',** graft; **C,** endarterectomy; **C',** direct suture and patch graft reconstruction; and **D,** bypass graft. (Redrawn from Fairbairn, J.F., Jurgens, J.L., Spittell, J.A.: Peripheral vascular disease, Philadelphia, 1972, W.B. Saunders Co.)

Nursing intervention for the patient having arterial reconstruction

1. Check color, temperature, sensation, and quality of peripheral pulses hourly for first 8 hours
2. Record blood pressures
3. Administer vasopressor or vasodilator drugs as prescribed
4. Observe for untoward reaction such as myocardial infarction, which may occur because of underlying disease process
5. Allow out of bed when permitted:
   a. Caution against sharp flexion in area of the graft
   b. Caution against leg crossing and prolonged extremity dependency
6. Check for signs of infection in incisional areas: redness, swelling, purulent drainage

---

plasty (widening of the origin of the femoral artery with a vein patch), and *endarterectomy* (stripping arteriosclerotic plaques from the intima and inner media using balloon catheters or other instruments). Postoperative nursing assessment and interventions are outlined here.

AMPUTATION. Although a partial or complete amputation of an extremity may be necessary as a result of sarcoma or trauma, the majority are necessitated by atherosclerosis obliterans. The surgery may be necessary at any age. The level of the amputation is determined by the extent of diseased tissue removal needed to preserve functioning extremity.

TYPES OF AMPUTATION

Below-the-knee (BK) amputations make up about one third of all amputations for peripheral vascular disease. This amputation is usually done in the middle third of the leg, leaving a stump at 12.5 to 17.5 cm (5 to 7 inches) below the knee. This type of amputation is preferable for younger persons who will remain physically active, because preservation of knee function permits a more natural gait. Also, the lower the level of amputation, the less energy and balance will be required for walking.

Nursing intervention for patient having amputation surgery

Preoperative intervention

1. Accept patient's reaction of distress, anger or grief, and discouragement
2. Coordinate essentials of patient care among patient, nurses, physician, and physical therapist
3. Discuss with patient and family:
   a. Information about the surgical procedure
   b. What to expect with the rehabilitative program and the use of the prosthesis
   c. Postoperative routines: positioning, exercises to strengthen thigh muscles and prevent knee and hip contractures
   d. Exercises to strengthen arm muscles such as push-ups and weight lifting
   e. Crutch walking
   f. Amputation dressings and the use of a cast over the residual limb (The cast reduces edema, hastens stump shrinkage, and provides for attachment of metal pylon.)
   g. Phantom limb sensation as a normal occurrence following amputation

Postoperative intervention

1. Check plaster cast over the stump; in the base of the cast is a metal socket to which a pylon will be attached for weight bearing (Fig. 27-8)
2. Observe for signs and symptoms of a pulmonary embolus
3. Monitor vital signs
4. Observe stump dressing for signs of hemorrhage; mark outside of the dressing so rate of bleeding can be quickly assessed
5. Avoid hip and/or knee contractures
6. If traction has been applied to the stump to prevent retraction of skin and muscle away from the surgical incision, provide for position changes without disturbing pulleys and weights

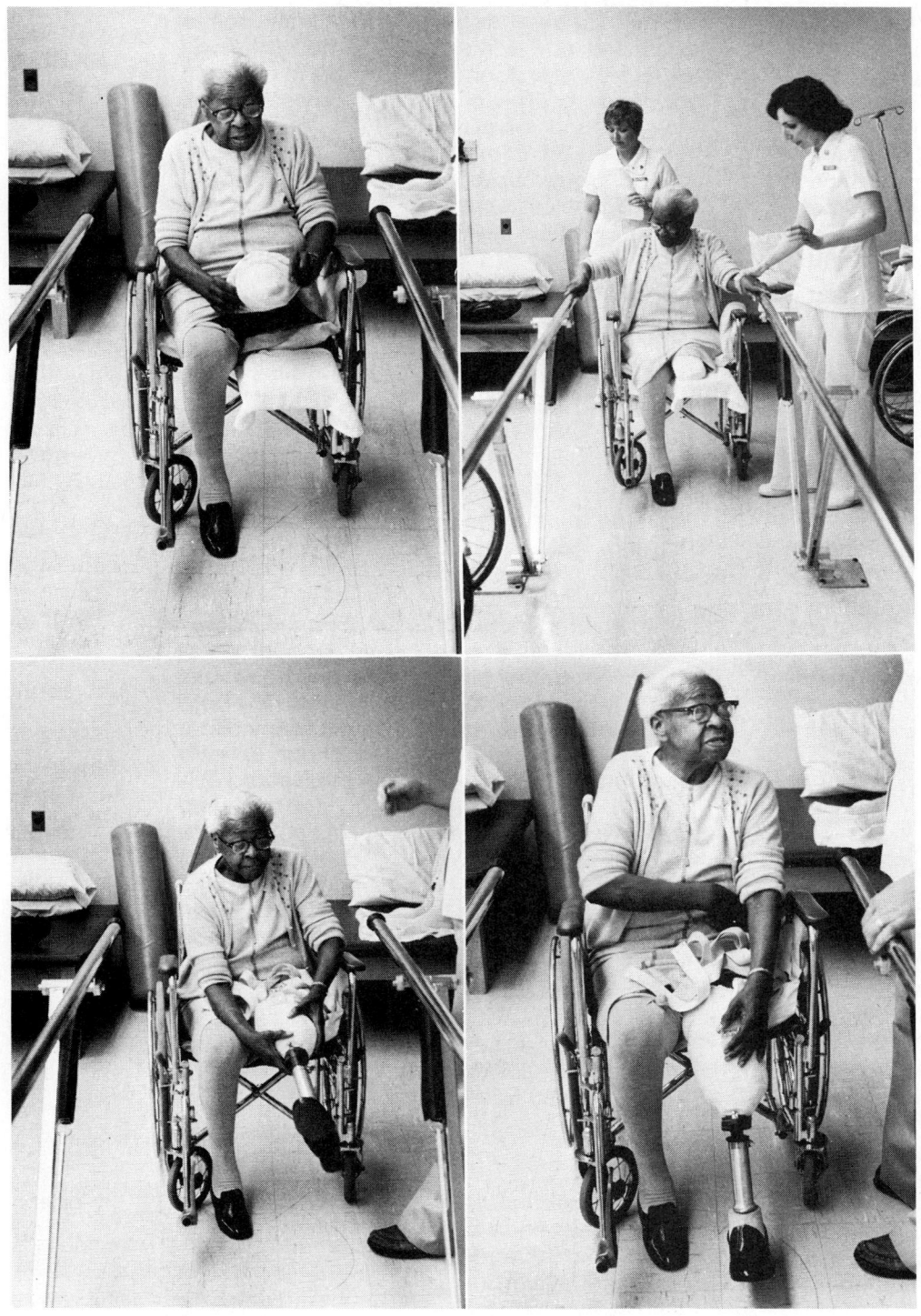

Fig. 27-8. Patient with cast on stump with metal pylon attached for weight bearing.
Continued.

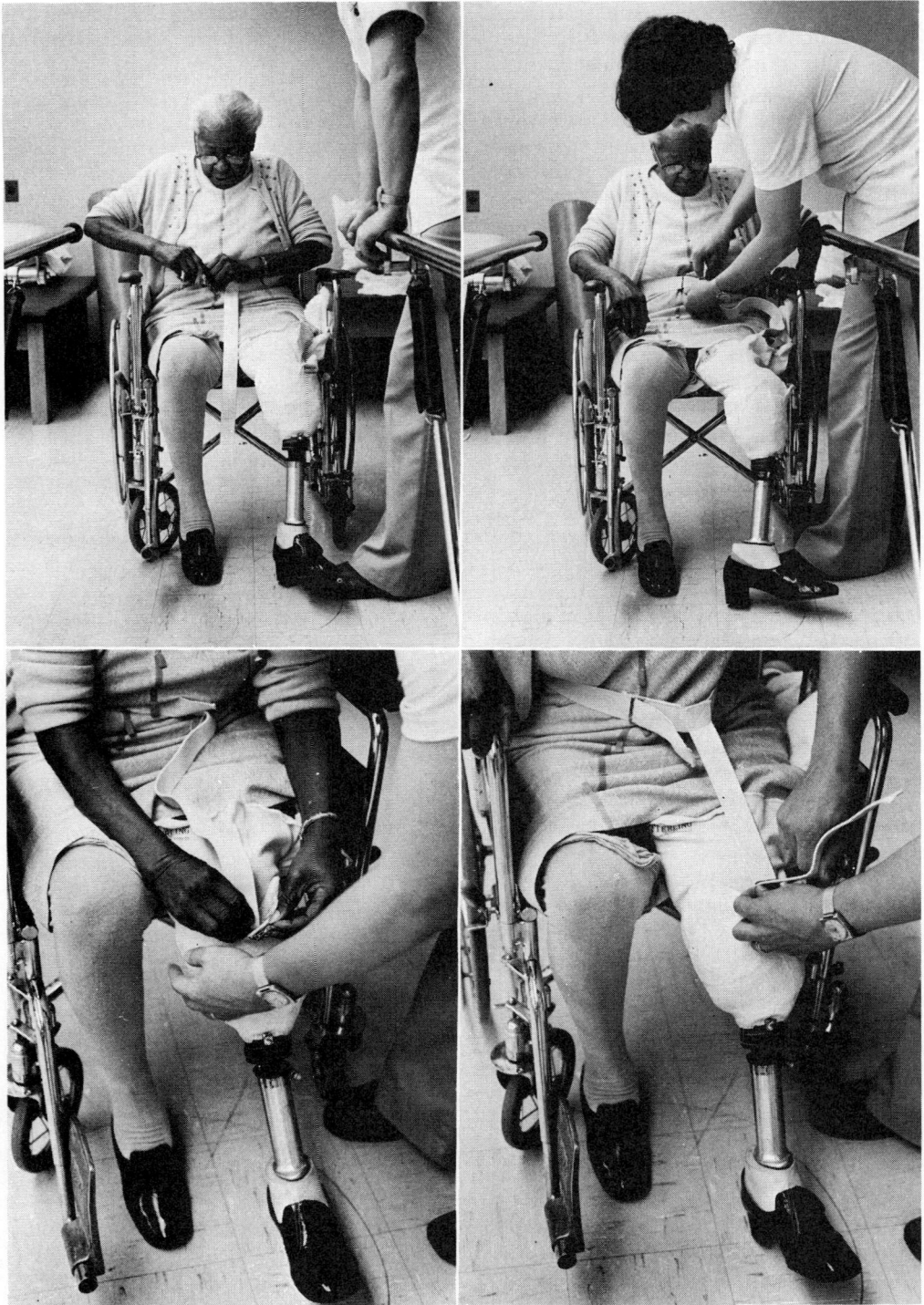

Fig. 27-8, cont'd. Patient with cast on stump with metal pylon attached for weight bearing.

Above-the-knee (AK) amputations are frequently necessary because of the extent of disease. The most important factor in determining the level of amputation is the adequacy of arterial blood supply, and although the BK amputation is preferred for rehabilitation, the AK procedure has been found to require reamputation less frequently, and it heals more successfully. The AK amputation is usually performed between the lower third to the middle of the thigh. In amputating a limb the surgeon attempts to leave a stump that permits satisfactory use of prosthesis.

COUNSELING AND TEACHING

1. Exercises
   a. Range-of-motion exercises are started early to prevent flexion contracture of the hip and knee.
   b. In bed, use overhead trapeze bar for self-help in moving. This strengthens the biceps muscles; most imporant for crutch walking.
   c. Out of bed, begin self-care activities such as rising from a chair and standing. Pushing up from a chair strengthens the triceps muscles. Teach patient to preserve center of gravity and balance

with remaining leg under him or her when rising. The nurse can assume a position in front of or behind the patient with firm grip on his/her waist.

2. Stump care
   a. Inspect for redness, blisters, or abrasions.
   b. Give daily care to the stump: bathe with mild soap, rinse, and pat dry. Do no soak, use alcohol, oils, or creams.
   c. If bandage is used, remove bandage twice daily; give care as described previously and reapply in firm, even bandage. (Bandage dressing is used to reduce swelling and to shape the stump [Fig. 27-9].)
   d. If stump sock is used, change daily and more often if needed. Wash in warm water with a mild soap, rinse in warm water, lay it flat on a towel to dry. Stump sock is worn to absorb perspiration and protect the skin from contact with the prosthetic socket. The stump sock must fit smoothly without wrinkles. Do not repair sock; the repaired area will cause pressure.

3. Remaining extremity: care of the remaining foot and

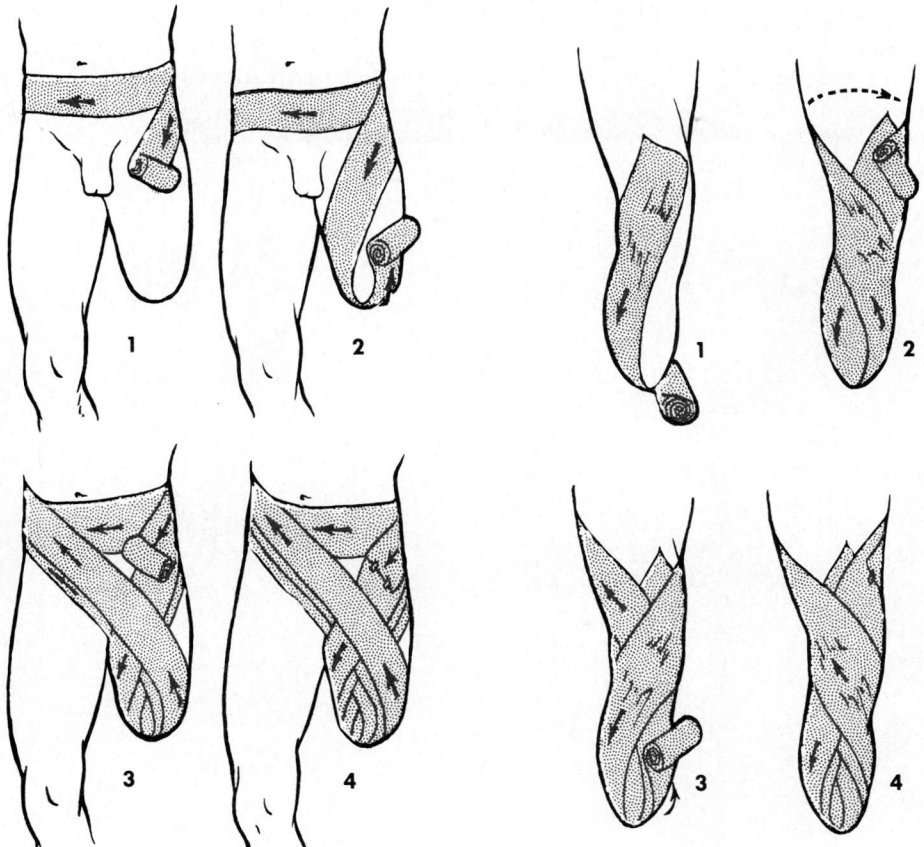

Fig. 27-9. Left, correct method of bandaging midthigh amputation stump. Note the bandage must be anchored around patient's waist. Right, correct method for bandaging midcalf amputation stump. Note that bandage need not be anchored about waist.

leg is particularly vital. Arterial supply must be maintained by exercises and skin care (p. 709).

4. Crutch walking: teaching the patient crutch-walking gaits often becomes the responsibility of the nurse if a physical therapist is not available.

ESSENTIALS OF CRUTCH WALKING

Crutches should be measured for each patient. In *method 1,* the patient lies on the back with the arms at sides. The measurement is taken from the axilla to a point 15 cm (6 inches) out from the side of the heel. This is the length of the crutch minus 1.9 cm (¾ inch) for crutch tips. In *method 2,* the patient is measured from 5 cm (2 inches) below the level of the axilla to the base of the heel. In *method 3,* 40 cm (16 inches) is subtracted from the patient's total height. Even with careful measurement, alterations may have to be made after the crutches are used. Posture, for example, may change, altering the length needed. The crutches should not cause pressure on the axillae, and the patient is taught not to rest the weight on the axillary bars more than a few minutes at a time. Pressure on the axillae causes pressure on the brachial plexus, which can lead to severe and sometimes permanent paralysis of the arms ("crutch paralysis"). The patient is taught that weight should be borne on the palms of the hands.

Before attempting crutch walking, the patient is assisted out of bed and should stand with help to get the feel of normal balance. A walker or parallel bars may be used until the patient feels secure (Fig. 27-10). At this time the patient begins to practice correct standing posture with head up, chest up, abdomen in, pelvis tilted inward, a 5-degree angle in the knee joint, and the foot straight. Practice in front of a mirror is very helpful. The patient is encouraged not to look toward the foot. Next the patient should practice standing while supported by crutches to get the "feel" of them. The nurse should be sure that the patient begins at this time to bear weight on the palms and not on the axillae (Fig. 27-11). Before the patient begins to try to use crutches, the proper hand and arm position and gait should be demonstrated. This will help the patient understand what is to be done. In all crutch walking the patient is taught to concentrate on a normal rhythmic gait, such as the *three-point gait* (Fig. 27-12).

The first gait that the patient wil use is the *swing-through* (Fig. 27-13, *A*) or *swing-to gait* (Fig. 27-13, *B*), which require no carefully guided instruction if the patient knows how to bear weight and has been taught to check posture, balance, and rhythm. In this gait the amputated limb and the crutches both advance either to or beyond the level of the normal limb and are followed by the normal leg. This is a simple, fast gait that gives little leg exercise but is useful for rapid maneuvers such as are needed in crossing streets. The patient may use this gait when beginning to walk with one prosthesis.

When the patient with double amputations has been fitted with prostheses, the *four-point gait* (Fig. 27-13, *C*) may be taught. This gait is taught to the count of four as follows: right crutch, left foot, left crutch, right foot.

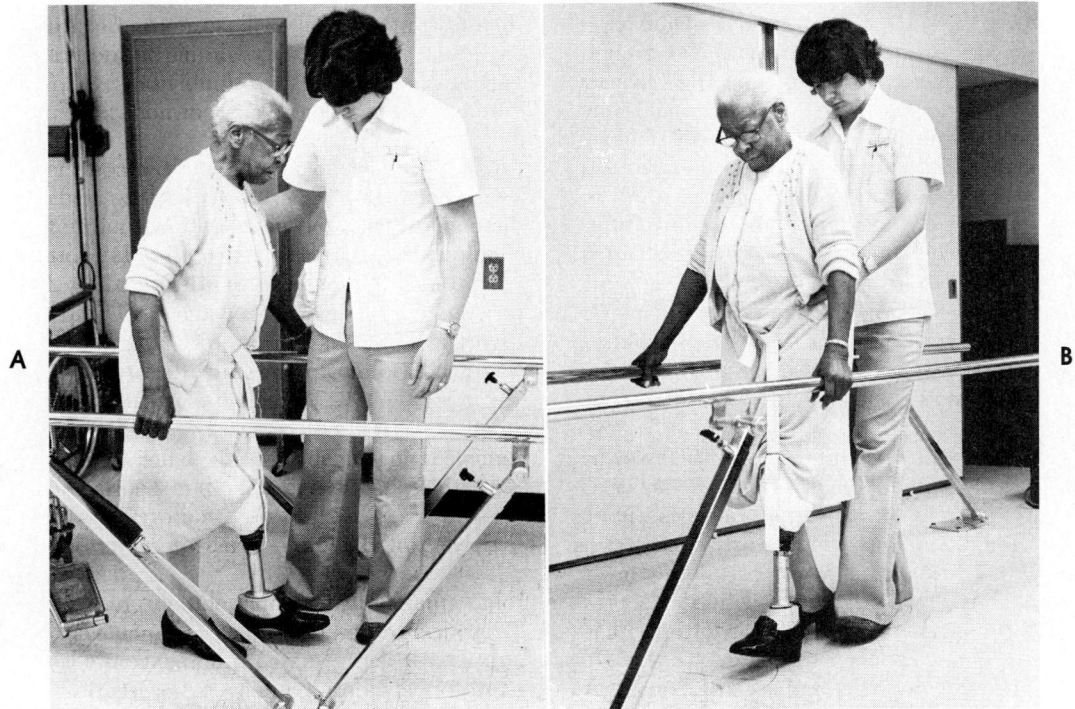

Fig. 27-10. A, Patient steps forward on the prosthesis while using the bars for stability. **B,** walking behind the patient enables the therapist to assess her gait.

Some patients with bilateral amputations must always use this gait (which is also widely used by those with involved neuromuscular disabilities and poor balance). It is a safe gait because the patient always has three points of contact with the ground at any time. Most patients progress to the *two-point gait,* in which the foot and the opposite crutch move together and then the prosthesis and the opposite crutch. It is often taught to the count of two as follows: left crutch and right foot (one) and right crutch and left foot (two). The two-point gait is much faster and is easier to maintain in a rhythmic pattern than the four-point gait.

The patient with one prosthesis may progress to one crutch and then to a cane, which should be abandoned eventually. The crutch or cane should be held in the hand on the side *opposite* the prosthesis because, as the patient normally walks, the arm on the opposite side of the body alternately swings forward. Holding the cane or crutch on the same side as the prosthesis results in an awkward, unrhythmic gait.

It is important for the nurse to know which gait the physical therapist is teaching the patient so that he/she may be reminded not to revert to a previous gait. It is to be expected that the patient with a double amputation will learn to manage much more slowly than a patient with a single amputation. Persons with AK amputations also take much longer to learn to walk and otherwise manage their movements than persons with BK amputations.

EMBOLECTOMY AND ENDARTERECTOMY. Unresponsiveness to the medical therapy will necessitate choice of a surgical procedure. Surgery may be necessary within a few hours to prevent muscle necrosis and loss of the extremity. *Embolectomy* is the treatment of choice when a large artery has been occluded. The blood vessel is opened, and the clot is removed. *Endarterectomy* or *"reaming"* may be done. This is the removal of the clot and substances adhering to the vessel wall and also a part of the lining of the vessel (Fig. 27-7).

REMOVAL OF ANEURYSM AND CLOSURE OF FISTULA. The blood vessel may be ligated unless the procedure is incompatible with the life of tissues distal to the lesion. Homografts (a section of the patient's vein) or Teflon or Dacron grafts may be used in larger blood vessels of the extremities either to replace the portion of the artery that contains the aneurysm or to bypass the abnormality.

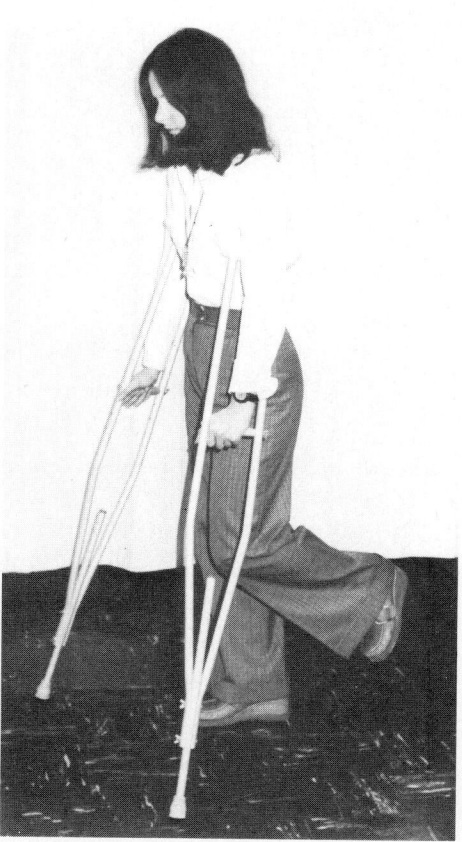

Fig. 27-11. Axillary crutches are ambulatory aids best used by young persons or persons with good motor ability, particularly if patient is non-weight bearing on one leg. Here patient has good balance and erect posture.

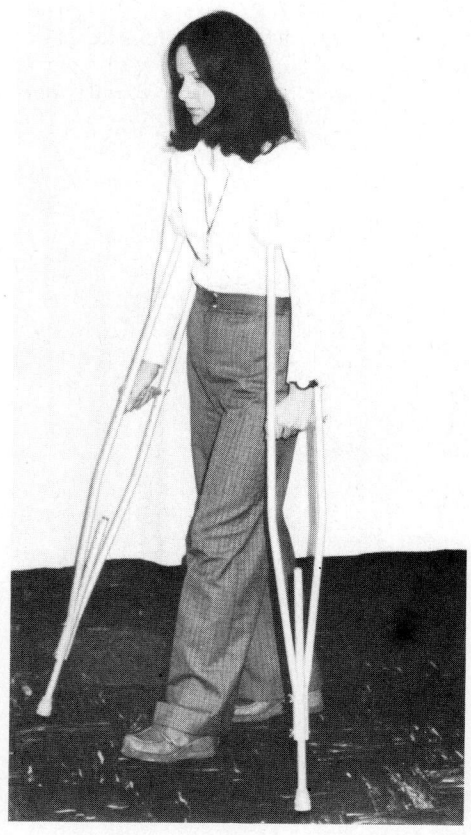

Fig. 27-12. Three-point is more stable crutch gait and can be used by most patients who can use walker. It provides for greater mobility than walker, so patient may also negotiate stairs.

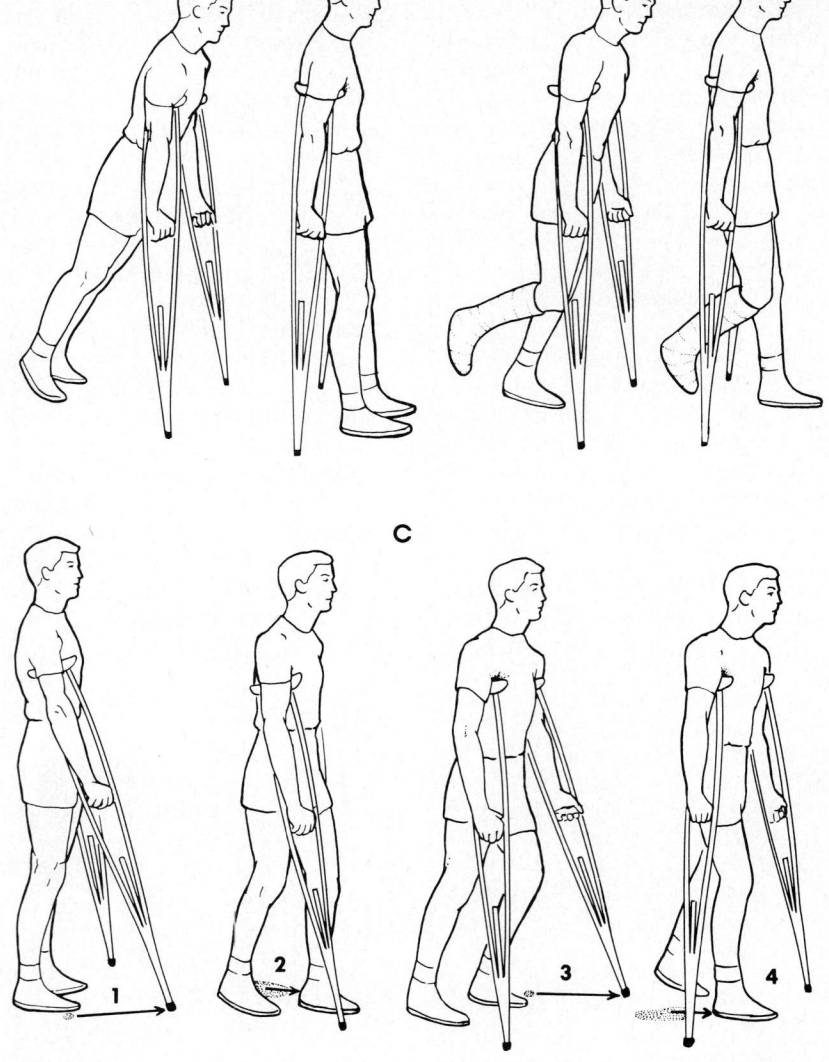

Fig. 27-13. A, Swing through gait. **B,** Swing to gait. **C,** Four point gait.

Nursing care of the patient having surgical removal of a thrombus

Preoperative nursing intervention

1. Maintain bed rest
2. Keep extremity flat in bed
3. Provide warmth and freedom from bed linen weight
4. Administer medications as prescribed
5. Observe and record blood pressure, pulses, skin and extremity changes
6. Record pain, site, intensity, and measures that relieve pain
7. Observe and record any untoward effects to other parts of the body

Postoperative nursing intervention

1. Encourage movement of extremity as prescribed to stimulate circulation
2. Assess surgical wound for evidence of hemorrhage
3. Assess and record pulses, especially the distal pulses
4. Record blood pressures; compare to preoperative status
5. Begin health teaching appropriate to patient's health history and findings on physical examination

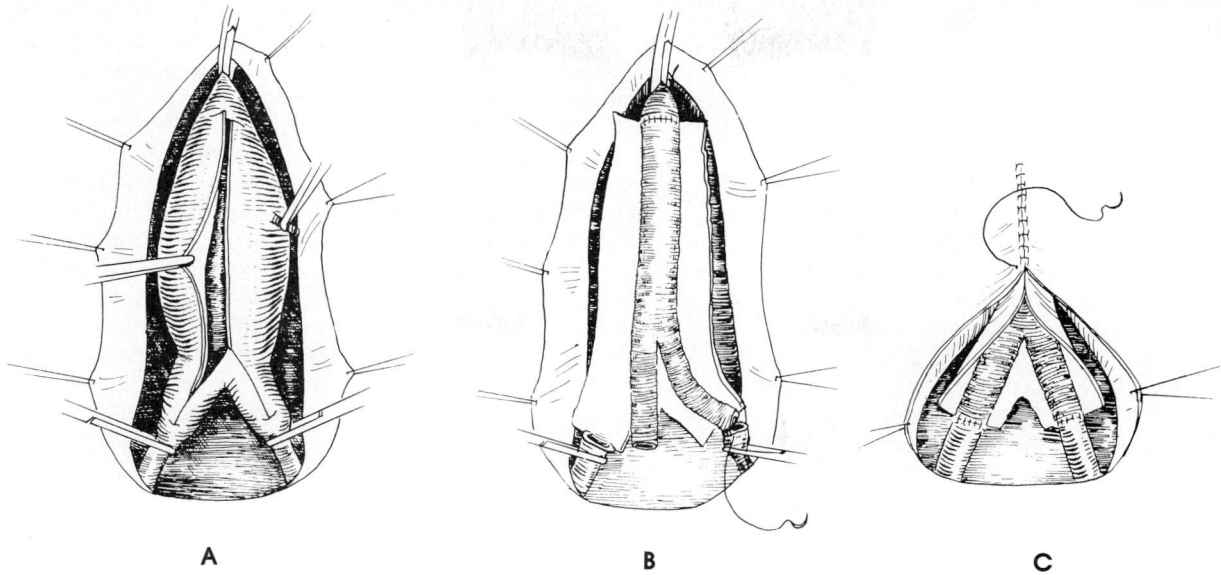

A   B   C

Fig. 27-14. Abdominal aneurysm. **A,** Aneurysm of the aorta and iliac arteries. **B,** Bifurcation graft used to replace the excised aneurysm. **C,** Closure of the posterior peritoneum over the graft and suture line. (Redrawn from Crawford, E.S., et al.: Surg. Clin North Am. **46:**963-978, 1966.)

Fig. 27-14 illustrates the excision of an aneurysm and its replacement with a synthetic graft. Popliteal function is better at the flexion crease when the patient's own vein is used.

Preoperative and postoperative nursing assessment and nursing care are similar to that for the patient having surgery for removal of a thrombus.

Teaching the patient with arterial disorders

Patient education is important in preventing exacerbations of symptoms and arterial occlusion. Preventive health teaching is described in detail in the earlier part of the chapter. The following topics should be included in the teaching program:

1. Avoidance of smoking
2. Need to keep the extremities warm and to avoid cold and trauma
3. Need for moderate exercise within limits of discomfort
4. Prevention of infection and skin breakdown
5. Avoidance of leg massage
6. Diet to avoid or control atherogenic disease
7. Need to report changes in temperature and skin color of extremities or increase in pain
8. Need for medical follow-up

EVALUATION

Evaluation is based on expected patient outcomes. Questions to ask may include the following:

1. Is patient able to increase activity without added discomfort?
2. Has injury been avoided?
3. Can the patient describe the nature of the disorder and the treatment regimen?
4. Can the patient describe ways to prevent exacerbations of symptoms?
5. Is patient continuing with follow-up care?

VENOUS AND LYMPH DISORDERS

The veins transport blood from the capillary beds back to the heart. The walls of the veins are thinner and less muscular than those of the arteries, thus allowing for greater distensibility with changes in pressure. Veins of the extremities carrying blood against gravity are equipped with valves. The effectiveness of the valves and the competency of the veins are important in the prevention of venous disease. The etiology, signs and symptoms, and medical therapy for thrombophlebitis and varicose veins are described in Table 27-2.

Thrombophlebitis

PATHOPHYSIOLOGY

Thrombophlebitis or venous thrombosis is inflammation of the vessel wall with formation of a clot. Venous thrombosis is most frequent in the veins of the lower extremities in both deep and superficial veins. The most frequent veins affected are the saphenous, the femoral, and popliteal veins and the small veins of the calf.

The thrombus can grow larger with successive layering of platelets, fibrin, white blood cells, and red blood cells. The greatest danger to the patient is the breaking off of

Table 27-2. Venous disorders

Disease	Etiology	Signs and symptoms	Medical therapy
Thrombophlebitis	Venous stasis from heart failure, shock, immobility Conditions reducing blood flow return to lower abdomen: pregnancy, malignant tumors, obesity Trauma to venous walls: fractures, intravenous drugs or hypertonic intravenous solutions or presence of a catheter Increased coagulability of blood caused by blood dyscrasias such as polycythemia, severe anemia, oral contraceptives Abrupt withdrawal of anticoagulant medications	Entire limb may be swollen, pale, and cold Area along the vein may be reddened and feel warm to touch Homans' sign: pain in calf on dorsiflexion of the foot Superficial veins feel hard and thready, and are sensitive to pressure	Bed rest with activity as ordered Warm moist packs may be ordered for deep and superficial thrombophlebitis (ice packs may be preferred) Elevation of extremity Heparin and coumadin as ordered (p. 704) Vasodilators (p. 704) to combat arterial spasms and improve circulation Streptokinase to resolve the thrombus
Varicose veins	Congenitally defective venous valves Hereditary weakness of the vein walls Prolonged standing, placing strain on valves in addition to lack of muscle action to help return of blood Poor posture with sagging abdominal organs Pregnancy and abdominal tumors interfering with good venous return Chronic systemic disease causing poor venous return to the heart: Heart disease Cirrhosis of the liver Infection in and trauma to the veins leading to thrombophlebitis and eventual varicosities when the valves become incompetent or destroyed	Veins appear as darkened, tortuous raised blood vessels; more pronounced on prolonged standing Feeling of heaviness in the legs Fatigue Pain and muscle cramps Edema	Conservative treatment: Elevate feet for short time at least every 2 to 3 hours Wear elastic stocking Weight reduction nutrition program Posture improvement Surgical treatment (p. 716)

a portion of the thrombus, producing signs of an embolus (Fig. 27-15). Emboli being carried back to the heart can lodge in the coronary arteries or elsewhere. The most common are pulmonary emboli.

ASSESSMENT

Subjective data

1. First symptom noted by patient
2. Pain: when first occured, activity that produces pain, intensity, site
3. Changes noted in extremity

4. Presence of edema
5. Pain in calf on dorsiflexion of foot (Homans' sign)

Objective data

1. Observe for redness, differences in size of extremities (measure and record)
2. Observe for prominent and superficial veins
3. Palpate for warmth and tenderness from groin to toes
4. Palpate femoral, popliteal, posterior tibial, and dorsalis pedis pulses
5. Elicit Homans' sign with dorsiflexion of the foot
6. Obesity: weigh and record past and present weight

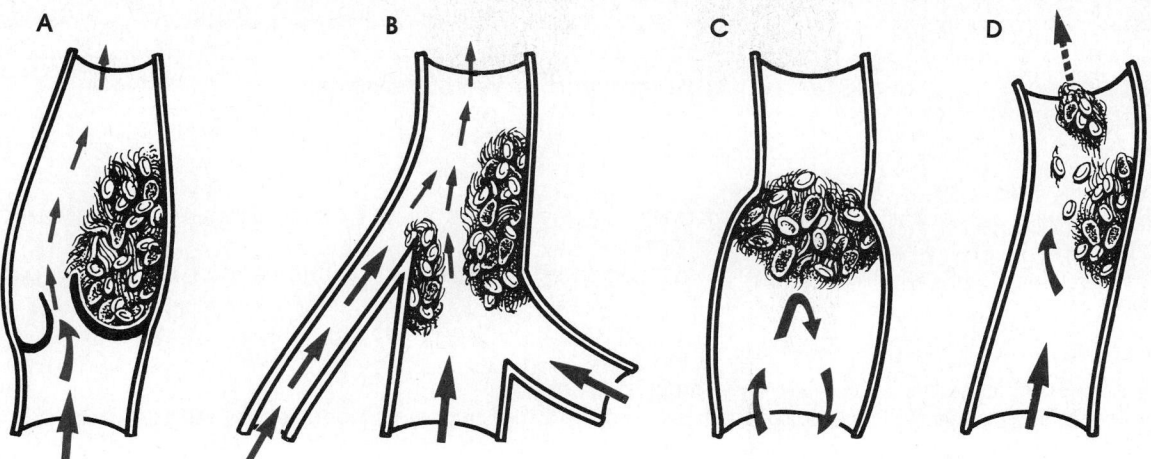

Fig. 27-15. Development of thromboemboli with arrows indicating direction of blood flow. **A,** Thrombus in a valve pocket of a deep vein with blood flowing beside thrombus. **B,** Thrombi tend to form at bifurcations of deep veins with some slowing of blood flow. **C,** Complete occlusion of vein by thrombus forcing back flow of blood. **D,** Embolus which has broken off from thrombus and is floating in blood stream. Could migrate to lungs and cause pulmonary embolus.

Diagnostic tests

Venography (phlebography)

Radioactive isotopes may be used to confirm the presence or absence of deep vein thrombosis. A substance that will become incorporated into the thrombus, such as *fibrinogen* or *urokinase,* is administered intravenously, and the area is scanned by x-rays. An increased uptake of the radioactive material indicates the presence of a thrombus.

The injection is made through a foot vein. This test may not be done, since it does cause a brief vein inflammatory reaction.

Doppler ultrasonography

Ultrasound is used to detect aneurysms and to measure flow through vessels. In *Doppler ultrasonography,* a flow probe or electronic stethoscope is placed over the patient's femoral and popliteal veins. The flow probe directs an ultrasound beam at the involved areas; the beam is reflected off the red cells circulating through the blood vessel back to the probe. The reflection varies according to the rate of flow in the vessel. This change in the frequency of reflected sound according to velocity of the flow is referred to as the Doppler effect (Fig. 27-16). Both extremities are compared for diminished or absent readings over the veins.

Trendelenburg test

The *Trendelenburg test* is the simplest test for varicose veins. The patient lies down with the leg raised until the vein empties completely. A tourniquet is then applied above the knee. The patient stands and the vein is observed as it fills. A normal vein fills from below; a varicose vein fills from above because the valve fails to retain

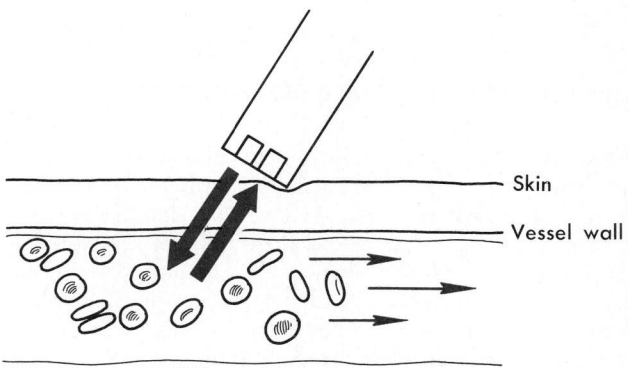

Fig. 27-16. Doppler effect showing red blood cells reflecting sound.

the blood that has drained into the portion of the vessel above.

DATA ANALYSIS AND PLANNING

Nursing diagnoses

Possible nursing diagnoses for the person with thrombophlebitis may include the following:
Mobility, impaired physical
Comfort, alteration in: pain in inflamed extremity
Alteration in nutrition: more than body requirements
Knowledge deficit
Tissue perfusion, alteration in: peripheral

Expected patient outcomes

The patient will be:
1. Free of pain.

Care of the person with a venous surgery

Preoperative nursing assessment and care
1. Palpate and record all peripheral pulses
2. Continue with anticoagulant therapy as ordered by physician; observe for spontaneous bleeding anywhere in the body, for example gastrointestinal or genitourinary system
3. Observe patient for sudden embolus to another part of the body such as the heart or pulmonary vascular system

Postoperative nursing assessment and care
1. Continue with observations as were done preoperatively
2. Avoid stasis and edema in the extremities; begin program of activity as permitted by the physician

---

2. Able to ambulate.
3. Able to describe nutritional plans for body requirements.
4. Able to demonstrate knowledge of medications, exercise, and walking program.
5. Able to demonstrate application of elastic stocking (to be covered under patient teaching).

IMPLEMENTATION

Assisting with achievement of therapeutic goals
Bed rest

Superficial thrombophlebitis is usually treated by rest; however, physicians differ in regard to the amount of activity that is allowed. Some believe that the clot is sufficiently adherent to the vein wall to make its release unlikely and that moving about helps to improve general circulation and to prevent further congestion of blood in the veins. Others believe that complete immobilization is necessary to prevent a part of the thrombus from breaking away and becoming an embolus. The patient who has thrombophlebitis of large and deep vessels, however, usually is kept quiet. Care must be taken that the patient is not frightened by being kept quiet; explanations from both the physician and the nurse will be helpful in reassuring the patient.

Application of moist warm packs

Continuous applications of warm moist heat are often used for both deep and superficial thrombophlebitis. However, some physicians believe that heat increases the risk that emboli will be released, because it induces vasodilation. These physicians order ice packs for their patients, especially for those with deep vein thrombosis. When warm packs are used they are usually ordered to cover the entire extremity. Heating pads permanently set on "low" may be used to keep the packs at a consistently safe temperature.

Elevation of extremity

Many physicians prefer that the affected limb be elevated slightly to reduce edema and to prevent stasis distal to the thrombus. It may also relieve pain. Other physicians believe that the danger of an embolus being released is greater if the limb is elevated. Therefore the nurse will need to determine the procedure to be followed in the care of each patient.

Surgery

If conservative measures such as bed rest and anticoagulation are not successful, if the thrombosis is extensive and recurrent, or if embolization is recurrent, surgery may be necessary. The involved vein, such as the superficial femoral vein, may be ligated, or the vena cava may be interrupted by ligation or by placement of a vena caval umbrella or grid that impedes blood flow (Fig. 27-17).

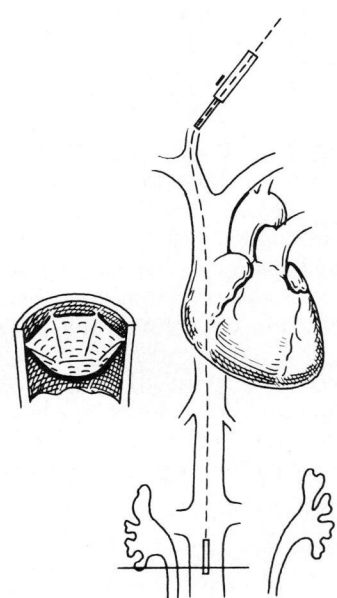

Fig. 27-17. Transvenous method of vena caval interruption using caval prosthesis of umbrella design. Insert illustrates open umbrella. (Redrawn from Fairbairn, J.F., Jergens, J.L., and Spittell, J.A.: Peripheral vascular disease, Philadelphia, 1972, W.B. Saunders Co.)

These procedures are referred to as *ligation* or *plication of the vena cava.*

Counseling and teaching

Following thrombophlebitis in a lower extremity and regardless of treatment that has been chosen, the patient may need to wear an elastic stocking or elastic bandage when up and about.

The elastic stocking or elastic bandage is used to compress the superficial veins, increase flow through the deep veins and prevent venous pooling or stasis.

Activities for prevention of recurrent thrombophlebitis of the lower extremities are encouraged. The physician is consulted as to steps that the nurse will include in the teaching plan.

Patient teaching for use of elastic stocking

1. Measurement must be individualized: check with hospital supply person or with department store for correct method
2. The length of elastic stocking, whether to below the knee or to the groin, must be ordered by the physician
3. Patient is taught to roll stocking on from foot upward before getting out of bed
4. Special skin care daily (p. 698)
5. Stocking may be removed at bedtime
6. Stocking should be laundered as necessary; a second pair should be on hand

---

Patient teaching for activity and exercise

Purpose of teaching is explained to the patient: to decrease venous pressure and promote blood flow by contraction of extremity muscles
1. Begin dorsiflexion of both feet while sitting or lying down
2. Walk daily; increase distance as tolerated
3. Swim several times weekly if possible
4. Use stationary bicycle
5. Begin daily exercises of all parts of the body

EVALUATION

Based on expected patient outcomes, the quetions to be asked may include the following:
1. Is patient able to ambulate without discomfort?
2. Can the patient describe nutritional plans for body requirements and weight maintenance?
3. Can the patient discuss medications, exercise, and walking program?
4. Can the patient demonstrate application of elastic stocking?
5. Is patient continuing with follow-up visits to clinic or physician's office?

Varicose veins
PATHOPHYSIOLOGY

Varicose veins are abnormally dilated veins with incompetent valves, occurring most often in the lower extremities and the lower tunk. In the lower limbs the great and small saphenous veins are most often involved. At least 20% of the total population is affected by varicose veins. The highest incidence is in the third, fourth, and fifth decades of life.

The precipitating factor in varicose vein formation is simply a weakening of the vein wall. Because the vessel wall is weak, it does not withstand normal pressure and dilates with pooling of blood. As the vessel dilates, the valves become stretched and incompetent. This results in the inability to support a column of blood and more venous pooling (Fig. 27-18).

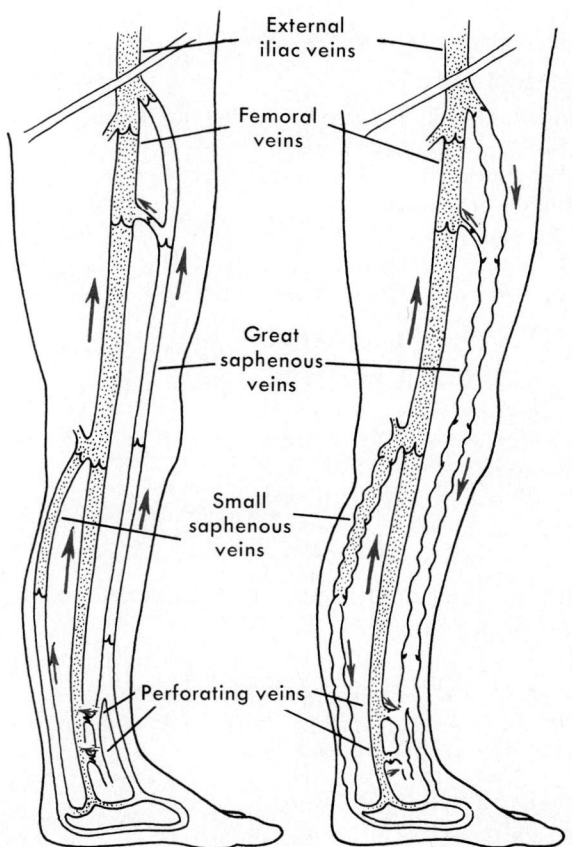

Fig. 27-18. Left, venous flow in normal veins. Right, venous flow in varicose veins. (Redrawn from Fairbairn, J.F., Jurgens, J.L., and Spittell, J.A.: Peripheral vascular disease, Philadelphia, 1972, W.B. Saunders Co.)

ASSESSMENT

Subjective data

Questions that may be asked include the following:
1. When did symptoms first appear and how have the extremities changed in appearance?
2. What is the person's occupation? Amount of standing or sitting on the job?
3. Is there past history of thrombophlebitis?
4. Pregnancies? How did the extremities appear during pregnancy?
5. Does patient have history of heart disease? What is present condition and medical therapy?

Objective data

1. Observe and record appearance of both extremities
2. Palpate pulses in both extremities
3. Palpate vessels for signs and symptoms listed in Table 27-2
4. Assess presence of edema

Diagnostic tests

The tests listed below are described on p. 715.
a. Trendelenburg test
b. Venography
c. Doppler ultrasonography

DATA ANALYSIS AND PLANNING

Nursing diagnoses

Possible nursing diagnoses include the following:
Comfort, alteration in: pain
Tissue perfusion, alteration in: peripheral
Activity intolerance
Nutrition, alteration in: more than body requirements (in presence of obesity)
Self-concept, disturbance in: body image

Expected patient outcomes

The patient will be:
1. Free of pain.
2. Able to walk and be active physically.
3. Able to describe the treatment regimen.
4. Able to describe plans for follow-up care.

IMPLEMENTATION

Assisting with achievement of therapeutic goals

Conservative approach

Rest periods with elevation of feet every 2 to 3 hours
Application elastic stocking during the day
Appropriate daily activity to promote circulation
Beginning weight reduction plan

Surgical intervention

Surgical treatment for varicosities consists of ligation of the vein above the varicosity and removal of the varicosed vein distal to the ligation, provided the deep veins are able to return the venous blood satisfactorily (Fig. 27-19). The great saphenous vein is ligated close to the fem-

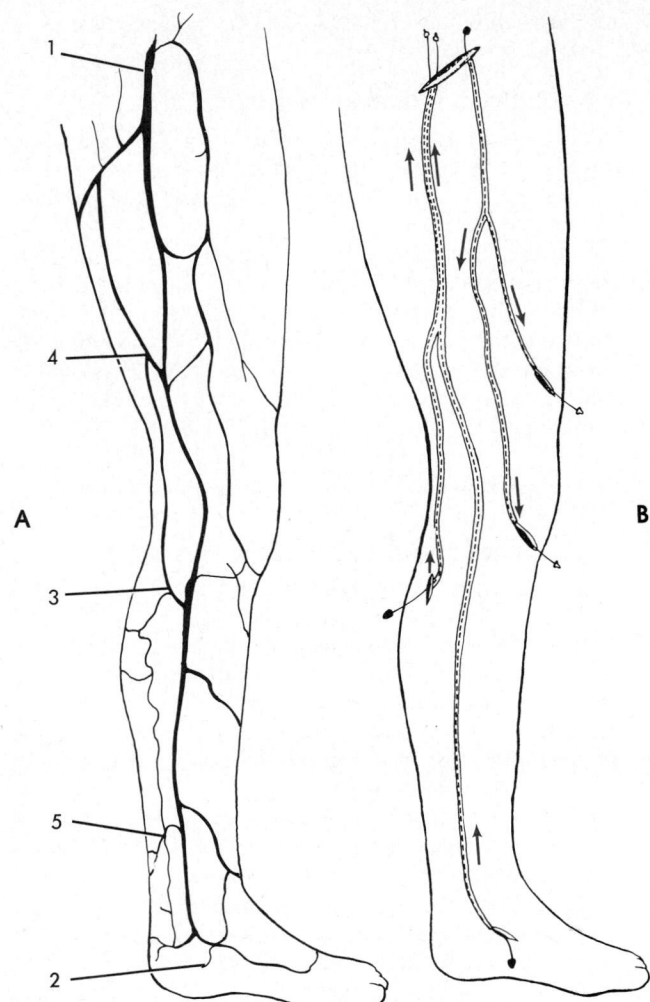

Fig. 27-19. A, Outline of incompetent great saphenous system, with numerals indicating main tributaries. **B,** Passing of strippers in preparation for removal of incompetent veins.

oral junction if possible, and the great and small saphenous veins are then stripped out through small incisions at the groin, above and below the knee, and at the ankle. Sterile dressings are placed over the incisions, and an elastic bandage extending from the foot to the groin is applied firmly. The postoperative care is listed in box on p. 719.

Postoperatively the patient should know that varicose veins may recur, since large superficial collateral vessels may develop and in turn become varicosed. The general teaching plan after surgery remains the same as for the patient being treated conservatively for varicose veins.

Counseling and teaching

1. Avoid tight garters or constricting girdle or pantyhose.
2. Avoid crossing the legs at the knee.
3. Avoid standing or sitting for long periods of time.

Postoperative nursing care for venous ligation

1. Patient is assisted out of bed to walk about beginning on the day of surgery to prevent thrombi in other veins.
2. Analgesics are given for the first 24 to 48 hours for pain and discomfort.
3. Elastic bandage is checked several times a day to avoid looseness and exposure of the incisions.
4. Observe for bleeding, especially on the first postoperative day. If bleeding occurs, elevate the leg, apply pressure over the wound, and notify the surgeon.

Causes of secondary lymphedema

Mastectomy with excision of lymph nodes
Trauma
Malignant tumors
Tissue inflammation
Filariasis (transmitted by mosquitoes)

---

4. Examine occupation and need for modification
   a. Allow for getting up and walking for several minutes every hour.
   b. Dorsiflex the feet at the ankles frequently (at least for a few minutes every hour).
   c. Elevate the legs if possible at the work situation.
   d. Wear elastic stockings.
5. Maintain prescribed daily caloric intake.
6. Avoid poor posture when sitting or standing.

EVALUATION

Based on expected patient outcomes, the questions to be asked may include the following:
1. Is patient able to be free of pain with daily activities, for example, walking?
2. Can the patient describe the treatment regimen?
3. Can the patient describe avoidance of exacerbations of symptoms?
4. Does the patient exhibit improved self-concept?
5. Is the patient continuing with follow-up care?

Lymphedema

PATHOPHYSIOLOGY

Lymphedema occurs primarily as a result of (1) increase in the quantity of lymph, (2) absence of lymphatics, (3) partially or completely blocked lymphatics, or (4) incompetency of the transport system. Lymphedema may be primary (congenital or developing at puberty as a result of hypoplastic development of lymph vessels), or it may be secondary.

SIGNS AND SYMPTOMS

Lymphedema of the lower extremities begins with mild swelling on the dorsum of the foot, usually at the end of the day, which gradually extends to involve the entire limb. The condition is aggravated by the following:
1. Prolonged standing
2. Pregnancy
3. Obesity
4. Warm weather
5. Menstrual period

MEDICAL THERAPY

Treatment is conservative. The goal is to improve lymph drainage. Therapy includes physical therapy, thiazide diuretics, active and passive exercises. This conservative plan of treatment is included in the counseling and teaching section.

ASSESSMENT

Subjective data

1. When first observed and changes since first episode of swelling
2. History must include pregnancies, history of varicosities, weight changes, occupational requirements

Objective data

1. Observe both extremities for edema
2. Palpate peripheral pulses

Diagnostic tests

The lymphography test, in which radiopaque contrast medium is injected into the lymph channels is helpful in differentiating lymphedema from venous disease.

DATA ANALYSIS AND PLANNING

Nursing diagnoses

Possible nursing diagnoses include the following:
Comfort, alteration in: pain
Injury, potential for
Mobility, impaired physical
Self-concept, disturbance in: body image and self-esteem
Skin integrity, impairment of: potential

Tissue perfusion, alteration in: peripheral
Anxiety
Social isolation

Expected patient outcomes

The patient will:
1. Know measures to take to relieve edema (elevating foot of bed, not wearing restrictive clothing).
2. Be free of pain.
3. Be able to be physically active.
4. Have knowledge to alleviate anxiety.

IMPLEMENTATION

Assisting with achievement of therapeutic goals

1. Physical therapy: light manual massage in the direction of the lymph flow is followed by prescribed active and passive exercises to help transport flow into the bloodstream
2. Thiazide diuretics: given to remove the protein from the tissue spaces and allow the fluid to enter the capillaries
3. Nutrition: avoid salty or spicy foods that increase thirst and predispose to fluid retention and edema
4. Continue long-term antibiotics for control of recurrent cellulitis and infection

Assisting with comfort and ADL

1. Wear elastic stockings
2. Avoid constricting clothing
3. Elevate affected extremity when sitting
4. Avoid prolonged standing
5. Walk for short distances daily
6. Daily light massage in the direction of lymph flow[1]
7. Sleep with foot of bed elevated (4 to 8 in)

Counseling and teaching

1. Prepare a teaching plan from material included under prevention and health education (pp. 696-697)
2. Encourage and support
   a. Help patient with emotional reaction to disfigurement
   b. Help patient through depression, social rebuffs, or difficulties encountered in job environment
3. Prepare patient for surgery

Surgical intervention

Surgery is performed to accomplish the following:
Reduce size of extremity
Improve appearance of extremity
Reduce incidence of inflammatory episodes
Limit secondary skin changes associated with chronic lymphedema
Surgery removes hypertrophied lymph channels and edematous subcutaneous tissue, and a bypass is formed to allow lymph flow. The procedure uses skin grafts from other parts of the body.

EVALUATION

The questions to be asked would include the following:
1. Is the patient able to be physically active without discomfort?
2. Does the patient exhibit improved self-image and decreased anxiety?
3. Does the patient see improved social relationships with peers and others?
4. Is the patient able to describe the nature of the disorder and the treatment regimen?

HYPERTENSION

Hypertension is often considered in conjunction with peripheral vascular diseases, since it is a major risk factor in atherosclerosis, the largest single cause of peripheral vascular disease.

Hypertension has been defined as persistent levels of blood pressure above the one accepted by the World Health Organization: "Hypertension is persistent levels of blood pressure in which the systolic pressure is above 140 mm. Hg and the diastolic pressure is above 90 mm. Hg."[55]

Using this definition, it has been estimated that 20 million Americans have hypertension. Of these, about one half remain undiagnosed, and of those in whom the disease has been diagnosed, one half are receiving inadequate or no treatment or have ceased to comply with their treatment regimen.

PATHOPHYSIOLOGY

Blood pressure is determined by two factors: flow and resistance. Blood flow is in turn determined by cardiac output (strength, rate, rhythm of heart beat, and blood volume). The resistance to flow is primarily determined by the diameter of blood vessels and, to a lesser degree, by the viscosity of the blood. Increased peripheral resistance as a result of narrowing of the arterioles is the single most common characteristic in hypertension. Dilation and constriction of peripheral arterioles may be controlled by several mechanisms.

Renal regulation is an essential component of blood pressure control. Fig. 27-20 illustrates the normal steps in the renin-angiotensin system. Note that, as with most natural control mechanisms, this system has a negative feedback loop to prevent excessive response.

Stimulation of the sympathetic nervous system causes the release of the catecholamines epinephrine and norepinephrine. This stimulation can be the result of environmental stressors, adrenal hormones, or autonomic nervous system activity (for example, impulses from the carotid sinus). Epinephrine is an inotropic agent that increases the force of cardiac contraction while narrowing the passageway, causing the blood pressure to increase. Parasympathetic stimulation has the opposite effect, causing relaxation of the smooth muscle of the vessels.

With prolonged hypertension the elastic tissue in arterioles is replaced by fibrous collagen tissue. The thick-

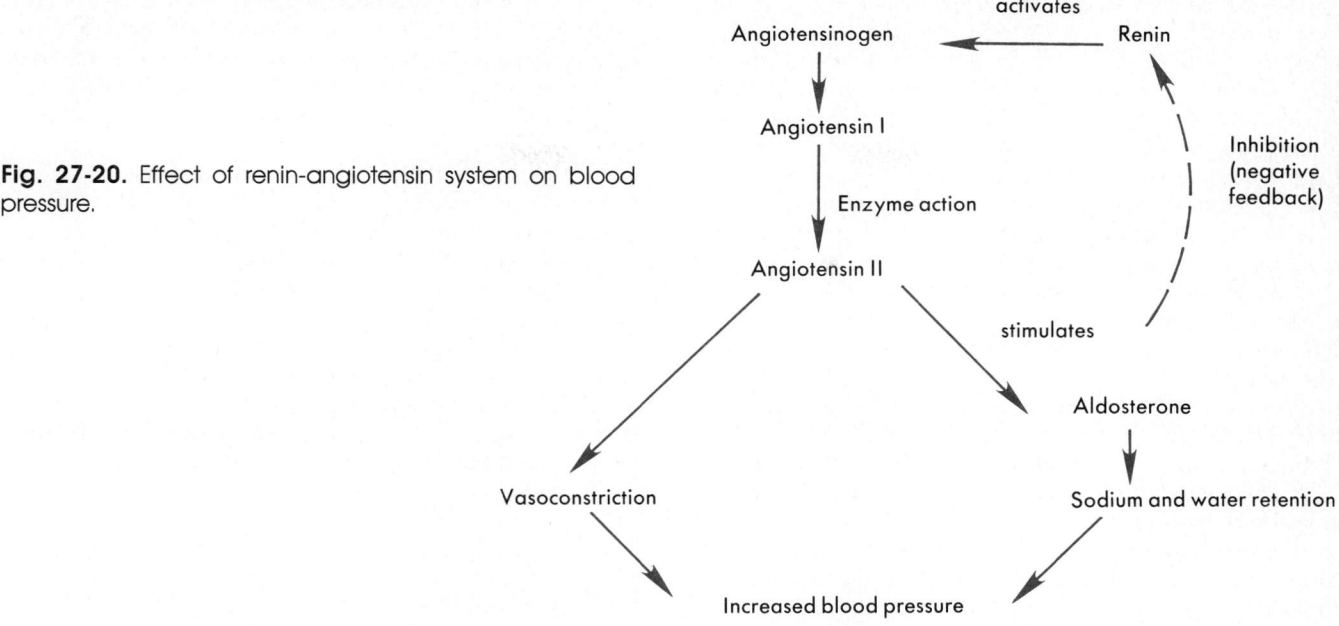

Fig. 27-20. Effect of renin-angiotensin system on blood pressure.

Table 27-3. Hypertension

Etiology	Signs and symptoms	Medical therapy

Primary (essential)
  Risk factors
  Positive family history
  Abnormal sodium retention and water retention
  Sensitivity to the renin-angiotensin system, which regulates both vasoconstriction and sodium retention
  Obesity
  Hypercholesteremia and increased serum triglycerides
  Smoking
  Continuous emotional disturbances
 	
Secondary hypertension
  Coarctation of the aorta
  Adrenal gland: pheochromocytoma, a catecholamine-secreting tumor; Cushing's disease
  Kidney disease; chronic glomerulonephritis (most common known cause)
  Toxemia of pregnancy
  Thyrotoxicosis
  Increased intracranial pressure from tumors or trauma
  Collagen diseases
  Secondary to the effects of certain drugs such as oral contraceptives
	In the early stages, hypertension is essentially asymptopatic. When symptoms do occur, they include:
	1. Headache: occipital and commonly present in the early morning
	2. Vertigo and flushed face
	3. Spontaneous epistaxis
	4. Blurring of vision or scotomas with retinal changes
	5. Nocturnal frequency caused by increased pressure and not by renal disorder
	6. Eventually as consequence of prolonged hypertension:
	  a. Coronary insufficiency and occlusion
	  b. Congestive heart failure
	  c. Renal failure
	  d. Cerebrovascular accident (stroke)
		Antihypertensive drugs (Table 27-4)
		Nutrition:
		1. Reduced caloric intake
		2. Reduced salt intake
		Weight control
		Exercise program

ened arteriole wall then becomes less distensible, offering even greater resistance to the flow of blood. The left ventricle then must exert more force to empty completely; it becomes more distended as it fails to eject a normal stroke volume, and the muscle fibers stretch (hypertrophy) in an attempt to increase the strength of contraction. Inadequate blood supply through the coronary arteries may cause angina pectoris, or a myocardial infarction may occur. Eventually, the hypertrophy of the left ventricle results in congestive heart failure.

Outside the heart itself, the changes in the arteriolar walls may result in permanent damage to organs. The kidney is especially susceptible, and when fibrinoid necrosis occurs in the afferent arteriole, the glomerulus is deprived of its blood supply; permanent kidney damage and possible renal failure result. Cerebral vessels are also frequently affected; neurologic changes or frank stroke may result either from hemorrhage from a leaky vessel or from thrombosis.

Hypertension may be *primary* (essential), having no known cause, or it may be *secondary* to other conditions (Table 27-3).

Age is a major factor in primary hypertension. Arterial blood pressure rises gradually throughout the life span. After the age of 60, peripheral vascular resistance increases at about 1%/year. What constitutes normal blood pressure for the aged and what should be considered hypertension in the elderly continues to be debatable. There is general agreement that regardless of age, the higher the systolic or diastolic pressure, the higher the morbidity and mortality.

Malignant hypertension refers to hypertension that is severe and rapidly progressive. It is most common in black men under age 40. Unless medical treatment is successful, the course is rapidly fatal, and most persons die within 2 years. Death is secondary to the changes that occur in the kidney, heart, or brain and the patient dies from uremia, myocardial infarction, congestive heart failure, or cerebrovascular accident.

ASSESSMENT

Subjective data

1. Past or present history of renal or cardiovascular disease
2. History of headache, edema, nocturia, bleeding from unexpected sites, for examples, the nose
3. Visual changes
4. When symptoms first noticed (relate to age or other physical condition in the patient's own words)
5. Weight changes
6. Dietary habits, especially salt intake
7. Occupation and stressors
8. Pain on walking or exercising (intermittent claudication)

Objective data

1. Blood pressure in both arms; also supine and erect position readings
2. Palpation of arteries in neck and wrists and in femo-

ral, popliteal, posterior tibial; and dorsalis pedis (Fig. 27-6)
3. Examination of eyes for evidence of vascular changes; the nurse may need to rely on the findings of the physician

Diagnostic tests

1. Urinalysis; complete blood count, including serum sodium, potassium, chloride, and so forth
2. Pheochromocytoma: urinary test for catecholamines
3. Cushing syndrome test of urine: 17-ketosteroids, serum corticoids
4. Intravenous pyelogram for renal disease
5. Electrocardiogram to assess cardiac function
6. All other probable causes are evaluated from the thorough history and physical examination and further tests done, for example, history of diabetes

DATA ANALYSIS AND PLANNING

Nursing diagnoses

Possible nursing diagnoses would include the following:
Comfort, alteration in: pain
Knowledge deficit
Noncompliance
Nutrition, alteration in: more than body requirements
Tissue perfusion, alteration in: cerebral, cardiopulmonary, renal gastrointestinal and peripheral
Anxiety

Expected patient outcomes

The expected outcomes for the patient with hypertension are as follows:
1. Patient maintains blood pressure within as close to normal range as possible.
2. Patient will show no evidence of progression of renal, visual, or circulatory symptoms.
3. Patient will adhere to therapeutic outcome:
   a. Understands medications and reasons for taking them; describes side effects.
   b. Is less anxious with more knowledge of hypertension related to self.
   c. Maintains dietary regimen with understanding of restrictions; salt, cholesterol, calories.
   d. Takes own blood pressures and keep record.
4. Weight loss to normal weight for individual will be achieved.
5. Patient relates need for continued professional follow-up.

IMPLEMENTATION

Assisting with achievement of therapeutic goals

Drug therapy is currently the only successful means of treating hypertension with the exception of hypertension secondary to a cause such as coarctation of the aorta, in which surgery is the immediate recourse. Important drugs used for the control of hypertension are summa-

Table 27-4. Oral drugs used in hypertension

Drug	Trade name	Mode of action	Side effects
Diuretics			
Thiazide derivatives			
Chlorothiazide	Diuril	Block sodium reabsorption in cortical portion of ascending tubule; water is excreted with sodium, producing decreased blood volume	↑ BUN
Hydrochlorothiazide	Hydrodiuril		↑ Uric acid
	Esidrix		↓ Potassium
	Oretic		↑ Blood glucose
Trichlormethazide	Naqua		↑ Calcium
	Metahydrin		Less common: sensitivity reactions, gastrointestinal tract irritation, rashes, anemia, thrombocytopenia, purpura, pancreatitis
Methylchlorthiazide	Enduron		
Benzthiazide	Exna		
	Aquatag		
Polythiazide	Renese		NOTE: Thiazides are ineffective in renal failure
Cyclothiazide	Anhydron		
Furosemide	Lasix	Block sodium reabsorption in medullary portion of ascending tubule; same action as thiazides	Same as for thiazides; more likely to result in hypovolemia and dehydration
Ethacrynic acid	Edecrin		
Chlorthalidone	Hygroton	Same action as thiazides	Same as for thiazides; more likely to result in hypovolemia and dehydration
Quinethazone	Hydromax		
Potassium sparing			
Spironolactone	Aldactone	Antagonizes the effect of aldosterone on tubular cells; sodium is excreted in exchange for potassium	Hyperkalemia, gynecomastia, hirsutism, irregular menses, rash, drowsiness, confusion
Triamterene	Dyrenium	Acts directly on sodium pump to excrete sodium in exchange for potassium	Hyperkalemia, diarrhea, nausea, vomiting, rash, photosensitivity
Combination drug			
Spironolactone-hydrochlorothiazide	Aldactaside		
Drugs acting on central nervous system			
Rauwolfia compounds			
Reserpine	Sandril	Depletion of catecholamines in sympathetic postganglionic fibers	Drowsiness, lethargy, nasal congestion, bradycardia, depression, gastric hyperacidity
	Serpasil		
	Reserpoid		
Whole root	Raudixin		
Alseroxylon fraction	Rauwiloid		
Deserpidine	Harmonyl		
Guanethidine	Ismelin	Blocks norepinephrine release from adrenergic nerve endings	Orthostatic hypotension (very common), diarrhea, impotence or loss of ejaculation
			NOTE: Poor, inconsistent absorption from gastrointestinal tract
Methyldopa	Aldomet	Metabolized into a false neutrotransmitter displacing norepinephrine from its receptor sites; sympathetic activity reduced	Orthostatic hypotension, drowsiness, fever, liver damage, anemia, impotence
			NOTE: Drug of choice in presence of renal disease
Propranolol	Inderal	β-Adrenergic blocker at peripheral autonomic site	Gastrointestinal tract disturbance, thrombocytopenia, rash, congestive heart failure, aggravation of asthma, fever; increase in conduction disturbance

Continued.

Table 27-4. Oral drugs used in hypertension—cont'd

Drug	Trade name	Mode of action	Side effects
Drugs acting on central nervous system—cont'd			
Metoprolol	Lopressor	Same action as propranolol	Same as for propranolol
Nadolol	Corgard		
Timolol	Biocadren		
Phenoxybenzamine	Dibenzy-line	α-Adrenergic blocker at peripheral autonomic site	Nasal congestion, blurred vision, tachycardia, gastrointestinal tract disturbance
Phentolamine	Regitine	Same action as phenoxybenzamine	Same as for phenoxybenzamine; produces direct vasodilation
Pentolinium	Ansolysen	Block both parasympathetic and sympathetic nerve transmission at ganglia	Orthostatic hypotension, dry mouth, blurred vision, constipation, urinary retention
Mecamylamine	Inversine		
Trimethaphan	Arfonad		Hypotension, urinary retention, angina
Clonidine	Catapres	Stimulates α-adrenergic receptor in brain; causes inhibition of sympathetic vasoconstriction	Orthostatic hypotension, dry mouth, sedation, headache, constipation, fatigue
Vasodilators			
Hydralazine	Apresoline	Direct relaxation of arteriolar smooth muscle causing vasodilation	Headache, tachycardia, nausea, weakness, angina, rash, dizziness, fever
Prazosin	Minipres		
Sodium nitroprusside	Nipride	Same action as hydralazine	Hypotension, gastrointestinal disturbance, tachycardia, cyanide toxicity
Diazoxide	Hyperstar	Same action as hydralazine	Hypotension, sodium and water retention, angina, gastrointestinal disturbances

rized in Table 27-4. The thiazide diuretics are used most often and have been found to be effective in about 50% of patients. Drugs acting on the central nervous system are given with the thiazides when the thiazides are ineffective alone.

Counseling and teaching

Because of the alarming statistics regarding this disease, the importance of detecting persons with hypertension becomes as imperative as the treatment that would follow. Fig. 27-21 diagrams recommended steps in a screening program of detection and confirmation.

Follow-up care

1. Nutrition
   a. Explanations of restrictions such as salt and cholesterol
   b. Diet plan illustrating 24-hour caloric intake
2. Medications
   a. Dosage, hours, expected action, and side effects to report to physician
   b. Reasons for continuing with prescribed drugs even when patient feels symptom free

3. Blood pressure readings—whenever possible the patient or family member learns to take blood pressures and keep a daily record
4. Plan a program of regular physical exercises with the patient
5. Review stress factors with the patient and discuss coping mechanisms
6. Emphasis on supervision by health professionals for the rest of patient's life
   a. Refer to Fig. 27-22 for follow-up recommendations.

EVALUATION

Questions to be asked include the following:
1. Is patient keeping blood pressure within "normal" range by taking medications and maintaining nutritional (dietary) and activity (exercises) therapy?
2. Can patient speak of follow-up renal, visual, and other examination findings?
3. Is patient's anxiety diminished or eradicated by having knowledge about hypertension and the life-long follow-up needed?

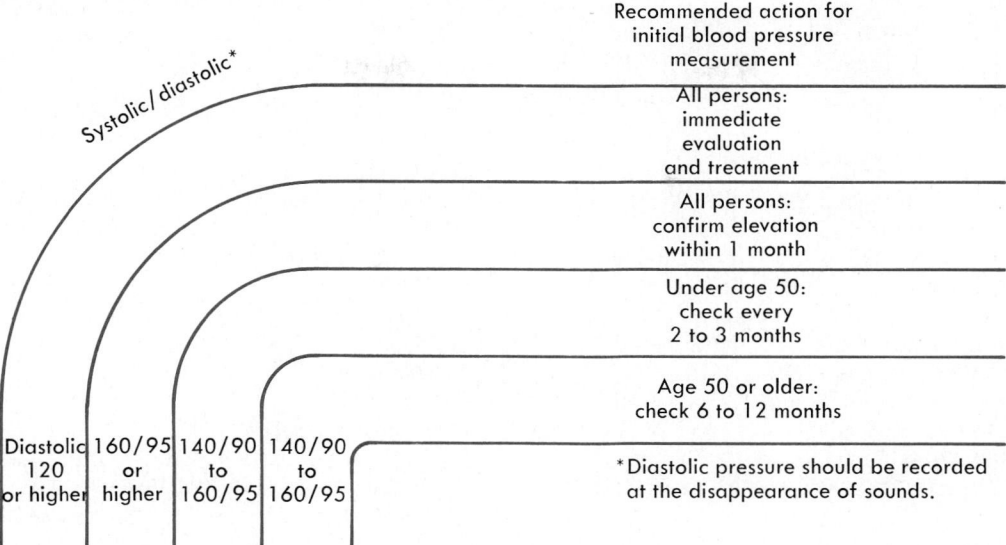

Fig. 27-21. Detection and confirmation of high blood pressure. (From U.S. National High Blood pressure education programs, Recommendations of the Joint National Committee on Detection, Diagnosis and Treatment of High Blood pressure, Bethesda MD, 1973, National Institute of Health.)

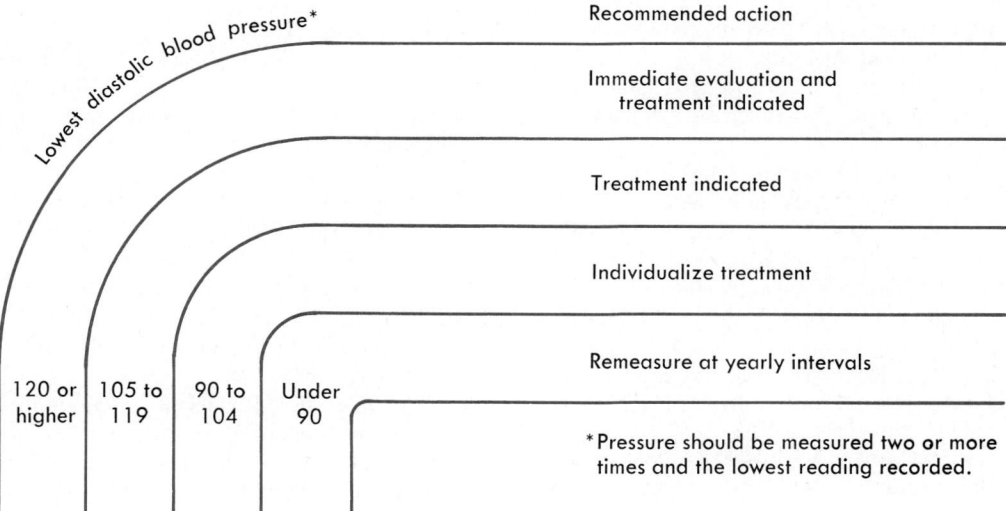

Fig. 27-22. Follow-up recommendations for persons with high blood pressure. Patient education begins when blood pressure is measured initially. Without alarming patient, person taking pressure should inform patient of blood pressure reading and carefully communicate importance of following recommended action. Patients not requiring evaluation or treatment are to be reassured and importance of annual blood pressure measurement strongly emphasized. (From U.S. National High Blood Pressure Education Programs. Recommendations of the Joint National Committee on Detection, Diagnosis, and Treatment of High Blood Pressure. Bethesda, Md., 1973, National Institutes of Health.)

4. Is patient abstaining from tobacco, caffeine, and alcohol?
5. Is patient losing weight as prescribed?
6. Is patient taking and recording own blood pressure?
7. Is patient continuing with clinic or other appointments on follow-up basis?

REFERENCES AND SELECTED READINGS*

1. Abramson, D.I.: Vascular disorders of the extremities, ed. 2, New York, 1974, Harper & Row, Publishers, Inc.
2. Albrechtson, U., et al.: Streptokinase treatment of deep venous thrombosis and the post-thrombotic syndrome, Arch. Surg. **116**:33-37, 1981.
3. Alderman, D.B.: Surgery—and schlerotherapy—for varicose veins, RN **39**:OR-1, OR-4, OR-6, 1976.
4. Alderman, M.H., and Schoenbaum, E.E.: Detection and treatment of hypertension at the work site, N. Engl. J. Med. **293**:65-68, 1975.
5. *Atchison, J.S., and Murray, J.; Post-vascular surgery, Nurs. 78 **8**:36-39, 1978.
6. Baird, R.N., and Abbott, W.M.: Vein grafts: an historical perspective, Am. J. Surg. **134**:293-296, 1977.
7. Barnes, R.W., et al.: Prediction of amputation wound healing, Arch. Surg. **116**:80-83, 1981.
8. Borhani, N.O.: Epidemiology of hypertension as a guide to treatment and control, Heart Lung **10**:245-253, 1981.
9. Conn, H.F.: Current therapy, Philadelphia, 1983, W.B. Saunders Co.
10. *Craven, R.F., and Curry, T.D.: When the diagnosis is Raynaud's, Am. J. Nurs. **81**:1007-1009, 1981.
11. *Cudkowicz, L., and Sherry, S.: Current status of thrombolytic therapy, Heart Lung **7**:97-100, 1978.
12. DePalma, R.G.: Atherosclerosis in vascular grafts. In Gotto, A.M., and Paoletti, R.: Atherosclerosis reviews, vol. 6, New York, 1979, Raven Press.
13. *Doyle, J.E.: If your patient's legs hurt, the reason may be arterial insufficiency, Nurs. 81 **11**:74-79, 1981.
14. *Eddy, M.E.: Teaching patients with peripheral vascular disease, Nurs. Clin. North Am. **12**:151-159, 1977.
15. *Engstrand, J.L.: Rehabilitation of the patient with a lower extremity amputation, Nurs. Clin. North Am. **11**:659-669, 1976.
16. *Fagin-Dubin, L.: Atherosclerosis: a major cause of peripheral vascular disease, Nurs. Clin. North Am. **12**:101-108, 1977.
17. *Fahey, V.A.: An in-depth look at deep vein thrombosis, Nurs. 84 **14**:33-41, 1984.
18. *Falotico, J.B.: Pulmonary embolism, Crit. Care Update **8**:5-15, 1981.
19. *Fenn, J.E.: Reconstructive arterial surgery, for ischemic lower extremities, Nurs. Clin. North Am. **12**:129-142, 1977.
20. *Finnerty, F.A., Jr.: Treatment of hypertensive emergencies, Heart Lung **10**:275-284, 1981.
21. *Frank-Stromberg, M., and Stromberg, P.: Test your knowledge of managing the patient with hypertension, Nurs. 81 **11**:56-59, 1981.
22. Hahn, A.B., Barkin, R.L., and Oestreich, S.J.K.: Pharmacology in nursing, ed. 15, St. Louis, 1982, The C.V. Mosby Co.
23. *Hartshorn, J.C.: What to do when the patient's in hypertensive crisis, Nurs. 80 **10**:36-45, 1980.
24. *Haughey, C.W.: Understanding ultrasonography, Nurs. 81 **11**:100-104, 1981.
25. Helgeland, A.: Treatment of mild hypertension: the five year Oslo study, Am. J. Med. **69**:725-732, 1980.
26. Hill, M.N., and Foster, S.B.: High blood pressure, Nurs. 82 **12**:72-75, 1982.
27. Hobbs, J.T., editor: The treatment of venous disorders: a comprehensive review of current practice in the treatment of varicose veins and the post-thrombotic syndrome, Philadelphia, 1977, J.B. Lippincott Co.
28. Jasinkowski, N.: The unique needs of a distal bypass patient, RN, **45**:44-47, 1982.
29. Jones, A.F., and Kempczinski, R.F.: Aortofemoral bypass grafting, Arch. Surg. **116**:301-305, 1981.
30. *Jones, L.N.: Hypertension: medical and nursing implications, Nurs. Clin. North Am. **11**:283-295, 1976.
31. Juergens, J.L., Spittell, J.A., and Fairbairn, J.F.: Peripheral vascular diseases, ed. 5, Philadelphia, 1980, W.B. Saunders Co.
32. Kessro, B.: Peripheral arterial insufficiency: postoperative care, Nurs. Clin. North Am. **12**:143-149, 1977.
33. Leonard, A.R., Igra, A., and Hawthorne, A.: Status of high blood pressure control in California, Heart Lung **10**:255-268, 1981.
34. *Loustau A., and Blair, B.J.: A key to compliance, Nurs. 81 **11**:84-87, 1981.
35. *Lowther, N.B., and Carter, V.D.: How to increase compliance in hypertensives, Am. J. Nurs. **81**:963, 1981.
36. Mancini, M., et al.: Role of diet in atherosclerosis. In Hegyeli, R.: Atherosclerosis reviews, vol. 7, New York, 1980, Raven Press.
37. *Maschak-Carey, B.J., and Moore, K.: Anticoagulation therapy, Crit. Care Update **8**:5-16, 1981.
38. *Mitchell, E.S.: Protocol for teaching hypertensive patients, Am. J. Nurs. **77**:808-809, 1977.
39. Porter, J.M., Baur, G.M., and Taylor, L.M.: Lower extremity amputations for ischemia, Arch. Surg. **116**:89-98, 1981.
40. *Quinless, F.: Peripheral vascular disease, physiology, signs and symptoms, Nurs. 84 **14**:52-53, 1984.
41. Rodman, M.J.: Thromboembolic disorders. I. Venous thrombosis, RN **39**:81-82, 85-86, 1976.
42. Rodman, M.J.: Thromboembolic disorders. II. Arterial thrombosis and embolism, RN **39**:61-66, 1976.
43. Roon, A.J., Moore, W.S., and Goldstone, J.: Below-knee-amputation: a modern approach, Am. J. Surg. **134**:153-158, 1977.
44. Ross, R., and Glomset, J.: The pathogenesis of artherosclerosis. I. N. Engl. J. Med. **295**:369-377, 1976.
45. Ross, R., and Glomset, J.: The pathogenesis of artherosclerosis. II. N. Engl. J. Med. **295**:420-425, 1976.
46. Ryzewski, J.: Factors in the rehabilitation of patients with peripheral vascular disease, Nurs. Clin. North Am. **12**:161-168, 1977.

*References preceded by an asterisk are particularly well suited for student reading.

47. *Sexton, D.L.: The patient with peripheral arterial occlusive disease, Nurs. Clin. North Am. **12:**89-99, 1977.

48. *Walter, J.: Coping with leg amputation, Am. J. Nurs. **81:**1349-1352, 1981.

Classic

49. *Bosanko, L.A.: Immediate postoperative prosthesis, Am. J. Nurs. **71:**280-283, 1971.

50. Burgess, E., et al.: Immediate postsurgical prosthetics in the management of lower extremity amputees, Washington, D.C., 1967, Department of Medicine and Surgery, Veterans Administration.

51. *Garrett, J.F., and Levine, E.S., editors: Psychological practices with the physically disabled, New York, 1962, Columbia University Press.

52. *Gordon, T., and Kennel, W.B.: Predisposition to atherosclerosis in the head, heart, and legs: the Framingham study, JAMA **221:**661-66, 1972.

53. *Jackson, B.S.: Chronic peripheral arterial disease, Am. J. Nurs. **72:**928-934, 1972.

54. Laughlin, E., Stanford, J., and Phelps, M.: Immediate postsurgical prosthetics fitting of a bilateral, below-elbow amputee: a report, Artif. Limbs **12:**17-19, 1968.

55. National Heart and Lung institute Task Force on Arteriosclerosis:Arteriosclerosis, vol. II, U.S. Department of Health, Education and Welfare, NIH no. 72-219, 1971.

56. *Plaisted, L.M., and Friz, B.R.: The nurse on the amputee clinic team, Nurs. Outlook **16:**34-37, 1968.

57. *Rose, M.A.: Home care after peripheral vascular surgery, Am. J. Nurs. **74:**260-262, 1974.

28

The Patient with Hematologic Problems

ROSEMARIE M. HOGAN and DEANNA MELTON XISTRIS

STUDY QUESTIONS

- What are the normal cellular constituents of blood? Where are blood cells formed? How are they destroyed? What are the normal RBC count, WBC count, hemoglobin and hematocrit levels for men and women?

- Trace the successive processes that occur when blood clots. What are blood coagulation factors?

- From your understanding of physiology, explain why the patient who is anemic may have dyspnea, tachycardia, and fatigue.

- Why does WBC count increase during infection? Why is a person with leukopenia (WBC count below 5000) more susceptible to infection?

Disorders related to the hematologic system are usually the result of problems in the normal production, development, and function of the components of blood or alterations in the rate of blood cell destruction. The illness can be either chronic or acute or a combination of both.

ANATOMY AND PHYSIOLOGY

The hematopoietic system includes blood and its components as well as the reticuloendothelial system (RES), which is located throughout the body. Its function is phagotizing foreign materials and lysing (breaking down) red blood cells.

Components of the hematopoietic system

BLOOD

Blood is an aqueous solution (plasma) that contains proteins, electrolytes, and inorganic and organic constituents. Solids make up 7% to 9% of the blood.

The cell components of blood include erythrocytes or red blood cells (RBC), leukocytes or white blood cells (WBC), and thrombocytes or platelets (Table 28-1). All normal cells are derived from a single stem cell that can divide into lymphoid and blood stem cells, which in turn become progenitor cells that divide along a specific single pathway (Fig. 28-1). This process is known as *hematopoiesis* and takes place in the bone marrow of the skull, vertebrae, pelvis, sternum, ribs, and proximal epiphysis of long bones. Production may take place in all the long bones during periods of increased demand, such as with hemorrhage or during cell destruction (hemolysis).

Table 28-1. Normal values of cellular blood components

Type	Normal values
Red blood cells	Male: 4.6-6.2 million/mm³
	Female: 2.4-5.4 million/mm³
White blood cells	4000-10,000/mm³
Neutrophils	51%-67%
Eosinophils	1%-4%
Basophils	0%-1%
Monocytes	2%-6%
Lymphocytes	25%-33%
Platelets	150,000/mm³
Hematocrit	Male: 45%-52%
	Female: 37%-48%
Hemoglobin	Male: 13-18 g/dl
	Female: 12-16 g/dl
Mean corpuscular volume (MCV)	80-90 µm
Mean corpuscular hemoglobin concentration (MCHC)	32%-36%

For the differential blood count items (Neutrophils through Lymphocytes): Differential blood count—totals 100%

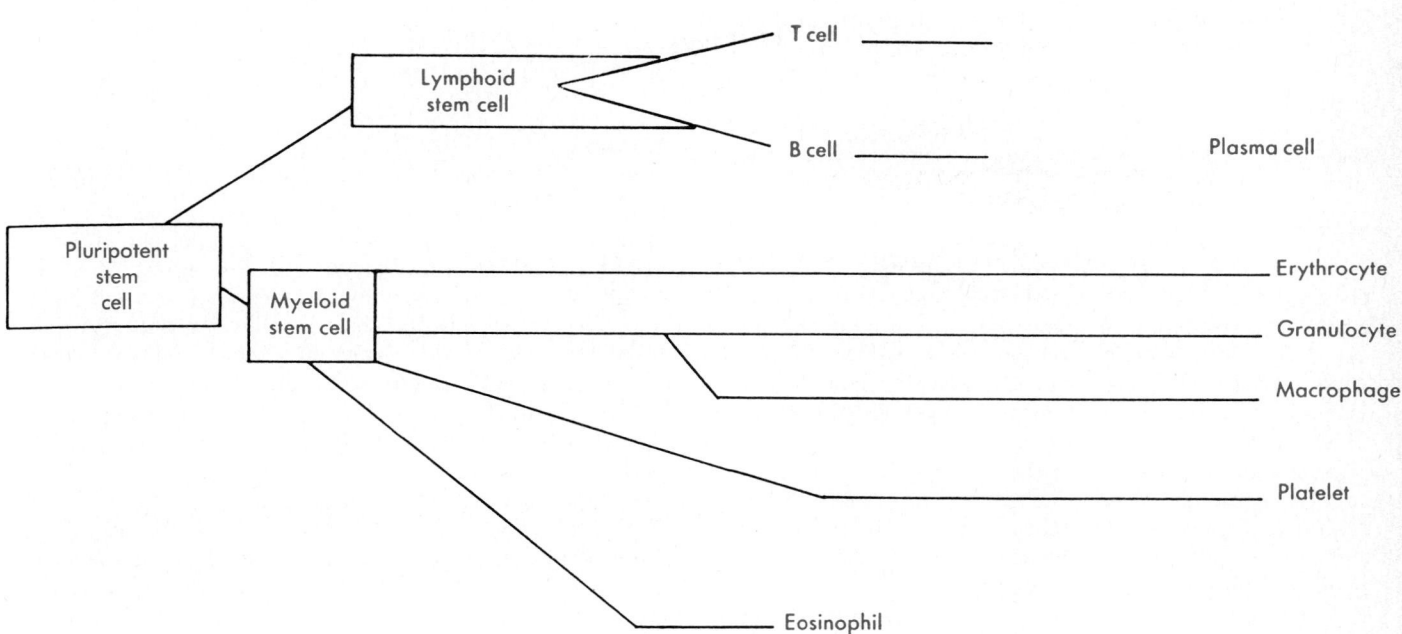

Fig. 28-1. Scheme of stem cell differentiation showing common progenitor cell for erythrocytes, granulocytes, and platelets. (Adapted from Clinc, M., and Golde, D.: Blood, **53:**157-164, 1979.)

Red blood cells

An RBC is a nonnucleated biconcave disc that is soft and pliable, which enables it to change its shape during passage through the microcirculation. The RBC's major component is hemoglobin (Hb), a protein that transports oxygen and carbon dioxide and maintains normal pH through a series of intracellular buffers (see Chapter 10). The Hb molecule contains globin (two pairs of polypeptide chains) and four heme groups, each one containing an atom of ferrous iron. Maturation of RBCs requires adequate amounts and use of vitamin B_{12}, folic acid, proteins, enzymes, and minerals (for example, iron, copper).

RBCs circulate for 120 days and are then destroyed by the macrophages of the RES. Energy in the form of ATP is required to maintain cell membrane integrity, the relatively low sodium and high potassium content of the red

Table 28-2. Laboratory tests for hematologic assessment

Blood cell	Function	Diagnostic test
RBCs	Mediate the exchange of oxygen and carbon dioxide between lungs and tissue	RBC, hemoglobin, hematocrit, reticulocyte count Blood indices: Mean corpuscular hemoglobin concentration (MCHC), mean cell volume (MCV), mean corpuscular hemoglobin (MCH) Red cell fragility Morphologic description in stained smear
Platelets	Platelet plug; promotion of thrombin production	Platelet aggregation Platelet count Bleeding time

WBCs
  Granulocytes
    Neutrophils
    Eosinophils
    Basophils
  Lymphocytes
  Monocytes
	
	Phagocytosis
	
	Allergic and immunologic responses
	Formation of imunoglobulins
	Phagocytosis
		WBC
		WBC with differential

cell, and as a defense against oxidation and other environmental stressors.

White blood cells

WBCs may be classified into two groups as follows: *granular leukocytes* (also called *Polymorphonclear* [PMN] *leukocytes*) consisting of neutrophils, eosinophils, and basophils; and *nongranular leukocytes* consisting of monocytes and lymphocytes. The granulocytes contain enzymes that kill and digest bacteria upon degranulation of the cells.

Neutrophils are present in the circulation or along the capillary walls (the margination pool). They move into the tissues and mucous membranes and serve as the body's primary defense against bacterial infection through the process of phagocytosis (see Chapter 6).

Monocytes are larger than neutrophils and have one large folded or indented nucleus. They leave the circulation and become tissue *macrophages,* which also have phagocytic action, removing dead and injured cells, cell fragments, and microorganisms.

Lymphocytes are mononuclear with a round or oval nucleus. They originate primarily in lymphoid tissue (lymph nodes) but also in the bone marrow. There are two types of lymphocytes, the long-lived circulating T-lymphocytes (from the thymus) and short-lived noncirculating B-lymphocytes. T-lymphocytes initiate the cellular immune reponse, while B-lymphocytes (immunoglobulins) initiate the humoral immune response (see Chapter 6).

Laboratory tests have been developed to measure the amounts and functioning of all cellular components of the blood (Table 28-2).

Platelets

Platelets (thrombocytes) are not cells but are granular, disc-shaped, nonnucleated cell fragments. One-third of platelets are in the spleen as a reserve pool and the remainder in circulation. Platelets are also derived from the stem cells and are essential to hemostasis and coagulation. Hemostasis results from the adhesion and aggregation capabilities of platelets to plug small breaks in blood vessels. Platelets also release thromboplastin (factor III), which, in the presence of calcium ions, convents prothrombin into thrombin in the first step of the coagulation mechanism (Fig. 28-2). In the second step of the coagulation mechanism, thrombin promotes the conversion of fibrinogen (a soluble plasma protein) into fibrin (an insoluble strand). Step one require coagulation factors IV, V, VIII, IX, X, XI, and XII; whereas step two requires factors IV and XIII.

RETICULOENDOTHELIAL SYSTEM

The RES, also called the mononuclear phagocyte system or macrophage system, includes circulating monocytes and their precursor cells in the bone marrow. It also includes more or less fixed mononuclear phagocytic cells found in blood channels in the spleen and liver (Kupffer cells), in the lymphatic system, in serosal cavities of the body, in the lungs, in general connective tissue, and in the bone marrow.

In addition to phagocytosis, the RES processes the Hg of RBCs that have reached the end of their life span, splitting Hb into an iron-containing substance and bilirubin (see Chapter 31).

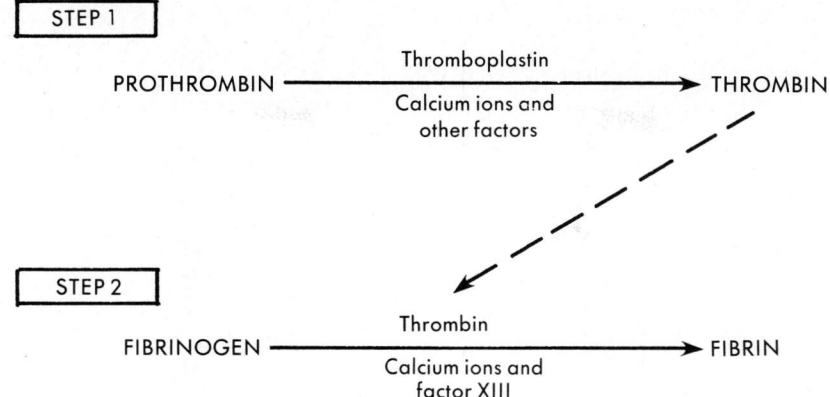

Fig. 28-2. Basic steps in coagulation process.

Coagulation factors

Factor I	Fibrinogen
Factor II	Prothrombin
Factor III	Thromboplastin, tissue thromboplastin
Factor IV	Calcium
Factor V	Proaccelerin, labile factor
Factor VI	(Not assigned)
Factor VII	Serum prothrombin convension accelerator (SPCA)
Factor VIII	Antihemophilic globulin (AHG) Antihemophilic factor (AHF)
Factor IX	Plasm thromboplastin component (PTG), Christmas factor
Factor X	Stuart factor
Factor XI	Plasma thromboplastin antecedent (PTA)
Factor XII	Hageman factor
Factor XIII	Fibrin-stabilizing factor

Physiologic changes with aging

The effect of aging on hematopoiesis is still being studies with findings that are sometimes ambiguous or of questionable clinical significance. There is evidence from studies of mouse marrow that stem cells have a limited capacity to proliferate. Findings from animal studies suggest that changes related to aging do not have clinical significance.[46] The cellularity of human marrow decreases with age, but this may be the result of an increase in fat from osteoporosis rather than a decrease in hematopoietic cells.

In humans, the total number of leukocytes and differential counts show no variation through middle age and no gross changes in old age. In general the leukocyte count does not rise as high in response to infection, and studies suggest that the elderly have a diminished marrow granulocyte reserve.

The Hb level decreases after middle age although the decrease in women seems to be relatively less than that in men. Unexplained anemia in the elderly has been noted, but iron absorption is not impaired; however, use of orally administered iron is reduced. This anemia does not appear to be related solely to age.[46] Serum iron and iron-binding capacity decrease in the elderly, and low serum vitamin B_{12} and folic acid levels occur in a significant proportion of elderly people but without anemia.

No age-related changes in platelets have been reported. RBC sedimentation rate increases significantly, but this rate is of limited value in detecting disease in the elderly. Some of the plasma coagulation factors have been reported to increase with age (factors I, V, VII, and IX). Partial thromboplastin time may be shortened.[18]

PREVENTION AND HEALTH EDUCATION

Exposure to certain chemicals and drugs place individuals at high risk for hematologic disorders, especially aplastic anemia and the leukemias. Individuals with inadequate dietary intake of iron and vitamins (for example, folic acid and B_{12}), alcoholics, and others with poor dietary habits because of inadequate knowledge or low income, are particularly susceptible to anemia. Women who have long-term blood loss because of heavy menstrual bleeding (menorrhagia) are also at risk for anemia, as are other persons with long-term slow blood loss.

Other diseases such as sickle cell anemia, the thalassemias, and hemophilia are hereditary; therefore, marriage between carriers of defective genes may result in children with the disease.

Health teaching involves identifying persons at high

risk and ways in which the risk factors can be mitigated. Occupational health nurses are involved in identifying industrial chemicals or processes that place workers in danger and in working with companies to minimize those risks. Nurses in all settings teach about dietary needs for iron and other vitamins. An important facet of this teaching is helping those persons with low incomes to identify inexpensive sources of the vitamins and minerals necessary for hematologic health. Nurses also may become politically active in order to ensure that there is adequate government funding for food stamps and other low-cost nutritional programs for those persons who have marginal incomes.

One of the most difficult and sensitive roles for nurses is that of genetic counselor, communicating to individuals with hereditary problems the risk factors involved and possibility of having children with severe hematopoietic disease. The persons are allowed to make their own decisions after information has been shared with them, a decision that can be devastating to the individual no matter what it is.

Major health problems related to blood and lymph systems

Disorders associated with the hematopoietic system are diverse in their underlying pathologic manifestations, disease course, and response to treatment. Most often, the symptoms manifested are the result of interference with the normal development and function of the blood components and with altered hematopoiesis (blood cell production). Normally homeostasis is maintained through a balance between the rate of production of normal blood cells and the rate of destruction. Disorders of the blood are manifested when this hemostatic balance is lost. Disturbances in the coagulation mechanism also result in blood disorders.

In addition to primary hematologic disorders, secondary effects from disease of another body system may also manifest themselves in abnormal hematologic findings. For example, the anemia that is associated with azotemia is the consequence of disease existing outside of the hematopoietic system.

Major health problems include the following:
1. RBC disorders
   a. Anemias
   b. Erythrocytosis: polycythemia
2. Coagulation disorders
   a. Platelet disorders: thrombocytopenia, platelet function disorders
   b. Hemophilia
   c. Disseminated intravascular clotting (DIC)
3. WBC disorders: agranulocytosis, leukemia
4. Lymph system disorders: lymphadenopathy, lymphomas (Hodgkin's and non-Hodgkin's)

DISORDERS ASSOCIATED WITH ERYTHROCYTES

Anemia and erythrocytosis are the general categories of red cell disorders. *Anemia* refers to a deficiency of RBCs as reflected in a decreased Hb level, packed cell volume (hematocrit), and red cell count. Anemias may be divided into those that are the result of blood loss, impaired production of RBCs, increased destruction of RBCs, or nutritional deficiency.

Anemia may also be differentiated by examining the size of a red cell and the amount of Hb contained. The suffix *-cytic* refers to RBC size and *-chromic* refers to amount of hemoglobin.

Anemia secondary to blood loss
PATHOPHYSIOLOGY

Anemia associated with blood loss may be acute or chronic. Acute anemia is the direct result of the decrease in a large amount of circulating RBCs. An adult of average build can lose 500 ml of blood (out of a total of 6000 ml) without serious or lasting effects. Losses of 1000 ml or more can cause acute consequences (Table 28-3). The severity of symptoms depends on the severity of blood

---

Causes of anemia

1. Blood loss: acute or chronic
2. Impaired RBC production: aplastic anemia
3. Increased RBC destruction (hemolysis)
   a. Congenital: hereditary spherocytosis, sickle cell anemia, thalassemia, enzyme deficiency
   b. Acquired: autoimmune, drug induced
4. Nutritional deficiency
   a. Iron deficiency
   b. Megaloblastic anemia: B_{12} deficiency, folic acid deficiency

---

Descriptive cell characteristics in anemia

Size	Macrocytic (large)
	Normocytic
	Microcytic (small)
Hemoglobin	Normochromic
	Hypochromic (decreased)

loss. Increased cardiac output, pulmonary function, erythropoietic activity, and compensatory peripheral vasoconstriction to shunt blood to vital organs are responsible for some of the signs and symptoms.[47]

Chronic anemia secondary to blood loss is the most common cause of iron-deficiency anemia (p. 741). The body has remarkable adaptive powers and may adjust fairly well to a marked reduction in RBCs and Hb, provided the condition develops gradually. An individual may remain asymptomatic even though the total RBC count may drop to almost half of its normal level (4.5-5 million/cu mm) or the Hb level to below 7 g/dl (normal is 12 to 18 g/dl). When blood loss is continuous and moderate in amount, the bone marrow may be able to keep up with the losses by increasing RBC production. If the cause of chronic blood loss is not found and corrected, eventually the bone marrow will not be able to keep pace with the loss, and symptoms of anemia will appear.

ASSESSMENT

With acute blood loss, in addition to the signs of hypovolemic shock, the patient will experience weakness and may be short of breath if sufficient RBCs have been lost. Weakness and fatigue may also be experienced with chronic blood loss. Patients are monitored on a continuing basis for futher signs of bleeding.

Decreased Hb and hematocrit serum levels are diagnostic tests of particular significance with acute anemia, although these signs will not be evident until several hours after the blood loss. With chronic anemia, RBC counts, Hb and hematocrit levels, mean corpuscular volume (MCV), and mean corpuscular hemoglobin concentration (MCHC) are important diagnostic tests and measures. All indices are usually below normal (see Table 28-1) for normal values).

DATA ANALYSIS AND PLANNING

Nursing diagnoses specific to the anemia resulting from blood loss, not including those associated with hypovolemic shock, may include the following:
1. Impaired gas exchange
2. Alteration in tissue perfusion (cerebral, cardiopulmonary)
3. Potential for physical injury (related to weakness and fatigue)

Expected patient outcomes include the following:
1. Patient is alert and oriented
2. Patient is relaxed and comfortable
3. No injuries have occurred from falls

IMPLEMENTATION

Nursing interventions for acute blood loss are the same as those for hypovolemic shock (Chapter 11). Since transfusion of whole blood may be used to replace both plasma and RBC loss, nurses are alert for signs of transfusion reactions (Chapter 39).

If patients are weak, dizzy, or in any way confused because of severe anemia, they are supervised in ambulation to prevent exertional dyspnea, fatigue, and falls. Rest periods are provided. If oral iron preparations are prescribed, patients are taught to take them with meals to avoid gastric irritation.

EVALUATION

Questions to ask may include the following:
1. Does the patient state that fatigue is controlled?
2. Is the patient comfortable?
3. Has the patient been free from falls?

Anemia secondary to impaired production of RBCs: aplastic anemia

PATHOPHYSIOLOGY

The defect leading to aplastic anemia is most likely injury or destruction of a common stem cell (Fig. 28-1), affecting all subsequent cell populations. It is characterized not only by impaired RBC production but also by depression or cessation of activity of all blood-producing elements. There is a decrease in white cells (leukopenia) and a decrease in platelets (thrombocytopenia).[16] Signs and symptoms and medical therapy for aplastic anemia are listed in Table 28-3.

ASSESSMENT

Subjective data include the person's history of exposure to chemicals (insecticides, benzene) and drugs, plus the family history of any similar anemia. Physical examination is often normal. A hemogram characteristically reveals pancytopenia (a marked decrease in the numbers of all cell types). The reticulocyte count is low. The patient is monitored for signs of infection (from the leukopenia) and bleeding (from the thrombocytopenia).

Diagnostic tests include peripheral blood smears and bone marrow examination, which provides the definitive diagnosis. Examination of the peripheral blood smear allows for determination of the morphology of the cells (type, origin), the extent of cell maturity, and the ratio of the various cell types to each other.

Drugs that may cause aplastic anemia

Chloramphenicol
Colchicine
Mephenytoin
D-penicillamine
Phenylbutazone
Sulfonamides
Trimethadione

Table 28-3. Disorders of red blood cells

Disorder	Etiology	Signs and symptoms	Medical therapy
Anemias			
Secondary to blood loss			
Acute	Hemorrhage	Hypovolemic and hypoxemic symptoms (weakness, stupor, irritability, cool moist skin, hypotension, tachycardia, ↓ Hb and Hct, pallor)	IV fluids, whole blood or packed cells; identify source of loss; administration of iron
Chronic	GI or other malignancy, slow bleeding ulcer, bleeding hemorrhoids, menorrhagia	Depends on degree of ↓ in Hb; if less than 8.0 g/dl: weakness, fatigue, ↑ pulse, pallor, exertional dyspnea	Packed cells, iron; identify source of loss
Aplastic anemia	Drugs, chemicals, radiation, chemotherapy, virus, congenital	As in chronic anemia plus those related to ↓ WBC and platelets (ecchymoses, petechiae, GI, GU, CNS bleeding, increased risk of infection)	Removal of causative agent; supportive care until bone marrow is regenerated: transfusions, laminar air-flow room, androgen to stimulate erythropoiesis, bone marrow transplantation, antilymphocyte-globulin therapy
Hemolytic anemia			
Congenital			
Sickle cell	Genetic	↓ Hb; ↓ Hct; pain (bones, joints, back); generalized, localized or migratory; vomiting; fever; infections; chronic leg ulcers; cardiomegaly; mumurs; CHF; delay in growth and sexual maturation; swollen hands and feet (dactylitis); jaundice	No specific therapy; analgesics, oxygen, adequate hydration, treatment of infection, polyvalent pneumococcal vaccine to prevent pneumococcal infections, antisickling agents (experimental), therapeutic apheresis
		Thrombotic crisis: severe pain in abdomen and musculoskeletal system	Adequate hydration, exchange transfusions (replacing person's blood with packed red cells, unit for unit)
		Aplastic crisis: rapid ↑ in anemia	
Thalassemia	Decreased synthesis of one of the globin chains of Hb	Thalassemia minor: mild anemia	No therapy required; transfusions with severe symptoms or to maintain Hb near normal
		Thalassemia major: severe anemia	
Enzyme deficiency	Genetic defect in pathways that metabolize glucose	Anemia when person exposed to oxidant drugs (aspirin, sulfonamindes, antimalarial)	Cessation of causative drug

Acquired hemolytic anemia	Drug (alpha methyldopa, penicillin), autoimmune response, idiopathic or secondary to lymphocytic lymphomas or chronic lymphocytic leukemia	Same as with other anemias	Corticosteroids, splenectomy in those who do not respond to drug therapy
Nutritional anemia Iron deficiency anemia	Inadequate dietary iron, chronic blood loss	Gradual development; may have few signs; fatigue, exertional dyspnea, severe anemia, brittle spoon-shaped (concave) nails with longitudinal ridges, atrophy of tongue papillae, smooth shiny tongue, cheilosis (cracks in corner of mouth); low serum iron, pallor, weakness	Determine and correct cause Oral iron administration (ferrous sulfate); parenteral iron if oral not tolerated or not absorbed via GI tract; adequate balanced diet
Megaloblastic anemia	Vitamin B_{12} deficiency caused by absence of intrinsic factor (pernicious anemia) or interference with absorption in ileum	Low serum B_{12} and folate levels, neurologic abnormalities (peripheral neuropathies, loss of balance), symptoms associated with underlying disease and anemia	
Erythrocytosis Polycythemia vera (primary)	Stem cell abnormality, cause unknown	Absent in early stages; headache, tinnitus, blurred vision, reddened skin, nosebleeds, ecchymoses, GI bleeding caused by platelet dysfunction, thrombosis, hepatomegaly, splenomegaly, ↑ total RBC volume, ↑ or normal plasma volume	Periodic phlebotomy (removal of blood), radioactive phosphorus, chemotherapeutic agents such as busulfan
Secondary polycythemia	Hypoxia, renal tumors, living in high altitudes	↑ RBC, ↑ Hct; symptoms may be similar to but less severe than those in polycythemia vera	Correct underlying condition
Pseudopolycythemia	Stress: occurs in middle aged, obese, highly anxious males; cigarette smoking exacerbates symptoms	As above; is self-limiting; symptoms are mild	Stress reduction

Bone marrow aspiration

Aspiration is the most common procedure for obtaining a bone marrow sample. The procedure is possible because normal bone marrow is soft and semifluid and can therefore be removed by aspiration through a needle. Bone marrow aspiration is also used in the diagnosis of acute leukemia and thrombocytopenia.

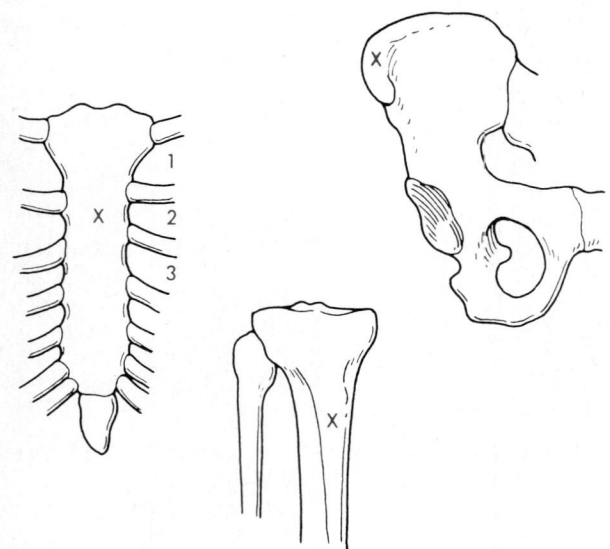

Fig. 28-3. Sites for bone marrow aspiration: sternum, iliac crest (most common), and tibia.

Procedure

The skin surrounding the puncture site (Fig. 28-3) is shaved, if necessary, and cleansed with an antiseptic such as povidone-iodine complex (Betadine). Sterile towels are placed around the site. The skin and periosteum are anesthetized to avoid pain. First, the most superficial layer of the skin is infiltrated with procaine. After a few seconds the needle is further advanced until bone is touched. Procaine is then injected to anesthetize the periosteum.

The marrow aspiration needle is inserted, and when the marrow cavity is entered, the marrow stylet is removed from the needle and a sterile syringe is attached. The syringe plunger is drawn back until marrow appears in the syringe. As the plunger is drawn back the person will experience a brief, sharp pain, sometimes described as a burning sensation. The pain is caused by the suction exerted as the plunger is pulled back. Some persons may complain of tenderness at the aspiration site for a few days. Most often no pain or discomfort is experienced following the procedure.

Attempts at bone marrow aspiration may yield a "dry tap" because of hypocellularity and a decrease in active marrow, and bone marrow biopsy is often necessary.

Nursing care with bone marrow aspiration

1. Explain procedure to patient, stating that there may be brief discomfort when the marrow is aspirated.
2. To prevent movement, place hands on patient's shoulders and instruct patient to remain still at the time of aspiration.

Fig. 28-4. Bone marrow biopsy needle showing shape and size.

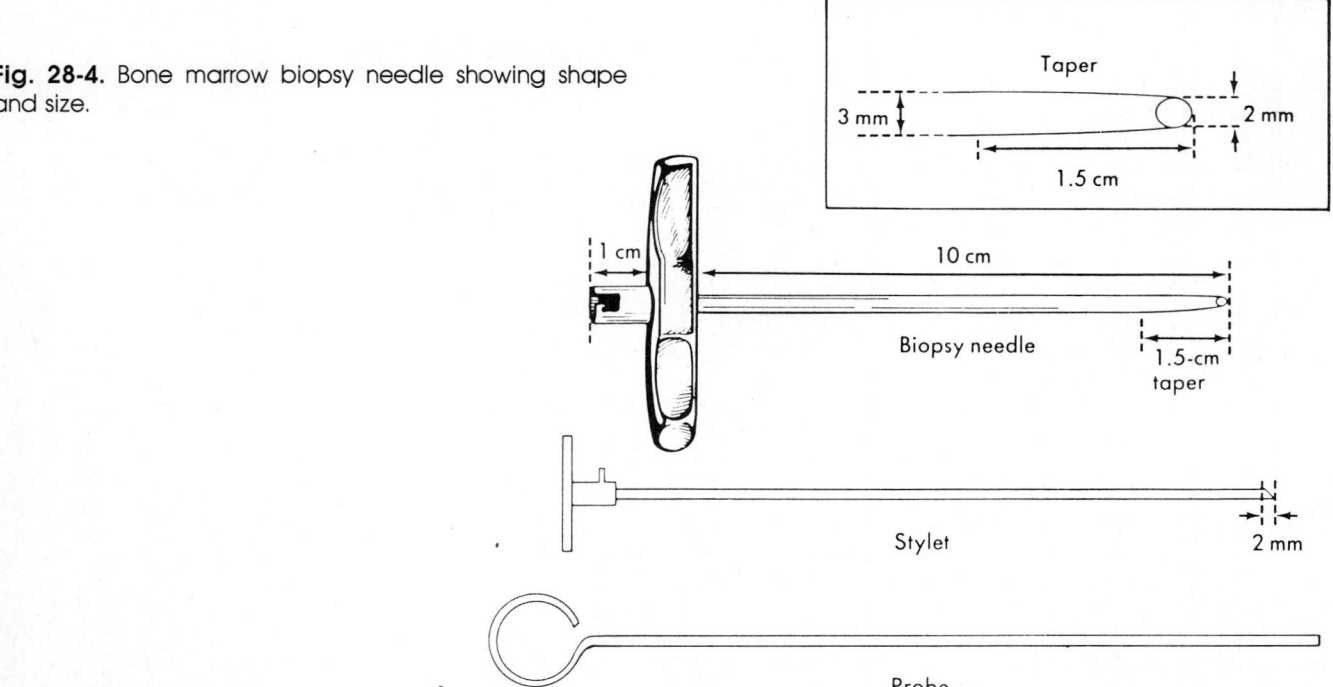

3. Apply pressure over aspiration site after needle is removed to prevent bleeding; apply pressure for 3 to 5 minutes if patient is thrombocytopenic.
4. Assess for bleeding from aspiration site.
5. Provide comfort measures to help patient relax.

Bone marrow biopsy

A bone marrow biopsy is indicated when a large sample of bone marrow is needed. Persons also likely to undergo a bone marrow biopsy are those with pancytopenia, metastatic tumor, lymphoma, and multiple myeloma.

The most comon site for bone marrow biopsy is the posterosuperior iliac spine, although the sternum may also be used. The initial steps in the biopsy procedure are similar to those outlined for bone marrow aspiration. The use of a Jamshidi needle allows for a core of marrow to be collected (Fig. 28-4). Nursing care following a bone marrow biopsy is similar to that of bone marrow aspiration.

From microscopic examination of the bone marrow, iron stores can be determined, as can the morphology of the progenitor cell. Megaloblastic (RBC precursor) changes and the absence of cells may be observed. Infiltration with leukemic cells may also be determined by bone marrow biopsy.

DATA ANALYSIS AND PLANNING

Because the levels of all of the blood cells are decreased, the individual is prone to severe and life-threatening complications, primarily infection and bleeding. (The nursing care of persons with decreased WBC and platelet count is discussed on pp. 740 and 750).

Nursing diagnoses related to anemia from blood loss apply also to aplastic anemia, depending on the severity of the disease. Additional nursing diagnoses include the following:
1. Infection: Potential for
2. Injury: Potential for bleeding
3. Knowledge deficit

Expected patient outcomes may include those for anemia from blood loss as well as the following:
1. The patient is free of nosocomial infections.
2. Bleeding is controlled.
3. The patient can explain measures to prevent infection and hemorrhage.

IMPLEMENTATION

Assisting with implementation of therapeutic goals

Nursing care depends on the severity of symptoms. The patients may be critically ill. If bone marrow transplantation is attempted, prevention of infection while bone marrow elements are suppressed by radiation and chemotherapy is essential (p. 750).

Preventing infection

1. Place patient in private room; avoid contact with visitors and staff who have infection.
2. Place patient in protective isolation or laminar air flow room (see Chapter 14), if necessary.
3. Provide meticulous hygiene, including daily bath, careful oral hygiene, perineal care; use antiseptic creams.
4. Avoid catheterization.
5. Use povidone iodine skin cleansing for 1 minute be-

Teaching the person with aplastic anemia

1. Infection prevention
   a. Good handwashing technique
   b. Avoiding contact with those who have infections
   c. Avoiding the sharing of eating utensils and bath linens
   d. Daily baths with meticulous perineal care
   e. Good oral hygiene, avoiding gum injury
   f. Clean environment
   g. Recognition of signs and symptoms of infection and need to report these to physician
   h. Avoiding eating raw meats, fresh fruits and vegetables.
2. Teach hemorrhage prevention
   a. Observing for bloody urine, stool, petechiae, and so on, reporting these to physician
   b. Using soft toothbrush or swab for mouth care
   c. Keeping mouth clean and free of debris
   d. Avoiding enemas or other rectal insertions
   e. Avoiding picking or blowing nose forcefully
   f. Avoiding trauma, falls, bumps, cuts; avoiding contact sports
   g. Avoiding use of aspirin or aspirin preparations
   h. Use of electric razor
   i. Using adequate lubrication and gentleness during sexual intercourse

fore parenteral injections (or other preparation as ordered).

6. Maintain a clean environment.
7. Provide emotional support for anxiety when infection occurs.

Preventing hemorrhage

1. Assess all sites for bleeding.
2. Test urine (hemastix) and stool for blood (guaiac).
3. Keep venipuncture and intramuscular injections to a minimum.
4. Apply pressure to venipuncture sites for 5 minutes, arterial sites for 10 minutes.
5. Use soft toothbrush or swab for mouth care.
6. Keep mouth clean and free of debris with normal saline rinse if bleeding occurs.
7. Avoid taking rectal temperatures, administering rectal medication, and giving enemas.
8. Avoid invasive procedures.

Teaching

All persons with aplastic anemia need to know how to protect themselves from infection and excessive bleeding. Points to emphasize are listed in box on p. 737.

EVALUATION

Questions to ask may include the following:
1. Have infections been prevented?
2. Are breath sounds normal?
3. Are body secretions normal in color, odor, and consistency?
4. Has hemorrhage been prevented?
5. Does the patient know how to prevent infection and hemorrhage?

Anemia secondary to increased destruction of RBCs: hemolytic anemia

PATHOPHYSIOLOGY

Hemolytic anemia results when the red cells are destroyed at such a rapid rate that the bone marrow is unable to compensate for the loss. The severity of the anemia is determined by the degree of lag between the rate of RBC destruction (hemolysis) and the rate of bone marrow production of red cells (erythropoiesis). Hemolytic anemias may be congenital or acquired. The signs and symptoms and medical therapies for hemolytic anemias are listed in Table 28-3.

Congenital hemolytic anemias

Congenital hemolytic anemias include hereditary spherocytosis, the hemoglobinopathies, thalassemia, and enzyme deficiency. *Hereditary spherocytosis,* an inherited autosomal dominant trait, is characterized by a membrane abnormality that leads to osmotic swelling of the red cell and susceptibility to destruction by the spleen. It is most

Table 28-4. Phenotypes for sickle cell

Genetic relationship	Hemoglobin alleles	Sickle cell disease
Homozygous dominant	Hemoglobin A Hemoglobin A	No disease
Heterozygous	Hemoglobin A Hemoglobin S	Sickle cell trait
Homozygous recessive	Hemoglobin S Hemoglobin S	Sickle cell anemia

commonly detected in childhood but may become manifest initially in adulthood. Diagnosis depends on observation of spherocytes on the peripheral blood smear and by demonstration of increased osmotic fragility of the red cells in the laboratory. It is almost invariably corrected by splenectomy.

Hemoglobinopathies refer to a group of diseases in which there is substitution of one or more amino acids in the globin chain of the Hb molecule, leading to the formation of abnormal Hb (for example, hemoglobins S and C). Their diagnosis and differentiation are facilitated by Hb electrophoresis. The most common hemoglobinopathy is Hb S disease, or sickle cell anemia.

Sickle cell anemia

Sickle cell anemia occurs predominantly in the black population. Approximately 8% of American blacks are heterozygous for Hb S and therefore have *sickle cell trait* (Table 28-4). They produce both Hb S and normal Hb A. Sickle cell trait is a benign disorder, often asymptomatic, with no anemia and a normal life span. Genetic counseling and screening may be suggested to inform affected individuals that marriage to another person who is also heterozygous for Hb S may lead to offspring with sickle cell disease.

Individuals who are homozygous for Hb S can only produce the defective Hb S. It is these individuals who have sickle cell disease and are affected with a chronic hemolytic anemia, episodes of painful "crisis," and an anticipated shortened life span.

The basic abnormality lies within the globin (protein) fraction of the Hb, where a single amino acid is substituted for another in one of the polypeptide chains. This single amino acid substitution profoundly alters the properties of the Hb molecule. The tendency toward sickling is dependent on both the relative quantity of Hb S in the RBCs and the levels of oxygen tension within the tissues of the body.

The clinical manifestations of the disease result from the sickling phenomenon. Sickling occurs when red cells containing Hb S are deoxygenated; it is the result of the poor solubility of the Hb S, which crystallizes in the RBCs. The sickle shape represents conformity of the red cell membrane to the spindle cell aggregates of the sickle Hb (Fig. 28-5). Sickling is always present to some extent in the patient with sickle cell anemia.

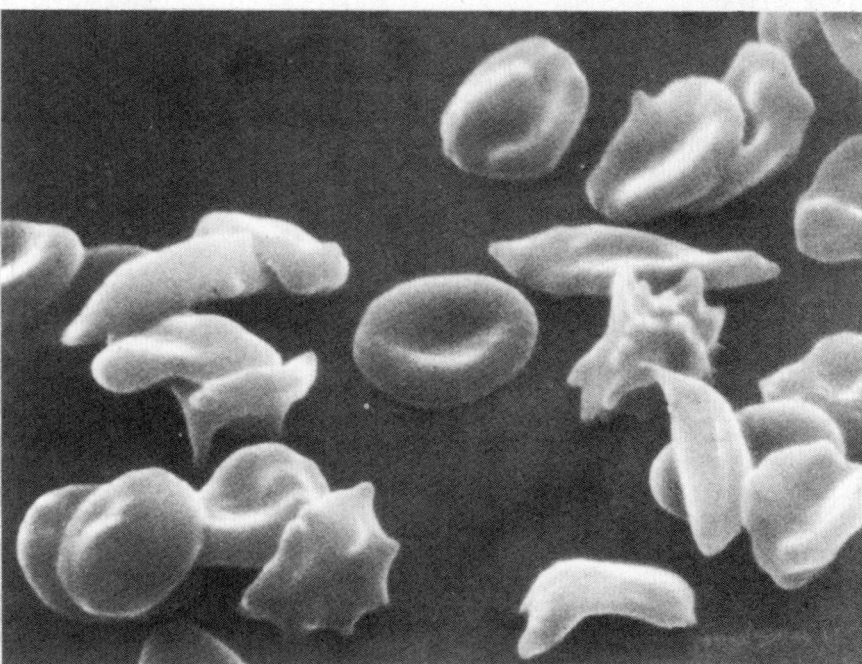

Fig. 28-5. Sickled red cells.

SICKLE CELL CRISES. Basically, any event that increases the body's need for oxygen or that alters the transport of oxygen may lead to the exacerbation of symptoms called *crisis.* Symptoms may be exacerbated by pregnancy, infection, surgery, trauma, and dehydration. Sickle cell crises are primarily thrombotic or aplastic.

Thrombotic crisis is the most common type, and is caused by the occlusion of blood vessels by the sickled cell. Pain, which may be severe, is the primary symptom, and often involves the abdomen and musculoskeletal systems.

Aplastic crisis is secondary to infection and is a temporary decrease in erythropoiesis. The anemia rapidly becomes worse.

Thalassemia

Thalassemia is an inherited disorder characterized by a decreased synthesis of one of the globin chains of Hb. The beta (β) chain is most often affected (β-thalassemia). As a result, there is a decreased synthesis of Hb as well as an accumulation in the erythrocyte of the unaffected globin chain. These alterations result in decreased red cell production and a chronic hemolytic anemia. The red cells are characteristically hypochromic (low MCH) and microcytic (low MCV). Hb electrophoresis is diagnostic.

There are two types of thalassemia, thalassemia minor, which is usually asymptomatic; and thalassemia major, which is characterized by severe anemia. Life span is significantly shortened, and frequent transfusion therapies may produce iron overload, a problem that can be ameliorated by use of an iron-chelating drug such as deferoxamine.

Enzyme deficiency

Deficiency of enzymes in the pathways that metabolize glucose and generate ATP frequently leads to premature red cell destruction. The most common clinically significant enzyme abnormality is that of *glucose-6-phosphate dehydrogenase.* This disorder is common in a mild form among the black population in the United States and in the Mediterranean area and may cause chronic hemolytic anemia. When an oxidant drug puts the cells under stress, acute hemolysis results.

Acquired hemolytic anemia

Hemolytic anemia may be drug induced or may be caused by an autoimmune disorder. In the latter case an antibody develops that is directed against an antigen on the individual's own RBCs. The antibody-coated red cells are destroyed prematurely by reticuloendothelial cells, particularly in the spleen. Diagnosis is confirmed by demonstrating the presence of the antibody on the red cells (antiglobin or Coombs' test).

Drugs produce hemolysis in a variety of ways. Alpha methyldopa (Aldomet) is associated with production of an autoantibody and a positive Coombs' test in approximately 20% of patients. More rarely, high-dose penicillin produces hemolysis through production of an antibody that requires the presence of penicillin on the red cell membrane for its effects to occur. This disorder is often fatal, in part because transfusion is often made difficult and dangerous by the fact that the autoantibody reacts not only with the patient's red cells but also with all donor cells.

DATA ANALYSIS AND PLANNING

Nursing diagnoses would include those associated with anemia from blood loss (p. 733), if hemorrhage has occurred. Additional nursing diagnoses might include the following:

Alteration in comfort: pain in joints
Ineffective individual/family coping
Knowledge deficit

Expected patient outcomes include the following:

1. Patient states feeling comfortable
2. The person/family can do the following:
   a. Describe signs and symptoms requiring immediate medical intervention
   b. Describe ways to prevent excessive bleeding
   c. State awareness of community resources for hemophiliacs and genetic counseling services
   d. State plans to carry medical identification information
   e. State plans for follow-up care

IMPLEMENTATION

Assisting with achievement of therapeutic goals

Bleeding disorders may require local treatment such as ice bags, manual pressure or dressings, immobilization, and elevation of a body part. Joint aspiration may be necessary. Muscle stretching exercises are begun after pain and bleeding have subsided (usually within 3 to 5 days). Active range of motion exercises are encouraged when swelling has subsided.

In major hemorrhages, careful monitoring is necessary to avoid fluid overload if large plasma volumes are given. Concentrates (Table 28-7) have been developed to provide the deficient factors and to prevent fluid overload and fewer side effects (for example, urticarial or febrile reactions) in some patients. High cost and contamination with the virus of serum hepatitis are drawbacks, however, to the use of some of the concentrates. Factor replacement therapy may be given on an outpatient basis, either in a clinic or in the home. Home infusion programs have gained interest and are seen as a way of controlling bleeding episodes more quickly, thereby decreasing the need for hospitalization and a long absence from school or work.

The outlook for the person with hemophilia has been greatly improved by the availability of transfusion therapy. In the past many persons with factor VIII deficiency died in the first 5 years of life. Today persons with moderate or mild hemophilia may live normal, productive lives.

Counseling and teaching

Threat of spontaneous bleeding episodes and pain control are ongoing stressors the individual must confront. Important points for teaching are listed in the box. Those individuals who are able to meet the demands of their illness and adapt their life-styles accordingly are able to live productive lives as individuals, spouses, parents, and employees.

Genetic counseling, aimed at explaining the pattern of inheritance of hemophilia, may be of great value to adults

---

Teaching the person with hemophilia

1. Nature of the disease, genetic basis
2. Prevention of hemorrhage (p. 738)
3. Possibility of bleeding after dental extraction
4. Avoidance of contact sports
5. Importance of carrying a card or wearing a Medic-Alert tag with name, blood type, physician's name and phone number, and diagnosis
6. Community resources (National Hemophilia Foundation)
7. Family planning techniques if desired
8. Need for medical follow-up

Table 28-7. Blood factor replacement therapy for hemophilia

Type	Clotting factors	Comments
Fresh frozen plasma	All	Thawed to 37° C; allergic reactions are common; fluid overload possible, especially in older persons
Cryoprecipitate	VIII, fibrinogen	Thawed to 37° C before infusion; occasional allergic reactions; low risk of hepatitis transmission
Lyophilized factor VIII concentrate	VIII	Stable at room temperature; possible hemolytic reactions for persons with blood types A, B, AB when given over prolonged period; allergic reactions rare
Vitamin K dependent complex	VII, IX, X, prothrombin	Keep refrigerated; higher risk of hepatitis transmission and thrombus formation (heparin usually given concurrently)

contemplating parenthood. Such counseling can assist potential parents in evaluating realistically their ability to raise a child afflicted with hemophilia and to anticipate ways to meet the demands placed on both of them and the child.

The National Hemophilia Foundation* is an organization established for persons with hemophilia and their families. The basic function of the national organization is hemophilia research. In addition, it publishes literature, produces films, and promotes health care legislation in Washington. Local chapter services include special camps for children with hemophilia, counseling and group therapy sessions, and a newsletter that reports on advances in hemophilic care. A chapter may function as a liaison agent between hospitals and families with insurmountable bills for blood.

EVALUATION

Questions to ask the patient may include the following:
1. Is the person comfortable?
2. Is the person/family able to deal with the stresses associated with the disorder?

---

*25 West 39th St., New York, NY 10018.

3. Does the person know the nature of the disease, ways to prevent hemorrhage, available resources?

Disseminated intravascular coagulation

DIC is a pathophysiologic response of the body's hemostatic mechanisms to disease or injury. DIC is a complicated and potentially fatal syndrome that is characterized initially by clotting and secondarily by hemorrhage. It almost always occurs in response to a primary disease, massive trauma, or surgery (especially prostatic, orthopedic, or open-heart).

PATHOPHYSIOLOGY

DIC is essentially an imbalance between the processes of coagulation and anticoagulation. The normal balance of clotting factors and fibrinolytic factors, which under normal conditions prevent bleeding while maintaining the fluidity of the blood, are altered.

The primary disease or injury causes the initiation of the clotting process. This response is generalized and occurs throughout the vascular system, creating a state of

---

Nursing care of the person with DIC

1. Monitor continually for new bleeding sites or changes in amount of bleeding (especially if heparin therapy is given)
2. Assess and record amount of drainage from chest and nasogastric tubes and oozing from incisions
3. Monitor fluid rates; be alert for signs of fluid overload (increased pulse rate, distended jugular veins, and increased CVP)
4. Provide care for the critically ill patient (see Chapter 41)
5. Explain to family what is occurring and provide opportunities for expressions of feelings

---

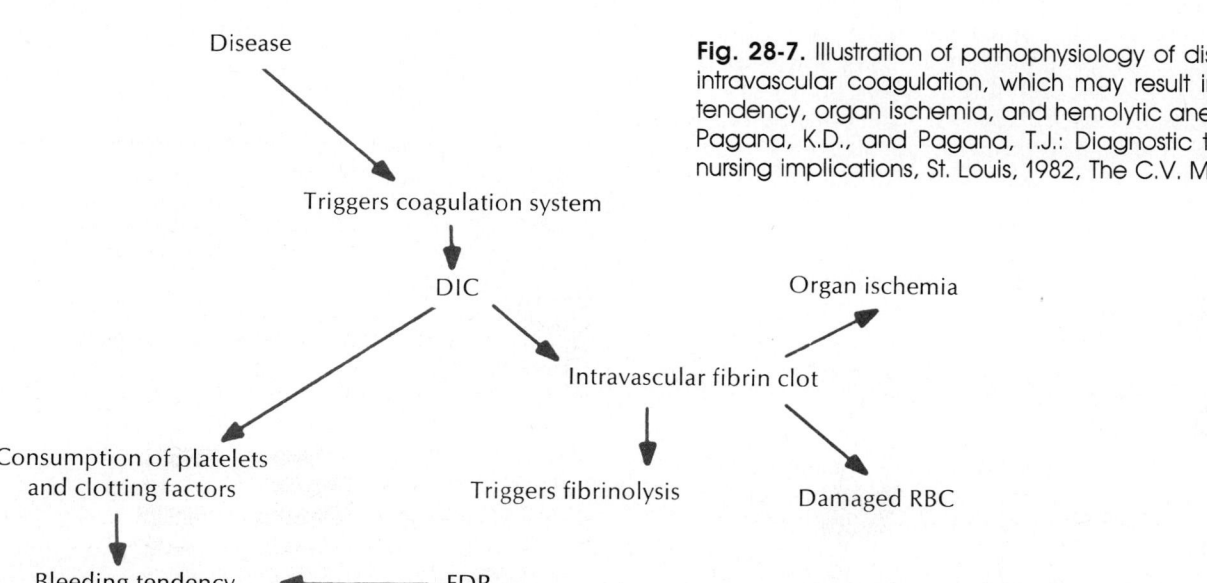

Fig. 28-7. Illustration of pathophysiology of disseminated intravascular coagulation, which may result in bleeding tendency, organ ischemia, and hemolytic anemia. (From Pagana, K.D., and Pagana, T.J.: Diagnostic testing and nursing implications, St. Louis, 1982, The C.V. Mosby Co.)

hypercoagulability. The fibrinolytic processes, which normally operate to limit clot extension and dissolve clots, are then stimulated (Fig. 28-7). As clotting factors are depleted and fibrinolysis continues, a state of *hypocoagulability* develops.

The most common sequela of DIC is hemorrhage. This paradox is caused by decreased platelets and the depletion of clotting factors II, V, VIII, fibrinogen and the production of fibrin degradation products (FDP) through fibrinolysis. The FDP acts as anticoagulants, which increase the hemorrhagic tendency.

ASSESSMENT

The first signs and symptoms (Table 28-6) may be those of hemorrhage (oral, vaginal, rectal, after injection and venipuncture, petechiae, and ecchymosis). Pain may be present from joint bleeding.

Laboratory findings, which may be the only indications of the syndrome in the early stages, include the following:
1. Decreased circulating platelet count
2. Prolonged PT
3. Prolonged PTT
4. Decreased factors V and VIII
5. Decreased fibrinogen levels
6. Increased fibrin split products (fibrinolysis)
7. Abnormal RBCs on peripheral blood smear

DATA ANALYSIS AND PLANNING

Nursing diagnoses include those related to fluid deficit. Expected patient outcomes are those for acute blood loss (p. 733).

IMPLEMENTATION

Nursing intervention in the care of the patient with DIC is extremely challenging. The person is critically ill and frequently has numerous sites of bleeding before DIC becomes evident. Frequently the patient is comatose, and the presence of purpura, numerous intravenous lines, and drainage tubes makes the patient's appearance especially upsetting to the family. Most of the primary conditions associated with DIC are of a sudden nature, and the family requires help in understanding this catastrophic occurrence and support during the long period of treatment.

DISORDERS ASSOCIATED WITH WHITE BLOOD CELLS

Changes in number of white cells

NEUTROPENIA

Neutropenia is defined as a neutrophil count of less than 2000/cu mm. It may occur as a primary hematologic disorder but is seen more often in association with other disorders, including malignant disease of the bone marrow, aplastic anemia, megaloblastic anemia, use of che-

motherapeutic agents, starvation, and viral infections. The degree of susceptibility to infection is in direct proportion to the degree of neutropenia. Individuals with marked neutropenia are at risk for contracting a life-threatening infection.

Agranulocytosis is an acute disease in which there is a sudden decrease in the number of WBCs, usually as the result of chemicals or drugs (sulfonamides, propylthiouracil, chloramphenicol, and bone marrow depressant drugs such as chemotherapeutic agents). Clinical signs include infection, malaise (discomfort, headache, lassitude, muscle aches), ulceration of mucous membranes, chills, and fever. A sepsis may develop, which may lead to death. Care is directed toward removal of the causative agents and resolving infection. If bone marrow is not destroyed, the prognosis for recovery is good.

NEUTROPHILIA

Neutrophilia is defined as a neutrophil count greater than 10,000/cu mm. Such an increase is a normal response to infections, primarily bacterial. It may also increase with strenuous exercise. Prolonged elevation of the neutrophil count, especially in the absence of an apparent cause, is a reason for a diligent search for the underlying cause. Persistent elevated neutrophil counts are associated with leukemia, polycythemia vera, myeloid metaplasia, and a variety of systemic and inflammatory disorders. Treatment consists of therapy for the primary condition.

Leukemia

PATHOPHYSIOLOGY

Leukemias are malignant disorders of the hematopoietic system involving the bone marrow and lymph nodes; they are characterized by uncontrolled proliferation of leukocytes and their precursors. The large number of cells accumulate first at the site of origin (granulocytes in the bone marrow, lymphocytes in the lymph nodes), then spread to hematopoietic organs, leading to organ enlargement (splenomegaly, hepatomegaly). The proliferation of one type of cell often interferes with the normal production of other hematopoietic cells, leading to the development of immature cells and to cytopenias (decreased numbers). The immaturity of the white cells leads to decreased immunocompetence with increased susceptibility to infections.

The cause of leukemia is unknown. An increased incidence of leukemia in siblings has led to hypotheses of genetic predispositions or viral origins. Radiation and chemicals (including antineoplastic drugs) have also been implicated.

CLASSIFICATION OF LEUKEMIAS

The leukemias are classified as acute or chronic and further subdivided according to cell type or maturity of the cell (Table 28-8).

Table 28-8. Characteristics of different leukemias

Type	Peak age (years)	WBC level	Bone marrow cell predominance
Acute lymphocytic leukemia (ALL)	2 to 4	Decreased (granulocytopenia)	Lymphoblasts
Acute myelogenous leukemia (AML)	12 to 20; after 55	Normal or decreased	Myeloblasts
Chronic lymphocytic leukemia (CLL)	50 to 70 males	Increased 20,000 to 100,000	Lymphocytes
Chronic myelogenous leukemia (CML)	30 to 50 males	Increased 15,000 to 500,000	Granulocytes, Philadelphia chromosome

Table 28-9. Leukemias

Type	Etiology	Signs and symptoms	Medical therapy
Acute lymphocytic leukemia (ALL)	Genetic predisposition; environmental factors (ionizing radiation); chemicals (benzene, arsenic, chloramphenicol, antineoplastic agents); immune deficiency states	Respiratory infections, anemia, bleeding of mucous membranes; proliferation of lymphoblasts in bone marrow, lymph nodes, spleen; hepatomegaly; splenomegaly; bone pain; CNS symptoms (headache, vomiting, seizures)	Combined chemotherapy, radiotherapy and immunotherapy; drugs: vincristine, prednisone, L-asparaginase
Acute myelogenous leukemia (AML)	Same as above	Same as above	Chemotherapy with daunorubicin, cytarabine, doxorubicin, 6-thioguanine
Chronic lymphocytic leukemia (CLL)	Same as above	Painless and massive lymphadenopathy and splenomegaly; hepatomegaly with disease progression; anemia; thrombocytopenia; fatigue; weakness; pruritic vesicular lesions	Chemotherapy with alkylating agents (chlorambucil) and glucocorticoids (only when symptoms appear)
Chronic myelogenous leukemia (CML)	Same as above	Fatigue, weakness, anorexia, weight loss; blastic (accelerated) phase: anemia, thrombocytopenia, fever, adenopathy, splenomegaly with sensation of abdominal fullness	Chemotherapy with agents used in AML; also vincristine, busulfan

Acute leukemias

Acute leukemias involve immature cells and are classified according to the predominant cell in the bone marrow, either lymphoblasts (acute lymphocytic leukemia) or myeloblasts (acute myelogenous leukemia). Acute leukemias have a rapid onset and a short course, ending in death if untreated. The immaturity of the white cells leads to numerous infections, such as ulceration of the mucous membranes, pneumonias, and septicemias. Early symptoms include fever, lymphadenopathy, pallor, and fatigue from anemia, and ecchymoses (Table 28-9). The WBC count may be normal or decreased.

Acute lymphocytic leukemia (ALL)

ALL arises from a single lymphoid stem cell (Fig. 28-1) with impaired maturation and accumulation of the malignant cells in the bone marrow. It is common to find different stages of lymphoid development in the bone marrow from very immature to almost normal cells. The degree of immaturity is a guide to prognosis; the more immature cells, the poorer the prognosis. Leukocytes in the bloodstream are predominantly in the blast form. The WBC count is often decreased but a blood smear will show immature lymphoblasts. It is primarily a disease of children, but adults may develop it.

Acute myelogenous leukemia (AML)

AML arises from a single myeloid stem cell (Fig. 28-1) and is characterized by the development of immature myeloblasts in the bone marrow. The WBC count is usually in the low ranges of normal, and bone marrow aspiration reveals an increased number of myeloblasts. In the untreated patient or the person who is nonresponsive to therapy, the median survival time (MST) is approximately 2 to 3 months. Complete remission occurs in 50% to 75% of treated patients, and there is an MST of approximately 2 to 3 years. Approximately 20% of patients are in complete remission at 5 years and are capable of prolonged disease-free periods (remissions).

Chronic leukemias

Chronic leukemias are classified according to the predominant mature white cell, either lymphocytes (chronic lymphocytic anemia) or granulocytes (chronic myelogenous leukemia). Chronic leukemias have a more insidious onset and an MST of 3 to 4 years. Initially there are fewer infections than in acute leukemias because of the maturity of the white cells in the chronic disorder, but eventually infections of the skin and pneumonias result from decreased immunocompetence. Early signs of chronic leukemias include fatigue, weakness, anorexia, and weight loss characteristic of a hypermetabolic state. An enlarged spleen and liver can usually be palpated. The WBC count is usually elevated.

Chronic lymphocytic leukemia (CLL)

CLL is characterized by a proliferation of small, abnormal, mature B-lymphocytes, leading to decreased synthesis of immunoglobulins and depressed antibody response. The accumulation of abnormal lymphocytes begins in the lymph nodes, then spreads to other lymphatic tissues. There is a marked increase in the number of both leukocytes and mature lymphocytes. At the time of diagnosis the bone marrow is often filled by lymphatic infiltrations. The WBC count is elevated to a level between 20,000 and 100,000. Bone marrow biopsy shows infiltration of lymphocytes.

Chronic myelogenous leukemia (CML)

The primary defect in CML is an abnormal stem cell leading to an uncontrolled proliferation of the granulocytic cells. As a result of this proliferation, there is a marked increase in the number of circulating granulocytes. In most cases, a characteristic chromosomal abnormality, the *Philadelphia chromosome,* is present. Diagnosis of CML is made on the basis of an elevated WBC count of 15,000 to 500,000, granulocytes on the peripheral blood smear that range in maturity from blast cells to mature neutrophils, granulocytic hyperplasia in the bone marrow, and the presence of the Philadelphia chromosome.

DATA ANALYSIS AND PLANNING

Nursing diagnoses

Nursing diagnoses will be based on collected data and may include the following:

Potential for infection
Activity intolerance
Anxiety
Coping, ineffective family
Oral mucous membranes, alterations
Sexual integrity, impairment of
Altered nutrition, less than body requirements

Many of the interventions for these diagnoses are discussed in Chapter 14.

Expected patient outcomes

The person or significant other can describe the following:
1. The nature of the disease
2. The chemotherapeutic program
3. Symptoms requiring immediate medical follow-up
4. Available community resources

IMPLEMENTATION

Assisting with achievement of therapeutic goals

Leukemia, by its nature, is a diverse illness. The varied courses and response or lack of response to treatment also add to the diversity. Complete remission of the disease is the goal of medical therapy since cure is not possible at this time. Complete remission exists when all tests are normal and all symptoms have disappeared. Partial remission occurs when symptoms have disappeared but the disease remains in the bone marrow.

Chemotherapy

Chemotherapy is the primary treatment modality. The first phase of chemotherapy is termed *induction chemotherapy* and consists of combination chemotherapy (use of more than one chemotherapeutic agent, see Chapter 14). Commonly used agents used in the treatment of leukemias are listed in the box below. Bone marrow studies are conducted 2 and 3 weeks following initiation of therapy. A different drug regimen will be given if evidence of disease in the marrow is still present after 3 weeks.

Chemotherapeutic agents commonly used in leukemia therapy

L-Asparaginase
Chlorambucil
Cyclophosphamide
Cytarabine
Daunorubicin
Doxorubicin
6-Mercaptopurine
Methotrexate
Prednisone
6-Thioguanine
Vincristine

During induction therapy, the patient is at high risk for hemorrhage or infection. Nursing care of the patient during this phase includes the following:

1. Monitor vital signs every 4 hours
2. Use of bleeding precautions
   a. Use soft toothbrush or swabs for mouth
   b. No rectal temperatures, medications, or enemas
   c. Use of electric razor
   d. Avoidance of aspirin
3. Monitor for signs of bleeding (observation of skin, testing urine with hemastix and stool for guaiac)
4. Give antibiotics on time to maintain blood levels if fever occurs
5. Monitor administration of whole blood or blood component therapy, if given
6. Assess intravenous site of chemotherapy for redness, swelling, tenderness, extravasation of drugs
7. Provide immediate care of extravasation of chemotherapeutic drugs (discontinue infusion, apply ice to area, infiltrate subcutaneous area with sodium bicarbonate or steroids)[6]
8. Provide emotional support to patient and family
   a. Time for them to talk, share fears and concerns, ask questions
   b. Carefully explain therapy and planned activities
   c. Include family in all aspects of care

Maintenance therapy, the second phase of therapy, is usually required to maintain a complete remission. This therapy is often given on an outpatient basis. Appropriate duration of therapy in patients who continue free of disease varies, depending on the type of the disease and the patient's response to therapy.

Bone marrow transplantation

Bone marrow transplantation, using HLA-identical bone marrow, has been used with increasing frequency and promises to have an increasing impact on the progress of AML. In addition to leukemia, bone marrow transplantation is being used for patients with lymphoma, aplastic anemia, thalassemia, and immunodeficiency disorders.

Pretransplant preparation is necessary for bone marrow transplantation. It has two goals, *immunosuppression* to allow acceptance of an immunologically nonidentical graft and *cytoreduction* to kill all tumor cells. This is accomplished by chemotherapy followed by total body irradiation.

The procedure comprises taking 500 to 800 ml of blood and marrow cells from the donor, mixing it with heparin and tissue culture media, and then straining the mixture through a stainless-steel screen to break up marrow particles.[40] The marrow is then placed in a blood transfusion bag and administered intravenously through a Hickman catheter at the same rate as RBC administration (about 4 hours).

About 40% to 50% of patients develop severe acute graft-vs-host reaction, which involves severe skin, liver, and GI symptoms and death[31] or veno-occlusive disease of the liver.[13] One approach being used to prevent graft-vs-host reaction is treatment of the donor marrow with mono-

---

Teaching the person with leukemia

1. Nature of the disease process and its effects
2. Prevention of infection
3. Drug regimen: name, side effects (see Chapter 14)
4. Method of arranging for chemotherapy administration and periodic blood counts
5. Symptoms requiring immediate medical attention (fever, bleeding)
6. Available community resources (American Cancer Society, Leukemia Society*)
7. Need for continual medical follow-up

*211 East 43rd St. New York, NY 10017.

---

clonal antibodies before transplantation; this removes mature T-cells, which cause the reaction, but leave immature T-cells for prevention of infection.

Nursing care is focused on prevention of infection and on providing emotional support; skin care; and maintenance of fluid, electrolyte, and nutritional balance.

Counseling and teaching

Each individual with leukemia responds in a different way. It cannot be predicted for certain if an individual will respond to a prescribed treatment or how long a remission will last. Likewise, how the individual incorporates the illness into life is also unique to each person. Nursing has the key role in patient education. Of utmost importance in learning is the ability of the person to identify the body's signals that blood abnormalities exist. Bone pain, often severe, may signal blast crisis (acute proliferation of immature cells).

Individuals whose illness runs the course of several months to years often become very knowledgeable about their disease, blood components, related symptoms, and specific chemotherapeutic drugs. These persons sometimes discuss their progress in terms of changes in their blood counts. Over time many individuals become attuned to how such changes affect them. For example, they often can predict their count by how they feel. Many such persons respond well to being included in their plan of care during hospitalization and in preparation for discharge.

Time set aside for patient teaching also allows for a sharing time with the individual. This time may provide the foundation for an honest nurse-patient relationship from which emotional support may be given.

EVALUATION

Questions to ask the patient may include the following:
1. Is the patient knowledgeable about the disease, its effects, and the treatment regimen?
2. Can the patient describe symptoms that require medical intervention?

3. Can the patient state importance of and schedule for chemotherapy and periodic blood tests?
4. Are the laboratory tests showing improvement toward normal values with therapy?

DISORDERS ASSOCIATED WITH THE LYMPH SYSTEM

Lymphadenopathy

Lymph node enlargement (lymphadenopathy) may be caused by infection in the area drained by the lymph vessel containing the node or by systemic infection. Enlargement of the node, which in this situation is usually painful, is a positive sign indicating immune responsiveness to the invading microorganisms. Lymphadenopathy may also occur when the node is invaded by cells normally not present (leukemic cells, cancer cells) and is a pathophysiologic sign with lymphomas, such as Hodgkin's disease.

Lymphangiography is a radiologic technique used for evaluation of lymph nodes to detect the presence of disease. This procedure is especially valuable in the assessment of those nodes that are anatomically too deep to allow for evaluation by palpation. For this procedure a small incision is made on the dorsal surface of each foot so that the small lymph glands are made accessible. A dye is slowly instilled over several hours, filling all lymph chains and nodes. Radiographs are usually done immediately after the dye is absorbed and again at intervals of 24 and 48 hours after the procedure. In addition, because the dye remains in the lymph nodes for as long as 6 months after the initial study, disease status and response to therapy can be periodically evaluated with routine abdominal x-ray films.

Lymphomas

Lymphomas are malignant disorders of the lymph system. Hodgkin's disease is considered separate from other lymphomas.

Staging of Hodgkin's disease

Stage	Definition
I	Single abnormal lymph node
II	Two or more abnormal lymph nodes on the same side of the diaphragm
III	Abnormal lymph node regions on both sides of the diaphragm, which may also be accompanied by involvement of the spleen
IV	Diffuse or disseminated involvement of one or more extralymphatic organs or tissues with or without lymph node involvement

---

PATHOPHYSIOLOGY

Hodgkin's disease

Hodgkin's disease, which was considered fatal until fairly recently, is now potentially curable. Although the cause is unknown, it is thought that viruses may be implicated. The person has *defective cellular immunity (T-cell disease)* and is therefore at high risk for infections. Four pathologic variants of Hodgkin's have been recognized: *lymphocyte predominant, nodular sclerosis, mixed cellularity,* and *lymphocyte depletion.* The lymphocyte predominant and nodular sclerosis types have the best prognosis and lymphocyte depletion the worst. Hodgkin's disease is usually characterized by the presence of the Reed-Sternberg cell, a large macrophage-derived cell.

The most important prognostic indicator is the stage of disease at the time of diagnosis. Accurate staging (see box) is crucial to the subsequent treatment regimen:

All stages are subclassified further, as follows:

A No symptoms
B Presence of weight loss, fever, profuse night sweats

Non-Hodgkin's lymphoma

Non-Hodgkin's lymphomas (NHL) include a broad spectrum of lymphoid malignancies with different histopathologies, disease courses, and responses to therapy. Accurate identification of the histopathology is crucial to the determination of the treatment plan. NHL can be categorized as *lymphocytic, histiocytic,* or *mixed cell types.* A lymphocytic cytology has the most favorable prognosis, and the histiocytic has the least favorable. Immature lymphocytes are produced, leading to impaired B-cell (humoral) immune response. These patients, therefore, are also at high risk for infections.

ASSESSMENT

Subjective data include the following:
1. Knowledge of the disorder
2. Effect of fatigue on the ability to carry out ADL
3. Discomfort from night sweats or pruritus
4. Appetite and present nutritional status

Objective data includes weight and condition of skin from scratching (for example, excoriations).

Diagnostic tests for lymphomas may include a chest x-ray film to identify a mediastinal mass and lymphangiography to evaluate the retroperitoneal nodes. The liver and spleen are evaluated by radionuclide scanning or by computed tomography (CT scan). A staging laparotomy may be performed to obtain a biopsy specimen of retroperitoneal lymph nodes and of both lobes of the liver and to remove the spleen. The diagnostic workup is often arduous and difficult, and explanation of the diagnostic procedures helps provide the patient with the emotional support so often needed during this time.

Slides are often sent to major cancer centers for consultation regarding the classification of the disease. Once the diagnosis is made, the extent of the disease (staging) must be determined for planning the treatment regimen.

DATA ANALYSIS AND PLANNING

Nursing diagnoses may include the following:
Comfort, alteration in: pruritus, night sweats
Skin integrity: potential for impairment of
Knowledge deficit
In addition, side effects of chemotherapy and radiation therapy may provide data for alterations in nutrition and bowel elimination.

Expected patient outcomes may include the following:
1. The patient states feeling more comfortable
2. Skin breakdown from scratching is minimal
3. The patient can describe the following:
   a. The nature of the disorder
   b. The therapeutic regimen
   c. Resources in the community

IMPLEMENTATION

Assisting with achievement of therapeutic goals

Chemotherapy and radiation therapy are the primary treatment modalities for the lymphomas (Table 28-10). For Hodgkin's disease, treatment yields a cure rate of approximately 90% for stage I and 80% for stage II. Combination chemotherapy is the treatment of choice for stages IIIb and IV. The most commonly used combination is the MOPP regimen (see chapter 14). It is administered in a 2-week course each month with prednisone added during the first and fourth course. The drugs are administered for at least 6 months or for two or three courses following the attainment of complete remission. Complete remissions are achieved in approximately 80% of these patients, and long-term, disease-free remissions and probable cures occur in half of this group.

When nodal radiation is used, only those areas of the body to be irradiated are exposed; the other areas are protected by a mantle (Fig. 28-8).

Varying approaches are used for non-Hodgkin's lymphomas. Either single alkylating agents, such as chlorambucil, or combination chemotherapy may be used. Either local or total nodal radiation therapy may be given. Explanation of the treatment regimen is important to ensure patient understanding and compliance to achieve the therapeutic goals.

Promotion of comfort and safety

Fever, pruritus, and profuse night sweats may lead to general discomfort. Comfort measures for pruritus (for example, baths, antipruritic medication [see Chapter 37]) may be instituted. Frequent changes of night clothing or bed linens may be necessary and a high fluid intake is encouraged.

Counseling and teaching

Hodgkin's disease most often affects young adults, therefore special attention needs to be given to minimize the impact of the illness and its treatment on their lives, not only during the treatment period but beyond. Before the initiation of treatment, therapy-induced sterility should be discussed.[21] For young women receiving radiation therapy alone, surgical relocation of the ovaries outside the field of radiation may be performed. Sterility frequently occurs in association with chemotherapy. For women this is often temporary, and the ability to conceive and bear normal children often returns after therapy is completed. For men, sterility is more frequently permanent. For this reason the option of sperm banking should

Table 28-10. Disorders of the lymph system

Disorder	Etiology	Signs and symptoms	Medical therapy
Hodgkin's disease	Unknown	Lymph node enlargement (firm, nontender, painless), fever, weight loss, night sweats, pruritus, fatigue	Radiation therapy for stages IA and IIA, radiation and chemotherapy for stage IIIA, combination chemotherapy for stages IIIB and IVB
Non-Hodgkin's lymphoma	Unknown, viruses implicated	Nontender "bulky" lymphadenopathy, moderate hepatomegaly and splenomegaly, fever, night sweats, weight loss	Initial localized radiotherapy; total nodal radiation and chemotherapy for multifocal lesions
Multiple myeloma	Lymphoproliferative disorder of plasma cells (malignancy)	Severe disabling bone pain (especially in weight-bearing areas), hypercalcemia, renal failure, anorexia, CHF, bleeding tendency, coma	Radiation for bone pain, chemotherapy, hydration, ambulation, blood transfusions for anemia, analgesics

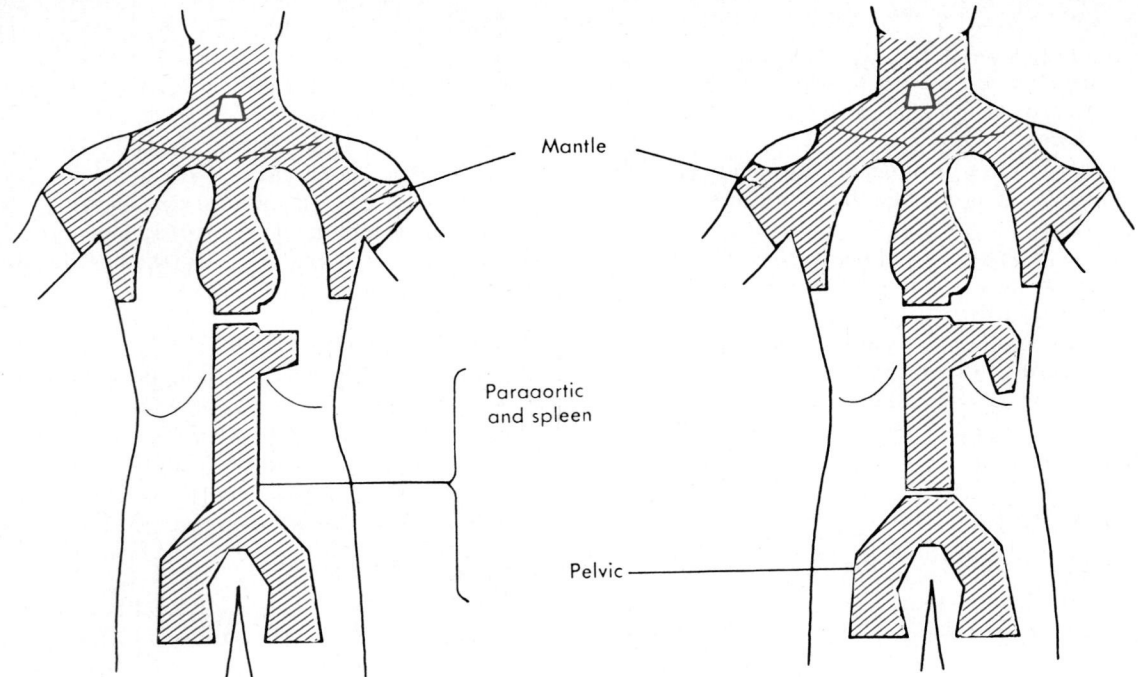

Fig. 28-8. Diagram of mantle and inverted Y fields used in total lymphoid radiotherapy of Hodgkin's disease. (From Rosenberg, S.A., and Kaplan, H.S., Calif. Med. **113:**23, 1970).

be discussed before beginning either radiation or chemotherapy.

To allow for work and career development, every effort should be made to schedule treatment at those times and days of the week that least interfere with work and other important events in the person's life. The nurse has a crucial role in assisting individuals to develop a realistic approach to the illness and in successfully meeting the demands and limitations imposed by the illness and its treatment.

Individuals with lymphomas may have periods of remission and recurrence. Such peaks and valleys are stressful and disruptive. Many patients describe subsequent courses of treatment following a recurrence as more stressful than the initial treatment. Comments include, "Is it worth it? I don't have the same faith." Other patients, realistically encouraged by the initial response to treatment, are able to express an optimistic outlook, "It worked the first time. It will work again." Recognition of the stress involved in therapy requires that support systems be available to the individual. The health care team can provide some of the needed support and guidance as the individual learns to incorporate the illness into daily life.

Teaching the patient includes the following:
1. Nature of the disorder
2. Importance of the extensive work-up in identifying the treatment plan
3. Effects of therapy on sterility
4. Need for periodic blood counts
5. Side effects of radiation and chemotherapy and how to cope with them (see Chapter 14)
6. Need for continued medical follow-up
7. Community resources (American Cancer Society)

EVALUATION

Questions to ask may include the following:
1. Is the person relatively comfortable?
2. Is the skin free of avoidable excoriations?
3. Can the person describe the nature of the disease and the effects of therapy?
4. Can the patient state times and dates for follow-up care or have written information for guidance?
5. Does the person know where to turn for assistance if needed?

REFERENCES AND SELECTED READINGS*

1. Barber, S.M.: Blood cell products in the supportive care of patients with acute leukemia, Nurs. Times **76**:152-154, 1980.
2. Buetler, E.: Iron. In Goodhart, R., and Shiels, M., editors: Modern nutrition in health and disease, Philadelphia, 1980, Lea & Febiger.
3. Bick, R.: Disseminated intravascular coagulation and related syndromes, etiology, pathophysiology, diagnosis, and management, Am. J. Hematol. **5**:265-282, 1978.
4. *Brown, M.: Standards of care for the patient with "graft-vs-host disease" post bone marrow transplant, Ca. Nurs. **4**:191-198, 1981.
5. Buickus, B.A.: Blood therapy: administering blood components, Am. J. Nurs. **79**:937, 1979.
6. *Campbell, V.B., Preston, R., and Smith, K.Y.: The leukemias: definition, treatment and nursing care, Nurs. Clin. North Am. **18**(3):523-542, 1983.
7. Carter, S., Glatstein, E., and Livingstone, R.: Principles of cancer treatment, New York, 1982, McGraw-Hill Book Co.
8. Cline, M., and Golde, D.: Controlling the production of blood cells, Blood **53**:157-164, 1979.
9. Curry, A.: Protective isolation study: practice corner, Oncology Nurs. Forum **8**:42, 1981.
10. Dietz, K.: Radiation therapy: programmed instruction, Ca. Nurs. **2**:127-138, 1979.
11. Diggs, L.W., Sturm, D., and Bell, A.: The morphology of human blood cells, ed. 4, Chicago, 1978, Abbott Laboratories.
12. Flynn, K.T.: Iron deficiency anemia among the elderly, Nurs. Pract. **3**:20-24, 1978.
13. *Ford, R., McClain, R.N., Cunningham, B.A.: Veno-occlusive disease following marrow transplantation, Nurs. Clin. North Am. **18**(3):563-568, 1983.
14. Gibbons, P.T.: Transfusion therapy in sickle cell disease, Nurs. Clin. North Am. **18**(1):201-205, 1983.
15. *Godwin, M., and Baysinger, M.: Understanding antisickling agents and the sickling process, Nurs. Clin. North Am. **18**(1):207-214, 1983.
16. Goldstein, M.: Aplastic anemia, Hosp. Pract. **15**:85-96, 1980.
17. Haskell, C.: Cancer treatment, Philadelphia, 1980, W.B. Saunders Co.
18. Herbert, C.: Folic acid and vitamin B_{12}. In Goodhart, R., and Shiels, M., editors: Modern nutrition in health and disease, ed. 6, Philadelphia, 1980, Lea & Febiger.
19. *Hutchison, M.M.: Aplastic anemia: care of the bone-marrow failure patient, Nurs. Clin. North Am. **18**(3):543-552, 1983.
20. Hutchison, M.M., and King, A.H.: A nursing perspective on bone marrow transplantation, Nurs. Clin. North Am. **18**(3):511-522, 1983.
21. Kaempfle, S.: The effects of cancer chemotherapy on reproduction: a review of the literature, Oncology Nurs. Forum **8**:11-18, 1980.
22. Kaye, D., and Rose, L.F.: Fundamentals of internal medicine, St. Louis, 1982, The C.V. Mosby Co.
23. Kenny, M.W.: Sickle cell disease, Nurs. Times **76**:1582-1584, 1980.
24. Knobf, M., and others: Cancer chemotherapy treatment and care, Boston, 1981, G.K. Hall & Co.
25. Lamberg, L.: Genetic screening: learning what you never wanted to know, Today's Health **54**:28-31, 1976.
26. Lopez, J.A., and Hausz, M.: Therapeutic apheresis, Am. J. Nurs. **82**:1572-1578, 1982.
27. Massie, R., and Massie, S.: Journey, New York, 1976, Warner Books, Inc.
28. Miller, V.G.: The sickle cell anemia patient in surgery, AORN J. **30**:1083-1090, 1979.
29. Nausef, W.M., and others: A study of the value of simple protective isolation in patients with granulocytopenia, N. Engl. J. Med. **304**:448-452, 1981.
30. Owen, H., and others: Bone marrow harvesting: nursing implications, Ca. Nurs. **4**:199-205, 1981.
31. Parker, N., and Cohen, R.: Acute graft-vs-host disease in allogenic marrow transplantation, Nurs. Clin. North Am. **18**(3):569-578, 1983.
32. Price, S.A., and Wilson, L.M.: Pathophysiology, New York, 1982, McGraw Hill Book Co.
33. Refkind, R., and others: Fundamentals of hematology, Chicago, 1976, Year Book Medical Publishers, Inc.
34. Rooks, Y., and Pack, B.: A profile of sickle cell disease, Nurs. Clin. North Am. **18**(1):131-138, 1983.
35. Rossman, M., Slavin, R., and Taft, E.: Pheresis therapy: patient care, Am. J. Nurs. **77**:1135-1141, 1977.
36. *Rozzell, M.S., Hijazi, M., and Pack, B.: The painful episode, Nurs. Clin. North Am. **18**(1):185-199, 1983.
37. *Scott, D.W., Goode, W.L., and Arlin, Z.A.: The psychodynamics of multiple remissions in a patient with acute nonlymphoblastic leukemia, Ca. Nurs. **6**:201-206, 1983.
38. Smith, I.E.: Hodgkin's disease drug therapy: working toward a cure for all, Nurs. Mirror **147**:37-39, 1978.
39. Spears, L.: The morbidity of sickle cell trait, a review of the literature, Am. J. Med. **64**:1021-1036, 1978.
40. Thomas, E.D.: Bone marrow transplantation; present states and future expectations. In Isselbacker, K.V., and others: Harrison's principles of internal medicine, New York, 1982, McGraw Hill Book Co.
41. Thomas, S.: Transfusing granulocytes, Am. J. Nurs. **79**:942-945, 1979.
42. *Varricchio, C.: The patient on radiation therapy, Am. J. Nurs. **81**:334-342, 1981.
43. Victor, H.: The nutritional anemias, Hosp. Pract. **15**:65-89, 1980.
44. Walters, I., and others: Complications of sickle cell disease, Nurs. Clin. North Am. **18**(1):139-184, 1983.
45. Welch, D.: Thrombocytopenia in adult patients with leukemia, Ca. Nurs. **1**:463-466, 1978.
46. *Williams, I., Earles, A.N., and Pack, B.: Psychological considerations in sickle cell disease, Nurs. Clin. North Am. **18**(1):216-230, 1983.
47. Williams, W., Bentler, E., Erslev, A., and Lichtman, M.: Hematology, New York, 1983, McGraw-Hill Book Co.
48. Syngaarden, J.B., and Smith, L.H.: Textbook of medicine, ed. 16, Philadelphia, 1982, W.B. Saunders Co.

*References preceded by an asterisk are particularly well suited for student reading.

UNIT VIII
Metabolic and Endocrine Problems

29   The Patient with Diabetes Mellitus

30   The Patient with Endocrine Problems

31   The Patient with Hepatic, Biliary, and Pancreatic Problems

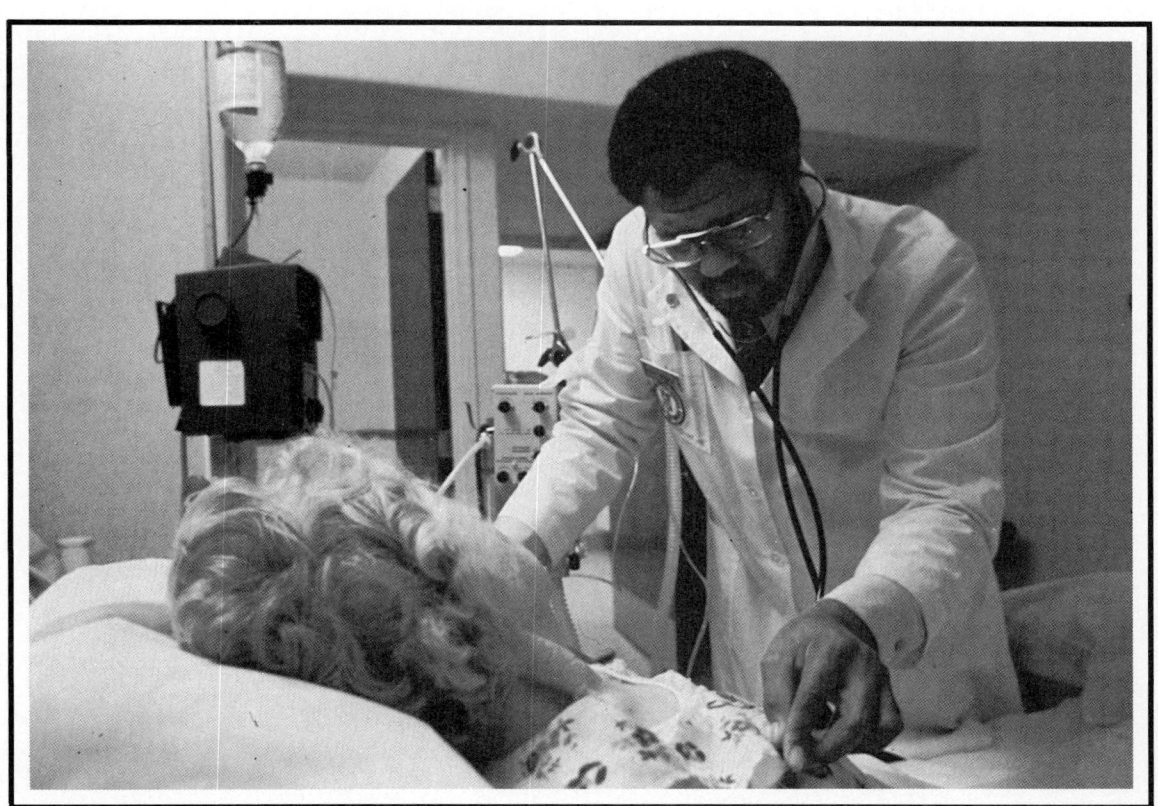

29

The Patient with Diabetes Mellitus

DOROTHY BLEVINS and VIRGINIA L. CASSMEYER

STUDY QUESTIONS

- Review the anatomy and physiology of the pancreas.

- Compare the prices of some of the insulin preparations and of disposable syringes. If a patient is taking a daily dose of 30 U NPH insulin, how long will a bottle last? What will be the monthly cost?

- What are the differences in preparation and procedures of the blood tests for diabetes mellitus?

- Why are the paper impregnated strips and tapes more reliable than Clinitest tablets for urine testing for diabetes mellitus?

- Ms. P. is a 25-year-old computer technician with newly diagnosed insulin-dependent diabetes mellitus (IDDM, type 1). She will be hospitalized for 3 more days and is motivated to learn how to care for herself.
  Outline an *initial* teaching plan, to be accomplished before Ms. P. is discharged.
  Outline a second teaching plan to be carried out by the community health nurse after Ms. P. is discharged.

Diabetes mellitus is a complex chronic disease involving (1) disorders in carbohydrate, protein, and fat metabolism and (2) the development of macrovascular, microvascular, and neurologic complications. It is classified as an endocrine or hormonal disease because of its central feature of hyperglycemia, which results from a deficit in production or utilization of insulin.

ANATOMY AND PHYSIOLOGY

Persons with normal metabolism are able to maintain blood glucose levels of 60 to 110 mg/dl (euglycemia) under markedly different conditions of food intake. In nondiabetic persons, blood glucose levels may rise to 120 to 140 mg/dl after eating (postprandial), but these then rapidly return to normal.

Hormonal regulation of blood glucose

Of the five hormones involved in the regulation of blood glucose levels, the pancreatic hormone, *insulin*, is the only one that lowers blood glucose. (Glucagon, growth hormone, epinephrine, and glucocorticoids all raise blood glucose levels.) Research is ongoing to determine the effect of other hormones and neurotransmitters on insulin and blood glucose levels.

The pancreas is both an exocrine and an endocrine gland. It lies retroperitoneally behind the stomach, with its head and neck in the curve of the duodenum, its body extending horizontally across the posterior abdominal wall, and its tail touching the spleen. More than 1 million islet cells are located throughout the organ.

The three types of endocrine cells are alpha (α), which secrete glucagon, beta (β), which secrete insulin, and

759

	Actions of insulin	
Hypoglycemic	Decreases blood glucose level overall
	Increases uptake and utilization of glucose by adipose and muscle cell
	Increases phosphorylation of glucose by liver
	Increases glycogenesis
Suppresses fat metabolism	Increases lipogenesis
Promotes protein synthesis	Increases amino acid incorporation into protein

Table 29-1. Diagnoses of diabetes mellitus and other categories of glucose intolerance

Disorder	Description	Criteria for diagnosis
Diabetes mellitus Insulin dependent (IDDM), type 1	Insulin deficient due to islet cell loss; often associated with specific HLA types, predisposition to viral insulitis or autoimmune phenomenoa; *ketosis prone;* occurs at any age, common in youth	Unequivocal elevation of plasma glucose ($\geq$200 mg/dl) and classic symptoms of diabetes (polydipsia, polyuria, polyphagia, weight loss) Fasting plasma glucose (FPG) $\geq$140 mg/dl on two occasions FPG <140 mg/dl and 2 hr plasma glucose $\geq$200 mg/dl with one intervening value $\geq$200 mg/dl after a 75 gm glucose load (OGTT)
Noninsulin dependent (NIDDM), type 2	*Ketosis resistant;* more frequent in adults, but occurs at any age; majority of patients overweight; familial tendency; may require insulin for hyperglycemia during stress	
Diabetes associated with certain conditions or syndromes	Hyperglycemia occurring in relation to other disease states: pancreatic disease, drugs or chemicals, endocrinopathies, insulin receptor disorders, certain genetic syndromes	
Impaired glucose tolerance	Abnormality in glucose levels intermediate between normal and overt diabetes; may progress to diabetes, improve to normal, or remain unchanged	FPG <140 mg/dl and 2 hr plasma glucose $\geq$140 mg/dl and <200 mg/dl with one intervening value $\geq$200 mg/dl after a 75 gm glucose load
Gestational diabetes (GDM)	Glucose intolerance with recognition of onset during pregnancy	Two or more of following plasma glucose concentrations met or exceeded using a 100 gm glucose load: FPG 105 mg/dl; 1 hr, 190 mg/dl; 2 hr, 165 mg/dl; 3 hr, 145 mg/dl

Adapted from C. R. Shuman and I. L. Spratt: Office guide to diagnosis and classification of diabetes mellitus and other categories of glucose intolerance, Diabetes Care **4(2)**:335, 1981. With permission from the American Diabetes Association, Inc.

Older terms used to describe diabetes mellitus

Juvenile onset *Usually* in younger individuals; IDDM (type 1).
Maturity onset *Usually* in older persons; NIDDM (type 2).
Latent No symptoms present, but hyperglycemia can be detected by laboratory examination.
Subclinical Under normal circumstances, results of fasting blood glucose tolerance test are normal; during stress, patient demonstrates impaired glucose tolerance.
Secondary Another disorder causes hyperglycemia.

Table 29-2. Comparison of insulin dependent and noninsulin dependent diabetes mellitus

	Insulin-dependent DM (IDDM, type 1)	Noninsulin-dependent DM (NIDDM, type 2)
Age of onset	More often in persons <40 years	More often in persons >40 years
Insulin	Absolute deficit	Relative deficit
Ketosis	Prone	Resistant
Complications	More often affects small blood vessels in eyes and kidneys	More often affects large blood vessels and nerves
Treatment	Insulin, diet, exercise	Diet and exercise; may be supplemented by hypoglycemic agents (about 30%)

delta (Δ), which secrete gastrin and pancreatic somato-statin.

Insulin is necessary for the transport of glucose, amino acids, potassium, and phosphate across cell membranes, especially those of adipose and resting muscle cells. Insulin is also needed to activate enzymes that promote intracellular metabolism. It seems to function by a fixed receptor model; that is, it combines with a receptor on the plasma membrane of the cell and initiates a sequence of postreceptor cellular activities that are coordinated by a second messenger, most probably cyclic guanosine 3,5-monophosphate (CGMP).[10] (The reader is referred to a physiology text for further detail on the action of insulin.)

It should be apparent that when there is a deficit of insulin, as in diabetes mellitus, *hyperglycemia, increased fat metabolism,* and *decreased protein synthesis* occur.

CLASSIFICATION OF DIABETES MELLITUS

The new classification system of glucose intolerance is described in Table 29-1. This system is gaining rapid acceptance throughout the country.[41] In addition to the five diagnoses of glucose intolerance shown in the Table, two others are specified:

1. Potential abnormality of glucose tolerance (in persons with known risk factors)
2. Previous abnormality of glucose tolerance (in persons who have had transient hyperglycemia).

This new system is designed to promote better compari-son of research studies and to decrease the ambiguity of previously used terms. The reader needs to be familiar with other terms still in use by patients and health care providers.

Table 29-2 compares the essential features of the two types of diabetes mellitus (DM): insulin-dependent diabetes mellitus (IDDM, type 1) and non-insulin-dependent mellitus (NIDDM, type 2).

A major characteristic of *type 1 DM (IDDM)* is the therapeutic need for insulin for survival. This insulin deficit is often termed absolute, in comparison with a relative deficit of insulin in *type 2 DM (NIDDM)*. Because of the complete dependency on exogenous insulin, persons with type 1 disease tend to have more severe and unstable glucose intolerance. In addition, they are prone to acute metabolic complications of ketosis and ketoacidosis (p. 765). Note that both forms of the disease may occur at any age; however, IDDM (type 1) is more typically found in children, whereas NIDDM (type 2) is more commonly associated with onset after age 25 years. Both forms of the disease are associated with vascular and neurologic complications; however, they differ in the organs most frequently affected. NIDDM is associated with high levels of circulating insulin that is ineffective at the insulin receptor site and for postreceptor function.

Gestational diabetes mellitus (GDM) has its onset during pregnancy. If glucose tolerance remains impaired after the pregnancy, the disease is reclassified as IDDM or NIDDM. Pregnancy stresses glucose tolerance in all women, particularly in the latter half of pregnancy when a growth hormone, human chorionic somatomammotropin (HCS), is secreted in increasing amounts. This hormone increases the supply of amino acids and glucose to the infant and diminishes the effectiveness of insulin. There is a direct correlation between mean blood glucose levels and infant mortality and morbidity. The presence of any type of DM in pregnancy requires careful medical management if optimal health of the infant and mother is to be achieved. Close control of blood glucose is recommended prior to conception as well as during pregnancy.

Glucose intolerance associated with certain conditions or syndromes is seen in persons who develop hyperglycemia as a complication of another disease or as a result of treatment. Commonly used drugs that can induce hyperglycemia include furosemide (Lasix) and thiazide diuretics, glucocorticoids, epinephrine, dilantin, and nicotinic acid.

PREVENTION AND HEALTH EDUCATION

Diabetes mellitus is probably not a single entity but a heterogenous group of diseases with diverse causes that are incompletely understood.[26] Both genetic and environmental factors have been implicated and are under study. Although these are still incompletely understood, high-risk factors have been identified by epidemiologic studies.

Primary prevention

Currently, avoidance of obesity and, if necessary, reduction of weight under medical supervision are the ma-

jor foci in primary prevention of NIDDM (type 2). Because of the strong association of NIDDM with hypertension, heart disease, and atherosclerosis, health practices that diminish risk factors for these diseases are recommended for the general population, for those identified at high risk for diabetes, and for persons with diagnosed diabetes (Chapter 26).

The role of heredity is now believed to be strongest in NIDDM, but genetic counseling is not appropriate because the pattern and mode of genetic transmission is not understood well enough to predict which offspring will develop the disease. This does not deny familial history as a risk factor for diabetes mellitus.

Autoimmunity may be a factor in the development of some diabetes. Scientists are studying whether there can be safe clinical application in humans of recent discoveries that suggest that onset of diabetes may be related to immunologic changes. Some studies have shown that persons with certain histocompatibility antigens (HLA antigens) are at increased risk of developing IDDM (type 1). Mumps, rubella, and Coxsackie virus B have been associated with development of IDDM. Fig. 29-1 illustrates a postulated interaction between viral agents and the pancreatic beta cells.

Risk factors for diabetes mellitus

Obesity
Family history of diabetes mellitus
Delivery of a baby weighing >9 lb.

Table 29-3. Glucose tolerance with aging (plasma glucose in mg/dl)

Age (yr.)	Normal			Probable diabetes, 2 hr	Diabetes, 2 hr
	Fasting	1 hr	2 hr		
0-30	110	185	165	166-185	>185
30-40	112	191	175	176-195	>195
40-50	114	197	185	186-205	>205
50-60	116	203	195	196-215	>215
60-70	118	209	205	200-235	>235
70-80	120	215	215	216-245	>245

From Andres, R., adapted from Prout, T.E.: *Diabetes mellitus*, ed 4, New York, 1975, American Diabetes Association.

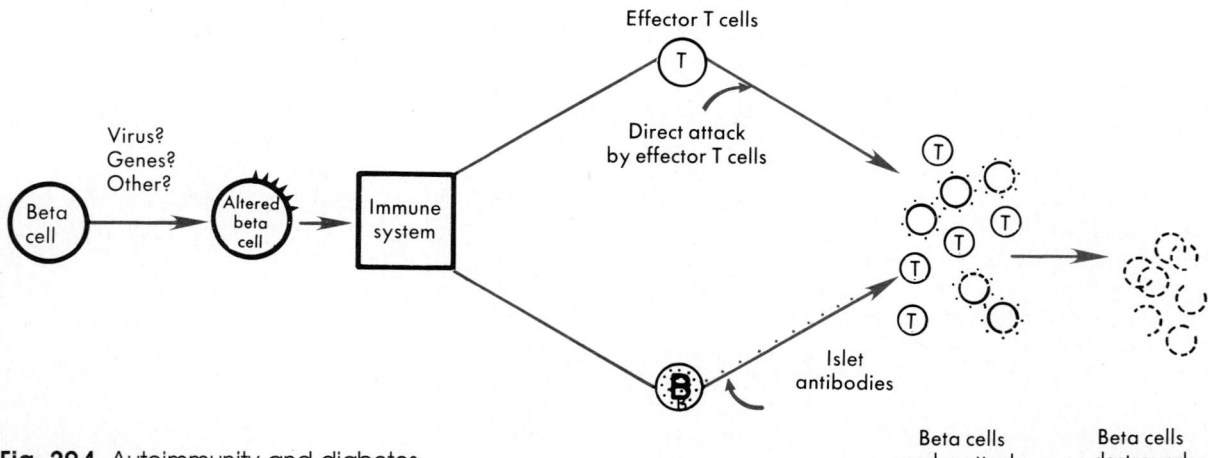

Fig. 29-1. Autoimmunity and diabetes.

Table 29-4. Urine tests for glycosuria

Test	Procedure	Interpretation
Clinitest tablets	Obtain freshly voided urine. Use only "fresh" whole tablets (off-white with blue specks) that completely dissolve. Use only the Clinitest dropper. Do not shake the tube during the reaction. Place required drops of urine (2 or 5) and *10* drops of *water* in a clean test tube. Drop 1 tablet into tube. Wait 15 sec after boiling has stopped to compare urine color with the proper color chart.	Clinitest is based on copper reduction of sugars, including glucose; thus false positive results can occur in the presence of other sugars. Other false positive results can occur if patient takes large doses of vitamin C, more than 6 tablets of aspirin per day, and certain drugs (gantrisin, levodopa, Benemid, Isonizid). Cephalosporins (for example, Keflex) may cause color reactions that make Clinitest results difficult to read.
2-drop method	Use *2* drops of urine and the 2-drop color chart. *Watch* the color reaction *during* the 15 sec waiting period.	Differentiates glucose content of 0.5%, 1%, 2%, 3%, and 5%. Large amounts of sugar may cause a "passthrough" reaction in which the color of the urine quickly changes from 5% to a lesser number.
5-drop method	Use *5* drops of urine and the 5-drop color chart.	Differentiates glucose content of 0.25%, 0.5%, 0.75%, 1%, and 2%.
Plastic, paper-impregnated strips and paper tape	All strips and tape should be held in air for reading; dip the test strip or tape quickly in and out of urine.	These strips and tapes show a reaction of urine and glucose oxidase, thus are specific for glucose. Inaccurate findings can occur if patients are taking ascorbic acid, pyridium, salicylates, or levodopa. More convenient and more costly than tablets.
Diastix, Keto-Diastix	Read after 30 sec with proper color chart on container.	Differentiates urine glucose content of 0.1%, 0.25%, 0.5%, 1%, and 2%.
Clinistix	Read in 10 sec with Clinistix color chart.	Estimates glucose presence as light, medium, and dark, thus most imprecise of all tests.
Tes-Tape	Tear 1½ inch from Tes-Tape roll; dip in urine and *read in air* after 1 or 2 min: 1 min, yellow-green, 0.25% 2 min, dark green, $\geq$ 0.5%; green-black, $\geq$ 2%.	Differentiates urine glucose content as 0.1%, 0.25%, 0.5%, and 2%

Secondary prevention: detection of DM

The majortiy (90%) of persons with diabetes mellitus have NIDDM (type 2). It is estimated that more than 10 million persons in the United States have diabetes mellitus; 40% to 50% of these individuals have mild hyperglycemia and glucose intolerance and are relatively asymptomatic, and the disease is undiagnosed. However well they feel, they are at risk for developing more severe glucose intolerance and vascular and neurologic complications. NIDDM is a risk factor for heart disease, amputation, stroke, and hypertension. Although in some patients diabetes is diagnosed only when vascular or neurologic complications ensue, increasing evidence points to a relationship between duration of disease and metabolic control of blood glucose and the development of long-term complications of diabetes.[39]

SCREENING PROGRAMS

Screening programs are directed chiefly toward detection of NIDDM (type 2) for two reasons: (1) the incidence of NIDDM is greater, and (2) screening programs are not effective in identifying IDDM (type 1) before the actual onset, which is very sudden and severe. Many authorities believe screening of high-risk populations (elderly, poor, nonwhite, pregnant women) to be a better use of resources than screening of entire populations.

The diagnosis of diabetes mellitus in the elderly is based on age-specific norms for fasting blood glucose levels and for glucose tolerance tests.[43] After the age of thirty years, these norms increase (Table 29-3). In addition, renal threshold (the blood glucose level at which glycosuria occurs) increases in the elderly, and urine tests for glycosuria may not give positive results even in the presence of significant elevations of blood glucose.

A basic principle of screening programs is that adequate follow-up is available for persons with positive findings. Plans for screening for diabetes mellitus must take into consideration that the elderly, the poor, and the nonwhite populations are medically underserved; community or neighborhood screening programs must involve the local health care providers in planning for adequate follow-up.

Educational and case finding programs can be carried

Table 29-5. Blood tests for diabetes mellitus

Test	Procedure and preparation	Interpretation
Fasting blood sugar (FBS)	NPO after midnight	Normal level 70-110 mg/dl (serum)
2 hr postprandial blood sugar	Blood sugar measured 2 hr after heavy meal or 2 hr after receiving loading of 100 gm of sugar	Normal level < 140 mg/dl
Oral glucose tolerance test (OGTT)	10 Hr fasting samples of blood and urine collected at beginning of test; patient is given 150 gm of glucose to drink; blood and urine collected at intervals of ½, 1, and 2 hr (2 hr GTT); samples may be collected at 3, 4, and 5 hr intervals (5 hr GTT)	Values between time zero and 2 hr 200 mg/dl; patients with hypoglycemia may have drop in blood sugar level much below normal and must be monitored for signs of hypoglycemia (see Table 29-2 for age-referenced values). OGTT should be performed only in patients who have been on unrestricted diet and physical activity 3 days before test; not recommended for (1) fasting hyperglycemia; (2) persons taking thiazides, Dilantin, propranolol, Lasix, thyroid, estrogens, birth control pills, steroids; (3) hospitalized patients or acutely ill or inactive patients. The patient should remain seated and not smoke during the test.
Intravenous glucose tolerance test (IGTT)	Same as for OGTT	Performed when OGTT contraindicated (see OGTT) or in presence of gastrointestinal disorder that interferes with glucose absorption
Cortisone-glucose tolerance test	Performed similar to GTT except that cortisone is administered at start of test	Used when GTT results are inconclusive; cortisone causes an abnormal increase in blood glucose level and decreased peripheral utilization of glucose in persons predisposed to diabetes; blood glucose level of 140 mg/dl at end of 2 hr is considered positive result.

out in health departments, neighborhood clinics, outpatient clinics, physicians' offices, local diabetes associations, industry, or in the community at health fairs or in mobile health units.

SCREENING METHODS

Tests for glycosuria, hyperglycemia, and impaired glucose tolerance are used to detect diabetes mellitus. Tables 29-4 and 29-5 describe the several tests used on urine and blood, the procedures and preparation for each, and the interpretation of findings. In the order listed, each succeeding test is more reliable but more costly and discomforting to patients. For screening purposes, Tes-Tape and Diastix urine tests are more reliable than Clinitest because they are specific for glucose, whereas Clinitest tablets show reactions to all sugars.

PATHOPHYSIOLOGY

Hyperglycemia

Normally, when insulin is present, glucose intake (or glucose production) in excess of caloric needs is stored as glycogen in the cells of the liver and muscle. This process of glycogenesis prevents *hyperglycemia* (blood glucose concentrations > 110 mg/dl). When *insulin deficit* is present, four metabolic derangements lead to hyperglycemia:

1. Transport of glucose across cell membranes is diminished.
2. Glycogenesis is diminished and excess glucose remains in the blood.
3. Glycolysis is increased; thus glycogen stores are reduced and "liver"glucose is added to the blood continually rather than when needed.
4. Gluconeogenesis is increased and more "liver" glucose is added to the blood from the breakdown of amino acids and fat.

CELLULAR STARVATION

Increased gluconeogenesis occurs particularly in IDDM (type 1). Blood glucose concentration is high in uncontrolled diabetes mellitus, yet cells are subjected to starvation conditions. Fatigue, loss of weight, and loss of strength can occur, with stunting of growth in children. Cellular starvation and changes in insulin and in other hormones lead to the increased mobilization and metabolism of fats. There is a resultant production of ketones (highly acidic, intermediate metabolites of fat). *Ketosis* is the condition of ketone excess in the blood. If severe enough, ketosis can lead to a form of metabolic acidosis and coma, *diabetic ketoacidosis*.

In NIDDM (type 2), ketosis is usually absent. There seems to be enough effective insulin to suppress the breakdown of fats and proteins, but not enough or not enough effective insulin to control blood glucose at normal levels. Although high levels of insulin can be present in the blood, this insulin is ineffective at receptor sites

---

Signs of dehydration
Dry mucous membranes
Loss of skin turgor
Soft or sunken eyeballs
Red, parched lips and tongue
Tachycardia
Hypotension

and for postreceptor function. Obesity is often present in these persons; however, if the glycosuria is severe enough, loss of weight can occur.

HYPEROSMOLALITY

A major pathophysiologic alteration associated with hyperglycemia is hyperosmolality. Blood glucose concentrations of 60 to 100 mg/dl correlate with normal blood osmolarity values of 280 to 290 mosmols/dl. Hyperglycemia increases blood osmolality. Increases in blood glucose content and blood osmolality lead to *dehydration* by two mechanisms:

1. Glycosuria and osmotic diuresis ensue when blood glucose concentrations exceed the renal threshold. There can be losses of large amounts of calories, water, and electrolytes.
2. Fluid shifts from the intracellular compartment to the more highly concentrated extracellular compartment, resulting in intracellular fluid deficit.

The osmotic diuresis results in increased urine volume (*polyuria*). Thirst is stimulated, and the patient drinks large amounts of fluid (*polydipsia*). Because of the calorie loss and cellular starvation, the appetite is increased and the person eats more (*polyphagia*). When combined with *loss of body weight* and *fatigue,* the "three p's" (polyuria, polydipsia, and polyphagia) are the classic signs of hyperglycemia. These symptoms are usually less severe in NIDDM, but the risks of dehydration are still present.

Hyperglycemic, hyperosmolar, nonketotic coma

Blood glucose levels may exceed 1000 mg/dl, urinary glucose may be 5% to 10%, and serum osmolality may exceed 370 to 380 mosmols/dl in the absence of blood ketones. Coma in these circumstances is termed hyperglycemic, hyperosmolar, nonketotic coma (HHNC) and occurs in NIDDM (type 2 disease). Most frequently, HHNC occurs in the elderly or in persons suffering from other illnesses, such as acute infections. So long as persons with hyperglycemia and glycosuria can respond to thirst and replete fluids lost by glycosuria, the risk of HHNC is diminished. Often, HHNC develops slowly over a period of days, and patients or caregivers may not

Table 29-6. Summary of differences between DKA and HHNC

Factors	DKA	HHNC
Onset	Slow	Slow
Precipitating factors		
Food	Excessive	Excessive
Complications	Infection	Infection
Insulin	Too little	Too little
Exercise	Too little	Nonsignificant factor
Symptoms		
Thirst	↑	↑
Vomiting	Frequent	Frequent
Hunger	Absent	Absent
Abdominal pain	Frequent	Not a major complaint
Vision	Dim	Dim
Signs		
Temperature	↑	↑
Respirations	Hyperpnea (Kussmaul breathing, acetone odor to breath)	Depressed
Blood pressure	Lowered, may be in hypovolemic shock	Lowered, may be in hypovolemic shock
Skin	Hot, dry flushed	Hot, dry
Dehydration	Loss of skin turgor, sunken eyeballs	Loss of skin turgor, sunken eyeballs
Neurologic signs	Lethargy → coma	Multiple, major signs
Laboratory findings		
Urine		
Glycosuria	5%	5%
Ketonuria	Highly positive	Usually negative
Blood sugar	↑ Above 200 mg/dl	↑ > 1000 mg/dl
Ketones	↑	Usually negative
Electrolytes	↓ Except serum, Na + K$^+$, which will ↓ as treatment begins	↑ Cl$^+$,Na$^+$ because of loss of ECF K$^+$ normal to ↑; as H$_2$O replaced, Na$^+$ and Cl$^-$ return to normal
Treatment	↑ Insulin, fluids, electrolytes	↑ Insulin, fluids, electrolytes

identify the need for increased fluid intake. The elderly have less accurate thirst sensations, and they and persons who are acutely ill may not have access to fluids for oral ingestion.

HHNC may also develop in nondiabetic persons receiving enteral or parenteral nutrition if hyperglycemia is induced. Adequate fluid intake and prompt recognition and treatment of hyperglycemia reduce the risk of HHNC in these persons. The mortality of HHNC is reported to be as high as 40% to 60% in some studies.[57]

Blood hyperosmolality, marked dehydration, and resultant fluid shifts decrease intracellular fluid volume. Cerebral dysfunction reflects cell dehydration and is manifested by changes in neurologic parameters. Laboratory findings reflect the fluid deficit and hyperosmolar state: normal to high serum sodium and chloride concentrations, elevated potassium concentration, and elevated blood urea nitrogen level. Table 29-6 compares the features of HHNC with those of diabetic ketoacidosis (DKA).

Signs of hyperglycemic, hyperosmolar, nonketotic coma (HHNC)

Fluid deficit	**Neurologic changes**
Dehydration	Sensory deficits
Hypotension	Motor deficits
Anuria	Focal seizures
Circulatory collapse	Aphasia
Elevated body temperature	Coma

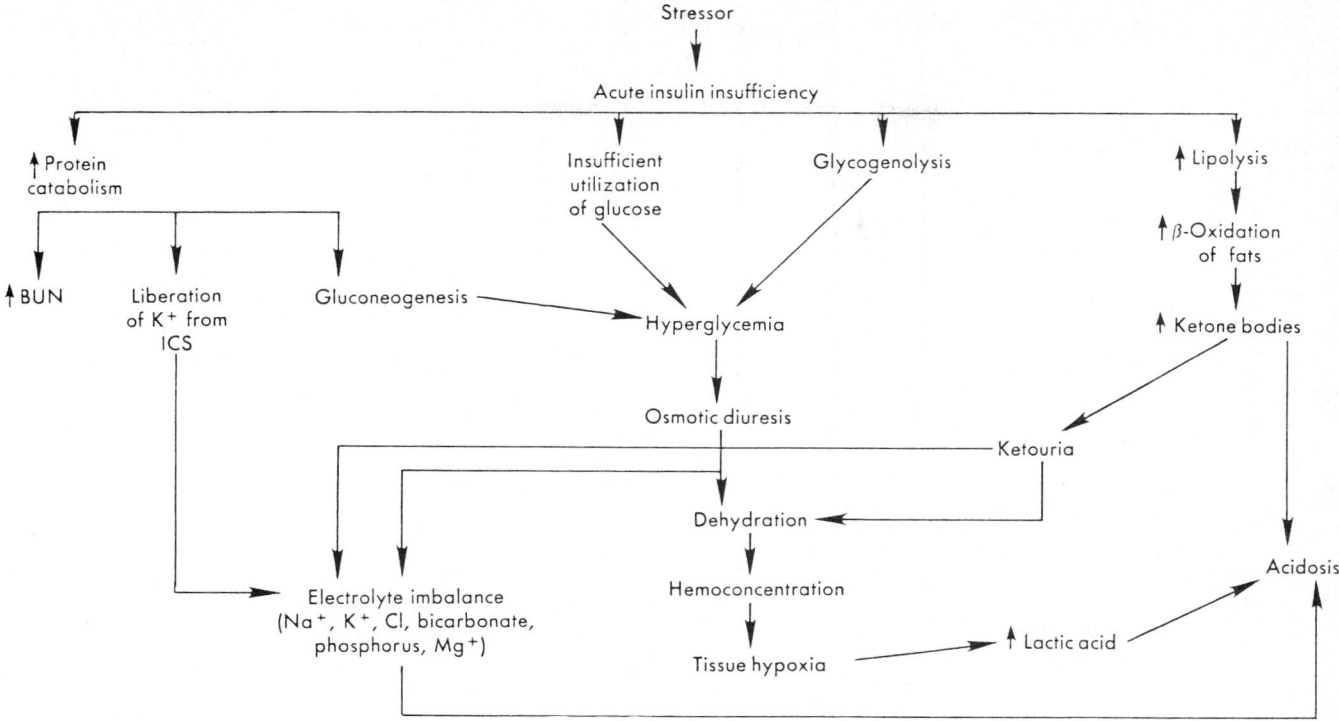

Fig. 29-2. Summary of metabolic alterations in diabetic ketoacidosis.

Signs of diabetic ketoacidosis
Dehydration Lethargy leading to coma Kussmaul breathing Flushed face Fruity breath odor Nausea and vomiting

Diabetic ketoacidosis

Diabetic ketoacidosis (DKA), a severe metabolic disorder, is characterized by hyperglycemia, hyperosmolality, and *metabolic acidosis.* It also results from insulin deficit and produces dehydration. In addition to the signs of dehydration, five clinical signs are characteristic of DKA.

Diabetic ketoacidosis is considered preventable and treatable. Mortality of 100% in the preinsulin era have steadily decreased, so that now death from DKA is rare. It is most frequently seen in persons with IDDM (type 1) but can occur in other types. It is usually precipitated in the known diabetic by stressors that increase insulin needs, although it may occur when diabetes is out of control because of noncompliance with prescribed therapy.

The most frequent precipitating factor is an *infection,* such as those of the urinary or respiratory tracts. Other major stressors that can precipitate diabetic ketoacidosis are surgery, trauma, major illnesses, therapy with steroids, and emotional upset. Occasionally diabetic ketoacidosis is the initial symptom in adults with undiagnosed diabetes, and it is often the initial problem in children with diabetes.

The metabolic alterations of DKA are illustrated in Fig. 29-2. The detection of symptoms of hyperglycemia, urinary ketones, sleepiness, "air hunger," nausea, and vomiting can alert patients to seek medical help early so that prompt treatment can be given.

Macrovascular changes

Diabetic persons develop *atherosclerotic changes* in larger arteries; these changes are the same as those seen in nondiabetics. It is well known, however, that diabetics are prone to develop atherosclerosis at an earlier age, that the disease progresses faster, and that it is more severe and extensive in diabetics than in nondiabetics. Diabetes is associated with various atherogenic factors: abnormal lipid metabolism, changes in platelet adhesion, and hormonal changes (Chapter 27).

Insulin plays a major role in the metabolism of fats and lipids. *Lipid disorders* are frequently found in persons with diabetes mellitus. The hyperlipoproteinemia seen in diabetes is usually identified as type 4 or type 5 and is often the result of an excess of very-low-density lipoproteins. In addition, diabetes is considered to be a contributing factor in the development of *hypertension,* which can accelerate atherosclerosis.

Decreased lumens of large blood vessels compromise the delivery of oxygen to tissues and can cause tissue ischemia, resulting in *cerebrovascular disease, coronary artery disease, renal artery stenosis,* and *peripheral vascular disease.* Approximately three fourths of all cerebrovascular accidents are related to diabetes; and myocardial infarction is the most common cause of death among older diabetics.[9] The course and treatment in diabetics with these problems are the same as in nondiabetics; however, the underlying diabetes must be controlled for the best recovery from the cardiovascular complications. Likewise, the cardiovascular complications will make the diabetes more difficult to control.

Microvascular changes

Microvascular changes are characterized by thickening and damage to the basement membrane of the capillaries. These changes do not occur in nondiabetics. The causes of these changes are unknown but are thought to be related to uncontrolled diabetes. Various factors, such as the role of protein fractions, glycoproteins, lipids, and lipoproteins, have been studied, but no conclusive evidence is yet available about the relationship between these factors and the microvascular changes seen in persons with diabetes.

NEPHROPATHY

One of the major results of microvascular changes is alterations in renal structure and function. Four types of lesions can occur: pyelonephritis, glomerular lesions, arteriosclerosis of the renal arteries and the afferent and efferent arterioles, and tubular lesions.

The progression of renal disease varies from person to person. An early sign of a glomerular lesion is *proteinuria* that gradually increases in severity. As renal insufficiency develops, the serum creatinine concentration and urea increase and other signs and symptoms of renal insufficiency and failure appear (Chapter 33).

Diabetes is present in approximately one fourth of all patients treated for end-stage renal disease in the United States. Each year about 4000 more diabetics require treatment for end-stage renal disease, at a cost of about

---

Factors accelerating renal disease with diabetes

Uncontrolled hyperglycemia
Hypertension
Urinary tract infection
Nephrotoxic drugs
Radiologic contrast dyes

$250 million. The incidence is much higher in patients who develop diabetes before age 20 years. After a duration of 20 years, the chance of a diabetic person developing renal disease is estimated at 50% in those with diabetes diagnosed before age 20 years, and 2% to 4% in those with diagnosis after age 20.[39] Attention is directed toward control or prevention of factors known to increase the progression of renal disease in diabetic persons.

The treatment and nursing care of renal insufficiency in diabetes are similar to that in nondiabetics. It is important to remember that as renal insufficiency develops, the patient receiving insulin may require *less* insulin because it will be excreted more slowly. Renal transplantation is the treatment of choice, because diabetic complications progress rapidly in many patients who receive dialysis. At some centers pancreatic transplantation is also done at the time of kidney transplantation.

DIABETIC RETINOPATHY

Blindness in the diabetic person is primarily a result of microvascular changes in the retina. After 10 years, half of all patients have some diabetic retinopathy. Diabetes is the leading cause of blindness in persons between the ages of 20 and 65 years. In addition to retinopathy, the diabetic person is also subject to increased *cataract* formation. Cataracts may be caused by prolonged hyperglycemia that results in swelling of the lens and opacity formation.

The early retinal lesion is a microaneurysm of the retinal vessels. Microinfarction and exudate formation follow. These early retinal changes may progress to a more serious stage, *proliferative retinopathy,* in which there is formation of new blood vessels on the retina (neovascularization). As these new vessels form, they shrink and cause traction on the retina. Retinal detachment and hemorrhage into the vitreous can result.

There are no symptoms of early retinal changes. Patients with diabetes are encouraged to have yearly eye examinations, preferably by an ophthalmologist. Efforts should be made to detect and control hypertension, because it is associated with increased incidence and rate of advance of diabetic retinopathy.[39]

Treatment of severe proliferative retinopathy has included adrenalectomy and hypophysectomy. Considerable evidence now indicates that *laser photocoagulation* controls retinopathy and decreases the risk of blindness. Photocoagulation uses thermal energy to seal capillary leaks, destroy new vessels, and cause adherence of the retina to the choroid. It is often performed on an outpatient basis.

Vitrectomy, the removal of vitreous humor that has been infiltrated by hemorrhage, is another treatment for retinopathy. The removed vitreous humor is replaced by saline solution. Improved vision does not always result.

Neuropathy

Diabetes may affect peripheral nerves, the autonomic nervous system, the spinal cord, or the central nervous system. Multiple and varied symptoms may result.

Neuropathies unique to diabetics may result from altered metabolism that results in accumulation of sorbitol (a highly osmatic particle) in nerve cells and in fluid shifts with swelling, and consequent rupture and destruction of the cell. Altered myelin synthesis may also be involved. Diabetics (as well as nondiabetics) may develop neuropathies as a result of vitamin deficiencies and electrolyte disturbances.[18] In diabetic neuropathies, sensory fibers are usually affected first, then motor fibers.

The diabetic may develop neuropathies that affect the autonomic nervous system. There may be gastric motility changes that lead to irregular food absorption; incontinence or impotence; or inability to detect early symptoms of hypoglycemia.

Most persons who develop peripheral diabetic neuropathy have both sensory and motor dysfunction. Treatment of acute hyperglycemia results in improved nerve velocities.[18] Diabetic neuropathy may be compounded by alcoholic or other peripheral neuropathy.

Lower extremity changes

The macrovascular changes, microvascular changes, and neuropathies all cause changes in the lower extremities. Diabetics develop gangrene considerably more often than nondiabetics. A significant change is anesthesia from loss of sensory nerve function; this contributes to minor trauma and undetected infections that result in gangrene. The infections start in cracks in hypertrophied skin, ingrown toenails, corns, and calluses as well as in traumatized areas. It is estimated that proper foot care could result in a 50% to 75% reduction in the need for amputations.[65]

A *neurotrophic ulcer* is one that is insensitive and often develops under corns or calluses. Pain in a neuropathic ulcer generally means infection with involvement of bone. The prognosis is not good.[38]

The interrelationships of vascular and nerve changes in diabetic foot lesions, which often result in amputation because of gangrene, are illustrated in Fig. 29-3. Gangrene may be dry or wet. *Dry gangrene* occurs when tissue death is not associated with inflammatory changes. Autoamputation (spontaneous detachment) of toes affected with dry gangrene is the treatment of choice. The area is kept dry during the process. Close monitoring for signs of infection in proximal tissues is necessary.

Wet gangrene is gangrene coupled with inflammation. *Septicemia* and *septic shock* may occur. Bed rest, antibiotic therapy, appropriate cleansing and debridement, and continuous monitoring for signs of extension are the preliminary treatment. Various diagnostic tests to determine the extent of the lesion, status of circulation, and presence of bone involvement are done before amputation is considered (Chapter 27).

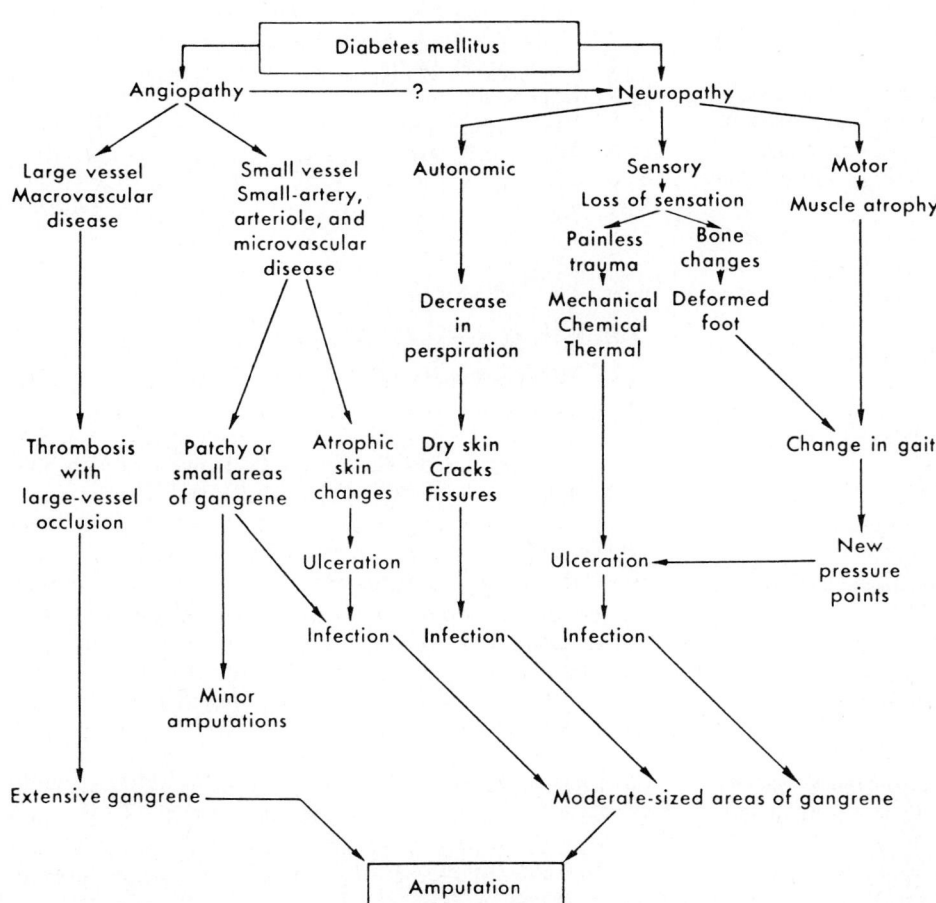

Fig. 29-3. How foot lesions of diabetes can lead to amputation. (Adapted from Levin, M.E.: Medical evaluation and treatment. In Levin, M.E. and O'Neal, L.W. editor: The diabetic foot, ed. 2, St. Louis, 1977, The C.V. Mosby Co.)

Classic signs of hyperglycemia

Polydipsia
Polyuria
Polyphagia
Weight loss
Fatigue

ASSESSMENT

Subjective data

Subjective data includes the presence and extent of classic signs of hyperglycemia. A thorough history should be taken to determine whether any conditions are present that affect blood glucose concentrations:

1. Food intake in excess of caloric requirements
2. Infection or other acute illness
3. Stress related to psychologic or social factors
4. Drugs or other treatments that affect blood glucose
5. Omission of required insulin or oral hypoglycemic agent

In addition, the nurse interviews the patient for evidence of the knowledge and skills necessary for effective self-care. Because education is an integral part of the treatment, the *learning needs* related to self-care of all patients who are diabetic are assessed. This assessment must be done early in the hospitalization in order to increase the time available for teaching. Unfortunately, many patients who have had diabetes for a long time may have inadequate knowledge, skills, or attitudes to manage their diabetes at optimal levels. The development of vascular or neurologic complications may require learning modifications of self-care measures. The last section of this chapter discusses the teaching needs of diabetic patients.

Objective data

Objective data to be collected include the following:

1. Level of consciousness
2. Blood and urinary glucose concentrations
3. Blood and urinary ketone concentrations
4. Blood urea nitrogen
5. Blood pressure, pulse, and respiratory pattern
6. Body temperature
7. Body weight
8. Urinary volume (per timed period)
9. Appearance of mucous membranes and skin
10. Skin turgor
11. Breath odor

When an acute metabolic crisis is suggested by the patient's clinical findings, further assessment is related to *metabolic acidosis* (p. 767) and *fluid imbalance* (p. 765). Table 29-6 compares the signs and symptoms of the two metabolic crises: hyperglycemic, hyperosmolar, nonketotic coma (HHNC) and diabetic ketoacidosis (DKA).

Assessment of any adult patient with diabetes mellitus also includes data for identifying *abnormalities related to vascular or neurologic changes*. Measures directed toward prevention or treatment of these complications may be required. In addition, the patient often needs assistance with activities of daily living and modification of diabetes self-care activities. Assessment should always include attention to the *lower extremities, vision, cardiovascular-renal,* and *neurologic status.*

DATA ANALYSIS AND PLANNING

Nursing diagnoses

Common nursing diagnoses for patients with diabetes mellitus include the following:

Fluid volume deficit, actual or potential
Knowledge deficit
Noncompliance
Alteration in nutrition: more than body requirements
Self-care deficits

Expected patient outcomes

1. Blood glucose level is at optimal level.
2. Ideal weight is maintained or achieved.
3. Hydration is adequate.
4. The patient has accurate information about diabetes mellitus and measures for its control.
5. The patient is able to perform required monitoring tests and interpret results.
6. The patient is able to implement self-care activities.
7. The patient can recognize and treat hypoglycemic reactions.
8. The patient knows when to seek medical assistance.

IMPLEMENTATION

Assisting with achievement of therapeutic goals

PROMOTING NUTRITION

Diet is considered to be the keystone of therapy in both IDDM (type 1) and NIDDM (type 2).

Dietary recommendations

1. There should be sufficient calories to promote normal growth and activity in the child and to maintain *ideal* weight and activity in the adult.
2. Calorie intake should be provided as follows:
   a. Protein, 20%
   b. Carbohydrate, 50%
   c. Fat, 30%
3. Most of the calories from carbohydrate (CHO) should be of starches from the sugars in milk, fruits, and vegetables.
4. No more than 10% of calories from fat should be of

saturated fats and the remainder from unsaturated fats.

5. There should be sharp limitations in the use of refined or concentrated sugars.

6. Consistency in timing and the distribution of calories, carbohydrates, protein, and fat for each meal is most important in IDDM.

7. Control of weight is most important in obese persons with NIDDM; balanced meals at consistent times will aid in achieving this goal.

8. A new dietary approach is a high-fiber, high-CHO diet, which has been shown to decrease insulin requirements, fasting and postprandial glucose levels, and cholesterol levels. A recommended diet is 55% to 60% CHO, 20% proteins, 20% to 25% fats, and 25 to 30 g plant fiber/1000 kcal.[2]

Principles of dietary planning

Should a nutritional history reveal that the patient's food intake and patterns of eating incorporate the above recommendations, few changes would be recommended. It is often said that the diet needed by a diabetic person is that needed by all persons. However, most Americans find it necessary to change dietary habits to reduce hyperglycemia and maintain ideal weight. Recommendations need to be made with awareness of the difficulty with which people change established eating habits.

Dietary planning should include considerations of the following factors:

1. The patient's personal, cultural, or religious food preferences

2. Lifestyle: working hours, family composition, financial resources

3. Activity: activity patterns; timing and level of exercise; periods of exercise, work, and sleep

4. Hypoglycemic drugs; onset, duration, and peak activity of insulin or oral hypoglycemic agents (p. 777)

5. Other modifications needed in consistency or nutrient content

Systems for learning dietary requirements

There are several systems by which dietitians and nurses help patients learn dietary requirements.[40] The simplest system is providing patients with *sample diet plans* for each meal that can be used until they are able to learn and choose more options. For example, the plan for breakfast could be as follows:

4 Oz orange juice
1 C cooked or dry cereal
1 Slice toast with 1 tsp butter
1 C 2% milk
Coffee

Other systems are developed around specific dietary components. One of these is the *points system,* in which foods are divided into categories: calories, carbohydrates, proteins, and fat.[58] Points are prescribed in terms of both calories and carbohydrates for the daily allowance of foods. meat, milk, and fat are included at each feeding.

Another system involves learning how to plan dietary intake to meet prescribed *percentage of carbohydrate* in common foods. For example, in this system the patient is directed to choose 130 g of a 3% (100 g of a 6%, or 7 g of a 9%) fruit or vegetable.

An even more complex system is used when the patient is asked to calculate and plan food intake on the basis of the *content of carbohydrate, fat, and protein* in specific foods.

The *food exchange system* has been widely used throughout the United States because of its ease in teaching. The exchange lists consist of seven groups of food divided on the basis of similar amounts of *carbohydrates and fats.* Patients can learn to exchange foods within one list to obtain a variety of food intake. Some of the common foods in each of the food groups are listed in Table 29-7.

Information about the food exchange system is available from hospitals, clinics, and physicians' offices and in diabetic educational literature. Standardized diet plans have been developed for various levels of calorie intake and can serve as guides; however, these should not be used without attention to individual requirements. The dietitian translates the diet prescription into numbers of food exchanges and food distribution throughout the day that will meet the patient's nutritional requirements. An example of a meal plan for a day using the food exchange system is given in Table 29-8.

Additional nursing activities related to dietary control include:

1. Assisting the patient to eat according to the diet plan

2. Monitoring and recording food intake

3. Obtaining substitutes for foods not desired or refused

4. Coordinating care so that patient's food is not delayed or omitted.

PROMOTING EXERCISE

Exercise is the second treatment modality of hyperglycemia in diabetes mellitus. Glucose can enter *active* muscle cells without the action of insulin, and can then be oxidized to carbon dioxide and water; thus *exercise has a hypoglycemic action.* Exercise also decreases insulin resistance and promotes weight loss in the obese diabetic.

Those persons receiving insulin or orally administered hypoglycemic agents should understand that diet and medications are planned around the usual activity level and pattern of exercise. Changes in activity level require changes in diet or medication (Table 29-9).

Strenuous activity undertaken without a decrease in hypoglycemic agent or an increase in food is a common cause of hypoglycemic reaction in patients receiving such medications. Patients are instructed to eat a quick-acting form of glucose just before an activity that is more strenuous than usual and to repeat this if the activity is lengthy (> 1 hour). Such a glucose source should always be available for treatment if hypoglycemic reaction occurs.

There is a greater chance of hypoglycemia when the

Table 29-7. Examples of food exchanges

Food product	CHO (gm)	Fat (gm)	Equivalents
Milk and milk products	12	Trace	1 C skim or nonfat milk 1 C yogurt ½ C evaporated milk
Vegetable Nonstarchy	5	2	½ C asparagus, carrots, eggplant, collards, tomatoes, and such
"Free" (lettuce, endive)	—	—	*As desired
Fruit	10	—	1 Small apple ⅓ C apple sauce ½ Banana ½ Grapefruit
Breads and starchy vegetables	15	2	1 Slice bread ½ Bagel 1 Tortilla (6 in) ½ Hamburger bun 2 Graham crackers 15 Potato chips ¾ C unsweetened cereal ¼ C cottage cheese (dry)
Meat Lean	—	3	1 Oz lean beef or fish ¼ C tuna
Moderate fat	—	15	1 Oz ground beef (15% fat) or boiled ham ½ C cottage cheese (creamed) 2 Tbs peanut butter
High fat	—	20	1 Oz ground beef (20% fat) Pork ribs or deviled ham 1 Oz cheddar cheese 1 Oz frankfurter
Fats	—	5	1 Tsp margarine or butter 1 Strip crisp bacon 1 Tbsp French dressing
Other	—	—	Calorie-free beverages, unsweetened gelatin, and such: as desired

Adapted from American Diabetes Association, Inc.: American Diabetes Association and National Institutes of Health, U.S. Public Health Service exchange lists for meal planning, Chicago, 1976, The Association.

Table 29-8. Sample of two menu plans using the exchange list*

	Menu 1	Menu 2
Exchanges	**Breakfast**	**Breakfast**
1 Fruit	½ Glass orange juice	¼ Cantaloupe
1 Milk (low fat)	1 Glass skim milk	1 Glass skim milk
1 Meat	1 Egg poached	1 Scrambled egg
3 Bread	2 Toast, ½ C oatmeal	1 English muffin, ½ C bran flakes
2 Fat	1½ Tsp margarine	1½ Tsp margarine
	Lunch	**Lunch**
1 Fruit	1 Peach	½ Banana
1 Milk (low fat)	1 Glass skim milk	1 Glass skim milk
2 Meat	Tuna salad sandwich (¼ C tuna with celery,	1 MacDonald's cheeseburger
2 Bread	2 slices bread, 3 tsp mayonnaise, and	(2 bread, 2 meat, 1 fat)
	lettuce)	1 Lettuce salad with 2 Tbsp
		French dressing
	Afternoon snack	**Afternoon snack**
1 Bread	6 Thin round crackers	Pretzels
1 Fruit	1 Apple	Grapes
	Dinner	**Dinner**
1 Fruit	¾ C strawberries	½ C pineapple
2 Vegetable B	1 C green beans	Sliced tomatoes
4 Meat	4 Oz round steak	4 Oz ham (boiled)
1 Milk (low fat)	1 Glass skim milk	1 Glass skim milk
2 Bread	1 Small baked potato	2 slices bread
	1 Roll	
3 Fats	1 Tbsp sour cream/2½ tsp butter	1 Tsp mayonnaise
	Evening snack	**Evening snack**
1 Bread	3 Rye wafers	6 Salt crackers
1 Meat	1 Oz low-fat cheese	¼ C low-fat cottage cheese

Adapted from American Diabetes Association, Inc.: American Diabetes Association and National Institutes of Health, U.S. Public Health Service exchange lists for meal planning, Chicago, 1976, The Association.
*Diet distributed over three meals and two snacks. Diet based on 2000 calories with 45% CHO (225 g); 35% fats (78 g); and 20% proteins (100 g).

Table 29-9. Effect of exercise on need for medication and food

	Increased exercise	Decreased exercise
Hypoglycemic agent	Decreased need	Increased need
Food	Increased need	Decreased need

peak action of the patient's insulin (or oral agent) and exercise coincide than when postprandial hyperglycemia and exercise coincide. Injections of insulin should be made into the abdominal tissue rather than the extremities before exercise of the legs and arms because exercise increases the speed of absorption.

MEDICATIONS

Insulin

Insulin is necessary for the survival of patients with IDDM (type 1). It is also used to treat NIDDM (type 2) in some patients in whom other measures have not achieved a desired level of blood glucose control.

The current trend in treatment is to achieve the best control of blood glucose possible for each individual, that is, to achieve blood glucose levels near normal limits if this can be done without significant hypoglycemia.

Properties of insulin

Four properties of insulin preparations may comprise the prescription: (1) type of action, (2) strength, (3) species source, and (4) purity.

TYPE OF ACTION. All insulins are hypoglycemic, but they differ in the speed with which they begin to act (*onset*), the period of time they have the strongest action (*peak*), and how long they act *(duration)*. Insulins are classified as short, intermediate, and long acting. Table 29-10 gives the characteristics of eight standard insulin preparations. Nurses need to know the characteristics of each in order to coordinate food and activity with insulin action. This coordination is necessary so that (1) insulin is available when food is taken for optimal metabolism, and (2) food is available while insulin is acting to prevent hypoglycemic reactions.

Three principles are useful in coordinating food and hypoglycemic medications:

1. Food must be taken after insulin (or oral agent) within the time of onset; for example, with regular insulin, food must be taken within 1 hour after injection.
2. Intermediate- or long-acting insulins require that a supplemental feeding be given, timed to match the peak action of the insulin, for example, a 3:00 PM feeding if NPH insulin given at 7:00 AM.
3. With intermediate- or long-acting insulin a bedtime feeding is required so that glucose is available through the night.

STRENGTH. Insulin preparations vary in the concentration of insulin units in 1 ml volume. U-100 insulin, or 100 units/ml, is the strength most frequently used. A few patients requiring very small doses may use U-40 insulin because it is easier to measure small doses accurately. In *insulin resistance*, a rare condition in which daily insulin doses exceed 100 units, U-500 insulin may be ordered.

It is very important that the insulin concentration and the insulin syringe calibration match in units per milliliter to prevent errors in dosing (Fig. 29-4).

Table 29-10. Action of insulin preparations

Type of insulin	Time of onset (hr)	Peak of action (hr)	Duration of action (hr)	Insulin appearance
Rapid acting				
Regular	< 1	2-4	4-6	Clear
Crystalline zinc	< 1	2-4	5-8	Clear
Semilente	< 1	4-7	12-16	Cloudy
Intermediate acting				
NPH	1-2	8-12	18-24	Cloudy
Globin zinc	2-4	6-10	12-18	Clear
Lente	1-4	8-12	18-24	Cloudy
Slow acting				
Protamine zinc	4-8	16-18	36+	Cloudy
Ultralente	4-8	16-18	36+	Cloudy

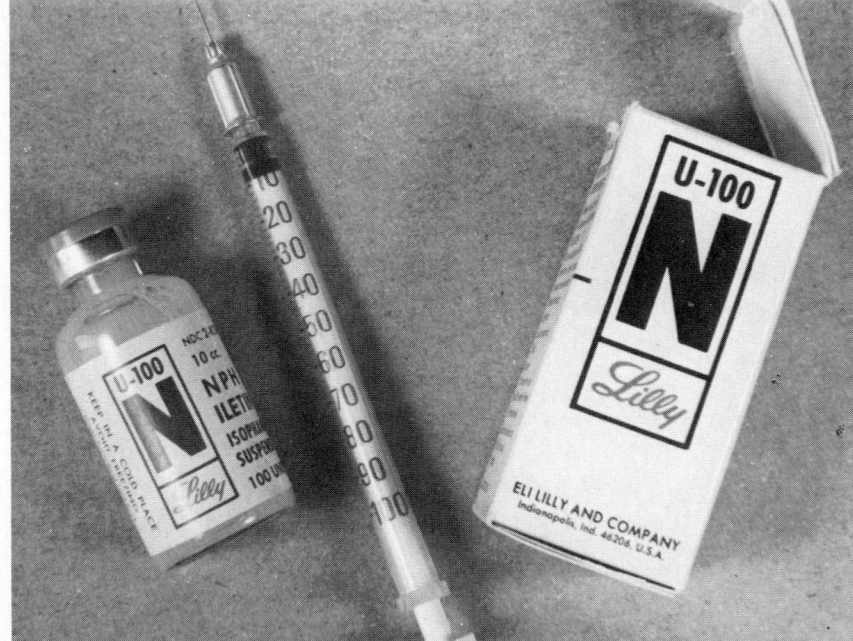

Fig. 29-4. U-100 insulin and disposable U-100 insulin syringe.

SPECIES. Insulin antigenicity can decrease insulin receptor effectiveness.[36] In the past, most insulin was prepared from a combination of beef and pork pancreas. Single-species insulin (usually pork) could be obtained for patients with beef-insulin allergy or antibodies. (Pork insulin most closely resembles human insulin and is considered the least antigenic animal insulin.) Recently several single-species pork or beef preparations have been marketed and are used to decrease insulin antibody formation.

"Human" insulin is now available for use in the United States; it is either porcine (pork insulin modified enzymatically to structurally resemble human insulin) or bacterially produced by recombinant DNA techniques. Human insulin has less antigenicity than animal insulin, and it greatly expands the insulin resources of the world.

PURITY. Over time, manufacturers have improved the purity of insulin preparations. Even so, standard insulins (single-peak insulins) may contain significant amounts of pro-insulin-like substances and other antigenic substances (for example, glucagon-like, pancreatic polypeptides). Insulins labeled "highly purified" (single component) are now being marketed and are recommended for use in persons with newly diagnosed diabetes, insulin allergy, or insulin lipodystrophy and when intermittent insulin therapy is required.[24]

Because of the many changes being made in insulin preparations, the nurse must clarify the insulin prescription if the type, strength, purity, or species is unclear. A change in any one of these properties may lead to significant differences in action. When the insulin prescription is changed, careful patient monitoring is necessary to identify the extent of clinical effect.

Insulin administration

Insulin therapy plans may include the following:
1. One intermediate insulin injection each day
2. Injections of regular insulin at each mealtime
3. Injection of a short-acting insulin and long- or intermediate-acting insulin morning and evening, respectively (split dose)

Increasingly, physicians are attempting to simulate the normal bodily secretion of insulin that occurs in nondiabetics, that is, a continuous basal level of insulin that rapidly increases with food intake. The most appropriate method for the individual patient is selected by evaluating response to a given method by blood glucose testing.

The insulin type and dosage is ordered in anticipation of food, activity, and other factors that balance or affect the insulin requirements. The following information is necessary before administering insulin:
1. Time of onset, peak, and duration of the insulin
2. Availability of food or adequate glucose at these times of action
3. Plans for treating hypoglycemia should it occur

Thus if a patient were ordered nothing by mouth for several hours, insulin should not be given until provision is made for an intravenous infusion of a dextrose solution.

ROTATION OF NEEDLE INSERTION SITES. The sites of injection must be rotated to assure proper absorption of insulin. Lipodystrophy can occur with repeated injections and can cause poor absorption of the medication. The major areas for injection of insulin are the arms, legs, buttocks, and abdomen. Each of these areas has multiple sites (Fig. 29-5).

Two forms of *lipodystrophy* can occur: hypertrophy and atrophy. *Hypertrophy* is thickening of an injection site because of the development of fibrous scar tissue from repeated injections in the same site. A hypertrophic area is usually devoid of nerve endings, and the patient likes to reuse it because injections are painless. Absorption from this area is slow and erratic.

Atrophy is loss of subcutaneous fat. The cause is unknown. It is thought to result from repeated injections in the same site, faulty injection technique, or impurities in the insulin. Some researchers have successfully treated

---

Guidelines for insulin administration

1. Always use an insulin syringe calibrated in the same units as the insulin.
2. Select insulin according to type, strength, species, and brand name as specified by the prescription.
3. Rotate or gently roll the bottle if it is other than regular or Globin insulin.
4. Examine *intermediate-* and *long-acting* insulin vials for suspension of insulin (cloudy appearance); do not use if it is not cloudy.
5. Check for and remove any air bubbles after insulin is drawn into the syringe (do not use an air bubble to clear the needle after injection).
6. When mixing insulins, do not vary the sequence in which two insulins are drawn into the same syringe; usually air is injected into both bottles (regular and intermediate); the insulin is withdrawn first from the regular vial and then from the longer acting insulin vial.
7. Use an injection site that has not been used in the past month.
8. Insert the needle into fatty tissue *closer to muscle than to skin*; if there is little subcutaneous tissue, "pinch" up the skin and use a 45-degree angle and a ⅜ or ½ in needle; use a 90-degree angle when the fat pad is large.

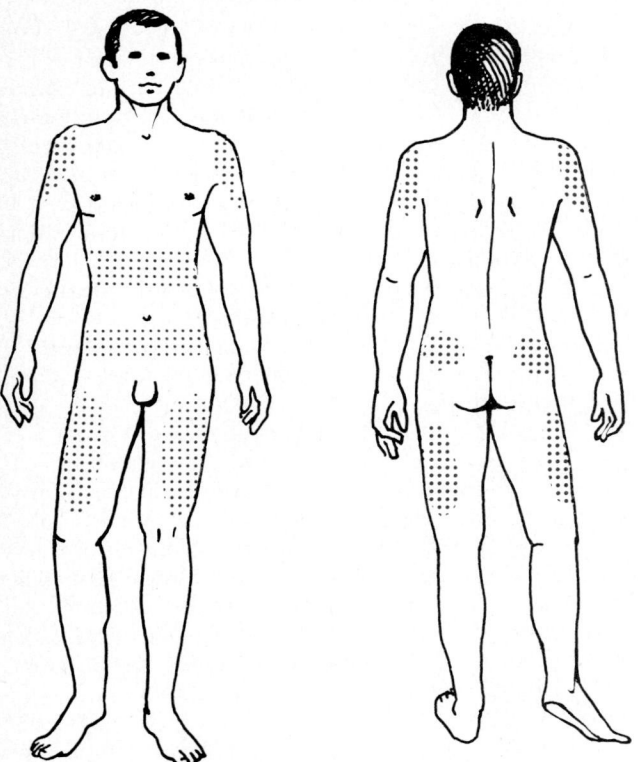

Fig. 29-5. Rotation of sites for insulin.

atrophy by injecting purified insulin into atrophic areas. A major nursing role is to ensure that the patient rotates the sites and gives the injections deep enough.

INSULIN PUMPS. Very close control of blood glucose can be achieved for some patients with IDDM by use of an insulin infusion pump. Insulin pumps, which are battery operated and portable, deliver regular insulin at a basal rate (continuously) and a bolus dose at meal times. The insulin is delivered from a reservoir through tubing to a needle placed in subcutaneous tissue (Fig. 29-6). Projected for the future is the closed-loop insulin delivery system, which will combine a pump, a blood glucose sensor, and a calculator to determine rate of delivery.

Insulin pumps now in use are open-loop systems. Although multiple insulin injections are avoided, patients must monitor blood glucose levels and manually set the insulin delivery rate. The pump is only disconnected to change the needle (every 2 or 3 days), while bathing or swimming, and during sexual activity.

About the same size as a small calculator, the pump can be worn on a belt at the waist or in a pocket. For each brand of insulin pump, the patient requires considerable education to ensure safe and effective insulin delivery. Complications include hypoglycemia, infection at the site of needle insertion, and rapid onset of ketoacidosis if the pump becomes disconnected.

Insulin pumps are expensive; however, insurance reimbursement of initial and maintenance costs is becoming more common. A recent policy statement by the American Diabetes Association[31] cautions that the use of portable infusion devices be prescribed and managed by diabetologists trained and skilled in their use.

Fig. 29-6. Insulin infusion pumps. (Courtesy Cardiac Pacemakers, Inc., St. Paul, Minn.)

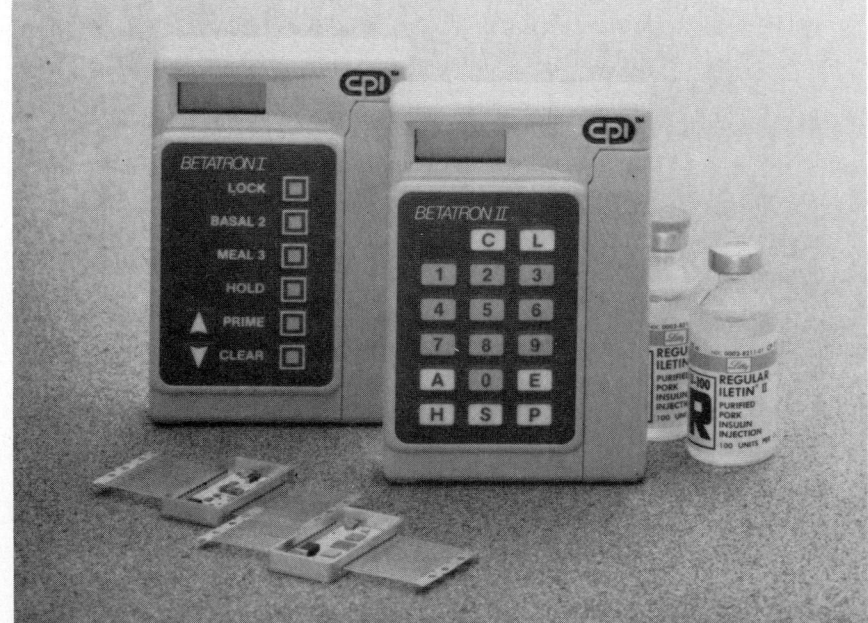

Oral hypoglycemic agents

Four orally administered agents are now available for use in controlling blood sugar levels in persons with diabetes mellitus; all are sulfonylurea compounds (Table 29-11). Two new sulfonylurea drugs are in FDA review, glypizide (Glucotrol) and glyburide (Micronase).[13] These are more potent than the first-generation compounds, thus doses will be smaller. It is hoped there will be fewer drug-drug interactions, because they are not so easily displaced (unbound) from albumins by other drugs.

The sulfonylurea compounds are thought to act primarily by increasing the ability of the islet cells of the pancreas to secrete insulin, although other methods of action are being studied. These agents have proved effective in the treatment of stable diabetes in adults. The drugs are not hormones, and it is a misnomer to refer to them as insulin.

All sulfonylurea drugs are metabolized in the liver. Diabetic patients with liver dysfunction must be monitored carefully for hypoglycemia because the action of sulfonylureas may be prolonged.

Physicians vary in their use of these agents because of the controversial study conducted in the 1970s by the University Group Diabetes Program (UGDP). The FDA recommends that orally administered hypoglycemic agents be limited to persons with symptomatic adult-onset non-ketotic diabetes mellitus that cannot be adequately controlled by diet or weight loss alone and in whom the administration of insulin is impractical or unacceptable. This recommendation was based on the report of the UGDP study that the death rate from cardiovascular disease was two and one half times higher in persons receiving tolbutamide as in those receiving a placebo. These results have been challenged by numerous groups.

Recent evidence indicates that some of the hypoglycemic agents increase insulin-receptor function as well as stimulating some insulin secretion in obese persons with NIDDM (type 2).[33] The medications are most effective in older persons; they are not used to treat IDDM or in pregnant women. They are useless in the treatment of diabetic ketoacidosis.

Persons taking oral hypoglycemic medications need to be as careful about taking the prescribed dosage, following the prescribed diet, maintaining the usual amount of exercise, testing the urine for sugar, and taking general health precautions as do persons taking insulin.

HYPOGLYCEMIA

Hypoglycemia (plasma glucose level <60 mg/dl occurs in at least two circumstances in diabetes mellitus. By far the most frequent occurrence is in the patient receiving insulin or an oral hypoglycemic agent, when there is an insulin excess relative to food intake or energy expenditure. Hypoglycemia in this situation occurs for the following reasons:

1. Too large a dosage taken in relation to the need for insulin
2. Too little food taken (meals delayed or omitted) or delayed gastric emptying
3. Exercise excessive in relation to food intake and hypoglycemic agent
4. Emotional stress
5. Vomiting, diarrhea, or decreased food absorption.

A less common instance is hypoglycemia occurring in the early phase of NIDDM, when a sluggish release of insulin allows peak insulin activity to occur hours after food has been ingested.

A *hypoglycemic reaction* can occur when hypoglycemia is present or when blood glucose level falls rapidly; that is, the blood glucose level may be >60 mg/dl but the patient experiences the symptoms of hypoglycemia. Symptoms of hypoglycemic reaction can vary among patients and from time to time in one patient.

Complications of oral hypoglycemic agents

Hypoglycemia
Allergic skin reactions
Gastrointestinal complaints
Hematologic disorders
Water retention and dilutional hyponatremia (with chlorpropamide)

Table 29-11. Oral hypoglycemic agents

Agent	Proprietary name	Usual daily dose	Divided dose per day
Acetohexamide	Dymelor	250 mg to 1.5 g	1 to 2
Chlorpropamide	Diabinese	100 to 750 mg	1
Tolazamide	Tolinase	100 mg to 1 g	1 to 2
Tolbutamide	Orinase	0.5 to 3 g	2 to 3
Second generation			
Glyburide	Micronase	2.5 to 30 mg	1 to 2
Glipizide	Glucotrol	2.5 to 40 mg	1 to 2

Signs and symptoms of hypoglycemia

Sympathetic nervous system activity

Pallor
Piloerection
Tachycardia
*Nervousness
*Weakness

*Perspiration
Hunger
Palpitation
Irritability
Trembling

Central nervous system activity

Headache
Diplopia
Emotional
   changes
*Mental confusion
Convulsions

Blurred vision
Incoherent speech
Fatigue
Numbness of lips,
   tongue
Coma

*Four signs most commonly reported by patients.[42]

Carbohydrates (10 to 15 g) for relief of hypoglycemia

½ C fruit juice
½ C cola drink
½ C gelatin dessert
4 Cubes sugar
2 Packets sugar
2 Squares Graham crackers

Symptoms of sympathetic nervous system (SNS) activity usually precede those of the CNS and are related to epinephrine action. Signs of cerebral dysfunction reflect hypoglycemia that interferes with the oxygenation of nerve cells. Repeated or prolonged attacks can cause brain damage.

For some patients, a disturbing development is a diminished ability to perceive hypoglycemic symptoms, particularly the early SNS symptoms. This dysfunction is associated with duration of disease, development of neuropathy, and use of certain drugs that affect the SNS (for example, beta blockers). Patients find this loss frightening because they no longer are able to intervene early in the reaction, but only when signs of cerebral dysfunction alert others or themselves to a more severe hypoglycemic reaction. If a hypoglycemic reaction is suspected, a blood glucose level should be obtained if it can be done quickly, in hospitalized patients or in those persons who test their own blood glucose levels.

To facilitate prompt treatment for unconsciousness, di-

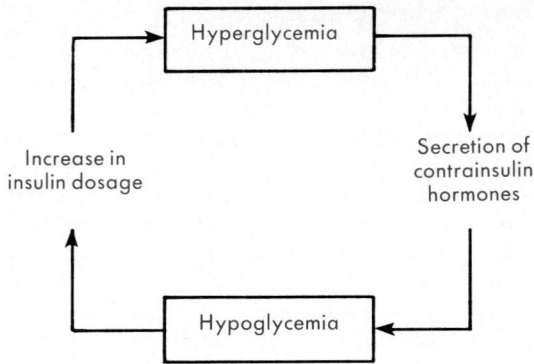

Fig. 29-7. Sequence of events in Somogyi phenomenon.

abetic persons should carry identification cards with the insulin or hypoglycemic agent and dosage listed. Medic-Alert bracelets or necklaces can also alert others to the diabetic status.

The treatment of hypoglycemia in a conscious patient is administration of a quickly absorbed sugar; 10-15 g carbohydrate should be given promptly. With this amount of food, the patient usually feels better within 5 to 10 minutes. Should symptoms not decrease, another feeding should be given after this time. With unconsciousness or severe hypoglycemia, a bolus of 50% dextrose is given intravenously.

SOMOGYI PHENOMENON

Some patients have great difficulty in stabilizing blood glucose levels. One cause of instability is the Somogyi phenomenon, a sequence of increasing peaks and valleys in blood glucose levels. It is often triggered by an insulin dosage in excess of true insulin requirements. The sequence of events is depicted in Fig. 29-7.

Very frequently the signs and symptoms are not obvious enough to be detected. In many instances the hypoglycemia occurs at night and is undetected. The hyperglycemia is recognized in the early morning, and it is assumed that the patient needs higher doses of insulin, but this treatment just makes the problem worse.

The signs and symptoms of the Somogyi phenomenon can be those normally seen with hypoglycemia, but frequently they consist only of nighttime sweats, nightmares, and a headache on arising. There may be weight gain in the presence of glycosuria, no glucose but ketone bodies in the urine (counterinsulin hormones stimulate lipolysis and β-oxidation of fats), and wide fluctuations in blood and urine glucose levels unrelated to meals.

Treatment consists of decreasing the insulin dosage. A primary nursing role is to document complaints of hypoglycemia, glucose intake, and laboratory results, and in particular to look for complaints of night sweats, nightmares, and early morning headaches. Correlating these complaints and laboratory results with the time of meals will also help to identify the phenomenon.

Indices of insulin deficit

pH value <7.35
Blood glucose level
Degree of ketonemia
Clinical findings, including degree of coma

CORRECTING ACUTE METABOLIC CRISES

Diabetic ketoacidosis (DKA) and hyperosmolar nonketotic coma (HHNC) are medical emergencies that require intensive nursing care. Therapy is directed toward correction of the hyperglycemia, dehydration, electrolyte imbalances, acidosis, and precipitating factors. All of these interventions are carried out simultaneously. Intense monitoring is necessary to evaluate the effects of treatment. Review Table 29-6 for the differences in symptoms of DKA and HHNC.

Insulin

Insulin replacement is based on one or a combination of several indices of insulin deficit.

Usually little insulin is needed to treat HHNC; in most instances patients are very sensitive to insulin and require small doses (5 to 15 units initially, with a total insulin dose of 25 to 50 units).

High-dose insulin therapy is the traditional treatment of DKA. It is effective and includes the use of subcutaneous or intravenous injections of regular insulin. *Regular insulin is the only insulin that may be given intravenously.* In this method, an adult patient with ketoacidosis might be given an initial dose of 50 to 150 units by bolus intravenously, then doses of 50 to 100 units every 1 to 2 hours until the acidosis is corrected. Or the patient might be given an initial bolus of 50 to 100 units of regular insulin intravenously and a similar dose subcutaneously, both of these doses repeated every 2 to 6 hours until the acidosis is corrected. Often adults may require 300 to 500 units of insulin in the first 24 hours of treatment. In children, dosage is more likely to be based on units per kilogram body weight.

In the last decade, a *low-dosage insulin* system of treatment has been used in DKA and is also effective. It may include the use of intramuscular, or intramuscular and intravenous infusion of insulin. In this system, 0.2 U/ml regular insulin may be infused in 5% dextrose in water at a rate of 1 ml/min (10 to 12 U/hr). (Thus the solution might be 200 U regular insulin added to 1000 ml 5% dextrose in water.) Often 10 to 12 U (50 ml) is injected in an intravenous bolus to initiate treatment.[46]

Regardless of the method of insulin replacement, as blood glucose level decreases, and nears 200 to 300 mg/dl, close attention must be given to preventing and detecting the onset of hypoglycemic reaction. The nurse should be more alert at this time for the symptoms of hypoglycemia and expect changes in insulin dosage that reflect the decreasing blood glucose levels.

Fluid and electrolyte replacement

The patient with HHNC may have a fluid deficit of 8 to 12 L, and the patient with DKA a deficit of 3 to 5 L. To correct the *dehydration and sodium deficit,* normal saline solution or 0.45% saline (half-strength normal saline) solution is given intravenously. Initially, the solution is infused rapidly and may be started at a rate of 1 to 3 L/hr or more in adults without cardiac or renal failure. When the urine output is 1 to 2 ml/min and the blood pressure is stable, the rate is reduced to 1 L in 2 to 4 hours. When the blood glucose level falls to 300 mg/dl, 5% glucose solutions are used. The patient must be monitored very carefully for signs of fluid overload.

Potassium is not initially added to the intravenous fluids because the patient's potassium serum level is usually *elevated* at the beginning of therapy. With correction of the dehydration, acidosis, and insulin deficit, potassium moves back into cells and hypokalemia results. Potassium as potassium chloride is then added. Serum potassium levels and ECG tracings are monitored continuously to determine the amount of potassium needed.

The administrations of fluids and insulin usually corrects the acidosis in DKA so that bicarbonate administration is seldom needed. Bicarbonate is not usually given unless the serum bicarbonate is 5 mEq/L and the blood pH is < 7.

An additional electrolyte imbalance that may develop during ketoacidosis is *hypophosphatemia*. Without adequate phosphorus, decreased peripheral oxygen delivery and additional tissue anoxia may result. Phosphorus in the form of potassium phosphate may be given.

Nursing interventions planned for the patient depend on the severity of the clinical findings and the prescribed therapy. In all patients, careful and frequent monitoring of the following is necessary:

1. Vital signs
2. Level of consciousness
3. Intake and output
4. Resolution of other signs of dehydration and acidosis
5. Signs and symptoms of fluid overload
6. Urine and blood glucose and ketone bodies

The nurse must make sure that the specimens are collected as ordered and that the appropriate tests are done. It is important that the results of the tests be documented. The assessments made by the nurse and the results of laboratory tests will be used to make appropriate adjustments in therapy. A flow sheet with all pertinent laboratory and assessment data is instituted so that all changes in the patient's status are displayed in a readily comprehensible manner.

Treatment of precipitating condition

As therapy of acute metabolic imbalance is begun (insulin, fluid and electrolyte replacement), attention is given to detecting and treating concurrent illness. Sometimes the precipitating factor is not determined until treatment is well under way and the patient recovered from coma sufficiently to give a history of preceding events. Sometimes family members can give insight into possible etiologic factors. A comon cause of DKA is infection. Antibiotic therapy should begin after specimens for culture and sensitivity of urine, sputum, wound drainage, or blood are obtained.

Should lack of knowledge or of compliance be implicated in DKA, institution of a teaching plan is appropriate as soon as the patient has recovered enough to be comfortable and is feeling well enough to learn.

Promoting safety and well-being

The patient with severe insulin deficit is critically ill and requires excellent nursing. Skilled care involves attending to the following:

1. Required monitoring (as discussed previously)
2. Prescribed therapeutic measures
3. Maintenance of airway in an unconscious patient
4. Frequent turning and skin care
5. Side rails and hand restraints if necessary to maintain intravenous lines
6. Attention to discomforts of abdominal pain, nausea, and vomiting that are usually present in the conscious patient

7. Maintenance of nutrition
   a. Fluids first when able to take something by mouth
   b. Solid foods as soon as possible to improve gastric tone
8. Maintenance of the flow sheet

MINIMIZING DISRUPTION OF DIABETES TREATMENT

Effective self-care of diabetes mellitus should be enhanced at every opportunity. Blood glucose control is increased when there is consistency of food intake, exercise, and medication from day to day. Mutual planning by patient and nurse can be done soon after admission of the conscious patient to determine the following:

1. Self-care practices that will be continued by the patient
2. Practices that need to be done by the nurse
3. Timing of insulin and medications that coincides with that at home

CARE DURING SURGERY AND DIAGNOSTIC TESTS

When fasting is necessary, caution must be used to avert hypoglycemia in the person who takes insulin or an oral hypoglycemic agent. Orders must be clarified as necessary to ensure that glucose is available while insulin is

---

Management of the person with diabetes during the perioperative period

1. Diabetics who receive insulin
   a. Preoperative
      1. Intravenous infusion of glucose on morning of surgery
      2. One-half usual insulin dose subcutaneously
   b. Intraoperative
      1. Monitoring of blood sugar levels if surgery is lengthy
      2. Additional insulin or glucose as needed
   c. Postoperative
      1. Intravenous infusion of glucose until food can be taken orally
      2. Insulin given subcutaneously in equally divided doses over 24 hours or added to intravenous fluids
      3. Urine or blood glucose monitored every 4 to 6 hours
      4. Additional insulin given if indicated from monitoring
2. Diabetics not normally given insulin
   a. Preoperative
      1. Intravenous infusion of glucose on morning of surgery
   b. Postoperative
      1. Blood sugar and urine glucose and ketone levels monitored every 4 to 6 hours
      2. Insulin given if indicated from monitoring
3. All diabetics
   a. 125 to 250 g CHO/day until normal diet resumed
   b. Normal regimen reinstituted as soon as possible before patient is discharged
   c. Continued monitoring of blood or urinary glucose and ketone levels even after usual diet resumed (increased insulin may be needed because of catabolism from surgery).

acting. Sometimes insulin administration is delayed until the patient finishes a specific test.

It is routine to schedule diabetic patients early in the morning for diagnostic tests or surgery to minimize the amount of disruption of their regimen.

Effects of surgery on the person with diabetes

Surgery is a physical and psychologic stressor for anyone. For the person with diabetes mellitus there are additional risks. The stress of surgery can result in disruption of metabolic control. Persons with diabetes are at increased risk for the following:

1. Decreased resistance to infection
2. Impaired wound healing
3. Age-related complications (many persons with diabetes are elderly)
4. Macrovascular and microvascular complications that may be present

The person with diabetes mellitus is at risk for developing *hypoglycemia or hyperglycemia* during the perioperative period. During this period, patients usually are not given anything by mouth and are given fluids intravenously. This decreases total caloric intake and may also decrease insulin needs. However, the effects of surgery on contrainsulin hormonal changes may increase the need for additional insulin. The stresses of surgery cause the release of ACTH, glucocorticoids, and catecholamines, all of which elevate serum glucose levels.

Management of the diabetic person undergoing surgery

Many methods are available for use in the person with diabetes during periods of fasting. To minimize the disruption in metabolic control, the patient's metabolism should be thoroughly regulated before surgery. The normal food, fluid, and medication routine is maintained until the night before surgery.

Teaching directed toward self-care

An integral part of the treatment of diabetes mellitus is education of patients so they can assume responsibility for required self-care, including seeking medical advice or treatment when needed. Teaching should begin at the time of diagnosis and continue until the patient is competent in maintaining on optimal level of wellness. The American Association of Diabetes Educators has proposed that 10 components comprise the educational program.

The Association further proposes that educational programs for diabetic persons be planned in three phases:

1. *Initial management,* in which the knowledge and skills needed to survive are emphasized
2. *Home management,* in which patients learn to be self-sufficient in the daily management of the disease
3. *Improvement of life-style,* in which patients learn how to enrich their lives by gaining flexibility in management, insight, and self-determination

---

Components of diabetes education

Definition of disease
Nutrition
Activity
Medication
Monitoring glucose control
Hypoglycemia
Illness
Psychologic adjustment
Hygiene and foot care
Follow-up

DEFINITION OF DISEASE

The three phases of definition of disease are illustrated in Table 29-12. Each phase is specified by objectives and the requisite knowledges, skills, and attitudes.

It is important that the nurse set priorities in teaching and begin with the most basic information. Too much information overwhelms patients, who often find the diagnosis emotionally disturbing. The resultant anxiety usually diminishes as patients learn they can perform the self-care measures and experience living with the disease and its treatment. Efforts are made that all those involved in the educational program have congruent goals and that plans are coordinated to avoid conflicts or discrepancies that confuse the patient and family.

Many diabetic patients are given initial instruction in the ambulatory setting, and further education is given at repeat visits, Initial instruction for a hospitalized patient with newly diagnosed diabetes should be planned with consideration of three factors:

1. Expected length of stay
2. Specific referrals for further teaching
3. Other concerns and teaching needs not related to diabetes self-care

NUTRITION

A dietary consultation should be initiated early in the educational program. The nurse and other health care professionals should not underestimate the difficulty with which persons change food habits. There is no substitute for a careful dietary history and mutual planning by patient and dietitian (or nurse) about those changes necessary to control blood glucose levels or weight. The nurse can assist the patient in selecting foods in the hospital, in planning menus for home, and in reinforcing the dietary instruction.

The diabetic diet does not require the use of special or dietetic foods. Persons with diabetes must be warned about being misled by the word *dietetic*. Dietetic may refer to low sodium content rather than to low sugar content. Dietetic candies and foods labeled light (or Lite) also

Table 29-12. Phases of diabetes education

Initial management	Home management	Improvement of life-style
Survival knowledge and skills	Self-sufficiency in daily management of diabetes	Enrichment of life by flexibility in management, insight, and self-determination

Objectives for the component definition of diabetes

States need for insulin in body	Lists symptoms of diabetes	Identifes significance of hyperglycemia in relation to other metabolic problems and long-term complications
Describes what happens in body when insulin is deficient	Explains relationship of symptoms to insulin deficiency	States significance of hyperglycemia and glycosuria, or vice versa, relative to changes in renal threshold
States simple working definition of diabetes	States how diagnosis of diabetes is made	Lists main differences between insulin-dependent and non-insulin-dependent diabetes
States role of food, activity, and medication in treatment of diabetes	IDDM: States relationship of undernutrition to insulin deficiency	States current knowledge of hereditary aspects of diabetes
	NIDDM: States relationship between state of overnutrition, inactivity, and relative insulin deficiency	Verbalizes concerns about diabetes in other family members

From A Joint Task force for the American Diabetes Association and the American Association of Diabetes Educators, Spring 1979, American Diabetes Association.

must be used with care. Dietetic foods are not necessarily low in calories and may have high fat content. Sugar substitutes can be used and still are available despite the controversy about the possible carcinogenic effects of saccharin.

Some persons who develop diabetes are accustomed to having an alcoholic beverage daily. With approval of the physician, the diabetic may have small amounts of alcohol. Because alcohol is a high-calorie food, it must be exchanged for fat calories in the diet. The combination of alcohol and chlorpropamide should be avoided because of a severe Antabuse-like reaction.

Four strategies are useful in helping patients learn to manage blood glucose levels by diet:

1. Weighing of meat and measuring of other foods acquaint patients with portion size.
2. Written instruction should accompany verbal discussion of the meal plan.
3. The patient's record of food intake can be correlated with records of blood or urine, glucose tests, food intake, exercise, and medication.
4. Patients should be helped to apply dietary knowledge by doing exercises in which the person chooses foods from hospital and restaurant menus or from a variety of food items (models, pictures).

ACTIVITY

All persons with diabetes benefit from regular exercise as part of treatment. Plans need to be reasonable and take into account previous activity level, cardiopulmonary sta-

tus, mobility, and interests. For example, an elderly hemiplegic patient could be encouraged to do range-of-motion and leg-raising exercises, and a younger person with no disabilities could be encouraged to develop interest in a specific exercise or sports program. Sports that are contraindicated for patients receiving insulin include those in which the dangers of hypoglycemia increase the hazard of the sport (for example, scuba diving or sky diving).

In addition to stressing the importance of exercise, the nurse can assist the patient in planning how to incorporate regular exercise into the life-style after discharge. Optimal timing of exercise would be during periods of greater hyperglycemia when blood glucose is less than 300 mg/dl. A greater chance of insulin reaction occurs when peak actions of insulin coincide with unanticipated exercise in the patient receiving insulin or oral hypoglycemic agents. The benefits of exercise as part of the overall treatment should be emphasized to persons who are obese and have NIDDM (type 2) as well.

MEDICATION

Insulin knowledge

Patients should be able to name their prescribed type of insulin and the dosage. They do not need to know all the insulin varieties, but they must be able to do the following:

1. Identify their prescribed insulin
2. Check the expiration date
3. Prepare and give the accurate dose
4. State they will never change the insulin (type, pu-

rity, species, strength) without the physician's direction

Self-injection of insulin

Most persons are fearful of self-injection and would prefer to postpone learning this task; yet repeated practice is necessary if they are to safely administer an accurate dose with sterile technique. The nurse must teach this skill early and with attention to the patient's fear, whether that fear is or is not expressed.

One study supports the belief that adults can learn this skill most readily and cope best if the first self-injection is not delayed for practice with equipment.[15] The nurse should firmly encourage the patient to hold the syringe, cleanse and pierce the skin, and inject the ordered insulin (or an equivalent dosage of sterile saline) from the syringe previously prepared by the nurse. Verbal encouragement and a guiding hand may be necessary for the patient to self-inject successfully. After adults experience self-injection, they are better able to focus on preparation of the insulin syringe (see p. 775 for guidelines in insulin administration).

Most patients prefer disposable syringes and needles. Patients should be helped to determine the quantity of supplies needed for at least a month. Prescriptions are not necessary for insulin or for syringes and needles. Cotton balls purchased in bulk and a bottle of 70% ethyl alcohol, as compared with individually wrapped alcohol pledgets, can reduce costs (91% alcohol is recommended if skin redness or irritation develops).

Typical trays for injection at home can be set up for use in demonstrations and for patients to use in practice. The nurse can discuss boxes or trays that can be used at home to keep all equipment together. The equipment should be stored on a shelf or closet, out of reach of children and out of sight.

Storage of insulin

Patients should be taught to give insulin at room temperature to decrease the risk of lipodystrophy and to decrease the antigenicity of the insulin. The current practice is to keep the currently used vial at room temperature and refrigerate additional vials, even though insulin vial labels direct the refrigeration of all insulin. It is known that regular insulin will remain stable for 12 months at 37° C (modified insulins for 24 months). Travelers are taught to carry insulin with them rather than to pack it in baggage that might be subjected to extreme temperatures in car trunks or cargo compartments of planes or trains.

Refrigeration is recommended when prefilled syringes are used, to decrease the potential bacteria growth from contamination.

Measures to assist the visually impaired diabetic

Blind patients or those with hand disability may be able to self-inject if the syringes are prepared for them. Often a 1-week supply of syringes are prefilled by a family member or neighbor who has been taught by a home-care

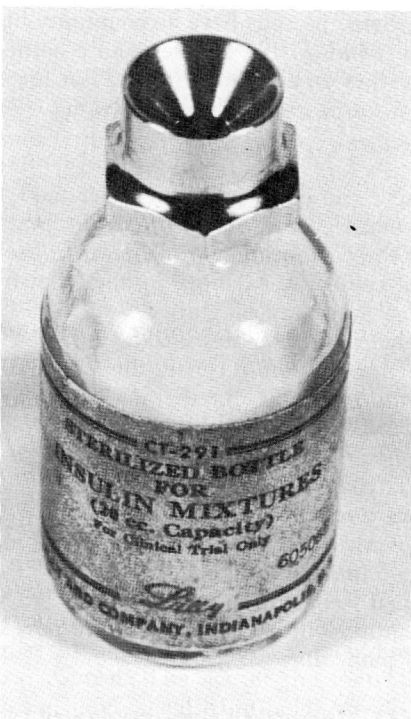

Fig. 29-8. Insulin needle guide that fits over top of insulin vial. Patient cleans stopper and guide with alcohol before placing guide on vial. Needle is laid in V of guide, and vial is pushed toward it. (Courtesy American Foundation for the Blind, Inc., New York, N.Y.)

nurse. It is important that the patient gently rotate the prefilled syringe before administering the insulin and allow it to come to room temperature.

In addition to prefilled syringes, the visually impaired patient may be able to see the darker and larger markings on a "low dose" syringe (volume 0.5 ml, scale U-100). This syringe can only be used for doses of <50 units U-100 insulin. Similarly, a magnifier that clamps on the insulin syringe may aid the patient in withdrawing an accurate dosage. Fig. 29-8 shows a needle insertion guide, which directs the needle into the rubber portion of the vial top.

Many other aids for the visually impaired diabetic are advertised in publications for diabetics or are available from the American Foundation for the Blind.* Special syringes with plunger locks or attachable devices for locking the plunger, and devices for measuring predetermined dosage can be purchased.

Persons with poor vision risk drawing air instead of insulin into the syringe. They must be cautioned to invert the bottle completely and to insert the needle only a short distance. Often they are advised to use only about two thirds of the bottle of insulin and to have on hand another

---

*American Foundation for the Blind, Inc., 15 West 16th St., New York, NY 10011.

axillae and groin). It is therefore very important that persons with diabetes carry out hygienic measures for prevention of infection.

Foot care

Prevention of ulcers, trauma, and infections of the lower extremities is the key to prevention of amputation. Ulcers, injured areas, and infections heal very slowly.

FOLLOW-UP

The many teaching needs of the person with diabetes mellitus have been discussed. The nurse is usually responsible for seeing that the person with diabetes mellitus gains the information, skills, and attitudes necessary for accurate self-care. Teaching is usually begun at the time of diagnosis, but the nurse must be aware that everything cannot be learned during the first contact. Priorities need to be set: the person should be taught the skills necessary to meet immediate needs, and then be referred to a community health nurse or diabetic teaching program. Follow-up might take place in a clinic, physician's or nurse's office, or in a program sponsored by the local diabetes association or a local hospital.

In addition to securing follow-up education appointments, the nurse can do the following:

1. Reinforce the value and need of continued learning
2. Encourage family members to participate
3. Give the patient written instructions and educational literature
4. Ensure that the patient has a resource person to call if assistance is needed before the next appointment

EVALUATION

Questions that guide the nurse's evaluation are derived from an understanding of potential effects of diabetes mellitus on physical well-being, the importance of education for self-management of blood glucose control, and the psychologic impact of this chronic disease and its treatment. Specific goals or objectives for each patient identify the intended outcomes of health care.

Specific questions may include the following:

1. What level of blood glucose control has been achieved?
2. Is the patient equipped with knowledge and skills to make decisions about food, exercise, medications, and when to seek medical advice?
3. Has the patient developed sufficient skill to be independent and safely carry out self-management of the disease in terms of administration of insulin injections or oral hypoglycemic agents, treatment of hypoglycemic reactions, and foot care?
4. Is the patient committed to prevention of short- and long-term complications (follow-up, self-management)?
5. Is the patient coping with diabetes self-care measures, fears and concerns, and life-style changes?

REFERENCES AND SELECTED READINGS*

1. American Diabetes Association and American Dietetic Association: A guide for professionals: the effective application of "exchange lists for meal planning," New York, 1977, American Diabetes Association.
2. Anderson, J.W., Midgley, W.R., and Wedman, B.: Fiber and diabetes (review), Diab. Care 2(4):369-379, 1979.
3. Anderson, J.W.: Newer approaches to diabetes diet: high fiber diet, Med. Times 1108:41-44, 1980.
4. Blevins, D., editor: The diabetic and nursing care, New York 1979, McGraw-Hill Book Co.
5. Bernstein R.K.: Role of glycosylated hemoglobin in diabetic vascular disease, Arch. Intern. Med. 140:442, 1980.
6. Bistrian, B.R.: The medical treatment of obesity, Arch. Intern. Med. 141:429-430, 1981.
7. *Boyles, V.A.: Injection aids for blind diabetic patients, Am. J. Nurs. 77:1456-1458, 1977.
8. Bray, G.A.: The overweight patient, Adv. Intern. Med. 21:267-308, 1976.
9. Bodhan, S.T., and Jans, K.: A new diabetic with complications, Nurs. Clin. North Am. 12:393-406, 1977.
10. Breckbill, V.: Physiological alterations in diabetes. In Blevins, D.: The diabetic and nursing care, New York, 1979, McGraw-Hill Book Co.
11. Boden, G., et al: Monitoring metabolic control in diabetic outpatients with glycosylated hemoglobin, Ann. Intern. Med. 92:357-360, 1980.
12. Bondy, P., and Rosenberg, L.: Metabolic control and disease, Philadelphia, 1980, W.B. Saunders Co.
13. Bonheim, R.: The second generation, Diab. Forecast 36:29-31, April-May, 1983.
14. Cahill, G., and McDevitt, H.: Insulin-dependent diabetes mellitus: the initial lesion, N. Engl. J. Med. 304:1444-1464, 1981.
15. Carlyon, P.E.: Diabetic self-injections: analysis or two teaching/learning approaches, unpublished thesis, Kent, OH, 1980, Kent State University.
16. Check, W.A.: Bacterially produced human insulin given therapeutically, JAMA 4:322-323, 1981.
17. *Christiansen, C., and Sasche, M.: Home blood glucose monitoring, Diab. Educator 6:13-21, Fall 1980.
18. Danowski, T.S., et al: Diabetic complications and their prevention or reversal, Diab. Care 3:94-99, 1980.
19. Danowski, T.S., et al: Parameters of good control in diabetes mellitus, Diab. Care 3:88-93, 1980.
20. Diabetes mellitus, vol. 5, New York, 1981, American Diabetes Association.
21. Dudley, J.D.: The diabetes educator's role in teaching the diabetic patient, Diab. Care 3:127-133, 1980.
22. *Dupuis, A.: Assessment of the psychological factors and responses in self-managed patients, Diab. Care 3:117-120, 1980.
23. Friedman, E.A.: Diabetic renal-retinal syndrome, Arch. Intern. Med. 140:1149-1150, 1980.
24. Gallaway, J.A., and DeShazo, R.D.: The clinical use of insulin and the complications of insulin therapy. In Ellen-

---

*References preceded by an asterisk are particularly well suited for student reading.

berg, H., and Rifkin, H.: Diabetes mellitus: theory and practice, ed. 3, Garden City, N.J., 1983, Medical Publishing Co.

25. Ganda, O.P., and Soeldner, S.S.: Genetic, acquired, and related factors in the etiology of diabetes mellitus, Arch. Intern. Med. **137:**461-469, 1977.
26. Ganda, O.P.: Pathogenesis of macrovascular disease in the human diabetic, Diabetes **29:**931-942, 1980.
27. *Garber, R.: The use of a standardized teaching program in diabetes education, Nurs. Clin. North Am. **12:**372-391, 1977.
28. Graf, R.J., et al: Nerve conduction abnormalities in untreated maturity-onset diabetes: relation to levels of fasting plasma glucose and glycosylated hemoglobin, Ann. Intern. Med. **90:**298-303, 1979.
29. Guthrie, D.W., and Guthrie, R.A.: Nursing management of diabetes mellitus, ed. 2, St. Louis, 1982, The C.V. Mosby Co.
30. *Hayter, J.: Fine points in diabetic care, Am. J. Nurs. **77:**594-500, 1977.
31. Indications for use of continuous insulin delivery systems and self-measurement of blood glucose: policy statement, American Diabetes Association, Diab. Care **5**(2):141-142, 1982.
32. Isaf, J.J., and Alogna, M.T.: Better use of resources equals better health for diabetics, Am. J. Nurs. **77:**1792-1795, 1977.
33. Jackson, J.E., and Bressler, R.: Clinical pharmacology of sulfonylurea hypoglycemic agent drugs, **22:**211-245, 1981.
34. Jovanovic, L, and Peterson, C.: The clinical utility of glycosylated hemoglobin, Am. J. Med. **70:**331-338, 1981.
35. *Judd, S., and Sonksen, P.H.: Teaching diabetic patients about self-management, Diab. Care **3:**134-139, 1980.
36. Kolterman, O.G., Scarlet, J.A., and Olefsky, J.M.: Insulin resistance in noninsulin-dependent type II diabetes mellitus, Clin. Endocrinol. Metab **11**(2):363-388, 1982.
37. Lief, P.: Renal impairment in diabetes mellitus. *In* Diabetes mellitus, vol. 5, New York, 1981, American Diabetes Association.
38. Levin, M.E., and O'Neal, L., editors: The diabetic foot, St. Louis, 1983, The C.V. Mosby Co.
39. National Diabetes Advisory Board: The prevention and treatment of five complications of diabetes (monograph), Charles M. Clark, Director, Diabetes Research and Training Center, Indiana University School of Medicine, Indianapolis, IN.
40. Neville, J.: Management by nutrition. *In* Blevins, D, editor: The diabetic and nursing care, New York, 1979, McGraw-Hill Book Co.
41. Office guide to diagnosis and classification of diabetes mellitus and other categories of glucose tolerance, Diab. Care **4**(2):335, 1981.
42. Paulk, L.H.: Hypoglycemic reactions: from the diabetic's perspective, unpublished thesis, Kent, OH, 1983, Kent State University.
43. Prout, T.E., editor: Diabetes mellitus, ed. 4, New York, 1979, American Diabetes Association.
44. *Rossini, A.A.: Self against self, Diab. Forecast **36:**26-28, 1983.

45. Roth, J.: Insulin receptors in diabetes, Hosp. Pract. **15**(5):98-103, 1980.
46. Sachs, M.: Management of diabetes by pharmacological agents. *In* Blevins, D.: The diabetic and nursing care, New York, 1979, McGraw-Hill Book Co.
47. Scott, F.B., Fishman, I.J., and Light, J.D.: An inflatable penile prosthesis for treatment of diabetic impotence, Ann. Intern. Med. **92:**340-342, 1980.
48. Service, F.J., and Nelson, R.L.: Characteristics of glycemic stability, Diab. Care **3:**58-62, 1980.
49. Shapiro, B., et al.: A comparison of accuracy and estimated cost of methods for home blood glucose monitoring, Diab. Care **4:**396-403, 1981.
50. Siperstein, M.D., et al: Control of blood glucose and diabetic vascular disease, N. Engl. J. Med. **296:**1060-1063, 1977.
51. Skillman, T.G.: Diabetic ketoacidosis, Heart Lung **7:**594-602, 1978.
52. Skillman, T.G.: More than one insulin injection per day improves control, Med. Times **108:**104-118, 1980.
53. Skyler, J.S., et al: Blood glucose control during pregnancy, Diab. Care **3:**69-76, 1980.
54. *Skyler, J.S.: Complications of diabetes mellitus: relationship to metabolic dysfunction, Diab. Care **2**(6):499-509, 1979.
55. Skyler, J.S., and Cahill, G.: Diabetes mellitus: progress and directions, Am. J. Med. **70:**101-104, 1981.
56. *Slater, N.: Insulin reactions vs ketoacidosis: guidelines for diagnosis and interventions, Am. J. Nurs. **78:**875-877, 1978.
57. *Sneid, D.S.: Hyperosmolar hyperglycemic nonketotic coma, Crit. Care Q. **2:**29-43, 1980.
58. Stucky, V.: The meal plan, *In* Guthrie, D.W., and Guthrie, R.A., editors: Nursing management of diabetes mellitus, St. Louis, 1977, The C.V. Mosby Co.
59. Sulway, M., et al: New techniques for changing compliance in diabetes, Diab. Care **3:**108-111, 1980.
60. Symposium on home blood glucose monitoring, Diab. Care **3:**57-149, 1980.
61. Tchobroutsky, G.: Relation of diabetic control to development of microvascular comlications, Diabetologia **15:**143-152, 1978.
62. Teller, J.: Vegetarian meal planning for the diabetic, Diab. Educator, **5**(2):12-20, 1979.
63. Unger, R.H., and Orci, L.: Role of glucagon in diabetes, Arch. Intern. Med. **137:**482-491, 1971.
64. U.S. Department of Health and Human Services: The treatment and control of diabetes: a national plan to reduce mortality and morbidity. A report of the National Advisory Board, NIH Publication No. 81-2284, Washington, D.C., 1980, U.S. Government Printing Office.
65. *Ventura, E.: Foot care for diabetics, Am. J. Nurs. **78:**886-888, 1978.
66. *Vranic, M., and Berger, M.: Exercise and diabetes mellitus, Diabetes **28:**147-163, 1979.
67. Walesky, M.E.: Diabetic ketoacidosis, Am. J. Nurs. **78:**872-874, 1978.
68. Wyngaarden, J.B., and Smith, L.H.: Textbook of medicine ed. 16, Philadelphia, 1982, W.B. Saunders Co.

Classic

69. Arieff, A.: Nonketotic hyperosmolar coma with hyperglycemia, Medicine **51:**73-94, 1972.
70. Gabbay, K., and O'Sullivan, J.: The sorbitol pathway: enzyme localization and content in normal and diabetic nerve and cord, Diabetes **17:**239-243, 1968.
71. Gerich, J.E., et al: Characterization of the glucagon response to hypoglycemia in man, J. Clin. Endocrinol. Metab. **1:**77-82, 1974.
72. Gerich, F.E., et al: Clinical and metabolic characteristics of hyperosmolar nonketotic coma, Diabetes **20:**228-238, 1971.
73. Pyke, D., and Pease, J.: Diabetic ketosis and coma, J. Clin. Pathol. **22:**57-61, 1969.

30

The Patient with Endocrine Problems

DOROTHY BLEVINS and VIRGINIA L. CASSMEYER

STUDY QUESTIONS

- Where is each of the endocrine glands located? Review the hormones secreted by each gland.

- Review the functions of the anterior and posterior pituitary, thyroid, and parathyroid glands. For each function, consider the effect on the body of excess or lack of secretion of the gland.

- Review the physiology of stress (Chapter 8). What is the role of the adrenal gland in the stress response?

- In what way does giving a large amount of a hormone (such as cortisone) to a patient who already is producing a normal amount affect production of the hormone? Why does this reaction take place?

- How would you explain to a patient who has a high basal metabolic rate (such as occurs with hyperthyroidism) that increased amounts of nutrients are needed?

- Review in your nutrition text foods high and low in calcium and phosphorus. What vitamin is essential for the body to use calcium effectively?

The endocrine system functions as the regulator of multiple body processes, primarily through the actions of hormones. Hormones are chemical compounds that are synthesized in glands under genetic control and then secreted into the blood. They affect specific target cells in the body and control diverse physiologic functions. Alterations in the function of the endocrine glands, hormones, or target cellular activities usually result in a wide variety of effects. Many endocrine diseases have a slow and subtle onset of symptoms; yet, since many of the functions controlled by the endocrine system are vital, dysfunction can be serious and even fatal.

Research is advancing the knowledge of complex cellular activities that result from the presence of hormones. Fig. 30-1 illustrates a simple schema of the components of the endocrine system, that is, the series of processes that are now considered integral to the endocrine system. This chapter will discuss the health problems related to the hormones of four endocrine glands: pituitary, adrenal, thyroid, and parathyroid. The endocrine functions of the pineal and thymus glands are poorly understood. The gonads are discussed in Chapter 35, and pancreatic beta cell dysfunction is discussed in Chapter 29.

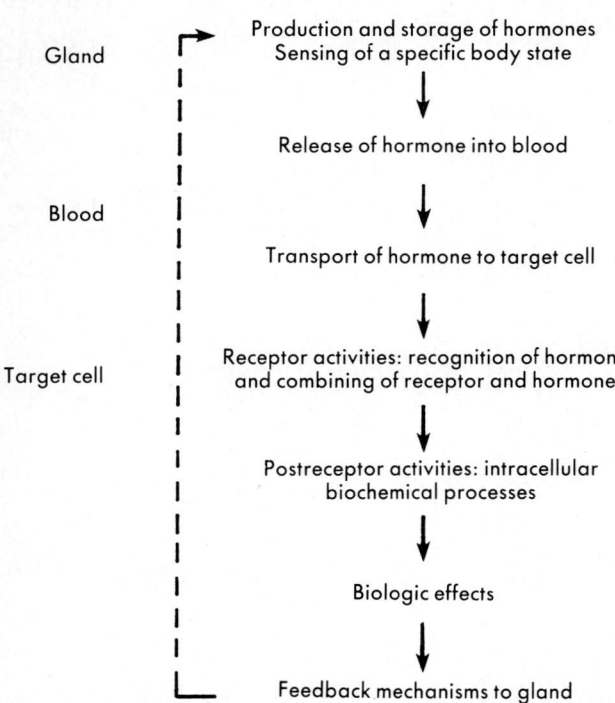

Fig. 30-1. Processes of endocrine system.

ANATOMY AND PHYSIOLOGY

Pituitary gland

The pituitary gland (hypophysis) is approximately 1 cm in size and weighs 500 mg. It lies in the sella turcica of the sphenoid bone at the base of the skull and is separated from the oral cavity by the sphenoid bone (Fig. 30-2.) The sella turcica is close to the optic chiasma. The pituitary gland is actually two glands, the larger anterior pituitary or adenohypophysis and the posterior pituitary or neurohypophysis. The anterior pituitary is often called the master gland because of its major influence on other glands and thus on the entire body.. It is known that five kinds of cells can be differentiated in the anterior pituitary lobe, and it is believed that each kind of cell secretes a specific hormone.

PITUITARY HORMONES

The small size of the pituitary gland should not be misleading. Five major hormones are secreted by the anterior lobe and two by the posterior lobe, all of which produce changes on far distant target cells. Thyroid-stimulating hormone (TSH), adrenocorticotropic hormone (ACTH), and the gonadotropic hormones are called tropic hormones because they stimulate other glands to secrete active hormones, which in turn effect changes on specific body cells. The other pituitary hormones exert their influence directly on body cells (nontropic).

Pituitary hormones

Anterior pituitary

Thyroid-stimulating hormone (TSH)	Stimulates thyroid to secrete thyroxin
Adrenocorticotropic hormone (ACTH)	Stimulates adrenal cortex to secrete cortisol
Gonadotropic hormones	
Luteinizing hormone (LH)	Induces ovulation and stimulates formation of corpus luteum and progesterone secretion in female
Follicle-stimulating hormone (FSH)	Stimulates follicle growth in ovary and secretion of estrogen in female
Interstitial cell–stimulating hormone (ICSH)	Stimulates secretion of testosterone in male
Growth hormone (GH) (somatotropin, STH)	Stimulates body growth; influences protein, carbohydrate, and fat metabolism
Prolactin	Stimulates mammary gland development

Posterior pituitary

Antidiuretic hormone (ADH)	Effects changes in kidney tubular membrane to increase water absorption; stimulates smooth muscle of intestines and blood vessels
Oxytocin	Stimulates uterine contractions and breast milk ejection

RELATIONSHIP BETWEEN HYPOTHALAMUS AND PITUITARY GLAND

The hypothalamus serves as a vital link between the neurologic and hormonal regulatory mechanisms. The hypothalamus exerts control over the anterior pituitary gland and thus over other glands and body cells. The hypothalamus (located in tissues around the third ventricle) and the anterior pituitary lobe are connected by the hypothalamus-hypophyseal portal blood system, by which neurosecretory releasing factors (RF) and neurosecretory inhibiting factors (IF) are carried from the hypothalamus to the pituitary. It is believed that for each anterior pituitary hormone there is an RF and an IF that stimulates or inhibits the release of that hormone. Fig. 30-3 summarizes the interactions between the hypothalamus, anterior pituitary gland, and other endocrine glands and target organs.

The hypothalamus is structurally connected to the posterior pituitary gland. ADH and oxytocin are actually produced in the hypothalamus in the paraventricular and su-

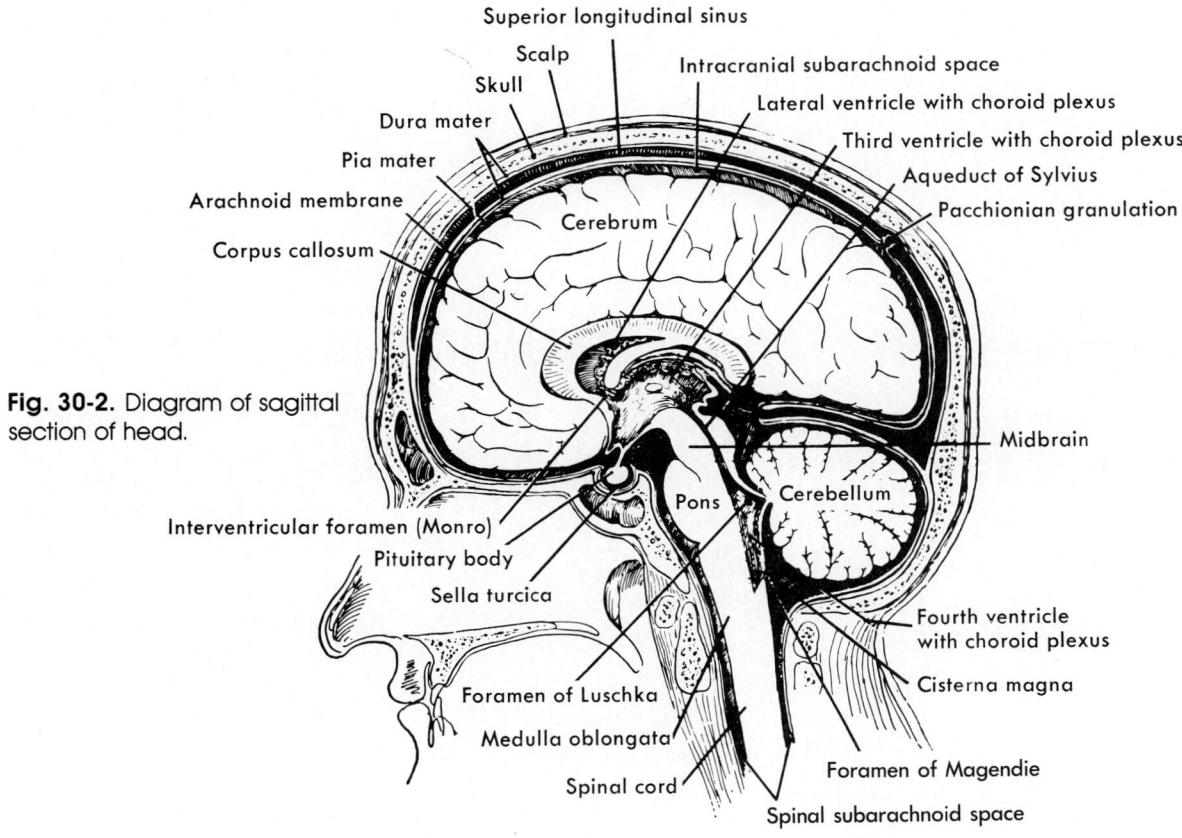

Fig. 30-2. Diagram of sagittal section of head.

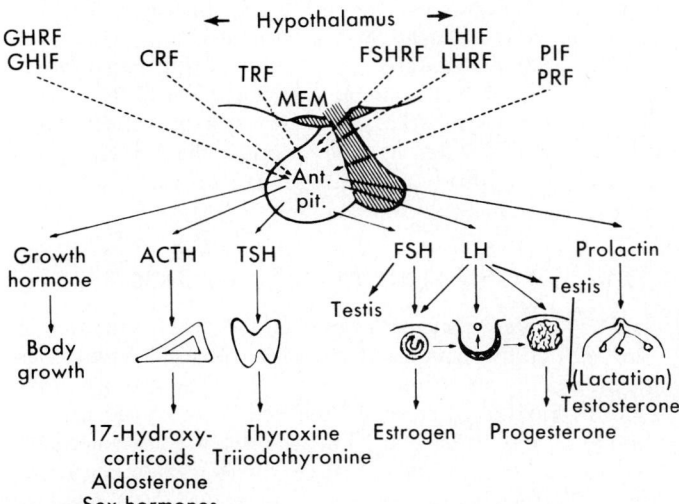

Fig. 30-3. Releasing factors that control output of hormones from anterior lobe of pituitary gland and ultimate hormone release from peripheral glands. *GHRF,* Growth hormone releasing factor; *GHIF,* growth hormone inhibitory factor; *CRF,* corticotropin-releasing factor; *TRF,* thyrotropin-releasing factor or hormone; *FSHRF,* follicle-stimulating hormone releasing factor; *LHRF,* luteinizing hormone releasing factor; *LHIF,* luteinizing hormone inhibitory factor; *PIF,* prolactin inhibitory factor; *PRF,* prolactin inhibitory factor; *MEM,* median eminence. (Modified from Mountcastle, V.B., editor; Medical physiology, vol. 1, ed. 14, St. Louis, 1979, The C.V. Mosby Co.)

Fig. 30-4. Nerve tracts from hypothalamus to posterior lobe of pituitary gland. (From Anthony, C.P., and Thibedeau, G.A.: Textbook of anatomy and physiology, ed. 11, St. Louis, 1982, The C.V. Mosby Co.)

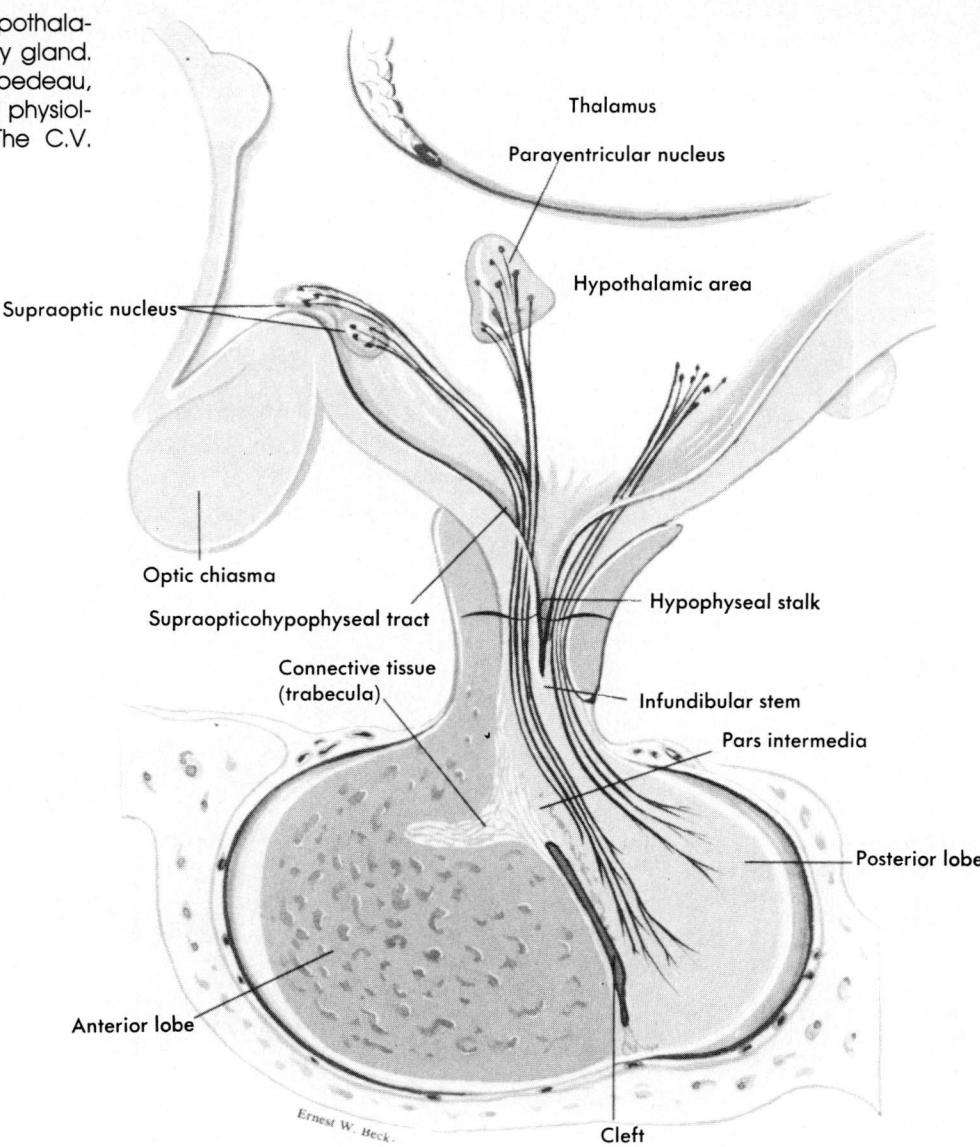

Thalamus

Paraventricular nucleus

Hypothalamic area

Supraoptic nucleus

Optic chiasma

Supraopticohypophyseal tract

Hypophyseal stalk

Connective tissue (trabecula)

Infundibular stem

Pars intermedia

Posterior lobe

Anterior lobe

Ernest W. Beck.

Cleft

praoptic nuclei and are carried down neurons by axonal transport to the terminal branches that are located in the posterior pituitary lobe (Fig. 30-4). There they are stored and then released.

Adrenal glands

The two adrenal organs lie in retroperitoneal tissue, each capping the upper pole of a kidney. There are two glands in each adrenal organ: the adrenal cortex or outer layer and the adrenal medulla or central portion. The *adrenal cortex* secretes two groups of hormones that are necessary for life: the glucocorticoids of which cortisol is the major hormone, and the mineralocorticoids of which aldosterone is the major hormone. The third group of hormones secreted by the cortex in both men and women are the two sex hormones, androgen and estrogen. This source of sex hormones is an important consideration in

certain pathologic conditions or when treatments require the absence of a particular sex hormone.

The *adrenal medulla* secretes epinephrine and norepinephrine, which augment the neurotransmitters produced by the sympathetic nervous system. These catecholamines secreted by the adrenal medulla are not necessary for life, but, in excess, are responsible for serious hypertension.

Thyroid and parathyroid glands

The thyroid gland is located in the anterior aspect of the neck and weighs about 20 gm. It consists of two lobes connected by an isthmus and lies just below the larynx. The thyroid gland stores iodine and secretes the thyroid hormone and calcitonin. The thyroid hormone actually consists of two hormones, thyroxin (tetraiodothyronine, T_4) and triiodothyronine (T_3). These hormones regulate

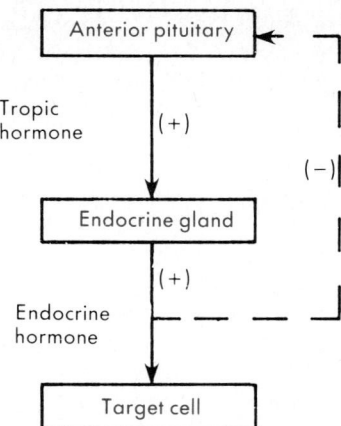

Fig. 30-5. Negative feedback system. Excess amounts of endocrine hormone will inhibit pituitary activity and thus stop development of more endocrine hormone.

the metabolic rate and the processes of growth and tissue differentiation. Calcitonin helps to maintain serum calcium levels.

The *parathyroid gland* consists of four minute glands that are variously located on the posterior aspect of each thyroid lobe. Parathyroid hormone regulates calcium and phosphorus metabolism.

Hormonal regulation

The amount of hormone available to receptors is critical for health. Current diagnostic practice relies heavily on measurement of circulating hormone levels by radioimmunoassay. The amount of hormone is kept within definite limits by a number of factors. One factor, the closed-looped negative feedback system, is illustrated in Fig. 30-5. In this system gland A produces tropic hormone X, which stimulates organ B to produce substance Y; substance Y then inhibits the secretion of hormone X by gland A. An extensive feedback loop exists between the hypothalamus, pituitary gland, and other endocrine glands.

Other factors influencing secretion patterns of hormones include sleep-wake patterns, age, and growth and development. Hormones are not secreted at a uniform rate, but are released in bursts rather than a steady flow. Some hormones have cyclic rhythmic patterns of secretions, and thus rhythmic patterns of serum hormone levels can be noted; for example, cortisol has a diurnal pattern and estrogen has a monthly cycle. Other hormones are secreted in response to blood levels of specific substances, for example, insulin, glucagon, and aldosterone.

The rate of excretion of metabolic inactivation also affects the levels of circulating hormones and prevents hormonal excess. Usually hormones have a very short activity period before they are degraded.

Receptor activity

It is hypothesized that hormones initiate cellular activity in one of two ways. In the *moblie receptor* method the hormones are believed to cross the plasma cell membrane and combine with receptors in the cytoplasm of the cell. They cross the nuclear membrane and react with particular proteins in the chromatin of the nucleus or bind with deoxyribonucleic acid (DNA). In general, steroid hormones, such as adrenal steroids, and androgen, estrogen, and progesterone act in this manner. Thyroid hormone may also react in the same way.

In the second method or the *fixed receptor* method, the hormone combines with a receptor on the plasma membrane of the cell and initiates a sequence of events coordinated by a second messenger causing the cell to initiate whatever activity it is equipped to do. ACTH, TSH, glucagon, parathyroid hormone, and the catecholamines initiate cellular activity in this manner.

Hypersecretion and hyposecretion

Regardless of the process involved in pathology, endocrine disorders are characterized by an alteration in *amount* of effective hormone, either an excess or a deficiency. Hormonal alterations may result from the following:
1. Change in the integrity of glandular tissue
2. Dysfunction of regulating mechanisms
3. Decrease in excretion or inactivation of hormones
4. Peripheral resistance to the action of the hormones

Etiologies of endocrine glandular disorders are classified as primary, secondary, or iatrogenic:

Primary: disorder of the gland

Secondary: disorder of a target gland because of disorder in the pituitary gland

Iatrogenic: disorder in a gland that occurs because of treatment

Hyposecretory states may occur when there is absence of glandular tissue or when there is hypoplasia. Atrophy and hypoplasia often occur together. Hypersecretory states may occur when there is hyperplasia or a tumor. For example, pituitary hyperplasia might be a response to hypothalamic stimulation. Hypertrophy is not always accompanied by an increased secretion of hormone. One pathologic cause of hypersecretory states is tissues secreting hormones in quantities not related to body needs.

Terms denoting glandular changes

Hypoplasia	Decrease in amount of functioning tissues
Hyperplasia	Increase in active secreting cells
Hypertrophy	Increase in gland size
Atrophy	Decrease in gland size

These tissues are not responsive to the regulating mechanisms, for example to the negative feedback loops or to the tropic hormone stimulation or lack of stimulation. This topic will be explained more specifically in each section describing dysfunction of a particular gland.

PREVENTION OF DISEASE AND HEALTH EDUCATION

Primary prevention

Few primary endocrine diseases can be prevented at this time. *Simple goiter,* a disease characterized by an enlargement of the thyroid gland, is an exception. This condition occurs because of a lack of ingested iodine. The nurse can participate in primary prevention by teaching the importance of eating foods that contain iodine, such as seafoods and leafy vegetables. In places where there is a known deficiency of iodine in the natural water (for example, the Great Lakes region), persons are encouraged to use iodized salt.

Although the relationships involved in hypernutrition and endocrine dysfunction are complex and not completely understood, prevention and control of obesity are helpful in reducing the risk of at least one endocrine disease, type II diabetes mellitus (Chapter 29).

Secondary prevention

Malignant tumors of the endocrine gland are less prevalent than other forms of cancer. The thyroid gland can be easily palpated, and people should be encouraged to have yearly physical examinations to help in early detection of thyroid carcinoma. This cancer appears in all age groups and especially in those with a past history of irradiation to the neck structures. In recent years, there has been a concerted search in the United States for adults who received irradiation of the thymus gland as children. These individuals are urged to seek medical attention for detection of thyroid cancer.

Heart disease can be induced or aggravated by certain hormonal alterations. Thyroid and adrenocortical dysfunctions are two examples in which early detection and treatment can minimize cardiovascular disease.

The nurse can assist in the early detection of these disorders by encouraging persons to seek medical attention for persistent vague complaints of decreased well-being that may include the following:
1. Fatigue
2. Altered nutritional intake
3. Changes in skin and hair appearance and condition
4. Changes in excretory patterns

While endocrine disease is not the only cause of these symptoms, it is true that these are early symptoms of many endocrinopathies.

Tertiary prevention

A major contribution of the nurse to patients with diagnosed endocrinopathies is that of assisting them to learn self-management of their chronic diseases. The progression of many hormonal deficiency diseases can be halted or slowed by patients who are educated and motivated to follow prescribed regimens of hormonal replacement. Hormonal replacement, when necessary, is an important method of treatment that must be handled by the patient over a long period of time. Failure to maintain adequate hormonal replacement results in illness and death.

Major health problems of the endocrine system

This chapter will use the approach of hyposecretion or hypersecretion of hormones to organize the information. Only those endocrine problems encountered most frequently will be discussed; these are listed in Table 30-1. The most frequent endocrine disorder in the United

Table 30-1. Health problems of the endocrine system

Gland	Hyposecretion	Hypersecretion
Pituitary	Panhypopituitarism, hypopituitarism, dwarfism, pituitary Addison's disease, hypoprolactinemia, diabetes insipidus	Hyperpituitarism, acromegaly, gigantism, pituitary Cushing's disease, hyperprolactinemia, syndrome of inappropriate ADH secretion (SIADH)
Thyroid	Hypothyroidism, cretinism, myxedema	Hyperthyroidism, Graves' disease
Parathyroid	Hypoparathyroidism, tetany	Hyperparathyroidism
Adrenal cortex	Addison's disease	Cushing's syndrome, hyperaldosteronism
Adrenal medulla		Pheochromocytoma
Pancreas (endocrine)	Diabetes mellitus	Hypoglycemia

States is diabetes mellitus, which is discussed in Chapter 29. The next most frequent disorder is hyperthyroidism (Graves' disease). All of the disorders can lead to significant health problems in individuals.

ANTERIOR PITUITARY DYSFUNCTION

The functions of the anterior pituitary gland are based on the function of the respective hormones, TSH;

ACTH; GH or STH; LH, FSH, and ICSH; and prolactin. Hyposecretion or hypersecretion of these hormones produces different effects (Table 30-2).

PATHOPHYSIOLOGY

Hypersecretion

Hyperpituitarism is the oversecretion of one or more of the hormones secreted by the pituitary gland and usually

Table 30-2. Anterior pituitary dysfunction

Alteration in secretion	Etiology	Signs and symptoms	Medical therapy
GH excess	*Primary* Pituitary tumors, pituitary hyperplasia	Gigantism in children; acromegaly in adults: growth of soft tissues, cartilages, bones; enlargement and coarsening of facial features; enlarged tongue; visceral enlargement: liver, spleen, heart, kidneys; warm, moist, coarse skin; husky voice; prominent muscle development; insulin resistance	Removal of tumor: adenectomy, hypophysectomy; medications that suppress GH: estrogen, medroxyprogesterone, chlorpromazine, bromocriptine mesylate
GH deficiency	*Primary* Hemorrhage; aneurysm; infection; granuloma; Trauma; congenital; tumor	Dwarfism in children; sensitivity to insulin; fasting hypoglycemia; hypoglycemia	Growth hormone replacement in children
ACTH excess	*Primary* Pituitary tumors; pituitary hyperplasia *Secondary* Nonpituitary secreting tumor; stimulation of the hypothalamus *Iatrogenic* Bilateral postadrenalectomy	Similar to Cushing's syndrome (adrenocortical excess) (Table 30-7)	Pituitary ablation: adenectomy, radiation, hypophysectomy; surgical removal of ectopic source of ACTH
ACTH deficiency	*Primary* Same as GH deficiency *Iatrogenic* Suppression of hypothalamic-pituitary-adrenal axis by endogenous corticosteroids	Similar to Addison's disease (adrenocortical deficit) (Table 30-7) asthenia (weakness); nausea, vomiting; hypotension; hypoglycemia; hyponatremia; hyperkalemia	Cortisone or cortisone derivative (see Table 30-7 for other treatment)
TSH excess	*Primary* Pituitary tumor; pituitary hyperplasia	Same as hyperthyroidism (thyroid hormone excess) (Table 30-14)	Hypophysectomy
TSH deficit	Same as GH deficit	Same as hypothyroidism (thyroid hormone deficit) (Table 30-14); cretinism in newborn; myxedema in adult	Thyroid hormone replacement

Continued.

Table 30-2. Anterior pituitary dysfunction—cont'd

Alteration in secretion	Etiology	Signs and symptoms	Medical therapy
Prolactin excess	*Primary* Pituitary tumor *Secondary* Hypothalamic dysfunction *Iatrogenic* Side effect of certain drugs	Amenorrhea; galactorrhea; depressed libido; infertility; impotency; change in secondary sex characteristics	Pituitary surgery; drugs to suppress prolactin (bromocriptine)
Prolactin deficit	Same as GH deficit	Failure of lactation postpartum	
Gonadotropic hormone excess		Precocious sexual development in children; changes in secondary sex characteristics; hirsutism	
Gonadotropic hormone deficit	Same as GH deficit	Delayed sexual development in children; in adults: female—amenorrhea, infertility; male—impotence; In both—changes in secondary sex characteristics	Replacement of sex hormones in cyclic pattern

---

Types of anterior pituitary adenomas

Type	Hormone secreted
Chromophobic	Prolactin (most common), GH, ACTH
Acidophilic	Prolactin, GH
Basophilic	ACTH, TSH (rare)

---

refs to anterior pituitary hormones. The most common cause of hyperpituitarism is pituitary adenomas.

Pituitary adenomas account for 5% to 10% of all intracranial tumors, and they most frequently arise in the anterior pituitary lobe. The factors responsible for their development is unknown. These adenomas have been classified according to the staining qualities of the cells of the tumors (chromophobic, acidophilic, or basophilic) and by the hormone-secreting characteristics of the cells. Approximately 75% of all anterior pituitary adenomas are of the chromophobic type, whereas basophilic tumors are the least frequent. Pituitary adenomas almost never secrete FSH or LH.

Pituitary tumors cause two clinical problems depending on the size, the location, and the secreting capacity of the tumor. These are (1) neurologic alterations resulting from pressure on surrounding nervous system structures and (2) hypersecretion of one or more anterior pituitary hormones.

Neurologic alterations

Since the pituitary lies in the cranial vault, abnormal growth will cause neurologic signs and symptoms. The major neurologic alteration is caused by pressure on the optic chiasma and optic nerves. Patients experience progressive loss of vision, and, if untreated, permanent blindness results. Most adenomas cause midline pressure and damage the fibers subserving vision in the upper temporal fields, causing a *bitemporal hemianopsia* (loss of vision in one half of the visual field of both eyes). Often the visual defect is asymmetric. Visual acuity is commonly spared, and the nasal field defects are rare.

Other symptoms include headaches that are characteristically bitemporal and bifrontal and result from pressure on the sella turcica.[2] Confusion and impaired memory may occur but are rare. Symptoms of increased intracranial pressure are also rare.

Endocrine alterations

The clinical picture may be the result of excessive secretion of prolactin, GH, ACTH, or TSH. The signs and symptoms of increased secretion of ACTH and TSH are discussed in the sections of this chapter on adrenal problems and thyroid problems, respectively.

PROLACTIN EXCESS. Prolactin excess is almost always caused by pituitary adenomas, usually microadenomas. Women usually seek help for endocrine dysfunction before neurologic signs and symptoms are present. They

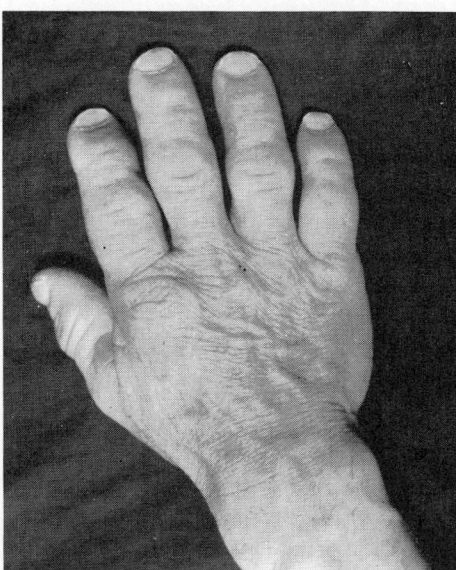

Fig. 30-6. Hand showing characteristics of acromegalic condition. (From Schottelius, B.A., and Schottelius, D.D.: Textbook of physiology, ed. 18, St. Louis, 1978, The C.V. Mosby Co.)

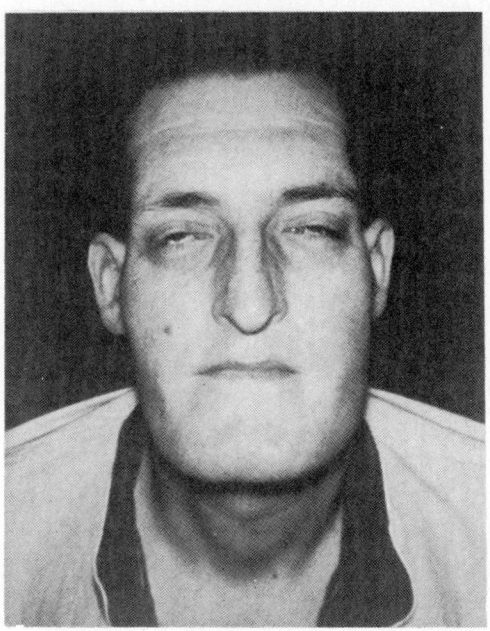

Fig. 30-7. Acromegaly. Note large head, exaggerated forward projection of jaw, and protrusion of frontal bone. (From Rimoin, D.L.: N. Engl. J. Med. **272:**923, 1965.)

may complain of amenorrhea or galactorrhea. They often complain of depressed libido. Men frequently will seek help for neurologic complaints. They may give a history of depressed libido, infertility, or impotence. Other signs of hypogonadism, such as changes in secondary sex characteristics, may be present.

GROWTH HORMONE EXCESS. An excess of GH is almost always caused by a secreting pituitary tumor, although occasionally there is no distinct tumor.[2] Hypersecretion of GH that occurs in children before fusion of the epiphysis results in *gigantism*. Such children reach enormous proportions because of massive growth in both the length and width of bones. Soft tissue enlarges along with the skeleton.

Hypersecretion of GH that occurs after the fusion of the epiphysis results in acromegaly. This disorder affects men and women equally and most frequently begins between the second and fourth decade. The changes are slow and progressive and frequently go unrecognized for some time. Table 30-2 lists the characteristic signs of acromegaly. The person may note an increase in ring, shoe, glove, and hat size. The hands become spadelike in appearance (Fig. 30-6). The enlargement of the mandible causes an under bite and increased spacing of the lower teeth. The forehead and orbital ridges become prominent (Fig. 30-7). Widening of spaces between joints occurs with increased cartilage growth. This leads to osteoarthritis with pain and limitation of joint motion. Changes in the spine may cause nerve root and cord compression.

There are many systemic changes that can result from excess in growth hormone:

Disorders of hyposecretion of anterior pituitary

Adrenal insufficiency
Growth hormone lack
Hypogonadism
Hypothyroidism

---

1. Increased metabolic rate
2. Increased sweating and sebaceous gland activity
3. Glucose intolerance (50% of patients) and insulin resistance that can lead to diabetes mellitus
4. Hypertension (25% of patients) and cardiomegaly can lead to congestive heart failure (CHF)

Many patients with GH excess eventually develop the neurologic defects discussed earlier. Frequently they do not seek help until then.

Hyposecretion

A number of diseases can interfere with the function of the anterior pituitary and cause hyposecretion of one or more hormones (hypopituitarism). Occasionally, panhypopituitarism occurs with a deficiency of all anterior pituitary hormones. The hormonal deficiencies usually occur in the order listed in the box above.

Table 30-2 lists the characteristic signs and symptoms, etiology, and treatment for hyposecretion of each of the

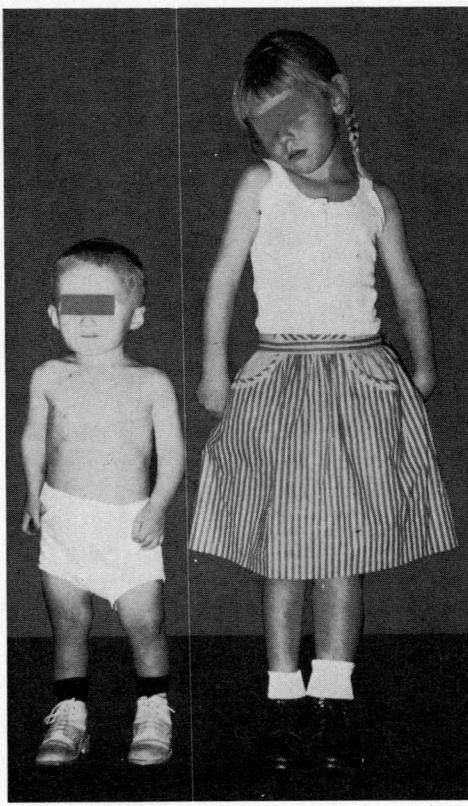

Fig. 30-8. Hypopituitary dwarfism in a 4-year-old boy whose height is 25 inches. Girl is also 4 years old and has a normal height of 39 inches. Dwarf has normal face, as well as head, trunk, and limbs of approximately normal proportions. (From Brashear, H.R., and Raney, R.B.: Shand's handbook of orthopaedic surgery, ed. 9, St. Louis, 1978, The C.V. Mosby Co.)

anterior pituitary hormones. The clinical picture will vary depending on the hormonal deficit present and the cause of the deficit.

If a tumor is present, the patient will have neurologic alterations similar to those seen with secreting pituitary adenomas. If the tumor arises from regions surrounding the pituitary, the neurologic signs and symptoms may be more severe. Signs and symptoms of increased intracranial pressure, such as hydrocephalus and papilledema are usually present.

Deficiency of GH in the adult is usually not significant. Congenital deficiency of growth hormone in the child results in short stature. *Dwarfism* is a rare disorder and is characterized by short stature that is apparent at about 4 years of age (Fig. 30-8). The child typically appears immature and has increased truncal fat. Bone age and height age are usually approximate, and as the child matures, the body proportions approach those of an adult.

TSH and ACTH deficiency are discussed in later sections in more detail. Refer to Table 30-2 for summary information.

ASSESSMENT

The application of the nursing process to patients with anterior pituitary dysfunction will focus on patients with pituitary surgery and hormonal imbalances related to lack of ACTH and GH. Many of the descriptions of assessment, data analysis, and planning discussed in this section can be applied to later sections in the chapter. There are some common clinical problems that are seen in several endocrine disorders:

1. Fatigue
2. Nutritional alterations
3. Fluid and electrolyte imbalances
4. Cardiovascular changes
5. Changed body characteristics
6. Intolerance to stress

Common assessment parameters for persons with endocrine dysfunction include the following:

1. Extent of the hormonal imbalance
2. Clinical problems present
3. Resources needed by the patient and family to cope with the disorder, diagnostic tests, and treatment measures
4. Symptoms of crisis (persistent headache, visual changes, polyuria, syncope)
5. Patient's perceptions of health problems, their management, and assistance needed

Assessment of psychologic and social factors is important because the diagnostic process can be lengthy, frightening, and costly. Stress in the patient with hormonal imbalances should be avoided as much as possible, since stress places an additional burden on the impaired endocrine function. Body image changes and physical problems may influence the person's goals, activities of daily living, and relationships with others. The person's coping abilities may also be diminished.

Subjective data

The collecting of information regarding changes in body characteristics is not only important in helping to define the physiologic problem, but also in identifying potential or present emotional or psychologic problems. Some of the changes that occur with endocrine disorders are irreversible even when the physiologic problem is controlled. Body characteristics are part of the identity of the person, and the patient may have problems dealing with the changes.

The patient's description of the following factors help define the needs for assistance:

1. Fatigue, rest, and sleep patterns
2. Eating patterns (frequency of food intake)
3. Fluid intake and output patterns
4. Cardiovascular history
5. Special hygiene or grooming needs (hirsutism, perspiration, obesity)
6. Discomforts
7. Medication usage
8. The endocrine disorder and its treatment

Table 30-3. Tests of anterior pituitary function

Test	Procedure	Interpretation
Hormonal radioimmunoassay TSH, ACTH, Prolactin, FSH, LH (ICSH), GH	Blood sample, no special preparation in most cases Glucose may be administered before blood collection	Used to measure circulating hormonal levels; for homones secreted in diurnal pattern (ACTH, GH), best obtained in early AM and at intervals throughout day to determine cyclic pattern
Provocative tests TSH stimulation	All require basal rate established by pretest assay; stimulant is given and the hormonal levels repeatedly measured	Normal serum TSH begins to rise at 10 min and peaks at 45 min; subnormal values reflect decreased pituitary reserve
ACTH stimulation		Normal response of serum cortisol is 7 μg/ml from normal baseline; subnormal values reflect pituitary or adrenal deficiency
GH stimulation	IV glucose may be given before stimulant	Normal response is a peak in GH levels approximately 60 min after stimulation
Suppression tests ACTH suppression	Collection of 24-hr urine for 17-hydroxycorticosteroids (OHCS) and of plasma for ACTH	A normal response is an increase in ACTH levels and 17-OHCS; no increase reflects decreased pituitary reserve
Cortisol suppression	Collection of 24-hr urine for 17-OHCS	Dexamethasone normally suppresses ACTH secretion; less than normal suppression can reflect pituitary or ectopic hypersecretion

Objective data

Initially, inspection is used to assess the patient's body growth and developmental status and should include the following:

1. Height and weight
2. Body proportions
3. Amount and distribution of muscle mass
4. Fat distribution
5. Skin pigmentation
6. Hair distribution

A great variation exists in the general population and often changes will not be obvious. Inspection of family members for like characteristics will provide information as to whether the characteristics seen in the pateint are caused by hereditary or pathophysiologic alterations. The patient's alertness and speech patterns can be assessed when the history is being collected. Physical assessment (Chapter 3) should be thorough in these patients because of the wide spectrum of bodily effects that occur with pituitary dysfunction.

Follow-up data includes monitoring the following:

1. Weight
2. Vital signs every 4 hours
3. Intake and output every 8 hours
4. Signs of infection

Diagnostic tests

It is now possible to measure the serum levels of GH, TSH, ACTH, prolactin, and gonadotropins by radioimmunoassay. Often on the basis of clinical findings the physician will use these measurements to confirm the excess or the deficit of a particular hormone. The determination of the etiology of the hormonal alteration is then investigated. This may involve the use of a stimulant or suppressant of the hormone and measurements of the effects on hormonal serum levels. Table 30-3 lists the most common tests of pituitary function, the procedures and explanations, and interpretations of the findings. Note that target organ function is also studied.

Skeletal roentgenograms can assess changes in bone structure, and skull roentgenograms can assess the size of the pituitary gland. Computed tomography (CT) scanning may be used to demonstrate the presence of intrasellar masses. In some instances pneumoencephalograms may be necessary to define the size of the mass or to exclude empty sellar syndrome. Visual field checks and an ophthalmoscopic examination are performed.

DATA ANALYSIS AND PLANNING

Nursing diagnoses

Nursing diagnoses for persons with pituitary dysfunction could conceivably include a majority of those proposed by the Nursing Conference Group because of the pituitary's role of master gland and its influence on health status. However, some more common diagnoses include the following:

Anxiety

Self-concept, disturbance in body image, self-esteem, role performance, personal identity

Coping, ineffective individual or family

Activity intolerance

Sleep pattern disturbance

Fluid volume, deficit or excess

Nutrition, alteration in: more or less than body requirement

Urinary elimination, alterations in patterns

Knowledge deficit

Expected patient outcomes

Expected patient outcomes for the person in hormonal imbalance as follows are:

1. Patient will have restoration of physiologic wellbeing, as evidenced by:
   a. Stable blood pressure and pulse within optimal limits
   b. Desired weight
   c. Balance of intake and output
   d. Prompt recovery from crisis
   e. Absence of infection
   f. Absence of signs of excess or deficit of specific hormones
2. Patient or significant others will demonstrate requisite knowledge, skill, and resources for selfmanagement of treatment measures:
   a. Describe the hormonal deficit and relate to signs and symptoms
   b. Explain the planned treatment measures and effects of treatment
   c. Explain the prescribed medication program
      (1) Awareness of the need for lifelong replacement therapy
      (2) Drugs, dosage, and frequency of therapy
      (3) Desired effects and side effects of therapy
      (4) What to do when signs and symptoms of undertreatment or overtreatment occur
   d. Describe the times when extra hormonal therapy is necessary
   e. Describe need to obtain Medic Alert symbol to wear
   f. State plans for regular follow-up care

IMPLEMENTATION

Assisting with achievement of therapeutic goals

Pituitary tumor (adenoma) is the most frequent cause of hyperpituitarism, and the most frequent treatment is surgery. If possible, pituitary tissue is not disturbed. Following an adenectomy, hormonal levels are expected to return to normal immediately. External radiation or *yttrium* (^{39}Y) implantation may also be used for treatment of a hormone-secreting pituitary tumor or pituitary hyperplasia, but hormonal levels are slow to return to normal with these therapies.

Certain drugs suppress GH: estrogen, medroxyprogesterone, chlorpromazine, and bromocriptine mesylate (Parlodel). Parlodel can also suppress hyperprolactinemia; however, symptoms recur when its administration is stopped.

Sometimes the treatment of hypersecretion of a gland results in a state of hyposecretion. When a total hypophysectomy (removal of the pituitary) is performed, panhypopituitarism results. Even though panhypopituitarism is not expected after a partial hypophysectomy, ^{39}Y implantation, or drug therapy, it can occur as a complication. All patients with these treatments are monitored for hormonal deficiencies.

Radiation therapy or cranial surgery is frightening to most patients and their families, and they need time to share concerns, fears, and questions with the nurse. All questions are answered as honestly and completely as possible.

The patient needs to be aware that the surgery or irradiation will remove excess hormone levels. Some of the coarsening features may disappear because soft tissue swelling will decrease, glucose intolerance will disappear, and visceral enlargement may decrease; but most of the physical changes associated with excessive GH are irreversible.

Surgery

TRANSSPHENOIDAL SURGERY. The transsphenoidal approach is most frequently used to resect an adenoma. The sella turcica is entered through the sphenoid sinus, and the tumor is removed with the aid of a surgical microscope (Fig. 30-2). The incision is made between the gums and upper lip. This approach may also be used to implant ^{39}Y. The opening made in the dura mater on entering the sella turcica is frequently patched with a piece of fascia taken from the leg; thus the patient must be prepared for the leg incision. The patch is to prevent a cerebrospinal fluid (CSF) leak. Leaking of CSF may occur for a few days postoperatively but should then stop. The nose may be packed and a gauze sling placed under it to absorb drainage.

Monitoring for the presence of a CSF leak is important. The following data are noted:

1. Complaint of a postnasal drip
2. Constant swallowing
3. Evidence on the nasal sling or gauze pads of a "halo ring" (clear CSF fluid marking around a darker center of serous fluid)

4. Testing the nasal drainage for glucose

CSF fluid contains glucose, whereas nasal drainage does not. If the glucose test is positive, a specimen should be sent to the laboratory for confirmation.

If a persistent leak occurs, bed rest with the patient's head elevated to place pressure against the patch is prescribed. Most often CSF leaks will heal spontaneously, but occasionally surgical repair is necessary. Activities that increase intracranial pressure should be avoided.

Headache may be present and is treated with nonnarcotic analgesics or codeine. Persistent headache or nuchal rigidity (neck stiffness) may indicate the presence of meningitis and is reported immediately. Because of the risk of infection, prophylactic antibiotics may be ordered preoperatively or postoperatively.

Other nursing interventions for the patient with transsphenoidal surgery include the following:

1. Encourage oral fluids and a clear liquid diet as soon as the patient is alert and no longer nauseated from the anesthesia.
2. Increase the diet as tolerated (anorexia may result from a decreased sense of smell).
3. Reassure the patient that the loss of smell is temporary and should improve as soon as the nasal packing or sling is removed.
4. Provide oxygen and humidity as ordered to keep the nasal and oral mucous membranes moist.
5. Provide mouth care:
   a. Avoid toothbrushing to prevent disruption of the suture line.
   b. Use soft cotton swabs to cleanse the teeth.
   c. Offer mouth rinses frequently.

TRANSFRONTAL SURGERY. When the pituitary tumor extends beyond the boundaries of the sella turcica (extrasellar), craniotomy is used to obtain adequate surgical exposure. (The care of the patient with a craniotomy is discussed in Chapter 20.) Other intracerebral tumors, disease, or trauma of structures lying near the pituitary may result in temporary or permanent pituitary dysfunction.

Assisting with correction of hormonal imbalance

The patient with panhypopituitarism requires lifelong replacement of cortisol, thyroid, and in most instances, sex hormones, whether the hormonal deficits are caused by disease, trauma, hypophysectomy, or irradiation. The exception to replacement of sex hormones following hypophysectomy is the patient with cancer whose pituitary was removed to eliminate gonadotropic stimulation of tumor growth.

ACTH deficiency and thus glucocorticoid deficiency will occur immediately if the total pituitary has been removed and may occur as temporary deficits after removal of an adenoma. When the total pituitary is removed, an intramuscular or intravenous cortisone preparation will be given preoperatively and immediately postoperatively. Oral replacement therapy using cortisone acetate, prednisone, or another synthetic preparation will be started as soon as oral intake can be tolerated. If a temporary deficit

---

Activities that increase intracranial pressure
Coughing
Sneezing
Blowing the nose
Bending over
Straining

Signs of adrenocortical insufficiency
Nausea, vomiting
Prolonged lethargy
More fatigue than expected
Slower recovery than expected
Mild hypotension

Signs of addisonian crisis
Hypotension
Dehydration
Hyponatremia
Hyperkalemia
Hypoglycemia

---

occurs, the patient is treated with replacement therapy as long as necessary. Plasma levels of cortisol will be checked before discharge to make sure that the deficit has been corrected.

To detect adrenocortical deficiency and to determine adequacy of cortisol replacement, frequent monitoring of any patient with potential for adrenocortical insufficiency is necessary. Actions include the following:

1. Taking vital signs every hour after surgery until stable, then every 4 hours
2. Tabulating intake and output every 8 hours
3. Weighing patient daily

Electrolyte studies will be ordered at least daily or more often to monitor sodium and potassium levels. Signs of insufficient cortisol replacement are usually vague and nonspecific.

The symptoms listed above should be reported and carefully evaluated. Progression of symptoms can be rapid and an *addisonian crisis* with profound shock can develop. There are five classic signs of adrenocortical deficiency. The treatment of addisonian crisis is discussed on p. 811. The critical treatment measure is the replacement of cortisol.

Teaching the patient requiring hormonal replacement

1. Never omit a dose of the drug.
2. Notify physician if a dose is not taken or not retained.
3. Wear an identification bracelet.
4. Carry information concerning:
   a. Name and dosage of drug to be given in case of an emergency.
   b. Name and phone number of physician to be notified in an emergency.
5. Carry an emergency supply of a rapid-acting cortisone preparation with directions for use (for example, hydrocortisone 100 mg in a sterile syringe).
6. Report to physician any signs and symptoms of adrenocortical deficiency (p. 803).
7. Avoid stress when possible.
8. Notify physician when illness, injury, or emotional crises occur.
9. Maintain regular medical follow-up.

DIABETES INSIPIDUS FOLLOWING PITUITARY SURGERY. The removal of the pituitary gland or edema of surrounding tissue can precipitate the sudden onset of *diabetes insipidus*. Disruption in the hypothalamic secretion of ADH can also result in ADH alterations.

Diabetes insipidus occurs frequently in patients following irradiation. It is usually not permanent, even if all of the pituitary gland has been removed, because ADH is produced in the hypothalamus and adequate amounts can be released from there.

Monitoring for patients who may develop diabetes insipidus includes the following:
1. Intake and output tabulated every 4 hours
2. Specific gravity determined on each urine specimen (continuously dilute urine with specific gravity of 1.000 to 1.005 are signs of diabetes insipidus)

Fluid intake must be maintained to balance the urinary volume, since polyuria is usually present. When diabetes insipidus occurs, thirst is a frequent complaint. It can usually be managed by providing ice chips and adequate water intake. If fluid deficit is severe, vasopressin (Pitressin) is administered by intravenous route.

LIFELONG HORMONAL REPLACEMENT
CORTISOL REPLACEMENT

The daily replacement of cortisol in patients with adrenocortical insufficiency is critical; it is necessary for life to continue. Cortisone is the drug of choice, and it is given to correlate with the patient's activity and to mimic the usual diurnal pattern. Since cortisone is ulcerogenic, it should always be given after meals or with milk. Antacids may be prescribed. If an adrenocortical derivative with glucocorticoid properties, such as prednisone, is prescribed, the dosage will be equivalent to the antiinflammatory potency of hydrocortisone (p. 810).

THYROID AND GONAD HORMONE REPLACEMENT

Deficiency of TSH and of thyroid hormones usually does not occur on a temporary basis, and it is not seen immediately even after the total pituitary has been removed, since the thyroid stores enough hormone to last for several weeks. If the total pituitary has been removed, the patient will eventually require thyroid replacement.

Gonadotropin deficiency requires lifetime therapy. To maintain libido, secondary sexual characteristics, and well-being, men will be given testosterone and women will receive estrogen-progesterone preparations. If childbearing is desired, the gonadotropins (LH and FSH) must be replaced.

Teaching patients about hormonal replacement

Nurses make an important contribution to patients with hypopituitarism when patients are helped to understand the prescribed regimen for hormonal replacement. The serious nature of adrenocortical insufficiency should be stressed. Specific points to include in the teaching are listed here.

POSTERIOR PITUITARY DYSFUNCTION

The two hormones of the posterior pituitary are oxytocin and ADH. Refer to obstetrical nursing texts for further information about oxytocin. The two alterations of ADH secretion, ADH excess and deficit, are described in Table 30-4.

PATHOPHYSIOLOGY

Hyposecretion of ADH

The secretion of ADH is an important and normal response to states of stress or hyperosmolality. ADH effects changes in the kidney tubular membrane to increase water absorption to dilute the hyperosmolality and to provide an adequate blood volume during stress. In the presence of ADH, the urine is concentrated. When ADH is absent, water is not reabsorbed in the tubules and a large amount (15 to 24 L/day) of dilute urine is produced.

When the posterior pituitary does not release ADH or

Table 30-4. Alterations in ADH (posterior pituitary) secretion

Alteration	Etiology	Signs and symptoms	Medical therapy
ADH excess: SIADH	Diseased lung and pancreatic tissue (for example, oat cell carcinoma); skull fractures, intracranial lesions, surgery; positive pressure breathing; drugs: chlorpropamide, morphine, thiazides; nephrogenic diseases	*Dilutional hyponatermia:* Serum Na below 130 mEq/L; weakness; lethargy; confusion; convulsions; weight gain; edema	Surgical removal of ADH secreting tissue (pituitary or nonpituitary); water restriction of 800 to 1000 ml/day; hypertonic saline; demeclocycline
ADH deficit: Diabetes insipidus	Head trauma, intracranial surgery or lesion; pituitary disorder; hypophysectomy	Polyuria, polydipsia, dilute urine (specific gravity 1.000 to 1.005); if fluid intake is insufficient: dehydration, vascular collapse; weakness, anorexia	Fluid intake to balance fluid output; vasopressin replacement: Pitressin, Lypressin, (deamino-D-arginine vasopressin nasal spray or drops; surgical removal of tumor; drug therapy: thiazide, diuretics, chlorpropamide

the hypothalamus does not secrete ADH in response to a hyperosmolar state, diabetes insipidus results. The potential is great for severe dehydration and vascular collapse if the patient does not replenish fluids lost by the excessive urination. The three classic symptoms that should alert the nurse to diabetes insipidus are polyuria, dilute urine, and polydipsia.

Often the patient complains of insatiable thirst. Ice water is preferred, although the reason for this is unknown. Voiding may occur so often that there is interference with sleep and the patient complains of tiredness.

Hypersecretion of ADH

In the syndrome of inappropriate antidiuretic hormone (SIADH), the patient is unable to excrete dilute urine and therefore retains water. Normally, ADH secretion is self-limiting; in SIADH, there is a continual release of ADH unrelated to plasma osmolality. Hemodilution results in depressed levels of solutes and electrolytes. Central nervous system (CNS) dysfunction occurs as a result of the hypo-osmolar state in which fluid shifts between intracerebral fluid compartments.

ASSESSMENT

A history of polydipsia and polyuria should always be explored further. If the patient with diabetes insipidus is able to replenish lost fluids, few other symptoms will be noticed. There can be a severe and sudden onset of dehydration and hyperosmolar fluid imbalance if oral intake is decreased.

Most symptoms of ADH excess (Table 30-4) are non-specific. Mental status changes can occur with either hyperosmolar or hypo-osmolar fluid imbalances. The patient who is unconscious, such as after intracranial or pituitary surgery, cannot relate feelings of discomfort or thirst nor can the nurse assess mental changes. Careful documentation of patterns of fluid intake and output can help alert caregivers to fluid imbalances in these patients.

Subjective data can be obtained from the conscious patient. Data to collect include the following:
1. Fluid intake and output patterns
2. Use of pitressin: frequency and side effects
3. Presence of thirst

Objective data center around fluid and electrolyte monitoring:
1. Mental status
2. Daily weight
3. Fluid intake and output every 8 hours or more frequently if risk of imbalance is high
4. Urine osmolality, specific gravity, and sodium content
5. Serum sodium and serum osmolality
6. Blood pressure

Diagnostic tests

Primary diabetes insipidus is rare, but secondary or iatrogenic diabetes insipidus is seen fairly often. Before diabetes insipidus is conclusively diagnosed, the patient must be shown to have a deficit in ADH and the patient's kidneys must be able to respond to ADH to rule out nephropathy. (Table 30-5 lists vasopressin and other tests.)

Another diagnostic problem is the differentiation of ADH deficiency from neurogenic polydipsia (compulsive

Table 30-5. Tests of ADH function

Test	Procedure	Interpretation
Radioimmunoassay	Blood sample	Clinical findings, sodium content and osmolality of blood and urine more commonly used
Water deprivation test	Water withheld until 2%-5% of body weight is lost; collect urine and serum samples for osmolality and sodium pretest and at ordered intervals; measure intake and output every 1-2 hr, weigh every 8 hr	Normal response is an increase in osmolality and sodium content and decrease in urine volume; in diabetes insipidus, no changes occur
Vasopresor stimulation	Baseline urine osmolality obtained pretest and after administration of vasopressin	Urine osmolality rises after vasopressin; confirms renal responsiveness to vasopressin and rules out nephrogenic origin

water drinking). A water deprivation test demonstrates ADH deficiency if urine output continues with no change in urinary osmolality and sodium content when the patient is deprived of water. Close monitoring of vital signs is necessary to detect significant changes before vascular collapse occurs. In neurogenic polydipsia, the water-deprived patient will need continual emotional support to endure the test and may exhibit extreme behavioral responses.

Usually laboratory studies of electrolytes and osmolality confirm the diagnosis of SIADH. A search for an extrapituitary source of ADH hypersecretion would include x-ray films of the skull, chest, and abdomen.

DATA ANALYSIS AND PLANNING

Nursing diagnoses

Nursing diagnoses for patients with ADH hyposecretion might include the following:

Fluid deficit, potential or actual (related to insufficient fluid intake or inadequate hormonal replacement)

Knowledge deficit (hormonal replacement rationale or methods)

Nursing diagnoses for patients with ADH hypersecretion might include the following:

Fluid excess, potential or actual (if evidence indicates excessive fluid intake is contributing to hypo-osmolar state)

Potential for injury (related to mental status changes)

Expected patient outcomes

Expected patient outcomes would include demonstrated fluid and electrolyte balance (Chapter 10). Expected patient outcomes for the patient with diabetes insipidus include the following:

The patient or significant others can:
1. Describe medication regimen.
2. State plans to obtain medication card or Medic Alert bracelet or necklace.
3. Describe symptoms requiring medical consultation.
4. State plans for regular medical follow-up care.

IMPLEMENTATION

Assisting with achievement of therapeutic goals
Maintaining fluid balance

Frequent monitoring of these patients and early detection of problems assists in achieving fluid and electrolyte balance. High priority nursing actions that ensure adequate intake for patients with diabetes insipidus include the following:
1. Provide access to and assistance with oral fluid intake, if permitted.
2. Notify physician if fluid intake is inadequate.
3. Maintain ordered flow rates of intravenous infusions.

Water restriction is the key therapeutic measure for SIADH-induced hyponatremia. Fluids may be restricted to as low as 500 ml/24 hr. During changes in electrolyte levels, thirst can be discomforting to the patient. The nurse can assist the patient's comfort and adherence to fluid restriction by
1. Moistening the patient's mouth frequently by offering ice chips rather than water to allow more frequent intake
2. Offering mouth rinses to the patient
3. Planning with the patient and dietitian the most satisfactory fluid distribution

The use of hypertonic saline solution is usually reserved for patients who have severe hyponatremia, dis-

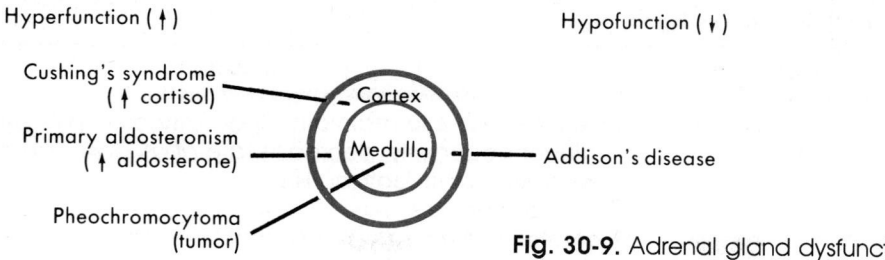

Fig. 30-9. Adrenal gland dysfunctions.

turbed sensorium, or convulsions. Appropriate safety measures are provided for the level of mental confusion.

A review of Table 30-4 indicates other medical treatments that may be necessary.

Assisting with ADH replacement

The key therapeutic measure for diabetes insipidus is the administration of *pitressin*. For immediate treatment of a crisis, vasopressin injection is used. Pitressin tannate in oil is only given intramuscularly; it is often painful and swelling may occur. It is best to warm the vial and to shake it vigorously to disperse the active ingredient.

For maintenance doses of pitressin, the patient learns to determine the dosage of sprays or drops in response to polyuria and thirst. The patient is cautioned about overdosage and its symptoms. (Table 30-4 lists the various preparations.) Overdosage of any pitressin medication results in symptoms of ADH excess

1. Weight gain
2. Edema
3. Abdominal cramping
4. Hypertension

Rhinopharyngitis may interfere with the absorption of nasal drops, sprays, or powders. For this reason, patients are taught to report this condition to the physician. Pitressin "snuff" is not frequently used now because of its irritating qualities.

Teaching the patient with ADH dysfunction

1. Knowledge of medication therapy
   a. Dosage and side effects of prescribed medication
   b. Correct use of prescribed pitressin nasal spray or drops (Chapter 24)
   c. Signs and symptoms (polyuria, polydipsia) that indicate the need to take prescribed medication
2. Need to report signs of rhinopharyngitis (runny nose and red, painful mucous membranes) to physician
3. Need to seek immediate medical follow-up if symptoms become worse or are not relieved by prescribed medications
4. Need to carry at all times an identification card or a Medic Alert bracelet or necklace indicating the nature of the disorder
5. Probable requirement for lifelong replacement therapy with diabetes insipidus
6. Need for regular medical follow-up care

EVALUATION

Evaluation is based on the expected patient outcomes. Key questions are

1. Is fluid and electrolyte balance achieved?
2. Is the patient able to maintain fluid and electrolyte balance by self-care measures?
3. Does the patient know the prescribed medication plan?

ADRENAL GLAND DYSFUNCTION

Dysfunction of the adrenal gland can be manifested as an increased or decreased function of the cortex or an increased function of the medulla (Fig. 30-9). The three major hormones of the adrenal cortex are cortisol, aldosterone, and androgens. The adrenal medulla produces epinephrine and norepinephrine (Table 30-6). The etiology, signs and symptoms, and medical therapy for adrenal gland dysfunctions are listed in Table 30-7.

PATHOPHYSIOLOGY

Hypersecretion
Cortisol excess

The most common causes of cortisol excess are bilateral hyperplasia of the adrenal gland and hypersecretion of cortisol as a result of excessive ACTH stimulation by the anterior pituitary. Approximately 25% of patients with cortical excess, however, have adrenal tumors.

The term *Cushing's disease* is used for pituitary-induced cortical excess, whereas the term *Cushing's syndrome* is used for all other causes of cortisol excess: adrenocortical tumors, ectopic tissue sources, and exogenous corticosteroid drugs (iatrogenic). Excesses of cortisol, aldosterone, and androgens are often found when there is adrenal hyperplasia from ACTH excess.

Whether the cause is pathologic or iatrogenic, excessive cortisol has widespread effects (Table 30-7). The changes in body appearance may be quite striking:

1. The *adipose deposition* is classic in its distribution to trunk, facies (moon face), and intrascapular areas.
2. *Muscle wasting* is most obvious in the extremities, which results in thin legs.
3. Pale, purplish *striae* result from thinning of skin and weakening of collagenous fibers that expose subcutaneous tissue.

Table 30-8. Comparison of antiinflammatory and mineralocorticoid potency of derivatives of adrenocorticosteroids

Drug	Antiinflammatory potency	Mineralocorticoid potency†
Hydrocortisone (Cortef)	1	0.03
Cortisone acetate (Cortone, Cortogen)	0.8	0.03
Prednisone (Deltasone, Meticorten)	4	0.04
Methylprednisolone (Medrol)	6	0.02
Triamcinolone (Aristocort, Kenacort)	5	None
Dexamethasone (Decadron)	30	None
Desoxycorticosterone (DOCA)	None	1
Fludrocortisone (Florinef)	10	4.2

*Potency relative to hydrocortisone, whose potency = 1.
†Potency relative to DOCA, whose potency = 1.

tivity (Table 30-8). The metabolic side effects of glucocorticoids do limit the dosage employed over time; however, these side effects are often necessary if adequate treatment is achieved. The side effects are medically managed when it is necessary to continue the corticosteroids.

Beside the problems caused by corticosteroid therapy (cortisol excess), the patient is also at risk for an episode of *adrenocortical insufficiency* (cortisol deficit) should the medication be stopped suddenly or should severe stress occur.

Aldosterone excess

The etiology, symptoms, and medical therapy of aldosterone excess are listed in Table 30-7. Three major effects of aldosterone excess are *hypertension, hypokalemia,* and *hypernatremia.* Hypertension results from the increased blood volume as a result of sodium reabsorption. As the sodium is retained, potassium is excreted and results in hypokalemia. Severe muscle weakness and electrocardiogram (ECG) abnormalities reflect potassium depletion.

With adrenal hyperplasia from ACTH excess (Cushing's disease), hypersecretion may be combined with metabolic alkalosis and with cortisol excess. When the cause of the aldosterone excess is an aldosterone-secreting adrenal adenoma, the resultant primary aldosteronism is not associated with other hormonal excesses. If untreated, cardiovascular disease and renal insufficiency occur.

Androgen excess

Frequently, excess adrenal androgen secretion occurs simultaneously with excess cortisol secretion. In females, this results in changes in sexual characteristics: a deepening of the voice, baldness, dark and coarse hair growth, and clitorial enlargement.

Although a small amount of estrogen is secreted by the adrenal gland, estrogen excess from this source is not significant. Bilateral adrenalectomy may be done to eliminate this hormone in the treatment of estrogen-sensitive tumors, such as certain breast tumors.

Catecholamine excess

Catecholamines secreted by the adrenal medulla are not essential for life because the sympathetic nervous system also produces these hormones. The functions of epinephrine and norepinephrine are listed in Table 30-6.

Although rare, the most common cause of excess catecholamines in adults is *pheochromocytoma,* a catecholamine-producing tumor of the adrenal medulla (Table 30-7). Similar tumors are sometimes found in the abdomen around the adrenal medulla or anywhere along the sympathetic nervous system trunk.

The prominent sign of catecholamine excess is hypertension, which may be labile, depending on blood levels of the catecholamines, or the blood pressure may stay persistently elevated. Most patients have an elevated blood pressure reading at least 50% of the time.[51] Headache is abrupt, severe, throbbing, and generalized; it usually has a short duration. If hypertension is long standing, the patient may have hypertensive retinopathy.

Frequently there is a history of paroxysmal attacks that are precipitated by multiple factors. Postural changes (especially flexion or bending of the body), sneezing, abdominal pressure, sexual activity, eating, urination, Valsalva maneuvers, exercise, pain, and changes in environmental or body temperature are some of the major precipitating factors.

In pheochromocytoma, the levels of catecholamines and their metabolites in the urine are increased.

Hyposecretion

The adrenal cortex is essential to life. Without its hormones, cortisol and aldosterone, the body's metabolic processes would respond inadequately to even minimal physical and emotional stressors, such as changes in temperature, exercise, or excitement. Severe stressors, such as those caused by serious infections or extreme anxiety, could result in shock and death.

Adrenocortical insufficiency

The inability to secrete glucocorticoids, mineralocorticoids, and androgens may occur as a result of atrophy, disease, or destruction of the adrenal gland. Conversely, when there is hypoplasia secondary to decreased ACTH secretion, usually only cortisol secretion is decreased. This occurs because ACTH has minimal influence on aldosterone secretion, which is under control of the renin-angiotensin system. ACTH has no direct influence on androgens. Androgen deficit has few symptoms.

A review of Table 30-6 will explain many of the signs and symptoms that occur with the lack of cortisol because of changes in protein, carbohydrate, and fat metabolism.

Gastrointestinal symptoms are often the reason that the person initially seeks help. Symptoms of adrenocortical insufficiency most often have a gradual onset and are vague. Asthenia (weakness) is a cardinal complaint, the intensity of which is out of proportion to other overt symptoms. It is usually more severe at times of stress and eventually may require the patient to stay in bed.

Hyperpigmentation with bronzelike coloration of skin and mucous membranes is a common sign in primary adrenal insufficiency. This is caused by increased levels of melanocyte-stimulating hormone (MSH) in the anterior pituitary. In normal persons, cortisol causes negative feedback inhibition of the anterior pituitary. This lack of cortisol in adrenal insufficiency allows the MSH level to increase. Persons with secondary insufficiency do not usually have hyperpigmentation because their levels of ACTH and MSH are low.

Iatrogenic adrenocortical insufficiency results from adrenal atrophy induced by corticosteroid therapy. An elevation in serum cortisol levels inhibits the secretion of ACTH, and thus the stimulation of the adrenal cortex cells is decreased. An abrupt cessation of corticosteroid therapy produces this serious side effect. To prevent adrenocortical insufficiency, corticosteroid drug dosages are gradually tapered down so the adrenal gland can hypertrophy gradually in response to higher ACTH levels. The ACTH increases as a result of the decreased cortisone levels. An alternative method is to administer ACTH before the withdrawal of glucocorticoid therapy.

Hypotension, hyponatremia, and hyperkalemia are characteristically seen in patients with primary adrenocortical insufficiency because of a lack of mineralocorticoids. These patients are subject to changes in cardiovascular status because of fluid and electrolyte alterations. A low circulating blood volume and a decreased heart size develop. ECG changes may occur with hyperkalemia.

ADDISONIAN CRISIS (ADRENAL CRISIS). Adrenal crisis is a severe and sudden exacerbation of adrenal insufficiency. It can quickly lead to death unless it is treated promptly.

Adrenal crisis can be precipitated by the following situations:

1. Stress conditions that require more adrenocortical hormones than are available
2. Sudden cessation of corticosteroid therapy
3. Surgery, trauma, or disease of the adrenal or pituitary gland

ASSESSMENT

Subjective data

Common considerations in assessing patients with pituitary dysfunction (p. 800) are also pertinent for adrenal dysfunction because of the effect of the anterior pituitary on the adrenal glands. The nurse can gain insight into patient needs by means of the following data:

1. Extent of fatigue
2. Patient's perception of body image changes
3. Mood changes
4. Ability to tolerate stress
5. Need for assistance with activities of daily living
6. Sleep patterns
7. Eating patterns
8. Knowledge of the adrenal dysfunction and its treatment
9. Medication regimen
10. Presence of discomforting symptoms

Objective data

Ongoing patient assessment should include the following:

1. Daily weight
2. Temperature and blood pressure every 4 hours
3. Intake and output every 4 hours
4. Skin integrity
5. Activity level
6. Food intake
7. Early signs of infection

For the patient with cortisol excess, the nurse should expect to monitor blood glucose levels and glucose and ketone levels in the urine. Patients with adrenal dysfunction are often very ill. A thorough physical examination can detect abnormalities that require attention.

Diagnostic tests

Diagnosis in adrenocortical dysfunction relies heavily on measurements of serum and urinary levels of hormones and metabolities (Table 30-9). There is usually no special preparation needed for tests of blood hormonal values unless provocative agents are used to test response of the adrenal gland to a stimulant or depressant. Provocative agents could be drugs, diet, or any stimulus that elicits a known response. For example, an upright position or sodium loading could test aldosterone secretion. When such tests are performed, special care must be taken to clarify any questions and avoid the need to reschedule that test. For example, the cortisone suppres-

---

Symptoms of adrenal crisis

Hypotension
Shock
Coma
Hyperpyrexia

Table 30-9. Comparison of laboratory findings in hyposecretion and hypersecretion of adrenal gland

Substance	Hyposecretion	Hypersecretion
Adrenal cortex		
Plasma levels		
Cortisol	Low in all cases of adrenal cortex insufficiency	High in all cases of adrenal cortex hypersecretion
Aldosterone	Low in primary adrenal insufficiency	High in adrenal hyperplasia or aldosterone-secreting tumors
Androgen	Low in primary adrenal insufficiency	High in adrenal hyperplasia or androgen-secreting tumors
ACTH	Low in pituitary hyposecretion of ACTH	High in pituitary hypersecretion of ACTH
	High in primary adrenal deficiency resulting from lack of feedback inhibition by cortisol	Low in primary adrenal hypersecretion because of inhibition of cortisol
MCH	High in primary adrenal insufficiency resulting from lack of feedback inhibition by cortisol	Normal
Electrolytes/solutes		
Sodium	≤130 mEq/L	Normal or 154 mEq/L
Potassium	≥5 mEq/L	3.5 mEq/L
Sodium/potassium ratio	30:1	Normal
Glucose	50 mg/dl	120 mg/dl
BUN	20 mg/dl	
Urinary excretion of cortisol metabolites	All are low in primary adrenocortical hyposecretion	All are high in primary adrenocortical hypersecretion
17-Ketogenic glucocorticoids (17-KGS) 5 to 23 mg/24 hr (m) 5 to 18 mg/24 hr (f)		
17-Hydroxycorticosteroids (17-OHCS) 3-10 mg/24 hr		
17-Ketosteroids (17-KS) (androgens) 5 to 18 mg/24 hr	17-KS may be normal with pituitary lack of ACTH	17-KS may be high in androgen-secreting tumors or enzymatic deficiency
Aldosterone and 18-glucoronide 16 mg/24 hr		Aldosterone elevated in hyperaldosteronism
Adrenal medulla		
Plasma levels		
Epinephrine		All are increased in pheochromocytoma
Norepinephrine		
Total catecholamines		
Urinary excretion		
Total catecholamines		All are increased in pheochromocytoma
Epinephrine		
Norepinephrine		VMA is end product of catecholamine metabolism
Metanephrine		Metanephrine is a urinary metabolite of epinephrine
Vanillylmandelic acid (VMA)		

Table 30-10. Tests of adrenocortical function

Function test	Procedure and preparation	Interpretation
ACTH stimulation test (various tests available)	Synthetic ACTH given in 500-1000 ml of normal saline at 2 units/24 hr; then 17-OHCS and plasma cortisol levels are measured; alternative way is to infuse 25 units of ACTH over an 8 hr period on 2-3 days and measure 17-OHCS and plasma cortisol levels on these days	Normally 17-OHCS excretion increases to 25 mg/24 hr and plasma cortisol increases to 40 μg/100 ml or greater; in patients with secondary adrenal insufficiency, the 17-OHCS rate is 3-20 mg/24 hr and the cortisol level is 10-40 μg/dl
Screening ACTH stimulation test	ACTH, 25 units, is given IM and plasma cortisol level is measured before and 30 and 60 min after tests	Normally plasma cortisol increases 7 μg/dl
Cortisol suppression test	Twenty-four-hour urine specimen for 17-OCHS is collected for baseline; dexamethasone, 0.5 mg, is given every 6 hr for 2 days; 24 hr urine is collected for these 2 days	Dexamethasone suppresses pituitary secretion of ACTH but does not change steroid excretion; normally by second day of desamethasone, 24-hr urinary level of OHCS should drop more than 50% below baseline, patients with adrenocortical excess (primary) will show decrease in 24 hr urine levels; patients with secondary adrenocortical excess will have drop, but less than 50%
Screening suppression test	Dexamethasone 1 mg, given at 12 PM, at 8 AM cortisol level is drawn	Normally cortisol should be less than 5 μg/dl
Mineralocorticoid suppression test (various tests are available)	IV infusion of saline 500 ml/hr for 4 hr Alternative: patient placed on normal sodium diet (100 mEq) or high sodium diet (200 mEq), after patient is in sodium balance, DOCA (10 mg every 12 hr) administered IM for 3-5 days	Normally saline infusion depresses plasma aldosterone to < 8 μg/dl if patient has been on a sodium-restricted diet and to < 5 μg/dl if the patient has been on a normal sodium diet Normal persons on a sodium diet of mEq/day will have a 70% decrease in aldosterone

sion test has a sequence of 5 days' testing. Failure to collect the 24-hour urine on the fourth or fifth day can result in a diagnostic delay of several days at a significant cost to the patient. Tests of adrenocortical function are described in Table 30-10.

Special care must be taken if provocative agents are used to test catecholamine secretion in suspected pheochromocytoma; histamine, which depletes catecholamines, may precipitate a hypertensive crisis. Regitine, an adrenergic-blocking agent, may induce severe hypotension. These agents are used infrequently today.

When urinary hormones and metabolites are to be measured, timed specimens are collected. Important nursing actions include the following:

1. Start and stop the urine collection at the specified times; this is necessary if the pattern of diurnal secretion is to be analyzed correctly.

2. Obtain the specimen container and preservative required by the hospital laboratory; icing the specimen may be necessary.

3. Instruct the patient and involved staff in the procedure recommended by the laboratory.

4. Ensure that all urine voided in the time period is collected.
   a. Just before starting the collection, the patient should void and that urine be discarded.
   b. The last urine collected should be of a voiding at the time the collection ends.

Additional tests that the physician may order include

1. Glucose tolerance test
2. Renal function tests (Chapter 33)
3. Roentgenograms of kidney or abdomen
4. Adrenal arteriograms

DATA ANALYSIS AND PLANNING

Multiple nursing diagnoses might be determined in patients with adrenal gland dysfunction because of the widespread effects of adrenal hormonal imbalance. The most probable nursing diagnoses are the same as those for patients with pituitary dysfunction (p. 802).

It is important that there be mutual planning with patients about care needs. The responses to body image changes, the potential of emotional lability, and the fatigue experienced by patients may overwhelm their ability to cope effectively with hospitalization.

Expected patient outcomes

1. Patients with *adrenocortical excess* can
   a. Describe dietary and fluid restrictions.
   b. Explain ways to avoid infections and describe what to do if infections occur.
   c. Describe any therapeutic regimens prescribed for hypertension or diabetes mellitus, if appropriate.
   d. Explain reasons to seek medical attention.
   e. State need at all times to carry identification stating name of drug, dosage frequency, and physician's name and phone number.
2. Patients with *adrenocortical insufficiency* can
   a. State why medications must be taken daily as prescribed.
   b. Explain the effects of stress on the need for medication.
   c. Identify stressors in own life and ways to control them.
   d. State awareness of the need for additional medication in times of severe stress.
   e. State need at all times to carry identification stating name of drug, dosage frequency, and physician's name and phone number.
   f. State plans for regular follow-up care.

IMPLEMENTATION

Supporting patients with adrenal dysfunction

Certain nursing measures are appropriate regardless of the type of adrenal dysfunction. The *maintenance* of medication regimens is a high priority. Other primary approaches include the following:

1. Provision of adequate rest
2. Regulation of blood pressure within desired limits
3. Maintenance of fluid and electrolyte balance
4. Maintenance of adequate nutrition to maintain or achieve desired weight and to keep blood glucose levels within normal limits
5. Provision of an environment that is as restful and as anxiety free as possible

The patient needs considerable support to deal with the changes in body image and the resulting changes in self-concept. Some of the body changes are reversible with successful treatment. Patients should be encouraged to accentuate the positive physical attributes, and as they recover, patients should be helped to see their self-worth. Emotional lability and the inability to handle emotional stressors should be anticipated. Stressors should be decreased as much as possible. A consistent routine should also be maintained.

Education of the patient and significant others is a major need. The patient needs to learn about the diagnostic tests, the treatment planned, and the potential complications of treatment.

The patient with Cushing's syndrome

It can be seen in Table 30-11 that patients with Cushing's syndrome may need assistance with the following:

1. Calorie and sodium restrictions
2. Potassium supplements
3. Diuretics and other antihypertensive agents
4. Protection against infection
5. Avoidance of stress
6. Safety measures to prevent pathologic fractures or bruising
7. Control of hyperglycemia

Persons with Cushing's syndrome are at particular risk of nonsocomial infection because of their immunosuppressed state. Immunosuppression combined with metabolic imbalance and obesity impairs wound healing. Careful use of handwashing and aseptic technique are essential. Patients must not be exposed to infections, and they should be isolated from other patients with infections. Staff members who have *any* signs or symptoms of infections should not care for these patients.

Women with facial hair (hirsutism) may prefer to keep depilatories or shaving equipment unobtrusively available. If the woman has a masculine appearance, the nurse can tactfully clear up misconceptions of others (for example, roommates) about the gender identity.

Table 30-11. Comparison of clinical problems of Cushing's syndrome and Addison's disease

Category	Cushing's syndrome	Addison's disease
Blood pressure	Hypertension	Hypotension
Blood sugar	Hyperglycemia	Hypoglycemia
Blood volume	Hypervolemia	Hypovolemia
Potassium balance	Hypokalemia	Hyperkalemia
Special features	Immunosuppression	Intolerance to stress
	Osteoporosis	

The patient with Addison's disease

Nursing activities for patients with adrenocortical insufficiency include the following:

1. Administering and teaching hormonal replacement
2. Ensuring frequent and adequate food intake with normal to increased protein content
3. Ensuring normal (or increased) sodium and fluid intake
4. Treatment of hypoglycemia
5. Avoidance of stress
6. Frequent rest periods

The patient with pheochromocytoma

The primary treatment of pheochromocytoma is surgical removal of the tumor. The priority in preoperative care is control of activities related to hypertensive crisis. During the hypertensive crisis phase, the patient should be in an intensive care unit. Cardiac monitoring and frequent monitoring of vital signs are necessary. During nitroprusside or phentolamine therapy, the blood pressure is taken every 15 minutes. These drugs are given by a controlled infusion pump at a rate that keeps the blood pressure at a prescribed level. When the blood pressure is at the desired level, the drugs will be gradually decreased. The blood pressure is closely monitored during this time.

Hypotension occurs as soon as the tumor is removed. This is usually treated with plasma or a plasma substitute. Volume expanders administered appropriately usually control the hypotension, and vasopressors are not necessary.[51]

On the first postoperative day, hypertensive episodes are common and are caused by the response to pain and the hypervolemia resulting from the treatment of hypotension following surgery. At this time the most effective therapy is a rapidly acting diuretic such as furosemide (Lasix) or ethacrynic acid (Edecrin).

The patient with primary aldosteronism

Successful surgical excision of tumors or resection of hyperplastic glands reverses the hypertension in about two thirds of the patients. In preparation for surgery, spironolactone, an aldosterone antagonist, is given daily. Supportive nursing activities include the following:

1. Monitoring blood pressure, daily weight, vital signs, and intake and output
2. Administering and observing effect of spironolactone
3. Sodium restriction
4. Preoperative preparation

Adrenal surgery

Adrenal surgery is often combined with suppressant drug therapy. Also, because of the known incidence of pituitary tumor developing after bilateral adrenalectomy, pituitary irradiation may follow this surgery.

After bilateral adrenalectomy, the patient has increased ACTH levels, and there is a life-threatening absence of glucocorticoids and mineralocorticoids. Immediate and lifelong replacement of these hormones is absolutely necessary for life. Bilateral adrenalectomy is most commonly used for treatment of pituitary-induced adrenal hyperplasia. In some instances, when the site of ectopic ACTH is not found or cannot be resected, a bilateral adrenalectomy will be used to reduce the cortisol levels.

Preoperative hormonal administration

In some instances during the preoperative period and during surgery, the physician will use drugs that suppress excessive secretion of the particular hormone. Of special concern during anesthesia and surgery is the patient with catecholamine excess and whose tumor may secrete bursts of hormone during manipulation. Conversely, patients with Cushing's syndrome may have intravenous infusions of hydrocortisone begun preoperatively (if suppressant drugs were used) and during surgery to prevent the sudden cortisol deficit that occurs with removal of adrenal tissue.

If antihypertensive drugs are being used preoperatively, they are discontinued before surgery, since the surgery may cause a rather severe drop in blood pressure. Sedation may be given at this time.

Postoperative care

Nursing care for patients undergoing adrenal surgery is administered with the understanding that

1. There is a sudden inability to secrete glucocorticoids and mineralocorticoids. Adrenal crisis is a major risk as evidenced by:
   a. Hypotension
   b. Cardiovascular collapse
   c. Hypoglycemia
   d. Hyperpyrexia
2. There is instability of the cardiovascular system.
3. Preoperative hormonal excess may have resulted in cardiovascular and renal dysfunction.

CARE DURING ADRENAL CRISIS. Early detection and reporting of the signs of adrenal crisis ensure more adequate treatment. The immediate care in adrenal crisis includes the following:

1. Administering prescribed high doses of hydrocortisone intravenously or with intravenous glucose, often combined with cortisone given intramuscularly.
2. Administering intravenous infusion of normal saline solution.
3. Maintaining absolute inactivity for the patient; all movement is done for the patient.
4. Eliminating all stimuli such as loud noises and bright lights.
5. Monitoring vital signs every 15 minutes and temperature every hour.
6. Maintaining intravenous lines for infusion of whole blood or albumin and vasopressor drugs as needed for severe hypotension.
7. Providing ice bag for headache.
8. Assisting with other therapy as indicated (for example, antimicrobial therapy for infection or intravenous glucose for hypoglycemia).

9. Protecting patient from infection; reverse isolation may be used.

HORMONAL CONTROL AND MONITORING. Immediately after surgery, replacement of corticosteroids is started. Hydrocortisone is given by intravenous drip, and the dosage is adjusted at intervals according to changes in blood pressure, electrolyte balance, and blood glucose level. The patient needs to be given constant nursing attention until hormonal stability is regained or a maintenance regimen established. Vasopressors may need to be given. Frequent blood pressure readings will be necessary to determine medication dosage needs.

The patient is also observed carefully for signs of hypoglycemia. This condition is most likely to occur if the patient had diabetes mellitus as a symptom, but it can occur in any patient who has adrenal gland surgery. Intravenous solutions containing glucose are usually ordered. If the patient is able to eat, the nurse should check to see that all food on the tray is eaten. Hypoglycemic reactions are most likely to occur in the early morning, and they may follow any unusual physical activity or emotional upset;.

ASSISTING WITH AMBULATION. The patient with adrenal surgery requires assistance when first ambulating, since hypotension may occur. Measures to minimize hypotension include the following:
1. Using Ace bandages or elastic stockings.
2. Monitoring blood pressure in lying, sitting, and standing positions; a drop of 10 mm Hg in diastolic pressure is considered significant.
3. Accompanying the patient when ambulating.
4. Checking blood pressure every 15 minutes when patient is first ambulating.
5. Accompanying the patient back to bed if the blood pressure drops.

Teaching hormonal replacement after surgery

When there is a cortisol-producing tumor of one of the adrenal glands, the increase in corticosteroids produced by that tumor will cause suppression of ACTH (by negative feedback) and subsequent atrophy of the nontumorous adrenal tissue. When resection of the tumor or a unilateral adrenalectomy is performed, replacement cortisol is given until adrenal hypertrophy and thus secretion of cortisol by remaining tissue is adequate. Following bilateral adrenalectomy lifelong hormonal replacement is required.

Lifelong hormonal replacement

Tapering cortisone to maintenance doses of glucocorticoids may take 1 to 3 weeks. Doses are planned individually for the patient day by day. Mineralocorticoids are not usually needed until cortisone levels are below 50 mg/24 hr. (Cortisone and hydrocortisone have sodium retention effects.)

Usual maintenance dosages for the patient with bilateral adrenalectomy are cortisone 37.5 mg/24 hr with 25 mg given at 8 AM and 12.5 mg at 4 PM. Administration at a later hour may interfere with the patient's sleep. Mineralocorticoids will also be required for survival.

Teaching the patient about adrenocortical insufficiency and the importance of hormonal replacement was discussed previously for the hypophysectomy patient (p. 804). It is not unheard of for patients to be admitted to the hospital in adrenal crisis because they did not understand the need to take their medication as ordered

EVALUATION

Evaluation will be based on the expected patient outcomes. Some questions to consider include the following:
1. Were patient and family assisted to use resources to cope satisfactorily with hospitalization?
2. Were complications minimized and crises detected and treated promptly?
3. Were the following outcomes achieved:
   a. Blood pressure regulation?
   b. Blood glucose regulation?
   c. Weight at desired level?
   d. Fluid and electrolyte balance?
4. Is patient able to manage self-care regimens?
5. Is patient aware of need for hormonal replacement?

PARATHYROID DYSFUNCTION

Parathyroid hormone (PTH) is primarily involved with maintenance of calcium and phosphorus levels by the following:
1. Increasing bone resorption
2. Increasing calcium absorption from gastrointestinal tract (needs vitamin D)
3. Decreasing urinary excretion of calcium
4. Increasing urinary excretion of phosphorus.

The management of hypocalcemia and hypercalcemia is discussed in Chapter 10.

PATHOPHYSIOLOGY

Parathyroid hormone (PTH) excess

Primary hyperparathyroidism (Table 30-12) results from increased secretion of PTH, usually by a parathyroid adenoma. Normally, a low serum calcium level stimulates secretion of PTH, whereas a high serum level inhibits its secretion. In primary hyperparathyroidism, PTH does not become suppressed with the elevated serum calcium level (dysfunctional negative feedback system), thus leading to hypercalcemia.

Secondary hyperparathyroidism develops from chronic hypocalcemic states, such as renal failure. Hyperplasia of the parathyroid glands develops with an increase in PTH. In some of these patients, the parathyroid glands become autonomous and lose their responsiveness to serum calcium levels (tertiary hyperparathyroidism).

Hyperparathyroidism results in *hypercalcemia* and *hypophosphatemia*. There is increased urinary excretion of both calcium and phosphorus with the following effects:
1. Inability of the kidney to concentrate urine
2. Polyuria
3. Increased risk of renal calculi with subsequent urinary obstruction or infection

Table 30-12. Parathyroid dysfunction

Etiology	Signs and symptoms	Medical therapy

PTH hormone excess
Primary
  Adenoma, carcinoma,
    idiopathic hyperplasia
Secondary
  Renal failure, rickets, PTH-
    resistant nephropathy,
    vitamin D intoxication
Ectopic
  PTH-like secreting tumor
	Hypercalcemia and hypophos-
	  phatemia:
	Anorexia, nausea, vomiting,
	  fatigue, depression, polyuria,
	  polydipsia, dehydration;
	  bone pain, muscle hypo-
	  tonia and hyporeflexia; con-
	  stipation
		Hydration, normal saline
		  infusion
		Furosemide (Lasix)
		Phosphate infusion or oral salts
		Calcitonin
		Mithramycin
		Dialysis
		Surgical excision or tumor or
		  parathyroidectomy

PTH hormone deficiency
Excision of glands, autoim-
  mune disease, idio-
  pathic
	Hypocalcemia:
	  Paresthesia, Chvostek's sign,
	  Trousseau's sign, carpopedal
	  spasm, marked anxiety, sei-
	  zures, laryngeal stridor, dys-
	  pnea, cyanosis, arrhythmias
	Hyperphosphatemia:
	  Soft tissue calcifications; nau-
	  sea, vomiting, abdominal
	  pain; Dry scaling skin, brittle
	  nails; patchy, thin hair
		Calcium salts: give with food
		  but not with diary products;
		  calcium gluconate, calcium
		  chloride
		Vitamin D supplements: Hytak-
		  erol, calciferol
		Dietary calcium and vitamin D
		Antacids (phosphate-binders)

4. Calcification of renal tubules

Calcium is lost from bone leading to demineralization of the bone, pathologic fractures, or cystic bone disease causing bone pain.

Most of the symptoms are a result of the hypercalcemia. Nausea, vomiting, and anorexia lead to weight loss and fatigue. The effect of increased calcium on the muscles leads to hypotonicity of skeletal muscles, tendon reflexes, and gastrointestinal muscles. Muscle weakness and fatigue are thus common findings. Mental changes may vary from confusion to depression or psychosis. Relatively small elevations of calcium may cause major mental changes, especially in elderly persons.

When the serum calcium level rises above 16 to 18 mg/dl, acute hypercalcemic crisis occurs. Severe intractable vomiting leads to dehydration and electrolyte imbalances. Fever, severe mental changes, or coma may result, ending in death if untreated.

Parathyroid hormone lack

The most common cause of hypoparathyroidism is the surgical removal of the parathyroid glands or an interference with the blood supply. With a diminished level of parathyroid hormone, there is increased bone resorption and the serum calcium level falls. Since parathyroid hormone is involved in the renal clearance of phosphate, serum phosphate levels increase. The decreased level of serum calcium results in neuromuscular irritability.

Acute hypocalcemia (tetany) is life-threatening, and

Signs of latent tetany

Paresthesia in fingertips and around mouth
Chvostek's sign (facial contraction on tapping facial nerve near jaw angle)
Trousseau's sign (carpal spasm after compression of upper arm with a cuff)
Carpopedal spasm (spasm of wrist and fingers and/or feet and toes)

---

the signs of latent tetany should always be promptly reported to the physician (Chapter 10).

It is important for the nurse to recognize that the clinical findings of hypocalcemia are more reliable than the serum total calcium level, which measures (1) the ionized (unbound) blood calcium, which is the active metabolic calcium, and (2) the nonionized (bound) calcium, which does not affect neuroactivity. Symptoms of hypocalcemia can progress to laryngospasm, bronchospasm, cardiac arrhythmia, and seizures. Changes in electroencephalographic (EEG) patterns may be present, and a prolonged Q-T interval is frequently seen on the cardiac monitor.

In chronic hypocalcemic states, some patients will develop calcifications of tissues (neurologic, visceral, and soft tissues).

ASSESSMENT

The signs and symptoms of calcium excess and deficit are priority observations when patients are treated for parathyroid dysfunction.

The following subjective data are obtained from the patient:

1. Presence of discomfort (bone pain), fatigue, or paresthesia
2. Elimination patterns (constipation, polyuria)
3. Medication usage
4. Dietary history
5. Knowledge of condition

Objective data include the following:

1. Mental status (signs of behavior changes)
2. Intake and output every 8 hours
3. Weight everyday
4. Muscle weakness
5. Electrolyte levels (calcium, phosphorus)
6. Condition of skin, hair, and nails

Diagnostic testing

Since the maintenance of normal calcium and phosphorus metabolism involves multiple systems besides the parathyroid (skeletal, gastrointestinal, and urinary), when parathyroid function is being assessed, the patient will also have diagnostic tests of these other systems. This is necessary to determine whether the problem with calcium and phosphorus metabolism is caused by parathyroid metabolism or other disease states. In addition, ECG, EEG, and sometimes nerve conduction studies may be done to detect hypotonicity or neuromuscular irritability.

Tests of parathyroid function are shown in Table 30-13.

DATA ANALYSIS AND PLANNING

Nursing diagnoses

Nursing diagnoses that might be determined for the patient with parathyroid dysfunction include the following:

Table 30-13. Diagnostic tests for parathyroid function

Test	Procedure	Interpretation
Serum		
Total calcium 4.8-5.2 mEq/L 9.6-10.4 mg/100 ml	Blood sample No preparation	Measures both bound and ionized calcium; increased in primary hyperparthyroidism; decreased in hypoparathyroidism
Phosphorus 1.3-1.75 mEq/L	Blood sample	Decreased with hypercalcemia and elevated in hypocalcemia and in renal failure
Alkaline phosphatase 2-5 Bodansky units	Blood sample	Increased in states of demineralization, liver disease, and by certain drugs
Parathyroid hormone (PTH) by radioimmunoassay	Blood sample	Elevated in hyperparathyroidism and decreased in hypoparathyroidism
Urine		
Calcium	Collect single specimen	Decreased in hypoparathyroidism
Quantitative	24-hr collection	Elevated in hyperparathyroidism
Phosphorus	24-hr collection	Elevated in renal failure, hypocalcemic states, and PTH excess; decreased with PTH lack
Function tests		
Ellsworth-Howard excretion test (PTH infusion test)	Fasting required; 200 units of PTH extract administered IV; hourly urine collections	Normal response is 5-6 times increased urinary phosphate excretion; an increase of 10 times is found in hypoparathyroidism
Phosphate tubular reabsorption test (TRP)	Blood sample for serum calcium and phosphate; four 24-hr urine collections	Normally 85-90% of phosphate is reasborbed by renal tubules; less than 85% indicates hyperparathyroidism
Response of serum calcium to calcium infusion, cortisone, phosphate deprivation	Baseline TRP test; provocative agent given; remeasure of TRP test	Used in differential diagnosis

Anxiety

Breathing pattern, ineffectual

Bowel elimination, alteration in: constipation

Comfort, alteration in: pain in bone

Injury, potential for

Knowledge deficit

Nutrition, alteration in: less or more than body requirements (vitamin D, calcium)

Urinary elimination, alteration in patterns

Expected patient outcomes

The patient with *hyperparathyroidism* can

1. List signs and symptoms of calcium imbalance.
2. Describe symptoms requiring medical follow-up.
3. Explain planned medication regimen, if appropriate.
4. Describe plans for follow-up care.

The patient with *hypoparathyroidism* can

1. Explain the prescribed drug therapy (calcium, vitamin D).
2. State reasons for lifelong calcium and vitamin D therapy, if total parathyroid function is lost.
3. Plan a diet high in vitamin D.
4. Describe symptoms of tetany or hypercalcemia that require immediate attention.
5. State plans for ongoing follow-up care.

IMPLEMENTATION

Assisting with achievement of therapeutic goals
Correction of hyperparathyroidism

Before definitive therapy for hyperparathyroidism is undertaken, the altered electrolyte levels must be normalized. This involves hydration followed by a potent diuretic, such as furosemide (Lasix), for the excretion of several grams of calcium per day. This therapy can only be used in patients with adequate renal function. Intake and output must be monitored closely in all patients receiving this treatment. Oral phosphate (salts or liquid) may be ordered, as well as a low calcium–high phosphate diet.

Calcitonin salmon (Calcimar) may be given in acute hypercalcemia. It has a rapid action and causes an abrupt inhibition of bone resorption. Sensitivity skin testing may be performed with 1 MRC unit applied to the forearm. A rapid fall in serum calcium level may occur following injection.

When serum calcium laboratory results are assessed, the serum protein level must also be assessed. If patients have decreased serum protein content (hypoalbuminemia), less calcium is bound, more is ionized, and thus patients may exhibit signs of hypercalcemia more readily.

The patient with hyperparathyroidism may exhibit other problems related to hypercalcemia. Nursing care includes

1. Monitoring for signs of renal calculi (Chapter 33)
2. Preventing fecal impaction by careful attention to elimination patterns and use of dietary fiber, fluids, and activity, and use of stool softeners, laxatives, or enemas as required

3. Providing symptomatic relief and adminstering prescribed agents for bone pain or gastrointestinal distress
4. Preparing patients for treatments and surgery to decrease anxiety
5. Providing rest periods to minimize fatigue

PARATHYROID SURGERY. Partial parathyroidectomy is usually the treatment of choice in primary hyperparathyroidism. The usual surgery involves removing three glands totally and part of the fourth gland. An alternative approach involves removing all four glands and implanting some of the removed tissue into the muscle of the forearm. Implantation avoids vascular failure and death of residual parathyroid tissue left in the neck.[24] If no glandular abnormality is found at the time of surgery, extensive exploration of the neck and surrounding areas for additional glands that could be the source of the symptoms is necessary.

The serum calcium level will decrease within 24 hours after successful surgery. The patient must be monitored carefully for signs of tetany. Parathyroid function usually returns to normal in 5 to 7 days. By this time the remaining parathyroid tissue resumes normal secretion. If mild hypocalcemia occurs, oral calcium is given. If hypocalcemia is severe, calcium gluconate or calcium chloride at a concentration of 1 mg/ml in 5% dextrose will be given intravenously. Calcium replacement will be continued until serum calcium level is returned to normal, usually within a few days. If signs and symptoms of hypocalcemia continue to be present, calcium and/or vitamin D replacement therapy in the same amount as that used to treat hypoparathyroidism will be necessary. While patients are on replacement therapy, they must be monitored carefully for signs and symptoms of hypercalcemia.

If total parathyroidectomy is performed, hypoparathyroidism will develop, and the patient will need the same treatement as any other patient with hypoparathyroidism.

Care of the patient with tetany

When the patient has a known risk of tetany, nursing interventions include the following:

1. Frequent assessment of signs of latent tetany (p. 817)
2. Prompt reporting to physician of any signs of hypocalcemia
3. Maintenance of emergency equipment (tracheostomy set and intravenous calcium) at bedside
4. Administering ordered calcium and vitamin D replacement with antacids to patient with hyperphosphatemia
5. Maintaining a quiet, nonstressful environment

The symptoms of hypoparathyroidism are more severe in patients with alkalosis because alkalosis causes more of the dissolved calcium to bind to serum albumin. If more calcium is bound, less is ionized, and hypocalcemic symptoms occur more readily. Attention to acid-base balance would include the prevention and treatment of causes of alkalosis: hypokalemia and respiratory alkalosis (hyperventilation). Caution should be used with agents that promote alkalosis, such as certain drugs and gastrointestinal intubation.

Providing a nonstressful environment for this patient is a major nursing responsibility. Actions might include the following:

1. Controlled visitation
2. Discussion with family members to avoid disturbing discussions
3. Explanations of treatments geared to patient's level and concerns
4. Frequent contacts by nursing staff

If tetany develops, the nurse assists as needed in emergency treatment of airway obstruction, cardiac arrhythmia, and seizures. Interventions for these conditions are discussed elsewhere in the text.

Teaching

Vitamin D appears to be the principal regulator of the level of calcium ions in the body and therefore increases the absorption of calcium. A diet high in vitamin D will need to be followed by the person with hypoparathyroidism. The amount of calcium and vitamin D is gradually adjusted until serum calcium level is normal. During re-

duction, recognition of early symptoms of hypoparathyroidism, such as numbness or tingling of fingers or toes, is important so that adjustment in dosage can be instituted. Hypercalcemia is a continuous hazard during therapy, and serum and urinary calcium levels are evaluated at regular intervals (every 6 to 12 months).

Teaching whould include the following:

1. Relationship of symptoms of hypocalcemia/hypercalcemia to
   a. Disease
   b. Medication usage
   c. Complications
2. Importance of medical care at prescribed intervals and when untoward signs develop
3. Importance of informing health care providers of the health problem
4. Consistent dietary inclusion of vitamin D and calcium-rich foods (excepting dairy foods that are high in phosphates)
5. Awareness that dietary intake alone is insufficient to maintaim calcium levels in the absence of PTH
6. Need of lifelong management of calcium balance by replacement planned on results of serum calcium levels

Table 30-14. Thyroid gland dysfunction

Etiology	Signs and symptoms	Medical therapy
Thyroid hormone deficit *Primary* Congenital, idiopathic; iodine deficiency; chronic thyroiditis; thyrotoxin *Secondary/tertiary* Pituitary or hypothalamic dysfunction *Iatrogenic* Radioactive iodine; surgery of thyroid; antithyroid drugs	Hypothyroidism (early signs): Weight gain, sluggishness, sleepiness, slowed mental process, slurred speech; intolerance to cold; constipation; dry skin, dry sparse hair; menorrhagia in young women Myxedema: Lethargy, coma; periorbital puffiness; nonpitting edema of feet and hands; large tongue; dull facies; pale, cool, rough, "doughy" skin	Replacement therapy of thyroid hormones: Thyroid Levothyroxine sodium Liothyronine sodium Thyroglobulin Liotrix
Thyroid hormone excess *Primary* Toxic diffuse goiter (Graves' disease) Thyroiditis Toxic nodular goiter Thyrotoxicosis Cancer of thyroid *Secondary/tertiary* Pituitary or hypothalamic hyperfunction	Graves' disease: Goiter, exophthalamus, hyperthyroidism Hyperthyroidism Nervous system: nervousness, irritability, fatigue, fine tremors Cardiovascular system: tachycardia, increased blood pressure, angina, arrhythmias, cardiac hypertrophy Muscle and bone changes: muscle weakness, atrophy, osteoporosis Skin changes: warm, moist skin, intolerance to heat, fine hair Sexual changes: amenorrhea, decreased libido Enlarged thyroid	Reduction of thyroid hormone Antithyroid drugs; sodium iodide, propylthiouracil, methimazole Radioactive iodine Surgery: subtotal or total thyroidectomy Thyroid crisis: Antithyroid drugs; oxygen, hypothermia to reduce fever, IV fluids, steroids, sedatives, cardiac drugs as necessary

EVALUATION

Questions that the nurse can use to evaluate the nursing care of the patient with parathyroid dysfunction include the following:

1. Were complications prevented by early detection and reporting of signs and symptoms?
2. Is patient prepared to manage treatment measures at home?
3. Is patient aware of need for lifelong replacement therapy, if indicated?

THYROID DYSFUNCTION

PATHOPHYSIOLOGY

Alterations in the thyroid gland may be associated with hyperthyroid, hypothyroid, or euthyroid metabolic states (Table 30-14).

Goiter

Any enlargement of the thyroid gland is spoken of as a goiter. A goiter may be caused by various disorders that prevent the synthesis of normal quantities of thyroid hormones. If the impairment is severe enough, the goiter may be associated with hypothyroidism.

Goiter occurs because of an impairment in hormonal synthesis associated with a reduction of the thyroid hormones T_3 and T_4. This reduction prevents the normal feedback inhibition of TSH. The TSH level is increased,

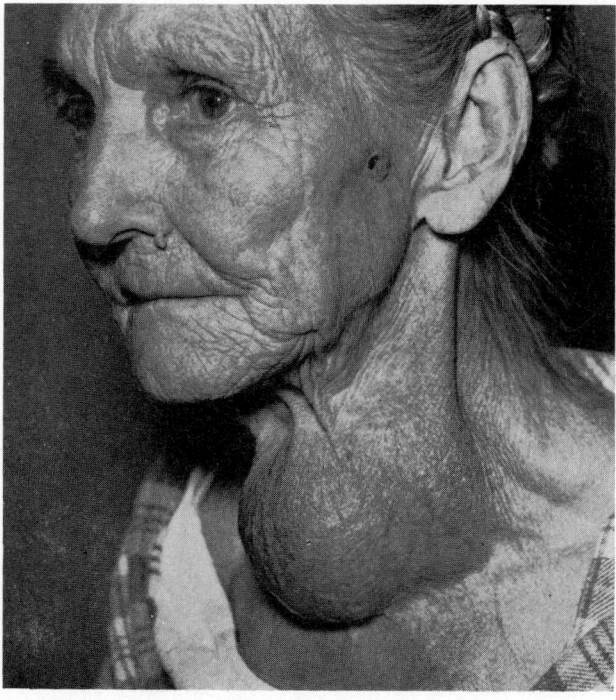

Fig. 30-10. Simple goiter. (From Prior, J.A., Silberstein, J.S., and Stang, J.M.: Physical diagnosis: the history and examination of the patient, ed. 6, St. Louis, 1981, The C.V. Mosby Co.)

which in turn causes an increase in thyroid mass. The thyroid enlargement (Fig. 30-10) may produce hyperplasia and be sufficient enough to allow for adequate hormonal synthesis.

Simple goiter may result from the following:

1. Iodide deficiency
2. Congenital metabolic defects preventing synthesis of thyroid hormones
3. Blocking of hormone synthesis by chemical agents (for example, substances in cabbage, turnips, soybeans)
4. Blocking of hormone synthesis by drugs (for example, thiocarbamides, sulfonylureas, and lithium

Simple goiter is frequently seen in females, appearing at puberty when the metabolic rate is highest and the body's need for thyroid hormone is greatest. It may disappear spontaneously after the age of 25 years.

Thyroiditis

Inflammation of the thyroid gland may be acute, subacute, or chronic and is characterized by painful swelling of the thyroid gland. Acute thyroiditis occurs when there is an infection of the thyroid gland. It is not common and is treated symptomatically. Subacute thyroiditis may last weeks or months, but the majority of persons become asymptomatic and return to normal thyroid function in time.

The most common form is Hashimoto's thyroiditis, in which the thyroid is infiltrated with lymphocytes and plasma cells. Autoimmunity is the most common cause. Early in the disease, during exacerbations of chronic thyroiditis, when functioning thyroid tissue is still present, excessive thyroid hormone may be released resulting in signs and symptoms of hyperthyroidism. As the disease progresses, the thyroid gland may be destroyed, and signs and symptoms of hypothyroidism may be present.

Hypothyroidism

The most common cause of hypothyroidism is destruction of the thyroid gland by surgery or radioactive iodine therapy. It may be secondary to pituitary failure and TSH lack or from hypothalamic disease that causes a deficiency of thyroid-releasing hormone. In hypothyroidism caused by a congenital developmental defect (cretinism, Fig. 30-11) or destruction of the gland by radiation or surgery, there is no tissue for TSH to act on. In hypothyroidism resulting from pituitary or hypothalamic problems, TSH is depressed and no hyperplasia occurs.

Regardless of the cause, the clinical findings are the same. The signs and symptoms result from a deficiency of T_3 and T_4, leading to a decrease in the normal metabolic functions that are under the control of T_3 and T_4.

The picture presented by the person with hypothyroidism will vary with the age of onset and the severity of the deficiency (Table 30-14). Myxedema is a term used to refer to a severe form of hypothyroidism in adults accompanied by an accumulation of hydrophilic mucopolysaccharides in certain tissues around the eyes and in the skin (Fig. 30-12).

Thyroid hormone functions

Hormones	Functions
Thyroxine (T_4) Triiodothyronine (T_3)	Regulates protein, fat, and carbohydrate catabolism in all cells
	Regulates metabolic rate of all cells
	Regulates body heat production
	Insulin antagonist
	Maintains growth hormone secretion, skeletal maturation
	Affects CNS development
	Necessary for muscle tone and vigor
	Maintains cardiac rate, force and output
	Maintains secretion of gastrointestinal tract
	Affects respiratory rate and oxygen utilization
	Maintains calcium mobilization
	Affects RBC production
	Stimulates lipid turnover, free fatty acid release, and cholesterol synthesis
Thyrocalcitonin	Lowers serum calcium and phosphorus levels
	Decreases calcium and phosphorus absorption in gastrointestinal tract

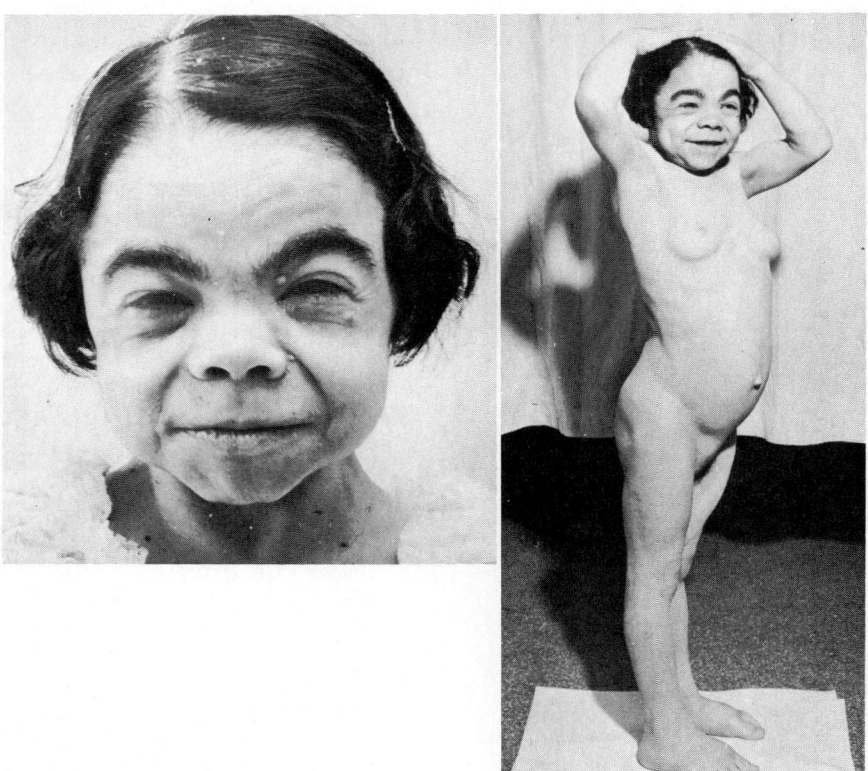

Fig. 30-11. Adult cretin (33 years old, untreated). Note characteristic cretinoid features, dwarfism (height of 44 inches), absent axillary and scant pubic hair, poorly developed breasts, potbelly, and small umbilical hernia. (From Schneeburg, N.G.: Essentials of clinical endocrinology, St. Louis, 1979, The C.V. Mosby Co.)

Cardiovascular dysfunction is a serious outcome of untreated hypothyroidism. Besides bradycardia, there may be elevation of diastolic blood pressure and possibly pericardial effusion. Pleural effusion and ascites may also be present. The heart is enlarged. In addition, all body functions are slowed. Deep tendon reflexes are diminished, and there may be joint effusion. Despite these marked changes, some individuals do not seem to be aware of the changes in their physical functioning, appearance, or behavior.

Myxedema crisis occurs as the myxedema worsens. The patient becomes less responsive and may go into a coma. An infection such as pneumonia, cellulitis, or pyelonephritis may precipitate the coma. There is decreased blood flow to the brain.

Hyperthyroidism

Hyperthyroidism is more common in women than in men, and there is a higher incidence between 20 and 40 years of age. It often appears after emotional trauma, infection, or increased stress and occurs frequently in persons who have had other endocrine disturbances.

Hyperthyroidism, or thyrotoxicosis, results from excessive secretion of thyroxine (T_4) or triiodothyronine (T_3). The most common causes are toxic diffuse goiter (Graves' disease) and toxic nodular goiter.

The clinical picture in hyperthyroidism is the same regardless of the cause. Some patients will have obvious signs and symptoms, but frequently these are insidious and nonspecific. The signs and symptoms are related to the increased metabolic rate, increased cardiac stimulation, increased nervous system activity, and interference with reproductive hormones (Table 30-14).

The cardiovascular system is seriously affected by hyperthyroidism because of the increased metabolic rate and the direct effects of thyroid hormones on the heart.

Graves' disease

Graves' disease, which is characterized by a triad of symptoms—*goiter, hyperthyroidism,* and *exophthalmos* (abnormal protrusion of the eyes, Fig. 30-13)—is thought to be an autoimmune disease. The thyroid-stimulating activity or sera in persons with Graves' disease is the result of thyroid-stimulating immunoglobulins (TSI), also called long-acting thyroid stimulator (LATS). The cause of the abnormal development of the immunoglobulins is unknown, but the effect of the stimulation is longer than that of the normal TSH.

Thyroid storm

Thyroid storm (thyroid crisis) may occur in persons with uncontrolled hyperthyroidism. It is believed that in a thyroid storm, increased amounts of hormones are released into the bloodstream and metabolism is markedly increased. It may be precipitated by infection, stressors, or thyroid surgery undertaken on a patient who was not adequately prepared with antithyroid drugs. The onset often occurs spontaneously. The patient's temperature may rise to 41° C (106° F) as the body becomes unable to release the heat formed with increased metabolism. The pulse may be rapid, and there is marked respiratory distress, apprehension, restlessness, irritability, and prostra-

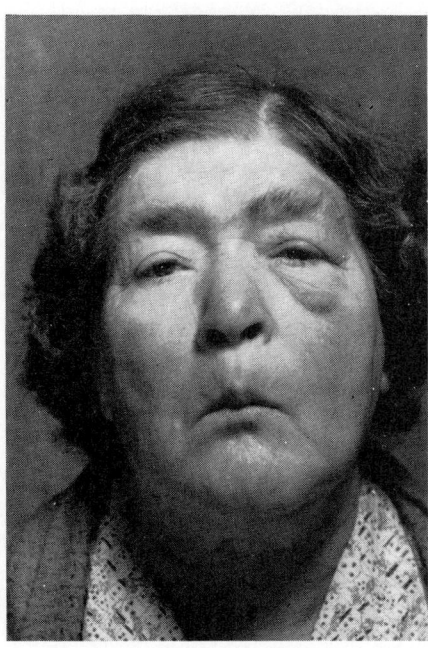

Fig. 30-12. Person with myxedema. (From Schottelius, B.A., and Schottelius, D.A.: Textbook of physiology, ed. 18, St. Louis, 1978, The C.V. Mosby Co.)

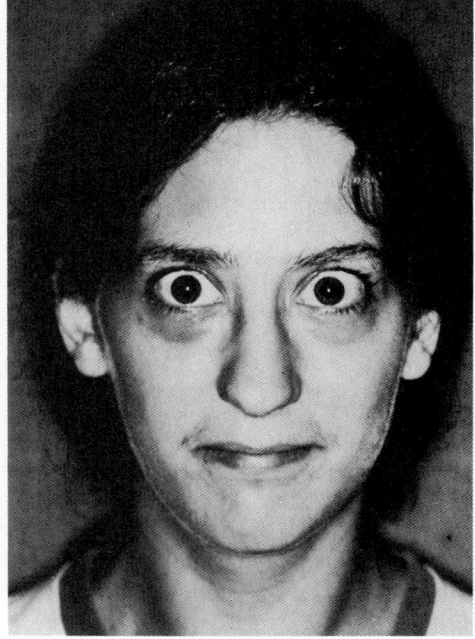

Fig. 30-13. Ophthalmopathy of Graves' disease. (From Kaye, D., and Rose, L.F.: Fundamentals of internal medicine, St. Louis, 1983, The C.V. Mosby Co.)

tion. The patient may becomes delirious and finally comatose, with death resulting from heart failure.

ASSESSMENT

Subjective data

Hypersecretion or hyposecretion of the thyroid gland has marked effects on the patient's ability to function, as well as on physiologic processes. The nurse collects data from the patient or a family member concerning past and present

Energy level

Mood and mental ability

Ability to carry out activities of daily living

Ability to manage stress

Intolerance to heat or cold

Food intake

Elimination patterns

The interview should help the nurse determine the patient's or family's understanding of the disease and its treatment, and about the care needs of the patient.

Objective data

Initial physical examination should provide baseline information about the patient's

Mental status (ability to follow directions)

Nutritional status

Cardiovascular status

Body characteristics

Skin appearance and texture

Hair quality and sparsity

Eye appearance and extraocular motion

Presence and location of edema

Neck appearance and range of motion

Abdominal girth

Extremities

Diagnostic tests

Testing for thyroid function can be made at the hypothalamic, pituitary, thyroid, serum, or peripheral tissue levels. Table 30-15 presents the major test procedures and preparations and the interpretations. The most commonly used tests are serum T_4 and T_3 concentrations and T_3 resin or RBC uptake. An elevated T_4 level often confirms clinical findings of overt hyperthyroidism, whereas T_3 testing is more sensitive in discerning mild hyperthyroidism. TSH radioimmunassay and stimulation testing can help differentiate primary and secondary hypothyroidism.

DATA ANALYSIS AND PLANNING

Nursing diagnoses

Nursing diagnoses for patients with thyroid dysfunction could include the following:

Bowel elimination, alteration in

Comfort, alteration in tolerance to heat, cold, stress

Cardiac output, alteration in: decreased

Coping, ineffective individual or family

Home maintenance management, impaired

Knowledge deficit

Nutrition, alteration in: less or more than body requirements

Self-care deficit

Sleep pattern disturbance

Expected patient outcomes

The person with *hyperthyroidism* on antithyroid drugs can

1. Explain the medication program.
2. Describe plans for a quiet, restful environment.
3. Plan meals to meet energy requirements.
4. State plans for follow-up care:
   a. State symptoms requiring immediate follow-up (signs of remission, thyroid crisis, hypothyroidism).
   b. State plans for regular medical appointments.
5. Describe eye care if exophthalmos is present.

The person with *hypothyroidism* can

1. Explain the prescribed medication program.
2. State reason for lifelong replacement therapy.
3. State plans for follow-up care:
   a. State symptoms requiring immediate follow-up of hypothyroidism or hyperthyroidism.
   b. State plans for regular medical appointments.

IMPLEMENTATION

Providing support to patient with thyroid dysfunction
Hyperthyroidism

Since the advent of antithyroid drugs and the trend toward early treatment, most persons with hyperthyroidism can be cared for at home. Although these persons usually are not particularly hyperactive, they are likely to be nervous and irritable. It is important that family and friends understand that extreme sensitivity and excessive irritability are part of the disease; otherwise, they may become upset with the individual and aggravate the situation. It may be necessary to do small things for these persons that they may seem physically able to do for themselves, and they need to understand why they are being helped.

The following interventions by nurses or caregivers at home are indicated for the person with hyperthyroidism:

1. Maintain a cool, quiet environment.
2. Assist patient to obtain sufficient rest.
3. Encourage quiet activities that require gross motor movements (for example, weaving, reading).
4. Assist with tasks requiring fine motor coordination for patient (for example, sewing, dishes).
5. Provide a high calorie, high protein diet; snacks between meals may be necessary to maintain weight and meet energy requirements.
6. Encourage the use of decaffeinated drinks.
7. If exophthalmos is present:
   a. Dark glasses will afford some protection from wind, sun, and dust.

Table 30-15. Diagnostic tests of thyroid function

Function test	Procedure and preparation	Interpretation
Tests related to serum levels of thyroid hormone		
Thyroxine-binding globulin (TBG)	Blood sample, no special preparation	Measures levels of TBG; TBG can be elevated or depressed by other conditions unrelated to thyroid problems; helpful in determining amount of bound and active T_3 and T_4
Serum T_4 concentration	Blood sample; test determines ability of T_4 extracted from serum to displace radioactive T_4 from T_4-binding proteins; not affected by iodides and dyes that elevate PBI and depress RAIU	Measures circulating thyroxine that is bound to TBG and free T_4; normal, 3-7 μg/100 ml; increased TBG such as occurs in pregnancy, and estrogen therapy causes increased T_4 values; decreased TBG as seen with glucocorticoid therapy and hypoproteinemia caused decreased T_4 values
Serum T_3 concentrations	Radioassay of blood sample; no special preparation	Measure circulating T_3 that is bound to TBG and free T_3; normal values are 100-170 ng/100 ml and are elevated in T_3 thyrotoxicosis; variations in thyroxine-binding globulin (TBG) can influence test results as they do for serum T_4
Triodothyronine (T_3) resin uptake	Blood sample drawn; in laboratory resin and radioactive T_3 are added to sample of blood; radioactive T_3 will bind to unoccupied sites of thyroxine-binding globulin (TBG); radioactive counts are done on blood and resins to determine amount of T_3 (radioactive) bound to resin	Normally 25-30% of radioactive T_3 will bind to resin; in hyperthyroidism, where there are increased amounts of endogenous thyroid hormone, value will be increased; in hypothyroidism T_3 resin uptake will be low; this is not a measure of the patient's endogenous T_3 level; test is affected by total amount of TBG; in wasting diseases where amount of TBG may be decreased, reading may be falsely elevated; in conditions such as pregnancy and estrogen therapy abnormal amounts of TBG may be available and a false-low T_3 may be obtained; phenytoin (Dilantin) and salicylates compete with thyroxine for TBG sites and may give false-negative T_3 resin uptake
Free T_4 and free T_3	Blood sample, special laboratory procedures	Measures unbound metabolically active T_4 or T_3; is a difficult test and is not used frequently; instead FT_4I is calculated; FT_4I varies directly with FT_4
Free T_4 index (FT_4I)	Serum T_4 and T_3U measured	Free T_4I is product of serum T_4 and T_3U; changes in TBG causes reciprocal alterations in serum T_4 and T_3U, so that FT_4I stays normal

Continued.

Table 30-15. Diagnostic tests of thyroid function—cont'd

Function test	Procedure and preparation	Interpretation
Protein-bound iodine test (PBI)	Serum blood sample; results of test are invalidated if patient has high exogenous sources of iodine; cough syrups, x-ray media, estrogens, and enriched iodine foods may cause false-high levels and should be avoided for 1 wk before test; mercury causes abnormally low readings	Test indirectly measures circulating T_4 concentration; normal range is 4-8 μg/100 ml of serum, decreased PBI indicates hypothyroidism; increased PBI indicates hyperthyroidism; test is being used less frequently because of availability of more specific tests
Thyroid antibody tests	Blood sample; in laboratory RBCs are latex coated with thyroid globulin and mixed with blood	Test may differentiate cause of thyroid enlargement; if antibodies are present, agglutination occurs
Tests related to peripheral effects of thyroid hormone		
Basal metabolism rate (BMR)	Patient at rest; amount of oxygen used while at rest is calculated; patient's oxygen use is compared with established norms for people of same sex, age, and size; results expressed in percentage above or below normal; patient receives nothing by mouth (NPO) the night before test, should have 8 hr of sleep, and should stay in bed morning of test; no food or smoking is allowed; anxiety will increase BMR, so patient needs explanation of what to expect	Normal range is − 15% to + 15%; in hyperthyroidism patient's BMR will be greater than + 15%; in hypothyroidism patient's BMR will be less than − 15%; BMR is less accurate than other tests described above but may be used to observe patients on thyroid therapy
Serum cholesterol level	Blood sample; patient placed on NPO list night before	Normals vary from laboratory to laboratory; high levels found in hypothyroidism and low levels found in hyperthyroidism; data augment other tests
Achilles tendon reflex recording	Electrodes from recording drum attached to patient's ankle; while ankle tendon is tapped, recording is done	Slow, sluggish jerk indicates hypothyroidism; rapid jerk indicates hyperthyroidism
Thyroid function tests		
Hypothalamus level test TRH stimulation test	TRH is given IV and then serum TSH levels are repeatedly measured	Normal serum TSH begins to rise at 10 min and peaks at 45 min, subnormal tests reflect diminished TSH reserve; supranormal response occurs in patients with hypothyroidism of thyroid origin; no response occurs in most patients with thyrotoxicosis except when it is caused by excess TSH

Table 30-15. Diagnostic tests of thyroid function—cont'd

Function test	Procedure and preparation	Interpretation
Pituitary level test TSH radioimmunoassay	Blood sample, no special preparation	Directly measures TSH levels, measurement aids in differentiating primary and secondary hypothyroidism; values are elevated in primary hypothyroidism because of loss of negative feedback
Thyroid stimulating hormone (TSH) stimulation test	Baseline levels of radioactive iodine uptake (RAIU) and protein-bound iodine (PBI) are taken, TSH injection is given and repeat RAIU and PBI levels are taken	Assists in differentiating between primary and secondary hypothyroidism; in primary hypothyroidism repeat level of RAIU and PBI stays the same; if they become normal, this indicates hypothyroidism caused by too little TSH (secondary)
Thyroid level test Radioactive iodine uptake (RAIU)	A tracer dose of radioactive iodine (^{131}I) is given by mouth. At 2, 6, and 24 hr following administration, scintillation detector is placed over neck in region of thyroid and amount of accumulated radioactive iodine is measured; excess iodine in any foods, cough medicines, x-ray media, other medications, and enriched iodine foods affect test by giving low readings; diarrhea, causing decreased absorption of tracer dose, gives low readings, renal failure, causing decreased excretion, can cause elevated readings; no radiation precautions are necessary	Normal thyroid will take up 5% to 35% of tracer dose; increased uptake occurs in hyperthyroidism; excess tracer dose is excreted in urine and can be measured; urine is collected for 24 hr; decreased amounts in urine indicate hyperthyroid state
Thyroid scan	Dose of ^{131}I is given, and scintillation scan is done: scanner is moved over thyroid, and a picture of distribution of radioactivity is recorded; no radiation precautions necessary	Size, shape, and anatomic function of gland assessed; areas of increased or decreased uptake noted
Thyroid suppression test	RAIU test and serum T_4 levels are done, patient given thyroid hormone for 7-10 days, RAIU and serum T_4 repeated	If euthyroid (normal), repeat RAIU and serum T_4 will be low; failure of hormone therapy to suppress RAIU and serum T_4 indicates hyperthyroidism

b. Soothing eye drops, such as methylcellulose, 0.5% to 1%, may provide comfort.

Hypothyroidism

The patient's slowed mental functioning requires understanding and patience on the part of caregivers. A thorough explanation of the cause of the changes in the patient's physical and mental responses should be given to family or friends. As the thyroid hormone levels return to normal, the patient's physical and mental states will return to their pre-illness levels.

During the time the patient is hypothyroid, nursing care includes the following:

1. Minimize environmental stressors, since the patient is unable to respond to them.
2. Administer replacement therapy and monitor pa-

tient for effectiveness of the therapy and for side effects.

3. Provide complete care at first and gradually increase patient's self-care.
4. Prevent constipation and fecal impaction by use of fluids, fiber, and stool softeners and encourage activity.

Assisting with achievement of therapeutic goals
Correction of the thyroid dysfunction

MEDICATIONS. Medications may be used to treat goiter, hyperthyroidism, or hyperthyroidism.

IODINE REPLACEMENT

If goiter is a result of iodine deficiency, iodine replacement therapy will be given. One drop of saturated solution of potassium iodide (SSKI) each week usually provides enough additional iodine for the thyroid gland to produce adequate thyroid hormones, and the hyperplasia

---

> ## Replacement therapy for hypothyroidism
>
> Thyroid (combination of T_4 and T_3)
> Levothyroxine sodium (synthetic T_4)
>   Synthroid
>   Levothroid
> Liothyronine sodium (synthetic T_3)
>   Cytomel
>   Trionine
> Liotrix (synthetic combination of T_4 and T_3)
>   Euthroid
>   Thyrolar

---

will gradually decrease. Using iodized table salt is an easy and inexpensive way of ensuring sufficient iodine intake, since the average adult can obtain more than twice the daily requirement from the amount of salt normally used.

ADMINISTRATION OF THYROID HORMONE FOR HYPOTHYROIDISM

The drugs used most commonly to treat hypothyroidism are listed in the box. It is important that dosages be increased gradually because a sudden increase in metabolic rate can cause death from cardiac failure. The daily maintenance dose of thyroid hormones varies widely. The correct dose is determined by a remission in the symptoms of hypofunction.

Adults with hypothyroidism respond quickly to the administration of thyroid hormones. Changes in appearance and physical symptoms occur within 2 to 3 days. Treatment must be continued throughout life, and the individual must be taught that failure to take the prescribed medication will result in an exacerbation of the disease. Medication dosage may need periodic adjustments to avoid symptoms of hyperthyroidism or hypothyroidism.

ANTITHYROID DRUGS

One approach to reduce the output of thyroid hormone in hyperthyroidism is the use of antithyroid drugs. Lugol's solution, propylthiouracil, and methimazole are the more commonly used drugs (Table 30-16). Usually a trial of antithyroid drugs is used before ablation of thyroid tissue by surgery or radioactive iodine.

The patient usually is started on a relatively large dose of an antithyroid drug, and then the dosage is gradually reduced to a level sufficient to maintain the euthyroid state. When antithyroid drugs are used as the primary therapy, they commonly are continued for 6 to 18 months or longer. Some patients will stay in remission without further therapy. Others will require longer drug therapy, additional therapy, or lifelong therapy. The patient should see the physician at regular intervals after drugs

Table 30-16. Antithyroid drugs

Drug	Actions	Interventions
Lugol's solution (sodium iodide)	Rapid action, blocks synthesis and release of thyroid hormone; less sustained action; reduces vascularity of the thyroid gland thus often used in preparation for surgery; saturates thyroid with iodide thus radioactive iodine studies or treatment of thyroid cannot be done	Explain to patient that compliance with dosage schedule is necessary; give through a straw to avoid staining of teeth; give in milk or fruit juice; teach patient to report toxic symptoms: brassy taste, sore teeth and gums
Propylthiouracil (Propacil) Methimazole (Tapazole)	Blocks synthesis of thyroid hormone, not the release of stored hormone	Explain to patient that 2-4 weeks are necessary before improvement is noticed; teach patient to report toxic symptoms: fever, sore throat, skin eruptions, leukopenia or pancytopenia

are discontinued so that early signs of recurrence will be noticed. It is important to give the drugs at regularly spaced intervals, since their blood levels are reduced in about 8 hours. Continued use of antithyroid drugs may not be tolerated by some persons.

RADIOACTIVE IODINE. Radioactive iodine is the ablative procedure of choice for older persons. A radioactive isotope of iodine, ^{131}I, is given by mouth, is absorbed rapidly in the stomach, and becomes concentrated in the thyroid. Usually, a single dose is given in a radioactive "cocktail." If an unusually large dose of radioactive iodine is given, hospitalization for several days may be necessary. Patients receiving usual amounts of the isotope may go directly home, and no special precautions are advised. It takes about 3 weeks for the symptoms of hyperthyroidism to subside, and over 2 months for thyroid function to become normal. Occasionally, remission is not achieved with one dose, and the treatment is repeated after an interval of several months.

Radioactive iodine is not used in pregnant women because of the potential effect on the fetus, since the placenta transports iodine easily. Some physicians to not use it in the childbearing years because of the potential for destruction of the gonads.

Patients who receive radioactive iodine for hyperthyroidism need to have the treatment explained to them with special care, and they usually need repeated reassurance that the radioactive properties are quickly dissipated. Since they may be more emotional than other persons, they sometimes think they are experiencing reactions to the drug long after this is possible. Permanent hypothyroidism is a potential complication of this therapy.

SURGERY. Surgery of the thyroid is the procedure of choice for removal of goiters causing pressure, cancer of the thyroid, and hyperthyroidism in persons under age 40.

Part or all of the thyroid gland may be removed surgically. Total thyroidectomy (complete removal of the thyroid) may be performed for cancer of the thyroid, and the patient must then take thyroid hormones regularly for the remainder of life. Hyperthyroidism may be treated surgically by removing approximately five sixths of the gland (subtotal thyroidectomy). In most cases this operation permanently alleviates symptoms, while the remaining thyroid tissue provides enough hormones for normal function. The remaining tissue can hypertrophy, however, and hyperthyroidism can recur.

Before thyroid surgery is undertaken, a normal (euthyroid) state is produced by drug therapy. An ECG is made before surgery to detect evidence of heart damage. Persons with heart damage are preferably treated with radioactive iodine.

Preoperative teaching includes teaching the patient to support the neck by placing both hands behind the head when positioning self in bed, getting out of bed, or coughing. This action avoids flexion and hyperextension of the neck during moving or coughing to protect the suture line from strain.

POSTOPERATIVE COMPLICATIONS

The complications following thyroid surgery are extremely serious and if they are not recognized and treated at once, they can result in death.

The dressing is observed for signs of hemorrhage for the first 12 to 24 hours postoperatively. Since blood may drain back under the patient's neck and shoulders, the nurse's hand should be slipped gently under the patient's neck and shoulders each time the dressing is checked. If signs of hemorrhage are present, the dressing should be loosened at once and the surgeon notified. If loosening the dressing does not relieve the respiratory difficulty and medical assistance will not be immediately available, the surgeon may instruct the nurse to remove the clips or sutures from the wound to relieve the pressure on the trachea. The surgeon may need to perform an emergency tracheostomy, and the patient must be taken to the operating room for retying of the blood vessels and resuturing the wound.

Although slight hoarseness is normal, the patient is observed for any increase in hoarseness and accompanying respiratory difficulty. To recognize early symptoms of recurrent laryngeal nerve injury, patients are asked to speak as soon as they have reacted from anesthesia and at intervals of 30 to 60 minutes.

Injury to the parathyroids is uncommon but may occur. Surgery or inflammation may block the normal release of parathyroid hormone and symptoms of calcium deficiency,

---

Possible complications following thyroid surgery

Complication	Signs and symptoms
Hemorrhage	Bright red blood on dressing
	Choking sensation
	Difficulty coughing and swallowing
	Tightening of dressing sensation
Edema about vocal cords and larynx	Hoarseness
	Dyspnea
Laryngeal nerve injury	Difficulty speaking
	Dyspnea
	Hoarseness (injury to one vocal cord)
	Respiratory obstruction (both vocal cords injured)
	Crowing sound
	Retraction of neck tissue
Injury to parathyroids	Tetany

Nursing interventions following thyroid surgery

1. Monitor for postoperative complications (bleeding, respiratory difficulties, hoarseness, dysphagia, tetany).
2. Maintain equipment at bedside for treatment of laryngeal obstruction (tracheostomy set) and tetany (calcium gluconate).
3. Encourage high-carbohydrate fluids by mouth and a soft diet as tolerated.
4. Use prescribed analgesic throat lozenges or gels 30 minutes before meals to ease swallowing.
5. Use a humidifier to decrease and thin secretions, if appropriate.
6. Encourage activity that does not put tension on suture line until sufficient healing (5 to 7 days) has occurred; then encourage gradual range of neck motion.
7. Teach patient about required drugs (dosage, side effects) and importance of medical follow-up.

---

tetany, may appear from 1 to 7 days postoperatively. Serum calcium levels are usually monitored, and hypocalcemia is treated by replacement of calcium gluconate intravenously. Daily oral doses of calcium chloride are then given until normal function returns. If not all the glands were destroyed by injury, the remaining glands hypertrophy and function returns. If all were destroyed, the patient must have lifetime therapy to manage calcium levels.

Postoperative nursing intervention are summarized in box above.

EVALUATION

Evaluation is based on expected patient outcomes. Questions useful in evaluation nursing care of patients with thyroid dysfunction may include the following:

1. Is patient prepared to manage self-care regimens at home?
2. Were complications prevented or promptly identified and treated?
3. Is patient able to achieve desired
   a. Weight?
   b. Energy level and activity?
   c. Sleep and rest?

REFERENCES AND SELECTED READINGS*

1. Beland, I.L., Rice, V.H., and Power, L.: Metabolic crises. In Meltzer, L.E., Abdella, F.G., and Kitchell, J.R.: Concepts and practices of intensive care for nurse specialists, ed. 2, Philadelphia, 1976, The Charles Press Publishers.
2. Bondy, P., and Rosenberg, L.: Metabolic control and disease, Philadelphia, 1980, W.B. Saunders Co.
3. Camunas, C.: Pheochromocytoma, Am. J. Nurs. **83:**887-891, 1983.
4. Cataland, S.: Hypoglycemia: a spectrum of problems, Heart Lung **7:**459-462, 1978.
5. *Clancey, J., and Abruzzi, L.: Pituitary tumors, growth disease: nursing intervention of patients with pituitary tumor, J. Neurosurg. Nurs. **10:**24-28, 1978.
6. Cooperman, D., and Malarkey, W.B.: Pituitary apoplexy, Heart Lung **7:**450-454, 1978.
7. Costen, G.: Endocrine disorders associated with tumor of the pituitary and hypothalamus, Pediatr. Clin. North Am. **26:**15-31, 1979.
8. DeGroot, L., and others: Endocrinology, vol. 1-3, New York, 1979, Grune & Stratton, Inc.
9. DeLuca, H.T.: Vitamin D endocrinology, Ann. Intern. Med. **85:**367-377, 1976.
10. *Evangelisti, J.T., and others: Thyroid storm: a nursing crisis, Heart Lung **12:**184-194, 1983.
11. Fairchild, R.S.: Diabetes insipidus: a review, Crit. Care Q. **2:**111-118, 1980.
12. Fass, B.: Glucocorticoid therapy for nonendocrine disorders: withdrawals and "coverage," Pediatr. Clin. North Am. **26:**251-256, 1979.
13. Fauci, A., and others: Glucocorticosteroid therapy: mechanisms of action and clinical considerations, Ann. Intern. Med. **84:**304-315, 1976.
14. Geola, F., and Chopra, I.: Hyperthyroidism and hypothyroidism, Med. Times **108:**64-69, 73-74, 1980.
15. *Gillies, D.A., and Alyn, I.B.: Caring for patients with thyroid disorders: how good are your skills? Nurs. 77 **7**(10):71-80, 1977.

---

*References preceded by an asterisk are particularly well suited for student reading.

16. *Gotch, P.M.: Teaching patients about adrenal corticosteroids, Am. J. Nurs. **81:**78-85, 1981.

17. Hahn, A.B., Barking, R.L., and Oestreich, S.J.K.: Pharmacology in nursing, ed. 15, St. Louis, 1982, The C.V. Mosby Co.

18. *Hallal, J.: Thyroid disorders, Am. J. Nurs. **77:**418-432, 1977.

19. Hamburger, S., and Rush, D.: Syndrome of inappropriate secretion of antidiuretic hormone, Crit. Care Q. **2:**119-129, 1980.

20. Hays, R., and Levine, S.: Antidiuretic hormone, N. Engl. J. Med. **295:**659-665, 1976.

21. Hellman, R.: The evaluation and management of hyperthyroid crises, Crit. Care Q. **2:**77-92, 1980.

22. Hoffman, J.T.: Syndromes of ectopic hormone production in cancer, Nurs. Clin. North Am. **15:**499-509, 1980.

23. *Hoffman, J.T., and Newby, T.B.: Hypercalcemia in primary hyperparathyroidism, Nurs. Clin. North Am. **15:**469-480, 1980.

24. Honigman, R.E.: Deciphering diagnostic studies: thyroid function tests, Nurs. 82 **12**(4):68-71, 1982.

25. Isselbacher, K., and others: Harrison's principles of internal medicine, ed. 9, New York, 1980, McGraw Hill Book Co.

26. Kaplan, S.: Disorders of the adrenal cortex. I, Pediatr. Clin. North Am. **26:**65-76, 1979.

27. Kaplan, S.: Disorders of the adrenal cortex. II, Pediatr. Clin. North Am. **26:**77-89, 1979.

28. Koppers, L.E.: Pheochromocytoma—critical care, Crit. Care Q. **2:**93-97, 1980.

29. *Krueger, J., and Ray, J.: Endocrine problems in nursing, St. Louis, 1976, The C.V. Mosby Co.

30. *Kubo, W.M., and Grant, M.: The syndrome of inappropriate antidiuretic hormone, Heart Lung **7:**469-472, 1978.

31. LaFranchi, S.: Hypothyroidism, Pediatr. Clin. North Am. **26:**33-51, 1979.

32. Lee, W.N.: Thyroiditis, hyperthyroidism, and tumors, Pediatr. Clin. North Am. **26:**53-64, 1979.

33. Lukert, B.P.: Hypercalcemia, Crit. Care Q. **2:**11-18, 1980.

34. Mannix, H., and others: Hyperparathyroidism in the elderly, Am. J. Surg. **139:**581-585, 1980.

35. McFadden, E.A., Zaloga, G.P., and Chernow, B.: Hypocalcemia: a medical emergency, Am. J. Nurs. **83:**227-230, 1983.

36. *Nemeroff, D.R.: Transphenoidal hypophysectomy, J. Neurosurg. Nurs. **13:**303-312, 1981.

37. O'Dorisio, L.M.: Hypercalcemic crisis, Heart Lung **7:**425-434, 1978.

38. Rush, D.R., and Hamburger, S.C.: Drugs used in endocrine metabolic emergencies, Crit. Care Q. **2:**1-9, 1980.

39. Sanford, S.J.: Dysfunction of the adrenal gland: physiologic considerations and nursing problems, Nurs. Clin. North Am. **15:**481-498, 1980.

40. Schimke, R.N.: Adrenal insufficiency, Crit. Care Q. **2:**10-27, 1980.

41. Schwartz, S.: Principles of surgery, ed. 4, New York, 1984, McGraw-Hill Book Co.

42. *Smith, J.: Nursing management of diabetes insipidus, J. Neurosurg. Nurs. **13:**313-317, 1981.

43. *Solomon, B.L.: The hypothalamus and the pituitary gland: an overview, Nurs. Clin. North Am. **15:**435-451, 1980.

44. Sowers, D.K., and Sowers, J.R.: Pituitary emergencies, Crit. Care Q. **2:**45-54, 1980.

45. Stephens, G.J.: Pathophysiology for health practitioners, New York, 1980, Macmillan Publishing Co., Inc.

46. Stillman, M.J.: Transphenoidal hypophysectomy for pituitary tumors, J. Neurosurg. Nurs. **13:**112-122, 1981.

47. Urbanic, R.C., and Mazzaferri, E.L.: Thyrotoxic crisis and myxedema coma, Heart Lung **7:**435-447, 1978.

48. VanLoon, G.: New drugs in the treatment of pituitary disorders, Primary Care **4:**721-737, 1977.

49. Vorhess, M.: Disorders of the adrenal medulla and multiple endocrine adenomatosis, Pediatr. Clin. North Am. **26:**209-222, 1979.

50. Wake, M.M., and Brensinger, J.F.: The nurse's role in hypothyroidism, Nurs. Clin. North Am. **15:**453-467, 1980.

51. Wyngaarden, J.B., and Smith, L.H.: Textbook of medicine, ed. 16, Philadelphia, 1982, W.B. Saunders Co.

31

The Patient with Hepatic, Biliary and Pancreatic Problems

DOROTHY R. BLEVINS and VIRGINIA L. CASSMEYER

STUDY QUESTIONS

- Review the functions of the liver. Explain the symptoms that may occur when the various functions are impaired.

- Review the anatomy of the biliary system. What are the important constituents of bile? What is its function in digestion?

- List some drugs that you have learned are toxic to the liver.

- Review the blood vessels leading to and from the liver. How does portal circulation differ from other venous systems?

- Review isolation procedures and precautions for enteric and blood/body fluids.

- What is the physiologic basis for color changes in the skin and sclerae with jaundice?

- Review the nature of alcoholism (see Chapter 9). What resources are available for alcoholics in your community?

The liver, biliary system, and pancreas are affected by a variety of pathologic processes that may severely affect digestion and normal metabolic processes. Many of the disorders are chronic and require that the patient make changes in life-style to keep the problem under control. These patients need nursing support in adapting to their chronic health problem and in learning the necessary self-management skills.

ANATOMY AND PHYSIOLOGY

Hepatic system

The hepatic system is a major system involved in regulation of body functions. The liver is one of the largest organs of the body and consists of two lobes located in the right upper quadrant of the abdomen under the diaphragm. It extends up under the ribs. The gallbladder lies under the inferior surface of the liver (Fig. 31-1).

The liver is made up of small liver lobules (Fig. 31-2) composed of hepatic cellular plates. Each hepatic cellular plate is usually two cells thick, and between these cells run biliary canaliculi. Hepatic sinusoids, which receive blood from both the portal vein and the hepatic artery, lie on the opposite sides of the hepatic cells. After flowing through the hepatic sinusoids, blood is emptied into the

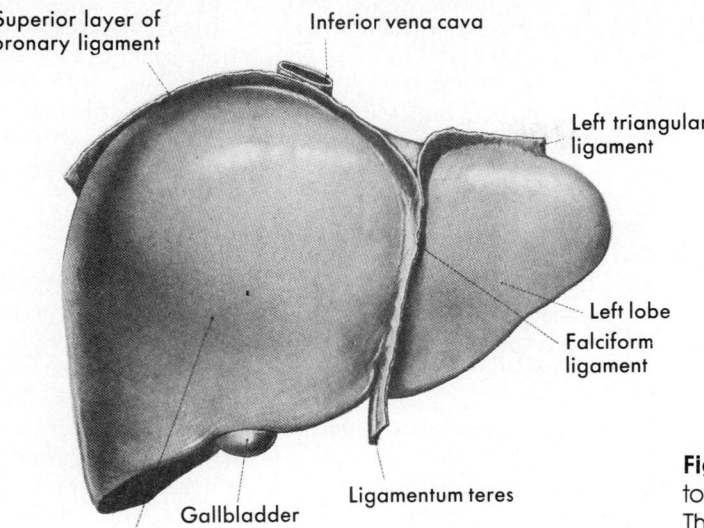

Superior layer of coronary ligament

Inferior vena cava

Left triangular ligament

Left lobe

Falciform ligament

Ligamentum teres

Gallbladder

Right lobe

Fig. 31-1. Anterior view of liver. (From Hamilton, W.J., editor: Textbook of human anatomy, ed. 2, St. Louis, 1976, The C.V. Mosby Co. By permission of Macmillan, London & Basingstoke)

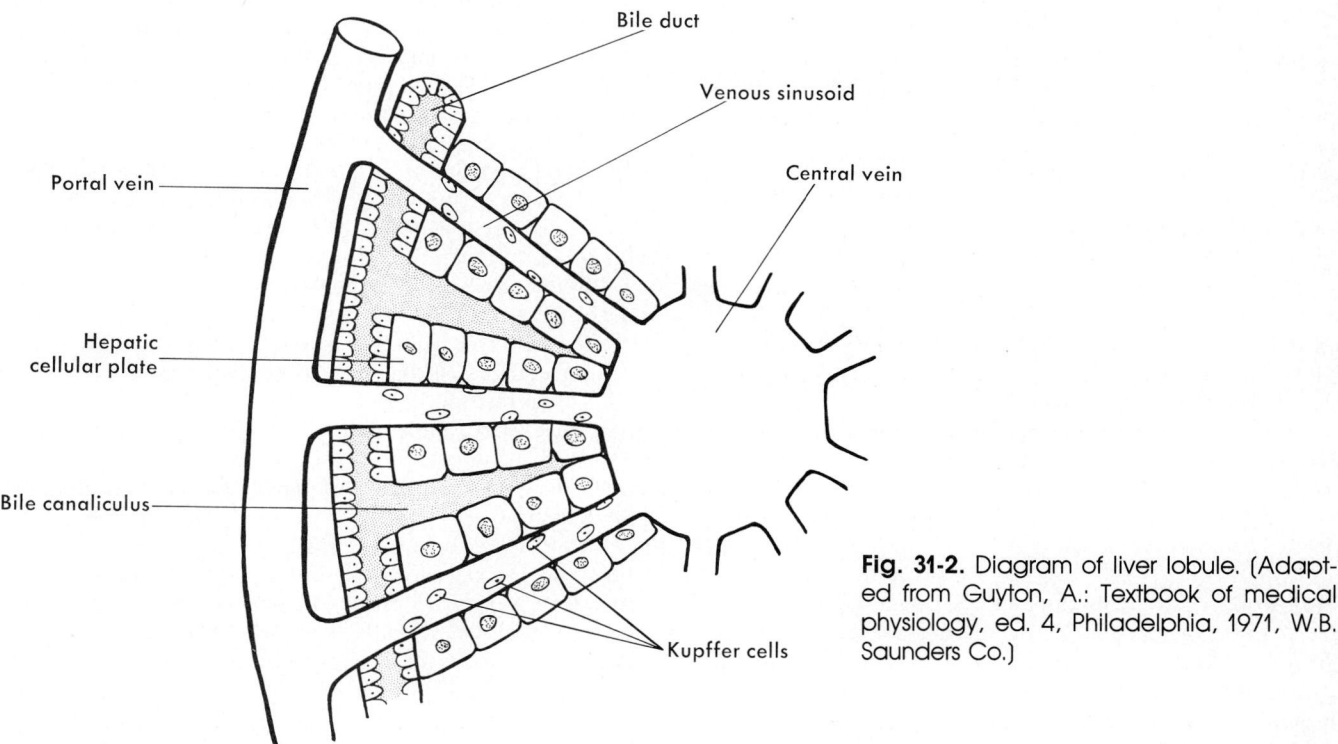

Bile duct

Venous sinusoid

Central vein

Portal vein

Hepatic cellular plate

Bile canaliculus

Kupffer cells

Fig. 31-2. Diagram of liver lobule. (Adapted from Guyton, A.: Textbook of medical physiology, ed. 4, Philadelphia, 1971, W.B. Saunders Co.)

central vein and from there flows into the hepatic vein. The hepatic sinusoids are lined with Kupffer's cells, which are reticuloendothelial cells that phagocytize bacteria and other foreign products.

The liver is ideally structured to receive large supplies of blood to carry out its multiple functions, such as participation in carbohydrate, protein, and fat metabolism; bilirubin metabolism; and detoxification.

CARBOHYDRATE, PROTEIN, AND FAT METABOLISM

The liver plays a major role in the metabolism of the three major food nutrients. Through various enzymatic activities, the liver can oxidize carbohydrates, proteins, and fats for energy or use these nutrients to produce compounds that can be stored for future use or to manufacture needed compounds.

Role of liver in metabolism

Carbohydrate metabolism

Glycogenolysis: splitting up of glycogen to yield glucose

Gluconeogenesis: synthesis of glucose from amino acids or glycerol

Metabolism of galactose

Protein metabolism

Synthesis of albumin, globulin, blood clotting factors (fibrinogen, prothrombin)

Production of urea from deamination of proteins

Fat metabolism

Production of phospholipids, lipoproteins, cholesterol

Formation of ketone bodies

The liver is the only source of albumin, which is necessary for the maintenance of osmotic pressure, and of prothrombin. Normal production of prothrombin is dependent on the following four factors:

1. Ingestion of foods that can undergo synthesis in the intestines
2. Presence of bile in the intestines for production of vitamin K
3. Absorption through the intestinal wall of the vitamin K
4. Use of the vitamin K by the liver in the formation of prothrombin

The waste product of protein deamination, ammonia, is converted to urea by the healthy liver through the Krebs-Henseleit cycle. Urea is then excreted by the kidney.

BILIRUBIN METABOLISM

Bilirubin is a by-product of the heme portion of red blood cells and is released when red blood cells are destroyed. The bilirubin at this point is not water soluble (unconjugated) and is carried in the blood attached to protein. The liver is responsible for picking up this unconjugated bilirubin, for conjugating it into a water soluble form, and for secreting conjugated bilirubin into the bile. The bilirubin in bile is emptied into the duodenum and is broken down by bacteria into urobilinogen. Some of the urobilinogen is excreted with the feces, giving the stool its brown color. Some is eliminated in the urine, and the remainder returns to the liver and is reconverted to bilirubin.

DETOXIFICATION

The liver has a prime role in detoxification of both exogenous and endogenous substances. It also has a major role in the detoxification of many drugs. All barbiturates (except phenobarbital and barbital) and many other sedatives are inactivated by the liver. The status of the liver plays an important role in the effectiveness or toxicity of these and other drugs. The liver also detoxifies corticosteroids, aldosterone, and estrogen.

Biliary system

The biliary system consists of the gallbladder and its associated ductal system (Fig. 31-3). The ductal system provides a pathway for the bile that is formed in the liver to reach the intestine and also functions to regulate bile flow. The liver produces up to 1 L of bile per day. As it is formed, bile is excreted into the hepatic ducts, where it passes into the cystic duct to be stored in the gallbladder.

The capacity of the gallbladder is usually 50 ml but can increase in size under normal conditions. In the gallbladder, bile is concentrated to a solution that is five to 10 times as concentrated as that produced in the liver.

Neural and hormonal mechanisms control the secretion of bile from the gallbladder. Food, particularly lipids in the duodenum, causes the release of cholecystokinin (CCK) from the mucosa of the duodenum. CCK is released into the blood and travels to the gallbladder. One of its activities is to stimulate the gallbladder musculature to contract. At the same time it causes the muscle of the sphincter of Oddi (at the end of the common bile duct) to relax and permit entry of bile into the duodenum. Gastrin, another gastrointestinal hormone, and vagal stimulation can also cause the gallbladder to contract.

Bile acids are predominantly composed of a cholesterol derivative, and they function in the intestinal metabolism of fats and other substances as follows:

1. Facilitate fat digestion by emulsifying fats for action by intestinal lipases
2. Facilitate absorption of fats, fat-soluble vitamins, iron, and calcium
3. Activate the release of pancreatic and intestinal enzymes

Mixed in with bile are waste products such as bilirubin; thus the release of bile into the duodenum is one way in which wastes are excreted from the body. Because bile can be released directly from the liver into the duodenum, the removal of the gallbladder has no long-term consequences.

Pancreatic system

The pancreatic system includes the exocrine glands of the pancreas (acinar cells) and a ductal system (Fig. 31-3). (The endocrine functions of the pancreas are described in Chapter 29.) Acinar cells release their secretions into ducts that converge to form the main pancreatic duct (duct of Wirsung). In most persons, the pancreatic duct merges into the common bile duct at its entry into the duodenum, but in some persons the common bile duct and pancreatic duct do not merge.

The acinar cells of the pancreas secrete two substances: one is an iso-osmolar solution with a high con-

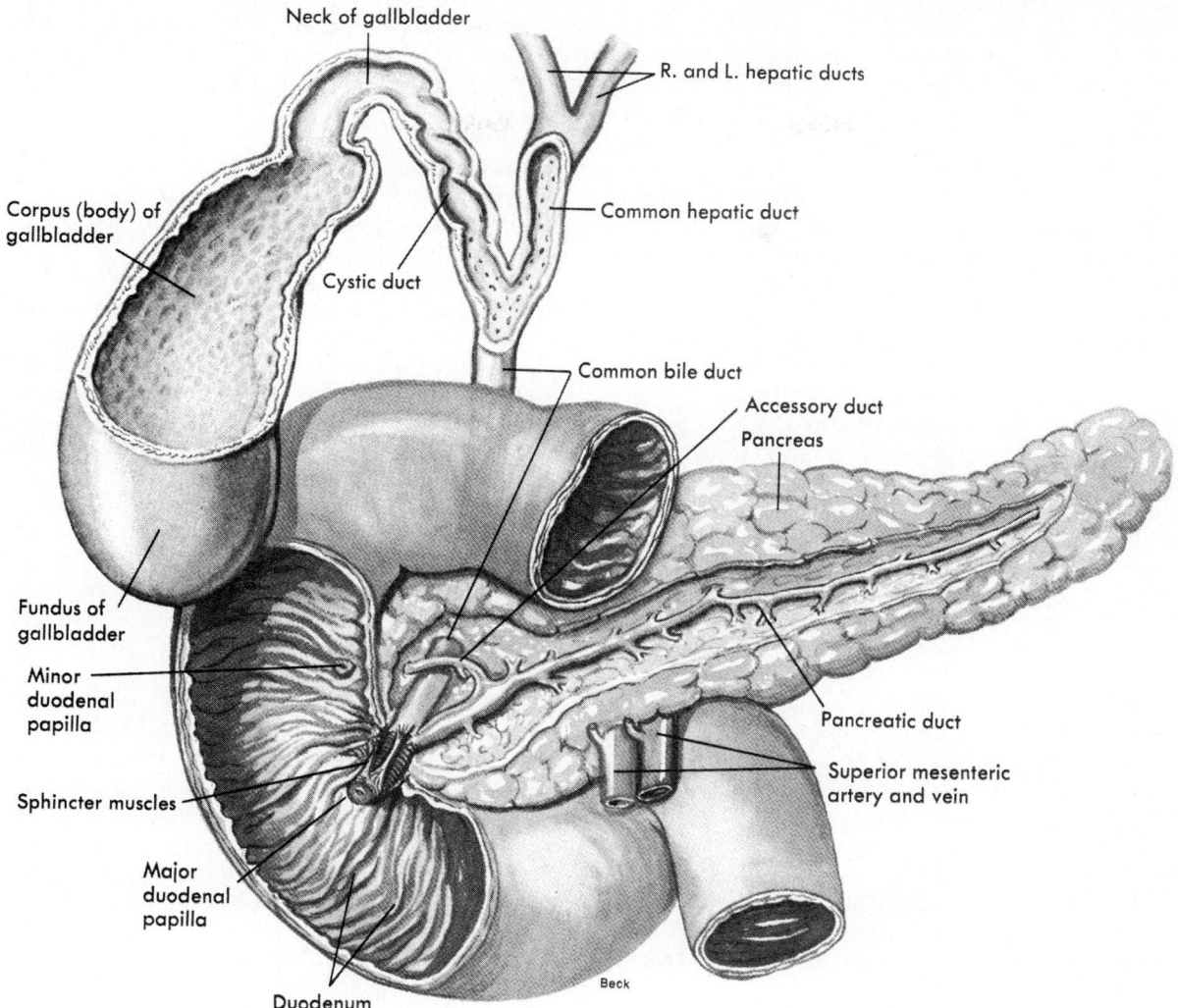

Neck of gallbladder

R. and L. hepatic ducts

Corpus (body) of gallbladder

Common hepatic duct

Cystic duct

Common bile duct

Accessory duct

Pancreas

Fundus of gallbladder

Minor duodenal papilla

Pancreatic duct

Sphincter muscles

Superior mesenteric artery and vein

Major duodenal papilla

Duodenum

Beck

Fig. 31-3. Anatomic schemata of biliary and pancreatic ductal systems. Note head of pancreas surrounds common bile duct. (From Anthony, C.P., and Thibodeau, G.A.: Textbook of anatomy and physiology, ed. 11, St. Louis, 1983, The C.V. Mosby Co.)

centration of bicarbonate, and the other contains multiple digestive enzymes.

1. Proteolytic enzymes: trypsinogen, chymotrypsinogen, and procarboxypeptidase
2. Amylotic enzyme: amylase
3. Lipolytic enzymes: lipases
4. Nucleolytic enzymes: ribonuclease and deoxyribonuclease

The pancreatic exocrine secretions are released under the influence of the vagus nerve and secretin, cholecystokinin-pancreozymin, and gastrin during digestion. Gastrin is released during the gastric phase and stimulates the release of bicarbonate-rich solution. The entry of chyme and acids into the small intestines stimulates the release of secretin and cholecystokinin-pancreozymin. Secretin then stimulates further secretion of the pancreatic bicarbonate-rich solution, and cholecystokinin-

pancreozymin stimulates the release of the pancreatic enzyme-rich solution.

PREVENTION AND HEALTH EDUCATION

Primary prevention

HEPATITIS

Certain diseases of the hepatic system can be prevented. For example, the spread of viral hepatitis can be halted if the public is taught to use good hygienic practices and proper sterilization techniques.

Toxic hepatitis also can be prevented if the public is informed about precautions in the use of toxic substances. Since cleaning agents, solvents, and related substances sometimes contain substances that are harmful to the liver, the public should read instructions on labels and should follow them explicitly. Dry-cleaning fluids may contain carbon tetrachloride, which can cause liver injury if warnings to avoid inhalation of the fumes and to keep windows open are not heeded. If people must use these agents inside the home, a good practice is to open the windows wide, to use the cleaning materials as quickly as possible, and then to vacate the premises for several hours, leaving the windows open.

Many solvents used to remove paint and plastic material and to stain and finish woodwork contain injurious substances and should be used outdoors—not in the basement—since dangerous fumes may spread throughout the house. Cleaning agents and finishes for cars should be applied outdoors or in a garage with the door open. Nurses in industry have a responsibility to teach the importance of observing regulations to avoid industrial hazards, such as exposure to nitrobenzene, tetrachloroethane, carbon disulfide, and dinitrotoluol.

Some drugs that are known to cause mild damage to the liver must be used therapeutically. A safe rule to follow is to avoid taking any medication except that specifically prescribed by a physician for a specific ailment.

CIRRHOSIS OF THE LIVER

Cirrhosis of the liver as a cause of death in the United States now ranks fifth in persons between the ages of 45 and 64 years of age, with more men and nonwhites in the higher risk groups. Programs aimed at the prevention of cirrhosis are designed primarily to control the ingestion of alcohol. Prevention of alcohol addiction and early intervention in the disease of alcoholism are two important measures in reducing the incidence and severity of pancreatitis, alcoholic hepatitis and cirrhosis, and selected gastrointestinal disorders.

GALLSTONES

It is not possible at this time to prevent gallstones, the most prevalent disorder of the biliary tract. Populations that are at higher risk are people who are obese and those with certain metabolic and hemolytic disorders. Patients who tend to form stones in the ducts are usually advised to be careful of their fat intake and to drink generous amounts of fluids.

Secondary prevention: detection of disease

Early detection of disease is always important if treatment is to be most beneficial. This is well illustrated by several disorders to be discussed in this chapter. For example, nonspecific gastrointestinal distress may be noticed by patients long before specific symptoms of tumors of the liver, the pancreas, and bile ducts become apparent. Nurses can encourage persons who complain of vague but persistent symptoms to seek medical evaluation. The use of home remedies or over-the-counter preparations can also delay proper diagnosis of serious illnesses.

VIRAL HEPATITIS

Viral hepatitis is by far the most important infection attacking the liver. It is a reportable disease in all states. Centers for Disease Control (CDC) statistics indicate that viral hepatitis is one of the four most frequently reported infectious diseases in the United States. It is well accepted that the figures for any given year may be grossly underestimated, since persons with subclinical manifestations are often not reported as having active disease.

There are three types of viral hepatitis, type A (HAV); type B (HBV); and type non-A, non-B (Table 31-1). Other terms used in the past for the types of hepatitis reflect differences in incubation period and mode of transmission. Several tests using serologic markers have been developed to detect infection by HAV and HBV. (Non-A, non-B hepatitis is identified by exclusion.) The four most commonly used tests are described in Table 31-2. HBsAg (formerly called Australian antigen) is the first test performed; if this test is positive, no further tests are done. The tests are used when there is reason to believe hepatitis is clinically present.

A simple test is available as a screening test for bilirubinuria. The test is done by placing 5 drops of urine on the Icotest reagent tablet. Since bilirubin is present in the urine of the person who has viral hepatitis before clinical signs appear, it has been suggested that as part of a disease detection program this test be done on anyone exposed to hepatitis, on all schoolchildren, on hospital patients and employees, on blood donors, on employees in public institutions and industrial plants, and on food handlers. Early recognition of the disease would make control of its spread easier.

An important step in prevention of hepatitis has been the mandatory screening of blood donors for HBsAg. This has greatly reduced the incidence of type B hepatitis, but type B hepatitis can occur if the donor's level of HBsAg is below detectable levels. There is no screening test for the non-A, non-B virus.

Immunization

Three agents are now available for postexposure prophylaxis of hepatitis. The most current CDC guidelines should be used to determine which is most appropriate in a given situation.

1. Immune serum globulin (ISG) provides temporary and passive immunity; modifies the severity of hepatitis infection
2. Hepatitis B immune globulin (HBIG, Anti-HBs, hyperimmune serum globulin) provides temporary and passive immunity, specific for HBV; used when the source of contact is known to have a positive test for HBsAg
3. Hepatitis B vaccine (HbVac, inactivated hepatitis B) has been available since 1981 for stimulating active immunity for HBV in high-risk populations.

Table 31-1. Characteristics of different types of viral hepatitis

Characteristic	Hepatitis A	Hepatitis B	Hepatitis non-A,non-B
Previous names	Infectious Epidemic Short-incubation	Serum Homologous serum Long-incubation	None
Onset	Abrupt, febrile	Insidious, seldom febrile	Insidious, often non-icteric
Incubation period			
Onset	10-40 days	45-180 days	14-150 days
Average	30	90	50
Incidence	50% of cases	25% of cases	25% of cases
Primary sources	Fecally contaminated food, water, milk, shellfish	Blood, serum, plasma	Blood, serum, plasma
Primary route of infection	Fecal-oral	Percutaneous, sexual	Percutaneous, sexual
Mortality	Less than 0.5%	1-5%	1-3%
Populations:			
Posttransfusion	No	10% of cases	90% of cases
Age	Younger	Older	Older
High risk	Low income, overcrowded, institutionalized	Health care workers, patients and staff in dialysis units, laboratory workers, homosexuals, drug users	Recipients of blood transfusions or blood components
Carrier state	Does not occur	Occurs	Occurs
Prophylaxis	Gamma globulin (ISG) ameliorates severity	Hepatitis B immune globulin (HBIG) at 1 week, repeated at 1 month reduces risk of infection Hepatitis B vaccine (HbVac)	Not available
Major preventive measures	Sanitation controls (food, water, milk, sewage), pollution control of lakes and rivers; "enteric" precautions with diagnosed cases	Screening of blood donors for HBsAg or history of jaundice; use of volunteers who donate blood rather than those who receive pay; use of disposable and individual equipment for parenteral administration; avoidance of blood products from pooled sources; blood/body secretions precautions with diagnosed cases	

Table 31-2. Serologic tests for hepatitis antigens and antibodies

Test*	Hepatitis A (HAV)	Hepatitis B (HBV)	Hepatitis non-A, non-B
HAV-Ab/IgM	Positive test, develops early in the disease, 4-6 weeks after infection	Not positive	Not positive
HBsAg	Not positive	Positive test, develops 4-12 weeks after infection; it is also positive in chronic infections of HBV and in carrier states	Not positive
HBcAb	Not positive	Develops 2-16 weeks after infection; indicates past infection with HBV	Not positive
HBsAb	Not positive	Develops 2-10 months after infection; reflects clinical recovery and immunity	Not positive

*Ab, Antibodies; Ag, Antigens; s, Surface marker (viral coating); c, Core viral material (Dane particle).

The effectiveness of immunization is increased when post exposure prophylaxis is started early. Health care workers should promptly report to the agency health service any contamination by needle-pricks or other skin-penetrating wounds.

Anyone who has been exposed to viral hepatitis should be urged to report this fact to the physician. This is especially important for a woman in the second or third trimester of pregnancy. Although the role of transplacentally transmitted viral hepatitis in causing injury to the liver in newborn infants has not been determined, the disease is believed to increase the likelihood of abortion, stillbirth, and congenital abnormalities.

It is also recommended that persons planning to travel to areas where hepatitis A is endemic receive immune serum globulin. The dose for an adult is approximately 2 ml (0.01 ml/lb body weight) injected intramuscularly.

Preventing transmission

There is no specific treatment for viral hepatitis and no adequate immunization for type A or type non-A, non-B at this time; therefore, it is only by making use of what is known about the viruses that control can be accomplished.

Data on the physiochemical and biologic characteristics of the viruses are accumulating slowly. The hepatitis viruses are extremely resistant to such antimicrobial measures as drying, chlorination, disinfectants, heat, ultraviolet light, radiation, and freezing. The viruses are especially refractive to such measures when protected by the presence of serum proteins. At boiling temperatures the viruses can survive for about 20 to 30 minutes. Autoclaving is the best method to ensure destruction of the viruses on contaminated articles. When boiling is the only available way to sterilize needles and other equipment, everything placed in the water sterilizer is *covered completely and boiled for at least 30 minutes.*

CDC guidelines

CDC guidelines for isolation differentiate control measures needed for type HAV and for types HBV and non-A, non-B hepatitis (the latter two types are treated similarly). HAV is assigned the category *enteric precautions* to prevent transmission of the disease by direct or indirect contact with feces. HBV and non-A, non-B hepatitis are classified as *blood/body fluid precautions* to prevent transmission of the disease by direct or indirect contact with blood and body fluids.

The following guidelines are recommended for use with *all* patient *not* designated as having hepatitis to prevent the nurse from contacting hepatitis from persons who are unidentified as contagious or who are carriers and from transmitting the virus to others.

1. Handwashing before and after patient contact is essential.
2. Disposable needles, syringes, and other equipment in contact with blood are placed in rigid containers that are later incinerated.
3. Disposable gloves are suggested for use when handling soiled urinals, catheters, bedpans, or commodes or when the patient or bed linens are soiled by body excreta or secretions.
4. Containers for body secretions should be plastic or waterproof.
5. All patients should have their own thermometer if disposable equipment is not used.
6. Good housekeeping practices should be mandatory in areas where food is prepared or served and in bathrooms.

Hepatitis type A

The presence of HAV in stool and blood is highest during the incubation period and in the early symptomatic phase. It is not necessary to isolate the patient with HAV for the entire icteric period; usually isolation can be removed one week after the onset of jaundice. CDC guidelines contain the most current details for enteric isolation for HAV. A carrier state is not known for HAV. Patients with HAV require no special directions if they are discharged after the communicable period.

Hepatitis types B and non-A, non-B

Less is known about non-A, non-B hepatitis than the other two types. Current practice is to use similar precautions for HBV and non-A, non-B hepatitis. The viruses for these two types remain in the blood for much longer periods of time than for HAV; thus isolation may be used for the entire hospitalization period. CDC guidelines contain the most current details for blood/body fluids precautions for these two types of hepatitis. A carrier state is recognized when the HBsAg test remains positive for 6 months; asymptomatic carriers can be a source of infection.

Patients with HBV or non-A, non-B hepatitis are instructed to prevent transmission of the disease to others. Specific instructions for at home include the importance of the following:

1. Handwashing before eating and after use of toilet
2. Separate equipment for hygiene (razor, toothbrush, drinking glass, and so on)
3. Avoiding mucous membrane contact (kissing, sexual contact) until the physician recommends otherwise as based on laboratory results
4. Cleanliness of bathroom and kitchen areas
5. Use of detergents with bleaching agents and hot water cycle for laundry
6. Use of hot water for dishwashing

Special attention in homegoing instruction is given when unusual exposure to feces, blood, or secretions is expected (for example, incontinent patients, hemodialysis patients). Disposable gloves should be used by caregivers. (Although fecal-oral transmission is considered negligible in these two types of hepatitis, feces can be contaminated by blood from lower gastrointestinal mucosal sites and the virus transmitted through breaks in skin.)

Major health problems

Disorders that are encountered in the liver, the biliary system, and the pancreas include not only those caused by infectious organisms but also abnormalities from changes in structure and function. The more common disorders are outlined below.

1. Disorders of the hepatic system
   a. Focal hepatocellular disorders
      1. Liver abscess
      2. Trauma to the liver
      3. Tumors of the liver
   b. Diffuse hepatocellular disorders
      1. Hepatitis

2. Cirrhosis of the liver
3. Hepatic coma
2. Disorders of the biliary system
   a. Cholecystitis
   b. Cholelithiasis
   c. Carcinoma of the biliary system
3. Disorders of the pancreas
   a. Pancreatitis
   b. Tumors of the pancreas.

DISORDERS OF THE LIVER

A variety of pathologic states can affect the liver. Diseases of the liver may be classified in several ways. In this chapter, disorders secondary to focal damage and disorders secondary to diffuse damage will be discussed.

PATHOPHYSIOLOGY

Focal hepatocellular disorders

The three most common focal disorders of the liver, their etiologies, signs and symptoms, and medical therapies are listed in Table 31-3. Each disorder will be discussed briefly.

Liver abscess

Liver abscesses may result from a variety or organisms. The most common pyogenic organisms are *Escherichia coli* and *Staphylococcus aureus*. In pyogenic abscesses the bacteria cause pus formation and a pus-filled cavity. *Entamoeba histolytica* is also an important worldwide cause of amebic liver abscess and dysentery. In amebic infections the vegetative form of the organism moves from the gut to the small portal canaliculi in the liver, where it becomes activated, releasing enzymes that cause local tissue destruction. Multiple abscesses occur. The clinical manifestations of liver abscess are often nonspecific.

Trauma to the liver

Because of its location and size, the liver is frequently subjected to trauma. If the injury is severe, rupture of the liver may occur with severe internal hemorrhage. Injury to the liver may occur with trauma to the chest or abdomen.

Severe lacerations or rupture of the liver has a mortality estimated to be about 30%. Death that occurs shortly after the injury is caused by uncontrollable hepatic hemorrhage. This happens in part because the walls of the hepatic veins are thin, the liver is highly vascular, and the bile mixing with the blood interferes with clotting. Deaths occurring later after injury may be caused by biliary peritonitis, shock, or infections.

Small lacerations or ruptures of the liver, except for temporary peritoneal irritations from blood oozing into the peritoneal cavity, usually heal and leave a subcapsular scar. In some instances the hematoma may become infected, with abscess formation complicating the healing process. Hepatic cysts may also develop. Trauma that causes severe contusions may result in subsequent degen-

Table 31-3. Focal disorders of the liver

Disorder	Etiology	Signs and symptoms	Medical therapy
Liver abscess	Infection complication, of obstructed biliary tract, contiguous viscera, intestinal tract, septicemia; traumatic injury to liver, amebic abscess	Fever, chills Vague abdominal discomfort, tenderness over liver, palpable liver Jaundice, leukocytosis ↑ serum alkaline phosphatase ↑ SGOT	Surgical incision and drainage Broad spectrum antimicrobial therapy for pyogenic abscess Amebic abscess: emetine hydrochloride, chloroquine, metronidazole
Trauma to liver	Penetrating stab wounds Blunt wounds (automobile accidents or falls)	Variable signs: pain, shock, abdominal rigidity Blood or bile with peritoneal tap	Drainage Suture and drainage Resection Blood volume management Antimicrobial therapy
Carcinoma of liver	Primary risk factors: hepatitis, cirrhosis, hepatotoxins, trauma Metastasis from any site but commonly from carcinoma of abdominal viscera, breast, lung, kidney, ovary, testes, skin	Weight loss, weakness Jaundice, anemia Ascites, edema Upper right quadrant pain, hepatomegaly Unexplained fever Elevated liver enzymes (SGOT, SGPT) Elevated sedimentation rate	Surgical excision Chemotherapy: methotrexate, 5-fluorouracil, doxorubicin (Adriamycin), mitomycin C; often administered by hepatic artery perfusion Homotransplantation Decompression of biliary tract

eration of the injured hepatic cells. The prognosis depends on the amount of tissue damaged, and the final outcome for the patient may not be known for many years after the initial injury.

Tumors of the liver

Tumors of the liver may be either malignant or benign. Benign lesions include hemangiomas, cysts, and rarely adenomas. These benign tumors occasionally enlarge enough to become symptomatic and present problems in differentiation from a malignant tumor. If the latter occurs, surgical intervention may be required.

Malignant tumors may be metastatic or primary. *Metastatic tumors* are common; they occur 20 times more frequently than primary tumors and rank second to cirrhosis as a cause of fatal liver disease.[16] Metastatic carcinoma of the liver varies from a few small nodules to large nodes. Adjacent nodes may eventually grow together and compress the surrounding liver tissue. Usually different parts of the liver are uniformly involved so that liver biopsy may be a useful diagnostic aid.

Primary hepatic carcinomas may arise within the liver (hepatocellular) or the bile duct cell (cholangiocellular) or may be of mixed origin. Hepatocellular tumors are the most common. Primary liver cancer accounts for only 1% to 2% of malignant tumors found at death in the United States. They are more common in men and usually occur in the fifth and sixth decades of life.

Primary lesions may be multiple or singular, diffuse or nodular, and may spread to only a lobe or to the entire liver. The cancerous cells appear to compress the surrounding normal liver cells and to spread quickly by invading the portal vein branches. Spread may be by direct extension to surrounding tissue. Primary cancers also tend to cause hemorrhage and necrosis. The most common site for metastasis of the primary liver lesion is the lung, but it may metastasize elsewhere. Primary lesions tend to grow rapidly, sometimes without signs or symptoms, and the patient may live only a short time after onset.

Jaundice and ascites are signs that the metastic or primary process is quite far advanced. Extreme weakness is also usually an outstanding symptom. Ascites occurs secondary to compression of the portal vein. Gastointestinal bleeding may also be present and may confuse the diagnosis. A special blood test that may be used to help diagnose primary liver carcinoma is the high serum concentrations of alpha-fetoprotein (AFP).

Diffuse hepatocellular disorders

Regardless of the specific pathologic condition, disorders secondary to diffuse parenchymal damage present the patient with common problems. These problems will be discussed before the specific disorders of *hepatitis,* acute inflammation of the liver, and *cirrhosis,* chronic fibrotic disease of the liver, are discussed.

Table 31-4. Bile pigment metabolism: jaundice

Types of liver cell dysfunction	Serum bilirubin (conjugated)	Serum bilirubin (unconjugated)	Total serum bilirubin (conjugated and unconjugated)	Urine urobilinogen	Urine bilirubin	Stool	Jaundice (icterus)
Normal	<0.2 mg/dl	<0.2 mg/dl	+	±	0	Brown	0
Hemolytic	<0.2 mg/dl	>0.2 mg/dl	+ +	+ + + +	0	Dark brown	Light reddish yellow
Familial	<0.2 mg/dl	>0.2 mg/dl	+ +	±	0	Brown (normal)	Reddish yellow
Hepatitis	+	>0.2 mg/dl	+ +	+ + +	+ +	Light brown	Deep reddish yellow
Cirrhosis	+	>0.2 mg/dl	+ +	+ + +	+ +	Light brown	Deep reddish yellow
Incomplete biliary obstruction	+ +	>0.2 mg/dl	+ + +	Variable and fluctuating	+ + +	Light	Light to deep greenish yellow
Complete biliary obstruction	+ + +	>0.2 mg/dl	+ + + +	0	+ + +	Clay colored	Deep greenish

Common manifestation of diffuse hepatocellular disorders

JAUNDICE. Jaundice is a symptom complex caused by a disturbance of the physiology of bile pigment and is present in many diseases of the liver, pancreas, and biliary system. There is an excess of bile pigment in the blood, which eventually is distributed to the skin, mucous membranes, and other body fluids and body tissues, giving them a yellow discoloration.

Jaundice, caused by faulty liver function as a result of disease of the hepatic cells, is described as *hepatocellular*. This type of jaundice results from acute, diffuse response of the liver cells to injury by viruses or toxins (hepatitis) or as part of the chronic syndrome of cirrhosis.

When jaundice results from intrahepatic or extrahepatic obstruction that interferes with the flow of bile, it is described as *obstructive*. Intrahepatic obstruction is illustrated by cholestasis (suppression of bile flow), a side effect that may result from certain drugs, for example, phenothiazines. The site of pathology is the canaliculi or the small biliary ductules. Frequent causes of extrahepatic obstruction are gallstones lodged in the common bile duct, pancreatitis, and carcinoma of the head of the pancreas. Fig. 31-3 illustrates how pancreatic enlargement can compress the common bile duct.

Jaundice may also be caused by destruction of great numbers of blood cells *(hemolytic)*, which results in the production of excessive amounts of bilirubin and the inability of the liver to excrete the bilirubin as rapidly as it forms.

Regardless of the type of jaundice, the following effects are observed:

1. Increase in plasma concentration of bilirubin
2. Increase in excretion of conjugated bilirubin
3. Increase or decrease in the amount of bilirubin that reaches the intestines
4. Alteration in amount of urobilinogen excreted in the urine

The results of interference with bile flow or bilirubin production are summarized in Table 31-4. The presence of bile pigment in the skin causes *pruritus* (itching) in about 20% to 25% of the patients who have jaundice.

BLEEDING TENDENCIES AND ANEMIA. Bleeding tendencies and anemia are common complications of liver disease. They may occur in persons with advanced hepatitis, cirrhosis, and biliary duct obstruction. These tendencies are a result of deficiencies in the formation of clotting factors, thrombocytopenia, and a deficiency of erythrocytes. In patients with obstructive jaundice and liver disease, the synthesis of various clotting factors is impaired. If the patient's bile duct is obstructed, absorption of fat and vitamin K (fat-soluble) is reduced. Even if vitamin K is absorbed, severely damaged liver cells cannot synthesize adequate amounts of these factors, especially prothrombin. Other vitamin deficiencies (A, B complex, D) may also result from decreased absorption of fat-soluble vitamins and the inability to store the vitamins.

The patient with liver disease may also develop an enlarged spleen as a result of portal hypertension. This is believed to be responsible for the resulting thrombocytopenia and increased red blood cell destruction.

Various other factors contribute to the anemia, including blood loss from gastrointestinal bleeding and decreased red blood cell production secondary to folic acid deficiency and poor protein intake. In addition, alcohol has a direct toxic effect on bone marrow.

INFECTION. The patient with diffuse hepatocellular disease is at risk for infection. Depressed protein synthesis, lymphatic obstruction of the splanchnic organs, impaired Kupffer cells, and depressed bone marrow all play a part. Leukopenia may be present.

FLUID AND ELECTROLYTE ALTERATIONS. Fluid volume deficit results when body losses exceed body gains and should be considered when the following symptoms are seen:

1. Vomiting
2. Anorexia with decreased intake
3. Hemorrhage
4. Diarrhea
5. Bilary or pancreatic drainage

It is important that nurses understand that patients with *hypoalbuminemia* (serum level below 4.0 g/dl) may have a contracted intravascular volume, even in the presence of edema and ascites. This phenomenon is seen most often in cirrhosis and results from the decreased production of albumin and the continued loss of this protein into the peritoneal cavity. As a result, the colloidal osmotic pressure of the blood is decreased (leading to increased fluid filtration through the capillary wall) while the return of fluid to the capillary is impaired. The patient is less able to maintain adequate perfusion of tissues should blood volume decrease further.

The several factors that lead to *ascites* (accumulation of serous fluid in the peritoneal cavity) are illustrated in Fig. 31-4. The sequence of these mechanisms and how they interact to intensify ascites is not well established. A vicious cycle is established as the albumin lost into the peritoneal cavity further decreases the patient's serum albumin level.

Hydrothorax and ankle and presacral edema may accompany the ascites. The patient with cirrhosis frequently retains abnormal amounts of water and sodium. Although total body sodium and water excess occur, *hyponatremia* is frequent and reflects the disproportional retention of water in comparison to sodium.

Renal function is also believed to affect fluid and electrolyte balance in patients with liver disease. Alterations in renal function may occur because of decreased blood volume, portal hypertension, and increased circulating hormones. Decreased excretion of water, sodium, and metabolic wastes is common. Oliguria and azotemia (nitrogen wastes in the blood) may occur abruptly and signal hepato-renal syndrome. Although renal medullary bloodflow is maintained in this condition, there is a marked decrease in renal cortical bloodflow. Precipitants of this condition, which has a mortality rate of nearly 90%, are:

1. Diuretic therapy
2. Parecentesis
3. Gastrointestinal hemorrhage

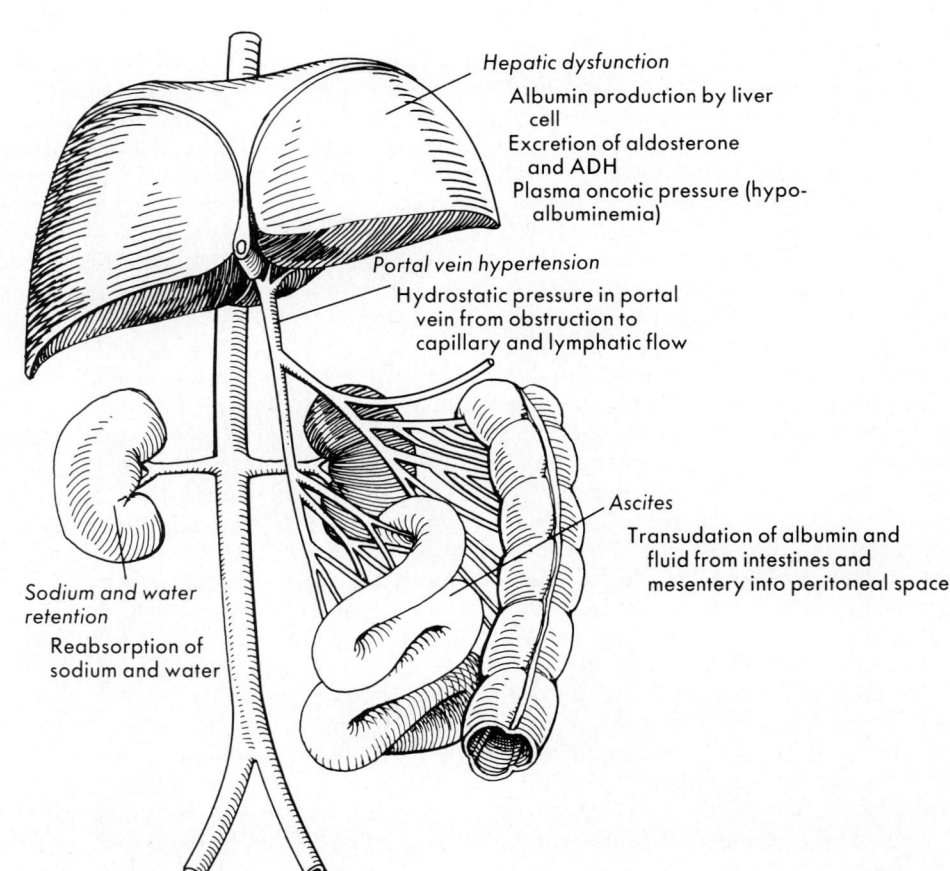

Hepatic dysfunction
Albumin production by liver cell
Excretion of aldosterone and ADH
Plasma oncotic pressure (hypo-albuminemia)

Portal vein hypertension
Hydrostatic pressure in portal vein from obstruction to capillary and lymphatic flow

Ascites
Transudation of albumin and fluid from intestines and mesentery into peritoneal space

Sodium and water retention
Reabsorption of sodium and water

Fig. 31-4. Factors contributing to ascites in hepatic disease.

Hepatitis

Hepatitis may be defined as any acute inflammatory disease of the liver. Although the term *hepatitis* is most commonly used in conjunction with viral hepatitis, the disease can be caused by toxic injury to the liver, viruses, or bacteria (Table 31-5).

TOXIC HEPATITIS. The pathologic changes in the liver will depend on the toxic agent (see box below). For example, necrosis and fatty infiltrates are present when the causative agent is carbon tetrachloride, whereas cholestasis with portal inflammation is seen when the toxic agent is chlorpromazine.[16]

Two types of chemical hepatotoxicity occur: direct toxic and idiosyncratic. In direct toxic hepatitis, the agent causes toxicity with predictable regularity and is dose dependent. In idiosyncratic toxic hepatitis the reactions are sporadic and is not dose dependent, suggesting host idiosyncrasy.

Common hepatotoxins

Drugs: chlorpromazine, isoniazid, tetracycline, thiazide, thiouracil, acetaminopyhen
Organic solvents: carbon tetrachloride, methylenedianiline (MDA)
Phosphorus, heavy metals
Plant poisons
Alcohol

VIRAL HEPATITIS
ACUTE VIRAL HEPATITIS

Viral hepatitis causes diffuse inflammatory infiltration of hepatic tissue. With typical viral hepatitis, there is no collapse of lobules, no loss of lobular architecture, and minimal or no fibrosis. Inflammation, degeneration, and regeneration may occur simultaneously, distorting the normal lobular pattern and possibly creating pressure about the portal vein. Laboratory findings include elevations in serum levels of transaminase (SGOT), prothrombin time, alkaline phophatase, and bilirubin. Because the pathologic process is usually distributed evenly throughout the liver, biopsy in most cases is diagnostic for viral hepatitis.

In most instances of nonfatal viral hepatitis, regeneration begins almost with the onset of the disease. The damaged cells are removed by phagocytosis and enzymatic reaction, and the liver returns to normal.

The outcome of viral hepatitis may be affected by such factors as the following:

1. Virulence of the virus
2. Amount of hepatic damage sustained before exposure to the virus
3. Natural barriers to damage and disease of the liver
4. Supportive care patient receives when symptoms appear

The majority of patients recover normal liver function, but the disease may take several courses; different terms describe each of them (see box, p. 845).

The three types of viral hepatitis are described on p. 837. Symptoms of the various types are not clinically distinctive from each other except that acute symptoms may be more severe in hepatitis A. Symptoms usually appear from 4 to 7 days before jaundice is apparent. Anorexia is

---

Table 31-5. Diffuse disorders of the liver

Disorder	Etiology	Signs and symptoms	Medical therapy
Viral hepatitis	Hepatitis virus A (HAV) Hepatitis virus B (HBV) (see Table 31-1)	Preicteric stage: Anorexia, nausea and vomiting, chils and fever, arthralgia, right upper quadrant tenderness, fatigue	Rest Diet: high calorie, high protein, low fat Avoidance of toxins
		Icteric stage: Jaundice (yellow sclera and skin), dark urine, light colored stools Post-icteric stage: fatigue	Vitamin K
	Atypical course (see box, p. 845)	Signs of liver failure similar to those seen in cirrhosis	Treatment based on dysfunction Corticosteroids may be used Dialysis

Continued.

Table 31-5. Diffuse disorders of the liver—cont'd

Disorder	Etiology	Signs and symptoms	Medical therapy
Cirrhosis of the liver	Alcohol, malnutrition, hepatotoxins, biliary obstruction, congestive heart failure, metabolic problems, infectious diseases, gastrointestinal diseases	Malaise Gastrointestinal symptoms: anorexia, indigestion, nausea, vomiting, flatulence, altered bowel function Malnutrition: muiscle wasting, muscle weakness, loss of weight Fluid retention: edema, ascites, abdominal distention, hydrothorax (often on right), weight gain Jaundice: pruritus, hypoprothrombinemia, steatorrhea, light colored stools, dark urine Hepatomegaly, splenomegaly Hyperestrinism: palmar erythema, gynecomastia, spider angiomas, sparse body hair, testicular atrophy Portal hypertension: caput medusae, hemorrhoids, esophageal varices, edema of lower extremities Gastrointestinal bleeding Esophageal varices, gastric or duodenal ulcers Bleeding tendencies purpura, hematuria, gingival bleeding, epistaxis, melena, hematemesis Anemia: Pallor, fatigue, ↓ RBC, hematocrit and hemoglobin	Rest Diet: high calorie, normal to high protein (unless ammonia toxicity is present), low fat, vitamin supplement (A, B, C, D) Bile salts Abstinence from alcohol Serum and water restriction Furosemide, spironolactone Albumin infusion (salt-poor) Peritoneal-jugular shunt (PJS) Paracentesis Antihistamines, tranquilizer, Vitamin K (Hykinone) Bile salts Surgical procedures that shunt blood away from liver Fresh blood transfusion, plasma expanders, normal saline (IV) Esophageal tamponade Iced saline lavage Pitressin (IV) Measures to prevent hepatic coma Vitamin K Transfusions of whole blood, plasma, platelets High protein diet with supplements of vitamins and folic acid Splenectomy
Hepatic coma	Precipitating factors: Infection, high protein intake, GI bleeding, blood transfusions, hypokalemia, alkalosis	Prehepatic coma: Impaired attention span, impaired concentration, apathy, insomnia, slurred speech, yawning, asterixis, fetor hepaticus Coma: muscular rigidity, hyperreflexia, myoclonus seizures	Protein-free diet Enemas, cathartics Lactulose, neomycin Dialysis, exchange transfusion Corticosteroids Amino acid (arginine) or levodopa replacement Colon by-pass Liver transplant

one of the most frequent symptoms. This preicteric stage lasts for approximately 1 week and then subsides as hepatocellular jaundice occurs.

The icteric stage usually reaches its intensity in 2 weeks and may last from 4 to 6 weeks. The *posticteric* or convalescent stage begins with the disappearance of jaundice and may last from a few weeks to several months. Complete recovery is usually expected in 6 months. The disease may relapse during this stage, with recurrence of previous symptoms but to a milder degree.

Atypical courses of hepatitis

Submassive hepatic necrosis	Destruction of substantial group of adjacent cells but without destruction of the greater part of a lobule
Massive hepatic necrosis	Destruction of whole lobule
Fulminant viral hepatitis	Sudden and severe degeneration of the liver
Subacute fatal viral hepatitis	Slower severe degeneration of the liver

---

CHRONIC VIRAL HEPATITIS

Chronic hepatitis can occur in all types but is seldom seen with hepatitis A. Chronic hepatitis occurs in 10% of patients with HBV and 25% of those with non-A, non-B. *Chronic active hepatitis* is characterized by signs and symptoms of liver disease or abnormal liver function tests for periods greater than 6 months. During this time there is extension of the necrosis with loss of normal structure and function. Very frequently the disease progresses to cirrhosis. If left untreated, most patients will die within 4 to 5 years; about 75% respond well to corticosteroid treatment.

Chronic persistent hepatitis is characterized by abnormal liver function tests, fatigue and hepatomegally for greater than 6 months, but there is no necrosis and no increase in mortality.

Cirrhosis of the liver

Cirrhosis of the liver refers to several diseases that are characterized by diffuse inflammation and fibrosis of the liver that result in drastic structural changes and significant loss of liver function. The basic processes leading to cirrhosis are liver cell death with scar tissue formation and regeneration of cell mass that causes distortion of the structure with a resultant change in circulation. Destruction of the lymphatic system and the capillary bed (sinusoids) retards the portal vein bloodflow and thereby increases the volume and pressure of blood in the portal vein.

The major types of cirrhosis are described in Table 31-6. Postnecrotic cirrhosis from infectious disease is the most common type on a worldwide basis. More rare non-

---

Table 31-6. Types of cirrhosis

Type	Etiology	Description
Laennec's cirrhosis (nutritional, portal, or alcoholic cirrhosis)	Alcoholism, malnutrition	Massive collagen formation; liver in early fatty stage is large and firm; in late state it is small and nodular
Postnecrotic cirrhosis	Massive necrosis from hepatotoxins, usually viral hepatitis	Liver is decreased in size with nodules and fibrous tissue
Biliary cirrhosis	Biliary obstruction in liver and common bile duct	Chronic impairment of bile drainage; liver is first large then becomes firm and nodular; jaundice is major symptom
Cardiac cirrhosis	Right side congestive heart failure (CHF)	Liver is swollen and changes are reversible if CHF treated effectively; some fibrosis with long-standing CHF
Nonspecific, metabolic cirrhosis	Metabolic problems, infectious diseases, infiltrative diseases, gastrointestinal diseases	Portal and liver fibrosis may develop; liver is enlarged and firm

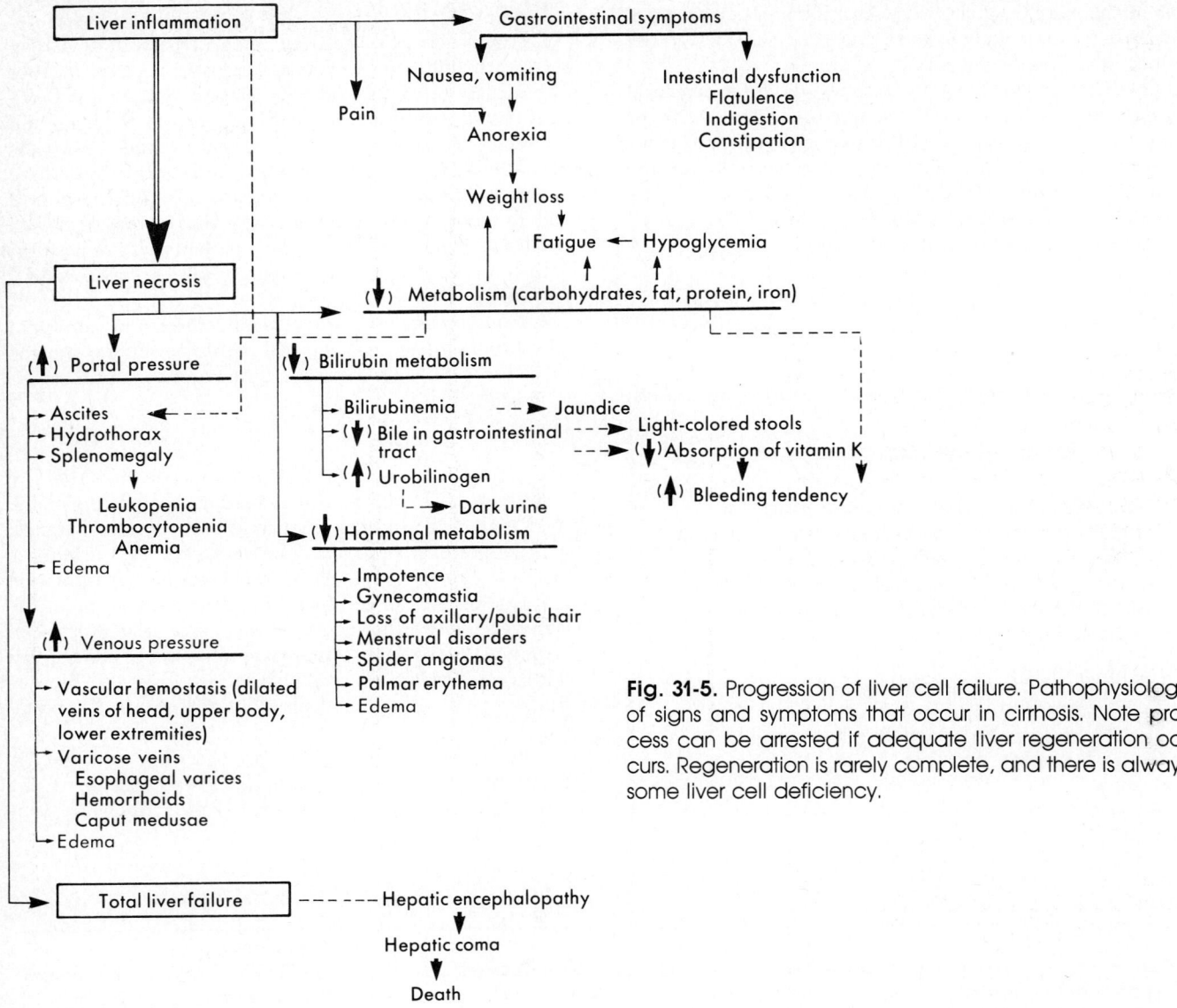

Fig. 31-5. Progression of liver cell failure. Pathophysiology of signs and symptoms that occur in cirrhosis. Note process can be arrested if adequate liver regeneration occurs. Regeneration is rarely complete, and there is always some liver cell deficiency.

specific types account for about 10% of deaths resulting from cirrhosis.

In Laennec's cirrhosis, the most common type in North America, chronic alcoholism is a frequent cause; it may also be caused by malnutrition associated with other diseases such as pancreatitis, diabetes mellitus, and ulcerative colitis. Alcoholics who develop liver disease first develop fatty degeneration of the liver. These fatty changes are usually reversible if appropriate treatment is instituted. If the degenerative process continues, acute inflammation (*alcoholic hepatitis*) and then *alcoholic cirrhosis* follow.

The signs and symptoms seen in cirrhosis are similar regardless of the cause and result from the progressive destruction of hepatic cells. Regeneration and proliferation of fibrous tissue cause obstruction of the portal vein. Cirrhosis is manifested clinically by the following several

alterations, discussed previously: portal hypertension, jaundice, bleeding tendencies and anemia, decreased resistance to infection, ascites, and edema.

Once the disease is established, it usually advances slowly to death. Many people, however, can be helped to live for years if they follow instructions. The liver has remarkable powers of regeneration. Sometimes sufficient collateral circulation can be established and sufficient repair of hepatic tissue can be accomplished so that symptoms subside for long periods. Unfortunately, at other times rapid deterioration occurs. Two crises are often responsible: hepatic coma and bleeding esophageal varices. Fig. 31-5 summarizes the numerous alterations that occur in cirrhosis of the liver.

As the cirrhotic process continues, the patient is prone to develop many life-threatening complications. Death may occur from total liver failure, bleeding esophageal

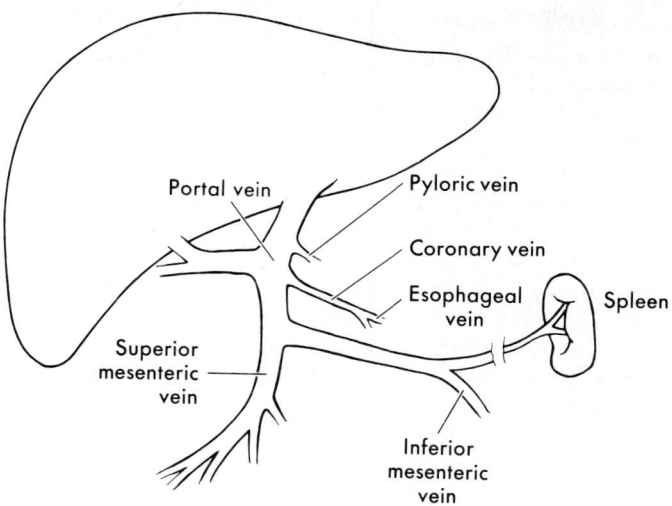

Fig. 31-6. Splanchnic veins. Venous drainage of splanchnic organs. When portal hypertension develops, other vessels can become engorged, leading to stasis and hypoxia of respective organs. (From Groër, M.E., and Shekleton, M.E.: Basic pathophysiology: a conceptual approach, ed. 2, St. Louis, 1983, The C.V. Mosby Co.)

varices, hepatic coma, or renal failure. Severe ascites and jaundice; neurologic symptoms; and decreased prothrombin, albumin, and sodium levels indicate a poor prognosis.

PORTAL HYPERTENSION. As circulation in the portal system becomes impaired because of sturctural changes in the liver, portal hypertension occurs (Fig. 31-6), producing splenomegaly and increasing edema of the lower extremities. As pressure increases in the portal veins, a back flow of blood into the veins emptying into the portal veins occurs. These veins in turn develop collateral channels of circulation. Collateral channels are most likely to occur in paraumbilicus veins, the hemorrhoidal veins, and the veins at the cardia of the stomach that extend into the esophagus. These veins become distended and tortuous because they are not anatomically equipped to handle large volumes of blood. This results in hemorrhoids, esophageal varices, and a ring of varicosities surrounding the umbilicus (caput medusae).

BLEEDING ESOPHAGEAL VARICES. Bleeding esophageal varices (Fig. 31-7) occur in approximately 30% of all patients with cirrhosis of the liver.[28] These small vessels become tortuous and fragile and may be affected by mechanical trauma from ingestion of coarse food and acid pepsin erosion, which may result in bleeding. Bleeding may also occur as a result of coughing, vomiting, sneezing, straining at stool (Valsalva's maneuver), or any physical exertion that increases abdominal venous pressure. Bleeding is frequently abrupt and without pain. Severe hematemesis and resultant shock may follow, requiring emergency treatment.

Hepatic coma

Hepatic coma (hepatic encephalopathy) is metabolic encephalopathy of the brain associated with liver failure.

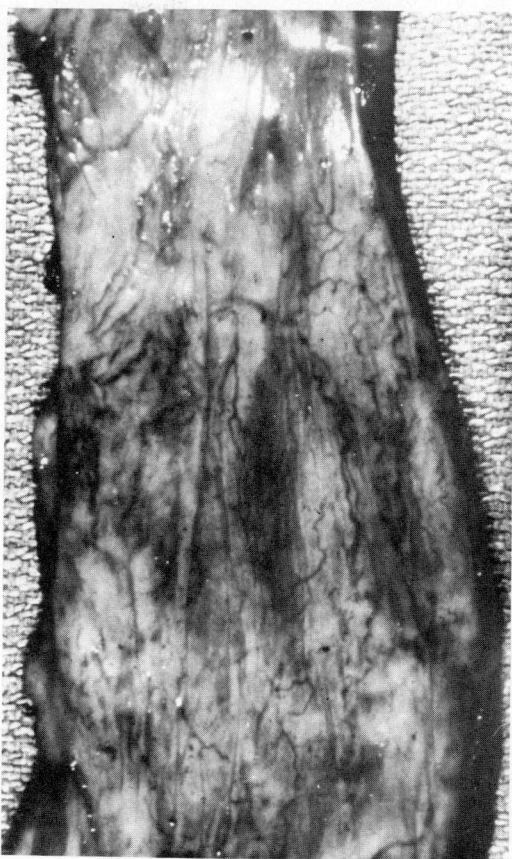

Fig. 31-7. Esophageal varices. Swollen varices and extensive collateral circulation are evident in segment of esophagus from patient with Laennec's cirrhosis. (From Groër, M.E. and Shekleton, M.E.: Basic pathophysiology: a conceptual approach, ed. 2, St. Louis, 1983, The C.V. Mosby Co.; Courtesy department of pathology, University of Tennessee, Knoxville).

Factors precipitating hepatic coma

Gastrointestinal ammonia (old blood in bowel from gastrointestinal hemorrhage)

High-protein intake

Transfusion, especially with stored blood

Thiazide diuretics and acetazolamide (Diamox)

Hypokalemia, secondary to thiazide diuretics or to potassium loss from the bowel

Shunting of blood into systemic circulation without passing through hepatic sinusoids (natural collateral bypass of blood or surgical bypass)

Alkalosis secondary to hyperventilation and hypokalemia

Hyperbilirubinemia (serum bilirubin greater than 35 mg/dl)

This dysfunction of the central nervous system is thought to be precipitated by elevated ammonia concentrations. Many patients with hepatic coma have an increase in blood ammonia concentration. Normally, ammonia, which is formed in the intestines from the breakdown of protein by intestinal bacteria, is converted to urea in the liver. When liver failure occurs, ammonia is not converted into urea and ammonia concentration in the circulating blood is increased. Factors that may precipitate hepatic coma are summarized in the box, p. 847.

ASSESSMENT

Subjective data

The patient's description of complaints or symptoms and course of illness yields useful data for the nurse who is planning care for the patient with liver disease. Among the potential symptoms, the following are explored:

1. Level of fatigue and amount of rest needed
2. Extent of pruritus and measures used to relieve it
3. Severity of anorexia; food intake patterns and likes and dislikes
4. Nausea or vomiting
5. History of ankle edema or ascites
6. Changes noted in mood, alertness, and mental ability
7. Pain: onset, location, measures used to relieve it
8. Episodes of bleeding, lightheadedness, or syncope
9. Known allergies or toxic agents

When viral hepatitis is a potential medical diagnosis, the past history often contributes clues as to the time and type of contact (blood or sera, polluted water, food, shellfish, and so on). The past history is also vital in determining the injurious agent in toxic hepatitis. The patient's description of the course of illness in chronic hepatitis or cirrhosis can be helpful in giving the nurse insight into the patient's understanding of the disease, its prognosis, and whether the patient believes there is control over its progress.

When alcohol ingestion is a factor, data from the patient should include the patient's knowledge of the effect of the alcohol and the person's desire to abstain from drinking (see Chapter 9).

Objective data

A thorough physical assessment is required on admission to obtain data for baseline comparisons. There is a possibility that any of the manifestations listed in left box below will be present in a patient with a liver disease; in the patient with cirrhosis, these manifestations will be chronic in nature and subject to progressive worsening.

The patient with liver dysfunction can deteriorate rapidly, and many factors can depress liver function. It is helpful to have the same nurse responsible for documenting changes in mental functioning that can occur as liver dysfunction worsens (see box below).

Asterixis (liver flap) is a characteristic sign elicited by asking the patient to dorsiflex the wrist while the arm is extended. The patient's hand has a peculiar flapping tremor. *Fetor hepaticus* is a sweet but fetid breath odor. Asterixis, fetor hepaticus, and decreasing consciousness indicate progressing hepatic encephalopathy.

Ascites and edema are monitored for changes in size of the abdomen or extremity. All patients with abdominal wounds or bleeding tendencies are monitored for signs of internal hemorrhage (shock).

The following list serves as an observational guideline:

1. Body weight
2. Vital signs
3. Intake and output
4. General appearance: muscle mass, nutritional status, color of skin and sclera
5. Mental status
6. Breath sounds and respiratory effort
7. Abdomen, including abdominal girth
8. Skin: color, presence of spider angiomas, bleeding sites, excoriations, palmar erythema
9. Extremities: edema
10. Color of urine and stools

Examination of the liver

The liver may be examined while examining the abdomen. The abdomen is first observed for the following signs:

1. Striae caused by stretching of skin with ascites
2. Engorged veins caused by obstruction of portal flow
3. Abdominal distention caused by ascites

Common manifestations of liver disease

Ascites and edema
Bleeding tendencies
Esophageal varices with gastrointestinal bleeding
Malnutrition
Jaundice
Hepatic encephalopathy (hepatic coma)

Parameters of mental functioning

Attention span
Ability to concentrate
Irritability
Apathy
Restlessness
Writing patterns
Speech patterns
Level of consciousness

Auscultation of the abdomen for bowel sounds is done before percussion or palpation. To percuss the liver, start at an area below the umbilicus in the midclavicular line and percuss upward until dullness is heard. Then start at about the fourth intercostal space, midclavicular line, and percuss downward. The vertical span of liver dullness should be approximately 6 to 12 cm in width. If this percussion reveals an enlarged liver, the liver can be percussed in the same manner at the midsternal line. At this point it normally is 4 to 6 cm in width (Fig. 31-8). Lung consolidation or right pleural effusion can obscure the upper border dullness, while gas in the colon can obscure the lower border dullness.

Percussion is also used to check for the presence of *shifting dullness*. Ascites causes dullness and bulging of flanks when the patient is supine (Fig. 31-9); tymphony may be found centrally. If the patient is turned to the side, the bulging and dullness is shifted to the dependent side.

While the patient is lying supine, the abdomen can be examined for presence of a *fluid wave*. In performing this test, the edge of the patient's hand is placed on the midline abdomen to prevent transmission of wave through abdominal wall. One hand of the examiner is placed on the patient's right flank and the opposite hand sharply strikes the left flank. A sharp wave will be felt by the examiner's hand in the presence of a significantly large amount of fluid (ascites).

The liver may also be palpated by deep palpation (Fig. 31-10). The liver edge, if palpable, presents a firm,

Fig. 31-8. Percussion of liver. Vertical span of liver dullness should measure approximately 6 to 12 cm at midclavicular line, *A,* and 4 to 8 cm at midsternal line, *B.*

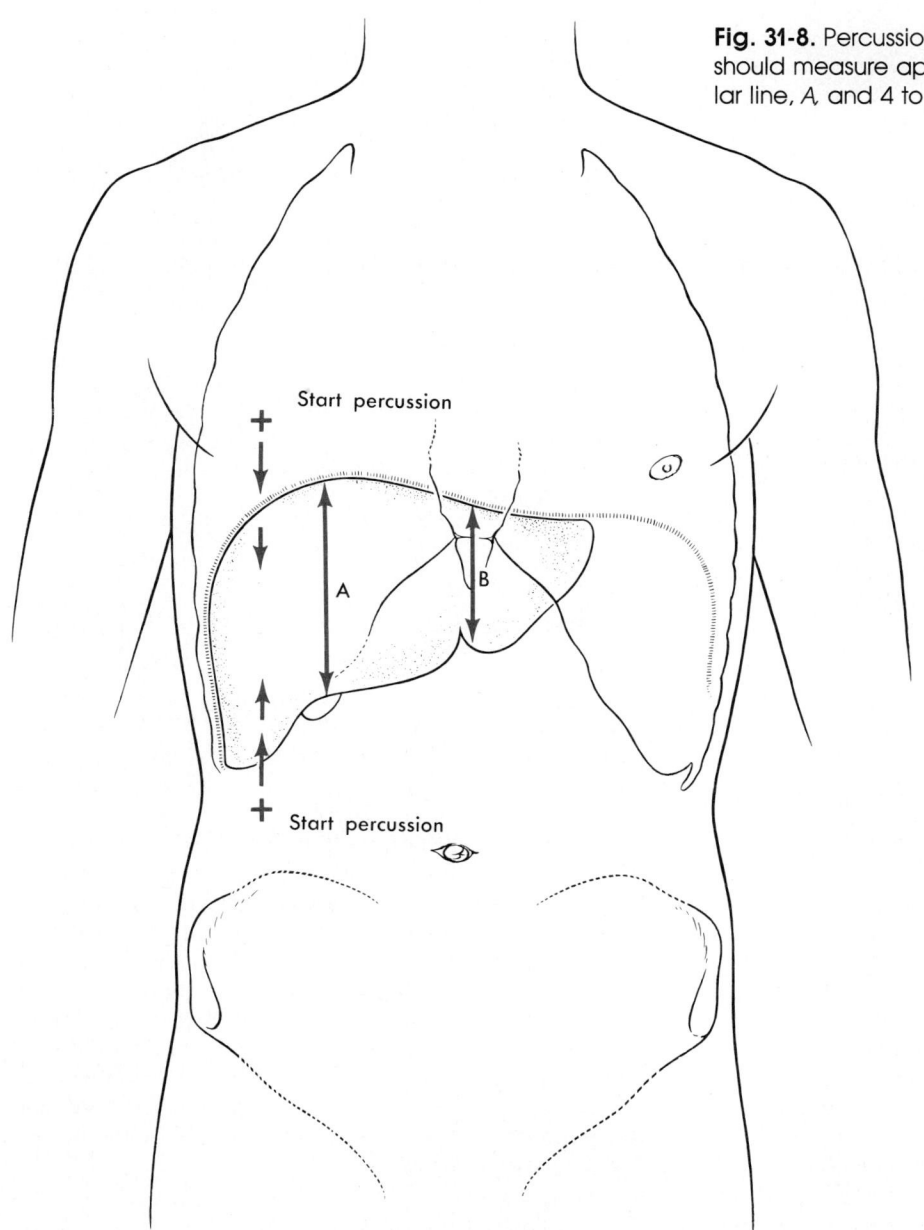

Start percussion

A   B

Start percussion

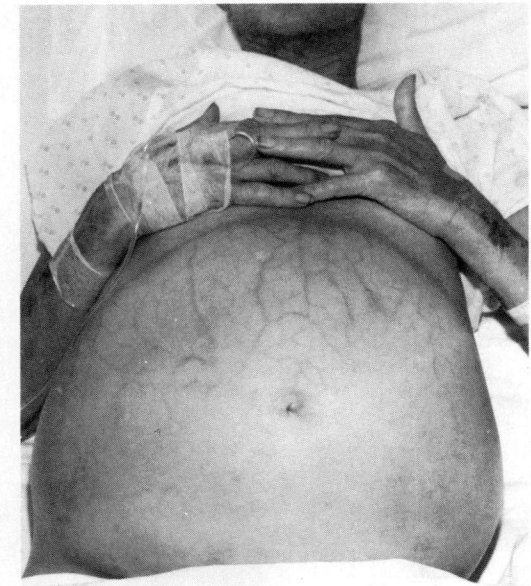

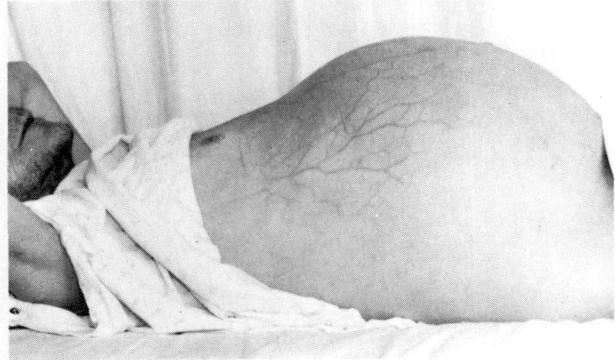

Fig. 31-9. Massive ascites. Note bulging flanks, dilated upper abdominal veins, and everted umbilicus (From Prior, J.A. Silberstein, J.S., and Stang, J.M.: Physical diagnosis: the history and examination of the patient, ed. 6, St. Louis, 1981, The C.V. Mosby Co.)

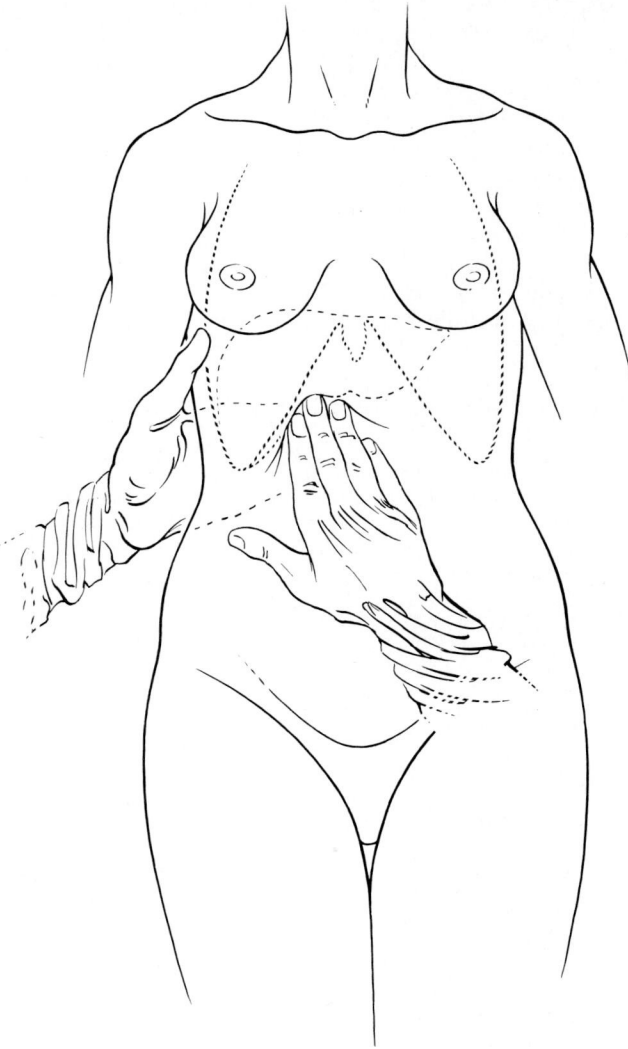

Fig. 31-10. Correct placement of hands for palpating liver.

sharp, regular ridge with a smooth surface. It is considered abnormal when felt more than 1 cm below the costal margin.

Diagnostic tests

Multiple tests may be necessary to determine the extent and seriousness of heaptic disease. Some of the laboratory tests are listed in Table 31-7. Additional studies may include abdominal films, barium swallow and barium enema, and endoscopic examinations. A liver scan, liver ultrasound, or CAT scan may also be peformed (Table 31-8). The diagnostic workup will frequently include one or several tests for examination of the biliary tract (p. 863).

LIVER BIOPSY. Biopsy of the liver presents the risk of hemorrhage because of the vascularity of the liver and the bleeding tendencies that often occur with liver disease.

The procedure may be open or closed. The open procedure is done in the operating room, and the usual preoperative procedure is required.

The closed procedure is often done in the patient's bed. This procedure is contraindicated if the patient has an infection of the right lower lobe of the lung, ascites, or a blood dyscrasia, or is unable to cooperate by holding a breath. The procedure consists of inserting a specially designed needle through the chest or abdominal wall into the liver and removing a small piece of tissue for study. Movement by the patient may tear the liver covering. No physical preparation is necessary for a closed procedure but written consent is usually required and food and fluids may be withheld after midnight the night before. Nursing activities include the following:

1. *Preprocedure*
   a. Explain procedure to patient

Table 31-7. Laboratory tests of liver function with possible changes in hepatocellular and biliary disease

Test	Normal	Hepatocellular disease	Biliary disease
Fat metabolism			
Serum total cholesterol	150-250 mg/dl	Decreased	Increased
Cholesterol ester	70%	Decreased	Decreased
Serum phospholipids	150-380 mg/dl	Decreased	Increased
Protein metabolism			
Total serum protein	6-8 g/dl	May be normal	
Albumin	3.2-4.5 g/dl	Decreased	
BUN	10-20 mg/dl	Varies	
Serum prothrombin time	12-15 sec	Increased	Increased
Blood ammonia	75 μg/dl	Increased	
Bilirubin metabolism			
Total bilirubin	0.1-1.0 mg/dl	Increased	Increased
Conjugated (direct)	0.1-0.3 mg/dl	Increased	Increased
Unconjugated (indirect)	0.2-0.8 mg/dl	Increased	
Urine bilirubin	None	Increased	Increased
Urine urobilinogen	0.1-1.0 Ehrlich U/dl	Increased	Decreased
Fecal urobilinogen	90-280 mg/day		Decreased
Serum enzymes			
SGOT	5-40 IU/L	Increased (nonspecific)	
Serum glutamic pyruvic transaminase (SGPT)	5-35 IU/L	Increased	
Lactic dehydrogenase (LD)	90-200 IU/L	Increased (nonspecific)	
Gamma-glutamyl transpeptidase (GGT)	Men: 10-38 IU/L Women: 5-25 IU/L	Increased	
Alkaline phosphatase	30-85 IU/L	Increased (slightly)	Increased
Excretory function			
Bromsulphalein (BSPO excretion)	< 5% retained after 45 min	Increased	

Table 31-8. Radiography and scintography of the liver

Procedure	Preparation	Interpretation
Radiosiotope scanning ^{131}I rose bengal ^{99}Tc colloidal technetium ^{67}Ga gallium citrate Risa^{131} radioionated serum albumin ^{198}Au colloidal gold	Injection of radioisotope A scintilloscope detects, amplifies, and records radiation No preparation necessary except for ^{67}Ga, for which enema and laxatives will be ordered to prevent absorption by GI tract	The liver will be outlined by radiosiotope scanning techniques to help identify tumors, cysts and abscesses (Fig. 31-11); hepatocellular abscesses and carcinomas show as areas of heavy radioactivity with ^{67}Ga; decreased areas of radioactivity usually are those of nonfunctioning tissue
Ultrasonic hepatography (liver ultrasound)	Preparation includes enema and/or laxatives and sometimes dietary preparation to decrease intestinal gas (low carbohydrate, no carbonated beverages) Barium studies should be done after ultrasonic exams or 48 hours before	Use of sound waves to bombard liver and surrounding areas; images caused by differences in sounds reflected by solid tissue, air-filled cavities, and fluid-filled cavities; can help in determining focal or diffuse liver disease
Computerized axial tomography (CAT scan)	No preparation needed; patient must lie still Sometimes dye studies of the biliary system are done at the same time; barium studies should be done after CT scan	Use of CAT scan is becoming more available and provides radiographic visualization of liver and surrounding structures; a computer handles the complex calculations used to analyse the multiple images of serial sections of tissue

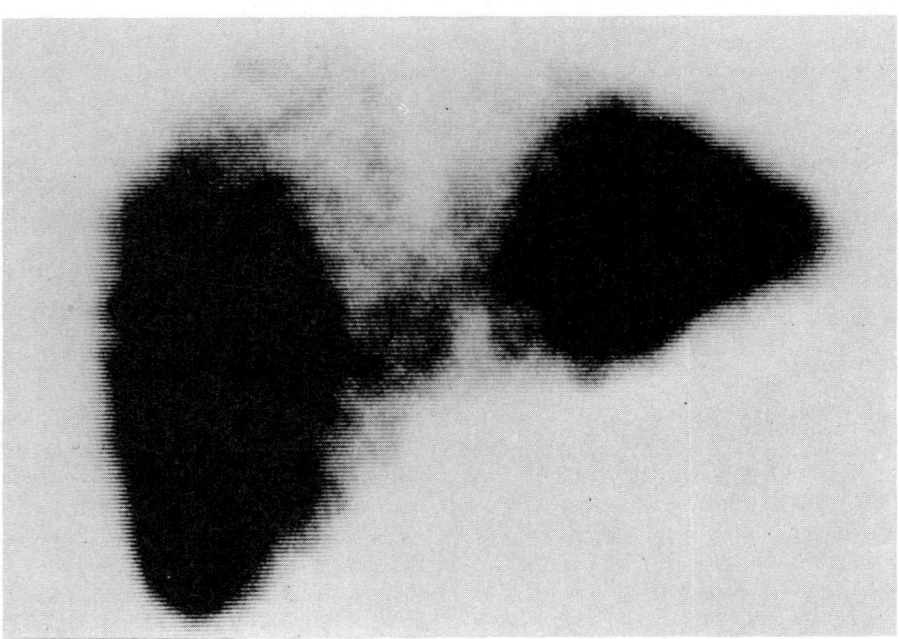

Fig. 31-11. Liver scan showing metastasis to liver (light area on right) or carcinoma of colon. (Courtesy Abbas M. Rejali, M.D., Department of Radiology, Case Western Reserve University, Cleveland, Ohio)

   b. Explain need to hold breath during the procedure; help patient practice holding breath and maintaining a sustained exhalation

   c. Report inability of patient to hold breath on command

   d. Give vitamin K as prescribed

2. *Postprocedure*

   a. Maintain bedrest for prescribed period (8 to 24 hours)

   b. Turn patient on *right* side for first few hours with pillow placed against the abdomen for pressure on liver

   c. Monitor patient

     1. First hour

       a. Observe site for hemorrhage every 15 minutes

       b. Monitor vital signs every 15 minutes

     2. Up to 24 hours, take vital signs hourly

     3. Report signs of hemorrhage (increased pulse, decreased blood pressure, cold clammy skin) and peritonitis (increased temperature, pain in lower abdomen)

   d. Provide analgesics as prescribed for mild right upper quadrant or right shoulder pain

DATA ANALYSIS AND PLANNING

Nursing diagnoses

Numerous nursing diagnoses may be identified for persons who have hepatic dysfunction. Some of the most common diagnoses include the following:

Comfort, alteration in: pain, pruritus, abdominal distention

Nutrition, alteration in: more or less than body requirements (calories, protein, vitamins, fat, carbohydrates, sodium)

Activity intolerance

Sleep pattern disturbance

Breathing pattern, ineffective

Tissue perfusion, alteration in (edema)

Fluid excess

Skin impairment: actual or potential

Self-care deficit

Knowledge deficit

Expected patient outcomes

When patients have acute health problems related to liver disease or injury, the following patient outcomes may be appropriate:

1. Improvement in signs and symptoms
2. Free of complications of disease or treatment
3. Free of avoidable stressors
   a. Avoidable discomfort
   b. Infections
   c. Complications of bedrest
   d. Activity in excess of energy level

As patients recover from acute processes or crises, outcome criteria reflect the increased responsibility of the patient for self-care for further recovery and for the prevention of relapse. Patient education and counseling become important in this phase of the patient's illness. Expected patient outcomes may include the following:

1. Can explain the disorder and relationships to relevant symptoms and treatment
2. Able to describe plans for self-care (activity, rest and sleep, food and fluid intake, medications, wound care if surgery performed)
3. Can describe signs and symptoms to be reported to physician
4. Able to explain way to avoid toxins or injurious agents
5. If alcoholic, able to make conscious decision about use of services such as Alcoholic Anonymous

IMPLEMENTATION

Focal liver disease

Treatment of liver abscess consists of incision and drainage of the abscess or abscesses and treatment with broad-spectrum antibiotics for pyogenic abscesses. The prescribed medications for amebic abscesses may have to be taken for long periods, and the patient should know that the abscess can rupture and cause the infection to spread. The patient is instructed to report any new signs and symptoms of infection. Portal hypertension occurs in rare instances from scarring of the liver as part of the healing process. These patients require close follow-up after discharge from the hospital.

If trauma to the liver has occurred, blood volume replacement is usually required. Emergency surgery may be needed to suture the ruptured liver and local pressure applied to stop the bleeding. Removal of necrotic tissue may also be indicated as well as drainage of any bile that may be leaking from the liver surface. The patient may require long-term follow-up to check for signs and symptoms of residual liver damage. Nursing care in the acute period is the same as for any patient requiring abdominal surgery as a result of trauma. The type of monitoring required will depend on the extent of the patient's injuries.

In most instances there is no corrective medical surgical treatment for metastatic or primary carcinoma of the liver because the disease is too far advanced when first diagnosed. Chemotherapy may be used in an effort to regress tumor growth, although the results are still poor. Patients are usually alert at this time and will know the prognosis. The patient and family are assisted to live with the prognosis and to do the things they wish to do in the time remaining for the patient (see Chapter 14). Various interventions, similar to those for the patient with cirrhosis, will be needed to manage physical changes that occur as liver failure progresses.

In a few patients with primary tumors, surgery may be possible. If the tumor is limited to a single lobe and there is no evidence of metastases elsewhere, a hepatic lobectomy may be done to remove metastatic as well as primary carcinoma. The remarkable regenerative capacity of the liver permits resection of 70% to 80% of the organ.

Homotransplantation of the liver has been performed in a few medical centers, but the survival rate has been poor. The liver must be transplanted rapidly because of difficulty preserving the organ. Death occurs as a result of rejection or infection secondary to depression of immune response by immunosuppressive therapy. Rapid advances in technology and pharmacologic agents are occurring; however, availability of donor organs and high costs are major limitations.

Surgery of the liver

PREOPERATIVE CARE. The following special considerations are necessary in the preoperative period:

1. If the prothrombin level is low, vitamin K is given.
2. If the patient has upper respiratory disease or infection, vigorous respiratory therapy is given; because of the thoracoabdominal approach and postoperative splinting, postoperative atelectasis and pneumonia are more frequent complications.
3. If malnourishment is present, protein hydrolysates are given by total parenteral nutrition (TPN) in addition to blood transfusions and glucose infusions in an effort to protect the liver from further metabolic insult.
4. Bowel preparation with antimicrobials is sometimes used as for intestinal surgery.
5. Salt-poor albumin may be given to increase blood colloidal pressure and blood volume.

POSTOPERATIVE CARE. Postoperatively the patient is acutely ill and requires constant attention. Central venous pressure (CVP) and pulmonary capillary wedge pressure (PCWP) are usually monitored hourly for at least 24 hours. Blood volume and serum glucose and albumin are markedly decreased after surgery. Possible postoperative complications are listed in box below.

Postoperative nursing care includes the following:

1. Monitor the patient continuously for the following:
   a. Hemodynamics (see Chapter 11)
   b. Intake and output
   c. Vital signs
   d. Abdominal girth
   e. Mental status
   f. Sugar in urine
   g. Dressing for bleeding or drainage
2. Maintain patency of gastrointestinal tubes (NPO is usually maintained for several days)
3. Maintain intravenous flow rates as ordered
4. Encourage deep breathing and turn patient frequently
5. Report signs of complications promptly
6. Administer treatments ordered to control hepatic dysfunctions or to treat complications

Following surgery of the liver, the patient may be out of bed by the third postoperative day but must be attended constantly; pulse, blood pressure, and respiratory rate are monitored before, during, and after any exertion, since complications such as hemorrhage and hypovolemia may still occur. Cortisone may be prescribed to prevent fibrosis and to enhance liver regeneration.

Food is usually started by the fifth postoperative day, and the patient must be monitored for ability to handle protein nitrogen waste products (BUN levels, mental status). Patients given preoperative TPN have increased endogenous insulin capacity. This may prolong the postoperative hypoglycemia response, and additional glucose intake may be required for 2 to 3 weeks.

Diffuse liver disorders

There is no specific treatment for diffuse hepatocellular disorders; therefore, therapy is primarily supportive. A primary goal is to aid the repair and regeneration of hepatic tissue after acute processes. Rest and diet are primary modes to achieve this goal and to prevent further liver damage.

Therapeutic management is also directed toward control of specific syndromes presented by the patient, as described earlier. Management therefore includes the following:

1. Prevention or control of edema and ascites
2. Control of bleeding tendencies and anemia
3. Control of gastrointestinal bleeding (esophageal varices)
4. Relief of portal hypertension
5. Management of hepatic coma

Supportive care

PROMOTING REST AND COMFORT. Rest of the liver can best be provided by decreasing metabolic demands of activity, of infection, of catabolism, and of stress response. Great care must be taken to avoid exposure to infection or hepatotoxins.

The physician usually prescribes the desired amounts of rest and activity. In hepatitis, serum enzyme levels may indicate necrosis and may serve as a guide (the higher levels indicate a need for more rest and restricted activity). It is believed that activity and maintaining an upright position decrease hepatic bloodflow, thus preventing optimal circulation to the already compromised liver.[30] Relapses are frequently attributed to premature increases in activity.

Possible complication following hepatic surgery

Hemorrhage, coagulation defects

Hypovolemia

Hypoglycemia

Hypoalbuminemia

Infection: wound, subdiaphragmatic

Atelectasis or pneumonia

Fluid and electrolyte imbalance (dilutional hyponatremia, metabolic alkalosis)

Hepatic coma

During the first few days after onset of symptoms in acute disease, the patient feels ill, and maintaining bed rest may not be difficult. Bed rest is encouraged during the acute phase, and the patient may become restless when symptoms begin to abate. Activity is increased as the acute phase subsides.

Since the liver is directly involved in the metabolism of nutrients for energy and the production of elements necessary for the formation of red blood cells to carry oxygen, disease of the liver will change the patient's energy level. As recovery begins, many patients will complain of not being able to do their usual activities. Boredom often occurs and ways can be suggested to encourage activities that are interesting but that require little energy. Rest periods are necessary. It is important to assess the person's energy level and to use this as a guide for helping plan activities of daily living. Recurrence of anorexia, enlargement or tenderness of the liver, or lack of progress as indicated by laboratory studies indicate a need to return to bed rest.

Patients with ascites may experience dyspnea resulting from pressure being exerted upward on the diaphragm. A high Fowler's position may assist respiratory efforts. Skin care may present another problem since these patients are often emaciated despite edema. The use of alternating pressure mattresses and flotation pads may be helpful. When edema is severe, the skin may "weep" as the accumulation of fluid seeps through the pores. Frequent change of bed linen will be necessary.

RELIEF OF PRURITUS

Itching caused by the accumulation of bile acids in the tissues can be uncomfortable. Measures to promote comfort for the patient with pruritus (see Chapter 37) are used. In addition, cholecystyramine resin (Questran, Cuemid), which is an exchange agent, may be prescribed

---

General nursing measures for patients with diffuse liver disease

1. Promote rest and comfort
   a. Encourage bed rest during acute phase
   b. Encourage increasing activity and rest periods as liver tests return to normal
   c. Intervene if the patient is having prolonged visits or frequent visitors who interfere with adequate rest
   d. Use measures to relieve pruritus
2. Promote nutrient intake
   a. Encourage diet high in calories, proteins, and vitamins A, B complex, C, D, and K
   b. Encourage fluids, up to 3000 ml/day, for persons with acute typical hepatitis
   c. Restrict sodium and fluids, as prescribed, for persons with cirrhosis or fulminant hepatitis when ascites and edema are present
3. Prevent infection
   a. Use frequent handwashing and good medical and surgical asepsis to prevent nosocomial infection
   b. Prevent skin excoriations and resultant infection from scratching in patients with jaundice
   c. Prevent skin breakdown in patients who are malnourished, edematous, ascitic, and less mobile
   d. Report signs of incipient infection to physician
4. Prevent bleeding
   a. Arrange with the laboratory to minimize number of venipunctures
   b. Start infusions (IVs) when blood samples are drawn
   c. Apply pressure for 5 to 10 minutes to sites of venipunctures or injections
   d. Suggest patient use a soft toothbrush or cotton swabs for teeth brushing to prevent bleeding gums
   e. Serve the patient with esophageal varices only soft foods (for example, bread rather than toast)
   f. Avoid taking temperatures rectally, and use gentle pressure and well-lubricated enema tips if hemorrhoids are present
5. Teaching the patient
   a. Take frequent rest periods until liver returns to normal
   b. Eat a diet high in calories; protein (unless restricted); and vitamins A, B complex, C, D, and K
   c. Check for weight gain and increased abdominal girth (if edema and ascites are possible complications)
   d. Avoid persons with upper respiratory infections
   e. Avoid over-the-counter drugs that may be hepatotoxic
   f. Report for weekly liver function tests until abnormal results show a downward trend toward normal levels
   g. Report signs of recurring illness as evidenced by liver tenderness, jaundice, increasing fatigue, and anorexia

to increase fecal excretion of bild acids. The powder is dissolved in juice, milk, or water and given with meals. This medication should not be given with other drugs, since it binds (inactivates) acids. Gastric distress, constipation, skin reaction, and bleeding tendencies have been noted with prolonged treatment. Vitamin K and other fat-soluble vitamins may have to be given intramuscularly for absorption. It may take up to 1 week for cholecystyramine to develop full antipruritic effect, and pruritus may return when the drug is discontinued.

PROMOTING NUTRITIONAL INTAKE. The liver's ability to excrete toxins and to carry on its many other functions may be seriously hampered by inadequate intake of protein and vitamin B. If liver damage has occurred, the organ's ability to store glycogen and vitamins A, B complex, C, and D may also be decreased. The patient may be in much greater need of regular intake of complete foods than before the illness. Oral bile salts may improve the digestion and absorption of fats and fat-soluble vitamins.

A diet high in calories, protein, and vitamins; fairly high in carbohydrates (unless weight reduction is desired); and with moderate amounts of fat is often ordered for patients with liver disease. Because alcohol is thought to interfere with hepatic conversion of folic acid to its active metabolites, many persons with cirrhosis have a folic acid deficiency anemia that usually responds well to treatment with oral doses of folic acid. Other nutritional anemias requiring nutritional supplements include vitamin B_{12} and iron deficiency anemias (see Chapter 28).

High levels of protein may be prescribed, but it is exceedingly difficult for patients to eat these amounts. Foods that are especially high in protein such as meat, fish, poultry, eggs, and dairy products are recommended. The person is often anorexic, and it can become a challenge for the nurse to identify ways to encourage the person to eat the prescribed diet. It is good to remember that the nurse is the health team member who provides this direct assistance to the patient.

Up to 3000 ml/day of fluids are encouraged for patients with acute hepatitis. Frequent drinks of fruit juices and milk drinks will provide needed nutrients in addition to the necessary fluid.

PREVENTION OF INFECTION AND INJURY. Persons with liver dysfunction have decreased resistance to infection. There is also a tendency to bleed when injury occurs. Selected measures to decrease the risk of infection and bleeding are listed in box on p. 855.

Assisting with specific medical therapies

REDUCTION OF EDEMA AND ASCITES. Sodium restriction and bed rest are usually the first approach to reduce edema. These measures and an adequate diet often result in a spontaneous diuresis that reflects improved hepatic function. The amount of sodium restriction may be based on 24-hour urinary excretion of sodium and is generally not less than 1 g daily. The lack of salt in food makes it less palatable, and the patient may not consume adequate protein and calories. Inadequate intake is reported to the

---

Assessment parameters for patients with edema or ascites
Daily weights Intake and output Measurement of abdominal girth Blood pressure Mental status

physician and dietitian since adjustments may need to be made in sodium restriction. Salt substitutes such as potassium gluconate may be permitted.

A second intervention that may be used is fluid restriction. Fluids may be restricted to as little as 500 ml/day and will usually not exceed 1500 ml/day. The fluid restriction may affect the patient's food intake. The patient is encouraged to assist in planning the distribution of fluid intake.

Nursing assessments to monitor fluid and electrolyte balance in patients with edema or ascites are listed in the box above.

DIURETIC THERAPY

Diuresis in cirrhosis often occurs slowly. Its complications include hypokalemia, oliguria, azotemia, and encephalopathy. Physicians are more cautious in this disease than in others in the use of aggressive measures of producing diuresis. Hypoalbuminemia, a contracted intravascular volume, and dilutional hyponatremia contribute to decreased mobilization of ascitic fluid and to complications.

Furosemide (Lasix) and/or spironolactone A (Aldactone A) are commonly used diuretic agents. Fluid and electrolyte levels must be carefully monitored during the initial administration of diuretic therapy. Hypokalemia may be treated with a potassium supplement.

Infusions of salt-poor albumin in 25 g units to promote retention of an adequate vascular volume may be given to avert azotemia and encephalopathy during diuresis. Effects of albumin infusion are short-term. It is often used to improve the patient status during acute crises or to prepare the patient for surgery. The administration of salt-poor albumin may expand the blood volume rapidly. During and following administration, the patient is monitored carefully for signs of pulmonary edema.

PARACENTESIS

A peritoneal tap may be done to obtain fluid for laboratory study but paracentesis places the patient at risk for complications such as shock, hypovolemia, azotemia and encephalopathy. Although once a standard mode of therapy, paracentesis is now used with caution and usually only as a last resort in patients with severe and chronic liver disease.

If the abdomen is taut with fluid and is producing dyspnea and anorexia, paracentesis may be necessary. In general, only small amounts of fluid are removed; this decreases the risk of rapid fluid shifts and additional protein loss. One liter of ascitic fluid contains as much protein as 200 ml of whole blood. Salt-poor human blood albumin may be administered following this procedure to counteract the loss of fluid and protein.

PERITONEOJUGULAR SHUNT

In chronic and resistant ascites caused by cirrhosis, a LeVeen peritoneojugular shunt (PJS) may be used. The LeVeen PJS allows for the continuous reinfusion of ascitic fluid back into the venous system through a silicone catheter with a one-way pressure sensitive valve. One end of the catheter is implanted in the peritoneal cavity, and the tube is channeled through subcutaneous tissue to the superior vena cava where the other end is implanted. The valve opens when there is a pressure differential greater than 3 mm of water between the abdominal cavity and the thoracic vein, allowing fluid to move from the peritoneal cavity into the superior vena cava.

Persons treated with the LeVeen PJS may also receive furosemide therapy, and the two together have been successful in relieving ascites in some patients. Persons who have a LeVeen PJS may still have severe problems, including disseminated intravascular coagulation, bleeding varices, and congestive failure.[27]

A modification of the PJS, the Denver shunt, is sometimes used when ascites is marked and is the result of malignancy. Malignant ascites may contain a lot of particulate matter that can stop the flow of ascitic fluid through the tubing. The Denver shunt has a subcutaneous pump that can be compressed manually to irrigate the tubing. Increased comfort and improvement of renal and respiratory function have been reported.[18]

When shunts are first implanted and functioning, there can be dramatic changes such as hemodilution of intravascular fluid, decrease in abdominal girth, and increased renal output. As peritoneal fluid is removed, less of a pressure gradient exists between the peritoneal fluid and the jugular vein. To force the valve open, deep breathing is encouraged at regular intervals with the patient in supine position.

MINIMIZING ANEMIA AND BLEEDING TENDENCIES. Anemia that is not of nutritional origin is treated by measures that control blood loss. Hemorrhage may be a major problem in diseases of the hepatic system. Because the jaundiced person may have a low prothrombin level, the prothrombin and coagulation time of the blood may be prolonged, and the person may bleed easily. For this reason the person is a poor surgical risk and may bleed from minor procedures.

Urine and stools are checked for either old or fresh blood, and if bleeding is suspected, specimens are saved. Steady oozing of blood from hemorrhoids is not unusual in severe jaundice. Incisions heal more slowly when jaundice is present, and dressings are inspected frequently for bleeding. The patient's activity may be restricted until wounds have healed completely. Other nursing measures to minimize bleeding are listed in the box on p. 855.

Therapy for bleeding tendencies is aimed at the restoration of clotting factors. If a decreased prothrombin level is identified, vitamin K will be given parenterally. This will not help if liver cell damage is the cause of reduced prothrombin formation. If this is the case, whole blood or plasma may be given to replace clotting factors at least temporarily. If the patient has a reduced platelet level, platelet transfusion may be given.

CONTROL OF GASTROINTESTINAL BLEEDING. The risk of gastrointestinal bleeding is much increased in the presence of portal hypertension and jaundice. Table 31-5 lists the treatment measures used with bleeding esophageal varices. This hemorrhage is often massive and life-threatening. If the hemorrhage is considered to be minor, introduction of a nasogastric tube and administration of an antacid may be sufficient to control the hemorrhage. Esophagogastric tamponade is the most widely used therapy for massive hemorrhage. Intravenous injection of vasopressin (Pitressin) is given to reduce portal pressure and bloodflow by constricting the splanchnic arterioles and to decrease the blood supply to the liver.

ESOPHAGEAL TAMPONADE

The esophagogastric tube (Blakemore-Sengstaken) is a three-lumen tube with two balloon attachments. One lumen serves as a nasogastric suction tube, the second is used to inflate the gastric balloon, and the third is used to inflate the esophageal balloon (Fig. 31-12). The tube is passed through the nose into the stomach with the balloons deflated. When the tube is in the stomach, the gastric balloon is inflated and the lumen clamped; the tube is then pulled out slowly so that the balloon is held tightly against the cardioesophageal junction. A cube of foam rubber (nasal cuff) is placed between the tube and the nares and secured to the face with pressure-sensitive tape. The nasal cuff absorbs excess nasal secretions, reduces trauma to the nostril, and provides traction to maintain the tube in proper position.

If bleeding continues after the gastric balloon is inflated, the esophageal balloon, which is connected by a Y tube to a manometer, is inflated to the desired amount of pressure and then clamped. To stop the bleeding, the pressure must be greater than the patient's portal venous pressure. If bleeding is from esophageal varices, blood will no longer be aspirated from the stomach. If there is still blood present, the stomach may be lavaged with a small amount of ice water or a solution of iced alcohol and water may be circulated through the balloon to provide vasoconstriction as well as pressure.

The nasogastric lumen is usually connected to intermittent gastric suction, which permits easy appraisal of cessation of bleeding and also keeps the stomach empty. It is important to remove all blood from the stomach because the presence of it may precipitate hepatic coma from ammonia produced from the digested blood.

The esophageal balloon can be left inflated up to 48 hours without tissue damage or severe discomfort. The

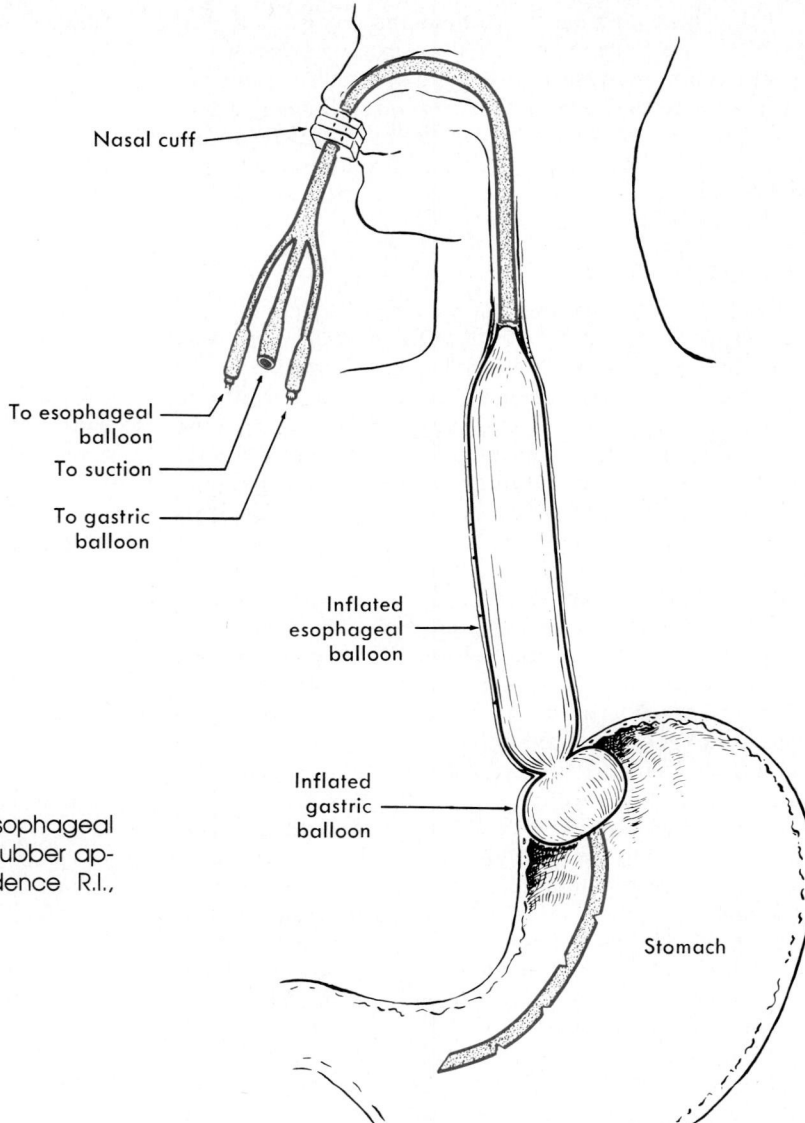

Nasal cuff

To esophageal balloon

To suction

To gastric balloon

Inflated esophageal balloon

Inflated gastric balloon

Stomach

Fig. 31-12. Blakemore-Sengstaken tube with esophageal and gastric balloons inflated (Redrawn from Rubber appliances in surgery and therapeutics, Providence R.I., Davol, Inc.)

fully inflated gastric balloon with traction exerted on it, however, compresses the stomach wall between the balloon and the diaphragm, causing ulceration of the gastric mucosa and severe discomfort. To offset the possibility of necrosis, the physician may release the traction and balloon pressures periodically. If the gastric balloon ruptures (and the patient is not intubated), the entire tube may move up and obstruct the airway; if this happens, the esophageal balloon is deflated at once and the entire tube is removed.

The nurse will be assisting with the following therapeutic measures when the esophageal balloon is in place:

1. Administering prescribed fresh whole blood and intravenous infusions (Fresh blood avoids increased ammonia and citrate and has relatively more coagulation factors.)
2. Administering saline cathartics through the naso-

gastric tube to hasten expulsion of blood from the gastrointestinal tract; enemas may also be ordered to decrease gut contents and bacterial action on the blood
3. Administering lactulose or neomycin to decrease bacterial effect on digested blood in the intestines in an effort to prevent hepatic coma

Nursing care of the patient with esophageal tamponade includes the following:

1. Explain procedure and provide continued support to patient during the procedure
2. Monitor vital signs until blood pressure is stable
3. Ensure that patient does not pull at the tube
4. Provide mouth and nares care every 1 to 2 hours
   a. Provide patient with tissues, and encourage spitting of saliva into a receptacle
   b. Have patient rinse mouth well to remove any

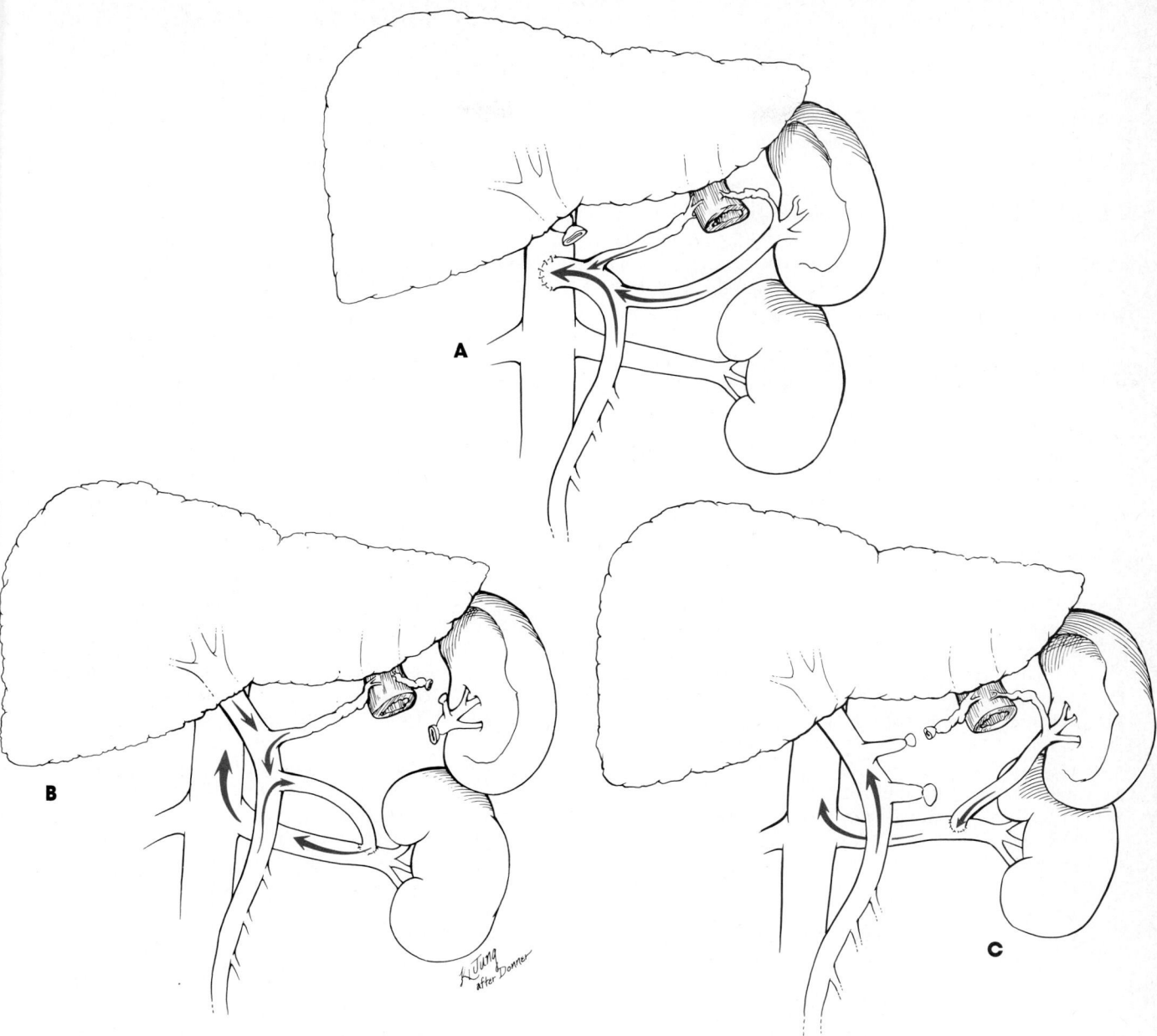

Fig. 31-13. Decompression operations for portal hypertension. **A,** End-to-side porta-caval shunt. **B,** Splenorenal shunt. **C,** Distal splenorenal shunt.

old blood; a Water Pik under low pressure may be helpful
c. Gently suction mouth and throat if patient is weak
d. Keep nostrils clean and lubricated with water-soluble jelly
5. Measure and record pressure of esophageal balloon every hour; maintain pressure at prescribed level
6. Maintain transfusions and infusions at prescribed rate
7. If iced solutions are used in the balloons, report patient chilling to the physician who may then order a warming blanket

8. Record intake and output; test gastrointestinal output for occult blood (guaiac)
9. Consult physician concerning permissible patient movement; passive range of motion is usually allowed
10. Provide comfort measures (for example, rub back, change patient's position)

RELIEF OF PORTAL HYPERTENSION. The only way to achieve permanent lowering of portal pressure is by surgical treatment to reduce bloodflow through the obstructed portion of the portal system. Depending on the location of the obstruction, various operative procedures may be employed (Fig. 31-13). It must be remembered that the patient with liver damage severe enough to cause bleeding esophageal varices is not a good operative risk. Preoperative criteria for a portacaval shunt include the following:

1. At least one hemorrhage from esophageal varices
2. Absence of ascites and hepatic coma
3. Bilirubin level below 1.5 mg
4. Albumin level above 3 g/100 ml

It is generally felt that a prophylactic shunt is not justified. The patient is usually apprehensive about the recommended operation; yet in selected cases it is known that the operative risk is much less than the risk from recurring hemorrhage. Vitamin K, antibiotics, and transfusions are usually given preoperatively.

Postoperatively the patient needs close observation and constant nursing attention as to the following:

1. Give narcotics for pain (amounts are usually guarded)
2. Avoid sedative drugs because of their toxic effects on the diseased liver
3. Observe patient carefully for impending hepatic coma (beginning signs include mental confusion, slowness in response, generally inappropriate behavior)
4. Encourage patient to breathe deeply and cough hourly
5. Record fluid intake and output accurately, and report any lessening of output (renal function sometimes decreases for a time following surgery)
6. Monitor patient carefully for hemorrhage (signs of shock)
7. Monitor patient for signs of thrombosis at site of anastomosis (pain, distention, fever, nausea)
8. Encourage activity within the prescribed limits; leg and arm exercises are often started on the first postoperative day
9. Monitor lower extremities for signs of edema; elevation of the lower extremities may be ordered to prevent edema formation (edema may form from the sudden increase of bloodflow into the inferior vena cava)

Regional heparization may be employed to prevent thrombosis of the portal vein. A fine polyethylene catheter is inserted into the right gastroepiploic vein during surgery, brought out through the wound, and attached to a continuous drip of heparin and saline solution. The surgeon determines the rate of flow. The catheter must not be obstructed or subjected to tension in any way during the period of insertion, up to 5 to 7 days. If activity is limited during this period, active range of motion of the lower extremities is encouraged.

After shunting procedures, less of the venous blood passes through the liver, and protein end-products are not completely detoxified. For this reason the patient is usually placed on a low protein diet. Intestinal antibiotics may be given so that fewer bacteria remain in the bowel to break down protein and to increase the production of ammonia.

MANAGEMENT OF HEPATIC COMA. Treatment of hepatic coma centers around finding and treating the precipitating cause (Table 31-5), providing general supportive measures, and avoiding additional trauma to the liver. Many of the therapeutic measures previously discussed can precipitate hepatic coma. The patient is very ill and is vulnerable to any increase in stress. The meticulous nursing care required for any patient who is unconscious is necessary. Particular care should be taken to protect the patient from infection.

Measures to decrease ammonia levels include the following:

1. Eliminating protein completely from the diet for several days
2. Giving carbohydrates by mouth or through nasogastric feedings
3. Administering intestinal antibiotics (for example, neomycin) and other agents (such as lactulose) that destroy or alter bacteria in the intestines and subsequently reduce the amount of ammonia formed
4. Giving enemas and cathartics (for example, magnesium sulfate) to empty the bowel and to prevent further ammonia formation

Some physicians prefer to rely on cathartics and cation exchange resins to help remove toxic substances from the bowel rather than to give antibiotics. Antibiotics destroy bacteria, which are active in the manufacture of vitamin K, and the absence of bacteria causes diarrhea and other symptoms that may worsen the patient's condition. Other measures used for some patients with hepatic coma are described in Table 31-5.

Many patients in hepatic coma die of renal failure secondary to an inadequate circulating blood volume (hypovolemia). In some patients renal function progressively deteriorates without any apparent cause. The treatment of hepatic coma requires careful balancing of fluid administration to maintain adequate perfusion of the kidney without creating an excessive load on the cardiovascular system. Nursing activities include the following:

1. Monitor desired flow rate very closely
2. Observe patient for signs of cardiovascular overload (dyspnea, moist respirations, coughing frothy sputum, distended neck veins, restlessness)
3. Monitor urinary output from indwelling catheter
4. Monitor changes in CVP readings that are suggestive of either hypervolemia or hypovolemia

Since most narcotics and sedatives must be detoxified by the liver, they are contraindicated in patients with impaired liver function. If a sedative is necessary, drugs such as chlordiazepoxide or phenobarbital may be used, which are excreted by the kidney.

The patient who has had definite or threatened hepatic coma may be kept indefinitely on a low-protein diet. When protein is added to the diet, it is added gradually and often does not exceed 40 g/day (average intake in the United States is 70 to 80 g/day). In addition, the patient may receive neomycin or lactulose daily. Patients with chronic liver disease may go in and out of coma; therefore, they are monitored for any change in behavior that would indicate early coma. The patient and family are taught to be alert to subtle changes in the patient's behavior and to seek medical assistance when this occurs.

EVALUATION

Evaluation will be based on the identified patient outcomes. For the person with acute liver dysfunction, questions to ask might include the following:

1. Are signs and symptoms returning to normal?
2. Have complications (infection, bleeding, skin breakdown) been avoided?
3. Is the patient getting sufficient rest?

For persons with chronic liver dysfunction, do the patient and family know the following:

1. The nature of the disorder and need for continued medical follow-up?
2. Measures to prevent exacerbations and complications?
3. Signs and symptoms to be reported to the physician?

DISORDERS OF THE BILIARY SYSTEM

Inflammation, stone formation, and carcinoma are the major disorders of the biliary system. The signs and symptoms and medical therapy are listed in Table 31-9.

PATHOPHYSIOLOGY

Cholecystitis

Cholecystitis, inflammation of the gallbladder, may be acute or chronic and is usually associated with gallstones or other obstructions of the bile passage. A large variety of organisms may contribute to acute disease. Cholecystitis is more common in women than in men. Sedentary, obese persons are affected more often, and the incidence is highest in the fifth and sixth decades of life.

In acute cholecystitis, the gallbladder is usually very enlarged and resembles a distended sac. Inflammation occurs, and the wall of the gallbladder becomes thickened and edematous. Impaired circulation, edema, and disten-

Table 31-9. Biliary tract disorders

Disorder	Etiology	Signs and symptoms	Medical therapy
Cholecystitis	Often associated with cholelithiasis	History of intolerance of fatty foods, gaseous eructations after meals, flatus, diarrhea, abdominal distention Nausea, vomiting Pain: right upper quadrant, referred to right scapula Fever, tachycardia Leukocytosis	Conservative: NPO, nasogastric intubation, IV infusions, meperidine hydrochloride, spasmolytics (papaverine, amyl nitrate), anticholinergics (chronic condition), antibiotics Surgery: cholecystectomy, cholecystostomy
Cholelithiasis	Persons at high risk: obese, pregnant, or has diabetes mellitus, cholecystitis, ileitis, hypothyroidism, hemolytic disease	As for cholecystitis Biliary colic: intense spasmodic pain with diaphoresis, tachycardia and prostration Jaundice Elevated serum bilirubin Prolonged prothrombin time	Conservative: meperidine hydrochloride, amyl nitrate, papaverine, dilaudid, atropine, nasogastric intubation, vitamin K Surgery: cholecystotomy, choledochostomy, choledocholithotomy, cholecystectomy, ERCP (endoscopy), EPT (endoscopic papillotomy), sphinctertomy, or sphincteroplasty
Carcinoma	High risk in persons with history of cholelithiasis	Jaundice, weight loss, pain, right upper quadrant mass	Cholesytectomy Choledochoduodenostomy Choledochojejunostomy Cholecystoduodenostomy Biliary drainage

ASSESSMENT

Subjective data

Some patients with biliary tract disease will be admitted for surgery while their disease is quiescent, whereas others will be in an acute stage of the disease. Potential and actual problems may therefore be present in individual patients. Minimum data to collect include the following:

1. Presence of discomforting symptoms (pain, jaundice, vomiting, diarrhea): onset, severity, location, factors that aggravate or alleviate symptom
2. Food intake patterns
3. Understanding of disease
4. History of respiratory problems
5. Expectations related to diagnostic or therapeutic measures
6. Use of medications

Objective data

Data is collected on admission to determine extent of present alterations and to serve as a baseline for future comparison. The following data are collected:

1. Mental status
2. Vital signs
3. Body weight
4. Abdominal assessment for distention
5. Breath sounds
6. Signs of jaundice

Intake and output measurements are started if patients have any unusual fluid losses or are acutely ill. Urine and stool are examined for color. Dark brown urine, caused by the presence of bilirubin, and a light colored stool, resulting from an absence of bile, may be noted. A dipstick test on urine for bilirubin and blood can be done quickly and easily.

Diagnostic tests

It is not unusual for patients with symptoms of biliary tract disease to have numerous diagnostic tests performed on the liver, pancreas, and biliary tract. See Table 31-7 for tests of serum bilirubin, urine bilirubin, urine urobilinogen, and fecal urobilinogen, and Table 31-4 for findings of these tests in obstructive and hepatocellular jaundice. The absence of urinary urobilinogen represents a highly significant finding for suggesting obstructive jaundice (a history of antibiotic therapy may influence the test results).

Other diagnostic tests are listed in the box, p. 863. The most frequent test of the biliary tract is an oral cholecystogram. If nonvisualization of the gallbladder is found, the test may be repeated the next day. Barium studies should follow gallbladder studies to prevent a barium-filled colon from obscuring the gallbladder.

Some patients find the oral dye of the oral cholecystogram to be very irritating; diarrhea is not uncommon, and nausea and vomiting can occur. Vomiting soon after ingestion of the tablets is reported, and directions are sought about further dosage. Intravenous injection of the dyes may cause allergic reactions in susceptible persons such as dyspnea, chills, diaphoresis, faintness, and tachycardia. Patients are queried about allergies or reactions to x-rays in the past. Some patients report temporary dysuria following the test.

DATA ANALYSIS AND PLANNING

Nursing diagnoses

Patients vary in their physiologic responses to biliary tract disorders as well as in their behavior; however, the following diagnoses might be identified in this group of patients:

Bowel alteration
Comfort, alteration in: pain, pruritus
Nutrition: more or less than body requirements
Knowledge deficit
Self-care deficit

For patients undergoing surgery with high abdominal incisions, the diagnosis of potential ineffective breathing patterns should always be made.

Expected patient outcomes

1. Person with acute disease:
   a. Pain and pruritus are relieved
   b. Wound heals without complications
   c. No other complications occur
2. Person with chronic disorders, for promotion of self-care abilities:
   a. Describes nature of the disorder
   b. Describes foods to be avoided or limited
   c. Explains any medications to be taken at home
   d. Explains therapeutic follow-up care

IMPLEMENTATION

Assisting with achievement of therapeutic goals

The treatment of choice for most patients with biliary tract disease is surgery. The decision as to when to operate depends largely on the age and condition of the patient and the response to treatment. Although some surgeons favor conservative treatment until acute infection has subsided, others believe that the danger of perforation of the gallbladder with subsequent peritonitis is so great that immediate surgery is advisable. Removal of the gallbladder is recommended when the acute condition has subsided. Infection may spread to the hepatic duct and liver, causing inflammation of the ducts (*cholangitis*) with subsequent strictures that may cause obstruction of bile flow, which are exceedingly difficult to correct surgically.

Food is withheld until acute symptoms subside. If vomiting persists, a nasogastric tube is passed and attached to suction. Meperidine hydrochloride may be given for pain and is preferred because its spasmogenic effect of the biliary tract is less than that which occurs with opiates. The inhalation of amyl nitrite may diminish intestinal and biliary spasms. When food is tolerated, a reducing diet (if appropriate) and careful avoidance of too much fat usually are recommended.

Endoscopic retrograde cholangiopancreatography (ERCP)

Advances in technology have allowed some patients with obstruction to have treatment through the use of fiberoptic endoscopy. Dilation and/or cautery of the sphincter of Oddi may be used to relieve stenosis or to remove a stone in the bile duct. The box below lists the therapeutic procedures possible with direct visualization of the duct. ERCP is usually done in the radiology department rather than in surgery.

Heparin instillation into a T-tube placed in the common bile duct can dissolve some cholesterol stones. Experimental trials with chemical dissolution of cholesterol stones using chenodeoxycholic acid (CDCA) or ursodeoxycholic acid (UDCA) appear to be effective in nonobese persons over age 40 with a functioning gallbladder and unobstructed biliary tract. It usually takes 2 years for the stones to dissolve completely.

Surgery

The terminology used to indicate specific biliary tract surgery is self-explanatory once common terms are understood. *Cholecyst* refers to the gallbladder, *choledocho* refers to the common bile duct, and *lith* refers to a stone (see box below). Biliary tract anastomoses are palliative operations to provide biliary drainage to the intestine through bypass of an obstructed area.

PREOPERATIVE CARE. Preoperative preparation of the patient with biliary disease is the same as that carried out for any patient having abdominal surgery (Chapter 32). Deep breathing and coughing postoperatively is particularly important because of the high abdominal incision, which makes these activities very painful and which predisposes the patient to right lower lobe pneumonia or atelectasis. An explanation of the types of drainage tubes that may be in place postoperatively may also be helpful. Vitamin K injections are administered if the prothrombin time is prolonged.

POSTOPERATIVE CARE. On recovery from anesthesia, the following guidelines are appropriate for most patients with cholecystectomy:

1. Place patient in low Fowler's position, but assist patient to change position frequently
2. Urge patient to cough and deep breathe at regular intervals (every 1 to 2 hours) until ambulating well

3. Monitor frequently for signs of hemorrhage (shock) the first few hours preoperatively (hemorrhage is rare, but may occur when the inflamed gallbladder was adherent to the liver and difficult to remove)
4. Give analgesics fairly liberally the first 2 to 3 days
5. Maintain a dry, intact dressing; usually a drain is inserted near the stump of the cystic duct; some serous fluid drainage is normal initially
6. Encourage progressive ambulation when permitted
7. When food is permitted, gradually increase diet to regular with low fat content or fat content as tolerated (appetite and fat tolerance may be diminished if there is external biliary drainage)

BILIARY DRAINAGE

External biliary drainage is provided by a catheter inserted into the gallbladder (cholecystostomy) or by a T-tube inserted into the common bile duct (choledochostomy) (Fig. 31-15). Usually stab wounds are used to bring these tubes through the skin. The T-tube is inserted to maintain patency of the common bile duct and to ensure drainage of bile out of the body until edema in the common duct has subsided enough for bile to drain into the duodenum normally. Cholangiograms (op-grams) are commonly performed in the operating room to ensure patency of the common bile duct; radiopaque dye is inserted through the T-tube.

Nursing actions for the patient with external biliary drainage include the following:

1. Connect any biliary drainage tubes to closed gravity drainage
2. Attach sufficient tubing so the patient can move without restriction
3. Explain to patient the importance of avoiding kinks, clamping, or pulling of the tube
4. Monitor the amount and color of drainage frequently; measure and record drainage at least every shift
5. Report any signs of peritonitis (abdominal pain or rigidity, fever) to the physician immediately
6. Monitor color of urine and stools (see Table 31-4); stools will be a light color if bile is flowing out a drainage tube but the normal color should gradually reappear as drainage diminishes and disappears

At first the entire output of bile (normally 500 to 1000

Surgeries of the biliary tract

Cholecystectomy	Removal of gallbladder
Cholecystostomy	Creation of an opening into gallbladder for drainage
Choledochotomy	Incision into common bile duct
Choledocholithotomy	Incision into common bile duct to remove a stone
Choledochoduodenostomy	Anastomosis of common bile duct with duodenum
Choledochojejunostomy	Anastomosis of common bile duct with jejunum
Cholecystogastrostomy	Anastomosis of gallbladder with stomach

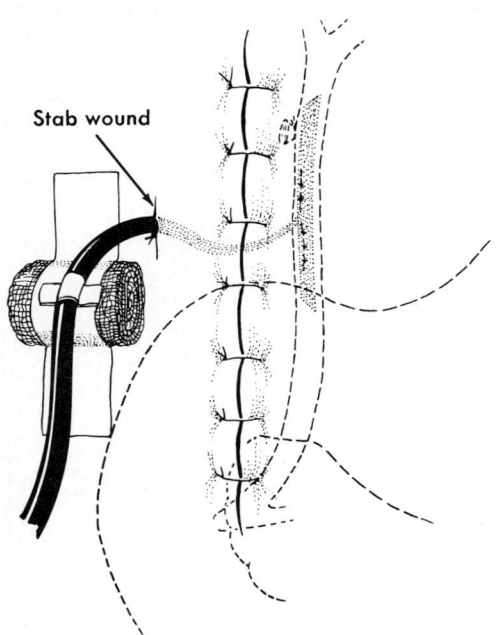

Fig. 31-15. Section of T tube emerging from stab wound may be placed over roll of gauze anchored to skin with adhesive tape to prevent its lumen from being occluded by pressure.

ml/day) may flow through the T-tube, but within 10 days most of the bile will be flowing into the duodenum. If bile is not flowing out the tube or through into the duodenum, it can be assumed that drainage is obstructed and that bile is being forced back into the common bile duct into the liver. The patient is observed closely for jaundice, particularly in the sclerae.

Occasionally with prolonged external biliary drainage, feeding of bile will be used to improve digestion. This is generally done through a feeding tube. Opaque containers should be used; tomato or grape juice can change its appearance.

Before the T-tube is removed, the patency of the common bile duct must be assessed. The tube is clamped for variable intervals and the patient monitored for signs of distress. If distress occurs, the tube is unclamped immediately and the physician informed. A cholangiogram is usually performed to confirm patency of the duct before the tube is removed. Following the removal of the T-tube, the patient may have chills and fever caused by edema and a local reaction to the bile; these symptoms usually subside within 24 hours.

Supportive care

Patients with prolonged illness, as with biliary tract fistula or metastatic carcinoma, will need supportive care and instructions related to specific symptoms. Common

---

Teaching the patient with a biliary system disorder

Postoperative

1. The patient to be sent home with dressings or drainage tube should be informed of the following:
   a. Expected amount of biliary drainage
   b. Frequency of dressing change or emptying of drainage bag
   c. Need to keep dressings dry and skin clean (soap and water is sufficient by time of discharge)
   d. Technique of dressing change and availability of supplies
   e. Signs to report to physician: excessive drainage, leakage, obstruction (jaundice, light-colored stools)
2. Resuming normal activities in about one month and sexual activities when desired; avoidance of heavy lifting for 6 weeks

Long-term care for chronic condition

1. Dietary restrictions
   a. Low-fat diet if fat is poorly tolerated
   b. Low calorie diet if weight reduction is necessary
2. Drug therapy, if appropriate
   a. Importance of medication in preventing recurrence of symptoms
   b. When and how to use medications such as anticholinergics or antispasmodics
3. Follow-up care
   a. Signs and symptoms to be reported to health care provider (pain, fever, jaundice, dark urine, pale stools, pruritus)
   b. Plans for follow-up care

problems encountered by these patients include the following:

1. Infection
2. Malnutrition
3. Fluid and electrolyte imbalance
4. Jaundice
5. Pain
6. Grieving

Teaching

The essential points to include in teaching the patient with a biliary system disorder are listed in box on p. 866.

EVALUATION

Evaluation is based on expected patient outcomes. Questions to ask may include the following:

1. Is patient comfortable?
2. Is jaundice decreased?
3. Is the wound healing?

4. Have complications been avoided?
5. Does patient know how to care for self at home, for example, as to diet, medications, care of any drainage systems or dressings?
6. Does patient know when and what to report to the physician?

DISORDERS OF THE PANCREAS

PATHOPHYSIOLOGY

Nonendocrine disorders of the pancreas consist primarily of inflammation (pancreatitis) and tumors. The endocrine pancreatic disorder of diabetes mellitus is discussed in Chapter 29.

Pancreatitis

Pancreatitis, an inflammatory disorder, may be acute or chronic. Table 31-10 lists the etiology, signs and symptoms, and medical therapy for these conditions.

Table 31-10. Disorders of the pancreas

Disorder	Etiology	Signs and symptoms	Medical therapy
Pancreatitis	Biliary obstruction Alcohol Idiopathic Tumors Infection Trauma Drug toxicity (chlorpormazine, chlorothiazide, isoniazide corticosteroids)	*Acute pancreatitis:* Epigastric pain, abdominmal tenderness Nausea, vomiting Shock, dehydration Fever, tachycardia Jaundice Abdominal rigidity Hyperglycemia Hypocalcemia Serum amylase greater than 300 Somogyi units *Chronic pancreatitis:* Recurring episodes of acute pancreatitis diarrhea, steatorrhea, weight loss, malnutrition, diabetes mellitus, jaundice	Fluid deficit: hydrating fluids, albumin, blood or plasma, electrolyte replacement Inhibition of pancreatic activity: NPO, propanthelamine (ProBanthine) or methantheline (Banthine), nasogastric suction, antacids Pain: meperidine hydrochloride, sympahetic nerve blocks, epidural anesthesia Paralytic ileus: Miller Abbot intubation Antacids Diet: high calorie, high protein, low fat Pancreatic enzyme replacement: pancreatin (Viokase), pancrelipase (Cotazym) pancrease Fiberoscopy with cannualization and sphincterotomy of sphincter of Oddi Pancreatic surgery
Tumors	Cystadenoma Duct cell adenoma Carcinoma of head of pancreas Islet cell tumors: Beta cell Nonbeta cell	Anorexia, nausea and vomiting, weight loss Pain Jaundice Hyperglycemia Hypoglycemia Peptic ulcer, diarrhea, steatorrhea	Surgery: pancreatic-duodenal resection (Whipple), cholecystojejunostomy or other bypass operation Chemotherapy Pancreatic resection Pancreatic resection and gastrectomy, cimetadine

Acute pancreatitis

Acute pancreatitis may be a single episode or there may be recurrent attacks (relapsing acute pancreatitis). The many causes of acute pancreatitis result in the response of the pancreas to injury or insult with diffuse inflammation. The most frequent causes are biliary system disorders, alcoholism, and idiopathic causes. Several mechanisms may explain the effect of alcohol such as the following:

1. Direct toxic effect of alcohol on acinal cells
2. Spasms of the sphicter of Oddi or pancreatic duct, permitting reflux of duodenal contents
3. Dietary deficiencies
4. Deposits of proteinaceous material in the small ducts

Pathologic changes appear to be produced by premature activation of proteolytic enzymes that are normally activated only in the duodenum. Activation of the enzymes may result from the following

1. Specific factors such as endotoxins, exotoxins, or ischemia
2. Reflux of duodenal contents through the pancreatic duct
3. Failure of enzyme inhibition

The activated enzymes digest pancreatic and surrounding tissues. Regardless of the pathogenic mechanism, severe destruction of the pancreas may result.

Acute pancreatitis may be divided into three stages, edematous or interstitial, hemorrhagic, and necrotizing. The mortality rate for the edematous stage is 10% to 15% and increases with each succeeding stage. Acute attacks usually occur suddenly.

Pain may result from distention of the pancreatic capsule, from obstruction of bile flow caused by compression of the common bile duct, and from peritoneal irritation. The pain may radiate to the back, flanks, and substernal area and may be more intense when the person is lying supine. Difficulty in breathing and cyanosis may accompany the severe pain. Vomiting at first relieves but continued vomiting worsens the pain. The patient often assumes a flexed posture to relieve pain.

Fluid and electrolyte abnormalities result from vomiting, local edema, ascites, or calcium precipitation into the inflamed pancreas. Hypovolemic shock may ensue if there is severe fluid loss. Shallow respirations may reflect metabolic alkalosis (induced by loss of gastric contents), limited diaphragmatic excursion, or ascites. Decreased breath sounds may be the result of atelectasis or pleural effusion. Rales may be present. Transient hyperglycemia may result from hypersecretion of glucagon in the edematous stage.

Chronic pancreatitis

In chronic pancreatitis there is permanent residual deficit, and relapses may occur in which there are episodes of acute inflammation superimposed on previously injured areas (chronic relapsing pancreatitis). Residual defects are fibrotic changes in the ducts (which become distorted and obstructed) and in the acinar cells (which atrophy and are replaced by scar tissue).

Pain is often harder to manage, and the disease may progress to the point where pain is constantly present. Between attacks the pain may disappear or may be only a vague discomfort. Fluid and electrolyte problems are not as severe as in acute pancreatitis, and shock does not occur.

Both pancreatic exocrine and endocrine insufficiency usually occur. Exocrine insufficiency leads to malabsorption and malnutrition, with the following symptoms: diarrhea, steatorrhea, and weight loss. Insulin insufficiency may result in diabetes mellitus. Calcification of the pancreas worsens.

Tumors of the pancreas

Tumors of the pancreas may be malignant or benign. Benign tumors are usually adenomas or cystadenomas and are relatively rare. Malignant tumors occur more frequently and are most often found in the head of the pancreas. Men are affected far more often than women, usually after middle age. Cancer of the pancreas is the fourth most common cause of cancer mortality in men.

Most malignant tumors of the pancreas appear to begin in the ductal areas, causing eventual blockage and resulting in chronic pancreatitis. Direct extension of the lesion may cause its spread to the posterior wall of the stomach, duodenum, colon, and common bile duct. The tumor may be diffusely spread over the entire gland, or it may be a well-defined growth. It usually grows rapidly, is highly invasive, and metastasizes frequently. Many patients live only 3 to 6 months after diagnosis is confirmed. Symptoms usually occur late in the course of the disease. Pain occurs in about 85% of patients. Jaundice occurs from common bile duct obstruction but is seldom a primary sign.

Islet cell tumors give rise to particular syndromes (Table 31-10) that are important in the differential diagnosis of hypoglycemia and peptic ulcer. These tumors may be benign or malignant. *Beta-cell pancreatic adenoma (insulinoma)* results in hyperinsulinism and episodes of hypoglycemia. Attacks are precipitated by fasting or exercise, and symptoms are relieved by glucose ingestion or infusion. *Nonbeta-cell tumors* result in peptic ulceration of the duodenum or jejunum. Hypersecretion of gastric acid is extremely severe in this Zollinger-Ellison syndrome (see Chapter 32). The patient often gives a history of severe diarrhea and steatorrhea.

ASSESSMENT

Subjective data

The nursing history should be thorough and should carefully document the course of symptoms, particularly pain and vomiting. The use of any medications, alcohol, and home remedies are explored. When alcohol use is a factor in pancreatitis, data are collected about the person's present perception of drinking as a problem for which help is needed (see Chapter 9). Baseline data about food intake patterns and likes and dislikes can help the nurse and dietitian plan for patients with malnutrition on anorexia.

Table 31-11. Laboratory tests for pancreatic disease

Test	Normal	Increased	Decreased
Amylase, serum	60 to 150 Somogyi units	Acute pancreatitis Chronic relapsing pancreatitis	Advanced chronic pancreatitis
Amylase (urine, 24 hr specimen)	35 to 260 Somogyi U/hr	Acute pancreatitis	
Lipase	0 to 1.5 U/ml	Acute pancreatitis Cancer of pancreas (early) Obstruction of pancreatic duct	Cancer of pancreas (early)
Calcium	4.5 to 5.75 mEq/L 9 to 11 mg/dl		Acute pancreatitis
Bilirubin (direct conjugated)	0.1 to 0.3 mg/dl	Cancer of pancreas Acute pancreatitis Chronic relapsing pancreatitis	
Glucose	90 to 120 mg/dl	Acute pancreatitis Chronic relapsing pancreatitis	

Objective data

The physical examination should be complete. Special attention is directed to the abdomen to elecit signs of ascites, guarding, or tenderness. Dehydration is usually found in acute pancreatitis. Although unusual, hypocalcemia may occur, therefore the patient is monitored for the presence of Chvostek's sign and Trousseau's sign (p. 817). Baseline abdominal girth can help determine further abdominal distention.

A brief listing of important data include the following:
General appearance and posture
Mental status
Body weight
Vital signs
Breath sounds
Abdomen: girth, tenderness, guarding
Chvostek's and Trousseau's signs
Urinalysis for sugar and acetone
Urinary intake and output

Diagnostic tests

Of the greatest value in establishing a diagnosis are measurements of enzyme levels (Table 31-11). A serum amylase level of greater than 300 Somogyi units in the presence of symptoms usually establishes a diagnosis of acute pancreatitis. There is no apparent relationship between the severity of the disease and the enzyme levels. With pancreatic trauma, a peritoneal tap may reveal an increased amylase level in the peritoneal fluid. When elevations of SGOT, alkaline phosphatase, and leucine aminopeptides occur, there is usually obstruction of the common bile duct or liver disease present. Laboratory findings consistent with dehydration may be present. In very severe cases, serum glucose levels may be elevated and serum calcium and protein levels may be decreased. Stool specimens may be examined for fat and fiber content.

An x-ray film of the pancreas is taken to identify structural abnormalities and calcium implantation. Often the biliary tract is extensively studied by radiographic methods. The pancreatic duct may be directly visualized by fiberoptic endoscopy, ERCP (p. 863).

DATA ANALYSIS AND PLANNING

Nursing diagnoses

There are multiple nursing diagnoses for the patient with a pancreatic disorder. Common nursing diagnoses, either actual or potential, may include the following:
Bowel elimination, alteration in: diarrhea
Comfort, alteration in: pain
Fluid volume deficit
Nutrition, alteration in: less than body requirements
Grieving, anticipatory
Knowledge deficit
Noncompliance
Self-care deficit

Expected patient outcomes

Patient outcomes will depend on individual patient data and identified nursing diagnoses. The following outcomes serve only as guidelines.
1. Patient has the following:
   a. Relief of pain
   b. Weight within normal range
   c. Absence of complications
2. Patient explains rationale of treatment measures and ways to implement these at home—diet, medications, avoidance of toxins.
3. Patient knows the significance of return of symptoms and reports these to physician promptly.

Signs of complications of acute pancreatitis

Paralytic ileus
Shock
Pulmonary edema
Hypocalcemia
Hyperglycemia
Jaundice

---

4. Patient and family have access to supportive services for long-term control of alcoholism or for hospice services when the prognosis for pancreatic carcinoma is poor.

IMPLEMENTATION

Assistance with achievement of therapeutic goals

Pancreatitis

Rest of the pancreas during the acute phase is achieved by measures that reduce stimulation of the exocrine secretions such as the following:
1. NPO status
2. Nasogastric suction
3. Anticholinergic drugs
4. Antacids

These measures decrease stimulation of the vagus nerve, and thus of hydrochloric acid, and decrease secretion of the enzymes secretin, gastrin, and pancreoenzyme-CCK, thereby reducing the inflammatory response. Antibiotics are not usually administered in the edematous stage or in the absence of complications. Atropine-like drugs are contraindicated in the presence of paralytic ileus and shock. There is some question of their efficiency in treating pancreatitis, and they are not always used.

Pain relief is usually achieved with meperidine hydrochloride rather than morphine or codeine, since it is less spasmogenic on the sphincter of Oddi. Some patients find that the pain is decreased if they assume a sitting position with the trunk flexed or with their knees drawn up to the abdomen in a side-lying position.

As soon as the acute attack passes, oral fluids and foods are started. Patients are placed on a low-fat bland diet distributed over five to six small feedings per day. When eating starts, the patient is observed carefully for pain, nausea, and vomiting, which indicate continuing inflammation and the need to return to a NPO status.

All patients with acute pancreatitis have the potential for developing chronic pancreatitis and should be monitored for the following signs and symptoms of complications (see box above).

The following nursing interventions are used depending on the presence or extent of dehydration and the presence of complications of acute pancreatitis:
1. Maintaining intravenous fluid replacement (blood, albumin, plasma, fluids) and electrolytes as ordered
2. Monitoring vital signs and central venous pressure
3. Monitoring intake and output every 1 to 4 hours
4. Administering vasopressors and other measures for shock
5. Maintaining patency of the gastrointestinal tube
6. Monitoring for glucosuria, ketonuria, Chvostek's and Trousseau's signs, and increasing abdominal girth
7. Encouraging deep breathing and coughing

Chronic pancreatitis

Therapy for the acute phase of chronic pancreatitis is the same as for acute pancreatitis. Pancreatic enzyme replacement durgs contain amylase, lipase, and trypsin. They are taken at mealtimes to aid digestion and to facilitate the absorption of fat-soluble vitamins. The patient should observe stools for the presence of steatorrhea, which should be reported immediately to the physician.

If diabetes mellitus is present, it is treated as described in Chapter 29. The patient needs to understand the relationship between pancreatitis and diabetes and needs to monitor for signs and symptoms on a continual basis. If signs and symptoms occur, they must be reported to the physician.

Pain control between acute exacerbations is a major nursing challenge. The dietary restrictions, if followed, will help to control pain. If appropriate and if patient is interested, behavioral control methods such as relaxation therapy may be taught. The patient will need to know why narcotics should be avoided.

Surgery

An exploratory laparotomy may be performed in acute pancreatitis when a diagnosis cannot be established and the possibility of general peritonitis, perforation of an organ, or a bowel obstruction cannot be excluded. If biliary obstruction is present, a surgical or endoscopic procedure may be done to divert or increase bile flow at the sphincter of Oddi and thereby reduce regurgitation of bile into the pancreatic duct.

Stenosis from intraductal calcification or strictures can lead to cyst or abscess formation. For the treatment of pseudocysts in pancreatitis, the surgeon may employ external drainage, construct anastomoses between the pancreas and gastrointestinal tract (for example, pancreaticojejunostomy), or resect part or all of the pancreas.

Exploratory surgery is often necessary to diagnose pancreatic tumors. Various techniques may be used when pancreatic tumors are present or to relieve pancreatic duct obstruction. Procedures to relieve obstructive jaundice are sometimes helpful in providing comfort (for example, cholecystostomy, choledochojejunostomy). Often malignant tumors of the pancreas are inoperable by the time diagnosis is made.

Pancreatoduodenal resection is sometimes done when the carcinoma is localized with no evidence of metastasis. The Whipple procedure involves resection of the antrum of the stomach, duodenum, varying amounts of pancreas, and often the gallbladder. Anastomoses are constructed between the stomach, common bile duct and pancreatic

---

Teaching the patient with pancreatic disorders

1. After pancreatic surgery
   a. Self-care as to dressings, tubes, medications
   b. Need for low-fat, high calorie diet, as appropriate
   c. Need for continued medical follow-up care
2. After acute pancreatitis
   a. Prevention of further attacks (avoidance of alcohol, narcotics, and abdominal injury; medical care when ill)
   b. Reporting symptoms indicating relapse or complications
      1. Pain
      2. Nausea and vomiting
      3. Abdominal distention
      4. Steatorrhea
      5. Polyuria, polydipsia, polyphagia
      6. Weight loss
      7. Fever
   c. Maintaining low-fat, bland diet with several small feedings per day and vitamin supplements
   d. Avoiding rich foods to keep pancreatic secretions at a minimum
   e. Continuing medication therapy (pancreatic enzymes, bile salts, oral hypoglycemic agents, or insulin)— scheduling, rationale, dose, side effects
   f. Need for continued medical follow-up care

---

ducts, and the jejunum. Malabsorption syndrom follows total pancreatectomy (protein, fat, iron, calcium, phosphate, vitamin B_{12}) as does diabetes mellitus.

The patient with extensive pancreatic surgery or disease may have a prolonged postoperative course. Malnourishment, postoperative complications (hemorrhage, fistulas, anastomotic leak, infection) and metabolic derangements may occur. Hemorrhagic and hypovolemic shock can lead to renal failure. Wound care must be meticulous. Drains are usually employed, and dressings should be inspected frequently and changed as often as necessary to maintain dryness. Severe tissue breakdown can occur if pancreatic fistula develops as pancreatic enzymes digest skin and underlying tissue. Measurement of biliary or pancreatic drainage is carefully recorded.

Teaching and counseling

After pancreatic surgery the patient may require teaching directed toward self-care (see box above) as well as counseling directed toward acceptance of chronic disease or malignancy. Not all patients with pancreatitis have alcoholism as a contributing factor, but those that do are encouraged to seek appropriate services (see Chapter 9).

EVALUATION

The expected patient outcomes serve as the basis for evaluating the extent to which patient status was improved. Questions to ask may include the following:
1. Were symptoms relieved?
2. Did serum amylase return to normal?
3. Was there prompt detection and treatment of complications?

4. Was patient adequately prepared to manage the treatment regimen at home?
5. Were patient and family referred to appropriate supportive services?

REFERENCES AND SELECTED READINGS*

1. Aach, R.: Viral hepatitis A to E, Med. Clin. North Am. **62:**59-69, 1978.
2. *Bates, B.: A guide to physical examination, ed. 3, Philadelphia, 1983, J.B. Lippincott Co.
3. *Belinsky, S.: Visualizing the pancreatic and biliary ducts, Am. J. Nurs. **76:**936-937, 1976.
4. *Bell, J.: Just another patient with gallstones? Don't you believe it, Nurs. 79 **9**(10): 26-33, 1979.
5. *Boyer, C.A., and Oehlberg, S.M.: Interpretation and clinical relevance of liver function tests, Nurs. Clin. North Am. **12:**275-290, 1977.
6. Burke, M.D.: Hepatic function testing, Postgrad Med. **64:**177-182, 1978.
7. Byrne, J.: Liver function studies. I. Introduction and bilirubin, Nurs. 77 **7**(7):12-14, 1977.
8. Byrne, J.: Liver function studies. II. Conjugation and excretion tests, Nurs. 77 **7**(9):88-90, 1977.
9. *Dougherty, W.M.: Serum bilirubin, Nurs. **82**(11):138-139, 1982.
10. *Fredette, S.L.: When the liver fails, Am. J. Nurs. **84:**64-67, 1984.
11. Frukes, J.T.: Physiological considerations in the medical management of ascites, Arch. Intern. Med. **140:**620-623, 1980.

---

*References preceded by an asterisk are particularly well suited for student reading.

12. Greenberger, N.J.: Gastrointestinal disorders: a pathophysiologic approach, ed. 2, Chicago, 1981, Year Book Medical Publishers, Inc.

13. Guenter, P., and Slocum, B.: Hepatic disease: nutritional implications, Nurs. Clin. North Am. 18(1):71-80, 1983.

14. Harvey, A.M., and others: The principle and practice of medicine, ed. 20, Englewood Cliffs, N.J., 1980, Prentice Hall, Inc.

15. Howes, R.M.: Our approach to acute pancreatitis, Resident Staff Phys. 23(3):51-56, 1977.

16. Isselbacher, K., and others: Harrison's principles of internal medicine, ed. 9, New York, 1980, McGraw-Hill Book Co.

17. Kelber, M.B.: Pancreatic enzymes: deciphering diagnostic studies, Nurs. 82 12(12):65-67, 1982.

18. Klopp, A.: Shunting malignant ascites, Am. J. Nurs. 84:212-213, 1984.

19. Kosel, K., and others: Total pancreatectomy and islet cell autotransplantation, Am. J. Nurs. 82:568-571, 1982.

20. Leery, C., and Kanagasundaram, N.: Alcoholic hepatitis, Hosp. Pract. 13:115-123, October. 1978.

21. Mahood, W.H., Dill, J.E., and Dill, R.P.: Hepatic failure. In Meltzer, L.E., Abdellah, F.G., Kitchell, J.R., editors: Concepts and practices of intensive care for nurse specialists, ed. 2, Bowie, MD, The Charles Press.

22. *Mar, D.D.: Drug-induced hepatotoxicity, Am. J. Nurs. 82:124-126, 1982.

23. Mountcastle, V.B., editor: Medical physiology, ed. 14, St. Louis, 1981, The C.V. Mosby Co.

24. *Peterson, A.: Acute viral hepatitis, Nurse Pract. 13(4):9-11, 1979.

25. Pierce, L.: Anatomy and physiology of the liver in relation to clinical assessment, Nurse. Clin. North Am. 12:259-273, 1977.

26. Quinless, F.: Portal hypertension: physiology, signs and symptoms, Nurse. 84 14(1):52-53, 1984.

27. Resnick, R.H.: Cirrhosis. In Conn, H.R., and others, editors: Current therapy 1984, Philadelphia, 1984, W.B. Saunders Co.

28. Sabiston, D.C., editor: Davis-Christopher textbook of surgery, ed. 12, Philadelphia, 1981, W.B. Saunders Co.

29. Schumann, D.: Correction of ascites with peritoneovenous shunting: a study of clinical management, Heart Lung 12:248-257, 1983.

30. Schiff, L.: Diseases of the liver, ed. 5, Philadelphia, 1982, J.B. Lippincott Co.

31. Schwartz, S.I., and others: Principles of surgery, ed. 4, New York, 1984, McGraw-Hill Book Co.

32. Seybert, P., Gardon, K.M., and Jackson, B.S.: The Leveen shunt: new hope for ascites patients, Nurs. 79 9(1):24-31, 1979.

33. Shahinpour, N.: The adult patient with bleeding esophageal varices, Nurs. Clin. North Am. 12:331-343, 1977.

34. Sherlock, S.: Diseases of the liver and biliary system, ed. 6, Philadelphia, 1981, F.A. Davis Co.

35. Stephens, G.J.: Pathophysiology for health practitioners, New York, 1980, MacMillan Publishing Co.

36. Taylor, D.L.: Gallstones: physiology, signs and symptoms, Nurs. 83 13(6):44-45, 1983.

37. Taylor, D.L.: Jaundice: physiology, signs and symptoms, Nurs. 83 13(8):52-54, 1983.

38. *Taylor, P.D.: Liver transplantation, Am. J. Nurs. 81:1672-1673, 1981.

39. *Thompson, M.A.: Managing the patient with liver dysfunction, Nurs. 81 11(11):100-107, 1981.

40. *Thorpe, C., and Caprini, R.: Gallbladder disease: current trends and treatment, Am. J. Nurs. 80:2181-2185, 1980.

41. U.S. Public Health Service, Centers for Disease Control: Isolation techniques for use in hospitals, ed. 3, Washington, D.C., 1983, U.S. Public Health Service.

42. Widmann, F.: Goodall's clinical interpretation of laboratory tests, ed. 9, Philadelphia, 1983, F.A. Davis Co.

43. Williams, S.R.: Essentials of nutrition and diet therapy, ed. 3, St. Louis, 1982, The C.V. Mosby Co.

44. Wyngaarden, J.B., and Smith, L.H.: Textbook of medicine, ed. 16, Philadelphia, 1982, W.B. Saunders Co.

Classic

45. Berk, R.N.: Radiology of the gallbladder and bile ducts, Surg. Clin. North Am. 53:973-1005, 1973.

46. Netter, F.: The Ciba collection of medical illustrations. III. Digestive system, vol. 3, Summit, N.J., 1964, Ciba Pharmaceutical Co.

47. Rutherdale, J.A., and others: Hepatitis in drug users, Am. J. Gastroenterol. 58:275-287, 1972.

48. Simmons, S., and Givens, B.: Acute pancreatitis, Am. J. Nurs. 71:934-939, 1971.

UNIT IX
Problems of Digestion or Elimination

32   The Patient with Gastrointestinal Problems
33   The Patient with Urinary Problems

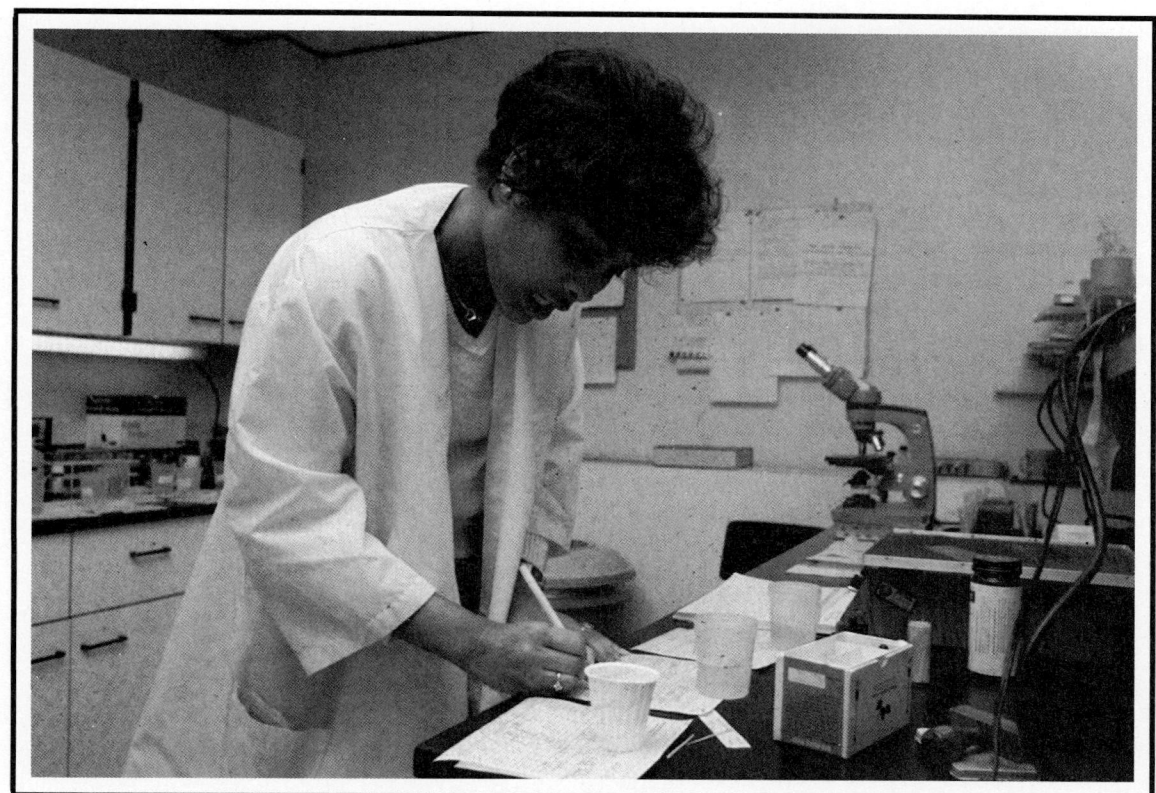

32

The Patient with Gastrointestinal Problems

BARBARA C. LONG

STUDY QUESTIONS

- Review the anatomy and physiology of the gastrointestinal system. What are some factors that stimulate gastrointestinal motility?

- What enzymes are present in the small bowel, and what is their action on normal skin?

- How can electrolyte balance be affected by excessive vomiting and persistent diarrhea?

- Review the medications that are used to control motility of the gastrointestinal tract.

- Examine written instructions given at your hospital to patients scheduled for diagnostic gastrointestinal tests and x-ray examinations. How could you use these tools most effectively?

- Practice testing a stool sample for occult blood (guaiac test).

ANATOMY AND PHYSIOLOGY

Maintenance of adequate nutrition and elimination requires an intact and functioning gastrointestinal tract. Normally, food and fluids are placed in the mouth, chewed (if solid), pushed to the pharynx by the tongue, and swallowed by automatic reflex activity down the esophagus into the stomach. Digestion starts in the mouth and terminates in the small intestine, although fluids continue to be reabsorbed in the colon. The anatomical structures of the gastrointestinal tract are illustrated in Fig. 32-1.

Mouth and esophagus

SALIVATION

The cortical thought of food initiates saliva production from the salivary glands. The salivary secretions are made up of *serous secretion,* containing ptyalin for starch digestion, and *mucus* secretion for lubrication. These two secretions account for one half of the upper gastrointestinal tract secretions.

MASTICATION

The teeth serve the function of initial food breakdown. No other part of the gastrointestinal tract can perform this function if the teeth are missing. Enzymes can act only on the exposed surfaces of the food particles. Very fine particulation prevents excoriation of the lining of the tract, and the rate of digestion is dependent on the total surface area of food particle exposed. General health teaching for children and adults should stress the reason behind thorough mastication of all food substances that are ingested.

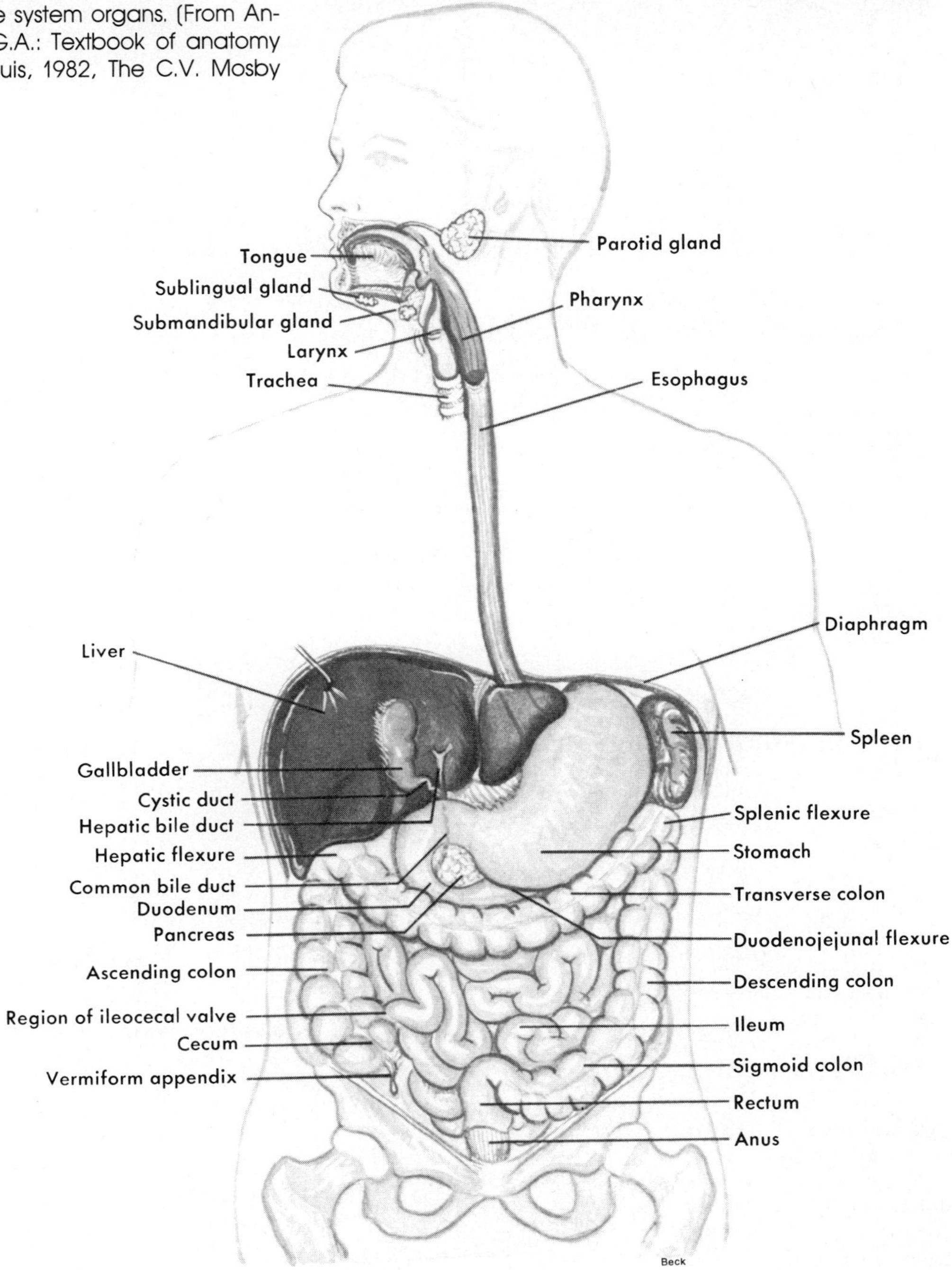

Fig. 32-1. Location of digestive system organs. (From Anthony, C.P., and Thibodeau, G.A.: Textbook of anatomy and physiology, ed. 11, St. Louis, 1982, The C.V. Mosby Co.)

SWALLOWING

Swallowing must be accomplished without compromising respiration. The tongue forces the bolus of food into the pharynx, from which point the food moves to the upper esophagus then down into the stomach. Food is prevented from passing into the trachea by the closing of the epiglottis over the trachea and the opening of the esophagus.

The esophagus is a hollow tube. The upper one third is composed of skeletal muscle and the remainder of smooth muscle. It is lined with mucous membrane, which secretes a mucoid substance for protection. The bolus of food arrives at the cardiac sphincter of the stomach usually within 5 to 10 seconds of ingestion.

The cardiac sphincter prevents reflux of stomach contents back into the lower esophagus. This area is heavily layered with mucoid glands. The secretions adhere to the food particles and prevent actual contact with the wall mucosa. The coated particles adhere to each other, forming a bolus for digestion. These secretions act as a pro-

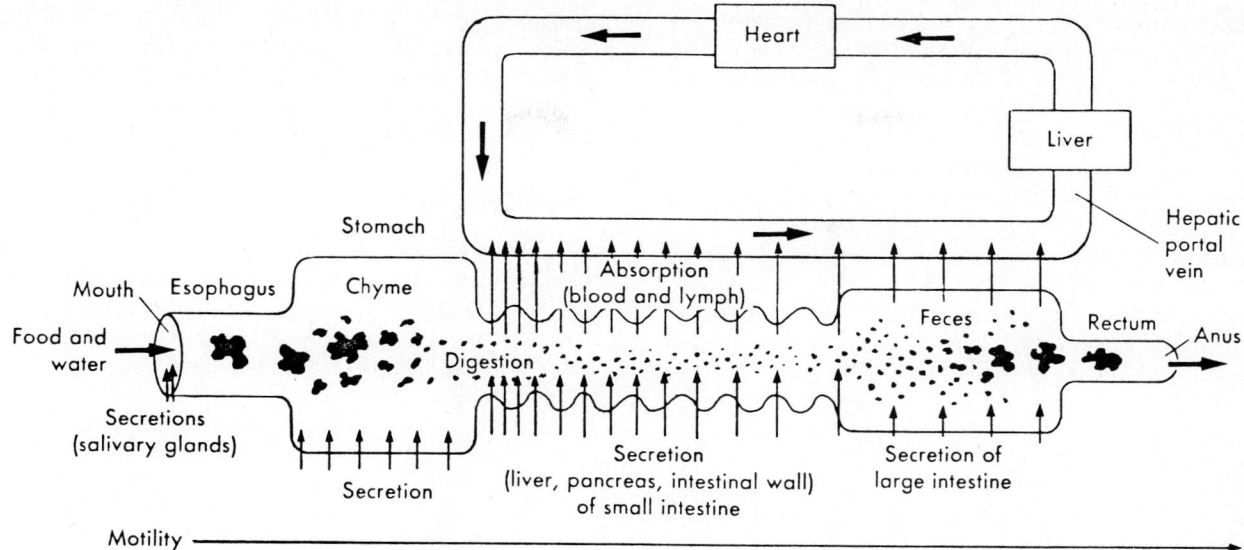

Fig. 32-2. Summary of gastrointestinal activity involving motility, secretion, digestion, and absorption. (From Human physiology, ed. 3, by Vander, et al. Copyright © 1980 by McGraw-Hill Book Co. Used with the permission of McGraw-Hill Book Co.)

tective mechanism for the sphincter zone, since they themselves are strongly resistant to digestion.

Stomach

The food bolus enters the stomach, the largest dilated portion of the tract. There is relatively little muscular tone, allowing for increased distention. Movement of food through the stomach and intestines is by *peristalsis*, the alternate contraction and relaxation of the muscle fibers that propels the substance in a wavelike motion.

The mucous membrane lining the stomach is arranged in thick folds known as *rugae* that provide an increased surface area for exposure and contain the openings of the gastric glands. The gastric secretions are clear and colorless and contain water, salts, enzymes, and hydrochloric acid. The amount of enzymes produced is in direct proportion to the amount needed, and the actual food substance stimulates the release of a particular enzyme. The gastric mucosa releases gastrin, which stimulates the production of *pepsinogen* (the precursor of pepsin), *rennin*, and *lipase*. Pepsin and rennin digest protein, and lipase splits fats. The production of hydrochloric acid (HCl) does not appear to be dependent on the presence of any particular food.

As the food moves toward the pyloric sphincter at the distal end of the stomach, peristaltic waves increase in force and intensity. The fluid bolus now becomes a substance known as *chyme*. Chyme is pumped through the pyloric sphincter into the duodenum. Emptying of stomach contents is regulated by two factors: consistency of the fluid chyme and the receptiveness of the duodenum.

The average length of time food remains in the stomach after a meal is 2 to 6 hours.

Intestines

The small intestine has three parts: the *duodenum*, which connects to the stomach, the *jejunum* or middle portion, and the *ileum*. The large intestine also has three parts: the *cecum*, which connects to the small intestine, the *colon*, and the *rectum*. The primary function of the intestines is to receive the chyme from the stomach and move the chyme forward to facilitate proper absorption of water, nutrients, electrolytes, and bile salts (Fig. 32-2). Secondary functions include secreting mucus and serving as a storage area before waste discharge.

MOVEMENT

Contents of the small intestine are propelled toward the anus by peristaltic movements that mix the intestinal contents. Chyme moves slowly and normally takes 3 to 10 hours to move from the stomach to the ileocecal valve (see Fig. 32-1). In the colon, the fecal contents are pushed forward by mass movements that occur only a few times each day. These mass movements are stimulated by gastrocolic reflexes initiated when food enters the duodenum from the stomach, especially after the first meal of the day. This is therefore the most fequent time of the day for defecation to occur.

The defecation reflex occurs when feces enter the rectum. Afferent impulses are transmitted to the sacral segments of the spinal cord, from which reflex impulses are transmitted back to the colon and rectum, initiating relaxation of the internal anal sphincter.

SECRETION

Secretions of the small intestine provide for the final digestion of food. As chyme enters the small intestine, gastric secretion of hydrochloric acid is slowed and *secretin, pancreozymin,* and *cholecystokinin* are released. Mucus secretion throughout the tract increases food adhesion, prevents contact of the food with the wall of the mucosa, enhances free passage of the food, neutralizes the small amounts of acid or alkali, and makes some particles more resistant to digestion.

ABSORPTION

Ninety percent of absorption occurs within the small intestine, either by active transport or diffusion. Many nutrients, such as amino acids, monosaccharides, sodium, and calcium, are transported by active transport, requiring metabolic energy expenditure. Other nutrients, such as fatty acids and water, diffuse passively across the cell membrane. Pancreatic lipase and conjugated bile salts must be present in the intestinal lumen for hydrolysis of fats into fatty acids to permit diffusion across the cell membrane.

Approximately 450 ml of chyme reaches the cecum per day. The transit time in the large bowel is slow, taking about 12 hours for material to reach the rectum. Reabsorption of water, electrolytes, and bile salts occurs predominantly in the ascending colon. The colon has the capacity to absorb 6 to 8 times more fluid than is delivered to it daily. Approximately 100 ml of fluid contents remains to be mixed with the residue of feces. Normally, this residue (feces) is evacuated on a fairly regular schedule. The evacuation schedule differs for each individual and may vary from 1 to 3/day to once every 3 to 4 days.

FLUID AND ELECTROLYTE BALANCE

Pathological alterations occur with the loss of particular segments of small or large bowel or when reabsorption is impaired. The loss of small bowel contents precipitates metabolic acidosis and hypokalemia. This problem may occur with drainage of small bowel contents through a suction tube or fistula or with persistent vomiting of the intestinal contents. Losses from the large intestine comprise mainly loss of water, sodium, and to a lesser extent chloride, resulting in dehydration and hyponatremia. This occurs in conditions in which the rate of peristalsis is increased.

BACTERIA

In addition to its role in nutrition, the intestinal tract supports bacterial growth that enhances digestive processes and has a role in antibody formation. Most of the organisms are in the large bowel. The organisms are responsible for the production of vitamin K, which is necessary for blood clotting. Antibiotic enemas decrease the number of organisms, thus interfering with vitamin K synthesis. Conditions that inhibit intestinal motility may lead to bacterial overgrowth in the intestines.

Physiologic changes with aging

Changes in the gastrointestinal tract structure and function may occur with aging but vary among individuals and may or may not cause altered functioning.

In the mouth, aging teeth become darker and may loosen from loss of supporting bone and gums. Teeth may become uneven or develop fractures, and circulation of the gums is reduced. Gum changes affect the fit of dentures. Salivary gland output decreases, leading to increased dryness of mucous membranes and making them more susceptible to breakdown. Dryness of the mouth may also interfere with chewing.

Changes in the ability to digest and absorb foods are related to decreased secretion of most digestive enzymes and bile production. Absorption of fats and fat-soluble vitamins becomes impaired. The increased residue resulting from decreased digestion and absorption may lead to increased flatulence. Gas-forming foods may be less well tolerated than when the person was younger.

Decreased intestinal motility may result from decreased peristalsis, decreased muscular tone of the intestinal wall, and decreased abdominal muscle strength. Decreased anal sphincter tone may also be present. These changes contribute to the increased occurrence of constipation in the older person.

PREVENTION AND HEALTH EDUCATION

Disorders of the digestive system are among the most commonly encountered health problems. Symptoms produced by digestive disorders are numerous and often lead to decreased employment productivity. Gastrointestinal symptoms, such as nausea and vomiting or diarrhea, often result from disorders of other body systems. Interference with functioning of the gastrointestinal system leads to temporary or long-term nutritional imbalances.

Primary prevention: prevention of disease

Since the cause of many gastrointestinal disorders is unknown, prevention may not be possible. However, some health practices are either known to be or are thought to be helpful in preventing some disorders (p. 879).

Secondary prevention: early detection

Early detection of major gastrointestinal health problems can prevent serious complications, such as a ruptured appendix with peritonitis. Persons at high risk for

Prevention of gastrointestinal problems: health teaching

Oral hygiene
1. Brush teeth after meals with fluoridated toothpaste
2. Use denture floss between teeth
3. Rinse mouth after eating sweets
4. Have regular dental checkups
5. Replace misfitting or broken dentures
6. Strengthen gums under dentures by rubbing with fingers or rinsing with alternating warm and cold liquid

Nutrition
1. Plan meals based on Basic four food groups (Chapter 7)
2. Substitute high-vitamin fruits for sweets, especially at end of meal (for example, apples, apricots, peaches, pears)
3. Avoid *excessive* amounts of foods that are found to irritate the oral mucosa (for example, raw tomatoes, hot peppers)
4. Avoid foods the person finds irritating to stomach, such as highly seasoned foods, large amounts of alcohol, or coffee
5. Include high-fiber foods (vegetables, fruits, whole-grain cereals) in the diet
6. Avoid foods that may cause food poisoning: unrefrigerated mayonnaise; cream-filled foods; inadequately cooked eggs, poultry, or meat (especially pork); improperly canned foods.

Smoking
1. Avoid constant exposure of lips to hot pipe
2. Avoid chewing tobacco
3. Discontinue cigarette smoking, if possible

Stress
1. Identify and remove cause of stress, if possible
2. Use measures to reduce stress response when stress occurs; for example; relaxation exercises (see Chapter 8)
3. Get adequate sleep on a regular basis

Early detection of major gastrointestinal disorders

1. *Signs requiring immediate medical follow-up*
   a. *Mouth*
      1. A sore that bleeds easily and does not heal
      2. A lump or thickening
      3. A persistant red or whitish patch
      4. Difficulty chewing, swallowing, or moving tongue or jaws
   b. *Abdomen*
      1. Persistent heartburn, indigestion
      2. Abdominal pain, especially if accompanied by nausea and vomiting
   c. *Elimination*
      1. Change in bowel habits
      2. Blood in the stool
2. *American Cancer Society recommendations for screening for cancer of colon and rectum*
   a. Digital rectal examination by physician every year after age 40
   b. Stool guaiac test done by patient at home every year after age 50
   c. Proctoscopic examination every 3 to 5 years after age 50; following two initial negative tests, 1 year apart.

cancer of the colon need careful screening to detect early signs of cancer, since the cancer may be in a more advanced stage before any symptoms occur. Guidelines for early detection are listed in lower box on p. 879.

Major health problems of the gastrointestinal system

There are several ways in which health problems can interfere with functioning of the gastrointestinal system: (1) interference with movement of food through the system, (2) interference with function because of inflammation, ulceration, or ineffective absorption, and (3) interference with passage of food, chyme, or feces through the system because of obstruction. Listed here are some common gastrointestinal disorders.

1. Interference with gastrointestinal motility and control
   a. Common dysfunctions: vomiting, flatulence, constipation, diarrhea, fecal incontinence
   b. Esophageal disorders: achalasia, esophageal diverticuli, gastroesophageal reflux, hiatal hernia
   c. Dumping syndrome (after gastrectomy)
   d. Paralytic ileus
2. Inflammatory disorders
   a. Mouth: stomatitis, gingivitis, dental caries
   b. Stomach: gastritis
   c. Intestines: enteritis, appendicitis, peritonitis, chronic inflammatory bowel disorders (ulcerative colitis, Crohn's disease, diverticulitis), parasitic infections (amebiasis, trichinosis)
   d. Rectum: anal fissures, abscesses, and fistulas; inflamed hemorrhoids
3. Peptic ulcers: gastric, duodenal, stress ulcers
4. Malabsorption disorders: lactase deficiency, disorders that decrease pancreatic secretions or bile salts, subtotal gastrectomy, small bowel disease, radiation enteritis
5. Obstructive disorders: tumors, hernias, adhesions, intussusception, volvulus

INTERFERENCE WITH GASTROINTESTINAL MOTILITY AND CONTROL

Common dysfunctions

Interference with gastrointestinal motility may lead to several common problems:
1. Vomiting: gastric hypermotility or delayed gastric emptying
2. Flatulence: intestinal hypomotility
3. Constipation: hypomotility of bowel or delayed bowel emptying
4. Diarrhea: intestinal hypermotility
5. Fecal incontinence: loss of anal control

VOMITING

Pathophysiology

Vomiting is often preceded by nausea but may occur alone. It may be a symptom of a disease process (such as infection or uremia) or a response to drugs, visceral injury, pain, psychic trauma, radiation, or motion. Vomiting is initiated by the vomiting center in the brain. It is reverse peristalsis. Vomiting can be defined as forceful ejection of stomach contents. If the pyloric end of the stomach is obstructed, the vomitus will project away from the person (projectile vomiting).

Prolonged and severe vomiting will interfere with nutrition and cause fluid and electrolyte imbalance, specifically dehydration and metabolic alkalosis with loss of potassium, chloride, and hydrogen ions. The act of vomiting produces a strain on the abdominal muscles, and in some postoperative patients it may cause wound dehiscence or bleeding. Vomiting is especially dangerous for anesthetized patients, persons in coma, and infants because they are likely to aspirate the vomitus into the lungs. Aspiration may cause asphyxia, atelectasis, or pneumonitis, especially in the elderly person whose nasopharyngeal reflexes are less acute than those of a younger person.

Assessment

Subjective data: onset of vomiting, patient's perception of cause

Objective data: examination of vomitus
1. Greenish yellow: bile
2. Bright red: overt bleeding of recent origin
3. Brownish "coffee-ground": blood that has been in the stomach for a period of time and is partly digested
4. Fecal odor: intestinal contents from an intestinal obstruction

Vomiting of blood is termed *hematemesis.* It is important to ascertain whether the content expelled from the mouth has been vomited from the stomach or coughed up from the lungs. Bloody sputum usually has a more frothy appearance than hematemesis. "Dry" emesis or retching may occur when the stomach is empty.

Implementation

1. Assisting with achievement of therapeutic goals
   a. If vomiting is anticipated (such as with radiation or motion), give prescribed antiemetic 30 minutes before the event
   b. If vomiting is present, give prescribed antiemetic by suppository or *deep* intramuscular injection
2. Assisting with comfort
   a. Provide a calm environment to decrease anxiety
   b. Suggest deep breaths through the mouth if nausea or gagging occurs
   c. Remove vomitus as soon as possible and provide oral hygiene
   d. Provide fluids in small amounts after vomiting subsides; ginger ale and other effervescent drinks are usually well tolerated.
   e. Provide solid foods (after vomiting subsides) that

are well tolerated, such as crackers, baked potato, apple

FLATULENCE

Pathophysiology

Gas collects in the gastrointestinal tract as a result of swallowed air, as gas formed by the action of intestinal bacteria, and as carbon dioxide formed by the action of bicarbonate with hydrochloric acid or fatty acids. Normally the gas is either reabsorbed or is expelled. When gastrointestinal motility is decreased, the gas collects in the stomach or intestines, causing abdominal distention and pain.

Assessment

"Gas pains" can cause severe abdominal discomfort. The abdomen is distended over the entire area (as differentiated from lower abdominal distention occurring from a full bladder). The abdomen has a drumlike sound if tapped.

Implementation

Some of the following interventions may help to decrease the intestinal gas volume when a pathologic condition is not present:
1. Avoid activities that increase repetitive swallowing of air
2. Maintain an erect position after meals to facilitate gas rising to the fundus of the stomach and being expelled
3. Eat a low-fat diet to decrease carbon dioxide production
4. Take antacids containing hydroxide and simethicone (Maalox Plus, Mylanta) 1 hour after meals to neutralize acid and reduce flatus
5. Avoid gas-forming carbohydrates that the person identifies as producing more discomfort (for example, selected vegetables, fruit, or bran)
6. Ambulate to increase peristalsis to move the gas through the intestinal tract, if discomfort is present

CONSTIPATION

Pathophysiology

Constipation may result from decreased motility of the colon or from retention of feces in the lower colon or rectum. In either case, since water is reabsorbed in the colon, the longer the feces remain in the colon the greater the reabsorption of water, and the dryer the stool becomes. The stool is then more difficult to expel from the anus.

Occasional constipation is not detrimental to health, although it can cause a feeling of general discomfort or abdominal fullness, anorexia, and anxiety in some persons. Habitual constipation leads to decreased intestinal muscle tone, increased use of Valsalva maneuver (bearing down using a closed glottis) as the person attempts to pass

---

High risk factors for constipation/fecal impaction

Nutritional depletion
Dehydration
Radiographic examinations using barium
Prolonged bedrest or inactivity
Prolonged use of constipating medications (aluminum-based antacids, anticholinergics, antihistamines, antidepressants, narcotics, phenothiazines, salts of bismuth, calcium, iron)

---

the hardened stool, and increased incidence of hemorrhoids.

Assessment

Constipation is identified by defecation of a hard, formed stool or a frequency considerably less than the person's usual pattern. The person may also report feelings of rectal pressure or fullness and may experience straining at stool. If the stool is permitted to remain in the colon until it becomes exceedingly hard, a *fecal impaction* occurs. Digital examination by means of inserting a gloved finger in the rectum may identify a fecal impaction. Hardened stool may be palpated in the lower left abdominal quadrant. Some persons are at high risk for developing constipation and fecal impaction (see box).

Implementation

1. Assisting with achievement of therapeutic goals
   a. Encourage a diet containing adequate high-fiber foods (raw or cooked vegetables and fruits, whole-grain cereal products)
   b. Encourage a fluid intake of at least 2000 to 2400 ml/day (8 to 10 glasses) unless contraindicated
   c. Encourage all hospitalized patients to be as active as possible within the limits of their activity prescription
   d. Facilitate change of a constipating antacid with one that has a more laxative effect in high-risk persons (p. 972)
   e. Use suppositories to initiate defecation in persons who lack innervation of rectum (paraplegics)
   f. Encourage use of prescribed laxatives after extensive barium studies
2. Teach the patient
   a. Effect of diet, fluids and activity in preventing constipation
   b. Planning of daily schedules to permit time for defecation after breakfast and dinner
   c. Avoiding use of laxatives on a regular basis (decrease muscle tone and mucus production; may lead to water and electrolyte imbalances)

DIARRHEA

Pathophysiology

The definition of diarrhea is based on the consistency of the stool and not on the number expelled per day. Diarrhea results primarily from pathologic disorders that increase the fluid content of the stool or that increase intestinal transit time. The end result is a watery stool.

Severe diarrhea can lead to excessive losses of water, sodium, potassium, and bicarbonate, leading to dehydration, hyponatremia, hypokalemia, and metabolic acidosis (see Chapter 10). Distention of the intestines and frequent contractions from the rapid motility lead to abdominal cramping, although discomfort may be absent (such as with diarrhea caused by stress). Increased peristalsis may produce high-pitched bowel sounds occurring at frequent intervals (borborygmi).

Assessment

The stool is monitored for consistency (soft to liquid) and amount. Abdominal cramping may occur only immediately before and during defecation, or it may occur irrespective of time and situation. Perineal irritation may result from the frequent defecation.

Implementation

1. Assisting with achievement of therapeutic goals
   a. Facilitate rest of the bowel
      (1) Administer medications as prescribed (see Table 32-1). If diarrhea occurs primarily after meals, give antidiarrheal medications 30 to 60 minutes before meals for maximum effectiveness.
      (2) Diet: control food intake to decrease intestinal stimulation and prevent irritation of inflamed mucosa
         (a) Give only fluids for 24 to 48 hours for severe diarrhea
         (b) Give high-protein, high-calorie, low–dietary fat diet when foods are permitted
   b. Assist with fluid and electrolyte replacement
      (1) Monitor for signs of fluid and electrolyte imbalance (thirst, dry mucous membranes, decreased skin turgor, headache, muscle weakness, fatigue, abdominal cramps, distention)
      (2) Monitor and facilitate parenteral fluids and electrolytes as prescribed by physician for severe diarrhea
      (3) Give oral fluids for moderate diarrhea; fluids high in sodium and potassium, such as fruit juices and bouillon, are recommended.
2. Assist with comfort
   a. Provide for personal hygiene after *each* loose stool
   b. Provide rest periods if fatigue is present

FECAL INCONTINENCE

Pathophysiology

Voluntary emptying of the rectum occurs when the external anal sphincter (under cortical control) relaxes and the abdominal and pelvic muscles contract. Conditions that interrupt transmission of messages to and from the brain (cortical lesions, spinal cord lesions), cause injury to the sphincter (trauma, fistulas, abscess), or cause perineal muscle relaxation (childbirth, perineal surgery, aging) may lead to fecal incontinence.

Common causes of diarrhea

Increased fluid content of stool

Intestinal infections
Chronic bowel disorders
Malabsorption disorders
Biliary tract disorders
Postgastrectomy syndrome
Saline laxatives
Antacids (magnesium based)
Caffeine

Increased motility

Stress
Gastric or intestinal resection
Surgical intestinal bypass
Antibiotics

Table 32-1. Drugs commonly prescribed for diarrhea

Drug	Action
Systemic effect	
Diphenoxylate (Lomotil, Colonil)	Decrease intestinal motility; side effects: constipation, sedation
Camphorated tincture of opium (paregoric)	
Loperamide (Imodium)	
Local effect	
Bismuth salts (for example, Pepto-Bismol)	Binds with bacterial toxin; side effect: black stool
Kaolin with pectin	Limited value; may protect the irritated, inflamed intestinal wall

Assessment

Fecal incontinence is characterized by involuntary passage of stool. Data to be collected include the following:
1. Frequency of defecations
2. Nature of the stool
3. Awareness of need to defecate
4. Ability to contract abdominal and perineal muscles
5. Willingness of person to participate in exercise or bowel control program.

Implementation

1. Assisting with achievement of therapeutic goals
   a. Provide a high-fiber diet to facilitate a formed stool.
   b. Provide a fluid intake of about 3000 ml/day to promote a soft stool.
   c. Administer a stool softener daily, if necessary, to keep the stool soft.
   d. Plan a bowel training program to prevent incontinence if control is not feasible. Within a few days the patient will probably defecate only once a day when stimulated. If the stool remains soft, the program may be changed to every other day. Consistency in carrying out the plan is important for success (see box below).
   e. If fecal incontinence is uncontrollable, the defecation pattern is identified. Place the patient on the toilet or commode at the time that defecation is anticipated. Protective disposable pants are available to provide the person with a sense of security and dignity.
2. Assisting with comfort
   Assist the person to cleanse the anal and perineal areas as soon as possible after fecal incontinence to eliminate odor and prevent skin breakdown.
3. Counseling and teaching
   a. Provide empathic communication. The person may have feelings of regression, inadequacy, or uncleanliness as a result of the loss of control. The person needs to feel accepted as an adult and accept the condition as a situational physical condition and not personal inadequacy.
   b. Encourage patients to participate in all or some of their own management to the extent that is possible, thus providing them with a sense of control.
   c. Teach perineal exercises for weak perineal muscles (Chapter 33).

Esophageal disorders

TYPES OF DISORDERS

There are a number of esophageal disorders that delay motility in the esophagus. Some of these disorders are described in Table 32-2.

PATHOPHYSIOLOGY

Esophageal motility may be impaired by physiologic dysfunction or lack of persitalsis (achalasia), by lack of structural integrity (diverticulum), or by irritation of the esophageal lining, particularly at the gastroesophageal junction (gastroesophageal reflux, hiatal hernia). Tumors may partially obstruct the lumen.

Varying degrees of *achalasia* can exist. In severe conditions the portion of the esophagus above the achalasia dilates and the person may have difficulty swallowing food and fluids past that point (Fig. 32-3).

An *esophageal diverticulum* is a bulging of the esophageal mucosa and submucosa through a weakened portion of the esophageal muscle (Fig. 32-4). As food is ingested, some of it may collect in the pouch formed by the weakened area. After a sufficient amount of food has collected in the pouch, it overflows into the esophagus and is regurgitated. There is always danger that some of the regurgitated food may be aspirated in the trachea during sleep.

Gastroesophageal reflux occurs when the lower esophageal sphincter (LES), at the junction of the esophagus and stomach, becomes incompetent and permits reflux of gastric material back into the esophagus. The acidity of the gastric juice irritates the esophageal mucosa, creating a muscle spasm. Chronic reflux may lead to stricture of the LES (as a result of fibrosis from the inflammatory process), delaying passage of food into the stomach. An incompetent LES may be idiopathic (no known cause) or may be exacerbated by anticholinergic drugs, caffeine,

---

Bowel training program

1. Include patient and family/friend in the planning
2. Determine when bowel evacuation usually occurs (most frequent times are after breakfast or dinner)
3. Determine whether a morning or evening program is more suitable for patient
4. Insert glycerine or bisocodyl (Dulcolax) *suppository* 30 minutes before expected time of defecation; give suppository at *same time every day*
5. Have patient sit on toilet if possible for defecation
6. If necessary, massage abdomen toward the sigmoid area (left lower quadrant) to encourage defecation; digital rectal stimulation may also stimulate defecation.

Table 32-2. Esophageal disorders

Disease	Etiology	Signs and symptoms	Medical therapy
Achalasia (aperistalsis of esophagus)	Unknown	Dysphagia for liquids and solids, weight loss, substernal chest pain Later: regurgitation	Forceful dilation of lower esophageal sphincter with pneumostatic or mechanical dilators
Esophageal strictures	Swallowing of caustic substances	Dysphagia	Esophageal dilation, resection of stricture
Esophageal diverticulum (pouch in mucosa)	Weakened esophageal wall	Dysphagia, fetid breath	Surgery for severe symptoms (excision of herniated sac)
Gastroesophageal reflux	Incompetent lower esophageal sphincter	Heartburn	High protein, low fat diet; avoidance of smoking, foods containing caffeine, chocolate, and alcohol
Hiatal hernia (diaphragmatic hernia)	Contributing factors: obesity, trauma, aging	50% asymptomatic, heartburn, dysphagia	No treatment for asymptomatic Heartburn: high-protein, low-fat diet; antacids Surgery for incarcerated hernias through thorax or abdomen

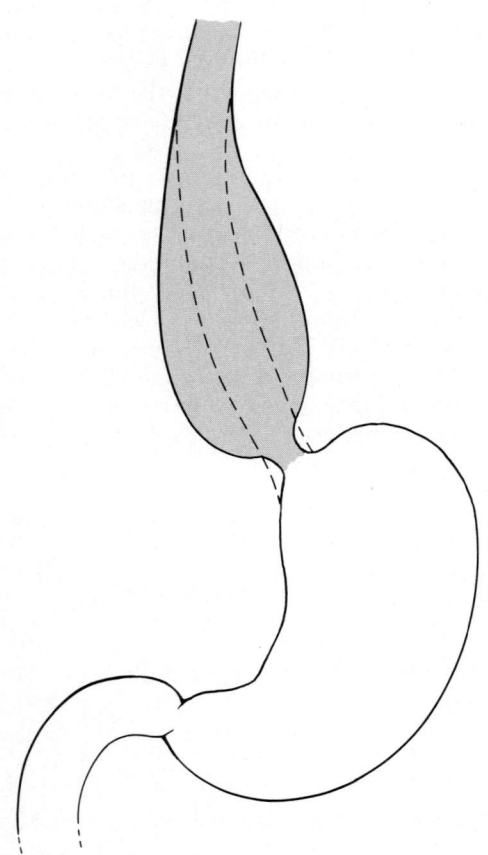

Fig. 32-3. Achalasia.

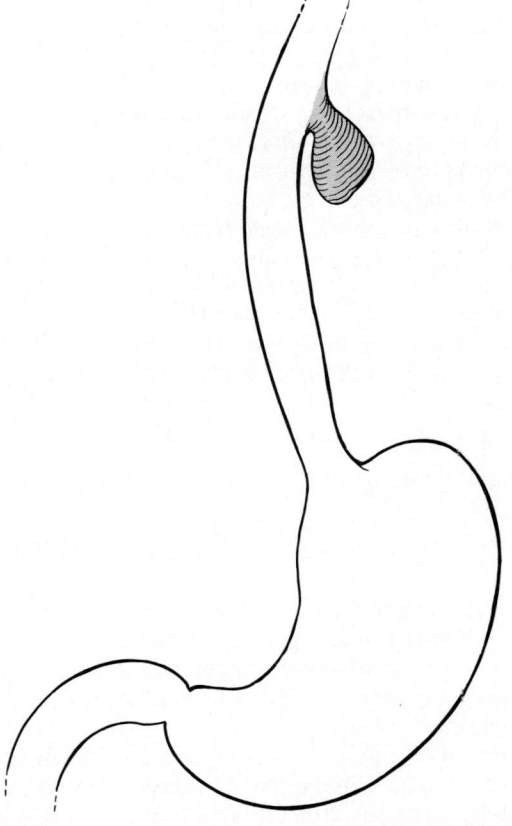

Fig. 32-4. Esophageal diverticulum.

theobromine (chocolate), ethyl alcohol, or smoking. Gastroesophageal reflux may also occur with *hiatus hernia*, a protrusion of part of the stomach through the diaphragm into the thoracic cavity (Fig. 32-5). Obesity and aging are contributing factors to the development of hiatal hernias.

ASSESSMENT

Subjective data

Dysphagia is a primary symptom of esophageal disorders. Esophageal dysphagia of motor origin characteristically produces dysphagia for both solids and liquids. This differs from dysphagia that results from paralysis of neurologic origin (difficulty swallowing liquids) or dysphagia caused by obstruction of the esophageal lumen (difficulty swallowing solids). If the patient has had dysphagia for a period of time, it is helpful to know what approaches to eating the person has found most useful.

The patient who experiences *regurgitation* is asked if this occurs at night (staining of the pillow may have been observed), and if there is a foul odor of the regurgitated material (seen with esophageal diverticulum).

Heartburn is a substernal "burning" sensation resulting from gastroesophageal reflux. The pain may be referred to the neck or back if severe. It is frequently accompanied by a sour regurgitation of gastric contents but is not accompanied by nausea.

Objective data

The ability to swallow is assessed by placing three fingers over the thyroid cartilage of the larynx (Adam's apple) and asking the person to swallow or by observing the movement of the larynx. If movement is limited, the gag reflex can be elicited by touching the posterior tongue or pharynx lightly with a tongue blade. A further assessment can be made, if necessary, by placing 1 to 2 ml of water in the oropharynx and asking the patient to swallow.

Diagnostic tests

The diagnosis of esophageal disorders is facilitated by x-ray films of the esophagus taken after barium swallow. The patient may be placed in Trendelenburg's position during the x-ray examination or fluoroscopy to identify gastroesophageal reflux.

A water siphon test is a fluoroscopic examination in which barium is swallowed followed by plain water. If the LES is incompetent, the barium will be seen to reflux back into the esophagus. Overnight pH recordings measured from swallowed glass electrodes will demonstrate periods of increased gastric reflux.

DATA ANALYSIS AND PLANNING

Possible nursing diagnoses for the person with an esophageal disorder include the following:

Alteration in comfort: pain (heartburn)

Alteration in nutrition: less than body requirements

Expected patient outcomes include the following:

1. The person has a nutritionally balanced intake.
2. The person describes any recommended dietary changes.
3. The person states he/she is feeling comfortable.
4. The person describes body position and activity requirements.

IMPLEMENTATION

Assisting with comfort and ADL

Persons with esophageal disorders who experience *dysphagia* have difficulty swallowing both solids and liquids. Frequent small feedings are suggested. Some patients drink large amounts of fluid while swallowing solids to increase esophageal pressure, thus pushing the food into the stomach. Eating with the head elevated encourages movement of food through the esophagus by gravity. Regurgitation of food may occur several hours after eating,

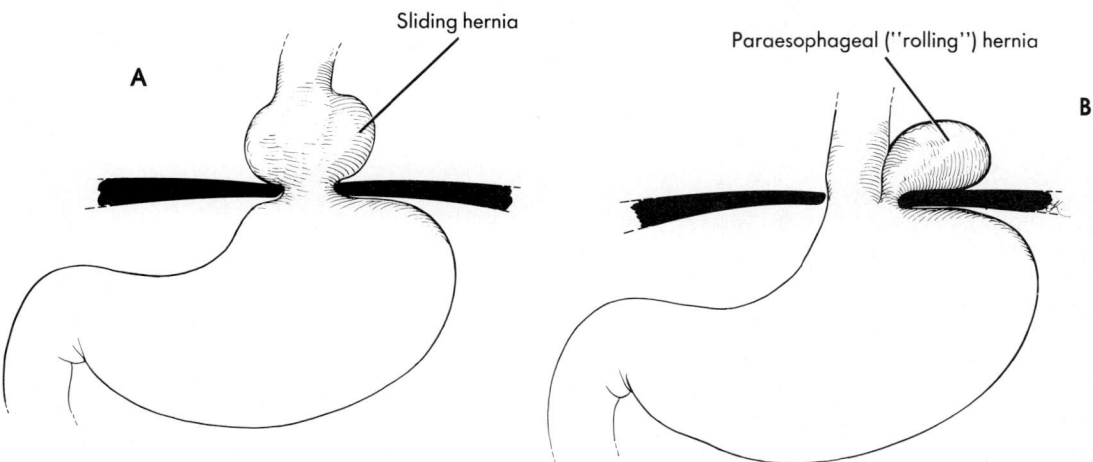

Fig. 32-5. Hiatal hernias. **A,** Sliding. **B,** Paraesophageal.

Patient teaching for heartburn

1. Eat a high-protein, low-fat diet to prevent esophageal regurgitation
2. Avoid foods containing caffeine (coffee, tea, colas), chocolate, and alcohol
3. Eat small frequent feedings to prevent gastric distention and increased gastric acid secretion
4. Avoid smoking
5. Avoid lying down or bending over for 2 hours after eating to prevent regurgitation
6. Avoid lifting or wearing tight belts or girdles after eating to prevent abdominal pressure
7. Sleep with head elevated

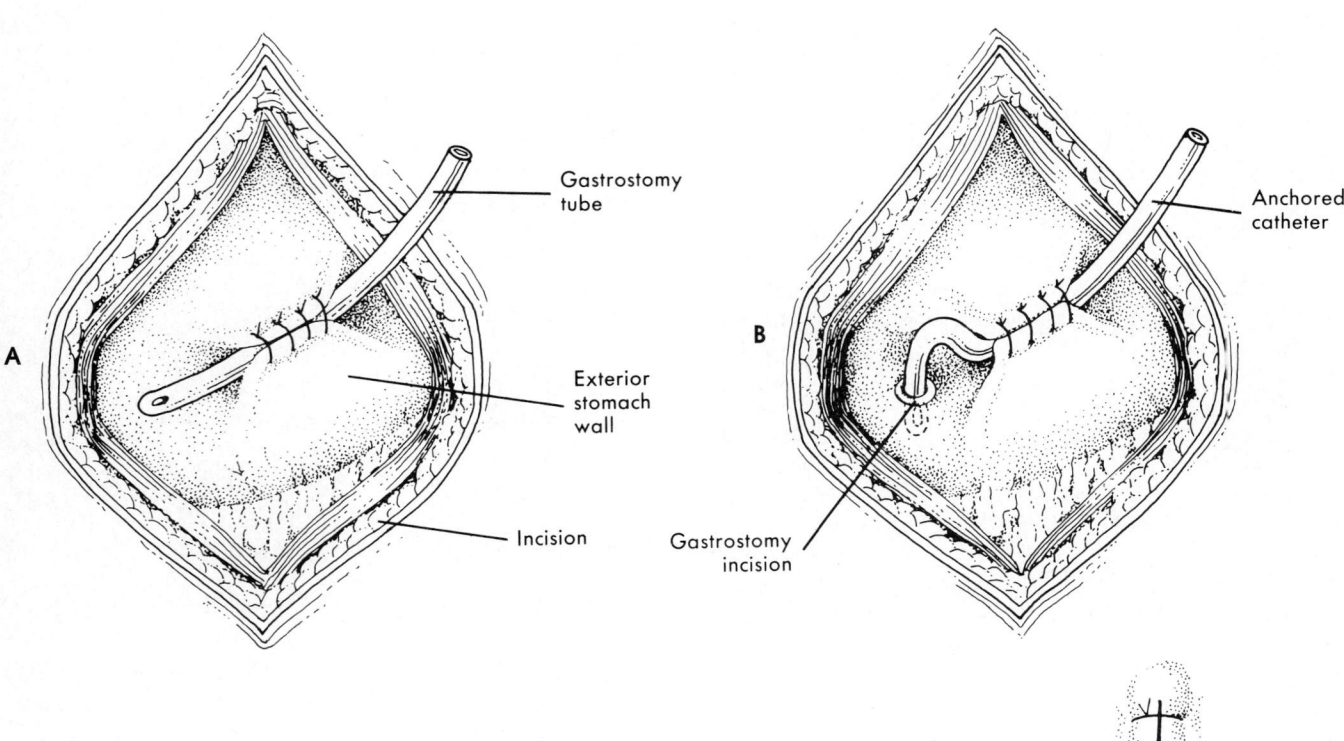

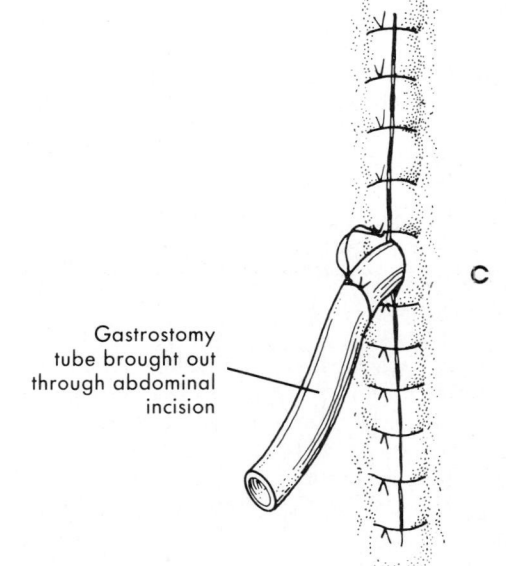

Fig. 32-6. Gastrostomy with tube. **A,** Catherer is laid on greater curvature of exterior stomach wall and sutured to secure it in place. **B,** Anchored catheter is then inserted into stomach. **C,** Abdomen is closed, and gastrostomy tube is sutured in place. A separate stab wound may be made for tube rather than bringing it out through incision line. (From Broadwell, D.C., and Jackson, B.L.: Principles of ostomy care, St. Louis, 1981, The C.V. Mosby Co.)

especially at night when the body is horizontal (therefore eating is avoided for at least 2 hours before bedtime).

Discomfort from heartburn can be decreased by administration of 30 ml of a liquid antacid 1 hour after meals, at bedtime, and whenever heartburn occurs. Gaviscon, which is a mixture of antacids with alginic acid, has been found to be effective in alleviating heartburn. Two to four tablets, when *chewed* thoroughly and then swallowed, produce a viscous antacid foam that coats the esophagus and floats on the gastric contents. If antacids are not effective, medications that increase LES contraction may be prescribed; these include bethanechol chloride (Urecholine) or metoclopramide (Reglan) to be taken 30 minutes before meals and at bedtime. Anticholinergic medications are avoided, because they decrease gastric emptying.

Patient teaching

Prevention is the best approach to treatment of heartburn. Key points for patient teaching are listed on p. 886.

Esophageal dilation

The physician may dilate the esophagus by the use of dilators (bougies) or inflatable bags. The procedures may be performed under fluoroscopy to prevent damage to the mucosa. In the postoperative period the patient is monitored for *chest pain* as a result of esophageal perforation. Fluids and soft foods are indicated when swallowing produces pain. Most patients will require pain medication in the early postoperative period.

Gastrostomy

Gastrostomy is an alternative approach to nasogastric tube feedings when the person is unable to swallow for a long period of time. The procedure is often performed under local anesthesia. A small incision is made in the left upper abdominal quadrant, and the stomach is exposed. A catheter is laid on and sutured to the exterior surface of the greater curvature of the stomach (Fig. 32-6). The tip of the anchored catheter is then inserted into the stomach and secured with a circle of sutures pulled tightly around the catheter (purse string sutures) to prevent leakage. The connecting end of the catheter is brought to the surface through either the incision or a separate stab wound. The incision is closed and the catheter is sutured and taped to the skin.

Immediately after surgery the gastrostomy tube is attached to low intermittent suction to prevent buildup of gas and gastric juices in the stomach. When bowel sounds become active and gastric drainage is less than 300 to 400 ml/day, the surgeon may order the tube to be clamped.

The initial meal, consisting of a small amount of tap water or glucose in water, is given, followed by an increasing amount of fluids every 4 hours. If there is no leakage of fluid around the tube and if the patient appears to tolerate the clear fluids, foods blended into a mixture are then added through the tube. A large-lumen tube is required for blenderized food.

The meals may be a special formula, elemental diet formula (Chapter 7), or regular food blended so that it will pass through the tube. The use of regular foods helps to maintain the patient's nutritional state, prevent diarrhea that often accompanies the use of specially prepared tube feedings that are high in fat, and make food preparation easier at home. Solid and liquid foods are blended into a mixture with a food blender, fork, or egg beater and are strained. Water is given through the tube between feedings so that approximately 2500 to 3000 ml of fluid is received daily.

The psychologic trauma of not being able to eat normally is usually severe. The patient may become depressed and need a great deal of encouragement. Most patients, however, as they become proficient in feeding themselves, gradually accept this method of obtaining nourishment as inevitable and adjust remarkably well. The patient is encouraged to sit at the family dinner table for family socialization.

The care of the patient with a gastrostomy is summarized in box on p. 888.

Esophageal surgery
Preoperative care

The *nutritional status* of the patient may need to be improved before surgery. A high-protein, high-calorie diet is prescribed when food and fluids can be taken orally. If severe dysphagia is present, inhibiting oral intake, total parenteral nutrition (TPN) (Chapter 7) may be necessary. Occasionally a temporary gastrostomy is performed to supply food in the preoperative or early postoperative period.

Mouth care is important, since the breath may be foul. The patient may raise a mixture of pus, blood, or decomposed food. If mouthwashes are used, they may need to be varied from time to time, since the flavor of the mouthwash may become identified with the unpleasant taste.

Patient teaching includes the care of the patient experiencing chest surgery (Chapter 25) if this is appropriate. A nasogastric tube will be in place after surgery.

Postoperative care

The immediate postoperative care centers on *prevention of respiratory complications* and *maintenance of chest and gastric drainage systems*. Small amounts of bright red blood may drain from the nasogastric tube for 6 to 12 hours after surgery. The color of the drainage then changes to greenish yellow. The nasogastric tube is not disturbed to prevent traction on the suture line.

When oral fluids are permitted after the nasogastric tube is removed, small amounts of clear fluid are given at frequent intervals until well tolerated. Soft foods are introduced gradually until the patient is receiving several small meals of bland food daily.

If part of the stomach has been pulled up into the thoracic cavity, the patient may complain of a feeling of fullness in the chest or difficulty in breathing after eating. Smaller, more frequent meals may alleviate this problem.

Nursing care of the patient with a gastrostomy

Promoting skin integrity

1. Inspect skin around gastrostomy for leakage.
2. Wash skin around catheter at least twice a day with soap and water. Dry well.
3. Apply a protective ointment (zinc oxide, karaya paste, Stoma-hesive) around tube opening if irritation or leakage is present.
4. Cover skin around tube.

Promoting gastric function

1. Attach tube after surgery to low intermittent suction.
2. Monitor tubing for patency (free of kinks, draining).
3. Check tube length each shift. Report changes to physician.
4. Measure and record gastrostomy drainage each shift.
5. Monitor for return of peristalsis (bowel sounds, flatus).
6. Monitor for decreased gastric function (nausea, vomiting, feelings of abdominal fullness, abdominal distention) when tube is clamped by order of physician.

Promoting nutrition

1. Giving the feeding
   a. Before each feeding, unclamp tube and aspirate gastric contents. Delay giving feeding if a residual of 75 ml or more is present, and report findings to physician.
   b. Give feeding with patient in high Fowler's or sitting position to prevent esophageal regurgitation.
   c. Warm feeding to room temperature.
   d. Dilute feeding with water if too thick.
   e. Use feeding tube to introduce the liquid into the catheter.
   f. Give 50 ml of water before feeding.
   g. Let prescribed feeding (usually 200 to 500 ml) flow in by gravity over a 10 to 15 minute period.
   h. Flush tube with 50 ml of water after feeding to maintain patency of tube.
   i. Clamp tube when feeding is completed.
   j. Keep patient's head elevated for 30 minutes after the feeding.
2. Monitor intake and output until gastrostomy feedings are well tolerated.
3. Weigh patient daily until weight becomes stable.
4. Monitor for signs of dehydration (dry mucous membranes, thirst, decreased skin turgor).

Promoting comfort

1. Provide mouth care.
2. Encourage patient to express feelings regarding not being able to eat normally.
3. Encourage patient to participate in giving the feeding.

Patient teaching

1. Preparation of food (blenderized food, special formula)
2. Positioning for eating
3. Method of giving the feeding
4. Washing equipment well after feeding; storing equipment in a clean place
5. Maintenance of skin integrity
6. Making plans for returning to usual activities
7. Need for medical follow-up
8. Symptoms requiring immediate medical attention (tube dislodgement, tube occlusion, bleeding, infection, leakage of fluid around opening)

If the esophageal sphincter has been removed or made incompetent, the patient may experience heartburn from gastric reflux. This problem may be prevented by the patient remaining upright for 2 hours after meals and sleeping with the head elevated. (See p. 885 for care of the person with heartburn.)

EVALUATION

The care of specific patients with esophageal disorders is evaluated on the basis of the expected patient outcomes. General questions to be asked are: Is the patient receiving a balanced nutritional input? Is the patient comfortable? Does the patient know (1) how to achieve comfort and a nutritional intake when at home, (2) medication dosage schedule and side effects, and (3) what signs and symptoms need to be reported to the physician?

Paralytic (adynamic) ileus

PATHOPHYSIOLOGY

Failure of peristalsis may result from disturbances in neural stimulation of the bowel (paralytic ileus) or from obstruction of the gastrointestinal tract (p. 918). When peristalsis ceases, the involved intestinal area becomes distended by gas and fluid. Approximately 8 L of fluid are secreted into the stomach and small intestines per day; most of this fluid is normally reabsorbed in the colon. When peristalsis ceases, much of the fluid remains in the stomach and small intestine. The retained fluid increases pressure on the mucosal wall and, if not removed, results in ischemia, necrosis, bacterial invasion, and eventually peritonitis. Loss of the fluids leads to hypovolemia (shock) and dehydration. Loss of sodium and chloride ions causes a shift of potassium from the cells, leading to hypokalemic alkalosis.

ASSESSMENT

Abdominal distention is a major symptom and can be assessed by measuring abdominal girth with a tape measure. The abdomen is always measured at the same site (usually across the umbilicus). The patient is monitored for signs of fluid and electrolyte imbalance (thirst, dry mucous membranes, decreased skin turgor, hemoconcentration, oliguria, muscle weakness) and for signs of shock. Bowel sounds will be absent when peristalsis has ceased, and bowel movements will not occur (obstipation).

The physician may order x-ray films, which will show air-fluid filled loops of intestines and stomach.

IMPLEMENTATION

Paralytic ileus can be prevented if treatment is initiated by the physician in high-risk situations, such as following gastrointestinal surgery. When the ileus is caused by other factors, treatment of the underlying condition is initiated. The major treatment is decompression of the stomach or intestines by intubation.

GASTROINTESTINAL INTUBATION

Intubation of the gastrointestinal tract is performed for a variety of reasons. The major reason for intubation for paralytic ileus is decompression of the stomach or intestines. Different types of tubes are used depending on the location to be drained.

Types of tubes

A nasogastric *Levin tube* (Fig. 32-7) is most commonly used for gastric intubation; however, because it is a single-lumen tube, damage to the mucosa may result even with intermittent suction. A less traumatic approach is the use of the double-lumen Salem *sump tube*. The larger lumen of the sump tube drains the area, while the smaller lumen provides a continuous flow of air at atmospheric pressure, thus maintaining the suction at a

---

Causes of paralytic ileus

Manipulation of abdominal viscera during abdominal surgery
Peritoneal irritation (peritonitis)
Pain of thoracolumbar origin
    Rib or spinal fractures
    Myocardial infarction
    Pneumonia
    Pyelonephritis
    Ureteral or biliary calculi
    Retroperitoneal hemorrhage
Sepsis
Hypokalemia causing decreased muscle tone of bowel
Intestinal ischemia

Reasons for gastrointestinal intubation

Gastric

Tests of gastric analysis
Tube feedings
Decompression of the stomach
Removal of gastric contents (gastric hemorrhage, perforation)

Intestinal

Intestinal decompression

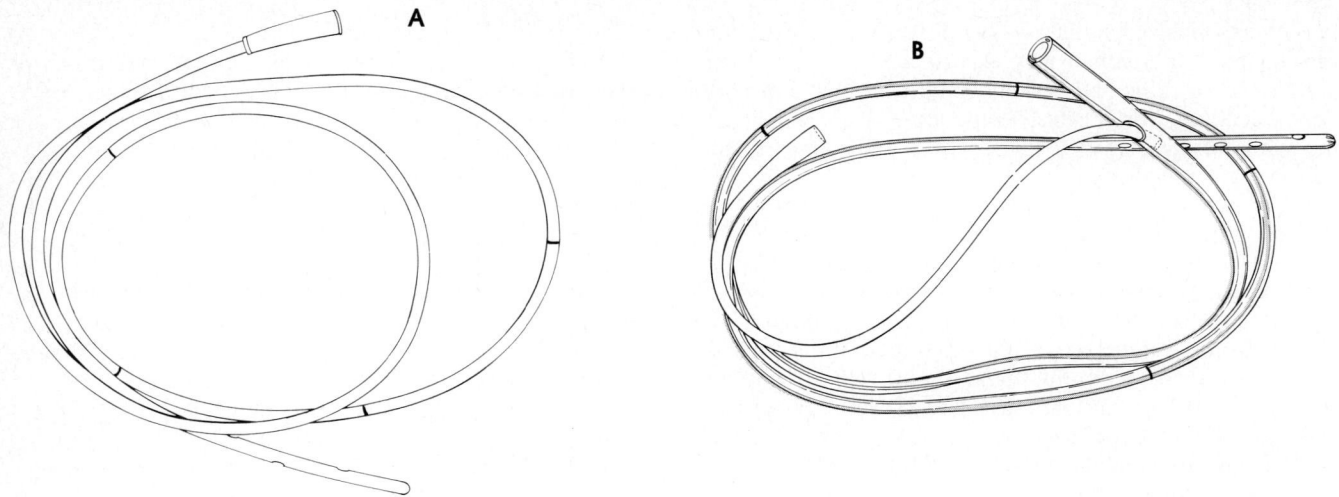

Fig. 32-7. Nasogastric tubes. **A,** Levin tube. **B,** Salem sump tube.

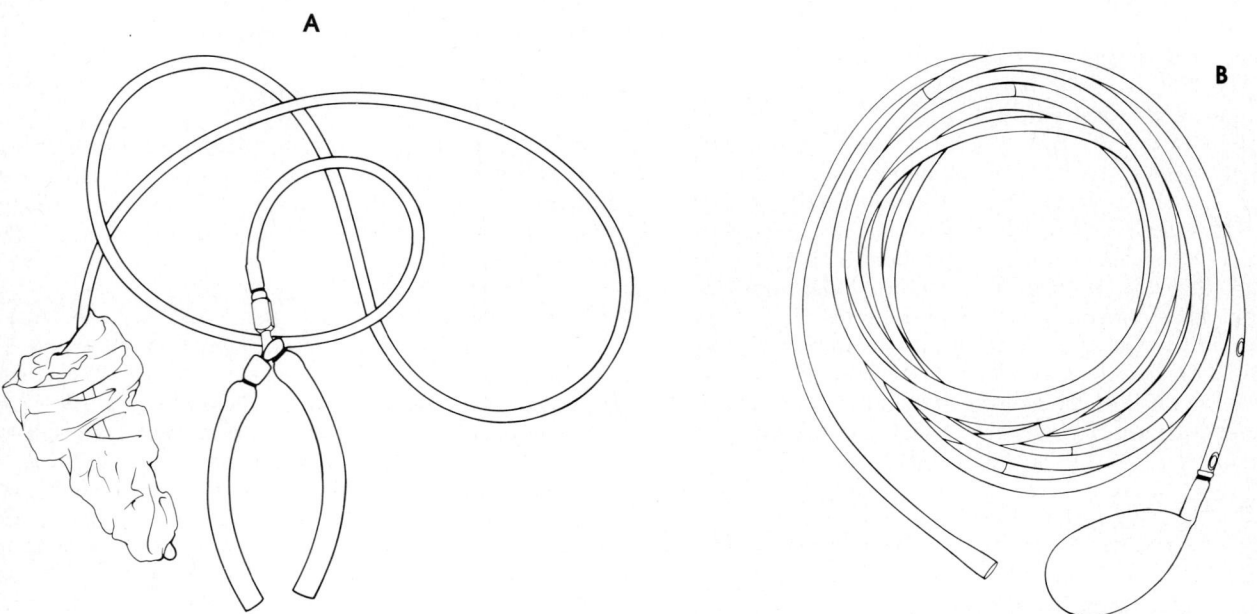

Fig. 32-8. Intestinal tubes. **A,** Miller-Abbott tube. **B,** Cantor tube.

lower level and preventing adherence of the tube against the tissue wall.

The tubes most often used for intestinal decompression are the Miller-Abbott tube and the Cantor tube. The length of these tubes permits their passage through the entire intestinal tract. There is a small balloon on the tip of each, which, when inflated with air or injected with water or mercury, acts like a bolus of food. This balloon stimulates peristalsis, which advances the tube along the intestinal tract. If peristalsis is absent, the weight of the mercury in the balloon will usually carry it forward. When a Miller-Abbott tube is used, the mercury is inserted into the balloon of the tube after the tube is passed.

The choice of tube depends on the physician's preference. The Miller-Abbott tube is a double-lumen tube. One lumen leads to the balloon, and the other has openings along its course, permitting drainage of intestinal contents and irrigation. The external end of the tube contains two openings, one for drainage of secretions and the other for inflating the balloon (Fig. 32-8). In irrigating this tube, the nurse must be careful that the correct opening is used—the one marked "suction." The other opening is for inflating or deflating the balloon. It should be clamped off and labeled "do not touch."

The Cantor tube, which is used less often, is a single-lumen tube with only one opening used for drainage. Before the tube is inserted, the balloon is injected with mer-

Insertion of nasogastric tube

1. Measure tube to mark desired length of insertion: distance from ear lobe to bridge of nose to xiphoid process. Mark tube with adhesive tape.
2. Place tube on ice for 5 minutes before insertion to stiffen it for easier insertion
3. Place patient in sitting postion with head slightly flexed. Protect clothing and provide patient with tissues
4. Lubricate tip of tube with water-soluble lubricant
5. Insert tube slowly and steadily through nose into pharynx; ask patient to swallow repeatedly while tube is advanced to marked site on tube
6. Ascertain location of tube in stomach by one of the following methods;
   a. Aspirate gastric contents; test with litmus paper for acidity
   b. Instill 20 ml of air into tube while listening to abdomen with a stethoscope; a roar will be heard if tube is correctly placed in stomach
7. Secure tube to nose with adhesive tape (Fig. 32-9)
8. Connect tube to suction:
   a. Levin tube to intermittent suction set at "low" pressure
   b. Sump tube to intermittent suction at "high" pressure or continuous suction at "low" pressure

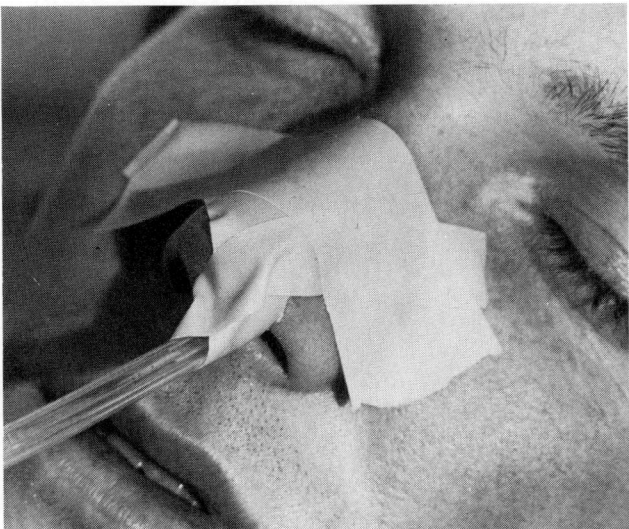

Fig. 32-9. Nasogastric tube secured by crossing tape over patient's nose and applying a second piece of tape over the bridge of the nose. (From Hirsch, J. and Hannock, L., editors: Mosby's manual of clinical nursing procedures, St. Louis, 1981, The C.V. Mosby Co.)

cury with a needle and syringe. The needle opening is so small that the globules of mercury cannot escape through it. The mercury can be pushed about so that the balloon is elongated for easy insertion.

Insertion of tubes

Nasogastric tubes may be inserted by either the nurse or the physician. *Intestinal* tubes are more difficult to insert because of the addition of the balloon. The intestinal tube can be mechanically inserted only into the stomach. Its passage along the remainder of the gastrointestinal tract is dependent on gravity and peristalsis. The weight of the mercury in the balloon helps propel the tube through the intestines.

The intestinal tube is passed in the same manner as the nasogastric tube. After the intestinal tube reaches the stomach its passage through the pylorus into the duodenum is facilitated by positioning and activity.

1. Encourage the following patient positions;
   a. Right side for 2 hours, then
   b. Lying on back with head elevated for 2 hours, then
   c. Left side for 2 hours
2. Encourage patient ambulation following passage of tube into the pylorus (often assessed by x-ray film)
3. Advance the tube 2 to 10 cm (1 to 4 inches) at specified intervals to provide slack for peristaltic action
4. Secure tube to face when desired point has been reached; coil extra tubing on bed or pin to clothing

The intestinal tube is usually monitored daily by x-ray film for signs of coiling or telescoping of the tube. Telescoping is movement of bowel along with the tube resulting in intussusception (p. 918), a serious complication.

Facilitating drainage

Since the gastric or intestinal fluid must move against gravity to be removed, suction is required. *Intermittent suction* is used for single-lumen tubes; constant suction could damage the mucosal wall if a section of the wall were to be pulled continually against the drainage holes of the tube. Intermittent suction permits the wall to drop away from the tube when suction is not occurring. The Gomco machine (Fig. 32-10), which has a "high" pressure and a "low" pressure setting is commonly used for intermittent suction. A *low* pressure is used for the Levin and the intestinal tubes; high pressure is used only with the sump tube. Constant suction is usually preferred for the sump tube.

Methods of assessing functioning of gastrointestinal tubes

1. Check the suction machine
   a. Light is blinking off and on
   b. Machine is plugged in and turned on
   c. Tubing connections are tight
2. Check tubing to identify kinks in the tubing or tubing clamped off by pressure of patient's body
3. Insert 20 ml of air through tubing while listening with stethoscope for "roar" sound at abdomen
4. Irrigate tube with 30 to 60 ml normal saline; a free flow of fluid into the tube and return of fluid mixed with gastric or intestinal contents indicates a patent tube

---

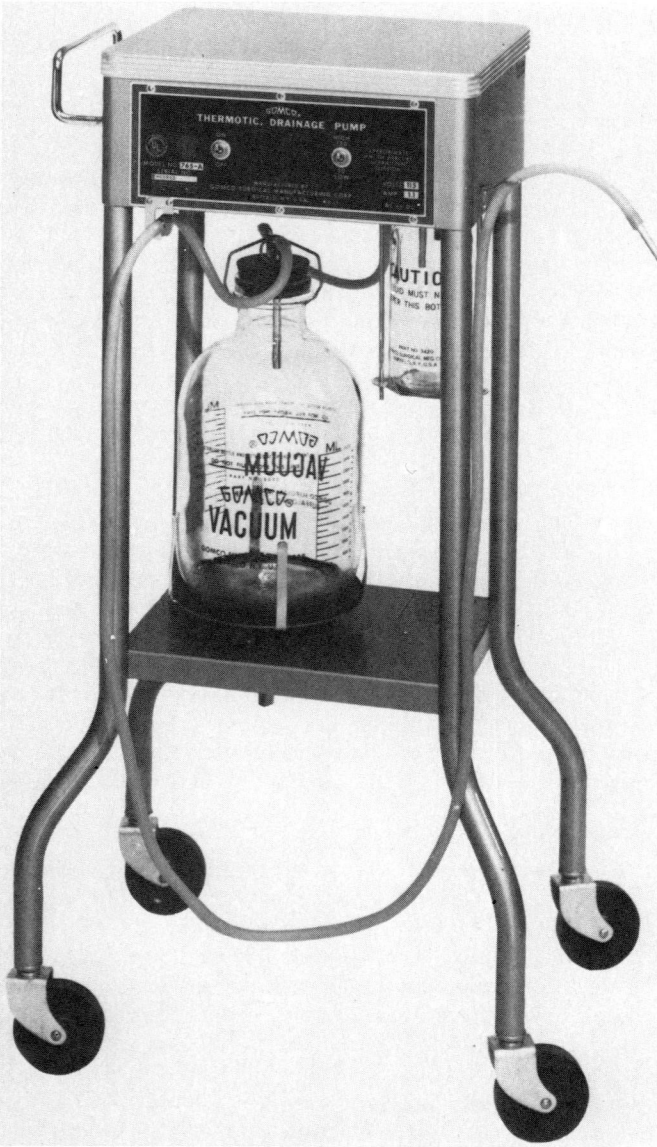

Fig. 32-10. Intermittent suction machine (Gomco). (Courtesy Chemetron Medical Products Co., St. Louis.)

Functioning of the suction apparatus is checked if no visible drainage is occurring or if the patient has nausea, vomiting, or abdominal discomfort.

Normal saline is used to *irrigate* the tube, since a hypotonic solution such as water would increase electrolyte loss.

Prevention of injury

To prevent necrosis of the nares from constant pressure, the tube is taped securely so that it does not press against the nostril or obstruct vision (Fig. 32-9). It is then pinned loosely to the clothing to support the weight of the tube and to permit free movement of the head.

The oropharyngeal mucosa or the parotid glands may become inflamed as a result of dry mucous membranes from oral breathing (nares plugged) or from gastrointestinal bacteria that travels up the tube by capillary action. Oral inflammations can be prevented by mouth care given every 4 hours or by sucking hard candy (sour balls) to stimulate flow of saliva. Ice chips should be used sparingly, since large amounts may result in hypotonic fluid ingested into the stomach with subsequent electrolyte loss through suction.

Promotion of comfort

The presence of the tube in the nasopharynx causes local discomfort, and the patient may complain of a lump in the throat, difficulty in swallowing, sore throat, hoarseness, earache, or irritation of the nostril. Excess secretions around the nares are removed, and a *water-soluble* lubricant, such as K-Y jelly, is applied to the tube and to the nostril to prevent crusting of secretions. Warm saline solution gargles may relieve dryness and soreness of the throat, and throat lozenges may be prescribed. Phenylephrine (Neo-Synephrine) 0.25% nose drops are sometimes helpful in relieving nasal stuffiness.

Frequent changing of the patient's position helps to relieve pressure from the tube on any one area in the throat. Unless contraindicated, elevation of the head of the bed to 30 degrees helps to prevent esophageal reflux and subsequent esophagitis.

Irrigation of nasogastric tubes

1. Irrigation of Levin tubes
   a. Check tube placement before irrigation
   b. Instill 30 to 60 ml of normal saline in tube
   c. Aspirate instilled fluid; if no fluid returns, reconnect tube to suction and watch for return drainage; add to fluid intake sheet
   d. If fluid does not flow easily into tube or return by aspiration or suction, try one or all of the following:
      (1) Rotate tube
      (2) Move tube in and out approximately 2 to 3 cm (1 to 1½ inches) unless prohibited by medical orders
      (3) Ask patient to turn on opposite side (tubing may be lodged against stomach wall)
   e. If tubing remains blocked, consult physician
2. Irrigation of sump tube
   a. Instill 30 to 60 ml normal saline through
      (1) Drainage lumen, or
      (2) Smaller vent lumen without interrupting suction
   b. When irrigation is completed, inject air through the vent lumen during suction to ensure air patency

---

INFLAMMATORY DISORDERS OF THE GASTROINTESTINAL SYSTEM

Inflammatory disorders may occur in the mouth, esophagus, stomach, intestines or rectum (Fig. 32-11). The inflammations may be acute or chronic.

Inflammatory disorders of the mouth

The mouth is an excellent barometer of general health, reflecting general disease and debility as well as good health. Specific diseases of the mouth most often occur when general nutrition and oral hygiene are poor, when people neglect their teeth, when smoking is excessive, and when broken teeth irritate the tissues.

In the mouth, inflammation may occur on the mucous membranes, gum, or tongue. Medical treatment depends on the site and causative factor (Table 32-3).

PATHOPHYSIOLOGY

Several factors contribute to the development of oral inflammatory disorders: (1) poor oral hygiene, (2) stress, (3) nutritional deficiencies, (4) debilitating diseases, (5) heavy smoking, and (6) chemotherapy. Poor oral hygiene leads to mouth debris, which can irritate the mucous membranes. Other irritants include smoke, broken teeth, and irritating foods. Stress, malnutrition, and chemotherapy interfere with the body's immune response, leading to breakdown of body defenses.

Inflammation of the mucous membranes often result in small, painful ulcerations. Scarring rarely occurs, as only the mucous membrane is usually involved. Inflammation of the gums may cause teeth to loosen.

Thrush may result when antibiotics are given over a period of time to control other infections. It is thought

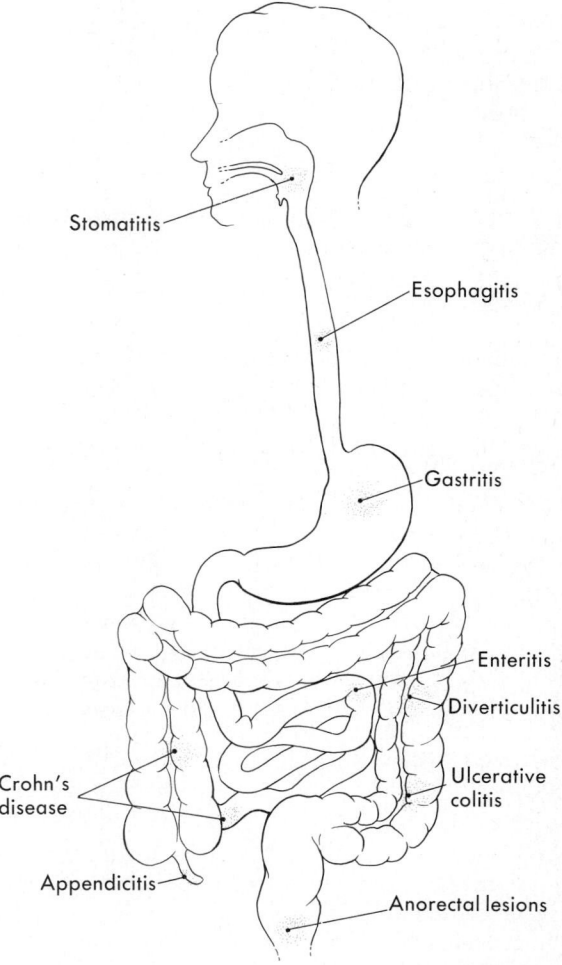

Fig. 32-11. Inflammatory conditions of gastrointestinal system.

Table 32-3. Inflammatory disorders of mouth

Disease	Etiology	Signs and symptoms	Medical therapy
Aphthous stomatitis (canker sores)	Biting cheek, virus	Ulcer on mucous membranes becomes covered with opaque material; pain	Triamcinolone acetonide in emollient dental paste (Kenalog in Orabase)
Herpetic stomatitis (cold sore, fever blister)	Herpesvirus type 1	Initial burning sensation, vesicle formation on junction of lips to mucosa, secondary infection, crusting	Symptomatic treatment: 70% alcohol initially for drying; petrolatum after vesicular stage; rest; avoidance of stress
Vincent's angina (ulceromembranous stomatitis)	Fusiform bacillus and a spirochete	Malaise, acute painful bleeding gums, fetid breath, ulceration on margins of gums, dysphagia	Gentle debridement by dentist; mouthwashes with warm normal saline or 3% hydrogen peroxide; rest; antibiotics if severe
Thrush	*Candida albicans* (fungus)	White patches (like milk curds) over inflamed membranes	Nystatin oral suspension
Gingivitis (gums)	Bacterial plaque, malocclusion, food impaction, vitamin deficiency	Red inflamed gums, bleeding with minimal injury, swelling of interdental spaces	Good oral hygiene and dental care
Periodontitis (loss of bone supporting teeth)	Same as for gingivitis	Same as for gingivitis, loose teeth, recession of gums, possible abscess formation	Dental care, dental surgery

that the elimination of bacteria permits growth of the existing fungus, causing thrush.

ASSESSMENT

In patients at high risk of developing infections, the mouth is assessed daily for developing or healing inflammations.

Subjective data

The patient is questioned about the presence and extent of the following symptoms: (1) pain in the mouth, (2) loss of appetite, (3) nausea, (4) foul taste in the mouth, and (5) increase or decrease of salivation. The pain is caused by the inflammatory response, and it restricts ability or desire to keep the teeth and mouth clean. This leads to the foul taste and loss of appetite. Swallowing of inflammatory debris may produce nausea.

Objective data

1. Mouth inspection
   a. Cleanliness
   b. Condition of teeth (caries, loose teeth, debris)
   c. Signs of inflammation (redness, edema, ulceration, or white curdlike patches of thrush)
   d. Bleeding of mucous membranes or gums
2. Ability of patient to carry out oral hygiene
   a. Mental status (decreased consciousness or confusion

   b. Ability to open mouth (pain may limit mouth movement)
   c. Cleanliness of mouth after oral hygiene
3. Ability to ingest and swallow food

DATA ANALYSIS AND PLANNING

Nursing diagnoses

Possible nursing diagnoses for the patient with an oral inflammation include the following:
Alterations in oral mucous membranes
Alteration in comfort: pain in mouth
Potential alteration in nutrition: less than body requirements
Potential alteration in fluid volume: deficit

EXPECTED PATIENT OUTCOMES

1. The patient's mouth is clean.
2. The patient
   a. States mouth feels comfortable.
   b. Eats a balanced diet.
   c. Remains hydrated (good skin turgor, moist mucous membranes).
   d. States the action and side effects of medications to be taken at home, including the need to complete antibiotic therapy.
   e. Describes risk factors to be avoided to prevent recurrence of an oral inflammation.

IMPLEMENTATION

Assisting with achievement of therapeutic goals
Medications

If antibiotics are ordered, they are given on time on a regular schedule to maintain blood levels. If the patient has difficulty swallowing tablets, they are crushed, if possible, or the antibiotics may be given intramuscularly or intravenously.

Mouth care

Thorough and frequent mouth care is a must.
1. Frequency
   a. Mild stomatitis: at least every 4 hours
   b. Severe stomatitis: at least every 2 hours[20]
2. Types of solutions
   a. Alkaline mouthwashes, such as sodium bicarbonate or sodium perborate
   b. Hydrogen peroxide diluted 1:4 with normal saline (mix immediately before use to prevent decomposition)
   c. Lidocaine rinses may be prescribed for stomatitis resulting from chemotherapeutic drugs
3. Removal of dentures if causing pain
4. If the toothbrush causes pain, gently wipe gum and teeth with moistened gauze wrapped around a tongue blade; rinse with solution followed by water

Assisting with comfort and ADL
Relief of pain

Pain may be partially relieved by good oral hygiene. Smoking is contraindicated. Cold drinks or sucking on frozen Popsicles may be soothing. Analgesic drugs may be necessary, and lidocaine may be applied to provide topical anesthesia.

Facilitating eating

If the mouth is very sore and painful, eating may be difficult, and the patient may need considerable encouragement. Soft foods, including strained meats and fish, pureed vegetables and fruits (except citrus), cooked cereals, soups, flavored gelatin, and ice cream, are best tolerated. Hot spicy foods are to be avoided; cold drinks may be soothing. High-protein, high-calorie drinks such as eggnog serve both nutritional and fluid needs.

Teaching

Persons at high risk for developing recurrent oral infections need to know about contributing factors that may be controlled, such as poor oral hygiene, poor nutrition, irritating foods, heavy smoking, and stress (see preventive measures, p. 879).

EVALUATION

Evaluation is based on the expected patient outcomes. Interventions may have to be modified based on the severity of the oral infection. The mouth is assessed daily for cleanliness and extent of healing and comfort.

Acute inflammatory disorders of stomach and intestines

Gastritis (inflammation of the stomach) and *enteritis* (inflammation of the intestines) may occur separately or together (*gastroenteritis*). Gastroenteritis of viral origin is a common occurrence. Some foods per se may cause irritation of the gastric or intestinal mucosa leading to mild symptoms of belching, abdominal discomfort, and diarrhea. Bacteria and parasites may also cause intestinal inflammations (Table 32-4).

PATHOPHYSIOLOGY

In acute gastritis or enteritis of viral origin, the mucosa appears red, inflamed, and edematous. The disease is usually self-limiting with renewal of the mucosal lining. Frequent ingestion of irritating substances, such as salicylates or alcohol, can cause gastric bleeding from capillary erosion. Gastritis may occasionally become chronic with atrophy of the mucosa predisposing to pernicious anemia or gastric carcinoma.

Acute gastroenteritis can be caused by direct bacterial or viral infection or by the effect of neurotoxins produced by bacteria. This produces either an increased secretion of water and salt into the gut lumen or an increase in motility, causing large amounts of undigested food and fluid to be excreted. In the latter case, large amounts of gas and foul smelling stool result.[36] With profuse diarrhea, large amounts of fluid and electrolytes may be lost, leading to dehydration, hyponatremia, hypokalemia, and metabolic alkalosis (see Chapter 10).

ASSESSMENT

Subjective data include presence of *anorexia, nausea,* and presence and extent of *abdominal discomfort.* If food poisoning is suspected, the person is questioned concerning possible sources of food contamination. Abdominal pain is usually diffuse except if acute appendicitis is present, in which case the pain may become localized over McBurney's point (midpoint between umbilicus and right anterior iliac spine).

Objective data to be collected includes the following:
1. Emesis—frequency, amount, presence of blood
2. Stools—frequency, character, amount if liquid, presence of foul odor
3. Flatulence
4. Signs of fluid and electrolyte imbalance (thirst, dry mucous membranes, hemoconcentration, oliguria, muscle weakness)

DATA ANALYSIS AND PLANNING

Nursing diagnoses

Possible nursing diagnoses may include the following:
Alteration in bowel elimination: diarrhea
Alteration in comfort: abdominal pain
Fluid volume deficit

Table 32-4. Acute inflammatory disorders of stomach and intestines

Disease	Etiology	Signs and symptoms	Medical therapy
Gastritis	Chemical irritants: alcohol, salicylates Bacteria: viruses Allergies (for example, shellfish) Corrosive substances: acids, lyes	Anorexia, epigastric fullness, nausea and vomiting, epigastric discomfort, hematemesis or melena; shock and esophageal strictures with corrosives	Mild: antacid, rest Severe: correction of fluid/electrolyte imbalances, sedatives, antacids Administration of specific antidote with corrosives
Gastroenteritis	Virus	Abdominal cramps, nausea and vomiting, diarrhea, headache	Nothing by mouth until nausea and vomiting subside, then fluids and bland diet; rest
Food poisoning	*Staphylococcus aureus:* enterotoxin in fish, meats, unrefrigerated mayonnaise or cream-filled foods; skin and respiratory tract of food handlers	Nausea and vomiting, abdominal pain, decreased temperature; diarrhea is variable	Bed rest, fluids
	Salmonella: inadequately cooked pork, poultry, eggs	Nausea and vomiting, abdominal pain, chills, fever, weakness	Bed rest, fluids
	Clostridium botulinum: improperly canned or smoked foods	Nausea and vomiting, double vision, flaccid paralysis of face and throat, dryness of skin and mucous membranes	Botulinum antitoxin, maintenance of ventilation and oxygen, parenteral fluids
Appendicitis	Appendiceal kinking or occlusion, obstruction by fecalith, infection by colon bacillia or streptococcus	Sudden onset, pain in mid-epigastrium becomes localized in right lower quadrant, nausea and vomiting, low grade fever, leukocytosis	Appendectomy when diagnosis confirmed
Amebiasis	Parasite found in tropical climates where sanitation is poor	Early: abdominal cramps, intermittent diarrhea/constipation, flatulence Late: frequent liquid stools containing blood, mucus; fever, colicky abdominal pain	Amebicidal drugs
Trichinosis	Roundworms transmitted by inadequately cooked food, especially pork	Edema of eyelids, muscle stiffness, weakness, fever, pain on eye motion, dyspnea	Symptomatic: bed rest, analgesics, steroids, thiabendazole

Expected patient outcomes

1. Stools are decreased in number and are of normal consistency.
2. Patient is hydrated.
3. Patient with gastritis describes substances that could cause recurrence of the condition and should therefore be avoided.

IMPLEMENTATION

Assisting with achievement of therapeutic goals
Initial care for appendicitis

When appendicitis is suspected, the patient usually is hospitalized at once and placed on bed rest for observation and the necessary diagnostic procedures (serum WBC, urinalysis, flatplate abdominal x-ray film) that must be performed. Since an operation may be performed shortly after admission, the patient is not given anything by mouth while reports of the blood count are awaited. Parenteral fluids may be given during this time. Narcotics are not given until the cause of the pain has been determined, since they would mask signs or symptoms. Sometimes an ice bag to the abdomen is ordered to help relieve pain. *Heat is contraindicated.* A rectal examination is performed by the physician to help establish the diagnosis, and the patient is given an explanation of why the procedure is necessary. Surgery consists of an appendectomy (removal of the appendix).

Maintaining hydration

When nausea and vomiting are present, the person is given nothing by mouth until symptoms subside. With severe vomiting, fluids and electrolytes will be replaced intravenously and a sedative such as sodium phenobarbital or an antiemetic such as prochlorperazine (Compazine) or trimethobenzamide (Tigan) will be given parenterally or by suppository. When vomiting subsides, tea, broth, and ginger ale are given orally every hour. Bland feedings of custard, gelatin, and cream soups are usually tolerated after 2 to 24 hours. Intake and output are carefully measured and recorded.

Assisting with comfort

Abdominal cramping from diarrhea may be relieved by constipating agents containing an opiate, such as paregoric, or diphenoxylate (Lomotil) which is chemically related to meperidine (Demerol) (see Table 32-1). Belching and defecation also often relieve the discomfort, If appendicitis is ruled out, heat to the abdomen may offer some relief.

Environmental control

If a parasite is identified as the cause of the inflammation (such as in amebiasis), excretion precautions may be observed. Cleanliness is stressed, and patients should know that it is important to wash their hands well after bowel movements and before meals to prevent spread of infection.

Chronic inflammatory bowel disorders

Ulcerative colitis and Crohn's disease (regional enteritis) are chronic nonspecific inflammatory disorders of the bowel. These disorders are often confused with each other but are different entities (Table 32-5). Both disorders may become exacerbated by stress. Many theories

Table 32-5. Comparison of Crohn's disease and ulcerative colitis

	Crohn's disease	Ulcerative colitis
General appearance	Usually normal	May feel and look ill
Age	Bimodal: 20 to 30 years and 40 to 50 years	Mostly young adults
Area affected	Mainly terminal ileum, cecum, and ascending colon (right side)	Colon only, primarily the descending colon (left side)
Extent of involvement	Segmental areas of involvement	Continuous, diffuse areas of involvement
Inflammation	Mosty submucosal	Mostly mucosal
Mucosal appearance	Cobblestone effect; granulomas	Ulcerations
Cancer potential	Normal incidence	Increased incidence
Character of stools	No blood; may have some fat; three to four semisoft per day	Blood present; no fat; frequent liquid stools
Reasons for surgery	Fistulas; intestinal obstruction	Poor response to medical therapy; hemorrhage; perforation
Complications	Fistulas; perianal disease; strictures; vitamin and iron deficiencies; fistulas to other organs	Pseudopolyps; hemorrhage; toxic megacolon; cachexia; perforation less often, causes peritonitis

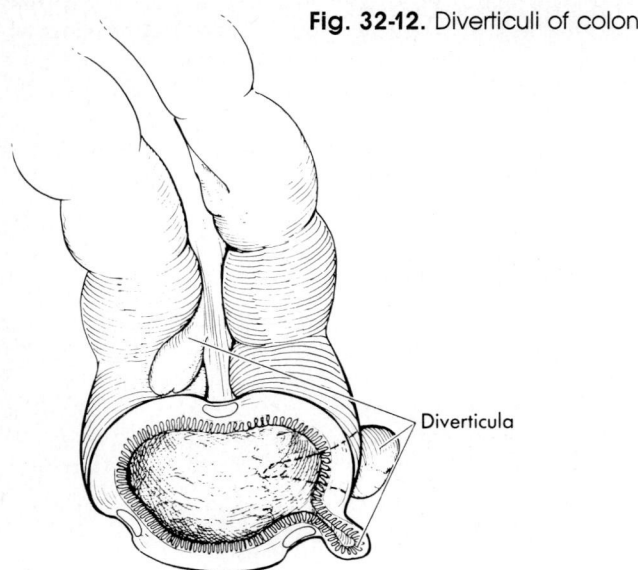

Fig. 32-12. Diverticuli of colon.

Diverticula

have been suggested about the possible causes of these two disorders; more recent studies are exploring the immunologic mechanisms as possible etiologic factors.

Diverticulitis is a focal bowel disorder involving inflammation of diverticula (outpouchings in the colon wall), especially the sigmoid colon (Fig. 32-12). Diverticula occur more commonly in elderly persons.

The etiologies, signs and symptoms, and usual medical therapies of chronic bowel inflammatory disorders are listed in Table 32-6.

PATHOPHYSIOLOGY

Ulcerative colitis and Crohn's disease differ in terms of location and type of lesions. Ulcerative colitis starts in the rectosigmoid colon and spreads upward. Crohn's disease can affect both the small and large intestines, and the areas of inflamed tissue are often separated by normal tissue. The lesions of ulcerative colitis are mucosal ulcerations that bleed easily. As the lesions advance, the bowel

Table 32-6. Chronic bowel inflammatory disorders

Disease	Etiology	Signs and symptoms	Medical therapy
Crohn's disease	Unknown	Periods of exacerbation and remission Acute: colicky or steady right lower quadrant pain, malaise, moderate fever, mild diarrhea, mucus or pus in stool Chronic: weight loss, anemia, fistula formation, intestinal obstruction	Diet: high-calorie, high-protein, high-vitamin Sulfonamides, azathioprine (Imuran) Surgery for fistulas or intestinal obstruction (colectomy or colostomy)
Ulcerative colitis	Unknown	Periods of exacerbation and remission Severe diarrhea (15 to 20 stools/day containing blood, mucus, pus) anorexia; weight loss; anemia; low grade fever Severe: weakness, debility, cachexia, dehydration, hypokalemia, hypoproteinemia	Diet: high-calorie, high-protein, high-vitamin (avoid milk) Sulfonamides, adrenocorticosteroids Surgery for refractory disease or complications (total colectomy with permanent ileostomy)
Diverticulitis of colon (inflamed mucosal pouches)	Older age, low intake of dietary fiber	May be asymptomatic Intermittent lower left quadrant pain aggravated by emotional tension or eating Constipation alternating with diarrhea	Diet: high in vegetable fiber, unprocessed bran Bulk stool additives; analgesics (pentazocine [Talwin]); anticholinergics (dicyclomine [Bentyl], propantheline [Pro-Banthine]) Bed rest, sedation and parenteral or oral fluids for severe episode Surgery for complications of perforation or obstruction (colectomy, temporary colostomy)

mucosa becomes edematous and thickened with scar formation. The colon may lose its elasticity and absorptive capability. The lesions of Crohn's disease are granulomatous ulcers that may involve deeper structures. The ulcers may perforate and form fistulas. Scar tissue may lead to intestinal obstruction.

The loss of absorptive capability in both ulcerative colitis and Crohn's disease leads to anorexia, weight loss, malaise, and diarrhea. Fluid loss from severe diarrhea leads to dehydration, hypokalemia, and hypoproteinemia.

Diverticula are formed when weakened areas of the colon are pushed outward into pouches by increased pressure within the colon. The cause is thought to be a low intake of dietary fiber, often found in the diet of persons living in industrialized societies. The nonsymptomatic condition is called *diverticulosis*. Symptoms appear when the diverticula become inflamed (*diverticulitis*), creating painful spasms. Bowel motility may be slow, leading to constipation because of the insufficient fiber, or fast, leading to diarrhea because of the inflammation.

ASSESSMENT

Both subjective and objective data are collected about the patient's knowledge of the disorder, the nutritional status, pattern of elimination, comfort, and ability to cope with stress.

Subjective data

1. Patient's understanding of the disorder
2. Awareness of any precipitating factors, such as stress, and usual coping patterns
3. Measures found helpful to relieve symptoms
4. Weight changes
5. Nutrient intake: appetite, type and amount of food/ fluids in a typical day, recent changes in dietary intake
6. Pattern of bowel elimination: character, frequency, amount, presence of unusual substances (blood, mucus, pus)
7. Pain: site, frequency, character
8. Fatigue

Objective data

1. Weight
2. Temperature
3. Observable eating patterns
4. Signs of dehydration with severe ulcerative colitis (decreased skin turgor, dry mucous membranes)
5. Stool: number, character, amount, presence of blood (overt, positive guaiac test), pus, mucus
6. Condition of perianal skin with severe diarrhea
7. Behavior: signs indicating stress or anxiety (for example, restlessness, pacing, twisting hands, verbal comments indicating concerns)

Information about the patient's understanding of the nature and precipitating factors are helpful for planning necessary teaching. The diet of the person with ulcerative colitis or Crohn's disease is analyzed in terms of nutritional adequacy. The person's usual daily intake can be compared to the basic four food groups to determine

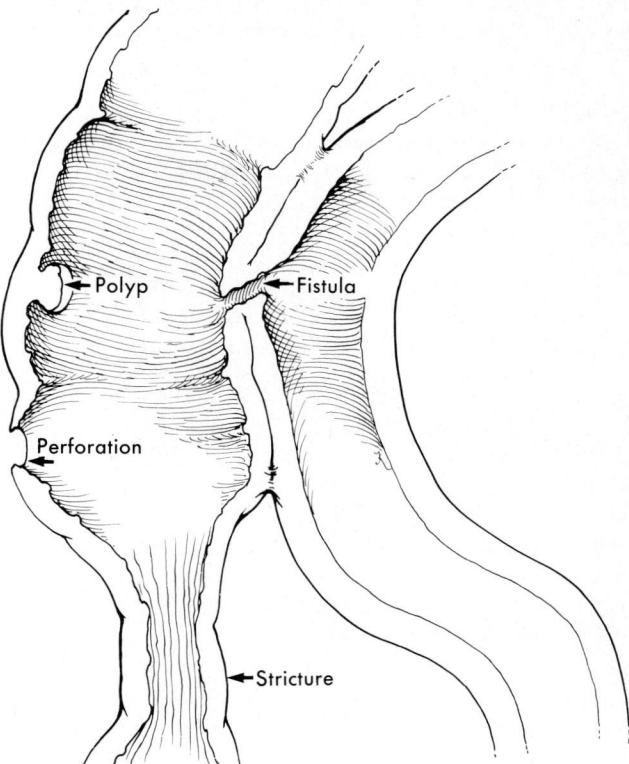

Fig. 32-13. Selected complications of chronic inflammatory bowel disorders.

quality of nutrient intake. Anorexia and intolerance to milk products are characteristic of ulcerative colitis. With severe ulcerative colitis or Crohn's disease, there is weakness from loss of weight because of the decreased nutrient intake and decreased absorption. Cachexia may result. The diet of the person with diverticulitis is assessed for intake of dietary fiber (fruits and vegetables, whole grain cereals).

The pattern of bowel elimination for the person with chronic bowel inflammation may vary as follows:

Ulcerative colitis	Severe diarrhea (15 to 20 stools/day); stool may contain blood, pus, mucus
Crohn's disease	Mild diarrhea; stool may contain mucus, fat or pus; no blood
Diverticulitis	Constipation or constipation alternating with diarrhea; stool may contain blood

With ulcerative colitis, abdominal cramps may occur with or without bowel movements. The colicky right lower quadrant abdominal pain of Crohn's disease and the left lower quadrant abdominal pain of diverticulitis are often relieved by a bowel movement. The pain of diverticulitis may be aggravated by eating.

Symptoms of chronic inflammatory bowel disorders may be exacerbated by stress or tension. Knowledge of the patient's perception of the effect of stress on the onset of symptoms and of the patient's usual coping patterns are useful for planning measures to relieve or reduce effects of stress.

Diagnostic tests

Chronic inflammatory bowel disease is diagnosed by means of radiographs, sigmoidoscopy or colonoscopy, and biopsy. Laboratory tests are conducted for the presence of anemia and for blood in the stools.

Radiographs

The *barium enema,* also called a lower GI series, helps to identify the lesions of chronic inflammatory bowel disorders, as well as complications such as fistulas, strictures, polyps, megacolon, or perforation (Fig. 32-13).

Endoscopy

The lower portion of the colon may be visualized by a 30 to 65 cm flexible fiberoptic sigmoidoscope, a rigid 15 cm proctoscope, or a rigid 30 cm sigmoidoscope. The flexible fiberscope is better tolerated by the patient. The upper portion of the colon requires a 105 to 185 cm fiberoptic colonoscope.

Stool examination for occult blood

Occult blood may be identified by one of three tests: guaiac (Hemoccult), benzidine, or orthotoluidine (Occultest). The *guaiac* test is the least sensitive but does not require special preparation. With the *benzidine* or *orthotoluidine* tests, false readings may be obtained by the ingestion of meat (false positive) or vitamin C in quantities greater than 500 mg/day (false negative). Patients are questioned about taking these substances before the benzidine or orthotoluidine tests are performed.

DATA ANALYSIS AND PLANNING

Nursing diagnoses

Significant data for the person with a chronic inflammatory bowel disorder may indicate the following possible nursing diagnoses:

Alteration in bowel elimination: diarrhea
Alteration in comfort: abdominal pain
Ineffective coping
Fluid volume deficit
Knowledge deficit
Alteration in nutrition: less than body requirements
Potential impairment in skin integrity

Barium enema

Purpose

Visualization of the structure of the colon by means of insertion by enema of radioopaque barium

Preparation of patient

1. Diet: nothing by mouth after midnight
2. Cleansing of colon: enemas, laxatives and/or rectal suppository (colon must be free of fecal matter for better visualization)
3. Patient teaching
   a. Explain procedure
   b. Time: approximately 30 to 45 minutes
   c. Sensation: similar to tap water enema
   d. May be tiring

Procedure

1. Instillation of barium in rectum (a rectal tube with a balloon may be used to help patient retain the barium)
2. Fluoroscopy then films to observe and record the barium flow and filling
3. Air insufflation to outline lesions when ulcerative colitis or polyps are suspected
4. Films also taken when barium is expelled to check for barium retention

After procedure

1. Provide food and fluids after test is completed
2. Observe stools for expulsion of barium
3. Assess patient for possible fecal impaction (absence of stools, hard mass in rectum, small amount of thick, liquid stool)
4. Give prescribed laxative or enema to remove residual barium
5. Plan a rest period for debilitated or elderly patient

Sigmoidoscopy

Purpose

Visualization of sigmoid colon

Patient preparation

1. Diet: light supper, light breakfast
2. Bowel preparation: enemas or rectal suppositories (omitted for ulcerative colitis or Crohn's disease)
3. Patient teaching
   a. Explanation of procedure
   b. Time: approximately 10 to 15 minutes
   c. Sensation: urge to defecate and some light abdominal cramping may be experienced

Procedure

1. Position: knee-chest (side-lying for elderly or debilitated persons)
2. Scope inserted and advanced to sigmoid flexure
3. Air insufflation for better visualization
4. Swabbing or suctioning of retained feces

After procedure

1. Clean anus of lubrication
2. Allow rest period
3. Monitor patient for sudden severe abdominal pain (bowel perforation is a rare complication)

Colonoscopy

Purpose

Direct visualization of entire colon

Patient preparation

1. Diet: clear liquid for 3 days, nothing by mouth for 8 hours before examination
2. Bowel preparation: laxatives 1 to 3 days before examination, enemas until clear the night before
3. Consent form signed
4. Patient teaching
   a. Explanation of procedure
   b. Time: ½ to 2 hours
   c. Sensations: discomfort is minimal with analgesic medication; feelings of pressure may be experienced

Procedure

1. Premedication: IV infusion of diazepam (Valium) and meperidine (Demerol)
2. Scope is inserted and advanced to cecum
3. Air insufflation for better visualization
4. Biopsy taken if indicated

After procedure

1. Observe stools for gross blood (hemorrhage)
2. Monitor for abdominal pain (perforation)
3. Monitor vital signs for 4 to 6 hours
4. Plan a rest period

Expected patient outcomes

1. Abdominal pain is decreased.
2. The patient is hydrated.
3. Skin of elbows, sacrum, and rectal area is intact.
4. The patient can describe:
   a. Diet to be followed.
   b. Measures to decrease bowel motility.
   c. Measures to promote rest.
   d. Symptoms requiring medical followup.

IMPLEMENTATION

Assisting with achievement of therapeutic goals
Promoting nutrition

A high-protein, high-calorie, high-vitamin diet is encouraged for the person with ulcerative colitis or Crohn's disease. Milk or milk products may be poorly tolerated. Encouraging a well-balanced diet may be challenging when anorexia and malaise are present. Fad diets are to be avoided, because they are usually not well balanced. When anemia is present, iron dextran (Imferon) is given by Z-track injection, since oral intake of iron is ineffective. Total parenteral nutrition may be necessary for the cachectic patient. Fluids are encouraged when diarrhea is present to prevent dehydration.

Either intravenous fluids or a clear liquid diet is prescribed for the person with acute diverticulitis to allow the bowel to rest. When the inflammation has subsided and the person becomes asymptomatic, a diet high in vegetable fiber (fruits and vegetables, whole grain cereals) is encouraged. Unprocessed wheat bran may be added to foods but should be started in small amounts and increased slowly over a 4 to 6-week period to 10 to 25 g/day.[1] Bran initially causes abdominal distention and excess flatus. The purpose of the high-fiber diet is to increase stool bulk and bowel transit time, thus increasing the diameter of the colon and leading to decreased intraluminal pressure.

Reducing bowel motility

When severe diarrhea is present, therapy is directed toward decreasing the bowel motility. It is crucial that a record be kept of the number, amount, and character of the stools, and that stool specimens be sent to the laboratory as requested. Antispasmodic drugs such as belladonna preparations may be given to slow peristalsis. Medications such as kaolin and bismuth (bismuth subcarbonate) may be used to help coat and protect the irritated intestinal mucosa and to give better consistency to the stools. Paregoric or diphenoxylate (Lomotil) may be used to lessen the frequency of stools. With diverticulosis, psyllium seed (Metamucil) or methylcellulose may be prescribed to increase stool bulk.

Promoting rest

Since stress and emotional tension may precipitate an exacerbation of chronic bowel disease, measures are taken to facilitate relaxation and rest. Relaxation techniques (see Chapter 8), planned rest periods, and regular sleeping hours may prove helpful.

If ulcerative colitis is of long duration, the patient is usually thin, nervous, and apprehensive and is inclined to be preoccupied with physical symptoms. Insecurity, dependency, and depressed or hostile behavior may be present, and empathic communication over time is usually needed to establish effective nurse-patient relationships. The patient needs to be included in the planning of care, which should incorporate those activities the patient has found helpful in the past.

Assisting with comfort and ADL

Bed rest may be prescribed for the acutely ill patient, and care must be taken for thin persons that bony prominences are protected by pressure-reducing devices, such as an alternating-pressure mattress, foam pad, or sheepskin.

The commode or bedpan should be emptied as often as it is used, even when the bowel movement is small. Room deodorizers may be used to dispel unpleasant odors. The commode or bedpan can be padded if the patient spends much time sitting on it.

The perineal area is washed as necessary, at least several times a day when profuse diarrhea is present. An analgesic ointment such as dibucaine (Nupercaine) may be applied to the anus to relieve discomfort. Sitz baths three times a day are beneficial to the skin and circulation and to provide rectal comfort.

Counseling and teaching

If symptoms of chronic inflammatory bowel disorders increase when stress occurs, the person is assisted in exploring the adequacy of usual coping strategies. Other types of coping strategies may be necessary (Chapter 8).

Teaching is an important nursing intervention in the care of the person with a chronic bowel disorder (see box).

Surgery

Ulcerative colitis can be treated by surgery. The trend is toward earlier surgical intervention for the acutely ill person and for persons experiencing frequent exacerbations. Surgery is clearly indicated when complications are present, including massive hemorrhage, perforation of the colon, strictures, and medically unresponsive toxic megacolon (dilation and hypertrophy of the colon).

Two types of surgery may be performed. The most common procedure is removal of the diseased colon and rectum, with the end of the ileum being brought out through the abdominal wall (ileostomy). If the rectum is only mildly diseased, an ileorectal anastomosis may be performed with preservation of rectal function.

A different type of surgical approach is the "continent ileostomy" or ileal pouch (Fig. 32-14). An intraabdominal reservoir with a nipple valve is formed from the distal ileum to provide continence. The capacity of the pouch increases slowly over months until it can hold approximately 500 ml. Contents of the pouch are removed several times a day by catheterization. Difficulties have occurred with valve failure and in keeping the ileal contents from becoming too thick and plugging up the stoma. At this time, only selected persons are considered suitable

Teaching for the patient with a chronic bowel disorder

1. Diet
   a. Ulcerative colitis or Crohn's disease: high-protein, high-calorie,, high-vitamin diet (avoid milk products with ulcerative colitis)
   b. Diverticulitis
      1. High-fiber foods (fruits and vegetables, whole grain cereals)
      2. Add unprocessed wheat bran slowly over a 4- to 6-week period
2. Elimination
   a. Take medications as prescribed to decrease bowel motility (Lomotil, paregoric) or to increase bulk (Metamucil, methylcellulose)
   b. Increase fluid intake if diarrhea or constipation is present
   c. Keep rectal area clean; use analgesic rectal ointment or take sitz bath for anal discomfort.
3. Promotion of rest
   a. Use relaxation measures (such as breathing exercises) when emotional tension is present
   b. Identify a source for an ongoing supportive relationship
   c. Maintain a regular sleep schedule
   d. Schedule daily activities to avoid fatigue; take rest periods as necessary
4. Health maintenance program
   a. List signs indicating possible exacerbation or complications (abdominal pain, increasing diarrhea or constipation, presence of blood or pus in the stool, fever, progressive weight loss)
   b. Plan for regular follow-up care.

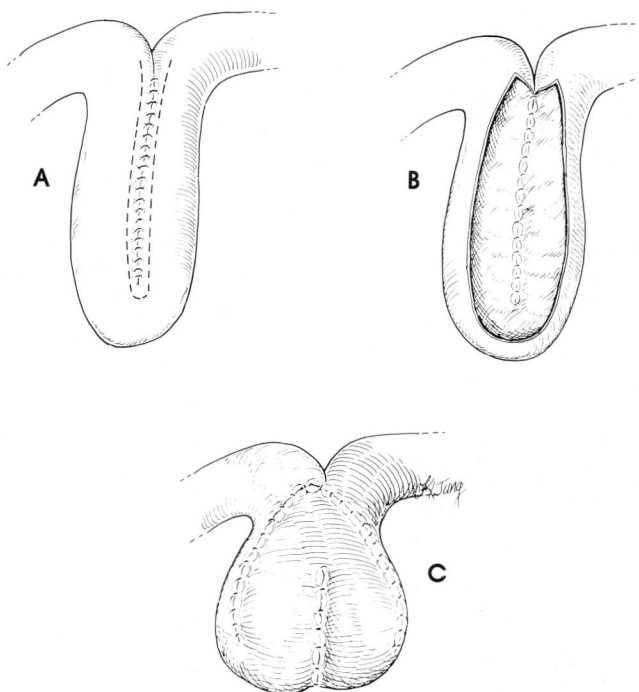

Fig. 32-14. Continent ileostomy. A reservoir is made by, **A,** suturing a loop of bowel together and then cutting around sutures; **B,** opening out incised area; and **C,** folding open area end-to-end and suturing. Distal end of ileum is brought out through abdominal wall.

candidates for this type of procedure. The procedure eliminates the need for wearing an external ileostomy bag.

Ileostomy care

The general care of the patient with an ileostomy is similar to that of the patient with a colostomy (p. 931).

Fecal drainage from the ileostomy stoma begins within 72 hours. It is liquid and may be constant. Commonly, patients will have approximately 1500 ml/day of drainage, although it may go slightly higher. Within 10 to 15 days, the ileostomy output will be a soft, slightly formed stool. The terminal ileum adapts to the loss of the colon and begins to reabsorb water. Patients with ileostomies have "toothpaste" consistency stools within 3 to 6 months after the adaptation of the ileum. Drainage usually occurs 2 to 4 hours after a meal, although there may be a small amount of output intermittently throughout the day.

Exceptions to this pattern of ileostomy elimination are seen in patients who have had previous bowel resections or resections of the ileum for Crohn's disease. The more small intestine that is lost, the greater the chance of a high volume of very liquid output with resultant dehydration.

Maintaining fluid and electrolyte balance

An excessive loss of fluid through the stoma may occur during the initial period after surgery, as a result of unabsorbed medications, or with diarrhea. Diarrhea for a person with an ileostomy is defined as very "hot" liquid output, in which the pouch must be emptied hourly or

---

Specific teaching for the patient with an ileostomy

1. Promoting fluid and electrolyte balance
   a. Look for signs of dehydration (dry skin and mucous membranes, thirst)
   b. Increase fluid intake if stool output markedly increases or if signs of dehydration occur. Drink fluids containing electrolytes (for example, Gatorade, bouillon)
   c. Avoid routine laxatives
   d. Monitor closely for increased fecal output when taking antibiotics
   e. When traveling, drink bottled water and avoid uncooked fruits and vegetables
2. Promoting nutrition and absorption
   a. Start with bland low-residue foods
   b. Introduce new foods (especially high-fiber foods) slowly
   c. Avoid several high-fiber foods at one meal to prevent blockage
   d. Chew foods thoroughly
   e. Avoid foods that cause problems such as gas or obstruction (these may include coconut, corn, celery, Chinese foods)
   f. Avoid foods that cause odors (these may include onions, cabbage, fish, spicy foods)
   g. Use liquid or chewable medications rather than enteric coated, time-released, or hard tablets, if possible.

---

more frequently.[17] During these periods the person is monitored for signs of fluid and electrolyte imbalance. The patient is taught how to promote fluid and electrolyte balance.

Promoting nutrition

The patient may be kept on a low-residue diet for 6 weeks to decrease the amount of bulky and undigested foods as the intestinal tract recovers from the surgical intervention. As the person begins to add foods, it is recommended that only one high-fiber food be added at a time and that the person chew the food well. Foods should not be eliminated from the diet unless the person is unable to tolerate them after two or three trials.

Food blockage (a large mass of undigested food, especially high-fiber foods) may occur with an ileostomy. The food becomes lodged at a kink, or narrowing, in the bowel and blocks the lumen. The result is a mechanical bowel obstruction. Blockage most commonly occurs when a person eats several high-fiber foods in one meal or does not chew the foods properly.

If the ileostomy becomes blocked, the person should get into a knee-chest position and gently massage the area below the stoma. Stomal edema will develop with a food blockage, and the pouch should be changed to accommodate the swelling. Diarrhea usually follows the removal of the obstruction, and the patient will need fluid replacement. Abdominal pain in the peristomal area is generally present for 3 to 5 days after obstruction. If the obstruction is not passed following the use of the knee-chest position, the patient should notify the physician.

EVALUATION

Evaluation is based on expected patient outcomes. Data is collected concerning the patient's comfort and knowledge about diet, elimination, rest, and need for medical follow-up.

Anorectal lesions

PATHOPHYSIOLOGY

The anorectal area may develop fissures, abscesses, or fistulas (Table 32-7). A *fissure* is usually the result of trauma caused by passage of hard-formed stool that overstretches the anal lining. It does not heal readily. An *anal abscess* may develop in an anal fissure, and if the sinus tract draining the abscess does not close, a chronic draining *fistula* may develop.

Hemorrhoids occur frequently as a result of congestion in the veins of the hemorrhoidal plexus. Heredity, occupations requiring long periods of standing or sitting, the erect posture assumed by human beings, structural absence of valves in the hemorrhoidal veins, increase of intraabdominal pressure caused by constipation, straining at defecation, and pregnancy are factors that predispose to development of hemorrhoids. Hemorrhoids may be internal (above the internal sphincter) or external (outside the anal sphincter). Many persons have both internal and external hemorrhoids.

ASSESSMENT

Pain and bleeding are the two major symptoms of hemorrhoids. Data to be collected include the following:
1. Pain
   a. Onset: with defecation, sitting, or walking
   b. Character: constant or episodic; sharp or throbbing
2. Bleeding: presence, amount, color (bright or dull red)

Table 32-7. Common anal lesions

Lesion	Description	Symptoms	Treatment
Anal fissure	Slitlike ulceration in epithelium of anal canal	Pain with defecation; bleeding; constipation	Stool softeners; analgesic ointments; sitz baths; surgical removal of fissure if medical therapy ineffective
Anal abscess	Abscess in tissue around anus	Persistent throbbing anal pain with walking, sitting, defecation; systemic signs of infection	Incision and drainage of abscess
Anal fistula	Hollow track leading through anal tissue from anorectal canal through skin near anus	Purulent discharge near anus	Fistulectomy or fistulotomy
Hemorrhoids	Varicosities of lower rectum and anus	Bleeding with defecation; pain if thrombosed	Analgesic ointments for mild discomfort; injection, ligation, or hemorrhoidectomy for severe discomfort

Table 32-8. Treatment of hemorrhoids

Procedure	Description	Comments
Incision	Drainage of blood from thrombosed hemorrhoid	Dry dressing for 12 to 24 hours
Injection	Sclerosing solution injected into submucosal area	Bleeding stops in 24 to 48 hours
Ligation	Constriction of hemorrhoids by rubber bands	Destroyed tissue sloughs off within 1 week
Hemorrhoidectomy	Excision of hemorrhoids	Preoperative: stool softener Postoperative: dressings may be omitted; stool softeners; first defecation is painful; monitor for excessive bleeding.

3. Stool: consistency (hardness), streaked with blood or pus

Bleeding is usually bright red because of the close proximity of the bleeding site. Internal hemorrhoids often bleed with defecation, whereas external hemorrhoids rarely bleed. Rectal bleeding must not be confused with menstrual bleeding in women.

DATA ANALYSIS AND PLANNING

Nursing diagnoses

Possible nursing diagnoses for the person with an anorectal lesion include the following:

Alteration in bowel elimination: constipation
Alteration in comfort: pain in rectal area

Expected patient outcomes

1. Rectal pain is decreased
2. Stool is soft and formed

IMPLEMENTATION

Assisting with achievement of therapeutic goals

Promoting normal stools

Chronic constipation may precipitate anal lesions. Once the lesion is present, defecation may initiate rectal spasms such that the person may delay defecation. This leads to formation of a hard stool as water is reabsorbed in the colon, causing further discomfort. Measures are therefore instituted to promote passage of a soft stool, including activity, adequate fluids (at least 2000 ml/day), and dietary fiber. A stool softener may be prescribed.

Promoting healing

Abscesses are incised and drained. Dressings containing purulent drainage must be changed frequently to protect the skin. Hemorrhoids may be incised, injected, ligated, or excised (see Table 32-8).

Gastroscopy

Purpose

Direct visualization of stomach by means of insertion of a fiberoptic gastroscope

Preparation of patient

1. Diet: Food and fluids withheld 6 to 8 hours before examination
2. Eyeglasses and dentures removed to prevent their damage
3. Ask patient to void before examination
4. Patient teaching
   a. Explain procedure
   b. Speaking will not be possible when scope is in position
   c. Time: approximately 15 minutes
   d. Sensation: feelings of pressure but no pain
   e. Hoarseness and sore throat may be present for several days after examination

Procedure

1. Topical anesthesia (spray or gargle) applied to throat
2. Valium given parenterally to relax patient
3. Gastroscope inserted through mouth with patient sitting or lying down
4. Air insufflated through scope to visualize mucosa
5. Biopsy may be obtained
6. Scope is removed; patient is asked to sit up immediately and to deep breathe, cough, and expectorate

After procedure

1. No food or fluids until gag reflex returns (2 to 4 hours)
2. Monitor vital signs every 30 minutes for 2 hours
3. Monitor for dyspnea, dysphagia, abdominal pain, fever, bleeding
4. Maintain safety precautions until effect of sedative wears off

Diagnostic tests

The diagnosis of peptic ulcer is made from the patient's history, a gastrointestinal series, gastric analysis, and stool examinations for occult (hidden) blood (p. 900). Direct visualization of the ulcer by endoscopy differentiates gastric ulcer from gastric carcinoma.

Selective *angiography* is becoming useful in the diagnosis and evaluation of treatment of gastric hemorrhage when angiography is combined with endoscopy. With angiography a contrast medium is injected through an arterial catheter for better visualization of bleeding areas and for differentiation between normal and tumor vessels. Following the procedure, the femoral insertion site is observed for signs of bleeding, and vital signs are taken at frequent intervals.

DATA ANALYSIS AND PLANNING

Nursing diagnoses

Possible nursing diagnoses for the patient with a peptic ulcer include the following:

Alteration in comfort: abdominal pain
Coping, ineffective individual
Knowledge deficit

Expected patient outcomes

The patient will be able to do the following:
1. State pain is decreased, minimal, or absent.
2. Describe medication program to be followed.
3. Describe factors that contribute to healing of ulcers and decreased recurrence.
4. Describe plans for follow-up care.

IMPLEMENTATION

Assisting with comfort and healing

Medications

The majority of peptic ulcers heal by drug therapy. *Cimetidine* (Tagamet) has been the drug of choice in recent years to promote healing by inhibiting the action of histamine (though it is not an antihistamine drug but a histamine-2 blocker). It also decreases both day and night pain, thus decreasing the use of antacids (Table 32-10). Ulcers heal within 8 weeks of cimetidine therapy.

The drug sucralfate (Carafate) has recently been introduced as an alternative to cimetidine. Sucralfate binds to the ulcer, forming a protective shield so that the ulcer may heal. It is not absorbed into the bloodstream and therefore has fewer side effects than cimetidine.

Table 32-10. Drug therapy for peptic ulcer

	Cimetidine	Antacids	Anticholinergics
Action	Decrease secretion of gastric acid	Decrease gastric acidity	Decrease gastric secretions, delay gastric emptying
Therapeutic effect	Promote healing, decrease pain	Decrease pain	Decrease nocturnal pain
Administration	Give 30 to 60 minutes *before* meals and at bedtime	Give 1 to 2 hours *after* meals for best effect (may be given as often as every 30 to 60 minutes)	Give 30 to 60 minutes *before* meals for best effect; do not give with antacid (decreased absorption)
Side effects	Muscle pain, transient diarrhea, dizziness, rash	Relatively none	Dry mouth, blurring of vision, headache, constipation, urinary retention
Comments	Therapy may last 8 weeks even when symptoms have subsided	Liquids are more effective than tablets; tablets should be chewed completely	Less effective than antacids or cimetidine; side effects usually occur with therapeutic doses

The pain of peptic ulcer is directly related to periods of the day when gastric acidity is high, particularly several hours after meals and at bedtime when acid secretion is high and the stomach is empty. *Antacids* are the most effective therapy for relief of peptic ulcer pain and act by decreasing gastric acidity. Antacids of choice are the non-systemic antacids (Table 32-11), which are poorly absorbed from the stomach and therefore do not alter the pH of the blood or interfere with normal acid-base balance. Sodium bicarbonate is readily absorbed and therefore should be avoided as an antacid for relief of ulcer pain. Also, the reaction of sodium bicarbonate and hydrochloric acid forms carbon dioxide, which may cause distention.

Antacids may be administered frequently, and if symptoms are severe it may be necessary to give them as often as every 30 to 60 minutes. When given in a fasting state, the buffering power is usually transitory. For maximal effectiveness, antacids should be given 1 hour *after* meals; this produces a buffering effect that lasts approximately 3 to 4 hours. Aluminum hydroxide becomes less reactive over time and should not be given with anticholinergic drugs or with tetracycline, since it interferes with absorption of these drugs.

Anticholinergic drugs are less effective than cimetidine or antacids but may be useful in decreasing nocturnal pain by delaying emptying of the evening snack. When given to relieve ulcer pain, anticholinergic drugs are usually prescribed in dosages that produce side effects (Table 32-10).

Food

Food, especially protein, acts as a buffer against the gastric acid but the effect is not long lasting. Eating frequently at regular intervals is therefore more effective for preventing pain than eating three large meals. Eating meals slowly helps prevent overdistention and reflux of the acid gastric contents back into the esophagus. Alcohol increases gastric acid secretion and is best avoided, especially on an empty stomach. Eating food at bedtime should also be avoided; the food will lead to increased gastric acid secretion without further buffering during the night and thus increase nocturnal pain.

Spices such as pepper or roughage foods such as bran have not been shown to be ulcerogenic, although they may not be tolerated by some persons. Substances that have been demonstrated to increase acid secretions are caffeine-containing beverages such as coffee, tea, or cola drinks. Persons are advised to avoid any foods that they tolerate poorly.

Special diets are no longer prescribed for persons with uncomplicated peptic ulcers except that the diet should be one that is well tolerated by the patient. Over the years many diet prescriptions have been suggested for treatment of peptic ulcer. One such diet was the Sippy diet which consisted of initial hourly feedings of half milk–half cream followed after a period of days by bland foods added gradually. This diet is unpalatable. There is no experimental evidence that special diets accelerate healing of an uncomplicated peptic ulcer.

Table 32-11. Commonly used antacids

Trade name	Drug composition	Comments
Maalox	Magnesium and aluminum hydroxide	Preferred antacid Good buffering effect Good taste Nonconstipating Low sodium content Can cause hypermagnesemia in persons with renal failure
Maalox Plus	Magnesium and aluminum hydroxide Simethicone	Same as above Antiflatus
Mylanta	Magnesium and aluminum hydroxide Simethicone	Same as Maalox Plus
Amphogel	Aluminum hydroxide gel	Constipating Can interfere with absorption of anticholinergic drugs Contains sodium Decreases absorption of phosphate Good antacid effect Give with water so that medication reaches stomach Can be given by continuous drip (1 part Amphogel to 2 or 3 parts water)
Gelusil	Magnesium trisilicate Magnesium and aluminum hydroxide	Slower buffering effect Gelatin effect in stomach to coat and protect the ulcer Nonconstipating
Riopan	Magaldrate (chemical combination of magnesium and aluminum hydroxide)	Rapid antacid action High acid-buffering effect No acid rebound Nonconstipating Low sodium content Can cause hypermagnesemia in persons with renal failure
Marblen	Magnesium and calcium carbonate Aluminum hydroxide Magnesium trisilicate	Neutralizes more acid than other antacids Nonconstipating Low sodium content
Alka-2	Calcium carbonate	Rapid neutralization of acid Constipating May cause hypercalcemia May cause acid rebound Not suitable for long-term therapy

Counseling and teaching

Ulcer pain typically appears in a cyclic manner, with periods of days to weeks of pain interspersed with periods of little or no pain.. Patients therefore need to know what to do at home to prevent or modify the pain. A summary of patient teaching related to pain relief is given in the upper box on p. 913.

In addition to knowing measures for relief of pain, the person with a peptic ulcer needs to understand about factors that contribute to healing and to prevention of ulcer recurrence. These factors include prevention of stress, avoidance of irritating substances that are poorly toler-

ated, avoidance of smoking, and maintenance of the medical regimen.

Stress plays a role in the pathogenesis of peptic ulcers, probably by means of the increased acid secretion from vagal stimulation.[57] Thus actions that avoid stressful situations or minimize the effect of stress can be beneficial for healing or for prevention of a recurrence. If removal from stressful environmental influences is impossible, the person must learn to cope with the stressful situations without reactivating the ulcer. (Measures to decrease stress are described in Chapter 8.) Occasionally the person is advised to obtain psychologic counseling for better

---

Patient teaching for relief of peptic ulcer pain

1. Take medications at prescribed times (cimetidine 30 to 60 minutes before meals, antacids 60 minutes after meals).
2. Have pain-relieving medications (antacids) available at all times.
3. Know when to anticipate increased need for antacids (during stress and for dietary indiscretions).
4. Avoid self-medication with systemic antacids such as bicarbonate of soda.
5. Avoid ulcerogenic drugs such as salicylates, corticosteroids, and phenylbutazone; use acetaminophen (Tylenol) or aspirin with magnesium hydroxide (Ascriptin) for relief of mild pain.
6. Know dosage, action, and possible side effects of medications (antacids have few side effects; cimetidine's side effects include muscle pain, transient diarrhea, rash).
7. Eat frequently at regular intervals.
8. Eat small meals slowly.
9. Avoid alcohol when possible, especially on an empty stomach.
10. Avoid bedtime snacks.

Patient teaching to promote healing of peptic ulcer

1. Avoid factors found to increase symptoms, if possible.
2. Structure home and work environment to keep stressors at a reasonable level.
3. Learn methods for reducing the effects of stress (for example, relaxation response, exercises).
4. Avoid stressful situations around mealtimes.
5. Plan for a quiet time (restful) after meals.
6. Stop smoking, or at the very least, cut down on the amount smoked.
7. Avoid foods found to be poorly tolerated (by patient).
8. Follow the medical regimen (for example, take cimetidine for the prescribed length of time even when symptom free).

---

understanding of the problems and for development of more effective coping behaviors.

Since there seems to be a relationship between *smoking* and irritation of a peptic ulcer, most physicians believe that the person who has a peptic ulcer should give up smoking permanently. To do so is sometimes very difficult, since often the person's life and work situations as well as personality are such that a change of this sort is a major one. Those few persons whose ulcers are reactivated when they attempt to give up smoking are urged at least to moderate the habit.

A summary of patient teaching related to promotion of healing is given in lower box above. If every consideration is given to adjusting the prescribed regimen to fit the appropriate physical, economic, and social pattern, the person with an ulcer will be better able to follow the medical treatment.

Surgery

Emergency surgery is necessary when a peptic ulcer perforates and causes peritonitis or erodes a blood vessel, causing severe hemorrhage. Elective surgery may be per-formed if the ulcer does not respond to the medical regimen and continues to produce symptoms, if it causes pyloric obstruction, or if a chronic recurring gastric ulcer is thought to be precancerous. The basic surgical procedures for treatment of peptic ulcers are subtotal gastrectomy, vagotomy, and pyloroplasty. Subtotal gastrectomy is now rarely performed alone but is usually combined with a form of vagotomy. Pyloroplasty is also combined with a vagotomy. The several common surgical combinations are listed in Table 32-12.

Subtotal gastrectomies are described in Table 32-13. The Billroth II (Fig. 32-1, *B*) is usually preferred for duodenal ulcers because of decreased duodenal recurrence. The duodenal stump is preserved to permit bile flow into the jejunum to mix with the food.

Part of the vagus nerve innervating the stomach is severed in a *vagotomy* for the purpose of decreasing gastric acidity. There are three types of vagotomies currently in use: truncal, selective, and proximal (Fig. 32-17). With both *truncal* and *selective* vagotomies, gastric emptying is inhibited; thus a pyloroplasty or antrectomy (removal of antrum or lower portion of stomach) must be performed

Table 32-12. Comparison of different types of surgery for peptic ulcer

Type of surgery	Advantages	Disadvantages
Truncal vagotomy with pyloroplasty	Low operative mortality and morbidity	High recurrence rate
Selective vagotomy with pyloroplasty	Preservation of vagal innervation of viscus. Fewer side effects than truncal vagotomy	More difficult to perform than truncal vagotomy
Proximal vagotomy	Preserves gastric emptying; low recurrence rate; fewer side effects; no intrusion of gastrointestinal tract	Newer procedure; requires experienced surgeon
Vagotomy with antrectomy	Lower recurrence rate than for vagotomy with pyloroplasty	Higher operative mortality. Greater side effects

Table 32-13. Comparison of subtotal gastrectomy procedures

	Gastroduodenostomy	Gastrojejunostomy
Common term	Billroth I	Billroth II
Procedure	Removal of lower part of stomach (antrectomy) with anastomosis to remaining segment of duodenum (Fig. 32-16, A)	Removal of lower part of stomach (antrectomy) with anastomosis to side of the proximal jejunum (Fig. 32-16, B)
Common use	Gastric ulcer	Duodenal ulcer
Side effects	Decreased gastric capacity, rapid emptying with decreased effect of pancreatic enzymes (malabsorption)	Same as Billroth I. Stasis with subsequent infection in the blind duodenal loop

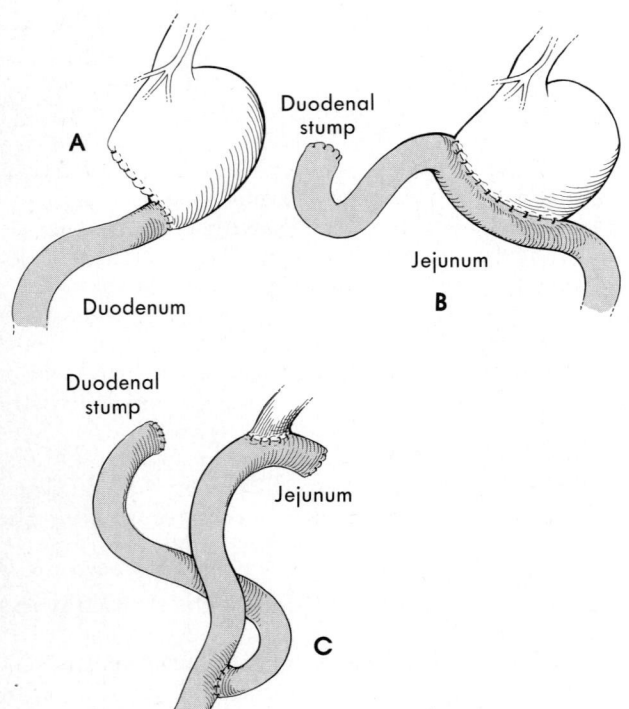

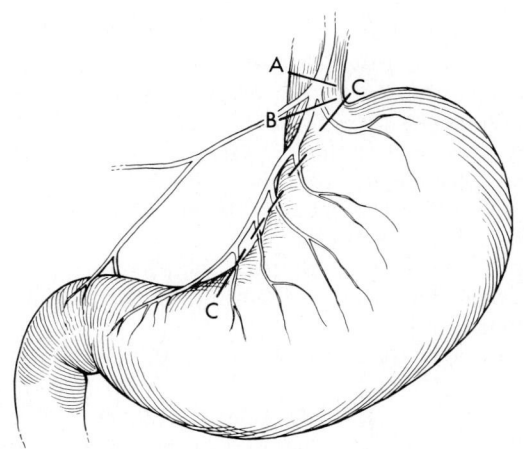

Fig. 32-17. Different types of vagotomies. *A,* Truncal. *B,* Selective. *C,* Proximal or parietal cell.

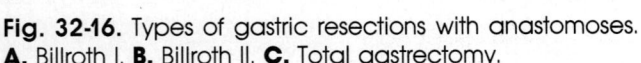

Fig. 32-16. Types of gastric resections with anastomoses. **A,** Billroth I. **B,** Billroth II. **C,** Total gastrectomy.

to prevent gastric stasis by enlarging the pyloric opening. The *proximal* vagotomy severs only the branches of the gastric portion of the vagal nerve that innervate the upper two thirds of the stomach, thus maintaining effective gastric emptying. Since a pyloroplasty or antrectomy is unnecessary with a proximal vagotomy, there is no intrusion into the gastric lumen, and side effects, especially diarrhea, are reduced.

A *pyloroplasty* or drainage procedure widens the pyloric outlet. It is performed with a truncal or selective vagotomy to prevent gastric stasis. One type of pyloroplasty is the Heineke-Mikulicz procedure (Fig. 32-18).

Care of the patient experiencing gastric surgery is described on p. 925.

COMPLICATIONS OF PEPTIC ULCER

A peptic ulcer may perforate a major blood vessel and cause hemorrhage, perforate the stomach or duodenal wall, or cause an obstruction at the pyloric end of the stomach.

Hemorrhage

Peptic ulcer is the most common cause of massive upper gastrointestinal bleeding. Duodenal ulcers have a higher incidence of bleeding than gastric ulcers. In some cases bleeding is slight and the only symptoms are tarry stools and a developing iron deficiency. When a major blood vessel erodes, bleeding is massive.

The medical management of hemorrhage is summarized in Table 32-14. Surgery is indicated for uncontrolled bleeding or for recurrence of hemorrhage. Vagotomy with pyloroplasty is preferred to gastrectomy. The drainage from the nasogastric tube is usually dark red for 6 to 12 hours after surgery but should turn greenish yellow within 24 hours. The patient may continue to pass tarry stools for several days postoperatively, but this is usually because the blood from the hemorrhage before surgery has not yet completely passed through the gastrointestinal tract. Stools may be guaiac positive for several days after bleeding stops.

Nursing interventions during the phase of *severe gastric bleeding* include the following actions:

1. Assisting with achievement of therapeutic goals
   a. Monitor vital signs and urinary output for response to shock therapy
   b. Monitor nasogastric drainage, emesis, and stools for amount of blood loss (stools may be red or tarry depending on the length of time required for passage)
   c. Test stools daily for occult blood (guaiac) until bleeding has clearly stopped
   d. Assist with medical treatments (blood transfusions, iced gastric lavage) and monitor patient's response
   e. Prepare patient for surgery if indicated
2. Assisting with patient comfort
   a. Provide special mouth care after vomiting (a weak solution of hydrogen peroxide will help remove blood from the oral mucosa)
   b. Administer prescribed sedative/narcotic regularly to decrease apprehension
   c. Remove all evidence of bleeding as quickly as possible
   d. Tell patient rationale for blood transfusion
   e. Tell patient that rest and quiet will help stop the bleeding
   f. Maintain a calm approach
   g. Restrict activities only to those deemed necessary until massive bleeding has slowed down or stopped

Perforation

Perforation is an erosion of a peptic ulcer through the muscular wall, providing an opening from the gastrointestinal tract into the peritoneal cavity. Most perforated ulcers are located on the anterior duodenal wall. Immediately on perforation a chemical peritonitis results from contact with the gastrointestinal contents, and bacterial peritonitis results within 12 hours. Symptoms and medical management are listed in Table 32-14. Persons taking corticosteroids may develop a peptic ulcer and perforation without exhibiting any of the usual symptoms.

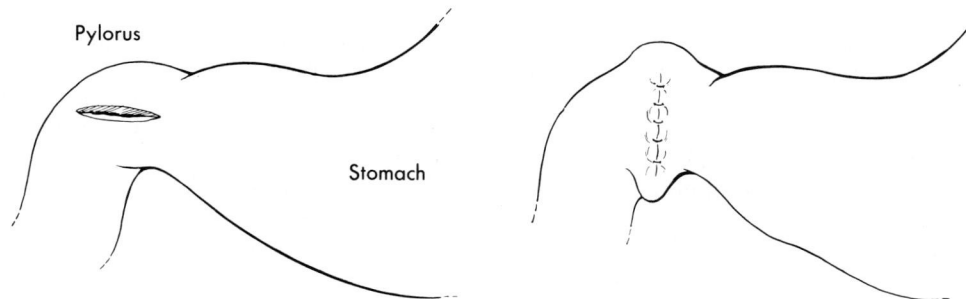

Fig. 32-18. Heineke-Mikulicx pyloroplasty. Longitudinal incision across pylorus is pulled apart and closed in transverse position to widen pyloric outlet.

decompression will ease the discomfort from the distention.

Since oral fluids are usually restricted, mouth care is important for prevention of infection in addition to comfort. If the patient is poorly nourished, measures to keep the skin soft and intact and free from pressure are indicated.

Surgery

Surgery is usually performed for relief of mechanical and vascular obstruction. The operative procedure varies with the cause and the location of the obstruction and the general condition of the patient. If constricting bands or adhesions are found they are cut, and it may be necessary to resect the occluded bowel and anastomose the remaining segments.

Care of the patient experiencing intestinal surgery is described on p. 928.

EVALUATION

Evaluation is based on expected patient outcomes. Questions to consider are; Is the patient hydrated? Has fluid overload been avoided? Have pulmonary and urinary complications been avoided? Is the patient relatively comfortable?

Hernias

Hernias account for a large number of intestinal obstructions. A hernia is a protrusion of an organ or structure from its normal cavity through a congenital or acquired defect. In addition to a loop of bowel, a hernia may contain peritoneal fat, a section of bladder, or a portion of the stomach, depending on its location.

Types of hernias

Inguinal
    Indirect   Loop of intestine passes through abdominal ring and follows course of spermatic cord into inguinal canal

    Direct   Loop of intestine passes through posterior inguinal wall

Femoral   Loop of intestine passes through femoral ring down into femoral canal

Umbilical   Loop of intestine passes through umbilical ring

Incisional   Loop of intestine or other organ protrudes through weakened scar

---

If the protruding structure of the organ can be returned by manipulation to its own cavity, it is called a *reducible* hernia. If it cannot, it is called an *irreducible* or *incarcerated* hernia. When the blood supply to the structure within the hernia becomes occluded, the hernia is said to be *strangulated*. Some types of hernias are described in box below.

A hernia that is not incarcerated can very often be reduced by the person lying down with the feet elevated or by lying in a tub of warm water and pushing the mass gently back toward the abdominal cavity.

Surgery is frequently performed for large hernias or when there is a high risk of incarceration. A *herniorrhaphy* consists of suturing the defect in the fascia. In the postoperative period following repair of an umbilical or large incisional hernia, a nasogastric tube may be used to prevent postoperative vomiting and distention with subsequent strain on the stuture line.

Because of postoperative inflammation, edema, and hemorrhage, *swelling of the scrotum* often occurs after repair of an indirect inguinal hernia. This complication is extremely painful, and any movement of the patient causes discomfort. Ice bags help to relieve pain. The scrotum is usually supported with a suspensory or is elevated on a rolled towel. Urinary retention may occur because of the discomfort in movement producing hesitancy in urination. Ecchymosis of the lower abdominal wall or upper thigh may occur after extensive manipulation during surgery. The ecchymosis fades in a few days. Sexual functioning is not affected.

The patient who has had elective surgery for a hernia is restricted from driving for at least 2 weeks. Physical activities should not include any heavy lifting, pulling, or pushing for at least 6 weeks.

CANCER OF THE GASTROINTESTINAL TRACT

Cancer may occur in any part of the gastrointestinal tract but is seen primarily in the stomach and colon/rectum (Table 32-16). General care of the person with cancer is described in Chapter 14.

Cancer of the mouth

PATHOPHYSIOLOGY

The lips, anterior tongue, and floor of the mouth are prone to develop malignant lesions. The cure rate for cancer of the *lips* is high because the lesion is easily apparent to the patient and to others. Metastasis to regional lymph nodes has occurred in 10% of persons when the case is diagnosed. In some instances a lesion may spread rapidly and involve the mandible and the floor of the mouth by direct extension.

Cancer of the *anterior tongue* and *floor of the mouth* may seem to occur together because their spread to adjacent tissues is so rapid. Metastasis to the neck has already

Table 32-16. Tumors of digestive tract

Place	Incidence	Contributing factors	Signs and symptoms	Medical therapy
Mouth				
Lips	4600	Smoking, alcohol	Fissure or painless indurated ulcer	Excision, jaw reconstruction if extensive
Anterior tongue and floor of mouth	14,700	Smoking, alcohol	Ulcer or growth	Local tissue perfusion with antimetabolites, Partial or total excision of tongue Radical neck dissection if extensive Radiation therapy instead of or following surgery
Esophagus	9000	Alcohol, heavy smoking	Dysphagia, regurgitation, aspiration of fluids, foul breath odor	Upper one third: radiation Middle one third: esophagogastrostomy Lower one third: esophagogastrectomy
Stomach	24,500	Low socioeconomic status; urban living; diet high in salted fish or starches or low in vegetables/fruits; pernicious anemia; genetic factors	Flatulence, gastric distress, anorexia, nausea, weight loss Late: abdominal pain cachexia	Subtotal gastrectomy, chemotherapy, radiation
Colon Ascending	126,000	Diet high in animal fat, protein, and refined carbohydrates; genetic factors; familial polyposis; ulcerative colitis	Occult blood in stool, anemia, nausea/vomiting, right upper quadrant pain, palpable mass	Right colectomy with anastomosis
Descending		Same as above	Gross blood in stool, progressive constipation, pencil-shaped stools	Left colectomy with anastomosis
Sigmoid colon and rectum		Same as above	Gross blood in stool, constipation alternating with diarrhea, sensation of incomplete bowel evacuation	Sigmoid: left colectomy with anastomosis Upper rectum: resection with anastomosis Lower rectum: abdominoperineal resection with colostomy

occurred in over 60% of persons when the diagnosis is made because of the tongue's abundant vascular and lymphatic drainage. The mortality is high. Lesions about the base of the tongue may go unnoticed by the patient and may be far advanced when treatment is started.

PREVENTION

Preventive measures include the following:
1. Avoid excess exposure to sun and wind on lips
2. Eliminate smoking or chewing tobacco or betel leaf
3. Maintain good oral hygiene and dental care
4. Consult physician for a mouth lesion that does not heal within 2 to 3 weeks

ASSESSMENT DURING RADIATION AND CHEMOTHERAPY

Condition of mouth: the intactness of the mucous membranes is threatened by chemotherapy or radiation

Eating patterns: changes may occur in the ability to cope with certain types of foods, especially solids, and with the ability to swallow. Patients may also have difficulty with choking and aspiration and with nasal returns and drooling when swallowing.

Verbal communication: the ability to speak will vary from some limitation to complete inability to speak, depending on the amount of tissue resected or destroyed.

Concerns: the person's facial appearance will also change depending on the extent of tissue removed or destroyed. Even with reconstructive changes, noticeable changes will be present.

DATA ANALYSIS AND PLANNING DURING THERAPY

Nursing diagnoses

Possible nursing diagnoses include the following:
Alteration in oral mucous membranes
Alteration in nutrition: less than body requirements
Impaired verbal communication
Disturbance in self-concept: body image

Expected patient outcomes

1. Incisions heal without infection.
2. Patient feeds self through appropriate means and consumes a nutritionally balanced fluid or soft diet.
3. Patient has a means of communication and is working to improve speech.
4. Patient interacts with others and states plans for gradual resumption of activities involving others.

IMPLEMENTATION

Surgery

The care of the patient experiencing surgery for cancer of the mouth is outlined on p. 923. The tongue may be partially excised (hemiglossectomy) or totally excised (glossectomy). If the lymph nodes are involved, a radical neck dissection (Chapter 24) may be performed.

Prostheses of the palate and jaw may be designed to replace portions of tissue that have been resected. If a prosthesis is to be made, impressions will be taken during the preoperative period; the prosthesis will be fitted when healing has occurred postoperatively. If a composite resection including a radical neck dissection is to be performed, reconstructive surgery will be done, if possible, during the initial procedure; it may also be performed at a later date.

The ability to speak is commonly lost for short or long periods after surgery, but if the vocal chords are intact, speech will eventually return. A magic slate may be used for communication; however, many patients have difficulty using this because of visual impairments. Conversation can be carried out so that the patient's responses can be limited to affirmative or negative gestures. Loud noises are disturbing to the patient since the oral tissue loss may create a channel that amplifies sound; therefore the patient should be addressed in a soft, clear voice. Speech retraining may be necessary, and a tape recorder may be useful for the patient to hear his or her own voice to work on improvements.

Radiation

Tumors of the mouth may be treated by radiation in various forms. Needles containing radium, radioactive cobalt, or other radioactive substances may be inserted and left in place for a prescribed time. Seeds containing emanations from radium or radioactive cobalt may be used and left in place indefinitely or else removed. External radiation treatment using x-rays or other radioactive substances may be prescribed.

Radiation therapy produces secondary effects in the mouth that include mucositis, dryness, dental decay, and tightening of the jaw muscle. Some of the changes may be permanent. The initial reaction is an inflammation of the mucous membrane. Sloughing of the tissues may occur and cause a fetid odor. Dentures are not tolerated for some time thereafter because of the sensitivity of the tissues. Dryness of the mouth begins 1 to 2 weeks after radiation is started and may persist throughout life. The dryness makes the mouth feel uncomfortable and gives an unpleasant taste.

Decreased salivary secretion and altered pH of the saliva contribute to rapid dental decay, especially at the gingival margins. An active dental control program is started before radiation therapy is initiated. Fluoride treatments to the teeth may be given and a conscientious toothbrushing regimen is instituted.

The general care of the patient receiving radiation therapy is discussed in Chapter 14. Specific considerations for the patient receiving radiation of the mouth include the following:
1. Provide good oral hygiene
2. Remove dentures at night; check dentures for fitness

Care of patient experiencing mouth surgery for cancer

Preoperative care

1. Clarify patient's knowledge of expected changes after surgery
2. Explain expected postoperative measures (including suctioning, nasogastric tube)
3. Provide openings for patient to begin to express feelings about changes in body image

Postoperative care

1. Monitoring
   a. Assess facial movement for facial nerve damage (if parotid gland excised): ask patient to raise eyebrows, frown, smile, show teeth, pucker lips
   b. Assess degree and character of drainage
      (1) Amount of drainage and presence of blood should be minimal
      (2) Hemorrhage may occur with wide resection of tongue
2. Promoting drainage
   a. Side-lying position initially
   b. Fowler's position when fully alert
   c. Suctioning of mouth (except for lip surgery)
   d. Gauze wick may be used to direct saliva into an emesis basin
   e. Maintain patency of drainage tubes, if used
3. Promoting oral hygiene and comfort
   a. Clean involved areas of mouth with cotton applicator moistened with hydrogen peroxide and saline
   b. Mouth irrigations
      (1) Use sterile equipment
      (2) Use solution of sterile water, diluted hydrogen peroxide, normal saline, or sodium bicarbonate (avoid commercial mouthwashes)
      (3) Protect any dressings from getting wet
      (4) A catheter may be inserted along the side of cheek and the solution injected with gentle pressure; a spray may also be used
      (5) Give analgesics as indicated (pain is usually mild)
4. Promoting nutrition
   a. Tube feedings will be used initially with hemiglossectomy
   b. Oral fluids: place in back of throat with Asepto syringe or feeding cup with attached tubing
   c. Eating soft foods
      (1) Encourage patient to feed self when possible
      (2) Teach patient to follow all meals with clear water to cleanse mouth
      (3) Avoid using fork, which may traumatize new tissue
   d. Foods
      (1) Avoid long-term use of commercial preparations such as instant breakfast drinks (may cause diarrhea or constipation)
      (2) Fruit-flavored yogurt preparations are less irritating than gelatin preparations and easier to swallow
      (3) Avoid very hot or cold foods (hot foods irritate new tissue; cold foods may cause facial pain or paralyze oral functions)
5. Promoting speech
   a. Limit patient responses initially to yes-no questions that can be answered by gestures
   b. Encourage patient when speech returns to speak slowly
   c. Listen carefully and validate communication before initiating action on requests
   d. Speak in a soft clear voice
   e. Refer patient to speech therapist if necessary
6. Encourage socialization with others

3. Encourage fluid intake of at least 2500 ml/day unless contraindicated
4. Encourage chewing sugar-free gum or lozenges to stimulate salivation
5. Provide humidity in air for added moisture and comfort
6. Avoid very hot or cold foods, dry bulky foods, or smoking to decrease irritation of sensitive mucous membranes.

Counseling

The person with cancer of the mouth faces two threats: threat to life and possible disfigurement. Because the face and neck are readily visible to others, one of the major problems that the person will have to cope with and adapt to is the change in body image. The impact of the loss may be slightly minimized when the grieving process begins early. The full emotional impact of the loss, however, occurs after therapy.

Withdrawal because of not wanting to be viewed by others or because of foul breath odor is often observed in these patients. The patient needs to experience acceptance by health professionals. The family members may need help in understanding patient behavior and in coping with their own feelings concerning the patient's appearance. Patients are encouraged to identify their feelings and are provided with support and explanations as appropriate. Patients are encouraged to mingle with others as soon as clues indicating readiness are observed.

Cancer of the stomach

Almost all gastric tumors are malignant. The incidence of cancer of the stomach has decreased dramatically over the past 50 years; nevertheless, gastric cancer is the seventh most common cause of cancer-related death. It occurs more frequently in men than women, and in Blacks and Orientals than Whites. It rarely occurs under the age of 40 and is most frequent between the ages of 50 and 70. Contributing factors, symptoms, and usual medical therapy are summarized in Table 32-16.

PATHOPHYSIOLOGY

Cancer may develop in any part of the stomach but is found most often in the distal third. Gastric cancer may spread directly through the stomach wall into adjacent tissues, to the lymphatics, to the regional lymph nodes of the stomach, to other abdominal organs, or through the bloodstream to the lungs or bones. Involvement of the regional lymph nodes occurs early, followed by involvement of the more distal nodes. There is a tendency to-

Table 32-17. Surgeries of the stomach

Name	Description	Comments
Esophagogastrostomy	Anastomosis of esophagus and stomach	Usually involves removal of lower one third of esophagus; tissue graft may be used
Esophagojejunostomy	Removal of stomach (total gastrectomy) and anastomosis of esophagus to jejunum	Two portions of jejunum meeting esophagus are sometimes joined to form a reservoir for food
Gastrectomy	Removal of part (subtotal) or all (total) of stomach	Remaining portions are anastomosed to small intestine
Gastrostomy	Insertion of tube through abdominal wall into stomach	Permits esophageal bypass allowing for nutritional feedings into gastrointestinal tract
Gastroduodenostomy	Formation of new opening between stomach and duodenum	In Billroth I surgery (Fig. 32-16, A) part of stomach is removed and remaining portion is anastomosed to duodenum
Gastrojejunostomy	Anastomosis of stomach with jejunum	In Billroth II surgery (Fig. 32-16, B) duodenal stump is closed after excision of lower part of stomach
Antrectomy	Removal of entire antrum (lower portion) of stomach	Usually followed by gastroduodenostomy
Pyloroplasty	Repair of pyloric opening of stomach	To enlarge opening and facilitate emptying of stomach
Gastric partitioning	Stapling of stomach to reduce size	Staples applied in two rows partially across stomach for control of massive obesity

ward intraperitoneal seeding, particularly to the peritoneal cul-de-sac. Prognosis depends on the depth of invasion and extent of metastasis.

SURGERY OF THE STOMACH

There are a number of different surgical procedures that may be performed on the stomach (Table 32-17). The word form -ostomy means "an opening into," thus gastrostomy refers to an opening into the stomach. If only one prefix precedes the term -ostomy, then the surgical opening is made from the exterior, such as gastrostomy. When two prefixes precede -ostomy, the surgery consists of an opening made between two organs (anastomosis); for example, a gastroenterostomy is an anastomosis of a portion of the stomach (gastro-) with a portion of the small intestine (entero-). The surgical procedures more commonly used for cancer of the stomach are gastroduodenostomy (Billroth I) and gastrojejunostomy (Billroth II).

Preoperative care

If the nutritional status of the patient is poor, an attempt is made preoperatively to improve nutrition. Total parenteral nutrition or a temporary gastrostomy (p. 887) may be necessary. If the patient is to have surgery for an ulcer, any special dietary prescriptions are continued through the preoperative period.

The major focus of nursing care is teaching the patient. Since the incision for gastric surgery is high in the abdomen, special emphasis is placed on teaching the patient breathing exercises preoperatively (see Chapter 17). The patient should know that a nasogastric tube may be in place for several days postoperatively because of decreased peristalsis from manipulation of the gastrointestinal tract organs during surgery and to prevent trauma or pressure on suture lines.

Postoperative care

The care of the patient after gastric surgery centers on promotion of pulmonary ventilation, nutrition, and comfort, and teaching the patient. Specific nursing care is listed on p. 926.

Pulmonary ventilation

Patients with high abdominal incisions are at high risk of developing postoperative pulmonary complications because they are inclined to lie still and breathe shallowly to limit incisional pain. Measures to encourage movement and deep breathing take high priority.

Gastric drainage

Drainage from the nasogastric tube after surgery usually contains some blood for the first 6 to 12 hours, but bright red blood, large amounts of blood, or excessive bloody drainage is reported to the surgeon immediately. If the nasogastric tube stops draining, the surgeon is also notified, since a buildup of gas or fluid can cause pressure on the suture line resulting in rupture or dislodgement of the sutures. It is the responsibility of the surgeon to adjust the placement of the nasogastric tube so that inadvertent dislodgement of the sutures is prevented. Signs of return of gastrointestinal functioning (auscultation of bowel sounds, passage of flatus) are reported to the surgeon.

Nutrition

Until the nasogastric tube is removed and the patient is able to drink enough nutritious fluids, fluids are given parenterally. The average patient is given about 3500 ml of fluids intravenously each day (2500 ml for normal body needs plus enough to replace fluids lost through the gastric drainage and vomitus).

Fluids by mouth are restricted for about 12 to 24 hours after the nasogastric tube is removed. Fluids are then introduced slowly until well tolerated. Small amounts of bland food may be added until the patient is able to eat six small meals a day and to drink 120 ml of fluid every hour between meals. The dietary regimen must be adapted to the individual, since some persons tolerate increasing amounts of food and fluids better than others. Vitamins are usually prescribed until the patient is eating a full, well-balanced diet.

Early satiety and regurgitation after meals are common problems after gastric surgery. Eating less food more slowly and chewing thoroughly is usually effective. Persistent early satiety or regurgitation may be caused by edema of the suture line. A nasogastric tube may need to be reinserted until the edema subsides.

Dumping syndrome

After a gastric resection, the dumping syndrome sometimes occurs. It may also occur in patients who had a vagotomy, antrectomy, or gastroenterostomy. The onset may occur during the meal or from 5 to 30 minutes after the meal. The attack may last 20 to 60 minutes. The patient complains of weakness, faintness, palpitations of the heart, and diaphoresis. Other symptoms include a feeling of fullness, discomfort, nausea, and diarrhea.

The symptoms are thought to be caused by the entrance of food directly into the jejunum without undergoing usual changes and dilution in the stomach. The food mixture, more hyperosmolar than the jejunal secretions, causes fluid to be drawn from the bloodstream to the jejunum. The reaction appears to be greater after the ingestion of sugar, since sugar is the most osmotically active food. The symptoms are also attributed to the sudden rise in blood sugar (hyperglycemia), with the entrance of glucose into the bloodstream and the subsequent fall in the blood sugar level. The rapid gastric emptying and the propulsion of chyme into the small intestine are felt to initiate an intensive gastrocolic reflex and cause diarrhea and a feeling of fullness and discomfort.

Teaching for the patient who experiences dumping syndrome includes the following:
1. Eat a low-carbohydrate, high-fat, high-protein diet
2. Drink fluids only between meals
3. Avoid eating large amounts of food at one time
4. Rest after meals (recumbent position for 30 minutes)

Nursing care of the patient experiencing gastric surgery

Preoperative care

1. Teach breathing exercises
2. Explain special postoperative measures: nasogastric tube and parenteral fluids until peristalsis returns

Postoperative care

1. Promoting pulmonary ventilation
   a. Encourage patient to turn, deep breathe, and cough at least every 2 hours or less until patient is ambulating well
   b. Give pain medication before activities to encourage active patient participation (thus increasing ventilation)
   c. Position patient to promote chest expansion (mid- or high Fowler's)
2. Promoting nutrition
   a. Measure nasogastric tube drainage accurately for determination of fluid and electrolyte replacement
   b. Monitor patient for signs of leakage of the anastomosis (dyspnea, pain, fever) when oral fluids are initiated
   c. Add small amounts of bland food at frequent intervals until foods are well tolerated
   d. Monitor patient for early satiety and regurgitation
   e. If regurgitation occurs:
      (1) Tell patient to eat less food at a slower pace
      (2) Report persistent regurgitation to physician
   f. Report signs of dumping syndrome (weakness, faintness, palpitations of heart, diaphoresis, feeling of fullness, nausea, diarrhea) to physician
   g. Monitor weight
3. Providing comfort
   a. Provide good mouth care until oral fluids are resumed
   b. Provide adequate analgesic medications during first few days to prevent pain
   c. Splint incision before patient coughs
   d. Encourage ambulation
4. Patient teaching
   a. Gradually increase amount of food each meal until able to eat three meals a day, if possible
   b. If discomfort occurs after eating, decrease size of meals and amount of fluids with meals and eat more slowly
   c. Avoid stress, if possible, during and immediately after meals; plan a rest period after eating
   d. Elevate head when lying down (if cardia of stomach removed) to prevent gastroesophageal reflux (heartburn)
   e. Use measures to modify effects of stress (see Chapter 8)
   f. Monitor weight regularly
   g. Report signs of complications to physician (vomiting after meals, increasing feeling of abdominal fullness, increasing weakness, hematemesis, tarry stools, pain, persistant diarrhea)

---

5. Take anticholinergic drugs before meals as prescribed

Total gastrectomy

Total gastrectomies are now rarely performed. The nursing care of the patient who has had a total gastrectomy (esophagojejunostomy) differs in some ways from that of patients undergoing other types of gastric surgery. A thoracic approach is used, and the nursing care will be the same as that for the patient who has had chest surgery. Drains are usually inserted from the site of the anastomosis, and there may be serosanguineous drainage.

There is little or no drainage from the nasogastric tube because there is no longer any reservoir in which secretions may collect, and there is no stomach mucosa left to secrete.

Following a total gastrectomy the maintenance of good nutrition is difficult because the patient can no longer eat regular meals and because the food that is taken is poorly digested and therefore poorly absorbed from the intestines. Since the patient also becomes anemic, ferrous sulfate, folate, and vitamin B_{12} are often prescribed. These patients rarely regain normal strength. Most of them are semiinvalids as long as they live.

Cancer of the bowel

Malignant tumors of the colon and rectum are among the most commonly occurring malignancies in the United States, second only to cancer of the lung in men and cancer of the breast in women. The incidence of bowel cancer is significantly higher in developed countries whose inhabitants are of Northern European descent, and it is lower in Japan, India, Africa, and some Latin-American countries. Two thirds of the malignancies occur in the sigmoid colon and rectum. Contributing factors, symptoms, and usual medical therapy are summarized in Table 32-16.

PREVENTION

Since dietary factors have a significant role in the incidence of bowel cancer, a diet that is high in dietary fibers and low in animal protein, fats, and refined carbohydrates may offer some protection against bowel cancer.[62] Although colorectal cancer cannot be prevented, early diagnosis and treatment offer a fairly good chance for cure. Anyone who develops a change in bowel patterns such as constipation, diarrhea, or alternating constipation and diarrhea, a change in the shape of the stool, or the passing of blood should consult a physician. Home testing kits for testing of occult blood are available for early detection of intestinal bleeding.

The American Cancer Society guidelines for early detection of colon or rectal cancer are listed on p. 879.

PATHOPHYSIOLOGY

Cancer of the colon may develop as a polyp growing into the lumen of the colon or as a mass on the wall that encircles the colon and narrows the lumen. There is usually no obstruction with lesions in the ascending colon because the fecal contents are still liquid and flow past the growth. Partial or total obstruction may result in the lower colon from formed stool unable to pass through the narrowed lumen. Ulceration of lesions leads to intestinal bleeding.

Cancer of the colon may spread by direct extension or through the lymphatic or circulatory systems, seeding at distant points in the peritoneum or at distant points in the colon. The liver is the major organ of metastasis.

DIAGNOSTIC TESTS

Diagnosis of cancer of the colon is made by physical examination, sigmoidoscopy, colonoscopy, and barium enema examination. Cancer of the rectum can be accurately diagnosed by pathologic examination of a biopsy specimen of the lesion taken during a proctoscopic examination. Stools are examined for occult blood.

Carcinoembryonic antigen monitoring

Carcinoembryonic antigen (CEA) is an antigen seen in fetal life. It was originally isolated from patients with colonic cancer but it is also seen in persons with ulcerative colitis, cirrhosis, and other forms of cancer and in chronic cigarette smokers.

The CEA test is not useful as a screening test for colonic cancer; however, it is useful as an indicator of the effects of therapy. For example, a drop in CEA level would suggest effectiveness of therapy. A continued high level or rise in level would suggest recurrence or spread of the tumor.

MEDICAL THERAPY

The treatment of cancer of the colon is always surgical, and the tumor, surrounding colon, and lymph nodes are resected. If the cancerous growth is such that it is not resectable or if the growth has caused an obstruction with accompanying inflammation an opening may be made into the cecum (cecostomy) or into the transverse colon (transverse colostomy) as a palliative measure to permit the escape of fecal contents. When the edema and inflammation around the tumor subside, the growth is resected, the bowel sections are anastomosed, and the cecostomy or colostomy is closed.

Other forms of therapy may be used in addition to surgery. Preoperative radiation retards cell growth so that cells that may be accidentally dislodged during surgery do not seed themselves at other locations. Combinations of chemotherapeutic drugs may be used, especially 5-fluorouracil and methyl-CCNU. Bacillus Calmette-Guérin (BCG) may be given to combat the immunosuppresive effect of surgery.

BOWEL SURGERY

Surgery of the bowel is usually performed in one of the following ways; (1) the diseased portion of the bowel is removed (resected) and the remaining ends are joined together (anastomosis); or (2) the diseased portion of the bowel is removed, and the functioning end is brought out onto the abdominal surface forming a "stoma".

Resection with anastomosis is the preferred surgical procedure, since this permits elimination through the rectum. Growths above the middle third of the rectum are usually resected and anastomosed. Growths in the middle and lower third of the rectum usually require removal of the entire rectum (abdominoperineal resection, p. 929) resulting in a permanent colostomy (p. 931). The normal continuity of the intestine is interrupted in this situation and feces are eliminated through the stoma instead of the rectum.

A newer approach is the anterior colonic resection with a stapled anastomosis that permits resections lower in the rectum. The procedure is performed with the use of a stapler gun that is inserted through the rectum after resection of the diseased portion of the colon through an abdominal incision. The two cut ends of the colon and rectum are stapled together by a double row of stainless steel staples and the stapler gun is then withdrawn. In very low resections or when blood supply is poor, a proximal temporary colostomy may be performed to prevent leakage during healing. The colostomy is subsequently closed in about 6 weeks. The major complication in the early postoperative period is leakage of intestinal contents into the pelvic cavity with development of a pelvic abscess. Care of the patient is the same as with other bowel surgery.

Preoperative care

Preoperative care consists primarily of preparing the bowel so that it will be free of stool, and of decreasing the intestinal bacteria. This is accomplished by (1) a low-residue diet for several days followed by clear liquids the day before surgery, (2) bowel cleansing by means of enemas and laxatives for several days before surgery, and (3) oral antibiotic therapy. The antibiotic chosen is one that is not absorbed through the intestinal tract, has low toxicity, and has broad-spectrum activity against colonic bacteria. Vigorous mechanical cleansing or purging may be poorly tolerated by some persons, such as the acutely ill or elderly; therefore these approaches may be modified.

An intestinal tube may be used in place of a nasogastric tube. As the intestinal tube passes through the small intestine, the bowel becomes "threaded" on it, and thus is compactly held together and shortened while the operation is performed. Use of the intestinal tube prevents pressure of fluid and gas on the suture line.

Postoperative care

Extensive handling of the gastrointestinal organs during surgery causes a marked inhibition of peristalsis. Care during the early postoperative period is directed at (1) preventing a buildup of fluid and gas by the use of gas-

---

Care of the patient experiencing bowel surgery

Preoperative care

1. Preventing infection
   a. Give low-residue diet several days before surgery
   b. Give clear liquids day before surgery
   c. Give prescribed antibiotic
   d. Give prescribed enemas and laxatives
2. Teaching
   a. Special postoperative procedures (for example, nasogastric intubation, parenteral fluids for several days)
   b. Deep breathing and coughing exercises
   c. Use of side rails to facilitate turning in bed without exerting pull on abdomen

Postoperative care

1. Promoting oxygenation
   a. Encourage turning and deep breathing exercises
   b. Encourage patient to be active
2. Maintaining fluid and electrolyte balance
   a. Maintain patency of gastrointestinal tube
   b. Record amount of drainage accurately
   c. Maintain prescribed flow of parenteral fluids
   d. Monitor for signs of fluid loss (dry skin and mucous membranes, decreased skin turgor)
3. Promoting elimination
   a. Monitor for signs of returning peristalsis (passage of flatus, return of bowel sounds)
   b. Encourage increasing ambulation
   c. Monitor character of initial stools
4. Promoting comfort
   a. Give good oral hygiene until oral fluids are taken freely
   b. Lubricate nares with water-soluble lubricant
   c. Use measures to maintain moisture of oral mucous membranes (rinse mouth, chew gum, suck hard candy)
   d. Give analgesics on a fairly regular basis during the first 48 hours to prevent severe pain
5. Teaching
   a. Drink at least 2000 ml of fluid daily to avoid constipation
   b. Avoid use of laxatives without medical approval; stool softeners or Metamucil may be used
   c. Avoid heavy lifting for at least 6 weeks after surgery

trointestinal intubation, (2) preventing pulmonary complications, (3) maintaining fluid and electrolyte balance, (4) promoting elimination, and (5) promoting comfort.

Atelectasis and pulmonary embolism may result from decreased respiration and circulation. Incisional pain may limit chest expansion and the patient may require much encouragement to move, ambulate, and breathe deeply. There is a high risk of pulmonary embolism after perineal resection. Venous congestion in the pelvic veins leads to stasis of circulation; platelets adhere to the vessel walls, especially at bifurcation of pelvic blood vessels, leading to formation of blood clots with possible embolism.

The length of time required for peristalsis to return depends on the extent of bowel manipulation. Presence of bowel sounds and passage of gas signals the return of function. It is not unusual after a resection of the bowel for diarrhea to occur after peristalsis returns. Usually it is temporary and soon disappears. When the stool becomes normal, the patient is advised to avoid becoming constipated, because a hard stool and straining to expel it could possibly injure the anastomosis, depending on its location.

The care of the patient experiencing bowel surgery is summarized in box on p. 928.

Care of the patient with an abdominoperineal resection

Preoperative care

1. Prepare patient as for other bowel surgery
2. Prepare patient for a stoma (p. 932)
3. Prepare patient for a perineal incision: wound may be open and, if so, will take longer to heal

Postoperative care

1. Provide care as for other bowel surgery
2. Preventing complications
   a. Shock: monitor for early signs and institute shock measures
   b. Hemorrhage
      (1) Check perineal dressing frequently: initial drainage is profuse and serosanguineous
      (2) Reinforce initial dressings as necessary
      (3) Report excessive bleeding to physician
   c. Thrombophlebitis/pulmonary embolism
      (1) Encourage leg exercises (Chapter 17) until patient is ambulatory
      (2) Encourage use of elastic stockings with elderly patients or those with poor leg circulation
      (3) Encourage ambulation when permitted
3. Promoting healing
   a. Maintain low continuous suction of sump catheters, if present
   b. Change perineal dressing frequently as needed after first 24 hours
      (1) Record precise directions for dressing change on nursing care plan
      (2) Irrigate wound with normal saline solution by use of catheter, hand-held shower massage, or Water Pik
      (3) Cover with dry dressings and hold in place with a T-binder (the T "top" is wrapped around the waist and the T strap is brought up between the legs)
   c. Substitute sitz baths for irrigation when patient is ambulatory; maintain free flow of water on perineal wound in sitz tub (rubber ring may be helpful)
   d. Provide stoma care (p. 933)
4. Promoting urinary elimination
   a. Mantain patency of indwelling catheter
   b. Monitor for residual urine when catheter is removed
      (1) Keep accurate intake and output records
      (2) Monitor for lower abdominal distention, patient discomfort, restlessness
   c. Use measures to encourage voiding if patient has inability to initiate stream
5. Promoting comfort
   a. Assist patient to find a comfortable position in bed: side-lying is usually preferred
   b. Assist patient to turn frequently
   c. Try a foam pad under buttocks for supine position
   d. Give narcotics at regular intervals until severe pain decreases (about 3 days postoperatively)

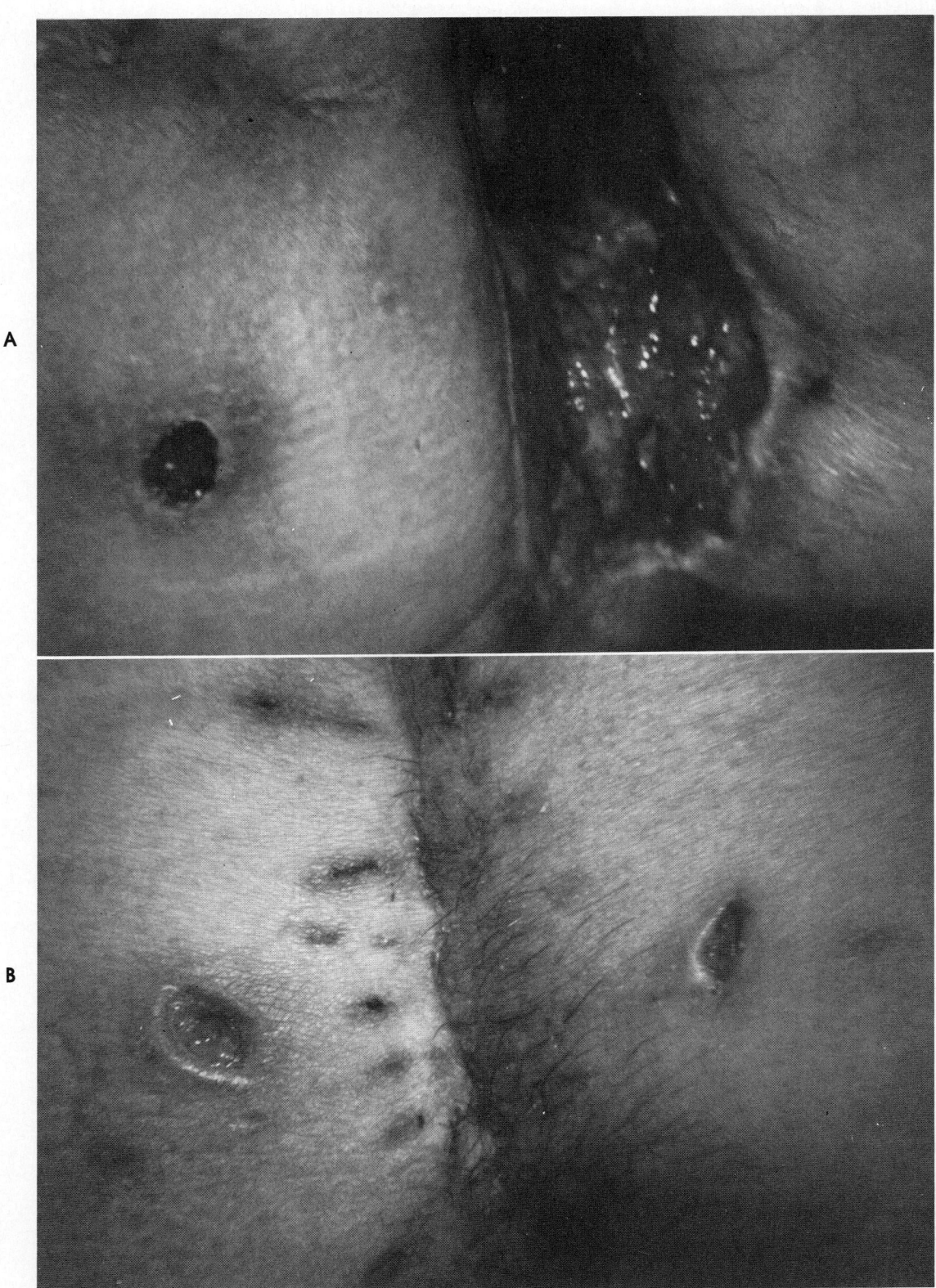

Fig. 32-20. Perineal wound following an anteroposterior resection for cancer in rectum. **A,** Postsurgical wound; note site of sump drain to left of wound. **B,** Following healing; perineum is completely closed; shape of buttocks looks normal.

Abdominoperineal resection

Malignant growths in the lower two thirds of the rectum are removed by means of an abdominoperineal resection. The operation is performed through two incisions: a low midline incision of the abdomen and a wide elliptic incision about the anus. Through the abdominal incision, the sigmoid colon is divided and the lower portion is freed from its attachments and temporarily left beneath the peritoneum of the pelvic floor. The proximal end of the sigmoid is then brought out through a small stab wound on the abdominal wall and becomes the permanent colostomy. Through the perineal incision, the anus, rectum and distal portion of sigmoid are removed. The perineal wound may be closed around Penrose drains, or it may be left wide open to heal slowly from the inside outward (Fig. 32-20). The open perineal wound will take longer to heal than a usual incision. Care of the patient with an abdominoperineal resection is summarized on p. 929.

Many patients complain of *phantom rectal sensations* and of feeling the necessity to defecate. An explanation of cortical perception and transmission of nerve impulses often helps the patient cope with these sensations.

Urinary retention is a common occurrence following rectal excision, with approximately 50% of men experiencing some degree of adynamic bladder paralysis after the Foley catheter is removed.[7] Factors that influence urinary retention include loss of pelvic support, chronic urinary tract infection, enlarged prostate, or nerve injury. Loss of pelvic support increases problems with micturition when the patient is supine; thus micturition may improve with ambulation. If nerve injury is present, problems with urinary retention and urinary tract infections may persist for 6 to 8 months with partial resolution of retention but with urinary incontinence experienced at night.[7]

Sexual difficulties may occur in about 40% of males following abdominoperineal resection. Difficulty with ejaculation is more commonly seen than impotence (difficulty with erection), but they may occur together.

Convalescence after an abdominoperineal resection is prolonged and may require many months. During this time the individual should remain under close supervision.

FECAL DIVERSION: STOMAS

Diversion of the fecal stream through the abdominal wall may be performed for gastrointestinal diseases or for trauma. The diversion may be temporary or permanent. In a *temporary diversion,* the fecal stream is rerouted to allow the gastrointestinal tract an opportunity to heal or to provide an outlet for the stool when an obstruction is present. A *permanent diversion* implies that the intestine cannot or will not be reconnected; thus a return to a normal elimination mode will not occur.

Surgical sites

When the small bowel (ileum) is the site of diversion, the ostomy is called an *ileostomy.* The surgical diversion of the large colon will result in a *colostomy.* The anatomic location of the colostomy will determine the name, that is, *ascending colostomy, transverse colostomy,* or *sigmoid colostomy.* The effects are different for each type of ostomy (Table 32-18).

Surgical procedures

There are three types of surgical procedures: an end stoma, a loop stoma, and a double-barreled ostomy.

When an *end stoma* is created surgically, the functioning proximal bowel is brought out through the abdominal wall to form a single stoma. The stoma is formed by bringing the intestine through an opening in the abdominal wall. The bowel is then folded on itself forming a cuff) and sutured (Fig. 32-21). The stomal surface is the mucosal lining layer of the intestinal wall; it is an absorbing surface. An abdominoperineal resection is done with removal of the rectum and anus.

The *loop stoma* is created by bringing the bowel through an abdominal incision, sliding a support under the bowel, and opening the upper wall of the bowel. The posterior wall remains intact. There is one stoma, but there are two openings: proximal and distal. The loop ostomy is generally a temporary procedure.

The *double-barrel ostomy* is created by bringing both the proximal and distal bowel through the abdominal wall, creating two stomas. This may be done as a planned temporary procedure for an inflamed or diseased bowel to permit the distal portion to "rest" or heal.

Common reasons for ostomy surgery

Ileostomy	Ulcerative colitis
Temporary colostomy	Trauma: gunshot wounds, stab wounds
	Complications of diverticulitis, volvulus, bowel ischemia, perforation
Permanent colostomy	Cancer of colon and rectum

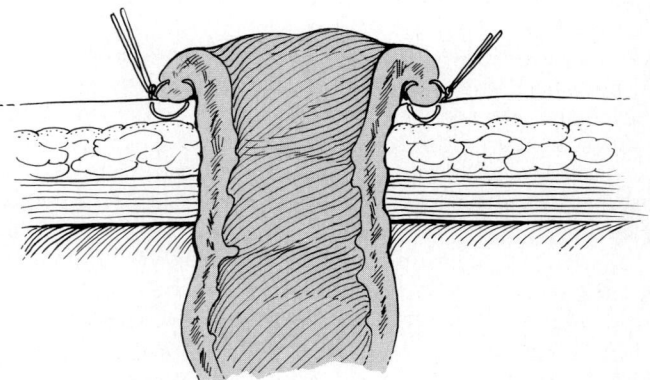

Fig. 32-21. Formation of an end stoma.

Table 32-18. Comparison of ileostomy and colostomies

	Ileostomy	Ascending colostomy	Transverse colostomy	Sigmoid colostomy
Location	Ileum (terminal end of small intestine)	Ascending colon	Transverse colon	Sigmoid colon
Type of drainage	Initial: liquid; 3 to 6 months "toothpaste" consistency	Liquid to soft	Soft	Formed
Bowel regulation	No	No	No	Yes
Fluid and electrolyte imbalance	Occurs frequently with illness and diagnostic procedures	Same as for ileostomy	Less possibility than with ileostomy but may occur more readily than normal	No different from a person with intact colon
Skin irritation	Irritation occurs easily from digestive enzymes	Same as for ileostomy	Some skin irritation from constant moisture	Irritation may occur occasionally
Other complications	Stricture or inversion of stoma; diarrhea with antibiotic therapy; food blockage	Stricture or inversion of stoma	Stricture or inversion of stoma	Stricture or inversion of stoma

Patients who do not receive adequate bowel preparation before a loop or double-barreled procedure may have a bowel evacuation through the rectum. Patients should be told this may occur. Mucus may continue to be passed through the rectum.

Psychologic response to ostomy surgery

When the physician first tells the person of the probable need for an ostomy, the immediate reaction is likely to be shock and disbelief. Whether the ostomy is to be temporary or permanent, it is difficult for most people to accept. It is not unusual for the person to be sad, withdrawn, and depressed after learning of the need for ostomy surgery.

Removal of any part of the body involves a sense of loss. Thus the person facing ostomy surgery may experience grief and mourning over the lost part, which includes shock, denial, anger, and depression. (See Chapter 16 for a discussion of these reactions.) In addition, because the surgery results in fecal contents being expelled through an unnatural opening in the abdomen, the patient will experience changes in body image. Usually the formation of the stoma is viewed as mutilating surgery, but for some individuals the surgery may be a relief or release from coping with chronic pain, diarrhea, or debility. No matter what reaction is expressed, patients need time and the support of others to work through their feelings.

Preoperative care

Counseling and teaching are important aspects of preoperative care. The patient and family/friends are assisted in identifying their feelings and reactions to the proposed surgery.

The patient's knowledge about the surgery is assessed, and a decision is made about how much to tell the patient. Some patients definitely benefit from discussing the care, reading materials, seeing equipment, and talking to persons who are living normal lives following ostomy surgery. Other patients find this approach upsetting. Asking patients what they would like to know will indicate how much information to give. Some suggested information is listed in upper box on p. 933.

Postoperative care
Stoma drainage

The stoma is assessed regularly for color and to ensure intactness of the stoma-skin suture line. A pink color denotes viability. A stoma that has impaired circulation will appear dark bluish red.

The stoma secretes mucus immediately following surgery and will continue to do so. During the first 24 to 48 hours, the stomal drainage is mucoid and serosanguineous. As the intestinal function returns, flatus will be produced. Flatus can be contained in an odor-proof pouch that can be emptied regularly from the bottom. Pinholes

Suggested preoperative teaching for patient requiring a stoma

1. Simple explanation with drawings of anatomy of the gastrointestinal tract
2. Explanation of surgery
   a. Areas to be removed
   b. Effect on bowel function
3. Definition of terms: colostomy (or ileostomy), stoma, pouch
4. Availability of nurse/enterostomal therapist after surgery to teach patient the care of the stoma
5. Availability of Ostomy Visitor

Stomal skin care

1. Primary prevention: protection
   a. Clean skin gently; pat dry
   b. Use a skin barrier to protect the skin exposed by pouch opening
   c. Use a skin sealant to:
      (1) Seal in powder or paste under pouch
      (2) Protect skin under tapes
   d. Change pouch when pouch seal leaks; do not add tape (leaking feces will irritate skin)
2. Secondary prevention: early management of skin breakdown*
   a. Erythematous skin
      (1) Change bag every 24 to 48 hours
      (2) Cleanse skin gently with warm water; pat dry
      (3) Apply heat (60-watt bulb at 12 to 16 inches from stoma) to uncovered skin for 20 minutes
      (4) Cover skin with skin barrier (wafer) cut exactly to size and shape of stoma (test skin barrier first for sensitivity)
      (5) Use a different pouch if original pouch caused sensitivity
   b. Eroded skin
      (1) Change bag every 24 hours
      (2) Use same approach as for erythematous skin, *except:*
         (a) After cleansing skin, apply aluminum acetate (Burow's solution) compresses for 30 minutes
         (b) After exposing skin to heat, apply Orabase to eroded areas

*Adapted from Broadwell, D.C. and Jackson, B.S.: Principles of ostomy care, St. Louis, 1982, The C.V. Mosby Co.

in a pouch will destroy its odor-proof quality, and there will be a constant odor in the room. This can be upsetting for a person who is undergoing so many new experiences. Odor is common when a bowel movement occurs or a pouch is emptied.

Fecal drainage is initially liquid for all ostomies. Drainage from a colostomy may then change quickly depending on its location (Table 32-18).

Protecting the skin

Fecal drainage from the stoma can be very irritating to the skin surrounding the stoma; therefore the skin needs protection. *Skin barriers* are substances that are applied to protect the skin. The most commonly used barriers are 4 × 4 inch squares or pectin-based *wafers* that are cut to

fit snugly around the stoma. *Pastes* are useful to fill in creases or folds in poor locations and to supplement wafers for a longer seal. Pastes and powders must be covered with a *sealant* (spray, liquid, gel, wipe) before a pouch can be applied.

Peristomal skin infections may be bacterial or fungal. The most common is a yeast infection from *Candida albicans.* The skin becomes bright red with papular lesions in an irregular area; secondary skin changes occurs as the process continues, and dry, scaling areas develop. Treatment involves the use of nystatin (Mycostatin) powder (unless the skin is moist) sealed with a skin sealant.

Care of the skin surrounding a stoma is summarized in lower box above.

fully for years may develop irregular results with irriga-   bathroom. The patient may wish to sit on a chair with a

---

Colostomy irrigation

1. Remove old pouch
2. Clean skin and stoma with water
3. Apply irrigating sleeve and belt
4. Fill bag with desired amount of warm water (250 to 1000 ml)
5. Hang bag so bottom of bag is at shoulder height
6. Remove air from tubing
7. Gently insert irrigating cone snugly into stoma, holding it parallel to floor
8. Let water run in slowly until patient identifies need to expel stool
9. Remove cone and allow solution to drain into container
10. When most of stool is expelled (about 15 minutes) rinse sleeve with water and close up bottom end
11. Encourage activity to complete bowel emptying (about 30 to 45 minutes)
12. Remove sleeve and apply clean pouch

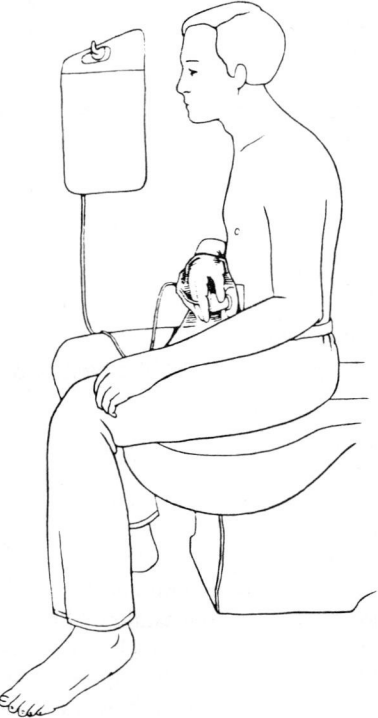

Fig. 32-23. Position for colostomy irrigation.

pillow and face the commode until the perineal wound heals. Subsequently the patient sits on the toilet (Fig. 32-23). Cramping during an irrigation may be caused by inserting the water too rapidly or from water that is too cold. Rate of flow varies with the pressure (height of the bag) and caliber of the tube.

There are many closed-end security pouches with a deodorizing gas release valve that may be worn by a person with a regulated colostomy. Since flatus cannot be eliminated or controlled, most people with colostomies prefer these small odor-proof pouches to a dressing.

Promoting nutrition

The diet of a person with a colostomy should not be restricted. People know which foods cause them to have more gas, diarrhea, or constipation. Persons have the right to choose whether or not they will eat gas-forming foods and have gas. Patients may be kept on low-residue diets for 6 weeks to decrease the amount of bulky undigested foods as the intestinal tract recovers from the surgery. The patient then begins to add foods to the diet.

Following a colostomy or ileostomy, persons tend to notice undigested foods that pass through the stoma. Seeds, kernels, peanuts, and other undigested residue usually do not alarm patients if they know this is normal.

Promoting return to normal activity

For most persons whose condition warrants it, optimal recovery is achieved within 3 months, and they can return to their normal activities, including work. Questions about activities need to be discussed before the patient goes home. Traveling is possible for the ostomate. Preparations to be considered are listed on p. 937. With careful planning the ostomate can participate in activities enjoyed before the surgery.

Promoting sexuality

The opportunity for the patient and significant other to ask questions regarding the return to normal sexual functioning needs to be provided. It is most often the nurse who hears cues such as,"I guess I'll never be able . . . ," or, "I wonder what my spouse . . . ." The nurse takes this opportunity to clarify this concern with the person. Arrangements can be made, if desired by the patient, for the significant other to be present when a frank discussion of sexual functioning is carried out by the nurse or physician. Many persons will not verbalize their concerns about sexuality so that a deliberate meeting must be planned to facilitate expression of these concerns. The patient and sexual partner can be assisted to consider sexual positions that may be more facilitating and less problematic if a bag is worn.[63]

Teaching for the patient with a stoma

Promoting nutrition and elimination

1. Eat a balanced diet. Avoid foods that cause diarrhea or constipation.
2. Drink at least 2500 ml of fluids daily (6 glasses).

Promoting return to normal activities

1. Participate in activities enjoyed before surgery.
2. Avoid direct contact sports such as football. Activities such as swimming, tennis, and planned exercise programs are all possible.
3. When traveling:
   a. Wear seat belt above or below stoma.
   b. Hand-carry regular ostomy supplies to facilitate care if baggage is misplaced.
   c. Use disposal bags.
   d. Carry plastic bags for disposal of used supplies.
   e. Take extra supplies for unexpected events requiring extra days.
   f. Eat moderately. Use restraint when eating new foods.
   g. Use caution about water intake in areas where "traveler's diarrhea" is a high risk.

Promoting sexuality

1. Allow time to ease into sexual relations
2. Resume sleeping in bed with partner if this was habit before surgery
3. Talk with partner about the stoma
4. Empty the pouch before intercourse
5. Use an attractive cover over the pouch
6. Tape pouch to abdomen or groin
7. Experiment with different positions

Preventing complications

Report the following symptoms to physician or nurse enterostomal therapist:
1. Changes in configuration, color, consistency, or odor of stool
2. Bleeding through stoma or rectum
3. Persistent diarrhea or lack of stool evacuation despite medications, treatment, fluids, diet, and exercise program
4. Persistent skin irritation despite treatment
5. Changes in contour of stoma (prolapse, inversion) or signs of infection
6. Persistent leakage around appliance
7. Signs of dehydration and electrolyte imbalance

About 15% of male ostomates have decreased sexual activity that may be related either to nerve injury or to psychologic reasons. The successful return to sexual activity depends on psychosexual functioning before surgery and adaptation and coping following surgery. Counseling may be helpful if nerve injury is not present and sexual difficulties are being experienced. Female ostomates have a decreased incidence of nerve injury because of the larger pelvis. Ostomy surgery does not interfere with contraception, pregnancy, or delivery. A pamphlet entitled *Sex and the Ostomate* is available from the United Ostomy Association.*

---

*United Ostomy Association, 1111 Wilshire Blvd., Los Angeles, CA 90017.

Assisting with coping

During hospitalization, there are additional resources available to the patient and family or friends to assist in adapting and coping with the ostomy. A representative from the local "ostomy group" who has been through the same experience may be helpful during both the preoperative and the postoperative period and will visit the patient if requested to do so. The enterostomal therapist, social worker, clinical nurse specialist, dietitian, and clergy may all be consulted as the needs are presented.

The patient and family should also be informed of the United Ostomy Association. The patient may become a member and through group sharing learn how others in the local community are effectively dealing with their alteration. The American Cancer Society will also provide assistance with information about home supplies, medications, and transportation.

Closure of colostomy

If the colostomy was performed to relieve obstruction or to divert the fecal stream to permit healing of a portion of the bowel, the person will be readmitted to the hospital at a later date for a further examination and for possible resection of the diseased portion of the bowel. The opening may subsequently be closed.

In preparation for a resection of the bowel and closure of the colostomy, the physican may order irrigations of both openings in the loop. Fluid, usually normal saline solution, is instilled into each opening; the solution into the distal loop will be expelled through the rectum. Mucus and shreds of necrotic tissue may be passed. The returns should be inspected before being discarded. A nonabsorbable sulfonamide dissolved in a small amount of water may be prescribed to be instilled slowly into the distal loop after the irrigation. The patient should retain this antibiotic solution as long as possible to lessen the risk of postoperative infection. The patient will be unable to retain any solution inserted into the proximal bowel. Oral sulfonamides are also given before surgery.

EVALUATION

Questions to ask concerning evaluation of the nursing care of the new colostomate may include the following:
1. Does the patient know:
   a. How to care for the colostomy?
   b. Where to obtain supplies?
   c. What symptoms or problems should be reported to the physician or nurse enterostomal therapist?
   d. Types of foods to include or avoid in diet and need for adequate fluid intake?
   e. Activities that can be resumed?
   f. Methods of promoting sexual relations?
   g. Measures to take when traveling?
2. Has the patient had opportunities to express feelings and concerns about the colostomy?
3. Is the patient beginning to assume some of the ostomy care by the time of hospital discharge?

REFERENCES AND SELECTED READINGS*

1. Almy, T.P., and Howell, D.A.: Diverticular disease of the colon, N. Engl. J. Med. **302**:324-330, 1980.
2. Andrysiak, T., Carroll, R.M., and Ungerleider, J.T.: Marijuana for the oncology patient, Am. J. Nurs. **79**:1396-1398, 1979.
3. American Cancer Society, Inc.: 1983 Cancer facts and figures, New York, 1983, The Society.
4. Arnelli, I., and Nassberg, B.R.: A clean, quick way to administer a barium enema through a colostomy, Nurs. 81 **11**(2):33-35, 1981.

---

*References preceded by an asterisk are particularly well suited for student reading.

5. Arvanitakis, C.: Diet therapy in gastrointestinal disease: a commentary, J. Am. Diet. Assoc. **75**:449-453, 1979.
6. *Auld, L.S.: Pseudo-ostomy: an experiment, Am. J. Nurs. **78**:1525, 1987.
7. Bartizal, J., and Slosberg, P.: Combined abdominoperineal resection, Surg. Clin. North Am. **57**:1253-1261, 1977.
8. Baum, M.E.: Enterostomal therapy in the hospital, Sup. Nurse **7**:11-14, 1976.
9. *Beart, R.W., and Curlee, F.: Intestinal stomas: managing the unmentionable, Geriatrics **33**(11):45-48, 1978.
10. *Beber, C.R.: Freedom for the incontinent, Am. J. Nurs. **80**:483-484, 1980.
11. *Beck, M.L.: Three common GI tests and how to help your patient through each, Nurs. 81 **11**(4):34-35.
12. *Beck, M.L.: Two intestinal tests: one oral, one anal, Nurs 81 **11**(7):20-25, 1981.
13. *Black, C.D., Popovich, N.G., and Black, M.C.: Drug interactions in the GI tract, Am. J. Nurs. **77**:1426-1429, 1977.
14. Block, P.L.: Dental health in hospitalized patients, Am. J. Nurs. **76**:1162-1164, 1976.
15. Bond, J.H., and Levitt, M.D.: Gaseousness and intestinal gas, Med. Clin. North Am. **62**:155-163, 1978.
16. Bowman, H.E.: Colon-rectal cancer: health organizations and government regulations, Surg. Clin. North Am. **58**:633-636, 1978.
17. Broadwell, D.C., and Jackson, B.S.: Principles of ostomy care, St. Louis, 1982, The C.V. Mosby Co.
18. *Broadwell, D.C., and Sorrells, S.L.: Loop transverse colostomy, Am. J. Nurs. **78**:1029-1031, 1978.
19. *Brunner, L.S.: What to do (and what to teach your patient) about peptic ulcer, Nurs. 76 **6**(11):27-31, 1976.
20. *Bruya, M., and Madeira, N.: Stomatitis after chemotherapy, Am. J. Nurs. **75**:1349-1342, 1975.
21. *Burkhart, C.: Upper GI hemorrhage: the clinical picture, Am. J. Nurs. **81**:1817-1820, 1981.
22. Cancer of the colon and rectum, CA **30**:208-215, 1980.
23. Chapman, M.L.: Peptic ulcer: a medical perspective, Med. Clin. North Am. **62**:39-49, 1978.
24. *Cullen, P.P.: Patients with colorectal cancer: how to assess and meet their needs, Nurs. 76 **6**(9):42-45, 1976.
25. *Curtis, C.: Colonoscopy: the nurse's role, Am. J. Nurs. **75**:430-432, 1975.
26. *Daly, D.M.: Oral cancer: everyday concerns, Am. J. Nurs. **79**:1415-1419, 1979.
27. *Dericks, V.C., and Donovan, C.T.: The ostomy patient really needs you, Nurs. 76 **6**(9):30-32, 1976.
28. *Didich, J.M.: How to gauge abdominal girth accurately, Nurs. 81 **11**(7):32-33, 1981.
29. Dyer, E., Monson, M.A., and Cope, M.J.: Dental health in adults, Am. J. Nurs. **76**:1156-1159, 1976.
30. Gerguson, J.A., editor: Symposium on colon and anorectal surgery, Surg. Clin. North Am. **58**:457-654, 1978.
31. Gisher, R.S., and Cohem, S.: Gastroesophageal reflux, Med. Clin. North Am. **62**:3-20, 1978.
32. Gowler, E., Jeter, K.F., and Schwartz, A.A.: How to cope when your patient has an enterocutaneous fistula, Am. J. Nurs. **80**:426-429, 1980.
33. Geels, W., et al.: The enterocutaneous fistula: supplanting

surgery with meticulous nursing care, Nurs. 78 8(4):52-55, 1978.

34. Given, B., and Simmons, S.: Gastroenterology in clinical nursing, ed. 4, St. Louis, 1983, The C.V. Mosby Co.

35. Griggs, B.A., and Hoppe, M.C.: Update: nasogastric tube feeding, Am. J. Nurs. 79:481-485, 1979.

36. Groer, M.W., and Shekleton, M.E.: Basic pathophysiology: a conceptual approach, ed. 2, St. Louis, 1983, The C.V. Mosby Co.

37. *High fiber diets and colonic disease, Am. J. Nurs. 77:255, 1977.

38. Holt, R.W., and Wherry, D.C.: Why flexible fiberoptic sigmoidoscopy is important in the geriatric patient, Geriatrics 34:85-87, 1979.

39. *Hongladarom, G.C., and Russell, M.: An ethnic difference—lactose intolerance, Nurs. Outlook 24:764-765, 1976.

40. *Hyman, E.: The pouch ileostomy, Nurs. 77 7(9):44-47, 1977.

41. Kagawa-Busby, K.S., et al.: Effects of diet temperature on tolerance of enteral feedings, Nurs. Res. 29:276-280, 1980.

42. *Kratzer, J.B., and Rauschenberger, D.S.: What to teach your patient about his duodenal ulcer, Nurs. 78 8(1):54-56, 1978.

43. *Lamanske, J.: Helping the ileostomy patient to help himself, Nurs. 77 7(1):34-37, 1977.

44. Lambert, M.L.: Drug and diet interactions, Am. J. Nurs. 75:402-406, 1975.

45. *Lamphier, T.A., and Lamphier, R.A.: Upper GI hemorrhage: emergency evaluation and management, Am. J. Nurs. 81:1814-1817, 1981.

46. Lieberman, T.R., and Barnes, M.: Gastointestinal fibroptic endoscopy: diagnostic and therapeutic aspects, Surg. Clin. North Am. 59:787-795, 1979.

47. *Literte, J.W.: Nursing care of patients with intestinal obstruction, Am. J. Nurs. 77;1003-1006, 1977.

48. *Long, G.D.: GI bleeding: what to do and when, Nurs. 78 8(3):44-47, 1978.

49. Mahoney, J.M.: Guide to ostomy care, Boston, 1976, Little, Brown & Co.

50. *McConnell, E.A.: Ensuring safer stomach suctioning with the Salem sump tube, Nurs. 77 7(9):54-57, 1977.

51. McKechnie, J.D.: Outdated and updated diets for GI disease, Consultant 18(9):82-86, 1978.

52. *McNamara, J.P.: Esophageal cancer, Nurs. 82 12(3):64-65, 1982.

53. Mendeloff, A.I.: Dietary fiber and gastrointestinal disease, Med. Clin. North Am. 62:165-171, 1978.

54. *Nortridge, J.S.: Helpful hints for assessing the ostomate, Nurs. 82 12(4):72-77, 1982.

55. Painter, N.: Diverticular disease of the colon: a bane of the elderly, Geriatrics 31:89-94, 1976.

56. Phipps, W.A., Long, B.C., and Woods, N.F.: Medical-surgical nursing: concepts and clinical practice, ed. 2, St. Louis, 1983, The C.V. Mosby Co.

57. Price, S.A., and Wilson, L.M.: Pathophysiology: clinical concepts of disease processes, ed. 2, New York, 1982, McGraw-Hill Book Co.

58. *Ramos, L.Y.: Oral hygiene for the elderly, Am. J. Nurs. 81:1468-1469, 1981.

59. Roderick, M.A.: Botulism, Nurs. 82 12(6):59, 1982.

60. *Rosenberg, F.H.:Lactose intolerance, Am. J. Nurs. 77:823-824, 1977.

61. Samborsky, V.: Drug therapy for peptic ulcer, Am. J. Nurs. 78:2064-2066, 1978.

62. Sherlock, P., Lipkin, M., and Winawer, S.J.: The prevention of colon cancer, Am. J. Med. 68:917-931, 1980.

63. *Simmons, K.N.: Sexuality and the femal ostomate, Am. J. Nurs. 82:409-411, 1983.

64. Stahlgren, L.H., and Morris, N.W.: Intestinal obstruction, Am. J. Nurs. 77:999-1002, 1977.

65. Stromberg, M.F., and Stromberg, P.: Test your knowledge of caring for the patient with peptic ulcer, Nurs. 81 11(5):66-69, 1981.

66. *Sweiger, J.L., Lang, J.W., and Sweiger, J.W.: Oral assessment: how to do it, Am. J. Nurs. 80:654-657. 1980.

67. Talbott, T.M., and MacKeigan, J.M.: Colon endoscopy in perspective, Surg. Clin. North Am. 58:459-468, 1978.

68. *Trowbridge, J., and Carl, W.: Oral care of the patient having head and neck irradiation, Am. J. Nurs. 75:2146-2149, 1975.

69. United Ostomy Association, Inc.: Sex, courtship, and the single ostomate, Los Angeles, 1976, The Association.

70. United Ostomy Association, Inc.: Sex and the male ostomate, Los Angeles, 1976, The Association.

71. United Ostomy Association, Inc.: Sex, pregnancy, and the female ostomate, Los Angeles, 1977, The Association.

72. Vukovich, V., and Grubb, R.D.: Care of the ostomy patient, St. Louis, ed. 2, 1977, The C.V. Mosby Co.

73. *Watt, R.: Irrigation—yes or no? Am. J. Nurs. 77:442-444, 1977.

74. *Watt, R.: Ostomies: why, how and where—an overview, Nurs. Clin. North Am. 11:393-404, 1976.

75. Wentworth, A., and Cox, B.: Nursing management of the patient with a continent ileostomy, Am. J. Nurs. 77:1424-1428, 1976.

76. What's a continent ileostomy? When Karen found out, so did we, Nurs. 81 11(11):84-89,1981.

77. *Wilpizeski, M.D.: Helping the ostomate return to normal life, Nurs. 81 11(3):60-64, 1981.

78. Winship, D.H., editor: Symposium on inflammatory bowel disease, Med. Clin. North Am. 64:1021-1231, 1980.

79. Wyngaarden, J.B., and Smith, L.H.: Textbook of medicine, Philadelphia, 1982, W.B. Saunders.

80. Yahle, M.: An ostomy information clinic, Nurs. Clin. North Am. 11:457-467, 1976.

81. Zenk, B.A., and Fidler, R., Sr.: Deciphering diagnostic studies: carcinoembryonic antigen, Nurs. 81 12(9):42-43, 1981.

33

The Patient with Urinary Problems

H. FRED FARLEY and PAULA LAMBRECHT MILLER

STUDY QUESTIONS

- Review the anatomy of the male and female urinary systems.

- Review the physiology of urine formation.

- Review the relationship between the location of renal pathology and alterations in serum electrolytes.

- Review the procedure for catheterization of the urinary bladder. What nursing actions can help prevent urinary tract infections?

- What foods are high in the following:
  Potassium?
  Sodium?
  Protein?

- Review common dietary restrictions prescribed for patients with renal failure.

- Review the criteria used for selection of the type of dialysis prescribed for specific patients with renal failure.

- What community resources are available in your area for patients with end-stage renal disease?

- Review the procedure used in your community for organ recovery used for renal transplantation.

Life depends on an organism's ability to convert raw materials into energy. This process is known as *metabolism*. Maintaining homeostasis or the state of equilibrium of the internal environment is essential for life. There must be a means to excrete metabolic wastes. Furthermore, the body must regulate fluid volume, electrolyte composition, and acid-base balance. The kidneys and other structures of the urinary system (Fig. 33-1) play a major role in the regulation of the internal environment.

The kidneys maintain the composition of body fluids and electrolytes within critical limits, provide a vehicle by which metabolic wastes are excreted from the body, and are also the primary organs for maintaining the acid-base balance in the body. In addition to these regulatory functions, the kidneys are involved in control of blood pressure, RBC production and calcium-phosphate metabolism. The multiple functions of the kidneys are summarized in Table 33-1.

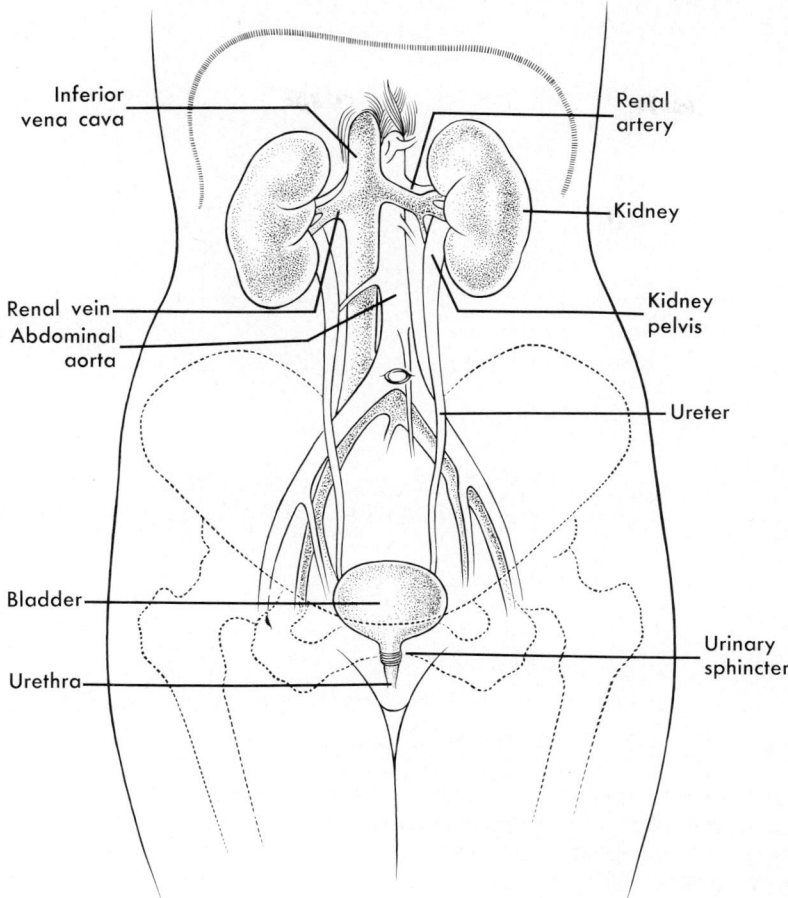

Fig. 33-1. Kidneys and other structures of urinary system.

Table 33-1. Major functions of the kidneys

Homeostasis of internal environment

Fluid volume control
Electrolyte regulation
Acid-base balance
Excretion of metabolic wastes, toxins, and drugs

Regulation of body processes

Regulation of blood pressure
Stimulation of RBC production
Regulation of calcium-phosphate metabolism

ANATOMY

The kidneys are two bean-shaped organs that lie behind the parietal peritoneum at the costovertebral angle. The organs are composed of nephrons, a vascular system, an interstitium, and the kidney pelvis. The *nephron* is the functional unit of the kidney, and each kidney contains approximately one million of these units. The structures of the nephron involved in the process of urine formation include the glomerulus and Bowman's capsule, the proximal convoluted tubule, the loop of Henle, the distal convoluted tubule, and the collecting tubule (Fig. 33-2). Bowman's capsule and both convoluted tubules lie in the cortex of the kidney, whereas the loop of Henle and collecting tubules are in the medulla. Urine from many collecting tubules drains into larger tubules that form the pyramids in the medulla and then drains into the kidney pelvis.

The ureters arise as extensions of the kidney pelves and empty into the bladder in an area called *the trigone.* These small tubes are composed of smooth muscle; their function is to propel urine from the kidneys into the bladder. Spasm and severe colic-type pain result from obstruction of the ureters. The bladder situated behind the symphysis pubis, can retain urine until an appropriate time for urination arises. This voluntary control is based on the learned inhibition of reflex pathway messages arising from the bladder walls. The urethral sphincter operating under voluntary control allows the urine to pass into the urethra for discharge from the body.

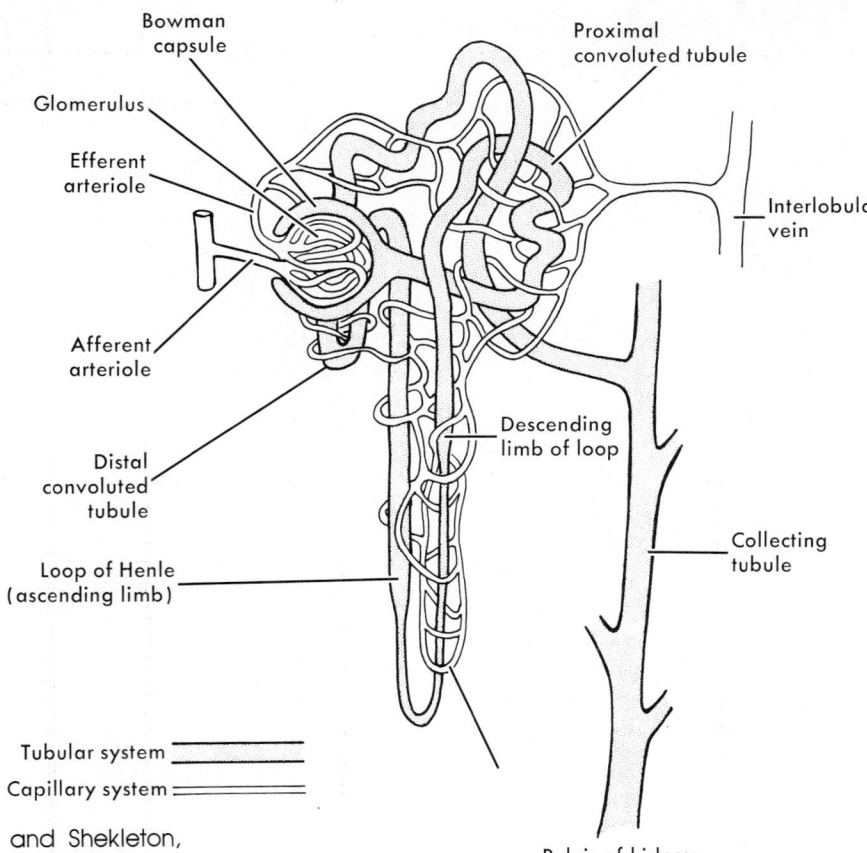

Bowman capsule

Glomerulus

Efferent arteriole

Afferent arteriole

Distal convoluted tubule

Loop of Henle (ascending limb)

Proximal convoluted tubule

Interlobular vein

Descending limb of loop

Collecting tubule

Tubular system

Capillary system

Pelvis of kidney

Fig. 33-2. Nephron. (From Groër, M.E., and Shekleton, M.E.: Basic pathophysiology; a conceptual approach, ed. 2, St. Louis, 1983, The C.V. Mosby Co.)

PHYSIOLOGY

A clear understanding of the physiology of the kidneys is essential to master the constellation of physiochemical changes that occur with renal failure. A short review of renal physiology follows.

The ultrafiltrate arising from the glomerular capillaries (*glomerular filtrate*) approximates 180 L/day. The amount of glomerular filtrate in a given time period is called the *glomerular filtration rate* (GFR). The GFR in an average-sized man is approximately 125 ml/minute (7.5 L/hour) or the equal in 1 day of about 60 times the plasma volume. The average GFR in a woman is about 10% less. The same forces that affect fluid transport between vascular and interstitial spaces in other parts of the body also affect filtration in the golmerular capsule. The GFR is affected by changes in hydrostatic pressure (for example, with decreased renal bloodflow in shock or with arteriolar constriction from sympathetic stimulation or medications) or by changes in osmotic pressure (for example, with hypoproteinemia).

The kidneys receive 25% of the cardiac output, and renal bloodflow approximates 600 ml/minute. This blood supply to the kidneys is basic to the formation of glomerular filtrate, or beginning urine, and to the nutrition and respiration requirement of kidney cells. Severe and pro-

longed problems with maintaining cardiac output and renal perfusion have profound effects on the formation of urine and the viability of the cells responsible for maintaining consistency in the internal environment.

After passing through a series of progressively smaller arteries, the blood enters the afferent arteriole that branches into the glomerular capillaries. The glomerulus, located in Bowman's capsule, is the first functional portion of the nephron. When blood enters the glomerular capillaries at a pressure not less than 60 to 70 mm Hg, an ultrafiltrate of plasma is formed. This ultrafiltrate (primitive urine) contains approximately the same concentration of the elements of plasma minus the proteins. This ultrafiltrate then passes through the remainder of the nephron for modification into actual urine.

Were it not for some conserving mechanism in the kidneys, a person would be depleted of fluid and salts within 3 to 4 minutes. The proximal convoluted tubule reabsorbs up to 85% to 90% of water in the ultrafiltrate; up to 80% of filtered sodium; and the majority of filtered potassium, bicarbonate, chloride, phosphate, glucose, and protein.

Dehydration would still occur if the body did not have an additional mechanism within the kidneys to conserve filtered water. This mechanism allows urine to be concentrated to less than 1% of the daily filtered volume.

The kidneys can vary the amount of fluid excreted so precisely that intake over that required for normal fluid balance is excreted and intake under that required for normal fluid balance leads to further concentration of the urine. The mechanisms responsible for this increased urine concentrating ability and precision in excreting appropriate urine volume exist in the loop of Henle and the distal convoluted and collecting tubules. The *loop of Henle* reaches into the medullary portion of the kidney, which is highly hypertonic in comparison to the filtrate. In the descending portion of the loop, sodium diffuses into the filtrate as the tubule passes deeper into the medullary area, and water moves out of the primitive urine in response to the high sodium concentration. The result is a reduction in volume of the glomerular filtrate and a dramatic increase in its osmolality. In the ascending limb of the loop of Henle, sodium is reabsorbed into the interstitium, but the loop is impermeable to the movement of water either into or out of the tubule. The primitive urine now presented to the distal convoluted and collecting tubules is greatly reduced in volume but hypotonic because of the reabsorption of sodium. The influence of antidiuretic hormone (ADH) on these last two segments of the tubule allows water to be reabsorbed into the interstitium in an amount compatible with maintenance of proper fluid balance. The reabsorption of water from the forming urine increases osmolality and results in the excretion of a hypertonic urine.

Electrolyte balance is achieved mainly in the distal convoluted and collecting tubule portions of the nephron. As with fluid, the major conservation site for electrolytes is the *proximal convoluted tubule* where the vast majority of all filtered electrolytes are reabsorbed, thus preventing rapid depletion of these substances. The precise regulation of body electrolyte composition occurs in the distal tubular segments. Depending on the concentrations of electrolytes presented to the tubular cells in the primitive urine and the concentrations of these substances in the interstitium, tubular cells secrete or further reabsorb electrolytes into the urine.

Acid-base balance is maintained partially through the reabsorption of bicarbonate in the proximal tubule. More precise control of acid-base status is achieved through the regeneration of bicarbonate and secretion of hydrogen ions into the urine during passage through the collecting tubule.

Metabolic wastes are excreted in the glomerular filtrate. Creatinine is little modified in its passage through the nephron; creatinine contained in the glomerular filtrate is excreted unchanged in the urine. Other wastes, such as urea, are excreted unchanged in the glomerular filtrate but undergo reabsorption during passage through the nephron. The amount of waste material excreted in urine in such an instance is only a fraction of that originally contained in the glomerular filtrate.

Excretion of drugs by the kidneys occurs through both filtration at the glomerular level and secretion into the urine by distal tubular cells. Penicillin is an example of a drug secreted by tubular cells.

Renal regulation of blood pressure is controlled by the renin-angiotensin-aldosterone system. *Renin* is a hormone released by the juxtaglomerular apparatus in response to sodium depletion, renal artery hypoperfusion, or stimulation of the renal nerves through the sympathetic pathway. *Angiotensinogen,* which is produced in the liver, is activated to *angiotensin I* in the presence of renin. An enzyme in the lungs converts angiotensin I to the active form, *angiotensin II.* Angiotensin II is a powerful vasoconstrictor and also stimulates the release of aldosterone. The combined effect of these two mechanisms is an elevation in blood pressure. The systemic hypertension associated with renal disease results from the inappropriate activation of the renin-angiotensin-aldosterone system.

RBC production is controlled by the kidneys. *Erythropoietin* is a hormone that is secreted by the kidneys. Erythropoietin stimulates bone marrow to produce RBCs. Persons with chronic renal failure often have serum hematocrit values of 18% to 30% (normal values are 42% to 47%). This decrease in hematocrit values is the result of decreased secretion of erythropoietin from the diseased kidneys compounded by bone marrow toxicity, decreased life span of RBCs and increased bleeding, all of which are associated with the altered metabolic state present in chronic renal failure.

Calcium-phosphate metabolism is also controlled by the kidneys. Vitamin D prohormone is converted to its active form by the kidneys. Active Vitamin D regulates not only GI absorption of calcium but also its depostition within the bone matrix as well as the metabolism of calcium and phosphorus.

A constellation of signs and symptoms arises in patients with chronic renal failure that cannot as yet be explained. This leads one to believe there may be some functions of the kidneys that we are not yet aware of. Because of this, nephrology remains an area rich with research questions.

Physiologic changes with aging

A direct relationship exists between blood supply to the kidneys and renal function. The rate of bloodflow to the kidneys is about 5 to 10 times greater than that to the heart, liver, and brain. Glomerular capillary pressure, which is the force that promotes ultrafiltration, is controlled by bloodflow to the kidneys. Therefore, physiologic alterations in the vascular bed can lead to changes in renal function.

Arteriosclerotic changes in renal arteries are the most common form of renal vascular pathology.[10] Arteriosclerotic changes occur to some extent in most normal individuals with aging. The degree of morphologic change experienced depends on the specific arteries affected and the extent of involvement.

Aging is also known to cause predictable increases in both systolic and diastolic blood pressure.[17] This slow increase in blood pressure begins at birth and continues through adulthood. This relationship between aging and increasing blood pressure is so well accepted that normal

Continuum of renal function

| Normal renal functioning | Diminished | Renal insufficiency | Renal failure |

Fig. 33-3. Continuum of renal function.

Factors contributing to the development of hypertension

High sodium intake
Family history of hypertension
Advanced age
Race (Black)
Obesity
Stress
Drugs, such as amphetamines, alcohol, nicotine

---

blood pressure is commonly described as 100 mm Hg plus the individuals age. Although this definition is not entirely accurate, it does suggest the effect of aging on blood pressure. Untreated hypertension further accelerates the development of atherosclerosis, which can lead to renal failure.

Prostatic hypertrophy is a common physiologic change associated with aging and will be discussed in full detail later in this chapter.

PREVENTION AND HEALTH EDUCATION

Renal function can be described as being on a continuum (Fig. 33-3). At one end of the continuum is normal renal function, while at the other end is renal failure at which point the patient exhibits signs and symptoms. Two other points on this continuum include decreased renal reserve and renal insufficiency. Decreased renal reserve exists when renal function has diminished to the point where additional physiologic or psychologic stress results in signs and symptoms of renal failure. The signs and symptoms usually resolve once the stress is removed. Renal insufficiency is defined as the reduced capacity of the kidney to perform its functions. Renal insufficiency is generally experienced when the GFR is 20% to 40% of normal. The patient with renal insufficiency typically requires symptomatic management by the physician.

Renal dysfunction can be somewhat elusive. An individual can be experiencing decreased renal function without signs or symptoms of an illness. Regular physical examinations, including serum chemistries, can aid in the detection of changing renal status.

Hypertension remains a major cause of renal disease. Early detection and treatment of hypertension can prevent or arrest renal complications. Persons at high risk for hypertension should be screened regularly. Factors

contributing to the development of hypertension are listed in the box on the left.

Urinary tract infections (UTI) are a significant source of morbidity in the United States. These infections contribute to illness during the active stage but also can lead to the development of chronic renal failure. Although the vast majority of UTI's clear spontaneously, there remains a portion significant enough to warrant consideration as a health problem. Early detection and treatment of a UTI decrease the probability of renal complications. The box below summarizes health care practices helpful in prevention and treatment of a UTI.

Urinary tract infections

Prevention
1. Cleanse perineal area properly; a shower is more desirable than a bath.
2. Drink adequate volume of fluid, 3 to 4 L/day.
3. Void frequently during waking hours, every 2 to 3 hours during day.

Treatment
1. Seek prompt medical attention for symptoms.
2. Continue with drug therapy even though symptoms abate.
3. Follow steps 1 through 3 listed above.
4. Follow-up care with repeated urine cultures are essential.

ASSESSMENT OF RENAL FUNCTION

Whenever a urinary tract disorder is suspected, a complete assessment of renal functioning is made. A guideline for the assessment follows:
1. Person's perception of illness
   a. Factors leading person to seek health care
   b. Knowledge of health status care needs
   c. Expectations regarding current health care
   d. Significant other's knowledge about person's health status
2. Previous or concurrent illness
   a. Other chronic health problems
   b. Medications currently taken
3. Social needs
   a. Resources for assistance as needed

  b. Current occupation; capacity to continue present work
4. Fluid balance
  a. Subjective
    (1) Shortness of breath (relate to position of comfort; activity tolerance)
    (2) Visual changes
    (3) Headaches
  b. Objective
    (1) Apprehension
    (2) Blood pressure (related to normal levels for the person; postural blood pressure)
    (3) Central venous pressure
    (4) Respirations (rate; depth)
    (5) Breath sounds
    (6) Pulse irregularities
    (7) Pericardial friction rub
    (8) Peripheral edema (location and extent)
    (9) Weight (direction of change; rate and extent of change)
    (10) Output (amount per hour; amount per day; released to intake)
    (11) Urine specific gravity
5. Electrolyte balance
  a. Subjective
    (1) Lethargy
    (2) Memory function
    (3) Paresthesias
    (4) Vague muscle weakness
  b. Objective
    (1) Behavior (observe for changes)
    (2) Level of alertness and orientation
    (3) Kussmaul's respirations
    (4) Blood pH
    (5) Serum electrolytes
    (6) ECG pattern
6. Nutrition
  a. Subjective
    (1) Anorexia, nausea, or vomiting
    (2) Aids to food tolerance
    (3) History of special diets
    (4) Knowledge of diet restrictions
    (5) Normal meal pattern
  b. Objective
    (1) Diet order (Na^+; K^+; protein)
7. Elimination
  a. Subjective
    (1) Bowel pattern
    (2) Laxative use
    (3) Nocturia
    (4) Symptoms of UTI
  b. Objective
    (1) Urinalysis
    (2) Urine culture
    (3) Serum creatinine value
    (4) Serum urea nitrogen
    (5) Stool guaiac
8. Skin and hygiene habits
  a. Subjective
    (1) Bathing pattern
    (2) History of dental care
  b. Objective
    (1) Lesions (skin, mucous membranes)
    (2) Moisture (skin, mucous membranes)
    (3) Parotitis
    (4) Condition of teeth
9. Comfort; rest; sleep
  a. Subjective
    (1) Puritus (extent, relief measures)
    (2) Sleep pattern (adequacy of rest)
    (3) Pain (nature, extent, and so on)
    (4) Breath odor (control measures)
  b. Objective
    (1) Scratching
    (2) Sleeping during day
    (3) Nonverbal signs of pain
    (4) Fever
10. Mobility; functional ability
  a. Subjective
    (1) Fatigue (extent; recovery with rest)
    (2) Weakness of an extremity
    (3) Numbness; tingling
  b. Objective
    (1) Balance
    (2) Gait
    (3) Muscle tone
    (4) Decreased sensation
11. Sexuality
  a. Subjective
    (1) Menses (pattern)
    (2) Concerns regarding sexual function and reproduction
  b. Objective
    (1) Behavior with significant others

Subjective data

Specific questions are directed at eliciting the presence of abnormal findings. *Dysuria* (painful urination) is usually described as "burning with urination" and is usually associated with frequency and urgency when a UTI is present. *Frequency* of urination is voiding at frequent intervals, either in small or large amounts; therefore, the approximate amount must be ascertained when this symptom is present. Small amounts may be caused by infection. Large amounts may be the result of an increased fluid intake or the effect of a diuretic. If frequency is associated with suprapubic discomfort and sense of fullness but not with dysuria, the cause may be retention of urine in the bladder with fequent overflow of the excess amounts. *Urgency* refers to the need to void immediately. It commonly accompanies frequency in persons with a UTI. A person with *nocturia* awakens at night with the need to urinate. Additional data include the number of times this occurs per night, the amount of fluid intake over 24 hours, and whether this is a change in the usual pattern.

Hesitancy refers to difficulty in initiating voiding. This

Possible causes of urinary symptoms

Dysuria	UTI
Frequency of urination	UTI, retention with overflow, excess fluid intake
Urgency	Bladder irritation as a result of inflammation, trauma, tumor
Nocturia	Increased fluid intake, diuretics, enlarged prostate gland, early renal disease
Hesitancy	Partial urethral obstruction
Decreased force and flow of urinary stream	Partial urethral obstruction, weakened perineal muscles
Urinary incontinence	Stress, spinal cord damage, CNS disease, UTI, urethral obstruction, injury during childbirth or prostatectomy

---

is often accompanied by a decrease in the force and flow of the urinary stream. Persons with difficulties in this area are asked if they have to strain to start or maintain the urinary flow. In men the most common partial obstruction is an enlarged prostate whereas in women there may be weakened perineal muscles or meatal stenosis.

Urinary incontinence is assessed by determining the specific nature of the problem: whether it occurs continually or only with stress, the presence of a sensation of fullness before voiding, health conditions associated with the incontinence, and the person's awareness of feelings regarding the incontinence. methods used by the person or family for controlling incontinence are identified.

Pain resulting from urinary disorders is located in different areas depending on the organ involved. Pain from the kidney is usually experienced over the kidney site in the back between the twelfth rib and the iliac crest (costovertebral angle). Pain from the ureters may begin over the kidney area but then radiate to the front along the course of the ureter and down into the groin. Pain from the bladder is usually suprapubic. Any discomfort from prostatic disease is usually felt in the perineum.

Objective data

URINARY OUTPUT

Most persons have a urinary output approximately equal to their fluid intake (see Chapter 10). *Polyuria* (urinary output greater than 2500 ml/day) may occur with an intake greater than 2500 ml/day, uncontrolled diabetes mellitus, or renal disease. *Oliguria* (urinary output less than 400 ml/day) may be the result of *suppression* of urine formation by the kidney (prerenal or renal factors) or to *retention* of urine in the bladder (postrenal factors). When urinary retention is present, the person experiences suprapubic discomfort and the enlarged bladder may be palpated above the symphysis pubis. Small amounts of urine being voided frequently is often a sign of retention with overflow. *Anuria* (urinary output less than 100 ml/day) is associated with renal failure.

Obtaining an accurate assessment of urinary output is often difficult in a hospital setting because urine is some-times discarded inadvertently or the patient voids into the toilet. When an accurate assessment is urgent, such as with shock or acute renal failure, an indwelling urinary catheter is usually inserted.

URINE CHARACTERISTICS

The urine is inspected for gross changes. Normal urine color varies from pale to deep yellow depending on the specific gravity. A very dark shade suggests that the urine may be concentrated (high specific gravity) or that there may be an increased excretion of bilirubin. Certain medications and foods may change the color of urine.

Hematuria, blood in the urine, may be detected overtly or may be present microscopically without visual signs. If blood is observed in the urine of a woman having her menstrual period, the vaginal orifice can be blocked with cotton balls and an additional specimen obtained to ascertain the source of the blood. Hematuria without pain is usually caused by disease of the kidney, bladder, or prostate. Hematuria with pain may be the result of calculi, a clot from renal bleeding, or bladder infection.

Cloudy urine may result from precipitation of phosphate salts in an alkaline urine or from bacterial growth. A urinary or vaginal discharge may also give the urine a cloudy appearance. (The method used to collect urine specimens is described under the section on diagnostic tests.

Possible causes of urinary symptoms are summarized in the box above.

Diagnostic tests

Special examinations of the urinary system are performed to identify the location and nature of existing disease. The accuracy of findings in many of the following tests is dependent on the assistance of the person in restricting or augmenting intake of fluids or in collecting specimens at designated time intervals. The person is given clear, precise directions; written instructions are a valuable supplement to verbal directions. Some examinations are performed under sedation. If the person is to

Urinalysis

Test	Normal	Abnormal
Color	Amber-yellow	Red indicates hematuria (possible urinary obstruction, renal calculi, tumor, renal failure)
Clarity	Clear	Cloudy: debris, bacterial sediment (urinary infection)
pH	4.6-8.0 (average 6.0)	Alkaline on standing or with UTI Increased acidity with renal tubular acidosis
Specific gravity	1.003-1.035	Usually reflects fluid intake; the less the fluid intake, the higher the specific gravity If specific gravity remains low (1.010-1.014), renal disease is suspected
Protein	0-8 mg/dl	Proteinuria may occur with high-protein diet and exercise (particularly prolonged) Seen in renal disease
Sugar	0	Glycosuria occurs after a high intake of sugar or with diabetes mellitus
Ketones	0	Ketonuria occurs with starvation and diabetic ketoacidosis
Red blood cells	0-4	Injury to kidney tissue (see hematuria)
White blood cells	0-5	UTI
Casts	0	UTI, renal disease

return home after such a procedure, prior discussion includes making arrangements for someone to accompany the person home following the procedure.

EXAMINATION OF THE URINE

Urinalysis

In identifying disease of the urinary tract, one of the first tests performed is urinalysis. This test yields information about probable locations and causes of urinary disease and some information as to the extent of the illness. Urinalysis is a test that assists in establishing tentative diagnoses and predicting additional tests and observations required to make precise diagnoses. Urinalysis also indicates abnormalities of nonrenal and nonurologic origin (for example, diabetes mellitus). The box above indicates possible normal and abnormal findings.

Clean-catch specimens

Ideally, the urine specimen is collected from the first voiding of the day. This sample is preferable because it is concentrated and abnormal constituents are more likely to be present. The person is given a clean container in which to catch urine. Cleansing the meatus before collecting the specimen decreases likelihood of external contamination; mild soap followed by water or a special antiseptic solution may be used. At least 50 to 100 ml of urine is collected for the test to ensure a sufficient amount to determine specific gravity in addition to microscopic analysis. If analysis of the urine cannot be performed immediately, the specimen must be refrigerated to retard bacterial growth.

Composite specimens

A specimen of all the urine excreted over a specific period of time is often required for urologic diagnosis. The duration of urine collections may vary from 2 to 24 hours. Specimens are examined for sugar, protein, sediment (blood cells and casts), 17-ketosteroids, electrolytes, catecholamines, and breakdown products of protein metabolism. These tests provide information on (1) the ability of the kidneys to excrete and conserve various solutes; (2) the production in the body of excessive hormones that are excreted in the urine; (3) changes in the body's regulation of glucose metabolism; (4) identification of organisms difficult to recognize through routine urine cultures; and (5) presence of abnormal cells and debris in the urine.

The accuracy of findings in this type of test is in most instances entirely dependent on cooperation of the patient. Whether the specimen is to be obtained in the hospital or in the home, the person needs to be told exactly how to collect it. Instructions for a composite urine specimen are found in the upper box on p. 948.

Composite urine tests may also involve collecting urine from multiple sources from the body. For instance, the person may pass urine from the urethra and also have a nephrostomy tube from which urine drains. Ureteral catheters may also be in place, with urine being collected from each kidney separately. Depending on the function of the test, whether the purpose is to measure the identified element in the urine as a whole or to measure separately the excretion of this element from each kidney, the urine collected from each source may be combined into one specimen container or collected into separate appropriately labeled containers.

Instructions for composite urine specimen

1. The bladder is emptied and the urine *discarded* at the appointed time to start the test.
2. Urine from *all* subsequent voidings is saved.
3. Specific directions for storing the urine should be given. Some specimens need to be kept cold during the collection period; some need preservatives added; some need no special care.
4. The person should void into a separate receptacle before defecation to prevent contamination of the specimen.
5. The bladder is emptied and the urine *added* to the collection at the appointed time to end the test.
6. The designated amount (properly labeled) is sent to the laboratory.
7. If an aliquot (5 to 10 ml sample of the total specimen) is the designated amount, the total amount collected is (1) measured and recorded on the specimen requisition and (2) mixed well before the aliquot is selected.

Directions for collecting a midstream urine specimen

Equipment needed

Sterile container for the urine
Three sponges (cotton or gauze) saturated with cleansing solution

General directions

Only outside of collecting container is touched
Urine is collected in container well after urinary stream is started

Special directions

Female
  Labia are kept separated throughout procedure
  Meatus is cleansed with one front-to-back motion with each of the three cleansing sponges
Male
  Foreskin is retracted if man is uncircumcised
  Glans is cleansed with each of the three cleansing sponges

Urine culture

Urine cultures are used to confirm suspected infections, to identify causative organisms, and to determine appropriate antimicrobial therapy. Cultures are also obtained for periodic screening of urine when the threat of UTI persists.

Urine in a properly collected and stored sample is considered to be normal if it contains 10,000 or fewer organisms per milliliter. Organisms of this magnitude are the result of normal urethral flora and do not signify UTI. A UTI is diagnosed when bacterial counts in a properly collected and stored sample reach 100,000 or more organisms per milliliter and the organisms are of one or very largely one bacterial type.[26] Contamination of the urine specimen during collection is most likely when bacterial counts include predominant colonies of *Staphylococcus,* *Streptococcus,* and diphtheroids, when two or more organisms contribute significantly to the total bacterial count,

or when repeated cultures yield differing results. All of these results are indicative of a need to repeat the culture, paying particular attention to the collection of the specimen and to its handling.

Specimens for urine culture may be obtained either by catheterization or by midstream voiding. It should be made clear, however, that *urethral catheterization should never by used routinely in collecting urine for culture because of the risk of introducing additional bacteria into the bladder.* Catheterization may be necessary to obtain a sterile urine specimen when the person is unable to void after being adequately hydrated or if the person is incontinent of urine. When a catheter is passed, meticulous attention is given to nontraumatic aseptic technique. After urine flow from the catheter is established, 5 to 10 ml of urine should be collected directly into a sterile specimen container. Care must be taken to ensure that the rim and the inside of the container are not touched by the catheter or by the hands. If a culture tube with a cotton plug is used as specimen container, care must be taken to keep the tube upright to prevent moistening the cotton and thereby contaminating the specimen. Cultures may also be ordered on the urine taken from the renal pelvis during ureteral catheterization or when ureterostomy or nephrostomy tubes are in place.

In collecting a voided specimen for culture, the nurse must decide if the patient is capable of independently obtaining the specimen or if nursing or medical personnel will need to collect a midstream specimen. Most persons who are ambulatory and are given precise and unhurried direction will be able to collect their own midstream urine specimen.

The first voided specimen of the day should be used whenever possible because bacteria will be more numerous. If the specimen is not cultured immediately, refrigeration is mandatory to prevent growth of organisms in the specimen.

EVALUATION OF BLADDER FUNCTION

Measurement of residual urine

Normally the bladder contains little or no urine after voiding; however, certain disease states inhibit the bladder from emptying completely. Some common conditions in which incomplete emptying of the bladder occurs are benign prostatic hypertrophy, urethral strictures, and interruptions in bladder innervation. Urine left in the bladder after voiding is called *residual urine*.

One way to determine the amount of residual urine is to *catheterize* the person immediately after voiding. This may be ordered by the physician on a one-time or on a repeated basis. Before catheterizing the person, the physician is consulted regarding the plan for establishing urinary drainage. If a large amount of residual urine is suspected, the physician may wish the catheter to be left in place in the bladder. *Residual urine volumes of 50 ml or less indicate near normal or returning bladder function.*

To avoid passing a catheter to measure residual urine volumes, x-ray examination of retained urine may be performed. In this procedure a radiopaque substance excreted by the kidneys is injected intravenously. As the dye is excreted in the urine, it passes into the bladder. A sufficient amount of urine containing the radiopaque material is allowed to accumulate in the bladder before the person is instructed to void. Immediately after voiding an x-ray film is taken. Any urine retained in the bladder will be visualized on the radiograph. This means of determining residual urine is used in conjunction with other studies requiring visualization of the urinary tract.

Cystometrogram

Cystometric examination is performed to evaluate bladder tone. In general, the examination is indicated when incontinence is present or when there is evidence of neurologic dysfunction of the bladder. A Foley catheter is inserted before the examination. After the person assumes a supine position, a liter bottle of normal saline or

Normal values of selected serum electrolytes	
Sodium	135 to 140 mEq/l
Potassium	3.5 to 5.0 mEq/l
Chloride	98 to 102 mEq/l
Bicarbonate	24 to 28 mEq/l
Calcium	9 to 22 mg%

sterile distilled water and a cystometer are connected to the catheter. Fluid is instilled at a constant and specified rate; measurements of the pressure exerted onthe fluid by the bladder musculature are recorded after the instillation of every 50 ml of fluid. The person is asked to report feelings of fullness, the need to void, and any urgency or discomfort. Fluid is instilled until urgency occurs or it is determined that the sensation is absent. During cystometric examination, bethanechol chloride (Urecholine) may be administered to determine its effect on enhancing the tone of a flaccid bladder, or an anticholingeric medication may be given to assess relaxation in a hyperactive bladder. There is no specific care required after cystometric examination.

Electromyography may be used to evaluate sphincter tone and intactness of nerve pathways.

EVALUATION OF RENAL FUNCTION

When findings of the general physical examination or urinalysis suggest renal disease, tests of renal function are conducted. A summary of renal function tests is found in the box on pp. 950-951. It should be remembered that the best overview of the patient's clinical condition is obtained by comparing the results of a number of tests. Therefore, it is common for a series of renal function tests to be ordered for an individual.

Serum electrolytes do not give conclusive results in terms of renal function. Many factors influence serum electrolytes. In renal failure, the serum electrolytes may be normal, elevated, decreased, or any combination of these. Serum electrolyte levels are monitored closely in patients with renal failure so that their level can be adequately regulated. The normal ranges for the most commonly measured electrolytes are shown in the box above.

VISUALIZATION OF THE URINARY TRACT

Technologic advances in the last several years have made it possible to visualize the urinary tract by both direct and indirect means. These tests allow for assessment of both structure and function of the organs and tissues of the urinary tract. Visualization of the urinary tract is used not only for diagnosis but also to evaluate the patient's response to therapy over a period of time.

Selected renal function tests

Test	Normal results	Purpose/significance	Nursing implications
Specific gravity of urine	1.010-1.026	Measures ability of kidneys to concentrate urine	First morning void is usually in the high normal range in healthy individual False high is caused by presence of radiographic dyes.
Osmolality of urine	400-600 mosm/kg	Excellent indication of renal function Osmolality is total concentration of particles in solution	No special preparation
Fishberg concentration test	Urine volume 300/ml/12 hrs Specific gravity of 1.024 or greater Urine osmolality of 850 mosm or greater	Used to determine ability of kidney to conserve fluid As differential diagnosis for diabetes insipidus and psychogenic polydipsia	No fluid can be taken during test period Test period of 8-12 hours usually during night First morning void assures maximum concentration Three hourly urine specimens are collected for volume, specific gravity, and osmolality following test period Patient should be observed for signs of vascular collapse
Urine chemistries	Sodium: 130 to 220 mEq/L Potassium: 39 to 90 mg/24 hrs Calcium: 100 to 300 mg/24 hrs	Urine electrolytes reflect ability of kidney to excrete and reabsorb electrolytes	Abnormal results may be caused by diseased processes other than renal disorders, for example, elevated urine calcium in hyperparathyroidism or prolonged immobilization
Creatinine clearance	Men: 100 to 150 ml/min Women: 85 to 125 ml/min	Clearance is rate at which a substance is excreted in terms of plasma concentration Because diet and metabolic state have little influence on it, serum creatinine is excellent for determining glomerular filtratation rate.	Procedure 1. Patient empties bladder and time is noted 2. *All* urine is saved for 24 hours 3. Exactly 24 hours after start of procedure the patient voids and specimen is saved 4. Total urine volume and urine creatinine is measured 5. Serum creatinine is determined at end of 24 hour period

Selected renal function tests—cont'd

Test	Normal results	Purpose/significance	Nursing implications
			6. Creatinine clearance is then calculated by formula: Clearance: $\dfrac{UV\dagger}{P\dagger}$ *U = Urine creatinine concentration *V = Urine volume *P = Plasma creatinine concentration
Serum creatinine	Men: 85 to 1.5 mg/dl Women: .70 to 1.25 mg/dl	Indicated ability of kidneys to excrete nitrogenous wastes	No specific preparation for test Diet and metabolic rate have little effect on serum creatinine
Blood urea nitrogen (BUN)	5-20 mg/dl	Indicates ability of kidneys to excrete nitrogenous wastes BUN gives a rough estimate of GFR	BUN can be affected by high protein diet, blood in GI tract, catabolic state (injury, infection, fever, poor nutrition)
Phenolsulfonphthalein excretion test (PSP)	30-50% of PSP dye excreted in 15 minutes	Measures tubular secretion rates	Procedure 1. Patient drinks 8 to 10 glasses of water 2. 1 ml PSP dye is given intravenously 3. Urine specimens are collected at 15-, 30- and 60-minute intervals 4. The exact time the urine specimen is collected must be recorded to calculate excretion rates

Cystoscopy

Cystoscopy is the direct examination of the bladder using an instrument called a cystoscope (Fig. 33-4). The cystoscope relies on a flexible optic fiber to provide illumination into the urinary tract. The instrument is attached to the illuminating source then slowly passed through the urinary tract, thus enabling direct visualization of the urethra, ureteral orifices, and bladder.

The cystoscopic examination may be performed with or without anesthesia. General anesthesia is required for cystoscopy when the person is quite apprehensive or when much manipulation is anticipated. In these instances, anesthesia reduces the possibility of trauma to the urethra or perforation of the bladder caused by sudden vigorous movement of the patient during the examination. Children are usually given a general anesthetic for this procedure.

Much of the discomfort felt during this procedure is the result of contraction or spasm of the bladder sphincters; this can be decreased through deep-breathing exercises and general relaxation on the part of the patient. A sedative such as diazepam (Valium) and a narcotic such as morphine or meperidine hydrochloride (Demerol) are usually given an hour before the examination.

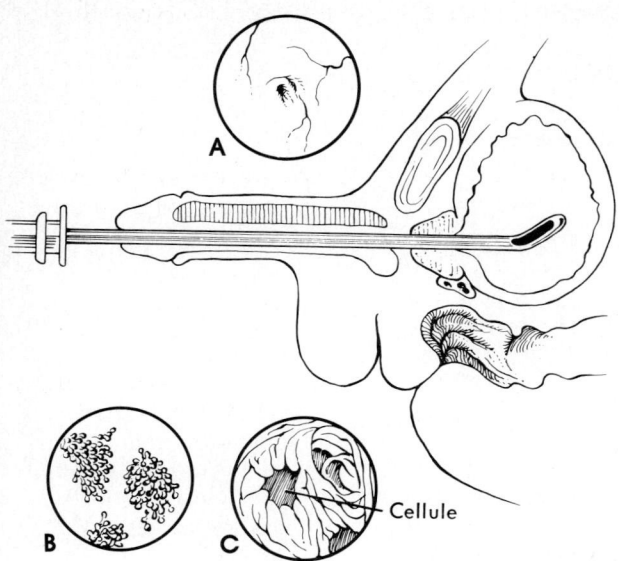

Fig. 33-4. Cystoscope inserted for examination of bladder. **A,** Appearance of normal ureteral orifice as seen through cystoscope. **B,** Appearance of papillomas of bladder as seen through cystoscope. **C,** Appearance of trabeculated bladder as seen through cystoscope. Note formation of cellules.

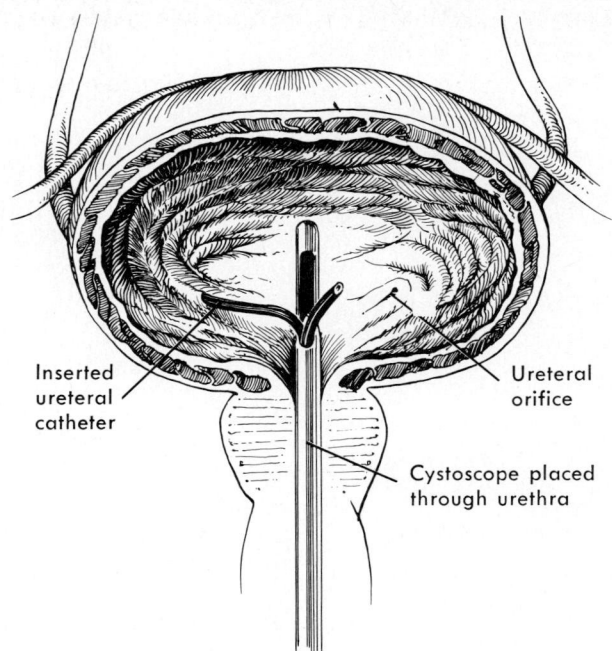

Fig. 33-5. Ureteral catheterization through cystoscope. Note ureteral catheter inserter into left orifice. Right ureteral catheter is ready to be inserted.

If the patient is relatively comfortable, the cystoscope should be passed with little pain, provided there is no obstruction in the urethra. A local anesthetic such as procaine (usually 4%) may be instilled into the urethra before insertion of the cytoscope.

When the patient is awake, passing the instrument will be followed immediately by a strong desire to void. This occurs as a result of the pressure the instrument exerts against the internal sphincter. During the examination the bladder is distended with distilled water to make visualization more effective. As the bladder becomes increasingly distended, the urge to void increases.

During cystoscopy a number of tests may be performed on the urinary system. Cystography involves the injection of a radiopaque dye such as methiodal (Skiodan) or air as a contrast medium to visualize the bladder and determine its size, shape, and any irregularities. Bladder capacity may be measured through instillation of distilled water. A *voiding cystourethrogram* can reveal reflux of urine into the ureters on voiding, a bladder malfunction that can lead to pyelonephritis.

Ureteral catheterization (with a nylon, radiopaque, size 4 to 6 Fr catheter) can be performed through the cystoscope. The catheter is inserted into the ureteral opening in the bladder, into the ureter, and into the renal pelvis (Fig. 33-5). This procedure may involve one or both ureters. It is performed (1) when culture and analysis of urine from individual kidneys is required; (2) when tests of renal function are to be performed on the kidneys separately; and (3) when visualization of the urinary tract is desired and intravenous pyelogram visualization has been inadequate, obstruction is present, or sensitivity to intravenous radiopaque material is noted.

Care should be taken that the person does not stand or walk alone immediately after cystoscopy. Blood that has drained from the leg while in the lithotomy position will flow back into the vessels of the feet and legs as standing is assumed. Accidents caused by dizziness and fainting can occur from the sudden change in distribution of blood.

Three complications of cystoscopy that need to be monitored are bleeding, perforation of the bladder, and spread of infection throughout the urinary tract or into the bloodstream (sepsis). Observation for frank bleeding (pink-tinged urine is normal) is necessary. Urinary output and voiding pattern are monitored to detect obstruction, and fluid intake is increased to prevent stasis. Mild analgesics are given for discomfort, and warmth is provided if the patient complains of being chilly. Vital signs are monitored as necessary.

Most hospitals require a signed permit before cystoscopy is performed after the person is given an explanation of what is to occur. Fluids are usually forced for several hours before the procedure. This ensures a continuous flow of urine in the event specimens need to be collected and aids in preventing multiplication of bacteria that may be introduced during the procedure. If general anesthesia is to be used, fluids may be administered intravenously. If radiographs are to be taken during the procedure, bowel preparation may be ordered.

Common radiologic examinations of the urinary tract

Test	Purpose	Procedure	Nursing implications
Retrograde pyelography	Visualization of urinary tract	1. Ureteral catheterization required 2. Radiopaque material (Hypaque, Renografin) gently injected 3. Radiographs are taken of the renal collecting structures	Patient may experience discomfort in region of kidneys as dye is injected Pain may be experienced if too large a volume of dye is injected and renal pelvis becomes distended
Intravenous pyelography (IVP)	Determine size and location of kidneys Demonstrate precence of cysts or tumors Outline filling of renal pelvis Outline ureters and bladder	1. Radiograph of abdomen (KUB) is taken to identify size and position of kidneys 2. Radiopaque dye is given intravenously 3. Radiographs of the kidneys are taken at 3-, 5-, 10-, and 20-minute intervals	Bowel cleansing required Fluids are often withheld for up to 8 hours to produce slight dehydration The patient should be informed that a feeling of warmth, flushing of the face, and a salty taste in the mouth may occur as the dye is injected The patient should be observed for signs and symptoms of a reaction to the dye including respiratory distress, diaphoresis, urticaria, instability of vital signs or unusual sensations. Cardiopulmonary resuscitation equipment and emergency medications should always be available for immediate use.
Kidney, ureters and bladder (KUB) radiograph	Gross visualization of kidneys, ureters, and bladder Calcifications and stones can be located	Radiograph of abdominal region obtained	Bowel cleansing may or may not be ordered
Urethrography	Visualization of urethral size and shape	Radiography of urethra taken after instilling 20 ml of radiopaque water-soluble lubricant	No special preparation
Computed tomography (CT)	Visualization of kidneys and renal circulation	Whole body CT scanner segments kidneys Can be done with IV contrast dye	If dye is used same implications apply as listed for IVP

Continued.

Common radiologic examinations of the urinary tract—cont'd

Test	Purpose	Procedure	Nursing implications
Renal angiography	Visualization of renal circulation Particularly useful in evaluating renal artery stenosis	Procedure is similar to IVP, however, the contrast dye is often injected directly into the femoral artery by passing a catheter through the artery to the level of the renal arteries	Nursing implications are the same as in IVP Patient must be observed for bleeding at arterial puncture site, especially within first 4 hours. The pressure dressing should be checked for fresh bleeding. The puncture site should be checked for tenderness or swelling. Vital signs and distal pulses must be assessed frequently (q 15 min × 4 hours). Bed rest should be maintained for 8 hours after the procedure.
Renography	Visualization of urinary tract Measures renal blood-flow Measures renal tubular and excretory function	Involves scintillation scanning or photography Radioactive isotope such as iodohippurate sodium tagged with I^{131} or I^{125} is injected intravenously Scintillating probes placed over the kidneys record the photographs	Since only trace doses of bound isotopes are used, no special precautions are necessary
Ultrasound	Used to distinguish between abnormal fluid collections and solid masses. Used to identify obstructions and detect abscesses. Often used to diagnose abscesses, ureteral leaks, and obstructions in renal transplant recipients	Sound waves are used to outline internal body structures. The procedure is accomplished by computer interpretation of tissue densities	Procedure is painless and noninvasive. A full bladder assists in outline structures

Radiologic examination

A number of radiologic examinations are used to visualize the urinary tract. Since the kidneys lie retroperitoneally, any accumulation of flatus or feces in the intestine can obstruct the view on the radiograph. To assure adequate visualization, bowel evacuation ir necessary before the radiographs are taken.

Radiographs of the urinary tract may be ordered in conjunction with other abdominal studies. Problems may arise in visualizing the urinary system if barium studies have been recently carried out. This problem can be prevented by scheduling tests so that examination of the urinary tract precedes barium contrast radiographs of the GI tract.

RENAL BIOPSY

Renal biopsy is potentially the most accurate diagnostic test for determining both the type and the stage of progression of renal pathologic conditions. Specifically, this test aids in differentiating diagnoses, in following the progression of disease, in choosing therapy most beneficial to the patient, and in determining prognosis of the illness. The biopsy can be performed either through a skin puncture (closed biopsy) or through an incision (open biopsy).

Inherent in taking a biopsy specimen of this vascular tissues is a potential threat of hemorrhage. Throughout the procedure, care is given to prevent and to detect early loss of blood. Before biopsy is performed, a thorough medical evaluation with particular attention to detection of any abnormality in bleeding or coagulation time is carried out. The patient's blood is usually typed and crossmatched with 2 units of blood; the blood is held for the patient until any threat of bleeding has passed.

An open biopsy carries less risk of hemorrhage and provides better visualization of the kidney; however, the risk of infection is increased, and a longer period of recovery is required.

Preparation before biopsy includes discussing the procedure with the patient. Topics covered include the necessity for the examination, the procedure itself, the care to be anticipated, and any questions of concern to the patient. The preparation of the patient is shared by the physician and nurse. In most institutions it is necessary to have the patient sign a special permit before having the biopsy performed. The biopsy may be carried out in the patient's room, in the radiology department, or in the operating room.

The procedure for *percutaneous (closed) biopsy* is as follows: Before the biopsy, the patient is taken to the radiology department for localization of the kidney. This is accomplished with a plain film, a dye contrast film, or fluoroscopic location. The position of the kidney in relation to body landmarks is marked on the skin in ink. The lower pole of the kidney is located, this being the site for biopsy, since it contains the fewest number of large vessels. The patient is then transported to the area where the biopsy will be performed. Sedation is usually not required except for children or adults who are restless and unable to relax sufficiently to follow necessary instructions during the test. The patient is placed prone over a sandbag or firm pillow and an additional soft pillow. The body should be bent at the level of the diaphragm, with the shoulders on the bed and the spine in straight alignment. Blood pressure and pulse rate are determined at this point and are recorded. Cleansing of the skin is carried out to remove as many surface contaminants as possible. The physician identifies the location for biopsy, and a local anesthetic agent is injected. As the biopsy is being taken, the patient is instructed to hold his or her breath. Pain may be felt in the kidney region as the tissue sample is taken. The needle is withdrawn immediately, and direct pressure is applied to the site for 20 minutes. A pressure bandage is then applied, and the patient is turned supine and is kept flat (one small pillow may be used under the head) and motionless for the next 4 hours. Coughing and any activity that increases abdominal venous pressure is to be avoided during this time. Blood pressure and pulse should be taken each 15 minutes for 1 hour, every 30 minutes during the next hour, and every

hour for an additional 2 to 3 hours. The patient should remain in bed for at least 24 hours. All urine is observed for hematuria, and bed rest is maintained until the urine is clear. Initially, the patient's urine is likely to demonstrate blood, but this rarely continues after a 24-hour period. Once out of bed, the patient should be cautioned against any heavy lifting for a period of 10 days.

Major health problems of the urinary system

The major health problems of the urinary system include (1) congenital disorders, (2) inflammatory disorders, (3) vascular disorders, and (4) obstructive disorders. The following are some common urinary disorders for each of these major categories.
1. Congenital disorders
   a. Structural malformation of urinary collecting system
   b. Agenesis of one or both kidneys
   c. Hypoplasia of one or both kidneys
   d. Dysplasia of one or both kidneys
   e. Polycystic disease
2. Inflammatory disorders
   a. UTI
   b. Chemical induced nephritis
   c. Glomerulonephritis
   d. Nephrotic syndrome
   e. Pyelonephritis
3. Vascular disorders
   a. Nephrosclerosis
   b. Renal artery stenosis
   c. Diabetic nephropathy
4. Obstructive disorders
   a. Calculi
   b. Neoplasms
   c. Prostatic hypertrophy
   d. Urethral strictures

Two other major health problems of the urinary tract, which will be discussed in this chapter, are: urinary incontinence and trauma to the urinary tract.

Nurses can assist in significantly reducing the morbidity of disease of the urinary system. This can be achieved through increasing public awareness of preventive measures, assisting in early detection of signs and symptoms of disease, and providing long-term care to the growing population of chronically ill individuals with urinary tract disease. This section defines common problems of the person with disease of the urinary system and identifies nursing implications of these disorders.

CONGENITAL DISORDERS

Structural malformations of the urinary collecting system occur in about 10% to 15% of the population.[9] These deviations range in severity from minor anomalies that do

---

Congenital malformations of the urinary tract

Duplication of the ureters
Hydroureters
Exstrophy of the urinary bladder
Epispadias
Hydrospadias

---

not require correction to those that are incompatible with life. Some of the congenital malformations that have a potential influence on the urinary function in adult life are listed in box above.

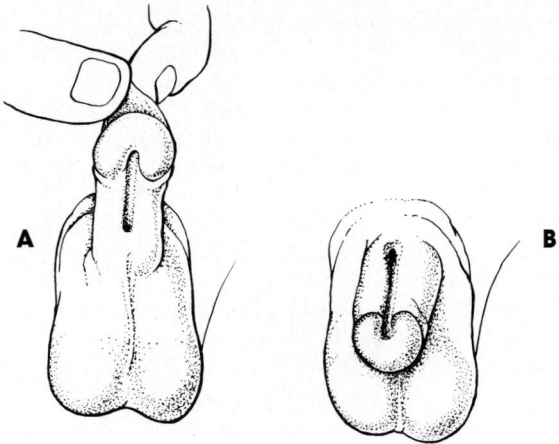

Fig. 33-6. A, Hypospadias. **B,** Epispadias.

Pathophysiology

Partial or complete duplication of the ureters is a relatively common anomaly of the urinary tract. Unilateral duplication occurs in about one in 200 births, while bilateral duplications occurs about one in 1200 births.[9] This defect includes duplication of the renal pelvis as well as the ureters. A *complete duplication* refers to the occurrence of two separate ureters from one kidney. More common is a *partial duplication* in which the duplicate ureters unite at some point between the kidney and bladder. The clinical significance of duplication of the ureter is dependent on the presence of obstruction or reflux. Obstruction at the point where the two ureters join or reflux from one ureter into the other in a partial duplication may led to dilation of the ureter, hydronephrosis, and a persistent or recurrent UTI. In the case of complete duplication, the ureter draining the upper pole of the kidney may open either into the bladder or into the vulva, urethra, or seminal vesicle. If the ureter drains ectopically (outside the bladder), incontinence and obstruction are generally present. Surgical intervention when necessitated by obstruction or reflux may include reimplantation of an ectopic ureter into the bladder, resection of the duplicated ureter, resection of the hydronephrotic portion of the kidney, or nephrectomy if severe renal damage has occured. *Triplication of the ureters* occurs infrequently, and management is the same as for duplication.

Hydroureter (dilatation of the ureter) may result from obstruction in the lower urinary tract, from vesicoureteral reflux, or from an atonic lower ureteral segment, all of which may be congenital. In some cases of severe ureteral dilation, peristalsis in the lower ureter is decreased secondary to atony. Urinary diversion for a time may allow the ureter to become amenable to future repair and reimplantation into the bladder. If such attempts fail, urinary diversion is permanent. Congenital deficiency of abdominal musculature, or prune belly syndrome, is rare and includes extreme hydronephrosis and dilated ureters. Treatment usually necessitates permanent urinary diversion.

Exstrophy of the bladder and *epispadias* are developmental anomalies that ofter occur together. They result from

failure of the midline to close adequately during fetal development and may vary a great deal in their severity.

Epispadias is a failure of closure on the dorsal surface of the penis and may extend from the glans to the perineum (Fig. 33-6, *B*). The defect often extends to the urinary sphincter, causing incontinence. If surgical correction involving the urinary sphincter is not successful, urinary diversion may be performed.

Exstrophy of the bladder, which occurs in approximately 1 in 40,000 births, may comprise only a small fistula leading to the surface of the abdominal wall that drains urine, or it may be so extensive that most of the interior of the bladder is everted on the outer abdominal wall. Usually the sphincter muscles of the urethra are faulty and epispadias is present. The muscles below the umbilicus are separated, and the pubic rami are not joined. Operations for exstrophy of the bladder may include attempts to reconstruct sphincter muscles of the urethra and to close the bladder and abdominal walls. If satisfactory repair cannot be made, as is frequently the case in complete exstrophy, permanent urinary diversion may be necessary. If untreated, the bladder wall undergoes squamous metaplastic changes that predispose the patient to adenocarcinoma in later life.

Hypospadias is a common anomaly in which the urethra opens in the male at any ventral point on the penis between the glans and perineum (Fig. 33-6, *A*). It is almost always accompanied by *chordee,* fibrous bands that cause curvature of the penis. In the female the urethra opens into the vagina. Very slight anomalies require no intervention; when treatment is indicated, surgical reconstruction of the urethra (and release of chordee in the male) is done. Postoperative strictures may occur, which require further treatment.

Congenital defects of the kidneys can include developmental defects as well as metabolic and enzyme defects that affect tubular transport, such as cystinuria. The discussion in this chapter will be limited to developmental defects that may have implications in adulthood.

Agenensis (absence) of both kidneys is rare and incompatible with life. However, unilateral agenesis is not uncom-

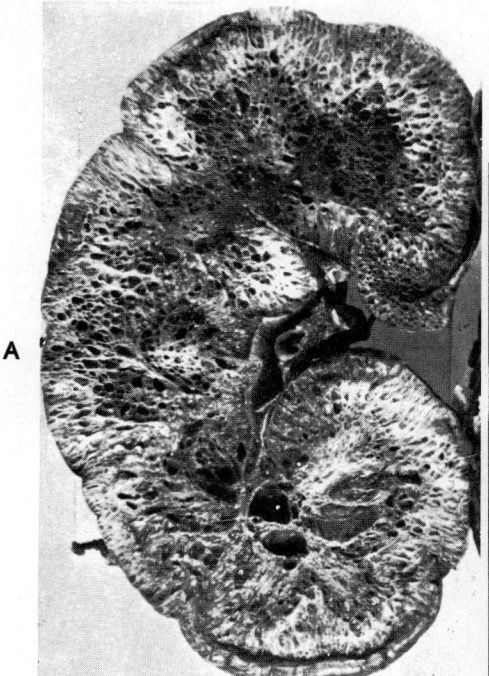

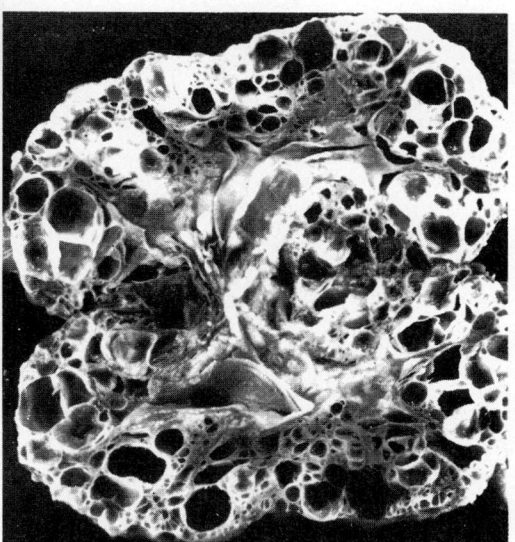

Fig. 33-7. Polycystic disease of kidney. **A,** Newborn infant. **B,** Adult. (From Anderson, W.A.D., and Kissane, J.M.: Pathology, ed. 7, St. Louis, 1977, The C.V. Mosby Co.)

mon. A person with this defect is often unaware of it as long as the remaining kidney remains functional. Unilateral agenesis is sometimes detected on radiographs taken for diagnosis of other problems. *Hypoplasia* is when the kidneys fail to develop to normal size, most commonly affecting only one side. However, when both kidneys are affected, there is a progressive development of renal failure.

Horseshoe kidney refers to fusion of the kidneys, usually at their lower poles. The incidence varies between 1 in 600 and 1 in 1800 births.[9] Potential problems that may arise because of anterior angulation of the ureters include stasis, hydronephrosis, and possible calculus formation. When indicated because of obstruction, surgical treatment comprises division of the fused part. Cases uncomplicated by obstruction or calculi are generally not treated surgically.

Dysplasia is the most common renal developmental disorder. Dysplasia results from the abnormal development of renal tissue during embryonic development. Renal dysplasias account for approximately 20% of urinary tract malformations and are often associated with other congenital defects of lower urinary tract.

Assessment

The initial assessment of a congenital malformation of the urinary system is often made at birth or shortly thereafter. Malformations of the external genitalia are usually detected on the initial physical examination. Each newborn is assessed for urinary drainage by monitoring initial voiding and regularity of voiding thereafter. Partial malformations often go undetected unless noted on diagnostic studies later in life.

Diagnostic tests

A complete series of radiographs may be ordered to determine the extent of the malformation. This would include IVP, retrograde pyelography, KUB, and ultrasound.

DATA ANALYSIS AND PLANNING

Possible nursing diagnoses for the patient with congenital disorders of the urinary system include the following:
Coping, ineffective individual
Fluid volume, alteration in: excess
Grieving, dysfunctional
Self-concept, disturbance in: body image
Sexual dysfunction
Urinary elemination, alteration in patterns

IMPLEMENTATION

Details of the nursing implementation for congential malformations can be obtained from a pediatric nursing textbook.

Polycystic disease

Polycystic disease is an inherited defect that involves the kidneys bilaterally. The kidneys are usually enlarged and filled with cysts. Polycystic disease is categorized into two groups, infantile and adult. Infantile polycystic disease is an autosomal recessive trait. The infant usually develops symptoms and dies within a few moths after birth. Adult polycystic disease is an autosomal dominant trait affecting about 1 in 500 persons. Adults with this disorder generally develop symptoms in the third to fourth decade of life. End-stage renal disease is usually reached 10 to 15 years after symptoms arise.

There is no preventative care for polycystic disease. However, early detection and medical care can prevent and control infection of the diseased kidneys and retard the development of end-stage renal failure.

PATHOPHYSIOLOGY

As polycystic disease progresses, cysts in the kidneys enlarge and rupture (Fig. 33-7). The ruptured cysts become infected and scar tissue develops, thus decreasing the number of functioning nephrons. The size of the cysts also increases gradually, creating pressure on the surrounding parenchyma and causing ischemic atrophy.

ASSESSMENT

Subjective data

The patient is questioned about the presence and extent of discomfort and pain in the flank. Colicky pain may be experienced when clots are passed down the ureter. Symptoms of uremia may be present when renal function has deteriorated to the point of end-stage renal disease. Fever, chills, and general malaise may be experienced by the patient.

Objective data

Hematuria and hypertension are each (independently) present in approximately 50% of all cases of polycystic disease. It is common for both hematuria and hypertension to be present in the same individual. On physical examination, the enlarged kidneys appear as large palpable abominal masses. Serum and urine electrolytes and creatine clearance tests provide accurate data about renal function. A urine culture is obtained to determine the presence of UTI.

Diagnostic tests

While a retrograde pyelograph and KUB can give valuable data about the size of the kidneys, the IVP is most often used to confirm the diagnosis of polycystic disease.

DATA ANALYSIS AND PLANNING

Nursing diagnosis

Possible nursing diagnoses for the patient with polycystic disease include the following:
Pain in flank
Ineffective individual and family coping
Alteration in fluid volume: excess or deficit
Alteration in tissue perfusion: renal
Alteration in patterns of urinary elimination
Alteration in nutrition: potential for more than body requirements

Expected patient outcomes

The person or significant other can state or describe the following:

1. Signs and symptoms of infection and blood loss requiring medical attention
2. Plans for follow-up health care
3. Appropriate health screening and follow-up care for children

IMPLEMENTATION

Assisting with achievement of therapeutic goals

Interventions for the patient with polycystic disease centers largely on preventing infection and bleeding. Infection is difficult to eradicate in persons with polycystic kidneys, and when infection is uncontrolled it leads to further destruction of kidney tissue. Frequent culture of the urine is performed and instrumentation and catheterization of the urinary tract are avoided whenever possible. Antibiotic therapy is often instituted. When antibiotics are ordered, they should be given on time and on a regular schedule to ensure adequate blood levels. The patients urinary output must be closely monitored.

Assisting with comfort and ADL

Analgesic drugs may be necessary in control of flank pain associated with enlarged kidneys.

When bleeding from ruptured cysts becomes severe enough to turn the urine from pink to red, bed rest is usually instituted. At these times the patient will require assistance with ADL. Otherwise independence in ADL should be encouraged.

Counseling and teaching

The patient will need to be instructed to be alert to signs and symptoms of infection and bleeding. The emotional overtones of this illness can be severe for both the individual and the family. Challenges exist in helping the person deal with an illness on an individual basis when relatives have died of the same disease and children have not yet developed symptoms. Counseling regarding family health care and the individaul's role in passing on a potentially fatal disease to children will, at times, be required. The patient should be instructed to monitor urinary output and report changes to their physician.

EVALUATION

The evaluation of nursing care of patients with polycystic disease is made on the basis of the identified nursing diagnoses. General questions to ask include the following: (1) Can the patient state signs and symptoms of infection and bleeding; (2) Can the patient state plans for follow-up health care; (3) Is the patient dehydrated or fluid overloaded; (4) Is the patient receiving a balanced nutritional input; and (5) Is the patient comfortable.

INFLAMMATORY DISORDERS

The kidneys are susceptible to inflammation caused by bacterial infection, altered immune responses, drugs and other chemicals, toxins and radiation. Inflammation may be acute or chronic. This section will address the most common inflammatory disorders of the urinary system.

Urinary tract infections

UTI is a significant source of morbidity in the United States and also is significant in the development of chronic renal failure. Infection occurs in both acute and chronic stages in all portions of the urinary tract.

Table 33-2 summarizes factors contributing to infection of the urinary tract. Although the great majority of noncomplicated urinary infections are asymptomatic and clear spontaneously, there remains a portion significant enough to warrant consideration as a health problem. There is no controversy among those practicing preventive health care regarding the question of the need for screening of asymptomatic infections; however, there exists difficulty in identifying the specific risk groups in which the detection and treatment of these infections yield significant improvement in the person's health. As the health care of our population becomes more oriented toward prevention of health problems, specific target populations will be better defined and the number of screening programs for asymptomatic UTI will increase.

Females seem more predisposed to UTI than males. Factors postulated in their higher infection rates include a shorter urethra close to the rectum and the lack of prostatic fluid protection present in the male. Infection rates for females approximate 1% of school-aged girls and 4% of women through the childbearing years.[6] Incidence of infection in females increases directly with sexual activity and with aging. Pregnancy does not seem to increase infection rates, although spontaneous clearing of infections is decreased during pregnancy, and there is a higher incidence of acute kidney infections progressing upward from the lower urinary tract.

Structural and functional abnormalities of the urinary tract, obstruction of the flow of urine, and impaired bladder innervation promote infection of the urinary tract. Mechanisms involved include stasis of urine, which provides a culture medium for bacteria; reflux of infected urine higher into the urinary tract; and increasing hydrostatic pressure.

Certain chronic health problems predispose persons to UTI by changing the metabolism of tissues, creating extrarenal obstructions, and altering the function and structure of kidney tissue. Common among these health problems are diabetes mellitus, gout, hypertension, polycystic kidney disease, multiple myeloma, and glomerulonephritis.

Instrumentation of the urinary tract is associated with high rates of infection. Catheterization, even when performed without breaks in asepsis, results in significant infection of the bladder. *Nosocomial infections* account for a sizeable percentage of all UTIs. Drug-resistant strains of *Staphylococcus* and *Pseudomonas,* along with various other organisms commonly found in hospitals, are frequently those involved in nosocomial UTIs. Prevention and control of all urinary tract infections can be most significantly influenced through a lowering of this nosocomial infection rate.

Infections of the lower urinary tract involve the urinary bladder (*cystitis*) and the urethra (*urethritis*). In the upper urinary tract, infection involves the kidney (*pyelonephritis*). The etiologic factors and general preventive and management principles are the same for infections anywhere in the urinary tract.

Three considerations are important in preventing infection of the lower urinary tract: (1) preventing or minimizing morbidity, which can accompany these infections; (2) preventing recurrence of the infection; and (3) preventing renal damage from untreated or inadequately treated ascending infection. Since individuals with a lower UTI seek medical attention as a result of symptoms or are identified through routine urinalysis or screening of populations at high risk, both education of the public and community health case finding assist in decreasing UTI and its complications.

The symptoms that bring the person to medical attention typically include urgency, burning on urination (dysuria), and slight to gross hematuria. Most persons, however, are asymptomatic or minimally symptomatic, the infection being identified only on routine examination of the urine. Bacteriuria and positive urine cultures serve as the basis for diagnosing a lower UTI. Growth of a single pathogen in excess of 1×10^5 organisms/ml of urine in a properly obtained and stored midstream specimen indicates infection.

Treatment goals for a lower UTI include sterilizing the urine and identifying any illness or urinary tract abnormality that may be contributing to the infection. After culture and sensitivity studies a 10- to 14-day course of antibiotic therapy is instituted. It is crucial that urine culture be obtained before initiating drug therapy to en-

Table 33-2. Risk factors associated with development of UTI

Risk factor	Common examples
Female	Short urethra
Structural abnormality	Strictures
	Incompetent ureterovesical junction anomalies
Obstruction	Tumors
	Prostatic hypertrophy
	Calculi
	Iatrogenic causes
Impaired bladder innervation	Congenital spinal cord malformation
	Spinal cord injury
	Multiple sclerosis
Chronic disease	Gout
	Diabetes mellitus
	Hypertension
	Sickle cell disease
	Chronic renal disease
Instrumentation	Catheterization
	Diagnostic procedures

sure appropriateness of antimicrobial medication and to decrease the development of resistant strains of organisms. The urine should be recultured every few months during the following year to reconfirm urine sterility.

A more extensive urologic workup including IVP and voiding cystogram may be performed for men and young children after a repeated or even first, UTI or when infection does not abate. This workup is performed on women when infection occurs repeatedly or cannot be cleared up with treatment. The rationale for this extensive workup is that a UTI is not common in men and children and that a significant portion of infections in these populations, and in women with persistent infection, involves abnormality of the urinary tract.

Medications commonly used in the treatment of a UTI include urinary antiseptics such as sulfisoxazole (Gantrisin) or nitrofurantoin (Furadantin) and systemic antibiotics. Sulfonamides are widely used; they are usually effective against the organisms causing a large percentage of UTIs, are safe, and are less likely than most systemic antibiotics to contribute to growth of resistant organisms. Urinary antiseptics that contain analgesic properties (Trimethoprim and sulfamethoxazole [Bactrim]) may be prescribed for the patient when burning is a problem.

Additional treatment includes increasing fluid intake to 3 to 4 L/day unless contraindicated. Increased fluids dilute the urine, which lessens irritations and burning, and provide a continual flow of urine to discourage stasis and multiplication of bacteria in the urinary tract. Sitz baths may provide comfort for individuals with urethritis. Patient education concerning the problem, the requirements for drug therapy, and follow-up care should facilitate early identification of recurrence and completion of drug regimens for eradication of bacteria. Success in both of these areas is directly dependent on patient follow-through and comprises the means by which the patient is able to assist in overcoming this health problem.

PATHOPHYSIOLOGY

Most infections of the urinary tract result from gram-negative organisms, such as *Escherichia coli, Klebsiella, Proteus, Enterobacter,* or *Pseudomonas,* that originate in the person's own intestinal tract and ascend through the urethra to the bladder. During micturition, urine may flow back up the ureters (*vesicoureteral reflux)* and carry bacteria present in the bladder up through the ureters to the kidney pelvis. Whenever stasis of urine occurs, such as with incomplete emptying of the bladder, renal calculi, or genitourinary obstructions, the bacteria have a greater opportunity to grow and a more alkaline media, which favors their growth and multiplication.

A UTI will occur primarily when host resistance is impaired. The major factors in preventing a UTI are tissue integrity and blood supply.[9] A break in the surface of the mucous membrane lining permits the bacteria to invade the tissue and cause infection. Breaks in tissue integrity result from erosions caused by tips of indwelling catheters or rough-edged renal stones, from neoplasms, or from invasion of the tissue by parasites such as *Schistosoma.* In the bladder, blood supply to the tissues can be compromised when the pressure within the bladder is markedly increased, as may occur with overdistention of the bladder, contracture of the bladder neck, or obstruction of the urethra by an enlarged prostate, metastatic growth, or urethral stricture.

ASSESSMENT

Subjective data

The subjective data should include assessment of symptoms of urgency and burning on urination (dysuria). Chills and fever may also be present. Data on predisposing factors, such as use of bubble baths or contraceptive jellies and a history of previous infections, should be collected.

Objective data

A urine culture should be obtained since bacteriuria serves as the basis for diagnosis of a lower UTI.

DATA ANALYSIS AND PLANNING

Nursing diagnoses

Possible nursing diagnoses for the patient with UTI include the following:
Alteration in comfort: pain on urination
Alteration in patterns of urinary elimination

Expected patient outcomes

The person will:
1. Have relief of symptoms
2. Show no further damage in kidney function; current damage is arrested
3. Have sterile urine or bacterial urine count of less than 1×10^4 to 1×10^5
4. Have identified or corrected any disease or abnormality that would contribute to reinfection or relapse

The patient or significant other can state or explain the following:
1. Signs and symptoms of lower UTI
2. When and how to take prescribed medication
3. Plan for follow-up care including urine cultures
4. Rationale and means of increasing fluid intake to 3 to 4 L/day

IMPLEMENTATION

Medications

1. If antibiotics are ordered, they must be given on time on a regular schedule to ensure adequate blood levels.
2. If the patient is to undergo instrumentation, the nurse should reinforce instructions about the specific procedure. Knowledge about potential sensations during instrumentation may relax the patient along with deep breathing exercises during the procedure.

Assisting with comfort and ADL

Individuals with urethritis may experience pain or itching in the perineum. Sitz baths may provide relief of these symptoms.

Teaching

Patient education concerning the problem, the requirements for drug therapy, and follow-up care should facilitate completion of drug regimens for eradication of bacteria and early identification of recurrence of infection. Success in both of these areas is directly dependent on patient follow through and comprises the means by which the patient is able to assist in overcoming this health problem. Female patients should be instructed in good perineal hygiene.

EVALUATION

The nurse's success in dealing with the patient with a UTI can be evaluated, in part, by the eradication of infection in the individual.

Chemical induced nephritis

Chemical induced nephritis is an idiosyncratic reaction that results in damage to the tubules and interstitium of the kidneys. This disease process was first noted in patients who were sensitive to the sulfonamide drugs. Many other substances are now associated with chemical induced nephritis including the following;

Solvents
   Carbon tetrachloride
   Methanol
   Ethyline glycol
Heavy metals
   Lead
   Arsenic
   Mercury
Antibiotics
   Kanamycin
   Gentamicin
   Amphotericin B
   Calistin
   Neomycin
   Phenazopyridine
Pesticides
Poisonous mushrooms

Signs and symptoms of nephritis include the following:
Fever
Eosinophilia
Hematuria
Mild proteinuria
Rash

Oliguria or output of 400 ml or less of urine in a 24-hour period occurs in approximately 50% of all cases.

Medical therapy usually includes immediate withdrawal of the suspected chemical. Hemodialysis may be instituted to facilitate the removal of nephrotoxins from the blood. Steroids may be administered for their anti-inflammatory response. A sodium restricted diet may be necessary to maintain fluid balance.

PATHOPHYSIOLOGY

Chemical induced nephritis usually begins within 15 days of exposure to the chemical. The inflammatory process disrupts the ability of the glomeruli to filter. Furthermore, the capillary membrane is altered to the extent that it becomes permeable to plasma proteins and blood cells resulting in proteinuria and hematuria.

ASSESSMENT

Subjective data

The patient should be questioned as to possible sources of chemicals such as new drug therapy, exposure to industrial chemicals, pesticides, or wild mushrooms.

Objective data

Urinalysis should be completed to assess for presence of protein and/or blood cells. Serum toxicology screening may yield the source of nephritis. Intake and output should be carefully measured. Daily weights are essential. The patient should be assessed for fluid status, including edema, blood pressure changes, and adventitious breath sounds.

DATA ANALYSIS AND PLANNING

Nursing diagnosis

Nursing diagnoses may include the following:
Alteration in fluid volume: excess
Alteration in patterns of urinary elimination

Expected patient outcomes

1. The person or significant other can explain the following:
   a. Rationale for therapy (maintenance of fluid balance)
   b. Nutritional restrictions (low sodium diet)
2. Edema and blood pressure are controlled.

IMPLEMENTATION

See acute renal failure (p. 994).

Glomerulonephritis

ACUTE GLOMERULONEPHRITIS

Glomerulonephritis is a disease that affects the glomeruli of both kidneys. Etiologic factors are many and varied; they include immunologic reactions (lupus erythematosus, streptococcal infection), vascular injury (hypertension), metabolic disease (diabetes mellitus), and disseminated intravascular coagulation (DIC). Glomerulonephritis exists in acute, latent, and chronic forms. The most common form of *acute glomerulonephritis* occurs

2 to 3 weeks after a streptococcal infection. Common sites of infection include the throat (tonsillitis, strep throat) and the skin (impetigo).

Children of preschool and grade-school age are most likely to develop the illness. Of all individuals developing acute poststreptococcal glomerulonephritis, approximately 1% to 2% will develop end-stage renal failure in which dialysis or transplantation is required to prevent death. Approximately 90% of children and 50% of adults with acute glomerulonephritis attain full recovery from illness, although recovery may require up to 2 years.[7] Little can be inferred from the severity of the acute episode regarding prognosis. Persons with mild illness may develop chronic disease, and those with severe illness may completely recover and have no recurrence of the illness.

Prevention of acute poststreptococcal glomeruolonephritis involves prompt medical treatment of sore throats and upper respiratory tract infections. Cultures should be obtained, and when indicated appropriate antibiotics prescribed.

Common complaints are shortness of breath, mild headache, weakness, and anorexia. Usual signs include proteinuria, hematuria, increased urine specific gravity, dependent edema, and an elevated antistroptolysin O titer. Additionally, signs of elevation in blood pressure, decreased urinary output, and elevation in serum urea nitrogen and creatinine levels may be present. Signs and symptoms reflect damage to the glomeruli with leaking of protein and red cells into the urine, varying degrees of decreased glomerular filtration with retention of wastes, and fluid overloading of varying severity.

Control of infection

Persistent infection is treated promptly to help further decrease antigen-antibody complex formation. Persons with poststreptococcal glomerulonephritis are given a prophylactic antibiotic; the drug of choice is penicillin. Rationale for this therapy is based on preventing further infections that could reactivate the nephritis. Prophylactic therapy may be continued for months after the acute phase of illness. Exposure to any infection must be avoided, since even mild infections may reactivate nephritis.

Activity

Bed rest is instituted until clinical signs disappear; this may involve a period of several months. Ambulation is allowed when blood sedimentation rates and blood pressure are normal and edema abates. If ambulation causes an increase in proteinuria or hematuria, bed rest is reinstituted. Since the period of bed rest may be long and the person usually does not feel ill, the nurse may need to continue reinforcing the importance of bed rest and assist in planning diversionary activities and the constructive use of time. For small children this can present no small problem. When bed rest is reinstituted after periods of ambulation, the person may become depressed. Helping the person to express concerns and feelings can serve as a basis for helping make realistic plans about the illness and its sequelae.

Maintenance of fluid balance

Edema and fluid overloading are anticipated and treated initially with dietary sodium restrictions. The amount of restriction depends on the severity of fluid retention, and it is maintained until dependent edema and circulatory overload are no longer a problem. Diuretics are generally reserved for managing severe fluid overload and pulmonary edema. The nurse is constantly alert for signs of fluid overload. Blood pressure elevation is treated with antihypertensive drugs only after fluid control has proved unsuccessful in contolling hypertension. Dietary protein is reduced only when blood urea nitrogen and creatinine levels are elevated. The diet should contain sufficient carbohydrate to prevent protein being used for energy. This helps maintain nitrogen balance.

Long-term care

Up to 2 years may be required for resolution of the illness. During this time proteinuria, hematuria, and cellular debris may exist microscopically. The person generally shows little to no change from normal in renal function. At this point normal activities may be continued, although fatigue, trauma, and infection need to be avoided as they exacerbate the illness. Good general health measures are stressed. Since these persons usually feel well, they often must be convinced of the need to continue prescribed treatment and to return to routine follow-up health care. They should understand which signs and symptoms are significant and indicate a need for medical attention. They need to be encouraged to pursue care even though they were thoroughly examined only a short time before.

PATHOPHYSIOLOGY

Acute poststreptococcal glomerulonephritis is a result of an antigen-antibody reaction with glomerular tissue that produces swelling and death of capillary cells. The antigen-antibody reaction activates the complement pathway, resulting in chemotaxis of polymorphonuclear (PMN) leukocytes with release of lysosomal enzymes that attack the glomerular basement membrane (GBM). The response in the membrane is an increase in the three types of glomerular cells (endothelial, mesangial, and epithelial), causing an increase in membrane porosity with resultant proteinemia and hematuria. Renal function is depressed by scarring in the glomerulus, which causes oliguria and retention of water, sodium, and nitrogenous waste products, leading to edema and azotemia.

Chronic glomerulonephritis

Although chronic glomerulonephritis (CGN) may follow the acute disease, the majority of persons give no history of the disease. In most instances no evidence of predisposing infection can be found. The course of chronic glomerulonephritis is extremely varied. Some persons with minimal impairment in renal function continue to feel well and show little progression of disease. With other individuals the progression of renal deterioration may be slow but steady and end in renal failure. In still other individuals the progression of disease is rapid.

Various symptoms of failing renal function, none of which may seem severe, may lead the person to seek health care. There may be a slow onset of recurrent dependent edema, or there may be mild headache, especially in the morning. Dyspnea on exertion or difficulty sleeping in a flat position may be noted. Blurring of vision may lead the person to an ophthalmologist, who may be the first to suspect chronic renal disease based on ocular vascular changes. *Nocturia* is a common complaint. Occasionally, chronic nephritis is discovered during routine physical examination or may be discovered by a school nurse who observes marked visual changes and lassitude in a student. Weakness, fatigue, and weight loss are common but nonspecific symptoms of chronic glomerulonephritis. Early in the disease urinalysis shows the presence of albumin, casts, and blood. At this point renal function tests may be normal. The ability of the kidneys to regulate the internal environment will begin to decrease as more and more glomeruli become scarred and the amount of functional renal tissue is reduced. Finally, when few intact nephrons remain, hematuria and proteinuria decrease, the specific gravity of the urine becomes fixed, and the nonprotein nitrogen level in the blood increases.

No specific therapy exists to arrest or reverse the disease process. with some forms of CGN steroid therapy may be attempted, although results of this therapy in arresting disease are not well documented. Care involves teaching the person to live healthfully: to avoid infections, to eat a balanced diet with moderate sodium intake if prescribed, to appropriately administer medications, and to maintain follow-up health care visits and report to the physician any exacerbations in signs and symptoms. Treatment of renal failure begins when the illness destroys so much kidney tissue that the individual's kidneys are no longer able to independently control his or her internal environment.

With any exacerbation of hematuria, hypertension, and edema, the person is put to bed, and treatment similar to that for acute glomerulonephritis is instituted. Signs of pulmonary edema and congestive failure are monitored for when caring for these persons. Treatment is symptomatic and supportive.

Women with CGN who become pregnant appear to be susceptible to toxemia and to spontaneous abortion. The woman who has had nephritis of any nature should be urged to see a physician if she plans on pregnancy. When pregnancy does occur, she should remain under close health supervision.

PATHOPHYSIOLOGY

CGN is characterized by slow progressive destruction (sclerosis) of glomeruli and gradual loss of renal function. The glomeruli have varying degrees of hypercellularity and become sclerosed (hardened). The kidney decreases in size; eventually there is tubular atrophy, chronic interstitial inflammation, and arteriosclerosis (Fig. 33-8).[9]

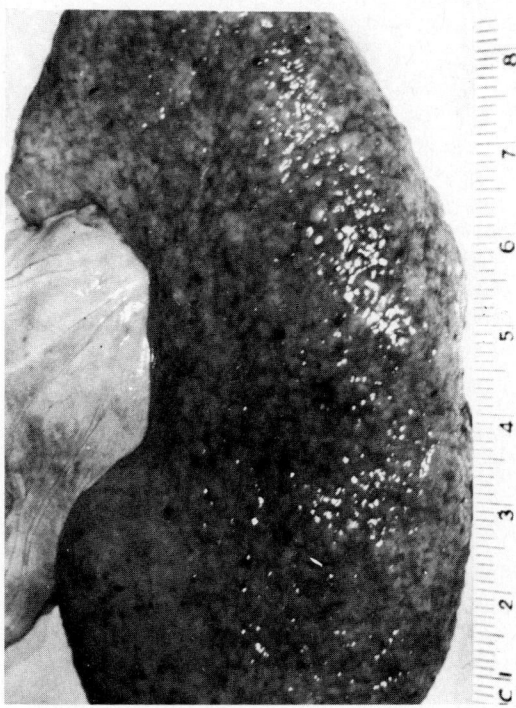

Fig. 33-8. End-stage chronic glomerulonephritis. Note pebbly surface corresponding to surviving hypertrophied nephrons amid atrophy. (From Anderson, A.W.D., and Kissane, J.M.: Pathology, ed. 7, St. Louis, 1977, The C.V. Mosby Co.)

ASSESSMENT

Subjective data

General questions to ask the patient would include (1) Have you experienced shortness of breath, headaches, weakness or anorexia? (2) Have you noticed a change in your pattern of urination, either frequency or volume? and (3) Do you recall a recent infection or symptoms of a virus?

Objective data

Objective data should include the following:
1. Frequent assessment of vital signs
2. Daily assessment for edema
3. Intake and output
4. Daily weights

Diagnostic tests

Urinalysis provides important data such as proteinuria, hematuria, and cell debris.

DATA ANALYSIS AND PLANNING

Nursing diagnosis

Possible nursing diagnoses include the following:
1. Alterations in nutrition: less than body requirements
2. Alterations in fluid volume: excess
3. Alterations in urinary elimination

Expected patient outcomes

The person or significant others can explain the following:

1. The rationale for therapy (prolongation of bed rest, maintenance of fluid blance)
2. Dietary changes (decreased sodium intake, adequate caloric intake, controlled protein intake if prescribed)
3. Medication program to be followed at home (prophylactic penicillin therapy)
4. Health maintenance program
   a. Measures to prevent further infection
   b. Signs that require immediate medical attention (hematuria, hypertension, edema, headaches)
   c. Plans for follow-up health care

IMPLEMENTATION

Assisting with achievement of therapeutic goals

1. Reinforce importance of bedrest during acute phase
2. Provide diversional activities for patient
3. Assist in maintaining adequate nutritional intake
4. Monitor signs of fluid and electrolyte balance

Teaching

A specific teaching plan should include the following:

1. Effects of diet and fluids on fluid and electrolyte balance
2. Explanation of medication regimen
3. Necessity of health follow-up must be stressed

EVALUATION

Evaluation is dependent on the specific nursing diagnoses relevant to the particular patient. Attention should be paid to evaluating the patients attainment of the outcome criteria.

Nephrotic syndrome

Nephrotic syndrome is not a single disease entity but is a constellation of symptoms. In nephrotic syndrome there is damage to the glomeruli and quantities of protein are lost in the urine. This condition has been associated with allergic reactions (insect bites, pollen, acute glomerulonephritis), infections (herpes zoster), systemic disease (diabetes mellitus, sickle cell disease), circulatory problems (severe congestive heart failure, chronic constrictive pericarditis), and pregnancy. Known glomerular disease is the most common precipitating event in adults; in children the syndrome appears frequently with no evidence of a causative factor. In approximately 25% of children and 50% to75% of adults who develop nephrosis the disease progresses to renal failure within 5 years.[2] In other individuals (particularly children) there may be remissions, or nephrosis may exist in a chronic form. Other than treating the underlying illess, little can be done to prevent a recurrence of nephrosis.

Clinical manifestations of the nephrotic syndrome include the following:

1. Severe generalized edema
2. Pronounced proteinuria
3. Hypoalbuminemia
4. Hyperlipidemia

Urine volumes and renal function may be either normal or markedly altered. Altered renal function and development of symptoms of renal failure occur as a result of progressing glomerulonephritis. Loss of appetite and fatigue are common. Women usually have amenorrhea or other disturbances in their reproductive cycle.

Treatment of nephrotic syndrome is directed toward reducing albuminuria, controlling edema, and promoting general health. Corticosteroids may be useful in controlling the illness, but the response to them will vary from remission of nephrosis to no response. Prednisone is the steroid preparation most frequently prescribed. The diet should contain normal to increased amounts of protein (1 g/kg body weight per day) and be high in calories. Periodic determination of proteinuria and measures of renal function enable the physician to monitor response to treatment and level of kidney function.

To control edema, sodium intake is reduced and diuretics are employed to increase excretion of fluid. When diuretics are administered over prolonged periods, hypokalemia usually results. Potassium may be supplemented through dietary intake; medication supplements should be initiated only after attempts to increase serum potassium through dietary means have failed. Bed rest is usually ordered when edema is severe; however, immobility is contraindicated for prolonged periods.

Persons with nephrosis need to direct particular attention toward preventing infection, since body defenses are impaired by urinary protein losses and edematous tissues are particularly susceptible to injury. When infection is suspected, it is important to give immediate attention to the problem. Culture and sensitivity studies are done and appropriate antibiotics are prescribed. The person is informed of the importance of prescribed medication and diet therapy and of the need for follow-up health care.

PATHOPHYSIOLOGY

The initial change in nephrotic syndrome is a derangement of cells in the glomerular basement membrane, resulting in increased membrane porosity with loss of large amounts of protein into the urine (proteinuria). As protein continues to be excreted, serum albumin is decreased (hypoalbuminemia), thus decreasing the serum osmotic pressure. The capillary hydrostatic fluid (push) pressure in all body tissues becomes greater than the capillary osmotic (pull) pressure, and generalized edema results (Fig. 33-9). As fluid is lost into the tissues, the plasma volume decreases, stimulating secretion of aldosterone to retain more sodium and water and decreasing the golmerular filtration rate to retain water. This additional fluid also passes out of the capillaries into the tissue, leading to even greater edema.

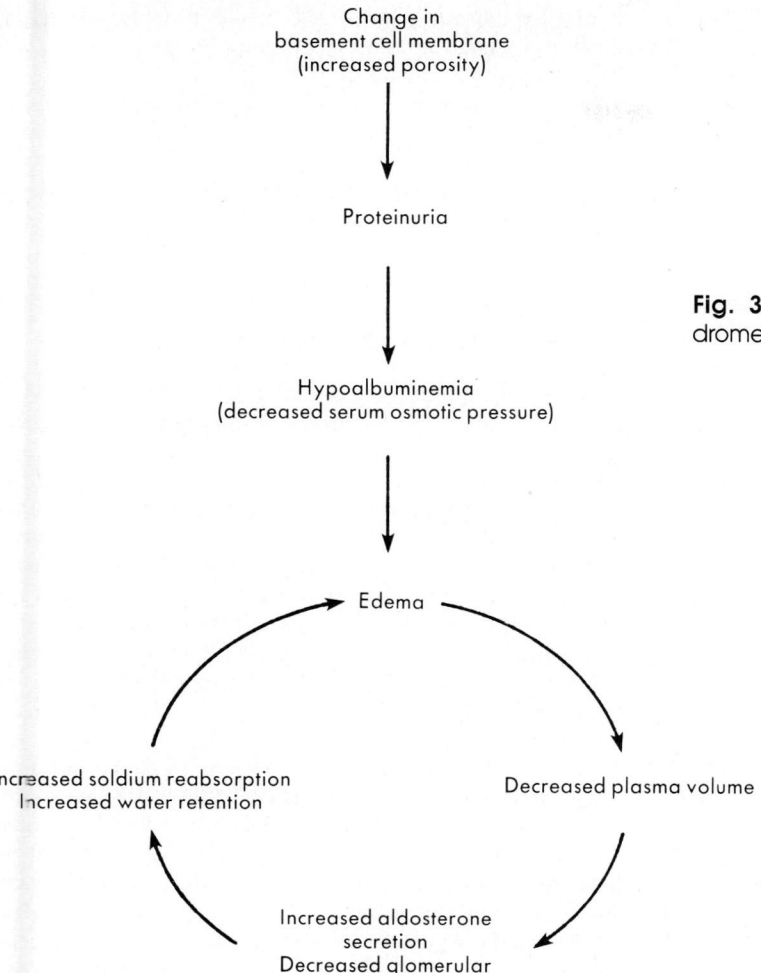

Change in
basement cell membrane
(increased porosity)

↓

Proteinuria

↓

Hypoalbuminemia
(decreased serum osmotic pressure)

↓

Edema

Increased soldium reabsorption
Increased water retention

Decreased plasma volume

Increased aldosterone
secretion
Decreased glomerular
filtration rate

Fig. 33-9. Pathophysiologic changes in nephrotic syndrome.

ASSESSMENT

Subjective data

The subjective data are the same as that collected on the patient with glomerulonephritis.

Objective data

Specific assessment should be directed to gather the following data;
1. Edema, amount and location should be recorded. Assessment of degree of pitting should be recorded. Record intake, output, weight, and abdominal girth daily
2. Condition of skin: severe edema may lead to skin breakdown
3. Respiratory status: pulmonary edema may develop
4. Signs and symptoms of infection

Diagnostic tests

Diagnosis is often made on the basis of clinical and laboratory findings. However, renal biopsy is sometimes used as a means of definitive diagnosis.

DATA ANALYSIS AND PLANNING

Nursing diagnoses

Possible nursing diagnoses include the following:
Alterations in comfort
Ineffective breathing pattern
Alteration in nutrition: less than body requirements
Impairment of skin integrity: potential
Alterations in patterns of urinary elimination
Alteration in fluid volume: excess
Outcome criteria for the person with nephrotic syndrome
1. Independence in ADL is maintained.
2. The person remains free of infection.
3. Edema and blood pressure are controlled; pulmonary edema and congestive heart failure do not occur.

The person or significant others can describe or state the following;
1. Measures to prevent infection
2. Name, dosage, frequency, and side effects of prescribed mediations (steroids, diuretics)
3. Dietary prescription (increased calories, adequate

protein, decreased sodium) and plan appropriate meals

4. Signs and symptoms requiring immediate attention (increase in edema, fatigue, headache, presence of infection)
5. Plans for follow-up health care

IMPLEMENTATION

Assisting with achievement of therapeutic goals

The nephrotic syndrome is usually complicated by periods of marked edema. During this time meticulous skin care is essential to prevent breakdown. Close monitoring of oral and parenteral fluid is necessary.

Steroids are often administered. Nursing assessment must include observing for side effects. Diuretics are usually required. The nurse should assess the patient's response and observe for over diuresis.

Usually a sodium and protein restricted diet is prescribed. This often results in a diet that is not appetizing to the patient. Appetite may also be diminished as a result of fluid overload. This all results in the potential for inadequate nutrition.

Assisting with comfort and ADL

The patient may tire easily and therefore require assistance with ADL. The patient should be encouraged to be independent but should not be allowed to overdo.

As edema increases, the patient becomes increasingly uncomfortable. Careful positioning and frequent changes in position may increase comfort while also protecting the skin. Males may develop edema in the scrotum, which can be particularly uncomfortable. A sling to support the scrotum will not only provide comfort but will also aid in reducing swelling.

Teaching

As the patient begins to convalesce the teaching plan should include the following:
1. Medication teaching
2. Nutrition teaching
3. Self assessment of fluid status including edema and weight gain

Pyelonephritis

Pyelonephritis refers to bacterial infection of kidney tissue. This infection usually begins in the lower urinary tract and ascends into the kidneys. A lower UTI may be asymptomatic, and kidney involvement may be the first indication of infection in the lower tract. Often the diagnostic workup of a person with pyelonpehritis reveals previously unknown urinary tract obstruction or the presence of other chronic kidney disease. *Escherichia coli* is the most common organism identified in pyelonephritis, and resistance to antibiotic therapy rarely results. Pyelonephritis is most commonly associated with (1) pregnancy; (2) obstruction, instrumentation, or trauma of the urinary tract; and (3) chronic health problems including diabetes, analgesic abuse, polycystic kidney disease, and hypertensive kidney disease.

The most significant efforts in preventing pyelonephritis are through early detection and adequate treatment of UTI.

Signs and symptoms of pyelonephritis include those associated with lower UTI as well as the following:
1. Fever
2. Chills
3. Malaise
4. Costovertebral tenderness
5. Leukocytosis

Signs and symptoms of renal failure may be present when nephron damage is extensive. Examination of the urine reveals white blood cells, white blood cell casts, and bacteria.

Optimal treatment includes early detection of the illness, antibacterial therapy based on urine cultures, and correction and treatment of any underlying systemic disease or urinary tract abnormality. Anyone with symptoms of dysuria, cloudy urine, or frequent small voidings should be examined for UTI and appropriately treated. Persons complaining of fever and costovertebral tenderness should be encouraged to seek medical attention.

The course of antibiotic therapy may extend over weeks, and the person may need to be reminded of the necessity to continue taking medication even when symptoms disappear and he or she begins to feel better. Continuing drug therapy to eradicate all infection and prevent development of resistant strains of organisms is stressed. The urine is recultured 2 weeks after drug therapy has been discontinued and every month thereafter for the next several months. Increasing fluid intake to 3 L/day in persons capable of excreting this amount of fluid is desirable to prevent stasis of urine and further bacterial growth. Should infection become chronic, drug therapy may continue indefinitely; the goal is to reduce and control the bacterial population of the urinary tract so that renal damage is prevented. Urine cultures should be repeated periodically, and the person should be instructed in the signs and symptoms indicating reactivation of infection and the need for medical attention.

PATHOPHYSIOLOGY

Infection of the kidneys occurs in both acute and chronic forms. Although acute pyelonephritis may temporarily affect renal function, rarely does this progress to a level of renal failure. Chronic pyelonephritis destroys renal tissue permanently through repeated inflammation and scarring. The process of developing chronic renal failure from repeated kidney infections occurs over a number of years or after several extensive and fulminant infections. It is estimated that pyelonephritis represents the original diagnosis in one third of all persons with chronic renal disease.

ASSESSMENT

Subjective data

1. Fever, chills
2. Nausea or vomiting
3. Flank pain
4. Frequency or urgency
5. Fatigue
6. Anorexia

Objective data

1. Assess quality of urine: urine becomes cloudy and concentrated
2. Assess temperature every 6 hours
3. Assess for tenderness over kidneys on palpation

Diagnostic tests

1. IVP
2. Cystoscopy
3. Urine cultures
4. Renal biopsy

DATA ANALYSIS AND PLANNING

Nursing diagnoses

Possible nursing diagnoses include the following:
Alteration in nutrition: less than body requirements
Alteration in fluid volume: excess
Alteration in pattern of urinary elimination

Expected patient outcomes

The person or significant others can state or explain the following:

1. Name, dosage, frequency, and side effects of antibiotic therapy
2. Rationale for continued antibiotic therapy even when symptoms are no longer present
3. Rationale and method for increasing fluid intake
4. Signs and symptoms of kidney infection and need to seek health care when symptoms recur
5. Plan for follow-up urine cultures and health care

IMPLEMENTATION

Assisting with achievement of therapeutic goals

1. Assess patient's temperature every 6 hours and report elevation to physician.
2. Promote rest during the acute phase.
3. Encourage an adequate diet within the prescribed restrictions.
4. Encourage fluid intake unless course of disease is complicated by renal failure.
5. Assess intake and output every 8 hours.
6. Assess for fluid overload by monitoring edema, daily weight, and blood pressure.
7. Assess for signs and symptoms of electrolyte imbalance, including:
   a. Changes in mentation
   b. Thirst
   c. Edema
   d. Heart rate and rhythm
8. Assess quality of urine including hematuria.
9. Administer antibiotic therapy as prescribed.

Assisting with comfort and ADL

1. Encourage rest during acute phase.
2. Assist with ADL as necessary and according to abilities of the individual patient.
3. Medicate, as prescribed, for flank pain. Back massages often provide short-term relief of discomfort.

Teaching

1. Instruct patient about need for continued antibiotic therapy after symptoms reside.
2. Instruct patient about monitoring urinary output.
3. Instruct patient about monitoring daily weight.
4. Instruct patient about need for on-going medical follow-up.

VASCULAR DISORDERS

Renal disease as a result of vascular disorders result from one of two processes. The first of these is disease of the main renal arteries or *renal artery stenosis*. The second disease process is sclerosis of renal arterioles or *nephrosclerosis*.

Renal artery stenosis

Renal artery stenosis is the cause of approximately 5% of all causes of hypertension.[11] Stenosis of the renal arteries is usually classified as either arteriosclerosis or fibromuscular dysplasia. In either case, the end result is a narrowing of the lumen of the arteries supplying the kidneys. Obstruction of the renal arteries can also be caused by aneurysms, thromboses, and emboli.

The signs of renal artery stensosis follow.

1. Hypertension
2. Disparity in size of kidneys
3. Delayed appearance of contrast medium in renal arteriograph
4. Hyperconcentration of contrast media in calyceal system on IVP
5. Lesion evidenced on renal arteriograph

Medical treatment will include vigorous antihypertensive therapy to control blood pressure. Prolonged hypertension will ultimately result in further renal involvement. When a well defined lesion exists in the renal artery, vascular surgery may be performed to remove the affected area.

PATHOPHYSIOLOGY

Renal stenosis results in a major reduction in circulation to the kidneys.[25] This change in renal perfusion results in increased secretion of renin and activation of the renin-angiotensin-aldosterone system. The end result is acceleration of hypertension, which if untreated leads to further pathologic changes in the kidneys.

Nephrosclerosis

Whereas renal artery stenosis results in hypertension, hypertension can cause nephrosclerosis. Hypertension is a major precipitating factor of renal disease. It is estimated that approximately 10% of individuals with essential hypertension develop severe renal damage, and approximately 1% will develop end-stage renal disease and die unless supportive care is provided.[14]

Preventive care includes greater screening efforts to detect persons with elevated blood pressure; adequate treatment and follow-up for those with hypertension; and education regarding the nature of the illness, the diet and medications, and the importance of periodic follow-up health care. Yearly blood pressure monitoring of persons with elevated blood pressure is a minimal preventive care measure.

By the time signs and symptoms indicating kidney involvement develop, the disease has progressed to an extreme point. Deterioration in renal function progresses gradually unless an acute or malignant phase of hypertension occurs to accelerate the process. Signs and symptoms are those of chronic renal failure.

Treatment of nephrosclerosis is directed toward early detection and treatment of hypertension. Causative factors are sought, and treatment to lower blood pressure is begun. When significant renal damage exists, stabilizing the person's current level of function or slowing deterioration of kidney tissue is the goal. Control of hypertension is continued, and management of end-stage disease and uremic symptoms provides for comfort and increased independence in daily living, although renal function may not improve.

PATHOPHYSIOLOGY

Peripheral vasculature is subject to adverse changes when subjected to hypertension. The kidney and brain circulation are most frequently affected.

Regardless of origin of hypertension (essential or renal), hypertension that is untreated over a period of time leads to the sclerosing of renal arterioles. The blood supply to glomeruli, tubules, and interstitium gradually decreases. Scarring and death of kidney tissue occur, and signs of renal insufficiency develop when damage to the kidneys has become extensive. *Nephrosclerosis* is the term given to this destructive process.

Diabetic nephropathy

Persons with diabetes develop vascular changes at a more accelerated rate than non-diabetic persons. These changes, which are a normal part of the aging process, result in chronic renal failure. This process of accelerated vascular change is most evident in patients with

Type I diabetes, which develops in childhood. In controlling the carbohydrate intake of the patient with diabetes, abnormal metabolism of fat occurs, resulting in elevated serum cholesterol levels. Immunofluorescent and electron microscopic studies of the renal vasculature suggests that large quantities of lipids leak into these blood vessels and precipitate on the vessel walls. The vascular changes caused by diabetes result in two distinct processes: glomerulosclerosis and nephrosclerosis. As described earlier, nephrosclerosis develops from sclerosing of the renal arterioles.[3] Glomerulosclerosis is the scarring of the capillary loops in the glomerulus. Pathologic changes occur in the basement membranes of the kidneys. The first indications of renal involvement in the patient with diabetes is proteinuria.

Assessment and implementation for vascular disorders

The nursing assessment and implementation for patients with renal involvement as a result of vascular disorders is the same as those outlined for chronic renal failure.

OBSTRUCTIVE DISORDERS

Urinary tract obstruction can occur in any portion of the urinary tract from the urinary calyces to the meatus.

Obstuction of any part of the urinary system from the kidney to the urethra will generate pressure that may cause functional and anatomic damage to the renal parenchyma. When any part of the urinary tract is obstructed, urine collects behind the obstruction producing a dilation of the structure. Muscles of the affected areas contract in an effort to push the urine around the obstruction. Partial obstruction may produce slow dilation of structures above the obstruction without functional impairment. As the obstruction increases, however, pressure builds up in the tubular system behind the obstruction causing a backflow or urine and dialtion of ureter (*hydoureter*). The urine backup eventually reaches the kidney causing dilation of the kidney pelvis (hydronephrosis). Pressure buildup in the renal pelvis leads to destruction of kidney tissue and eventual renal failure.

With obstruction urine flow is decreased even to the point of stagnation. This stagnant urine provides a good culture medium for bacterial growth, and rarely is obstruction seen without some infection. The specific effects that occur with obstruction depend on the location of the obstruction, the extent of obstruction (partial or complete), and the duration. Obstruction in the *lower* urinary tract causes bladder distension. If this is prolonged, muscle fibers become hypertrophied and *diverticuli* (herniated sacs of bladder mucosa) develop between the hypertrophied muscle bands. Since the diverticulum holds stagnant urine, infection often occurs, and bladder stones may form.

Obstruction of the *upper* urinary tract leads even more

quickly to hydronephrosis because of the small size of the ureters and kidney pelvis. Increased pressure causes partial ischemia of arteries between the renal cortex and medulla and dilation of the renal tubules leading to tubular damage. Stasis of urine in the dilated pelvis predisposes to infection and calculi, which add to the renal damage. Some urine can flow back up the renal tubule into the veins and lymphatics as a compensatory mechanism to prevent kidney damage. The unaffected kidney then takes on increased elimination of waste products. With prolonged obstruction the unaffected kidney hypertrophies and may function as effectively alone as both kidneys did before the obstruction. Obstruction of both kidneys leads to renal failure.

Hydronephrosis can occur without any symptoms as long as kidney function is adequate and urine can drain. An acute upper urinary tract obstruction will cause pain, nausea, vomiting, local tenderness, spasm of the abdominal muscles, and a mass in the kidney region. The pain is caused by the stretching of the tissues and by hyperperistalsis. Since the amount of pain is proportionate to the rate of stretching, a slowly developing hydronephrosis may cause only a dull flank pain, whereas a sudden blockage of the ureter such as may occur from a stone causes a severe stabbing (colicky) pain in the flank or abdomen. The pain may radiate to the genitalia and thigh and is caused by the increased peristaltic action of the smooth muscle of the ureter in an effort to dislodge the obstruction and force urine past it.

The nausea and vomiting frequently associated with acute ureteral obstruction are caused by a reflex reaction to the pain and will usually be relieved as soon as pain is relieved. A markedly dilated kidney, however, may press on the stomach causing continued GI symptoms. If the renal function has been seriously impaired, nausea and vomiting may be symptoms of impending uremia.

When the bladder is distended from lower urinary tract obstruction, the person will experience lower abdominal discomfort and a feeling of the need to void although voiding may not be possible. The bladder may be palpated above the symphysis pubis. With partial obstruction such as by benign prostatic hypertrophy the man first complains of increasing urinary frequency because the bladder fails to empty completely at each voiding and therefore refills more quickly to the amount that causes the urge to void (usually 250 to 500 ml), Nocturia may also be present.

When obstruction occurs the treatment consists of reestablishing adequate drainage from the urinary system. This may be temporarily accomplished by placing a catheter above the point of obstruction. Sometimes surgery must be performed to insert a catheter (nephrostomy, ureterostomy, suprapubic cystostomy). Later, definitive treatment is dependent on the cause. The infection is treated with antibiotics, fluids, and rest. Urinary antiseptics may also be given.

Causes of obstruction of the urinary tract are summarized in the box above.

Common causes of urinary tract obstruction

Lower urinary tract
  Bladder neoplasms
  Urethral strictures
  Calculi
  Tumors
  Benign prostatic hypertrophy (BPH)
Ureteral obstructions
  Calculi
  Trauma
  Nephroptosis ("floating" or "dropped" kidney)
  Enlarged lymph nodes
    Lymphosarcoma
    Reticulum cell sarcoma
    Hodgkin's disease
  Congenital anomaly
Kidney tubule or pelvis
  Calculi
  Ptosis
  Polycystic disease

The person with a sudden obstruction is usually acutely ill and may have severe colic but will not be able to remain in bed until the pain has been relieved. It is not unusual to see a person with acute renal colic walking the floor doubled up and vomiting. Narcotics such as morphine and meperidine and antispasmodic drugs such as propantheline bromide (Pro-Banthine) and belladonna preparations are usually necessary to relieve severe colicky pain. After narcotics have been given, the patient will be dizzy and must be protected from injury. As the pain eases, the patient can usually be made relatively comfortable in bed. As soon as the nausea subsides large amounts of fluids are urged.

Renal calculi

Urinary stones (*urolithiasis*) may develop at any level in the urinary system but are most commonly found within the kidney (*neprolithiasis*). Fig 33-10 illustrates the most common locations of calculi formation. At least 1% of the people in the United States will develop urolithiasis. About one-third of the individuals that have recurrent upper urinary tract calculi will eventually have the affected kidney removed.

Renal calculi (stones) are crystallizations of minerals around an organic matrix such as pus, blood, devitalized tissue or tumors. The mineral composition of renal calculi varies. About three fourths of the stones are calcium and oxalates; other stones are calcium phosphate, uric acid, and cystine.

No demonstrable cause can be found for over half of

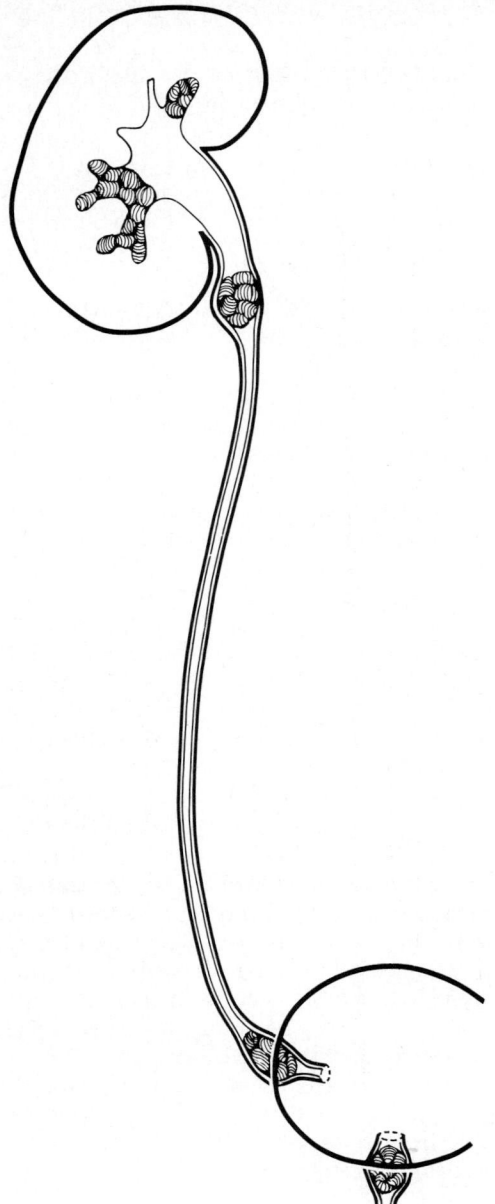

Fig. 33-10. Most common locations of renal calculus formation.

Renal calculus composition and contributing factors

Composition of stone	Factors contributing to stone formation
Calcium (oxalate and phosphate)	Hypercalcemia and/or hypercalciuria resulting from Hyperparathyroidism Vitamin D intoxication Multiple myeloma Immobilization Severe bone disease Renal tubular acidosis Prolonged intake of steroids
Uric acid	High purine diet Gout
Cystine	Cystinuria resulting from genetic disorder of amino acid metabolism

Table 33-3. Acid and alkaline ash food groups

Acid ash	Alkaline ash	Neutral
Meat	Milk	Sugars
Whole grains	Vegetables	Fats
Egg	Fruit (except	Beverages
Cheese	cranber-	(coffee,
Cranberries	ries,	tea)
Prunes	prunes,	
Plums	plums)	

From Williams, S.R.: Nutrition and diet therapy, ed. 4, St. Louis, 1982, The C.V. Mosby Co.

---

the renal stones that occur (idiopathic). A major predisposing factor is the presence of a UTI. Infection increases the presence of organic matter around which the minerals can precipitate and increases the alkalinity of the urine (by the production of ammonia), resulting in precipitation of calcium phosphate and magnesium ammonium phosphate. Stasis of urine also permits precipitation of organic matter and minerals.

Measures can be taken to decrease the potential for renal stones in persons at high risk. Adequate hydration (intake of 2500 ml/day or more unless contraindicated) will help to prevent urinary stasis that can lead not only to stone formation but also to a UTI. Persons restricted

to bed should be encouraged to turn and move frequently, exercising their arms if the legs are immobilized. Changing the body position of a bedfast patient by means of a CircOlectric bed or tilt table or by sitting up in a wheelchair (if permitted) can help to prevent urinary stasis. Even with exercises and the use of a wheelchair, however, paraplegics and quadriplegics often develop renal calculi. *Persons with indwelling catheters need scrupulous aseptic technique in catheter care to prevent infection and require adequate hydration and good catheter drainage to wash away minerals that can be deposited at the tip of the catheter.*

Persons at risk for developing calcium oxalate or phosphate or magnesium ammonium phosphate stones may be placed on an acid ash diet (Table 33-3) to promote excretion of an acid urine. Catheter irrigations using acetic acid solution or Renacidin help provide an acid environment and thus decrease precipitation of calcium and phosphates.

Pain (renal colic) is the primary symptom in an acute episode of renal calculi. The location of the pain depends on the location of the stone. If the stone is in the pelvis of the kidney, the pain is caused by hydronephrosis and is more dull and constant in character, occurring primarily in the costovertebral angle. As the stone moves along the ureter the pain can be excruciating and is intermittent in character. It is caused by spasm of the ureter and anoxia of the wall of the ureter from the pressure of the stone. Pain follows the anterior course of the ureter down to the suprapubic area and radiates to the external genitalia. Nausea and vomiting often accompany renal colic.

Gross hematuria may occur if the stone has rough edges, and microhematuria usually is present. Signs of UTI may also be present. Often a stone is "silent," causing no symptoms for years. This is especially true of very large renal stones. Extremely small smooth stones may be passed without the person's awareness.

Diagnostic tests are performed to determine the presence of one or more stones. Calcium stones are radiopaque, but uric acid stones usually cannot be visualized in radiographic studies. IVP may demonstrate dilation of the ureter above an obstructing stone. Very small stones may be washed away during the radiographic studies. Urinalysis will show the presence of red blood cells and sometimes the minerals involved in stone formation.

Because recurrence of renal calculi is common, additional studies are carried out after the acute episode has subsided. Successive determinations of serum calcium, phosphorus protein, electrolytes, and uric acid are performed to determine presence of underlying disease that can influence stone formation. The urinary pH should be measured with pH paper each time the person voids to ascertain the acidity or alkalinity. A nitroprusside urine test may be performed to check the presence of cystine. An accurate 24-hour urine collection is made to measure calcium, oxalate, phosphorus, and uric acid levels. The 24-hour urine collection may be made with the patient eating a normal diet or following a 3-day low-calcium, low-phosphorus diet.

ACUTE CARE

About 90% of urinary calculi are passed spontaneously. Therefore the urine of all patients with relatively small stones should be strained. Urine can be strained easily by placing two opened 4-inch × 8-inch gauze sponges over a funnel. The urine from each voiding is strained, and one needs to watch closely for the stone because it may be no bigger than the head of a pin and the patient may not realize that it has been passed.

Stones smaller than 5 mm have a good chance of being passed. If there is no infection or obstruction, the stone may be left in the ureter for several months. The person is observed closely but permitted to carry out usual activities. A person who is up and about is more likely to pass a stone than one who is in bed. Fluids should be taken freely (2500 ml/day or more) to promote passage of the stone and prevent infection.

Patients frequently have two or three attacks of acute renal colic before the stone passes. This is probably because the stone gets lodged at a narrow point in the ureter causing temporary obstruction. The ureters are normally narrower at the ureteropelvic and ureterovesical junctions and at the point where they pass over the iliac crest into the pelvis. If the stone is to pass along the ureter by peristaltic action, the patient will have some pain. The patient is involved in determining when pain medication is needed.

If the stone fails to pass, one or two ureteral catheters may be passed through a cystoscope up the ureter and left in place for 24 hours. The catheters dilate the ureter, and when they are removed the stone may pass into the bladder.

If there are signs of infection, an attempt is made to pass a ureteral catheter past the stone into the renal pelvis. If such an attempt is successful, the catheter is left as a drain. since pyelonephritis will quickly follow if adequate urinary drainage is not reestablished. When there is a catheter in each ureter, each catheter is labeled and should drain into a separate drainage bag. The catheters must be checked frequently to see that they are draining. Patients with ureteral catheters are usually confined to bed to prevent possible dislodgement of the catheters.

If the stone has passed to the lower third of the ureter, it can sometimes be removed by manipulation. Special catheters with corkscrew tips, expanding baskets, and loops are passed through the cystoscope, and an attempt is made to "snare" the stone. This procedure is performed with the patient under anesthesia. The aftercare of a patient on whom manipulation has been carried out is the same as that following cystoscopy. Any signs suggestive of peritonitis or a decreased urinary output are carefully watched for, since the ureter occasionally is perforated during manipulation.

Before discussing in detail the particular types of surgery used in the treatment of renal calculi, general principles of care of the patient requiring urologic surgery will be described.

PREOPERATIVE CARE

The focus of preoperative care is to prepare the patient for the impending surgery through instructions and to carry out the medical regimen including medications, shaving of the operative site, and preparation of the skin. Much of the patient's concern depends on the type of surgery and diagnosis. Since the surgery will temporarily or permanently alter urinary elimination, the person will be concerned about the degree of change that will be present.

Preoperative instructions include a discussion of the type and length of surgery, type of anesthesia, and the need for an intravenous line, catheter, or other drains. Instructions in coughing and deep breathing are crucial since adequate ventilation is a frequent problem postoperatively. The patient is informed of the pain medication routine—whether or not it will be offered or if it must be requested. A description of methods of decreasing pain, such as by splinting the incision, should be offered. The patient is assessed for understanding and acceptance of the surgery at the beginning and conclusion of instruction.

The evening before surgery the person may receive a shave, skin preparation, and/or a medicated shower, depending on the type of surgery. The woman patient may also receive a medicated douche to cleanse the perineal area. The person is given nothing by mouth after midnight. Persons having a urinary diversion will also require bowel preparation.

POSTOPERATIVE CARE

The basic needs of the patient requiring urologic surgery are the same as those of any other surgical patient. Special emphasis is placed on promotion of ventilation and adequate urinary output, prevention of distention and hemorrhage, and attention to drainage tubes and dressing.

Ventilation

Surgery of the kidney or upper ureters usually involves a flank incision that can influence respiratory status. Because the incision is directly below the diaphragm, deep breathing is painful and the patient is reluctant to take deep breaths or to move about. Splinting of the chest is common, and therefore atelectasis or other respiratory complications must be guarded against. In addiditon, because of the placement of the incision there is a greater incisional pull every time the person moves, as compared with an abdominal incision. The patient is often reluctant to turn in bed or to get up to ambulate. Most patients will be more comfortable turning themselves if they are given time, side rails to hold onto, and encouragement. Incisional pain usually requires a narcotic every 3 to 4 hours for 24 to 48 hours after surgery, and turning, ambulation, and deep breathing exercises can be planned so that these activities occur at the time the analgesic has the greatest effect. Patients may lie on the affected side unless a nephrostomy tube is in place. Even then they can be tilted to the affected side with pillows placed at the back for support. It must be ascertained that the tube is not kinked and that there is no traction on it.

Urinary output

The urinary output is monitored carefully for several days postoperatively to ascertain adequate renal functioning and drainage. The output should be at least 50 ml/hour, preferably greater, to prevent urinary stasis and subsequent infection. A urinary output of 20 to 30 ml/hour in a patient with satisfactory fluid intake (at least 1200 ml/day) and in the absence of signs of urinary retention is reported immediately to the physician. Urinary output includes drainage from nephrostomy or cystostomy tubes, urethral or ureteral catheters, and an estimate from urine-soaked dressings. Daily weights are compared with the preoperative weight and with each other to identify fluid retention.

Distention

Following kidney surgery most patients have some abdominal distention that may result in part from pressure on the stomach and intestinal tract during surgery. Patients who have had renal colic before surgery frequently develop paralytic ileus postoperatively. This condition may be related to the reflex GI tract symptoms caused by postoperative pain. Because of the problem of abdominal distention following renal surgery, food and fluids by mouth are often restricted for 24 to 48 hours postoperatively. By the fourth postoperative day most patients tolerate a regular diet. Fluids are then usually forced to 3000 ml/day.

Hemorrhage

Hemorrhage may follow such operative procedures as prostatectomy, nephrolithotomy, or nephrectomy. It occurs most often when the highly vascular parenchyma of the kidney has been incised. The bleeding may occur on the day of surgery, or it may occur 8 to 12 days postoperatively, during the period when tissue sloughing normally occurs with healing. The presence of bright red blood on the dressing or in the urine is reported immediately to the physician. The patient is observed for signs of shock. Since many patients with urologic disease have hypertension, the blood pressure may be relatively high but still represent a marked drop for the individual. Comparisons should therefore be made with baseline data.

If hemorrhage occurs, a pressure dressing is applied over the incision while awaiting the physician's arrival. Measures to prevent shock are instituted. Several liters of sterile physiologic saline solution for irrigation should be available.

Dressings

There may be large amounts of urinary drainage following urologic surgery except after nephrectomy. The drainage may be pink or dark red but should not be bright red. If the surgery involves a flank incision, drainage is usually the heaviest on the posterior edge of the dressing because of gravity flow. It is important therefore to turn the patient on the side opposite the surgery to examine the posterior edge of the dressing. When a suprapubic incision is present, drainage is heaviest on the side and in the inguinal region.

The dressings are usually held in place by Montgomery straps and must be changed frequently. Urinary drainage irritates the skin, has an unpleasant odor, and leads to discomfort. If a drain is present, the end of the drain should be placed over dressings, then covered with additional dressings to absorb the drainage. If a drainage tube is present, presence of large amounts of drainage on the dressing with little drainage coming from the tube indicates blockage of the tube. If a large amount of drainage is present, a disposable drainage bag used for urinary stomas may be applied over the drainage site.

Drainage tubes

A catheter is usually inserted during surgery to drain urine from the operative area and permit healing to occur. Different types of drainage tubes may be inserted, and each tube is connected to a separate drainage system. It is important to know the purpose of the catheter and the area to be drained.

Outcome criteria

The person will maintain the following:
1. Adequate urinary drainage
2. Clear breath sounds and normal respiratory rate and depth
3. Good skin integrity surrounding the surgical incision

The person or significant others can describe the following:
1. Maintenance of drainage and sterility of any indwelling drainage tube on discharge from the hospital
2. Plans for follow-up care

Removal of stones (calculi) blocking a ureter is termed *ureterolithotomy*. The root word "lith" refers to stones. Obstruction at the ureteropelvic junction is corrected by means of a *pyeloplasty* (plastic repair of the renal pelvis).

The bladder may be incised (cystotomy) for removal of calculi or as part of one method of prostate removal (suprapubic prostatectomy). A cystostomy (note the "s" in the middle of the word) is an opening made in the bladder for drainage, usually by means of a tube.

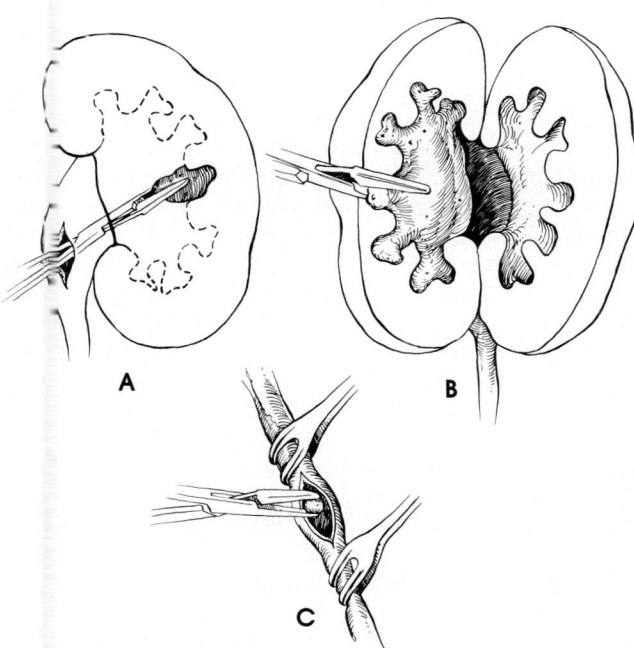

Fig. 33-11. Location and methods of removing renal calculi from upper urinary tract. **A,** Pyelolithotomy, removal of stone through renal pelvis. **B,** Nephrolithotomy, removal of staghorn calculus from renal parenchyma (kidney split). **C,** Ureterolithotomy, removal of stone from ureter.

SURGICAL INTERVENTIONS FOR RENAL CALCULI

Surgical intervention is indicated when a large stone (greater than 1 cm) is producing pain, obstruction, or infection. The operation for removal of a stone from the ureter is a ureterolithotomy (Fig. 33-11, C). A radiograph is taken immediately preceding surgery, since the stone may have moved, and it is desirable to make the incision into the ureter directly over the stone. If the stone is in the lower third of the ureter, a rectus incision is made. If it is in the upper two thirds, a flank approach is used. If the patient has a ureteral stricture that causes stones to form, a plastic operation to relieve the stricture may be carried out as part of the operation.

Removal of a stone through or from the renal pelvis is known as a pyelolithotomy (Fig. 33-11, A). Removal of a stone through the parenchyma is a *nephrolithotomy* (Fig. 33-11, B). Occasionally, the kidney may have to be split from end to end (a kidney split) to remove the stone. Patients in whom such a split is done may have severe hemorrhage following surgery.

Bladder stones may be removed through a suprapubic incision, or they may be crushed with lithotrite (stone crusher) that is passed transurethrally. This procedure is known as a *litholapaxy*. Following bladder stone removal, the bladder may be irrigated (intermittently or constantly) with an acid solution such as magnesium and sodium citrate (G solution) or Renacidin to counteract the alkalinity caused by the infection and to help wash out the remaining particles of stone. If there has been a suprapubic incision, the care of the incision is similar to that following a suprapubic prostatectomy. (See p. 977 for care of the patient requiring urologic surgery.)

Removal of a kidney (*nephrectomy*) may be indicated for some congenital anomalies or for irreparable damage to kidney tissue from trauma or diseases such as renal hypertension, tumor, multiple cysts, or kidney stones. Adequate waste removal can be maintained by the remaining kidney or by even less than half of one healthy kidney. In some instances only a portion of a diseased kidney is removed (*partial nephrectomy*). If an entire kidney is removed, a drain may be placed to remove serous fluid from the space previously occupied by the kidney. In this situation there will be no urinary drainage. Urinary drainage will occur with a partial nephrectomy.

Long-term care

Persons who have recurrent renal calculi benefit from ongoing prophylactic therapy, which is determined by the type of stone being produced. *All* persons with recurrent renal stones should drink fluids in sufficient quantity to produce very dilute urine and nocturia. This may amount to a daily intake of up to 4 to 5 L of fluid.[23] The purpose of the increased fluid intake is to rinse away any precipitates that can serve as a nidus for stone formation.

Any underlying identifiable cause of calciuria is treated to prevent recurrence of calcium stones. Hydrochlorothiazide (HCTZ) in doses of 50 mg twice a day may be prescribed for persons with hypercalciuria to decrease urinary excretion of calcium. Persons receiving HCTZ therapy must be monitored carefully for signs of electrolyte imbalances especially hypokalemia.

As previously stated, more than 50% of calcium stones are idiopathic. Foods high in calcium are sometimes restricted, but a very low-calcium diet is usually unsatisfactory because it is unpalatable. The solubility of oxalate salts is not pH dependent; therefore manipulation of pH is not useful. Sodium or potassium phosphate, 1.5 to 2.0 g/day, may be prescribed to decrease urinary calcium.

Phosphatic calculi develop in alkaline urine; thus their prevention depends on keeping the urine acid and preventing a UTI. Medications such as ascorbic acid or ammonium chloride may be given for a time to increase urine acidity.

The Shorr regimen has given beneficial results in the prevention of phosphatic calculi. A diet containing only 1300 mg of phosphorus daily is prescribed, and 40 ml of aluminum hydroxide gel is taken after meals and at bedtime. The aluminum combines with the excess phosphorus, causing it to be excreted through the bowel instead of through the kidney, thus decreasing the possibility of stone formation. Constipation frequently results from this regimen.

Prophylaxis for *uric acid* stones consists in alkalinizing the urine by the administration of sodium bicarbonate and acetazolamide (Diamox) sufficient to maintain a urine pH of 6.0 to 6.5 Allopurinol (Zyloprim) usually is prescribed to inhibit synthesis of uric acid.

Outcome criteria

The person or significant others can describe or state the following:

1. A plan to achieve a daily fluid intake of 4 to 5 L, sufficient to maintain a dilute urine
2. The need to be as active as possible and prevent long periods of immobilization
3. Menus to include any dietary restrictions
4. Name, dosage, desired action, and side effects of medications prescribed to acidify or alkalinize the urine
5. Plans for follow-up care
   a. Describe signs of recurrence of calculi (pain in costovertebral angle or radiating anteriorly to external genitalia)
   b. Describe assessment and prevention of a UTI

Renal neoplasms

Malignant renal tumors, primarily adenocarcinomas, account for 3% of all cancers. Small benign renal tumors (adenomas) may occur without causing significant damage or symptoms. Renal cell carcinomas rarely occur before the age of 40 years, are more commonly seen in the 50- to 70-year age range, and occur twice as often in men as in women.

Hematuria is the most frequent symptom of renal cell carcinoma. Unfortunately, the hematuria is often intermittent, lessening the person's concern and causing procrastination in seeking medical care. Any person with hematuria should have a complete urologic examination, since it is only by immediate investigation of the first signs of hematuria that there is any hope of cure. Other symptoms may include dull flank pain. flank mass, weight loss, fever, and polycythemia. Hypertension may result from stimulation of the reninangiotensin system.

An IVP may show a distortion of renal outline suggesting a kidney tumor. Small tumors in the parenchyma may not be apparent on a routine pyelogram but may be identified by CT scan. A CT scan is also useful in differentiating between renal cell carcinoma and a renal cyst. Angiography may also be performed to differentiate a cyst from a tumor.

Unless the person is a poor surgical risk or has extensive metastases, the diseased kidney is removed (*nephrectomy*) through a transabdominal, thoracoabdominal, or retroperitoneal approach. The first two approaches are preferred to secure the renal artery and vein and prevent any spread of malignant cells. (See p. 977 for care of the person requiring urologic surgery.)

Following surgery for a malignant tumor that is radiosensitive, the patient is usually given a course of x-ray therapy. Hospitalization is not always necessary during this time. Radiation may also be used over the metastatic sites as palliative treatment for the person with an inoperable tumor. Chemotherapy has not yet proved of value in the treatment of renal cell carcinomas. The survival rate after therapy depends on the extent of metastasis. The 10-year survival rate is very low, especially since many persons do not seek initial treatment until the disease is far advanced.

WILMS' TUMOR

Children under the age of 7 years may develop an embryonal type of highly malignant renal growth called Wilms' tumor. Most children with Wilms' tumor are under age 5, and half of them are younger than 3 years. Malignant renal tumors represent one of 20 cancers in children. Wilms' tumor metastasizes early. A mass in the abdomen may be the first sign, and later hematuria and anemia may occur. Excellent therapeutic results have been obtained by a combination of nephrectomy, radiation, and chemotherapy.

Renal carcinomas usually develop unilaterally but may be bilateral. In stage I the tumor margins are well defined (encapsulated) and compress the kidney parenchyma during growth rather than infiltrating it. The upper pole of the kidney is usually involved, and the tumor is usually large at the time of diagnosis. In stage II the tumor invades the fat surrounding the kidney. Stage III consists of local metastasis either through direct extension or through the renal vein or lymphatics (lymph node involvement). Distant metastases during stage IV are found primarily in the lungs or bone, but other areas, such as the liver, spleen, or brain, may also be involved.

TUMORS OF THE BLADDER

The most common site of cancer in the urinary tract is the bladder. Cancer of the bladder occurs three times more often in males than in females and multiple tumors are common, with about 25% of patients having more than one lesion at the time of diagnosis. This figure increases to about 50% in patients with papilloma, grade I carcinoma, over a 5-year period. Approximately 40% of the tumors involve the trigone, and an additional 45% involve the posterior and lateral bladder walls.

In the past 25 years, the incidence of bladder cancer in men has increased over 20% while the incidence in women has decreased over 25%. Known factors predisposing to bladder cancer are exposure to the chemicals beta-naphthylamine and xenylamine, infestation with *Schistoma haematobium,* and cigarette smoking.

Painless hematuria is the first symptom in the majority of bladder tumors. It is usually intermittent, and the individual may fail to seek treatment. Painless hematuria occurs also in nonmalignant urinary tract disease and in cancer of the kidney; therefore any hematuria should be investigated. Cystitis may be the first symptom of a bladder tumor, since the tumor may act as a foreign body in the bladder. Renal failure from obstruction of the ureters sometimes is the reason given for seeking medical care. Vesicovaginal fistulas may occur before other symptoms develop. The last two conditions indicate a poor prognosis because usually the tumor has infiltrated widely.

Cytologic examination of the urine may identify malignant cells before the lesion can be visualized by cystoscopy. The diagnosis is established by cystoscopic visualization of the bladder with biopsy. Clinical determination of the invasiveness of the tumor is important in establishing a therapeutic regimen and in predicting the prognosis. Any person who has had a papilloma removed should have a cystoscopic examination every 3 months for 2 years and then at less frequent intervals if there is no evidence of a new lesion. Repeated cystoscopies may seem unacceptable to patients who dread them. The necessity for frequent examination should be fully explained by the urologist and the explanation reinforced by the nurse. Emphasis should be placed on the necessity for repeated cystoscopies, since papillomas tend to recur without symptoms until they are far advanced tumors.

Tumors of the bladder range from small benign papillomas to large invasive carcinomas. Most of the neoplasms are of the transitional cell type since the urinary tract is covered with transitional epithelium. These neoplasms begin as papillomas; therefore all papillomas of the bladder are considered premalignant and are removed when identified. Squamous cell carcinoma occurs less frequently and has a poorer prognosis. Other neoplasias include adenocarcinoma (which is often inoperable) and rhabdomyosarcoma (seen in infants).

Grades I (well differentiated) and II (medially differentiated) bladder tumors are usually superficial, while grades III (poorly differentiated) and IV (anaplastic) tumors are usually invasive. Bladder cancers are *staged* according to the depth of invasiveness:

> Stage 0 Mucosa
> Stage A Submucosa
> Stage B Muscle

Stage C Per
Stage D I

The treatment for bla of the lesion and the dep

Surgery

Small tumors with minimal tissu may be adequately treated with *transureth excision.* A Foley catheter may or may not be ter aurgery. The urine may be pink tinge, b bleeding is unusual. Burning on urination may be lieved by forcing fluids and applying heat over the bladder region by means of a heating pad or a sitz bath. The patient is discharged within a few days after surgery.

If the tumor involves the dome of the bladder, a *segmental resection* of the bladder may be carried out. Over half of the bladder may be resected. A *cystectomy,* or complete removal of the bladder, usually is performed only when the disease appears curable. Complete removal of the bladder requires permanent urinary diversion.

Radiation

External cobalt radiation of large invasive tumors is often given before surgery to retard tumor growth. Supervoltage irradiation can be given when the patient physically cannot tolerate surgery. Radiation is not curative and has little value in patient management if the tumor is deemed inoperable. Internal radiation (radioisotopes or radon seeds) are rarely used since the introduction of better methods of external radiation.

Chemotherapy

Chemotherapy is primarily palliative. 5-Fluorouracil (5-FU) and doxorubicin (Adriamycin) are the most commonly used agents. Thiotepa may be instilled into the bladder as a topical treatment. The patient is dehydrated 8 to 12 hours before thiotepa treatment, and the drug remains in the bladder for 2 hours.

Benign prostatic hypertrophy

Benign prostatic hypertrophy or *hyperplasia (BPH)* is an adenomatous enlargement of the prostate gland. The prostate is an encapsulated gland weighing about 20 g that encircles the male urethra below the bladder neck. When the middle lobe of the gland enlarges, it causes narrowing of the urethra. More than half of all men over 50 years of age and 75% of men over 70 have some symptoms of prostatic enlargement. The cause is not known but appears to be related to the presence of male hormones.

One of the early symptoms of benign prostatic hypertrophy is nocturia (awakening at night to void) and urinary frequency in general. The man notices that the urinary stream is smaller and more difficult to start (hesitancy). The bladder muscle must contract more forcibly to push the urine past the partial obstruction, and the overworked muscles hypertrophy. Stagnant urine is held in trabeculae, or cellules, formed by sagging of the

ucous membranes between hypertrophied muscle
The bladder will not empty completely at each
g (residual urine); this urine becomes alkaline from
s and is a fertile medium for bacterial growth. The
an will then complain of symptoms of cystitis (frequency, urgency), and bladder stones may occur. Some
men develop hematuria from rupture of blood vessels that
have become overstretched. Destruction of renal function
can eventually occur from back pressure up the ureter to
the kidney. Acute urinary retention is not uncommon.

Enlargement of the lateral lobes of the prostate gland
may be palpated by digital rectal examination. Enlargement of the middle lobe is diagnosed by signs of partial
obstruction of the urethra and visualization of the obstruction and bladder trabeculae by cystoscopy.

Surgery is the primary treatment for benign prostatic
hypertrophy. During surgery the capsule of the prostate
gland is left intact, and the adenomatous soft tissue is
removed by one of four surgical routes: transurethral suprapubic, retropubic, or perineal. See Table 33-4 for a
comparison of the different approaches.

TRANSURETHRAL PROSTATECTOMY

Transurethral prostatic resection (TURP) is performed
when the major enlargement exists in the medial lobe
that directly surrounds the urethra. There must be a relatively small amount of tissue requiring resection so that
excessive bleeding will not occur and the time required to
complete the surgery will not be prolonged. A resecto-

Table 33-4. Comparison of types of prostatic surgery

	Transurethral resection	Suprapubic resection	Retropubic resection	Perineal resection	Radical perineal resection
Reason for surgery	Enlargement of medial lobe surrounding urethra	Extremely large mass of obstructing tissue	Large mass located high in pelvic area	Large mass located low in pelvic area	Cancer of prostate gland
Location of incision	No incision; removal by way of urethra	Low midline abdominal incision through bladder to prostate gland	Low midline abdominal incision into prostate gland (bladder not incised)	Incision between scrotum and rectum	Large perineal incision between scrotum and rectum
Drainage tubes	Three-way Foley catheter with 30-ml bag in urethra, constant irrigation for 24 hr	Cystotomy tube or drain through incision; Foley catheter with 30-ml bag in urethra	Foley catheter with 30-ml bag in urethra, constant irrigation for 24 hr	Foley catheter with 30-ml bag in urethra	Foley catheter with 30-ml bag in urethra; drain in incision
Bladder spasms	Yes	Yes	Few	Few	Few
Dressing	None	Abdominal dressing easily soaked with urinary drainage	Abdominal dressing; no urinary drainage	Perineal dressing; no urinary drainage	Perineal dressing; urinary drainage
Complications	Hemorrhage; water intoxication; incontinence	Hemorrhage; wound infection	Hemorrhage; wound infection	Hemorrhage; wound infection	Urinary incontinence; wound infection; impotence; sterility

scope (an instrument similar to a cystoscope but equipped with a cutting and cauterization loop attached to electric current) is passed through the urethra. The bladder is irrigated continuously during the procedure. The patient is grounded against electric shocks by a lubricated metal plate placed under his hips. Tiny pieces of tissue are cut away, and the bleeding points are sealed by cauterization (Fig. 33-12). A transurethral prostatectomy may be performed with the patient under general or spinal anesthesia.

Following a TURP, a large (24 Fr) three-way Foley catheter with a 30-ml balloon is usually inserted into the urethra. After the retention balloon of the catheter is inflated, the catheter is pulled down so that the bag rests in the prostatic fossa and provides hemostasis. Traction may be applied to the Foley catheter to increase pressure on the operative area to control bleeding. The large size catheter (24 Fr) is used to facilitate removal of clots from the bladder. Since the catheter retention balloon exerts pressure on the internal sphincter of the bladder, the patient continually feels the urge to void. If the catheter is draining properly, the stongest of these sensations usually passes momentarily. Attempting to void around the catheter causes the bladder muscles to contract and results in a painful "bladder spasm."

The nurse should discuss the physiology of the "need to void" with the patient preoperatively so that spasms will be seen as an expected event and not an abnormal complication. The patient is taught that the catheter produces the sensation of fullness and that *not* straining to pass urine around the catheter and drinking large amounts of fluids will reduce irritation and spasm. Narcotics are given to lessen the pain sensation; belladonna and opium suppositories are prescribed to relieve bladder spasms. As the nerve endings become fatigued, the frequency and severity of spasms decrease. This usually occurs by the end of 24 to 48 hours.

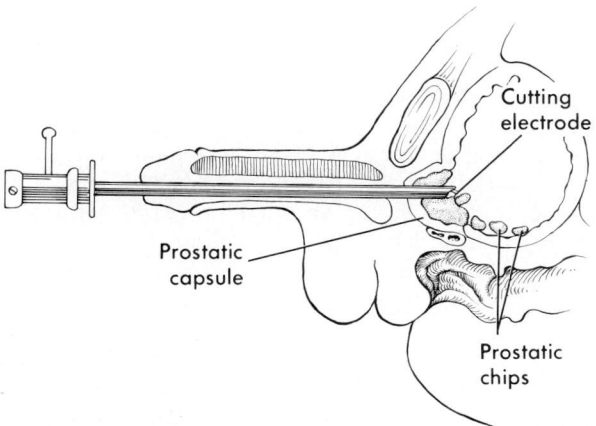

Fig. 33-12. Transurethral resection of prostate gland by means of resectoscope. Note cutting and cauterizing loop of instrument, enlarged prostate gland surrounding urethra, and tiny pieces of prostatic tissue that have been cut away.

The bladder is constantly irrigated by a three-way drip apparatus with normal saline or another solution prescribed by the surgeon. The purpose of constant irrigation is to keep the bladder free of clots that would block the drainage of urine.

A full bladder increases pressure on the outside of the prostatic fossa "milking" the bleeding vessels. Staining to have a bowel movement may also cause prostatic hemorrhage as can enemas, rectal tubes, and rectal thermometers, all of which are avoided for about a week postoperatively.

Persistent bladder discomfort, bladder spasms, or failure of a catheter to drain properly usually signifies one of the following serious complications, which require immediate medical attention: (1) hemorrhage and clot retention, (2) displacement of the catheter, or (3) unsuspected perforation of the baldder during surgery.

Sometimes patients develop *water intoxication,* formerly known as transurethral resection (TUR) syndrome, as a result of excessive irrigating solution being absorbed into the venous sinusoids during surgery. Cerebral edema may result. Confusion and agitation on the part of the patient may be the first signs of this condition.

Constant bladder irrigation is usually discontinued after 24 hours if no clots are draining from the bladder. The catheter may then be manually irrigated every 4 hours until removed, usually 3 to 5 days after surgery.

Following removal of the catheter, the patient should measure and record the time and amount of each voiding. The patient may not be able to void after removal of the catheter because of urethral edema. When this occurs, the catheter may need to be reinserted. Continence should also be assessed since the internal and external sphincters lie above and below the prostate gland, close to the operative area, and may have been disturbed during surgery.

About 2 weeks after TURP, when desiccated tissue is sloughed out, there may be a secondary hemorrhage. The patient, who probably is home at this time, must contact the physician immediately should there be any bleeding.

SUPRAPUBIC PROSTATECTOMY

The alternate methods of prostatectomy are open operations. In the *suprapubic resection* the prostate gland is removed from the urethra by way of the bladder; this type of resection is performed when a large mass of tissue must be resected. The usual method of draining urine following surgery is illustrated in Fig. 33-13, A. There will be some type of hemostatic agent placed in the prostatic fossa and urine will be drained by Foley catheter or cystotomy tube or both.

Hemorrhage is a possible complication, and the precautions are the same as those taken following TURP. Since there is some oozing of blood from the prostatic fossa, continuous bladder irrigations are usually ordered for the first 24 hours.

Cystotomy tubes are usually removed 3 to 4 days postoperatively; urethral catheters generally remain until the

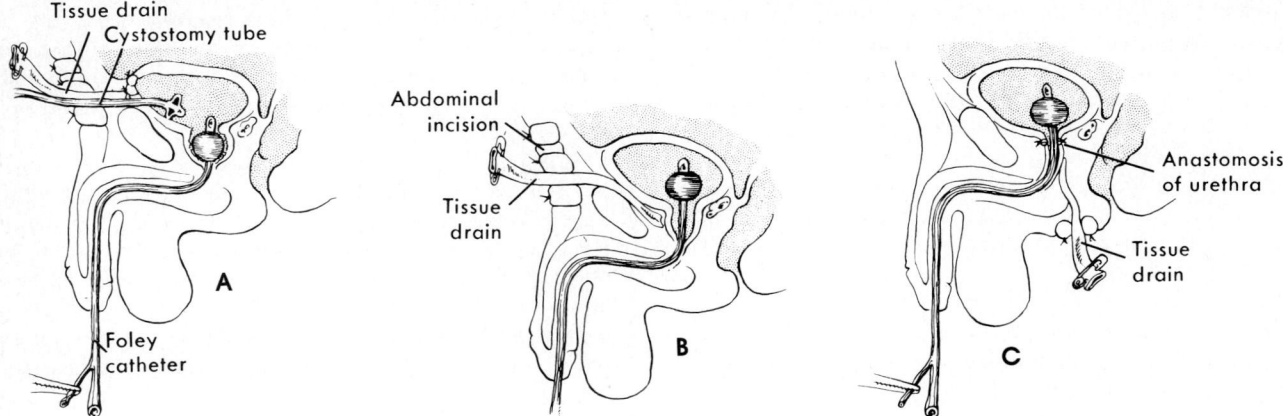

Fig. 33-13. Three methods of surgical removal of prostate gland. **A,** Suprapubic prostatectomy. Note placement of tissue drain, cystomy tube, and inflated Foley catheter in prostatic fossa. **B,** Retropubic prostatectomy. Note intact bladder, placement of tissue drain, and retention catheter. **C,** Radical perineal prostatectomy. Note placement of tissue drain in incision between scrotum and rectum and anastomosis of urethra made necessary by excision of prostate gland and its capsule.

suprapubic wound is healed. After the urethral catheter has been removed, the nursing care of the patient is similar to that for the patient undergoing transurethral resection. If the suprapubic wound should reopen and drain, a urethral catheter is usually reinserted.

RETROPUBIC PROSTATECTOMY

In a retropubic prostatectomy a low abdominal incision similar to that used for suprapubic prostatectomy is made, but the bladder is not opened. Rather, it is retracted and the adenomatous prostatic tissue is removed through an incision in the anterior prostatic capsule (Fig. 33-13, *B*).

Sphincter muscles are seldom damaged by retropubic prostatectomy, and there is no urine fistula. A large Foley catheter is inserted postoperatively, but bladder spasms are not usually a problem. When the Foley catheter is removed, the patient seldom has difficulty voiding. Hemorrhage from the prostatic fossa and wound infection may complicate the surgery; therefore precautions to prevent bleeding as discussed under TURP are taken. There should be no urinary drainage on the abdominal dressing. If urinary drainage on the abdominal dressing, purulent drainage, fever, or increased pain with ambulation occurs, the physician should be notified since these symptoms may indicate deep wound infection or pelvic abscess. Hospitalization generally is required for about 1 week after a retropubic prostatectomy.

PERINEAL PROSTATECTOMY

The perineal approach is used primarily for confirmed or suspected cancer of the prostate (Fig. 33-12, *C*). The incision is made between the scrotum and rectum. In addition to removal of the adenomatous prostate tissue, ad-

jacent tissue may be excised when cancer is confirmed. Preoperative and postoperative care is similar to that given a patient having radical perineal surgery.

PATIENT CONCERNS

Common to all patients undergoing prostatectomy are concerns regarding sexual functioning and the ability to be continent of urine. The nurse may need to provide an opportunity during interactions with the patient to promote expressions of these concerns by the patient. Impotence occurs physiologically when the perineal nerves are cut during a radical perineal prostatectomy and not with the other types of prostatectomies. If the man believes that the surgery will or may produce impotence, however, this may occur because of psychologic influences. Urinary incontinence frequently follows transurethral or suprapubic prostatectomy. Most men have some difficulty with continence after any type of prostatectomy. The patient should understand that this is normal for a period after surgery, and he should be taught perineal exercises to hasten recovery of control over voiding.

DISCHARGE PLANNING

The following points should be included in preparing the patient for discharge from the hospital: (1) Vigorous exercises, heavy lifting, and sexual intercourse should be avoided for about 3 weeks after returning home. (2) Driving during this period is also not advised. (3) Straining with defecation should be avoided; stool softeners or mild cathartics may be prescribed as home-going medication. (4) Fluids are encouraged to prevent stasis and infection and to keep stools soft. (5) The patient should be instructed to notify his physician should his urinary stream diminish. The urinary stream also will be checked on the patient's postoperative visit to the physician. This is important since urethral mucosa in the prostatic area is destroyed during surgery and strictures may form with healing.

OUTCOME CRITERIA

The patient or significant others can explain or describe the following:
1. Care of the catheter if discharged with an indwelling catheter
2. Perineal exercises if mild incontinence is present
3. Measures to prevent constipation
4. Signs of wound infection, urinary retention, or excessive bleeding requiring medical intervenion
5. Plans for medical follow-up
6. Activities to be avoided because of possible bleeding (sexual intercourse, heavy lifting, straining at stool) until medical permission to perform them is given (about 3 weeks)

Diagnostic tests

The following diagnostic tests are used in the diagnosis of benign prostatic hypertrophy:
1. Cystoscopy
2. IVP
3. Urethrograms, occasionally

It must be emphasized that any neoplasm developing in the abdominal space may result in obstruction of the urinary tract. The treatment is specific for the neoplasm, however, attention must also be paid to the renal obstruction.

Urethral strictures

A urethral stricture is a narrowing or constriction of the lumen of the urethra. Urethral strictures can be congenital or acquired. Congenital urethral strictures can occur in isolation or in combination with other urinary tract anomalies. Acquired urethral stricture can result from trauma secondary to accident or instrumentation, infection, muscular spasm, or pressure from the outside, by adjacent structures, or by growing tumors. Urethral strictures occur more often in men than women, primarily because of the length of the urethra. A common cause of strictures in the past was the instillation of silver nitrate in the male urethra for the treatment of gonorrhea. Although the treatment of choice for gonorrhea has changed, patients are still being hospitalized for this side effect. Urethral strictures are often repaired surgically by urethroplasty (Fig. 33-19).

Interventions for urinary retention

Interventions for urinary retention are aimed at reestablishment of urine flow. Some mechanical obstructions must be corrected by surgical intervention; others, such as that caused by an enlarged prostate, may require temporary urethral catheter drainage. If the person is having difficulty eliminating urine from the bladder in the absence of mechanical obstruction, measures that encourage voiding are attempted before catheterization is instituted. These measures may include assuring a position that facilitates voiding (positional stimuli), running water or blowing bubbles in water (auditory stimuli), or pouring water over the perineum or placing the hands in water (tactile stimuli). Sitting in lukewarm water may help relax the urinary sphincters. Bethanechol chloride (Urecholine) may be given to initiate voiding by stimulation of the detrusor muscle of the bladder. Persons having long-term problems may be taught to carry out intermittent catheterizations rather than maintaining an indwelling catheter.

Assisted urinary drainage is used in a variety of clinical situations in both acute and chronic care. Following are major reasons for catheter drainage of some part of the urinary system:
1. Relieve temporary anatomic or physiologic obstruction
2. Permit healing of various parts of the urinary system postoperatively
3. Permit accurate measurement of urinary output in severely ill patients
4. Relieve inability to void
5. Achieve continence
6. Prevent retention of urine in certain persons with neurogenic bladder dysfunction
7. Permit irrigation to prevent obstruction of urine flow

Reestablishment of the flow of urine is an immediate treatment goal. The type of catheter used to provide drainage in the presence of obstruction will depend on the location of the blockage.

Catheters are hollow tubes made of rubber, nylon, silk, plastic, metal, or glass. The circumference measurement is used to designate the size of the catheters and is specified in French units. One French (Fr) unit is equal to 1 mm in circumference. The size of the catheter to be used depends on the purpose for which it is used as well as the size and age of the patient. Appropriate urethral catheter sizes for adult men are 16 to 22 Fr, and for women, 14 to 20 Fr. Adult *ureters* are generally intubated with sizes 4 to 6 Fr.

Straight catheters include the following: (1) the *Robinson* catheter, which is made of rubber or plastic, has a hollow tip with two or more openings and is the catheter most frequently used for intermittent catheterizations (Fig. 33-14, *B*); (2) the *Coudé* catheter, which has a curved tip and is used for older men or when hypertrophy of the prostate is suspected to avoid trauma to the gland (Fig. 33-14, *D*); (3) the *whistle-tip* catheter, which has a whistle-shaped opening at the tip that is ideal for use when hematuria and blood clots are present (Fig. 33-14, *A*); and (4) the *filiform* catheter, which is a stiff catheter used when a urethral stricture is present.

Self-retaining, or indwelling, catheters are employed when continuous drainage is required. These cathaters are made of latex rubber, silicone-coated latex, or silicone. For short-term use, any of the three types is satis-

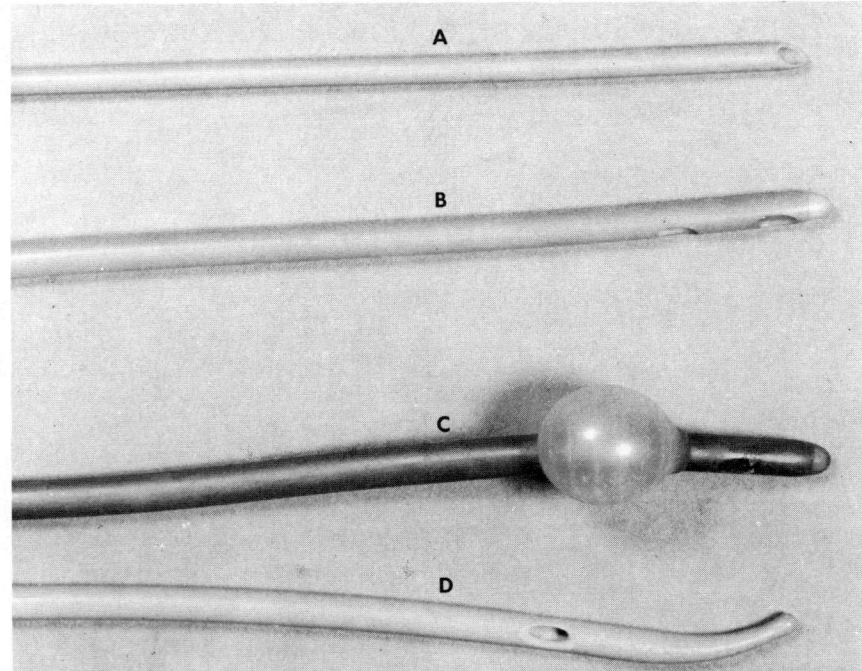

Fig. 33-14. Urethral catheters. **A,** Whistle-tip catheter. **B,** Many-eyed Robinson catheter. **C,** Foley catheter. **D,** Coudé catheter.

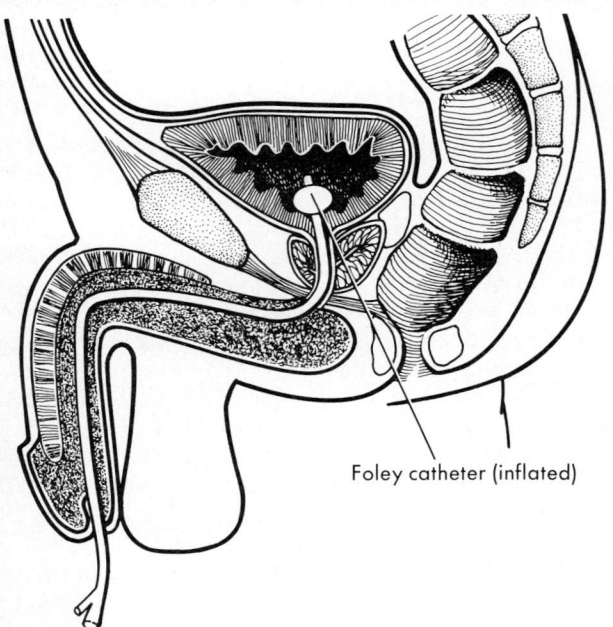

Foley catheter (inflated)

Fig. 33-15. Foley catheter in place with balloon inflated.

factory. For long-term use, silicone-coated or silicone catheters are preferred if encrustation is a problem. The *Foley* catheter is the most frequently used self-retaining catheter. It has a double lumen with an inflatable baloon at the distal end. The balloon is inflated with either normal saline or sterile water after it has been placed well within the bladder (Fig. 33-15).

Uretheral catheters must be securely anchored to prevent accidental dislodging of the catheter (Fig. 33-16). Proper anchoring will prevent accidental traction, which could result in injury to the baldder or urethra and yet keeps the catheter from moving in and out of the urethra causing irritation and infection.

Catheters that have been placed in the urinary system are usually allowed to drain by gravity. The procedure of connecting a catheter to a collecting device and allowing drainage to flow by gravitational force is called *straight drainage*. *Closed drainage* refers to the design of the collection set-up and indicates that the drainage tube is sealed to the collection container; this lessens the chance for contamination of the set-up and decreases the risk of a UTI. Most closed urinary drainage systems employ disposable plastic drainage bags and tubing.

Proper maintenance of the drainage system is a nursing function. Attention to the points outlined as follows will help to maintain drainage and decrease the entry of organisms into the system.

Since the purpose of the catheter is to promote drainage of urine, *patency* of the system must be ensured. The flow of urine from a catheter is checked hourly when urine is bloody and at least every 2 hours when there is no evidence of bleeding or disturbance in drainage. Common causes of obstruction of urine flow may be internal or external. Hemorrhage leads to formation of clots that may plug a catheter, and infection increases sediment in the urine that may clog the drainage system. Any evidence of bleeding or change in the amount of bleeding is reported to the physician. To detect the buildup of sediment in the drainage system, the catheter may be rolled between the fingers to detect gritty accumulation, and the

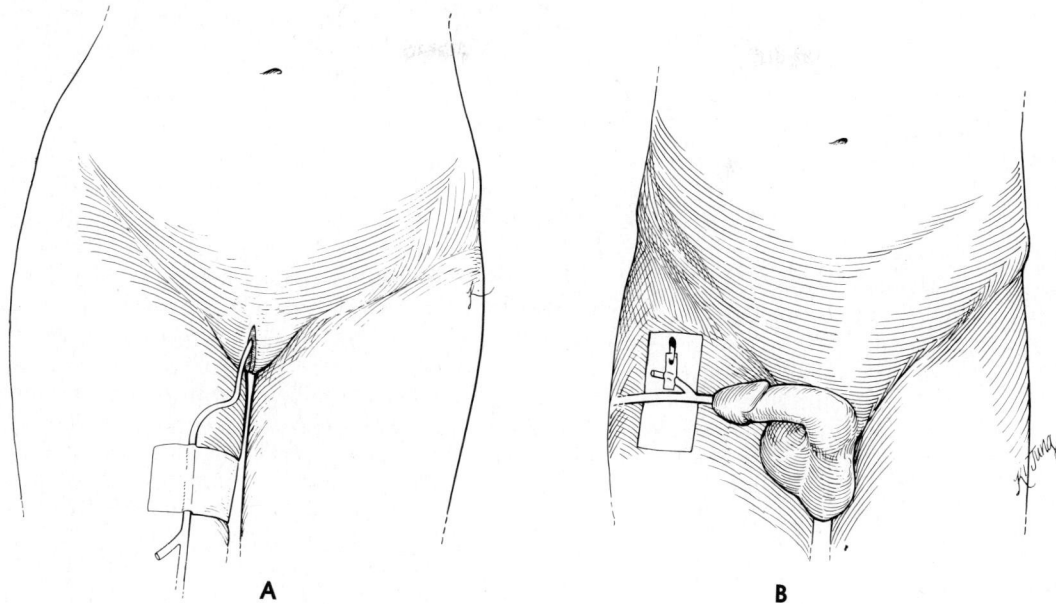

Fig. 33-16. Anchoring of Foley catheter. **A,** In female patient. **B,** In male patient. Proper anchoring prevents accidental traction that could result in injury to bladder or urethra and yet keeps catheter from moving in and out of urethra.

Maintenance of drainage system

Action	Rationale
Never disconnect the catheter except to irrigate	Prevent introduction of bacteria
Collect urine samples by inserting a small-bore needle into the drainage port that has been cleansed with alcohol or povidone-iodine (Fig. 33-17).	Maintain closed system and prevent introduction of bacteria
Never elevate drainage bag above level of the patient's bladder or cavity being drained; suspend bag from the bed frame when the patient is recumbent and from below the knee when the patient is ambulatory.	Prevent reflux of urine back into bladder; drainage bags are available with antireflux valves
Drainage bags and tubing should never be allowed to rest on the floor.	Prevent contamination of system
Observe tubing for kinks and loops.	Obstructions will result in reflux of urine
Empty drainage bag into a a measuring container that is used only for that particular patient; cleanse measuring container regularly.	Prevent cross-contamination of drainage system
Cultures of urine are usually ordered at regular intervals when a patient has an indwelling catheter.	Provides data on changing numbers and types of organism present in urine before symptoms appear
Observe collecting system daily for sedimentation and leaks.	Replace when sediment or leaks are present

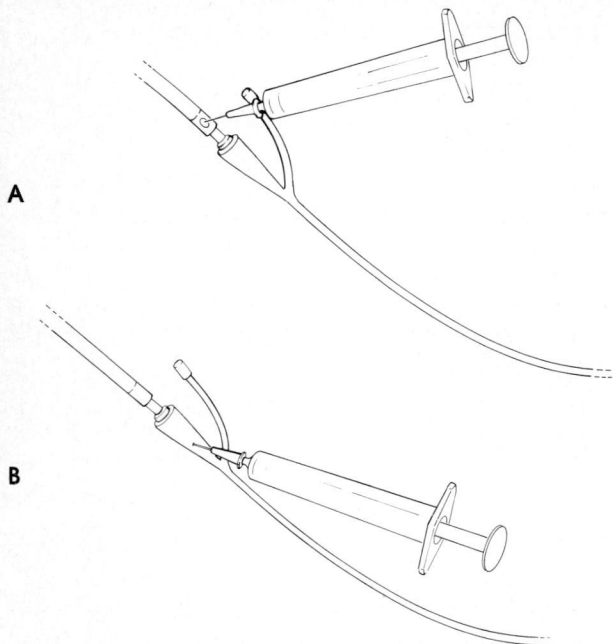

Fig. 33-17. Aspiration of sterile specimen from Foley catheter connected to closed drainage system. **A,** Aspiration from drainage port. **B,** Aspiration from Foley catheter.

drainage tubing is visually inspected. External causes of obstruction in urine flow include kinking and dependent loops in the tubing. If correction of these problems fails to restore the flow of urine, irrigation, if ordered, may be done. In the event that none of these measures restores the flow of urine, the physician is notified.

Catheters should be irrigated only with a physician's order. The physician should specify the quantity, frequency, and type of irrigating solution. When a catheter is to be irrigated, the size of the cavity into which the fluid is being instilled should be considered. *The renal pelvis of an adult should never be irrigated with more than 4 to 6 ml of fluid.* Commonly, 30 to 60 ml of fluid instilled two or three times is used to irrigate an adult urethral catheter.

The purpose of irrigation is to prevent obstruction of the catheter and the urine flow. All equipment used must be sterile, and asepsis must be maintained throughout the procedure. Therefore, opened irrigation sets cannot be reused for the next irrigation.

The solution usually ordered for irrigation is sterile normal saline, since it is nonirritating to tissues. Acetic acid or neomycin solutions may be ordered as irrigating substances. The ordered solution should be instilled gently to prevent trauma to the bladder or kidney. After instillation, the irrigating fluid is allowed to drain out by gravity. If fluid can be instilled easily but fails to return, a clot or small plug may be acting as a valve over the catheter opening. If this occurs in a catheter to the bladder, the bulb of the Asepto syringe can be depressed slightly and reattached to the tubing in an attempt to

withdraw the fluid and obstructing material. If fluid is not returned, the nurse can instill a small amount of fluid in an attempt to dislodge the clot. If the fluid again does not drain, the nurse should discontinue the irrigation and reconnect the tubing. If after a 10- to 15-minute period the catheter is not draining properly, the physician is notified.

When frequent irrigation of a urethral catheter appears necessary, intermittent bladder irrigation should be considered. This involves alternately instilling fluid from a reservoir (usually suspended above patient level) into the bladder through the catheter and allowing the solution to return freely to the collecting bag. Intermittent irrigation is not recommended for irrigation of the kidney because control of inflow in 4- to 6-ml amounts is difficult and instillation of larger amounts into the renal pelvis may lead to tissue damage.

Another variation in bladder irrigation involves the use of a three-way Foley catheter. Constant irrigation involves continuous and simultaneous inflow and outflow of irrigating solution for the bladder. The system is used more frequently after surgery of the bladder or prostate when bleeding is expected and clot formation with obstruction of the bladder outlet is a threat.

In calculating the patient's output when either intermittent or continuous irrigation of the bladder is employed, the amount of irrigating fluid is subtracted from the total volume of urinary drainage obtained in the same time period. the difference between these two values is the patient's actual urinary output.

If a ureter becomes obstructed, a catheter must be placed directly into the renal pelvis. This prevents renal damage that otherwise would occur as pressure in the kidney increases because of continued urine formation. When there is complete obstruction of a ureter, a *nephrostomy* or *pyelostomy* tube may be inserted surgically into the renal pelvis. The surgical incision is located laterally and posteriorly in the kidney region. Catheters used as nephrostomy or pyelostomy tubes are usually of the Pezzar (mushroom) or Malecot (batwing) types (Fig. 33-18). An alternate form of drainage for a ureteral obstruction is the surgical placement of a ureterostomy tube (a whistle-tip or many-eyed Robinson catheter, size 6 or 8 Fr) that is passed through an incision in the upper outer quadrant of the abdomen into the ureter above the obstruction. The catheter is then passed through the ureter to the renal pelvis.

If the ureter is unobstructed or partially obstructed, the renal pelvis may be drained by a ureteral catheter, which is passed up the ureter to the renal pelvis by a cystoscope (see Fig. 33-5). Ureteral catheterization is performed before gynecologic and lower abdominal surgery when there is danger of not recognizing and accidentally injuring the ureter during the operation. Ureteral catheterization is also used after surgery involving the ureters to prevent stricture as the ureter heals. When used for this purpose, the catheter is referred to as a *splinting catheter* (Fig. 33-19). Whether it is expected to drain urine will depend on its relation to other catheters used.

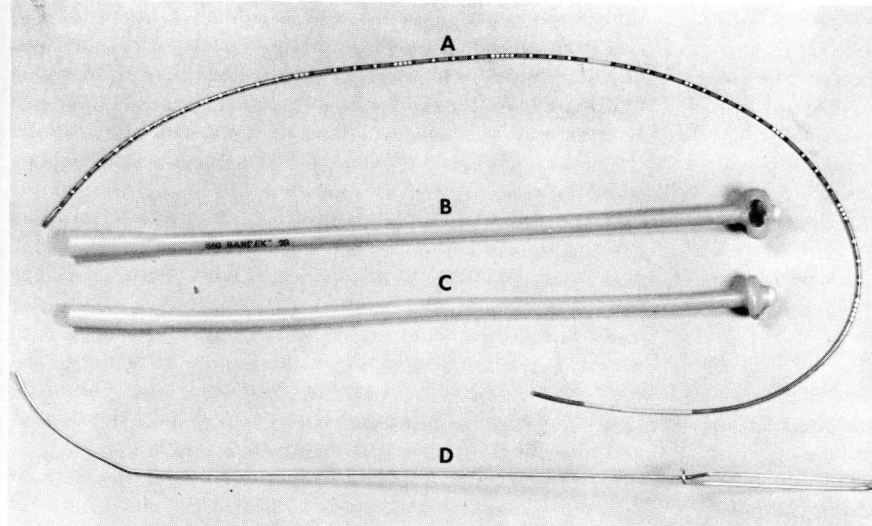

Fig. 33-18. A to C, Catheters used to drain renal pelvis. A, ureteral catheter. B, Malecote (batwing) catheter. C, Pezzer (mushroom) catheter. D, Stylet used to insert urethral catheter into male patient.

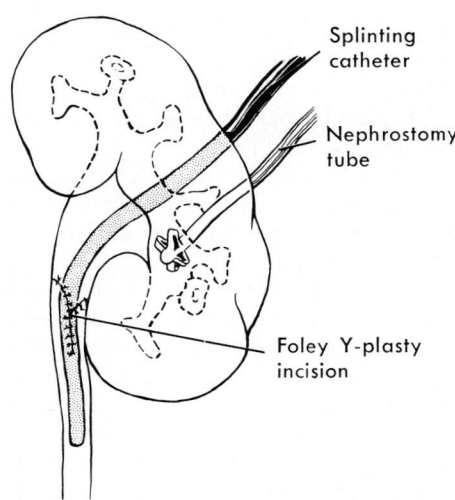

Fig. 33-19. Placement of splinting catheter after repair of ureteropelvic stricture. Note use of nephrostomy tube for drainage of urine during healing of anastomosis.

Adequate anchorage of nephrostomy catheters must be provided to prevent accidental dislodgment and trauma to the tissues in which they lie. The openings made for these tubes are essentially fistulas that rapidly decrease in size on removal of the catheter. Even 30 minutes after removal of this type of catheter it is often impossible to reinsert a similar-sized tube. When a catheter is inserted during surgery, it is usually sutured in place. In this case, additional anchorage consists of affixing the tube to the skin with adhesive tape after the skin has been cleansed. When the tube is not sutured in place, it should be anchored to the skin at *two points* using adhesive—with some slack in the tubing between the anchor points.

Free drainage of catheters leading to the renal pelvis is of the utmost importance. Since the normal renal pelvis

has only a 5- to 8-ml capacity, great pressure can be exerted on renal structures even when these catheters are obstructed for only a few minutes. Care must be taken to prevent kinking of the tubes while the patient is in the side-lying position in bed.

In some cases nephrostomy tubes may be left in place for several months, with the patient returning to the hospital later for their removal. Occasionally, the nephrostomy tube serves as a form of urinary diversion for long-term use. The person at home with a catheter draining the kidney pelvis must know how to obtain medical assistance quickly should the catheter obstruct or become dislodged.

When obstruction occurs below the bladder, constant drainage must be provided to prevent renal damage, which may occur because of inadequate emptying of the lower urinary system. One means of providing drainage is by the use of a cystostomy tube (usually a Foley, Malecot, or Pezzer catheter), which is placed directly into the bladder through a suprapubic incision. This method is usually used when the urethra is completely obstructed or when the prolonged use of a urethral catheter is to be avoided in a male patient. During some operative procedures both a cystostomy tube and a small urethral catheter will be inserted to drain the bladder. Both catheters must be monitored for patency. If patency is assured, it is not necessary to record the output from each catheter separately, since both tubes drain the bladder. The catheters will not necessarily drain equal amounts of urine. As is true with nephrostomy and ureteral catheters, secure anchorage of these catheters is also necessary.

Urethral catheterization is the most common means of draining the bladder, and insertion of this type of catheter is a nursing responsibility in many settings. The Foley catheter is most frequently used for this purpose.

Catheterization is a major cause of UTI, and strict asepsis should be practiced by anyone carrying out this procedure or assembling the drainage equipment. The need for urethral catheterization must be carefully evaluated; use of urethral catheter drainage only for nursing convenience is not appropriate.

When a female patient is catheterized, the supine or lateral position may be used; the male patient should be supine. The patient should be provided with a thorough explanation of the procedure before the catheterization. Privacy is maintained to help the patient feel less embarrassed and more relaxed. The patient is encouraged to take deep breaths during insertion to divert attention from the procedure and to increase relaxation of the bladder sphincters, making the procedure less uncomfortable.

If the nurse finds it difficult to pass the catheter, the procedure is discontinued and the physician notified. Traumatic catheterization predisposes the patient to a UTI and formation of urethral strictures. In patients who have urethral disorders, it is not unusual to be unable to pass a standard catheter; special equipment such as catheter directors, filiform catheters, or sounds may be needed. The introduction of such equipment into the urinary tract is not a nursing procedure; neither is catheterization of a patient in the immediate postoperative period following surgery of the urethra or bladder. (For specific information on the catheterization procedure refer to a fundamentals of nursing or a urologic nursing text.)

In addition to the previously discussed basic principles of catheter drainage maintenance, the meatal-catheter junction is gently cleansed twice a day with soap and water to prevent a UTI. Vigorous cleaning is avoided, since this predisposes the patient to infection by causing irritation and by removing protective micro-organisms. Irrigation of the catheter may be necessary when urine flow is sluggish but is not recommended on a routine basis.

Removal of the urethral catheter is a simple procedure. The adhesive anchor is removed. If a Foley catheter was used, the balloon is then deflated. The catheter is removed with a slow continuous pull. The patient may be asked to take a deep breath and hold it during withdrawal of the catheter.

It is normal to note some dribbling of urine for a few hours after a urethral catheter has been removed because of dilation of the sphincter muscles by the catheter. Dribbling of urine that persists longer than a few hours should be reported to the physician; this symptom may indicate damage to the sphincters. In determining the type of intervention necessary to reestablish bladder control, information about the nature of the incontinency is gathered. Incontinence is described as complete (constant dribbling) or occurring only on urgency or stress. It should also be observed whether incontinence is present in all positions (lying, sitting, standing). If muscular weakness of the sphincters is the major problem, incontinence is least likely to occur when the person is in a prone position and most likely to be a problem when standing or walking. Perineal exercises may help to regain control of voiding.

Another problem that may arise after removal of a catheter is the inability to void. The patient should be encouraged to drink fluids and then attempt to void. The nurse carefully assesses the patient's bladder for disten-

tion. Efforts are made to provide comfortable positioning and privacy to facilitate voiding. No patient with an adequate intake should go longer than 8 hours without voiding. It is not uncommon for a patient with edema of the bladder neck to require temporary reinsertion of a catheter to facilitate urinary output. It is the nurse's responsibility to accurately determine and record all spontaneous voidings of the patient until adequacy of output has been well established.

Color and consistency of the urine are noted. Cystitis (inflammation of the bladder) may develop after catheter removal because of incomplete emptying of the bladder as muscle tone is being reestablished. Any abnormalities in color, odor, or sediment in the urine are reported.

Education of the patient about signs and symptoms of urinary retention, changes in the color and consistency of the urine, and incontinence and dysuria is undertaken when bladder drainage is discontinued. Often the first indicators of dysfunction are subjective judgements offered by the patient. This information greatly increases the ability to detect early recurrence of urinary drainage problems and should be sought and clearly recorded.

Outcome criteria
1. Maintains free flow of urine through the catheter
2. Does not acquire a UTI

The person or significant others can explain or demonstrate the following:
1. The purpose and expected duration of the catheter
2. Aseptic technique in care of the catheter
3. How to arrange for reestablishment of urine flow should failure of adequate flow occur
4. Where to obtain needed supplies
5. Signs and symptoms of UTI requiring medical attention
6. Plans for follow-up care

It is not uncommon for patients to be discharged to home requiring catheter drainage on a temporary or permanent basis. The patient must be instructed in safely maintaining the urinary drainage system. Written instructions should be provided to supplement and reinforce this information. The services of a community health nurse may be indicated. The following areas must be included in home-going preparation of any person with indwelling catheter drainage:
1. Maintaining catheter patency
2. Prevention of UTI
3. Maintaining ADL
4. Dealing with catheter problems
5. Obtaining supplies
6. Continued urologic surveillance

The person (or care provider) must know how to check for kinks in the tubing and should be aware of the most appropriate way to secure the catheter to prevent kinking. An adequate fluid intake of 2 to 3 L of fluid per day should be encouraged unless contraindicated by the person's condition. Persons who will be irrigating their own catheters at home should practice this under supervision several times before discharge.

The person (or care provider) must be helped to understand the importance of cleanliness as a means of preventing complications. Instruction includes the necessity of good hand washing before and after working with the catheter. Instruction also includes cleanisng the meatal-catheter junction with soap and water twice daily. The person should be reassured that cleansing the meatal-catheter junction will not dislodge or pull out the catheter. Ideally, frequent disconnection of the catheter and drainage tubing should be avoided. However, the persons at home must disconnect the tubing at night to change from a leg bag to the overnight drainage bag and again in the morning to resume leg-bag drainage. To lessen the risk of contamination, the person is taught to wash the hands and then wipe the catheter and tubing with 70% alcohol before disconnection and reconnection. The disconnected ends of the drainage bags are protected with sterile gauze secured in place with a rubher band or a connector cap.

When equipment must be sterilized at home, instruction is given on how to do this properly. Before use, the equipment, which has been washed with soap and water, is boiled for a full 10 minutes in a pan of water. Other parts of the system such as collection bags and tubing should be kept as clean as possible by daily washing with soap and water followed by 15 minutes of soaking in a solution of equal parts of vinegar and water (half-strength vinegar). Teaching also includes the need to keep the drainage collection receptacle at a level lower than the cavity being drained.

The person needs to be well informed about the adaptations that can be made with the urinary drainage system to allow return to an optimal level of activity. A shower or tub bath with a catheter in place is generally permitted unless there is an unhealed surgical incision. The adhesive tape holding the catheter in place will need to be replaced after bathing. Leg bags are available in a variety of sizes and are concealed by clothing. There is no need for men or women to remove an indwelling catheter before intercourse—a question persons may be hesitant to ask. The male can fold the indwelling catheter over the penis to facilitate insertion during intercourse.[12] Questions pertaining to resumption of usual life-style activities should be encouraged so that the person can be as well prepared as possible for self-care at home.

The patient (or care provider) should be informed about how to handle problems such as obstruction of the catheter or displacement of the catheter. The person needs to know whether to contact the physician or to seek help through a clinic or emergency room. The amount of time that can safely elapse before obtaining help will depend on the type of catheter and its location.

At discharge the patient should be provided with adequate supplies for at least a few days. A list of names, addresses, and phone numbers of where additional supplies may be obtained and what resources are available to assist with payment if necessary should be given to the person before discharge. A written list of the specific supplies needed should be provided to aid the person, who is likely to be confused by the many products available.

The person with a urinary catheter of any type will need continued urologic surveillance. Instruction includes the need to contact the physician if back pain, fever, or other UTI symptoms are present and to plan for regular examination by the physician as well.

INTERMITTENT CATHETERIZATION

Intermittent catheterization of the urinary bladder is being used with increasing frequency in the treatment of neurogenic bladder dysfunction secondary to spinal cord trauma, birth defects, urinary retention, and some chronic diseases. Originally it was carried out only as a sterile procedure used in hospital settings. A clean, unsterile technique that facilitates home use of this method has been adapted by some urologists.[7]

Because periodic complete emptying of the bladder eliminates residual urine (an excellent culture medium for multiplication of bacteria) and maintains a good blood supply to the bladder wall by avoiding high intrabladder pressures, infections are often decreased, even when only a clean technique is used.

The goals of intermittent catheterization may vary from patient to patient but are generally to prevent urinary retention and its sequelae (UTI and renal damage) and to achieve continence. The patient should know exactly what is expected of the treatment plan to elicit full cooperation.

The hospitalized patient with intermittent catheter drainage of the bladder may be one for whom the treatment is temporary (as in the early phases of spinal cord trauma), one who is learning the technique for home use, or one who has been using intermittent catheterization before hospital admission. Even though the clean technique is suitable for home use, sterile technique is necessary during hospitalization to decrease the possibility of hospital-acquired infection when the catheterization is performed by hospital personnel. When hospitalized, the patient who customarily performs self-catheterization may continue to use clean technique if this method is used at home, but preferably a sterile catheter will be used each time or special precautions are taken to store the reusable catheter in a closed container. Specimens for culture must be obtained by the usual sterile catheterization technique to avoid contamination of the specimen. The patient is informed about the reasons why sterile precautions are necessary in the hospital setting.

A size 14 Fr Robinson catheter is generally used for an adult. The volume of urine obtained with each catheterization is recorded to ensure that schedule adjustments can be made if necessary. The adult bladder should not be permitted to hold more than 300 ml at any time, since greater amounts lead to overdistention of the bladder with greater susceptibility to infection. The frequency of catheterization is determined by the amount of residual urine (more than 200 ml) means that more frequent catheterization is necessary. Usually such individuals will need catheterization every 4 to 6 hours. A small amount of residual urine (less than 200 ml) after voiding means that the person will only need to do self-catheterization every 8 to 12 hours. Some persons eventually will be able to manage with once-a-day catheterization. Some individuals may also have to catheterize themselves at night if they have a large output of urine at night. It is important to realize that the person who normally does not perform self-catheterization at night at home may need to do so during periods where the fluid intake is greater than usual, as with intravenous fluid administration.

In some instances the physician will prescribe the frequency of catheterizations; in other instances, adjustment of the schedule may be a nursing judgment. If the nurse notes that excess volumes of urine are being obtained with a prescribed schedule, the physician is consulted about the need to alter the schedule.

Color, clarity, and odor of the urine are noted; and any symptoms of a UTI reported. Periodic urine specimens are obtained and sent for culture and sensitivity. Some individuals are given long-term antibiotic therapy prophylactically.

The person is helped to understand the rationale for intermittent catheter drainage, and the regularity of bladder emptying must be stressed. Basic anatomy of the genitalia and urinary tract is pointed out to aid the person to understand where the catheter is inserted and to alleviate fears of causing damage by misplacement of the catheter.

In most cases, clean (not sterile) catheterization technique is prescribed for home use. Hand washing is advised before each catheterization, and the meatal area is cleansed with soap and water. After inserting the catheter and draining the bladder, the catheter is removed and washed with soap and water before being stored in a clean, closed container for the next use. The catheter is reused until it becomes either too soft or too hard to be directed properly.

Most individuals require much support during the actual teaching but very quickly become comfortable with the procedure. Initially, a mirror is used to teach women where to place the catheter. The woman should learn to catheterize while sitting on the commode, using palpation to locate the urethral meatus. Men may sit or stand to catheterize themselves. It is important that men use generous amounts of lubricant to avoid urethral irritation; women generally do not require lubrication of the catheter.

If the person, because of age or physical limitations, is unable to perform self-catheterization, a care provider may be instructed in the technique. The individual or care provider must know where additional catheters may be obtained.

If sterile catheterization technique is needed for home use, more time and practice will be required to learn good sterile technique. Careful explanation of sterilization of equipment must be provided, and planning for adapting sterile intermittent self-catheterization to the individual's usual life-style must be worked out with the person.

If teaching of self-catheterization is performed on an outpatient basis or if hospitalization is short, follow-up for adjustment of schedule and other concerns of adaptation to home routine should be provided. This may be done by the primary nurse, by the physician, or by referral to a visiting nurse. Ongoing urologic care with periodic urine cultures is essential.

Outcome criteria

The person or significant others can state or demonstrate the following:
1. The reason for the intermittent catheter drainage
2. The need for regular, periodic, complete emptying of the bladder
3. Self-catheterization using clean technique unless sterile technique is prescribed
4. How to adapt the catheterization routine to the individual life-style
5. How to obtain needed supplies
6. Symptoms of a UTI requiring medical care
7. Plans for ongoing urologic care

Summary of tests used for diagnosis of obstructive disorders

	Renal calculi	Renal neoplasms	Prostatic hypertrophy	Urethral strictures
Cystoscopy	X	X	X	X*
Retrograde pyelography	X	X		
IVP	X	X	X	X*
KUB	X	X		
Urethrography			X	X
CT		X		
Renal angiography		X		
Renography				
Ultrasound		X		
Renal biopsy		X		

*Not always completed.

Assessment

SUBJECTIVE DATA

1. Pain and discomfort: ureteral stones can result in renal calculi bladder stones often result in a dull, heavy feeling in the suprapubic region
2. Nausea: often results from fluid overload and/or electrolyte imbalance
3. Voiding patterns
   a. Frequency
   b. Urgency
   c. Difficulty starting stream
   d. Dribbling at end of micturition
   e. Nocturia
   f. Burning on urination
4. History of obstructive disorders

OBJECTIVE DATA

1. Vomiting: result of fluid overload and/or electrolyte imbalance
2. Hematuria
3. Urinary output
4. Dyspnea
5. Edema
6. Palpable masses in abdomen
7. Bladder distention on palpation
8. Tenderness over kidneys or bladder on palpation

DIAGNOSTIC TESTS

The box on p. 986 provides a summary of the specific diagnostic tests used in the diagnosis of obstructive disorders. In addition to these diagnostic procedures, the patient would also undergo urinalysis and serum renal function studies.

Implementation

1. Assisting with achievement of therapeutic goals
   a. If vomiting is present, give prescribed antiemetic by suppository or deep intramuscular injection if not contraindicated.
   b. Assist in the maintenance of fluid and electrolyte balance by properly maintaining IVs and encouraging appropriate diet.
   c. Prevent urinary complications by maintaining urinary drainage; use aseptic technique in dealing with urinary drainage system.
   d. Assess intake and output at least every 8 hours.
   e. Encourage activity, as tolerated, to prevent urinary stasis
   f. Assess for bladder distention at least every 8 hours.
   g. Assess for hematuria.
   h. Assess for signs and symptoms of renal failure.
2. Assisting with comfort and ADL
   a. Maintain a calm environment to decrease anxiety.
   b. Administer prescribed pain medications as necessary.
   c. Administer antispasmodics as prescribed.
   d. Provide fluids in small amounts.
   e. Assist with ADL as necessary.
   f. Encourage self-care and independence as tolerated.
3. Teach the patient the following:
   a. Necessary diet and fluid restrictions
   b. Necessary care if patient is discharged with an indwelling catheter
   c. Need for follow-up care
   d. Necessity of following the prescribed medical regimen to prevent further problems

Evaluation

The following questions should be asked to evaluate the effectiveness of the nursing intervention:

1. Is adequate urinary drainage being maintained?
2. Is the patient's nutritional status adequate?
3. Is the patient maintaining maximum activity levels to prevent urinary stasis?
4. Can the patient describe action, dose, frequency, and side effects of all prescribed medications?
5. Can the patient describe signs and symptoms of recurrance of the obstructive disorder?
6. Can the patient state rationale for follow-up care?

URINARY INCONTINENCE

Urinary incontinence, the involuntary expulsion of urine, may be encountered in a number of temporary and permanent conditions. Inability to control urination is a problem that frequently leads to emotional distress and can seriously impair an individual's socialization patterns if not managed in a suitable manner. Incontinence must be managed either by the person or by others in a way that makes the person feel physically and emotionally comfortable and socially acceptable.

Persons with incontinence often present baffling management problems. Solutions require that the nurse understand the physiologic basis of incontinence.

Bladder sphincter control is necessary to have urinary continence. Such control requires normal voluntary and involuntary muscle action coordinated by a normal urethrobladder relfex. Understanding this coordinated sequence of nerve stimuli and muscle action will help the nurse understand how continence is maintained.

As bladder filling occurs, the pressure within the bladder gradually increases. The detrusor muscle (the three-layered bladder wall) responds by relaxing to accommodate the greater volume. When a certain point of filling is reached, usually 150 to 200 ml of urine, the parasympathetic stretch receptors located in the bladder wall are stimulated. The stimuli are transmitted through afferent fibers of the reflex arc to the reflex center for micturition. Impulses are then carried through the efferent fibers of the relfex arc to the bladder, causing reflex contraction of the detrusor muscle. The internal sphincter, which is normally closed, reciprocally opens, and the urine enters

Table 33-5. Major causes of urinary incontinence

Cause of urinary incontinence	Factors involved				Result
	Awareness of need to void	Cortical ability to inhibit voiding	Reflex arc	Bladder response to filling	
Cerebral clouding	Impaired	Impaired	Intact	Normal	Uncontrolled voiding because of reflex response
Infection	Intact	Intact, but overcome by strong reflex response	Abnormally stimulated	Heightened	Voiding because of strong reflex response (urgency)
Distrubance of CNS pathways (cortical lesions)	Diminished	Impaired	Intact	Heightened	Voiding because of reflex response
Disturbance of urethrobladder reflex					
Upper motor neuron lesion	Destroyed	Destroyed	Intact but deranged	Heightened	Voiding because of reflex response
Lower motor neuron lesion	Destroyed	Destroyed	Destroyed or impaired	Diminished to absent	Distention or incomplete emptying
Tissue damage	Intact	Intact, but not functional because of poor muscle response	Intact	Normal	Loss of control of voiding because of muscular impairment

the posterior urethra. Relaxation of the external sphincter and perineal muscles follows, and the bladder content is released. Completion of this reflex act can be interrupted and voiding postponed through release of inhibitory impulses from the cortical center, which results in voluntary contraction of the external sphincter. If any part of this complex function is upset, there is apt to be urinary incontinence.

The five major causes of urinary incontinence and the nature of the incontinence they cause are outlined in Table 33-5.

Cerebral clouding is most common in the aged. In many instances the elderly person is incontinent because of a lack of awareness of the need to empty the bladder. This type of incontinence is often not associated with any definite pathologic problem at the cerebral level. Cerebral clouding also occurs in acutely ill persons, who may be so ill that cerebration is dulled. They may not be able to think or may not have the energy to exercise voluntary control. Likewise a person who is comatose is incontinent because of loss of the ability to conrol voluntarily the opening of the external sphincter. As soon as urine is released into the posterior urethra, the bladder contracts and empties. This is the reason why voiding sometimes occurs under anesthesia.

Infection anywhere in the urinary tract may lead to incontinence, since bacteria in the urine cause irritation of the mucosa of the bladder and stimulate the urethrobladder reflex abnormally.

Disturbance of the central nervous system pathways may occur in diseases such as cerebral embolus, cerebral hemorrhage, brain tumor, meningitis, or traumatic injury of the brain. Adequate voluntary (cortical or cerebral) control of bladder function is prevented in these situations. Urgency incontinence may be present as a result of the inability to inhibit completion of the urethrobladder reflex by the higher centers.

Disturbance of the urethrobladder reflex may result from lesions of the spinal cord or damage to peripheral nerves of the bladder. This form of incontinence may be seen in persons with spinal cord malformations, injuries, or tumors, and those with compression of the cord caused by fractures of the vertebrae, herniated disk, metastatic tumor, or postoperative edema of the spinal cord. This type of difficulty can result in two types of responses known as *neurogenic bladder*. The person with a neurogenic bladder has no way of knowing when voiding is occurring.

Lesions above the S2 level of the spinal cord or impairment of the cerebrocortical centers do not destroy the reflex arc for voiding, although they may derange it. Such lesions destroy the potential for cortical control to inhibit the reflex. The result is an "upper motor neuron" or "automatic" bladder. The bladder is hypertonic and has a small capacity (less than 150 ml). The increased detrusor tone and increased sensitivity to small amounts of urine present in the bladder result in precipitous voiding and the potential for vesicoureteral reflux.

Damage to nerves in the cauda equina or sacral segments of the spinal cord may cause destruction of the reflex arc by interruption of its afferent, efferent, or central components. The result is a "lower motor neuron" or "flaccid" bladder. The bladder is hypotonic with capacities of 500 ml or more. Overflow incontinence, retention of residual urine, and the potential for vesicoureteral reflux are problems imposed by a hypotonic bladder.

Overflow incontinence is considered to be caused by pressure exerted on the distended bladder by the abdominal muscles. Residual urine, urine remaining in the bladder after incomplete emptying, provides a medium for the growth of bacteria, and a UTI is common.

Tissue damage to the sphincters of the bladder from instrumentation, surgery, or accidents, scarring following urethral infections, lesions involving the sphincter, or relaxation of the perineal structures may cause urinary incontinence. The latter cause of incontinence is seen occasionally following childbirth. The problem is local in nature and does not involve the nervous system.

Assessment
SUBJECTIVE DATA

The following questions should be asked:
1. What is the frequency of incontinence?
2. Can anything be associated with precipitating incontinence (stress, fear, laughing, exercise)?
3. Is pain or burning present with incontinence?
4. Is there a state of awareness to void before incontinence?

OBJECTIVE DATA

1. Volume of output
2. Characteristics of urine
3. Patient's ability to follow directions
4. Is there a physiologic reason for incontinence (for example, spinal cord injury)?

After all available data concerning incontinence have been collected and a reasonable cause for the incontinence determined, a program of appropriate management may be instituted. If the incontinence has been a long-standing problem well managed by the person or the family, continuation of usual methods of managment is facilitated. In these instances, particularly in a hospital or other institutional setting, the nurse should ascertain the method used by the person and provide whatever equipment or assistance is needed during the stay. Although the person may be managing well, additional suggestions may be offered by the nurse concerning newer equipment available, less costly equipment, and so on as appropriate. The patient may wish to try alternative methods even after discharge from the setting.

Control of urinary incontinence

No program of bladder retraining or management of uncontrolled incontinence is likely to be successful without the cooperation of the individual involved. The probable outcomes of the management program should be included in planning for implementation of the program.

Control of urinary incontinence is largely dependent on its cause. Measures include treatment of associated conditions, programs of bladder retraining, surgical procedures, or the use of internal or external drainage devices. Both the person and nurse need to know that rehabilitation may take weeks or months to accomplish. The person often becomes discouraged by recurring accidental voiding and needs a great deal of encouragement. It is often helpful to teach the physiology of voiding so that there is better understanding of the problem. Consistency in carrying out any plan for bladder control is often the key to success.

Intervention related to cause
SPHINCTER DYSFUNCTION

Repair of a sphincter that has been cut is almost impossible. When the *external sphincter* has been damaged, the person will be incontinent on urgency. A voiding schedule can be planned so that voiding occurs before the bladder is full enough to exert sufficient pressure to open the internal sphincter involuntarily. When the *internal sphincter* is damaged, there may be no acute feeling of the need to void. Here the problem is not one of incontinence but of retention. To assure regular emptying of the bladder, a regular voiding schedule is necessary. If both sphincters are damaged, there will be total incontinence.

STRESS INCONTINENCE

Urinary incontinence that occurs during coughing, straining, or heavy lifting is termed *stress incontinence*. It is seen primarily in women who have relaxed pelvic musculature, but it may also occur in men following prostatectomy. When bladder pressure is suddenly increased, urine enters the proximal third of the urethra then returns to the bladder when the pressure is decreased after exertion. Some of the urine escapes through the urethra. Usually the person is continent at night because bladder pressure is decreased in the recumbent position.

Perineal exercises are helpful in controlling mild stress incontinence. The exercises consist in tightening and relaxing perineal and gluteal muscles and can be performed in a number of ways. Much of the problem of incontinence caused by a relaxed perineum in women can be prevented if perineal exercises are taught before and following childbirth. These exercises also may be included as part of the health teaching of any woman. Following are different methods for performing perineal exercises.
1. Tighten the perineal muscles as if to prevent voiding. Hold for 3 seconds, then relax.

2. Inhale through pursed lips while tightening perineal muscles.
3. Bear down as if to have a bowel movement. Relax then tighten perineal muscles.
4. Hold a pencil in the fold between the buttock and thigh.
5. Sit on toilet with knees held wide apart. Start and stop the urinary stream.

Surgery may be indicated for severe stress incontinence. A *vesicourethropexy* (Marshal-Marchetti operation) consists of fixation of the urethra to the fascia of the rectus muscle of the abdomen with support given to the neck of the bladder. A suprapubic incision is usually made, but a transvaginal repair may be carried out if there is scar tissue around the urethra from vaginal surgery. A urethral catheter is inserted postoperatively and maintained for 5 to 6 days. The urine may be pink, but the urethral catheter is not irrigated as a rule. It is not uncommon for difficulty in voiding to be experienced immediately after the indwelling catheter is removed. The woman is observed for signs of vaginal bleeding. Straining and use of Valsalva's maneuver should be avoided until healing has occurred, and mild laxatives may be given to prevent straining from constipation. Surgeons differ in the amount of activity permitted in the early postoperative period.

URGENCY

Incontinence caused by UTI is generally temporary, responding to treatment of the infection by systemic antibiotics. Specific causes of infection such as obstruction must be identified and corrected where possible. Provision must be made for adequate fluid intake of 3000 ml or more per day unless contraindicated by the person's medical condition. Because of heightened bladder sensitivity to even small amounts of urine, urgency to void demands rapid response by the nurse to the request for help to void.

The person who has a brain tumor, meningitis, or traumatic injury to the brain that prevents adequate voluntary control of bladder function and causes urgency incontinence by inhibiting cortical control over the urethrobladder reflex may also respond to a bladder retraining program. If the person's condition or response prohibits such a program, an internal or external drainage device should be used.

NEUROGENIC BLADDER DYSFUNCTION

Persons with injuries of the spinal cord experience a transitory period of "spinal shock" in which urinary retention occurs. This is treated with continuous or intermittent catheter drainage that aims to prevent a UTI and overdistention of the bladder. Following this acute stage, further management depends on the exact nature of any residual neurogenic bladder dysfunction. Persons with a lesion above the sacral segments and who have an intact urethrobladder reflex may initiate voiding by pinching or stroking trigger areas of the thighs or suprapubic area. In persons with a lower motor neuron lesion the use of the *Credé method,* which consists of exerting manual pressure over the bladder, may be ordered to provide for more complete bladder emptying. The appropriateness of this technique must be determined by the physician as based on the person's complete urologic status. An increasing number of persons with neurogenic bladder dysfunction are being taught intermittent self-catheterization using clean technique to prevent infection and manage incontinence. Maintenance of a regular schedule is stressed, and the frequency of catheterization is determined on an individual basis.

Certain medications are sometimes used alone or in conjunction with an intermittent catheterization program in the management of incontinence related to neurogenic bladder dysfunction. Alpha adrenergic drugs such as ephedrine sulfate are used to increase urethral resistance. Anticholinergic drugs such as propantheline (Pro-Banthine) are prescribed to control the reflex bladder activity.

Bladder retraining

When incontinence is caused by dulled cerebration in the elderly, by confusion, or by acute illness, control can usually be established if a persistent retraining schedule is carried out. A voiding schedule is developed and strictly adhered to until the person gradually relearns to recognize and react appropriately to the feeling of having to void. A successful program of this type, leading to complete rehabilitation, or continence, requires mental competence of the individual. Otherwise someone else must always remind the person to follow the schedule.

People ordinarily void on awakening, before retiring, and before or after meals. If a diuretic such as coffee has been taken it is usually necessary to void about 30 minutes later. Using this knowledge, the nurse can begin to set up a schedule for placing the person on a bedpan or taking the person to the toilet. Then if a record is kept for a few days of the times the person voids involuntarily, it is usually possible to determine the normal voiding pattern. If the schedule based on the pattern of incontinence is not successful, toileting every 1 to 2 hours should be carried out on a 24-hour basis.

During the retraining program, *mobilization* of the individual, attention to the *position* assumed for voiding, and adequate *fluid intake* contribute to reduction of the possibility of infection. Complete emptying of the bladder eliminates the possibility of residual urine acting as a medium for bacterial growth, while a high fluid intake provides for internal bladder irrigation.

Elderly persons isolated from their families and familiar surroundings, confused by institutionalization, or suffering feelings of loss of self-esteem frequently respond well to mobilization in bladder retraining programs. Their circulation is enhanced by the imposed mobility, their awareness is increased, and they respond to the attention given them. In instances where nurses believe that it is easier to change bed linen than it is to establish an appropriate bladder retraining program, a disservice is done to the individual and more work is actually created for the nurse. The person becomes subject to UTI and skin breakdown, and feelings of worthlessness are increased. For those who can be continent, incontinence is an indignity.

When it is possible, toileting should be carried out in surroundings that will remind the person of the voiding function; that is, the person should be taken to the bathroom where the toilet can be used. If this is not possible, a bedside commode can be an adequate substitute. Many men can void into a urinal more easily if allowed to stand at the bedside. The use of a bedpan is unfamiliar and distasteful to most persons, but in instances where women must remain in bed, voiding into a bedpan can be facilitated if the head of the bed is rolled up as high as allowed. This kind of positioning is more consistent with the position normally assumed for voiding and facilitates complete emptying of the bladder. Few persons can void adequately in the supine position.

Providing adequate amounts of fluids, a minimum of 3000 ml per day, is necessary to ensure that there will be adequate amounts of urine produced and present in the bladder to stimulate the voiding reflex at the proper times. Fluids may be given at scheduled times, the largest portion being given during the day before 4:00 PM to decrease the frequency of voiding through the night. Persons on fluid restriction because of medical problems should, of course, receive no more fluids than the amount prescribed.

Urinary drainage for incontinence

Occasionally there are justifications for the use of an indwelling catheter for the incontinent patient. Such reasons include the need to protect a surgical incision or to permit healing of a decubitus ulcer in the area. Indwelling catheterization, however, presents many potential dangers, such as UTI, urethritis, epididymitis, and urethral fistulas. All other means to manage incontinence should be tried before resorting to catheterization. Proper catheter management is essential.

In males, external drainage can be easily accomplished by applying a watertight apparatus to the penis. The following is one method. Select a condom of the correct size. Puncture a hole in the closed end of the condom with an applicator stick. Attach the punctured end of the condom to a firm rubber or plastic drainage tube with either a 3-mm (1/8-inch) piece of rubber tubing or a strip of adhesive tape (Fig. 33-20). Before applying the condom, clean and dry the penis thoroughly and check it for edema, skin breaks, or discoloration. Invert the condom and roll it onto the penis. There should be no roll at the top that could cause constriction. At least 2.5 cm (1 inch) of the

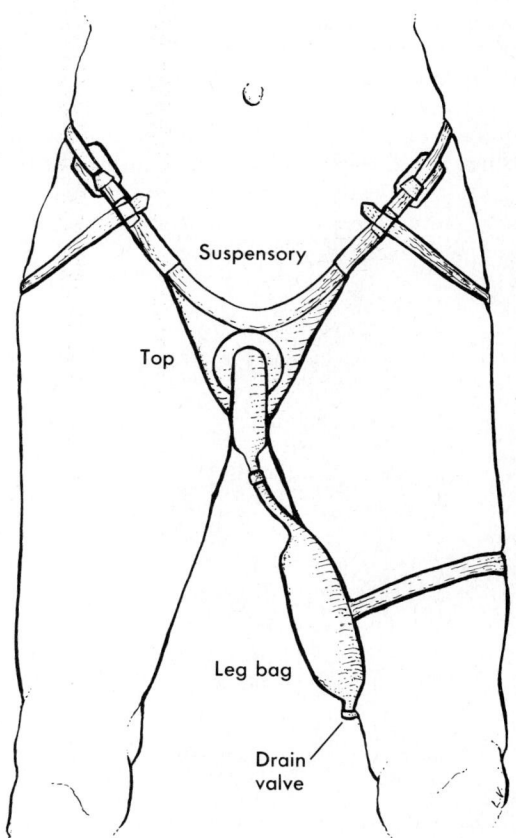

Fig. 33-21. Rubber urinary appliance. Note that it is supported by strap around waist and under buttock and is connected to drainage bag strapped to leg. Drain valve at bottom of bag is removed for emptying.

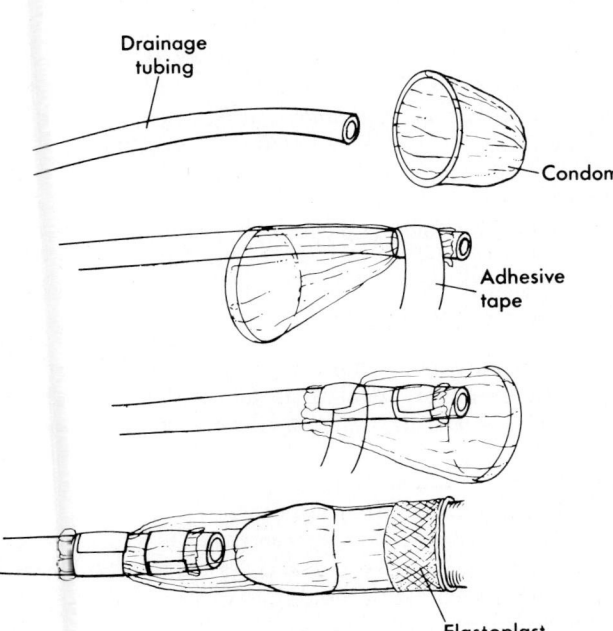

Fig. 33-20. One method of making external drainage apparatus.

condom should remain between the meatus and drainage tube to allow for penile erection. There should not be so much slack as to cause twisting and subsequent interference with drainage. Elastoplast is then applied over the condom and around the penis (never touching the skin). *Under no circumstances should adhesive tape be used.* The Elastoplast must not be constricting.

The external catheter should be removed daily, and the skin washed and checked. Frequent checking is necessary to determine whether edema or irritation is present and to ensure proper drainage. This is especially important in men with loss of sensation. The external device is attached to straight drainage or to a leg bag.

For persons who need external catheter drainage indefinitely, a rubber urinary appliance (sometimes called an incontinence urinal) may be used (Fig. 33-21). There are several models available, and the one best suited to the person's needs is selected. Two appliances are recommended to allow for cleaning and drying. They should be washed in mild soap, turned inside out, and thoroughly dried before using.

Most persons prefer to manage their own incontinence if they are at all able to do so. The nurse supports and encourages this, offering assistance as necessary and instruction in basic principles of skin care, equipment selection, and maintenance. The choice of management method should take into account the person's ability to manage as independently as is possible.

A relatively new surgical procedure, implanatation of an artificial urinary sphincter, can be used to achieve continence when other methods have failed. In this procedure a hydraulically activated sphincter mechanism is placed around the urethra or bladder neck. The sphincter is made to open and close at will by squeezing one of two bulbs implanted under the skin of the labia or scrotum (Fig. 33-22). Postoperative nursing care of the person with such an implant includes observation for and reporting of fever or pain on inflation of the device, swelling of the genitalia, and recurrence of incontinence. Complications of the procedure include erosion of the urethra, abscess, cellulitis, and mechanical malfunctions in the system. Men have had more success with the artificial sphincter than have women.

In some instances none of the above measures are appropriate or successful. Therefore, nursing goals of assisting the person to remain clean, free of odor, and free of decubiti may require external urinary protection; the type varies with the sex, functional status, and physical status of the person.

Data analysis and planning
OUTCOME CRITERIA

1. The person is free of perineal skin excoriation.
2. The person is free of urinary odor.
3. The person or significant others can describe or state the following:
   a. The relationship of adequate hygiene to the maintenance of skin integrity
   b. The relationship of adequate fluid intake to facilitate bladder training
   c. The bladder training plan
   d. How to care for minor skin problems if they occur
   e. How to obtain professional and community resources
      (1) Agencies that are available when necessary
      (2) How to obtain and maintain any needed supplies and equipment (drainage systems, commodes, protective padding, special beds)
      (3) Where and when to seek assistance if problems are encountered
   f. Plans for follow-up care

Nursing diagnoses

Possible nursing diagnoses for the patient with urinary incontinence follow. As in all disorders, the specific nursing diagnoses must be determined for each individual patient.

Comfort, alteration in: pain
Coping, ineffective individual
Home maintenance management, impaired
Knowledge deficit
Mobility, impaired physical
Self-care deficit: hygiene, toileting
Self-concept, disturbance in: body image
Skin integrity, impairment of: actual or potential
Urinary elimination, alterations in patterns

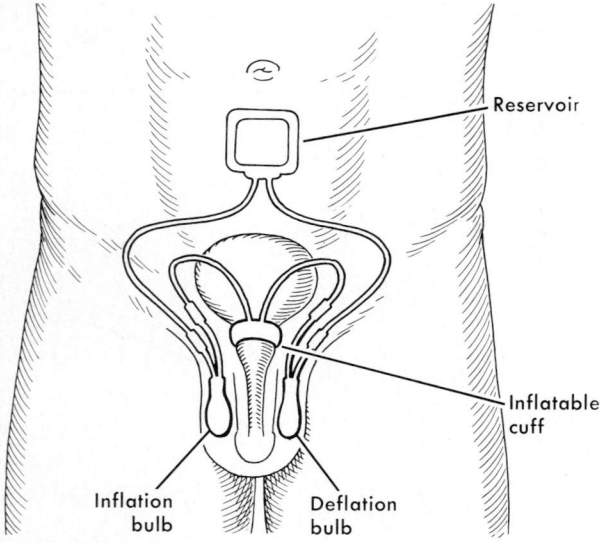

Fig. 33-22. Artificial bladder sphincter. Compression and release of inflation pump bulb inflates cuff surrounding urethra stopping urine flow. Compression and release of deflation pump bulb deflates inflatable cuff, returning fluid to storage reservoir. This releases urethral constriction, permitting urine to flow.

Implementation

ASSISTING WITH THE ACHIEVEMENT OF THERAPEUTIC GOALS

1. Encourage fluids to the limits of any prescribed restriction.
2. Use aseptic technique when handling the urinary drainage system.
3. Evaluate patient for participation in a bladder retraining program.
4. Encourage activity to prevent stasis of urine.
5. Meticulous skin care is essential to prevent breakdown.
6. Encourage self-care of incontinence, whenever possible.
7. Be supportive to patient by providing a relaxed atmosphere when providing care for incontinence.

COUNSELING AND TEACHING

The individual with urinary incontinence often experiences alterations in body image. The patient must receive adequate counseling to deal with this problem. The person should be encouraged to resume an active life-style whenever possible.

Teaching must include the following:
1. Care of any drainage systems that may be used
2. Perineal exercises for control of stress incontinence
3. Bladder retraining program whenever possible
4. Measures to maintain skin integrity
5. Signs and symptoms of UTI

Evaluation

Evaluation of the care of patients with urinary incontinency is based on the nursing diagnoses and goals. Questions to ask in this evaluation process include the following:
1. Is adequate urinary drainage being maintained?
2. Is the patient aware of professional and community resources available?
3. Can the patient state maintenance of necessary equipment?
4. Is the patient's skin free of excoriation?
5. Can the patient state plans for follow-up care?
6. Can the patient describe bladder training program?

TRAUMA TO THE URINARY TRACT

Assessing intactness of urinary tract structures must be part of the evaluation of any person with traumatic injury to the lower trunk. Injuries particularly related to urinary tract damage include fractures of the pelvis and sharp blows to the body.

TRAUMA OF THE LOWER URINARY TRACT

Pelvic fractures may result in *bladder perforation* and *ureteral* and *urethral tearing*. Following these injuries urinary output may be scant or absent, the urine may be bloody, and symptoms of peritonitis may appear. Treatment is directed toward stabilizing the patient and surgically repairing the perforation or laceration. After stabilizing the patient, a cystotomy may be performed to provide urinary drainage when injury involves the bladder or urethra.

KIDNEY TRAUMA

A sharp blow to the body, particularly to the lower back, may result in contusion, tearing, or rupture of a kidney. *Signs and symptoms include hematuria, pain, and tenderness of the upper abdominal quadrant and flank* on the involved side. Signs of shock may be present or absent depending on the extent of hemorrhage. Treatment includes control of bleeding, prevention of shock, and promoting drainage of the urinary tract. Vital signs, fluid balance records, and hematocrit levels are monitored to assess hemostasis. Complaints of pain may indicate developing ureteral colic, signifying obstruction of the ureter by a clot. Surgical intervention is required to control severe hemorrhage. Spontaneous healing of the kidney is otherwise permitted. Bed rest is maintained until gross hematuria clears; thereafter, activity is progressed according to continued absence of hematuria.

A kidney may become loosened and "float" or become displaced (*nephroptosis*). If symptoms of obstruction occur, the kidney may be sutured to its anatomic site (*nephropexy*). Postoperatively, the patient is positioned with the hips elevated to prevent tension on the suture line.

ASSESSMENT

Subjective data

1. Pain and discomfort
2. History of recent trauma, especially to lower abdomen
3. Voiding pattern, including time of last voiding

Objective data

1. Urine draining from open wounds
2. Incontinence
3. Hematuria
4. Diffuse abdominal pain on palpation
5. Distended abdomen on palpation

Diagnostic tests

1. KUB
2. Cystogram
3. IVP
4. Urinalysis

Data analysis and planning

The possible nursing diagnoses for the patient with trauma to the urinary tract depends on the nature and location of the injuries. Specific nursing care has been described in earlier sections of this chapter. Refer to the specific sections of this chapter for further information.

RENEL FAILURE

Renal failure indicates a state of total or nearly total loss of the kidney's ability to excrete waste products and to maintain fluid and electrolyte balance. Laboratory tests reflect the changes in the internal environment, and the person appears clinically ill. The person in renal failure cannot independently sustain life. Renal failure may be acute in onset or may develop slowly and progressively over a course of several years. When renal failure occurs suddenly, as within a few days, biochemical changes are often dramatic, and the person has little time to adjust to these changes. The person becomes very ill, and hospitalization, frequently involving placement in a critical care unit becomes necessary.

When renal failure occurs as the end result of a chronic kidney illness where kidney tissue is destroyed progressively over the course of several months or years, control of symptoms and preservation of functional abilities are achievable goals. Dietary adjustment, medications, and attention to preventing additional illnesses compensate for loss of kidney function in early stages of progressing renal failure. As renal function continues to deteriorate, dialysis or transplantation additionally becomes necessary to support life.

Acute renal failure

Acute renal failure occurs as a sudden and frequently reversible decrease or cessation of kidney function. It generally follows an identifiable trauma of either toxic or ischemic nature.[19] The health of the individual before the insult is usually good to adequate. Renal *ischemia* occurs when blood flow to the kidneys is reduced. The response of the normal kidney is vasoconstriction, which compounds the problem of reduced renal blood flow and increases renal ischemia. Perfusion problems affect both kidneys. When ischemia is prolonged, renal tubular tissue dies and frank renal failure develops.

A variety of substances are toxic to the cells of the renal tubules.[27] The kidney with its large bloodflow, ability to concentrate fluid in the medullary portion of the kidney (where the tubules are located) creates conditions in which exposure of tubular cells to toxins is maximized. The kidneys are affected bilaterally.

The major causes of ischemic and toxic injuries to the kidney that may lead to acute renal failure are listed in Table 33-6. Additionally, other conditions can precipitate acute renal failure: (1) acute glomerular disease, (2) acute severe infection of kidney tissue, (3) bilateral occlusion of the renal arteries, (4) mechanical obstructions in the urinary tract, and (5) hemoglobinemia and myoglobinemia. All of these conditions lead to massive and rapid destruction of kidney tissue.

Recovery from an episode of acute renal failure depends on the underlying illness, the condition of the patient, and the careful, supportive management given during the period of kidney shutdown. Mortality associated with acute tubular necrosis approaches 40%; these statistics largely reflect the deaths of severely ill persons in whom renal failure is a sequela to extensive underlying illness. Owing to the more widespread availability of dialysis, mortality directly attributable to decreased renal function from potassium intoxication, fluid overload, and acidosis has been reduced. The potential for recovery of renal function for those who survive the acute episode of tubular insufficiency is good. Although recovery statistics indicate that kidney tissue may regenerate more completely after toxic injury in comparison with ischemic injury, follow-up studies of persons years after episodes of acute tubular insufficiency show normal to near normal renal function.[15]

For those in whom acute renal failure has been caused by glomerular disease or severe infection of kidney tissue, the prognosis may not be as favorable. Return of renal function is determined by the extent of scarring and obliteration of functional renal tissue that has occurred during the acute episode of kidney failure. A significant number of adults who develop acute glomerulonephritis show some decrease in renal function, which may remain

Table 33-6. Conditions and substances that produce ischemic or nephrotoxic injury to the kidney

Ischemic*	Toxic†
Hypovolemia	Solvents (carbon tetrachloride, methanol, ethylene glycol)
Blood loss (surgery, trauma)	Heavy metals (lead, arsenic, mercury)
Plasma loss (burns, surgery, acute pancreatitis)	Antibiotics (kanamycin, gentamicin, polymyxin B, amphotericin B, colistin, neomycin, phenazopyridine)
Sodium and water loss (prolonged diarrhea or vomiting, GI tract drainage, sustained high fever)	Pesticides
Cardiac failure	Mushrooms
Myocardial infarction	
Cardiac arrhythmias	
Congestive heart failure	
Septic shock	

*Inadequate perfusion of the kidney.
†Injury to the kidney cells.

t a level not producing biochemical abnormalities or may progress to a chronic form of renal failure.

Signs and symptoms indicating the onset of acute renal failure appear rapidly and are a direct result of retention of fluids, electrolytes, and waste materials (Table 33-7). Typically, the person is acutely ill; in addition to the renal failure frequently being superimposed on an already severely compromised individual, biochemical changes occur rapidly and give the person little time to adjust to the altered internal environment. Either *oliguria* (urinary output below 400 ml/day) or *anuria* (urinary output below 100 ml/day) may be present, although oliguria is more common. Classically, the patient in acute renal failure shows a fall in urinary output within 1 to 2 days to between 50 and 400 ml/day. The specific gravity of the urine is low (1.010), and the osmolality of the urine approaches that of the person's serum (280 to 320 milliosmoles). Specific gravity and urine osmolality remain within this fixed range and reflect tubular damage with loss of concentrating ability. Additionally, the urine may show a higher concentration of sodium than would be expected in the case of dehydration or low circulating blood volume. This finding reflects the damaged kidneys' inability to conserve sodium ions and is an important consideration in diagnosing the existence of acute renal failure.

Fluid intake in excess of the diminished urinary output and insensible losses is retained in the body, resulting in edema. When fluid overload is excessive signs of congestive failure and pulmonary edema are present. Hypertension accompanies acute renal failure when the person is hypervolemic, although this is usually not a finding when fluid balance is controlled.

Retention of electrolytes and waste materials from cellular metabolism produces typical signs and symptoms often referred to as *uremia*. Serum potassium, urea nitrogen, and creatinine values rise sharply. In the person who has already sustained illness and trauma, urea nitrogen values may increase at a rate of 30 mg/100 ml/day. As urinary excretion of the acid end products of metabolism decreases, acidosis occurs, carbon dioxide values decline to 15 mEq/L or less, and Kussmaul's breathing occurs. Symptoms attributable to retained wastes and altered electrolyte balance include nausea, vomiting, drowsiness, fatigue, and shortness of breath with fluid overloading. Signs produced by these internal changes include confusion, convulsions, coma, GI tract bleeding, and asterixis.

Additional problems that may beset the person with acute renal failure are pericarditis and infection. Pericarditis is thought to develop as a result of pericardial irritation from accumulated metabolic wastes. It is diagnosed by the presence of a cardiac friction rub and pleuritic-like pain over the precordium. Fever often accompanies pericarditis. When fluid accumulates in the pericardial sac, the rub becomes less intense or absent and *pulsus paradoxus* (pulse weaker during inspiration) is likely to be present. Pericardial effusion can be confirmed by echocardiography. Infection frequently develops in response to lowered host resistance, multiple trauma, and immobility during the course of the illness.

When oliguria or rising creatinine and urea nitrogen values are noted, the physician must determine whether the decreased output and decreased renal function are the results of inadequate renal perfusion or of frank renal failure. This distinction directs treatment. In instances of poor kidney perfusion, restoring circulating volume by adding fluids and otherwise increasing cardiac output prevents death of kidney tissue and subsequent renal failure. In contrast, the treatment of true renal failure is supportive and is based on careful balance of input and output of fluid, electrolytes, and wastes. In addition to

Table 33-7. Symptoms caused by physiologic changes in acute renal failure

Symptoms	Physiologic effects	Findings
Oliguric phase		
Nausea; vomiting; drowsiness; confusion, coma; GI bleeding; asterixis; pericarditis	Inability to excrete metabolic wastes	Increased serum urea nitrogen, and creatinine levels
Nausea; vomiting; cardiac arrhythmias; Kussmaul's breathing; drowsiness; confusion; coma	Inability to regulate electrolytes	Hyperkalemia; hyponatremia; acidosis
Edema; congestive heart failure; pulmonary edema; hypertension	Inability to excrete fluid loads	Fluid overload; hypervolemia
Diuretic phase		
Urinary output of up to 4 to 5 L/day; postural hypotension; tachycardia	Increased production of urine	Hypovolemia; loss of sodium and potassium in urine
Increasing mental alertness and activity	Slowly increasing excretion of metabolic wastes	Initially, high BUN (fluid loss greater than solute loss); gradual return of BUN to normal

the urine sodium concentration as a diagnostic sign, the physician may wish to challenge the patient's ability to excrete fluid. In this instance usually 100 to 500 ml of fluid is given as rapidly as possible intravenously. A poorly perfused but intact kidney should respond with increased urinary output. During this treatment the patient must be closely monitored for signs and symptoms of congestive heart failure and pulmonary edema. The kidney in acute failure will be unable to produce a greater urine flow in response to this fluid challenge. The physician may give furosemide, 40 to 80 mg intravenously, in an attempt to produce a greater flow of urine. The test may be repeated if there is no response to the initial trial, although subsequent attempts to produce urine in this manner are contraindicated.

When the cause of a sudden acute decline in renal function cannot be identified, particularly when anuria is present, cystoscopy and retrograde pyelography may be used to detect the presence of any obstructive urinary tract disease.

The course of acute renal failure is usually characterized by *an initial oliguric phase followed in a number of days to a few weeks by a diuretic period.* Major patient care problems during the *oliguric phase* of illness include (1) inability to excrete metabolic wastes, (2) inability to regulate electrolytes, (3) inability to excrete fluid loads, (4) difficulty maintaining adequate nutrition, (5) increased potential for injury, and (6) discomfort. *Major patient care problems arising during the diuretic phase of the illness* include (1) inability to appropriately conserve fluid and (2) inability to appropriately conserve electrolytes.

Following the diuretic phase is a period of recuperation known as the *recovery phase.* During the recovery phase, renal function continues to improve. Gradually electrolytes and fluid status return to normal. The course of the recovery phase can last 3 to 12 months.

OLIGURIC PHASE

During the oliguric phase of acute renal failure, development of hyperkalemia, severe acidosis, severe fluid overload and pulmonary edema, infection, convulsions, or pericarditis connotes some urgency for control or resolution. Included among these problems are the major causes of death resulting from acute kidney failure.

Control and excretion of metabolic waste buildup

Because the patient's ability to excrete metabolic wastes (nonprotein nitrogen products and acids) cannot keep pace with production of these substances, alternative routes of excretion and control over production of these materials must be found. Means available to accomplish this include providing carbohydrate to spare protein stores, preventing additional tissue trauma, and increasing excretion of wastes through the lungs and through renal dialysis. Of these, dialysis is by far the most efficient and is the only true means available for controlling the internal environment of the severely ill hypercatabolic person. Daily laboratory tests will determine blood non-

protein nitrogens and bicarbonate levels, which serve as a guide for determining the frequency of dialysis.

Decreasing the production of metabolic wastes can be influenced through dietary means. Calories in the form of carbohydrates and fats provide energy and spare body protein stores, thus decreasing nonprotein nitrogen production. The body recycles urea to synthesize amino acids for protein building so that some regeneration of tissues can occur even though protein intake is curtailed.

Preventing infections and tissue breakdown decreases production of metabolic wastes. Aseptic technique should be rigorously pursued in all treatments performed on the patient. Indwelling lines and catheters are a common source of infection and are to be avoided when possible. *The patient should be isolated from anyone with an infection, including other patients, health care personnel, and visitors.* Detecting existent infections early so that treatment can be instituted promptly decreases tissue breakdown. When the patient is extremely weak and immobile, frequent turning and repositioning to prevent decubiti must be performed. Skin care for patients with edematous tissues should include observation and prevention of pressure and trauma; these tissues are particularly prone to breakdown.

Acidosis develops when hydrogen ion secretion and bicarbonate ion production diminish in the tubular cells. The pH of the blood decreases, the carbon dioxide content decreases, and central nervous system symptoms of drowsiness progressing to stupor and coma may appear. Although the lungs are unable to compensate totally for the increasing acid load, they help determine the rate at which acidosis develops and the frequency or need for dialysis. In compensating for increased metabolic acid loads, the lungs attempt to excrete more carbon dioxide. To maximize this pathway for acid excretion, pulmonary hygiene should be carried out. Preventing atelectasis and maintaining maximal lung expansion are goals of nursing care.

Regulation of electrolytes

Some common electrolyte disturbances occurring in acute renal failure are *hyperkalemia, hyponatremia (usually indicative of overhydration),* and increased body sodium content. The rate of accumulation of electrolytes varies greatly in acute renal failure; each patient must be managed individually. Daily or more frequent assessment of laboratory data and clinical signs and symptoms is needed to determine current electrolyte abnormalities and need for treatment.

Hyperkalemia

Patients in renal failure with extensive tissue trauma, infection, or bleeding are at a high risk of developing hyperkalemia. In the normal individual the potassium ion is exchanged in the distal convoluted tubule of the nephron for either sodium or hydrogen ions; for the healthy person there is no mechanism in the body to conserve the potassium ion. However, in the individual with acute renal failure in whom a large number of tubular cells are no longer functional, there exists no mechanism to remove potassium from the body. Hyperkalemia is said to exist when the serum concentration of this ion reaches a level of 5.5 mEq/L or higher. Serum concentrations of 7 to 10 mEq/L can be quickly reached in acute renal failure and are incompatible with normal cardiac function and life.

In monitoring for signs of potassium toxicity, electrocardiography and laboratory determinations of serum potassium are the most reliable indicators. Rarely does the patient become symptomatic, and pulse changes must not be relied on to indicate the degree of rise of potassium in the patient's system.

Interventions to control the rise of serum potassium and to prevent cardiac arrest include those that (1) decrease the intake of potassium, (2) decrease the liberation of potassium from body tissues, (3) protect the cardiovascular system, and (4) assist in removal of potassium from the body by nonrenal means.

Decreasing the intake of potassium is achieved by administering intravenous feedings or a diet in which the potassium content is very low or absent. All fluids and drugs that the patient receives intravenously should be checked for potassium content. Some medications (for example, most penicillin preparations) contain large amounts of this ion.

Controlling the breakdown of body tissues is extremely important in preventing a rapid rise in serum potassium.

Protecting the cardiovascular system from high levels of extracellular potassium (K^+) is essential. When high K^+ levels occur and the patient is exhibiting cardiovascular effects, renal dialysis is required. Because it takes several hours to get the dialysis treatment underway and for the K^+ to be reduced to safe levels other therapy is instituted. Hypertonic glucose (25%) may be given with 1 unit of regular insulin per 2 g of glucose. Over a 30-minute period, 200 to 300 ml of fluid is given to promote the movement of K^+ back into the cells. This lowers the serum K^+ level and reduces cardiac instability resulting from the high serum K^+ levels. The K^+ levels will begin to fall in 1 hour and will remain lowered for 4 to 6 hours.[6] In addition to hyperteonic glucose, calcium gluconate may be given intravenously to reduce the irritability of cardiac cells caused by the hyperkalemia.

To *promote the excretion of potassium* from the body when the kidneys are nonfunctional, an exchange resin such as polystyrene sodium sulfonate (Kayexalate) may be ordered for the patient as a temporary measure before a dialysis treatment when (1) the serum K^+ level is high and rising rapidly; (2) the serum K^+ level is rising, although at a controlled rate, and other metabolic disturbances do not necessitate dialysis; or (3) control of a rising serum K^+ is required before a patient's transfer to an acute care area where dialysis can be provided. This drug reduces serum potassium by exchanging sodium for potassium ions in the intestinal tract. It can be administered orally, through a nasogastric tube, or by enema. The medication is given orally when the patient's condition premits; oral daily doses range from 15 to 60 g/day. When sodium sulfonate is administered in enema form, the usual dose is 50 g of exchange resin for each enema; it may be repeated daily or as necessary to lower serum potassium. The medication is a powder that when mixed becomes a thick paste within a few seconds; therefore preparation should take place at the bedside just before administration. Often mannitol is used to mix the powdered sodium sulfonate, since it induces an osmotic shift of fluid into the bowel producing diarrhea, which helps to expel the medication, additional K^+ from the GI tract, and additional fluid from the hypervolemic patient. If spontaneous bowel movements do not occur, a cathartic or cleansing enema can be given to ensure the elimination of potassium from the bowel.

Hyponatremia

Hyponatremia in acute renal failure most commonly develops with overhydration of the patient. The oliguric patient cannot excrete large volumes of urine; when the administration of sodium-free or low-sodium intravenous or oral fluids continues in such an individual, the serum is diluted and the serum concentration of sodium falls.

In this situation hyponatremia is accompanied or caused by hypervolemia. In the very acutely ill, the situation commonly occurs when the patient receives numerous drugs and fluids in an attempt to treat coexisting life-threatening problems. When the volume of drugs and fluids cannot be reduced to a safe level, dialysis is required to remove the excess fluid and restore sodium balance.

Signs and symptoms of hyponatremia include warm, moist, flushed skin; muscle weakness, muscle twitching; and behavioral changes involving confusion, delirium, coma, and convulsions. Serum sodium concentrations will be below 130 mEq/L. The hematocrit and hemoglobin values suddenly fall without evidence of bleeding; this is caused by hemodilution.

Increased body sodium content

Increases in total body content of sodium also occur in acute renal failure. Commonly, this occurs when the patient is receiving medications high in sodium content and excess sodium in the diet. Edema and increasing blood pressure indicate retention of sodium and fluids even though the serum sodium concentration is normal or below normal.

Control of fluids

The oliguric or anuric patient is unable to excrete more than minimal amounts of fluid. Nursing care is directed toward three broad objectives: (1) monitoring for signs of fluid overload, (2) maintaining the patient's energy expenditure at a level compatible with the individual's state of health, and (3) controlling or helping the patient to control fluid intake.

All observations regarding the patient's state of hydration need to be recorded so that hour-to-hour and day-to-day comparisons can be made. Any finding indicating retention of fluids is reported to the physician. Edema can first be noted in dependent areas such as the feet and legs, in the presacral area, and around the eyes. The patient is observed carefully for signs of pulmonary edema and congestive heart failure. Central venous or arterial monitoring lines will help to provide data for short-term comparisons in managing the fluid balance of the critically ill person. Accurate recording of intake and output is extremely important as are daily weight records.

The patient in renal failure is unable to excrete fluid loads, and much energy is expended just to maintain current functional status. Positioning and activity are determined daily based on assessment of the energy level and ability to ventilate adequately.

Controlling fluid intake is essential when the ability to excrete fluid is limited. All fluid (parenteral and oral) must total only slightly more than daily output if severe overhydration is to be avoided. When the patient is neither to gain nor lose additional body fluid, the physician will calculate the patient's fluid replacement using the following as a guide: intake will approximate 500 ml/day plus urinary output and adjustments for additional fluid lost through fever, diarrhea, and wound drainage. Fortunately, when sodium intake is controlled, extreme thirst does not develop.

Devices that allow 50 to 150 ml of fluid to be isolated from the main intravenous solution container and drip chambers that allow precise control of fluids through administration of smaller drops of fluid are added safety measures when giving fluids parenterally to anuric or oliguric individuals. Accuracy in fluid balance records is essential. For the patient who is unable to take medications with small amounts of fluid, medications may be given in soft foods such as applesauce.

Maintenance of adequate nutrition

Most persons in acute renal failure are too ill to tolerate oral feedings either initially or for sustained periods of time. Some patients who are able to tolerate fluids orally find that eating food compounds the nausea they experience as a result of an altered biochemical environment and accompanying GI tract irrition. Intravenous hypertonic glucose in amounts of 100 g/day or more provides a temporary source of energy that slows the burning of the body's own protein stores. For patients who are severely ill or nauseated, maintaining positive nitrogen balance is not feasible. The total caloric intake for the patient on IV therapy will be influenced by the amount of fluids that can be tolerated in a 24-hour period.

If the patient is able to tolerate oral feedings, dietary protein and potassium are avoided unless dialysis has been initiated. In this case modest amounts of protein and potassium are allowed, thus increasing protein available for tissue building and increasing the palatability of the diet. Foods high in carbohydrate and fat content are encouraged. A total intake of 2000 calories per day is desired although often not achieved because of anorexia and nausea.

DIURETIC PHASE

After a period of oliguria or anuria, which may last a few days to 2 weeks, patients recovering renal function pass into another distinct phase of illness characterized by increased urinary output. Increased output indicates that the damaged nephrons are healing and are able to begin excreting urine. At first daily urine volume increases slowly, although within 1 to 2 days diuresis up to or exceeding 4 to 5 L/day may occur. Although fluid can be excreted, the kidneys are not yet healed. Often there is inability to excrete proportional amounts of waste materials, and serum concentrations of urea nitrogen may rise or remain elevated as urine volume increases. At times excessive excretion of sodium and potassium occurs during diuresis. Complete recovery of renal function is slow and requires anywhere from days to several months. Return of the renal function to normal or near normal levels is evidenced when the kidney can both conserve and dilute urine and when serum electrolytes and nonprotein nitrogen levels become normal.

Medical treatment during the diuretic phase is aimed at the symptoms. Electrolyte imbalances are likely to persist. These are treated as in the oliguric phase. Dehydration can become a potential problem when polyuria is present. Fluid replacement may become necessary.

ASSESSMENT
Subjective data
1. Voiding patterns
2. Weight gain
3. Nausea
4. Family history of renal disease
5. Recent history of flu-like symptoms
6. Medication use (nephrotoxins)

Objective data
1. Amount of urine excreted in 24 hours
2. Blood pressure, particularly postural changes
3. Daily weights
4. Fluid status
   a. Peripheral edema
   b. Auscultate breath sounds
   c. Skin turgor
5. Halitosis as a result of acidosis and/or ammonia secretion
6. Changes in mental status
7. Pulse rate and rhythm

Diagnostic tests
1. Serum chemistries
2. KUB
3. IVP

DATA ANALYSIS AND PLANNING
Nursing diagnoses
Fluid volume deficit, actual or potential
Fluid volume excess, actual or potential
Nutrition, alteration in: less than body requirements
Urinary elimination, alteration in patterns

Outcome criteria for the person in renal failure during the oliguric phase

The person demonstrates control of internal environment through the following:

1. Absence of pulmonary edema
2. Absence or control of peripheral edema
3. Control of blood pressure (range between 170/100 and 100/60 mm Hg)
4. Restored or maintained mental alertness
5. Control of electrolyte balance
   a. Sodium range of 125 to 145 mEq/L
   b. Potassium range of 3.0 to 6.0 mEq/L
   c. Bicarbonate above 14 mEq/L
6. Control of protein catabolism
   a. Urea nitrogen below 100 mg/dl
   b. Creatinine below 12 mg/dl
   c. Absence of skin breakdown
7. Absence of bleeding
8. Resolution or control of intercurrent illness (congestive heart failure, shock)

The person is free of the following:

1. Infection
2. Injury resulting from decreased level of awareness and strength
3. Toxicity from inadequately excreted medication

Outcome criteria for the person with renal failure during the diuretic phase

The person or significant others can state, identify, or describe the following:

1. Extent of recovery of kidney function
2. Any preventable environmental or health factor involved in generating the illness
3. A diet to maintain positive nitrogen balance and sufficient caloric intake
4. Signs and symptoms of dehydration and sodium and potassium loss
6. Plans for follow-up care

IMPLEMENTATION

Oliguric phase
Assisting with achievement of therapeutic goals

1. Fluid and electrolyte imbalance
   a. Assist in maintaining adequate nutrition.
   b. Assist patient in remaining within limitations of diet (protein, sodium, potassium, phosphorus, and fluid limits).
   c. Maintain fluid restrictions.
   d. Keep accurate records of intake and output.
   e. Weigh patient daily.
   f. Monitor vital signs frequently, including postural signs.
   g. Assess fluid status of patient.
   h. Administer phosphate binding medications as prescribed.
2. Activity
   a. Maintain strict bedrest in acute phase.
   b. Assist patient with ADL to conserve energy.
   c. Promote early ambulation.
   d. Maintain safe environment for patient.
3. Prevention and treatment of infection
   a. Assess patient for signs and symptoms of infection.
   b. If catheterization is required, asepsis must be maintained during insertion. Meticulous catheter care is essential.
   c. Maintain pulmonary hygiene while patient is on bedrest.
   d. Turn patient frequently.
   e. Administer antibiotics as prescribed.
4. Altered bleeding tendency
   a. Protect patient from injury.
   b. Administer stool softeners as prescribed.
   c. Instruct patient to use soft toothbrush.
   d. Assess patient for signs of bleeding
      (1) Bruising
      (2) Perform quaiac tests on stools, emesis, and NG returns
      (3) Changes in vital signs
5. Altered neurologic status
   a. Assess orientation at least every 8 hours.
   b. Assess level of concsiousness at least every 8 hours.
   c. Report any change in mental status to physician immediately.
   d. When ambulatory, assess patient's motor skills at least every 8 hours.

Assisting with comfort and ADL

1. Assist patient with ADL to conserve energy.
2. Instruct patient to deep breath when experiencing nausea
3. Provide fluid in small amounts; gingerale and other effervescent soft drinks are often tolerated better than other fluids.
4. Administer antiemetics as prescribed.
5. Provide patient with moist cloth to keep lips and mouth moist.
6. Meticulous mouth care is essential.
7. Meticulous skin care is essential.
   a. Assess skin for puritus and rashes.
   b. Bathe patient every day or more often if necessary, using super fat soap.
   c. Administer antipuritics (Benedryl, Periactin) as prescribed.

Control of environment

1. Protect patient from chilling.
2. Maintain a calm, supportive environment.
3. Reverse isolation may be instituted.
4. Use humidifier during dry months.

Diuretic phase

During the diuretic phase, nursing implementation is directed toward detection of fluid losses and electrolyte imbalances. Serious fluid and electrolyte depletion may occur. The care is the same as described in the oliguric phase with the exception of the following:

1. Fluid and electyrolyte imbalance
   a. Assess patient for adequate hydration.

b. Assess for changes in mental status indicative of low serum sodium levels.

c. Irregular apical pulses is indicative of hypokalemia.

2. Activity
a. Encourage independence in ADL as tolerated.
b. Encourage early ambulation as tolerated.

3. Coping with Illness
a. Encourage the development of a nurse-patient relationship that will assist the patient in expressing perceptions of illness.
b. Promote independence in patient.
c. Involve significant other in care of patient.

Teaching

During the diuretic phase the patient is usually ready for the start of the education process that is necessary for patients with kidney disease. These teaching plans must include the following elements:

1. Cause of renal failure.
2. Identification of preventable environmental or health factors contributing to the illness (for example, hypertension, nephrotoxic drugs).
3. Prescribed medication regimen.
4. Prescribed dietary regimen.
5. Signs and symptoms of returning renal failure.
6. Signs and symptoms of infections.
7. Need for on-going follow-up care.

PREVENTION OF ACUTE RENAL FAILURE

The incidence of acute renal failure can be reduced through identification and observation of populations at risk and identification and control of environmental risk factors. The greatest incidence of acute renal failure occurs in persons who have undergone major trauma, extensive burns, aortic surgery, massive blood loss, or severe myocardial infarction with or without associated arrhythmia. Acute renal failure also frequently occurs in patients with sepsis and in those having abnormal intravascular coagulation, such as DIC, since these acutely ill persons are prime candidates for inadequate kidney perfusion. Frequent monitoring of urinary output and detection of excessive losses of body fluid will help to identify instances of inadequate renal perfusion before development of renal failure.

Significant factors in preventive care for the general population include control of nephrotoxic drugs, increased medical supervision of persons with sore throats and upper respiratory tract infections, and increased case finding and treatment of individuals with bacteriuria and obstructive disease of the urinary system. Attempts to control the distribution and identification of nephrotoxic drugs and chemicals is largely accomplished through the Food and Drug Administration (FDA). Identification of nephrotoxic drugs and chemicals, enforced labeling of these substances, and drug dispensing by prescription only are examples of this agency's attempts to promote public health. Proper labeling and storage of potentially toxic drugs and chemicals in the home can reduce further the number of accidental ingestions of nephrotoxic substances.

Chronic renal failure

Chronic renal failure exists when the kidneys are no longer capable of maintaining an internal environment consistent with life and when return of function is not anticipated. For the majority of individuals the transition from health to a state of chronic or permanent disease is a slow one extending over a number of years. Recurrent infections and exacerbations of nephritis, obstruction of the urinary tract, and destruction of vessels from diabetes and long-standing hypertension lead to scarring of kidney tissue and progressive loss of renal function. Some individuals, however, develop total irreversible loss of renal function acutely; such loss of renal function usually develops in a matter of a few hours or days and follows a direct traumatic insult to the kidneys.

Chronic renal failure exists as a major health problem in the United States. Approximately 8 million individuals now have chronic kidney disease; approximately 60,000 persons die each year as the result of renal failure.[29]

PATHOPHYSIOLOGY

During chronic renal failure some of the nephrons (including the glomerulus and tubules) are thought to remain intact while others are destroyed (intact nephron hypothesis). The intact nephrons hypertrophy and produce an increased volume of filtrate with increased tubular reabsorption in spite of a decreased GFR. This adaptive method permits the kidney to function until about three fourths of the nephrons become destroyed. The solute load then becomes greater than can be reabsorbed, producing an osmotic diuresis with polyuria and thirst. Eventually, as more nephrons are damaged, oliguria occurs with retention of waste products.

PROGNOSIS

The individual with chronic renal failure can to some extent control and manage the symptoms of the disease. Although renal function that has been lost as a result of destruction of kidney tissue cannot be recovered, the life of the person can be maintained by limiting the intake of substances that require renal excretion and by providing alternative routes of excretion for waste products and electrolytes. By adhering to a prescribed management routine, albeit quite strict and demanding, life may be sustained. For some individuals medication and diet therapy alone may control uremic symptoms; other individuals may require dialysis or transplantation to control the symptoms of their disease.

PREVENTION

Obstruction and infection of the urinary tract and hypertensive disease are common and often asymptomatic causes of renal damage and renal failure. A significant reduction in the incidence of renal failure can be affected through increasing attention to general health promotion. Yearly physical examinations in which blood pressure is determined, urinalysis is performed, and the person is questioned about dysuria or pain in the urinary tract assist in early detection of diseases that may lead to renal failure.

General health maintenance can reduce the number of individuals progressing from renal insufficiency into frank renal failure. Care is aimed toward adequately treating medical problems and closely supervising the person's health status in times of stress (infection, pregnancy).

CLINICAL PICTURE

Although the clinical course of chronic renal disease varies from individual to individual, there are common features of the illness. Signs and symptoms result from disordered fluid and electrolyte balance, alterations in regulatory functions of the body, and retention of solutes. *Azotemia* (excess nitrogenous products in the blood), *anemia,* and *acidosis* are always present. Potassium and hydrogen ion excretion is impaired. Fluid and sodium balance is abnormal and may involve either abnormal retention or secretion of sodium and water; thus urinary volume can be decreased, normal, or increased. With end-stage renal disease, hyperuricemia is a common finding, although the varied serum levels of uric acid seem to have no definite relationship to the exact level of kidney function.[15] Increased levels of serum phosphate are characteristic, and calcium levels may be low or normal. These findings result from decreased renal excretions of phosphate and simultaneous reduction in ionized serum calcium. Through increased production of parathormone the body may reestablish a normal serum calcium level, although this is accomplished at the expense of the individual's bone matrix.

Hypertension may or may not be present. Often with the development of end-stage renal disease blood pressure is elevated and seems to be the result of increased total body water, a renally released vasopressor, or an inadequately secreted vasodepressor.[2] Glucose intolerance may be seen although usually not of sufficient severity to warrant treatment. The rising blood sugar level appears to be the result of an altered biochemical environment produced by the failing kidneys and does not signify the development of diabetes mellitus. As renal failure progresses the patient develops increased pigmentation of the skin; the skin becomes sallow or brownish in tone. With more advanced and insufficiently treated renal failure the patient may develop muscular twitching, numbness in the feet and legs, pericarditis, and pleuritis. These signs will disappear with restabilization of the patient with diet and medication or with the additional assistance of dialysis.

The symptoms of uremia usually develop so slowly that the patient and family often do not recall the time of onset of the illness. Symptoms generally noticed as uremia develops include lethargy, headaches, physical and men-

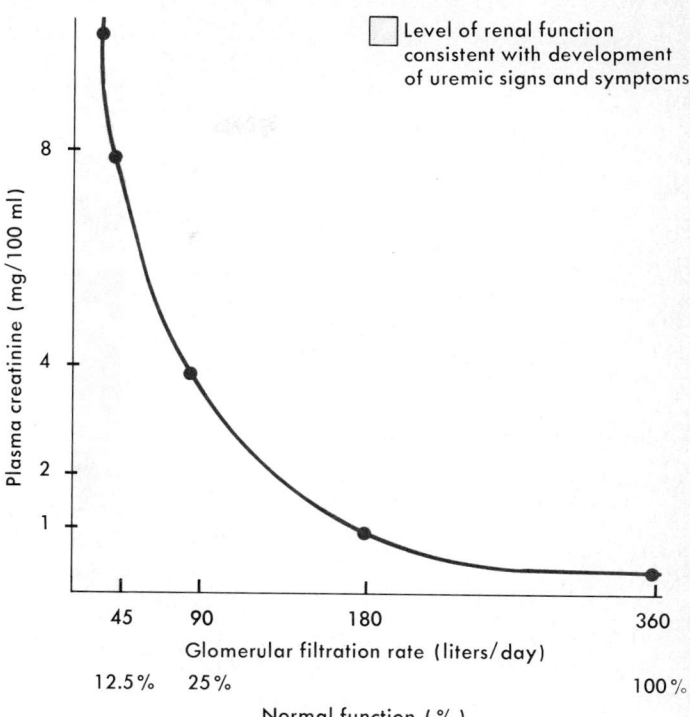

Fig. 33-23. Glomerular filtration and plasma creatinine levels.

tal fatigue, weight loss, irritability, and depression. Anorexia, persistent nausea and vomiting, shortness of breath on either mild or no exertion, and pitting edema are symptomatic of severe loss of renal function. Pruritus may be absent, mild, or severe.

The point at which the patient becomes obviously symptomatic and displays signs typical of renal failure occurs when approximately 80% to 90% of renal function has been lost (Fig. 33-23). At this level of renal function, creatinine clearance values will fall to 15 ml/minute or less.

Alterations in fertility

As end-stage renal failure develops, most women note changes in their menstrual cycle. Bleeding may occur at more widely spaced intervals, may be heavier or lighter in flow than normal, or may cease all together. This obvious change in reproductive cycle is usually accompanied by changes in fertility. Ovulation may occur normally or may occur only a few times a year. Pregnancy in uremic women is of much lower incidence than in the normal population. In men impotence may occur as chronic renal failure progresses toward end-stage disease. Dialysis or more vigorous treatment of uremia is indicated to return or maximize reproductive function. It should be stressed that sexual activity of some persons with chronic renal failure may remain quite normal even though changes in reproductive ability are present.

Table 33-8 summarizes the extent of organ system involvement experienced by patients with chronic renal failure.

Table 33-8. Summary of organ system involvement in patients with chronic renal failure

System	Manifestation	Cause
Integumentary		
Skin	Pallor	Anemia
	Gray/bronze pigmentation	Pigment retained
	Dry and scaly	Decreased size of sweat glands
		Decreased activity of oil glands
	Pruritus	Dry skin; phosphate deposits
Nails	Thin, brittle	Protein wasting
Hair	Dry	Decreased activity of oil glands
	Brittle	Protein wasting
Gastrointestinal		
Oral cavity	Halitosis (fetor uremicus)	Urea converted to ammonia by saliva
	Bleeding of gums	Change in platelet activity
Stomach	Nausea, vomiting, anorexia	Serum uremic toxins
	Gastritis, ulceration	Serum uremic toxins
Lower bowel	Constipation	Aluminum hydroxide given as phosphate binders
Cardiovascular	Hypertension	Fluid overload
		Renin-angiotensin mechanism
	Congestive heart failure	Fluid overload, anemia
	Arteriosclerotic heart disease	Chronic hypertension
		Calcification of soft tissues
	Pericarditis	Uremic toxins in pericardial fluid
		Fibrin formation on epicardium
Pulmonary	Uremic "lung" or pneumonitis	Uremic toxins in pleural space and lung tissue
Neurologic	Fatigue, headache, sleep disturbance	Uremic toxins
	Muscle irritability	Electrolyte imbalances
	Seizures	Cerebral swelling resulting from fluid shifting
Hematologic		
	Anemia	Suppression of RBC production
		Decreased survival time of RBCs
		Loss of blood through bleeding
		Loss of blood during dialysis
	Bleeding	Mild thrombocytopenia
		Decreased activity of platelets
Metabolic	Carbohydrate intolerance	Decreased sensitivity to insulin in peripheral tissues
		Delayed production of insulin by pancreas
		Increased survival time of insulin
	Hyperlipidemia	Increased production of serum triglycerides
		Increased output of glycerides by liver as a result of elevated insulin levels
Endocrine	Hyperparathyroidism	Elevated serum phosphate results in decreased serum calcium which stimulates parathyroid
	Infertility	Mechanism unknown
	Sexual dysfunction	Mechanism unknown

INTERVENTION

Major problems for the patient in chronic renal failure include (1) inability to appropriately control fluid balance; (2) inability to regulate electrolyte balance; (3) inability to excrete metabolic wastes; (4) inability to transport oxygen to cells; (5) inability to maintain normal rest and sleep patterns; (6) difficulty in maintaining adequate nutrition; (7) increased potential for physical injury; (8) discomfort; (9) alterations in fertility; and (10) changes in life-style, group membership, and feelings regarding self. Treatment goals for the person with chronic renal failure are listed in Table 33-9.

Control of fluid balance

The ability to excrete sodium and water in the urine varies considerably in chronic renal failure. Although volume problems for most patients with chronic end-stage renal disease involve hypervolemia resulting from a marked inability excrete sodium and water, some patients

Table 33-9. Treatment goals for the person with chronic renal failure

1. Stabilization of the internal environment as demonstrated by the following:
   a. Mental alertness, attention span, and appropriate interaction with the environment.
   b. Absence or control of peripheral edema, absence of pulmonary edema.
   c. Control of electrolyte balance:
      Sodium   125 to 145 mEq/L
      Potassium   3 to 6 mEq/L
      Bicarbonate   > 15 mEq/L
      Calcium   9 to 11 mg/dl
      Phosphate   3 to 5 mg/dl
   d. Serum albumin > 2 g/dl
   e. Control of protein catabolism and protein breakdown products
      Urea nitrogen   < 100 mg/dl
      Creatinine   < 15 mg/dl
      Uric acid   < 12 mg/dl
   f. Absence of joint inflammation and pain.
2. Infection and abnormal bleeding are not present.
3. Blood pressure is controlled at less than 160/100 mm Hg sitting and less than 30 mm Hg postural change on standing.
4. Anorexia, nausea, and pruritus are absent or controlled.
5. Intercurrent illness is resolved or controlled (heart failure, infection, dehydration).
6. There is no toxicity from inadequately excreted medication.
7. Nutrient intake is sufficient to maintain positive nitrogen balance.

are unable to conserve these substances and are subject to hypovolemic states. With either marked inability to excrete or conserve body fluid, the patient can develop severe fluid imbalances in a relatively short period of time. Care is directed toward identifying fluid imbalances and in providing an intake of sodium and water equivalent to the amounts of these substances excreted. The desired effect of this care is to maintain the patient in a normotensive, normovolemic state.

Controlling sodium intake can be an extremely challenging problem for both the nurse and the patient. Any sudden increase in weight indicates accumulating fluid, and the source of this fluid must be sought with the patient. Often when the person is not acutely ill and is responsible for control of intake, the problem can be traced to excess sodium ingestion, which produces thirst. In helping to avoid this cycle of thirst leading to increased fluid ingestion and overhydration, the patient is carefully taught the allowances of sodium and fluid in the diet and what restrictions are to be observed in purchasing commercially prepared foods. The words "sodium" and "salt" should be sought on food labels when the person is on a severely sodium-restricted diet, and these foods should be avoided. At times the person is unable to offer an explanation for increasing thirst and sodium ingestion. At this point the question of home self-medication (for example, sodium bicarbonate for indigestion) should be raised. After failure to uncover increased intake of either sodium or fluid to explain hypervolemia, the person is asked to list for a period of 3 consecutive days all foods and fluids ingested. This list can then be reviewed with the individual and used not only to uncover instances of dietary indiscretion but also as a teaching tool.

Regulation of electrolyte balance

Potassium and phosphorus retention occur in chronic renal failure. Signs of potassium intoxication and the role of cation exchange resins in the intestinal tract as an alternative route of excretion are discussed on p. 997. Serum potassium can be at least partially controlled in chronic renal failure by decreasing dietary and drug intake. Thorough diet teaching of the patient and all persons responsible for food preparation is essential. This teaching should help the patient identify the foods that are high in potassium and the methods of cooking that can reduce the potassium content of the diet. *Salt substitutes should be avoided by all patients with chronic renal disease since they contain large amounts of potassium.* Medications that are prescribed for the patient should be reviewed for potassium content.

Significant rises in serum potassium can be averted by preventing tissue breakdown. Potassium is largely an intracellular cation, and extensive tissue damage can liberate a lethal amount of this ion into the system of the patient with chronic renal failure. Patients should be advised to seek medical attention when symptoms of infection, GI bleeding, or other problems first appear.

When the kidneys fail, the ability to excrete phosphorus decreases. This leads to a vicious cycle whereby

Ca^{++} decreases, parathormone is stimulated, and bone demineralization occurs. Because the excess phosphorus is not excreted, calcium and phosphorus precipitate out in soft tissue. The serum phosphorus level again rises, the calcium level falls, and the cycle continues. Severe bone demineralization may develop, and if the problem continues unabated hyperparathyroidism can occur. Serum levels show elevated phosphorus with low to normal levels of Ca^{++}. Treatment is aimed at decreasing serum phosphorus levels. Aluminum hydroxide preparations that bind phosphorus in the intestinal tract and allow it to be eliminated are given in doses ranging from 1 to 5 g daily.

Aluminum hydroxide is best taken at mealtimes. It should not be taken with other medications because it can bind drugs in the intestinal tract. Aluminum hydroxide is constipating, and stool softeners or laxatives may have to be given to patients receiving large doses of it. Depressed serum levels of Ca^{++} may result not only from elevated levels of phosphorus but also from the inability of the diseased kidney to activate vitamin D. In the absence of vitamin D there is poor absorption of Ca^{++} from the intestinal tract. In some instances activated vitamin D or calcium supplements or both are prescribed.

Prevention of metabolic waste buildup

Azotemia and *acidosis* occur in all patients with chronic renal failure, although the severity of the problems and the degree to which the person has developed tolerance to the altered internal environment vary considerably.

Metabolic waste production can be significantly reduced by controlling dietary protein intake and by preventing catabolism of existing protein stores. The amount of protein allowed in the diet for the person with chronic renal failure can vary from 20 to 80 g/day. The specific level of protein intake prescribed depends on the presence of some means for clearing the products of protein breakdown from the patient's system. Dietary protein intake is more liberal for persons who have some ability to excrete wastes in their urine and for those being treated with dialysis. When restricting dietary protein, the quality of that allowed must be high. The persons must be taught to select foods that contain all of the essential amino acids. When calories are provided in the form of carbohydrate and fat for immediate energy needs, smaller amounts of protein can suffice for cellular growth and repair. Catabolism of existing protein stores liberates nitrogenous wastes. For this reason sources of potential infection such as indwelling catheters are avoided, and when infection is noted, it is immediately treated.

In chronic renal failure the kidneys are unable to excrete hydrogen ions and to manufacture bicarbonate. *Metabolic acidosis* results. On the basis of laboratory data acidosis may appear to be severe; however, persons with chronic renal failure adjust to lowered serum bicarbonate levels and often do not become acutely symptomatic even when bicarbonate levels reach values of 15 to 16 mEq/L. Because of this adjustment, treatment with bicarbonate is not routine. The lungs assume a prominent role in regulating acid-base balance, and helping the individual to maintain pulmonary function becomes an important objective for nursing care.

Determining patient tolerance of a state of acidosis that can fluctuate from moderate to critical levels (as additional stressors such as infection and blood loss occur) is important in the nursing care given the patient. Severe acidosis results in central nervous system depression.

Maintenance of oxygen transport to cells

Anemia universally accompanies chronic renal disease. Hematocrit values of 16% to 22% are not abnormal for these individuals. Anemia results from both a decreased production of red blood cells and a decrease in longevity of the cells in circulation. Although oral iron supplements may be tried, iron is not well absorbed by the GI tract in chronic renal failure, and in some individuals it may cause nausea and vomiting. Since dietary sources of folate (folic acid) may be restricted in chronic renal failure, and food preparation may further decrease the amount of folate ingested, this vitamin may be given as a medication. A sufficient dose is 1 mg/day. Transfusions are not generally given unless the hematocrit level becomes extremely low and the patient is grossly symptomatic. The reason for this is that when transfusions are given frequently, the patient's own stimulus to red cell production is decreased.

The severely anemic person complains of extreme fatigue and shortness of breath. Because of a lack of red cells there is an inability to transport sufficient oxygen to cells for energy production. Milder complaints of the anemic person include an inability to work or play without extended rest periods. Preventing the accumulation of excess fluid in a person with a very low hematocrit level allows energy to be used for ADL rather than for carrying extra fluid.

Other important nursing activities include helping the person to control blood losses. A soft toothbrush is recommended for oral care. Antacids taken at regular and frequent intervals can reduce GI tract bleeding. The person is instructed to observe for melena and to report this finding to the physician without delay. Anabolic steroids may be used, but their side effects of fluid retention, masculinization, and hirsutism may limit their usefulness.

Some degree of peripheral neuropathy occurs in almost all persons with chronic renal failure. Numbness, tingling, and burning of the extremities are common complaints. Treatment that is effective in controlling these symptoms consists of more intensive management of the uremic state.

Promotion of comfort, rest, and sleep

Rarely does the person with chronic renal failure have acute sharp pain; however, these individuals are subject to a wide variety of chronic discomforts. Most commonly these discomforts include pruritus, muscle cramping, numbness and tingling in the hands and feet, thirst, headaches, and irritation of the eyes. Most persons with end-stage renal disease develop pruritus. Patients relate that itching is of a deep sensation. Factors that seem to exacerbate the itching include increasing levels of serum phosphorus, dry skin, warm moist heat, and emotional stress. Itching is largely symptomatic, and measures that are effective in controlling it vary from individual to individual. Reducing levels of serum phosphorus with aluminum hydroxide preparations decreases itching for most patients. Keeping the skin moist and supple through use of lotions and bath oils, controlling the room temperature during sleep to prevent excessive warmth, emollient baths, and bathing with a vinegar solution are measures alone or in combination that may provide some relief from itching. Medications such as trimeprazine tartrate (Temaril) are also prescribed as necessary and for some individuals provide much relief from itching. Since emotional stress seems to increase the itching, helping the person verbalize feelings may provide for some resolution of conflict and help decrease itching. The urge to scratch the skin is acute in some persons. Because scratching is often vigorous injury to the skin with subsequent infection can result. Fingernails are trimmed closely. In preference to fingernails, a soft cloth should be used to scratch the skin.

Muscle cramping in the lower extremities and the *hands* is common in renal failure. Often cramping can be correlated with sodium depletion. Primary treatment for muscle cramping involves controlling the state of uremia and fluid and electrolyte balance. Temporary measures of heat and massage are effective for some persons.

Headaches in chronic renal failure result from a variety of causes. These include increasing blood pressure, progressing uremia, and rapid changes in osmotic gradients between cellular, interstitial, and intravascular compartments. Treatment of these problems has been discussed previously.

Ocular irritation in chronic renal failure is caused by calcium deposits in the conjunctiva that cause burning and watering of the eyes. Treatment involves controlling the plasma phosphate level through administration of oral aluminum hydroxide preparations. "Artificial tears" (methylcellulose) placed in the conjunctival sac every few hours also help to reduce irritation.

Insomnia and *chronic daytime fatigue* are common complaints of persons with chronic renal failure. This reversal of normal sleep patterns has been attributed to a variety of causes. These include (1) recurring occupation with thoughts concerning the disease state and resultant changes in life-style, (2) pruritus, and (3) the state of uremia itself. Reduction of high serum levels of urea nitrogen and creatinine through decreasing dietary intake of protein or dialysis may bring sleep patterns more toward normal. When control of uremia fails to cure insomnia, mild central nervous system depressants may be ordered.

General comfort at bedtime is needed to induce sleep at any time and is especially important whenever sleeping problems arise. Comfort measures can include warm baths, pursuing quiet activities an hour or two before bedtime, controlling itching, or anything the patient finds calming and soothing.

The individual who is awake a significant portion of the night may need to plan for rest periods during the day. These rest periods should be taken far enough ahead of bedtime to prevent compounding sleeplessness.

Maintenance of adequate nutrition

Maintaining a good nutritional intake can be difficult for persons with chronic renal failure. Anorexia, nausea, and vomiting frequently occur, and diets can be so severely restricted that they bear little resemblance to normal dietary patterns. In uremia, disturbances in fluid, electrolyte, and waste composition of body fluids occur and produce changes in osmotic gradients in all cells. When these changes occur in the cells of the GI tract and the central nervous system, anorexia, nausea, and vomiting result. Persons with uremia are prone to bleeding of the GI tract and the oral cavity. Urea is broken down to ammonia by the action of intestinal bacteria. Since ammonia is a mucosal irritant, ulceration and bleeding can occur. In addition to GI tract problems that lead to nausea and vomiting, there is a decreased salivary flow in persons with chronic renal disease. An ammonia smell and taste can accumulate in the mouth quickly and can further compound anorexia. Treatment includes administering antacids every 2 to 4 hours to decrease GI irritation. Dietary control of uremia, perhaps augmented by dialysis, should help to control disturbances in fluid, electrolyte, and waste composition of body fluids and thus help to control nausea and vomiting. Oral hygiene, especially before meals, is important to combat anorexia.

Modifying the diet as possible to the preferences of the individual can also help to maintain intake of food. Dietary teaching and meal planning can be approached according to an exchange system similar to that used for individuals with diabetes. With this approach there is greater ability to modify the diet according to personal preferences. The pattern of meals during the day is also a matter of personal preference. Some individuals prefer two or three meals a day. When eating patterns are known and used in dietary instruction and meal planning, intake of food is likely to increase.

Actual eating of prepared food can be promoted through attempting to decrease emotional tension at the dinner table. Periods other than mealtime should be used to discuss family and individual problems. Food that is attractively arranged and well flavored is likely to be more acceptable to the patient. Herbs and other flavorings can add variety to foods that are prepared without sodium. It is interesting that most persons relate that their taste for salt disappears once they have adhered to a low-sodium diet for several weeks. When the GI tract is ulcerated, bland foods may be tried in an attempt to increase ingestion of food.

Promotion of safety

Common injuries to the person in chronic renal failure include infection, accidents caused by decreased mental and visual awareness of the environment, and improper usage of medications. In chronic renal failure resistance to infection is decreased. Control of infection is essentially similar to that described in the section on care of the patient in acute renal failure. In addition, the person is counseled to avoid exposure to individuals with known infections and to avoid extreme fatigue, which lowers body resistance.

The buildup of osmotically active particles and fluid in the body that occurs in uremia produces changes in the cells of the brain that may lead to confusion and impairment in decision-making ability. In some instances convulsions and coma may result from the changed internal environment. Fluid accumulation and hypertension can produce visual changes. The patient's awareness of his or her environment also needs assessment.

At times the person may need to be helped in limiting activities to a level commensurate with mental processes and level of awareness. For instance, *blurred* vision and *delayed reaction time* contraindicate driving an automobile. *Convulsions* and *coma* may result from severe fluid, electrolyte, and waste imbalances. In most instances when the person is subject to developing these complications hospitalization is necessary. Individuals caring for the patient need to be aware of the possibility of seizure activity and take appropriate precautions. Correcting abnormal body chemistry is the most important measure for preventing coma or convulsions.

Education about medications is carried out with the person in the areas of both prescribed medications and over-the-counter or folk medicines. The use of common popular medications that are sold without prescription must be discouraged. All medications should be prescribed by the physician. Aspirin is dangerous because it is normally excreted by the kidneys and may rapidly build to toxic levels and prolong bleeding time. Ingestion of sodium bicarbonate (baking soda) or over-the-counter antacids containing sodium to treat indigestion can result in extremely large intakes of sodium. Many cold preparations also contain large amounts of sodium. Remembering to take prescribed medications can be a problem for the person who may have to take over two dozen pills each day. Correlating pill-taking times with major activities of the day is often helpful.

Coping with changes in life-style group membership, and feelings regarding self

Numerous alterations in life-style, group membership, and feelings regarding the self occur for the person with chronic renal failure. The numerous physical changes that occur often make it difficult to carry on activities that were once normally pursued. *Chronic fatigue* may make it impossible for the person to continue to be employed. Because the patient is often tired and not feeling well, it may be difficult to plan in advance for social events. The former roles of the sick member of the family must often be taken on by another. When roles cannot easily be changed or additionally assumed by other members of the family, serious threats to the organization of the family group occur. Physical appearance also changes

and is of much concern to most persons. As uremia progresses, the individual often becomes thin and weaker and appears sallow. Thoughts concerning death and the quality of life are common.

Denial often becomes a chief defense mechanism for the patient. With it the individual can periodically forget the constant threat of life. The use of this mental mechanism for the person with chronic renal failure can be quite appropriate as long as it is not manifested by maladaptive or harmful behavior. Inappropriate uses of denial involve continuous dietary indiscretion and failure to take prescribed medications.

Patients with chronic renal failure need the hope and encouragement that with treatment discomfort will be lessened and they will be allowed to pursue what seems most productive and important to them. Hope should not be focused on cure, but on learning to manage a new style of life. In managing the changes that occur as a result of chronic renal failure, the patients should be encouraged to be as independent and as active as possible. Patients should be taught to manage the treatment and should be given the responsibility of doing so. Nursing care should be provided as part of the team approach that assists patients in identifying problems and resources to meet them, and helps patients and their families adjust to the changes in their life-style.

ASSESSMENT

The nursing assessment of the patient in chronic renal failure is extremely complex. The assessment must include physical, psychologic, and social parameters. The initial nursing history and physical assessment must elicit adequate information to generate the appropriate nursing diagnoses. An example of a comprehensive nursing history is found in Fig. 33-24 and an example of a physical assessment in Fig. 33-25.

The extent of subsequent assessments will be determined by the medical regimen and nursing diagnoses for the individual patient.

DATA ANALYSIS AND PLANNING
Nursing diagnoses

Fluid volume deficit, actual or potential
Fluid volume excess, actual or potential
Nutrition, alteration in: less than body requirements
Urinary elimination, alteration in patterns
Noncompliance
Sexual dysfunction

This is not an exhaustive list. As the course of end-stage renal disease is run, most patients develop numerous complications, expanding the list of nursing diagnoses.

IMPLEMENTATION
Assisting with achievement of therapeutic goals

1. Encourage a diet high in carbohydrates and within the prescribed sodium, potassium, phosphorus, and protein limits.

Text continued on p. 1011.

HEMODIALYSIS NURSING NOTES
ADMISSION HISTORY

41   (Inpatient)/Patient Notes (Outpatient)

DATE	HOUR	
		I. Perception of Illness
		Why, initially, did you come to the hospital?
		What does the doctor plan for you while you are here?
		What do you expect is going to happen to you when you start dialysis?
		II. History of Past Illness (Include dates and hospitalizations).

		MEDICATIONS	DOSE	FREQUENCY	LAST DOSE TAKEN	REASON FOR TAKING

		Do you receive any special treatments or exercises?
		III. Activity
		Do you have difficulty walking or getting in and out of a chair?
		Can you climb stairs?
		Are you employed?
		What are your usual daytime activities?
		What are your recreational interests?

Fig. 33-24. Hemodialysis nursing notes: Admission history.

DATE	HOUR	IV.	Nutrition
			Are you on a special diet?
			Do you have difficulty following diet?
			How many meals do you eat a day?
		V.	Sleep Habits
			Do you sleep through the night at home?
			What helps in getting to sleep at night?
			What are your usual sleeping habits?
		VI.	Elimination
			How often do you urinate?
			Do you have any difficulty with urination?
			Frequency Pain on urination
			Urgency Other
			Have you ever had urinary tract infections?
			Twenty four hour urine output cc/24 hrs
			Color of urine?
			What are your usual bowel habits?
			Do you have difficulty with diarrhea or constipation?
			How often do you use enemas or laxatives?
		VII.	Reproductive System
			When was your most recent menses?
			Have you recently had a change in menses?
			Have you had any changes in sexual function recently?
			Do you have any concerns about reproductive or sexual functions?
		VIII.	Social
			Do you live with anyone?
			Upon whom do you rely when you need help?
			What type of dwelling do you live in?
			Do you have to climb stairs?

Admitting Nurse _____

Fig. 33-24, cont'd. Hemodialysis nursing notes: admission history.

HEMODIALYSIS NURSING NOTES
ADMISSION ASSESSMENT

41   (Inpatient)/Patient Notes (Outpatient)

DATE	HOUR	A) Vital Signs		
		Temperature		
		Pulses	Apical	
			Radial	
			Rhythm	
		Weight		
		Height		
		B) Cardiopulmonary		
		Vascular Access		
		Peripheral Pulses:	Right	Left
		Radial		
		Femoral		
		Popliteal		
		Pedal		
		Peripheral Edema?		
		Periorbital Edema?		
		Friction Rub?		
		Neck Vein Distention?		
		Cough? Sputum?		Smoking Habits?
		Adventitious Breath Sounds?		
		Shortness of Breath?		
		C) Neuromuscular		
		Orientation		
		Level of Alertness and Responsiveness?		
		Muscle Tone and Strength, Symmetry?		
		Weakness or Loss of Function of Extremities?		
		Balance		
		Numbness, Tingling or Tremors?		

Fig. 33-25. Hemodialysis nursing notes: Admission assessment.

DATE	HOUR	Patient Experiencing Difficulties with:
		Sight
		Speech
		Touch
		Taste/Smell
		D) Skin
		Color
		Turgor
		Temperature
		Lesions
		Condition of Nails
		E) General
		Presence of:
		Nausea
		Vomiting
		Headache
		Blurring of Vision

Admitting Nurse _____

Fig. 33-25, cont'd. Hemodialysis nursing notes: admission assessment.

2. Encourage the patient to remain within prescribed fluid restriction.
3. Medicate patient, as prescribed, for pain.
4. Promote meticulous skin care.
5. Protect confused patients from injury.
6. Assess intake and output every 8 hours.
7. Assess patient for fluid excess by palpating for edema, auscultating, breath sounds, and checking blood pressure at least every 8 hours.
8. Weigh patient every day.
9. Provide good oral hygiene.
10. Assess cardiac rhythm every 8 hours.
11. Assess level of consciousness every 8 hours.
12. Administer phosphate binding agents (Basoljel, Alternagel, Amphojel) with meals as prescribed.
13. In severely uremic patients, establish seizure precautions.
14. Provide calm supportive atmosphere.

Assisting with comfort and ADL

1. Medicate for pain as prescribed.
2. Encourage rest for fatigue, however, encourage self-care as tolerated.
3. Provide small quantities of fluid evenly spaced over the day to stay within fluid restriction.
4. Encourage use of damp cloth to keep lips moist.
5. Medicate with antipruritics as prescribed.

Teaching the patient

The patient with end-stage renal disease presents a unique opportunity for the nurse to promote optimum health through teaching and counseling. The patient will be discharged from the hospital and will be required to care for himself or herself. Every aspect of health care promotion related to end-stage renal disease must be conveyed to the patient. The following is a summary of that patient teaching.
1. Diet regimen including fluid restrictions
2. Medication teaching including action, dosage, and potential side effects
3. Explain relationships between diet, fluid restriction, medication, and blood chemistries
4. Symptoms that must be reported to physician
   a. Changes in urine output
   b. Edema
   c. Weight gain
   d. Dyspnea
   e. Infection
   f. Increased symptoms of uremia
5. Explain relationships between symptoms and their causes

Medical treatment of patients with end-stage renal disease

The medical management of patients with chronic renal failure can be classified as to the following:

1. Conservative management
2. Dialysis
3. Renal transplantation

CONSERVATIVE MANAGEMENT

Conservative medical management is primarily directed toward relief of symptoms. The focus is on the following:
1. Fluid and electrolyte regulation by control of diet and fluid intake
2. Blood pressure control by medication
3. Patient comfort

When progressive renal disease is present, conservative management may be adequate at first, but as renal function is diminished, more aggressive therapy may be necessary. When a patient is not an acceptable candidate for more aggressive therapy such as dialysis or renal transplantation, conservative management becomes the treatment of choice. The nursing implications of conservative management are the same as those discussed for chronic renal failure.

DIALYSIS

Dialysis involves the movement of fluid and particles across a semipermeable membrane. It is a treatment that can help restore normal fluid and electrolyte balance, control acid-base balance, and remove waste and toxic material from the body. It is a treatment than can sustain life successfully in both acute and chronic situations where substitution for or augmentation of normal renal function is needed. Specifically, dialysis is used to remove excessive amounts of drugs and toxins in poisonings of both an intentional and accidental nature, to correct serious electrolyte and acid-base imbalances, to maintain kidney function when renal shutdown occurs as a result of transfusion reactions, to temporarily replace renal function in persons with acute renal failure of various origins, and to permanently substitute for loss of renal function in persons with chronic end-stage renal disease.

Physiologic principles of dialysis

Dialysis is based on three principles: diffusion, osmosis, and ultrafiltration (Fig. 33-26). *Diffusion* involves the movement of particles from are area of greater to an area of lesser concentration. In the body this usually occurs across a semipermeable membrane. Diffusion is involved in the clearance of solute from the patient's body in both hemodialysis and peritoneal dialysis. Diffusion results in the movement of urea, creatinine, and uric acid from the patient's blood into the dialysate solution. This solution contains fewer particles to be removed from the bloodstream and higher concentrations of particles to be added to the blood (Fig. 33-27). Since the dialysate contains no protein waste products, the concentration of these substances in the blood will decrease because of random movement of the particles across the semipermeable membrane into the dialysate. The same principle applies

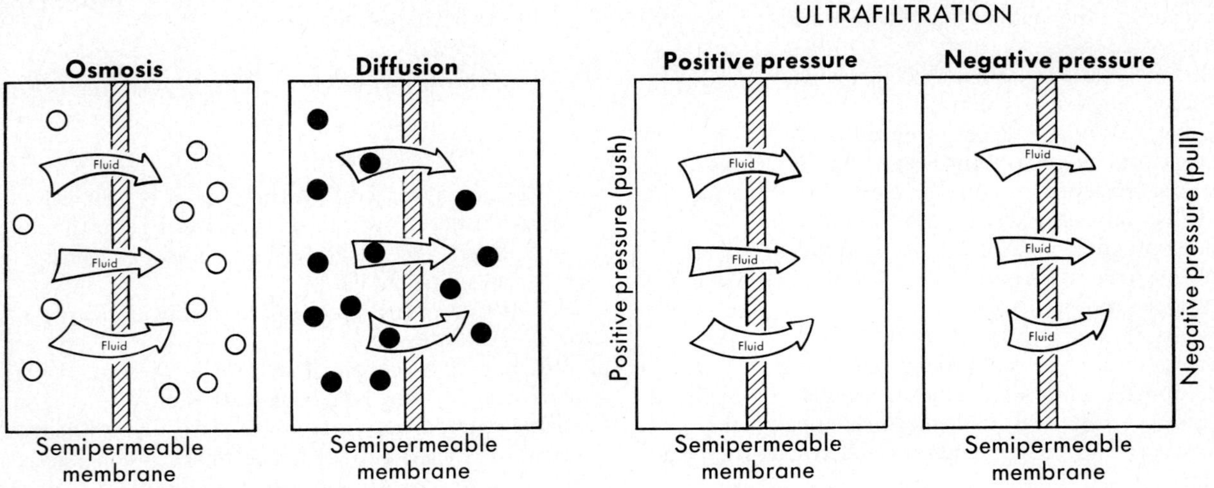

ULTRAFILTRATION

Osmosis **Diffusion** **Positive pressure** **Negative pressure**

Positive pressure (push)

Negative pressure (pull)

Fluid

Fluid

Fluid

Fluid

Fluid

Fluid

Fluid

Fluid

Fluid

Fluid

Fluid

Fluid

Semipermeable membrane Semipermeable membrane Semipermeable membrane Semipermeable membrane

Fig. 33-26. Dialysis is based on principles of **A,** osmosis, **B,** diffusion and ultrafiltration. Ultrafiltration occurs when either **C,** positive pressure, or **D,** negative pressure, is placed on system. Ultrafiltration can be maximized by exerting both positive and negative pressure on system simultaneously.

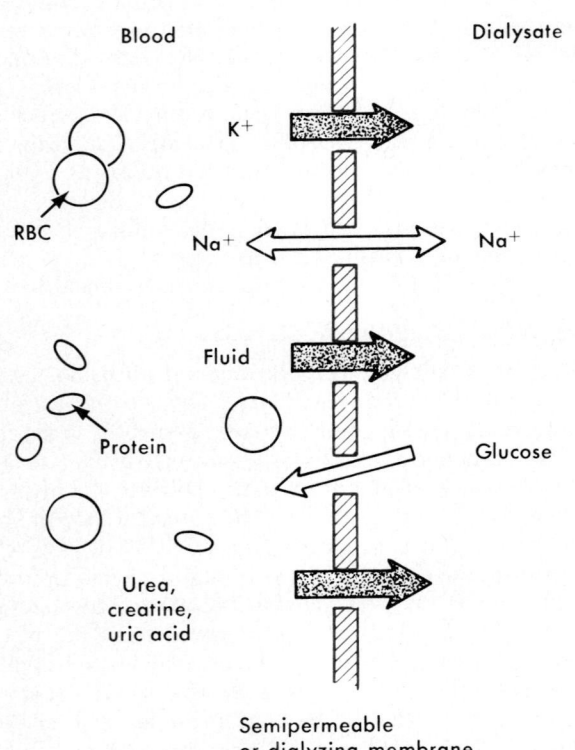

Fig. 33-27. Osmosis and diffusion in dialysis. Net movement of major particles and fluid is illustrated.

to the movement of potassium ions. Although the concentration of red blood cells and protein is high in blood, these molecules are quite large and do not diffuse through the membrane pores; hence they are not lost from the blood.

Osmosis involves the movement of fluid across a semipermeable membrane from an area of lesser to an area of greater concentration of particles. Osmosis is responsible for movement of extra fluid from the patient, particularly in peritoneal dialysis. Fig. 33-27 shows that glucose has been added to the dialysate to make its particle concentration greater than that of the patient's blood. Fluid will then move through the pores of the membrane from the patient's blood to the dialysate.

Ultrafiltration involves the movement of fluid across a semipermeable membrane as a result of an artifically created pressure gradient. Ultrafiltration is more efficient than osmosis for removal of fluid and is used in hemodialysis for this purpose. During dialysis, osmosis and diffusion or ultrafiltration and diffusion occur simultaneously.

Hemodialysis
Procedure

Hemodialysis involves shunting the patient's blood from the body through a dialyzer in which diffusion and ultrafiltration occur and back into the patient's circulation. To perform hemodialysis there must be access to the patient's blood, a mechanism to transport the blood to and from the dialyzer, and a dialyzer (area in which the exchange of fluid electrolytes and waste products occurs). Presently there are five major means for gaining access to the patient's bloodstream. These include the following:

1. Arteriovenous fistula (Fig. 33-28, *A*)
2. Arteriovenous graft (Fig. 33-28, *B*)

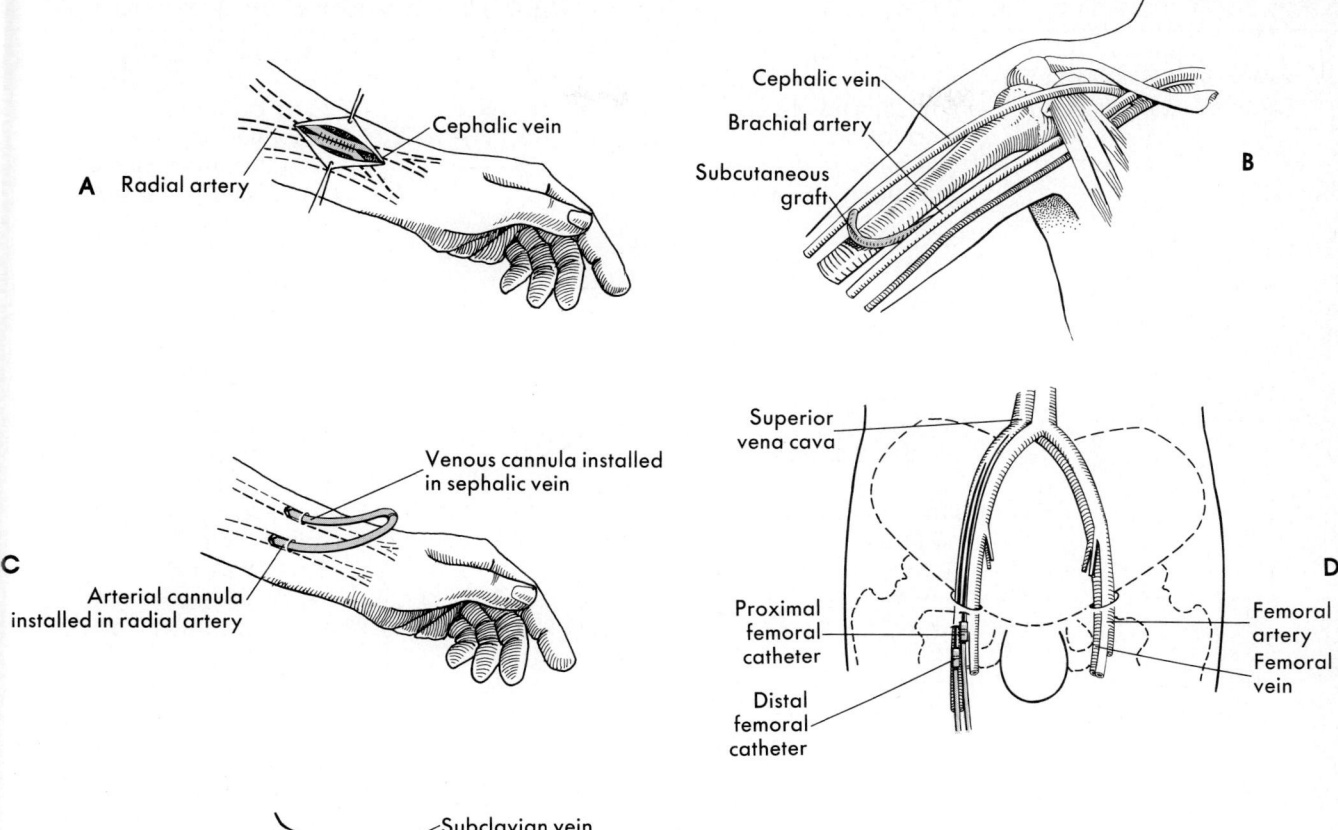

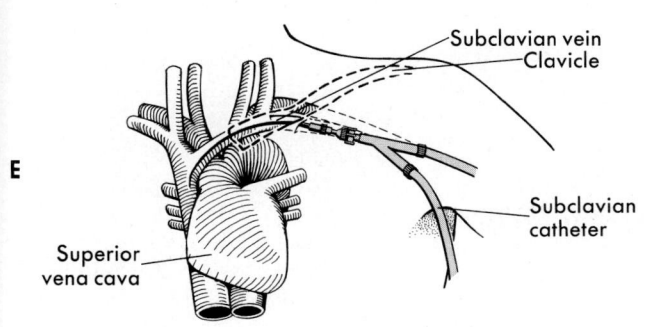

A Radial artery — Cephalic vein

B Cephalic vein — Brachial artery — Subcutaneous graft

C Venous cannula installed in sephalic vein — Arterial cannula installed in radial artery

D Superior vena cava — Proximal femoral catheter — Distal femoral catheter — Femoral artery — Femoral vein

E Subclavian vein — Clavicle — Subclavian catheter — Superior vena cava

Fig. 33-28. Frequently used means for gaining vascular access for hemodialysis includes **A,** arteriovenous fistula, **B,** arteriovenous graft, **C,** external arteriovenous shunt, **D,** femoral vein catheterization, and **E,** subclavian vein catheterization.

3. External arteriovenous shunt (Fig. 33-28, *C*)
4. Femoral vein catheterization (Fig. 33-28, *D*)
5. Subclavian vein catheterization (Fig. 33-28, *E*)

The indications and nursing implications for each access is summarized in Table 33-10.

Many persons expect to leave the dialysis treatment with a feeling of well-being. Few persons feel this way; most experience some minor discomfort that diminishes within several hours after dialysis. The greatest feeling of well-being seems to occur the day after dialysis.

Immediately before dialysis the patient is weighed, vital signs are taken, a sample of blood is drawn to determine the level of serum electrolytes and waste products, and the patient's physical status is assessed. Nursing care of the patient during hemodialysis should center around (1) monitoring the physical status of the patient before and during dialysis for evidence of physiologic imbalance and change, (2) comfort and safety needs of the patient, and

(3) helping the patient to understand and adjust to the care and changes in life-style. This latter objective involves educating the person as to the specifics of the treatment program (diet and medications in particular) and how these relate to altered kidney function. The person is encouraged to express concerns and feelings, and attempts must be made to help the individual work through these feelings. If dialysis is performed at home, the patient and back-up person must be able to institute all the care described.

Physiologic imbalances

Most physical problems that occur during dialysis are related to hypotension from removal of fluid and disequilibrium from a rapid reduction in extracellular electrolytes and wastes. *Hypovolemia* and *shock* can occur during dialysis as a result of rapid removal of fluid from the intravascular compartment. Since this can occur faster

Table 33-10. Indications and nursing implications for the major types of vascular access for hemodialysis

Type	Indications	Advantages	Nursing implications
Femoral vein catheterization	Immediate access Need for access seen as short duration	Ease of access Can be used immediately	Assess patient frequently for bleeding from insertion sites Requires frequent irrigation with heparin solution to maintain patency Sterile technique is essential when working with catheters
External shunt	Long term (weeks to months) needed for vascular access Access required within a few hours	Ease of access Can be used immediately	Assess patient frequently for bleeding at insertion site Assess patency of access frequently by observing continuous flow of blood through shunt Shunt is potential source of infection
Subclavian vein catheterization	Immediate access Short or long duration of vascular access	Does not restrict patient's activity Requires only one catheter	Assess patient frequently for bleeding from insertion site Sterile technique is essential when working with catheter Requires irrigation with heparin solution to ensure patency
Arteriovenous fistula and graft	Permanent access required	Is least likely of all the accesses to develop an infection Once maintained it provides easy access	Assess patency of fistula or graft by palpating or auscultating bruit Instruct patient to avoid compression of fistula by tight clothing or carrying objects with arm bent Patient must be instructed to assess fistula for signs and symptoms of infection including pain, redness, swelling or excessive warmth

than reequilibration of intracellular and intravascular volume relationships, the person may appear edematous and yet exhibit signs of shock. Signs and symptoms that indicate that the intravascular volume is being rapidly depleted are anxiety, restlessness, dizziness, nausea and vomiting, diaphoresis, tachycardia, and hypotension.

To avoid depleting the intravascular space and producing shock, the blood pressure and pulse rate are checked every 30 to 60 minutes, more frequently when the patient shows any of the previously mentioned signs and symptoms. Blood pressure readings should show only a slight gradual drop during the course of dialysis. Because the rate and pressure at which blood flows through the dialyzer are proportional to the rate and amount of fluid removed, blood flow and dialyzer pressure settings are carefully monitored. (A flow rate of 200 to 250 ml of blood per minute is a reasonable rate for an adult.) Unless the individual is severely hypertensive, rapid-acting antihyhertensive medications are usually withheld the morning of dialysis until after the treatment has been completed. Additionally, sedative drugs (analgesics, tranquilizers, hypnotics) and those primarily affecting the vasculature (nitroglycerin) predispose the patient to hypotensive episodes. Self-medication with these agents before and during dialysis must be carefully reviewed with each patient.

In treating a patient who shows signs of hypovolemia, initial nursing measures include determining the blood pressure and pulse, placing the head of the bed in a flat position, and raising the patient's feet. Administration of normal saline solution may be necessary to restore blood pressure. Throughout a hypotensive episode vital signs, level of consciousness, and any complaints offered are closely monitored. It is important for the nurse to know that vomiting frequently accompanies hypotension. Because an upper extremity must be maintained fairly immobile during the dialysis, it may be awkward for the patient to clear the mouth if vomiting should occur. The patient is helped to a safe position so that aspiration is avoided.

The patient is weighed before and after dialysis to determine amount of fluid loss during treatment. When the weight losses of several dialysis treatments are correlated with the patient's blood pressure, pulse, and other indications of hypovolemia, an individual pattern of the patient's tolerance to fluid removal can be determined. This trend or pattern can be used to help adjust the rate and overall effect of the dialysis in keeping with the patient's physiologic tolerance.

A *disequilibrium phenomenon* occurs for many dialysis patients. This syndrome occurs toward the end of or after dialysis. Disequilibrium results when excess solutes are cleared from the blood more rapidly than they can diffuse from the body's cells (particularly those of the central nervous system) into the vascular compartment. Hence, disequilibrium exists in the concentration of solute inside and outside the cells. Since particle content is greater inside the cells, water is taken in and edema results. Intracellular pH changes are also present. To some degree this process occurs with all patients with each dialysis procedure and helps to explain why patients do not feel their best immediately after treatment. *Severe disequilibrium or disequilibrium phenomenon* is most likely to be seen in the person whose blood chemistry values are exceptionally high before dailysis. Signs and symptoms of disequilibrium include *headache, restlessness, mental confusion,* and *nausea* and *vomiting.* Severe disequilibrium may result in convulsions, especially in children when blood urea nitrogen levels exceed the concentration of 100 mg/ml.

Treatment includes anticipation of severe disequilibrium. Often when a patient is beginning dialysis treatments, the procedures are kept short and may be spaced more frequently than normal during the first week. This allows solute to be cleared from the body without producing the extremely wide swings in body chemistry that would result in severe disequilibrium. Keeping the patient quiet, reducing environmental discomfort such as temperature extremes and bright lights, and closely supervising the patient to ensure physical safety are nursing care requirements. Mild analgesics may help to relieve headache. If disequilibrium becomes severe and the patient is still on dialysis, the therapy may be discontinued.

Care of the patient on dialysis should also include preventing *blood loss.* To prevent the patient's blood from clotting as it flows through the dialyzer, heparin is administered. Protamine sulfate is not generally given to the patient to counteract the effect of heparin. The patient is watched for signs of bleeding anywhere in the body. At the end of the treatment when dialysis needles are removed from the fistula, pressure dressings are applied to the puncture sites. They are observed at frequent intervals to detect hemorrhage. During and shortly after dialysis, treatments that cause tissue trauma should not be performed. These commonly include venipuncture and intramuscular injections. The patient who has had recent surgery, dental extractions, or recent trauma to soft tissues will have clotting times monitored frequently during dialysis to prevent hemorrhage. These patterns need to be closely observed for signs of bleeding.

Comfort

Nursing care should also include measures to increase the patient's physical comfort. Lying relatively immobile for even a few hours can produce pressure over bony prominences and general restlessness. Changing the patient's position increases tolerance to limited movement. Mouth care is required if the patient is nauseated and vomiting. Because an upper extremity is generally kept immobile during dialysis, the patient may need help with activities requiring the use of both hands.

PATIENT CARE DURING HEMODIALYSIS. Before the procedure, patients should have an opportunity to become familiar with the dialysis unit. They should be given an explanation of what will happen and what will be expected of them during the treatment. Patients often want to know (1) what types of pain will be experienced during the treatment, (2) how long and how often the dialysis will be, (3) what they should feel like during and after the treatment, (4) what they will be allowed to do during dialysis, and (5) if family members may be present during the therapy.

When the patient has an external shunt, no pain should be experience during initiation of dialysis. However, pain of a moderate degree may be present when venipuncture is performed in an arteriovenous fistula. A local anesthetic is used in most dialysis centers before insertion of the needles.

Patients should be told that they may experience some headache and nausea during the treatment and for a few hours afterward. Headache and nausea result from change in fluid, acid-base, and waste balance during dialysis. The symptoms should never be extreme, and relief should be attained from rest and sleep, mild analgesics, or antiemetics. Postural hypotension may also occur following dialysis; it is transitory in nature and caused by a relative depletion of intravascular volume secondary to fluid removal. The hypotension may produce dizziness and faintness. Relief should be obtained within a few hours with rest. The patient is assured that all of these symptoms will abate and that frequent monitoring during the procedure will help to control the degree of change that occurs during dialysis and the development of these symptoms.

A dialysis treatment lasts from 3 to 5 hours, depending on the type of dialyzer used and the time necessary to correct the fluid, electrolyte, acid-base, and waste problems that are present. Dialysis for an acute problem may be carried out daily or as often as the condition of the patient warrants. Hemodialysis for chronic renal failure is usually performed two or three times a week. Activity during dialysis is largely a matter of individual preference. Some persons sleep throughout their treatment; others read or carry on various activities.

Eating during dialysis is largely a matter of individual preference. Some individuals may become quite hungry, while for others the smell of food causes nausea. Patients may ask that they be allowed to eat foods not generally allowed during dialysis. Practice indicates that either allowing or discouraging eating freely during dialysis is a matter of individual unit philosophy. Because of the frequency of nausea, vomiting, and disequilibrium many patients experience during hemodialysis, it may be best to discourage eating to decrease the potential of aspiration.

Data analysis and planning

The following is a list of possible nursing diagnoses for the patient with end-stage renal disease being treated with hemodialysis. It should be emphasized that this is not intended to be an exhaustive list, but merely represents those diagnoses most often encountered.

1. Bowel elimination, alteration in: constipation
2. Comfort, alteration in: pain
3. Coping, ineffective, individual
4. Diversional activity, deficit
5. Knowledge deficit
6. Self concept, disturbance in
7. Urinary elimination, alteration in patterns
8. Fluid volume, alteration in:
   a. excess
   b. deficit

Outcome criteria for the person experiencing hemodialysis

The person or significant others can state, demonstrate, or plan the following:

1. The process of hemodialysis and relate to own body needs
2. Observations required of vascular access regarding infection and clotting as well as state means of obtaining care when these occur
3. Appropriate care of venous access
4. Common side effects of treatment, means for controlling mild symptoms, and means of obtaining medical attention for severe or persistant complications

5. Changes in medication schedule required before and after dialysis
6. A work and activity schedule as physical capabilities permit with minimal interference from scheduled dialysis time

Implementation
ASSISTING WITH ACHIEVEMENT OF THERAPEUTIC GOALS
A. Predialysis
   1. Record weight
   2. Obtain baseline vital signs
   3. Assess patient for fluid overload
      a. Pedal edema
      b. Periorbital edema
      c. Neck vein distention
      d. Adventitious breath sounds
   4. Assess vascular access for
      a. Patency
      b. Infection
B. Postdialysis
   1. Record weight
   2. Assess postural vital signs

For complete implementation refer to guidelines under chronic renal failure (see pp. 1018-1019).

Peritoneal dialysis

In peritoneal dialysis the dialyzing fluid is instilled into the peritoneal cavity and the peritoneum becomes the dialyzing membrane (Fig. 33-29). In comparison with hemodialysis treatments, which last 3 to 6 hours, peritoneal dialysis is maintained continuously for up to 36 hours. The procedure, once instituted, becomes largely a nursing responsibility. Peritoneal dialysis is used in treating acute and chronic renal failure. It can be performed in the hospital or at home.

Procedure

Access to the peritoneum is gained through introduction of a catheter into the peritoneal space. For acutely ill patients and those who are chronically ill and require sporadic dialysis, a sterile catheter is inserted for each procedure. For the chronically ill person treated on a rou-

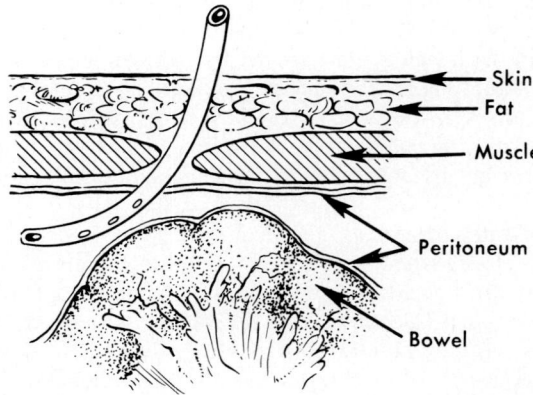

Fig. 33-29. Catheter in place in peritoneal cavity.

ne basis, a special catheter can be placed into the peritoneal space; the catheter remains until it malfunctions or another form of treatment is selected for the patient. These catheters present a continued potential entrance for organisms into the peritoneum. Each patient must be thoroughly instructed in the care of the catheter and the signs and symptoms indicative of local or peritoneal infection. These must be reported to the physician.

For all patients, weight, blood pressure, and pulse are recorded before initiating the procedure. These values serve as baseline information to assess changes in the patient's condition. For persons undergoing insertion of a peritoneal catheter before dialysis, assessment should be made of their knowledge of the procedure and their anxiety level. A mild sedative may help the severely anxious person to better tolerate the insertion of the catheter. it is important that these patients void just before catheter insertion; this decompresses the bladder and prevents accidental puncture during catheter placement.

To insert a peritoneal catheter, the physician cleanses the abdomen and anesthetizes a small area in the midline of the abdomen about 5 cm (2 inches) below the umbilicus. A small incision is made, and the many-eyed nylon catheter is inserted into the peritoneal cavity (Fig. 33-

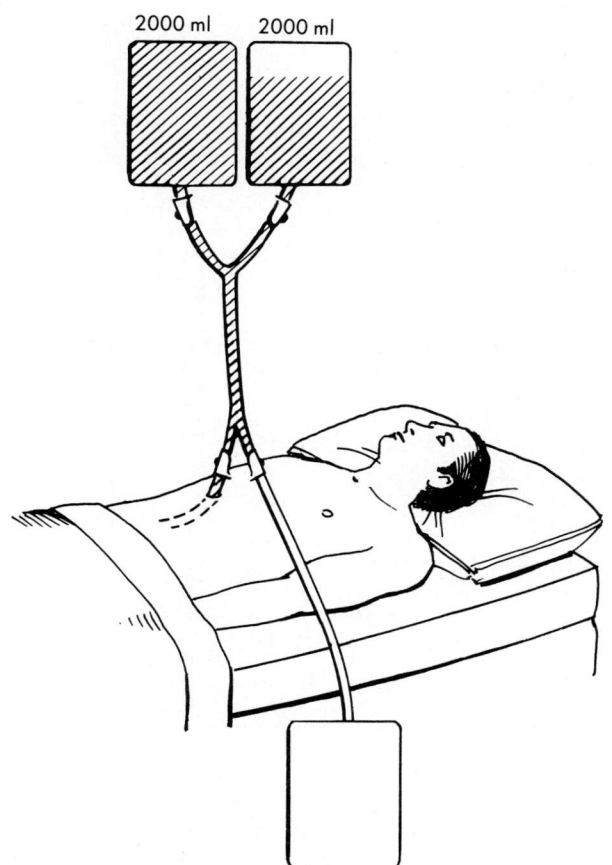

Fig. 33-30. Patient undergoing peritoneal dialysis. Dialysis fluid is being instilled into abdominal cavity.

30). A dressing is placed around the protruding catheter. Dialysis is initiated for the person with a permanent catheter by carefully cleansing the catheter and surrounding skin with a bactericidal agent before the catheter is connected to the dialysate line. Approximately 2 L of sterile dialysate warmed to body temperature is attached by tubing to the catheter and allowed to run into the peritoneal cavity as rapidly as possible. This usually takes about 10 minutes. The tubing is then clamped, and 10 to 30 minutes are allowed for osmosis of fluid and diffusion of particles into the dialyzing solution. At the end of the dwell time the tubing is unclamped and the fluid is allowed to flow by gravity from the abdomen. Fluid should drain in a steady stream. Drainage time should average about 10 to 15 minutes. The first drainage may be pink tinged as a result of the trauma of catheter insertion; however, this should clear with the second or third drainage. At no time should fluid draining from the abdomen appear grossly bloody. After fluid has drained from the abdomen, another cycle is started immediately. After the dialysis has been completed, the permanent catheter is again cleansed and a sterile cap is applied to the tip; the temporary catheter is removed, and the incision is covered with a dry sterile dressing. The small abdominal wound from the catheter should heal completely in 1 to 2 days.

Care during peritoneal dialysis

Complications most commonly associated with peritoneal dialysis include hypotension and hypovolemia, inadequate drainage of fluid from the peritoneal space, pain, atelectasis, respiratory distress, and peritonitis. As with hemodialysis, *hypotension* is most likely to result from rapid removal of fluid from the intravascular space. In addition to checking vital signs and observing the patient's behavior, records of fluid balance are crucial in determining the amount of fluid that has been removed. The net gain or loss of fluid from the abdomen should be determined at the completion of each cycle. To decrease the amount of fluid that is being removed from the vascular space, the physician may decrease the hypertonicity of the dialysate and may increase the rate at which fluid is administered through an intravenous line.

Drainage of fluid from the abdomen can be slow or impossible to start. Generally, this problem results when the tip of the catheter has become lodged against abdominal tissues. It may also result from plugging of the catheter with blood or fibrin that has accumulated as a result of tissue trauma. A small amount of heparin may be added to the dialysate to decrease the chance of a clot forming in the catheter. When the dialysate does not drain freely from the abdomen, the patient should be turned from side to side in an attempt to reposition the catheter in the peritoneal cavity. In addition, firm pressure may be applied to the abdomen with both hands and the head of the bed may be raised. If the flow of the dialysate does not increase, the physician is called to irrigate the catheter or reposition it.

Severe pain should not be experienced during perito-

Example of care plan for teaching the patient on hemodialysis

Date	Hour	Teaching/learning needs	RN signature
		Chronic renal failure being treated by hemodialysis	
Start	Stop	Plan	
		1. Introduce patient to hemodialysis unit using available printed material and a visit to unit when appropriate.	
		2. Explain normal kidney function	
		3. Explain kidney failure specific to patient's pathophysiology.	
		a. Types	
		b. Causes	
		4. Explain and reinforce medication regimen.	
		a. Purpose of each prescribed medication	
		b. Common side effects	
		c. Dosage and times of each medication	
		d. Prescription filling procedure	
		5. Reinforce dietary instructions.	
		a. Protein	
		b. Potassium	
		c. Sodium	
		d. Fluids	
		e. Calories	
		6. Instruct patient in necessity for and care of vascular access	
		a. Procedure for assessing presence of thrill and buit; who to notify if thrill or bruit is absent	
		b. Guarding against constriction of fistula, that is sleeping on arm or wearing tight clothing	
		c. Hygiene and removing dressing after dialysis	
		d. Signs and symptoms of infection, that is, redness, swelling, or tenderness	
		e. Measures to control hemorrhage should it develop while away from dialysis unit	

Example of care plan for teaching the patient on hemodialysis—cont'd

		7. Instruct patient about process of hemodialysis	
		a. Explain principles of dialysis in sufficient detail for learning level of patient.	
		b. Describe hemodialysis in full detail to patient	
		c. Explain common sights and sounds of dialysis unit to patient.	
		d. Describe common complications of hemodialysis to patient as well as usual treatments.	
		(1) Hypotension	
		(2) Nausea	
		(3) Vomiting	
		(4) Cramping	
		8. Instruct patient in interpretation of laboratory data and effects of hemodialysis, diet, and medications on these values.	
		9. Introduce patient to alternative modes of treatment of ESRD	
		a. Free-standing hemodialysis centers	
		b. Self-dialysis (home)	
		c. Peritoneal dialysis	
		d. Transplantation	
Date		Status of problems at discharge	
Date		Patient knowledge:	
Date		Follow-up plans:	
		RN signature _____	

neal dialysis. Moderate levels of pain are often experienced as fluid is instilled and withdrawn from the peritoneal cavity. Procaine hydrochloride may be instilled with the dialysate in an attempt to control the patient's discomfort. Mild analgesics may be ordered for administration at 3- to 4-hour intervals during the procedure.

When the patient is markedly overhydrated and shows evidence of congestive failure and pulmonary edema, respiratory difficulty may be encountered as the dialyzing fluid infuses. The quality and rate of respiration should be closely observed. The head of the bed can be raised to decrease the pressure of the dialysate on the diaphragm. The amount of dialyzing fluid used for each cycle may be decreased when respiratory distress becomes prolonged and severe. The patient, although encouraged to eat while being dialyzed, may find that this increases respiratory difficulty. To help overcome additional pressure created by a full stomach, frequent small meals may be provided.

Peritonitis is an ever present threat during peritoneal dialysis. Aseptic technique must be rigidly maintained during insertion of the catheter and throughout the procedure. Care should be taken to avoid contaminating the solution or the tubing when dialysate solution is hung. Cultures of the dialysate fluid are performed routinely to ensure continued attention to asepsis and to identify organisms if peritonitis should develop subsequently. The patient should be observed for signs of peritonitis. These include an elevated temperature and tenderness or pain of the abdomen.

Although the patient is generally confined to a recumbent position for the length of the dialysis, comfort and diversion can be provided. The patient may turn from side to side and move about in bed as desired as long as the catheter remains undisturbed. The patient may be provided assistance with oral care and bathing as needed. Visiting and other diversional activities should be encouraged when the patient's physical condition permits. If peritoneal dialysis is carried out at home, the patient and a backup person need to be able to do all steps described above.

Advances in the management of patients with chronic end-stage renal disease will likely reflect greater emphasis on independence for the patient. The technology for home dialysis and self-dialysis has been developed.[16,22] Continuous ambulatory peritoneal dialysis (CAPD) is one new development that should make self-dialysis safe, practical, and increasingly acceptable to patients. Basically, CAPD involves continuous contact of dialysate with the peritoneal membrane. Approximately 2 L of dialysate are maintained interperitoneally and exchanged by the patient through a permanent peritoneal catheter four to five times a day.[1]

The major advantages of peritoneal dialysis include the following:
1. Provides a steady state of blood chemistries
2. Patient can dialyze alone in any location without need for machinery
3. Patient can readily be taught process
4. Patient has few dietary restrictions; because of loss of protein in dialysate the patient is usually placed on a high protein diet
5. Patient has much more control over daily life
6. Can be used for patients that are hemodynamically unstable

Outcome criteria for the person experiencing peritoneal dialysis

The person or significant others can explain, demonstrate or plan the following:
1. The process of dialysis and relate work of dialysis to own body needs
2. Observation indicating infection of the peritoneal cavity or catheter and state means of obtaining care when these occur
3. Appropriate care of permanent peritoneal catheter
4. Common side effects of treatment, means for controlling mild symptoms, and means of obtaining medical attention for severe or persistent complications
5. Changes in medication schedule required before and after dialysis
6. A work and activity schedule as physical capabilities permit, with minimal interference from scheduled dialysis time

Implementation

1. Assisting with achievement of therapeutic goals
   a. Maintain strict sterile technique.
   b. Maintain strict intake and output during procedure.
   c. Monitor vital signs frequently, particularly at beginning and end of cycle.
   d. Weigh patient at beginning and end of treatment.
   e. Assess catheter site for signs of infection.
   f. Assess patient for edema.
   g. During cycles maintain accurate record of each cycle including the following:
      (1) Type of dialysate
      (2) Amount of dialysate infused
      (3) Amount of dialysate recovered
      (4) Time dialysate was left indwelling
      (5) Characteristics of recovered dialysate

Teaching the patient

The teaching requirements for the patient undergoing peritoneal dialysis is consistent with the teaching plan for hemodialysis. However, the patient will need to be instructed in the specifics of the process of peritoneal dialysis. If the patient will undergo CAPD, training should be accomplished in a home training center that is equipped to assist the patient in dealing with home care.

Kidney transplantation

Kidney transplants are being performed with increasing frequency in an effort to prolong the lives of persons with chronic renal failure. At present the ability to completely overcome the body's tendency to reject the grafted kidney has not been achieved. Persons undergoing kidney transplantation in essence exchange a program of chronic hemodialysis and its limitations for a new problem. Unless the kidney has been donated by an identical twin, the body senses the graft as a foreign tissue and attempts to destroy it (rejection).

DONOR SELECTION

Kidney allografts may be obtained from cadavers, matched family members, or an identical twin. Although more than half of the transplanted kidneys are from cadavers, better results are obtained from related donors. Currently, success rates 1 year after transplantation are 50% when a cadaveric kidney is used, 65% to 70% when a matched sibling or parent donates the kidney, and 90% when an identical twin is the organ donor.

Cadavers should be free of renal disease, neoplasms (excluding those of the central nervous system and skin), and sepsis. Permission for cadaver donation is given by next of kin or by persons who plan in advance to donate their organs.

The major requirement for the donated kidney is histocompatibility. Rejection occurs from a cell-mediated (type IV hypersensitivity) response or from a humoral (type II cytotoxic hypersensitivity) response. The important antigens are the human leukocyte antigen (HLA) and the ABO blood groups. For the ABO groups the same rules apply as for blood transfusions.

A new procedure currently being tested that researchers hope will significantly increase graft survival from living related donors is that of *donor-specific transfusion*.[21] Shortly before transplantation the recipient receives three transfusions of the donor's blood, each 2 weeks apart. After these transfusions, if the recipient and donor blood cross-match is still compatible, transplantation is performed. The purposes of donor-specific transfusion are (1) to identify those recipients who would respond unfavorably to the donated organ and (2) to desensitize the recipient to the donor's tissue. Preliminary results of this procedure are encouraging.[24]

Related donors must be in good health, be highly motivated to be a donor, have good mental health, and not be receiving drugs such as barbiturates, which depress reflexes and electrical brain activity. The donor is given a complete medical evaluation and in some cases may be referred to a psychiatrist for further evaluation.

Viability of the donor kidney must be maintained until the time of transplantation surgery. Preservation times of 24 to 72 hours have been reported with proper technique. Methods include washing out the formed blood elements and perfusing a heparinized electrolyte solution at 2° to 4° C. Use of a pulsatile flow pump and oxygenator helps to preserve the kidney beyond 6 to 12 hours.

PREOPERATIVE CARE

Nursing care of the patient in the preoperative phase includes physical and emotional preparation for the surgery. The patient and family should understand the outcomes expected from the surgery and the follow-up care that will be required. They should be prepared for the possibility of the kidney not functioning after transplantation.

The nature of the surgery and location of the transplant, the possible need for postoperative dialysis, the use of immunosuppressive drugs, and the need for infection prevention after surgery must be explained to the patient and family. As with any surgical patient, the individual should know if drainage tubes will be inserted during surgery, that medication will be given for relief of pain, and that moving about, coughing, and deep breathing will be necessary as soon as they awake from anesthesia.

Throughout the period from the patient's acceptance as a transplant candidate to the time of surgery, the concerns and anxieties of the patient and family regarding transplantation need to be identified. As appropriate, the nurse and other members of the health team are called on to help in dealing with these concerns and anxieties.

The patient must be in optimal physical condition for transplantation. Dialysis may be required before transplantation to ensure optimal fluid and electrolyte balance, acid-base balance, and removal of wastes. The integrity of the vascular access must be maintained. Before surgery the extremity containing the vascular access may be wrapped to draw attention to it and identify it as containing the patient's access for dialysis. This identification will help all individuals caring for the person to avoid using the affected extremity for blood pressure determinations, drawing of blood, or intravenous infusions.

SURGERY

During surgery the transplanted kidney is placed in the iliac fossa (Fig. 33-31).[21] Generally, the peritoneal cavity is not entered. The patient's own kidneys are not disturbed unless they are infected or are the cause of significant hypertension. The recipient undergoes bilateral

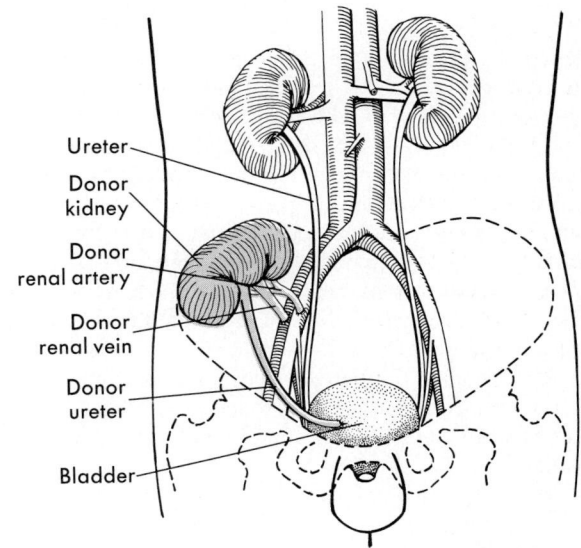

Fig. 33-31. Location of transplanted kidney showing anastomosis of renal artery, renal vein, and ureter.

Ureter

Donor kidney

Donor renal artery

Donor renal vein

Donor ureter

Bladder

nephrectomy before transplant surgery. The patient's kidneys are left intact whenever possible to maintain erythropoietin production, blood pressure control, and prostaglandin synthesis and metabolism. The donor ureter is used to the extent that is possible. If long enough, it is connected to the bladder in such a way as to prevent reflux of urine. If the ureter is short, a ureteroureterostomy may be performed. A catheter is placed in the wound to promote drainage of accumulating fluid.

POSTOPERATIVE CARE

Immediate postoperative care includes maintaining drainage of the urinary bladder hourly, assessing the adequacy of fluid and electrolyte balance, protecting the patient from infection, observing for signs and symptoms of rejection and other complications, and identifying the effects of medications that have been administered throughout the entire care cycle.[18] A free flow of communication must be maintained with the patient and significant others regarding the individual's progress.

In the operating room a Foley catheter is inserted into the bladder to promote drainage of urine and to prevent bladder distention and pressure on the newly anastomosed ureter. If gross hematuria or clots are noted in the drainage system, the physician should be notified immediately.

As with any surgical patient, the possibility of hemorrhage and hypovolemia exists. Blood pressure and pulse are determined frequently. Because the patient may have little or no urinary output for a number of hours to weeks after transplantation, fluid and electrolyte balance must be monitored carefully. Paramaters indicating disturbed fluid and electrolyte balance are listed in the discussion of care of the patient with chronic renal failure. Any drainage from dressing or tubes should be carefully calculated into the patient's fluid balance record.

REJECTION

Rejection, the leading cause of graft failure, may occur as a *hyperacute event,* as an *acute event,* or as a slow and *progressive decline* in renal function. In a hyperacute event, rejection occurs immediately after surgical implantation. Instantly following arterial anastomosis, circulating cytotoxic antibodies infiltrate and infarct the foreign tissue. The hyperacute rejected kidney is usually removed immediately to prevent further complications. Acute rejection typically begins within the first 2 weeks but may be seen 2 or more years after transplantation. Most transplant patients undergo at least one episode of acute rejection. Rejection is caused by a cell-mediated immune response. The delay in the ocurrence of the first attack is related to the time it takes for T-lymphocytes to become sensitized.

Signs and symptoms indicative of acute rejection are listed in Table 33-11.

Chronic rejection is a slow progressive process. It occurs secondary to both cell-mediated and humoral im-

Table 33-11. Signs and symptoms of acute rejection of a transplanted kidney

1. Decrease in urine output
   a. Oliguria
   b. Anuria
2. Fever greater than 37.7° C (100° F); may be masked by steroids
3. Pain or tenderness over grafted kidney
4. Edema
5. Sudden weight gain, 2 to 3 pounds in 24 hours
6. Hypertension
7. General malaise
8. Rise in serum creatinine value
9. Decrease in creatinine clearance

mune responses. The signs and symptoms are similar to those that occur in acute rejection, however, they occur more slowly. In most instances the patient will eventually lose all renal function as chronic rejection progresses.

Treatment of acute rejection usually consists of large doses of SoluMedrol (methylprednisolone) administered intravenously. Local graft irradiation may be used to destroy infiltrating lymphocytes.

As was stated earlier, rejection of the grafted kidney is a function of the recipient's immune system. Therefore, survival of such a graft depends on the suppression of the immune response. Several methods are used to immunosuppress patients. Antilymphocytes serum (ALS) and antilymphocyte globulin (ALG) are gaining widespread use. ALS and ALG work by coating the lymphocytes, thus making them more susceptible to phagocytic destruction by cells of the reticuloendothelial system.

Azathioprine (Imuran) is the most commonly used immunosuppressive drug. It functions by inhibiting DNA and RNA synthesis, thereby suppressing antibody synthesis. Cyclophosphamide (Cytoxan) functions like and is often used in conjunction with Imuran. Cytoxan also destroys circulating lymphocytes. Corticosteroids like prednisone and SoluMedrol are also used as immunosuppressives. Corticosteroids function by decreasing antibody production and inhibit antigen-antibody complex formation. They also prevent leukocyte infiltration of the graft.

Side effects of therapy with immunosuppressive medications as well as nursing interventions are listed in Table 33-12.

ASSESSMENT

The assessment of the patient following renal transplant is multifaceted. Areas of assessment must include the following:

1. Postoperative nursing management
2. Fluid and electrolyte balance
3. Signs and symptoms of acute tubular necrosis
4. Signs and symptoms of rejection
5. Signs and symptoms of side effects resulting from high-dose immunosuppression

Table 33-12. Common side effects of immunosuppressive therapy and nursing interventions

Side effect	Nursing intervention
Leukopenia	1. Observe for signs of infection 2. Reverse isolation 3. Antibiotic therapy as prescribed
GI irritation and bleeding	1. Perform guaiac tests on stool, vomitus, and NG aspirate 2. Administer antacids as prescribed 3. Provide calm, supportive environment 4. Assess postural vital signs
Increased appetite	1. Reinforce diet teaching 2. Encourage low sodium diet
Alopecia	1. Suggest use of wig 2. Encourage patient that hair will grow back 3. Provide emotional support
Acne	1. Encourage frequent bathing 2. Instruct in use of appropriate soaps
Delayed wound healing	1. Maintain sterile technique for dressing changes 2. Assess wound each dressing change for signs of infection 3. Encourage adequate protein in diet
Change in mental status (mood swings)	1. Observe patient for changes in behavior and report to physician 2. Provide calm supportive environment 3. Provide diversional activities

DATA ANALYSIS AND PLANNING

Outcome criteria

The person or significant others can state or demonstrate the following:
1. The prescribed diet and how it will be achieved.
2. The medication plan
   a. State name, dosage, frequency, rationale, and side effects of prescribed medications (immunosuppressives, antacids)
   b. State method of obtaining medications
3. Accurate taking and recording of oral temperature, 24-hour urine specimens, weight, fluid intake, and urinary output
4. Recommended preventive health care measures
   a. State measures useful in preventing infection.
   b. State plan for dental and gynecologic health care.
   c. State need to avoid immunization with live-virus vaccines
5. A program for continued health supervision
   a. Explain concept of immunosuppression and relate this to health care needs
   b. Describe signs and symptoms requiring immediate medical attention
   c. Relate appropriate information regarding sexual functioning and family planning.
   d. State need to preserve dialysis access.
   e. State resources available for assistance with illness and rehabilitative concerns and means of contact with resources.
   f. Explain specific plans for follow-up health care.

Nursing diagnoses

1. Immediate postoperative period
   Comfort, alterations in: pain
   Fluid volume, alteration in: excess
   Urinary elimination, alteration in
2. Long-term
   Knowledge deficit
   Urinary elimination, alteration in

IMPLEMENTATION

1. Assisting with achievement of therapeutic goals
   a. Immediate postoperative period
      (1) Maintain sterile technique in caring with wound and urinary drainage catheter.
      (2) Encourage early ambulation.
      (3) Administer medications as prescribed.
      (4) Assess patient for signs and symptoms of an infection both at surgical incision and systemically.
   b. Fluid and electrolyte balance
      (1) Maintain accurate intake and output.
      (2) Weigh daily at same time.
      (3) Monitor signs of fluid and electrolyte imbalance.
      (4) Monitor and regulate parenteral fluid replacement as prescribed by physician (usually 1 ml/ 1 ml).
      (5) Encourage oral intake as tolerated.
2. Assisting with comfort and ADL
   a. Promote rest periods when fatigue is present.
   b. Administer pain medication as prescribed.

c. Assist with ADL as necessary but encourage independence.
3. Control of environment
   a. Maintain calm reassuring environment.
   b. Reverse isolation may be required while patient is immunosuppressed.
   c. Restrict visitors with colds or other infections.
   d. Provide diversional activities.
4. Teaching the patient
   a. Instruct patient in actions, dosage, and potential side effects of medications.
   b. Instruct patient in signs and symptoms of graft rejection and information to report to physician.
   c. Instruct patient in signs and symptoms of infection and action to take.
   d. Instruct patient in maintaining accurate intake and output.
   e. Instruct patient in necessity of daily weights.
   f. Instruct patient in necessity to avoid trauma to graft site since it is superficially placed.
   g. Reinforce the need for medical follow-up following discharge.

REFERENCES AND SELECTED READINGS*

1. *Arenz, R.: Do-it-yourself dialysis, RN **44:**57-60, 1981.
2. Black, D.A.K.: Renal disease, ed. 4, Oxford, England, 1979, Blackwell Scientific Publications, Ltd.
3. Chambers, J.: Save your diabetic patient from early kidney damage, Nurs. 83 **13:**58-63, 1983.
4. *Cianci, J., and others: Renal transplantation, Am. J. Nurs. **81:**354-355, 1981.
5. Fennel, S.: Percutaneous renal biopsy, Am. J. Nurs. **75:**1292-1294, 1975.
6. Goldberger, E.: A primer of water electrolyte and acid-base syndromes, ed. 6, Philadelphia, 1980, Lea & Febiger.
7. *Hartman, M.: Intermittent self catheterization, Nurs. 78 **8:**75-77, 1978.
8. *Irwin, B.: Now—peritoneal dialysis for chronic patients too, RN **44:**49-52, 1981.
9. Lapides, J., editor: Fundamentals of urology, Philadelphia, 1976, W.B. Saunders Co.
10. Leaf, A., and Cotran, R.: Renal pathophysiology, Oxford, 1980, Oxford University Press.
11. Maxwell, M.H., and others: Comparative study of renovascular hypertension: demographic analysis of the study, JAMA **220:**1195, 1972.
12. Mooney, T.O., Cole, T., and Chilgren, R.: Sexual options for paraplegics and quadriplegics, Boston, 1975, Little, Brown and Co.
13. Pallay, V.: Clinical testing of renal functions, Med. Clin. North Am. **55:**231-241, 1971.
14. Papper, S.: Clinical nephrology, ed. 2, Boston, 1981, Little, Brown and Co.
15. Papper, S.: Renal failure, Med. Clin. North Am. **55:**335-357, 1977.
16. Popovitch, R.P., and others: Continuous ambulatory peritoneal dialysis, Ann. Intern. Med. **88:**449-456, 1978.
17. Porth, C.: Pathophysiology, Philadelphia, 1982, J. B. Lippincott Co.
18. *Prewit, D.: Post-operative complications: an overview, Nephro. Nurse **5:**27-32, 1983.
19. *Randolph, G.: Bringing them back out of renal shutdown, RN **44:**34-39, 108-112, 1981.
20. Report of the Coordination Committee: Research needs in nephrology and urology, Vol. 5, p. 3. National Institute of Health, National Institute of Arthritis, Metabolism and Digestive Disorders, Public Health Service, DHEW Publication No. (NIH) 78-1485 Washington, D.C., 1978.
21. Robbins, K., Richard, A., and Ronselli, M.: Donor specific transfusions as pre-treatment for living related donor transplants and nursing implications, Nephro. Nurs. **5:**4-8, 1983.
22. Robson, M.D., and Oroponlous, D.G.: Continuous ambulatory peritoneal dialysis: a orientation in the treatment of chronic renal failure, Dialysis Transplant. **7:**999-1103, 1978.
23. Rous, S.N.: Urology in primary care, St. Louis, 1976, The C.V. Mosby Co.
24. Salvatiena, O., and others: Deliberate donor specific blood transfusions prior to living related renal transplantation, Ann. Surg. **192:**543-552, 1980.
25. Schrier, R.: Renal and electrolyte disorders, Boston, 1980, Little, Brown and Co.
26. Stamm, W.: Guidelines for prevention of catheter-associated urinary tract infections, Ann. Intern. Med. **82:**386-390, 1975.
27. *Stark, J.: Acute renal failure, Nurs. 82 **12:**26-33, 1982.
28. Stroot, V.R., and others: Fluids and electrolytes: a practical approach, ed. 2, Philadelphia, 1977, F.A. Davis Co.
29. U. S. Department of Health Education and Welfare, Center for Disease Control: Outline for surveillance and control of nosocomial infections, Atlanta, 1974, The Department.
30. *Underwood, M.A.: Urinary tract infections, Crit. Care Q. **3:**63-70, 1980.

*References preceded by an asterisk are particularly well suited for student reading.

UNIT X
Sexual and Reproductive Problems

34   Sexuality in Health and Illness

35   The Patient with Reproductive Problems

36   The Patient with Problems of the Breast

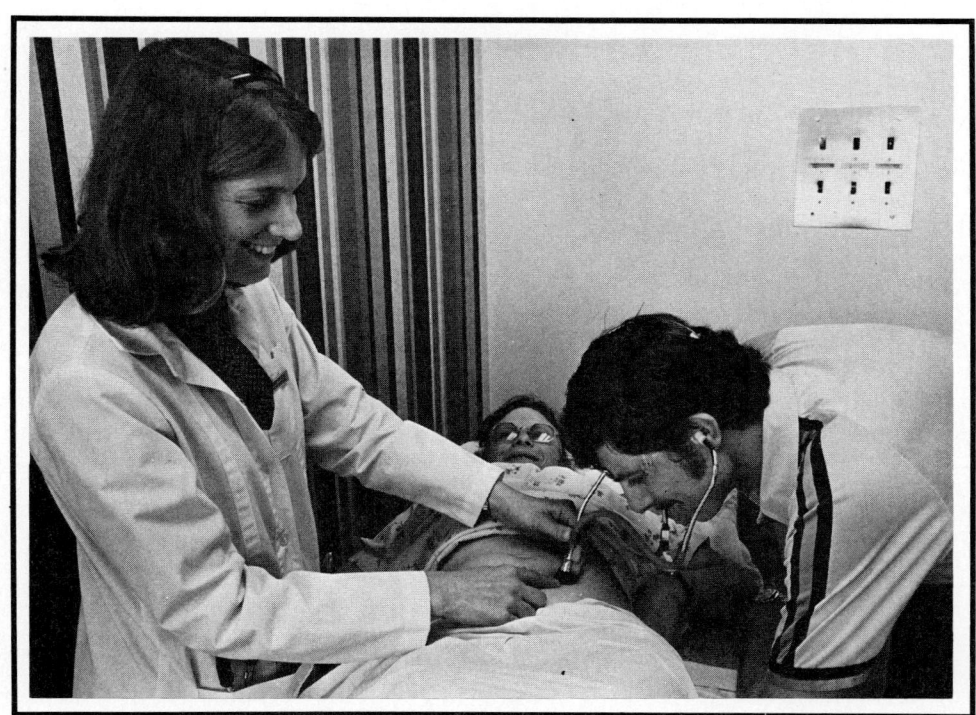

34

Sexuality in Health and Illness

NANCY FUGATE WOODS

STUDY QUESTIONS

- What instances in your own life shaped some of your feelings about yourself as female or male?

- What nursing behaviors would increase your comfort in describing your own sexual history?

- Examine your beliefs about homosexuality. In what ways might your beliefs help or hinder working with homosexual patients who have sexual concerns?

- Examine the list of diseases in Table 34-3 and the list of medications in Table 34-4. Have any of these conditions existed for patients for whom you have provided care recently? How might their sexual response have been affected? Did they express any concerns about their sexuality or sexual response? Discuss the nursing care that could have been offered.

SEXUALITY AND HEALTH

Human sexuality is not merely a biologic phenomenon, but one that pervades the total person. A complex interrelationship exists among biologic, psychologic, and sociocultural aspects of our sexuality. The very complexity of human nature makes it difficult to define sexuality, much less sexual health. Nevertheless, the recognition of the importance of sexuality as a component of health has led some groups, among them the World Health Organization, to risk such a definition:

Sexual health is the integration of the somatic, emotional, intellectual, and social aspects of sexual being, in ways that are positively enriching and that enhance personality, communication, and love.[28]

Evolution of human sexuality

The evolution of our sexuality illustrates the complexity and interrelationship of aspects of our sexuality. From the moment of conception a variety of factors come into play to influence our sexuality, not only as children but also as adults. In early embryonic life the X or Y chromosome from the paternal sperm sets in motion a process analogous to a relay race; that is, each component has control of the process for a time, eventually yielding control to another[38] (Fig. 34-1). The chromosomes tag the undifferentiated fetal gonads as male or female, thus setting in motion another process by which hormonal secretions of the testes in turn affect not only the appearance of the genitals but also pathways in the brain.

The appearance of the infant's genitals at birth initiates another series of events, those primarily dependent on socialization of the child. The behavior of other persons during infancy and early childhood and the appearance of the child's external genitals are instrumental in the evolution of childhood gender identity and role. In fact, gender identity seems to be well established by the time a person is 18 months of age. At puberty, biologic influences again come to the fore as hormones influence the genital structure and eroticism.

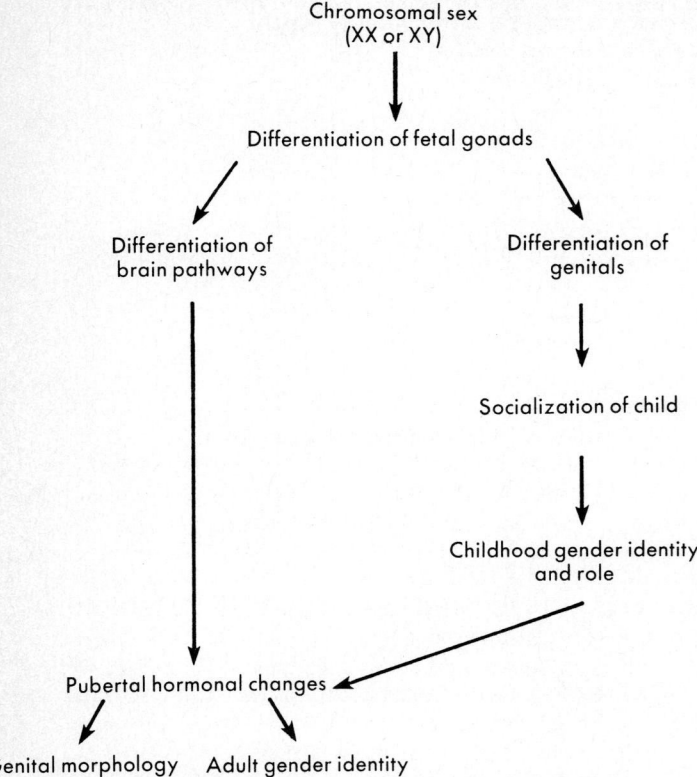

Fig. 34-1. Evolution of sexuality.

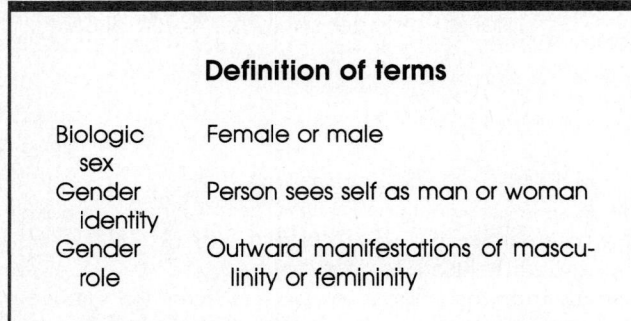

Definition of terms

Biologic sex	Female or male
Gender identity	Person sees self as man or woman
Gender role	Outward manifestations of masculinity or femininity

Thus from conception we are all sexual beings subject to multiple influences throughout life. If the previous processes proceed without interference, the person's biologic sex is congruent with gender identity and gender role.

This complex set of biologic and psychosocial variables begun at conception has a pervasive influence on the remainder of our lives. The biologic component of sexuality (sexual function or expression) constantly interacts with the psychologic components (gender identity, thoughts, and feelings), as well as with social factors (such as sanctioned role and mores and folkways regulating sexual expression). Such complexity mandates a holistic approach to conceptualizing a person's sexual problems and concerns.

Physiologic aspects of human sexuality

PHASES OF THE HUMAN SEXUAL RESPONSE

Masters and Johnson, pioneers in the scientific study of the physiologic aspects of sexual behavior, demonstrated that sexual response is a cyclic phenomenon consisting of four phases.[36]

The physiologic changes seen during human sexual response (Table 34-1) depend on two main principles: myotonia and vasocongestion. It is through the congestion of pelvic blood vessels and involuntary muscular contractions in the pelvic organs and other parts of the body that changes supportive of orgasmic experience are attained. It should also be noted that sexual response involves the total body.

Excitement phase

The excitement phase is the initial component of the cycle. It develops from sexually arousing stimuli such as touch; an increase in sexual tension is observed during this phase. Vasocongestive changes are seen in the external genitals and the breast in both women and men. In addition, a sex flush, which looks like a red, maculopapular rash, appears over the chest in some persons. An increase in both the heart rate and blood pressure is evident, paralleling the level of sexual excitement.

Plateau

The plateau phase is a consolidation period during which sexual tension becomes intensified. Vasocongestion continues. The uterus continues to elevate in the pelvis, which creates a tenting effect in the innermost portion of the vagina. The sex flush continues to spread, sometimes involving the neck, face, and arms. Hyperventilation occurs in both sexes, along with heart rates of 100 to 175 beats per minute. There is elevation of systolic blood pressure (20 to 60 mm Hg for women, 20 to 80 mm Hg for men) and diastolic blood pressure (10 to 20 mm Hg for women, 10 to 40 mm Hg for men).

Orgasm

Orgasm, the involuntary climax of sexual tension, involves only a small portion of the sexual response cycle. The climactic release of sexual tension is evident in contractions throughout the body. Uterine contractions are also noted in the female with orgasm, much like those characteristic of labor.

Resolution

During the resolution phase, an involuntary period, the changes involving the blood vessels, sexual organs, and muscular tension are reversed. The uterus and testes return to their normal positions. Cardiovascular and respiratory rates quickly return to normal. Occasionally a thin film of perspiration may appear over the entire body. Women may at this time begin another sexual response cycle immediately; men must observe an obligatory period during which they cannot be restimulated to higher levels of sexual tension.

Phases of the human sexual response

Phase	Description
Excitement	Increase in sexual tension evidenced by swelling of genitalia and vaginal lubrication
Plateau	Intensification of sexual tension with more pronounced genital swelling
Orgasm	Involuntary climax and release of sexual tension evidenced by muscle contraction
Resolution	Dissipation of muscle tension and swelling

Table 34-1. Sex organ changes during sexual response

Phase	Changes in the female	Changes in the male
Excitement	Vaginal lubrication Vagina becomes longer and wider Uterus begins to elevate in pelvis Clitoris becomes longer and wider Labia minora extend outward Nipples enlarge, areolae become engorged, breast size increases	Penis becomes erect Scrotal sac tenses Testes begin to rise toward perineum Nipples enlarge
Plateau	Clitoris retracts Labia and outer part of vagina (orgasmic platform) become congested Uterus continues to rise in pelvis	Diameter of penis continues to increase Testes increase in size to 50% and elevate close to perineum
Orgasm	Orgasmic platform contracts rapidly (throbbing sensation) Uterine contractions Rectal sphincter contractions	Expulsive contraction along entire urethra to expel semen Internal bladder sphincter contractions (prevent semen from entering bladder) Rectal sphincter contractions
Resolution	Vasocongestion decreases rapidly from vagina/labia and slowly from clitoris and breasts Uterus descends to usual position	Rapid loss of penis size to 1 to 1.5 times usual size Slower resolution of penis size to usual size Testes descend into scrotum

REQUIREMENTS FOR SEXUAL RESPONSE

The requirements for the physiologic sexual response include intact sexual organs, adequate vasculature to support the vasocongestive changes, functional innervation of the genital organs, and the appropriate hormonal milieu.[32] The changes of myotonia and vasocongestion are thought to be mediated by the autonomic nervous system. Perception of the sexual experience at cortical levels requires intact sensory pathways from the genitals and other peripheral structures to the cortex. The capacity to stimulate oneself or a partner sexually depends on the presence of intact motor pathways from higher centers to the effector muscles involved. It should also be noted that thoughts and feelings or visual, auditory, and olfactory-gustatory stimuli alone may result in arousal to orgasmic experience even in the absence of tactile perception.

Adequate hormonal milieu, with appropriate hormonal release, influences both the structure and function of the genitals; for example, the decreased estrogen levels during menopause are believed to be responsible for a decreased amount of vaginal lubrication. Finally, the presence of intact genital structures is usually thought to be a requisite for sexual response, but substitution of prosthetic devices for sexual organs is an option beginning to be explored. Although each of these components is important in sexual response, it is possible for humans to experience profound sexual pleasure even when one or more of these is absent.

TRIPHASIC CONCEPT OF HUMAN SEXUAL RESPONSE

Recently Kaplan[12] has suggested a triphasic concept of human sexual response. She delineates three phases—

desire, excitement, and orgasm—that are related components of sexual response but are governed by separate neurophysiologic systems. This notion is useful for understanding not only the physiology of sexual response, but also the consequences of pathophysiologic conditions, the etiology of sexual dysfunction, and appropriate therapies.

Desire phase

The desire phase refers to the experience of a sexual appetite or drive produced by the activation of a neural system in the brain. Sexual desire is experienced as sensations that move the person to seek sexual experiences. It is likely that the sexual centers of the brain have either neural or chemical connections with the pleasure and pain centers of the brain. The pleasure centers are stimulated when we have sex, which accounts for the pleasurable quality of sexual behavior. On the other hand, the pain centers can inhibit the sexual system. Some persons suggest that the pleasure center is stimulated by release of endorphins in sexual behavior. If a sexual object or situation produces pain, then it will cease to evoke desire.

Testosterone is important in mediating sexual desire in both men and women. Luteinizing hormone and the neurotransmitters serotonin and dopamine also may be important in mediating sexual desire. Bonding to another person and love are powerful stimuli to sexual desire. There seem to be many stimuli capable of evoking sexual desire, such as sight, smell, and other sensory cues, and some of these are conditioned by culture. Fear and pain, however, are potent inhibitors.

The connections between the sex center and other parts of the brain also make it possible for people to "turn off" sexual desire when other stimuli are more important or when it is not to the individual's advantage to pursue sexual activity. Hypoactive desire and inhibited sexual desire are common problems of the sexual desire phase.

Excitement phase

The excitement phase is similar to the excitement and plateau phases described by Masters and Johnson and is produced by reflex vasodilation of the genital blood vessels. This vasodilation causes the genitalia to swell and changes their shape to adapt to their reproductive function. The vasocongestion is primarily a parasympathetically mediated response, and an intense sympathetic response such as that produced by fear and anxiety can instantly lead to loss of erection. It is believed that erection is governed by two spinal reflex centers. The thoracolumbar center (psychogenic) appears to respond more to psychic stimuli, whereas the sacral center is stimulated from tactile input to the genitalia. It is believed that the spinal reflex centers and the higher neural connections are analogous in men and women. Disorders of the excitement phase include difficulty in attaining or maintaining erection in men and difficulty with swelling and lubrication in women.

Orgasm phase

The orgasm phase corresponds to orgasm as described by Masters and Johnson. It is also a genital reflex governed by spinal neural centers, but it consists of reflex contractions of certain genital muscles. Disorders of the orgasm phase include inadequate ejaculatory control (premature ejaculation) and retarded ejaculation in men and orgasmic dysfunction in women. Other disorders include painful intercourse and sexual phobias.

Sexuality and aging

Changes in sexual function become accentuated during middle age, although their onset is gradual and they probably begin long before they are perceived. Men need more time to attain an erection, and once attained, it is likely to be less full than in earlier years. The testes elevate more slowly with sexual excitement, and vasocongestive changes in the scrotum and testes are less noticeable. With prolongation of the plateau phase of the sexual response cycle, the middle-aged man actually achieves much better control over ejaculation than he had as a young adult.

Orgasm is perceived as happening more quickly, and feelings of ejaculatory inevitability may disappear entirely. Resolution of sexual tension becomes more rapid with age, and the obligatory refractory period (a period during which the man cannot be restimulated to orgasm) becomes longer. With aging, men actually gain better control of ejaculation, and because of reduced ejaculatory demand, they may be satisfied not to ejaculate with each intercourse.

In women, menopausal changes may lead to delay in production of vaginal lubrication and diminished expansion of the vaginal barrel. Changes in external genitals as well as the breasts are apparent. The woman's orgasmic experience becomes shorter, and resolution occurs more rapidly.

Studies of healthy aging individuals indicate that a decline in overall interest and activity is seen with age. However, men from each age range tend to report greater interest and activity than women in each respective age range. Several factors can influence sexual interest and activity in middle and old age. Level of sexual activity in youth appears to be related to that in older years.[17]

Factors that influence sexual interest and activity in middle and old age

Women	Men
Marital status: availability of a partner	Past sexual experience
Age	Age
Enjoyment of sex in earlier years	Objective and subjective health ratings
	Social class

As men age, an interest-activity gap appears; that is, they desire more sexual activity than they are able to experience. This gap grows as men age; however, it remains small for women. Women without a socially acceptable partner may adaptively inhibit their sexual interest. The wider interest-activity gap for men may reflect their socialization to express more interest in sex. Other social factors, such as the role loss associated with children leaving the parents' home and retirement, are likely to influence the older person's sexual interests.

Variations in sexual expression

Sexual behavior is a product of society and culture as well as our biology. Each culture has a set of norms that prescribes which behaviors are sexual and which are acceptable. In cross-cultural comparisons of sexual behavior, a wide variety of sexual expression is found. In Western society, sex is frequently equated with penis-in-vagina intercourse. Yet a wide range of behaviors exists encompassing sexual meaning (for example, talking, sharing thoughts and feelings, or just touching another person). This wide range of behaviors causes us to question what is "normal." Yet normal can refer to prevalence of a behavior, optimal function, a statistical distribution, or fashionable or socially acceptable behavior. Comfort[5] suggests that as professionals we do not restrict our definition of normal to what we, personally, admit to enjoying.

Sexual variations

Heterosexuality	Choice of adult sexual partner of opposite sex
Homosexuality	Choice of adult sexual partner of same sex
Bisexuality	Choice of adult sexual partners of same and opposite sex
Transvestism	Sexual satisfaction achieved by dressing in clothing of opposite sex
Incest	Sexual relations with close relative, for example, child
Zoophilia	Choice of sexual object is an animal
Fetishism	Sexual object is an inanimate object
Voyeurism	Sexual satisfaction achieved by watching others
Exhibitionism	Sexual satisfaction achieved by exposing genitals
Sadism	Sexual satisfaction achieved by inflicting pain
Masochism	Sexual satisfaction achieved by receiving pain

Instead he recommends that we consider the following questions:

1. What does the behavior mean to the individual?
2. Does the behavior enrich or impoverish the sexual life of the individual and those persons with whom sexual relations are shared?
3. Is the behavior tolerable to society?

Variation in sexual behavior is bounded only by one's imagination and to some extent by the culture. Different types of sexual expression are described in box below.

Sexual intercourse may be restricted to marriage or to a similar relationship in some socities. In others there may be legitimized extramarital rights, and in some, premarital sexual freedom is encouraged. The position for intercourse varies between cultures and within cultures. Usually the position assumed for intercourse reflects other aspects of the culture; for example, in cultures where families sleep in the same quarters, often side-to-side positions are used to afford some privacy from other occupants of the room.

Culture also dictates whether the woman plays an active or passive role in sexual activity and the duration of the act of intercourse. Precopulatory stimulation may be brief or lengthy, and the type used, such as kissing, painful acts, and manipulation of the breasts or genitals, varies with the culture. Sexual frequency may also be governed by norms, and in some cultures is prohibited during menses, lactation, pregnancy, or before hunts or battles.

Heterosexuality is the most prevalent form of sexual expression among adults of known societies, but it is rarely the only type of sexual behavior in which humans engage. Homosexual behavior is found in most species of mammals; in humans it is most common among adolescents and males.

Since "normal" sexual response may be determined by cultural norms as well as physiologic, phylogenetic, legal, statistical, moral, and social standards, it is impossible to state a hard and fast definition of the "normal state."

HOMOSEXUALITY

Homosexuality is the most common sexual variation, yet is poorly understood by health professionals. It has been viewed as an illness, a criminal offense, and a lifestyle in Western society. Recently the American Psychiatric Association removed homosexuality from the "illness" classification; however, the social climate remains less liberated. Although the majority of society still seems to subscribe to the definition of homosexuality as an illness, only a minority of homosexuals classify themselves as ill.

Kinsey[33,34] estimated that 13% of women and 37% of men had had at least one homosexual experience leading to orgasm. The extent to which these persons engaged in homosexual behavior varied greatly. Thus Kinsey suggested that a continuum existed on which the two poles represented exclusive heterosexuality (0) and homosexuality (6), and the five remaining categories (1 through 5) represented a combination of the two. Individuals in categories 1 and 5 had predominant heterosexual or homosexual orientations. Those in categories 2 and 4 still had a clear preference for heterosexual or homosexual relations, but retained an active interest in the other form. Category 3 represented persons who had equal heterosexual and homosexual interests.

The Institute for Sex Research[2] conducted a large-scale study of the sexual dimensions of homosexual experience in the San Fancisco Bay area. Although the authors of the report are careful to point out that their results may not mirror the entire homosexual population, the study did include men and women, both white and black. Results revealed that homosexuality encompasses more than the person's sexual tendencies. Although there was variability on the homosexual-heterosexual continuum for both male and female homosexuals, there was more heterosexuality in the feelings and behaviors of homosexual women than men.

Most of the homosexual men and women were relatively covert about their homosexuality. The mother and siblings were more likely to be aware of the individual's homosexuality than other family members. Families were more likely to be aware of the person's homosexuality than other members of society. In most cases friends, employers, and colleagues were aware of the person's homosexuality.

Homosexual men or women could not be stereotyped as sexually hyperactive or inactive; instead, the amount of activity varied with each individual. Public cruising (purposive search for a sexual partner) was infrequent among lesbians. Of those homosexuals involved in public cruising, most conducted their sexual activity in their own homes. Gay bars were the most popular cruising locales.

Homosexual men had many more sexual partners than did lesbians. There seemed to be more emphasis placed on sexual activity among males. This may be a function of lesbians' preference for relationships based more on emotions than on sex, or it may merely be a function of the problems male homosexuals experience in meeting partners. For both male and female homosexuals, a relatively steady relationship with a love partner was a meaningful event.

The male homosexual subculture seemed to place more emphasis on youth than did women. Social prestige did not seem to be a major determinant of sexual appeal.

A variety of sexual techniques was used. Male homosexuals most frequently employed fellatio, hand-genital stimulation, and anal intercourse. Female homosexuals most frequently engaged in masturbation with their partners and in cunnilingus. Men and women both specified receiving oral-genital sex as a preferred technique.

Sexual problems encountered included difficulty in meeting a suitable sexual partner, maintaining affection for the partner, and meeting the other's sexual request. There was a lower incidence of these problems among lesbians. Whereas almost two thirds of the male homosexuals had at some time contracted a sexually transmitted disease from homosexual sex, only one of the lesbians had done so. More women than men had considered stopping their homosexuality, but only a minority in each case had done so. At interview, more men than women regretted their homosexuality.

About 20% of the homosexual males had been married, and more than 33% of the white lesbians and almost 50% of the black lesbians had been married once. They did not perceive their homosexuality as having a particular affect on their children.

Homosexual men and women seemed to have more friends than their heterosexual counterparts. Their friends included both homosexuals and heterosexuals. Lesbians were more involved in activities outside the home or with others than were homosexual males. Men were more likely than women to have experienced social difficulties, but few had been arrested because of their homosexuality.

When homosexual respondents were compared with their heterosexual counterparts in terms of adult psychologic adjustment, it appeared that the dysfunctional and asexual homosexuals were less well off than those in the heterosexual group. However, homosexual adults who have come to terms with their homosexuality are no more distressed psychologically than heterosexual men and women.[2] Thus therapists would do well to consider why a person's homosexuality is problematic and examine ways to enhance the person's life rather than direct therapy at changing the person's sexual orientation.

SEXUALITY AND ILLNESS

People today seem to be more comfortable in expressing their concerns about their sexual health than has previously been the case. As a result of this increased comfort, nurses are increasingly expected to provide accurate information about sexuality and health, as well as to listen with comfort and understanding to the sexual concerns patients describe. Although many persons can openly describe their problems, others are too embarrassed or lack the vocabulary necessary to do so. For this reason it is important that nurses have a frame of reference to help them identify persons at risk for sexual problems or concerns.

There are many ways in which illness may affect sexuality and sexual function. Illness may influence sexuality through changes in body structure or function, use of certain medications, or alteration in the person's body image.

Changes in body structure

Changes in the structure of the nervous system, circulatory system, or genital organs may result in sexual health problems. Many examples of these structural changes and the probable mechanism by which they interfere with sexual health are given in Table 34-2. Anatomic disruptions are probably best exemplified by the spinal cord–injured person who has sustained irreversible

Table 34-2. Changes in body structure and sexual health

System	Probable mechanism of interference
Central and peripheral nervous systems	
Spinal cord injury	Disrupts integrity of peripheral nerves and spinal cord reflexes involved in sexual response (for example, erection)
Spinal cord tumors	
Herniated disk	
Multiple sclerosis	
Spina bifida	
Amyotrophic lateral sclerosis	
Tumors of frontal or temporal lobes	May interfere with function of centers controlling sexual drive
Cerebrovascular accident	
Trauma to frontal or temporal lobes	
Cardiovascular system	
Thrombus formation in vessels of penis	May interfere with blood supply to penis, thus interfering with erection
Leriche's syndrome	
Sickle cell disorders	
Leukemia	
Trauma to vasculature supplying sexual organs	
Reproductive/sexual system	
Prostatectomy, radical perineal	May destroy nerve supply, interfering with sensory and motor aspects of sexual response
Abdominal perineal resection	
Lumbar sympathectomy	
Rhizotomy	May result in disturbed ejaculation
Absence of penis or penile injury	May result in impotence as well as disturbed ejaculation
Penectomy	
Imperforate hymen	Precludes or discourages intromission
Congenital absence of vagina	
Pelvic exenteration	
Vaginectomy	
Obstetric trauma or poor episiotomy	Leaves gaping vaginal opening or painful scarring, thus discouraging intercourse
Damage to pubococcygeus muscle	

damage to neural pathways that interferes with some methods of sexual function (Chapter 20).

Changes in body function

Many illnesses alter physiologic processes esential to the sexual response, including nervous transmission, vasocongestion, hormonal metabolism myotonia, and perception of pleasurable sensation. Table 34-3 illustrates some illnesses that have the potential to interfere with sexual response and the hypothesized mechanisms by which they affect sexual response.

In general, it appears that the extent of a physiologic disorder and its chronicity determine relative frequency of sexual problems. Diabetic women experience a higher rate of difficulty with lubrication than do nondiabetic women, particularly women who have been diabetic for 6 years or longer and who have neuropathy.[23a] This relationship between chronicity and dysfunction is also observed in men with diabetes. A high incidence of impotence, however, is found among diabetic men during the first year after diagnosis. It is believed in this instance

that the lack of diabetic control (physiologic derangement) is responsible for the sexual dysfunction.[39]

For chronic illnesses as a group, it is easy to hypothesize a relationship between perception of health status, degree of fatigue, metabolic derangements, altered roles, fear of dying, and the demands of a chronic illness on the partner and changes in the sexual relationship.

Although some medical-surgical conditions do not interfere directly with sexual functions, their perceived seriousness or the presence of symptoms discourages persons from engaging in their usual sexual practices. One very common example is associated with cardiac disease, more specifically myocardial infarction. Although marital coitus probably does not demand a great energy expenditure, many persons are fearful of attempting intercourse after having a heart attack. One study of married men who had had myocardial infarctions demonstrated that heart rates with orgasm were much lower in this group than among the younger group studied by Masters and Johnson.[3] An active physical conditioning program did produce significant improvements in the frequency and quality of sexual activity for men who had had a myocar-

Table 34-3. Influence of changes in body function on sexual health

Physiologic interferences	Hypothesized mechanism of action	Physiologic interferences	Hypothesized mechanism of action
Systemic diseases		**Diseases of the genitalia—cont'd**	
Pulmonary disease	Debility, pain, and depression probably interfere with sexual desire as well as expression	Trauma to penis	
Renal disease		Vaginal infections	
Malignancies		Senile vaginitis	
Infections		Vulvitis	
Degenerative diseases		Leukoplakia	
Some cardiovascular diseases		Bartholin's cyst	
		Allergic response to vaginal sprays and deodorants	
Metabolic disruptions		Vaginitis following radiation therapy	
Cirrhosis	Hepatic problems in men result in estrogen buildup from inability of liver to conjugate estrogens; similar processes occur in women along with general debility	Pelvic inflammatory disease	
Mononucleosis		Fibroadenomas	
Hepatitis		Endometriosis	
		Uterine prolapse	
		Anal fissures, hemorrhoids	
Hypothyroidism	By depression of CNS function, general debilitation, and depression, libido may be decreased, and impaired erectile abilities in men may result	Pelvic masses	Local irritability, damage to genitalia, and consequent interference with reflex mechanisms involved in erection and ejaculation
Addison's disease		Ovarian cysts	
Hypogonadism		Prostatitis	
Hypopituitarism		Urethritis	
Acromegaly			
Feminizing tumors			
Cushing's disease		**Medical or surgical castration**	
Diabetes mellitus		Orichiectomy	Lowered androgen levels depress libido and lead to impotence, retarded ejaculation, or impaired sexual responsiveness
Diseases of the genitalia		Radiation therapy	
Priapism	Each of these problems involves damage to genital organs, which may result in painful intercourse	Oophorectomy, adrenalectomy	
Peyronie's disease			
Balantitis			
Phimosis			
Genital herpes			

Modified from Kaplan, H.S.: The new sex therapy, New York, 1974, Quadrangle Press.

dial infarction. This energy expenditure associated with sex seemed to be better tolerated by those who exercised regularly.

In general, the literature indicates that the postmyocardial infarction patient may return to regular sexual activity provided there are no symptoms of congestive heart failure. However, certain conditions that increase energy expenditure during coitus are to be avoided. These include having intercourse shortly after a meal or soon after alcohol consumption, since both increase the heart rate and metabolic demands. Extremes in temperatures and anxiety-provoking or secretive situations should also be avoided. The energy expenditure in climbing two flights of stairs appears to produce a greater increase in heart rate than does orgasm.[13]

Effects of pharmacologic agents

Pharmacologic agents that have the potential to affect sexual drive, as well as performance, are listed in Table 34-4. The relationship between extent of physiologic derangement and degree of sexual dysfunction may be demonstrated by pharmacologically induced changes. For example, alcohol induces transiently positive changes; in small doses it initially promotes relaxation and release of inhibitions, as do other psychoactive drugs. However, in larger doses, alcohol has negative effects on sexual function, leading to central nervous system depression and interference with motor activity.

Several categories of drugs have demonstrably negative effects on sexual function. These include antihypertensives, antidepressants, antihistamines, antispasmodics,

Table 34-4. Drug effects on human sexual behavior

Drug or drug category	Effect	Probable mechanism of action
Oral contraceptives	Positive	Permits separation of sexual activity from concern about conception
Antihypertensives Guanethidine (Ismelin) Reserpine (Serpasil) Mecamylamine (Inversine) Trimethaphan (Arfonad) Spironolactone (Aldactone)	Negative	Peripheral blockade of nervous innervation of sex glands
Antidepressants Imipramine (Tofranil) Desipramine (Norpramin, Pertofrane) Amitryptyline (Elavil) Nortriptyline (Aventyl) Protriptyline (Vivactil) Phenelzine sulfate (Nardil) Tranylcypromine sulfate (Parnate) Pargyline (Eutonyl)	Negative	Central depression; peripheral blockade of nervous innervation of sex glands
Antihistamines Diphenhydramine (Benadryl) Promethazine (Phenergan) Chlorpheniramine (Chlor-Trimeton)	Negative	Blockade of parasympathetic nervous innervation of sex glands
Antispasmodics Methantheline (Banthine) Glycopyrrolate (Robinul) Hexocyclium (Tral) Poldine (Nacton)	Negative	Ganglionic blockage of nervous innervation of sex glands
Sedatives and tranquilizers Chlorpromazine (Thorazine, Megaphen) Prochlorperazine (Compazine) Thioridazine (Mellaril) Mesoridazine (Serentil) Chlordiazepoxide (Librium) Diazepam (Valium) Benperidol Phenoxybenzamine (Dibenzyline) Chlorprothixene (Taractan)	Negative and positive	Central sedation; blockade of autonomic innervation of sex glands; suppression of hypothalamic and pituitary function Tranquilization and relaxation
Ethyl alcohol	Negative Transiently positive	Central depression; suppression of motor activity; diuresis Release of inhibitions; relaxation
Sex hormone preparations Cyproterone acetate Methandrostenolone (Dianabol) Nandrolone phenpropionate (Durabolin) Norethandrolone (Nilevar)	Negative	Antiandrogenic effects on sexual function; loss of libido; decreased potency
Potassium nitrate (saltpeter)	Questionable	Diuresis

From Woods, N.F.: Human sexuality in health and illness, ed. 3, St. Louis, 1984, The C.V. Mosby Co.   *Continued.*

Table 34-4. Drug effects on human sexual behavior—cont'd

Drug or drug category	Effect	Probable mechanism of action
Cantharis (Spanish fly)	Negative	Irritation and inflammation of genitourinary tract, systemic poisoning
Yohimbine	Questionable	Stimulation of lower spinal nerve centers
Narcotics and psychoactive drugs	Negative	Central depression; decreased libido and impaired potency
Morphine	Transiently positive	Release of inhibitions; increased suggestibility; relaxation
Heroin		
Cocaine		
Marijuana		
LSD		
Amphetamines		
L-Dopa and p-chlorophenylalanine	Questionable	Improvement of well-being
Amyl nitrite	Questionable	Vasodilation of genitourinary tract; sommoth muscle relaxation
Caffeine	Questionable	CNS stimulant
Vitamin E, selenium	Questionable	Supports fertility in laboratory animals

Table 34-5. Some health problems resulting in body image changes that may raise sexual concerns

Surgically induced	Traumatically induced	Others
Mastectomy	Burns	Dermatologic disorders
Ostomy	Lacerations, scarring	Obesity
Hysterectomy	Amputations	Congenital anomalies of sexual organs (for example, absence of penis, hypospadias)
Amputation of limb or limbs		Unusual breast size, including immaturity or hypertrophy

sedatives, and tranquilizers, ethyl alcohol, some sex hormone preparations, and some narcotics and psychoactive drugs.

Body image changes

The extent to which distortion of body image influences sexuality often depends on the perceptions of two persons: oneself and a significant other. Multiple variables may influence the body image of a woman who has had a mastectomy. Although one might suspect that the extent of surgery and pain in the operative area would be most important, the value she assigned to her breasts, her preoperative body image, and social factors such as the quality of her preoperative sexual relationship are also influential. In one study the quality of the relationship the woman had with her husband before the surgery was the most important determinant of her return to sexual functioning after surgery.[27]

The visibility of a defect plays an important role in sexual adaptation. Visibility of a disability seems to be just as disruptive of marital and family relations as it is of other social relationships.[27]

Finally, the meaning and significance one attaches to the changed body part may interfere with sexual behavior. The amputee who views the loss as castration, the

woman who sees her hysterectomy as a neutering surgery, and the person who equates an ostomy with loss of adult control are likely to experience problems with self-image and, in turn, sexual adjustment. Thus both society's perception of the person and the individual's concept of self can interfere with sexual health. Some common health problems resulting in body image change are listed in Table 34-5.

Several authorities believe that the interpersonal components of sexual problems are of primary importance. They advise that both partners be involved in the treatment of sexual problems.

Environmental restrictions

Environmental factors such as privacy, competing stimuli, and segregation interfere with sexual expression. Institutionalization rarely affords sufficient privacy for sexual expression. Many institutions segregate persons on the basis of sex. For whatever reason this may be done, the act of segregation may elicit a range of adaptation, including masturbation, homosexual activity, or withdrawal from human warmth.[37] Often these adaptive behaviors are punished, and those who resort to them are stigmatized. In some institutions staff members may assume an in lococ parentis stance, treating even aging perscns as if they required protection from their sexual inclinations.

SEXUAL CONCERNS, DIFFICULTIES, AND DYSFUNCTIONS

People experience a variety of sexual problems ranging from concerns about sexual phenomena to sexual dysfunctions. Each type of problem is the consequence of different antecedents, and each requires somewhat different therapeutic approaches.

Sexual concerns

Sexual concerns constitute a souce of worry, dissatisfaction, or discomfort for individuals but do not produce difficulty in sexual function, profound problems in the sexual relationship, or a greatly altered sexual self-concept. Sexual concerns often arise because of misinformation or lack of information, conflicting values, difficulty communicating about sexual issues, and anxiety or guilt about sexual phenomena.

These concerns are usually amenable to sex education strategies, such as permission giving, provision of limited information, values clarification exercises, rehearsal of communication, validation of normalcy, and provision of anticipatory guidance.

Sexual difficulties

Sexual difficulties create discomfort in the sexual relationship, may occasionally interfere with sexual function, and sometimes may challenge the person's sexual self-image. Sexual difficulties include the following:
1. Inability to relax
2. Disinterest in sexual activity
3. Sexual dissatisfaction
4. Inability to please or be pleased by a partner
5. Problems in the timing of sexual activities

These difficulties are amenable to counseling approaches, including relaxation training, exploration of alternatives in the sexual repertoire, provision of specific suggestions, and training in communication skills.

Sexual dysfunctions

Sexual dysfunctions usually result not only in disruption of sexual function but also in severe strains on the sexual relationship and a threatened sexual self-image. There are several types of sexual dysfunctions: disorders of sexual desire, disorders of arousal, disorders of orgasm,[12] and pain with coitus.

DISORDERS OF SEXUAL DESIRE

Disorders of the desire phase include hypoactive sexual desire and inhibited sexual desire. The person with hypoactive sexual desire loses interest in sexual matters, does not pursue sexual gratification, and is not likely to

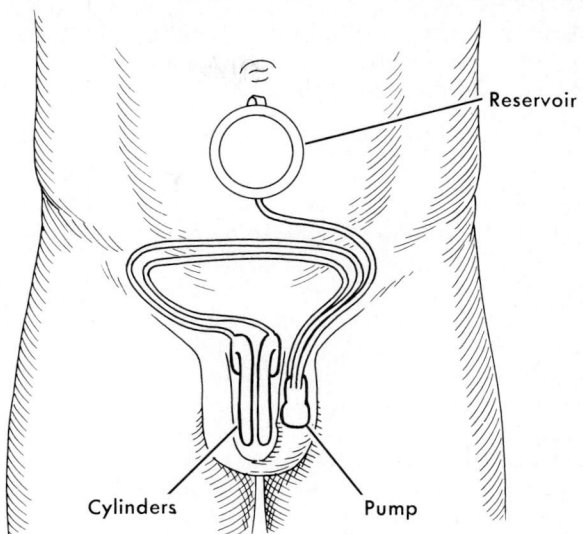

Fig. 34-2. Inflatable penile prosthetic implant. Reservoir is implanted under abdominal muscles, inflatable cylinders in each corpus cavernosum, and pump inside scrotum. Man can compress pump to fill cylinders from reservoir, producing penile erection. Small release valve in lower portion of pump bulb releases fluid to return penis to flaccid state.

participate in sexual opportunities. Individuals with inhibited sexual desire may be able to experience lubrication or erection but do not experience much pleasure.

DISORDERS OF AROUSAL

Disorders of arousal (the excitement phase) include inability to have an erection in men (erectile dysfunction, sometimes referred to as *impotence*) and difficulty with lubrication and swelling in women (*general sexual dysfunction*). Erectile dysfunction probably affects most men at least once in their lifetimes, and transient episodes are estimated to occur in 50% of all men. These fleeting episodes are considered within the range of normal. Impotence occurs in varying degrees; some men experience total inability to attain an erection of sufficient hardness. This frustrating, humiliating condition may lead to decreased self-esteem and consequent depression. Impotence is described as primary if the man has never been able to achieve or maintain an erection that would permit intercourse. Secondary impotence, a more common phenomenon, occurs situationally and is likely to be seen in conjunction with pathophysiologically and pharmacologically induced states.

The penile prosthetic implant has recently been devised as a method of treatment for organic erectile dysfunction in men. The inflatable penile prosthesis (Fig. 34-2) is implanted surgically and does not interfere with normal urinary elimination. The prosthesis is inserted through perineal and abdominal incisions. Penile edema is minimal, but scrotal edema may occur. Pain may be severe during the first week, and mild pain may continue for several weeks after surgery. As with any prosthetic device, there is a need to integrate it into the person's self-image and the relationship.

DISORDERS OF ORGASM

Disorders of the orgasmic phase include inadequate ejaculatory control or premature or retarded ejaculation in men and orgasmic dysfunction in women.

Premature ejaculation occurs when the man cannot inhibit his ejaculation for a long enough period of time to permit his partner to experience orgasm in at least half of their attempts at intercourse. This is thought likely to be a conditioned response to hurried circumstances and is treated quite successfully by means of the "squeeze technique." This technique requires the man or his partner to place the thumb and second and third fingers at the coronal ridge of the glans, exerting enough pressure over this area for 3 to 4 seconds to relieve the feeling of ejaculatory inevitability. *Retarded ejaculation,* also known as ejaculatory incompetence, implies that despite the amount and quality of stimulation of the penis, intravaginal ejaculation either does not occur or is so delayed that the couple experiences pelvic irritation and fatigue as a result.

Primary orgasmic dysfunction occurs in the woman who has not experienced orgasm with sexual activity, including intercourse or masturbation. Secondary orgasmic dysfunction is characterized by the inability to experience orgasm under certain conditions. The woman with secondary orgasmic dysfunction has experienced orgasmic sensations with one form of stimulation at some point in her life. This problem does not preclude the woman from experiencing sexual arousal and its physiologic accompaniments. Rather, only the orgasmic portion of the sexual response cycle seems impaired.

PAIN WITH COITUS

Vaginismus is a relatively rare sexual problem characterized by an involuntary, conditioned spasm of the vaginal outlet, thus causing it to shut tightly. This problem precludes sexual intercourse, but vaginismic women may be orgasmic with alternative methods of sexual stimulation.

Dyspareunia, or painful intercourse, may be attributable to a number of factors ranging from a full lower bowel to feelings of aversion toward sexual intercourse. It is sometimes experienced by women with steroid alterations, for example, the postpartum mother and the postmenopausal women.

Gender disorders

Although many gender disorders exist, they are encountered less often in medical-surgical practice than the problems discussed earlier. Recently the media have called attention to one gender identity problem, transsexualism, that may be encountered in some medical-surgical services.

Transsexualism refers to the condition of people who are convinced that they are "trapped in the body of the wrong sex." These persons believe that they belong to the opposite sex and desire the body, appearance, and social status of the opposite sex. Many actually live in the role of the opposite sex before treatment. Male-to-female transsexuals are usually treated initially with hormonal therapy, and later surgical revision of the genitals is performed. The surgery involves removal of the male genitals and revision of the scrotal and neighboring tissue to resemble the female genitals. Usually the surgery is cosmetically successful, and an artificial but functional vagina can be created. These women are, of course, sterile, since they have neither ovaries nor uterus.

The female-to-male transsexual has a less cosmetically effective and functional surgical transformation. In a series of procedures, the breasts and the vulva are revised and a phallus is created. Hormonal therapy is also used to effect the transformation. Often the creation of the penis requires extensive grafting and surgical revision, and the female-to-male transformation is consequently more difficult and usually less satisfactory. After the transformation these men are also sterile.

Both men and women electing transsexual surgery require considerable emotional support. They usually have careful psychologic assessments before and following the surgery. Because of their cultural conditioning, nurses sometimes find it difficult to relate appropriately to the transsexual. Often it is necessary to analyze one's attitudes and values carefully to be accepting of these patients.

Transsexualism should not be confused with *transvestism,* the act of dressing in the clothing of the opposite sex. Additionally, transsexuals are not homosexuals.

Hermaphroditism is a congenital condition in which the reproductive structures appear ambiguous. Early life experiences seem to have profound impact on our gender identities. It is important, therefore, that sexual assignment be correctly established early in life to prevent gender confusion later.

NURSING PRACTICE

Prerequisites for intervention

Three prerequisites are important before practitioners can help individuals with their sexual problems:
1. A knowledge base
2. Awareness of own value system
3. Ability to communicate genuinely and therapeutically with patients

KNOWLEDGE BASE

The knowledge base that is required is listed in the box on p. 1039. Without such knowledge the nurse has no basis for discriminating between normal and abnormal responses or the interpretation of patients' concerns, and thus no basis for education or counseling.

Knowledge base prerequisite for sexual counseling

Understanding of sexual response
Knowledge of the variety of sexual behaviors that exist in our society and their prevalence
Understanding of the types of sexual dysfunctions
Awareness of the relationship between age, life events, pathologic conditions, behavioral problems, pharmaceutic agents, and sexual function

---

AWARENESS OF OWN VALUE SYSTEM

In addition to an adequate knowledge base, an awareness of one's own value system, including the biases and beliefs about appropriate and inappropriate sexual behavior, is also important. Unless professionals can accept their own sexuality and are comfortable with their own behavior, it is difficult to convey comfort to others. Self-acceptance is seen as prerequisite to the development of a nonjudgmental and tolerant approach. Just as individuals have belief systems related to sexual phenomena, so do professionals. This does not imply that the sex educators or counselors must condone every variety of sexual activity. Rather, it is essential that they be aware of their own feelings and values and attempt to keep them in perspective by acknowledging them. This assists them in maintaining a supportive climate that encourages sharing of feeling by patients and simultaneously permits professionals to acknowledge the validity of their own beliefs.

Furthermore, there are some issues about which the professional has such strong beliefs that these values would interfere with effective intervention. An example encountered in practice is the health professional whose basic conviction is that homosexuality is an illness or deviation rather than a variation in sexual expression or orientation. No matter how extensive the professional's training, knowledge base, and therapy skills, such a strong basic belief is likely to interfere greatly with the ability to relate objectively to a homosexual's sexual problems. Often professionals need to acknowledge their inability to deal with sexual problems because of their own value systems. Topics likely to elicit biases among health professionals include abortion, alternative life-styles, and sexual variations.

THERAPEUTIC COMMUNICATION

Finally, the professional needs to be able to communicate genuinely and therapeutically with patients. Often this involves using the person's own language, which may be different from that of the health professional. Without the ability to interact accurately and empathetically with individuals, the most sophisticated knowledge base and objective attitudes are of little benefit.

Nurses frequently encounter behavioral problems that involve the individual's sexuality. One common problem is the patient who acts out sexually, for example, by making inappropriate sexual gestures, using explicit sexual language, or exposing the sexual organs. Two general principles are helpful in coping with such a situation:
1. Analyze what meaning this behavior might have for the patient.
2. Assert the right as a human being to establish limits that protect the nurse's integrity.

In responding to a patient who has exhibited sexual behavior that is deemed inappropriate, one can analyze why the behavior occurs and share this observation with the patient. Is the patient attempting to gain control in a situation in which he or she has little or no control? Is the patient trying to obtain validation of his masculinity or her feminity? Is the patient unaware that the behavior has sexual overtones or is making the nurse uncomfortable?

Nurses have the right to establish limits with patients to protect their own integrity. Violation of certain body boundaries, for example, touching the breasts or buttocks of the nurse or exposing one's genitals, is not behavior that nurses must tolerate to be "accepting of patients." Nurses' responses, however, can address three important points:
1. The inferred meaning of the behavior can be shared—"I know you feel helpless right now. . ."
2. The boundary can be established—"That's not acceptable behavior."
3. The patient's sexuality can be validated—"You're a good looking guy, but that's just not acceptable behavior."

Some patients cannot respond appropriately to these strategies, and in some instances the nurse may need to believe that not working with this patient is permissible.

Prevention of sexual problems

Nurses may prevent sexual problems among patient populations through three strategies: education of patient groups likely to have sexual concerns, provision of anticipatory guidance throughout the life cycle, and promotion of a milieu conducive to sexual health.

EDUCATION OF PATIENT POPULATIONS

Education of patient populations implies more than mere dissemination of information. Just as nurses are being educated to provide sex education, patients may also need assistance in exploring the attitudes and values that shape their sexual behavior and in developing the ability to communicate comfortably about sexual phenomena. Thus providing accurate knowledge about sex and sexuality is not synonymous with education for a healthy sexuality.

ANTICIPATORY GUIDANCE

Nurses are often in strategic positions to provide anticipatory guidance at sensitive points in the life cycle.

Adolescence and middle age are two life periods during which anxiety about sexuality is likely to surface. By informing individuals about the usual changes experienced at these points (for example, nocturnal emissions or concerns about masturbation in adolescents or worry about effects of menopause on the ability to function sexually among middle-aged persons), nurses can assist individuals to cope realistically with major changes in their bodies. Adults with young children can also benefit from anticipatory guidance regarding their children's sexuality.

PROMOTION OF A MILIEU CONDUCIVE TO SEXUAL HEALTH

Some approaches useful in developing a milieu conducive to sexual health include minimizing guilt experienced in conjunction with sexual thoughts, feelings, and behavior. This may be accomplished by assisting persons to examine objectively the consequences of their activities within a reality-oriented framework. Reduction of performance anxiety (for example, concern about how well one is able to function) can be facilitated by helping individuals to understand the relationship between being attentive to their own performance at the expense of losing touch with their sexual feelings. "Spectatoring" refers to the habit of watching oneself or a partner perform. Just as in athletics, one cannot be both spectator and a performer without minimizing the effectiveness of the performance.

Often individuals need to be advised to modify their environments to reduce competing stimuli. Use of anxiety-provoking settings or those settings prone to interruption can help establish dysfunctional patterns. (The relationship between anxiety and orgasmic dysfunction and premature ejaculation has been well established.)

Finally, maintenance of good general health facilitates optimum sexual functioning. Fatigue, pain, and malaise are stimuli that compete with sexual pleasure.

Assessment

THE SEXUAL HISTORY

Many health care providers may not be experienced in eliciting a sexual history and at first may be uneasy. No doubt this uneasiness is conditioned by social prohibitions about discussing intimate matters such as sexual experiences or behavior. However, health professionals are expected to be informed, willing to discuss sexual matters openly with patients, and prepared to educate and counsel them appropriately. Nurses who are hesitant to deal with sexual matters with patients are helped by working through their own feelings about sex and sexual matters. Seeking counsel from other nurses or health professionals who are comfortable with the topic is often helpful. Some nurses may find it helpful to attend a workshop on sexuality for nurses.

Although there is no single approach to taking a sexual history, application of certain principles facilitates both

---

Principles that facilitate obtaining a sexual history

Action	Effect
1. Obtain sexual history early in nurse-patient relationship	Legitimizes sexuality as part of health Provides permission for patient to discuss sexual concerns
2. Avoid overreaction or underreaction to patient's comments	Facilitates truthful data gathering
3. Use language patient understands	Facilitates accurate data gathering
4. Move from less sensitive to more sensitive areas	Facilitates patient-nurse comfort
5. Terminate sexual history by inquiring if patient has additional questions or concerns	Conveys a willingness by nurse to further explore sexual matters

---

the patient's and the nurse's comfort. Absolute requirements for history taking include the following:
1. Provision of privacy, such as in a closed room
2. An atmosphere of trust between patient and nurse, such as assurance of confidentiality for the patient
3. Comfort on the part of nurses with their own sexuality

Some principles for promoting patient-nurse comfort are listed above. The sexual history itself may be therapeutic. Within the context of obtaining the data, the nurse can provide permission for the patient to discuss concerns, provide limited information or suggestions, or validate the normalcy and acceptability of the patient's concerns and practices.

It may be necessary for both patient and nurse to define their terms. Street language may be unfamiliar to the nurse, and highly technical language may be confusing to the patient. The nurse may need to become familiar with some commonly used street language to be sure of what the patient is reporting.

The technique of moving from less sensitive to more sensitive areas paves the way for both the patient and nurse. For example, the nurse may explore a woman's sexual role before discussing her ability to have orgasm, her menstrual history before her experience with sexual variations, and her personal experiences with sex education before her actual sexual experiences. In all of these situations, the decision to pursue the topics depends on the cues presented by the patient that sexual concerns are present.

Brief sexual history

1. Has your (illness, pregnancy, or hospitalization) interfered with your being a (husband, wife, father, mother)?
2. Has your (abortion, heart attack, etc.) changed the way you see yourself as a (woman, man)?
3. Has your (colostomy, hysterectomy, etc.) changed your ability to function sexually (or your sex life)?

BRIEF SEXUAL ASSESSMENT

A brief assessment can be incorporated in the nursing history by means of three questions. The first of these questions deals with the person's role, the next with the affective-cognitive elements of sexuality, and the last with biologic aspects of sexual function. The questions may be modified to deal with illness, hospitalization, life events, or any other relevant entity that may influence or interfere with sexual health.

The questions may also be adapted to elicit the patient's expectations of changes resulting from procedures or hospitalization that he or she is about to experience. These brief items invite the patient to explore sexual concerns. Often it is unnecessary for the nurse to ask the second and third questions, since many patients proceed to state their concerns about masculinity, femininity, and sexual functioning without further prompting.

Promotion of sexual health

PRINCIPLES FOR PROMOTING SEXUAL HEALTH

Mims[16] cites some basic principles involved in the promotion of sexual health. The first of these principles acknowledges that there is no single set of appropriate sexual values in our society. Rather, the professional needs to accept that major conflicts of values exist. A second principle is that education (provision of accurate and adequate information) is more helpful than indoctrination. Although it is often tempting to impose one's own solutions or values on others, growth of the individual is more likely to be fostered by guidance rather than indoctrination. Finally, it is suggested that individuals be assisted to make their own informed choices rather than conform to guidelines established by a professional or an agency. It is the individual, and not the health professional, who will have to cope with the consequences of the individual's choice.

LEVELS OF INTERVENTION

Annon[30] presents an extremely useful distinction between the various levels of intervention possible for persons with sexual concerns or problems. He terms these levels permission, limited information, specific suggestions, and intensive therapy. These are listed in order of sophistication, with permission requiring the most basic preparation and intensive therapy requiring specific educational preparation in sex therapy techniques. Annon's contention is that sexual problems may be resolved on a variety of levels and do not always require counseling or intensive therapy.

Permission

Often individuals merely want to know that they are normal, acceptable, and not "perverted." They seek out the health professional for validation of their sexual normalcy. This type of intervention requires minimal preparation on the part of the professional. Permission may be applied to thoughts, fantasies, dreams, and feelings, as well as to overt sexual behaviors. At times nurses will be asked to provide individuals with permission not to engage in certain sexual behaviors if this is their choice. This may relieve individuals from feeling pressured to conform to someone else's standards for sexual behavior that are not necessarily their own.

People with disabling diseases that interfere with their usual forms of sexual expression may seek permission to discuss alternative approaches to sexual pleasure. For example, cord-injured persons may welcome the permission from staff members to discuss alternatives to penis-vagina intercourse. Women who do not experience orgasm with every act of intercourse may be seeking permission not to do so, even though some of their friends insist that "normal women do." A common concern among young married couples is the normalcy of oral-genital sex. Often these couples merely seek reassurance that this variation is not perverted or, on the contrary, that it is not mandatory to engage in this practice unless both partners are comfortable with it.

Limited information

The next level of intervention can also be therapeutic as well as preventive. It involves providing information to individuals that is directly relevant to their particular problems or concerns. Some common areas of sexual concern that may require only limited information include worry about breast and genital shape, configuration, and size; masturbation; sexual intercourse during menstruation; and oral-genital sex. A woman who is about to have a hysterectomy is often concerned that she will no longer be able to have intercourse or that she will have no more sexual desire. Informing the woman in advance of the surgery that this is not true may remove unnecessary barriers from the resumption of sexual activity. Similar information would be helpful to a man about to undergo a prostatectomy. Even though the man having a transurethral resection is likely to experience retrograde ejaculation, he may still have an erection and enjoy intercourse. Having this information before surgery may avert later sexual problems.

Specific suggestions

Before giving individuals specific suggestions regarding direct attempts to help change their behavior and reach a designated goal, it is essential to obtain a detailed sexual history including the following:

1. Description of the problem; its onset and course
2. The person's ideas about the cause of the problem and why it persists
3. Past attempts at treatment and their effectiveness
4. The patient's current goal for treatment

Some specific suggestions may relate to the conditions conducive to optimum sexual functioning, specific approaches to use given certain illnesses or surgeries, and directives for coping with some sexual dysfunctions. One specific suggestion often incorporated in sexual counseling is that a couple having difficulties with intercourse abstain from it for a specified period. This admonition is designed to reduce the "pressure to perform" perceived by a member of the dysfunctional couple.

Specific suggestions can be given to *cord-injured persons,* including positions most likely to be comfortable, care of the indwelling catheter before and during intercourse, and techniques available to stimulate the noninjured partner. Use of imagery (fantasy) can also be incorporated as a specific suggestion.

Ostomy patients often have concerns about accidents involving their appliances during intercourse. Specific suggestions might include emptying the appliance before initiating sexual activity, employing cosmetic covers for the stoma bag, or avoiding excess pressure over the stoma site until the ostomy incision is well healed.

Cardiac patients can be counseled to minimize their cardiac work load during sexual activity by avoiding intercourse in very hot or very cold rooms and within 3 hours of eating a big meal or drinking alcoholic beverages and by allowing plenty of time for rest after intercourse. Patients who have had myocardial infarctions are counseled to consult a nurse practitioner or physician if they experience chest pain or palpitations during or after intercourse, or if they feel extremely tired afterward.

Nurses can offer some rather simple directives for coping with specific sexual dysfunctions. The man whose problem is premature ejaculation can be taught to use the squeeze technique (p. 1038) or the partner may learn to apply it. Women who have inadequate lubrication and experience painful intercourse as a consequence of steroid starvation during the postpartum period or menopause may benefit from the use of a water-soluble lubricant such as K-Y jelly.

Intensive sexual therapy

The intensive sexual therapy approach combines techniques and concepts of psychotherapy with special approaches to intervention with individuals or couples having sexual problems. Usually the problems involved are one or more of the sexual dysfunctions discussed earlier. These forms of therapy usually require intensive preparation beyond that provided in most schools of nursing. However, an awareness of the sexual dysfunctions enables nurses to refer persons with complex problems to trained therapists.

REFERENCES AND SELECTED READINGS*

1. *Assey, J.L., and Herbert, J.M.: Who is the seductive patient? Am. J. Nurs. **83:**530-532, 1983.
2. Bell, A., and Weinberg, M.: Homosexualities, New York, 1978, Simon & Schuster, Inc.
2a. Bell, A., Weinberg, M., and Kiefer-Hammersmith, S.: Sexual preference: its development in men and women, Bloomington, Ind., 1981, Indiana University Press.
3. *Boyer, G., and Boyer, J.: Sexuality and aging, Nurs. Clin. North Am. **17**(3):421-427, 1982.
4. *Byers, J.P.: Sexuality and the elderly, Geriatr. Nurs. **4**(5):293-297, 1983.
5. Comfort, A.: The normal in sexual behavior: an ethnological point of view, J. Sex. Ed. Ther. **2:**1-7, 1975.
6. *Driver, J.D.: Elders and sexuality, J. Nurs. Care **15**(2):8-11, 1981.
7. Frank, E., Anderson, C., and Rubinstein, D.: Frequency of sexual dysfunction in "normal couples," N. Engl. J. Med. **299:**111-115, 1978.
8. *Fuentes, R.J., and others: Sexual side effects . . . what to tell your patients, what not to say . . . commonly prescribed drugs, RN **46**(2):34-41, 1983.
9. *Hogan, R.M.: Human sexuality: a nursing perspective, New York, 1980, Appleton-Century-Crofts.
10. Hogan, R.M.: Influences of culture on sexuality, Nurs. Clin. North Am. **17**(3):365-376, 1982.
11. Johnson, C.D., and others: Alcohol and sex: alcohol induced problems of sexual function, Heart Lung **12**(1):93-97, 1983.
12. Kaplan, H.S.: Disorders of sexual desire and other new concepts and techniques in sex therapy, New York, 1979, Simon & Schuster, Inc.
13. Larson, J.: Heart rate and blood pressure responses of coronary artery disease patients during sexual activity and a two-flight stair climbing test, master's thesis, Seattle, 1978, University of Washington.
13a. Lion, E.: Human sexuality in nursing process, New York, 1982, John Wiley & Sons, Inc.
14. *Marks, R.G.: Sexual side effects: how drugs can change fertility, RN **46**(3):61-63, 1983.
15. Masters, W., and Johnson, V.: Homosexuality in perspective, Boston, 1979, Little, Brown & Co.
16. *Mims, F.H.: Sexual health education and counseling, Nurs. Clin. North Am. **10:**519-528, 1975.
17. *Mims, F.H.: Sexual stress: coping and adaptation, Nurs. Clin. North Am. **17**(3):395-405, 1982.
18. Mims, F.H., and Swenson, M.: Sexuality: a nursing perspective, New York, 1980, McGraw-Hill Book Co.
18a. Moses, A., and Hawkins, R.: Counseling lesbian women and gay men: a life issues approach; St. Louis, 1982, The C.V. Mosby Co.
18b. Paul, W., and others: Homosexuality: Social, psychological, and biological issues, Beverly Hills, Calif., 1982, Sage Publications.

*References preceded by an asterisk are particularly well suited for student reading.

19. *Roberts, N.: Advising patients on sex after surgery, AORN J. **32:**55-61, 1980.
20. Savage, J.S.: Effect of crisis on female sexual identity, Issues Health Care Women **3:**151-160, 1981.
21. *Sex and aging: a game people play, Geriatr. Nurs. **3:**263-264, 1982.
22. *Spennrath, S.: Understanding the sexual needs of the elder patient, Canad. Nurse **78:**25-29, 1982.
23. Szasz, G.: Sexual incidents in an extended care unit for aged men, J. Am. Geriatr. Soc. **31:**407-411, 1983.
23a. Whitley, M.P., and Berke, P.: Sexual response in diabetic women. In press.
24. *Wood, R., and Rose, K.: Penile implants for impotency, Am. J. Nurs. **78:**234-238, 1978.
25. Woods, J.S.: Drug effects on human sexual behavior. In Woods, N.F.: Human sexuality in health and illness, ed. 3, St. Louis, 1984, The C.V. Mosby Co.
26. *Woods, N.F.: Human sexuality in health and illness, ed. 3, St. Louis, 1984, The C.V. Mosby Co.
27. Woods, N.F., and Earp, J.A.: Women with cured breast cancer: a description of women's experiences four years after mastectomy, Nurs. Res. **27**(5):279-285, 1978.
28. World Health Organization: Education and treatment in human sexuality: the training of health professionals, Tech. Rep. Series, No. 572, Geneva, 1975, The Organization.
29. Zalar, M.K.: Role preparation for nurses in human sexual functioning, Nurs. Clin. North Am. **17**(3):351-363, 1982.

Classic

30. Annon, J.: The behavioral treatment of sexual problems, Honolulu, 1974, Enabling Systems, Inc.
31. Hellerstein, H., and Friedman, F.H.: Sexual activity and the postcoronary patient, Arch. Intern. Med. **125:**987-999, 1970.
32. Kaplan, H.S.: The new sex therapy, New York, 1974, Brunner/Mazel, Inc.
33. Kinsey, A.C., Pomeroy, W.B., and Martin, C.W.: Sexual behavior in the human male, Philadelphia, 1948, W.B. Saunders Co.
34. Kinsey, A.C., and others: Sexual behavior in the human female, Philadelphia, 1953, W.B. Saunders Co.
35. Kolodny, R.C.: Sexual dysfunction in diabetic females, Diabetes **20:**557-559, 1971.
36. Masters, W., and Johnson, V.: Human sexual response, Boston, 1966, Little, Brown & Co.
37. Masters, W., and Johnson, V.: Human sexual inadequacy, Boston, 1970, Little, Brown & Co.
38. Money, J., and Ehrhardt, A.: Man and woman, boy and girl, Baltimore, 1972, The Johns Hopkins University Press.
39. Rubin, A., and Babbott, D.: Impotence and diabetes mellitus, JAMA **168:**498-500, 1958.

35

The Patient with Reproductive Problems

BARBARA C. LONG and GREER GLAZER

STUDY QUESTIONS

- Review anatomy and physiology of reproductive tract.

- Review the menstrual cycle. During which phase does ovulation occur? What is the relationship between estrogen and progesterone and the cycle?

- What are the main purposes of a douche? Review the procedure. What solutions are used most often?

- What is the incidence of sexually transmitted diseases (STD) in your community? What services are available for detection and treatment of STD? Are human sexuality and STD taught in your local schools? Are similar programs available for adults?

- Examine the chart of a woman who has had a hysterectomy. What was her psychologic response to removal of the uterus? How would you respond to a woman in this situation who was crying and saying that she felt "less than a woman"?

Professionals and lay people have become more enlightened about prevention of problems of the reproductive system. This increased awareness has led many persons to initiate requests for information about or treatment of reproductive system problems. Although men and women are better informed today about matters relating to reproductive health, many neglect preventive measures and ignore signs or symptoms of illness because of embarassment and the special significance that they attach to the reproductive organs.

In spite of advances in medicine, science, and technology, diseases and disorders of the genital system continue to threaten the lives and the physical and emotional health of men and women, sometimes needlessly. Many of these problems are preventable; many of them can be treated and cured.

ANATOMY AND PHYSIOLOGY

Female genital system

EXTERNAL STRUCTURES

The external genitalia of the female, or vulva, consist primarily of the labia majora, labia minora, and clitoris (Fig. 35-1). Two glands are located in this area: Skene's glands, opening into the urethral orifice, and Bartholin's glands, situated at each side of the vaginal opening near the base of the labia. These glands are common site of infection.

INTERNAL ORGANS

The female internal reproductive organs, consisting of the vagina, uterus, fallopian tubes, and ovaries, are

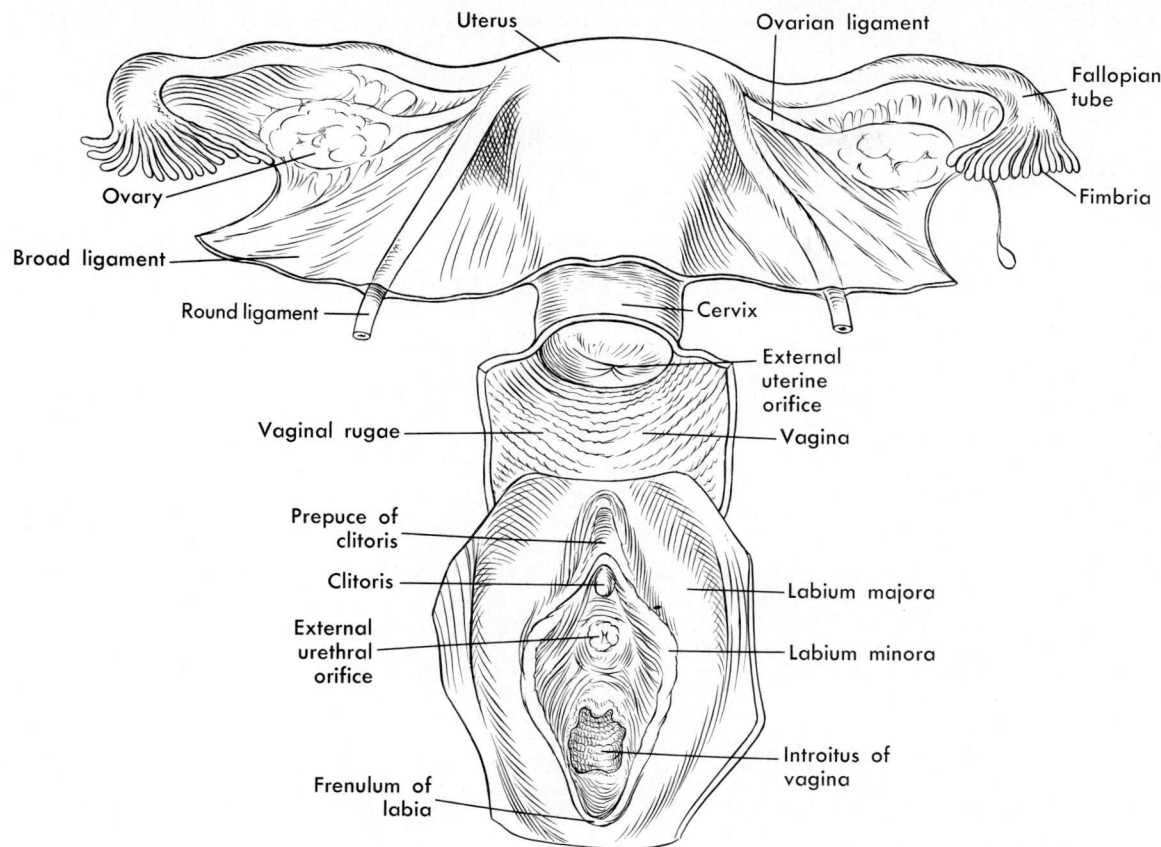

Fig. 35-1. Female internal organs of reproduction. Major ligaments are shown.

shown in Fig. 35-1. These organs are located within the cavity of the true pelvis unless their size is increased by disease or pregnancy.

Vagina

The vagina leads from the external structures to the uterus. The length of the vaginal canal varies, and the posterior wall is longer than the anterior wall. The uterine cervix protrudes into the upper vagina, creating recesses (fornices) around the margins of the cervix.

The vagina is lined with pink mucous membrane arranged in folds called rugae. Physiologic events (for example, pregnancy) and pathologic conditions (for example, infections) often alter the color of the vaginal mucosa because of congestion with blood. The membrane is lubricated by vaginal secretions that are normally acid during the years of ovarian function; neutral or alkaline secretions are normally found in postmenopausal women. An alkaline medium promotes growth of bacteria.

Uterus

The uterus consists of three portions: the fundus (upper crest), the main body (corpus), and the neck (cervix). In adult females the position of the uterus may vary. It is usually anteverted (tipped forward) and slightly anteflexed (bent forward at an angle), but it may also be ret-

roverted, retroflexed, or in midposition. During menopause the uterus decreases in size.

The uterus has three functional layers: parametrium or outer layer, myometrium or middle muscular layer, and endometrium or mucous membrane lining. The outer surface of the uterus is covered by the peritoneum. Reflection of the peritoneum posteriorly between the uterus and rectum creates a space known as the cul-de-sac of Douglas. This space is a common entry site for endoscopy or for surgical drainage of the peritoneal cavity.

Ovaries

The ovaries are endocrine glands as well as reproductive organs. Their functions are to store follicles, to produce mature ova, and to produce and secrete estrogen, progesterone, and androgens. Ovarian functions are readily disturbed by acute and chronic diseases. The functions can also be altered or interrupted by surgery, radiation, and the ingestion of drugs such as oral contraceptives. After menopause the ovaries undergo rapid regressive changes and decrease in size.

ENDOCRINE FUNCTIONS

The major hormones produced by the ovaries are estrogen and progesterone. *Estrogen* is the hormone responsible

Fig. 35-2. Hormone control of menstrual cycle.

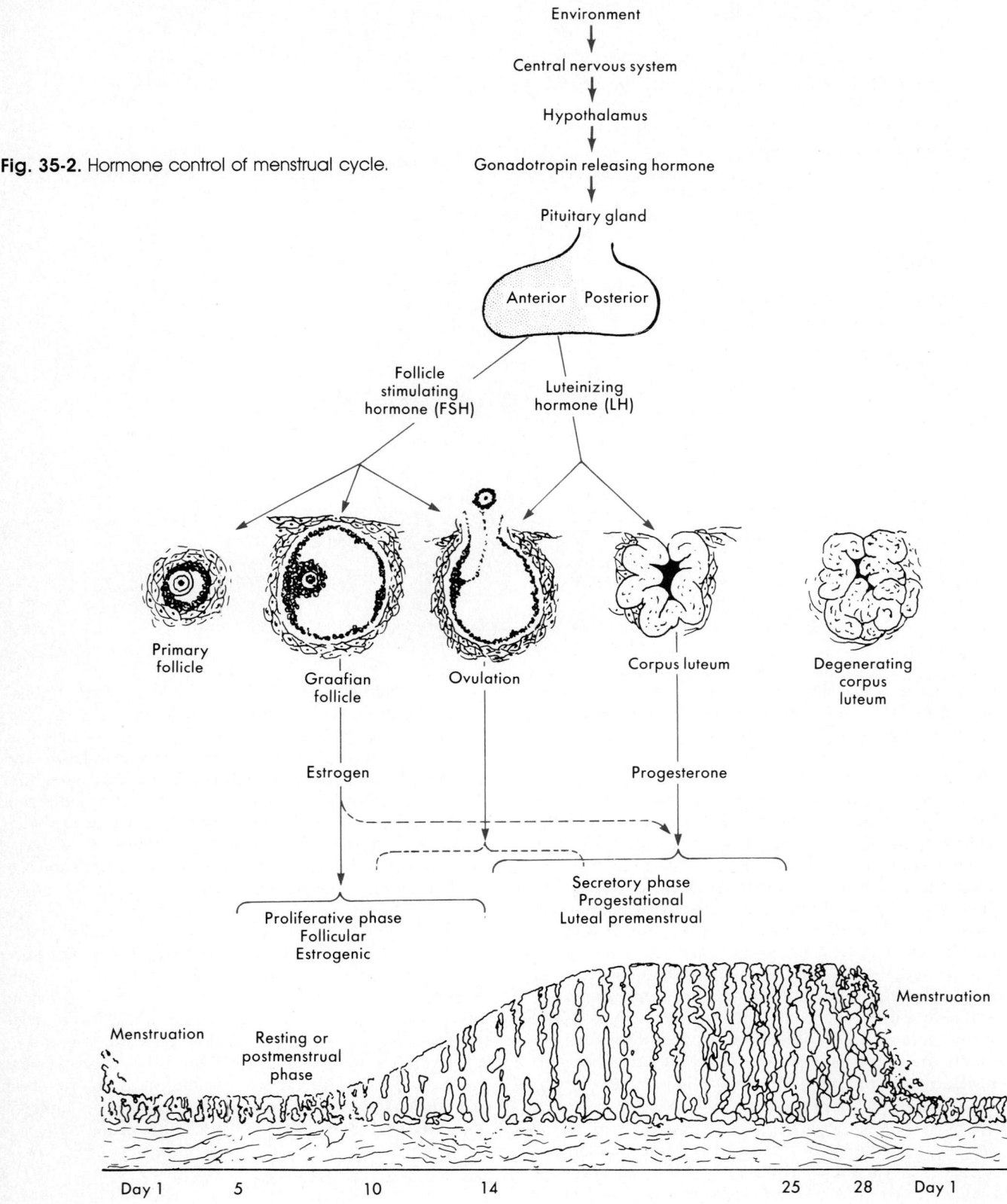

Environment

Central nervous system

Hypothalamus

Gonadotropin releasing hormone

Pituitary gland

Anterior   Posterior

Follicle stimulating hormone (FSH)

Luteinizing hormone (LH)

Primary follicle

Graafian follicle

Ovulation

Corpus luteum

Degenerating corpus luteum

Estrogen

Progesterone

Proliferative phase
Follicular
Estrogenic

Secretory phase
Progestational
Luteal premenstrual

Menstruation

Menstruation   Resting or postmenstrual phase

Day 1   5   10   14   25   28   Day 1

Menstrual cycle

Menstrual phase (menstruation): Day 1 to day 4
   Estrogen and progesterone withdrawn before onset of menstrual flow
   Shedding of endometrial lining
Proliferative (follicular) phase: Day 5 to day 14
   Regrowth of endometrial tissue
   Secretion of follicle-stimulating hormone (FSH) by the pituitary gland
   Development in ovary of a mature graafian follicle containing a mature ovum
   Secretion of increasing amounts of *estrogen* by graafian follicle
   Suppression of FSH when estrogen level becomes high, leading to secretion of luteinizing hormone (LH) by
      pituitary gland
Secretory (luteal) phase: Day 15 to days 25 to 28
   Rupture of graafian follicle releasing ovum (ovulation) starts the secretory phase
   Movement of ovum through fallopian tube to uterus
   Formation of corpus luteum at site of ruptured graafian follicle
   Production of *progesterone* by corpus luteum
   Stimulation by progesterone of endometrial cell growth
   Marked decrease in progesterone level if implantation does not occur; menstrual phase then begins again

for the development of secondary sex characteristics at the time of puberty. After puberty the primary function of estrogen is to cause development of the endometrium in preparation for implantation of a fertilized ovum. Estrogen causes the retention of calcium and phosphorus and thus promotes bone growth. After menopause the decline in estrogen levels may account for some of the symptoms that sometimes occur, such as hot flashes, osteoporosis (loss of calcium from bone), and vaginal atrophy. *Progesterone* enhances the action of estrogen on the endometrium. It also prevents muscular contractions of the myometrium as an aid for maintaining pregnancy should the ovum become implanted.

Secretion of ovarian hormones is cyclic, with each cycle requiring an average of 28 days. Unless stimulated by pituitary hormones, however, the ovaries do not fulfill their hormone-secreting and ovum-producing functions.

The phases of the menstrual cycle are illustrated in Fig. 35-2. The secretory (luteal) phase is the least variable part of the menstrual cycle. Irregular menstrual cycles are most frequently related to longer or shorter menstrual or proliferative (follicular) phases.

On the day of ovulation, about 25% of women experience pain in the lower abdomen on the side of ovulation. This pain (mittelschmerz) is probably a result of peritoneal irritation from follicular fluid or blood released from the ovary with the ovum. This sign rarely occurs with every cycle and is therefore an unreliable indicator of ovulation. If the pain occurs on the right side and is severe, it may be mistaken for appendicitis.

Male genital system

The male reproductive organs and associated structures are shown in Fig. 35-3. The male reproductive organs produce sperm, suspend the sperm in a liquid, and deliver the sperm into the vagina to fertilize an ovum. Another important function is secretion of male hormones, the androgens. Sperm are produced in the testes and are conveyed through the vas (ductus) deferens to the urethra. Semen consists of sperm with fluids from the seminal vesicles and the prostate gland. The prostate gland is important clinically because of its affinity for congestive, inflammatory, hyperplastic, and malignant disease. Because the prostate gland encircles the urethra, even benign enlargement (hypertrophy) may lead to obstruction of the urethra.

The male hormone *testosterone* is produced by the interstitial cells of the testes and is responsible for development of the genitalia during puberty and for maintaining the genitalia in a functional state during life. Androgenic hormones are also responsible for the development of secondary sex characteristics including growth of body hair and thickening of the vocal cords. Testosterone secretion is closely related to pituitary gland function, and the rate of secretion is determined by levels of luteinizing hormone (LH) in the blood. Secretion of testosterone decreases slowly with age.

Physiologic changes with aging

Menopause, which occurs in the middle-aged woman, results in physiologic changes from the hormonal decrease. When ovulation ceases, no progesterone is produced and estrogen diminishes. In the male, androgen production decreases steadily during adulthood to about age 60 years, then levels off.

The physiologic changes do not diminish the elderly person's ability to engage in sexual intercourse (see Chapter 34) but may lead to discomfort or complications. The

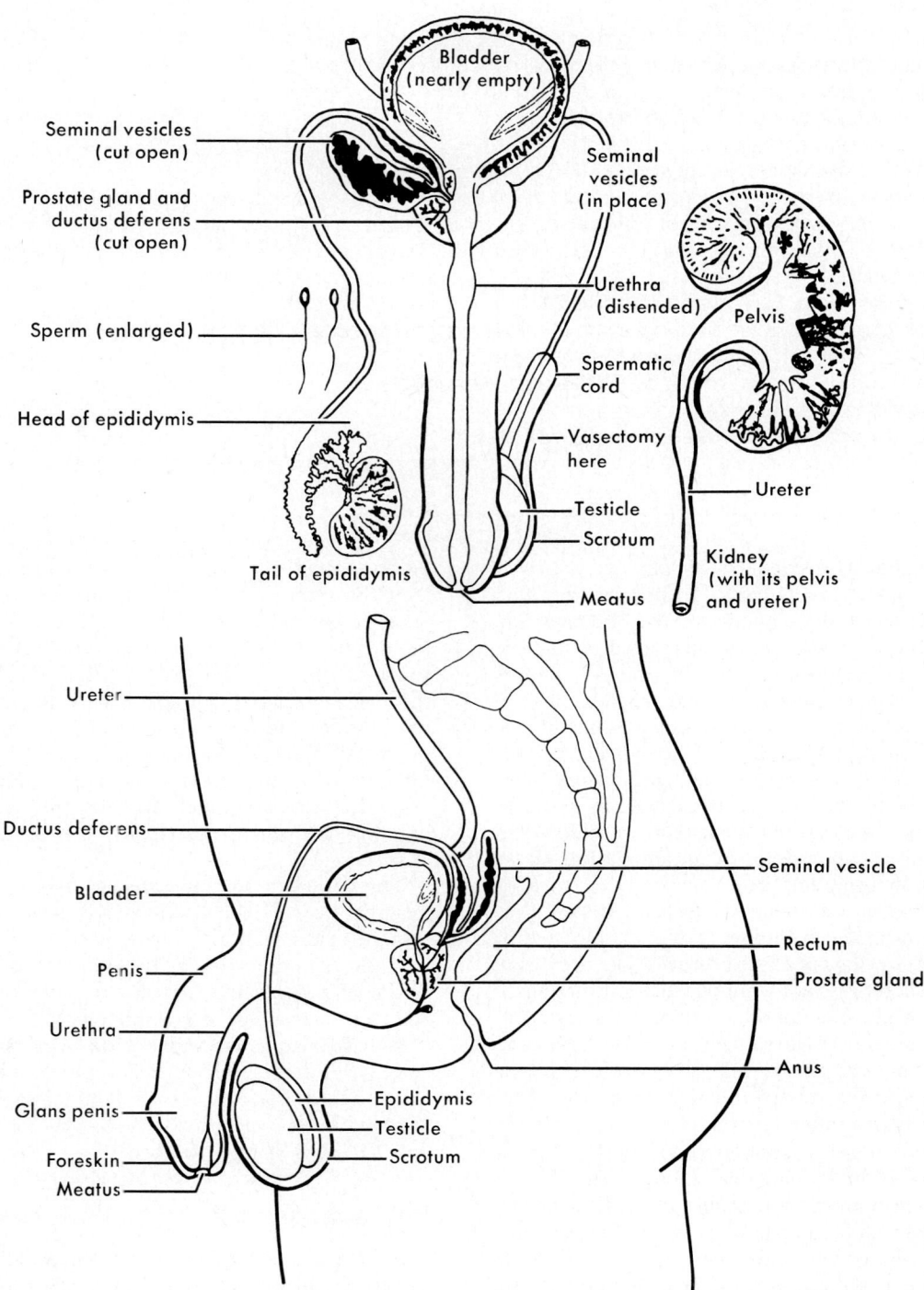

Fig. 35-3. Male organs of reproduction. Note relatively large size of seminal vesicle as compared with testicle.

Physiologic changes in reproductive tract with aging

Female

Uterus	Decreased size
Ovaries	Atrophy, with decreased size
Vagina	Decreased width and length
	Vaginal entrance (introitus) narrowed
	Vaginal secretions decrease and become more alkaline

Male

Testes	Decreased size and firmness
Seminal fluid	Decreased amount and viscosity
Prostate gland	Hypertrophy (enlargement)
Penile erection	Slower, decreased frequency of involuntary morning erections

vaginal dryness and narrowed introitus may cause dyspareunia (painful intercourse). Vaginal infections occur more readily in the alkaline medium. Muscle weakness may lead to cystocele, rectocele, or uterine prolapse.

PREVENTION AND HEALTH EDUCATION

Prevention of infection

Vaginal infections may result from the presence of large numbers of invading organisms or from decreased resistance to infection. Those women in whom the natural barriers to infection are at a minimum (low estrogen levels, thinness of the vaginal epithelium, or reduced acidity of the vagina) are at greatest risk.

Large numbers of organisms may invade the vagina or urethra from inadequate personal hygiene, from another person during sexual intercourse, or from use of unclean articles such as douche nozzles. Decreased resistance to infection may result from vaginal secretions becoming more alkaline, providing a more suitable medium for bacterial growth. Vaginal yeast infections may be a side effect of drugs such as the tetracyclines or oral contraceptives. Preventive measures include the following:

1. Wiping from front to back after bowel movements
2. Voiding shortly after intercourse to wash away organisms
3. Using a condom (male) during intercourse if either partner has been exposed to a genital infection
4. Recognizing signs of infection in the sexual partner and urging medical attention
5. Abstaining from intercourse if one partner has a genital infection
6. Avoiding douching (which may alter vaginal pH) unless advised by a physician for treatment

Risk factors for vaginal infections

Aging
Diabetes
Pregnancy
Allergies
Stress
Malnutrition
Inadequate perineal hygiene
Excessive douching
Use of vaginal inserts
Oral contraceptives
Broad-spectrum antibiotics
Intercourse with infected partner

Risk factors for uterine cancer

Cancer of the cervix

First sexual intercourse at early age
Multiple sexual partners

Cancer of the endometrium

History of infertility
Failure of ovulation
Prolonged estrogen therapy
Late menopause
Combination of diabetes, high blood pressure, and obesity

Examinations for prevention of uterine cancer as recommended by the American Cancer Society

1. Pap test once every 3 years after two initial negative tests 1 year apart
2. More frequent Pap tests for persons at high risk
3. Endometrial tissue sample at menopause for persons at high risk for endometrial cancer

7. Seeking immediate medical attention for early signs of vaginal infection (abnormal vaginal discharge, vaginal itching), especially in persons at high risk.

Early detection of cancer

Dramatic decreases in death from cancer are associated with early detection and treatment. The decline in deaths from cervical cancer is primarily the result of increased use of the Papanicolaou smear for mass screening, combined with more frequent and more thorough gynecologic examinations. Cancer of the cervix is easier to detect through the Pap smear than is cancer of the endometrium.

Health teaching for prevention of uterine cancer includes regular pelvic examinations that include a Pap smear.

Health teaching related to menstruation and menopause

MENSTRUATION

Menstruation occurs on an average of every 28 days; the normal range is 26 to 34 days. The menstrual flow usually lasts for 3 to 7 days (average 4 days). Normally 30 to 180 ml (average 50 ml) of menstrual fluid is lost during the period. One half to three fourths of the fluid is blood, and the remainder is mucus, fragments of endometrial cells, and desquamated vaginal epithelium.

Normally menstrual fluid does not clot unless it is retained in the uterus or vagina for a prolonged time. It is believed that the endometrium produces an anticoagulant that prevents clotting of blood in the uterus. An occasional very small clot may occur during the first 24 hours, and this is probably a particle of endometrial tissue. Large clots or pus in the menstrual flow are never normal.

During pregnancy menstruation ceases, and then returns within 6 to 8 weeks after delivery, although lactation suppresses the menses for varying periods of time. Unless disease occurs, the menstrual periods recur during adult life until menopause.

Before and during menstruation a variety of discom-

forts may be present and are considered normal. These may include the following:
1. Fluid retention (up to 2.5 kg weight gain)
2. Slight aching in lower back, legs, pelvis
3. Mild fatigue
4. Breast changes
   a. Sensation of fullness, tenderness, and increased size
   b. Changes start before menses begin, and last 1 to 2 days after flow begins
4. Constipation or diarrhea
5. Mood changes premenstrually

Menstruation is a manifestation of normal body function and should be treated as such. The "period" and "monthly period" are accurate terms to use if the woman does not wish to say "menstruating." Terms such as "being sick," "on the rag," or "having the curse" are to be avoided because of their negative connotation.

In order to become knowledgeable about the patterns of their menstrual cycles, women are encouraged to keep a written record. Establishing this habit makes it possible to predict the onset of the next menstrual period and to determine the range of cycles and duration of flow. Should it be necessary to seek the attention of a health professional for any reason, the date of onset of the last menstrual period (LMP) is known.

DYSMENORRHEA

Although menstruation is a normal physiologic process, some women experience varying degrees of discomfort (menstrual cramps). Studies have shown that dysmenorrhea is the greatest single cause of absenteeism by women

---

Health teaching for menstruation

1. Knowledge of the physiologic process
2. Factors that may alter the menstrual cycle: stress, fatigue, exercise, acute and chronic illness, changes in climate or working hours, pregnancy
3. Personal hygiene
   a. Wear pads during early period of heavy flow
   b. Change tampons frequently to decrease risk of toxic shock syndrome
   c. Consult a physician if tampons cause discomfort
   d. Take a daily bath for comfort (warm bath may relieve slight pelvic discomfort)
4. Exercise
   a. Exercise is not contraindicated and may help prevent discomfort
   b. Modify exercise if fatigue occurs
5. Diet
   a. Restrict salt intake if fluid retention is present
   b. Consult physician if fluid retention persists after menstruation
6. Discomfort (dysmenorrhea)
   a. For mild discomfort take aspirin or acetaminophen, apply warmth, rest
   b. For prolonged severe discomfort, consult physician.

from school or work. Dysmenorrhea may result from various causes (see box below). Primary dysmenorrhea often disappears after pregnancy or by age 25 years.

Dysmenorrhea cannot necessarily be prevented, but positive attitudes can be encouraged; a woman who regards menstruation as normal is less likely to experience it as an illness. Women who are consistently unable to engage in usual activities because of pain associated with menstruation should be urged to seek health care for diagnosis and treatment of any existing secondary dysmenorrhea. Posture and nutrition have not been found to affect the incidence of dysmenorrhea.

Discomfort from dysmenorrhea may be relieved by aspirin, acetaminophen, ibuprofen (Brufen, Motrin), naproxen (Naproxyn), or indomethacin (Indocin). Ovulation can be suppressed by oral contraceptives, with possible prevention of dysmenorrhea.

MENOPAUSE

Menopause, or the *climacteric,* is the transitional phase between reproductive and nonreproductive ability. Menopause is said to have occurred when there has been no menstrual flow for 1 year (although some women have periods even after 1 year of amenorrhea). During the climacteric, which usually lasts for 12 to 18 months, there is a gradual decline in ovarian function. The ovaries gradually cease to produce ova and estrogen, and as a result the menses become scanty, irregular, and farther apart, until they stop altogether.

Natural menopause may occur between 35 and 60 years of age (average age 51 years). Early menopause may be caused by a number of factors (see box below).

Menopause may be artificially induced by such procedures as irradiation of the ovaries, surgical removal of both ovaries, or hysterectomy. Each of these has one common consequence, namely, cessation of menstruation. However, surgical removal or irradiation of the ovaries results in menopause with all its physiologic changes, whereas ovaries left intact after hysterectomy will continue to function provided the age of climacteric has not yet been reached.

Physiologic changes in the genital organs as a result of loss of hormonal functioning are listed on p. 1049. Women can still enjoy sexual activity after menopause. There may be changes in the skeletal system; about 30% of women develop osteoporosis from the effect of lack of estrogen on calcium balance.

Health teaching

Most women have heard of the "change of life." The negative image of menopause is reinforced by the media, books, health professionals, and the general public. Depending on the climate in which they were reared and on their own changes in attitude toward normal functions of the reproductive organs, women may feel more or less free to discuss menopause and their feelings and concerns during this period of life. Because many problems related to the reproductive organs occur in this age group, and because it is important for mental health that women be helped to make menopause as comfortable as possible, it is important for nurses to identify women who can profit from interventions.

Education regarding menopause should precede its onset. Women approaching menopause, regardless of whether it is an event of normal aging or is artificially induced, need to know what menopause is, why it occurs, the effects menopause has on reproductive and sexual ability, what can be done to make menopause more comfortable, and those symptoms that require medical attention.

Many women go through the climacteric with little awareness of its occurrence. Some women, however, experience hot flashes (flushes), which are felt as waves of warmth accompanied by flushing of the skin, especially the face, neck, and arms, and perspiration. The hot flash is the perception of the spread of heat from an anatomic point of origin on the body to other areas of the body. Hot flashes may be so mild that they are hardly noticed or so severe that they produce distress. Estrogen may be prescribed by the physician for severe discomfort. During estrogen therapy women should be seen at least every 6 months for examination and for review of menopausal symptoms. The examination should include the breasts and reproductive organs, Pap smear, and blood pressure.

Feelings of depression and uselessness may occur, particularly among women who have been highly invested in

---

Causes of dysmenorrhea

Primary dysmenorrhea
High concentration of uterine prostaglandins

Secondary dysmenorrhea
Pelvic inflammatory disease
Endometriosis
Cervical stenosis
Retropositioned uterus

Factors associated with early menopause

Excessive exposure to radiation
Hard manual labor
Poor general health
Breast-feeding
Inadequate spacing between pregnancies
Frequent spontaneous or therapeutic abortions
Hypothyroidism with severe obesity

Health teaching for menopause

1. Knowledge about menopause
   a. Cessation of ovarian function with cessation of menstruation over 12 to 18 months
   b. Changes in reproductive ability
      (1) Conception still possible during the period of change
         (a) Contraception should be used for 1 year after last menstrual period
         (b) Rhythm method unreliable contraceptive method during this period
      (2) Ability to conceive ceases when menopause completed
   c. Sexual ability still present
   d. Physical symptoms vary from mild to severe; estrogen therapy may be given to relieve severe symptoms
2. Promotion of health and physical appearance
   a. Moderate exercise to maintain muscle tone and help prevent osteoporosis
   b. Dietary control to prevent weight gain
   c. Activities that encourage self-esteem and interest outside of self
   d. Peer support groups during menopause, if necessary
   e. Medical attention required for recurrence of bleeding or other vaginal discharge
3. Prevention of discomfort
   a. Prevention of dyspareunia: local application of lubricant or vaginal cream
   b. Relief of vaginal itching: vitamin E or estrogen therapy
   c. Relief of vasomotor reactions (hot flashes)
      (1) Moderation of factors identified by the person as exacerbating hot flashes (excitement, alcoholic beverages, heavy eating, excessive clothing, impairment of heat loss in hot weather)
      (2) Vitamin E or B complex vitamins

---

the maternal role. Peer support groups may be very helpful in these situations.

Publications that may help the woman during the climacteric include *Our Bodies Ourselves**, *The Menopause: A Positive Approach†*, and *Menstruation and Menopause‡*.

INTERFERENCES WITH REPRODUCTION

The ability to have children may be modified either to prevent conception or to terminate a pregnancy. Some persons are unable to procreate. The topics of contraception and abortion are covered in maternity nursing texts and are not repeated here.

Sterilization

Voluntary sterilization has become increasingly acceptable to both men and women as a method of preventing pregnancy. It is the most commonly used method of fertility control for married couples older than 30 years. Sterilization may also be performed in selected instances where pregnancy would create risks to the health or life of the woman or infant (for example, heart disease, severe diabetes, probable genetic defects in the infant).

Interferences with reproduction

Contraception	Process of temporary prevention of impregnation or conception
Sterilization	Process of making an individual incapable of reproducing, either permanently or until the process is reversed
Abortion	Termination of a pregnancy before the fetus is viable
Infertility	Inability to achieve a pregnancy within a stipulated time (at least 1 year) of unprotected sexual intercourse

---

*Boston Women's Health Book Collective: New York, 1980, Simon & Schuster, Inc.
†Reitz, R.: Philadelphia, 1979, Chilton Book Co.
‡Weideger, P.: New York, 1976, Alfred A. Knopf, Inc.

Table 35-1. Methods of sterilization

Method	Description	Comments
Female *Tubal sterilization* ABDOMINAL		
Minilaparotomy	Ligation or cutting of fallopian tubes under direct vision through small abdominal incision	Local or general anesthesia Complications: wound infection, hematoma, bladder injury Advantages: good chance for sterility reversal
Laparoscopy	Electrocoagulation of segment of fallopian tubes by laparoscopy through small abdominal incision	Local or general anesthesia Advantages: minimal discomfort, short procedure
VAGINAL		
Culpotomy	Ligation or cutting of fallopian tube through small incision in cul-de-sac of Douglas	Local, spinal, or general anesthesia Higher complication rate than laparoscopy (infection, hemorrhage)
Culdoscopy	Electrocoagulation of segment of fallopian tubes by culdoscope through small incision in cul-de-sac of Douglas	Local anesthesia Higher complication rate than laparoscopy
Male		
Vasectomy	Removal of a segment of vas deferens through small incision in scrotum	Local anesthesia Complications rare Bruising, mild edema, and mild discomfort common

Because sterilization may be a permanent method of contraception, it is absolutely necessary to obtain voluntary, informed consent. Patients receiving federal funds for sterilization must be at least 21 years old and mentally compentent.

METHODS OF STERILIZATION

Methods of sterilization are described in Table 35-1. The abdominal approaches are favored by some physicians because they are familiar with the female pelvic anatomy as viewed from the abdomen and because the fallopian tubes are free and suspended in this position, which makes them easy to see, manipulate, and ligate or cauterize.

Successful sterilization (conception prevented) is dependent on the technique used, the surgeon's experience in performing the procedure, and the length of the tube removed. The main causes of failure in the female are recanalization of the fallopian tube, erroneous ligation, and pregnancy resulting from tuboperitoneal fistula. In the male spontaneous recanalization (reanastomosis) may occur; the cause is unknown but duplication of the vas deferens has occasionally been noted.

EFFECTS OF STERILIZATION

Physiologic effects

Although tubal sterilization usually terminates a woman's ability to bear children, ovarian hormones and menstrual functiong are not altered and artificial menopause is not induced. Ability to derive satisfaction from sexual intercourse should not be impaired, and some women may experience greater enjoyment from intercourse free from fear of pregnancy.

Because vasectomy interrupts the continuity of the vas deferens, sperm are prevented from being ejaculated with other components of the semen. However, sperm are still produced and the ejaculate is not noticeably diminished in amount. Residual fertility lasting for a variable period is present because of sperm in the semen beyond the point of occlusion of the vas. Sperm *gradually* disappear from the ejaculate; thus conception is possible in the immediate postoperative period. Semen analysis will determine when sperm have finally disappeared.

Psychologic effects

Men and women who elect sterilization seem to have little or no regret after the surgery if they understand what to expect during and after the procedure and are able to express their feelings and have questions answered before the procedure. Persons with preexisting emotional problems have reported feelings of depression, loss of self-esteem, guilt, and difficulty in sexual adjustment after surgery.

PREOPERATIVE CARE

Preoperative counseling is indicated to identify men and women before surgery who may later have strong regrets and emotional problems. One aim of counseling before surgery is to confirm that the decision for sterilization is made as objectively as possible. Previous experience with other methods of contraception can be explored and reasons for dissatisfaction with the methods

determined. It may by that there is lack of knowledge about contraceptive methods, and with adequate information the couple might choose a means other than sterilization. The discussion of sterilization methods should be based on the federal government's informed consent guidelines.

POSTOPERATIVE CARE

Many of the sterilization procedures are performed on an outpatient basis, and the patient can be discharged when the effects of general anesthesia have worn off and vital signs are stable. If the patient expresses feelings of guilt or regret about having been sterilized, a review of the reasons for sterilization and positive effect on sexual relationships may need to be repeated.

Informed consent guidelines (federal) relating to sterilization

1. Choice is made by patient, without pressures (for example, loss of welfare benefits, wrath of health care provider).
2. Benefits and risks of sterilization are described:
   a. Benefits: permanent, no further costs or decision making.
   b. Risks: usual surgical risks, possibility of future pregnancy (not 100% effective).
3. Alternative contraceptive methods are described.
4. Patient is encouraged to ask questions.
5. Explanations are given about the entire sterilization procedure, costs, and possible side effects (effects on hormones, weight changes, menstrual changes, sexual response).
6. Written instruction and risk factors are explained to patient.
7. Written consent to the procedure is signed by patient and witnessed.

Teaching for the patient who has had a sterilization procedure

Woman

1. Rest for 24 to 48 hours after procedure
2. No heavy lifting or strenuous exercise for 1 week
3. Abstain from sexual intercourse
   a. Abdominal method: until wound is healed and no discomfort is present
   b. Vaginal method: 1 week
4. Report to physician signs of fever, persistent abdominal pain, or bleeding from incision

Man

1. Apply ice to scrotum, take sitz baths for minor discomfort and swelling
2. Wear scrotal support for 48 hours
3. Rest for 48 hours after procedure
4. No heavy lifting or strenuous exercise for 1 week
5. Abstain from sexual intercourse for 3 days
6. Use an alternate method of contraception until physician reports semen no longer contains sperm
7. Report to physician signs of fever, persistent scrotal pain, or profuse incisional bleeding

STERILIZATION REVERSAL

Requests for reversal of previous sterilization may be made because of divorce and remarriage, death of children, or change in economic status, as well as for other reasons. The chances of reversing the effects of sterilization are improving as a result of refinement of microsurgical techniques.

Reconstruction of the fallopian tubes involves an end-to-end anastomosis of the ligated or dissected tubes with or without insertion of plastic lumen. Success of restoration of tubal function is partly dependent on the original surgery performed, especially regarding the length of the tubal portion excised. Ligation of the tubes produces adhesions that must be dissected away to the point of tubal patency; this reduces the amount of remaining tubal structure. Also the length of the fallopian tube remaining after reconstruction may play a role in permitting adequate time for the fertilized ovum to undergo maturational changes in preparation for implantation.

In the male, reconstruction consists in attempting to rejoin the severed ends of the vas deferens. Success is measured by the presence of sperm in the semen after reconstruction. A notable point is that although sperm reappear in the semen, the pregnancy rate after reconstruction is low; the reason for this is unknown.

Infertility

It has been estimated that 10% to 15% of all couples in the United States are unwillingly childless. Approximately 50% of couples who undergo assessment and treatment for infertility are likely to conceive. Although infertility is most often attributed to women, in about 40% of infertile marriages the man is infertile.[38]

The fertility of a couple is affected by coital frequency and the age of the man and the woman. Increased coital frequency enhances fertility. Frequent ejaculation improves sperm motility unless ejaculation is excessive, resulting in depletion of available sperm. Fertility peaks at age 24 years in women and age 25 years in men.

CAUSE AND PREVENTION

There are many causes of infertility in men and women. Some are preventable or correctable, others are not. There is no known cause in 10% to 20% of infertility problems.

One of the most common preventable causes of infertility in women is infection of the pelvic organs, especially as a result of gonorrhea, which causes obstruction of the fallopian tubes. Such serious consequences are preventable through prophylactic use of penicillin for women exposed to gonorrhea and through early diagnosis and treatment of all vaginal and cervical infections.

Many of the ovarian and hormonal problems that cause infertility produce symptoms such a menstrual irregularities and ill health before a problem with conception is ever recognized. Many of these problems can be managed with hormone therapy, provided women seek help at an early age or as soon as deviations are noticed. Birth control pills should be avoided by women who have not established normal menses or have irregular menstrual cycles. Some authorities suggest a break from prolonged usage of birth control pills to reactivate the hypothalamic controls.

In males, bilateral undescended testes (cryptorchidism) should be corrected surgically before puberty. In later life cryptorchidism may produce sterility because of failure of the testes to develop their sperm-producing function, even if the condition is surgically corrected. Destruction of testicular tissue by infectious processes can be prevented through prompt treatment when symptoms first appear.

ASSESSMENT

It is important that couples who wish to have children seek medical advice if they are unsuccessful after about a year of trying to achieve pregnancy. Infertility evaluation often requires a long time.

Attempts to correct infertility are based on data obtained through a detailed history and physical examina-

---

Causes of infertility

Disorder	Effect
Female	
Obstructions of fallopian tubes	Interfere with transport of ovum
Diseases of body or cervix of uterus	Inhibit passage of active sperm
Hormonal deficiencies	Inhibit release of ovum
	Inhibit development of endometrium for implantation
Male	
Obstruction of vas deferns	Interfere with transport of sperm
Diseases of testes, undescended testes, hormonal deficiencies	Inhibit development of sperm

---

Examination for infertility

Tests	Data obtained
Male	
Multiple semen examination	Determine presence, number, and motility of sperm
Testicular biopsy if sperm count low or absent	Presence of sperm indicates obstruction of vas deferens
Female	
Basal body temperature chart	Determines that ovulation is occurring
Postcoital test of cervical secretions	Measure ability of sperm to penetrate cervical mucus and remain active, and quality of the mucus
Endometrial biopsy, serum progesterone and estradiol levels, laparoscopic inspection of ovaries	Determine whether ovulation is occurring (if in question)
Rubin test (uterotubal insufflation)	Determine patency of fallopian tubes
Hysterosalpingography (x-ray after insertion of contrast media)	Determine patency of uterus and fallopian tubes
Hormonal tests for males and females	Determine whether the problem is hormonal

---

tion as well as from laboratory tests and clinical studies. A sexual history is taken and sexual practices are reviewed. Suggestions about sexual intercourse are given if this seems to be the problem. The couple should attempt to attend the first interview together because they share responsibility for infertility, information is needed by both partners. and this may be their first opportunity to confront their feelings about being infertile.

Examination of the man

Many physicans prefer to carry out examination of the man first, because it is more easily accomplished and less time consuming. Stricture and varicoceles (dilated veins of the spermatic cords) may be corrected by surgery.

If sperm count and motility of sperm are low, thyroid extract and vitamins may be prescribed along with a well-balanced diet, rest, and moderate exercise. A lack of vitamins A and E in the diet may cause some atrophy of the sperm-producing structures. The couple are advised to have intercourse every other day during the fertile period (usually 12 to 16 days before the beginning of the next menstrual period). When the man is completely aspermatic, conception is impossible, and the couple should be counseled regarding the alternatives open to them.

Examination of the woman

If the man is found to be fertile, examination of the woman is carried out. If sperm are being destroyed by vaginal and cervical secretions, smears from these sites are studied. If the secretions are too acid or too alkaline, medicated douches may be prescribed. A douche with sodium bicarbonate taken just before intercourse has been found to increase the motility of sperm in many cases. Tubal strictures or obstructions are sometimes repaired by plastic surgery, but the rate of success in restoring tubal function is very low. Underlying metabolic diseases are corrected if possible.

COPING WITH INFERTILITY

Couples who wish to have children but find themselves unable to do so experience immeasurable emotional distress. Feelings of inadequacy are common, as are anger and guilt. The infertile couple must confront feelings about lack of control, self-image, self-esteem, and sexuality. Couples who are informed that they will never be able to have children experience a life crisis with all of its ramifications, and they have a strong need to grieve. For those who are told they are a normal, fertile couple, but for whom pregnancy does not result despite months or years of tests, studies, examinations, and advice, feelings of frustration alternating with hope are common.

All of these couples require emotional support, including encouragement to grieve, to express their anger and other feelings in order to regain objectivity and to avoid premature decisions and actions about alternatives. The urgent need for such support is reflected in the emergence of support groups organized by infertile individuals and couples.

ALTERNATIVE INFERTILITY APPROACHES

Infertile couples need to make choices from among available alternatives. The more common approaches are to try to adopt a child or to remain childless. Two more recent approaches include in vitro fertilization and surrogate mothers. *In vitro fertilization* consists of fertilization outside the mother's body, followed by placement of

Table 35-2. Inflammatory disorders of the female reproductive tract

Disorder	Cause	Signs and symptoms	Medical therapy
Vulvitis/vaginitis	*Candida, Trichomonas, Gardnerella,* coliform bacteria, *Gonococcus,* herpes simplex	Itching of vulva or vagina, vaginal discharge, dyspareunia	Antifungal agents, antibiotics (oral, topical, douches), sitz baths
Cervicitis	*Gonococcus, Streptococcus, Staphylococcus,* herpes virus, *Chlamydia*	Mucopurulent discharge, erosion of cervix	Cauterization of cervix, antibiotics
Pelvic inflammatory disease (salpingitis)	*Gonococcus, Chlamydia,* coliform bacteria, *Streptococcus, Mycoplasm,* anaerobic bacteria	Severe abdominal pain, lower abdominal cramps, intermenstrual spotting, dyspareunia, fever and chills, malaise, nausea and vomiting, foul-smelling purulent vaginal discharge	Penicillin, tetracycline; rest; heat to abdomen, analgesics, oral contraceptives, therapy for 3 months
Toxic shock syndrome	Toxin from *Staphylococcus aureus*	High fever, vomiting, watery diarrhea, sore throat, myalgia, erythematous rash with desquamation; if severe, impaired renal, hepatic, cardiopulmonary function	Antibiotics, rapid hydration, supportive therapy for septic shock

the fertilized ovum in the uterus. The success rate of this method is still low.

Surrogate mothers are women who contract to conceive by artificial insemination and give the baby to the semen donor after delivery. Many social, moral, psychologic, and legal implications surround this approach.

Artificial insemination is the placement of a few drops of donor semen in the cervicovaginal, intracervical, or intrauterine (more painful) area. It is simple, safe, inexpensive, and highly successful. Having intercourse around the time of insemination or mixing the partner's semen with the donor's may be emotionally satisfying for the couple.

The major indication for artificial insemination is male infertility. Loss of children because of Rh or ABO incompatibility or severe hereditary defects transmitted by the man are other indications.

Major health problems of the reproductive system

The major problems of the reproductive system include inflammation, structural disorders, tumors, and sexually transmitted diseases. The first three types of disorders are discussed separately for women and men because of the inherent anatomic differences. Sexually transmitted diseases are discussed as a separate topic because the

problems are common to both women and men. The various disorders that fall within the cited categories are as follows:

1. Female disorders
   a. Inflammatory disorders: vaginitis, cervicitis, pelvic inflammatory disease, toxic shock syndrome
   b. Structural disorders: relaxed vaginal outlet, uterine displacement, prolapse of uterus, fistulas
   c. Tumors: ovarian tumors and cysts, endometriosis, uterine fibroid tumors, cervical polyps, and cancer of the cervix, endometrium, and ovary
2. Male disorders
   a. Inflammatory disorders: urethritis, prostatitis, epididymitis, orchitis
   b. Structural disorders: hydrocele, spermatocele, varicocele, torsion of spermatic cord
   c. Tumors: cancer of the testes, prostate gland, penis
3. Sexually transmitted diseases: gonorrhea, syphilis, herpes genitalis, chlamydial infection, trichomoniasis

DISORDERS IN WOMEN

Inflammatory Disorders

TYPES OF INFLAMMATORY DISORDERS

Inflammations of the female reproductive tract are seen most commonly in the vagina, cervix, or fallopian tubes and adjacent areas (Table 35-2). Many of these infections can be prevented (p. 1049).

PATHOPHYSIOLOGY

Vulva and vagina

Normally the vagina is protected from infection by its pH and the presence of *Döderlein's bacilli*. If the vaginal pH is altered, if the invading organisms are numerous, or if the woman's resistance is decreased by aging, malnutrition, stress, disease, or the use of drugs, the risk of infection is increased. Yeast organisms grow best in an acid pH <4.7, whereas *Trichomonas* and organisms causing nonspecific vaginitis thrive in a pH >5 (more alkaline).

Organisms causing infection of the vulva and vagina are most often introduced from outside sources such as clothing, hands, douche nozzles, or other contaminated articles or during intercourse. In sexually active women reinfection may occur after treatment unless their sexual partners are also successfully treated.

Women of menopausal and postmenopausal age often develop vaginitis (sometimes referred to as atrophic or senile vaginitis). Increased alkalinity of the vaginal secretions is a contributing cause, and the pyogenic bacterial invasion of the thin vaginal mucosa produces symptoms of burning, pruritus, and *leukorrhea* (whitish-yellow vaginal discharge).

Inflammation may also occur in Bartholin's glands or less frequently in Skene's glands. The infection is usually unilateral but may be bilateral. With infection the duct from the gland becomes partially or completely obstructed, resulting in severe redness, enlargement of the gland, and edema of the surrounding tissues. The area becomes tender, and walking may become painful. The usual result of the infectious process is an abscess. Occasionally, acute bartholinitis subsides, leaving fibrotic or scar tissue. When this occurs, a Bartholin's cyst develops. The cyst may vary in size, from a few centimeters in diameter to the size of a hen's egg, is mobile, and nontender.

Cervix

Cervicitis, infection of the cervix, is the most common gynecologic disorder, affecting more than half of all women. There are two forms of cervicitis, acute and chronic, of which the chronic is the most frequent. Cervicitis usually progresses from the acute to the chronic form if not treated, and it may go undetected for a long time. In fact, the cervix may heal and appear quite healthy after the disease has spread upward. This condition presents few symptoms, and those symptoms that occur do not ordinarily lead women to seek medical attention. If the vaginal discharge is slight, the woman may not become concerned.

Cervicitis may follow childbirth or abortion or it may be caused by infection of a cervical laceration or erosion. In untreated cervicitis the tissues are constantly irritated, and there is some evidence that this irritation predisposes to cancer.

Fallopian tubes

Inflammation of the fallopian tubes, *salpingitis,* may be local or more often may spread to the ovaries, pelvic peri-

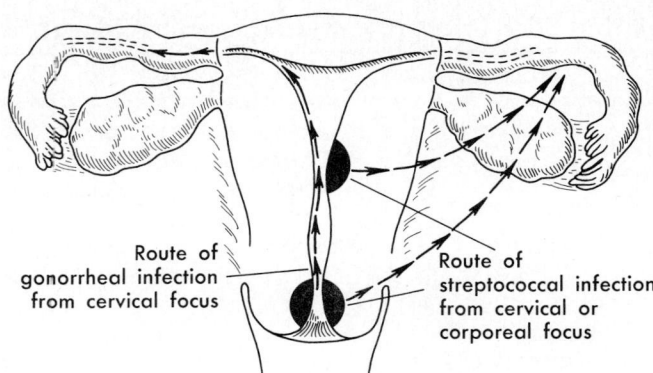

Fig. 35-4. Two chief routes of pelvic infection (From Novak, E.R., Jones, G.J., and Jones, H.W., Jr.: Novak's textbook of gynecology, ed. 9, Baltimore, 1975, The Williams & Wilkins Co.

toneum, pelvic veins, or pelvic connective tissue. This widespread inflammation is termed *pelvic inflammatory disease (PID)*. The pathogens may invade the pelvic organs during sexual intercourse, childbirth or the postpartum period of after abortion. PID is reported to occur five times more often among women using intrauterine devices (IUDs) for birth control than among women using other methods.

Pathogenic organisms are usually introduced from outside the body and pass up the cervical canal into the uterus. They seem to cause little trouble in the uterus but pass into the pelvis by way of the fallopian tubes, through thrombosed uterine veins, or through the lymphatics of the uterus (Fig. 35-4). The invaded structures become host to an acute or chronic inflammatory process.

Many of the pathogens causing PID lodge in the fallopian tubes. Purulent material collects in the tubes, adhesions form, strictures may occur, and sterility is a frequent result. Adhesions resulting from inflammation may cause such distress that complete removal of the uterus, fallopian tubes, and ovaries is necessary. Although generalized peritonitis can occur, the infection usually remains confined to the lower abdomen and pelvis. A severe inflammatory process may lead to dehydration, electrolyte imbalances, and prostration.

Toxic shock syndrome

Toxic shock syndrome, although not exclusively a reproductive disorder, occurs most commonly in menstruating females, especially among those using superabsorbent tampons. The syndrome has been associated with toxins produced by *Staphylococcus aureus*. It is suggested that the organism gains entry to the circulation through lesions in the vagina produced by tampons. Superabsorbent tampons provide a milieu favorable to bacterial growth because they can contain a large amount of menstrual blood and may be left in place several hours. Sepsis results from the effect of the toxins.

Types of vaginal discharges with inflammation

Inflammation	Discharge
Vaginitis	
Candida	White, curdlike, cheesy, sweetish odor
Trichomonas	Yellow to green, frothy, foul odor, copious
Gardnerella	Grayish white, fishy or foul odor, scanty
Cervicitis	Whitish yellow (mucopurulent), amount varies

Drugs commonly prescribed for inflammations of the female reproductive tract

Drugs	Route
Antibiotic	
Ampicillin	Oral
Procaine penicillin G	Oral
Tetracylcine	Oral
Antifungal	
Clotrimazole (Gyne-Lotrimin)	Vaginal, topical
Micronazole (Monistat)	Vaginal, topical
Nystantin (mycostantin, Nilstat)	Vaginal, topical, oral
Amebicide	
Metronidazole (Flagyl)	Oral

ASSESSMENT

Subjective data
Itching

Itching is a major symptom of vulvular or vaginal infection. The itching may result from irritation from the vaginal discharge or from end products of the inflammatory response. The degree of itching experienced is monitored for signs of decreasing intensity as the inflammation subsides. Itching is most intense with *Trichomonas* infections.

Causes of vulvar or vaginal itching other than infection include epithelial changes seen with menopause, high urinary sugar content as in diabetes mellitus, pediculosis pubis, scabies, allergies, pinworms, or cancer of the vulva. With severe pruritus there are usually excoriations of the skin caused by scratching, and secondary infection may result. Dysuria may occur as a consequence of local irritation of the urinary meatus.

Pain

Pain is primarily a symptom of PID. In *acute* PID there is usually severe cramping lower abdominal pain; in *chronic* PID the pain is typically dull and aching and may be located in the lower back as well as the lower abdomen. Occasionally women have been thought neurotic because of ongoing reports of the diffuse pain, only to have chronic PID diagnosed later.

Objective data
Vaginal discharge

Vaginal discharge is a major finding in most inflammations of the female genital tract. The *character* and *amount* of the discharge are monitored because these differ depending on the type and severity of the disorder. Normally, many women have a scant, thin, whitish vaginal discharge, primarily at the time of ovulation.

DATA ANALYSIS AND PLANNING

Nursing diagnoses

Nursing diagnoses for the woman with a gynecologic inflammation are based on collected data and may include the following:
Alteration in comfort: pain
Alteration in comfort: itching
Knowledge deficit
Sexual dysfunction: dyspareunia

Expected patient outcomes

1. Patient states feeling more comfortable.
2. The patient can:
   a. Describe how infections of the reproductive organs occur and spread
   b. Describe potentially undesirable effects of infections on the reproductive tract
   c. State signs that indicate improvement or lack of response to therapy
   d. Describe methods to prevent infection of sexual partner.

IMPLEMENTATION

Usual methods for medical therapy are given in Table 35-2. Some alternative therapies developed by women are included in Table 35-3.

Assisting with achievement of therapeutic goals
Medications

The major types of prescribed medications are antibiotic, antifungal, or amebicidal agents. The medications

Table 35-3. Alternative therapies for vaginitis

Infection	Intervention	Dosage	Administration
Monilia	Gentian violet	Few drops/qt water 0.25% to 2% (over-the-counter drug)	Douche or local application
	Vinegar (white)	1 tbsp/1 pt water	Douche every day for 5 to 7 days; twice daily for 2 days
	Acidophilus culture	2 tbsp/1 pt water	Douche twice daily
	Acidophilus yogurt Plain yogurt	1 application to labia hourly and as needed for symptom relief	
Trichomonas	1 handful chapparel chamomile	Steep in 1 qt water for 20 min	Douche 2 to 3 times/wk for 2 wk
Nonspecific vaginitis	Vinegar douche	5 tbsp/2 qt water	Every other day for 1 wk
	Salt (sea)	1 tbsp/1 qt water	Every other day for 1 wk
	1 tsp goldenseal and 1 clove minced garlic	Steep in 1 qt boiling water	Douche every day for 1 wk
	1 tsp goldenseal Povidone-iodine (Betadine) gel	Steep in 1 pt water; strain through cloth	Douche every day for 1 wk Twice daily for 1 wk

From Fogel, C.I., and Woods, N.F.: Health care of women: a nursing perspective, St. Louis, 1981, The C.V. Mosby Co.

should be used by the patient for the prescribed number of days. They may be prescribed to be taken orally, used topically, or as a suppository (to be placed in the vagina) or douche. Douching is also used to apply heat to promote healing by increasing circulation and for comfort. If both heat and topical medications are prescribed, the topical medication is applied after the douche.

Supportive therapy

Patients with severe PID are usually hospitalized for intensive therapy. They are usually placed on bed rest in mid-Fowler's position to provide dependent drainage so that abscesses will not form high in the abdomen where they might rupture and cause generalized peritonitis. Fluids are given intravenously to correct dehydration and acidosis.

Surgical procedures

Surgical intervention may be necessary in selected instances as described below.

INCISION AND DRAINAGE OF ABSCESS. An abcess of a Bartholin's gland may need to be incised and drained (I & D). After I&D a small amount of purulent drainage tinged with blood is expected, but any active, bright red bleeding should be reported to the physician. Relief from pain occurs almost immediately after I&D. The woman

may experience soreness or mild pain for about a day. Perineal irrigations or sitz baths serve the purpose of cleansing and giving comfort. Warm water can be used to cleanse the involved area after each voiding or bowel movement.

CAUTERIZATION OF CERVIX. When cervical lacerations or erosions are present, the area is usually cauterized. Silver nitrate sticks may be used to remove very small lesions. For larger areas requiring cauterization, an electric cautery unit is used. The woman is informed that a small, lubricated sheet of lead will be placed against the skin under the lumbar areas as a safety device for grounding electrical charges and that there will be slight bleeding, which will be controlled by a tampon or packing inserted by the physician. The odor of burning tissue when cautery is used is distressing to some patients. They are told to expect an odor but that the odor is insignificant and that the procedure is over quickly. Slight discomfort may be experienced.

Instructions for follow-up care vary, but usually include the following:

1. Leave the tampon or packing in place as long as the physician advises (usually 8 to 24 hours).
2. Report to the hospital or physician's office if bleeding is excessive (more than occurs during a normal menses).

Teaching the woman with an inflammation of the reproductive tract

1. Knowledge of spread of infection and its effects
2. Application of vaginal medication
   a. Wash hands before and after procedure
   b. Lie down after insertion to facilitate distribution of medication in vagina
   c. Do not douche after insertion of medication
   d. Wear a minipad
3. Sexual intercourse
   a. Abstain, if possible, to prevent discomfort and spread of infection to partner
   b. If abstention not feasible, advise male to use a condom
4. If repeated infections have occured:
   a. Use an alternative brand of birth control pill or alternative method of control
   b. Use only clean equipment if douches are used
   c. Restrict sexual intercourse
   d. Encourage sexual partner(s) to seek medical attention
5. Report signs of further infection (increased vaginal discharge, bleeding, pain, fever).

---

3. Do not douche or have sexual relations until the next visit to the physician unless specific instructions have been given for resumption of intercourse.
4. An unpleasant discharge caused by sloughing of destroyed cells may appear 4 to 5 days after cauterization; frequent warm baths will help this condition.

REMOVAL OF REPRODUCTIVE ORGANS. If a tubal abscess develops with PID, a salpingectomy (removal of the fallopian tubes) may be necessary. In severe chronic PID more reproductive organs may also need to be removed. Surgery of the reproductive tract is discussed on p. 1066.

Assisting with comfort

Itching is the primary discomfort with inflammations of the vulval and vagina. Frequent bathing and sitz baths may be helpful. Soothing lotions may be prescribed. Vinegar douches that decrease the alkalinity of the vagina may also relieve the pruritus.

Pain is the primary discomfort with PID. Heat (hot water bottle or electric heating pad) applied to the abdomen may promote circulation and ease the discomfort. Analgesics are often necessary to relieve the pain.

Dyspareunia (discomfort with intercourse) may be present as a result of the inflammation. Abstinence is advised until the inflammation subsides.

Counseling and teaching
Counseling

Women with PID are usually of childbearing age. If severe or chronic PID is present, infertility may result from adhesions in the fallopian tubes or from removal of reproductive organs. The woman needs opportunities to identify her feelings regarding potential or actual infertility (p. 1056).

Teaching

Many women with inflammations of the reproductive tract can be treated on an ambulatory basis. Women who are hospitalized will require further therapy at home (see box above).

Structural disorders
TYPES OF STRUCTURAL DISORDERS

Women may experience problems with relaxation of the vaginal outlet, displacement or prolapse of the uterus, or fistulas that may develop between the bladder or rectum and the vagina (Table 35-4).

PATHOPHYSIOLOGY

Most of the structural problems of the reproductive tract experienced by women result primarily from stretching and weakening of the ligaments supporting the uterus or of the muscles of the perineum. When the pelvic supporting tissues are relaxed, the urinary bladder may sag below the uterus and press against the vaginal wall *(cystocele)* (Fig. 35-5). This leads to stress incontinence (see Chapter 33). Similarly the posterior vaginal wall may weaken and the rectum may herniate into the vagina *(rectocele)*. The weakened rectal wall predisposes to constipation and hemorrhoids.

The uterus itself may be displaced, either flexed forward (anteflexion) or backward (retroflexion) or tilted backward (retroversion) (Fig. 35-6). In addition the uterus may lose its support and descend *(prolapse)* into the vaginal canal. With complete uterine prolapse, the cervix protrudes beyond the vaginal orifice. Cystoceles, rectoceles, and uterine prolapse are more commonly seen in older women.

Table 35-4. Structural problems of the female reproductive tract

Disorder	Cause	Signs and symptoms	Medical therapy
Relaxed vaginal outlet	Unrepaired childbirth lacerations, loss of pelvic muscle tone from repeated pregnancies or congenital weakness	Dragging pain in back and pelvis, stress incontinence, constipation, hemorrhoids	Plastic surgery
Uterine displacement	Congenital, PID, endometriosis, pregnancy, pelvic tumors, trauma	May be asymptomatic; dysmenorrhea, backache	Postural exercises, vaginal pessary
Uterine prolapse	Childbirth injuries, muscle relaxation due to age	Bearing down sensation, backache	Vaginal pessary, hysterectomy
Fistulas	Radiation of cervix, gynecologic surgery, trauma during childbirth	Vaginal leakage of urine, gas, or feces	Surgical removal of fistula (fistulectomy)

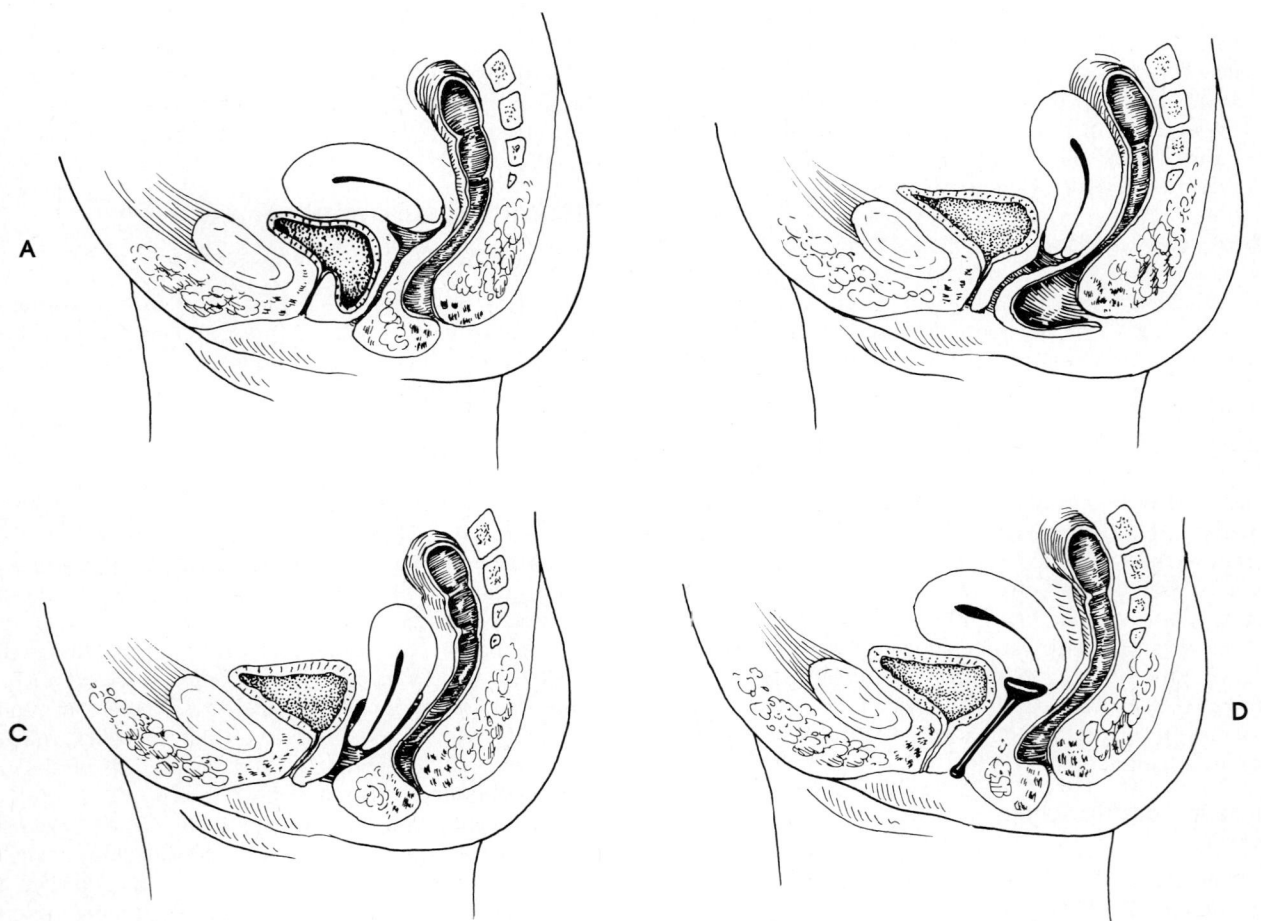

Fig. 35-5. Abnormalities of vagina. **A,** Cystocele: downward displacement of bladder toward vaginal orifice. **B,** Rectocele: pouching of rectum into posterior wall of vagina. **C,** Prolapse of uterus into vaginal canal. **D,** Stem pessary in place to maintain normal anatomic position of uterus.

Fistulas are abnormal passageways between two organs. *Vesicovaginal fistulas* are openings between the bladder and vagina and lead to leakage of urine through the vagina. Because the vagina does not have a sphincter, urinary incontinence results. *Rectovaginal fistulas,* which are less common, are passageways between the rectum and vagina. These lead to fecal incontinence and uncontrollable flatus expulsion. Both types of fistulas may close spontaneously but frequently need to be repaired surgically. If so, 3 to 4 months are required for the inflammation to subside before surgery can be attempted.

ASSESSMENT

Women with structural disorders of the reproductive tract often experience low-grade discomfort in the pelvic area and back. In addition, problems with urinary or fecal control may be present. Data to be collected if incontinence is present include the following:

1. Extent of incontinence
2. Pattern of incontinence: incontinence from a cystocele is intermittent, occurring mostly during stress (such as laughing or crying); incontinence from fistulas is continual seeping
3. Usual methods of coping (for example, use of pads, plastic pants, avoidance of fluids before social occasions)
4. Feelings regarding incontinence

DATA ANALYSIS AND PLANNING

Nursing diagnoses

Possible nursing diagnoses include the following:
Alteration in comfort: pain
Alteration in elimination: incontinence

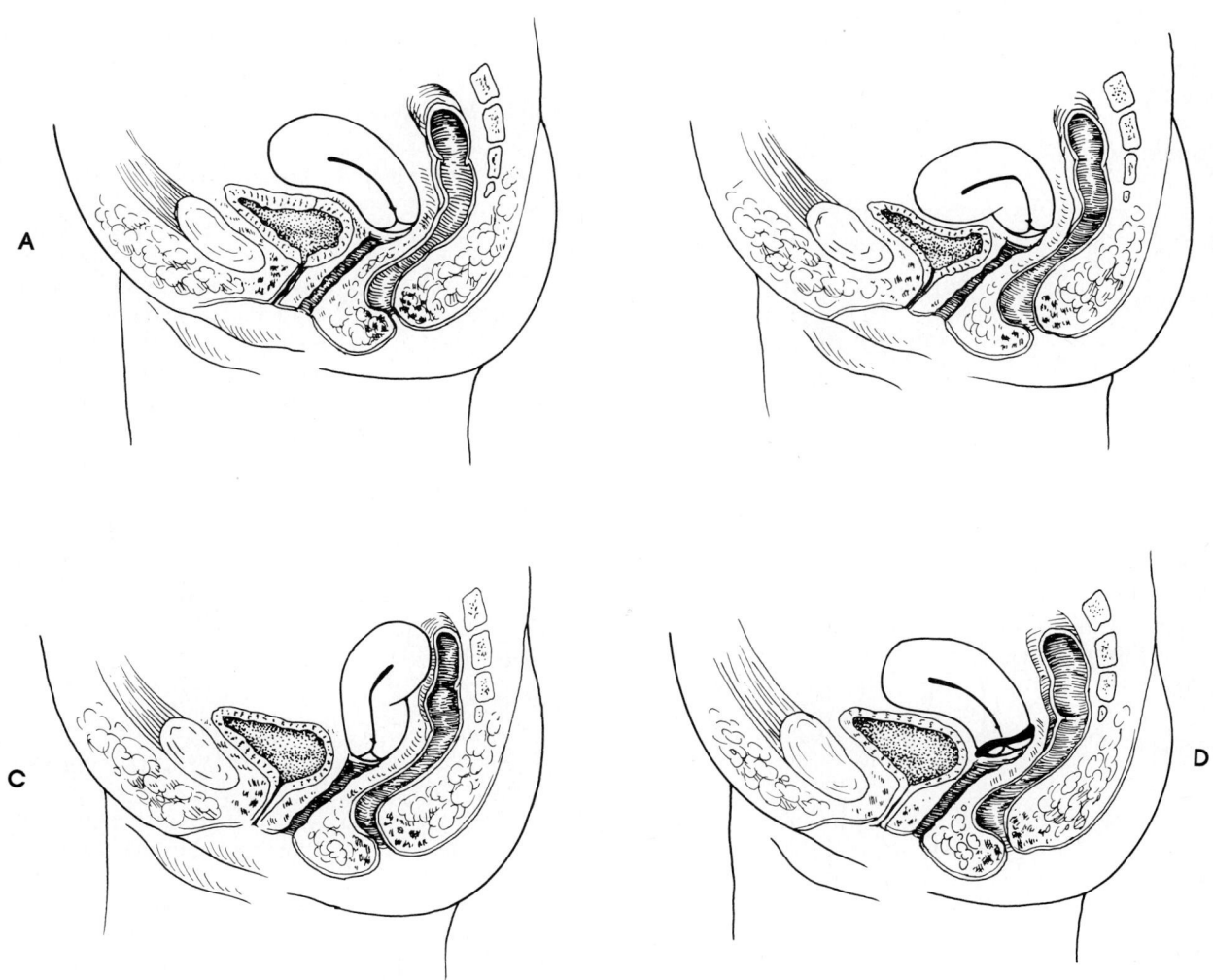

Fig. 35-6. Normal and abnormal positions of uterus. **A,** Normal anatomic position of uterus in relation to adjacent structures. **B,** Anterior displacement of uterus. **C,** Retroversion, or backward displacement, of uterus. **D,** Normal anatomic position of uterus maintained by use of rubber S-shaped pessary.

Fig. 35-7. A, Albert Smith pessary, **B,** Pessary in place to hold posterior vaginal fornix, and with it attached cervix, well backward and upward in pelvis. (From Beacham, D.W., and Beacham, W.D.: Synopsis of gynecology, ed. 10, St. Louis, 1982, The C.V. Mosby Co.)

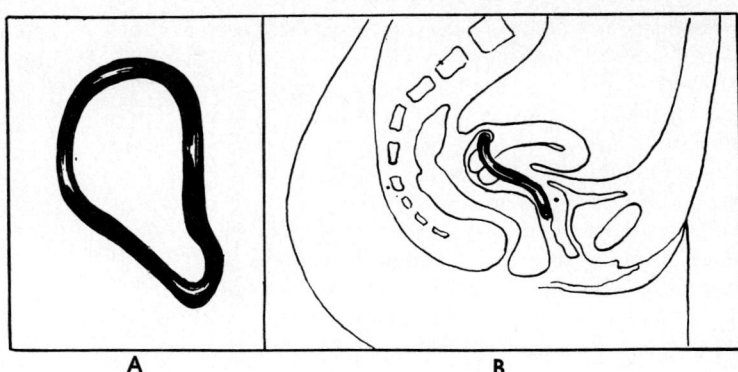

A   B

Surgeries for repair of structural problems

Anterior colporrhaphy	Repair of cystocele
Posterior colporrha-phy	Repair of rectocele
Marshall-Marchetti	Suspension of bladder in correct position
Fistulectomy	Removal of fistula

Expected patient outcomes

Expected patient outcomes are as follows. The woman:
1. States feeling comfortable
2. Performs self-care measures to manage the condition.
3. Seeks help from a health professional when appropriate.

IMPLEMENTATION

Assisting with achievement of therapeutic goals

If symptoms are severe enough to interfere with the woman's ability to function effectively, the primary medical therapies are the use of a *pessary* (plastic ring inserted to support the uterus [Fig. 35-7]) or *surgery* to repair weakened muscles and walls or fistulas (see box above).

Preoperative care

If the rectum is involved, preoperative laxatives and enemas are usually given to reduce bowel contents. Clear liquids are given 24 hours before surgery.

Postoperative care

Repair may be accomplished vaginally or through a suprapubic incision. In the latter method, a suprapubic tube may be inserted and maintained for several days to permit healing (see Chapter 33). An indwelling urethral catheter is inserted after anterior colporrhaphy to keep the bladder empty and to allow edema to subside to prevent pressure on the incision.

After surgery involving the rectum, laxatives may be given to prevent strain on the incision. Care of the patient after rectal surgery is described in Chapter 32.

Prevention of infection is effected by good perineal care after voiding or defecation. A heat lamp at the perineal area may be used for comfort and to promote healing.

Assisting with comfort

Pain from structural disorders is usually low grade. Aspirin and acetaminophen usually suffice as analgesics, if required.

Psychologic discomfort related to incontinence is usually more of a problem. The woman can be helped to explore her feelings about the incontinence and possible effects on sexual functioning. Before surgery is planned, alternative methods of keeping dry can be explored. For a vesicovaginal fistula, a menstrual rubber cap (Tassette) may be attached to a catheter and leg bag urinal. For stress incontinence, menstrual pads or padded plastic pants may be helpful.

Dribbling of fecal matter into the vagina from a rectovaginal fistula is particularly distressing and may be temporarily lessened by a high enema; this is useful prior to social situations. Constipating diets to decrease fecal leakage are not useful because they eventually cause pressure that may aggravate the condition and increase the size of the fistula.

Teaching

1. Before surgery
   a. Perineal exercise (Chapter 33) to strengthen weakened perineal muscles
   b. Pelvic exercises to assist in repositioning of uterus
      1. Knee-chest position for 5 minutes three times a day
      2. Lying on abdomen 2 hours per day
   c. Encouragement to seek medical consultation for symptoms of lower abdominal pain or incontinence
2. After surgery
   a. Use of douches or mild laxatives as prescribed (gentle insertion of douche nozzle)
   b. Avoidance of heavy lifting, prolonged standing, or

Table 35-5. Benign tumors of the female reproductive tract

Type	Signs and symptoms	Medical therapy
Ovarian tumors and cysts	Increased abdominal size; fatigue; sense of pelvic fullness	Oophorectomy
Endometriosis	Pain that increases in severity during menstruation, dyspareunia, irregular menstrual cycles	Antiovulation drugs (oral contraceptives, danazol), analgesics Surgery: younger than 35 years, resection of lesions; older than 35 years, total hysterectomy, salpingectomy, oophorectomy
Uterine fibroid tumors	Menorrhagia, low back pain, dysmenorrhea, constipation, irregular enlarged uterus	Small tumors: no treatment Severe symptoms or rapidly growing tumors: myomectomy or hysterectomy
Cervical polyps	Leukorrhea, abnormal vaginal bleeding	Surgical removal (polypectomy)

sexual intercourse until permitted (usually about 6 weeks)

c. Description of loss of vaginal sensation usually for several months (normal response)
d. Avoidance of enemas after rectal surgery until healing is complete
e. Reporting of signs of infection or pain to physician.

Tumors

BENIGN TUMORS

Many different types of benign neoplasms affect the female reproductive tract. The more common sites for these tumors are the ovaries or myometrium of the uterus (Table 35-5).

Ovarian tumors

Most ovarian tumors are benign and are often asymptomatic. There are numerous types depending on the site and tissue involved. Ovarian cysts occur frequently. Simple cysts are thin-walled structures containing serous fluid and are often seen during menopause. Corpus luteum cysts result from an exaggeration of the process of formation and resorption of the corpus luteum. Follicle cysts arise during the evolution or involution of the graafian follicle. Cysts do not become malignant. Severe pain may result if a cyst becomes twisted on its pedicle, and the symptoms may resemble appendicitis.

Polycystic ovarian disease (Stein-Levanthal) is characterized by enlargement of the ovaries, with numerous cystic follicles encased in a fibrotic capsule. Effects of these tumors are often not noted unless there is compression of a neighboring organ or blood supply, a menstrual disorder, or infertility.

Endometriosis

Endometriosis is a condition in which endometrial cells that normally line the uterus are seeded throughout the pelvis and occasionally extend to as distant a location as the umbilicus (Fig. 35-8). With each menstrual period

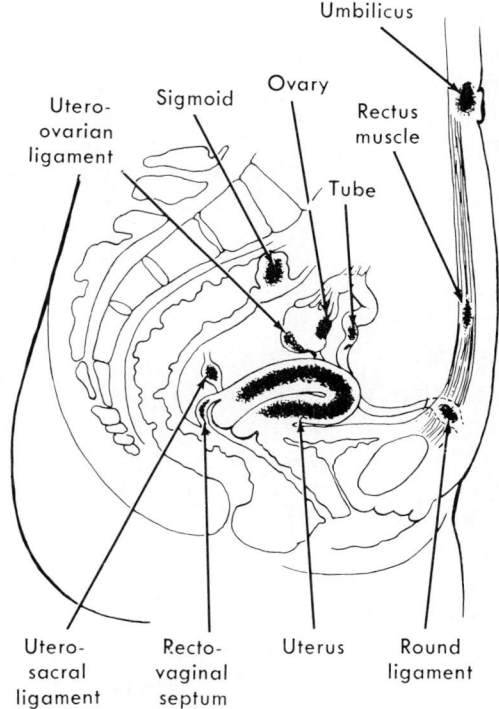

Fig. 35-8. Sites of endometrial implants.

the endometrial cells are stimulated by the ovarian hormones and bleed into the surrounding areas, causing an inflammation. Subsequent adhesions may be so severe that pelvic organs become fused together, occasionally causing a stricture of the bowel or interference with bladder function. Encased blood may lead to palpable tumor masses, which often occur on the ovary and are known as *chocolate cysts*. Occasionally these cysts rupture and spread endometrial cells still farther throughout the pelvis.

Usually endometriosis progresses gradually and does not produce symptoms until the age of 30 to 40 years.

Occasionally, however, symptoms appear when the woman is in her teens. Approximately half of the women with endometriosis are infertile, and endometriosis is sometimes first detected when a woman complains of inability to conceive.

If the woman is young and wants children, the treatment for endometriosis is usually as conservative as possible. Pregnancy is beneficial, because menstruation ceases during this time. If a young woman has endometriosis, she and her husband usually are advised to have their family early, because the fertility rate is low, sterility caused by adhesions may occur, and a hysterectomy may have to be done within a reasonable period of time. Nursing the infant is also recommended because it delays the onset of menstruation after delivery. Menopause stops the progress of this condition.

Uterine fibroid tumors

Fibroid tumors are the most common tumors of the female genital tract. They are discrete benign tumors of the uterine muscle and connective tissue. The sizes of myomas are variable. Most are found in the body of the uterus (corporeal) but some occur in the cervix or may involve the broad ligament. Submucous tumors may impinge on the blood vessels of the endometrium and produce bleeding. As they grow larger they may impinge on the opposite uterine wall and distort the cavity of the uterus. In some instances submucous tumors develop pedicles and may protrude through the vagina or cervix, resulting in infection or ulcerations.

Fibroid tumors of the uterus tend to disappear spontaneously with menopause. They rarely become malignant. Infertility may result from a myoma that obstructs or distorts the uterus or fallopian tubes. Myoma in the body of the uterus may cause spontaneous abortions, and those near the cervical opening may make the delivery of a baby difficult and may contribute to hemorrhage postpartally.

Cervical polyps

Cervical polyps form when an area of the mucosa proliferates. These growths are usually visible at the cervical os as bright red, vascular, fragile areas. They are most often pedunculated and appear to protrude from the cervical canal. Polyps may occur singly or in clusters.

Because of the vascularity of the polyp, bleeding is a common symptom. The bleeding is small in amount and occurs between menstrual periods and closely resembles that of early cancer of the cervix. Especially characteristic is the contact bleeding produced by coitus, by douching, or by vaginal examination.

The pedicle by which the polyp is attached is usually quite small, and the polyp can easily be removed by twisting the pedicle at its base or by biopsy. Tissue examination of removed polyps is essential because epidermoid cancer arises from cervical polyps in a small percentage of cases.

SURGERY OF THE REPRODUCTIVE TRACT
Types of surgery

Minor surgical procedures are performed primarily for diagnostic purposes. Major surgery involves removal of one or more reproductive organs (see box below).

Minor procedures
Preoperative care

Dilation and curettage is the standard procedure for investigating any irregular bleeding. In addition it may be performed to correct a cervical stricture or to treat dysmenorrhea. Cervical biopsy and conization of the cervix are done to test for the presence of malignancy. All of these procedures may be performed on an outpatient basis. Cervical biopsy does not require anesthesia, whereas local or general anesthesia may be used for D and C or

---

Surgeries of the female reproductive tract

Procedure	Description
Minor procedures	
Dilation and curettage (D and C)	Dilation of the cervix and scraping of uterine walls
Cervical biopsy	Punch biopsy of the cervix
Conization of cervix	Removal of cone-shaped portion of cervix
Major procedures	
Oophorectomy	Removal of ovaries
Salpingectomy	Removal of fallopian tubes
Hysterectomy (vaginal, abdominal)	Removal of uterus, either through the vagina or abdomen
Radical hysterectomy	Removal of uterus, upper vagina, and parametrium
Pelvic exenteration	Removal of pelvic viscera (bladder, rectosigmoid) and all reproductive organs

conization. The usual preoperative preparation is given; shaving is rarely required.

Postoperative care

VAGINAL BLEEDING. Bleeding is monitored every 15 minutes for 2 hours and then as necessary thereafter. The blood loss is best recorded in estimated milliliters. A blood loss of at least 60 ml is required to saturate a perineal pad. It is important to record each pad change as well as blood loss. Any excessive bleeding is reported to the physician. More blood is lost by conization of the cervix than with the other procedures, and oozing may be controlled by packing inserted at the time of surgery.

DISCOMFORT. Mild abdominal cramping may be experienced postoperatively. Mild analgesics such as codeine sulfate and acetylsalicylic acid are usually ordered to relieve pain. Abdominal pain after D and C that is continuous, sharp, and not relieved by analgesics should be reported immediately to the surgeon; this type of pain may indicate perforation of the uterus.

TEACHING
1. Rest more than usual for first 24 hours postoperatively.
2. Avoid heavy lifting or marked exertion for 4 weeks.
3. Leave tampon or packing in place as advised (usually 8 to 24 hours).
4. Report to physician bleeding that is more than usually experienced during normal menses.
5. No douches or sexual intercourse until advised by physician.

Major procedures
Preoperative care

Preparation of the patient for gynecologic surgery is similar to that for major abdominal surgery. Functioning of other systems within the pelvis (urinary, intestinal) is evaluated, particularly if there are any symptoms of dysfunction.

PSYCHOLOGIC PREPARATION. Removal of reproductive organs can significantly affect the woman emotionally, and time may be needed to help her adjust to the proposed changes. The reproductive organs are a major component of "womanhood," and loss of these organs creates a change in body image. Women see menstrual functioning as a symbol of femininity; therefore, with sudden cessation of menstruation some women state feelings of being "less of a woman."

Feelings of sexuality in terms of sexual relations are also threatened. Some women worry that sexual relations may be hindered or be less satisfactory. In actuality, many women find after hysterectomy that sexual relations are enhanced because fear of pregnancy has been removed. Except in rare instances of pelvic exenteration, sexual intercourse is possible after healing has occurred.

Women who experience some difficulties in adjusting may be those of childbearing age and those at menopause. The latter are still adjusting to life's changes and may be at a crisis period in their life. The nurse's role is to help the woman explore her feelings and to correct myths or misunderstandings before surgery to facilitate an easier recovery.

PHYSIOLOGIC PREPARATION. Close proximity of the urinary tract and bowel to the reproductive organs requires measures to prevent infection. Preoperative measures are also taken to prevent postoperative thromboembolism.
1. Antibiotics to treat or prevent infection
2. Bowel preparation if bowel will be involved
   a. Mechanical cleansing (laxatives, enemas)
   b. Liquid diet for 24 hours
3. Medicated douches if there is high risk of infection
4. Persons at high risk for thrombophlebitis (varicose veins, obesity, diabetes mellitus)
   a. Low-dose heparin
   b. Support stockings
   c. Discontinuation of oral contraceptives 3 to 4 weeks preoperatively.

Postoperative care

General care of the patient after major gynecologic surgery is essentially the same as that after abdominal surgery. Measures to prevent respiratory complications are important. Fluid and electrolyte balance is monitored carefully.

PREVENTION OF THROMBOEMBOLISM. Thrombophlebitis and pulmonary embolism are major postoperative complications after pelvic surgery as a result of venous stasis in the major pelvic veins. Symptoms may be absent until signs of pulmonary embolism occur (chest pain, hemoptysis) 1 week later. Because the involved veins are usually deep in the thigh, the only local symptoms may be pain and swelling in the thigh and a positive Homan's sign (pain with dorsiflexion of foot).

URINARY COMPLICATIONS. Urinary *retention* is a common occurrence after gynecologic surgery as a result of handling of the bladder during surgery. An indwelling urinary catheter is usually inserted for 3 to 5 days postoperatively until muscle function returns. Suprapubic drainage by means of a small polyethylene catheter introduced into the bladder by means of a large-bore needle or trocar may be used in place of the standard urethral catheter. Urinary *infection* (a common postoperative occurrence) is minimized with use of suprapubic drainage.

Urinary *fistula* may result despite careful surgical technique. It is identified by leakage of urine through the vagina. Many such fistulas close spontaneously. The woman may be placed on her stomach and gentle intermittent suction applied to the indwelling catheter to encourage healing of the fistula.[2]

GASTROINTESTINAL PROBLEMS. Gastrointestinal function usually returns 24 to 72 hours after surgery, depending on the extent of handling of the intestines. Persistent nausea and vomiting with severe abdominal distention may indicate ileus, and all oral intake is stopped and a nasogastric tube inserted. Most patients, however, have return of function. Abdominal distention with abdominal cramping may result from collection of gas in the sluggish bowel. Ambulation and heat encourage expulsion of the gas.

Nursing care of woman experiencing major gynecologic surgery

Preoperative care

1. Identify patient's understanding of planned surgical procedure and correct misunderstandings
2. Encourage and support self-exploration of feelings related to proposed surgery
3. Provide support stockings for persons at high risk for thromboembolism
4. Teach breathing and leg exercises.

Postoperative care

1. Monitor
   a. Fluid and electrolyte balance
   b. Breath sounds and respiratory excursion
   c. Abdominal distention
   d. Pain in abdomen
   e. Pain in thighs
   f. Dressing
   g. Signs of urinary tract infection
2. Encourage breathing exercises every 2 to 4 hours until patient becomes active
3. Urinary drainage
   a. Maintain patency of indwelling urinary catheter
   b. When catheter removed, monitor for leakage of urine in vagina (signs of urinary fistula)
4. Provide pain medication through third postoperative day on a fairly regular schedule, then as needed thereafter
5. For gas pains, apply heat (hot water bottle, electric heating pad) to abdomen, encourage ambulation, try a rectal tube
6. Prevent thrombophlebitis
   a. Teach patient not to keep knee or thighs sharply flexed; no pillows under knees
   b. Continue support stockings for patients at high risk
   c. Encourage leg exercises every hour while awake until ambulating freely
   d. Lower head of bed to flat postion for a short time every 2 hours for 24 hours, then every 4 hours until ambulating freely
   e. Encourage walking, increasing distance
7. Continue providing emotional support
8. Teach patient
   a. Resume home activities gradually
   b. Car riding permitted after first week at home, but no driving for 3 to 4 weeks, especially with standard shift car
   c. Avoid heavy lifting, riding over rough roads, walking swiftly, jogging, or dancing (activities that tend to cause pelvic blood congestion) for 6 to 8 weeks
   d. Resume preoperative sexual activities such as cuddling or closeness immediately
   e. Resume sexual intercourse in 4 to 6 weeks
   f. Report immediately to physician any signs of thromboembolism
   g. Return for postoperative medical evaluations as instructed

---

PSYCHOLOGIC SUPPORT. Postoperatively, almost all patients feel depressed for several days. The patient often is unable to explain why she is depressed and crying. Grieflike responses to loss of a body part may appear as they do after loss of other body parts. Feelings of guilt, shame, and remorse are common. Encouraging the woman to continue activities associated with being feminine, such as using makeup, arranging her hair, and wearing her own clothing, often helps the woman to regain her feminine perspective. During this time she needs understanding and empathic care. Families may need to be helped to accept these responses calmly, and a husband may need help in understanding her need for reassurance of his continued love and affection.

Cancer

Malignancies in the female reproductive tract occur primarily in the uterus (cervix and endometrium) and in the ovaries (Table 35-6); they may also occur, although less frequently, in the vagina or vulva. Cancer of the reproductive tract ranks second to cancer of the breast in females.[1]

Table 35-6. Cancer of the female reproductive tract

Site	Incidence	Usual age (yr)	Signs and symptoms	Medical therapy
Cervix	4%	30 to 50	Early: may be asymptomatic, vaginal discharge, spotting between menses Late: dark, foul vaginal discharge, pain	Conization of cervix for cancer in situ in young women; hysterectomy, radiation (internal, external)
Endometrium	9%	50 to 65	Early: postmenopausal bleeding Late: uterine enlargement, pain	Hysterectomy and bilateral salpingo-oophorectomy, radiation (internal, external), progestin for metastases
Ovary	4%	All ages	Early: asymptomatic Late: ascites, edema of legs, pain	Salpingo-oophorectomy; hysterectomy may also be necessary; chemotherapy, radiation

Table 35-7. Stages of cancer of female reproductive tract

Stage	Cervix	Endometrium	Ovary
0	Confined to epithelium	Confined to epithelium	—
I	Confined to cervix	Confined to corpus	Confined to ovary
II	Extends outside cervix but does not involve pelvic wall or lower third of vagina	Involves corpus and cervix	Involves ovaries with pelvic extension
III	Involves pelvic wall and lower third of vagina	Involves pelvic and vaginal wall (but not bladder or rectum)	Intraperitoneal metastases
IV	Involves bladder, rectum, or metastatic spread	Involves bladder, rectum, or metastatic spread	Involves metastatic spread

The death rate from cancer of the *cervix* has fallen steadily over the past 40 years. This decline has been attributed to early detection through annual examinations (including a Papanicolaou smear) and improved surgical and radiotherapeutic techniques. Cancer of the cervix identified and treated early at the preinvasive stage is 100% curable, thus *early detection* (p. 1049) *is vitally important.*

The incidence of *endometrial* cancer is rising slowly, partly because it is primarily a disease of postmenopausal women and women are living longer.

Cancer of the *ovary* has had a steady slow *increase* in incidence but appears to be leveling off.[1] Because it is asymptomatic in the early stages, it is often far advanced before diagnosis is made. The only effective means of assuring early diagnosis is a pelvic examination every 6 months, including careful ovarian palpation, and surgical exploration of any questionable ovarian growth.

PATHOPHYSIOLOGY

Cancer of the cervix

Most cervical cancers are squamous carcinomas that arise in the intraepithelial layers (preinvasive stage or carcinoma in situ). It usually takes 5 to 10 years for squamous cell carcinoma to become invasive beyond the basement membrane. Spread usually occurs by direct extension or by means of the lymph system. Therapy depends on the stage (extent of spread) (Table 35-7).

Cancer of the endometrium

Cancer of the endometrium is primarily a slow-growing adenocarcinoma. Because it occurs mostly in postmenopausal women, estrogen stimulation unopposed by progesterone is thought to be implicated. Prolonged use of estrogen during menopause increases the risk of endometrial cancer seven times.[41] Cancer of the endometrium is usually diagnosed when the postmenopausal woman seeks medical care for vaginal bleeding. Although the incidence is more than twice that for cancer of the cervix, the death rate is lower.

Cancer of the ovary

Ovarian cancer causes more deaths than cancer of the uterus. The pathophysiology of ovarian cancer is complex, and there are a great variety of tumors. The ovaries may be a site of metastasis from the gastrointestinal tract, breast, pancreas, or kidneys.

DIAGNOSTIC TESTS

Pelvic examinations

Pelvic examinations are useful for visualization of changes in the vulva, vagina, and cervix; for palpation of internal organs, especially the ovaries and surface of the uterus; and for obtaining Pap smears.

Women are advised to avoid douching and applying any vaginal preparation (medicinal or deodorant) for at least 24 hours before examination. They should void immediately before the examination, because an empty bladder makes palpation of the pelvic organs easier, decreases patient discomfort, and eliminates possible distortion of the position of pelvic organs caused by a full bladder. The technique for performing pelvic examinations is described in most physical examination texts.

After the pelvic examination a woman may need assistance in removing her legs from the stirrups and getting down from the table. Elderly women merit careful assistance after the pelvic examination because unnatural positions, such as the knee-chest and lithotomy positions, may alter the normal circulation of blood sufficiently to cause faintness.

Papanicolaou (Pap) test

The Pap test is a cytologic test that makes it possible to detect abnormal cells, not all of which are cancerous. However, the Pap test has made it possible through routine use to detect precancerous conditions and cancer of the cervix early enough to make treatment of these conditions almost 100% successful. For detection of atypical cells, the Pap test is 95% accurate. False negative reports are most frequently the result of an inadequate sample or improperly fixed slide.

The Pap test involves microscopic examination of cells collected from the vaginal pool, exocervix, and endocervical canal. Samples of cells are obtained by using a vaginal pipette with a rubber tip and a specially designed wooden spatula. Secretions containing exfoliated cells are preferably obtained from the cervix or external os.

Guidelines for Pap tests

1. Ideal time for a Pap test is 5 to 6 days after menstrual termination.
2. Avoid tub bath or douche for 48 hours before the test.
3. Delay a Pap test for at least 1 month after use of *topical* antibiotics (produce rapid, heavy shedding of cells).
4. Slight vaginal bleeding (spotting) after the test may occur; excessive bleeding should be reported to the physician.
5. Medications such as tetracycline or digitalis may alter the results.[13]

Glass slides should be labeled and ready for use. A solution of 95% alcohol and ether in a wide-mouthed jar is used because rapid fixation of the smear is essential. The secretions are collected, smeared on the glass slide, and immediately placed back to back in the fixative solution to prevent drying out and cell distortion.

Do-it-yourself Pap tests are available. These can be used by women who are reluctant or unable to visit a physician for examination.

Obtaining endometrial cells for study
Jet washings

Jet washings consist of inserting an irrigating device into the uterus and irrigating the uterine cavity with about 30 ml normal saline solution. The normal saline solution containing cells from the uterine cavity is returned by suction into a collecting chamber. The cells are then centrifuged out, stained, and examined microscopically.

Vacuum curettage of endometrium

The procedure and apparatus used for vacuum curettage are similar to those used in suction curettage for performing an abortion. The cervix is dilated, and the suction tip is inserted through the cervix into the uterus. Suction is applied, and the entire uterine cavity is suctioned to secure specimens for study.

Ultrasound

Ultrasound has become a useful diagnostic tool for gynecologic problems. It can be used to locate pelvic masses, IUDs, and ectopic pregnancies. The computed tomography (CT) scan is *not* widely used but may be helpful in identification of very small lesions.

Endoscopy

The pelvic organs and surrounding tissues can be visualized directly by endoscopy. Various procedures may be used depending on the organs or structures to be inspected. Maintaining asepsis throughout any of these procedures is important in preventing infection.

During the procedures, air may enter the abdominal cavity and cause discomfort. Placing the woman in a prone position with a pillow under the abdomen may decrease discomfort. Douching and intercourse should be avoided for about 1 week after a culdoscopy.

TREATMENT MODALITIES

Surgery

Total abdominal hysterectomy (TAH) with or without bilateral salpingo-oophorectomy (BSO) is the most common treatment for gynecologic cancer (Table 35-6). Care of the patient experiencing gynecologic surgery is described on p. 1067. The woman with cancer not only experiences the same feelings associated with loss of reproductive organs as other women but is at the same time facing the concerns related to cancer (see Chapter 14). This is therefore a period of high anxiety for the woman, and she requires considerable empathy and emotional support as she works through her feelings.

Radiotherapy

Intracervical, intrauterine, or external whole pelvic irradiation may be given preoperatively to shrink the tumor to facilitate safety of the operation. Radiation may also be used as adjunct therapy postoperatively. Guidelines for radiation therapy are described in Chapter 14. Premenopausal women who receive pelvic irradiation will lose their ovarian function.

Radiation of the pelvic organs may create problems in sexual functioning. Patients have reported lack of libido, marked pain or discomfort with intercourse, and feelings of a narrow or shortened vagina.[12] These problems may add to the woman's feelings of sexual inadequacy from interferences with reproductive function.

Intracavitary implant

Radium or cesium may be inserted through a tandem placed in the uterine cavity (Figs. 35-10 and 35-11). During an intracavitary implant, it is important that all normal tissues remain in their natural position and that the radioactive substance is not placed nearer than is anticipated and provided for by the protective materials used. Gauze packing is usually inserted into the vagina to push

---

Endoscopic procedures for visualization of pelvic organs

Colposcopy	Visualization of vagina and cervix under low-power magnification
Culdoscopy	Insertion of a culdoscope through posterior vaginal vault into cul-de-sac of Douglas for visualization of fallopian tubes and ovaries
Hysteroscopy	Insertion of a hysteroscope through the cervix for visualization of inside of the uterus
Laparoscopy	Insertion of a laparoscope (under local anesthesia) through small incision in abdominal wall (inferior margin of umbilicus), which is insufflated with carbon dioxide; permits visualization of all pelvic organs (Fig. 35-9).

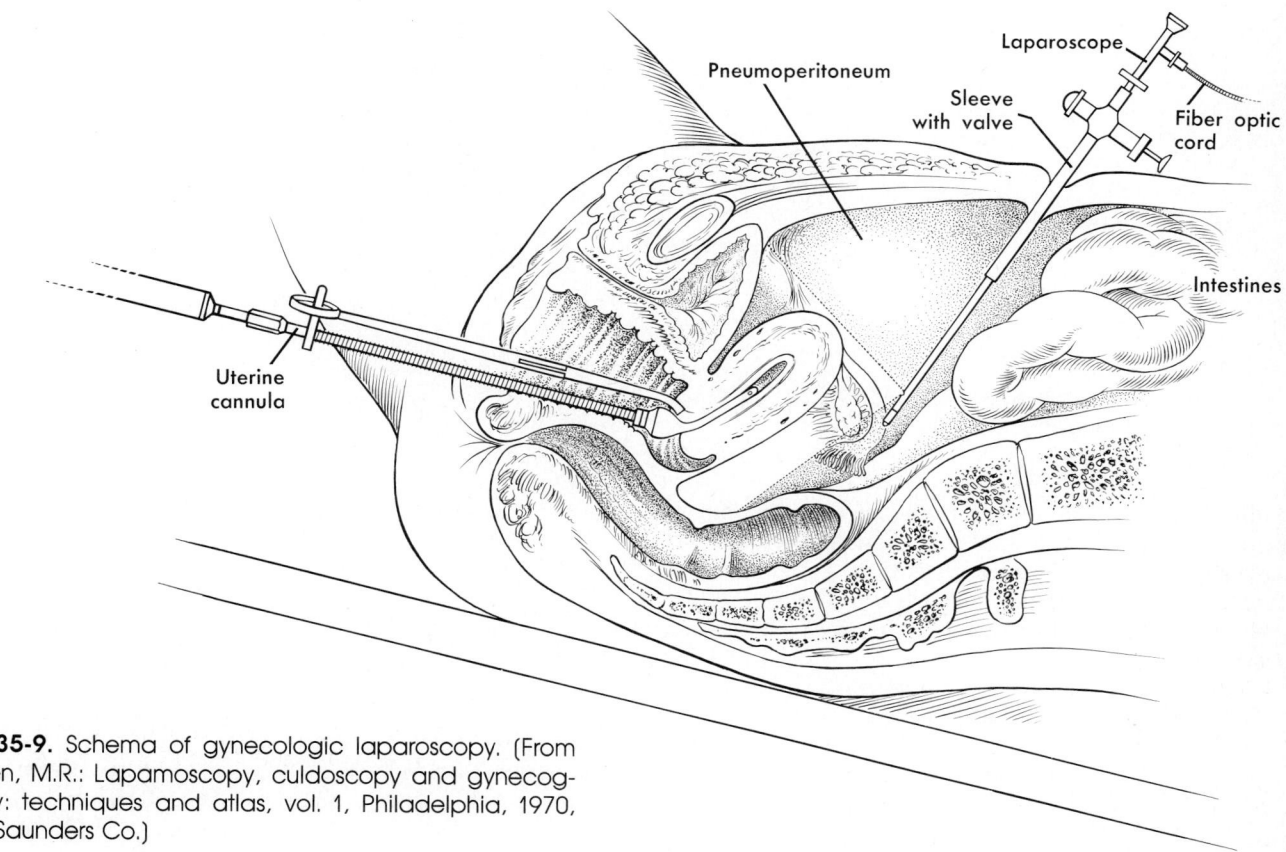

Fig. 35-9. Schema of gynecologic laparoscopy. (From Cohen, M.R.: Lapamoscopy, culdoscopy and gynecography: techniques and atlas, vol. 1, Philadelphia, 1970, W.B. Saunders Co.)

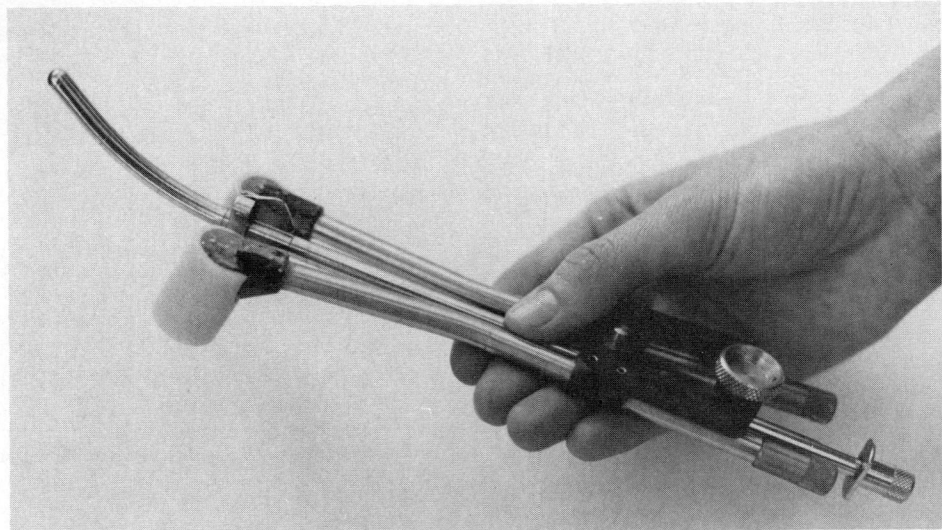

Fig. 35-10. Assembled configuration of tandem and colpostat before placement.

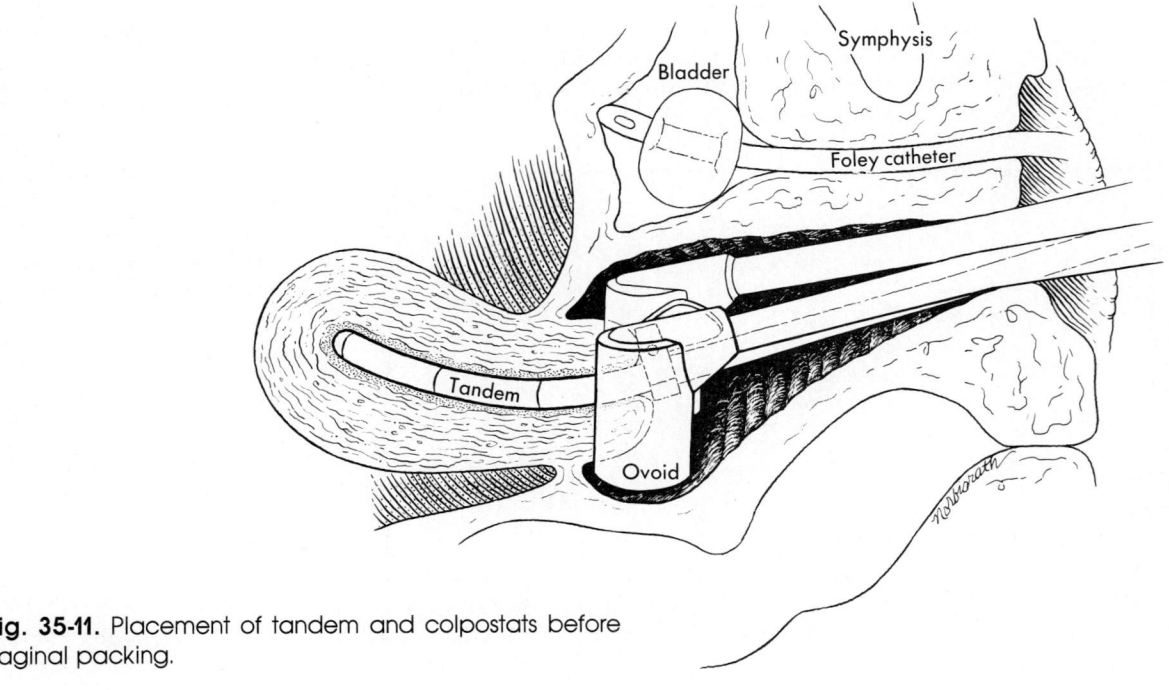

Fig. 35-11. Placement of tandem and colpostats before vaginal packing.

both the rectum and the bladder away from the area being irradiated. A urinary catheter is inserted before therapy to prevent bladder distention. Low-residue diet and cleansing enemas are given before therapy, and the enema is repeated after therapy to prevent bowel distention.

Nursing care consists of the following guidelines:
1. Keep patient flat in bed; may turn side to side
2. Provide analgesics for severe uterine contractions from dilation of cervix
3. Provide good perineal care; there will be foul-

smelling vaginal discharge from cell destruction; a deodorant is helpful
4. Encourage fluids to 3000 ml/day to maintain urinary adequacy
5. Follow general guidelines for internal radiation
6. Plan care that includes measures to decrease social isolation.

Radiation sickness may result as a systemic reaction to the breakdown and reabsorption of cell proteins. Local reaction may include cystitis and proctitis. Vaginal discharge will continue for some time after termination of

Table 35-8. Inflammatory disorders of the male reproductive tract

Disorder	Cause	Signs and symptoms	Medical therapy
Urethritis	*Chlamydia, trachomatis, ureaplasma, urealyticum*	Urgency, frequency, and burning with urination, purulent urethral discharge	Antibiotics
Prostatitis	*Chlamydia trachomatis, Neisseria gonorrhoeae*	Perineal pain, fever, dysuria, urethral discharge	Antibiotics, rest, hydration, analgesics, stool softener, sitz baths
Epididymitis	Same as for prostatitis	Sudden scrotal pain, scrotal edema	Antibiotics, injection of procaine around spermatic cord, bed rest with scrotal elevation, analgesics
Orchitis	Pyogenic bacteria, gonococci; may follow mumps or tuberculosis; may result from trauma or surgical manipulation	Same as for epididymitis; nausea and vomiting, pain radiating to inguinal canal	Same as for epididymitis

therapy, and the patient may need to take douches for as long as the odor and vaginal discharge persist. Some vaginal bleeding may occur for 1 to 3 months after irradiation of the cervix. The woman who is at home should report persistent rectal irritation to the physician. The patient is usually discharged from the hospital within a day or two after the applicators are removed, but may return for another course of radiation.

Complications to watch for after radiation of the uterus are vesicovaginal fistulas, ureterovaginal fistulas, cystitis, phlebitis, and hemorrhage. Each is caused by the radiation or by extension of the disease process. The patient is urged to report even minor symptoms to her physician.

Chemotherapy

Chemotherapy has not significantly improved cancer of the uterus and therefore is rarely used in this situation. Chemotherapy is used more often for cancer of the ovaries. Combinations of drugs such as cisplatin, doxorubicin, and cyclophosphamide may be given. The drugs are not curative, but some long-term remissions may result.[41]

DISORDERS IN MEN

Inflammatory disorders

Nonspecific pyogenic organisms as well as specific organisms such as the gonococci and tubercle bacilli may cause stubborn infections of the male reproductive system. Urethritis, prostatitis, epididymitis, and orchitis are the most common infections (Table 35-8). Infecting organisms may reach the genital tract by direct spread through the urethra, or they may be borne by blood or lymph.

PATHOPHYSIOLOGY

Prostatitis

Prostatitis is commonly associated with urethritis. It may be acute or chronic; recurrent episodes of acute prostatitis may cause fibrotic tissue to form. The fibrosis causes a hardening of the prostate gland, which may initially be confused with carcinoma. In the granulomatous form of prostatitis, the enlargement may take 3 to 6 months to resolve.

Epididymitis

Epididymitis is one of the most common inflammations of the male reproductive system. It is frequently a complication of gonorrhea or the first indication of tuberculosis of the genitourinary tract. It may follow instrumentation or prostatectomy.

Traumatic or chemical epididymitis is a sterile inflammation caused by direct injury or reflux of urine down the vas deferens. The chemical form is frequently seen in military recruits during basic training as a result of straining with a full bladder, which causes urinary reflux.

Bilateral epididymitis usually causes sterility. Untreated epididymitis leads rather rapidly to necrosis of testicular tissue and septicemia, which can be fatal.

Orchitis

When mumps are contracted after puberty, approximately 18% of the cases are complicated by orchitis (inflammation of the testes). Orchitis may also be caused by bacteria or it may follow septicemia. Usually both testes are involved, and if it is bilateral, sterility often results. Sterility does not occur with unilateral involvement.

PREVENTION

Because urethral infection spreads so readily to the genital organs, men should not be catheterized unless it is absolutely necessary. Because of the length and curvature of the male urethra, some trauma to the urethral mucosa is likely to accompany catheterization or the passage of instruments such as a cystoscope. The distal part of the urethra is not sterile, and trauma makes the urethra susceptible to attack from the bacteria present. Fluids should be given liberally after passage of instruments through the urethra.

Any postpubertal male who is exposed to mumps usually is given gamma globulin immediately unless he has already had the disease. If there is any doubt, globulin usually is given. Although gamma globulin may not prevent mumps, the disease is likely to be less severe, with less likelihood of orchitis developing and subsequent sterility.

DIAGNOSTIC TESTS

The site of the infection will influence treatment. The physician may obtain segmented bacteriologic localization cultures to make the determination. Four sterile culture tubes are used for collection. The patient must be well hydrated, have a full bladder, and be able to cooperate.

1. The first 5 to 10 ml of a voiding is collected.
2. After approximately 200 ml have been voided, a 5 to 10 ml midstream specimen is collected.
3. The patient is asked to stop voiding, and the prostate gland is massaged rectally until prostatic secretions are collected.
4. The next 5 to 10 ml of urine are collected, and the bladder is then emptied.
5. The specimens are refrigerated and taken to the laboratory for culture within 4 hours.

INTERVENTION

Assisting with comfort

Mild to moderate discomfort may be experienced by the man with an inflammation of the genital tract. *Heat* may be applied for prostatitis by means of sitz baths, but is *contraindicated for epididymitis or orchitis* because of possible destruction of sperm cells. *Cold* is applied in the latter cases for relief of swelling and discomfort. If an ice cap is used, it should be placed under the scrotum and should be removed for short intervals every hour to prevent ice burns. A plastic glove may be filled with crushed ice; with the palm of the glove placed under the scrotum, the fingers provide cold to the sides.

Swelling and discomfort of the scrotum can also be relieved by elevation of the scrotum, either on a folded towel or with adhesive strapping known as a Bellevue bridge (Fig. 35-12).

Counseling and teaching

The female nurse must be particularly sensitive to the reactions and feelings of male patients who have diseases

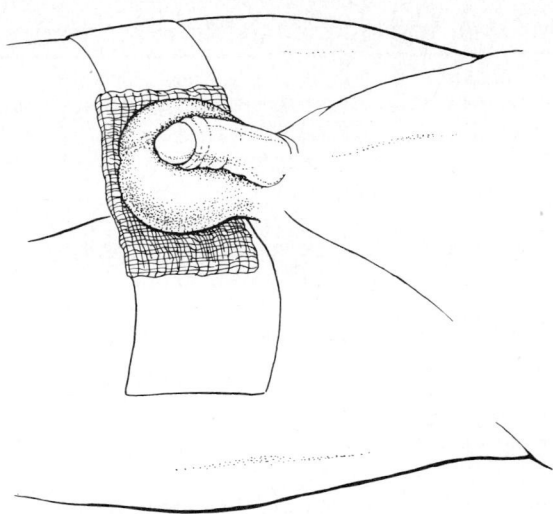

Fig. 35-12. Bellevue bridge.

Male reproductive disorders that may affect sexual functioning

Sterility	Impotence
Bilateral epididymitis	Radical prostatectomy
Severe bilateral orchitis	External radiation of pelvic floor
Torsion of testes	Total penectomy

---

of the reproductive system. The patient may feel more comfortable discussing his problems with a male nurse. However, it is incumbent on all nurses to provide a comfortable environment in which these patients can verbalize their concerns and feelings.

Patient comments with subtle sexual connotations may reveal concerns the patient has regarding his sexuality, and he often must be given permission to discuss these concerns. The patient may "try out" his sexuality on a female nurse. Rejections from her may be perceived by the patient as less threatening than rejection by a loved one.

Certain reproductive disorders in the male are accompanied by a high incidence of sexual dysfunction. The patient may be worrying needlessly about possible sterility (inability to conceive a child) or impotence (inability to have an erection). If the patient does have a condition in which the incidence of sexual dysfunction is high, the nurse needs to know the specific patient situation, because these dysfunctions do not always occur in each disorder (see box above).

Teaching includes the need to continue antibiotic therapy for the prescribed length of time (which may be lengthy in chronic prostatitis).

Table 35-9. Cancer of the male reproductive tract

Site	Incidence	Usual age (yr)	Signs and symptoms	Medical therapy
Testes	0.5%	18 to 35	Painless enlarged testis, gynecomastia	Surgery: orchiectomy; radiation, chemotherapy
Prostate gland	18%	>60	Urethral obstruction, low back pain, anemia	Surgery: radical resection of prostate gland, radiation, hormonal therapy
Penis	1%	50 to 70	Nodular growth on foreskin, fatigue, weight loss	Surgery: partial or total penectomy

---

Structural disorders of testes and scrotum

Hydrocele	Benign nontender collection of clear amber fluid within the outer covering of the testes, leading to scrotal swelling
Spermatocele	Benign nontender cystic mass attached to epididymis containing milky fluid and sperm
Varicocele	Dilation of spermatic vein, primarily on left side (due to longer left spermatic vein)
Torsion of spermatic cord	Kinking and twisting of spermatic cord and artery

---

Structural disorders

Structural disorders of the testes and scrotum may occur in some men (see box above).

Immediate medical attention should be sought for any swelling of the scrotum or the testes within it. Any acute swelling of sudden onset must be considered twisting (torsion) of the spermatic cord until proved otherwise.

Hydrocele is treated by aspiration of the fluid. Usually no therapy is needed for *spermatocele*, although aspiration or surgical excision may be done. *Varicocele* is often seen in men with low fertility. Ligation of the spermatic vein has been shown to improve semen quality.

Torsion of the spermatic cord interrupts the blood supply, leading to ischemia and severe pain that is not relieved and may be aggravated by scrotal elevation. Absence of pain indicates infarction and necrosis; gangrene may be a serious sequela. Unless the testis is gangrenous it is not excised, because it may still produce hormones even if spermatogenesis is destroyed. The testis is fixed surgically to the scrotal wall (orchiopexy). The contralateral testis is usually fixed prophylactically at the same time.

Body image distubances may include fears of castration, loss of masculinity, sterility, and impotence. The possibility of these fears being justified depends on the degree of insult to the testis and the functioning of the remaining testicle.

Tumors

Tumors of the male reproductive tract are usually malignant. The more common tumors involve the testes, prostate gland, and penis (Table 35-9).

PATHOPHYSIOLOGY

Cancer of the testes

Cancer of the testes is the second most common malignancy in men between the ages of 25 and 34 years and is the second most common cause of death from cancer in this age group. The causes are still unknown. Acquired causes being investigated are chemical carcinogens, trauma, and orchitis. Environmental factors are also being considered because there is a greater incidence of testicular cancer in rural than in urban areas. *Biopsy of the testis is contraindicated* because of the highly metastatic character of testicular carcinoma.

Cancer of the prostate gland

The prostate gland is the second most common site of cancer among men; it is responsible for 10% of all deaths from cancer in men. The cause is not known. It rarely occurs before the age of 50 years, incidence increases with age, and there is an increased familial risk. The younger the man the more lethal the disease. Although cancer may start anywhere in the prostate gland and may be multifocal in origin, it usually arises in the peripheral lobes, causing a palpable nodule, before progressing to an advanced, inoperable, and incurable stage. For this reason there is agreement that all men over age 50 years should have an annual rectal examination.

Cancer of the penis

The incidence of penile cancer is highly dependent on hygienic standards as well as cultural and religious practices. It almost never occurs in a male who was circumcised at birth. Circumcision after puberty does not decrease the risk of cancer when compared with the incidence among uncircumcised males. Circumcision removes the prepuce, or foreskin, which provides a haven for bacteria. The bacteria act on desquamated cells producing smegma, which is irritating to the tissue of the glans penis and the prepuce. This chronic irritation is considered to be carcinogenic. Trauma and sexually transmitted diseases are felt to be coincidental to penile cancer rather than causative.

PREVENTION

Regular testicular self-examination (TSE) is recommended to detect cancer of the testes in its early stages when it is most likely to be localized and most curable. *All young men should be taught testicular self-examination.* By performing TSE routinely, each man can get to know what is normal for him and more readily identify any lumps or abnormalities. Any swelling that is not normal

---

Testicular self-examination (TSE)

1. Perform TSE after a bath or shower when scrotum is warm and most relaxed
2. Grasp testis with both hands and palpate gently between thumb and fingers (Fig. 35-13):
   a. The testis should feel smooth, egg-shaped, and firm to touch
   b. The epididymis, found behind the testis, should feel like a soft tube

---

should be examined by a physician. Nine of ten testicular cancers are detected by the patient or his sexual partner.

DIAGNOSTIC TESTS

Diagnosis of cancer of the prostate gland is confirmed by *prostatic biopsy.* If the transrectal route is used, no bowel preparation is required. Vital signs are monitored for possible hemorrhage because of the high vascularity of the gland. Bleeding may be from the urethra or the bladder and may be internal. The patient is observed for fever, acute urinary retention, rectal bleeding, pain or swelling of the scrotum.

SURGERY

Surgery of the testicle

Orchiectomy consists of en bloc excision of the spermatic cord, the contents of the inguinal canal, and the testis with the tunica attached. The adjacent area is explored for metastases.

Preoperative care

In addition to usual preoperative care, psychologic preparation for surgery is important. The man will usually be concerned about the effects of castration. *Unilateral* removal of a testis will *not* demasculinize him or cause sterility. Prostheses are available to replace the removed testis.

Postoperative care

ACTIVITY. Bed rest may be instituted for 24 to 48 hours after extensive removal of tissue, but ambulation usually is begun within 12 hours after surgery. Leg exercises are important if bed rest is to be maintained. The scrotum is

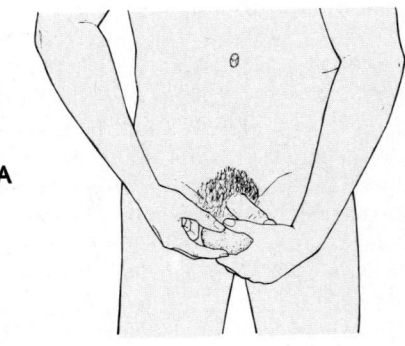

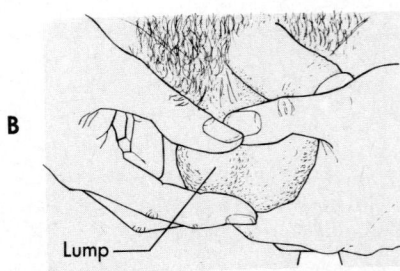

Fig. 35-13. Testicular self-examination. **A,** Grasp testis with both hands; palpate gently between thumb and fingers. **B,** Abnormal lumps or irregularities are reported to physician. (Adapted from Fred Hutchinson Cancer Research Center, Cancer Control Program: Self breast and testicular exam [grant no. 2 R18-Ca 16404], Seattle 1980, Cancer Control Program.)

elevated on a rolled towel, or the man may wear an athletic supporter while in bed. An athletic supporter or tight undershorts should be worn for support when the patient is ambulating.

POSTOPERATIVE COMPLICATIONS. The two major problems after scrotal surgery are edema and intrascrotal hemorrhage. *Edema* may be controlled by ice bags for the first 12 hours and a compression dressing for 3 to 5 days.[2] Ice is best applied by filling a rubber glove with crushed ice. Signs of hemorrhage or complaints of increasing discomfort are reported to the physician.

TEACHING

1. Avoid prolonged standing, which increases scrotal edema.
2. Wear athletic supporter or tight undershorts until healing is complete.
3. Take 20-minute tub baths three times per day for 1 week after discharge.
4. Avoid heavy lifting for 4 to 6 weeks.

Radical prostatic resection

In patients in whom a diagnosis of prostatic cancer is made before local extension of the cancer or distant metastasis, a radical resection of the prostate gland usually is curative. The entire prostate gland, including the capsule and the adjacent tissue, is removed. The remaining urethra is then anastomosed to the bladder neck.

Because the internal and external sphincters of the bladder lie in close approximation to the prostate gland, it is not unusual for the patient to have urinary incontinence after this type of surgery. The perineal approach is most used, but the procedure may be accomplished by the retropubic route (see Chapter 33).

Preoperative care

If the surgery is to be done via a perineal approach, the patient is given a bowel preparation (enemas, cathartics, antibiotics) and only clear fluids the day before surgery to prevent fecal contamination of the operative site. Postoperatively, when food is permitted, a low-residue diet may be given until wound healing is well advanced.

Radical prostatectomy results in physiologic sexual dysfunction from disruption of genital innervation. Ninety percent of patients lose emission, ejaculation, and erectile potency. Ten percent do have satisfactory erections, possibly because some nerves escape damage during surgery. Both the man and his sexual partner are made aware of this sexual dysfunction before surgery. The information is given by the physician, but the involved persons need opportunities to share their concerns about the proposed surgery.

Postoperative care

URINARY DRAINAGE. The patient returns from surgery with an indwelling urethral catheter. A large amount of urinary drainage on the dressing for a number of hours is not unusual. This can be managed by use of an ostomy bag around the dressing. Urinary drainage should decrease rapidly. There should not be the amount of bleeding that follows other prostatic surgery.

Because the catheter is not being used for hemostasis, the patient usually has little bladder spasm. The catheter is used both for urinary drainage and as a splint for the urethral anastomosis; therefore, care is taken that is does not become dislodged or blocked. The risk of blockage is greatest during the first hour. The catheter may be irrigated intermittently or continuously as ordered by the physician. The catheter is usually left in the bladder for 2 to 3 weeks.

FECAL CONTROL. Fecal incontinence may occur after surgery as a result of relaxation of the perineal musculature. Control of the rectal sphincter usually returns readily. Return of function can be facilitated by perineal exercises (Chapter 33) started within a day or two after surgery and continued after rectal sphincter control returns, to strengthen bladder sphincters (unless the bladder sphincters have been permanently damaged).

PSYCHOLOGIC SUPPORT. The patient with cancer of the prostate gland is often very depressed after radical prostatectomy because he suddenly realizes the implications of being impotent and perhaps permanently incontinent. At times the man may have difficulty talking to his sexual partner about his concerns and the effect of his impotence on their relationship. The nurse can encourage each person to share his and her feelings separately, then gently encourage and facilitate mutual sharing by the partners.

Penile surgery

If the cancer is confined to the prepuce, circumcision may be adequate. If the lesion is on the glans, partial penectomy or amputation of the penis is required. If the shaft of the penis is involved, total amputation may be necessary. The decision is based on the amount of penis remaining after excision with an adequate tumor-free margin. The remaining penis must be long enough for the patient to void standing, direct the stream, and not void on himself. If this is possible, the sexual function will probably be retained. If total amputation is required, a perineal urethrostomy is performed in which the urethra is redirected to an opening between the scrotum and the anus. With spread of the cancer to the scrotal contents, radical removal is required, either hemipelvectomy or hemicorporectomy.

Sexual counseling is indicated for the patient with a total penectomy. Some patients with a urethrostomy have experienced orgasm and ejaculation following stimulation of the perineal, scrotal, and testicular regions.

RADIATION

Although the normal testis is shielded during external radiation of an involved testis, it does receive radiation scattered from the abdomen and thighs. A period of 70 days is required to determine whether spermatogenesis has been affected. Spermatogenesis may be decreased for 7 months to 5 years of more. Although genetic defects are possible after irradiation, there is currently no evidence to cause serious concern. Genetic counseling may be helpful for those couples desiring children.

Sexually transmitted diseases

Type of organisms	Disease
Bacteria	Gonorrhea, chancroid, granuloma inguinale, *Gardnerella vaginalis*
Spirochete	Syphilis
Chlamydia	Nongonococcal urethritis, epididymitis, cervicitis, PID, lymphogranuloma venereum
Virus	Herpes genitalis, hepatitis B, cytomegalovirus, AIDS, genital warts
Protozoa	Trichomoniasis
Yeast	Candidiasis
Parasites	Pediculosis pubis, scabies

Radiation for prostatic cancer may be delivered by external beam or by implant. The testes are shielded during external radiation. Erectile dysfunction may occur.

Iodine 125 retropubic prostatic implantation may be used initially or after failure of external radiation therapy. Complications of iodine 125 implantation include blood loss from multiple needle punctures during implantation, deep vein thrombosis, pulmonary emboli, hematomas, and abscesses. Potency is retained. Risk of incontinence and serious rectal complications such as rectourethral fistulas increases with the size of the gland and the intensity of the implant seed.

HORMONE THERAPY

Estrogen therapy may be used for advanced prostatic cancer when metastasis has occured, especially to the bone. Bilateral orchiectomy to eliminate androgen may be combined with estrogen therapy. The estrogen given is usually stilbestrol. In males, estrogen frequently causes gynecomastia (enlargement of the breasts), loss of libido, arrest of spermatogenesis, and testicular atrophy.

Estrogen helps to decrease pain and reduce tumor size. The use of hormone therapy provides a longer symptom-free period but makes palliation more difficult when symptoms recur. If endocrine is delayed, symptoms recur earlier but longer palliation is possible.

SEXUALLY TRANSMITTED DISEASES

Sexually transmitted disease (STD) is *usually* or *can be* transmitted from one person to another with heterosexual or homosexual intercourse or intimate contact with the genitalia, mouth, or rectum. The former term *venereal disease* has been changed to encompass the many disorders that may be transmitted by sexual contact. Many of these disorders are discussed elsewhere in this text.

Epidemiology

Many of the newly recognized STDs have become epidemic or hyperendemic as a consequence of changing sexual behavior patterns. Not only has the incidence of many STDs increased, but for agents with multiple modes of transmission (for example, hepatitis B virus, enteric pathogens), the proportion of infections that are transmitted sexually has also increased.

All states require that each case of syphilis and gonorrhea be reported to the state or local health officer. Herpes genitalis, trichomoniasis, and candidiasis are not reportable in any state. The true incidence of STDs is therefore not known because of variable reporting requirements and also because many cases are not reported by clinicians.

Three major changes occurring in recent years are often given as reasons for the trends of reported cases of STDs. The first change is the use of antibiotics and the changes in antibiotic susceptibility of pathogenic organisms. The widespread, perhaps indiscriminate, use of penicillin and other antibiotics between the late 1940s and early 1950s parallels the decline in both syphilis and gonorrhea during that period (Fig. 35-14). Some of the organisms developed a greater resistance to antibiotics over time. There is no firm evidence to indicate a decrease in effectiveness of penicillin against syphilis, but the gonococcus tends to develop resistance to antibiotics.

A second explanation of the rise in incidence of STDs is that they are more likely to occur if the social system is permissive. During times of war and other catastrophes it is easier for agencies to control interpersonal behavior, whereas in times of peace and absence of national crisis, civil liberties tend to flourish. The incidence curve of syphilis and gonorrhea after World War II seems to support this thesis.

The third explanation centers around permissive sexual behavior. Concern has been particularly expressed about the prevalence of gonorrhea among adolescents who are considered to be promiscuous. In fact, rates for gonorrhea show young adults of 15 to 29 years of age to be at greatest risk for acquiring gonorrhea.

The above discussion makes an assumption of sexual promiscuity, and in doing so requires acknowledgement of advances in contraceptive technology, especially "the pill." The condom was the main method of contraception before the advent of antibiotics and oral contraceptives.

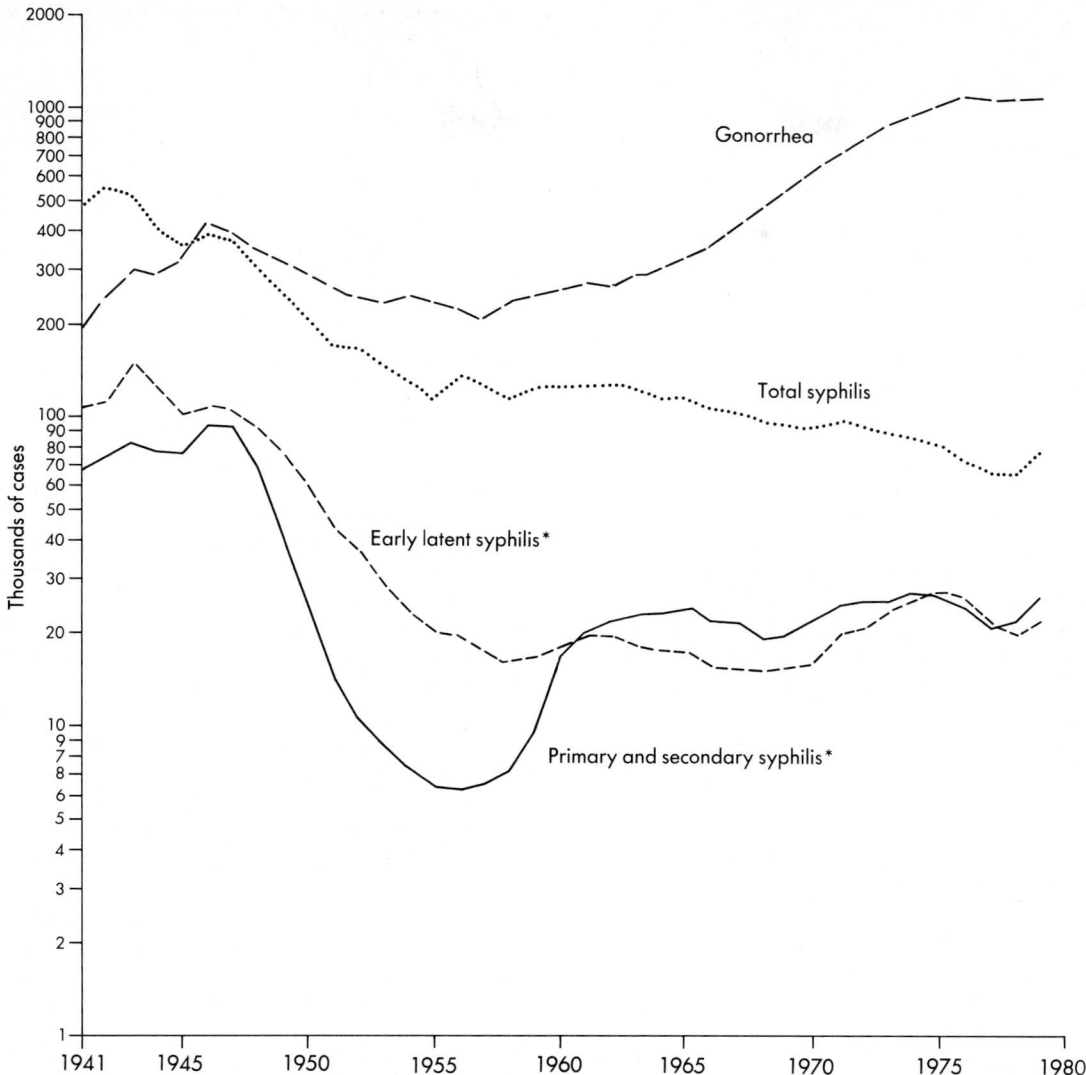

Fig. 35-14. Reported cases (by diagnosis) of syphilis and gonorrhea in the United States, 1941 to 1979. Asterisks indicate that incidence for 1941 to 1946 is for fiscal year (12-month period ending June 30). Figures for 1947 to 1979 are for calendar year.

The use of the condom may have discouraged spread of the STDs by providing a mechanical barrier to the organisms. With the advent of antibiotics and the pill, people began to lose fear of untreated STD and pregnancy, and thus sexual promiscuity increased significantly, leading to increased exposure to infection. Currently it is not unusual for the same person to have two or more organisms causing infection simultaneously.

Sexual transmission

The STDs are contagious diseases spread almost exclusively by contact during sexual intercourse, that is, when mucous membrane surfaces come in contact during geni-

tal, oral, or anal sexual activity. Because the causative organisms survive only very briefly outside a warm, moist environment, there is almost no way to contract STDs from toilet seats, towels, and bed linens.

Although STDs are not usually transmitted in public restrooms, conditions caused by fungi, bacteria, and lice can be transmitted from water in unclean toilet bowls. Women using a conventional toilet expose the vaginal and anal area to pathogens that can be introduced by the backsplash of contaminated toilet water.

There are some notable exceptions to sexual transmission. During pregnancy the fetus may become infected in utero by placental transmission, and the infant may acquire congenital syphilis or be stillborn. Infants of mothers with gonorrhea may contact infections of the eyes (ophthalmia neonatorum) during birth, and unless treated this can lead to permanent blindness.

Prevention and control

Prevention and control measures for STDs include the three levels of prevention. *Primary prevention* is directed at preventing the disease and includes the following:

1. Educating uninfected persons so that they can avoid contact with an infected person
2. Identifying and treating exposed persons who are asymptomatic
3. Interviewing patients with infection for identification of contacts
4. Examining and providing preventive treatment of contacts
5. Participating in educational programs for the public
6. Participating in programs of control

The goal of these efforts include eradication of the reservoir of disease in the population. *Secondary prevention* is directed toward prevention of complications (such as PID in the female with gonorrhea). *Tertiary prevention* focuses on decreasing the effects of complications such as sterility.

EDUCATION

Education of uninfected persons can be effected through schools and community groups frequented by adolescents and young adults. Because the highest incidence of STD occurs between ages 15 and 29 years, this is the population that needs information on the consequences of STD and how the diseases can be avoided. Many films are available from local and state health departments.

A clinic may be the person's first contact with the health care system. The patient is often young, fearful of pain, and unaccustomed to surroundings of a clinic. Young patients especially fear that their families and friends may learn they have an STD. Minors need to know that they can probably obtain treatment without parental consent. Presently more states permit physicians to treat STD in minors without obtaining parental consent.

For single persons, contracting an STD and securing help means they must admit to having sexual relations, and some of them may feel guilty about their sexual activity. Persons with an STD have not only a physical but a social, emotional, and perhaps economic problem as well. They need constructive and comprehensive help.

Teaching about treatment

Many lay persons know the treatment for syphilis and gonorrhea is penicillin, but they may not be fully informed about this and other aspects of treatment. Because some of the diseases respond to penicillin or other antibiotics, many people believe that all general infections can be cured simply, and this is not so. Some people be-

lieve they acquire an immunity after one infection, which is also a myth.

Persons receiving an antibiotic or other medication for STDs must be informed of the action of the drug, its duration of effectiveness, side effects, chances of cure, and the need for follow-up. They need to be advised that treatment failures do occur and that reinfection rates are high. Return visits should be encouraged whenever possible, because adequacy of treatment of all of the STDs is evaluated best by laboratory analysis for the specific organism.

Self-care

Effective self-care is based on knowledge about the condition and effect on others as well as self. Teaching may include the following major points:

1. Method of transmission
2. Possibility of reinfection
3. Possibility of infection of sexual partner(s)
4. Need for sexual partner to be checked for signs of infection, know what signs to look for, and have a culture done for asymptomatic infection
5. Need to abstain from intercourse, if possible; if not, the man should wear a condom

Self-care also includes information regarding care of self, which may include the following:

1. Frequent hand washing and bathing are indicated (many organisms are destroyed by soap and water)
2. Douching is contraindicated for women unless prescribed for the purpose of applying heat or medication
3. Cotton underwear that permits air circulation and does not trap moisture is advised
4. No unprescribed lotions, creams, or ointments should be applied to the lesions

CONTACT INVESTIGATION

Interviewing the patient for contacts is done at the time of the initial visit in the event that the patient does not return for follow-up. This interview is probably best done after the patient is examined, the type of infection is determined, and the treatment is prescribed. If assessment is accompanied by information giving, the patient should be better informed about STDs. It is hoped that the patient will be less concerned about self and more willing and able to give information about sexual contacts so that these persons may also obtain treatment if asymptomatic and thus prevent spread to others.

Interviewing for contacts involves two aspects. The patient is first asked to name sexual contacts. Second, the patient is interviewed for "cluster suspects," friends or acquaintances who may have been exposed to the same contacts or who have symptoms of a STD. Because one focus of STD control is on increasing self-referrals, the patient is asked to advise known contacts and cluster suspects to present themselves for examination and preventive treatment. Confidentiality is stressed.

There is reason to believe that patients do not name all

heir contacts at the time of the first interview and that another interview after the patient has reflected will usually result in additional names of contacts. Because of the understandable reluctance of many people to name their sexual contacts, in many areas the patient is given the responsibility of informing the contacts and advising them of their need for treatment. (The contacts are not named, but instead cards that permit both examination and treatment without identification are given to the contact by the patient.) The local health departments cooperate in locating, culturing, and treating these contacts as necessary.

If the sexual contacts do not have symptoms of infection at the time of the first examination, treatment is instituted to abort infection. Giving preventive treatment to contacts who have no clinical evidence of infection has gained popularity and acceptance in the United States, and indications are present that this same approach is being used more often in management of patients with the "minor" STDs.

Gonorrhea

Gonorrhea, often referred to as "GC" or "the clap" by lay people, is caused by *Neisseria gonorrhoeae*. It is the most commonly reported communicable disease in the United States. Gonorrhea is of great concern because of its epidemic rise, high reinfection rate, and seriousness of residual effects. The signs and symptoms and medical therapy for gonorrhea are outlined in Table 35-10.

DIAGNOSTIC TESTS

Gonorrheal infection may be suspected on the basis of history, symptoms, and clinical evidence obtained by physical examination. However, identification of the organism is necessary to confirm the diagnosis and to rule out other problems. In men the diagnosis is confirmed by gram-stained smear of the discharge from the penis. Culture of the discharge from the penis is usually reserved for those whose smears are negative in the presence of strong clinical evidence.

Gram-stained cervical smears are inadequate for diagnosing gonorrhea in women. These smears are negative in about 50% of women with gonorrhea and are falsely positive in some cases. Therefore cultures from the cervix, urethra, throat, and anus are usually taken.

GONORRHEA IN MEN

Because of the distress produced by symptoms, men usually present themselves for examination early in the disease. As a result, diagnosis is made and treatment instituted early, and complications and residual effects of gonorrhea are uncommon among men. Sterility from orchitis or epididymitis can occur as a residual effect, but this is rare.

The incidence of asymptomatic gonorrhea in men is believed to be low. However, there is an increasing awareness of the importance of asymptomatic infection in the transmission of gonorrhea.

GONORRHEA IN WOMEN

Women rarely have early distressing symptoms of gonorrhea. Early signs of slight discharge and a vague feeling of pelvic fullness are often disregarded by the woman. Medical assistance is generally sought if discomfort is present, such as occurs with bartholinitis.

Gonorrhea in women most often begins as asymptomatic cervicitis, and the infection can be present for extended periods without causing noticeable signs. Hence there are a high number of infected, asymptomatic women. These women do not receive treatment unless

Table 35-10. Selected sexually transmitted diseases

Disease	Incubation period	Signs and symptoms	Medical therapy
Gonorrhea	Men: 3 to 30 days Women: 3 days to an indefinite period	Men: purulent urethral discharge, dysuria, epididymitis, prostatitis Women: asymptomatic in early stages; cervicitis with purulent discharge, bartholinitis, salpingitis	Aqueous procaine penicillin G (IM) and probenecid (PO); or ampicillin and probenecid(PO)
Syphilis	3 weeks (9 days to 3 months)	Positive serologic tests, chancre in stage I	Penicillin
Herpes genitalis	3 to 14 days	Vesicles that rupture and form ulcerations, pain, inguinal lymph node enlargement, dysuria, flulike symptoms	Symptomatic; topical acyclovir
Genital warts	1 to 6 months	Horny papules on vulva, vagina, cervix, perineum, anal canal, urethra, glans penis	Weekly applications of podophyllum resin in tincture of benzoin; electrocautery

gonorrhea is diagnosed through screening or unless the woman is identified by the sexual partner and presents herself for treatment.

Frequently complications are the first indicators of gonorrhea in women. Salpingitis (PID) is the most common complication. During the course of treatment for salpingitis, many women are surgically sterilized. In cases of untreated gonorrhea, the residual effects of chronic pelvic inflammatory disease, infertility, and ectopic pregnancy are well known.

Other complications of untreated gonorrhea in both men and women include dermatitis, myocarditis, meningitis, and arthritis. The incidence of these complications is higher among women because of the prolonged period of infection with symptoms.

THERAPY FOR GONORRHEA

Therapy for gonorrhea presents a greater problem than for syphilis because the gonococcus tends to develop resistance to antibiotics. It also is believed that inadequate therapy is common. Several drug regimens are in use

with emphasis on single-dose treatment to avoid problems in follow-up and patient cooperation. Large dosages are used for the single-dose treatment.

Before initiating treatment with penicillin, it is important to screen for a history of previous reaction to penicillin. Symptom of life-threatening reactions such as anaphylaxis most often occur within 30 minutes after injection, and although such reactions are rare, it may be advisable to detain patients for this period of time after parenteral administration of penicillin.

In addition, some individuals may experience a procaine reaction, indicated by disorientation, agitation, a "high" feeling, hallucination, or combativeness. This reaction usually begins 5 minutes after the injection and resolves within 20 to 30 minutes. Monitoring the blood pressure and attempting to calm the individual are important.

Syphilis

Syphilis is caused by the spirochete *Treponema pallidum*, which gains entry to the body through either the

Table 35-11. Stage of syphillis

	Primary	Secondary	Latent	Late
Duration	2 to 8 wk	Appears 2 to 4 wk after chancre appears; extends over 2 to 4 yr	5 to 20 yr	Terminal if not treated
Clinical signs	Hard sore or pimple on vulva or penis that breaks and forms painless, draining chancre; may be a single chancre or groups of more than one; may be present also on lips, tongue, hands, rectum, or nipples; chancre heals, leaving almost invisible scar	Depends on site; low-grade fever, headache, anorexia, weight loss, anemia, sore throat, hoarseness, reddened and sore eyes, jaundice with or without hepatitis, aching of joints, muscles, long bones; sores on body or generalized fine rash; condylomata lata (venereal warts) on rectum or genitalia	No clinical signs	Tumorlike masses, gumma on any area of body; damage to heart valves and blood vessels; meningitis, paralysis, lack of coordination, paresis, insomnia, confusion, delusions, impaired judgment, slurred speech
Communicability	Exudates from lesions and chancre highly contagious	Exudates from lesions highly contagious; blood contains organisms	Contagious for about 2 yr; not contagious to others after that; blood contains organisms; may be transmitted placentally	Noncontagious; spinal fluid may contain organisms

mucous membrane or skin during intercourse. The organism is readily destroyed by physical and chemical agents including heat, drying, and mild disinfectants such as soap and water.

Although the total number of cases of syphilis has decreased steadily since about 1963 (Fig. 35-14), the number of reported cases of primary and secondary syphilis has increased since 1975. The highest incidence of syphilis is found among persons 20 to 24 years old. Many cases of syphilis, however, are unreported. Intensive screening of pregnant women and increased prenatal care have resulted in dramatic decreases in the incidence of congenital syphilis. It is felt that of all the methods by which syphilis can be acquired, congenital syphilis is the most preventable, yet cases continue to be reported.

If untreated, syphilis progresses through four identifiable stages: primary, secondary, latent, and late (Table 35-11). Latent and late syphilis are often classified as tertiary syphilis. Note the major complications listed among the clinical signs of late syphilis.

DIAGNOSTIC TESTS

Serologic testing is used for detecting syphilis. Two identifiable antibodies appear in the blood from 1 to 4 months after syphilis is contracted. The tests in common use require a sample of venous blood. Two types of tests, treponemal and nontreponemal, are presently available. The tests differ in the type of antibody measured and in the antigen used to detect antibodies.

The nontreponemal tests, commonly called serologic tests for syphilis (STS), measure an antibody-like substance called reagin. The Veneral Disease Research Laboratory (VDRL) test is the most frequently used serologic test for syphilis and is the test used most often for routine premarital and prenatal screening.

A reactive STS is confirmed by alternate serologic tests. For this purpose, the fluorescent treponemal antibody-absorption (FTA-ABS) test is most often used, because it is the most sensitive and specific test for syphilis available.

False negative test results may occur because antibodies are not present in the serum of the infected person until the organism gains entry into the circulation. Negative syphilis test results may also occur when an individual is taking antibiotics.

A false positive test result may occur with an STS test from hypersensitivity reactions, acute bacterial or viral infection, recent vaccination, or chronic systemic illness such as tuberculosis, collagen disease, or malaria. Follow-up testing with FTA-ABS is done when a positive STS result is obtained. Syphilis is therefore not diagnosed on the basis of the initial testing.

Once antibodies are present they do not completely disappear from the serum. Although treated and noninfected, the person may have a positive serology test result for an indefinite period. If successful therapy is given before antibodies develop, these tests results may never be positive unless the person again becomes infected and develops antibodies. Therefore serologic tests in use today do not always indicate an active syphilitic infection and only detect the presence of antibodies.

A presumptive diagnosis is made on the basis of suspect lesions, positive serologic test results, known exposure to infection, and involvement of regional lymph nodes.

THERAPY FOR SYPHILIS

Syphilis can be successfully treated at any stage of the disease, although treatment may have to be prolonged in latent and late syphilis. Although syphilis can be cured in late stages, the damage to the body is much less easily managed.

Because penicillin continues to be effective in the treatment of syphilis, it remains the drug of choice. All types of penicillin are effective, but penicillin G benzathine is preferred because it is long acting and can be given in a limited number of injections. Contacts are also given penicillin.

Herpes genitalis

Herpes genitalis (genital herpes) is caused by infection with *Herpesvirus hominis* type 2 (HVH-2). Herpes genitalis is the most important STD of the past decade. Its chronicity, frequent recurrences, and difficult treatment and prevention distinguish it from other STDs. Its peak incidence parallels the young age groups affected by other STDs.

Herpes genitalis is a lifelong disease once acquired and carries with it not only intense and recurrent discomfort but also anxieties about future childbearing, malignancy, and sexual and marital functioning. In early pregnancy women infected with herpes have an increased chance of miscarriage. Because genital herpetic lesions endanger the fetus during delivery, cesarean delivery is often required. Genital herpes has also been associated with cervical cancer. It is now generally accepted that HVH-2 is spread by sexual contact.

Following primary herpes, the virus persists in a latent or unrecognized form in most patients. It is believed that latent infections are localized in the ganglia of sensory nerves to the genitalia. When the host factors favor it, the latent infection becomes clinically apparent as recurrent herpes. Factors known to predispose to recurrent infection include fever, emotional upsets, premenstrual states, and overexposure to heat.

Unfortunately, about 75% of all patients have at least one recurrence. Fortunately, recurrent infections are usually milder and of shorter duration than primary infections and usually produce local rather than systemic reaction. The patient experiencing a recurrent infection often has prodromal signs of paresthesia and burning at the site where the lesion will erupt.

Signs and symptoms of genital herpes are listed in Table 35-10. Diagnosis is made by isolation of the virus from specimens obtained from lesions. Pap smears or fluid from vesicles collected in transport medium demonstrates cellular characteristics of viruses.

There is no known cure for genital herpes; therefore, treatment is symptomatic. The lesions may be washed with Burow's solution, hydrogen peroxide, or soap and water, then dried well. A hair dryer may facilitate drying. The skin is then dusted with cornstarch.

REFERENCES AND SELECTED READINGS*

1. American Cancer Society: 1984 cancer facts and figures, New York, 1984, The Society.
2. American College of Surgeons, Committee on Pre and Postoperative Care: Manual of preoperative and postoperative care, ed. 3, Philadelphia, 1983, W.B. Saunders Co.
3. Austin, J.M. Jr., Cain, M.G., Hicks, J., and Wolf, S.: The Gravelee method: an alternative to the pap smear? Am. J. Nurs. **83**:1058, 1983.
4. Barber, H.: Manual of gynecologic oncology, Philadelphia, 1980, J.B. Lippincott Co.
5. Berkus, M., and Daly, J.: Cone biopsy: an outpatient procedure, Am. J. Obstet, Gynecol. **137**:953-958, 1980.
6. *Brown, L.: Toxic shock syndrome, M.C.N. **6**:57-59, 1981.
7. *Brown, M.A.: Primary dysmenorrhea, Nurs. Clin. North Am. **17**(1):145-153, 1982.
8. Cosper, B., Fuller, S., and Robinson, G.: Characteristics of posthospitalization recovery following hysterectomy, J.O.G.N. Nurs. **7**:7-11, 1981.
9. Crosson, K.: A patient teaching aid for the pelvic exenteration patient, Oncol. Nurs. Forum **8**:53-56, 1981.
10. Darrow, W.W.: Approaches to the problem of venereal disease prevention, Prev. Med. **5**:165-175, 1976.
11. Ebersole, P., and Hess, R.: Toward healthy aging, St. Louis, 1981, The C.V. Mosby Co.
12. *Edlund, B.J.: The needs of women with gynecologic malignancies, Nurs. Clin. North Am. **17**(1):155-163, 1982.
13. Fischbach, F.: A manual of laboratory diagnostic tests, Philadelphia, 1980, J.B. Lippincott Co.
14. *Fogel, C.I., and Woods N.F.: Health care of women: a nursing perspective, St. Louis, 1981, The C.V. Mosby Co.
15. Fred Hutchinson Cancer Research Center, Cancer Control Program: Self breast and testicular exam (grant no. 2 R18 CA 16404), Seattle, 1980, Cancer Control Program.
16. Gardner, H.: Herpes genitalis: our most important venereal disease, Am. J. Obstet. Gynecol. **135**:553-554, 1979.
17. *Galt, P.L.: Taking your part in the fight against testicular cancer, Nurs. 81 **11**(5):45-50, 1981.
18. *Googe, M.C.S.: The inflatable penile prosthesis: new developments, Am. J. Nurs. **83**:1044-1047, 1983.
19. Herbert, P., et al.: Colposcopy: what is it? J.O.G.N. Nurs. **5**:29-33, 1976.
20. *Hogan, R.: Human sexuality: a nursing perspective, New York, 1980, Appleton-Century-Crofts.
21. Krupp, M.A., and Chatton, M.J.: Current medical diagnosis and treatment 1983, Los Altos, Calif., 1983, Lange Medical Publications.
22. Kuczynski, H.: Pros and cons of douching: the nurse's role in counseling, J.O.G.N. Nurs. **9**:90-93 1980.
23. Lovesky, J.: Menstruation: alternatives to pharmacologic therapy for menstrual distress, J. Nurse Midwife **23**:34-44, 1978.
24. *Lynch, J.M.: Helping patients through the recurring nightmare of herpes, Nurs. 82 **12**(10):52-57, 1982
25. Lytle, N.: Nursing of women in the age of liberation, Dubuque, Ia. 1977, William C. Brown Co., Publishers.
26. Martin, L.: Health care of women, Philadelphia, 1978, J.B. Lippincott Co.
27. *Menning, B.E.: The psychosocial impact of infertility, Nurs. Clin. North Am.**17**(1):155-163, 1982.
28. Miles, P.: Sexually transmissible diseases: fourteen sexually transmissible diseases currently recognized by the Centers for Disease Control, Atlanta, Georgia, J.E.N. **6**(3):99-106, 1980.
29. *Mims, F., and Swenson, M.: Sexuality: a nursing perspective, New York, 1980, McGraw-Hill Book Co.
30. Murray, R., Huelskoetter, M.M., and O'Driscoll, D.: The nursing process in later maturity, Englewood Cliffs, N.J., 1980, Prentice-Hall, Inc.
31. Novak, E.R., Jones, G.S., and Jones, H.W., Jr.: Novak's textbook of gynecology, ed. 9, Baltimore, 1975, The Williams & Wilkins Co.
32. Oill, P.: Herpesvirus type 2 infection of the genital tract, J.E.N. **6**(3):13-16, 1980.
33. Patient information: what you should know about infertility, Contemp. Obstet. Gynecol. **15**:101-105, 1980.
34. Pettyjohn, R.: Health care of the gay individual, Nurs. Forum **18**:366-393, 1979.
35. Renaer, M., et al.: Psychological aspects of chronic pelvic pain in women, Am. J. Obstet. Gynecol. **134**:75-80, 1979.
36. Sandelowski, M.: Women, health and choice, Englewood Cliffs, N.J., 1981, Prentice-Hall, Inc.
37. Seibel, M., Freeman, M., and Graves, W.: Carcinoma of the cervix and sexual function, Obstet. Gynecol. **55**:484-487, 1980.
38. Speroff, L., Glass, R.H., and Kase, N.: Clinical gynecologic endocrinology and infertility, ed. 2, Baltimore, 1978, The Williams & Wilkins Co.
39. *Tyson, M.D.: Let's talk about menopause, Nurs. 78 **8**(8):34-36, 1978.
40. U.S. Department of Health and Human Services, Public Health Service: STD fact sheet edition 35, HHS pub. No. (CDC) 81-8195, Atlanta, 1981, Centers for Disease Control.
41. Way, L.W.: Current surgical diagnosis and treatment, ed 6, Los Altos, Calif., 1983, Lange Medical Publications.
42. Woods, N.F.: Human sexuality in health and illness, ed. 2, St. Louis, 1979, The C.V. Mosby Co.
43. Yarborough, B.: Teaching plan for the patient undergoing total pelvic exenteration, Oncol. Nurs. Forum **8**:36-40, 1981.

*References preceded by an asterick are particularly well suited for student reading.

36

The Patient with Problems of the Breast

BARBARA C. LONG

STUDY QUESTIONS

- Review the anatomy of the breast and adjacent structures.

- What are some of the psychologic reactions to be expected when a patient faces the loss of a breast?

- How do you think you might feel if you discovered a lump in your breast?

- Review the normal range of motion of the shoulder. Make a list of daily activities that involve full use of this joint.

- Outline how you would teach self-examination of the breast to one woman or to a group of women.

- Check some of the clothing stores in your community for those selling breast prostheses. Compare types and prices of available prostheses.

The breasts are associated functionally with the reproductive system as an organ for milk production in the postpartum woman. The female sex hormones influence the development of the breasts and the production of milk.

The breasts are also associated with feelings of sexuality and are an integral component of sexual behavior. The development of the breasts in the female adolescent indicates to her the approach of womanhood and emphasizes her femininity. The breast, especially the nipples, which are erectile tissue, are erogenous areas in sexual activity. The advertising media emphasize the desirability of the female breast; femininity is typified by a fashion model's breasts, whereas masculinity is typified by the flat, expansive chest of the lifeguard. Diseases of the breast therefore evoke varied feelings and cause fears and concerns that influence the practice of breast self-examination or the seeking of diagnostic and therapeutic care.

The most common diseases of the breast are dysplasia (fibrocystic disease), fibroadenoma, cancer, and infections. Although these diseases occur primarily in women, *they can also occur in men*. Cancer requires the most extensive nursing care and is discussed in greater detail than the other diseases.

PREVENTION AND HEALTH EDUCATION

Avoidance of common breast problems

PREMENSTRUAL BREAST DISCOMFORT

Tenderness, discomfort, and swelling of the breasts before menstruation are normal functional changes in the breasts that respond to monthly cyclical changes in estrogen and progesterone. Water retention contributes to the swelling. Women who experience some of these problems can be taught to reduce dietary salt during the immediate premenstrual period. Increased physical activity during this time will improve cardiovascular dynamics and help reduce the tight, puffy feeling.

BREAST DISCOMFORT DURING PHYSICAL ACTIVITY

Bras provide support for the breast and help to prevent sagging and pulling on the underlying muscle. All but small-breasted women may find participating in physical activity uncomfortable unless a bra is worn. A "jogbra," which does not contain metal clips or fasteners and which has seams on the outside of the fabric away from the skin, may provide greater comfort for physical activity.

Early detection of malignancy
EXAMINATIONS OF THE BREAST

Mortality from breast cancer can be prevented in many instances through early diagnosis and treatment. The American Cancer Society recommendations for examinations of the breast include the following:
1. Monthly breast self-examination by *all* women over 20 years of age
2. Women 20 to 40
   a. Examination by a physician every 3 years
   b. One baseline breast x-ray examination between ages 35 and 40
3. Women 40 and over
   a. Examination by a physician every year
   b. Yearly breast x-ray examination after 50

Studies have shown that the groups of women who are least likely to have regular breast examinations by a physician are elderly, poorly educated, low-income, and black women. Some of the reasons are as follows:

Lack of knowledge
Low priority set on preventive measures
Lack of income
Fear of finding a tumor
Concern over possibility of breast removal
Fear of death
Possible life changes if breast cancer is found
Embarrassment
Examination considered too trivial for busy physician

Most breast cancers (about 90%) are discovered by self-examination. Breast cancer is usually curable when discovered early and treated immediately. All women, beginning at high school age, should know how to carry out breast self-examination.

BREAST SELF-EXAMINATION (BSE)

Nurses working in the hospital or community settings have the responsibility of teaching women how to examine their breasts and of explaining why it is necessary.

Guidelines for breast self-examination

1. Perform BSE regularly each month
   a. Premenopausal women: shortly after conclusion of the menstrual period
   b. Postmenopausal women: at a set time each month (such as the first day of the month)
2. Use a systematic approach (*one* of the three listed here
   a. Palpate in concentric circles beginning at outer rim of breast tissue and move toward nipple
   b. Divide breast into quadrants and examine area in each quadrant from outer perimeter toward nipple
   c. Palpate inner half then outer half of breast
3. Examine the entire breast tissue, including the tail (Fig. 36-1) and the nipple
4. Carry out examination in both the horizontal and vertical body positions (Fig. 36-2)
5. Use the flat parts of the fingers for palpation.

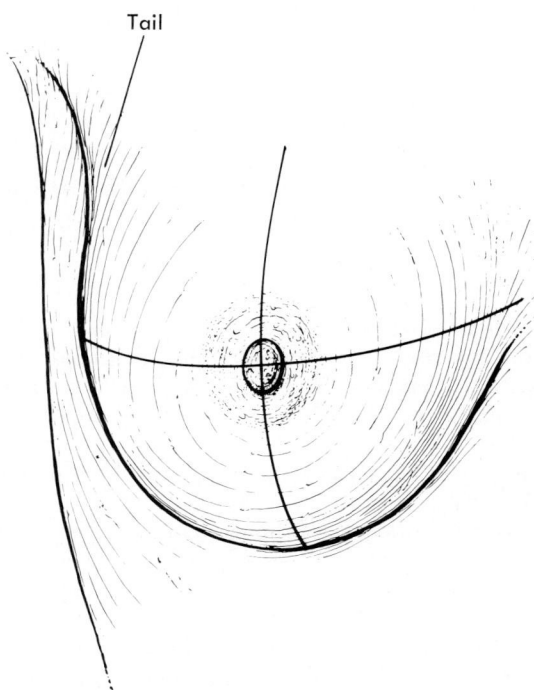

Fig. 36-1. Breast mass includes "tail" that extends from upper, outer quadrant toward axilla. (From Malasanos, L. et. al.: Health assessment, ed. 2, St. Louis, 1981, The C.V. Mosby Co.)

Patients can be asked during the admission history if they practice BSE, and necessary instructions can be given when feasible.

When working with groups of women, arrangements can be made with the American Cancer Society or the local health department for showing movies developed for the general public describing the traditional method of self-examination. Models of breasts are available for women to practice palpation of lumps.

Some women have engorgement of the breast premenstrually, and the breasts normally may have a lumpy consistency at this time. The condition usually disappears a few days after the onset of menstruation. Guidelines for BSE are listed in box on p. 1086.

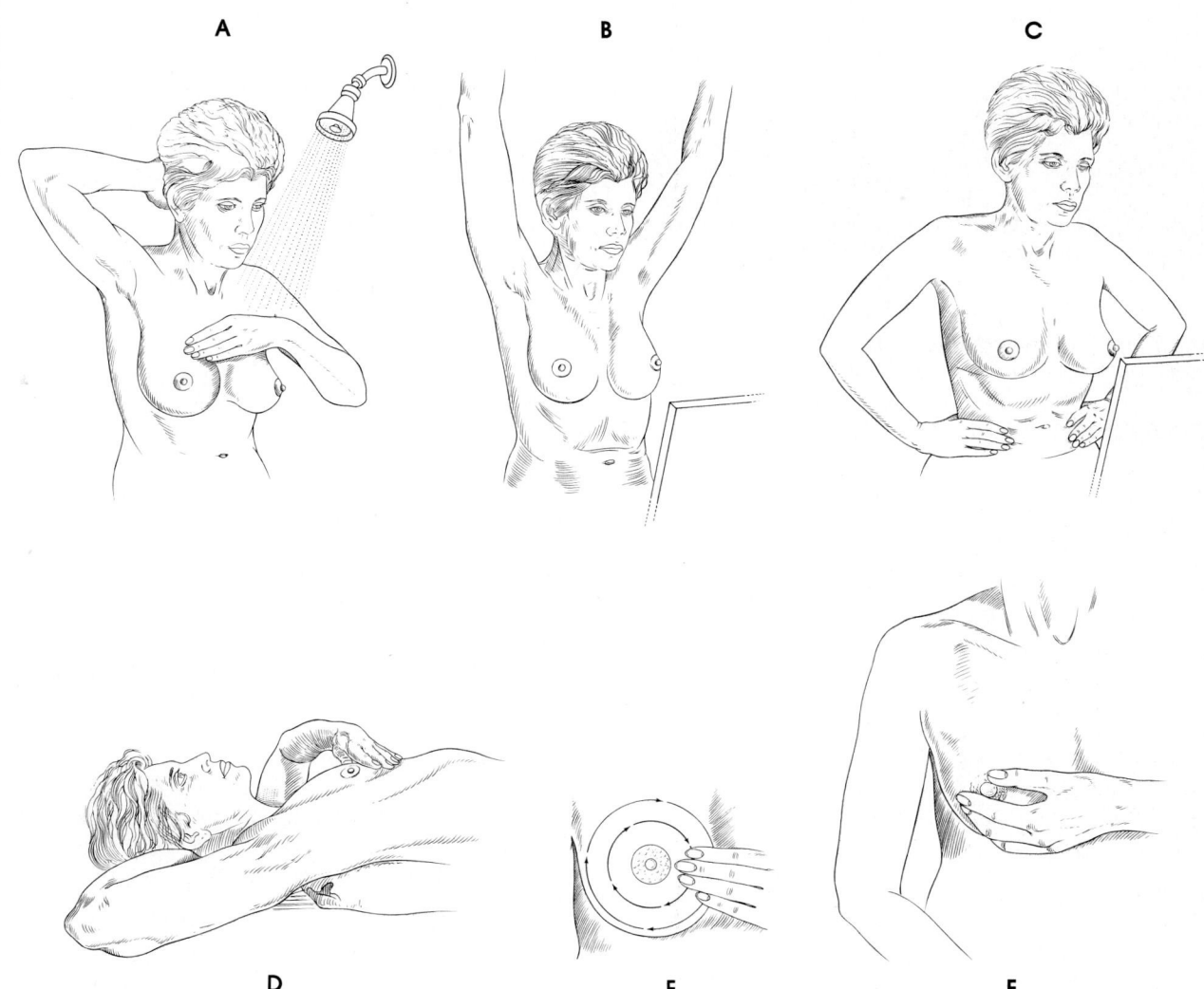

Fig. 36-2. Breast self-examination. **A,** Examine breasts during bath or shower since flat fingers guide easier over wet skin. Use right hand to examine left breast and vice versa. **B,** Sit or stand before a mirror. Inspect breasts with hands at sides then raised overhead. Look for changes in contour or dimpling of skin. **C,** Place hands on hips and press down firmly to flex chest muscles. **D,** Lie down with one hand under head and pillow or folded towel under that scapula. **E,** Palpate that breast with other hand using concentric circle method. It usually takes three circles to cover all breast tissue. Include tail of the breast and axilla. Repeat with other breast. **F,** End in sitting position. Palpate areola areas of both breasts, and inspect and squeeze nipples to check for discharge.

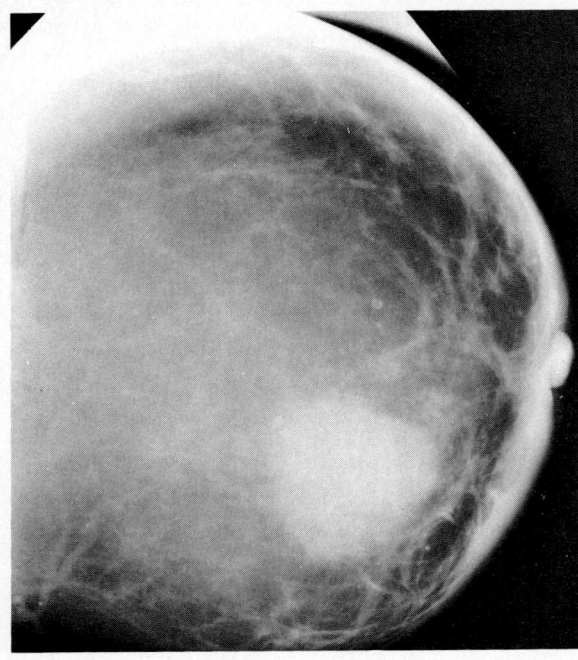

Fig. 36-3. Mammogram of patient with area of density indicating carcinoma. (From Cramer, L.N. and Lapayowker, M.S.: Applied anatomy of the female breast: surgical radiographic and thermographic. In Masters, F.W., and Lewis, J.R., Jr., editors: Symposium on aesthetic surgery of the face, eyelid, and breast, vol. 4, St. Louis, 1972, The C.V. Mosby Co.)

DIAGNOSTIC TESTS FOR BREAST EVALUATION

Radiographs

MAMMOGRAPHY

Mammography is an x-ray examination of the breast used to detect early lesions before they are palpable (Fig. 36-3). Mammography is about 85% accurate in detecting early breast cancer. It does have limitations, particularly in the penetration of dense breasts as in adolescents, young nulliparous women, or women with large breasts. A low energy x-ray beam is used to delineate the breast structures; this radiation dose is acceptable for use in frequent reexaminations. During the examination the breast is pressed firmly against the film holder and several films are taken of each breast.

XERORADIOGRAPHY

Xeroradiography is similar to mamography except that an aluminum plate with an electrically charged selenium layer is used in place of the familiar black and white mammogram x-ray film. The resulting film is blue and white (Fig. 36-4). Xeroradiography is thought to provide sharper contrast of blood vessel patterns and tissue densities.

THERMOGRAPHY

Increased metabolism and increased blood supply to a malignant lesion increase the skin temperature and vascularity of the breast. Thermography is a technique that measures and records the heat emissions coming from the breast. Thermography is used less frequently because of a high number of false-positive results. Its use is primarily as a screening device with follow-up of any positive results by mammography.

ULTRASONOGRAPHY

Ultrasound is currently being evaluated for its possible value in detecting lesions in the dense breasts of young women. Although ultrasound can differentiate the presence of a cystic mass, it does not indicate calcium deposits or tissue configurations, facts considered important in the diagnosis of malignant tumors.

Aspiration

Aspiration of an identified soft breast mass may be performed if a cyst is suspected. A large-bore needle is inserted into the mass and the contents withdrawn and sent to the laboratory for cytologic studies. The only discomfort is associated with insertion of the needle. If cytologic tests are positive, biopsy is performed. If the tests are negative and there are characteristics of cystic disease, no further tests are performed. If there are some doubts, despite the negative results, further radiographic studies may be performed.

Breast biopsy

Biopsy is the only way to determine conclusively whether a tumor is benign or malignant. Most lesions (80%) are found to be benign.

The procedure may be performed with the patient un-

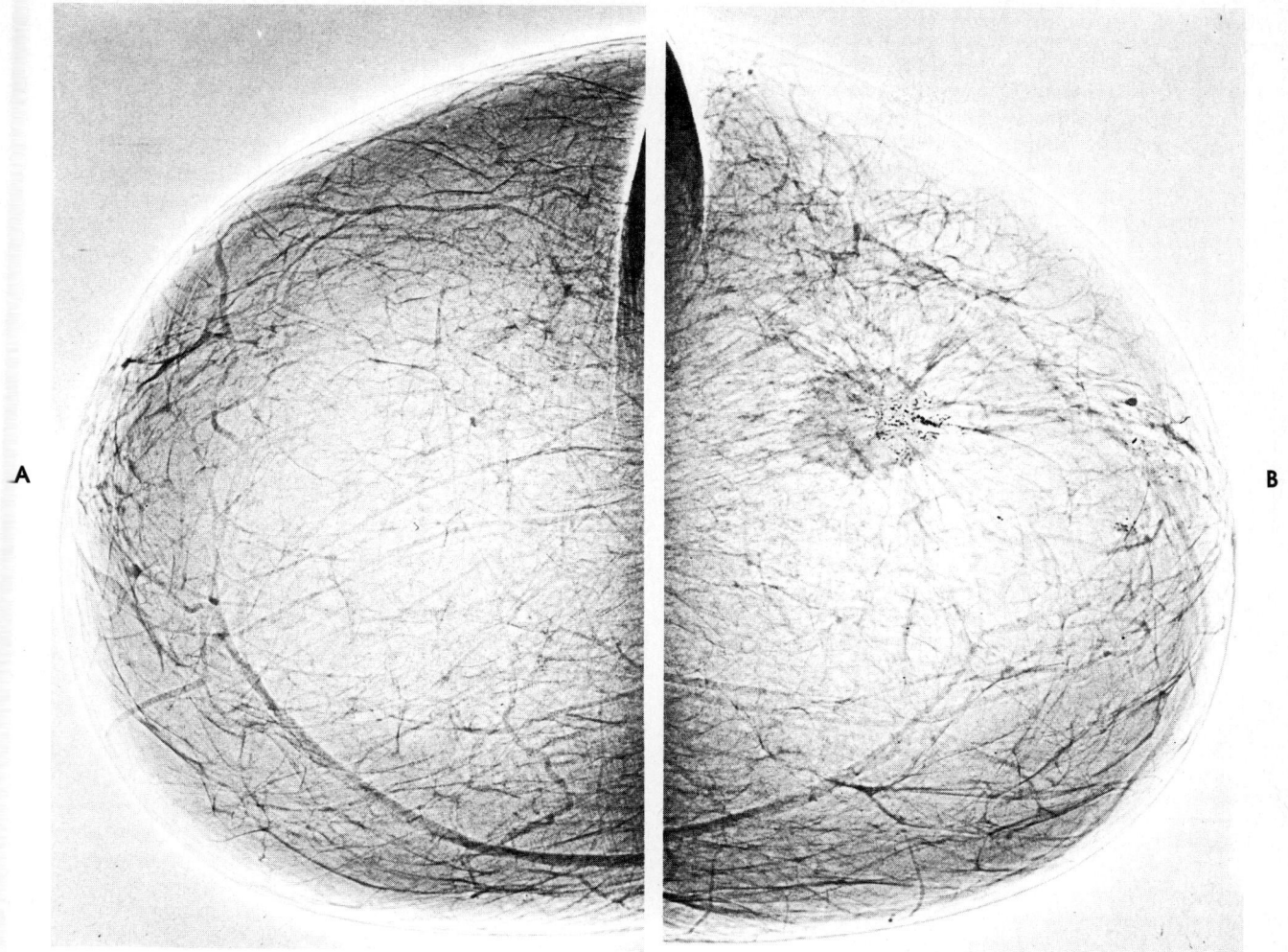

Fig. 36-4. Xeroradiographs. **A,** Normal left breast **B,** Right breast shows mass with spiculated margins characteristic of neoplasm. (Courtesy University Hospitals of Cleveland.)

der local or general anesthesia in an ambulatory surgical suite or as an inpatient. An incision is made and a portion of the mass (or the entire mass if it is very small) is removed and sent to the laboratory for examination. Following the procedure there may be mild discomfort. Results will be available immediately, if a frozen section is done, or within 48 to 72 hours.

Sometimes the small size makes location of the lesion difficult or uncertain when biopsy is attempted. Therefore to locate areas for surgical biopsy, a small methylene blue dye marker is made within the area of the breast using a syringe and needle during mammographic monitoring. This is done in the x-ray department a few hours before the surgical biopsy, and the marker is made while the patient is under local anesthesia. No color disfiguration is apparent on the breast surface as a result of this procedure, but the mark ensures that the biopsy tissue corresponds to the site identified by mammogram. This

procedure requires preinstruction of the patient and support in the x-ray department.

BENIGN BREAST DISORDERS

The major benign breast disorders are fibrocystic in nature (dysplasia), benign tumors (fibroadenomas), or infections (mastitis, with or without breast abscess) (Table 36-1).

PATHOPHYSIOLOGY

Benign breast disorders are usually characterized by one or more movable breast masses, often seen bilaterally. The nodularity may be discrete or diffuse. If tenderness is present, it usually occurs or is increased premenstrually. Any nipple discharge, which may be clear, green, or brownish (but not bloody), is usually sponta-

Table 36-1. Benign breast disorders

Disorder	Characteristics	Signs and symptoms	Medical therapy
Dysplasia (fibrocystic disease)	Refers to several cystic nodular disorders of the breast that become painful during menstruation; seen mostly in women age 30 to 50; estrogen hormone a causative factor	Painful, often multiple and bilateral soft masses in breast; may increase in size or remain the same	Aspiration of probable cyst; biopsy of doubtful cyst to confirm diagnosis; yearly mammograms; intermittent diuretics for premenstrual breast engorgement; symptomatic pain relief
Fibroadenoma	Fibroplastic tumors commonly seen in young women under age 25	Firm, round, freely movable, nontender mass in breast	Surgical excision with patient under local anesthesia on outpatient basis
Mastitis	Inflammation of breast, usually from cracked or infected nipples	Pain, redness, swelling of breast, fever	Systemic antibiotics; incision and drainage if an abscess forms; symptomatic pain relief

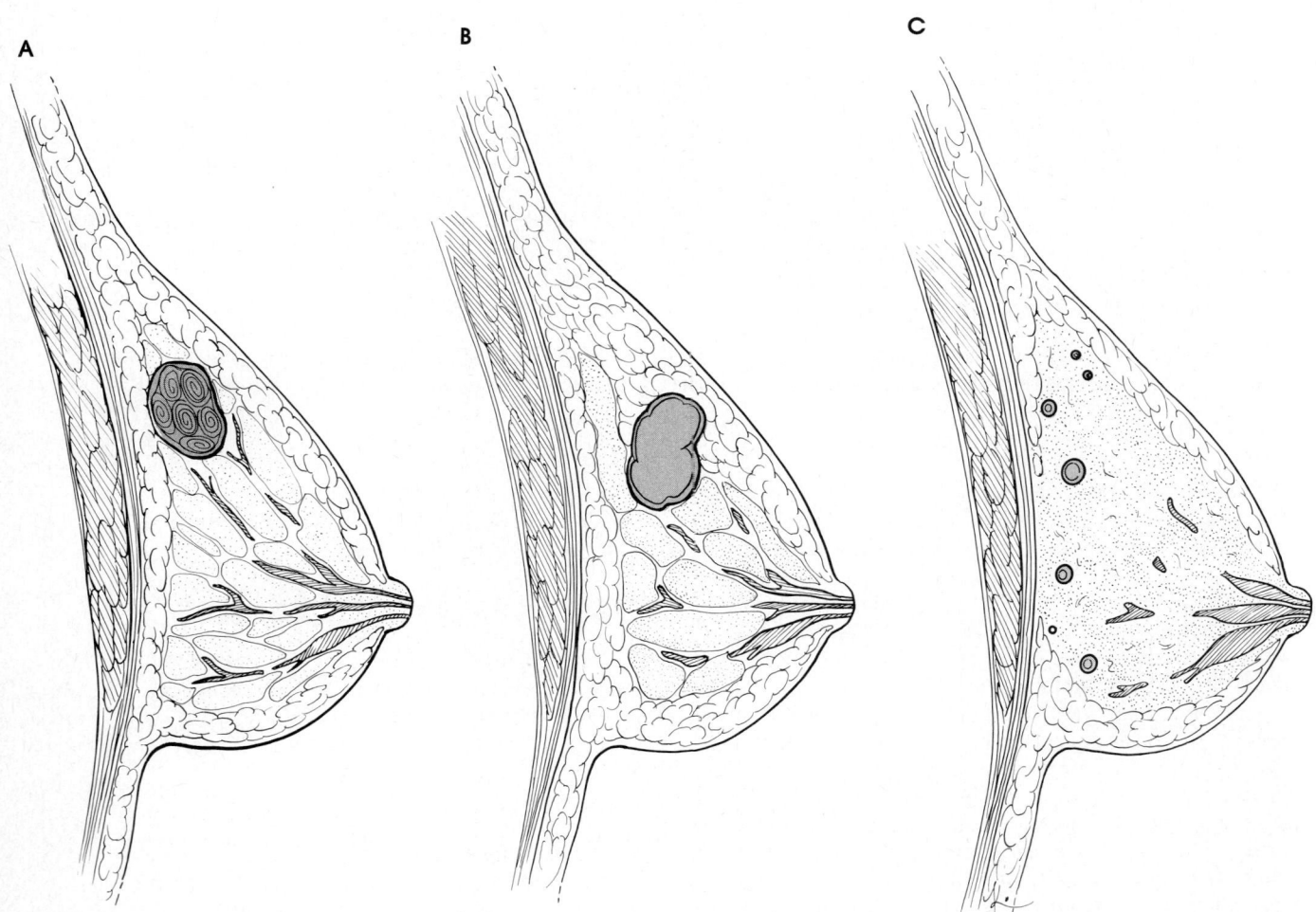

Fig. 36-5. Benign breast disorders. **A,** Fibroadenoma. **B,** Cyst. **C,** Adenosis (fibrocystic disease).

Table 36-2. Differences between benign and malignant breast masses

Benign	Malignant
Usually bilateral; may be unilateral	Unilateral
Found often in outer quadrants but may occur anywhere	Found most often in upper outer quadrant and tail or in central nipple portion
Single or multiple	Usually single
Well-circumscribed	Irregular
Soft or firm	Firm
Movable	Nonmovable
Usually have cyclic tenderness; may be nontender	Nontender
No skin changes	Later findings: skin thickened; dimpling
	Very late: ulceration
No palpable lymph nodes	Palpable lymph nodes except in early period
No nipple retraction; discharge usually bilateral, serous, or greenish	Nipple retraction; discharge usually unilateral and may be bloody

neous, especially just before menstruation. Women who take oral contraceptives may experience some nipple discharge that ceases when the "pill" is discontinued.

Males may have overdevelopment of breast tissue (gynecomastia) as a result of estrogen production during puberty or older age, adrenal or gonadal tumors, or certain drugs, for example, amphetamines, antidepressants (tricyclic), antihypertensive agents, antineoplastic agents, cimetidine, diazepam, digitalis, estrogen, human chorionic gonadotropin, isoniazid, and phenothiazines.

ASSESSMENT

Data are collected concerning the person's feelings and knowledge about the disorder, including the following:
1. Concerns about the mass
2. Knowledge of benign versus malignant tumors
3. Knowledge regarding breast self-examination
4. Presence of discomfort

DATA ANALYSIS AND PLANNING

Nursing diagnoses

Nursing diagnoses for the woman who has a benign breast disorder may include the following:
Anxiety
Alteration in comfort: pain in breast
Knowledge deficit

Expected patient outcomes

1. Breast discomfort is minimized.
2. The patient
   a. Can describe difference between benign and malignant breast disease.
   b. Plans to do monthly breast self-examination.
   c. Plans for yearly medical follow-up.

IMPLEMENTATION

Assisting with comfort

Breast discomfort may be decreased by mild analgesics (such as aspirin or acetaminophen), by application of heat or cold, or by breast support. Heat may be applied by application of a warm damp washcloth covered by a dry towel and heating pad or hot water bottle. Some persons experience relief from an ice bag or a washcloth wrung out in cold water.

Wearing a firm brassiere both day and night may also help to relieve breast discomfort. The brassiere should fit well and give good support, especially for the upper outer breast quadrant.[30]

Counseling and teaching
Reducing anxiety

Most women who identify a breast mass immediately think of cancer and are therefore usually very anxious before the diagnosis is verified. Even after being told that the condition is benign, some women continue to have some anxiety. *Mild* anxiety is useful as this acts as a stimulus for continuing medical follow-up.

The woman who is moderately or severely anxious needs an opportunity to express her concerns to an empathic listener. As the anxiety decreases, the woman is better able to deal with any discomfort and to continue her usual activities.

Teaching

The risk of breast cancer in women with mammary dysplasia is twice that for women in general. It is *very important*, therefore, that these women know how to perform accurate breast self-examination and how to recognize masses that differ from the masses of their dysplasia (Table 36-2). More frequent medical follow-up than that specified for asymptomatic persons is indicated.

The role of methylxanthines in the reduction of symptoms in benign breast disorders is controversial. Omission of coffee, tea, and chocolate from the diet may help some persons and is worth a try.

EVALUATION

Evaluation is based on expected patient outcomes. Questions to ask may include the following:
1. Is breast discomfort lessened?

2. Does the person know:
   a. The difference between benign and malignant disease?
   b. The method and frequency of breast self-examination?
   c. The frequency of medical follow-up?

CANCER OF THE BREAST

Cancer of the breast is the leading cause of cancer *mortality* in women as well as the leading cause of death in women age 40 to 50 years. It is estimated that 1 out of 11 women in the United States will develop cancer of the breast, and this probability increases with age.

PATHOPHYSIOLOGY

Breast cancer is not one disease but many, depending on the tissue of the breast involved, its estrogen dependency, and the age of onset. Premenopausal breast malignancy is different from postmenopausal malignancy. Treatment response and prognoses differ with various malignancies.

Some tumors are termed "estrogen dependent"; they contain receptors that bind estradiol, a type of estrogen, and their growth is stimulated by estrogen. These receptors are not present in normal breast tissue or in tissue with dysplasia. Presence of estrogen-dependent tumors is identified by an estrogen receptor assay test (ERA) that is performed on biopsied tissue. Postmenopausal women have a higher incidence of hormone-dependent breast cancers. These cancers respond to hormone treatment (endocrine chemotherapy, oophorectomy, or adrenalectomy).

Malignant breast tumors differ from benign tumors (Table 36-2). They are usually solitary, irregularly shaped, firm, nontender, nonmobile masses with a tendency to adhere to the pectoral muscles and to the skin, causing retraction or dimpling of the skin. The skin may become thickened, giving it an "orange peel" effect. Involvement of the lymph nodes is present in about two thirds of the women at the time of diagnosis. Favored sites for metastasis are the lungs, bone, liver, brain, adrenal glands, and ovaries.

Breast cancers are classified using the TNM classification (described in Chapter 14). T refers to tumor size, N to nodal involvement, and M to metastasis. The classification of breast cancer (Table 36-3) serves as a basis for prognosis and direction for treatment.

PREVENTION

Persons at risk

Cancer of the breast cannot be prevented, but cure is more likely if cancer is identified early and treatment started immediately. Most tumors are located by the woman herself; therefore all women should practice breast self-examination (p. 1086). Persons who are at high risk should know of their risk and are urged to have careful follow-up. A major factor that places the woman at risk is a long, uninterrupted time period of cyclic hormone changes, that is, early menarche, late menopause, and no pregnancy.

High-risk factors associated with breast cancer

Sex	Female (99% in women)
Age	Over age 50 (80% over age 35)
Familial history	Mother/sister, especially with premenopausal or bilateral breast cancer
Menstrual history	Menarche before age 11; menopause after age 50
Pregnancy	First live birth after age 30, or nullipara
Medical history	Primary breast cancer (risk increased 7 times for a second primary breast cancer); uterine endometrial cancer; mammary dysplasia

---

Table 36-3. TNM classification of breast cancers

Stage	Tumor size	Nodal involvement	Metastasis
I	Less than 2 cm (T1)	None (N0)	None (M0)
II	Less than 5 cm (T1 or T2)	Movable axillary nodes (N1)	None (M0)
III	Greater than 5 cm or invasion of skin or attached to chest wall	Movable or fixed axillary nodes (N1 or N2)	None (M0)
IV	Any size (any T)	Any nodes (any N)	Yes (M1)

PRETREATMENT PHASE

Assessment

If a malignant breast tumor is suspected or diagnosed as such, the following data are obtained as a baseline for planning:

1. Identification of family relationships and the existence and availability of support persons
2. Usual coping mechanisms
3. Feelings and thoughts about the woman's sexuality and the relationship of the breast to these feelings
4. Thoughts about feelings of the sex partner (if appropriate) concerning forthcoming diagnostic procedures or potential therapy options
5. Future goals, life expectancies, zest for living, and actual or perceived responsibility to others

If possible, data are obtained from the sex partner (if appropriate) regarding his feelings about the forthcoming surgery. This identifies possible conflicts in perceptions, the degree of support that can be anticipated from the sex partner, and the potential effects of the partner's feelings on the woman's adaptation and relationships.

During the pretreatment phase, numerous diagnostic tests (p. 1088) may be performed to determine the nature and extent of the tumor.

Assisting with coping with anxiety

Since much emphasis is placed on the breast as a symbol of attractiveness, the thought of losing a breast becomes almost intolerable to many women. This is particularly true of those who depend largely on physical attractiveness to hold the esteem of others and to secure gratification of their emotional needs. Psychologists have pointed out that there is a symbolic connection between the breasts and motherhood that is severely threatened when a breast must be removed. In addition, cancer of the breast often occurs at menopause or soon after when some women feel that they have lost much of their sexual attractiveness. Surgical removal of the breast may save a woman's life, but it also may cause her to feel less feminine.

Although she may try to conceal fear, any woman who is hospitalized for removal of a breast tumor is anxious, and some may be in a state of near panic. Most fears are related to sexual acceptance, social isolation, disfigurement, recurrence, and death. Many of these women have been unable to discuss their worries and feelings with their significant others, including their spouse. The nurse can help the patient to express feelings and to understand what breast surgery means to her as a person. The woman who is having breast surgery has a special need to feel understood and accepted by all persons who are providing care.

Simple explanations with repetition may decrease the patient's fears of the unknown. If it seems that the patient does not fully comprehend the physician's explanation, the nurse can repeat the explanation and report this to the physician, who in turn can talk with the patient again and clarify any misconceptions, alleviating needless anxiety. Since attention span, memory, and perception are limited when anxiety levels are high, it is helpful if the nurse can be present when information is given to the patient. The nurse can then repeat, reinforce, or clarify given information.

Assisting with decision making

When the diagnostic work is completed and the classification of the tumor has been made, the physician, often with the consultation of the hospital tumor board members (medical, surgical, and radiation oncologists), discusses and proposes the treatment protocol by which the tumor would be most successfully destroyed and which offers the best prognosis for the patient. The patient and family are often involved at this point in this treatment decision plan. If the patient is not involved, she should request to be made knowledgeable of the findings of the diagnostic measures and the reasons for the therapy plan now being described by her.

There are currently many treatments for breast malignancy; the primary therapies are surgery and radiation. If the malignancy is small, nonaggressive, and present in a young woman, she may, for instance, have several options for therapy that offer her a comparable prognosis with the knowledge available at this time. Every woman should realize, however, that the latest therapy found in magazines may or may not be *best* for her. Nurses have an advantage in assisting a patient to understand the factors involved in the decision making from the expertise of the medical professional but still taking into consideration the subjective hesitations of the woman.

In some instances, such as an inflammatory carcinoma that rapidly invades the mammary lymphatics, there may be only one treatment plan (immediate radiation). In this situation a nursing diagnosis of *powerlessness* may be identified from collected data because the woman has no alternatives from which to choose. Letting the patient make decisions about other aspects of her life and activities of daily living, whenever possible, helps the patient hold onto a sense of control of her life.

BREAST SURGERY

Type of surgery

Different types of surgery may be performed for removal of tumors with or without removal of the breast and underlying tissue. The type depends on the extent of the growth and degree of spread. Until the results of long-range studies are in, controversy remains pertaining to the best therapy that gives the optimum results with the least amount of deformity. At this time, modified radical mastectomy is the recommended primary procedure of choice for most patients with potentially curable breast cancer.[17] Radical mastectomy may be necessary in those cases where the tumor has invaded the muscle. Very small local tumors may be controlled by breast-sparing techniques (see box, p. 1094).

Preoperative care

Preoperative care includes helping the woman deal with her anxiety concerning loss of a breast. Breast re-

---

Types of surgery for removal of breast tumors

Lumpectomy	Simple removal of the tumor mass
Partial mastectomy	Removal of tumor mass and 2.5 to 7.5 cm (1 to 3 inches) of surrounding tissue
Subcutaneous mastectomy	Removal of all underlying breast tissue, leaving skin, areola, and nipple intact
Simple mastectomy	Removal of entire breast but not axillary nodes
Modified radical mastectomy	Complete removal of breast (with or without pectoralis minor) and removal of some axillary lymph nodes
Radical mastectomy	Complete removal of breast, axillary lymph nodes, pectoralis muscle (major and minor), and adjacent fat and fascia

---

construction at a later date is cited so the patient knows this may be a possibility (p. 1100).

The American Cancer Society sponsors a volunteer program, Reach to Recovery, in which the patient has an opportunity to visit with a woman who has had a mastectomy. This encourages the patient, and she will receive practical help from someone who has made a satisfactory adjustment to the same operation. Although most of the patient visits by the volunteer from Reach to Recovery occur during the postoperative period, preoperative visits may be very helpful to some women and can be requested.

Preoperative *teaching* should include the following information if a mastectomy is planned:

1. A catheter draining the incision and attached to suction may be used.
2. The arm on the affected side will be elevated.
3. Sitting up and turning in bed should be done by *pushing* up on the unaffected side, not pulling.
4. Postoperative exercises will be started early.

Telling the patient about the exercises helps to give her the feeling that there is something in the situation that she can control and contribute to, and thus she will begin to have a positive attitude toward rehabilitation.

Postoperative care
Wound care

Following the completion of the mastectomy and closure, a stab wound may be made and a catheter inserted and attached immediately to a low, constant suction, such as that provided by a Hemovac or other low suction system. The purpose of the catheter is to remove blood and serum that may collect under the skin flaps and that would prevent healing and predispose the tissue to infection. There is usually no drainage from around the incision when a catheter is draining properly. The catheter may be clamped for short periods of ambulation and is usually removed within 3 to 5 days or when the amount of drainage is less than 5 to 10 ml in 24 hours.

The dressing is checked often for the first few hours to detect hemorrhage or excessive serous oozing. The bedclothes under the patient must be examined for blood that may flow down from the operated region. Any evidence of bleeding is reported to the surgeon. Dressings may be re-

---

Early exercises for postmastectomy patient

Surgical day	Flex and extend fingers; pronate and supinate forearm
First postoperative day	Squeeze rubber ball
As soon as tolerated	Brush teeth and hair

---

moved in 24 hours, or they may not be changed for several days after the operation. The skin sutures are often removed on the sixth to eighth postoperative day. Usually this is after the patient's discharge from the hospital.

Postmastectomy activity and exercise

When the patient returns from surgery, she is placed in a semi-Fowler's position to decrease venous oozing. The arm is elevated to enhance circulation and prevent edema. The pillows are arranged so that the hand is higher than the arm and the arm is above the level of the right atrium. *No blood pressure readings, injections, or blood testing* should be done on the *affected* arm because of potential circulatory impairment or infection (to prevent lymphedema). A sign or tape should be placed on this side of the bed with this message.

Exercises are essential to prevent shortening of muscles, stiffness, and contracture of the shoulder girdle, and to preserve muscle tone so that the affected arm can be used without limitations. To prevent additional deformities, exercises should be bilateral ones with the patient using both arms simultaneously. The time to start specific postoperative exercises depends on the extent of the operation and whether skin grafting has been necessary (as with radical mastectomy).

Slings are to be avoided. Gentle exercises started early in the postoperative course help decrease muscle tension as well as regain muscle function more quickly. The patient must know what motion is intended in each exercise. For example, the patient may brush her hair with the arm on the affected side, but she may lower her head

---

Postmastectomy arm exercises

Exercise: Climbing the wall

1. Stand facing wall with toes close to wall.
2. Bend elbows and place palms of hands against wall at shoulder level.
3. Move both hands parallel to each other up the wall as far as possible until incisional pull or pain occur.
4. Move both hands down to starting position.
5. Goal is complete extension with elbow straight.
6. Activities that utilize the same action: reaching top shelves, hanging out clothes, washing windows, hanging curtains, setting hair.

Exercise: Arm swinging

1. Bend forward from waist, permitting both arms to relax and hang naturally.
2. Swing arms together left to right (motion comes from shoulder).
3. Swing arms in circles parallel to floor, clockwise and counterclockwise.
4. Stand up slowly.

Exercise: Rope pull

1. Attach a rope over a shower rod or hook.
2. Grasp each end of rope, alternately pulling on each end, raising affected arm to a point of incisional pull or pain.
3. Shorten rope over time until affected arm is raised almost directly overhead.

Exercise: Elbow spread

1. Clasp hands behind neck.
2. Raise elbows to chin level, holding head erect. Move slowly and rest when incisional pull or pain occur.
3. Gradually spread elbows apart. Rest when pull or pain occur.

From American Cancer Society: Reach to recovery, New York, The Society.

---

and hunch her shoulders in such a way that she does not get normal use of the shoulder girdle. The whole intent of the exercise may therefore be lost.

The patient is encouraged under close supervision to exercise each day more and more to the limits of incisional pulling and pain. A specific exercise schedule planned by nurse and patient together is imperative. It is an important aspect of nursing care for this patient.

Continuing exercises are as recommended by the American Cancer Society (see box above). With exercise, full range of motion will return; that is, both arms can be extended equally high above the head. This will not be achieved before the patient leaves the hospital; therefore the patient must learn and be motivated in the hospital so she will continue exercises at home on a regular basis. Following radical mastectomy, full muscle power for horizontal adduction may be less.

Promoting comfort

Pain in the operated area may be referred to the affected arm or shoulder. Sensations of numbness and tingling over the chest that are painful may cause the patient to take short, shallow breaths in the early postoperative period. She is kept comfortable with analgesics, and a deep breathing and coughing routine is started. Each chest excursion may painfully discourage compliance, and the patient may need considerable encouragement.

Phantom symptoms of the missing breast occur in those women who had painful breasts or nipples before the surgery. This can be very disconcerting to the woman, and reassurance may be needed that these sensations will eventually disappear.

The body requires increased energy for healing and for coping with the grief of the loss of the breast. Fatigue occurs not only in the early postoperative period but often for up to 6 weeks after surgery. The woman needs to know that this is a normal reaction and that she should plan for rest periods.

Providing psychologic support

After surgery, denial of the changes in body image may take the form of the woman speaking about "the cancer" and "the mastectomy" but never dealing with her loss or her fears on an emotional level. Denial here is a conservation of energy. If she is to express herself on an emotional level, she must have someone who is capable and responsible to support her according to *her* need. If she does not receive this professional assistance, the impact of her loss occurs at a later date when support systems may not be available.

Avoidance of looking at the dressing or incision can be expected initially. The incision is large, and the feeling experienced by most women is that of mutilation. Postponing looking at the incision delays the impact of the realization that the breast is indeed gone. Preparing the woman in advance concerning the size of the incision is helpful, but she still needs considerable support when viewing the incision and her new image. She is usually physically capable when she feels stronger and begins to socially respond to others. She is encouraged to look at the incision several times before discharge from the hospital, while health professionals are available for support.

Feelings of anger and resentment may occur and if present frequently are projected onto female staff or friends. Families may also express anger or anxiety and may complain without cause about the care the patient is receiving. Feelings of decreased self-worth and self-esteem on the part of the patient plus increased dependency needs often produce depression.

The feeling of being isolated and alone during this experience can be helped by interaction with others who have had the same experience, such as a visitor from the Reach to Recovery program. The Reach to Recovery volunteer holds the potential of motivating the patient, extending hope, and providing visible evidence that femininity, personality, and activity can be retained and proves to be a good resource person as the patient moves from hospital to community. Often whether or not the patient has the opportunity to use this resource depends on a nurse's initiating the contact.

After the patient is discharged, she may experience periods of depression if she perceives her recovery is slow or if she tries to reenter her previous activities and responsibilities sooner than her energy reserves return. She may have difficulty sleeping or concentrating if she is still acutely grieving with little recognition or little support. Although she will be aware of this, she usually will be unable to express her needs; significant others can be told of her continuing need for support and patience and can help to extend the kind of support needed.

Sexual adaptation

Woods[33] has identified a number of factors that can influence sexual adaptation following mastectomy (Fig. 36-6). Women with very small or very large breasts may have long-unresolved feelings about breast size and may also experience more difficulty in obtaining a satisfactory breast prosthesis. The woman who perceives the surgery as mutilating may withdraw from the sexual relationship, fearing rejection from her partner. Women who felt sexually inadequate before surgery may find these feelings enhanced postoperatively and use the surgery as a reason for withdrawing from sexual relationships.

The nurse can initiate a discussion with the patient concerning her thoughts and feelings about return to sexual activity (if appropriate) and can encourage the patient to talk about her concerns with her sexual partner. Sexual and marital counseling is helpful for couples who are unable to communicate their feelings openly with each other.

Breast prostheses and clothing

Information about breast prostheses is given to the patient whenever she asks about them or appears interested. The volunteer from Reach to Recovery is a good resource person for current information and suggestions concerning prostheses and clothing. She may accompany the patient as she shops for her first prosthesis, serving as a support person. Breast prostheses are not fitted until at least 6 weeks postoperatively or until the incision is healed and is no longer tender.

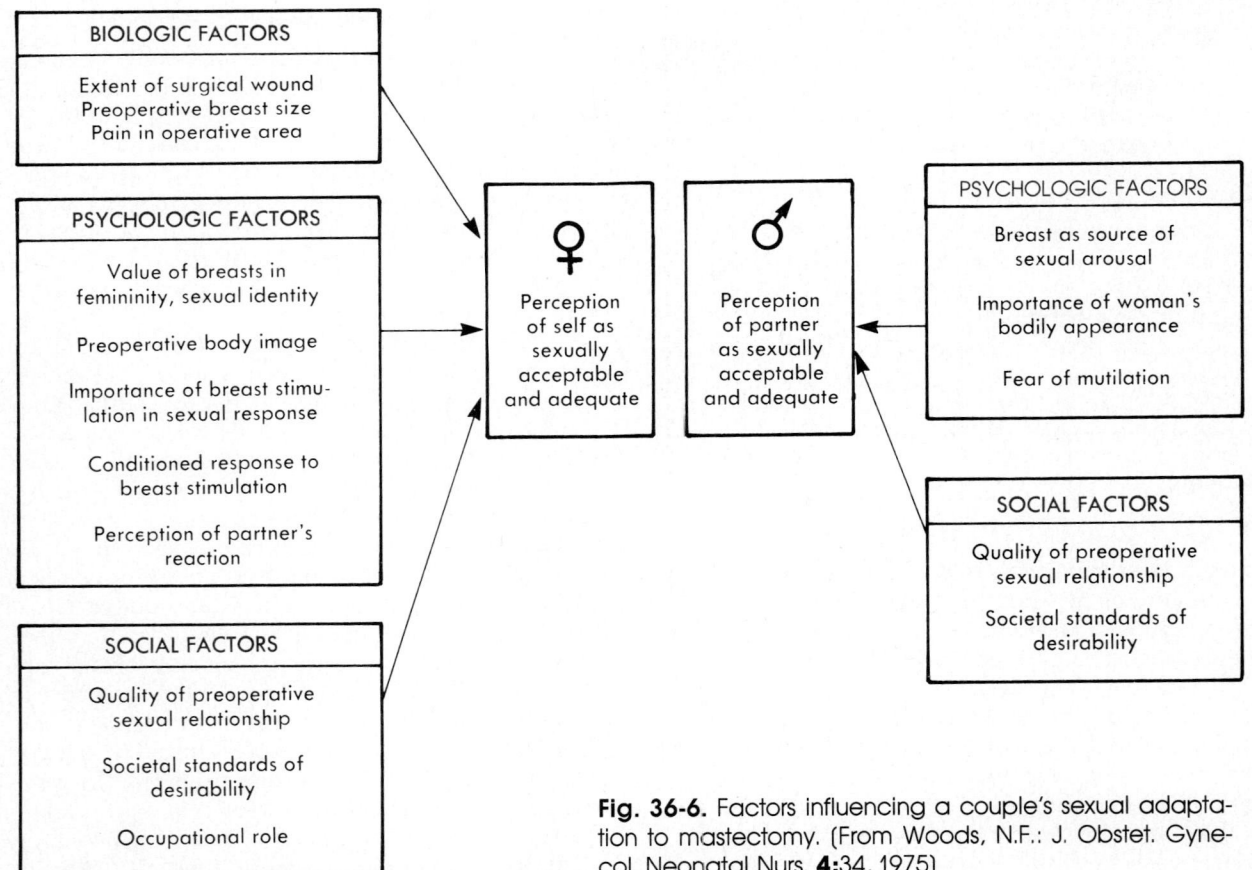

Fig. 36-6. Factors influencing a couple's sexual adaptation to mastectomy. (From Woods, N.F.: J. Obstet. Gynecol. Neonatal Nurs. **4:**34, 1975)

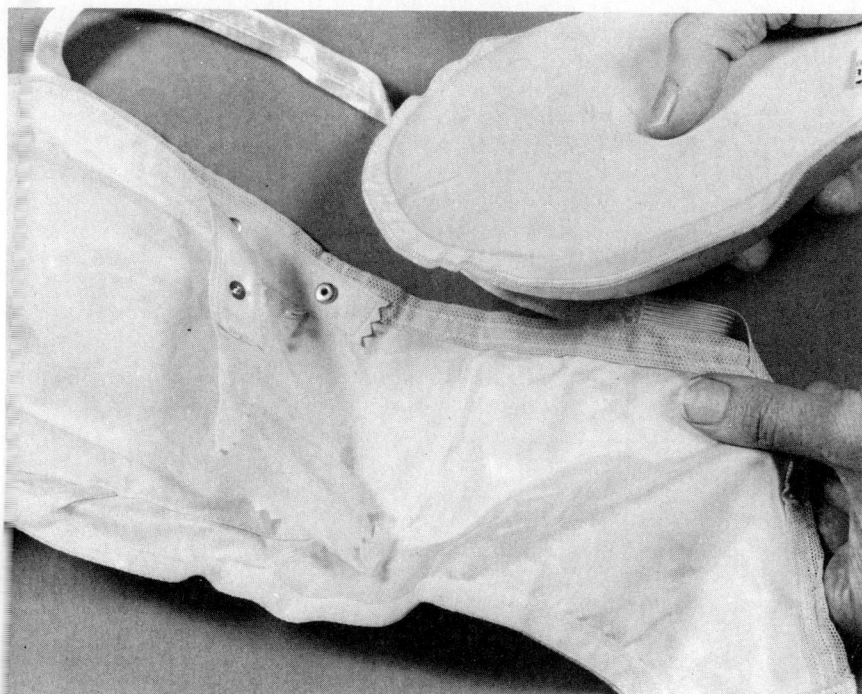

Fig. 36-7. Inner pocket that will hold padding or proshtesis securely can be made in patient's own brassiere. Note snaps that simplify removal of padding.

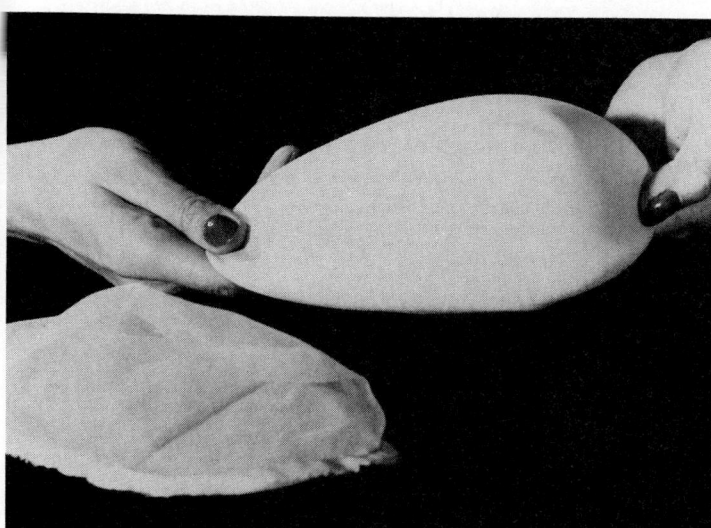

Fig. 36-8. Foam-covered, liquid-filled breast prosthesis. (Courtesy Camp International, Jackson, Mich.)

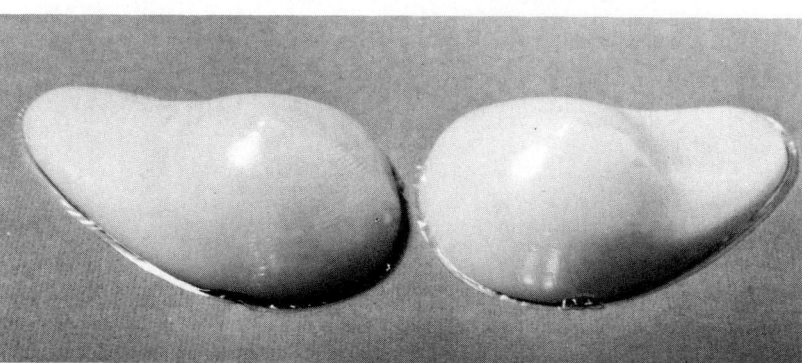

Fig. 36-9. Silicone-filled breast prostheses. (Courtesy Camp International, Jackson, Mich.)

Until the incision is well healed, the woman is advised to wear one of her own brassieres, which can be lightly padded with a soft, fluffy filling (Fig. 36-7) or a temporary soft prosthesis, available from Reach to Recovery, that will not shift and embarrass her. Opaque, loose-hanging gowns are usually most acceptable to the patient. All clothing should have wide armholes to prevent constriction of the underarm.

Breast prostheses vary in price, type, and weight (Figs. 36-8 and 36-9). Women want prostheses to make them look symmetric and *feel* bilaterally weighted. Even small-breasted women will change posture if weighting is not balanced. Firm, molded prostheses have a disadvantage of remaining elevated when the woman is lying supine, whereas fluid types have a more natural look.

Lymphedema

Many patients develop a slight edema of the upper arm that disappears within a week. A few patients, however, develop a severe edema that persists, that may become permanent, and that is caused by surgical interruption of lymph channels and nodes. The incidence is greater in persons who are obese, develop infections, or are subjected to irradiation. Some surgeons order an elastic sleeve that gives additional support to the vessels in the arm; this should extend from the wrist to the shoulder. It is similar to an elastic support stocking and usually may be removed when the patient is in bed. A diuretic such as chlorothiazide (Diuril) may be ordered to help relieve the edema.

Teaching

In addition to teaching points stressed earlier, the patient is taught to report symptoms indicating infection or poor healing of the incision. Since the woman is at high risk for developing cancer in the other breast, she needs to carry out monthly breast self-examination for early identification of another lesion. The points to be stressed in teaching are included in the summary of the care of the patient with a mastectomy listed in box below.

Care of the patient who has had a mastectomy

Preoperative care

1. Help patient explore feelings about loss of breast and fears related to cancer
2. Provide simple explanations; repeat as necessary
3. Teach patient:
   a. Expectation of catheter to drain wound
   b. Need for postoperative exercises

Postoperative care

1. Give immediate care
   a. Place patient in semi-Fowler's position
   b. Wound care:
      (1) Attach catheter to suction drainage
      (2) If Hemovac suction is used, empty when half-full to maintain suction
      (3) Check dressing and bed for signs of drainage
   c. Elevate arm on pillow
   d. Monitor circulation of arm on affected side; report signs of swelling and numbness of lower arm or inability to move fingers
   e. Avoid blood pressure readings, blood testing, or injections in affected arm
   f. Teach patient to sit up in bed by *pushing* up on elbow of *unaffected* side, rather than pulling up with arm
   g. Encourage deep breathing and coughing
   h. Give analgesics for comfort

2. Encourage postmastectomy arm exercises
   a. Start gentle exercises early (see p. 1094)
   b. Start special mastectomy exercises (see p. 1095) when prescribed
3. Encourage rest periods; monitor for fatigue
4. Provide emotional support
   a. Continue to help patient explore feelings
   b. Prepare patient in advance concerning size of incision and be with her, if possible, when she looks at incision
   c. Encourage patient to identify feelings about resuming sexual activities (if appropriate) and to discuss these feelings with sexual partner
5. Teach patient
   a. Wear a brassiere padded with a soft fluffy filling or temporary soft prosthesis until incision is healed
   b. Substitute a regular breast prosthesis later
   c. Avoid clothing that constricts the underarm
   d. Avoid injections and blood pressure measurements in affected arm
   e. Report symptoms indicating need for immediate medical attention:
      (1) Edema of affected arm
      (2) Redness or infection of scar
      (3) Breakdown of scar tissue
      (4) Mass in other breast or axillae
   f. Plan to do monthly breast self-examination on remaining breast

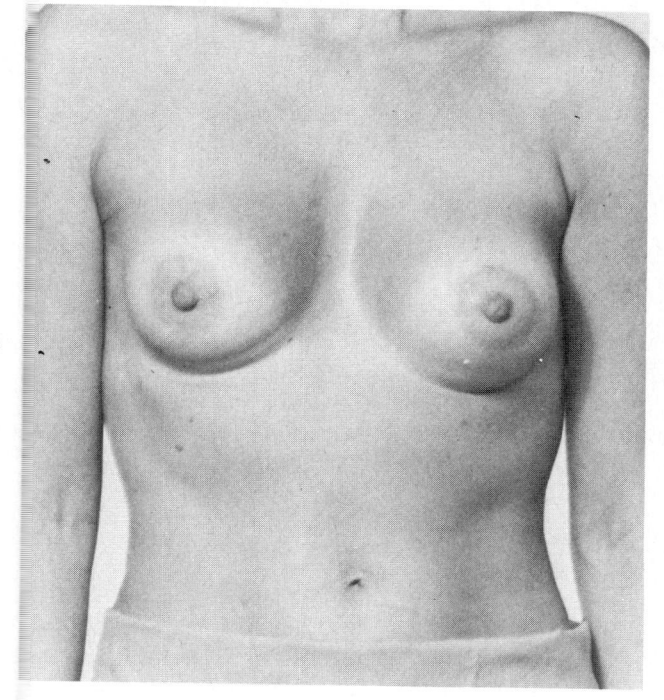

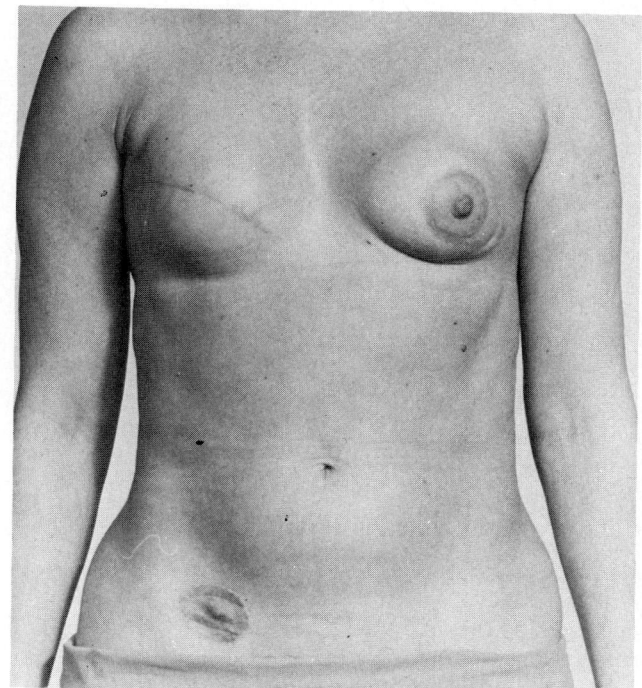

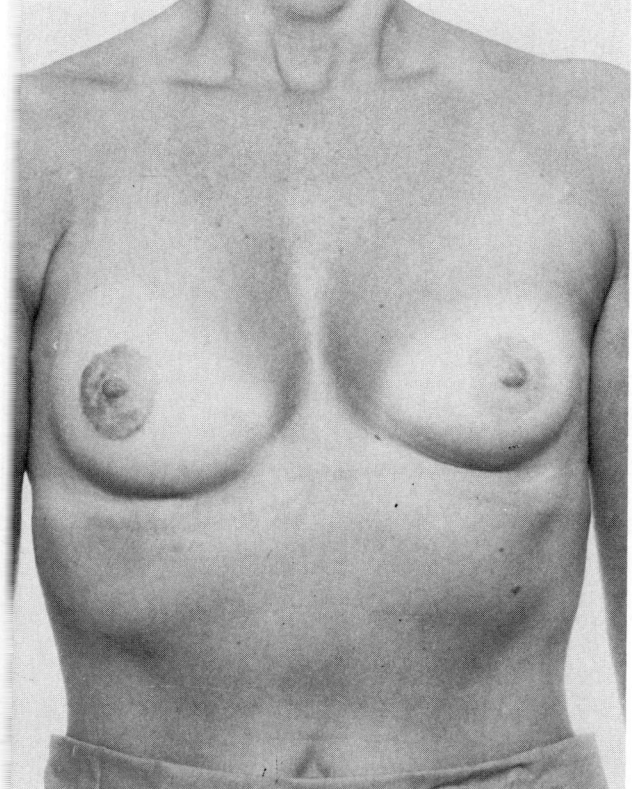

Fig. 36-10. Removal of early intraductal carcinoma in right upper quadrant with breast reconstruction. **A,** Preoperative view. **B,** 5 months postoperative with implant inserted 4 days after surgery; nipple-areola graft banked in inguinal area. **C,** 2 years after initial surgery.

BREAST RECONSTRUCTION

Reconstruction mammoplasty is a possibility for many women following a mastectomy. For some women, breast reconstruction is not essential to their positive self-image and esteem, femininity, or sexual experience. Many do not want the added surgery and attendant anesthesia, the costliness of time or money, or the pain. They are comfortable and active and successful without the added surgery. Other women consider it important for their self-esteem and continuing relationships with others. Breast reconstruction is contraindicated when there is an aggressive tumor, a probability that metastasis has occurred, a concern about adequate healing being impaired, or unrealistic psychosocial expectations.

Every woman should know about the options of reconstruction after mastectomy, whether it is appropriate for her stage of disease, as well as those facts that tell her what it can and cannot do. She should have the opportunity to talk and read about breast reconstruction so she can determine its meaning for her. An excellent pamphlet, "Breast Reconstruction Following Mastectomy for Cancer," is available free of charge from the American Cancer Society. This pamphlet is used to best advantage by nurses and patients speaking together and reading and interpreting the questions and answers in the brochure together.

Reconstruction can be performed at the time of mastectomy, or, as is preferred by most plastic reconstruction surgeons, the reconstruction can take place some months later after some psychologic readjustment, physical strength, and energy reserves have been achieved. Some women change their minds during the adjustment period.

Surgical procedure

The surgery consists of a Silastic implant filled with silicone or saline solution placed under the subcutaneous tissue. A nipple can be reconstructed if necessary from labial tissue or, in the absence of malignant cells, the patient's own nipple is sometimes banked on her inner thigh or inguinal area and salvaged at the appropriate time for reimplanting (Fig. 36-10). The nipple may become blackened in color in the immediate postoperative period, but this will fade. Drains are inserted into the surgical site for 2 to 3 days to prevent hematoma.

Nursing care

1. Monitor drainage for amount, color, and odor.
2. Monitor body temperature for presence of infection.
3. Change dressing only if prescribed; dressings over nipple grafting are left intact for 7 to 10 days.
4. Have patient wear a brassiere continuously to maintain implant position and alignment.
5. Encourage only prescribed activity and exercises; shoulder and arm movements may be restricted.

The American Cancer Society is adding a program on breast reconstruction to their rehabilitation visitation program, Reach to Recovery. It entails volunteers who have themselves had reconstruction because of cancer. This is an additional resource for patients and professionals.

RADIATION THERAPY

Radiation therapy may be performed, as primary therapy or following surgery, by external beam therapy or by interstitial therapy.

External beam therapy

External beam therapy is performed on an outpatient basis. Treatments are usually given daily for approximately 5 weeks. The patient may require assistance in transportation and can be made aware of the American Cancer Society Transportation Program.

The woman receiving external beam therapy will have an extended period of fatigue and depression from the catabolism and loss of breast tissue. In addition, she may experience nausea, heartburn from transient esophagitis, and cough from transient pneumonitis.

The patient needs the same considerations, emotional support, and teaching as she would have with surgery as primary therapy. A malignancy is present in her breast; it threatens her. Her breast may or may not ever look the same; it will not feel the same; she will mourn. All the teaching and precautions for lymphedema pertain to the patient receiving external beam therapy.

Interstitial therapy

Iridium (^{192}Ir) needles are implanted in the breast with the patient under general anesthesia. The patient is placed in a single room and experiences little discomfort after the implantation. Ambulation within the room is permitted. Radiation precautions of internal therapy (Chapter 14) are followed. The needles are removed by the physician after 3 days, and the patient is discharged. The patient's needs are similar to those of patients receiving other internal radiation therapy.

ADJUVANT THERAPY

There are many combination therapies given to women with breast malignancies. Since many of the therapy protocols are under study by regional cancer research groups, the specific cytotoxic agent or agents and dosage in chemotherapy or hormonal therapy may vary in different parts of the country. In general, chemotherapy may be given after surgery or after primary radiation therapy, or there may be a combination of all three modes of therapy. Hormonal therapy may also be used. Tamoxifen (an antiestrogen) has been found useful for some postmenopausal women whose tumors are estrogen dependent.

EVALUATION

Questions to be considered for women who have received therapy for cancer of the breast may include the following:

1. Has she had an opportunity to discuss her feelings and to begin to deal with her change in body image?
2. Has she identified support persons to turn to when she feels depressed?
3. Does she know the exercises that are to be continued at home?

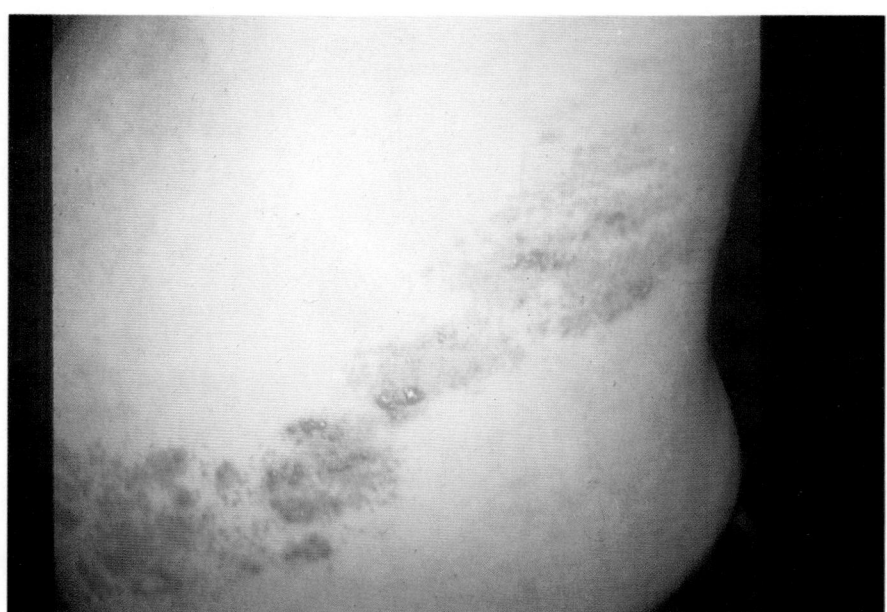

Plate 1. Herpes zoster. (Courtesy David Bickers, M.D., Cleveland, Ohio.)

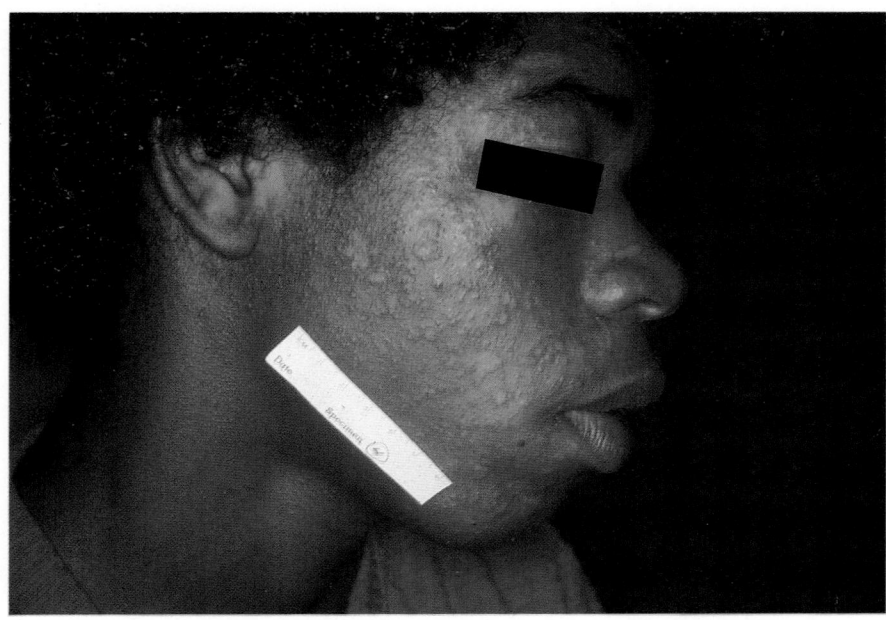

Plate 2. Contact dermatitis from hair preparations. (Courtesy David Bickers, M.D., Cleveland, Ohio.)

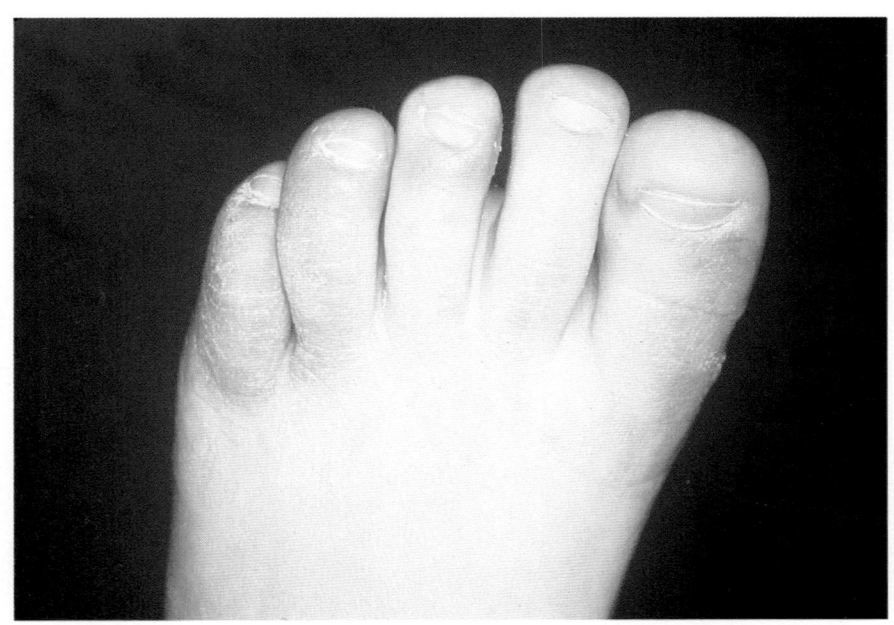

Plate 3. Dermatitis from shoes. (Courtesy David Bickers, M.D., Cleveland, Ohio.)

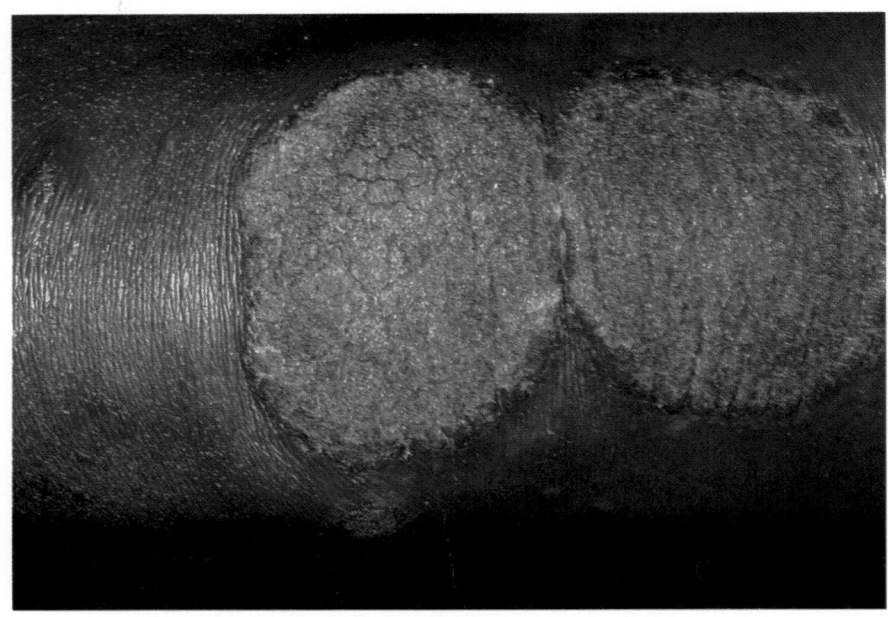

Plate 4. Scaling lesions of psoriasis. (Courtesy David Bickers, M.D., Cleveland, Ohio.)

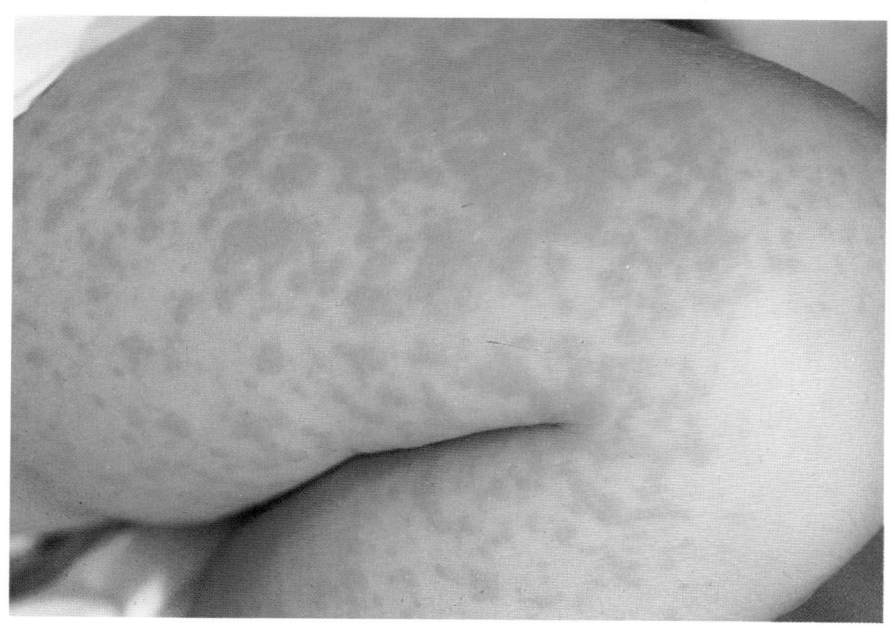

Plate 5. Maculopapular rash resulting from a drug allergy. (Courtesy David Bickers, M.D., Cleveland, Ohio.)

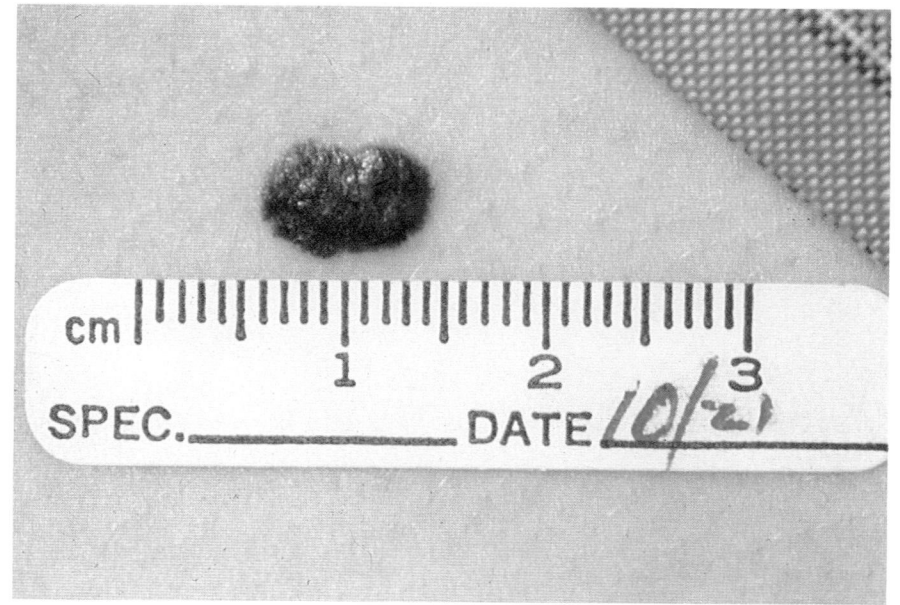

Plate 6. Malignant melanoma. (Courtesy David Bickers, M.D., Cleveland, Ohio.)

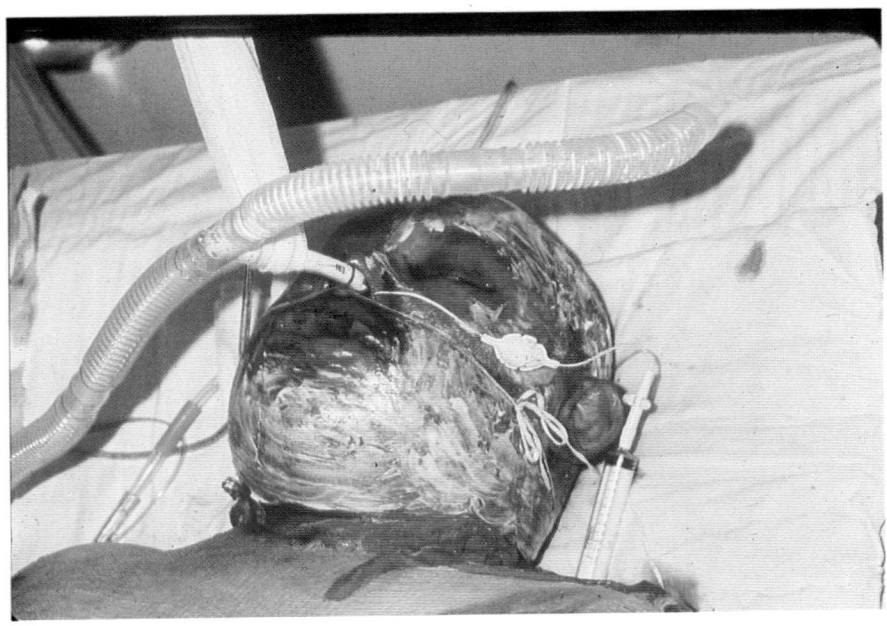

Plate 7. Endotracheal intubation for patient with severe edema 5 hours post-burn. (Courtesy Burn Center, Cleveland Metropolitan General Hospital.)

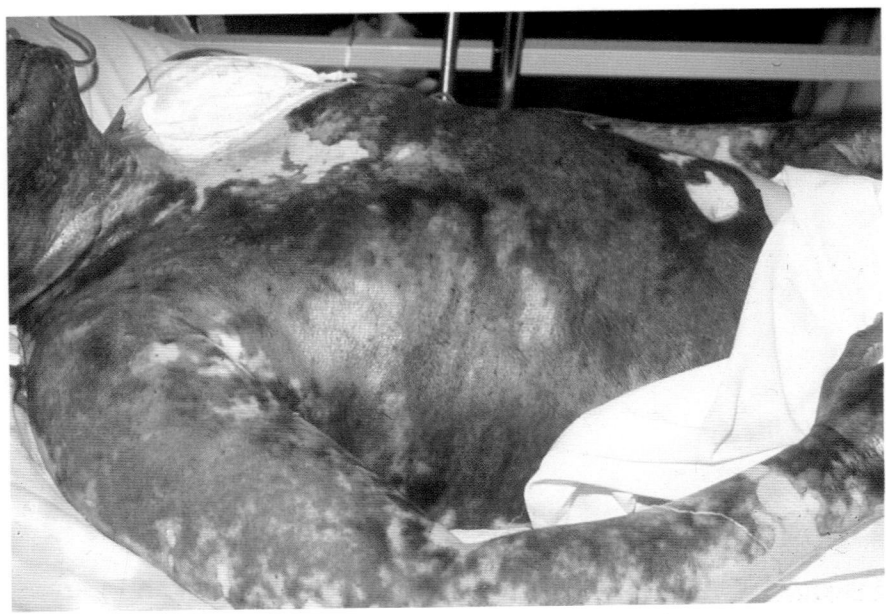

Plate 8. Postburn *Pseudomonas* infection (Courtesy Burn Center, Cleveland Metropolitan General Hospital.)

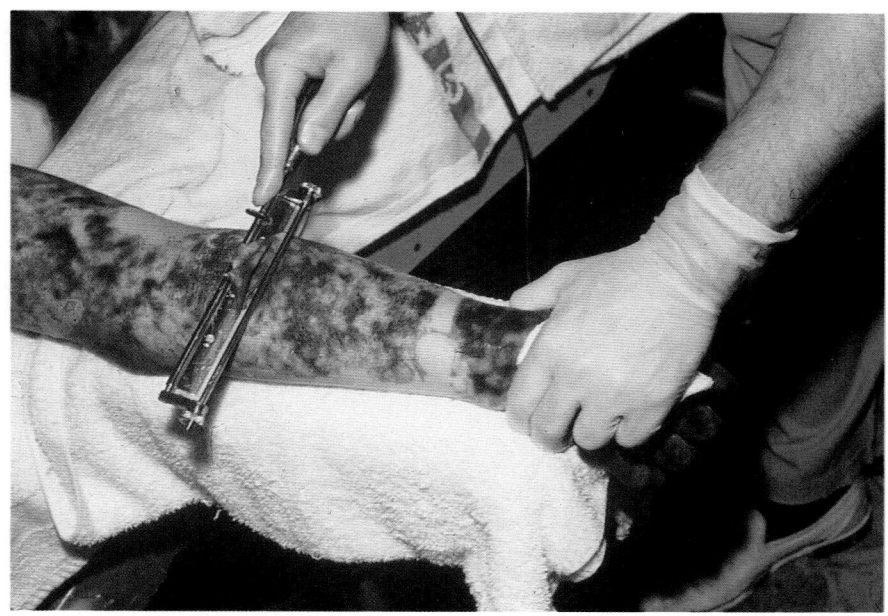

Plate 9. Debridement of a burn (Courtesy Burn Center, Cleveland Metropolitan General Hospital.)

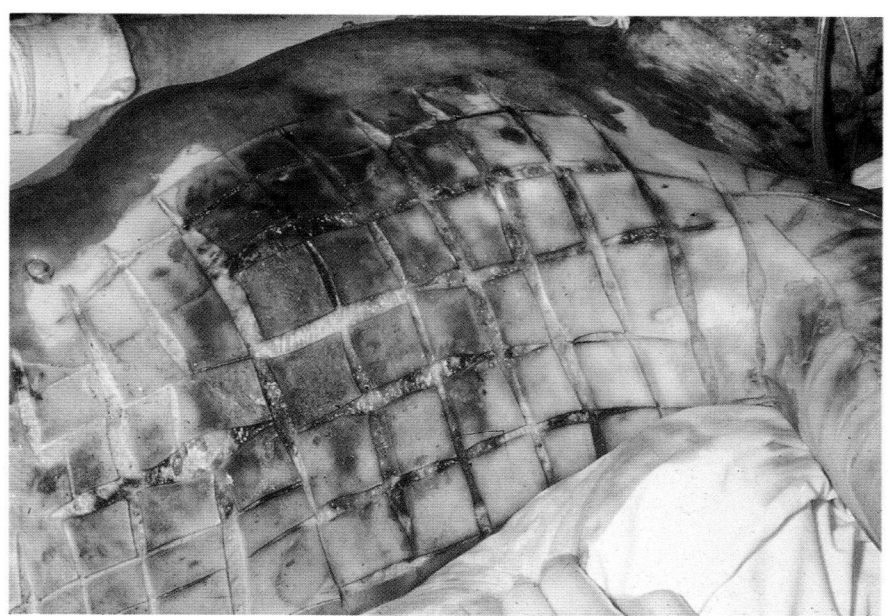

Plate 10. Grid escharotomy used to alleviate circulatory and pulmonary constriction. (Courtesy Burn Center, Cleveland Metropolitan General Hospital.)

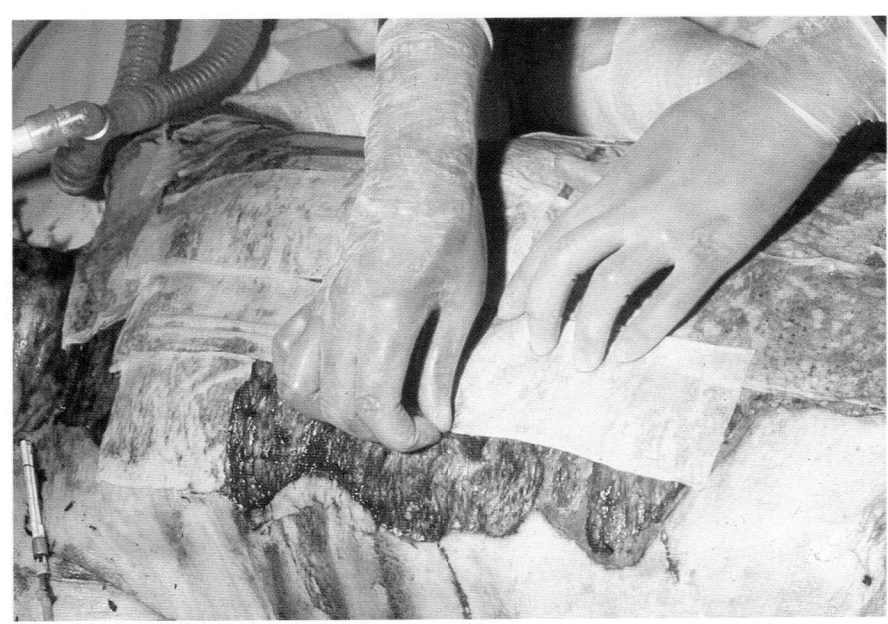

Plate 11. Application of a pigskin graft. (Courtesy Burn Center, Cleveland Metropolitan General Hospital.)

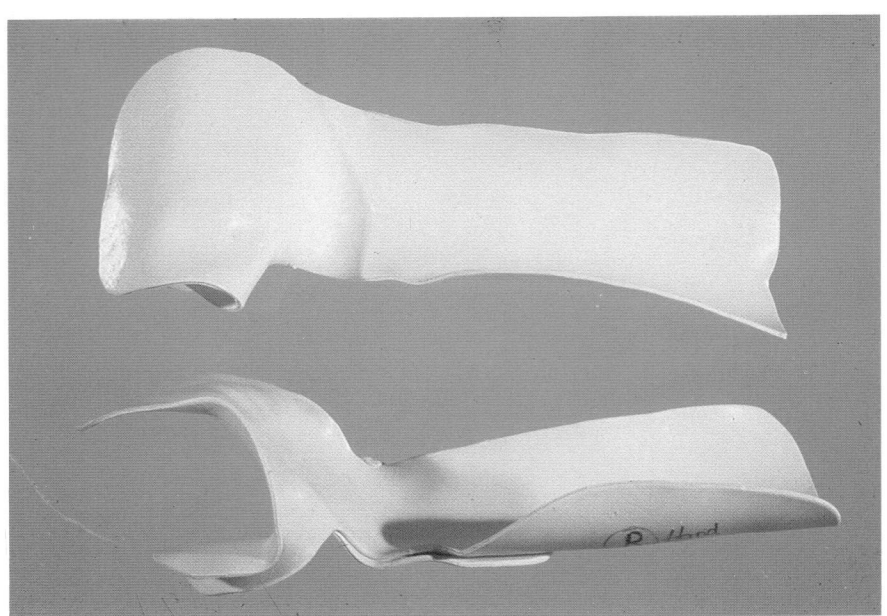

Plate 12. Hand splints for burns. (Courtesy Burn Center, Cleveland Metropolitan General Hospital.)

UNIT XI
Problems of Physiologic Defense Mechanisms

37   The Patient with Dermatologic Problems

38   The Patient with Burns

39   The Patient with Immunologic Problems

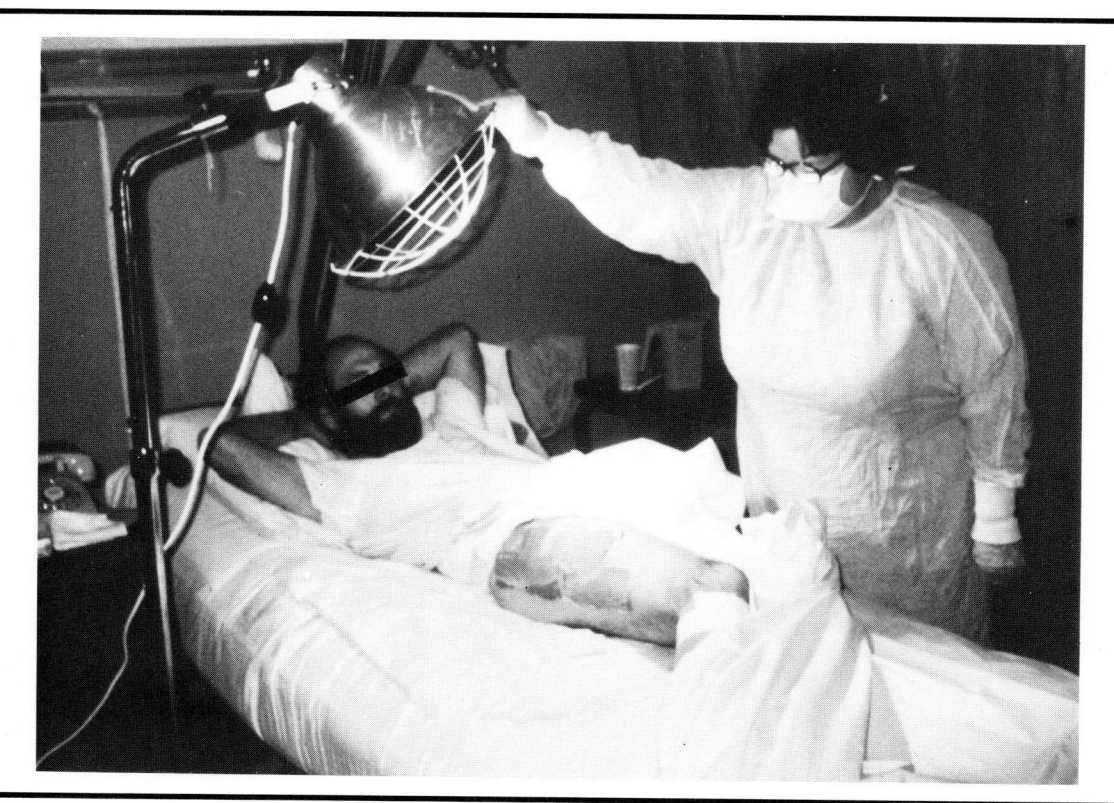

37

The Patient with Dermatologic Problems

BARBARA C. LONG

STUDY QUESTIONS

- Review the anatomy and physiology of the skin.

- Review assessment of the skin (see Chapter 3).

- Examine the skin of three of your patients. How do they differ? Describe any lesions in terms of color, shape, size (be specific), and distribution.

- Imagine that you have many scaly lesions over your face and arms. What changes do you think might occur in your life? How would you feel about these changes?

- You are a school nurse in an affluent community. You have discovered that several children have pediculosis (lice). Discuss with your classmates (1) problems that you might expect and (2) approaches you could use that would be most effective in eradicating the pediculosis.

- Go to a drugstore and examine the products advertised for psoriasis. Estimate the yearly cost of using some of these drugs on a regular basis.

The skin is the largest organ of the body. It is exposed to the external environment and provides the first line of defense of the body, yet at the same time it is affected by changes in the internal environment. General health maintenance requires maintenance of healthy skin. Skin changes may result from environmental changes (such as heat and cold, sunlight, and lack of moisture), from systemic disorders, and from disorders of the skin itself. In this chapter are discussed the major health problems of the skin and surgical correction of impairments of the skin and underlying tissue (plastic surgery). General assessment of the skin is discussed in Chapter 3.

ANATOMY AND PHYSIOLOGY

Anatomy

The skin is composed of two main layers, the epidermis and the dermis. The *epidermis* is composed of two parts, a thin layer of closely packed dead squamous cells covering a second layer of cells containing melanin, which gives skin its color. The dead cells are constantly being shed and replaced by deeper cells. Blood vessels do not reach into the epidermis (Fig. 37-1).

The second main layer, the *dermis,* is composed of bundles of collagen fibers that act to support the epidermis. It is well supplied with nerves and blood vessels and contains the sweat glands, sebaceous glands, and hair follicles.

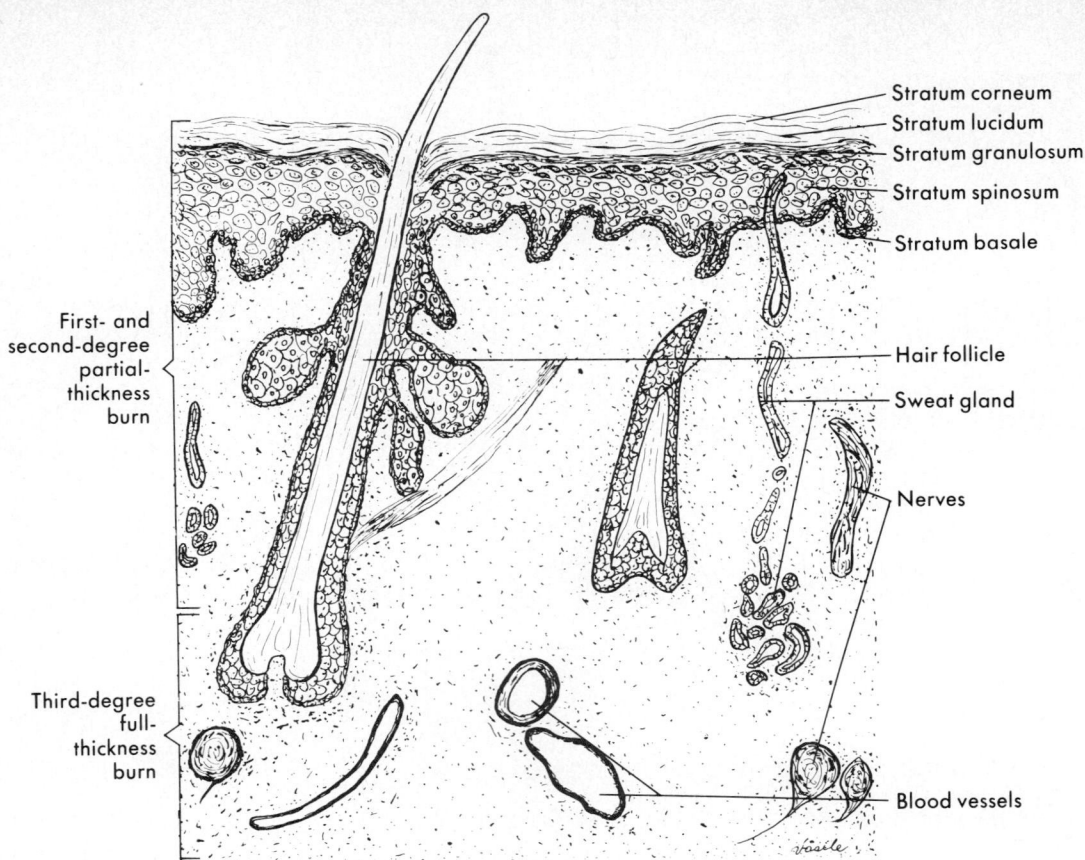

Fig. 37-1. Microscopic view of skin in longitudinal section.

The labels in the figure are:

Stratum corneum
Stratum lucidum
Stratum granulosum
Stratum spinosum
Stratum basale

First- and second-degree partial-thickness burn

Third-degree full-thickness burn

Hair follicle
Sweat gland
Nerves
Blood vessels

Functions of the skin

Protection from environment: pathogenic organisms, foreign substances, heat, rays

Heat regulation

  Conduction: transfer of heat by direct contact to other objects or air

  Convection: removal of heat by air currents on skin

  Evaporation: removal of heat by water loss from skin surface

Sensory perception: sensory receptors in skin

Excretion: removal of water and electrolytes

Production of vitamin D: effect of sunlight

Expression: communication of feelings

Below the dermis is the subcutaneous tissue, consisting of loose connective tissue and fat. It is loosely attached to underlying structures in most body areas.

Physiology

The skin has numerous functions. Fat-soluble substances can penetrate the skin by passing through the hair follicles and sebaceous glands. Atrophic or senile skin contains fewer hair follicles; thus permeability of fat-soluble substances through the skin is decreased in the elderly.

The epidermis can be weakened by scraping or stripping the surface, such as by dry razors or by removal of tape. Once the barrier has weakened, permeability to substances such as bacteria or drugs is increased. Large amounts of drugs can be absorbed by extensive denuded skin areas. Epidermis that becomes overdry may crack and lead to breaks in the surface. If it remains wet for long periods it becomes macerated and the moisture provides a medium for bacterial growth.

Blood vessels of the skin assist in control of body temperature by constriction in cold environments to promote conservation of heat and by dilation in warm environments to promote loss of heat by radiation. These mechanisms help maintain a constant internal body temperature.

Skin changes with aging

As people grow older changes occur in the skin and hair (Table 37-1) that make differentiating normal from abnormal changes more difficult. The changes result primarily from loss of subcutaneous tissue, degeneration of collagen and elastic fibers, loss of melanocytes, increased capillary fragility, decreased secretion of sweat glands, hormonal changes, and overexposure to environmental elements. The skin wrinkles and becomes looser, and spotty pigmentation develops on sun-exposed areas.

The elderly person is also more likely to have one or

Table 37-1. Normal skin and hair changes seen in elderly persons

Assessment parameters	Changes caused by aging
Skin	
Color	Hyperpigmentation in exposed areas
	Hypopigmented areas
Moisture	Dry skin (sometimes scaly)
	Decreased perspiration
Elasticity, turgor	Decreased elasticity
	Loose folds
	Decreased turgor
Texture	Some rough areas
	Thinner, more transparent skin
Lesions	Skin tags on face and neck
	Seborrheic keratoses
	Senile angiomas
	Stasis dermatitis
	Bruises (capillary fragility)
Hair	
Consistency	Thinner on head and body
	More bristly on face, in nose
Distribution	Loss of hair on head and body
	Increased hair on face

more chronic diseases and to be taking medications that can cause skin changes. Dry skin may cause itching and may lead to skin breakdown if scratched. Toenails become thicker and difficult to trim; fingernails become more brittle and develop longitudinal ridges. Body hair changes in consistency and distribution.

PSYCHOLOGIC EFFECTS OF DERMATOLOGIC PROBLEMS

There is a certain degree of "beauty orientation" in Western culture. Cosmetics to enhance good looks are extensively used by men and women. It is no wonder that skin diseases or physical defects that detract from "good looks" produce psychologic reactions.

A person's emotional reaction to a deformity or defect must not be underestimated. Pride in oneself, the ability to think well of oneself and to regard oneself favorably in comparison with others are essential to the development and maintenance of a well-integrated personality. Every person with a defect or handicap, particularly if it is conspicuous to others, suffers some threat to emotional security. The extent of the emotional reaction and the amount of maladjustment that follow depend on the individual's makeup and ability to cope with emotional insults. It is not unusual for the individual to withdraw from a society that is unkind. The defect may be used to justify failure to assume responsibility or to justify striking out against an unkind society.

Prevention of skin disorders

Maintenance of healthy skin
1. Avoid strong or harsh soaps or detergents.
2. Keep skin well hydrated; apply lubricating lotion or cream to dry areas after soaking in tub.
3. Avoid scraping or stripping skin surface by dry razors or removal of tape.
4. Dry damp areas (such as between toes) well to prevent maceration of skin.
5. Wear loose clothing on hot days to permit loss of heat by evaporation.

Avoidance of causative agents
1. Avoid agents that cause skin disorders in most persons, for example, poision ivy, excessive sunlight.
2. Avoid specific agents known to cause a skin disorder in self.
3. Use protective skin lotions when exposed to excessive sunlight.

Observation of skin changes
1. Note and report changes in size, color, or general appearance of pigmented skin areas, particularly moles.
2. Note and report changes in size and appearance of existing skin lesions.

Avoidance of self-treatment
1. Do not use previously prescribed prescriptions on new and different skin lesions.
2. Seek medical advice when skin conditions develop.

Skin diseases that produce marked disfigurement of visible body surfaces can therefore result in alterations in body image. Feelings of decreased worth by persons with large draining lesions or with severe disfigurement are reinforced during interactions with others. Some people are repelled by the sight of severe skin diseases, or may experience a threat to their own body integrity and physically withdraw to avoid interaction. Some persons may experience nonverbal messages of disgust when others view their disfigurement for the first time. This is markedly poignant when those nonverbal messages are sent by significant others or by health professionals.

In working with the person with severe skin disease the nurse first examines his/her own feelings that could be expressed nonverbally in a negative manner. The patient and family are assisted to cope with their feelings.

PREVENTION AND HEALTH EDUCATION

Prevention of dermatologic conditions not only relieves the patient of discomfort but is cost effective because many skin conditions are chronic. In addition, maintenance of intact healthy skin has a positive effect on a person's well-being. Prevention of dermatologic conditions includes maintenance of healthy skin, avoidance of causative agents (when possible), observations of skin changes, and avoidance of self-treatment.

Major health problems of the skin

There are numerous types of skin conditions, many of which occur only rarely. Some of the more common skin conditions discussed include the following:
1. Inflammatory skin conditions
   a. Bacterial infections: folliculitis, furuncles, and carbuncles
   b. Viral inflammations: herpes simplex, herpes zoster, warts
   c. Fungal inflammations: candidiasis, dermatophytoses
   d. Parasitic infestations: pediculosis, scabies
2. Dermatitis: contact, atropic, or stasis
3. Scaling papular disorders: psoriasis, pityriasis rosea, lichen planus
4. Tumors of the skin: keratoses, hemangiomas, premalignant lesions, malignant lesions
5. Skin disorders in blacks

INFLAMMATORY SKIN DISORDERS
TYPES OF INFLAMMATORY SKIN DISORDERS

The skin may become inflamed from bacteria, viruses, or fungi or by parastic infestation.

Bacterial skin infections

Most bacteria that normally inhabit the skin are nonpathogenic. Pathogenic bacteria that penetrate the outer skin layer may cause a superficial skin infection or superficial folliculitis or they may penetrate deeper, causing a deep folliculitis or a furuncle (Table 37-2).

Superficial folliculitis occurs most often with uncleanliness, maceration, exposure to oils and solvents, traction on the hair from tar therapy, or occlusion therapy. Furuncles and carbuncles occur most often in obese, poorly nourished, fatigued, or otherwise susceptible persons with poor hygiene, in debilitated elderly people, and in persons with inadequately treated diabetes mellitus.

Viral skin inflammations

Viruses may cause either simple or more serious skin inflammations (Table 37-3). One of the most common viruses found in humans is the *herpes simplex* virus (HSV). It occurs as two similar yet serologically different strands, type 1 and type 2. The type 1 virus is found primarily in lesions of the face and mouth (fever blister, cold sore), eye (keratitis), and brain (encephalitis). Type 2 is associated with lesions of the genitalia that can be transmitted by sexual contact (see Chapter 35). Factors that may precipitate recurrence of herpes simplex lesions include fever, upper respiratory tract infection, exhaustion, and stress. Lesions are also more common during the menses or after direct exposure to the sun's rays.

Herpes zoster (see Plate 1, following p. 1102) is caused by the same virus (V-Z) that causes varicella (chickenpox). Varicella is believed to be the primary infection in a nonimmune host, whereas herpes zoster is thought to be the response in a partially immune host. Although herpes zoster is far less communicable than chickenpox, persons who have not had chickenpox may develop it after exposure to the vesicular lesions of persons with herpes zoster. For this reason, susceptible persons should not care for patients with herpes zoster.

Herpes zoster can be serious in any adult and may even lead to death from exhaustion in elderly debilitated persons. It is one of the most drawn out and exasperating conditions found in elderly patients and leads to discour-

Table 37-2. Bacterial skin infections

Type	Description	Signs and symptoms	Medical therapy
Folliculitis	Infections of the hair follicles, primarily by *Staphylococcus;* occurs frequently after tar or occlusive therapy	Itching of hairy areas, pustules in hair follicles; abscess may develop	Saline or Burow's solution soaks; topical antibiotics
Furuncles (boil)	Deep folliculitis or nodule around hair follicle	Local swelling and redness; severe local pain; core turns yellow and "points" in 3 to 5 days; may rupture spontaneously	Systemic antibiotics; hot moist compresses (discontinued when drainage starts); incision and drainage (I & D); topical antibiotics after I & D
Carbuncle	Cluster of furuncles		
Cellulitis	Diffuse spreading infection of skin and subcutaneous tissue, usually resulting from cocci	Area is red, warm, swollen, painful with poorly defined borders; fever, malaise, leukocytosis	Hot moist dressings; systemic antibiotics; rest

agement and demoralization. Contrary to popular thought, one episode of herpes zoster does *not* provide immunity, and the disease may recur.[35] Herpes zoster often occurs in persons with Hodgkin's disease and in those with lymphoid and some bone cancers, because of reduced cell-mediated immunity.

Fungal inflammations

Fungi are larger and more complex than bacteria. They may be unicellular, such as yeast, or multicellular, such as molds. Fungi may cause common skin disorders (Table 37-4).

Yeasts thrive in warm, moist environments such as the

Table 37-3. Viral skin inflammations

Type	Description	Signs and symptoms	Medical therapy
Herpes simplex (fever blister, cold sore)	Infection by herpes simplex virus; may occur anywhere but seen primarily on lips, mouth, genitalia	Initial burning and itching; appearance of painful, small, grouped vesicles; crust forms, healing within 10 to 14 days	Primarily symptomatic; early application of 70% alcohol or moistened styptic pencil may help; analgesics
Herpes zoster (shingles)	Acute vesicular eruption by the V-Z virus along a nerve pathway	Cluster of skin vesicles along course of peripheral sensory nerves; usually one side, primarily on thorax or face; crust develops and drops off in 10 to 14 days; pain, malaise, fever, itching; neuralgic pain may persist	Primarily symptomatic; relief of pain, rest; calamine lotion for itching Postherpetic neuralgia: tranquilizers, vitamin E
Warts (verruca)	Benign growths from a viral infection; plantar warts on soles of feet grow inward; anogenital warts have a cauliflower appearance	Small, circumscribed, painless, hyperkeratotic papules, usually on hands, may disappear spontaneously; pain with plantar warts; itching with anogenital warts	Removal by electrodessication or cryosurgery

Table 37-4. Fungal skin inflammations

Type	Description	Signs and symptoms	Medical therapy
Candidiasis	Overgrowth of yeastlike fungus, primarily in mouth and vagina	Mouth: white spots like milk curd Vagina: cheesy discharge, itching	Oral griseofulvin, antifungal powder for vaginal infection
Dermatophytoses			
Tinea capitis	Fungal infection of scalp (ringworm of scalp)	Round lesion with erythema, slight scaling and some pustules around edge; temporary alopecia	Antifungal medication by shampoo or topical application
Tinea corporis	Fungal infection of non-hairy parts of body (ringworm of body)	Flat lesions with clear centers and red borders	Oral griseofulvin and topical application of antifungal medication
Tinea cruris	Fungal infection of groin (jock itch)	Brown to red lesion extending outward from groin, itching	Same as for tinea corporis
Tinea pedis (athlete's foot)	Fungal infection between and under toes	Cracks between toes, maceration, vesicular lesions; toenails may become thickened and discolored	Oral griseofulvin for weeks or months, antifungal topical medication

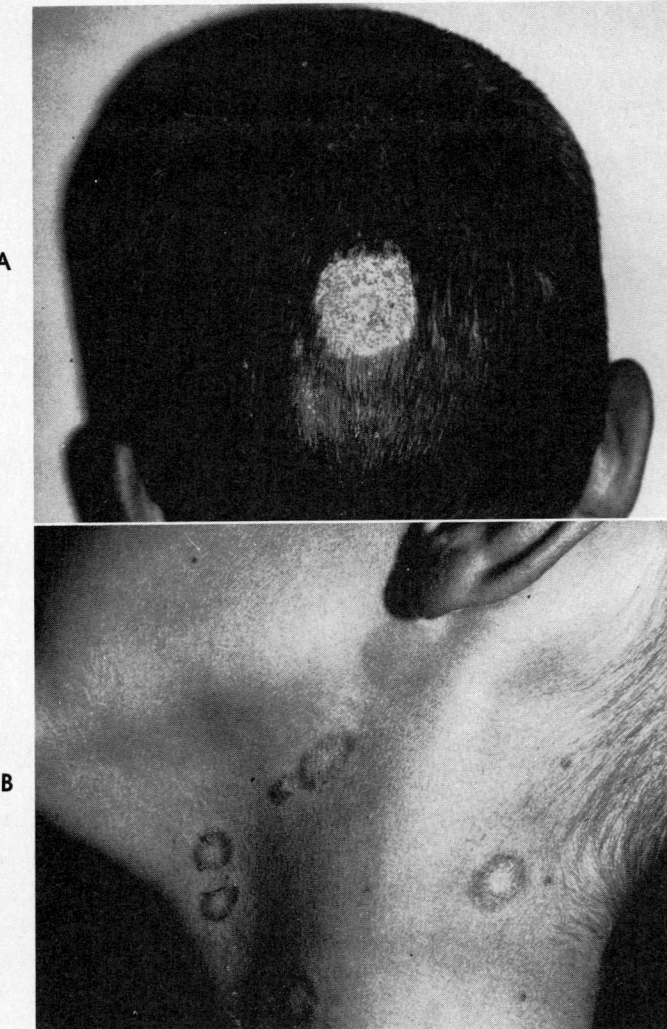

Fig. 37-2. **A,** Tinea capitis. **B,** Tinea corporis. (From Stewart, W.D., Danto, J.L., and Maddin, S.: Dermatology; diagnosis and treatment of cutaneous disorders, ed. 4, St. Louis, 1978, The C.V. Mosby Co.)

mouth and vagina. Problems occur when there is an overgrowth, commonly occurring with pregnancy, use of oral contraceptives, poor nutrition, antibiotic therapy, diabetes mellitus, other endocrine diseases, and immunosuppressed conditions.

The more common fungal infections are the dermatophytoses (tinea). Tinea *capitis* (Fig. 37-2) (inappropriately called ringworm of the scalp) is transmitted readily under crowded conditions where poor hygiene exists. Minor scalp trauma facilitates implantation of the spores; hence the infection can be spread by contaminated barber's instruments, combs, or sharp brushes. Tinea *cruris* (jock itch) occurs frequently in men, especially those who have tinea pedis and those who frequently wear athletic supporters or tight shorts, but it is being seen more frequently in women who wear tight pantyhose or slacks.

The most common dermatophytosis is tinea *pedis,* or

Facts about athlete's foot

1. It is seen mostly in young men.
2. Walking barefoot in gymnasiums or around swimming pools does not necessarily lead to infection.
3. Prophylactic foot baths are ineffective.
4. Wearing white socks does not affect the course of infection.
5. Susceptible persons will acquire athlete's foot regardless of their activities.

---

athlete's foot. There are many misconceptions about prevention and treatment of athlete's foot. It is often confused with other foot eruptions, such as contact dermatitis, psoriasis, or simple intertrigo (chronic bacterial infection of the areas between the toes, or intertriginous areas). Factors that may lessen infection include wearing sandal-type shoes or going barefoot (to decrease tissue moisture) and using good foot hygiene including washing the feet frequently and drying well between the toes.

Parasitic infestations

Parasites may live on the body or clothing (lice) or burrow under the skin (itch mite), causing inflammations of the skin (Table 37-5).

Lice obtain their nutrition by sucking blood from the skin. They leave their eggs on the skin surface attached to hair shafts, and this results in the transference from person to person. Control and treatment of pediculosis (lice infestation) can be hampered by persons of all incomes who refuse to admit that the lice exist among their family members.

Scabies is highly prevalent during periods of overcrowding, such as that seen in Europe during World War II or in other war-torn areas. During the 1950s and 1960s the incidence of scabies decreased, but during the 1970s there was a rise in the incidence of scabies worldwide. The reason for the pandemic is unknown and is thought to be multifactorial, including poverty, sexual promiscuity, increased worldwide travel, and ecologic changes.[15]

The itch mite penetrates the skin and lays eggs; the larvae mature in 10 days and move to the skin surface, where the female is impregnated; then the cycle is repeated. The incubation period varies, but often a long period elapses before symptoms are noted. Scabies occurs among all age groups and socioeconomic levels.

ASSESSMENT

Subjective data from persons with inflammations of the skin are centered on the extent of *itching* and *pain.* Data are collected concerning the site, intensity, duration, and methods found to be helpful in alleviation of the discomfort. Data are also collected concerning the person's

Table 37-5. Parasitic infestations

Type	Description	Signs and symptoms	Medical therapy
Pediculosis			
Head lice	Attach to hair shaft and lays eggs (nits); transmitted by direct contact	Itching of scalp, excoriation of skin, and secondary infection from scratching	Topical application of gamma benzene hydrochloride (Kwell) by shampoo, lotion, or cream; combing with fine-toothed comb to remove nits
Body lice	Found in seams of underclothing; transmitted by direct contact, clothing, linens	Same as for head lice	Topical application of gamma benzene hydrochloride by lotion or cream
Pubic lice	Resembles a tiny crab; nits are visible in pubic hair; transmitted by sexual contact, bed linen, towels	Same as for head lice	Same as for body lice
Scabies	Female itch mite burrows under skin and lays eggs; transmitted by prolonged contact	Severe itching; wavy brownish, threadlike lines seen mostly on hands, arms, and body folds and genitalia; secondary infections	Scabicides

Table 37-6. Comparison of vehicles for topical medications

Type	Base	Effect
Powder	Dry	Drying by absorbing moisture; cooling by evaporating moisture
Lotion	Powder suspended in water or oil	Protective, cleansing, cooling, antipruritic effect depending on drug and base used
Creams and ointments	Emulsions of oil and water	Occlusive covering over skin to prolong contact of medication with skin, good skin penetration; warming effect
Paste	≥50% powder in ointment base	Holds medication for longer period of time with slower skin penetration

knowledge of the type of infection, measures to control spread, and prescribed treatments to be carried out at home.

The skin is routinely assessed during physical inspection and whenever there is patient contact, such as while providing hygiene care, comfort measures, or prescribed treatments. Changes in previous lesions or occurrence of new lesions are reported.

DATA ANALYSIS AND PLANNING

Nursing diagnoses

Nursing diagnoses for the person with a skin inflammation may include the following:
Alteration in comfort: itching
Alteration in comfort: pain
Knowledge deficit.

EXPECTED PATIENT OUTCOMES

1. The patient states feeling comfortable
2. The patient can describe:
   a. Measures to prevent spread
   b. Prescribed treatment measures
   c. Plans for medical follow-up for severe inflammatory disorders.

IMPLEMENTATION

Assisting with achievement of therapeutic goals
Topical medications

Topical medications can be prepared in a variety of bases (Table 37-6). *Powders* are effective in reducing friction and moisture in intertriginous areas. They are first sprinkled into the hand, then applied to the skin to avoid releasing excess powder into the air and causing irritation to the mucous membrane. Powders are used sparingly to prevent caking and are not used on wet surfaces because this leads to caking. Cornstarch is *not* suggested, because it encourages growth of yeast, bacteria, and fungi.[20]

Lotions must be shaken well because the insoluble powder may settle out. Lotions with a water or alcohol base are applied by patting gently. (Alcohol increases the cooling effect of the lotion.) A gauze pledget may be used to apply extremely thin lotions. Lotions with an oily base are applied thinly and evenly with the palm of the hand. A small area of skin is often tested to determine whether the cream or lotion will be tolerated over the entire body. The topical medication is applied to a small area (silver dollar size) on the person's forearm. The time and exact location of the trial are recorded, and the skin response to the trial medication is observed after 24 hours.

Ointments do not usually leave an oily residue on the skin unless they have a petrolatum base. A nonporous covering such as plastic should not be used over an ointment unless so prescribed, because the heat retention may increase percutaneous absorption of the medication.

Ointments may be applied with gloved hands or with the bare palm, depending on the type of ointment used. If a dressing is to be applied, the ointment may be spread on the dressing with a tongue blade before application to the skin. Anthralin may be caustic to normal skin, so gloves should be worn. Crude coal tar is always applied in firm, long, downward strokes to prevent folliculitis, because tar is an irritant. Creams, as opposed to ointments, may be rubbed in.

Wet dermatologic dressings

Wet dressings are used frequently over various lesions for cooling, drying, antipruritic, vasoconstricting, or debriding effects. Plain tap water or physiologic saline solution may be used or medications may be added. An as-tringent effect may be obtained with the use of Burow's solution.

The type of dressing material used for a wet dressing should not have a cotton filling, because cotton leaves particles and a residue on the skin, which may cause irritation. Several layers of fine mesh gauze are ideal, and roller gauze or Kerlix may be used for extremities. A face mask may be designed by cutting openings for the eyes, nose, and mouth from several thicknesses of gauze. At home, muslin-type cotton material such as clean old sheets may be used; the materials need not be sterilized but are washed or discarded every 24 hours.

The best effects of wet dressings are obtained by several treatment periods spaced over the waking hours. The solution is applied at room temperature to prevent the marked vasoconstriction with subsequent vasodilation that occurs with cold solutions. Although the dressings can be kept wet by adding solution with the dressings in place, this usually leads to excessive dripping.

Promoting comfort

Pain with skin inflammations is usually minimal except in selected situations such as herpes zoster. In general, aspirin or acetaminophen usually suffice as analgesics, and the application of wet dressings and topical medications usually relieves most discomfort from pain.

Relief of pruritus

Pruritus (itching) is a major discomfort, to one extent or another, with skin inflammations.

PATHOPHYSIOLOGY OF PRURITUS. Pruritus is a cutaneous symptom that provokes the desire to scratch and is an underlying symptom of many disorders. It is a modified form of pain but is less tolerable. It occurs only in the skin, certain mucous membranes, and the eyes. The areas most sensitive to itching are the nostrils, mucocutaneous junction, external ear canal, and perineum.

One of the most common causes of pruritus is dry skin, sometimes occurring as a result of excessive bathing, particularly with bubble bath, which has a drying effect.

Application of dermatologic wet dressings

1. Prepare solution to apply at room temperature. Sterility is not required.
2. Soak dressing thoroughly in solution.
3. Protect bed or clothing with towel or bath blanket.
4. Wring out dressing (should be wet but not dripping).
5. Apply dressings in smooth layers (two to four layers); wrap fingers and toes separately; wrap joints so that they can bend.
6. Remove, soak, and reapply dressings every 3 to 5 minutes.
7. Continue treatment for 20 to 30 minutes.
8. Pat skin dry.

Common causes of itching

Dry skin
Skin irritants: plastic or glass fibers, wool, plant products
Insects
Drug reactions
Psychogenic reactions
Skin diseases: inflammations, dermatitis
Infectious diseases
Systemic diseases: obstructive biliary disease, uremia, diabetes mellitus
Neoplasia: Hodgkin's disease, leukemia, lymphoma

Factors that can intensify itching include vasodilation, tissue anoxia, and stasis of circulation.

Pruritus leads to the motor response of scratching. Persons with very intense itching may excoriate the skin severely by digging deeply into the skin with their fingernails when trying to alleviate the itch. Persons with generalized itching may be observed to be in almost constant motion—twisting, rubbing, and scratching.

GENERAL MEASURES FOR RELIEF OF PRURITUS

1. Apply cold to cause vasoconstriction.
2. Avoid soaps and detergents with dry skin; use a bath oil.
3. Hydrate in a tepid bath followed by application of an emollient lotion.
4. Use cool, light, nonrestrictive clothing or bedclothes.
5. Keep nails trimmed to avoid skin excoriation from scratching.

Guidelines for baths and soaks

1. The water temperature should be of comfort to patient (usually 32° to 38° C, or 90° to 100° F).
2. Medication should be completely dissolved while tub is filled.
3. The soak should last 20 to 30 minutes.
4. Persons are assisted out of the water when oils and such are added, to prevent slipping.
5. A rubber mat will help prevent slipping.
6. Skin is *patted* dry, not rubbed, to avoid skin irritation.
7. Creams or ointments are applied immediately after the bath to retain moisture.
8. After a medicated bath pour 1 cup bleach into used tub water; let stand 5 minutes; wipe sides and bottom of tub; drain tub and clean as usual.

---

6. Keep the room cool (about 20° C, or 68° to 70° F) and increase the humidity (30% to 40%).

BATHS AND SOAKS. Tub baths or soaks to a specific part of the body are soothing and antipruritic and are an effective means of rehydrating the skin. Substances may be added to the bath for special therapeutic effects (Table 37-7).

Teaching

Prevention of spread

Bacterial infections and parasitic infestations may spread to other persons, particularly caregivers and family members, if precautions are not instituted.

For *staphylococcal* infections in hospitalized patients, wound isolation procedures are instituted until drainge subsides. Hands must be washed thoroughly after contact with the patient. Gloves are usually worn when changing dressings.

It is not uncommon for entire families to have some type of staphylococcal infection after one member has had a boil. Teaching includes the following:

1. All family members should bathe and shampoo daily with bacteriostatic soap while infection lasts.
2. Razor blades are discarded after use.
3. Separate bath linens are used by each family member.
4. Bath linens are changed daily while infection lasts.
5. Contaminated wound supplies are discarded in two sealed plastic bags.

With *parasitic* infestations, all family members should take one treatment to prevent spread. Clothing, linen, and towels are washed, then dried in an automatic dryer or ironed after line drying, or are dry cleaned. Garments that have been stored for 1 month will not be infested. No special precautions are needed for other objects, because parasites do not live long away from the host.

Self-help skills

Many persons with skin inflammations will be carrying out treatments at home and therefore may need teaching

---

Table 37-7. Preparations commonly used for baths or soaks

Substance	Effect	Suggested actions
Colloids: oatmeal, cornstarch, soybean powder	Antipruritic, drying	Tub surfaces become very slippery; support person to prevent falls
Potassium permanganate	Antifungal, drying, deodorizing	Strain pulverized tablet through cheesecloth to prevent irritation; stains surfaces and linens
Burow's solution (aluminum acetate)	Antibacterial, drying	Commonly used for soaks
Sulfur bath suspension	Antibacterial	Rinse body with tepid water after bath to remove residual sulfur particles
Tar preparations	Antipruritic, moisturizing	Do not use soap with tar baths
Bath oils: Alpha-Keri, Jeri-Bath, Domol	Antipruritic, moisturizing	Tub surfaces may become slippery

about therapeutic measures. Written instructions are more likely to be followed correctly. Points to stress in teaching include:

1. Use medication only as prescribed.
2. Avoid harsh rubbing of the skin.
3. Avoid nonporous covering over dressing unless ordered.
4. Dissolve completely all solid medications added to baths and soaks.
5. Apply lotions and powders in thin layers.
6. Use old clean sheets, if desired, for wet dressings.

EVALUATION

Evaluation is based on expected patient outcomes. Questions to ask may include the following: Is the person comfortable? Does the person know how to care for the lesions at home?

DERMATITIS

Dermatitis, a superficial inflammation of the skin, refers to several different conditions resulting in the same type of lesions (Table 37-8). The term *eczema* is often used synonymously with dermatitis but frequently refers to the chronic type.

PATHOPHYSIOLOGY

Contact dermatitis may result from irritation of the skin from the substance itself (*irritant contact dermatitis*) (Plates 2 and 3, following p. 1102) or from a hypersensitivity immune reaction from contact with a *specific* antigen (*allergic contact dermatitis*) (Table 37-9). The sensitizing allergen may reach the site by direct contact; by indirect contact such as transmission by animals, from one part of the body to the other, by the hands, or on clothing; or by the air such as in smoke.

Summary of nursing care for inflammatory skin disorders

Bacterial infections

1. Cleanse skin well with soap and water or with hexachlorophene.
2. Use wet compresses to apply heat or as a medium for medication (for example, Burow's solution).
3. Apply prescribed antibiotic topical medication.
4. Elevate an extremity with cellulitis.
5. Teach family members how to prevent spread of staphylococcal infections:
   a. Avoidance of contamination from drainage
   b. Cleansing practices
   c. Disposal of contaminated articles.

Viral inflammations

1. Assist with relief of pain and pruritus:
   a. Loose clothing to minimize contact
   b. Analgesics as prescribed
   c. Warm moist compresses
   d. Spirits of camphor or camphorated lip ice to oral lesions of herpes simplex
   e. Neuralgia after herpes zoster:
      (1) Analgesics as prescribed (narcotics are usually avoided
      (2) Tranquilizers and sedatives as prescribed
      (3) Ethyl chloride spray for possible temporary relief
      (4) Other forms of pain relief measures (see Chapter 12) that might be helpful
   f. Calamine lotion over vesicular areas to relieve itching.

Fungal inflammations

1. Promote dryness of affected area:
   a. Area dried well after washing
   b. Powders applied lightly to prevent maceration and caking
   c. Clean loose-fitting clothing for aeration
   d. For athlete's foot, cotton socks, changed at least daily; sandal-type shoes when possible.
2. Promote healing:
   a. Prescribed topical medication
   b. Need for continuation of treatment for prescribed time (may be weeks or months).

Parasitic infestations

1. Wash area well before treatment.
2. Remove nits with a fine-toothed comb.
3. Apply a *thin* layer of prescribed lotion or cream.
4. Shampoo, shower, or bathe thoroughly after 24 hours to remove medication.
5. If eyelashes are involved, remove nits and apply petroleum jelly to smother lice.
6. Give analgesics or antipruritic agents as necessary.
7. Teach prevention of spread to all family members:
   a. Machine wash clothing and bed linens
   b. Dry clothing and linens in dryer or iron after line drying
   c. Dry clean clothing that cannot be washed
   d. Treat all family members if one is infested.

Atopic dermatitis is hereditary hypersensitivity of the skin that lowers the threshold to pruritus so that minor stimuli cause intense itching. Exacerbating factors include sudden changes in temperature or humidity; exercise; psychologic stress; fibers such as wool, fur, or nylon; detergents; and perfumes. There is a marked tendency toward vasoconstriction of superficial blood vessels, and the skin blanches readily. Adults with eczema often have had atopic dermatitis during infancy and adolescence.

Persons with atopic dermatitis are highly susceptible to viral infections, especially herpes, and to bacterial infections such as those caused by *Staphylococcus* or beta hemolytic *Streptococcus*. There is also an increased incidence of fungal infections such as tinea.

Table 37-8. Types of dermatitis

Type	Cause	Signs and symptoms	Medical therapy
Contact	External agents: irritants (mechanical, chemical, biologic) or allergens	Site and pattern of lesions depend on exposure pattern; erythema, local edema, vesicles, then oozing, crusting and scaling; pruritus Chronic: skin becomes brownish and thickened	Weeping uninfected lesions: wet dressings with Burow's solution; topical steroids; systemic antibiotics when infection present
Atopic	Hypersensitivity reaction, hereditary	Pruritus; lesions similar to contact dermatitis; become localized in adults to antecubital and popliteal areas, behind ears, under chin	Same as above
Stasis	Decreased circulation in legs	Skin reddened and edematous, pruritus, infection from excoriations with scratching	Elevation of legs; wet compresses for weeping lesions
Seborrheic (dandruff)	Unknown	Erythematous scaly lesions of scalp, face, ears, chest, or back	Selsun Blue shampoo for scalp; topical steroids for severe lesions

Table 37-9. Common causes of contact dermatitis of different areas

Area	Cause
Face	Cosmetics, hair sprays, hair dyes, airborne contactants
Earlobes	Nickel
Ears	
Pinnae	Photosensitizers
Canals	Medications
Eyelids	Cosmetics, airborne sensitizers, transfer by hands
Nose (bridge)	Metal or plastic spectacle supports
Lips and perioral area	Toothpaste, lipstick
Neck	Perfumes, clothing (especially wool)
Axillae	Deodorants, clothing, perfumes
Scapular area	Nickel in clasps on straps
Breasts	Elastic and other brassiere material
Waist	Elastic
Perianal area	Dibucaine (Nupercaine) and other medications, excessive use of cleansers
Arms and legs	Poison ivy and other plants
Wrists	Nickel, etc. in watchbands
Hands	Detergents and other cleansers, gloves
Feet	Medication for "athlete's foot," shoes

From Moschela, S.L., Pillsbury, D.M., and Hurley, H.J.: Dermatology, Philadelphia, 1975, W.B. Saunders Co.

ASSESSMENT

Subjective data

When acute lesions from contact dermatitis or exacerbation of eczema occur, it is important to identify the causative factors in order to avoid further contacts or to change, if possible, any exacerbating factor. Data to collect initially include the following:

1. Knowledge of causative factors and method of contact
2. Possible contacts with irritants in the home, at work, or during recreational activities
3. History of recurrent infections (possible decreased immune response)
4. New drug prescriptions, especially penicillin or sulfanilamide
5. Increase in stress noted by patient
6. Alleviating factors (physician or self-prescribed)
7. Extent of pruritus and alleviating factors

Objective data

The lesions are inspected daily for changes and presence of infections. Observations are also made concerning the extent of scratching of the lesions by the patient.

Diagnostic tests

Hypersensitivity to specific antigens can be tested in vivo by skin tests or by the use test (Chapter 39). In skin testing, the antigens are administered to the skin either through intradermal, scratch or patch tests, or an allergen may be instilled in the eye.

DATA ANALYSIS AND PLANNING

Nursing diagnoses

Nursing diagnoses for the person with dermatitis may include the following:

Alteration in comfort: itching
Knowledge deficit

Expected patient outcomes

1. The patient states itching is decreased
2. The patient can describe:
   a. Causative agents (if known), source of the agent, and method of control
   b. Measures to prevent further contact
   c. Problems of self-treatment
   d. Treatment measures to be carried out at home

IMPLEMENTATION

Assisting with achievement of therapeutic goals
Promoting healing of lesions

Weeping infected lesions respond rapidly to wet dressings with Burow's solution (p. 1112) for 20 minutes four times daily. Crusts and scales are not removed but are allowed to drop off naturally as the skin heals.

The major form of *topical* therapy consists of corticosteroid cream or ointment. Fluorinated corticosteroids may

---

Teaching for the person with dermatitis

1. Nature of the causative agent (if known) and method of contact; avoidance of agent
2. Avoidance of extremes of heat and cold
3. Avoidance of dry skin:
   a. No harsh soaps and detergents (use a mild soap such as Ivory)
   b. Soak in bath water (oil may be added) for 20 to 30 minutes
   c. Steroid cream directly after bath
4. Avoidance of wool, nylon, or fur fibers on sensitized skin
5. Use of gloves if necessary to handle irritant or allergenic substance
6. Limiting of strenuous exercise, especially in hot weather (leads to itching)
7. Exposure of affected areas to sunlight (improves condition)
8. Dangers of self-treatment (may lead to delay in healing and increase in infected lesions or to increased absorption through denuded skin areas)
9. Avoidance of other persons with infections (for those with atopic dermatitis)

---

be used for localized lesions in adults but are *never used on the face.* An occlusion wrap over the steroid in adults may enhance the steroid effect but may lead to folliculitis. The occlusion wrap consists of a nonpermeable covering, such as plastic wrap, over the dressing; it is only applied when prescribed by the physician.

Promoting comfort

The focus of care is relief of the pruritus in order to break the itch-scratch cycle that leads to lesions and discomfort. Measures to promote relief of itching are described on p. 1113. Application of the wet dressings and topical steroids helps to reduce the itching. Colloidal baths may be helpful. Sedation and tranquilizers are used judiciously to help decrease itching but not induce sleepiness.

Teaching

The more the person knows about the condition and what will affect it, the better the person can prevent further contacts and enhance recovery (see box above).

EVALUATION

Evaluation is based on expected patient outcomes. Questions to ask may include the following: Is itching decreased? Does the person know how to care for the skin at home and how to prevent further recurrence?

Table 37-10. Types of papulosquamous disorders

Type	Characteristic	Signs and symptoms	Medical therapy
Psoriasis	Common hereditary chronic disorder; not infectious or contagious; has periods of exacerbation	Elevated, erythmatous, sharply circumscribed, scaling plaques; occur mostly on scalp, elbows, and knees; mild pruritus; nails become yellowed and pitted	Wet dressings with acute flare ups; topical steroids with occlusive wraps; PUVA therapy; coal tar therapy followed by ultraviolet light
Pityriasis rosea	Common skin disorder in young adults, especially women; not contagious; lasts 6 to 8 weeks, rarely recurs	Starts with single lesion; oval, thin scaly border, yellowish center; multiple lesions appear later; pruritus	Topical steroids; systemic steroids in severe cases
Lichen planus	Common skin disorder; may resolve in 6 to 18 months or become chronic	Shiny flat-topped papules on flexor surfaces of wrists, ankles, trunk, and mucous membranes; severe pruritus; nails become distorted	Topical steroids with occlusive wrap; intralesional or systemic steroids

SCALING PAPULAR DISORDERS

Papulosquamous disorders are characterized by papular lesions with scaling borders. The most common of these is *psoriasis* (Table 37-10). There are no precipitating factors for psoriasis, but some persons may develop exacerbations after climatic changes, stress, trauma, or infection. Pregnant women often see a remission of symptoms.

PATHOPHYSIOLOGY OF PSORIASIS

The turnover time for normal skin is 28 days. After the cells in the basal layer of the skin divide, it normally takes them 14 days to reach the stratum corneum (outer skin layer) and an additional 14 days for the cells to be sloughed off. In psoriasis the time is accelerated to 4 to 7 days. Much of the scaling (see Plate 4, following p. 1102) seen in psoriasis is rapid shedding of the cells; treatment is therefore based on slowing the mitotic activity.

ASSESSMENT

Subjective data include the following:
1. Knowledge about the disease
2. Measures used for control at home
3. Concerns about appearance
4. Usual recreational and social activities.

Objective data include observations regarding changes in the lesions.

DATA ANALYSIS AND PLANNING

Nursing diagnoses

Nursing diagnoses for the person with psoriasis may include the following:

Self-concept, disturbance in: body image
Knowledge deficit

Expected patient outcomes

The patient can describe the following:
1. Nature of the disorder (noncurable, recurrence of symptoms)
2. Problems with self-medication
3. Prescribed treatment program
4. Plans for socialization with others

IMPLEMENTATION

Assisting with achievement of therapeutic goals
Application of occlusive wrap

Occlusive wraps are usually prescribed over topical steroid therapy for psoriasis. Plastic wrap or plastic bags may be used to cover large areas. The bags should not be rapidly flammable. If large areas must be covered for home therapy, a plastic exercise body suit can be worn, particularly for overnight therapy.

Crude tar therapy

Coal tar preparations may be applied as a topical medication, as a bath (Balnetar), or in combination with ultraviolet light (UVA). In the latter case the tar preparation is applied 12 hours before the UVA treatment. Estargel or Fototar are applied to the affected area for 5 minutes, then the excess is removed by patting with tissue to minimize staining. Areas treated with coal tar preparation should be protected from direct sunlight for at least 24 hours after application of the tar product. Folliculitis may result from coal tar therapy.

PUVA therapy

PUVA therapy consists of a combination of orally administered methoxsalen (Psoralen) and long-wave ultraviolet light (UVA), hence the name. Methoxsalen is a photosensitizing agent. The person is exposed to UVA 2 hours after ingestion of the methoxsalen. Some side effects of PUVA therapy include pruritus, erythema, localized blistering, a moderate flare-up of psoriasis, and transient nausea. Because the skin remains photosensitive until methoxsalen is excreted, persons receiving this treatment are warned to avoid exposure to the sun for at least 8 hours after ingestion of the medication.

Counseling and teaching

Because the lesions are commonly found on visible skin areas, persons with psoriasis are faced with a socially disabling disease. They may need help in identifying and coping with their feelings and with changes that may occur in their life-style. Arms and legs can be covered with clothing if the person is sensitive about appearance. Social contacts are encouraged.

Lesions may fade with treatment, only to recur eventually in the same area or elsewhere. The disease is not curable and may wax and wane continuously. Persons who are not aware of this may lose confidence in the physician and seek a quick cure. Because psoriasis is so common and so stubborn in response to treatment, manufacturers of patent remedies find a lucrative field for their products among persons with the disease. Self-treatment may lead to considerable expense for worthless products, increased discomfort, and delay in treatment of acute episodes. Persons with psoriasis are encouraged to consult a dermatologist as needed.

EVALUATION

Evaluation is based on expected patient outcomes. Questions to ask may include the following:

Does the person know the nature of the disease (incurable)?

Does the person plan to follow medical therapy (rather than self-treatment) when exacerbation occurs?

Is the person planning social activities with others?

SKIN REACTIONS FROM SYSTEMIC DISEASES

Changes in the skin may result from systemic conditions, most commonly dermatitis medicamentosa, erythema multiforme, and discoid lupus erythematosus.

Dermatitis medicamentosa

Skin lesions may result from toxic, metabolic, or allergic reactions to drugs (Table 37-11). Many of the reactions are hypersensitivity immune reactions and include fever, malaise, and vasculitis in addition to skin changes. The rash is often bright red, semiconfluent, macular papular (see Plate 5, following p. 1102) generalized, and bilateral. It can appear at any time, but the onset is usually sudden. Hypersensitivity occurs early when previous sensitization has taken place.

Persons are asked when admitted to the hospital if they have any known allergies. For drug allergies, a sticker indicating the drug is placed on every physician's order sheet to alert the physician or nurse not to order or give the drug to the patient. Sudden skin changes in patients receiving medications are brought to the physician's attention.

Teaching of the patient may include the suggestion that the patient wear a Medic-Alert bracelet specifying the drug to which the patient is allergic so that the drug is not administered unknowingly in an emergency situa-

---

Drugs that cause photosensitivity reactions

Antidepressants (tricyclic)
Gentamycin(topical)
Griseofulvin
Nalidixic acid (NegGram)
Phenothiazines
Thiazide diuretics

Table 37-11. Skin reactions to common medications

Reaction	Medication
Erythematous rash	Antibiotics, sulfonamides, thiazide diuretics, barbiturates, phenylbutazone
Purpura (ecchymosis, petechiae)	Thiazides, sulfonamides, barbiturates, anticoagulants
Mucocutaneous lesions (vesicles, bullae, ulcers)	Sulfonamides, penicillin, barbiturates, phenylbutazone
Urticaria	Penicillin, salicylates
Photosensitivity	Phenothiazines, thiazides, tetracycline, griseofulvin, sulfonamides

tion. Persons who are taking drugs that cause photosensitivity reactions are advised to avoid direct exposure to sunlight.

Erythema multiforme

Erythema multiforme is a skin condition believed to occur secondary to an underlying systemic disease such as an infection. The skin eruption is characterized by red to purple macules, papules, and vesicles and may be preceded by fever, chest pain, and arthralgia. The treatment is to seek out the underlying cause and eliminate it if

possible. Local treatment includes baths, soaks, and dressings. If the lesions appear in the mouth, special mouth care is indicated, including irrigations with warm salt solution.

Discoid lupus erythematosus

Lupus erythematosus occurs in two forms, systemic (SLE) (see Chapter 23) and discoid (DLE). DLE is a chronic, relatively benign skin condition seen in young adults, rarely after age 50 years. Precipitating factors include physical trauma and stress. There is no cure for DLE.

Table 37-12. Tumors of the skin

Tumor	Description	Medical therapy
Keratoses		
Corns	Thickened skin lesion with a center core that thickens inwardly	Corrective shoes; felt pad with a center hole for relief of pressure
Callus	Thickened horny skin layer in circumscribed lesions often seen on plantar surface of foot	Well-fitting shoes, moleskin and padding; scraping with emery board; salicylic acid plasters
Seborrheic keratosis	Benign tumors; resemble large, darkened, greasy warts	Do not require treatment; may be removed by curettage and electrodessication or cryotherapy
Actinic keratosis (senile, solar)	Benign round or irregular tumors; red-brown to gray in color, with a dry scaly appearance; 25% may become malignant	Removal by curettage and electrodessication or by cryotherapy
Premalignant		
Leukoplakia	Thickened white patch on mucous membrane of mouth or vagina; may develop into invasive squamous cell carcinoma	Small lesions removed by electrodessication; large lesions excised
Pigmented nevi (mole)	Circumscribed pigmented papules; brown moles with hair or evenly colored dark moles are usually benign	Excised for cosmetic reasons or if sudden change in size or color, or bleeding
Malignant		
Squamous cell carcinoma	Malignant tumor of surface epidermis; starts as a firm nodule, becomes indurated with an inflammatory base; may metastasize if on lip or ear (Fig. 37-3)	Removal by surgical excision, curettage with electrodessication, irradiation, or chemosurgery
Basal cell carcinoma	Malignant tumor primarily over hairy areas; tumors have a translucent appearance with indurated center; may be ulcerated with crusting; grow slowly and rarely metastasize	Same as above
Malignant melanomma	Most serious but relatively uncommon skin cancer; lesions vary in appearance and rate of growth; often have irregular pigmentation; metastasize frequently; early diagnosis leads to more favorable prognosis	Total wide excision with skin grafts to cover defects in many cases; chemotherapy, immunotherapy

popigmentation may result from atopic dermatitis and tinea. Some dermatologic disorders that are unique to blacks include traumatic alopecia and pseudofolliculitis barbae. Keloids are common.

Traumatic alopecia

Hair shafts in blacks are highly susceptible to breakage, and hair loss may result from some hair care practices such as tight hair curlers, corn-row braiding, hot combing, or the use of picks. Wetting or "softening" the hair before the use of a pick may help prevent trauma to the hair. The hair usually grows back when the specific practice is discontinued.

Pseudofolliculitis barbae

Hair follicles in blacks are curved rather than straight; therefore the hair curls back as it grows. After shaving, the sharpened point of the hair shaft (especially if a straight razor has been used) acts like a hook and reenters the skin, causing an inflammmatory response. The most commonly affected areas include the chin and upper anterior neck. The legs and axilla may also develop pseudofolliculitis from shaving.

The lesions consist of papules and pustules, with some postinflammatory hyperpigmentation. Treatment consists of growing a beard or shaving with a safety razor set at a coarse setting. As the beard is growing, a brush or rough washcloth may be used to dislodge ingrowing hairs. A mild depilatory may be used in place of shaving.

Keloids

Although keloids are seen in all races, they are much more prevalent in blacks. Keloids are hard, raised, shiny growths of collagen tissue that usually originate from a scar and then grow beyond the wound, often with clawlike projections. Keloids occur most often in young adults but may require many years to reach full growth. Highly susceptible areas for keloid growth include the sternum, mandible, ear, and neck. Keloids may recur after simple excision; therefore surgery is often followed by intralesional steroid therapy, radiation therapy, or electron beam therapy.

PLASTIC SURGERY

Plastic surgery is concerned with correction or reconstruction of deformities of body structures either present at birth or resulting from disease or trauma. Purposes of the surgery include restoration of function and improvement in appearance.

General care of the patient having plastic surgery

PREPARATION FOR SURGERY

It is believed that any plastic surgery for an obvious defect is justified if it helps people feel they have a better

---

> ### Types of plastic surgery
>
> Skin grafting
> Cosmetic surgery
>   Removal of skin marks
>   Dermabrasion
>   Medical tatooing
>   Nose straightening (rhinoplasty)
>   Face lifting (rhytidoplasty)
>   Breast reconstruction (mammoplasty)

---

chance for recognition among other persons. The plastic surgeon may reshape a nose or repair a deformed hand so that an emotionally stable person will have more assurance. It is foolish to assume, however, that reconstructive surgery alone will correct a basic personality problem. Some people blame an apparently trivial physical defect for a long series of failures in their lives when the major defect lies within their personalities. Because of this possibility, the person is usually studied before surgery is planned. It is necessary to know what the person expects the surgery to accomplish before the physician can decide whether such expectations are realistic and if surgery should be performed.

Before surgery the surgeon will tell the patient what probably can be done and what changes are possible. It is important to know what the patient has been told so that misunderstandings and misinterpretations can be avoided. Preparation is necessary for the normal appearance of skin grafts and reconstructed tissue immediately after surgery. Postoperative tissue reaction may distort normal contours, suture lines may be reddened, and the color of the newly transplanted skin may differ somewhat from that of surrounding skin. The appearance of the surgical area changes as the edema decreases and the suture line becomes less reddened and indurated. Six months after surgery the scar will be less noticeable than at 6 days or 6 weeks postoperatively.

The patient who is admitted to the hospital for plastic surgery may have extensive scarring and deformity and may be exceedingly sensitive to scrutiny. On the other hand, the patient may have little apparent deformity, and it may be difficult to understand why the patient wishes to have surgery. The nurse cannot know what the disfigurement means to the individual and should avoid judgment concerning the necessity of surgery.

MAINTAINING PSYCHOLOGIC COMFORT

Plastic surgery raises many of the same concerns of other surgeries. Specific concerns may include the following:

1. Economic
   a. Possible long hospitalization and convalescence for skin grafting

Table 37-13. Various types of skin grafts

Type of graft	Description	Use	Comments
Free grafts			
Split-thickness: thin	Epidermis and thin layer of dermis (0.25 to 0.30 mm)	Burns	Becomes vascularized quickly Survives transplantation readily Donor sites heal quickly Poor cosmetic results Considerable postgraft contraction Does not withstand trauma
Split-thickness: intermediate or thick	Epidermis and thicker layer of dermis (0.40 to 0.45 or 0.55 to 0.60 mm)	Widely used over large wounds	Less contraction Better cosmetic results Epithelialization of donor site occurs completely but more slowly
Full-thickness	Epidermis and all of dermis	For small areas where matching skin color and texture is important	Best cosmetic results No contraction Donor site must be sutured (no epithelialization) Limited donor sites Lowest transplantation survival
Flap grafts	Skin and subcutaneous tissue; one end remains attached to donor site for vascularization	Large areas of defect; over avascular areas	More complex, requires greater skill Bulky May introduce hair into nonhairy areas

---

Graft sources

Autograft	Tissue moved from one part of the body to another
Homograft	Tissue transplanted from another person
Heterograft	Tissue transplanted from another species

---

b. Elective cosmetic surgery may not be covered by medical insurance
2. Physical discomfort
3. Physical appearance in postoperative period
4. Final outcome of surgery

These concerns may result in anxiety and mild depression during the first few days after surgery.[6] Empathic communication by the nurse helps the patient identify and deal with concerns.

Skin grafting

Skin grafting consists of replacing damaged skin with healthy skin to prevent unsightly scars.

GRAFT SOURCES

Skin for grafting may be obtained from various sources. The most suitable form is the *autograft,* because it does not provoke an immune response with rejection of the graft. *Homografts* (which are temporary) may be necessary if the patient's condition is poor and if large areas must be covered, as with burns. The survival time of homografts varies from a few days to a number of weeks. Depending on the tissue used and the recipient site, the transplanted tissue will then die and slough or be absorbed and replaced by the host's own developing tissues. *Heterografts,* which are rejected quickly by the recipient, are used only in special cases, such as when homografts are not available and covering of the wound is essential.

TYPES OF GRAFTS

Plastic surgery may be performed by means of *free grafting,* which consists of cutting tissue from one part of the body and moving it directly to another part. It may also be done by leaving one end of the graft attached to the body to provide a blood supply for the graft until blood vessels form at the new place of attachment *(flap graft).*

The surgeon selects skin for grafting that is similar in texture and thickness to that which has been lost, and studies the normal lines of the skin and its elasticity to

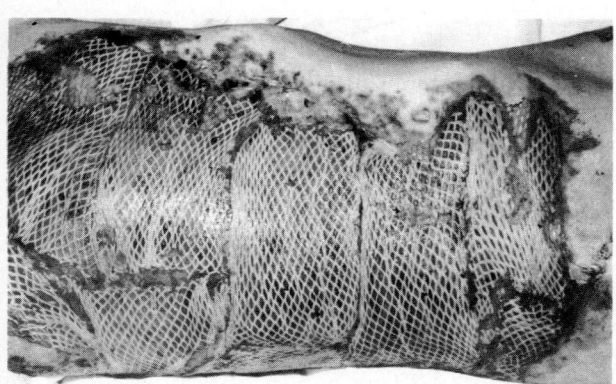

Fig. 37-5. Mesh graft covering full-thickness burn. (Courtesy Burn Unit, Cook County Hospital, Chicago.)

avoid noticeable scars. Scar tissue contracts with time, and in normal circumstances this is good because it produces a complete closure of the line of injury. However, in some cases scar tissue may contract in such a way that surrounding tissues are pulled out of normal contour, and distortion may result.

Free grafts

Free grafts are the most commonly used skin grafts. There are several types of free grafts, each with its advantages and limitations (Table 37-13). Split-thickness grafts consist of epidermis and varying thicknesses of the dermis. Full-thickness grafts include the entire dermis and epidermis (Fig. 37-1). The most widely used type is the intermediate or thick split-thickness graft. They can be cut into large pieces with a dermatome set to ensure a uniform thickness of the graft, and these can then be cut into smaller pieces to match the area to be grafted.

Meshed grafts are either thin or intermediate split-

Nursing care of patients with skin grafts

Preoperative care

1. Recipient site:
   a. Apply warm soaks and compresses under aseptic conditions (as prescribed)
   b. Apply prescribed topical antibiotics
2. Donor site: cleanse with germicidal soap as prescribed, usually the night before and the morning of surgery

Postoperative care of recipient site

1. Elevate graft site when possible
2. Protect graft site from pressure and motion (for example, place graft site uppermost, use cradle over bed)
3. Instruct patient not to lie on dressing
4. Apply warm moist compresses, if prescribed:
   a. Wash hands before changing dressings
   b. Use meticulous aseptic technique
   c. Warm compresses to no more than 40.5° C (105°F)
5. Compresses may sometimes be covered with a sterile petroleum jelly dressing and moistened by gently directing fluid from sterile syringe under edge of dressing
6. Report any signs of hematoma or fluid collection under graft

Postoperative care of donor site

1. Keep donor site covered for 24 to 48 hours until serum dries
2. Apply heat lamp with caution (denuded skin is sensitive) to hasten drying
3. Use a bed cradle, if appropriate, to allow more air circulation
4. Leave fine-mesh gauze, which is adherent to donor site, in place until it drops off (usually within 3 weeks)
5. Trim loose edges of mesh gauze as it loosens with healing
6. Give analgesics as necessary for discomfort

Postoperative care after flap grafts

1. Support body parts placed in awkward position from immobilization of flap graft
2. Assess graft as possible for circulatory insufficiency (sharp color demarcation, decreased temperature)
3. Maintain aseptic technique to prevent infection
4. Assist patient to be as self-sufficient as possible with activities of daily living
5. If hospitalization is prolonged, help patient plan diversionary activities

thickness grafts that have been placed through a perforating machine that creates a mesh. Meshed grafts are elastic and can be used to cover larger areas than the original size (Fig. 37-5). They also conform more easily to irregular surfaces and can be placed over less clean bases than regular split-thickness grafts. Cosmetic appearance is poor. Meshed grafts are used frequently to cover large burned areas.

Full-thickness grafts, for survival, must develop their own blood supply (which takes 2 weeks). If the graft dies, the skin is irretrievably lost to the body, because regeneration of skin at the donor site is not possible.

Flap grafts

Flap grafts are used to cover larger defects than can be covered by free grafts. Flap grafts are made by cutting along three sides of a flap (two long and one short side). There are basically two major types of flap grafts. The *transposed* graft is slid over to a nearby skin area to be covered and is sutured in place. The *tube pedicle* graft is formed by suturing the long sides of the graft together to form a tube and then suturing the end to another area of the body. An intermediary site may be used, such as the forearm, in a two-step procedure, to permit moving the tube to a farther site on the body. After the graft has taken, the original site is freed and the graft is sutured to the recipient site.

CARE OF THE PATIENT WITH A SKIN GRAFT

Four conditions are necessary for a graft to survive:
1. Adequate vascularization of the recipient site
2. Constant contact with the underlying tissue
3. Immobilization
4. Freedom from infection[7]

Anything that comes between the undersurface of the graft and the recipient area, such as a discharge caused by infection, excess serous fluid, or blood, will float the graft away from close contact and may cause it to die. To prevent floating, some surgeons insert drains at strategic spots along the edges of the graft, or a small catheter is

---

Teaching the patient with a skin graft

1. Keep surface of healed graft moistened daily with a skin lotion for 6 to 12 months. (Grafted skin does not sweat; it dries and cracks easily.)
2. Protect grafted skin from direct sunlight with a sunscreen lotion for at least 6 months.
3. Wear a strong elastic stocking for 4 to 6 months with grafts on lower extremities.
4. Report changes in the graft (hematoma, fluid collection) to physician.

---

inserted on the edge of the graft under the recipient skin and attached to suction to remove the fluid.

The area is inspected frequently to see if the skin is adhering to the underlying tissue. If fluid collects under the skin graft, it is removed by aspiration with a sterile needle and syringe or the fluid is rolled to the wound edge with a sterile applicator.

A wide variety of materials are used as dressings. The choice depends on the kind of graft and the surgeon's preference. Petrolatum, Adaptic gauze, or Telfa dressings are often selected. Often the graft is covered with a piece of coarse mesh gauze anchored to the adjacent skin edges with an elastic bandage to give firm, gentle pressure and to immobilize the area. The first dressing may be covered with a compress of sterile normal saline solution. Because the compress is moist, it fits the contour of the wound better. Continuous pressure is necessary to keep the graft adherent to the recipient bed, but pressure should not be so firm as to cause death of the graft.

Inner dressings on the recipient site are usually changed by the surgeon 1-2 days after surgery, and it is usually possible to know then whether the result of the operation is satisfactory.

Before patients with skin grafts are discharged, they need to know how to care for the recipient and donor sites at home until healing has occurred (see box below).

Cosmetic surgery

REMOVAL OF SKIN MARKINGS

Disfiguring marks of the skin may be removed by abrasive action (dermabrasion) or by changing the color through medical tattooing. Both procedures are painful.

Either local or general anesthesia is used for *dermabrasion*, which may be performed on an inpatient or outpatient basis. The skin is abraded with a wire brush or diamond fraise (Fig. 37-6). There is postoperative swelling, discomfort, crusting, and erythema, which may persist for several weeks. The procedure may be done in stages. A Telfa dressing with antiseptic solution and a pressure dressing are usually applied, although the area may be left uncovered if oozing is slight.

Medical tattooing is performed on an ambulatory basis; no anesthesia is used, although a sedative may be prescribed to be taken 1 hour before surgery. The procedure is done in several stages; pigment is impregnated into the skin with a tattooing needle. The skin is left exposed to air to dry and crust. An ice bag may be applied to relieve postoperative discomfort.

RHINOPLASTY

Reconstructive surgery of the nose can be done either to correct an anatomic problem (Chapter 24) or for cosmetic reasons (Fig. 37-7). A local anesthetic is usually used. The incision is usually made at the end of the nose inside the nostril so that it is not conspicuous. A nasal packing is inserted for 24 to 48 hours; the patient is cautioned not to sniff or blow the nose after the packing is

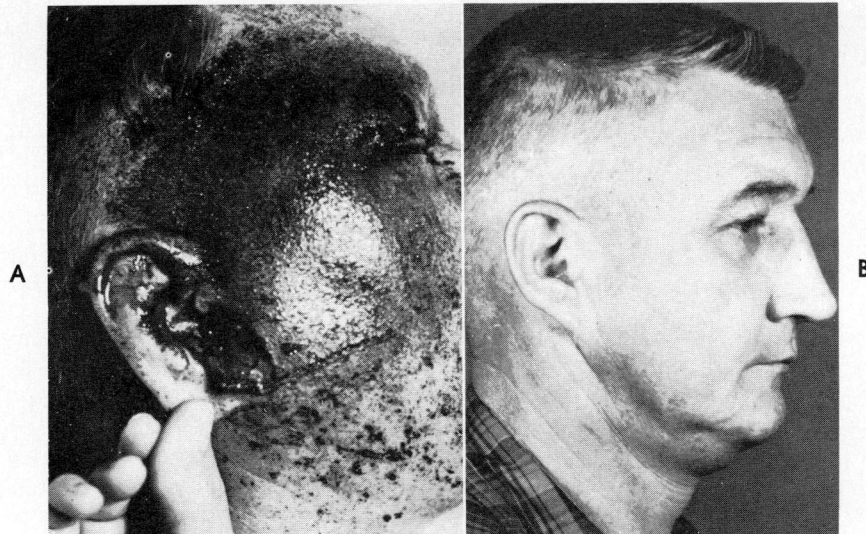

Fig. 37-6. A, Meticulous cleansing and dermabrasion were required to remove impregnated bits of galvanized metal. **B,** Postoperative veiw of patient 17 years after dermabrasion. (From Saunders, W.H., et. al: Nursing care in eye, ear, nose, and throat disorders, ed. 4, St. Louis, 1979, The C.V. Mosby Co.)

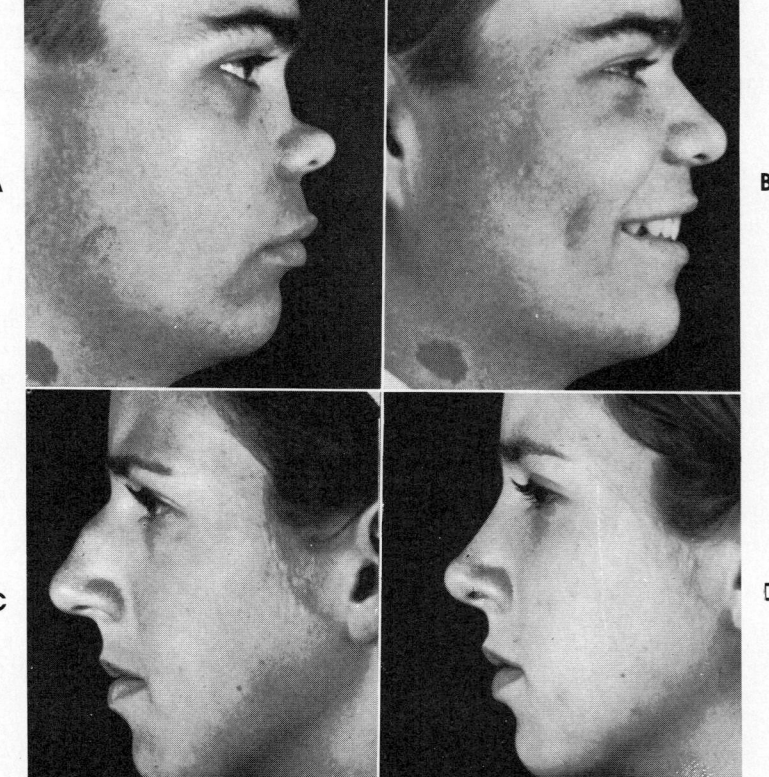

Fig. 37-7. A, Saddle nose after nasal infection at 8 years of age; **B,** it is repaired with Silastic nasal implant. **C** and **D,** Nasal convexity and chin retrusion repaired by combined rhinoplasty and chin augmentation. (From Saunders, W.H., et al.: Nursing care in eye, ear, nose, and throat disorders, ed. 4, St. Louis, 1979, The C.V. Mosby Co.)

removed, to prevent bleeding. A nasal splint may be applied for protection.

There will be ecchymosis (bruising) and swelling around the eyes and nose for 10 to 14 days after surgery; ice compresses and an ice bag may be used to hasten fluid reabsorption. The patient must anticipate waiting several weeks before evaluating the final result of surgery.

RHYTIDOPLASTY

For face lifting, an incision is made at the hairline, and excess skin is separated from its underlying tissue and removed. The remaining skin is pulled up and sutured at the hairline, thus removing wrinkles and giving firmness and smoothness to the face. A gentle pressure dressing is then applied and left in place for 24 to 48 hours. The patient frequently needs medication for pain in the postoperative period because of the extent to which the tissue has been undermined. The surgery may be repeated at a later date.

MAMMOPLASTY

Reconstructive breast surgery may be done to replace breast tissue removed by surgery (Chapter 36) or to improve the appearance of the breasts. Some women with conspicuously large and pendulous breasts may wish to have them reduced in size. Large breasts are embarrassing to some women and make it difficult for them to participate in sports, maintain good posture, and buy clothes that fit. Such women often respond to reconstructive surgery remarkably well. Cosmetic surgery of the breast may also be done to make unusually small breasts larger. A variety of plastic materials may be used for this procedure.

REFERENCES AND SELECTED READINGS*

1. *Acres, C., and Kraft, E.R.: Skin transplantation, Am. J. Nurs. **81:**1466-1467, 1981.
2. *Anders, J.E., and Leach, E.E.: Sun versus skin, Am. J. Nurs. **83:**1015-1020, 1983.
3. *Black skin problems, Am. J. Nurs. **79:**1092-1094, 1979.
4. *Choulinard, F.: Vigilant nursing care after reconstructive surgery, Nurs. 79 **9**(6):18-25, 1979.
5. Comer, J. B.: Amphotericin B: ten common questions, Am J. Nurs. **81:**1166-1167, 1981.
6. *Conlee, D.: Put a new face on your care of cosmetic surgery patients, Nurs. 81 **11**(11):90-95, 1981.
7. Dunphy, J.E., and Way, L.W.: Current surgical diagnosis and treatment, 1983, Los Altos, Calif, 1983, Lange Medical Publications.
8. Grazer, F.M., and Klingbell, J.R.: Body image: a surgical perspective, St. Louis, 1980, The C.V. Mosby Co.
9. *Hawkins K.: Wet dressings: putting the damper on dermatitis, Nurs. 78 **8**(2):64-67, 1978.
10. *Heckel, P.: Teaching patients to cope with psoriasis: the unshared disease, Nurs. 81 **11**(6):49-51, 1981.
11. Kaye, D., and Rose, L.F.: Fundamentals of internal medicine, St. Louis, 1983, The C.V. Mosby Co.
12. Larrow, L., and Noe, J.M.: Port wine stain hemangiomas, Am. J. Nurs. **82:**786-790, 1982.
13. *Mangieri, D.: Saving your elderly patient's skin, Nurs. 82 **12**(10):44-45, 1982.
14. Moschella, S.L., Pillsbury, D.M., and Hurley, H.J.: Dermatology, Philadelphia, 1975, W.B. Saunders Co.
15. Orkin, M., and Maibach, H.I.: Scabies, a current pandemic, Postgrad. Med. **66:**53-62, 1979.
16. Parrish, J.: Dermatology and skin care, New York, 1975, McGraw Hill Book Co.
17. Pillsbury, D.M.: A manual of dermatology, ed. 2, Philadelphia, 1980, W.B. Saunders Co.
18. Rees, T.D., et al.: Aesthetic plastic surgery, Philadelphia, 1980, W.B. Saunders Co.
19. Robinson, J.K.: Moh's surgery for skin cancer, Am. J. Nurs. **82:**282-283, 1982.
20. Schmidt, L.M.: Topical dermatologic therapy,, Pediatr. Clin. North Am. **25:**191-209, 1978.
21. *Schulmeister, L.: Screening for skin cancer: a necessary part of your assessment routine, Nurs. 81 **11**(10):74-78, 1981.
22. *Stuart, M.S.: Skin flaps and grafts after head and neck surgery, Am. J. Nurs. **78:**1368-1373, 1978.
23. *Topical therapy: choosing and using the proper vehicle, Nurs. 77 **7**(11):9-10, 1977.
24. *Uhler, D.M.: Common skin changes in the elderly, Am. J. Nurs. **78:**1342-1344, 1978.
25. Wyngaarden, J.B., and Smith, L.H.: Textbook of medicine, ed. 16, Philadelphia, 1982, W.B. Saunders Co.

*References preceded by an asterisk are particularly well suited for student reading.

38

The Patient with Burns

PENNY O'MALLEY

STUDY QUESTIONS

- From your knowledge of anatomy and physiology, what are the harmful effects of loss of a large area of skin?

- What is the effect on the body of loss of a large amount of circulating blood fluid (plasma)? Of loss of serum proteins?

- What is the effect on the body of a sudden increase in fluid to the circulatory system?

- Name some ways of helping a patient increase fluid intake.

- What foods are high in protein? What are some ways in which high-protein foods may be given to a critically ill patient?

- Think about the concerns you might have if today you experienced extensive burns over your body.

Burns are wounds caused by dry or moist heat, chemicals, electricity, radiation, and other rays such as X rays. The most common cause of burns is fire, which kills 13,200 and scars and injures 300,000 Americans each year, including 50,000 persons who must be hospitalized for periods of 6 weeks to 2 years. Many of these deaths can be prevented. Knowledge, patience, and understanding are needed in the nursing care of severely burned persons during the acute and long-term recovery phases. Principles of burn care are the same regardless of the cause.

PREVENTION AND HEALTH EDUCATION

Many injuries and deaths incurred from burns can be prevented either through changes in the environment or through health teaching concerning methods of prevention.

Environmental changes

Many groups have been involved in recent years in making environments safer from fire or in giving early warning of fire and smoke. The Flammable Fabrics Acts have regulated the use of flame-resistant fabrics, especially in children's clothing. Approximately 85% of all flame burns involve burning fabrics.[15] Laws requiring that industrial products known to be flammable be labeled and that new products be tested carefully for their flammable qualities before being marketed must be rigidly enforced.

Each year brings increased demand for careful inspection and regulation of places in which the ill and elderly are housed. Aged persons frequently are housed in old and poorly equipped structures, and many of them have burned to death. Nurses can bring necessary pressures to bear to ensure adequate protection and planned evacuation should a fire occur.

Laws require that doors in public buildings be hinged to swing outward, that draperies and decorations be fireproof, and that stairways with special fire doors be used. Stairway doors should never be propped open in any public building; this constitutes a fire hazard. All public and private buildings should have smoke detectors.

Health teaching

Nurses can help prevent accidental burns from occurring by participating in health education programs that stress fire prevention and the consequences of fires, such as burns, deformities, and death, and by promoting legislation that would control some people's thoughtless practices and make working and living environments safer.

A high incidence of burn injuries in adults are related to accidents while cooking or smoking or otherwise using matches. Burns commonly occur when the person is distracted while cooking or falls asleep while smoking. Complete elimination of smoking would provide for a safer environment.

Sunburn should be cautioned against, because even a relatively mild first-degree burn over a large part of the body can cause change in fluid distribution and kidney damage.

All persons should know what to do if clothing catches fire (drop to ground and roll). Families as well as institutions should hold regular fire drills and know what to do if a fire does occur:

1. Go to a safe area and call the fire department.
2. Doors that feel hot to touch should not be opened, because superheated air causes tracheal burns and asphyxiation.
3. Smoke should be avoided by crawling below it.
4. Fires on the stove should be extinguished by covering the pan with a lid or soda bicarbonate; do not use water to douse grease fires or attempt to move a burning pan.

PATHOPHYSIOLOGY OF BURNS

Classification of burns

Burns are classified as first, second, and third degree, depending on their depth (see Table 38-1). First and second-degree burns are also classified as *partial-thickness* burns, whereas third degree burns are *full-thickness* burns (Fig. 38-1). First- and second-degree burns are likely to be painful because nerve endings have been injured. During the healing phase the person experiences dryness and itching caused by increased vascularization of sebaceous glands, reduction of secretions, and decreased perspiration.

With third-degree burns nerves are destroyed, resulting in a painless wound. The destroyed tissue is unable to epithelialize; therefore these areas must be covered either by skin growing from normal skin around the edges of the burned area with scar formation or by skin grafts. Skin grafting is preferred for its esthetic advantages.

Pathophysiology of severe burns

As a result of burns normal skin function is diminished, with the following resulting physiologic alterations:

1. Loss of protective barriers against infection
2. Escape of body fluids
3. Lack of temperature control
4. Destruction of sweat and sebaceous glands
5. Decrease in number of sensory receptors.

The severity of these alterations depends on the extent of the burn and the depth to which damage has occured.

Three stages follow *severe* burns: the immediate hypovolemic stage, the diuretic stage, and the long-term re-

Table 38-1. Factors used in determining depth of burn injury

Degree	Depth	Sensation	Blisters	Color	Texture
First (minor) Second (partial thickness)	Epidermis only Involvement of epidermis and dermis	Painful Very painful	None Large, thick walled; usually will increase in size	Increased redness If vesicles are ruptured, skin may be mottled but demonstrates capillary refill on pressure	Normal Normal or somewhat firm
Third (full thickness)	Destruction of all layers of skin into subcutaneous tissue including fascia, muscle, and bone	Little or no pain	None, or if present, thin walled; do not increase in size	Skin may be charred, white, brown, or red; does not demonstrate capillary refill	Firm and leathery

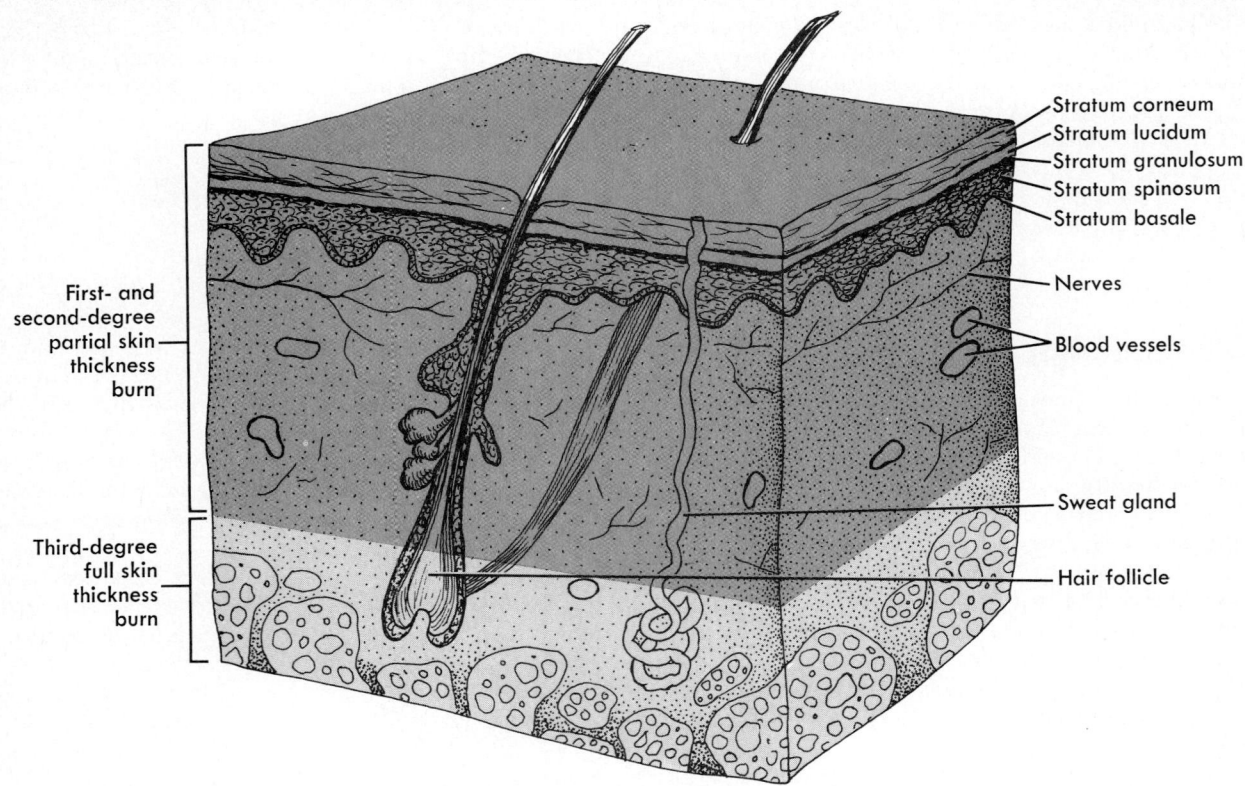

First- and
second-degree
partial skin
thickness
burn

Third-degree
full skin
thickness
burn

Stratum corneum
Stratum lucidum
Stratum granulosum
Stratum spinosum
Stratum basale

Nerves

Blood vessels

Sweat gland

Hair follicle

Fig. 38-1. Level of human skin involved in burns.

habilitative stage. Fig. 38-2 presents an overview of the pathophysiologic changes seen in severe burns.

HYPOVOLEMIC STAGE

Fluid shift, vascular to interstitial

The hypovolemic stage begins with the burn and lasts for the first 48 to 72 hours. It is characterized by a rapid shift of fluid from the vascular compartments into the interstitial spaces as a result of the immediate inflammatory response. Abnormally large amounts of extracellular fluid, sodium chloride, and protein pass into the burned area to cause blisters and local edema or escape through the open wound. Visible fluid loss is only a small part of the fluid lost from the circulating blood and other essential fluid compartments. Most of the fluid loss occurs deep in the wound, where fluid extravasates into the deeper tissues.

Burns of areas such as highly vascular muscle tissue or the face are believed to cause greater fluid shift than comparable burns on other parts of the body. Fully *one half of the extracellular fluid* of the body can shift from its normal distribution to the site of the burn.

Hypovolemic shock occurs, resulting in a tremendous drop in blood pressure and inadequate blood flow through the kidneys. This in turn leads to further shock and anuria, and death within a short time if treatment is not given promptly or is inadequate. These changes are summarized in Fig. 38-3.

Dehydration of the nondamaged tissue cells may result. More fluids and sodium are lost initially from the capillaries than is protein. This increases the capillary osmotic pressure, leading to dehydration with pronounced edema in the burned area. As protein continues to be lost because of the increased capillary permeability, *hypoproteinemia* results. The increased amount of protein in the tissue spaces is a further contributing factor to edema formation. Proteins may be lost through the open wound, and nitrogen is lost through the kidney from catabolism, leading to a significant negative nitrogen balance. With oliguria the blood urea nitrogen (BUN) concentration is elevated.

The loss of fluid from the vascular system causes *hemoconcentration*, and the hematocrit rises. Blood flow becomes sluggish in the burned area and cellular nutrition decreases. Large numbers of red blood cells become trapped in the burned area and are hemolyzed. Renal damage and hematuria may occur as a result of reduced blood volume and passage of the end products of the hemolyzed cells through the glomeruli. The decreased renal blood flow leads to *oliguria*.

Electrolyte imbalances

Potassium excess in the blood (hyperkalemia) results from injury to the tissue cells and red blood cells and from the diminished urinary output, and may lead to heart block and ventricular failure. Potassium may be encouraged to move back into the cells by the administration

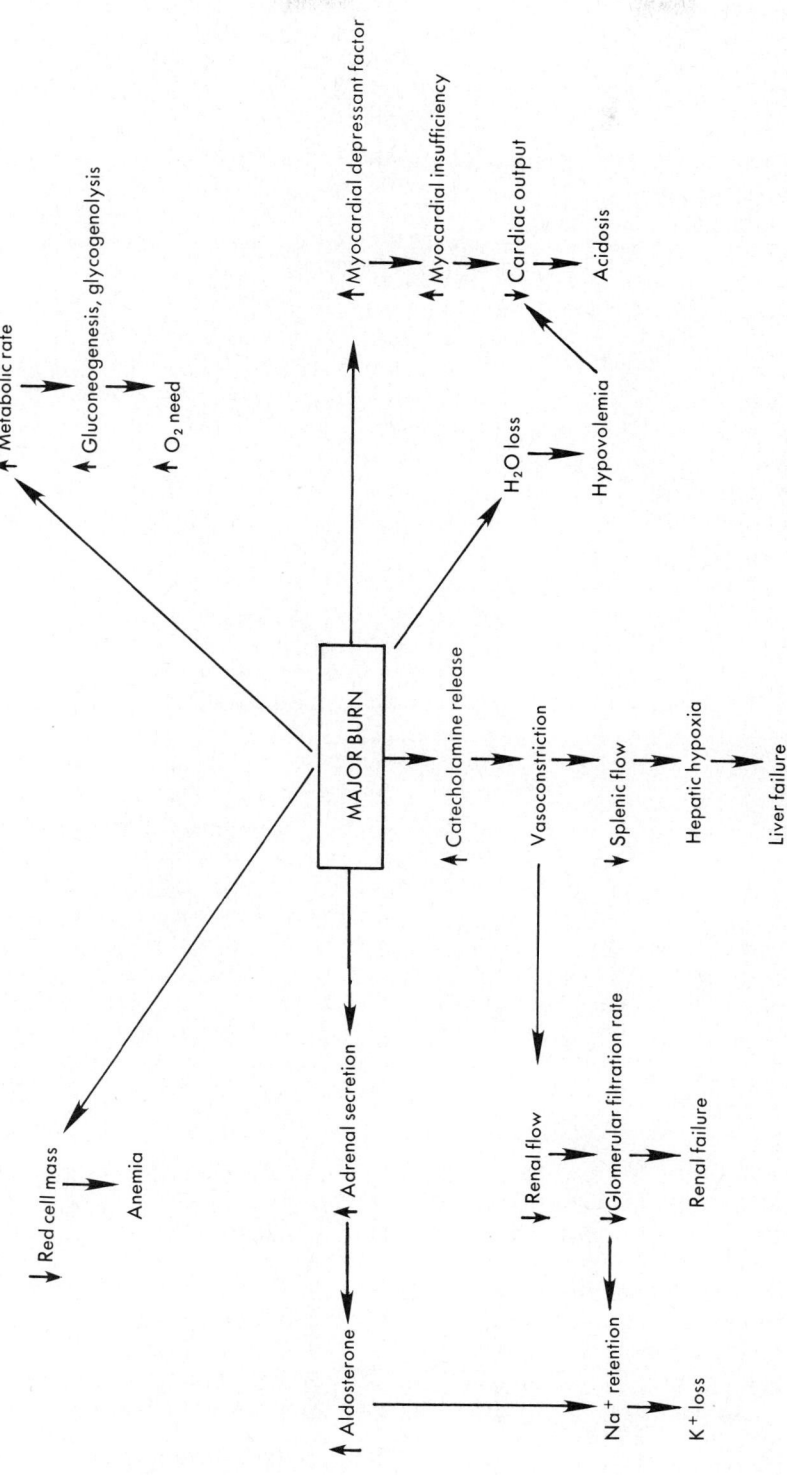

Fig. 38-2. Overview of pathophysiology of major burn.

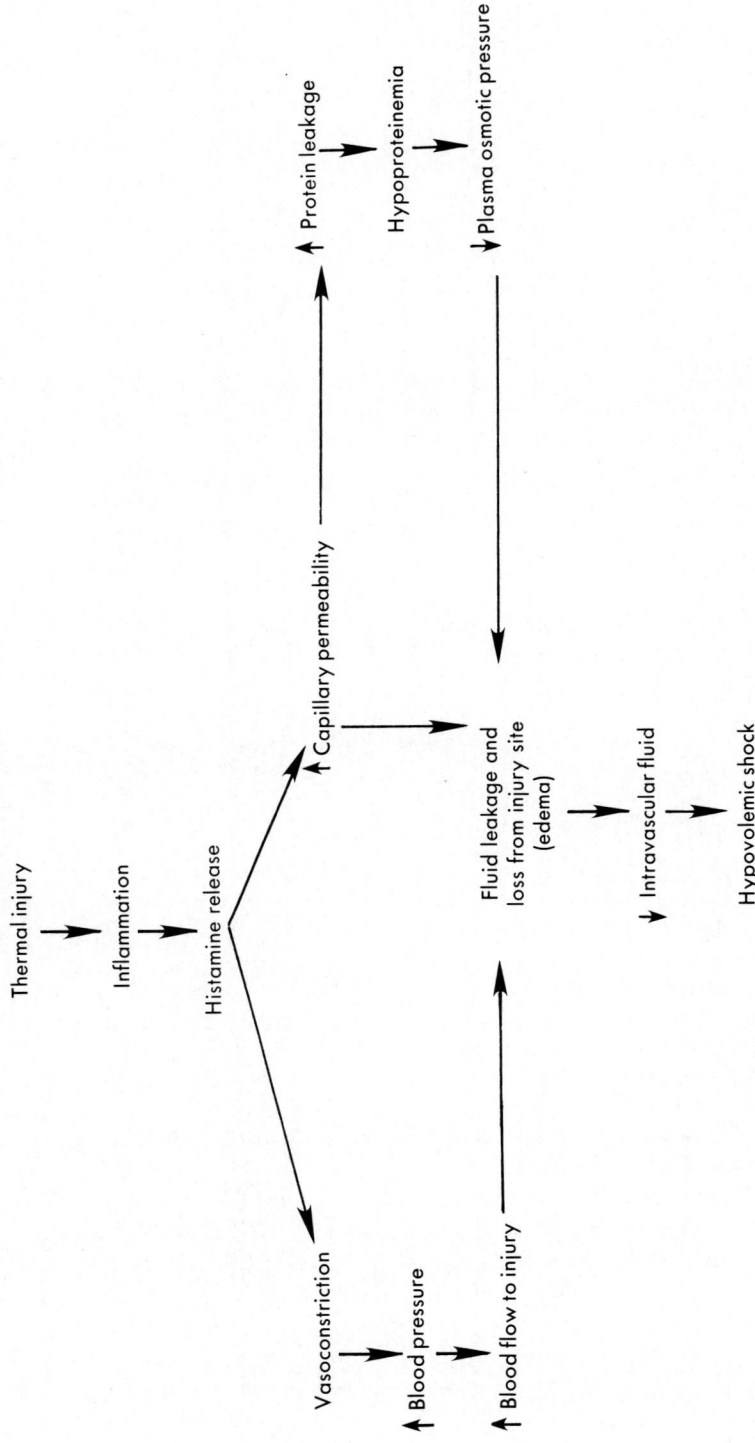

Fig. 38-3. Flow diagram of fluid shifts resulting in hypovolemic shock.

of insulin, because potassium is transported back into the cells along with glucose.

Sodium is retained by the body as a result of the endocrine response to stress. Aldosterone is increased, leading to sodium reabsorption by the kidney. This sodium, however, quickly passes into the interstitial spaces of the burn area with the fluid shift; therefore, despite the increased amount of sodium in the body, most of it is trapped in the edema fluid, and a *sodium deficit* occurs.

Inadequate tissue perfusion results in anaerobic metab-

olism, and the acid end products are retained because of the decreased kidney function. *Metabolic acidosis* may then develop.

DIURETIC STAGE

The diuretic stage begins about 48 to 72 hours after the person was burned, and the changes occur rapidly. The differences in changes occurring between the hypovolemic and diuretic stages are summarized in Table 38-2.

Table 38-2. Physiologic changes with burns

| Change | Hypovolemic phase | | Diuretic phase | |
	Mechanism	Result	Mechanism	Result
Extracellular fluid shift	Vascular to interstitial	Hemoconcentration	Interstitial to vascular	Hemodilution
Renal function	Decreased renal flow from decreased blood pressure and decreased cardiac output	Oliguria	Increased renal flow from increased blood volume	Diuresis
Sodium level	Na$^+$ reabsorption by kidneys *but* Na$^+$ lost in exudate and trapped in edema fluid	Sodium deficit	Na$^+$ loss with diuresis (becomes normal in 1 week)	Sodium deficit
Potassium level	K$^+$ released by tissue and red blood cell injury; decreased K$^+$ excretion from decreased renal function	Hyperkalemia	K$^+$ moves back into cells; K$^+$ lost by diuresis	Hypokalemia
Protein level	Protein loss into tissues by increased capillary permeability	Hypoproteinemia	Loss of protein during continued catabolism	Hypoproteinemia
Nitrogen balance	Tissue catabolism; protein loss in tissues; more nitrogen lost than taken in	Negative nitrogen balance	Tissue catabolism, protein loss, immobility	Negative nitrogen balance
Acid base balance	Anaerobic metabolism from decreased tissue perfusion; increased acid end products; decreased renal output (these lead to retention of acid end products); loss of serum bicarbonate	Metabolic acidosis	Sodium bicarbonate lost in diuresis; hypermetabolism with increased metabolic end products	Metabolic acidosis
Stress response	Occurs because of trauma	Decreased renal flow	Occurs because of prolonged nature of injury and psychologic threat to self	Stress ulcers

Fluid shift, interstitial to vascular

A fluid shift occurs in the opposite direction from the initial stage, and the edema fluid returns to the vascular system. Blood volume increases, leading to increased renal blood flow and diuresis unless renal damage has occurred. Serum electrolyte and hematocrit levels will be decreased because of the hemodilution. *Fluid overload* may occur as fluids shift from the interstitial spaces. *During this phase extreme caution in administration of intravenous fluids is mandatory.* The patient's vital signs, breath sounds, and urinary output are used to determine the amount of intravenous fluid replacement. *Dehydration* may occur if rapid urinary fluid losses deplete the intravascular reserve.

Electrolyte imbalances

Sodium is lost with diuresis, and a *sodium deficit* may occur. *Hypokalemia* results from potassium moving back into the cells or being excreted in the urine. Protein continues to be lost from the wounds. *Metabolic acidosis* remains a possibility because of the loss of sodium bicarbonate in the urine and the increased fat metabolism secondary to decreased carbohydrate intake.

Anemia and malnutrition

After the period of fluid shifts the patient remains acutely ill. *Anemia* develops from the loss of red blood cells. *Negative nitrogen balance,* which begins at the onset of the burn, continues throughout the acute period and is secondary to continued loss of protein from the wound, from tissue catabolism resulting from immobility, and from decreased protein intake. *Hypovitaminosis* may also occur from the decreased intake of vitamins. *Weight loss* results from increased metabolism after loss of water and heat from the wound, from loss of fluid during diuresis, and from catabolism during tissue breakdown.

REHABILITATIVE STAGE

The rehabilitative stage begins when the burned area is reduced to less than 20% of the body surface. The person is now in an *anabolic phase.*

ASSESSMENT

Assessment of the person who has sustained a severe burn depends on the cause and extent of burn injury.

Subjective data

Information is obtained from either the burn victim or other persons concerning how the burn occurred. If the burn was caused by heat or fire, data should include the following:
1. Duration of contact
2. Presence of smoke (possible respiratory damage)
3. Location (enclosed area suggests possibility of carbon monoxide poisoning)
4. Whether an explosion occured (other possible injuries).

The age of the patient is important in estimating the severity of the burn. In burns involving up to 30% of the body surface in persons under the age of 50 years, except infants and very young children, the mortality is low. As the age of the patient increases beyond 50 years the mortality rises even in burns of less than 30%. Elderly persons often have preexisting cardiovascular, pulmonary, or renal diseases that decrease their ability to cope with severe burns. Presence of these conditions in younger persons also delays recovery.

Objective data

The wound is inspected and loose debris removed if necessary. *Size* of the burn involves amount of body surface area (BSA) involved. The larger the BSA involved the greater the severity of threat to the individual (Table 38-3). For adults the "rule of nines" (Fig. 38-4) is one easy method of determining BSA.

Certain areas of the body are of special concern when burns occur because of high potential for loss of function or because of poor vascularization. Burns on the face, eyes, ears, neck, hands or feet, and genitalia are classified as major. Damage to the tracheobronchial tree through heat and smoke inhalation is also considered major.

Factors determining severity of burns

Age of patient
History of cardiac, pulmonary, renal, or hepatic disease
Injuries sustained at time of burn (for example, fracture, internal injuries)
Size of burn
Depth of burn
Body part involved

Identification of airway burns

Singed nasal hair
Burns of mouth or throat
Brassy sounding cough
Sooty expectoration
Respiratory distress

Further assessment is required for the severely burned person:

1. Evaluate respiratory status:
   a. Monitor respiratory excursion
   b. Monitor respiratory sounds
2. Monitor all vital signs for signs of hypovolemic shock; vital signs should stabilize when intravenous fluids are started
3. Check for circulatory competence with circumferential burns (assess peripheral pulses every 15 minutes during initial period)
4. Monitor urinary status (output 30 ml/hr)
5. Weigh patient as a baseline for evaluating fluid loss; monitor weight on an ongoing basis
6. Send blood samples to the laboratory for immediate evaluation (protein, RBC, and arterial blood gases)

Table 38-3. Classification of burns by depth and extent

Severity	Second degree	Third degree
Critical*	>25% BSA, adults >20% BSA, children	>10% BSA
Major	15% to 25% BSA, adults 10% to 20% BSA, children	2% to 10% BSA
Minor	<15% BSA, adults <10% BSA, children	<2% BSA

*Also included as critical are burns in persons younger than 18 months or older than 45 years or burns of critical areas (head, extremities, genitalia).

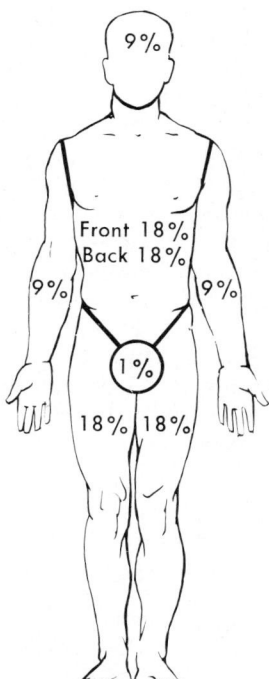

Fig. 38-4. "Rule of nines" is used to estimate amount of skin surface burned (adult).

DATA ANALYSIS AND PLANNING
Nursing diagnoses

Nursing diagnoses for the person with a severe burn depend on the identified data. Possible nursing diagnoses include the following:

Anxiety
Breathing pattern: ineffective
Fluid volume deficit
Potential for injury: infection
Potential for injury: contractures
Nutrition alteration: less than body requirements
Family processes, alterations in

Expected patient outcomes

1. The patient will:
   a. Be in a state of homeostasis (normal blood volume, normal serum electrolytes, vital signs at preburn levels)
   b. Be in a state of positive nitrogen balance
   c. Be free of infection
   d. Have intact integumentation
   e. Be free of contractures
   f. Be mobile and independent in self-care.
2. At discharge, the person can:
   a. Demonstrate care of the burn wound
   b. Demonstrate range of motion exercises to prevent contractures
   c. Describe plans to eat a diet high in protein, calories, vitamins, and minerals
   d. Describe injuries that can occur to the healing or graft and methods of injury prevention
   e. Describe plans for return to former activities (work, social activities)
   f. Describe plans for follow-up health care.

IMPLEMENTATION
Prehospital emergency care

If *flame* is involved and clothing is on fire, the victim's first reaction is to run, which only fans the flame. Rolling the burning person in a blanket on the ground to exclude oxygen, thereby putting out the fire, is one of the best procedures. Any water source can be used to extingish flames. The person whose clothing is aflame should never stand, because this increases the danger of inhalation burns, in which heat and smoke are drawn into the lungs. Once all flames are extinguished it is important that the burning agent be removed and the wound cooled.

Chemicals should be identified, and copious flushing with water is initiated. As much as 20 to 30 minutes of continuous flushing may be necessary to ensure complete removal of the destructive agent. Burns occurring about the eyes should also be lavaged with copious amounts of cool, clean water, and if the burn was caused by acids the procedure should be repeated in 10 to 15 minutes.

Persons who are burned on the *face and neck* or those

Initial care for major burns

1. Extinguish flame
2. Remove nonadherent *smoldering* clothing
3. Establish patency of airway. Assess for inhalation burns (singed nasal hair, mouth burns, sooty cough, dyspnea); give oxygen if available
4. Cool wound with copious amount of tepid water (or saline solution if available)
5. Assess and initiate treatment for injuries requiring immediate attention
6. Remove tight-fitting jewelry or clothing
7. Cover burn with moist sterile or clean cover
8. Cover unburned areas with warm dry cover to prevent heat loss
9. Transport victim to nearest medical facility.

Initial treatment of major burns in emergency room

1. Establish airway; administer humidified oxygen.
2. Initiate fluid therapy by intravenous catheters.
3. Insert indwelling catheter for hourly urine measurement.
4. Insert nasogastric tube to remove stomach contents and prevent aspiration.
5. Insert central venous pressure and pulmonary wedge pressure catheters.
6. Manage pain with intravenously administered narcotics.
7. Gather accurate baseline mental status.
8. Weigh patient for baseline measurement.
9. Observe circulatory competence of all extremities.
10. Initiate treatment of burn wounds.
11. Initiate tetanus prophylaxis.
12. Initiate protective isolation measures.

---

who have *inhaled* flame, steam, or smoke should be observed closely for signs of laryngeal edema and airway obstruction. Persons with airway burns should be transported immediately to a hospital or burn center if available. Often burns are more severe than they first appear to be.

The hospital or burn center should be notified so preparations can be made for the arrival of the patient, because a well-prepared and well-equipped team needs to be assembled to care for the severely burned person. Burn centers are located throughout the United States, many of them in major medical centers in urban areas. These centers are equipped with personnel expert in the care of burned patients.

While awaiting transportation to a medical facility the burned person is kept quiet and lying down. Pain and infection can be minimized by covering exposed burned areas with sterile dressings or the cleanest material available, such as clean sheets. These coverings may be soaked in cool water to ease the pain, reduce the edema, and prevent evaporation of body water. Ice should be avoided because sudden vasoconstriction causes severe shifting of fluid. *Oils, salves, and ointments should not be used on burns* because these materials hamper treatment. Pain is best controlled by gentle and minimal handling and by the application of dressings to exclude air from the burned skin surfaces. Deep, third-degree burns are usually painless because nerve endings have been destroyed, and for the first few minutes the person may appear not too badly affected. In most cases, however, first- and second-degree burns accompany third-degree burns, causing discomfort.

For obviously small burns fluids may be given by mouth with caution. Large burns are accompanied by decreased peristalsis; therefore nothing should be given by mouth. Patients with large burns or smoke inhalation may vomit, and particular attention is given to preventing aspiration of vomitus.

Assisting with achievement of therapeutic goals

COMPREHENSIVE TEAM APPROACH

Comprehensive care of the burn patient can best be provided by a multidisciplinary team approach. This is a desirable method designed to meet the complex and varied needs of the patient. The nurse's role in the team is to coordinate the interactions of the various disciplines and to incorporate the team's suggestions and approaches into an effective plan of care.

Because this type of care is most likely to be available in specialized burn units and centers, patients are frequently moved to these units when transportation can be effected safely. Generally accepted criteria for admission to these specialized care facilities include burns of the head, neck, and face; burns of the perineum or joints; burns that involve more than 25% of the body; and burns in children younger than 2 years and adults older than 60 years. When such specialized care is not available the nurse may be able to serve as a catalyst and suggest that as many disciplines as are available be actively involved in the care of the patient.

IMMEDIATE INPATIENT INTERVENTION

Rapid and efficient care can be provided by anticipation of patient needs and having an organized admission procedure to treat burns in the emergency room.

Airway maintenance

If any *respiratory distress* is present an airway should be established. Prophylactic intubation is initiated if any heat or smoke has been inhaled or if the head, neck, or face is involved (see Plate 7, following p. 1102). Inhalation injuries are best managed with controlled ventilation, because swelling of the upper airway can progress to obstruction. Endotracheal intubation is preferred over a tracheostomy because edema of the respiratory passages frequently subsides within a few days and avoidance of surgical trauma is desired. Depending on the severity of symptoms, emergency treatment may include oxygen, suctioning, and postural drainage.

Pain relief

Morphine sulfate or meperidine hydrochloride is often given intravenously to the patient with extensive burns. The intravenous route is used because of inadequate absorption at peripheral sites. Large doses of sedatives and analgesics are avoided because of the danger of respiratory depression and because they may mask other symptoms.

Initial wound care

All debris and loose skin are removed from the burn wound and the area is cleansed. Dressings with the selected topical preparation are applied. Tetanus prophylaxis is initiated.

REPLACING BODY FLUIDS

Replacement of fluids and electrolytes is an essential part of the treatment and is instituted as soon as the extent of the burn and the patient's condition have been determined. Ideally, fluid therapy is started within an hour after a severe burn. Insertion of a large-bore central venous line permits the rapid administration of fluids and electrolytes.

Three types of fluid are considered in calculating the needs of the patient:
1. Colloids (plasma, plasma expanders)
2. Electrolyte fluids (lactated Ringer's solution, normal saline or 0.5N saline solution, hypertonic sodium solution)
3. Nonelectrolyte fluids (glucose in water).

These types of fluids are used in different combinations depending on the extent of the burn and physician preference.

Fluids administered during the first 48 hours are given to *maintain circulating blood volume*. Additional fluids and electrolytes are added to replace loss from vomiting or from nasogastric drainage. The amount of fluid replacement required during the first 48 hours is determined by assessment of the following factors:
1. Urinary output
2. Serum electrolyte levels
3. Blood gas findings
4. Central venous pressure
5. Body weight
6. Hematocrit level (maintained at slightly above normal)
7. Level of consciousness
8. Vital signs.

Fluid needs for the first 24 hours are calculated from the time of the burn. The usual pattern of fluid replacement is as follows:

Hour 0 to 8	One half of total amount for first 24-hours
Hour 8 to 16	One fourth of 24-hour total
Hour 16 to 24	One fourth of 24-hour total
Hour 24 to 48	One half of total amount for first 24 hours

Monitoring of fluid needs and complications

A *central venous line* line will be required to permit fluid replacement and to monitor fluid volume. A *Swan-Ganz* catheter may be inserted to monitor pulmonary arterial and capillary wedge pressures in the severely burned patient, for identification of hypovolemia or hypervolemia, and to assist in evaluating fluid therapy. If fluids are permitted orally, accurate recording is important. Unlimited oral intake and failure to measure it may result in too much fluid in the circulating blood, resulting in water intoxication (see Chapter 10).

The rate of *urinary output* is a reliable measure of determining the adequacy of fluid therapy *during the first 48 hours*. Usually a retention catheter is inserted and drained into a calibrated container. The amount of urine is measured and recorded every hour. The urine is observed for color and analyzed for hematocrit level. The physician is notified of hematuria or a positive Hemastix reaction. Urine flow of 30 to 50 ml/hr is adequate for an adult. *If the urinary output rises above or falls below these figures, the physician is notified immediately.* Fluid therapy will need to be adjusted accordingly. Lack of urinary output may indicate insufficient fluids or acute tubular necrosis. All efforts must be taken to provide sufficient fluid to protect vital organs.

After the first 48 to 72 hours the urinary output is no longer a reliable guide to fluid needs, because water deprivation may occur even when the urinary output for adults is 100 ml/day or more (diuretic stage). Fluid needs are then determined by measuring *serum electrolyte levels*. Fluid replacement during the diuretic stage is based on individual assessment. Parenterally administered fluids may be discontinued if serum electrolyte levels return to normal. If dehydration occurs from diuresis, fluid replacement therapy may be continued until blood volume is stabilized. The patient is observed closely for signs of water intoxication or pulmonary edema.

Electrolytes

The hyperkalemia of the first (hypovolemic) stage can change to hypokalemia within a very few hours during diuresis or as the potassium moves back into cells. The serum levels of potassium are monitored closely, and potassium is replaced parenterally when hypokalemia results. Compromised renal function significantly complicates potassium management, because potassium is excreted by the kidney.

PREVENTING INFECTION

A major principle in the care of the burned person is the prevention of infection. Local and systemic infections

Table 38-4. Treatment methods for burned skin areas

Method	Approach	Comments
Open (exposure)	Burned area cleansed and exposed to air; no clothing or bedclothes over burned area Cradle over bed to protect burned area; cautious use of lights or heat lamp to provide warmth Isolation technique essential (gown and mask); sterile linen on bed Room kept at 29.5°C (85°F) and humidity at 40% to 50%	Used mostly for burns on face, neck, perineum, and broad areas of trunk Hard crust forms to protect wound; crust falls off spontaneously in 14 to 21 days as wound heals Monitor for pain or chills
Closed	Burned areas cleansed Dressing applied and changed one to three times per day	Monitor for signs of impaired circulation (numbness, pain, tingling) Monitor for signs of infection (odor on dressings, fever, tachycardia)
Hydrotherapy	Patient placed in hydrotherapy tub once or twice per day for 20 to 30 minutes Attendants wear gowns and gloves until patient's wounds healed Tub room kept at 26.5° to 32° C (80° to 90° F) to prevent chilling	More painless method of dressing removal Aids in wound cleansing by removal of loose eschar and other debris Facilitates range of motion exercises Treatment started after vital signs and fluid balance stabilized

(septicemia) are the most common complications of burns and are a major cause of death, particularly in burns covering more than 25% of the body (see Plate 8, following p. 1102). Autogenous sources are the primary sources of infection initially, although the wound is highly susceptible to infection from exogenous sources. The person's own bacteria become trapped under the crusty eschar, and agressive wound management is necessary. The skin should be shaved to decrease potential sources of bacteria.

The organisms that usually infect burn wounds are *Staphylococcus aureus, Pseudomonas aeruginosa,* and the coliform bacilli. In the past few years there has been a high incidence of fungal infections resulting from the use of broad-spectrum antibiotics. *Candida albicans,* which normally is found in the gastrointestinal tract, accounts for the majority of fungal infections. Cultures of matter from the patient's nose, throat, wound, and unburned skin and a punch biopsy specimen may be taken on admission and at biweekly intervals to determine the bacteria present and their sensitivity to antibiotics.

All persons who approach the patient should wear gowns and masks to prevent the introduction of their organisms into the wound. Persons with upper respiratory tract infections should not be permitted near the patient. Surgical aseptic technique and sterile gloves are used when applying dressings. Hydrotherapy tanks used for aggressive cleansing of burn wounds need particular attention to prevent infection of burn wounds when the tanks are used by different patients.

Different methods of treating the burned area (Table 38-4) may be used depending on the location of the burn,

its size and depth, the facilities available, and the patient's response to therapy. One method may be replaced with another during the course of treatment.

Wound care

The extent of local cleansing depends on the severity of the burn and the judgment of the physician. Detergents or antiseptic preparations, such as povidone-iodine (Betadine), are effective cleansing agents. Daily tubbing and mechanical debridement must be done to remove wound exudate and debris. Washing and friction removes build-up of debris and supports healthy tissue regeneration.

Eschar is a black, leathery, dead tissue covering over third-degree burns that results in 48 to 72 hours from dehydration of the wound. Loose eschar may be gradually removed through the use of whirlpool baths or debridement (see Plate 9, following p. 1102). Uninfected eschar acts as a protective covering. The danger of infection exists as bacteria proliferate beneath the eschar. Spontaneous separation, produced by bacterial action, occurs unless surgical debridement is performed first. An escharotomy (linear incision of constricting eschar) may be necessary when constriction of circulation or respiration is evident (see Plate 10, following p. 1102).

Topical agents (Table 38-5) are more effective in preventing local infection because impairment of the vasculature in the burn area prevents systemic antibiotics from reaching the wound. Antibiotics may be given prophylactically or may be withheld until an infection occurs.

Dressing change may be painful, and analgesics, if reqired, should be given 30 minutes before the procedure

Table 38-5. Topical medications used in burn therapy

Drug	Advantages	Disadvantages
Mafenide (Sulfamylon)	Effective bacteriostatic agent against many gram-negative and gram-positive organisms Highly stable drug	Metabolic acidosis if renal function impaired Discomfort initially after application Allergic manifestations
Silver sulfadiazine (Silvadene)	Broad antimicrobial activity against *Pseudomonas* and *Candida* organisms No electrolyte imbalances	Hypersensitivity reactions Wound may develop a slimy, grayish appearance simulating an infection despite negative cultures
Povidone-iodine (Betadine)	Broad antimicrobial activity against bacteria, fungi, yeasts, viruses, protozoa Nonirritating and nonsensitizing	
Silver nitrate	Bacteriostatic effect Lessens pain and eliminates odor Isolation technique not required with silver nitrate treatments	Dressings must be kept wet; dryness leads to precipitation of silver salts into wound Solution is hypotonic; leads to electrolyte loss, especially sodium Stains everything black (gown and gloves are used during application and splashing of environment is avoided)
Neomycin	Effective against most organisms	Serious toxic effects May cause irreversible hearing loss or kidney failure with prolonged use

for maximal effectiveness. Most dressing changes are performed after tubbing, because this facilitates dressing removal and less pain.

Wound coverings

The burn wound may be covered with dressings or grafts.

Dressings

The type of dressing usually applied consists of a single layer of fine-mesh gauze held in place by a wrapping of a coarse gauze such as Kerlix. Counterpressure wrappings (Ace bandages) may be applied. Large, bulky dressings are rarely used today for large burns except in selected instances, because infection control is more difficult. The purposes of applying some type of light covering include prevention of infection from exogenous sources, facilitation of debridement, maximal contact by topical agents, and prevention of fluid evaporation with loss of body heat.

Wet dressings may be used, such as with silver nitrate or normal saline application. A single layer of fine mesh gauze is usually placed over the wound, covered with thick gauze pads to maintain moisture, and held in place with a gauze wrapping. The dressings must be kept wet. Plastic wrap should *not* be used to cover the dressings, because this prevents any fluid evaporation, causes increased heat at the wound site, and results in patient discomfort and increased tissue destruction and infection.

Skin grafts

Skin grafts are applied to cover the burn wound and speed healing, to prevent contractues, and to shorten convalescence. Successful grafting reduces the patient's vulnerability to infection and prevents the loss of body heat and water vapor from the open wound or eschar.

Split-thickness mesh *autografts* (see Chapter 37) and free grafts are commonly used in the treatment of burns. *Homografts* (from skin of other persons) may be used; although these grafts are commonly rejected in 4 to 5 weeks, only about 10 days are required to cover a large granulating burn wound. *Heterografts* of materials such as pigskin (see Plate 11, following p. 1102) or a synthetic substitute are being used commonly to provide temporary protection to wounds, reduce pain, promote granulation, and reduce surface bacterial count.

PROMOTING NUTRITION

Metabolism is increased after moderate to severe burns as a result of stress, fluid loss, fever, infection, hypercatabolism, and immobility. Uninjured cells have increased metabolic activity initially as a result of decreased oxygenation because of hypovolemia. Nitrogen losses are great because of the protein loss through the burn wound in addition to the usual losses from trauma and immobility. The catabolic phase may last for more than a month in persons with extensive injury.

Table 38-6. Specific nutritional needs of adults following extensive burns

Nutrient	Daily requirements	
	Preburn	Postburn
Protein	0.8/kg body weight	2-4 kg/preburn body weight
Calories	1700 to 3000	3500 to 5000
Vitamin C	45 mg	1 to 2 gm
B complex vitamins		5 to 10 times normal requirements

Weight gain occurs initially because of fluid retention. After diuresis there is a marked loss of weight caused by loss of fluid and negative nitrogen balance. Profound weight loss may lead to death. The weight curve will level out at a point below the preburn weight, and weight gain does not begin until the wounds are nearly all grafted. Weight is monitored closely until recovery.

Promoting nutritional needs is therefore an important part of burn therapy. Attention is directed toward adequate intake of all nutrients. Those nutrients that have specific additional requirements are listed in Table 38-6. Note the large increases required for protein, calories, and vitamins C and B. Iron preparations are required for persons who develop anemia.

Ensuring the necessary nutrient intake is often difficult because of the following factors:
1. Paralytic ileus (neuroendocrine response)
2. Nausea and vomiting
3. Anorexia
4. Large quantity of required nutrients.

Initially, during the hypovolemic stage, the major concern is fluid and electrolyte balance. Fluids are give intravenously until fluid balance is achieved. Efforts are then directed to meet the increased nutritional requirements. If the person is unable to eat, total parenteral nutrition (TPN) or tube feedings (if gastrointestinal function is restored) are instituted.

As soon as nausea has subsided and the gastrointestinal tract is functioning, all efforts are made to encourage oral intake.
1. Carbonated beverages supply necessary electrolytes and sugar during the early period.
2. Salty solutions (for example, meat broth) help replace sodium chloride.
3. Broths and fruit juices containing potassium are withheld for 48 hours or until serum potassium levels decrease.
4. High protein powdered milk preparations increase protein intake.
5. A high-protein, high-calorie, high-vitamin diet is prescribed.
6. Iron preparations are required for persons who develop anemia.

7. Supplementary feedings facilitate increased nutrient intake.
8. High-fiber foods are encouraged to prevent constipation and fecal impaction.
9. Painful and disagreeable dressing changes and other treatments are avoided immediately before meals.

PREVENTING MOBILITY LIMITATIONS

Contractures are among the most serious long-term complications of burns. Two major types of contractures occur, those caused by *muscle and joint stiffening* and those occurring after *skin grafting*. Many patients must undergo painful reconstructive surgery that would not have been necessary if those in attendance had been alert to the prevention of contractures. Early skin grafting prevents many contractures by mobilizing the patient sometimes months earlier than would otherwise be possible.

Contractures from joint immobility develop primarily because of pain following the burn, fatigue, and depression. The patient must be helped to maintain range of joint motion. It is important that patients understand why ambulation or motion is necessary even though it is painful. Constant encouragement can be provided by setting short-term achievable goals.

Body positions
1. Encourage *prone* and *supine* positions for a definite time interval each day:
   a. Use of special beds (Stryker frame, Foster bed, CircOlectric bed) facilitates turning of patient with minimum handling
   b. Special beds are particularly useful for extensive burns on back and front of trunk, thighs, and legs.
2. Encourage frequent position changes:
   a. Avoid prolonged periods in semi-Fowler's position
   b. Turn bed at intervals so patient does not stay in a preferred position for long periods (patient will move)
   c. Move bedside table to opposite side of bed to encourage movement to opposite side.
3. Burns on *neck and chin:*
   a. Encourage position of neck hyperextension for part of day
   b. Place pillow under shoulders with bed flat for neck hyperextension.
4. Burns on *hand:*
   a. Consult physician and physiatrist (rehabilitation specialist) for recommended hand position
   b. Hands with *dorsal* surface burns are often positioned in a *flexed* position of function
   c. Hands with *palmar* surface burns are often positioned in *hyperextension*
   d. Total hand burns usually positioned as for dorsal burns
   e. Splints (see Plate 12, following p. 1102) may be used to position hand
   f. Open method of treatment may be used to encourage frequent exercises.

Emotional responses to severe burns

Patient response	Nursing approach
Regression (adapting a behavior of an earlier life time frame)	Acknowledge inability to cope Provide structure: allow patient choice in some instances Reward appropriate behavior
Depression (withdrawal into oneself)	Support patient Encourage verbalization of frutrations Encourage activity within clinical limitations
Paranoia (suspicion of intended harm)	Acknowledge complaints of manifestation of fear Investigate all complaints Support patient Provide reality orientation

---

Exercises

Exercises for prevention and correction of contractures are begun as soon as the patient's vital signs are stable. Supervision by a physical therapist is desirable. When burns are completely covered (by healing or by graft) exercises may be performed more easily in an occupational therapy or physical therapy department where the patient also may benefit from a change in environment.

In the department of physical medicine, exercises often are performed in water. A Hubbard tank may be used for this purpose. The occupational therapist may help the patient to improve range of motion in a satisfying and efficient fashion by teaching functional activities of daily living and crafts suitable for particular needs. The nurse must know what the patient is being taught by the physical therapist and the occupational therapist so that progress can be continued on the nursing unit.

Facial exercises are encouraged for burns on the face or neck to prevent scars from tightening as they form. Chewing gum and blowing up balloons provide exercise that helps to prevent facial contractures.

Contracture clinics are available for burn patients and are associated with some burn centers. If this service is not available, the nurse in the hospital or the community health agency may have to take responsibility for teaching the patient how to prevent contractures from developing.

Promoting comfort

Pain is a major problem in the care of the patient with burns. The acute pain syndrome is the primary response. During this period the following approaches can help to minimize the pain:
1. Provide analgesic medication 30 minutes prior to painful treatments.
2. Provide clear explanations to gain patient's cooperation.
3. Handle burned parts gently.
4. Use careful sterile technique (infection causes increased pain).

Fears following major burns

Death
Pain
Disfigurement
Prolonged hospitalization
Job security
Disruption of life-style
Reaction of family and friends

5. Encourage patient to participate in treatment whenever possible.
6. Use distracting activities and relaxation techniques when appropriate.

Pain may persist for a long time (chronic pain) (see Chapter 12). The effects of the chronic pain will depend on the persn's usual coping style, personality, availability of resources, and extent and complications of the burn.

Counseling and teaching
PROVIDING EMOTIONAL SUPPORT

The emotional impact of severe burns is enormous and reality based. During the first few days the patient is too ill to fully comprehend what has happened. Numerous fears then emerge.

Patients who are severely burned usually are exhausted and often demoralized by the pain, treatments, and frequent dressing changes. Defense mechanisms may be evident as the patient attempts to control pain. Care givers need to be supportive, although they may find the patient's behavior unacceptable. Support and understanding will allow the patient to develop more acceptable means of coping with the stressful situation. Diazepam (Valium)

Discharge instructions for burn patients

We on the burn team are happy to see that you are able to go home. To ensure you the speediest possible recovery, it is important that you are able to care for yourself and recognize problems that may interfere with your complete recovery.

If any of the following occur, please call the hospital and ask for the burn clinic. The nurse will be able to assist you.

1. Healed area breaking open; cover with clean dressing.
2. Formation of blisters.
3. Signs of infection:
   a. Fever, temperature >37.2°C (99°F).
   b. Redness, pain, swelling, hardness, or warmth in or around wound or any other part of body.
   c. Increased or foul-smelling drcinage from wound.
4. Problems with Ace bandages or Jobst garment, such as improper fit, formation of blisters, or opening of healed area underneath.

Your first clinic appointment will be on _____. If a family member can come with you they can register for you and you may go to the burn clinic waiting room.

Skin care for healed burn

These are your guidelines for your daily skin care of a healed burn. When you do your skin care, this is the time to look at the involved areas and note whether there are any changes that need to be reported.

1. Wash healed area every day with solution of 2 tbsp mild soap (Dreft or Ivory Snow) and water.
2. Wash gently with washcloth to remove dead skin.
3. Rinse skin well after washing.
4. Dry thoroughly.
5. Apply Nivea lightly twice a day and more frequently if the skin is dry and flaked.
6. Do not put Nivea on open areas.
7. You can purchase Nivea at your local drugstore

Care for burn wound

These are your guidelines for the care of your burn wound. When you do your care, this is the time to look at the involved areas and note whether there are any changes that need to be reported.

Procedure for burn wound care

1. Wash hands.
2. Remove dressing and dispose of in paper bag or wrap in newspaper.
3. Wash hands.
4. Wash open area with gauze using solution of mild soap (Dreft or Ivory Snow) and water. Add 1 tbsp soap to a basin of water, 2 tbsp if you use the bathtub. Use a clean towel and washcloth with each dressing change.
5. Rinse skin well.
6. Wash hands.
7. Apply dressing as described below.
8. Wear gloves. Wash basin or bathtub with a disinfectant such as Lysol.
9. Wash hands.

Care of clothing

When you are discharged, you may find that healed burn areas are sensitive to harsh detergents, fabric softeners, and clothing dyes. If you are sensitive, we suggest the following:

1. Launder new clothing before use by machine or hand with mild soap (Dreft or Ivory Snow).
2. Rinse clothes twice.
3. Do not use fabric softeners.
4. If you have open burns or a healed area opens, wash all clothes separately from those of other family members.
5. Scarlet red ointment will permanently stain clothing.
6. If dyes used in clothing cause irritation, wear white articles.

Ace bandages

You have been taught to put on your own Ace bandages while in the hospital, but if you do have a problem with this, please notify the burn clinic. It is also important that you know how to care for them and understand problems that occur.

1. If they are too loose they will be ineffective and must be rewrapped.
2. If they are too tight they will cause discomfort, numbness, tingling, and puffiness and must be rewrapped.
3. They must be worn for a long time, probably 6 to 12 mo, to be effective, so please do not stop wearing them until your doctor tells you to.
4. To care for your Ace bandages:
   a. Hand wash with mild soap (Dreft or Ivory Snow) in cold water.
   b. Towel dry.
   c. Lay flat or place over rod or clothesline.
   d. Do not use clothespins.

Jobst garment

You have been taught how to put on your Jobst garment while in the hospital, but if you have a problem with this, please notify the burn clinic. It also is important that you know how to care for it and understand problems that can occur.

1. If it is too loose it will be ineffective and you will require a new garment.
2. If it is too tight it will cause discomfort, numbness, and tingling. Do not wear it if this occurs, but notify the burn clinic as soon as possible.
3. To care for your Jobst garment:
   a. Hand wash with mild soap (Dreft or Ivory Snow) in cold water.
   b. Towel dry.
   c. Lay flat or place over rod or clothesline.
   d. Do not use clothespins.

Courtesy Cleveland Metropolitan General Hospital Department of Nursing Service.

may be helpful in decreasing anxiety and providing muscle relaxation.

If possible the patient should see facial burns only after being prepared for the experience. Support and understanding will be needed in order for the patient to cope with what will be seen in the mirror. The patient will exhibit readiness by asking to look in the mirror. Interaction with other burned patients who are further along in their healing process may help the patient feel that recovery is possible. In some instances the recovery is incredible, and although differences in skin pigmentation remain, the redness that accompanies burns and newly healed skin often fades considerably within a few months. Pigmentation problems are more acute for persons with brown or black skin; their skin may be a different shade, freckled, or whitish in color.

Clinical observation indicates that the burned individual experience concern about changes in body perceptions. Because the skin, peripheral blood vessels, and lymph vessels are damaged, the burned patient's sense of *body boundary* is frequently altered. Patients undergoing debridement after loosening of burn eschar describe sensations of having their skin torn away from them. It has been asserted that persons who perceive their body boundaries as being well defined tend to be more confident and have a higher goal and task completion drives. It is therefore possible that those who lose a part of that sense of definiteness will tend to take a more languid approach to life with less successful interactions with others.[32]

The patient should have an opportunity to talk about any problems and fears. Some patients may discuss these concerns with the nurse when they cannot express them to relatives, and the nurse must be prepared to listen and help the individual accept necessary changes in life-style. Relatives may be able to give information that will clarify the patient's needs and resources. Relatives and friends also may need support in accepting the patient's change in appearance, and help in planning for the patient's return to the home and community. Almost every burned patient and family need the help of the social worker. The nurse should recognize this need and initiate the referral.

TEACHING

Patients have a great need for education so that they may take increasing responsibility for their own care. Teaching includes the following:
1. Care of the healed burn wound
2. Nutritional needs
3. Prevention of injury
4. Recognition of signs and symptoms of complications
5. Methods of coping with resocialization.

Complete and comprehensive instructions followed by return demonstrations contribute to learning the necessary skills to be independent and prudent in self-care activities after discharge. Patients should not be discharged from the hospital until they can care for themselves physically and are prepared to meet the stresses involved in returning to their former living patterns. Accentuation of the individual's strengths and focus on effective coping mechanisms will overshadow limitations the person may be experiencing.

Teaching needs in the rehabilitative stage

Complete recovery and rehabilitation of the severely burned patient is a long and costly process. Many industries have compensation insurance to cover part of the cost.

There is a fairly high frequency of malignant degeneration of scar tissue after burns. This is particularly true when the burn is caused by electricity or by x rays. Patients who have been burned therefore should have medical checkups at regular intervals indefinitely and should be advised to report any unusual change in the burn scar at once.

EVALUATION

Evaluation is based on the expected patient outcomes. Questions to be considered include the following:
Is the patient comfortable?
Are there any signs of infection?
Are there any signs of beginning contractures?
Is a high-protein, high carbohydrate, high-fat diet being consumed?
Is the patient involved in the plans of care?
Is the patient mobile and independent in self-care?
Has the patient had opportunities to explore feelings and resolve problems?
Is the patient making plans for resocialization?
Does the patient know how to carry out required home treatments and when to seek medical care?

REFERENCES AND SELECTED READINGS*

1. Artz, C.P., Moncrief, J.A., and Pruitt, B.A.: Burns: a team approach, Philadelphia, 1979, W.B. Saunders Co.
2. *Busby, H.D.: Nursing management of the acute burn patient and nursing management of optimal burn recovery, J. Cont. Educ. Nurs. **10**:16-30, 1979.
3. Curreri, P.W., and Luterman, A.: Nutritional support of the burned patient, Surg. Clin. North Am. **58**:1151-1156, 1978.
4. *deTornay, R., and Doswell, W.M.: Nursing decisions: experiences in clinical problem solving, Series 2, No. 7: Kare A., a patient with burns, RN **40**(5):59-68, 1977.
5. Dyer, C.: Burn care in the emergent period, J. Emerg. Nurse **6**:9-16, 1980.
6. Emig, E., and Lloyd, J.R.: How to get burned children home sooner, RN **40**(7):37-39, 1977.
7. Feist, C.: Reprieve, Nurs. 79 **9**(10):144, 1979.
8. Fire in the United States, United States Department of Commerce, United States Fire Administration, National Fire Data Center, 1978.

*References preceded by an asterisk are particularly well suited for student reading.

9. *Gaston, S.F., and Schumann, L.L.: Burn wound management, Crit. Care Update **7**:5-17, 1980.

10. *Hadley, R.D.: Knowledge, understanding: keys to burn patient care, Am. Nurse **9**:9-10, 1977.

11. Hayter, J.: Emergency nursing care of the burned patient, Nurs. Clin. North Am. **13**:223-234, 1978.

12. Helm, P., et al.: Burn rehabilitation: a team approach, Surg. Clin. North Am. **58**(6): 1263-1278, 1978.

13. Jacoby, F.G.: Individualized burn wound dressings, Nurs. 77 **7**(6):62-63, 1977.

14. Jacoby, F.G.: Nursing care of the patient with burns, ed. 2, St. Louis, 1976, The C.V. Mosby Co.

15. Jones, C.A., and Feller, I.: Burn nursing is nursing, Crit. Care Q. **1**:77-78, 1978.

16. Jones, C.A., and Feller, I.: Burns: the home stretch. . . rehabilitation, Nurs. 77 **7**(12):54-57, 1977.

17. *Jones, C.A., and Feller, I.: Burns: what to do during the first crucial hours, Nurs. 77 **7**(3):22-31, 1977.

18. Kinzie, Y., and Lau, C.: What to do for the severely burned, RN **43**(4):46-51, 1980.

19. Marvin, J.A.: Acute care of the burn patient, Crit. Care Q. **1**(3):30-33, 1978.

20. Marvin, J.A.: Planning home care for burn patients, Nurs. 83 **13**(8):65-67, 1983.

21. *Nursing grand rounds: realistic goals don't mean failure, Nurs. 79 **9**(5):54-59, 1979.

22. *Nursing grand rounds: septic shock in a burn patient, Nurs. 76 **6**(1):39-43, 1976.

23. *Nursing grand rounds: severely burned patients: anticipating their emotional needs, Nurs. 80 **10**(8):47-50, 1980.

24. Rogenes, P.R., and Moylan, J.: Restoring fluid balance in the patient with severe burns, Am. J. Nurs. **76**:1952-1957, 1976.

25. Schumann, L., and Gaston, S.: Common sense guide to topical burn therapy, Nurs. 79 **9**(3):34-39, 1979.

26. Singletary, Y.: More than skin deep, J. Psychiatr. Nurs. **15**:7-11, 1977.

27. Twombly, M.: The shift into third space, Nurs. 78 **8**:38-39, 1978.

28. *Wagner, M.: Emergency care of the burned patient, Am. J. Nurs. **77**:1788-1791, 1977.

Classic references

29. Bowden, M.L., and Feller, L.: Family reaction to a severe burn, Am. J. Nurs. **73**:316-319, 1973.

30. Feller, I., and Archanbeault, C.: Nursing the burned patient, Ann Arbor, Mich., 1973, Institute for Burn Medicine Press.

31. *Williams, B.P.: The burned patient's need for teaching, Nurs. Clin. North Am. **6**:615-639, 1971.

32. Williams, B.P.: The problems and life-style of a severely burned man. In Bergersen, B., et al., editors: Current concepts in clinical nursing, vol. 2, St. Louis, 1969, The C.V. Mosby Co.

39

The Patient with Immunologic Problems

BARBARA C. LONG and E. RONALD WRIGHT

STUDY QUESTIONS

- Review the structure and function of the immune system (Chapter 6).

- Why has there been such recent concern in the news media about AIDS? What are some of the major problems of AIDS victims?

- What is the significance of leukopenia? What major nursing interventions are indicated for leukopenia?

- Review the procedure for blood transfusions.

- Examine the chart of a patient receiving blood transfusions. What was the purpose of the transfusion? What was the patient's response to the transfusion?

Immunologic alterations occur in a wide variety of diseases, and although knowledge concerning the immunologic bases of these diseases is expanding rapidly, much remains obscured. In some disorders the immunologic basis is clear-cut, such as in allergic disorders and immunodeficiency diseases. In some instances, as in systemic lupus erythematosus (SLE), immunologic response is known to have a role, but the relative significance of the immuologic factors is not clear. In still other disorders, such as neoplasias, the role of the immunologic response as the causative agent is even less well documented.

The structure and function of the immune response is discussed in Chapter 6. Because immunologic factors are operative in such a wide variety of disorders, much of the information about the disorders is found elsewhere in the text. This chapter will describe the various categories of immune disorders and will discuss in more detail those disorders not described elsewhere.

Major health problems of the immune system

Immunologic disorders occur when the immune response malfunctions. The disorders may be a result of immune deficiencies, abnormal production of immunoglobulins, excessive response to specific antigens, or immune response to self-antigens (Table 39-1). Each of these major categories will be discussed in this chapter. The majority of immunologic problems (other than the great variety of autoimmune diseases discussed throughout the text) are hypersensitivity disorders, so these disorders will be discussed in more detail.

IMMUNODEFICIENCIES
PATHOPHYSIOLOGY

Protection of the host depends on an intact immune system. Interference with development of cells and tis-

Table 39-1. Classification of immunologic disorders

Category	Immune response	Examples
Immunodeficiencies	Deficiencies in the proper expression of immune response system, part of the system, or specific cells	Primary deficiencies, deficiencies associated with other diseases, acquired immunodeficient syndrome (AIDS)
Gammopathies	Abnormal production of immunoglobulins	Multiple myeloma, hypergamma-globinemia
Hypersensitivities	Exaggerated or inappropriate response to specific antigen	Anaphylaxis, allergies, transfusion reactions, graft rejections
Autoimmunities	Immunologic attack on self-antigens	Rheumatoid arthritis, SLE, glomerulo-nephritis

sues of the immune response leads to immunodeficient disorders. Since the cells and tissues of the immune response system develop sequentially, if a defect in that development appears, the severity of the resulting deficiency reflects the stage of development at which the abnormality arose. Deficiencies may exist in immunoglobulin synthesis (B cell deficiency), cellular immune functions (T cell deficiency), or phagocyte defects.

Immunodeficiencies may be primary or secondary. Primary immunodeficiencies, those resulting from improper fetal development, are genetic disorders in children. Some primary immunoglobulin deficiencies may not become evident until the person is an adult, and these are termed *common variable immunodeficiencies* (CVI). Persons with CVI develop recurrent virulent infections and display a high incidence of malignancies, hematologic disorders, and autoimmune diseases.

Secondary immunodeficiencies are a nonspecific depression of the immune response as a result of some interference with the immune sytem. These deficiencies are present to one degree or another in most of the major disease conditions experienced by persons in addition to the normal response to aging. Thus when caring for a person beyond the age of 60 years or with any acute disease condition, the concepts of immunodeficiency must be considered. Situations in which immunodeficiency plays a major role are listed in the box above.

Major stress of any type may affect immune response as a result of increased corticosteroid production and alterations in protein metabolism. A form of immunodeficiency, immunosuppression, may result from or be deliberately created by the use of radiation, drugs, or antigens and antibodies (Table 39-2).

In recent years there has been an increased incidence of acquired immunodeficient syndrome (AIDS). Over two thirds of the reported cases have been among homosexual or bisexual males, but the disorder is not confined to this population. High-risk factors are thought to include genetic predisposition (Haitian ancestry), abuse of intravenous drugs, many sexual partners, and many episodes of sexually transmitted diseases.[2] The basis of the disease is unknown, but a virus is thought to be involved and the person becomes immunodeficient. The disorder begins insidiously with fatigue and upper respiratory infection.

Disorders influenced by immunodeficiencies

Protein-calorie malnutrition
Alcoholism
Infections (especially viral)
Cancer
Autoimmune diseases
Lymphomas (including Hodgkin's disease)
Allergies
Trauma
Transplantation

Purple patches appear on the skin. This is followed by enlarged nodes, fever with night sweats, rapid weight loss, and dyspnea. The person cannot respond immunologically to infection and death ensues.

ASSESSMENT

Subjective data

Subjective data to obtain from the person with immunodeficiency include the following:
1. Knowledge of the immunodeficiency
2. Knowledge of prevention of infection
3. Occurrence of recurrent infections (type)
4. Concerns related to the immunodeficiency
5. Availability of support persons for the person with AIDS

Recurrent viral or fungal infections are suggestive of T cell–mediated deficiencies, whereas recurrent bacterial infections may have an underlying B cell (immunoglobulin) deficiency.

Objective data

Objective data include monitoring for early signs of infection (fever, pain, nasal discharge, cough, and enlarged nodes). The skin is inspected daily for lesions.

Table 39-2. Induced immunosuppression

Method	Comments	Use
Antigen administration	Specific antigen administered in small amounts over time	Allergy desensitization
Antibody administration	Specific antibody administered to combine with antigen and block contact with immunocompetent cell	Obstetrics: prevent sensitive Rh-negative mother from responding to Rh-positive fetus during pregnancy
Antilymphocytic serum (ALS)	Prepared from serum of horse immunized with human lymphocytic tissue; when administered to humans produces lymphocytopenia, thus fewer cells available for immune response	Restricted use as a result of side effects (serum sickness, anaphylactic shock, nephritis)
Irradiation	Destroys lymphocytes, thus fewer cells available for immune response; total body irradiation affects hematopoietic system, gastrointestinal (GI) system, and central nervous system (CNS)	Local irradiation: renal allografts Total body irradiation: organ transplantation
Drugs	Corticosteroids impair T cell function and cause catabolism of immunoglobulins and lymphocytopenia Cytotoxic drugs destroy rapidly dividing immuologically stimulated cells	Diseases where immune disorder is unknown (for example, autoimmunities); tissue and organ transplantation

Diagnostic tests
T cell (cellular) deficiency tests

T cell function can be screened by delayed hypersensitivity skin testing to common antigens. Specific antigens, including purified protein derivative (PPD), *Candida,* mumps antigen, streptokinase, and streptodornase, are injected intradermally. Reactions are read after 24 and 48 hours to determine hypersensitivity. The test is to determine the hypersensitivity, not the presence of disease. A person who does not react to any of these antigens is said to be *anergic.*

B cell (humoral) deficiency tests

ELECTROPHORESIS. The movement of colloid (protein) particles in an electrical field is called electrophoresis. In an applied electrical field, different proteins migrate at different rates because of their different sizes and shapes, and this property can be used to analyze plasma protein content. The plasma proteins consist of albumin and globulins, which can be further divided into alpha globulins, beta globulins, and gamma globulins (immunoglobulins). The serum proteins are subjected to electrophoresis in a medium that stabilizes the migration so that the proteins can be stained and examined.

QUANTITATIVE IMMUNOGLOBULIN TEST. Three of the immunoglobulins—IgG, IgA, and IgM—can be measured quantitatively, whereas IgD and IgE are present in amounts too small to measure. Venous blood is collected; no special preparation is required.

DATA ANALYSIS AND PLANNING

Nursing diagnoses

Possible nursing diagnoses for the person with an immune deficiency may include the following:

Potential infection
Knowledge deficit
Anxiety

Expected patient outcomes

1. Infection is avoided or controlled.
2. The patient can describe:
   a. Measures to avoid infection.
   b. Signs dictating immediate medical attention.
   c. Need for continued medical follow-up.
3. Anxiety is minimized.

IMPLEMENTATION

Replacement therapy

Gamma globulin is used for replacement therapy in primary B cell deficiency disorders but is also given as prophylaxis against viral diseases. When giving gamma globulin intramuscularly, a large-bore (18 to 20-gauge) needle is recommended, and the solution is injected slowly. Large amounts need to be divided and given at separate sites. Plasma therapy is better tolerated by the individual than large doses of gamma globulin, and all five immunoglobulins are included in the plasma. Homologous serum hepatitis and transfusion reactions, however, are potential risks with plasma therapy.

Replacement therapy for T cell–mediated immune deficiencies is more complex. Transfer factor (extracted from lymphocytes of humans who have demonstrated delayed hypersensitivity reactions), thymosin (a thymic hormone), and bone marrow transplants have been used.

Protecting from infection

The most important factor in the care of the immunodeficient or immunosuppressed person is protection from infection. Care differs depending on whether the degree of immunosuppression is minimal, moderate, or severe:

1. Care for minimal immunosuppression
   a. Use good medical asepsis
   b. Avoid persons with infections
   c. Give meticulous cleaning and protect even minor skin breaks
   d. Avoid injections as much as possible
   e. Maintain nutrition at optimum level
   f. Maintain adequate fluid hydration (intake of more than 1200 ml/day)
2. Care for moderate immunosuppression
   a. May be placed in reverse isolation
      1. Single room with door closed
      2. All who enter wear mask and gown and carry out isolation technique
   b. If person is acutely ill, give mouth care, perineal care, and pulmonary hygiene to prevent infection
3. Care for severe immunosuppression
   a. Patient isolation by laminar air flow units or life islands (Chapter 14)
   b. Use same protective measures as for moderate immunosuppression

The patient with AIDS may be given special precautions regarding blood, oral secretions, urine, and stool.[2] If the patient has a concurrent pneumonitis, full isolation technique is presently being carried out (until further research establishes the exact nature of the disorder). Patients with early signs of AIDS should not be placed in the same room with patients with infections because of the immunodeficiency. Antibacterial drugs that contain trimethoprim and sulfamethoxazole (Bactrim, Septra) may be prescribed prophylactically.

Promoting comfort

Care of the person with rapidly advancing AIDS is primarily supportive. Measures that promote aeration and decrease pain and cough are instituted. Because of the profuse sweating, frequent linen changes may be necessary.

Counseling and teaching
Decreasing anxiety

Knowledge that an overwhelming infection can have serious consequences, being placed in protective isolation, or knowledge that the mortality is high can provoke anxiety in the person with AIDS. An empathetic, supportive approach can help the patient identify fears and concerns and reduce anxiety.

Support persons are vital to the person with AIDS. Some homosexual communities have established support groups. Some persons obtain more support from individuals, more often friends. It is helpful for the AIDS victim to identify and develop a supportive relationship with a person or group.

Teaching the person with immunodeficiency

1. Explain immunodeficiency, that is the inability of the body to fight infection.
2. Take measures to prevent infection.
   a. Avoid persons with infections (especially colds).
   b. Avoid bumping or breaking the skin.
   c. Inspect skin daily for lesions.
   d. Eat a balanced diet (Chapter 7).
   e. Drink at least 6 glasses of fluid per day.
   f. Avoid becoming fatigued.
   g. Get a regular amount of sleep each night.
3. Report signs of infection to physician immediately.
4. See physician on a regular basis as instructed.
5. For the person with AIDS:
   a. Be selective in sexual partners.
   b. Limit number of sexual partners.
   c. Avoid sexual contact with person with known infection.
   d. Avoid introduction of fecal organisms in mouth.
   e. Use condom for anal sex.

Teaching

People who are immunosuppressed or who have AIDS need to know about their condition and how to avoid infection (see box above).

EVALUATION

Evaluation is based on expected patient outcomes. Questions to ask may include the following:
1. Does the person know the nature of the immunodeficiency?
2. Does the person know how to prevent infection?
3. Has infection been prevented during hospitalization?
4. Has anxiety decreased?

GAMMOPATHIES
PATHOPHYSIOLOGY

Gammopathies, better termed *hypergammaglobulinemias*, are elevated levels of gamma globulin in the serum. The normal synthesis of an immunoglobulin is the result of the proliferation and plasma cell differentiation of a single clone of B cells in response to an antigenic signal. In gammopathies a single clone or multiple clones of plasma cells begin to overproduce immunoglobulin product in response to inappropriate antigenic stimulation.

Monoclonal (M-type) *gammopathies* involve a single B cell clone and are commonly referred to as plasma cell dyscrasias. A common monoclonal gammopathy is multiple myeloma.

Polyclonal gammopathies involve the overproduction of virtually all classes of immunoglobulins. The major causes are infectious diseases (especially chronic bacterial infections such as lung abscess and osteomyelitis), connective tissue diseases (such as SLE and rheumatoid arthritis), and chronic active liver disease. IgG and IgM are the most commonly involved immunoglobulins, and the degree of immunoglobulin level reflects the severity of the disease. The development of high levels of dysfunctional gamma globulins depresses the synthesis of normal immunoglobulins, which renders the person susceptible to infection.

Multiple myeloma

PATHOPHYSIOLOGY

Multiple myeloma is a monoclonal plasma cell malignancy seen in both men and women, occurring in middle and old age. It is characterized by widespread bone destruction, anemia, hypercalcemia, and hyperuricemia. These symptoms are traced to the proliferation of plasma cell tumors from the bone marrow into the hard bone tissue, causing an erosion of the bone. Frequent recurrent infections (especially of the respiratory tract) and spontaneous pathologic fractures occur because of the production of ineffective immunoglobulins, which, in turn, depress the production of normal antibodies. Renal failure may result from precipitation of urate and calcium crystals.

MEDICAL INTERVENTION

Radiation therapy may be given for palliative treatment of localized bone pain and pathologic fractures. Chemotherapy is the major treatment. Alkylating agents, specifically melphalan, are given in combination with adrenocorticosteroids. Several weeks may elapse between the initiation of therapy and signs of improvement. The average survival time is 3 years, but survival may be prolonged with periods of exacerbation and remission.

SUPPORTIVE NURSING CARE

Ambulation and adequate hydration are vitally important to prevent renal complications from the increased amounts of urates and calcium being excreted in the urine. Fluid intake should be sufficient to ensure a urinary output of a minimum of 1500 ml/24 hr. Ambulation may be difficult because of the skeletal pain and the possibility of fractures. A lightweight spinal brace and analgesics may facilitate ambulation.

Measures to prevent infection are instituted and include avoidance of persons with upper respiratory tract infections. Medical attention should be sought for any

---

> ### Factors influencing hypersensitivity responses
>
> Increased responsiveness of the host
> Increased amount of allergen
> Nature of allergen
> Entrance of allergen through appropriate site
> Short time period between contacts

---

signs of infection, and antibiotics are often given, since infections are usually caused by gram-positive organisms. Rest periods are planned if fatigue from anemia is present.

HYPERSENSITIVITY REACTIONS

PATHOPHYSIOLOGY

The immune response sytem that has been previously sensitized is designed to provide an immediate, effective, protective reaction to subsequent encounters with the sensitizing antigen. This of course is a positive factor in the provision of immunity; however, under a given set of conditions or because of an idiotypic reactivity to a particular antigen, the response of the immune system may produce detrimental effects. This inappropriate response is usually manifested as a tissue-damaging overreaction to the antigen; thus it is termed *hypersensitivity* or *allergy*. The antigenic stimulants invoking the reactions are referred to as *allergens*. Hypersensitivities, then, are classic expressions of the immune system, but they take place in inappropriate sites, in excessive amounts, or with inappropriate involvement of nonspecific tissues. Whether an allergic response occurs and to what degree depend on a combination of interrelated factors (see box above).

Hypersensitivities can be broadly divided into two categories based on the components of the immune system involved in mediating the hypersensitivity reaction: humoral or immediate response (B cell mediated) and cellular or delayed response (T cell mediated). The humoral response can be further subdivided into type I anaphylactic, type II cytotoxic, and type III immune complex (Table 39-3). Since type I, II, and III hypersensitivities are the result of interactions involving circulating antibodies, these reactions can be transferred from a sensitized host to a nonsensitized host by serum transfer. Type IV cell-mediated sensitivities can be transferred only by lymphocyte exchange.

Type I hypersensitivities

The type I hypersensitivities may take different forms depending on the type and amount of allergen and the degree of sensitization (Table 39-4). Anaphylactic shock

Table 39-3. Summary of hypersensitivity reactions

Property	Hypersensitivity type			
	Immediate (humoral)			Delayed (cellular)
	I Anaphylactic	II Cytotoxic	III Immune complex	IV Cell mediated
Immune system mediators	IgE (IgG) bound to mast cells	IgG or IgM (+ complement)	IgG or IgM + complement	T cells, macrophages
Allergens	Exogenous antigens	Foreign cells or alteration of cell surface antigens	Soluble antigens	Infectious agent, contact allergens, foreign tissues, cancer cells
Response to intradermal skin test	Wheal and flare within 30 min, edema	Not done	Erythema and edema within 3 to 8 hr	Erythema and induration within 24 to 48 hr
Pathophysiologic effects	Release of histamines, kinins, SRS-A from mast cells, which affect smooth muscle shock organs	Direct cytotoxic destruction of cells	Acute inflammatory reaction; primarily polymorphonuclear neutrophil leukocytes	Tissue destruction, primarily lymphocytes and macrophages
Examples	Systemic anaphylaxis, atopic allergies, hay fever, insect sting reactions	Hemolytic disease of the newborn (Rh), transfusion reactions	Serum sickness, Arthus reaction, glomerulonephritis	Tuberculin reaction, skin graft rejection, poison ivy

Table 39-4. Type I hypersensitivities (allergies)

Disorder	Etiology	Signs and symptoms	Medical therapy
Anaphylactic shock	Penicillin, heterologous antiserum, insect stings, pollen, x-ray contrast media, food	Initial itching and sneezing, apprehension. Edema of face, hands, and other body parts; dyspnea, wheezing, shock	Epinephrine subcutaneously; Benadryl intramuscularly; aminophylline to relax bronchial spasm; tracheal intubation for tracheal edema; control of shock
Urticaria (hives)	Foods, especially eggs, fish, and nuts; drugs such as penicillin. Chronic: stress, exposure to heat and cold	Skin lesions: pale pink elevated edge on an erythematous background (wheal). Pruritus	Self-limiting; epinephrine or antihistamines may be given
Atopic			
Allergic rhinitis (hay fever)	Pollens and spores of molds	Sneezing, itching, and watery eyes, running nose	Antihistamines; corticosteroids on a temporary basis for severe cases; desensitization (Chapter 24)
Allergic asthma	External antigens	Wheezing, coughing, dyspnea	Epinephrine, bronchodilators (for example, aminophylline) (Chapter 25)
Atopic dermatitis	Fibers in wool, furs, and nylon; detergents, soaps, perfumes, and cosmetics; changes in temperature; stress	Pruritus; vesicles, oozing, and crusting lesions; scaling	Wet dressings, topical steroids (Chapter 37)

is the most serious, life-threatening form and requires immediate medical intervention.

The less severe and more common forms of type I hypersensitivities are the atopic allergies, seen in about 15% of the population. *Atopic* refers to an inherited hypersensitivity. It is the tendency to become hypersensitive that is inherited, not the allergy to a specific substance. What persons become hypersensitive to is determined by the allergens to which they are exposed.

PATHOPHYSIOLOGY

Type I hypersensitivities are associated with the reactions mediated by the IgE class of immunoglobulins. The IgE immunoglobulins attach to the surface of mast cells and basophils, providing a site for allergens to bind to the cells. This causes the cell to release vasoactive substances, including histamine (Fig. 39-1).

Thus in type I reactions the detrimental symptoms are not at the site of the antigen-antibody reaction but at the site of the organs or tissues where the histamine and other mediators exert their action. If those mediators remain confined to a local area, the tissue reactions remain localized and are referred to as *local anaphylaxis*. The local hypersensitivity that most people demonstrate to a mosquito bite, the wheal-flare type of reaction, is the classic example of this type of reaction. The reaction may also become localized in the nose and eyes (hay fever), in the bronchial passages (allergic asthma), or in the skin (atopic dermatitis). If, however, the mediators become released systemically, the response is known as *systemic anaphylaxis*, which can produce anaphylactic shock (Chapter 11).

Histamine's three main effects are the following:
1. Constricts smooth muscle such as in the bronchi, resulting in bronchial spasm
2. Increases vascular permeability, resulting in urticaria (hives) or tissue edema
3. Increases mucous secretions, as occurs in hay fever and asthma

The symptoms will be determined by the organ affected.

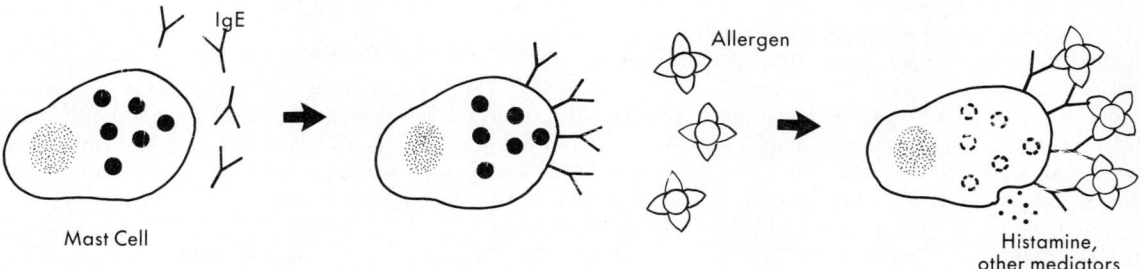

Fig. 39-1. Type I hypersensitivity. IgE binds to mast cell; allergen then binds to IgE, causing degranulation of mast cell with release of histamine and other mediators.

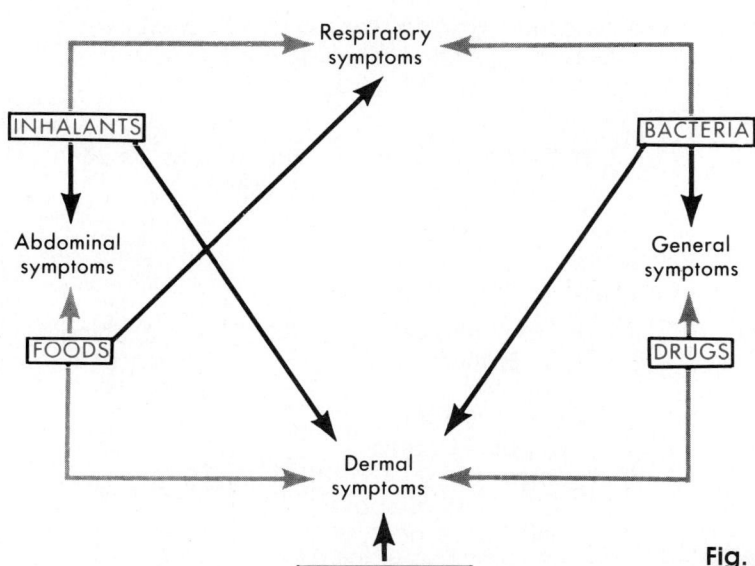

Fig. 39-2. Causes of allergic responses and symptoms produced.

Different etiologic factors cause different symptoms (Fig. 39-2).

For type I reactions to occur, the hypersensitive individual must initially come into contact with the allergen that triggers the synthesis of the specific antiallergenic IgE antibodies. This primary contact is known as a *sensitizing dose*. On subsequent contact with the allergen (termed the *shocking or challenging dose*), the individual exhibits the symptoms of type I sensitivity.

ASSESSMENT

All patients should be questioned about allergies and sensitivities to drugs before drug therapy is initiated. If there is any positive history, the physician is consulted before a new drug is given, and if it is given, the patient is watched closely for allergic responses.

It is usually possible to determine specific allergens to which a person is hypersensitive by taking a history that includes the following:

1. History of allergic reactions in the past (type, frequency, perceived cause)
2. Familial history of allergies
3. Recent exposure to sensitizing substances
4. Changes in living, working, or environmental conditions
5. Characteristics of present environment (house, clothing, plants and trees, or animals)
6. Increased stress in recent past
7. Types of symptoms: respiratory, dermal, or general
8. Alleviating factors, either prescribed by a physician or self-prescribed

Diagnostic tests
Skin testing

Skin tests are often used to determine whether a person has a sensitivity to certain substances in the external environment. Several methods of testing are used (Table 39-5). Occasionally 1 drop of a test extract is instilled into the eye to test for sensitivity (conjunctival test). Redness of the conjunctiva and tearing will appear within 5 to 15 minutes in an allergic person. Tests for allergenic substances are usually done in a series.

Use test

A person with a food allergy is asked to keep a food diary for at least a week. On the basis of this diary, suspect foods such as milk, wheat products, and eggs may be removed from the diet (elimination diet) until symptoms subside and then added one at a time in an attempt to identify the offending foods. Reaction to the use test may be immediate or over a period of time. Some persons become discouraged during the testing and may need encouragement to adhere to the testing schedule.

DATA ANALYSIS AND PLANNING
Nursing diagnoses

Nursing diagnoses will differ depending on the type of allergic disorder present and the data collected. Persons who have allergies that are related to environmental conditions necessitating changes in the home or occupation may have problems with *coping*. Many persons either lack information or have inaccurate information, therefore there may be a diagnosis of *knowledge deficit*.

Table 39-5. Allergy skin tests

Test	Method	Time of reading	Positive signs	Use
Intradermal	Allergens are injected intradermally at spaced intervals on forearm or intrascapular area; control tests with diluent alone done concurrently	15 to 30 min	Wheal with surrounding erythema	Allergies to pollen, feathers, animal dander, dust
Scratch	Skin cleaned with alcohol and allowed to dry; skin scratched superficially (1 to 4 mm long), and extract applied to scratch	30 min	Erythema	Same as for intradermal
Patch	Sensitizing substance applied to small (1-inch) gauze square and covered with tape	48 hr	+ Erythema only + + Erythema and papules + + + Erythema, papules, and vesicles + + + + All of above and bullae or ulceration	Allergies to clothing, detergents, perfumes, cosmetics

Expected patient outcomes

The patient can do the following:

1. Explain what substances are allergens and must be avoided.
2. Describe measures to be taken to control the environment (if pertinent).
3. Describe measures to prevent anaphylactic shock (if pertinent).

IMPLEMENTATION

Assisting with achievement of therapeutic goals

Preventing anaphylactic reaction

Persons with a history of allergies are at high risk for developing anaphylactic reactions from drugs or animal sera. Hospitalized persons who are sensitive to certain substances should be identified, and the information posted conspicuously outside of the room, on the medical order sheets of the patient's record, or in both places. In addition, many hospitals use a special color identification bracelet for the person who is sensitive to certain substances.

If immunization is necessary, animal sera should be avoided and another type given, if possible. When it is necessary to use animal serum, the individual should first be tested for sensitivity to the substance. An intradermal skin test preceded by a scratch or eye test is recommended. If animal sera, allergenic extracts, or contrast media containing iodide are given, a syringe containing 1:1000 epinephrine hydrochloride, an antihistamine such as diphenhydramine (Benadryl), and isoproterenol (Isu-

Table 39-6. Methods of decreasing environmental inhalant antigens

Area	Method
Floors	No wool carpets or felt rug pads; washable throw rugs over wood or tiled floors may be used
Furniture	No kapok stuffing; foam-stuffed furniture is preferable
Clothing	No wool; place closet garments in plastic bags
Bedding	
Pillows	No feathers; use foam or Dacron-filled
Mattress	Use foam mattress over a covered box spring; allergy-free covers
Blankets	Washable cotton
Pets	No fur-bearing pets
Cleaning	Daily damp dusting; no shaking of articles
Air	Air conditioning, if possible; electrostatic filters

prel) should be readily available. The patient is kept under surveillance for at least 20 minutes. Any reaction that occurs within a few minutes forewarns of an impending emergency.

Desensitization (immunotherapy)

An attempt may be made to slowly desensitize a person by injecting small but increasingly larger doses of the allergen at regular intervals (usually 1 to 4 weeks) over a long period. This treatment may take up to 5 years. It is about 80% effective against pollens causing hay fever but is less effective against asthma or dermatitis. It is essential that the person understand that desensitization is of little value until the environment is controlled; otherwise the constant exposure to allergens will only increase antibody response.

Control of environment

Persons whose allergies are caused by environmental inhalants will need a room free of house dust, animal dander, fungus spores, and other allergens. Because 90% of the airborne particles in the house (for example, house dust) are 5 μm or less in size, an electrostatic filter will be necessary. An electrostatic filter attracts particles by means of highly charged metal plates, which can be removed for cleaning. These filters come in portable models for room use or can be attached to the central heating system. Methods of decreasing environmental inhalant antigens are listed in Table 39-6.

Some hospitals have environmentally controlled rooms that may be used to remove a highly allergic person from the usual environment and thus facilitate the search for the substances to which the individual is sensitive. The room is kept free from substances most likely to be allergenic. Various articles used at home may be introduced one at a time to see if they cause symptoms. Only a limited number of staff members are allowed to enter the room, and they may be requested to avoid the use of cosmetics and to wear special gowns.

Teaching

There are several facts about allergens that are helpful to understand.

1. Persons who believe they have "rose fever" are really allergic to pollenating grasses; persons who believe they are allergic to goldenrod are really allergic to ragweed; both roses and goldenrod are insect pollenated.
2. Persons may be allergic to the pollen of one tree and not another; therefore there is a need to know which tree is pollenating at the time symptoms appear.
3. Persons who are allergic to pollenating grasses will have the same symptoms no matter which grass is pollenating. If they move from one geographic area to another, they will become sensitized to whatever grasses are present in that area.
4. Persons may be allergic to spores of molds and not realize it. Molds are most likely to be found inside

the house in warm, damp basements or in crawl spaces under the house. They are also found outside the house in leaves of certain trees, wheat, and corn.

5. For pollens and spores, the highest counts (amounts in the air) occur between 12 midnight and 8 AM.

Prevention of exacerbations requires knowledge of ways to avoid the allergens and when to seek medical as-sistance. Important points in the teaching of patients with allergies are summarized in box below.

EVALUATION

Evaluation is based on expected patient outcomes. Questions to consider include the following:

Teaching for the patient with allergies

1. Avoid allergens, when possible
   a. Seasonal inhalants
      (1) Air-condition the house, if possible.
      (2) Use electrostatic window filter if house is not air-conditioned.
      (3) Plan vacations outside the ragweed area during the peak of pollenating season, if possible.
   b. Environmental inhalants (Table 39-6)
   c. Drugs
      (1) Remind physician of allergy when new medication is prescribed.
      (2) Read all labels of nonprescription drugs before taking new drug.
      (3) Wear a MedicAlert bracelet indicating the known drug allergy.
   d. Food
      (1) Examine labels of new prepared food for presence of allergen.
      (2) Avoid eating unknown foods when travelling.
   e. Contact allergens
      (1) Use a nonallergenic soap or detergent and cosmetics and take these when travelling.
      (2) Use Ivory soap if allergic to most soaps and detergents.
2. If sensitive to insect stings
   a. Keep a sting emergency medical kit readily available.
   b. If sting occurs:
      (1) Swallow uncoated antihistamine tablet.
      (2) Place isoproterenol tablet under tongue.
      (3) Inject 1:1000 epinephrine hydrochloride. (A family member should also know how to do this.)
      (4) Seek medical help immediately.
3. Continue medical follow-up if medications are required

Table 39-7. Types of blood relacement

Component	Indications
Whole blood	Loss of blood volume (trauma, surgery)
Packed red cells	Anemias
	Liver and kidney disease
Washed red cells	Febrile reaction after receiving leukocyte-poor red cells
Leukocyte-poor red cells	Febrile transfusion reactions
Frozen red cells (leukocyte free)	Prospective transplant recipients
Platelet concentrate	Thrombocytopenia
Cryoprecipitate (antihemophilic factor)	Hemophilia
Gamma globulin	Prophylaxis for certain virus diseases
	Immunodeficiency disease
Plasma	Shock
Fresh-frozen plasma	Immodeficiency disease

1. Does the person know how to avoid the specific allergens?
2. Have plans been made to decrease contact with the allergen?
3. Does the person know when to seek medical help?

Type II hypersensitivities (cytotoxic)

PATHOPHYSIOLOGY

The underlying mechanisms of type II hypersensitivities involve the direct binding of IgG or IgM immunoglobulins to an antigen on the surface of a cell. This antibody labeling then triggers the destruction of the cell.

BLOOD TRANSFUSION REACTIONS

The type II hypersensitivity is classically illustrated by the reactions that occur in mismatched blood transfusion reactions. Blood replacement therapy is used when there has been excessive blood loss (whole blood or blood components) or in treatment of diseases of the hematopoietic system. Replacement therapy may be whole blood or one or more of the blood components (Table 39-7). Blood transfusions are not without dangers to the recipient; therefore the transfusion of 1 unit (500 ml) of blood for minor therapy is not usually recommended.

Pathophysiology

There are many antigens on the surface of red blood cells, but in terms of potential immunologic reaction the major clinically significant systems are the ABO and Rh systems.

ABO system

The four major human blood groups are listed here. Since type AB blood contains both antigens, persons with type AB may receive blood from any type (Fig. 39-3). Persons with type O may donate blood to other types, but since both antigens are absent in type O, they may not receive another type without experiencing a reaction.

Within the serum, individuals possess naturally occurring antibodies to the red blood cell (RBC) surface antigens of the ABO blood groups that are not present on their own RBCs. Thus a person with type A blood will possess anti-B antibodies within the serum. These antibodies, called *isohemagglutinins*, are usually of the IgM class. The antibodies are capable of cross-reacting with the A or B antigens on the surface of the "foreign" ABO types. On transfusion, mismatched blood will be immediately coated by the isohemagglutinins, causing agglutination of the introduced cells and the rapid lysis (breakdown) of the cells. The products released by the lysed cells are then dumped into the bloodstream.

Rh system

The Rh system is more complex because there are at least 27 different antigens in this system. The most immunogenic is the D antigen. Whe the term *Rh positive* is used, the presence of antigen Rh-D is implied; *Rh negative* indicates the absence of antigen D. Approximately 85% of the population have Rh-positive blood.

When the person with Rh-negative blood is first exposed to Rh-positive blood, Rh antibodies are formed. On subsequent exposures to Rh-positive blood, the Rh antibody binds to its corresponding antigen on the surface of the RBCs containing the Rh antigen. The Rh-antigen RBCs are then rapidly broken down by macrophages in the spleen with conversion of hemoglobin to bilirubin resulting in jaundice.

HLA system

Human leukocyte antigens (HLA) are found on many types of tissue cells and on blood leukocytes and platelets. The system is more complex than the RBC antigen systems, and there are literally thousands of combinations of the antigens that can occur. Sensitization may occur through pregnancy or through exposure to platelets and white blood cells (WBCs) during transfusions. Repeated transfusions of blood cells may lead to transfusion reactions.

Prevention of transfusion reactions

Prescreening of potential blood donors is essential. Blood received from volunteer donors through the American Red Cross Blood Service or hospital blood banks is preferable to that of paid donors, because paid donors may be less likely to report past or present diseases that may affect the recipient.

After the blood has been collected, the blood group and subgroups including Rh typing are identified and the blood is tested for syphilis and hepatitis. The blood must be cross-matched with blood from the recipient to determine compatibility and prevent an acute hemolytic reaction. Cross-matching consists of mixing samples of the donor's blood and the recipient's blood and examining for cell clumping or hemolysis.

Major blood groups

A	Antigen A is present
B	Antigen B is present
AB	Both antigens A and B are present
O	Neither antigen A nor B is present

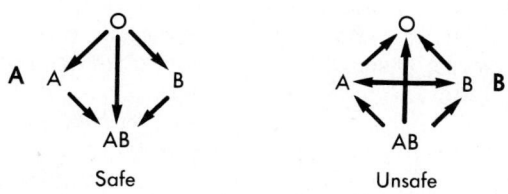

Safe   Unsafe

Fig. 39-3. Blood groups and the groups each can receive blood from and give blood to. **A,** Safe. **B,** Unsafe.

Most of the serious reactions that now occur during transfusions are the result of human error. Safeguards include the following:

1. Blood must be kept cold until ready to use.
2. Blood that has remained at room temperature for more than 30 minutes should not be returned to refrigeration for reissue.
3. Blood should be administered within a 4-hour period.
4. The unit of blood must be labeled with the patient's name, and the label must be checked against the patient's wristband before the blood is given.

5. All blood products should be administered through filters.
6. The patient must be monitored throughout the blood administration.

Complications of blood transfusions
Immunologic transfusion reactions

Several immunologic reactions can occur with blood administration (Table 39-8). The most serious reaction is the acute hemolytic reaction that occurs during administration of the first 50 ml of blood transfused. Several hours after a hemolytic reaction, the urine becomes red

Table 39-8. Immunologic reactions to blood transfusions

Reaction	Cause	Mechanism	Symptoms	Occurrence	Action
Acute hemolytic	Recipient has antibody with which transfused red cells are incompatible	Red cells agglutinate, rapid hemolysis Capillary plugging (type II hypersensitivity)	Headache Lumbar pain Constriction of chest Nausea, vomiting Chills, fever Hemoglobinuria Signs of shock, disseminated intravascular coagulation (DIC), renal shutdown	Shortly after initiation of transfusion	Transfusion stopped Saline solution continued intravenously Blood unit and blood sample from patient sent to laboratory for immediate testing Treat for shock, DIC, renal shutdown as they occur.
Delayed hemolytic	Anamnestic immune response	Slow hemolysis	Jaundice Anemia	Days to weeks after transfusion	Monitor adequacy of urinary output and degree of anemia
Allergic	Transfer of an antigen or a reaginic antibody from donor to recipient	Immune sensitivity to foreign serum protein (type I hypersensitivity)	Urticaria Wheezing Dyspnea Bronchospasm	Within 30 min after initiation of transfusion	Mild: give antihistamine, continue transfusion Severe: give aqueous epinephrine (0.5 ml of 1:1000 intramuscularly)
Pyrogenic	Reaction of antigen other than on RBC (leukocytes, platelets) Bacterial contamination	Leukocyte agglutination Bacterial pyrogens	Fever, chills Flushing Palpitations Tachycardia	Within 30 to 90 min after initiation of transfusion	Stop transfusion Treat symptomatically (antipyretics) after ascertaining that acute hemolytic reaction is not occurring Transfuse with leukocyte-poor blood or washed RBCs

(port-wine urine) and the urinary output is diminished. The urine contains RBCs and albumin. This reaction is thought to be caused by the release of a toxic substance from the hemolyzed blood that causes a temporary vascular spasm in the kidneys, resulting in renal damage, and blockage of the renal tubules by the hemoglobin precipitated out in the acid urine (hemoglobinuria). If the patient receives more than 100 ml of incompatible blood, irreversible shock with complete renal failure may occur, and death may follow.

As blood cells disintegrate (lyse), large amounts of potassium are released into the bloodstream; if renal function is impaired, hyperkalemia will develop. If this occurs, the patient may be treated with renal dialysis. Since fever is a sign of both acute hemolytic reaction and the less serious pyrogenic reaction, the transfusion is stopped until the diagnosis is made.

Nonimmunologic reactions

Complications other than those of immunologic origin include the following:
1. Fluid overload
   a. Occurs mostly in elderly persons and those with congestive heart failure or severe anemia (hemoglobin less than 5 g/dl)
   b. Can be prevented by use of packed cells
   c. If occurs, slow down or stop infusion (depending on severity of symptoms)
2. Air embolism
   a. Results when blood is administered under air pressure following severe blood loss
   b. If occurs, place patient in left side-lying Trendelenburg position (diverts air away from pulmonary artery)
3. Complications of massive blood replacement (exchange of one blood volume in 24 hours)
   a. Thrombocytopenia with abnormal bleeding (from platelet deterioration)
   b. Cardiac arrhythmias (from cold blood)
   c. Electrolyte level imbalances
      (1) *Hyperkalemia* (potassium released as RBCs break down)
      (2) *Hypocalcemia* (binding of sodium citrate from donor blood with recipient's serum calcium ions)

Type III hypersensitivities (immune complex)

PATHOPHYSIOLOGY

The type III hypersensitivities result from the union of soluble antigens with immunoglobulins of the IgM and IgG classes. The complexes that are formed are too small for phagocytosis, so rather than being removed by the reticuloendothelial system (RES), they are deposited in body tissues. This causes an inflammatory response, usually intravascular.

SERUM SICKNESS

A type III hypersensitivity of clinical significance is serum sickness, which can develop from 1 to 3 weeks after the administration of a large amount of "foreign" serum (for example, horse serum). It may also occur with the administration of certain drugs, particularly antimicrobials such as penicillin.

Itching and discomfort at the injection site are usually the first symptoms noted. These are followed by lymphadenopathy, fever, urticaria or erythematous rash, facial edema, and joint pain. Objective signs of arthritis may be present.

Serum sickness is a self-limiting disease. Mild symptoms respond well to antihistamines and salicylates. More severe symptoms are treated with a steroid such as prednisone, with relief of symptoms often obtained within hours. Epinephrine is given if an anaphylactic reaction occurs.

Type IV hypersensitivities (cell mediated)

PATHOPHYSIOLOGY

Type IV hypersensitivities are cell mediated (delayed type) involving T cells. Antigens identified as foreign to the body can cause a reaction in two ways, by direct or by indirect action. The T lymphocyte can destroy the antigen directly by attaching itself to the antigen cell wall, breaking down the cell membrane, and causing lysis and death of the cell. This direct action approach appears to be a major factor in transplant rejections. The indirect approach consists of activating nonspecific phagocytic cells (macrophages and polymorphonuclear leukocytes) through release of lymphokines by the sensitized T lymphocytes.

Clinical examples of type IV hypersensitivities are microbial hypersensitivity reaction, allergic contact dermatitis (Chapter 37), and tissue transplant rejection.

MICROBIAL HYPERSENSITIVITY REACTION

An example of microbial hypersensitivity is the body's reaction to the tubercle bacillus. The body does not react initially when the bacillus invades a nonsensitized host. However, as the cell-mediated response is activated, tissue destruction (cavitation) and general toxemia result. After the initial sensitization, subsequent contact with the tubercle bacillus will elicit a hypersensitivity reaction. This is the basis of the tuberculin skin test.

TISSUE TRANSPLANT REJECTION

The rejection of foreign cells and tissues by the body is a beneficial function of the immune system primarily mediated by a type IV hypersensitivity. If it were not for this mechanism, the human body would be a haven for the inappropriate establishment of growth of any animal cell that penetrated the external defense mechanisms;

however, this process is regarded as a disservice when it operates to prevent the positive aspects of the exchange of tissues between hosts.

Pathophysiology

The antigenic determinants of the tissues that lead to graft rejection are primarily found on the surface of the cells within the transplanted tissues. These antigens are known as *histocompatibility antigens* and are controlled by

---

**First-set rejection
of nonmatched allograft**

1 to 3 days	Skin becomes vascularized
6 to 10 days	Sensitized lymphocytes appear in regional lymph nodes; lymph nodes enlarge
12 to 14 days	Vascular bed begins to deteriorcte; graft becomes necrotic and is sloughed off

---

independently segregated genes within the chromosomal structure of the animal. They are also called human leukocyte antigens (HLA), as discussed previously.

Tissue typing

In preparation for a tissue transplant from another person (allograft), the closest match of donor-recipient transplantation antigens is sought. This is done by tissue typing for the major antigenic determinants (ABO, Rh, and HLA). The recipient's serum is then cross-matched with donor lymphocytes for compatibility.

Tissue response

When nonmatched skin is transferred to the new host, a first-set rejection occurs. If another skin graft is taken from the same donor and is transplanted to a different site on the same recipient, the graft rejection is more rapid. This accelerated reaction or second-set rejection is so rapid that the graft may never be vascularized before it is sloughed. Graft rejection can be minimized by induced immonosuppression (p. 1147).

Some allografts circumvent immunorejection because of their site in the body. Corneal and cartilage grafts survive without the need for immunosuppression because these sites are avascular. By some (as yet unknown) mechanism, the fetus developing within the uterus enjoys this same privileged status.

Table 39-9. Some diseases with autoimmune aspects

Disease	Autoantigen	Comments
Pernicious anemia	Intrinsic factors of parietal cells	Specific autoantibodies detectable
Autoimmune hemolytic anemia	Antigens on the surface of RBC	RBC surface antigens may be altered by drugs
Systemic lupus erythematosus	Nucleoproteins, DNA, many other antigens	Multiple autoimmune responses
Guillain-Barré syndrome	Myelin	
Glomerulonephritis	Cross-reactive streptococcal antigens	May also result from direct attack of glomerular basement membrane
Rheumatic fever	Cross-reactive streptococcal antigens	
Rheumatoid arthritis	Immunoglobulin G	Rheumatoid factor is IgM that reacts with IgG
Ulcerative colitis	Colon cells	
Myasthenia gravis	Skeletal and heart muscle	Thymectomy improves
Male infertility	Sperm cell	Agglutinins formed against sperm cells
Multiple sclerosis	Brain cells	Not proved to be autoimmune
Sympathetic uveitis	Uveal tissues	Release of sequestered uveal antigen
Autoimmune thyroiditis	Thyroid hormones and tissues	Autoantibodies and sensitized lymphocytes

AUTOIMMUNE DISEASES

Individuals sometimes respond immunologically to some of their own antigens. The chance that the control mechanisms will be lost increases with the age of the individual. The symptoms of such a self-attack are referred to as *autoimmune disease* or *autohypersensitivity*. For the most part, these self-reactions are not immunologically initiated; the causative agent lies outside the immune system, but the immune response serves as the pathogenic mechanism.

The autoimmune process may occur for the following reasons:

1. New antigens may result from genetic changes.
2. Existing antigens may be altered by injury, infection, or drugs (for example, methyldopa (Aldomet), penicillins, cephalosporins).
3. The immune apparatus itself may become altered.[1]

There is a higher incidence of autoimmune disease in women and in persons with a familial history of autoimmune disease.

Many diseases for which no etiologic agent could be identified have been classified as autoimmune, only to be removed from that category when some cryptic, latent, or slow-growing agent was identified within the cells or tissue under attack. Some of the diseases listed as autoimmune-associated diseases in Table 39-9 will probably be removed from that list as the initiating factor or microorganism is identified. The care of persons experiencing these diseases is discussed elsewhere in this text.

REFERENCES AND SELECTED READINGS*

1. Alexander, J.W., and Good, R.A.: Fundamentals of clinical immunology, Philadelphia, 1977, W.B. Saunders Co.
2. *Allen, J., and Mellin, G.: The new epidemic: immune deficiency, opportunistic infections, and Kaposi's sarcoma, Am. J. Nurs. **82**:1718-1722, 1982.
3. *Blood transfusions today: what you should know and do, Nurs. 78 **8**(2):68-72, 1978.
4. *Buickus, B.A.: Blood therapy: administering blood components, Am. J. Nurs. **79**:937-941, 1979.
5. *Cianci, J., and Lamb, J.: Organ transplantation: matching donors and recipients, Am. J. Nurs. **81**:544-545, 1981.
6. *Cullins, L.C.: Blood therapy: preventing and treating transfusion reactions, Am. J. Nurs. **79**:935-936, 1979.
7. Cunningham, B.A.: The structure and function of histocompatibility antigens, Sci. Am. **237**:96, 1977.
8. *Dharan, M.: Immunoglobulin abnormalities, Am. J. Nurs. **76**:1626-1628, 1976.
9. *Donley, D.L.: Nursing the patient who is immunosuppressed, Am. J. Nurs. **76**:1619-1625, 1976.
10. Ern, M.: Immunology: bone marrow transplantation, CA Nurs. **3**:387-400, 1980.
11. Fruth, R.: Anaphylaxis and drug reactions: guidelines for detection and care, Heart Lung **9**:662-664, 1980.
12. *Glasser, R.J.: How the body works against itself: autoimmune diseases, Nurs. 77 **7**(9):38-43, 1977.
13. Groenwald, S.L.: Physiology of the immune system, Heart Lung **9**:645-650, 1980.
14. Kaye, D., and Rose, L.F.: Fundamentals of internal medicine, St. Louis, 1983, The C.V. Mosby Co.
15. *Kazak, A.: Blood therapy: processing blood for transfusion reactions, Am. J. Nurs. **79**:935-936, 1979.
16. Krupp, M.A., and Chatton, M.J.: Current medical diagnosis and treatment, Los Altos, Calif. 1983, Lange Medical Publications.
17. *Leser, D.R.: Synthetic blood: a future alternative, Am. J. Nurs. **82**:452-455, 1982.
18. *Lind, M.: The immunologic assessment: a nursing focus, Heart Lung **9**:658-661, 1980.
19. McLeod, B.C.: Immunologic factors in reactions to blood transfusions, Heart Lung **9**:675-681, 1980.
20. *Nysanther, J.O., Katz, A.E., and Length, J.L.: The immune system: its development and functions, Am. J. Nurs. **76**:1614-1618, 1976.
21. *Parker, A.L.: Blood therapy: massive transfusion, Am. J. Nurs. **79**:944-948, 1979.
22. Rana, A.N., and Luskin, A.: Immunosuppression, autoimmunity, and hypersensitivity, Heart Lung **9**:651-657, 1980.
23. Rossman, M., Slavin, R., and Taft, E.G.: Pheresis therapy: patient care, Am. J. Nurs. **77**:1135-1141, 1977.
24. Rutman, R., and others: Blood therapy: screening donors and the phlebotomy procedure, Am. J. Nurs. **79**:926-930, 1979.
25. *Sophie, L.R.: Meeting the immunologic challenge of transplant nursing, Heart Lung **9**:690-694, 1980.
26. Tenczynski, J.: Leukapheresis: the process, Am. J. Nurs. **77**:1133-1134, 1977.
27. *Thomas, S.: Blood therapy: transfusing granulocytes, Am. J. Nurs. **79**:942-943, 1979.
28. Wyngaarden, J.B., and Smith, L.H.: Textbook of medicine, ed. 16, Philadelphia, 1982, W.B. Saunders Co.

*References preceded by an asterisk are particularly well suited for student reading.

UNIT XII
Emergencies and Disasters

40 Problems Encountered in Emergencies and Disasters

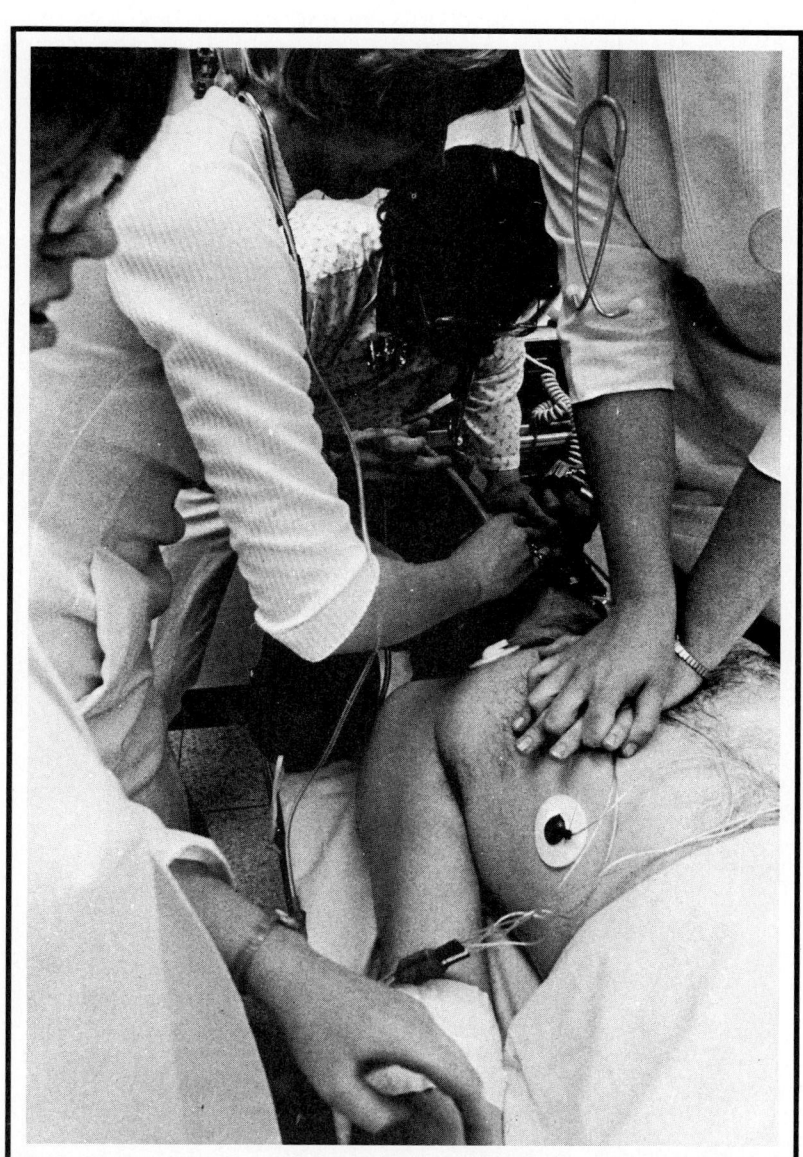

40

Problems Encountered
in Emergencies and Disasters

BARBARA C. LONG

STUDY QUESTIONS

- What is the most common cause of accidents in your community as noted in your newspapers?

- What are some precautions taken in your hospital unit to prevent patient accidents? Are there any additional measures that could be taken?

- What actions are taken in your hospital for the reporting of accidents within the hospital? What measures are taken to prevent further similar accidents?

- Draw a diagram of your hospital unit, noting the location of exits, placement of fire extinguishers, and fire doors.

- How are the personnel in your hospital alerted that a fire has occurred?

- What precautions could you take in your life to avoid rape?

- Examine the disaster plan for your hospital. As a nursing student, what actions should you take if the disaster plan were instituted? What actions would be expected if you were a staff nurse on your unit?

Nurses are frequently called on to provide emergency care in the community or in settings where medical help is not immediately available; therefore all nurses need to know the basics of emergency care. In this chapter are identified major points in the delivery of emergency care in the community, in assessment and intervention for common emergencies, and in principles of management in disasters.

PREVENTION OF ACCIDENTS

Accidents in the United States claim more than 100,000 lives each year, half from motor vehicle accidents. Accidents are the leading cause of death in persons younger than 45 years and are the third leading cause in those 45 to 64 years of age.

In terms of morbidity, approximately *60 million* persons, or about 30 of every 100, are injured in the United States every year. Billions of dollars are spent annually on medical expenses, property damage, and administrative costs related to accidents. Money lost from potential earnings or disability adds to this figure.

Accidents that result in injury or death involve human suffering that cannot be measured in dollars: pain, long-term rehabilitation, disabilities (temporary or permanent), loss and grief, and family disruption.

Accident prevention is a major public health goal, and both the Public Health Service and the American Public

Health Association (APHA) actively promote accident prevention. Community groups can be helpful in investigating accident statistics in their local area and in disseminating information to encourage accident prevention. Nurses have an important role in accident prevention, both through their roles as professionals and as residents of a community. The influence of nurses can be extended in many areas because nurses are represented in school, industry, community nursing programs, and hospitals.

Home

Accidents in and about the home are responsible for almost one third of all accidental deaths each year. Falls account for about half the number, and fires and poisonings for most of the remainder. Many aged persons who fall do so when walking from room to room. Some fall because of heavily waxed floors, loose rugs, poor lighting, scattered toys, and other conditions that could have been corrected. People fall from roofs, windows, high ladders, and steps; and are fatally burned or otherwise injured while using solvents and cleansing agents without proper knowledge of their hazards.

The number of electric appliances used in the home has increased the danger of electric shock and fire from overloaded circuits. Many persons die in fires caused by burning cigarette ashes dropped on furniture or rugs or discarded in waste containers and by cigarettes that are dropped when the smoker falls asleep. Attention needs to be given to teaching homeowners to have older heating systems checked periodically for gas leaks and other unsafe features. All persons in a household should be aware of what to do in the event of fire, and fire evacuation drills are encouraged. Homes should be equipped with smoke alarms in strategic places such as the kitchen, bedrooms, hallways, and basement.

Most accidental poisonings occur in children, but adults are not free from this risk. Nonpotable liquids should be kept in their original containers, tightly capped, and *never* placed in a soft-drink bottle, drinking glass, or cup. Medications should never be taken from unmarked or poorly marked bottles.

The community health nurse has an opportunity to assess safety hazards during home visits and to teach the family about general accident prevention as well as specific measures for the safety of the ill person.

Community

Community action can best be effected by group action, but it often takes persistence to interest and stimulate group action. Parent-teacher associations, recreational associations, and religious and social groups are usually interested in accident control. Phases of accident prevention that should be of community interest include the following:

1. Teaching of accident prevention in public schools
2. Better control and inspection of homes for the aged and prisons
3. Rigid enforcement of driving regulations
4. Improvement of street lighting and traffic signals at busy intersections
5. Periodic inspection of all automobiles
6. Promotion of laws pertaining to fire-proofing of buildings
7. Promotion of laws protecting the public from flammable clothing, potentially harmful toys, and similar items.

Hospitals

Assessing the need for safety in the general environment and for the safety of specific patients and taking measures to prevent injury are important functions of the nurse. The nurse can participate in policy making and

---

**Home safety features
for elderly persons**

Floors	Large rugs and carpets anchored
	Small rugs with nonskid backing
	Avoidance of floor wax (unless nonskid)
Stairs	Uniform height
	Nonskid treads
	Risers marked with contrasting color
	Strong handrails
	Adequate lighting
Bathroom	Handrail in tub or shower
	Skidproof bath mat
	Treads in tub or on shower floor
	Seat in shower

**Safety measures to prevent falls
of hospital patients**

1. Handrails in hospital corridors
2. Armchairs rather than armless chairs
3. Chairs in bathrooms or showers
4. Call systems in bathrooms and lounges as well as in patients' rooms
5. Hi-Lo beds (placed in low position when patient ambulating)
6. Night lights in patient rooms (especially elderly patients).

safety monitoring through membership on hospital safety committees.

FALLS

Falls are the major cause of hospital-incurred injuries. Hospitalized persons are in unfamiliar surroundings with strange furniture and equipment, may be weak for many reasons, or may become confused, all of which can contribute to falls. Elderly persons are at high risk for falls. All patients should be assessed for the potential of falling, and preventive measures should be instituted.

The use of side rails is a nursing decision. Side rails should be kept raised for all unconscious patients. A confused patient may attempt to climb over the side rail and thus have farther to fall; a jacket restraint may be more useful in this situation.

Patients who are weak may need frequent reminders to seek assistance before ambulating. Some patients do not want to "bother the nurse" and attempt to walk to the bathroom unaided, especially at night. All patients should use supportive slippers; paper slippers can be a hazard.

FIRE

All hospitals and nursing homes must have established fire prevention routines, and all personnel must be familiar with these routines. Participation in *fire drills* should be taken seriously, and evaluation should follow each drill.

Fires usually occur from smoking or faulty electrical equipment. Because smoking is also hazardous to health, many hospitals restrict smoking in patients' rooms and in many public areas. If smoking is permitted, ashtrays should be available and the patient and visitors instructed about not emptying them. If patients are careless smokers who may drop a cigarette or ash, their smoking should be monitored. Faulty electrical equipment is not used. Any questions about smoke should be investigated and reported immediately. If a fire should occur, the nurse in charge who is most familiar with the patients' conditions should be in charge of any evacuation.

DELIVERY OF EMERGENCY CARE

Community

The National Safety Act of 1966 requires each county to appoint an emergency medical care committee. The effectiveness of these committees varies greatly, influenced to a large extent by citizen interest and political activity. Every community needs an organized emergency care system with support and input from community health organizations and community political elements.

Many communities have emergency medical technicians (EMTs) or paramedics to respond to emergency calls. EMTs have had preparation beyond basic first aid training but do not carry out invasive procedures. Paramedics have had more training than EMTs and can carry out such skills as starting intravenous fluids, giving medications, defibrillation, and intubation. The preparedness of personnel responding to emergency calls and the responsibilities that are legally permissible vary among states and communities within each state.

The American Heart Association has been instrumental in developing a program to educate large numbers of persons who are certified to administer cardiopulmonary resuscitation (CPR). This increases the possibility of a trained person being available to initiate resuscitation early in a larger number of emergency situations.

Hospitals

Hospital emergency rooms are often overloaded with persons seeking assistance for nonacute health problems. Newer approaches to delivery of both emergency and nonacute health care, such as urgent care centers in the community, are being initiated.

Many emergency departments have direct radio communication with rescue personnel in the community. Treatment can be initiated at the scene of the accident under medical direction and hospital personnel can be better prepared to receive the injured. This helps to eliminate some of the delays in initiation of care.

The role of the nurse in the emergency department has changed considerably in recent years as a result of the

---

Fire safety approaches

1. Close doors and windows of all patient rooms until evacuation is necessary.
2. General precautions:
   a. Do not open a door that feels excessively hot
   b. Keep low as possible if air is hot and smoke-filled
   c. Use wet cloths around nose and mouth if air is hot (try not to inhale smoke or hot air).
3. If evacuation is advisable:
   a. Patients closest to fire are evacuated to opposite end of corridor (horizontal evacuation)
   b. Downward evacuation is effected (when instructed) by *stairway* (never by elevator)
   c. Ambulatory patients are evacuated first; patients are led by hospital personnel, if possible.

increased utilization of emergency departments by persons seeking medical attention and the increased sophistication of therapeutic management. Emergency department nurses are developing the following skills:

1. Assessment and triage (sorting patients to determine priority of medical attention)
2. Management of persons with high levels of anxiety
3. Specialized technical skills (initiating parenteral fluids, defibrillation, resuscitation, intubation, operating monitoring devices)
4. Interpreting selected laboratory findings and electrocardiograms and acting on these findings.

LEGAL ASPECTS OF EMERGENCY CARE

Nurses who intervene to assist victims in an emergency situation should be aware of the legal ramifications that can ensue as a result of their actions. Many states have enacted Good Samaritan laws in an effort to protect health personnel who aid accident victims. These laws vary in coverage among states as to the classes of people who are protected from liability, types of situations, geographic limits, and extent of immunity.

Good Samaritan laws serve to identify in statutory language those persons or situations that provide some degree of immunity from liability, many of which already exist by common law. Persons are judged as not liable unless they act willfully with gross negligence. Negligence is the key word. Damage must occur if negligence is to be proved, and the actions of the nurse must be the immediate cause of the damage.

"Reasonable care" provided by the nurse at the scene of an accident is usually judged as that care given by another similar nurse *under the prevailing situation.* Thus the care provided on a back road on a dark rainy night would not be judged the same as that given in an emergency room.

Nurses who work in hospital emergency departments need to be aware of legal implications of care provided in that setting, such as the care given to minors when parents are not present to give consent and actions that may be taken in helping police officers gather evidence.[6]

ASSESSMENT

When an emergency occurs or on arriving at the emergency scene, it is important to assess the situation, the patient, and the environment before initiating action. Some conclusions can be drawn from the immediate environment. If there is trauma to multiple victims, all should be assessed before any but lifesaving interventions are initiated. Overt clues such as an automobile accident, report of falling, or ingestion of poison can give direction to probable types of injuries. A complete head-to-toe assessment is carried out, if possible, before moving the victim so that additional injuries or conditions requiring intervention can be identified (see box, p. 1167).

Priority assessment

Airway

Presence of respirations
Presence of foreign body, vomitus, loose dentures in mouth

Breathing

Respiration rate, depth, character
Use of accessory muscles for breathing
Tracheal deviation

Circulation

Presence of carotid pulse
Pulse rate, strength, rhythm
Presence of hemorrhage
Skin color, temperature, moisture

Level of consciousness

Response to voice and touch (or painful stimulus)
Pupillary response
If unconscious, presence of Medic-Alert tag

Data collection

A person who is not breathing, who has no palpable pulse, or who is hemorrhaging needs immediate assistance. Obtaining data to identify these circumstances is the first priority in assessment. This is sometimes referred to as the ABCs of emergency assessment (Airway, Breathing, Circulation). Assessing the general level of consciousness can be done as the nurse approaches the victim. If pulse and breathing are absent, CPR is initiated (p. 1170). Hemorrhage is treated by direct pressure to the wound.

Before starting the head-to-toe assessment, observe the following and assess those areas first:

1. Victim's general position
2. Obvious signs of deformities or asymmetry
3. Any purposeful movements
4. Signs or symptoms of pain or discomfort.

During the overall assessment continue to monitor for changes in level of consciousness and respiratory status. Ask the victim or any relative or friends present to describe the preceding events; the presence of any medical conditions such as heart or lung disease, epilepsy, or diabetes; or any special medications taken by the victim that may have a bearing on the present situation.

If there is more than one person on the scene, the nurse or paramedic should remain with the victim while others are given directions to assess the environment for additional signs of danger and to call for any needed transportation.

Head-to-toe assessment

Head and neck

Assess airway

Assess pupils

Examine ears, nose, mouth for bleeding, other drainage, foreign body

Palpate* cervical spine for pain (do not move head)

Examine head for bleeding, lacerations, contusions, depression of skull

Palpate jaw for fracture (pain, deformity)

Ask about stiffness of neck (if no history of trauma, assess movement)

Examine neck for distended neck veins, presence of tracheal stoma, tracheal deviation

Chest and spine

Observe chest movements for symmetry of expansion and character of respirations

Palpate clavicles for fracture (pain, deformity)

Examine chest for external injury

Palpate ribs for fracture (pain)

Palpate spine for point tenderness (do not move victim)

Abdomen and pelvis

Palpate pelvis for pain in groin when pressure applied over pelvis

Ask about abdominal pain

Examine abdomen for external injury, rigidity, distention, penetrating objects

Extremities

Examine for signs of external injury

Ask about pain in extremities

If no obvious injury, ask victim to move each limb

Test for sensation in each limb

Assess presence and strength of peripheral pulses

*All palpations should be carried out gently.

Data analysis

RESPIRATIONS

The rate, depth, and character of respiration provide clues to the presence of ventilatory, central nervous system, or metabolic problems. Most trauma victims breathe a little faster than normal (18 to 24 breaths/min). If the person shows signs of respiratory effort (nasal flaring; suprasternal, intercostal, or substernal retractions), the airway may be partially obstructed. The type of sound accompanying respirations may indicate the degree and location of a partial obstruction. The following findings are suggestive of specific emergency care problems:

1. Rate
   a. Slow (<10 /min): ventilatory or CNS problem
   b. Rapid (>26/min): hypoxia, acidosis, shock
2. Depth
   a. Shallow; shock, chest pain
   b. Deep: hypoxia, hypoglycemia, metabolic acidosis
3. Sound
   a. Inspiratory stridor: upper airway obstruction (above tracheal bifurcation)
   b. Expiratory wheezes or stridor: lower airway obstruction
4. Frothy, blood-tinged sputum: lung injury, pulmonary edema, pulmonary embolus

SHOCK

In persons who sustain major trauma or a major stressor to the system, such as myocardial infarction, shock usually develops (see Chapter 11). Signs of shock include restlessness; pale cold moist skin, rapid thready pulse, and rapid shallow respirations. Nausea and vomiting may occur. With anaphylactic shock the victim may complain of itching or burning of the skin, tightness in the chest, and difficulty in breathing. Wheals may develop on the skin, and the face and tongue may develop edema.

SENSATION

Pain may result from trauma if there is soft-tissue injury, fracture, or visceral damage. Pain may also occur with tissue anoxia, such as with obstruction of blood vessels or frostbite. Data obtained from the patient include location (region), severity, quality, onset and duration, and provoking factors. For a further discussion of pain, see Chapter 12.

Loss of sensation may result from injury to peripheral nerves or injury to nerves in the central nervous system. Peripheral nerve injuries may occur with fractures, lacerations, penetrating wounds, or dislocations. Loss of sensation concurrent with loss of movement and absence of local tissue or bone injury indicates central nervous sytem injury, for example, spinal cord injury or cerebral hemorrhage.

LEVEL OF CONSCIOUSNESS

Level of consciousness is assessed by determining whether the person responds immediately to voice and touch, responds only to painful stimuli, or does not respond. Unconsciousness may be due to many causes (see box, p. 1168). Pupillary response differs depending on the underlying problem.

If there has been trauma to the brain it is important to ascertain level of consciousness at different times. Temporary loss of consciousness followed by alertness and equal pupils usually indicates a concussion. If there is no

---

Possible causes of unconsciousness

1. Hypoxia (decreased oxygen to brain)
   a. Respiratory insufficiency
      (1) Airway obstruction from foreign body, secretions
      (2) Pneumothorax
      (3) Spinal cord injury
   b. Shock
      (1) Cardiogenic: cardiac arrest
      (2) Hypovolemic: hemorrhage
2. Metabolic (chemical brain depressants)
   a. Extrinsic
      (1) Drugs: alcohol, narcotics, barbiturates, antihistamines, tranquilizers
      (2) Poisons: carbon monoxide, carbon tetrachloride, hydrocarbons, methane gas
   b. Intrinsic
      (1) Ketones: diabetic ketoacidosis, starvation
      (2) Glucose: hypoglycemia, hyperglycemia
      (3) Ammonia: liver failure
      (4) Urea: kidney failure
      (5) Hormonal hypofunction: hypothyroidism, Addison's disease
      (6) Electrolyte imbalance: sodium, potassium, calcium, hydrogen ions
3. Brain pathologic conditions
   a. Trauma: concussion, brainstem contusion, intracranial hematoma
   b. Seizures: epilepsy, tumors, idiopathology
   c. Cerebrovascular accident: cerebral hemorrhage, thrombosis
   d. Tumors: benign, malignant
   e. Infections: meningitis, encephalitis

Pupillary response in unconscious patients

Cause	Pupillary response
Shock or respiratory insufficiency	Equal, may be dilated
Drugs, chemicals	Equal, may be dilated or constricted
Intracranial hemorrhage, cerebrovascular accident	Usually unequal
Brain damage	Fixed, no response to light

skull fracture the patient is simply observed for 24 hours. *Alertness after injury followed by increasing loss of consciousness and unequal pupils* usually indicates an intracranial hematoma. Medical attention is urgent if an intracranial hematoma is suspected.

An unconscious person should be placed in a position that facilitates patency of the airway (side-lying position unless contraindicated) and the respiratory status constantly monitored.

OTHER DATA

Analysis of the data should include the following:
1. Type of injury or medical emergency that has probably occurred
2. Urgency of the need for medical attention
3. Availability of resources for carrying out necessary interventions
4. Availability of transportation
5. Time factor before medical attention can be obtained.

GENERAL INTERVENTIONS
Principles of management

Some principles of management of injuries or sudden illnesses serve as guidelines for giving first aid:
1. Remain calm and think before acting.
2. Identify oneself as a nurse to victim and bystanders.
3. Do a rapid assessment for *priority* data (airway patency, breathing (respiration), and circulation (pulse).

Concerns occurring during trauma

Fear of pain
Fear of death
Fear of unknown
Disability
Loss of time from work
Cost of medical care

Causes of asphyxia

Foreign body obstruction of airway
Tongue falling back in pharynx
Edema of respiratory tissues (smoke)
Laryngospasm
Near-drowning
Trauma to chest or lungs
Pulmonary diseases

---

4. Carry out *lifesaving* measures as indicated by the priority assessment.
5. Do a head-to-toe assessment before initiating *general* first aid measures.
6. Keep the victim lying down or in the position in which found (unless orthopnea is present), protected from dampness and cold.
7. If victim is conscious, explain what is occurring; assure victim that help will be given.
8. Avoid unnecessary handling or moving of the victim; move the victim only if danger is present.
9. Do not give fluids if there is a possibility of abdominal injury or if anesthesia will be necessary within a short time.
10. Do not transport the victim until all first-aid measures have been carried out and appropriate transportation is available.

Lifesaving measures (described on succeeding pages) are carried out first when the initial assessment indicates the presence of breathing or circulatory difficulties. After breathing has been reestablished and excessive bleeding controlled, other interventions are carried out when the head-to-toe assessment is completed.

The victim is kept in a supine or sitting position, depending on symptoms, until all necessary interventions are carried out. Wounds are covered and fractures splinted before the victim is transported. Because shock is a possibility when major injuries occur, the victim should be protected from chilling. On a cold day, protection may be needed underneath the victim and sufficient covering to prevent loss of body heat but not cause vasodilation. Fluids are given orally only to a conscious person showing signs of shock if there will be a considerable delay before medical care can be obtained and if abdominal injury is not present.

Psychologic support

People who experience trauma may have numerous anxieties. It is often easy to overlook the victim's need for emotional support when physiologic needs require immediate attention.

A calm, interested approach that conveys concern to the victim as a person is helpful. Giving information frequently during all phases of emergency care to both victim and family or friends will help them understand what is occurring and that help is being provided, thus decreasing some of the anxiety.

Varying levels of tolerance to stress are found in different individuals. Highly anxious persons may need someone to stay with them. At the scene of an accident a calm bystander can be helpful. Some hospitals provide selected volunteers for that purpose. All health personnel need to evaluate frequently their own effectiveness in assessing anxiety and in conveying understanding and emotional support to the victim and family during an emergency.

CARDIOPULMONARY PROBLEMS

For life to be maintained oxygen must be taken in by the lungs and pumped to the tissues; carbon dioxide must be returned from the tissues to the lungs and exhaled. Thus any obstruction that interferes with the diffusion of these gases, failure of the heart to pump, or inadequate blood to carry the oxygen to the tissues is a threat to life and demands immediate emergency intervention. Airway patency, breathing facilitation, and circulation maintenance are the ABCs of emergency care and take first priority in assessment and intervention.

Airway obstruction and breathing difficulties

ASSESSMENT

Asphyxia occurs for various reasons (see box above). Signs of asphyxia are related to the efforts made by the victim to take in air and to the decreasing oxygenation:

1. Dyspnea
2. Use of accessory respiratory muscles (prominent neck muscles, intercostal rib retractions, nasal flaring)
3. Wheezing or stridor from air moving through narrowed passageways
4. Rales or rhonchi if fluid is present in alveoli
5. Skin pale (ashen in blacks)
6. Cyanosis (late sign).

Heimlich abdominal thrust maneuver

1. Stand behind victim.
2. Encircle arms around victim's waist (Fig. 40-1).
3. Place one fist between umbilicus and sternum with thumb against abdomen.
4. Place second hand over fist.
5. Press on abdomen with quick upward thrusts.

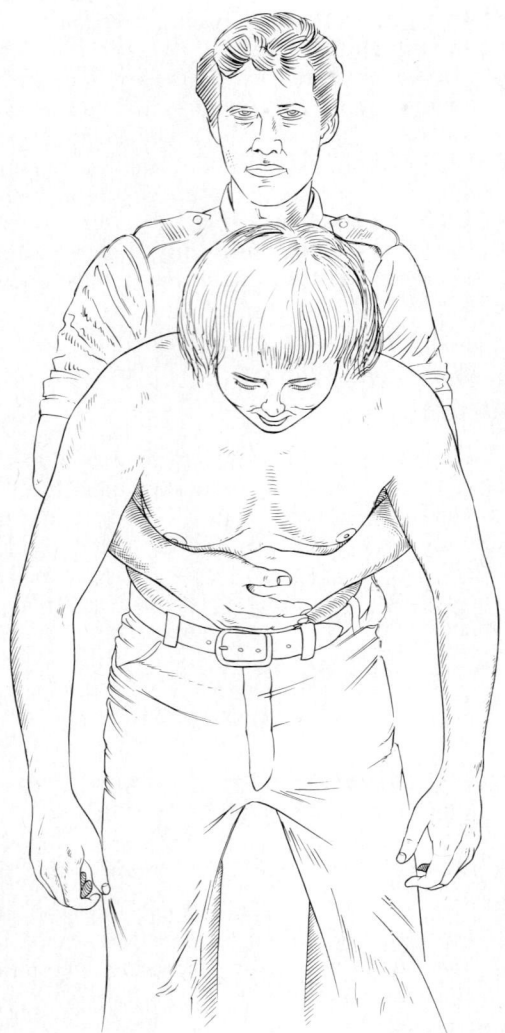

Fig. 40-1. Heimlich abdominal thrust maneuver. Rescuer places fist between umbilicus and xiphoid process with thumb pressed against abdomen.

INTERVENTION FOR ASPHYXIA

The first step in assisting a person who is having extreme difficulty in breathing is to position the person to ensure a maximal airway.

If the airway is obstructed by a foreign body the person may need assistance in its removal. Four forceful blows to the back between the shoulder blades may dislodge the object. If this is not effective, the Heimlich abdominal thrust maneuver may be attempted (see box).

If the person is unconscious and the tongue is blocking the airway, and if there is no trauma suggesting a neck fracture, the neck is hyperextended (Fig. 40-2). This maneuver alone may be enough to open the airway.

If extension of the head and neck does not initiate breathing, artificial ventilation must be initiated immediately (p. 1172). Failure of the chest to rise with ventilation indicates that the airway is obstructed by a foreign body. Actions to be taken include the following:

1. Turn victim on side and give four sharp blows between shoulder blades.
2. If foreign body is not dislodged, give four abdominal thrusts.
3. Check mouth quickly for dislodged foreign body; remove foreign body by sweeping a hooked finger across back of throat.
4. Repeat above maneuvers if normal breathing does not occur or chest expansion does not resume with artificial ventilation.

Cardiopulmonary resuscitation

Cardiopulmonary arrest is recognized by the cessation of breathing and circulation and signifies a state of clinical death. Immediate and definitive action must be instituted within 4 to 6 minutes after the arrest, or biologic death will occur.

Unresponsiveness, cessation of respirations, development of pallor and cyanosis, absence of heart sounds and blood pressure, loss of palpable pulse, and dilation of the pupils are present. (Pupillary response can be misleading in patients who are receiving drugs such as atropine or opium derivatives or in the presence of corneal pathologic conditions.) If a hospitalized patient is being monitored by means of an ECG machine or cardiac monitor, the electrocardiographic pattern of ventricular fibrillation or, less commonly, ventricular asystole will appear.

TECHNIQUES OF BASIC LIFE SUPPORT

Basic life support is an emergency procedure that consists of recognizing cardiopulmonary arrest and initiating proper CPR techniques to maintain life until the victim either recovers or is transported to a medical facility where advanced life support measures are available (Table 40-1). The sequence of CPR is listed on p. 1172.

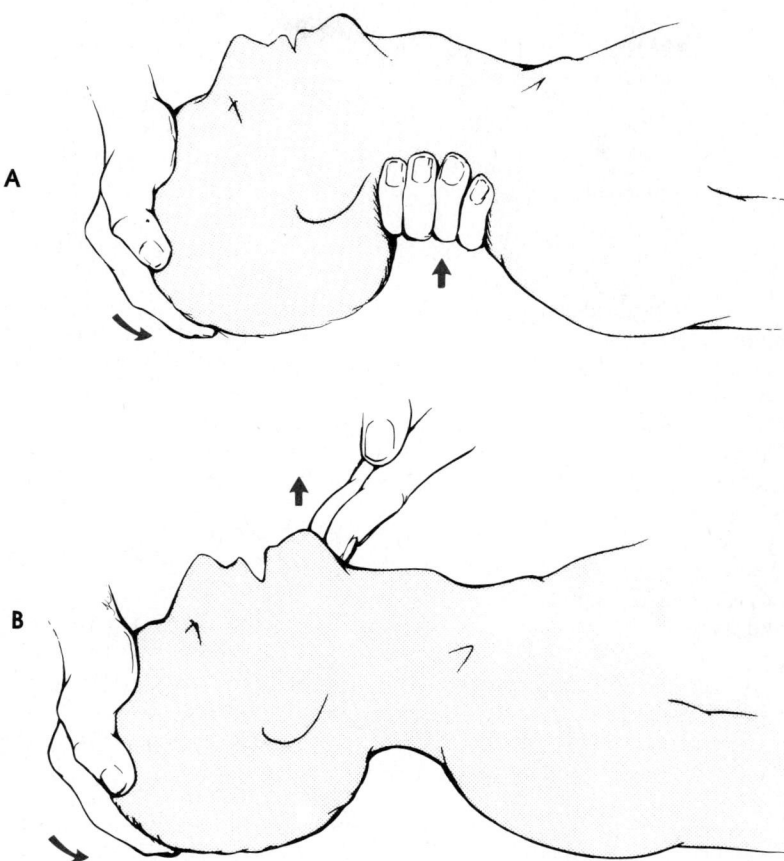

Fig. 40-2. Head tilt. **A,** Neck lift. Place one hand behind neck and other hand on forehead. Lift neck with one hand and tilt head backward by applying pressure to forehead. **B,** Chin lift. Place one hand on forehead and tips of fingers of other hand under lower jaw near chin. Bring chin forward while pressing forehead down.

Table 40-1. Life support measures in cardiac arrest

Findings	Action	ABCs of action
No response		
Absence of respirations; cyanosis; dilated pupils	Open airway	A—Open *Airway*
Respirations still absent	Initiate artificial ventilation	B—Restore *Breathing*
Carotid pulse not palpable	Initiate external cardiac compressions	C—Restore *Circulation*
ECG: ventricular fibrillation	Drug therapy; defibrillation	D—Provide *Definitive* treatment

---

Sequence of CPR in adults

Step 1: Assess level of consciousness
1. Shake victim's shoulder and shout, "Are you OK?"
2. If no response, summon help
3. Place victim supine on *firm* surface.

Step 2: Open airway
1. Hyperextend neck by head tilt or neck lift methods (Fig. 40-2)
2. Place ear over victim's nose and mouth
   a. Look to see if chest is moving
   b. Listen for air escaping during exhalation
   c. Feel for air movement against face
3. If patient is not breathing, proceed to step 3.

Step 3: Initiate artificial ventilation
1. Give four quick mouth-to-mouth breaths without allowing victim to exhale completely after each ventilation.

Step 4: Assess circulation
1. Palpate carotid pulse
2. If carotid pulse not palpable, proceed to step 5.

Step 5: Initiate external cardiac compressions
1. If only one rescuer:
   a. Do 15 cardiac compressions at a rate of 80/min
   b. Follow with two artificial ventilations
   c. Repeat sequence.
2. If two rescuers:
   a. One person does cardiac compressions, at a rate of 60/min without pause
   b. Second rescuer ventilates victim quickly after every five compressions.
3. Palpate carotid pulse after first minute of CPR to assess effectiveness, and subsequently every few minutes to check for return of spontaneous circulation.

Mouth-to-mouth ventilation

Mouth to mouth ventilation is performed as follows:
1. Maintain victim in head-tilt position.
2. Pinch nostrils.
3. Take a deep breath and place mouth around outside of victim's mouth, forming a tight seal.
4. Blow into victim's mouth.
5. Adequate ventilation is demonstrated by:
   a. Rise and fall of chest (1 to 2 in)
   b. Hearing and feeling air escape as victim passively exhales
   c. Feeling in own airway the resistance of victim's lungs expanding.

External cardiac compressions

External cardiac massage is the rhythmic compression of the heart between the lower half of the sternum and the thoracic vertebral column. This intermittent pressure compresses the heart, raises intrathoracic pressure, and produces an artificial pulsatile circulation. Correctly performed cardiac compressions can produce a peak systolic blood pressure of >100 mm Hg, but the diastolic pressure is close to zero and the mean blood pressure in the carotid arteries is approximately 40 mm Hg, or one-fourth to one-third normal.

The technique for performing external cardiac compressions is as follows:
1. Position yourself close to victim's sternum.
2. Place heel of one hand on sternum two fingerwidths above tip of coccyx, second hand on top of first hand with fingers parallel and pointing away from body.
3. Position shoulders directly over victim's sternum.
4. Keep elbows locked in a straight position.
5. Depress lower sternum 1½ to 2 inches.
6. Keeping hands in position, release pressure on sternum to allow heart to fill.
7. Repeat, depressing and releasing sternum.
8. Perform compressions regularly and smoothly.

Precordial thump

The precordial thump is a quick blow delivered to the middle portion of the sternum within 1 minute after cardiac arrest. The precordial thump has been found to be useful in cases of *witnessed* cardiac arrest and when a patient is being monitored. It generates a small low-voltage stimulus in the heart. In an anoxic heart that is still beating precordial thump could be hazardous because it may induce ventricular fibrillation.

The precordial thump maneuver may be used at vary-

Table 40-2. Drugs commonly used for cardiac arrest

Drug	Use	Action
Atropine sulfate	Slow pulse following cardiac standstill	Accelerates heart rate
Bretylium tosylate (Brety-lol)	Ventricular fibrillation, ventricular arrhythmias	Suppresses ventricular fibrillation and arrhythmias
Calcium chloride (10% solution)	Ventricular standstill	Increases myocardial contractility and conduction velocity
Dobutamine HCl (Dobutrex)	Refractory pump failure	Increases myocardial contractility
Epinephrine HCl (Adrenalin) 1:10,000 solution	Ventricular fibrillation	Positive inotropic (force of contractions) and chronotropic (regularity of beat) effect; peripheral vasoconstriction
Isoproterenol HCl (Isuprel)	Asystole, cardiovascular collapse	Positive inotropic and chronotropic effects that increase cardiac output
Metaraminol bitartrate (Aramine)	Shock	Potent vasopressor, increases peripheral resistance
Levarterenol bitartrate (Levophed)	Shock	Potent vasopressor, positive inotropic effect, increases peripheral resistance
Sodium bicarbonate (50 mEq)	Metabolic acidosis	Provides bicarbonate to return serum pH to normal
Lidocaine HCl (Xylocaine)	Arrhythmias	Shortens refractory period, suppresses automaticity of ectopic foci

ing times during CPR, depending on the circumstances surrounding the arrest. In the case of a witnessed cardiac arrest the precordial thump should be administered as soon as the absence of a pulse is discovered. If there is no immediate response to the thump CPR is initiated immediately.

CONTINUATION OF CPR

CPR should be stopped for no more than 5 seconds every 4 to 5 minutes to assess the return of spontaneous pulse and respiration. Rescuers should continue CPR until one of the following takes place:

1. Spontaneous circulation and ventilation return.
2. Another rescuer takes over basic life support.
3. Victim is transported to an emergency facility where qualified personnel assume the responsibility for CPR.
4. Victim is pronounced dead by a physician.
5. Rescuer is exhausted and unable to continue.

IN-HOSPITAL CARDIAC ARREST

Many hospitals have prepared teams of personnel, including physicians, nurses, anesthesiologists, and technicians, who can be called to give immediate and complete care in the event of a cardiac arrest. Most hospitals are equipped with a cardiac arrest tray or have access to a specially equipped cart on which all necessary emergency items are available: ECG machine, suction device, oxygen, defibrillator, airway and Ambu or other breathing bag, laryngoscope, a variety of endotracheal tubes, cut-

down set, fluids for intravenous administration, and tracheostomy set should this be necessary.

Medications usually administered during a cardiac arrest (Table 40-2) are generally available on the emergency cart. Supplementary *oxygen* is given after breathing resumes to treat the resultant hypoxemia. Oxygen is also given for other types of hypoxemia following trauma or stress such as with smoke inhalation, carbon monoxide poisoning, near-drowning, myocardial infarction, or chest injuries.

COMPLICATIONS OF CPR

The most common complication of external cardiac massage is fracture of the ribs. This may occur in some individuals even though the technique of external cardiac compressions is performed correctly. Other complications that can occur despite correct CPR technique include fractured sternum, costochondral separation, lung contusions, and laceration of the liver. Any indication of labored respiration, paradoxical pulse, muffled heart sounds, tachycardia, decreased breath sounds, or drop in blood pressure is reported to the physician immediately.

Special cardiopulmonary problems
MYOCARDIAL INFARCTION

The person suspected of experiencing a myocardial infarction needs immediate attention. The greatest risk of mortality occurs within the first 2 hours after onset. If the heart ceases to beat, CPR is instituted immediately.

The patient who is breathing may be more comfortable in a well-supported sitting position. Oxygen is given if available. A calm atmosphere is of utmost importance, and the patient should never be left alone; fear will add an additional stress to the already overburdened heart (see Chapter 26).

NEAR-DROWNING

Approximately 6000 people die from drowning in the United States every year, over half in home swimming pools. *Near-drowning* refers to asphyxiation or partial asphyxiation from a fluid medium, with the person either recovering spontaneously or resuscitated at least temporarily.[3] The three types of drowning are wet, dry, and secondary.[6] *Wet drowning* is the most common type and refers to asphyxiation from the aspiration of fluid into the lungs, inhaled as the person panics and gasps for breath. *Dry drowning* refers to asphyxiation from laryngospasm that prevents both air and water from entering the lungs. *Secondary drowning* is the recurrence of respiratory distress after recovery from the initial incident, and may occur a few minutes to several days later.

If the victim of near-drowning has ceased breathing, artificial ventilation is initiated as soon as possible, even before the victim has been completely removed from the water. Time should not be wasted trying to remove water from the lungs. If distention of the abdomen from swallowed water interferes with adequate ventilation, the victim can be rolled onto the stomach and lifted with pressure over the stomach to force the water out.

Persons who have experienced near-drowning should be observed closely for at least 24 hours, even if they indicate that they feel all right. Pulmonary edema can develop after several hours.

ELECTRICAL INJURIES

Electricity can cause injury in a number of ways:
1. Depression of respiratory center
2. Ventricular fibrillation (stimulation of heart at end of refractory period, even by low electric current)
3. Bone fractures and persistant muscle injury (from powerful muscle contractions)
4. Burns at entry and exit points.

The extent of injury from electricity depends on the point in the heartbeat cycle that is stimulated by the electricity, the intensity of the current, and skin resistance. Moisture decreases skin resistance, so greater damage occurs when skin is moist from water or perspiration.

The victim must be removed from the source of electricity, with the rescuer being careful to avoid contact with the electric charge. CPR is started immediately if breathing and pulse are absent, and continued even when there is no evidence of response. Defibrillation is indicated for ventricular fibrillation.

Causes of bleeding

External	Internal
Lacerations	Chest trauma
Crushing injuries	Abdominal trauma, for
Amputations	example, ruptured
Fractures	spleen
Nosebleeds	Trauma to thigh
	Esophageal varicies
	Peptic ulcers

Hemorrhage

PATHOPHYSIOLOGY

Considerable blood loss may result from external or internal bleeding. Internal bleeding is more difficult to identify.

When a blood vessel is severed there is immediate contraction of the vessel wall, reducing the size of the opening and decreasing blood loss. Platelets begin to adhere to the roughened edges until a platelet plug is formed. A clot begins to form within 1 to 2 minutes. By 3 to 6 minutes the clot has filled the end of the blood vessel, blocking blood flow. Arteries have thick walls, and large arteries have musculature that can produce considerable vasospasms. Amputation of a leg, for example, may produce minimal bleeding. Veins and capillaries have thinner walls.

ASSESSMENT

External bleeding, if excessive, will saturate the clothing and be readily visible. If the person is wearing bulky outer garments, bleeding may be concealed. The examiner should run the hands quickly over the entire body under the outer clothing, being sure to check underneath the victim. Saturated clothing may need to be cut away so that the area of bleeding can be examined. The scalp is very vascular, and what appears to be considerable bleeding may result from a small scalp laceration.

Three types of bleeding may be observed:
1. Arterial bleeding: spurting bright red blood
2. Venous bleeding: continuous flow of darker blood
3. Capillary bleeding: oozing of blood.

Internal bleeding may be difficult to identify. Bleeding into the thorax (hemothorax) may inhibit respirations, and chest pain may be present. Abdominal bleeding may be evidenced by rigidity of abdominal muscles and abdominal pain. Hemoptysis or hematemesis indicate pulmonary or gastrointestinal bleeding.

Shock occurs with severe internal or external bleeding. The victim is assessed for weak rapid pulse, slow shallow respirations, cold clammy skin, anxiety, restlessness, and

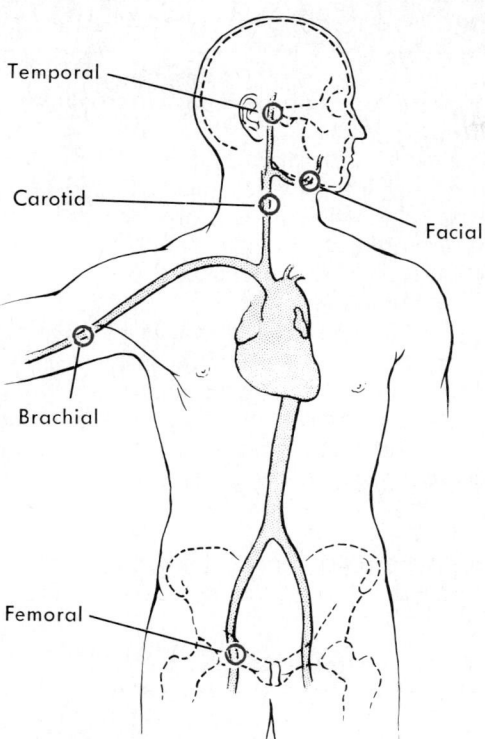

Fig. 40-3. Pressure points—locations at which large blood vessels may be compressed against bones to help control hemorrhage.

thirst. The pupils are equal, may be dilated, and respond slowly to light.

INTERVENTION

Actions for control of *external* bleeding include the following:
1. Apply direct pressure over site of bleeding.
2. Apply pressure over a pressure point (Fig. 40-3) if bleeding cannot be controlled by direct pressure.
3. Use tourniquet *only* in selected situations (massive uncontrollable arterial bleeding):
   a. Use blood pressure cuff or wide triangular bandage folded six to eight times
   b. Do not cover or release tourniquet
   c. Attach a notation to patient giving location of tourniquet and time of application.

For suspected *internal* bleeding, keep the person lying down and protected from dampness and cold. Prevent further hypotension and seek immediate medical attention.

POISONING

Poisoning in adults occurs for various reasons:
1. Not checking medication labels (overdose or wrong medication)
2. Lack of knowledge (for example, taking alcohol and sedatives together)
3. Taking an excess amount in an attempt to obtain a desired effect
4. As a suicide attempt

ASSESSMENT

A *rapid* assessment is made to determine whether poisoning or overdose has occurred so that immediate action can be taken to prevent or diminish the effects of the poison or drug. It is important to identify clues that poisoning is a possibility and the type and quantity of the poisonous agent.

The conscious victim is questioned about the type and amount of substance taken or the nature of the poisoning. When the victim is unconscious, not much time should be spent looking for needle marks. Identification of the poison or drug can be facilitated by asking others to look for clues while you examine the victim. Empty containers, spilled fluids, open medication bottles, or syringes may provide needed information. *All* potential agents should be gathered in their original containers and taken to the hospital with the victim. The physician may need to know the ingredients of the agent for those situations when an antidote is indicated.

COMMON ACCIDENTAL POISONING

Immediate action is necessary if poisoning is suspected; in some instances delay of a few minutes may make a difference between life and death. An *unconscious* victim must be transported *without delay* to the nearest medical facility.

If the victim is *conscious* identify the type, method, and estimated amount of poison or drug taken. Have someone call a physician immediately, if possible. Most large cities have *poison control centers* that maintain an extensive file on the most common substances and drugs. The telephone number is usually easily obtained from a list of emergency numbers in the front of the telephone directory.

Management consists of stopping absorption of the poisonous substance or drug. Poisonous substances can be inhaled, absorbed through the skin or mucous membranes, ingested, or injected. The type of intervention depends on the method by which the poison entered the system (Table 40-4).

If it is known exactly what poisonous substance or drug has been ingested, a specific antidote may be given in some cases by the physician. The use of a "universal antidote" has not proved effective.

BACTERIAL FOOD POISONING

Food poisoning occurs more frequently than is reported, because the majority of persons recover quickly without treatment. The incidence of food poisoning from

Table 40-3. Types of poisoning

Type	Examples	Therapy
Inhaled	Carbon monoxide, toxic gas	Remove victim from site to fresh air; give oxygen if available; give CPR if indicated; transport to medical center
Contact	Insecticides	Rinse skin with copious amounts of water
Ingested	Drugs, household chemicals, insecticides, lead	1. For noncaustic ingested substances, induce vomiting with syrup of Ipecac a. 30 ml in adults b. May be repeated once in 15 min c. Follow with small glass of fluid 2. For caustic substances: a. Give small amount of milk or water b. Seek immediate medical attention 3. For drugs, follow vomiting with 30 to 50 gm activated charcoal in 60 to 90 ml water 4. In the emergency room, lavage may be used to eliminate agent
Injected	Insect bites, drugs	1. Bee stings: a. Remove stinger with scraping motion b. Apply ice c. A paste of sodium bicarbonate and water or weak solution of ammonia may be applied 2. Ticks a. Remove tick by applying turpentine or gasoline b. Apply ice after tick removed 3. Drugs: a. Take victim to medical center b. See Chapter 9 for discussion of substance abuse

commercially prepared foods has become relatively uncommon in the United States, but food poisoning from home-cooked foods or improper handling of foods still occurs.

Bacteria such as *Staphylococcus aureus* or *Clostridium botulinum* can produce a toxin that acts as a poison, causing acute gastrointestinal tract upset. Because *S. aureus* toxin (the most common type) does not spread through the body, the symptoms are limited. The *C. botulinum* toxin does spread, and can be fatal (Table 40-4). *Salmonella* organisms introduced in food multiply in the intestines, causing acute gastrointestinal tract upset and infection.

Food poisoning is not caused by food that has spoiled or decomposed unless the food happens to contain disease-causing bacteria. Acute food poisoning can be prevented (see box).

Prevention of food poisoning

1. Can low-acid foods (foods other than tomatoes or fruits) under pressure to prevent botulism.
2. Discard any can that bulges.
3. Avoid slow cooling of meat or poultry dishes.
4. Use a meat thermometer when cooking extremely large pieces of meat (especially pork).
5. Keep meats, fish, poultry, mayonnaise, and cream-filled foods refrigerated.

Table 40-4. Bacterial food poisoning

Symptoms	Causative agent	Source	Comments
Nausea and vomiting, abdominal pain, lowered temperature, diarrhea is variable	*Staphylococcus aureus:* enterotoxin	Fish and meats (especially ham), dehydrated milk, unrefrigerated mayonnaise and cream-filled foods; skin and respiratory tract of food handlers	Mortality low Toxin heat stable Incubation 1 to 6 hr Symptoms last 8 to 24 hr Treatment: bed rest, fluids
Nausea and vomiting, diarrhea, abdominal pain, chills and fever, weakness	*Salmonella:* multiply in gut and produce toxin	Inadequately cooked eggs, poultry, meat (especially pork)	Mortality low Organism killed by heat Incubation 10 to 48 hr Symptoms last 2 to 5 days Treatment: bed rest, fluids (no antibiotics; they produce resistant strains)
Nausea and vomiting; double vision; flaccid paralysis of face, eyes, mouth, throat; dryness of skin, mouth, throat	*Clostridium botulinum:* exotoxin; spores germinate under anaerobic conditions and produce toxin	Improperly canned vegetables, meat (low-acid foods); spiced, smoked, vacuum-packed, or canned alkaline foods eaten without cooking	Mortality high Toxin heat labile Incubation 12 to 36 hr Death from respiratory failure

Table 40-5. Reactions to heat

Type	Cause	Signs and symptoms	Therapy
Heat cramps	Loss of sodium chloride in perspiration during strenuous exercise in hot weather	Severe cramps; pain in arms or legs	Salty fluids (for example, Gatorade) and food by mouth; extra water; rest in cool place
Heat exhaustion	Sodium and water depletion; fluids are replaced by some water, but inadequate salt	Vasomotor collapse: faintness, weakness; skin pale or ashen, cold, moist	Recumbent position in cool environment; fluids, preferable with salt; transport to medical center if severe
Heat stroke (sunstroke)	Failure of perspiration regulating mechanism; prolonged exposure to heat, especially in elderly, obese, or unacclimatized person	Skin dry, hot, flushed; faintness, dizziness; fever; unconsciousness	Reduce body temperature immediately by placing person in air-conditioned room; apply cool moist cloths, use fan; transport immediately to medical center
Burns	Direct heat, chemicals, electricity, radiation	First degree: erythema, pain Second degree: vesicles, pain Third degree: charred, coagulated, white skin	Apply cool water For specific care of severe burns, see Chapter 38

ENVIRONMENTAL INJURIES

Heat

Three types of general reactions to heat may occur (Table 40-5). *Heat cramps* can be prevented by taking extra salt and water before strenuous exercise in hot weater. The condition is self-limiting. *Heat exhaustion* is vasomotor collapse from the inability of the body to supply vessels adequately with sufficient fluid, usually from loss of sodium through perspiration. This usually occurs after vigorous exercise in hot weather, especially in the unacclimatized person.

Heatstroke is the most serious reaction to heat. It is caused by a failure of the perspiration regulating mechanism in the hypothalamus. It is typically seen during a heat wave, and elderly and obese persons are at high risk. The body retains heat rather than dissipating it through perspiration. Without treatment, most heatstroke victims die; the heat permanently damages the entire nervous system. Persons do not recover from heatstroke as quickly as from heat exhaustion, and may have faulty heat regulation for the rest of their lives. These individuals should avoid repeated long exposure to heat.

Cold

Excessive cold can lower body temperature, causing hypothermia, or can injure cells by direct exposure, causing frostbite.

HYPOTHERMIA

Hypothermia may result accidentally from exposure to cold weather. The extent of the cooling effect depends on the temperature and exposure time, the thermal conductivity of the environment, and the amount of air current present. Moisture is a good conductor, air is not. Wet clothing therefore contributes to increased cooling of the body. Several light layers of clothing to provide air insulation will keep a person warmer than one heavy layer. Air movement contributes to heat loss; thus lower environmental temperatures can be tolerated better in the absence of wind (windchill factor).

When the body is exposed to cold, shivering occurs to produce heat by increased metabolism. As the cold increases, shivering ceases and heat loss exceeds heat production. The individual becomes listless, apathetic, and sleepy and may become indifferent to the surroundings and not seek adequate protection. Pulse and respirations become slower as metabolism decreases. Freezing of the extremities, unconsciousness, and finally death result if help is not received.

The victim needs to be kept warm while being transferred to a medical facility. Wet clothing is removed immediately and warmed blankets applied. If a tub bath is given, the temperature should be approximately 40° to 42° C (104° to 108° F). Warmer temperatures can cause skin damage from the decreased circulation to the skin. Rubbing of the skin is to be avoided because this can also cause skin damage. Warm liquids may be given if the victim is conscious.

The person experiencing hypothermia is monitored closely during rewarming. Hypovolemic shock can occur from vasodilation. If fluids are given intravenously, overloading of the circulation is a potential complication. Vital signs are monitored for sudden changes. Cardiac monitoring may also be indicated for signs of ventricular fibrillation and cardiac arrest.

FROSTBITE

Cellular injury occurs with exposure to extreme cold. Cell water freezes, and the resulting ice crystals damage the cell. The degree of injury depends on the depth of freezing. Frostbite occurs most frequently in exposed areas such as the nose, cheeks, ears, and fingers and can be prevented by adequate covering with loose-fitting dry clothing. Toes are also susceptible because of dampness and tight pressure from shoes or boots. Persons with circulatory problems are more prone to develop frostbite.

Superficial frostbite is characterized by soft, whitened, or dull ashen skin that does not redden with pressure. The part can be rewarmed by contact with warm skin, covering, application of warm dry socks if toes are affected, or gently immersing the part in warm, not hot, water.

Deep frostbite is evidenced by hardness of the frozen tissue because of deep subcutaneous tissue injury. After thawing the skin becomes hyperemic and edematous with blister formation. The edema subsides in 24 to 48 hours, and tissue breakdown with necrosis results. The frozen part should be covered to warm it, and the victim should be taken to a medical center as soon as possible. Care is then similar to that for vascular disease of the extremities. Efforts are made to decrease the oxygen needs of the tissues while healing takes place, to improve blood supply by use of drugs, and to prevent infection of open lesions. Necrotic tissue may have to be debrided for healing to occur.

Radiation

Radiation injury is caused by exposure to gamma rays and neutrons from radioactive material. Persons can become contaminated by the rays through the air from unshielded radioactive material, or inhaled or swallowed on particles of contaminated dust or smoke. The amount of radiation that a person receives depends on various factors:

1. Strength of radiation source
2. Distance from the source
3. Duration of exposure
4. Area of the body exposed to the radiation source
5. Amount and type of shielding

PREVENTION

Rescue workers who must remove a victim from an area of radioactivity need to protect themselves from radiation exposure. Because radioactive particles can be carried on dust, all skin areas must be covered and a filtering mask worn by rescue workers after an explosion involving nuclear materials. The greater the duration of exposure, the greater the potential for injury; therefore the victim must be removed immediately to a less hazardous environment. Some of the basic principles of emergency care may have to be violated when there is danger of other explosions or when fires occur. The rescue worker should remove all contaminated clothing at the edge of the contaminated area, and any exposed skin areas are washed thoroughly. A shower should be taken as soon as possible as an additional preventive measure.

INTERVENTION

Radiation rays can cause a local inflammatory reaction of the skin, similar to a burn. The involved area may be washed gently with soap and water and a dry sterile dressing applied. No antiseptic or disinfectant solutions should be used, and no debridement should be attempted.

Radiation sickness will not become apparent until several days after exposure. There may be nausea and vomiting shortly after exposure, but this ceases spontaneously. Because radiation affects the body's immune response, later symptoms may include severe inflammation and sometimes sloughing and hemorrhage of the mucous membranes of the mouth and throat, bloody diarrhea, purpura (hemorrhagic spots under the skin), and alopecia (loss of hair). Severe leukopenia quickly follows exposure to large amounts of radiation.

There is no specific treatment for radiation sickness. The patient needs the same care as one who receives radiation treatment, including rest, protection from superimposed infection, good mouth care, fluid and electrolyte replacement, and a high-calorie diet (see Chapter 14).

MUSCULOSKELETAL INJURIES

Wounds

Injury to soft tissue may result in open wounds, which damage the skin, or in closed wounds, which damage underlying tissue but leave the skin intact (Table 40-6).

Suturing of lacerations and incisions should be carried out within the first few hours after injury to obtain maximal healing with fewer complications or scarring. If the

Table 40-6. Types of wounds

Type	Description	Therapy
Open wounds		
Abrasion	Scraping of skin surface (brush burn)	Wash well with soap and water; keep clean; no covering necessary
Laceration	Jagged cut through skin and underlying tissue	Wash well with soap and water; edges approximated by "butterfly" adhesive or by suturing
Incision	Straight cut through skin and underlying tissue by sharp knife	Same as for laceration
Puncture	Penetration of skin and underlying tissue by sharp-pointed object; skin quickly seals over when object is removed	Soak wound; encourage bleeding in small wound to wash out bacteria; monitor for signs of infection; tetanus prophylaxis
Stab	Form of puncture wound by large object such as a knife, stick, or piece of glass	Do not remove object; stabilize object to prevent further damage; control bleeding; seek immediate medical attention
Closed wound		
Contusion (bruise)	Injury by blunt object; blood vessels rupture, and blood seeps into tissue; edema from trauma to injured cells	Apply ice or cold compresses for 24 to 48 hours; analgesics for pain; rest of injured part

Table 40-7. Tetanus prophylaxis following injury*

Booster date	Wound size	Prophylaxis
Within past 10 yr	Small, moderate	0.5 ml toxoid†
	Severe or more than 24 hr old	0.5 ml toxoid
		250 units TIGH‡
More than 10 yr or none	Small	0.5 ml toxoid (start series)
	Moderate	0.5 ml toxoid (start series)
		250 units TIGH
	Severe	0.5 ml toxoid (start series)
		500 units TIGH

*Recommended by the American College of Surgeons.
†Absorbed tetanus toxoid.
‡Tetanus immune globulin (human).

Table 40-8. Some major injuries affecting chest wall and pleural cavity

Injury	Cause	Signs and symptoms	Initial emergency care
Rib fracture	Blow to chest	Pain on inspiration; local tenderness	Transport
Flail chest	Ribs fractured in more than one place; chest wall becomes unstable	Paradoxical respirations; respiratory distress; chest pain	Apply external pressure: sandbags, pillow, your hand; give oxygen; transport with flail side down
Open pneumothorax (open sucking wound)	Penetrating trauma to chest; loss of negative intrathoracic pressure as air moves in and out of wound	Sucking sound on chest wall during inspiration; tracheal deviation	Cover wound with occlusive dressing during exhalation; give oxygen
Simple pneumothorax	Laceration of lung, hyperinflation (blast injuries, driving accidents), loss of negative intrathoracic pressure	Sudden onset of chest pain; decreased breath sounds of affected area; dyspnea, tachypnea	Semi-Fowler's or Fowler's position; give oxygen
Tension pneumothorax	Complication of other types of pneumothorax; air enters pleural cavity but cannot escape	Respiratory distress; paradoxical chest movements; neck vein distention; tracheal deviation to unaffected side	Maintain airway and breathing; give oxygen (needle thoracotomy by trained person)
Hemothorax	Blunt and penetrating chest injuries; injuries to major blood vessels and heart; blood collects in pleural cavity	Decreased breath sounds; dyspnea (cyanosis and signs of shock if severe)	Treat for shock; give oxygen

wound is grossly contaminated the decision may be made to delay suturing for a few days to permit thorough cleansing. Healing then occurs by tertiary intention.

Puncture wounds are particularly vulnerable to infection, and bacteria such a *Clostridium tetani,* which thrive without air, may infect these wounds. Because anaerobic bacterial infections are extremely serious, a physician should be consulted if the puncture was made by a dirty object.

Tetanus prophylaxis for contaminated wounds depends on the size of the wound and the person's previous tetanus immunization (Table 40-7). (See chapter 13 for a discussion of active immunization with toxoid or passive immunization with immune serum globulin.) Tetanus (lockjaw) is highly fatal, and the only sure method of prevention is through immunization.

CHEST WOUNDS

Injuries to the chest may result in open chest wounds, fractured ribs, or injuries to the heart (cardiac tamponade) and lung (Table 40-8). These conditions are described in more detail elsewhere in the test.

Open wounds of the chest create a problem if there is intrusion into the pleural cavity. Air is drawn into the pleural space because of the existing negative pressure. The resultant positive pressure causes pneumothorax (collapse of the lung). A sucking noise is heard as the air is drawn in and respirations are impaired. Immediate action is indicated to cover the opening. A nonporous material must be used, because air can pass through a standard dressing or material. Plastic wrap, which is not only nonporus but tends to cling to the skin, is excellent. If a dressing is used it must be covered with petrolatum to create an air barrier. After the chest wound has been sealed, a pressure dressing is applied. Continual monitoring of respirations is indicated.

Persons with chest trauma are considered to have sustained serious injury until proved otherwise. Primary consideration in emergency management is maintenance of an open airway, breathing, and circulation. Oxygen is administered at high flow. Rapid transport after initial emergency measures is essential.

ABDOMINAL WOUNDS

Blows to the abdomen can rupture underlying organs. The spleen is often lacerated, and the intestines, liver, kidney, and bladder may also sustain injury. Symptoms may include abdominal pain and rigidity, nausea and vomiting, shock, and contusions on the abdominal wall. The victim may assume a position with knees drawn up toward the abdomen. If severe shock is present the use of antishock trousers (if available) is indicated before transport. The trousers extend from the ankle to below the lowest rib. After application the trousers are inflated to apply pressure on the lower half of the body, decreasing the size of the vascular system and redirecting blood flow to vital areas (Fig. 40-4).

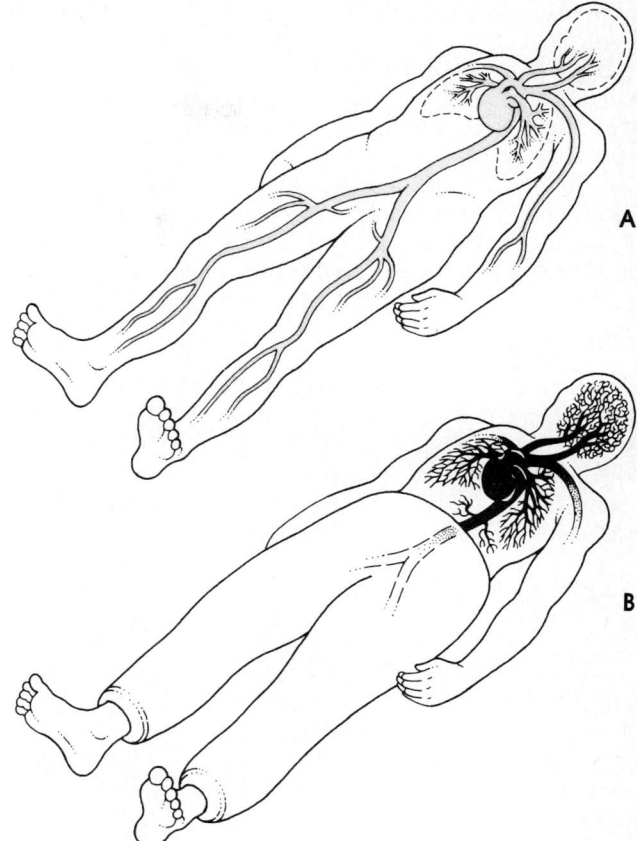

Fig. 40-4. In shock states, perfusion of vital organs is greatly enhanced by antishock trousers. **A,** Before application. **B,** After application. (From Budassi, S., and Barber, J.: Emergency nursing: principles and practice, St. Louis, 1981, The C.V. Mosby Co.)

If there is an open wound evisceration may occur. If the abdominal organs are exposed to the air and become dry, necrosis can result. The abdominal organs lying outside the abdominal cavity should therefore be covered by a warm, moist, preferable sterile covering. If a sterile dressing is not available it is better to cover the organs with a clean moist cloth and risk infection than not to cover the organs and risk loss of tissue.

AMPUTATIONS

Traumatic amputations are treated as other wounds by controlling hemorrhage and applying pressure dressings. Severe bleeding does not always occur. The amount of bleeding is dependent on the extent of trauma that occurs; the greater the amount of trauma, such as the amputation of a limb by a crushing injury, the greater will be the amount of muscle spasm in the arterial walls. This causes the artery to contract, and bleeding is decreased. A limb or appendage that is severed cleanly by a sharp object such as a knife will bleed more profusely. If a tourniquet is necessary it should be applied close to the site of the amputation to decrease potential injury to intervening tissue.

The amputated portion should be taken with the victim to the hospital because replantation is sometimes possible. The amputated part should be kept at about 5° C (40° F). It can be transported by immersion in a container filled with normal saline solution. The container can be kept cold by placing it in another container filled with ice. The amputated part should never be frozen, cleaned, disinfected, debrided, or perfused before transportation.

Fractures

Injury to the musculoskeletal system may result in fractures or dislocations of the bones, strained muscles, or torn ligaments (see Chapter 23 for a complete discussion of these injuries). Emergency care consists of assessment of injury and interventions to prevent further trauma until medical help is available.

ASSESSMENT

If pain is localized over a bone or joint it should be considered fractured until a definitive diagnosis is made. Obvious deformity can be either a dislocation (if at a joint) or a fracture. In a compound fracture the bone may protrude through the skin. The ability to move an extremity or digit does not negate a fracture, although the victim usually refrains from movement because of pain. Shock may occur with severe fractures, either from the stress of the trauma or from blood loss, such as the extravasation of blood in the thigh following injury.

Skull fractures may vary from a small linear fracture with few symptoms to severe depression of bone fragments into the brain. Basilar skull fractures may be accompanied by bleeding or draining serous fluid from the nose or ears or both. Fractures of facial bones may interfere with respiration if the air passages become blocked.

Pain or deformity at the *hip* can be caused by either a fracture or dislocation. The leg will be shortened in both instances but turned *outward* if there is a *fracture* and *inward* with a *dislocation*. Fractures of the extremities may be accompanied by loss of circulation or sensation if blood vessels or nerves are pinched by the bone fragment. Circulation distal to the fracture is assessed by observing skin color and presence of pulses. A neurologic check for sensation and circulatory system checks should be repeated after splinting and during transportation.

INTERVENTION

The general management of fractures is listed in box above.

Fracture of the spine

Any questionable injury to the head, neck, or back is treated as a fracture of the spine. The victim should not be moved when being examined for fracture of the spine (neck or back). The examiner slides a hand under the victim and checks for point tenderness along the length

---

General management of fractures

1. Do not move patient before splinting a fracture (unless there is danger of fire, explosion, or radiation).
2. Cover open wound before splinting.
3. Support fractured bone and move it as little as possible while splinting.
4. Splint fracture in the position it is found.
5. In *severely angulated* fractures of the *shaft* of the extremity bone:
   a. Decrease muscle spasm and prevent damage to blood vessels by straightening severe angulation of bone shaft
   b. Place one hand just below fracture and other hand farther down extremity
   c. Apply gentle traction to straighten extremity
   d. Maintain traction until extremity is splinted
6. *Never* straighten deformities of a joint (shoulder, elbow, wrist, knee).
7. Apply splints to include joint above and below fracture.
8. Pad rigid splints (boards) for comfort.
9. Reinforce soft splints (pillows) with a rigid material such as a magazine or board.
10. If using air splint:
    a. Inflate only by mouth to a point where the thumb leaves a slight dent
    b. Keep fingers and toes free for assessment of circulation.
11. Handle fractured part gently to prevent pain and shock.

---

of the spine. Bruises on the head may indicate that a force has been exerted that could cause a neck fracture. Bruises on the shoulder, back, or abdomen are frequently seen with back fractures, but a spinal fracture can be present in the absence of any bruises. If the spinal cord has been damaged there may be loss of movement or sensation to the extremities.

Two problems can occur from a fractured spine: damage to the spinal cord and neurogenic shock. If the cervical spine is fractured there may be interference with respiration, and respirations must be continually monitored. The victim may use diaphragmatic breathing for a short period but be unable to sustain this. Artificial ventilation is more difficult in that the neck cannot be hyperextended because this can cause further injury to the spinal cord. The head can be extended by gentle traction and the jaw pulled forward to open the airway. Traction must be maintained until the neck can be supported in this position. *The neck should never be flexed, twisted, or hyperextended if a fracture is suspected.* If the victim is not having difficulty with respiration, the neck can be splinted in the position in which it was found.

The person with a potential spine fracture must be transported on a firm base, preferably a back board. *Forward or backward flexion of the spine is to be avoided* to prevent further trauma to the spinal cord. The victim should be slid, not rolled, in straight alignment onto the back board. It takes several persons working together to move the victim safely. The victim remains on the back board during the initial diagnostic tests in the emergency room.

SEXUAL ASSAULT: RAPE

Rape is one of the violent crimes for which an increasing number of people, primarily women, are seeking help. Despite the increasing number of rapes reported, it is estimated that the incidence of unreported rape is from 200% to 300% higher.

It is difficult to obtain statistics concerning the sociologic variables relating to rape because of the large number of unreported cases. There are many misconceptions concerning rape; some *facts* include the following:

1. Rape occurs among persons of all social classes.
2. Rape is more commonly *reported* among the lower class.
3. Rape occurs mostly between persons of the same race.
4. A majority of rapes are committed by someone the victim knows.
5. Males, especially young boys, may also be rape victims; the attacker is usually another male.

Rape is a major problem in prisons in the United States. Some prison reform groups are actively addressing this problem, with the major emphasis on protecting the young and vulnerable from attack.

Rape crisis centers

Rape crisis centers are available in many large cities. These centers differ in their functions but usually provide one or more of the following:

1. Direct service to the rape victim
2. Service to professional agencies (health, law)
3. Community education

Service to health professionals and education of the community are efforts to help change the system for the rape victim.

The victim service consists of volunteers, many of whom have been raped themselves, who serve as victim advocates throughout the medical examination and police interview. Some form of follow-up service, such as counseling, may be available. Some rape crisis centers have volunteer attorneys who can offer the victim legal advice or representation.

Rape trauma syndrome

Rape is a traumatic event for the victim physically, psychologically, and socially. *Physical* force is often used; a weapon may be used either as a threat or to injure the victim, or the hands or fists may be used to beat the victim or threaten choking. Injury can also occur as the victim is attempting to defend self or is struggling on the ground or floor. The vagina and perineum may be injured by force used during the sexual attack, and the rectum may also be lacerated if anal sex has been attempted, more commonly in rape of males.

Psychologic trauma is usually severe; the rape victim is in a state of crisis. Fear is a dominant theme as the victim perceives the event as life threatening. Other feelings expressed by victims are depersonalization, shame, degradation, defilement, violation, guilt, humiliation, and anger. The victim has not only been under threat of harm but has also been subjected in many instances to multiple sexual assaults, some natural, some perverted, by one or more persons. Fellatio (oral sex) is frequently demanded by the rapist. Some rapists will urinate on the victim before leaving.

The person who has been raped goes through the same phases as any person facing a crisis situation. The initial phase is one of shock and disbelief. After the initial acute phase, there is a period of pseudoequilibrium when the victim rationalizes the event or attempts to suppress thoughts concerning the rape. Later there are periods of depression, phobic reactions, and nightmares.

The rape victim also experiences *sociologic* crisis. If the woman is married, marital relationships may be affected. If she is single she often fears repeated occurrences and may feel the need to move, especially if the attack occurred in her home or apartment. Decisions must be made concerning whom to tell about the incident, because loss of needed support of family and friends may occur. Job security or relationships with co-workers may be threatened. Sociologic problems take considerable time to resolve, but concerns related to these potential problems may occur in the initial emergency period.

Prevention and health care

All women need to know the measures they can take to help prevent rape from occurring (see box, p. 1184). It would also be helpful if every woman learned methods of self-defense. Some communities introduce both issues of rape and self-defense into secondary school curricula. Many YWCAs teach classes in self-defense. Rape crisis centers can provide information on availability of classes in the community.

Persons who are raped may seek medical help directly or call the police, who will then take the victim for medical examination. Some victims fear reprisal by the rapist or are unwilling for others to know about the rape and therefore do not seek medical attention. Victims need to be encouraged to report the incident.

Many hospitals have developed protocols for care of the rape victim in the emergency department. If such a protocol does not exist, it behooves the nurses in the emergency department to work toward development of one. Rape crisis centers can be helpful in this regard. The protocol may include some of the following:

1. High priority in triage
2. Provision for privacy without leaving the victim alone

may be in a position of being the only health care provider in a given area and be responsible for giving initial first aid treatment or supervising the activities of others. Because of their education and experience, professional nurses can be especially helpful in aiding victims to cope with their emotional reactions to the disaster. Nurses may also be asked to serve at emergency morgues for support of families experiencing loss of loved ones.

The American Red Cross, which assumes an active role during disasters along with governmental agencies, operates shelters for victims. They provide supplies and food as well as service personnel (shelter manager, nurses, physicians, food helpers). Nurses interested in serving during disasters at home or in other parts of the country may contact the local American Red Cross office. Other services provided by the American Red Cross include emergency services on an individual family basis and aid for recovery.

Community groups involved in disaster planning

Governmental	Political, law enforcement, fire
Health	Hospitals, physicians, nurses, pharmacists, social workers
Official	American Red Cross
Nonofficial	Telephone company, parent-teacher organization, religious organization

---

Prevention

Preparedness for disasters includes community planning to identify and, if possible, prevent disasters, and education of the public to minimize the number of casualties.

COMMUNITY PLANNING

Most states have disaster service agencies, which are outgrowths of civil defense organizations. These agencies act as coordinating agencies for the local agencies. Every community should have a disaster planning group as part of the emergency medical committee. There should be representation by all groups who will be active participants if a disaster occurs. The disaster planning committee has the following functions:

1. Identifying the types of disasters that may occur in the local community
2. Organizing a plan to be followed for different situations
3. Arranging for simulated drills to test the effectiveness of plans
4. Determining need for education or updating of necessary skills of participants

Nurses need to be active participants in the planning, implementation, and evaluation phases of community disaster preparedness.

During a disaster local hospitals become actively involved and need their own disaster plan to cope with the sudden influx of persons needing emergency care. Any time a large number of injured persons are in need of emergency care, hospital disaster plans are put into effect. Testing of hospital disaster plans at specified intervals by simulated drills is necessary for determining whether the plans are effective and what changes, if any, are needed.

Four-color coded triage system

0—Black: Dead

1—Red: Critical or life-threatening

These victims have a reasonable chance of survival only if they receive immediate treatment. Emergency treatment is initiated immediately and continued during transportation. This category includes victims with respiratory insufficiency, cardiac arrest, hemorrhage, and severe abdominal injury.

2—Yellow: Serious

These victims can wait for transportation after they receive initial emergency treatment. They include victims with immobilized closed fractures, soft-tissue injuries without hemorrhage, and burns on less than 40% of the body.

3—Green: Minimal

Victims in this category are ambulatory, have minor tissue injuries, and may be dazed. They can be treated by nonprofessionals and held for observation if necessary.

From Baker, F.J.: Topics Emerg. Med. 1:49-157, 1979.

PUBLIC EDUCATION

Public awareness of potential community disasters is needed for effective community preparedness. Disaster planning committees need support and participation of community members. Individuals need to know what they should do in the event of a disaster. Most radio and television stations regularly notify communities of potential disasters and give directions for preventive actions to be taken and for methods of obtaining further information should the disaster occur. Because electricity may be cut off, battery-operated radios should be available in all homes for continued communication.

All homes should have an emergency food cabinet with sufficient nonperishable foods to meet nutritional needs for several days. Supplies are rotated with current supplies to prevent food from spoiling or becoming outdated.

Assessment
TRIAGE

There are essentially two different approaches to triage during a disaster. The *military* triage system, which may be initiated during a mass casualty disaster, is based on the philosophy of doing the "best for the most with the least by the fewest." Victims with injuries of such magnitude that there is question of survival are given low priority for transportation. In this system the numbers of critically injured must greatly outnumber the health and transportation personnel available. Victims are reclassified as the emergency situation changes. Priority is then given to those victims with the greatest chance of survival.

The more commonly used *civilian* triage system is used with multiple patients or multiple casualties. Several victim sorting methods can be used for triage, but essentially all methods give most priority to life-threatening injuries and least priority to minimal injuries (see box, p. 1186).

DISASTER SYNDROME

The behavior of victims after the impact of disaster can be characterized as progressing through phases of shock, awareness, euphoria, and anger. The victims are experiencing loss; therefore the phases are similar to those experienced by others during any kind of loss (grieving).

The *shock phase* may last only a few minutes or up to several hours after impact. The victim is dazed, unable to comprehend what is occurring, and cannot follow even simple directions. Persons prepared to function in emergencies are less apt to spend much time in the shock phase.

The *awareness phase* may last up to several days. Victims become aware of survival and try to help others, minimizing their own injuries or losses. During this stage guilt feelings may arise because others died and they survived. The victim is highly suggestible, can follow simple directions, but cannot carry out problem solving effectively.

The *euphoria phase* may last for several weeks. The vic-

tim feels a sense of brotherhood with the community and participates willingly in helping others with plans for recovery.

Before resolution, the victim may go through the Why me? or *anger phase* that occurs because of the experienced loss. The anger is often projected against helping persons who were not personally affected by the disaster. It is especially important for nurses who may be assisting victims during the recovery phase to understand that the anger is part of the loss experience. As the victim copes with the losses incurred by the disaster and life returns to more normal patterns, the anger will disappear.

Intervention
EMERGENCY AID STATIONS

The number, size, and staffing of emergency aid stations depend on the type and extent of the disaster. One person in each aid station is designated for triage. One person must be designated the leader and is responsible for making decisions for maximal effectiveness of the unit. In the absence of a physician, a nurse assumes leadership of emergency care.

The types of injuries that occur will depend on the type of disaster. Common injuries and conditions requiring care include soft-tissue and bone injuries, respiratory insufficiency, cardiac arrest, and childbirth.

Victims are not transported until first aid care has been given, as in any emergency. If hemorrhage has not been controlled or fractures splinted, the victim may arrive at the medical center in shock that could have been prevented or minimized; surgical intervention will not take place until measures to treat shock are instituted and the patient's condition is stable. If first aid measures are instituted before transportation, the victim can be taken to surgery at the earliest opportunity. Records indicating all treatment given at an emergency aid center *must* accompany a victim who is referred or transported to a medical center or any other health care facility.

SHELTERS

Most shelters are set up in schools, which can house a large number of people. The role of the nurse in a shelter is to assess and provide for health needs of the shelter population. Some nursing functions include the following:

1. Isolating persons with suspected infectious diseases
2. Identifying persons with chronic illnesses and ascertaining whether prescribed drugs are available
3. Monitoring shelter occupants for signs of developing health problems
4. Identifying persons having problems coping with the disaster and providing emotional support and guidance as necessary
5. Making arrangements for care of pregnant women and infants
6. Assisting with necessary immunizations.

Assessment of safety factors in the environment is also

a nursing responsibility. The nurse is part of the shelter team and advises the shelter manager of any potential health hazards. The care of victims in a disaster is a team effort, and the nurse is an important member of this team.

REFERENCES AND SELECTED READINGS*

1. American College of Surgeons, Committee on Trauma: Early care of the injured patient, ed. 3, Philadelphia, 1982, W.B. Saunders Co.
2. *Bailey, M.: Emergency! First aid for fractures, Nurs. 82 **12**(11):72-81, 1982.
3. Barry, J.: Emergency nursing, New York, 1978, McGraw-Hill Book Co.
4. *Boyd, L.T., Shurett, P.H., and Coburn, C.: Heat and heat-related illnesses, Am. J. Nurs. **81**:1298-1302, 1981.
5. *Bucanan, L.: Emergency! First aid for spinal cord injury, Nurs. 82 **12**(8):68-75, 1982.
6. Budassi, S.A., and Barber, J.M.: Emergency nursing: principles and practice, St. Louis, 1981, The C.V. Mosby Co.
7. Cosgriff, J.H., Jr., and Anderson, D.: The practice of emergency nursing, Philadelphia, 1975, J.B. Lippincott Co.
8. *Crooks, L., Corn, M., and DeAtley, C.: Disaster planning: a team effort, AORN J **28**:395-410, 1978.
9. Czajka, P.A., and Duffy, J.P.: Poisoning emergencies: a guide for emergency medical personnel, St. Louis, 1980, The C.V. Mosby Co.
10. *DeLapp, T.D.: Accidental hypothermia, Am. J. Nurs. **83**:62-67, 1983.
11. *DeLapp, T.D.: Taking the bite out of frostbite and other cold weather injuries, Am. J. Nurs. **80**:56-60, 1980.
12. Eckert, C.: Emergency room care, ed. 4, Boston, 1981, Little, Brown & Co.
13. Farrell, J.: Illustrated guide to orthopedic nursing, Philadelphia, 1977, J.B. Lippincott Co.
14. Flint, T., and Cain, H.D.: Emergency treatment and management, ed. 6, Philadelphia, 1980, W.B. Saunders Co.
15. Foley, T., and Davies, M.: Rape: nursing care of victims, St. Louis, 1983, The C.V. Mosby Co.
16. *Fritz, C.P.: Emergency! First aid for wounds, Nurs. 82 **12**(10):68-75, 1982.
17. Furgurson, J.E., and Meislin, H.W.: Airway problems in the trauma victim, Topics Emerg. Med. **1**:9-28, 1979.
18. Furste, W.L., and Aguirre, A.: Preventing tetanus, Am. J. Nurs. **78**:834-837, 1978.
19. *Gaston, S.F., and Schumann, L.L.:Inhalation injury: smoke inhalation, Am. J. Nurs. **80**:94-97, 1980.
20. George, O.G.: Anatomy and physiology of CPR, AORN J **27**:992-996, 1978.
21. Gilroy, A., and Caldwell, E.:Initial assessment of the multiple injured patient, Nurs. Clin. North Am. **13**:177-190, 1978.
22. *Hargreaves, A.G.: Coping with disaster, Am. J. Nurs. **80**:683, 1980.
23. *Heimlich, H.J.: Death from food-choking prevented by a new life-saving maneuver, Heart Lung **5**:755-758, 1976.
24. Hendrix, M.J., LaGodna, G.E., and Bohen, C.A.: The battered wife, Am. J. Nurs. **78**:650-653, 1978.
25. *Holmstrom, L.L., and Burgess, A.W.: Assessing trauma in the rape victim, Am. J. Nurs. **75**:1288-1291, 1975.
26. Holmstrom, L.L., and Burgess, A.W.: The victim of rape: institutional reactions, New York, 1978, John Wiley & Sons, Inc.
27. *Jankowski, C.B.: Radiation emergency, Am. J. Nurs. **82**:90-95, 1982.
28. Kerr, A.: Orthopedic nursing procedures, ed. 3, New York, 1980, Springer Publishing Co., Inc.
29. Lanros, N.: Assessment and intervention in emergency nursing, Bowie, Md., 1978, Robert J. Brady Co.
30. Mancine, M.: Liability in the emergency room, Am. J. Nurs. **78**:1478-1482, 1978.
31. *Matheney, L.L: Emergency! First aid for cardiopulmonary arrest, Nurs 82 **12**(6):34-45, 1982.
32. *Meyd, C.J.: Acute brain trauma, Am. J. Nurs. **78**:40-44, 1978.
33. Miller, M.E.: Cycle trauma: nursing's three key roles, Nurs. 80 **10**(7):26-31, 1980.
34. Miller, R.H.: Textbook of basic emergency medicine, ed. 2, St. Louis, 1980, The C.V. Mosby Co.
35. *Monico, L.: The roles nurses play during a code, Nurs. 83 **13**(8):34-39, 1983.
36. *Niggemann, E.H.: Near-drowning, Nurs. 83 **13**(7):45, 1983.
37. *Palmer, E.L.: Student reactions to disaster, Am. J. Nurs. **80**:680-682, 1980.
38. *Pister, S.: Respiratory arrest: are you prepared? Nurs. 82 **12**(9):34-41, 1982.
39. *Rich, W., and Perchenbeger, M.: Managing flail chest: a matter of maintaining breath . . . and life, Nurs. 81 **11**(12):26-31, 1981.
40. Roderick, M.A.:Tetanus, Nurs. 82 **12**(7):63, 1982.
41. Rothstein, R.J.: Hemorrhagic shock in multiple trauma, Topics Emerg. Med **1**:29-40, 1979.
42. Schultz, L.: Rape victimology, Springfield, Ill, 1975, Charles C Thomas, Publisher.
43. Skeet, M.: Emergency procedures and first aid for nurses, St. Louis, 1981. The C.V. Mosby Co.
44. Standards for cardiopulmonary resuscitation and emergency cardiac care, J.A.M.A. **224**:453-508, 1980.
45. *Sumner, S.M., and Grau, P.E.: Emergency! First aid for choking, Nurs. 82 **12**(7):40-49, 1982.
46. Symposium on Trauma, Nurs. Clin. North Am. **13**:175-265, 1978.
47. *Talento, B.N., and Fernandez, J.C.: Nursing care for rape victims, AORN J **27**:1408-1418, 1978.
48. Warner, C., editor: Emergency care: assessment and intervention, ed. 3, St. Louis, 1982, The C.V. Mosby Co.
49. *Thompson, N.A.: Convert your assessment into a lifesaving care plan for the patient with abdominal trauma, Nurs. 83 **13**(7):26-33, 1983.
50. White, K.M.: Evaluating the trauma of gunshot wounds, Am. J. Nurs. **77**:1589-1593, 1977.

---

*References preceded by an asterisk are particularly well suited for student reading.

UNIT XIII
Critical Care Nursing

41 Care of the Patient in a Critical Care Unit

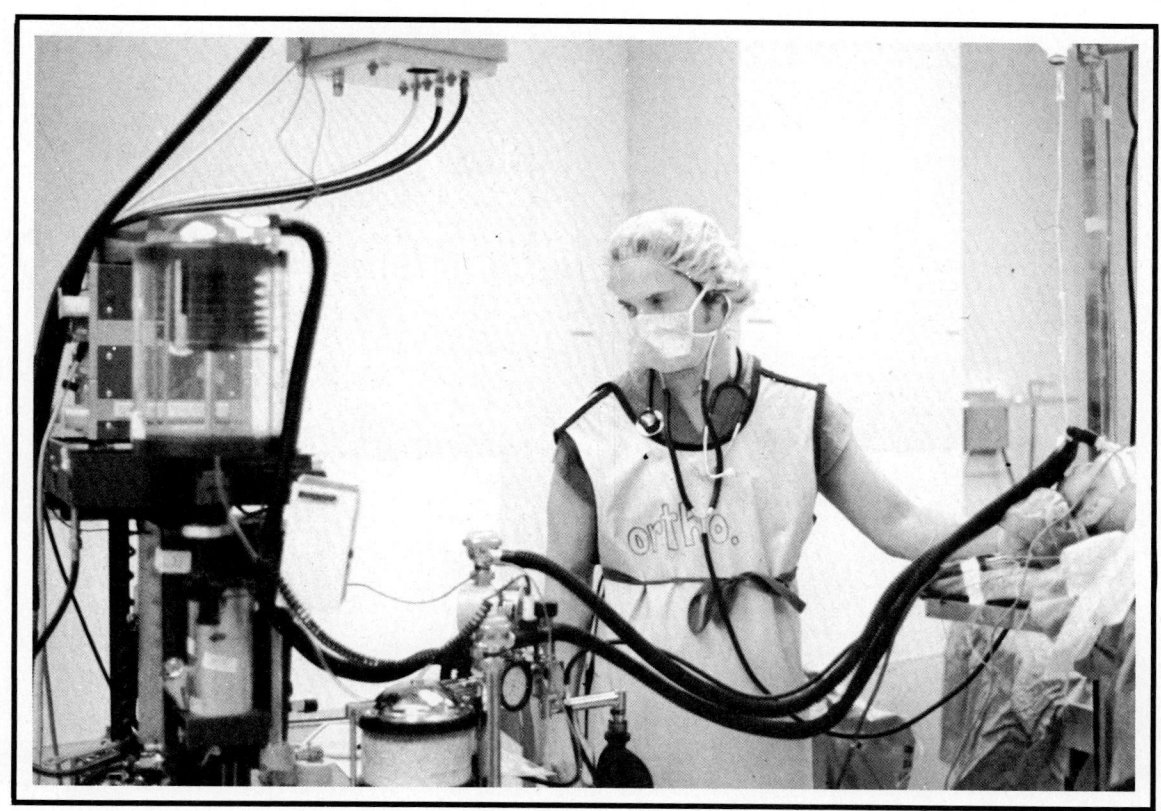

41

Care of the Patient in a Critical Care Unit

MAURA HOPKINS

STUDY QUESTIONS

- Examine the chart of a patient who spent time in a critical care unit. What patient parameters were monitored?

- Were any of the patient parameters below or above normal ranges? If so, what problems were identified and what actions were taken?

- Does the chart identify any psychologic stressors?

- If you were a relative of the patient, what information would you have wanted? What might have been your feelings about sitting for long periods in the waiting room, with patient visits of only a few minutes at stated intervals?

When "respirator centers" were developed in isolated locations nationally to combat the polio epidemic of the 1950s, the expectation was that the concentration of highly skilled personnel along with sophisticated medical equipment would positively influence the victims' survival. In addition to providing treatment these centers were dedicated to research, education, and training. They were, perhaps, the earliest form of the modern day intensive care unit (ICU).

Through the evolution of the coronary intensive care unit of the 1960s to the current nationwide availability of single- and multipurpose critical care units the role of the nurse in the care of the critically ill patient has remained the focal point of the success of these units. With vigilant observation of the patient's ever-changing condition, the critical care nurse is uniquely able to identify and initiate appropriate therapies, maintain complex treatment regimens, and intervene to prevent life-threatening situations.

In the 1980s nurses will find themselves working in a wide array of adult and pediatric critical care environments. These may be multipurpose ICUs or units specially designated for patients with a common type of problem, such as medical, surgical, coronary, cardiovascular (open heart), neurologic/neurosurgical, pulmonary, renal, neonatal, burn, and shock/trauma units. In all cases the goal of critical care nursing remains the same: to provide continuous, optimal nursing care to patients in life-threatening situations, remaining alert to the physiologic, psychologic, and social needs of the patient as an integrated being.

This chapter provides an overview of some of the common aspects of critical care nursing and the critical care environment. Effects of the critical care environment on patient, family, and staff are described. Assessment of the critically ill patient is followed by interventions designed to alleviate physical, psychologic, and social stressors experienced by critically ill patients.

Equipment commonly available within or near the ICU

Monitors

Cardiac
Hemodynamic (intraarterial, pulmonary artery)
Intracranial pressure
External arterial pressure

General equipment

ECG machine
Defibrillator
Intubation equipment
Emergency medications
Ventilator
Oxygen therapy equipment
Arterial blood gas analyzer
Hyper-hypothermia machine
Flouroscopy
Doppler flow detection device
Bed scale

Bedside equipment

Bed with removable headboard
Oxygen and manual ventilation device
Suction device
Intravenous infusion device

Supportive services (24 hour)

Pharmacy
Laboratory
Respiratory therapy
Radiology
Dialysis

ENVIRONMENT IN THE CRITICAL CARE AREA

Physical environment

The critical care unit is designed, equipped, and staffed to meet the anticipated needs of patients in life-threatening situations. The physical layout is frequently a modified circular design around a central nurses' station, allowing for direct visualization of all patients at all times. Patients may be separated in individual cubicles or be situated in a large open area with curtains as partitions. The advantage of direct nurse-patient visualization may accompany the disadvantages of limited patient privacy and patient exposure to frequent crisis intervention.

Supplies and equipment in critical care areas are highly sophisticated and must be readily accessible for all patients (see box above). Certain pieces of equipment are in constant use at each bedside (for example, cardiac monitor, oxygen, suction equipment), and others must be available within seconds (defibrillator, ventilator, ECG machine, emergency medications). Existing hospital space has often been converted to ICU use, and as the need for more specialized and sophisticated ICU equipment grows the critical care environment often becomes overcrowded.

Psychologic environment: stress on patient and staff

In the critical care environment advanced forms of technology and medical and nursing therapeutics are used in patients in extended crisis. Although aware of the special nature of this care, the patient and family focus on its appearance: flashing lights; buzzing machines; painful procedures; a noisy, brightly lit, crowded, hyperactive environment permeated by vague fears. The stressors on the patient and family are immense, heightened by those very treatment modalities that may prove lifesaving.

The stress on nursing staff in the critical care area stems in part from very high expectations: advanced knowledge of physiology related to all body systems, astute observational and physical assessment skills, and the technical ability to operate the highly sophisticated equipment. Critical care nurses must have excellent communication skills to deal with the patient and family's psychologic and social needs, continually incorporating interventions that the nurse might be tempted to assign a low priority in a critical situation.

Both the patient and the nurse are bombarded by continuous, varied stressors in the critical care environment. Low-level stress can be challenging and stimulating and may help to enhance creativity, production, and performance in any area. Continuous high-level stress can be devastating, both physically and psychologically. (Review Chapter 8 on Concepts of stress and adaptation for an in-depth analysis of the effects of stress.) It is very important for critical care nurses to understand how stress affects both the patient and family and to recognize that interactions will have to be modified to take this into account. In addition, nurses must be aware of their own stressors and the positive and negative effects of these stressors. They must safeguard their own physical and psychologic health and recognize how insufficient or ineffective coping mechanisms can lead to burnout.

The critical care unit is a powerful milieu that must

Stressors on patients/families and staff in the ICU

Patient/family

Unfamiliar environment, new faces
Noise, light levels
Interruption of sleep/wake cycles
Sensory deprivation/overload
Inaccessibility of family, friends
Lack of privacy
Lack of information/understanding of prognosis, care plan
Lack of information/understanding of policies, procedures
Anticipation of painful interventions
Confusion/disorientation related to physiologic factors
Impaired communication related to intubation
Observation of crisis intervention in other patients
Fear related to diagnosis
Fear of death

Staff

Expectations of self
Expectations of peers, supervisors
Intricate machinery and techniques
Closed, crowded work area
Constant contact with seriously ill, dying persons
Continual vigilance of multiple patients
Need for constant emergency readiness
Sustained high activity level
Limited breaks away from the high-stress unit
Limited communication with many patients related to intubation or altered level of consciousness
Limited opportunity to communicate with some families
Isolation from other nurses in the hospital
Ethical conflicts related to issues of resuscitation and use of life-maintenance equipment

---

be well understood by nurses who wish to take advantage of its environment to deliver truly advanced, comprehensive, patient-centered nursing care.

ASSESSMENT OF THE CRITICALLY ILL PATIENT

The nursing process is the same in critical care situations as in any other patient care setting. Management of critically ill patients requires establishing a data base, identifying real and potential problems, delineating priorities, defining outcome criteria, determining goals for intervention, executing the planned intervention, and modifying future goals and plans based on outcomes. Management of critically ill patients differs from management of other patients because of an ever-changing data base, a larger number of complex, interrelated problems, frequent reordering of priorities, and time limitations imposed by the rapidly changing condition of the patient.

The assessment process for the critically ill patient differs from the assessment of other patients only in terms of the number of supportive devices available to assist in data collection. The cardiac monitor, hemodynamic monitoring lines, and laboratory analyses provide data that must be incorporated into the total patient assessment. They are adjuncts to the direct observational data that the nurse gathers through careful history taking and physical examination. Monitored data is a useless string of unrelated facts and numbers until correlated to physical findings and integrarted into a meaningful analysis by the critical care nurse.

Nursing history

There are three main sources from which critically ill patients come to an intensive care unit: direct admission, transfer from another patient care division in the same or a different hospital, and postoperatively after certain planned operations. The patient admitted directly to the ICU (for example, in the case of a myocardial infarction) will often be accompanied by family or friends. Both the patient and family members are useful in obtaining a thorough and accurate history of the current illness and past illnesses/hospitalizations as well as a patient profile, the social information, and usual coping strategies. Although at the time of admission emphasis is on alleviating physiologic threats to survival, one member of the health team may take the opportunity to concurrently interview family members so that crucial facts about the patient's history can immediately be used in patient care. Even in the critical care setting, accurate and thorough history taking is vital to intelligent, individualized care planning and intervention.

When the patient is received in transfer from another nursing division, either directly or after surgery, consultation between the transferring and receiving nursing staffs is essential. The ICU nurses will benefit from the care plan developed by nurses who have had the opportunity to interact with the patient and family in a noncritical situation. Pertinent history, patient likes and dislikes, coping mechanisms, and family relations can all be relayed to the receiving nurses, enabling them to reduce the initial stress of the unfamiliar ICU environment. It is imperative that this type of pertinent history and care planning be shared among nurse colleagues to facilitate the patient's eventual recovery.

Physical examination

As with the assessment of any patient, history taking is followed by physical examination. The basic skills of inspection, palpation, percussion, and auscultation are used to elicit directly observed data from the patient. As in any other setting, explanations are given and patient cooperation is sought, even if the patient's comprehension of all that is said is questionable. (Refer to Chapter 3 on health assessment and to a physical assessment textbook for a thorough explanation on the use of these techniques.)

Monitored data

Nurses in all clinical settings use tools for isolated data collection from patients, for example, stethoscopes, sphygmomanometers, thermometers, and scales. Critical care nurses have the advantage of being able to use additional tools for continuous data collection, for example, cardiac monitors, hemodynamic pressure lines, and intracranial pressure monitoring devices. The explosion in critical care technology in the 1970s and 1980s is giving the critical care nurse amazing quantities of objective data with minimal time spent in system operations. Computerized monitoring systems are available that occupy less space and provide more capabilities than ever before. The most sophisticated of the "patient data management" systems take information from all the continuously monitored parameters (ECG, arrhythmias, pulmonary artery pressure, intraarterial pressure, central venous pressure, intracranial pressure, and body temperature) and combine it with manually entered data such as body weight, height, intake and output, and times of drug administration, and prepare a wide array of hemodynamic calculations and patient response trends for analysis by critical care practitioners. Certain types of continuous monitoring devices are in widespread use in nearly all critical care environments.

CARDIAC MONITORING

Cardiac monitoring involves placement on the patient's chest of conductive electrodes that recognize the electrical activity of the heart and relay it to a video display screen. Both the actual appearance of the patient's ECG and a numeric representation of the heart rate are displayed at the bedisde. Alarm limits are programmed by the nurse so that if the patient's heart rate rises above or falls below a safe range a tone sounds to alert the nurse. In monitoring systems with computerized arrhythmia analysis the monitor also recognizes specific rhythm abnormalities such as single or paired premature ventricular contractions, bigeminal rhythms, runs of ventricular tachycardia, ventricular fibrillation, or asystole. Variations in the audio or visual display of the alarm can alert the nurse to the relative seriousness of the arrhythmia, even from a distance. Cardiac monitoring is a noninvasive procedure and poses minimal risk to the patient.

HEMODYNAMIC MONITORING

Hemodynamic monitoring refers to invasive monitoring of the arterial or vascular system via a continuous electronic monitoring device. Table 41-1 lists the normal values of pressures found in the cardiovascular system, many of which are measured via bedside monitoring.

Table 41-1. Normal hemodynamic pressures

Area monitored		Normal presure (mm Hg)
Superior vena cava (SVC)	Mean	2 to 6 (3 to 10 cm H_2O)
Right atrium (RA)	Mean	2 to 6 (3 to 10 cm H_2O)
Right ventricle (RV)	Systolic	20 to 30
	Diastolic	0 to 5
	End diastolic	2 to 6
Pulmonary artery (PA)	Systolic	20 to 30
	Diastolic	10 to 20
	Mean	10 to 15
Pulmonary capillary wedge (PCWP)	Mean	4 to 12
Left atrium (LA)	Mean	4 to 12
Left ventricle (LV)	Systolic	100 to 140
	Diastolic	0 to 5
Aorta (Ao)	Systolic	100 to 140
	Diastolic	60 to 80
	Mean	70 to 90

Intraarterial monitoring

Intraarterial monitoring involves placement of a catheter into an artery, usually the radial or femoral artery. The catheter is connected to a high-pressure flush system normally filled with heparinized saline solution. The automatic flush, under pressure, delivers an average of 1 to 3 ml solution per hour through the catheter just to keep it patent. When a transducer is connected to the system and attached to the bedside monitor a waveform appears on the monitor that represents the fluctuation of the patient's blood pressure in the catheterized artery. A numeric display of the arterial pressure also appears on the monitor; in most patients this direct intraarterial pressure correlates very closely to external cuff pressure measurements.

Intraarterial pressure monitoring also provides direct access to arterial blood, which can then be easily obtained without further needle punctures for various laboratory tests, including arterial blood gas analysis. However, intraarterial cannulation is not without its complications. Nursing responsibilities include setup and safe, aseptic maintenance of the flush system and catheter insertion site; maintenance of a patent catheter with accurate waveform and pressure readings; and continuous patient observation to prevent the immediate life-threatening complication of hemorrhage.

Pulmonary artery monitoring

Pulmonary artery (Swan-Ganz) catheters are used to monitor cardiovascular function in critically ill patients. The catheter, which may have several openings along its length, is inserted into the superior vena cava, usually via the subclavian vein. It is threaded through the right side of the heart until the tip lies in the pulmonary artery. Pulmonary artery, central venous pressure (CVP), and pulmonary capillary wedge pressures can be obtained from the catheter once it is connected to a pressurized flush system and transducer-monitor system. In addition, cardiac output determinations can be performed. The pulmonary artery catheter is useful in providing data about left and right ventricular failure and in evaluating the effectiveness of vasopressor drugs, and is a significant tool in the management of severe cardiac failure and cardiogenic shock (see Chapter 26). (Table 41-2 lists the hemodynamic indices which can be computed from monitored data.) In addition the catheter serves as a central venous line for the infusion of fluids and potent medications. Pulmonary artery catheters are replacing the widespread use of single-purpose CVP lines because of the information they provide on left-sided heart function (wedge pressure, cardiac output) that cannot be obtained from a single CVP line.

In some cardiovascular ICUs it is common practice to forego using the pulmonary artery catheter and to insert a single line directly into the right atrium during open-

---

Complications of intraarterial monitoring

Bleeding

Thrombosis

Inflammation/infiltration

Infection

Air embolism

Paresthesias

Distal obstruction of the artery

Table 41-2. Normal hemodynamic indices

Measurement	Formula	Normal range
Cardiac output (CO)	Heart rate × Stroke volume	4.0 to 8.0 L/min
Cardiac index (CI)	$\dfrac{\text{Cardiac output}}{\text{Body surface area}}$	2.5 to 4.0 L/min/m²
Stroke volume (SV)	$\dfrac{\text{Cardiac output}}{\text{Heart rate}}$	60 to 130 ml/beat
Stroke index (SI)	$\dfrac{\text{Stroke volume}}{\text{Body surface area}}$	35 to 70 ml/beat/m²
Mean arterial pressure (MAP)	2/3 Diastolic + 1/3 systolic pressure	70 to 90 mm Hg
Pulmonary vascular resistance (PVR)	Mean pulmonary artery pressure − mean pulmonary capillary wedge pressure ÷ Cardiac output	<2 PVR units
Systemic vascular resistance (SVR)	$\dfrac{\text{Mean arterial pressure} - \text{central venous pressure (in mm Hg)} \times 80}{\text{Cardiac output}}$	900 to 1600 dynes/sec/cm⁻⁵

Complications of pulmonary artery (Swan-Ganz) monitoring

- Pulmonary artery rupture
- Infection
- Arrhythmias
- Thrombophlebitis
- Intracardiac knotting
- Balloon rupture with air embolism
- Pulmonary infarction

heart surgery, allowing direct monitoring of left-sided heart function. Other ICUs are beginning to use a newer type of fiberoptic pulmonary artery catheter that is able to perform continuous monitoring of pulmonary artery (mixed venous) oxygen saturation. Minute-by minute changes in systemic oxygen saturation can be monitored, reducing the frequency of arterial blood gas sampling while rapidly demonstrating the effects of various treatment modalities on systemic oxygenation. As with intraarterial pressure monitoring, pulmonary artery monitoring is not without risk. Nursing responsibilities are similar to those for arterial catheters, with the addition of continuous waveform observation to detect inadvertent catheter tip migration.

Surgical procedure: ______________________ 7 AM weight: ______ kg

	Vital signs										Set FI_{O_2}	Blood gases				
Date / Time	T	P	R	BP	CVP	MAP	PAP	MPAP	Wedge	CO	Meas. FI_{O_2}	pH	P_{CO_2}	P_{O_2}	HCO_3	Base / Sat.
8-hr total: 3 PM																
8-hr total: 11 PM																
8-hr total: 7AM																
24-hr total																

Fig. 41-1. Surgical intensive care unit flow sheet.

INTRACRANIAL PRESSURE MONITORING

Intracranial pressure (ICP) is frequently monitored in critically ill patients who have or are suspected of having intracranial disease or secondary increases in intracranial pressure. A catheter placed through the skull into the subarachnoid space allows intracranial pressure to be monitored directly via a transducer and tubing system. Intracranial pressure monitoring allows continued observation of the patient's response to therapies aimed at lowering intracranial pressure and immediately shows the patient's tolerance of nursing measures that can cause an unsafe rise in ICP (for example, turning, suctioning, changes in bed position). It also allows aspiration of cerebrospinal fluid for analysis or culturing or to relieve ex-

cess intracranial pressure unresponsive to other therapies. Nurses are responsible for obtaining accurate pressure measurements, analyzing trends and patient response to interventions, and preventing complications of monitoring. Scrupulous sterile technique is essential in handling the catheter or screw insertion site and all connections in the monitoring tubing system because of the direct avenue for microorganisms into the cerebrospinal fluid.

The preceeding are a few of the invasive monitoring techniques available to the critical care nurse for data collection. In all cases the nurse must be knowledgeable about maintaining these lines, about the normal appearance of the waveform associated with each line, of the

	Pulmonary function							Ventilator parameters		
Time	TV	V̇	VC	Qs/Qt	Vd/Vt	FRC	NIF	TV	V̇	Infla. pres.

Intake						Output				Chest tube			Patient notes
CVP line		Periph. IV					Sp. Gr.						
Type	Amt.	Type	Amt.	Oral	Amt.	Urine	SPOT			In	Out	Bal.	

Total intake: _____   Total output: _____

CARDIOVASCULAR

Apical HR _____ ECG rhythm _____

BP_____ CVP_____ PAP_____ PCWP_____

Pacer: Mode_____ Rate_____ MA_____

Heart sounds:_____

Skin color_____ Temp._____

Peripheral R: R_____ F_____ P_____ DP_____
pulses   L: R_____ F_____ P_____ DP_____

Specifics_____
_____
_____
_____

RESPIRATORY

Rate _____ Quality_____

Breath   R_____
sounds   L_____

FIO$_2$_____ Source_____

Mech. vent. TV_____ Rate_____ Mode_____

Chest tube(s)_____

Sputum_____ Cultures_____

Specifics_____
_____

FLUIDS/ELECTROLYTES

Last labs done:_____ Time_____

Abnormals:_____

Labs needed _____

        Time_____

IVs infusing (sol., amt., rate, site)

#1_____

#2_____

#3_____

#4_____

#5_____

        INTEGUMENT _____
        _____

NEUROLOGIC/PSYCHOLOGIC

LOC _____

Orientation _____

Affect_____

Pupils_____ ICP_____

Motor/sens._____

Resp. to environment_____

Social/emotional_____
_____

Specifics_____
_____

GASTROINTESTINAL

Abdomen _____

Bowel sounds_____

NG_____ Stool_____

Nutrition_____

Incisions/drains/ostomies_____
_____

Specifics_____
_____

GENITOURINARY

Urine: Amt._____ Color_____

Appearance_____

S/A_____ S.G._____ Voids_____

Catheter (type)_____

Skin condition_____

Renal function_____
_____
_____

Specifics_____
_____

Fig. 41-2. ICU on-shift assessment worksheet.

usual procedures necessary to prevent complications, and of the signs and symptoms of actual complications. The risk to the patient from invasive monitoring lines is significantly reduced when the lines are handled and cared for by knowledgeable personnel.

Baseline assessment

The complete history and physical examination is the necessary foundation for further ongoing data collection in the critical care setting, and the importance of accurate and thorough initial information cannot be overemphasized. But the multiple sources of data and the continually fluctuating stability of critically ill patients makes the constant reordering of priorities a necessity. The critical care nurse uses continual observation of the patient to update the data base in order to reformulate short-term goals and interventions.

Patient assessment must be thorough yet rapid. It must take into account the physical and psychologic reactions of an entrie organism under stress and not be limited by the usual or the expected. It must also be organized and repetitive so that small alterations or deviations from prior findings are noticed. Finally, it must be individualized so that time and attention can be given to particularly significant aspects of the assessment without losing sight of the whole.

Many intensive care units utilize some form of a systems approach to patient assessment. Frequently this consists of a complete head-to-toe systems review at the beginning of the shift, at which time the nurse gathers an initial data base. More time and depth are spent on the systems that present the greatest real or potential threat to the patient. When completed and documented the baseline systems assessment presents an accurate "status report" on the patient's condition, available for prior comparisons and future updating. Throughout the rest of the shift, the nurse charts the progress as the patient's condition improves or deteriorates from the baseline, keeping track of vital parameters on an ongoing flow sheet, such as is seen in Fig. 41-1.

Fig. 41-2 shows the outline of a basic beginning of shift assessment guide, which includes the main items to be assessed under each body system. Both routine parameters and individualized observations of specific problem areas can be elaborated on under the pertinent categories. The worksheet forms the outline of a repetitive assessment structure, which, once documented in the patient's record, makes information retrieval much easier.

Once patient assessment is completed, nursing diagnoses are established and nursing care plans formulated. Nursing interventions for critically ill patients are based on these care plans.

Throughout this text nursing interventions have been described for care of the patient with a particular type of physiologic impairment. These are interventions intended to improve the patient's physiologic functioning before the impairment reaches the critical stage. In some critically ill patients many of these interventions have already been

tried without success, and the patient's physiologic condition has deteriorated to the critical level, necessitating acute life-sustaining interventions. In other patients the initial illness is critical in itself (for example, acute myocardial infarction, severe trauma) and critical interventions are necessary immediately to sustain life.

The focus of the remaining three sections of this chapter is on physiologic, psychologic, and social interventions necessary in the individual who is critically ill.

INTERVENTIONS FOR THE CRITICALLY ILL PATIENT

Alleviation and prevention of physiologic and physical stressors

The ultimate goal of nursing intervention for any patient, regardless of the nature of the illness, is to promote, sustain, and restore optimum levels of physiologic, psychologic, and social functioning. However, in a critical care setting the immediate goal of ensuring a patient's survival initially determines the priorities for intervention; physiologic problems must be addressed first. Once life-threatening stressors have been alleviated, priorities are reordered and other problems can be addressed.

Physiologic priorities are determined by the degree of threat to the survival of the individual. Certain body systems are more prone to disorders that require intensive therapeutic interventions, and are frequently encountered in the critical care unit. These disorders are listed by system along with the specific interventions and additional interventions necessary to prevent complications of therapy.

RESPIRATORY SYSTEM

The highest priority in caring for a critically ill individual is the maintenance of a patent airway and adequate ventilation.

Acute respiratory failure

Acute respiratory failure may occur as a primary pulmonary deficit or as a result of a large number of other disorders that can affect the adequacy of ventilation or respiration. Crushing chest injuries, high-level spinal cord injury, neuromuscular diseases, extensive thoracic surgery, end-stage chronic obstructive pulmonary disease, sepsis, severe pneumonia, severe pulmonary edema, pulmonary embolus, congestive heart failure, sleep apnea, and shock are just come disorders that may be exhibited by patients in respiratory failure requiring intensive care.

Interventions in respiratory failure are first directed at establishment of an unimpeded airway, through endotracheal intubation via the nose or the mouth. Assisted ventilation may then be provided by a manual resuscitation device (Ambu or anesthesia bag), followed by continuous mechanical ventilation. Mechanical ventilation devices are classified by the method through which air enters the

---

Types of mechanical ventilators

Positive pressure	Negative pressure
Volume cycled	Whole-body chamber (iron lung)
Bennett MA-1, MA-2	Chest cuirass, chest shell
Bear	Phrenic nerve stimulator
Ohio	Direct diaphragm stimulator (investigational)
Servo	
Pressure cycled	
Bennett PR-2	
Bird	

---

lungs, that is, by either positive or negative pressure. Mechanical ventilatory support mandates observation of the proper functioning of the equipment and assessment of the impact of the support on the patient's status. Frequent arterial blood gas analyses may be used to evaluate the effects of this intervention and make appropriate changes in therapy.

Mechanical ventilation is a complex therapy and poses major risks for the critically ill patient, including pneumothorax, atelectasis, decreased cardiac output (especially if positive end expiratory pressure is used), gastrointestinal bleeding from a stress ulcer, and infection. Preventive interventions for the patient receiving mechanical ventilation include frequent assessment, position changes in bed, suctioning to remove secretions, intermittent deep ventilations (bagging or sighing), administration of antacids via nasogastric or gastrostomy tube, and scrupulous sterile technique in airway management to prevent a respiratory tract infection.

Adult respiratory distress syndrome

A particularly threatening respiratory complication that is prone to develop in critically ill patients is adult respiratory distress syndrome (ARDS). Also known as shock lung, set lung, wet lung, or post-pump lung, the predisposing factors for ARDS include a number of disorders seen in the critically ill: shock, trauma, disseminated intravascular coagulation (DIC), fat embolism, cardiopulmonary bypass, sepsis, cardiac arrest, and multiple blood transfusions. Damage to the alveolar-capillary membrane and increased capillary permeability leads to pulmonary edema and diffuse microatelectasis. ARDS is characterized by severe dyspnea, hypoxemia, diminished lung compliance, and a significant ventilation-perfusion defect.

The primary intervention for ARDS is mechanical ventilation with the addition of positive and expiratory pressure (PEEP). PEEP aids in reexpanding alveoli and preventing further alveolar collapse, thus improving oxygen transport. Nursing interventions for the patient with ARDS are the same as those for any patient with respi-

ratory failure who is receiving mechanical ventilation, and require a very high degree of skill. (See Chapter 25 for further discussion of respiratory failure and ARDS.)

CARDIOVASCULAR SYSTEM

Cardiovascular problems requiring intensive patient care are so frequently encountered that many insititutions have specific ICUs designed for the care of these patients (coronary care unit, postoperative cardiovascular unit). After support of ventilation, maintenance of cardiac function and systemic circulation is the highest priority in life-threatening situations. Disorders of the cardiovascular system that frequently require intensive observation and intervention include acute myocardial infarction, cardiogenic shock, congestive heart failure, open-heart surgery, and major vascular surgery.

The first line of intervention in severe cardiovascular disorders frequently is *drug therapy* aimed at improving cardiac function until more definitive measures can be instituted. Cardioactive and vasoactive drugs most often administered in a critical care setting are listed in Table 41-3. These highly potent medications often have a very small dosage margin between therapeutic and toxic levels, and the critical care nurse must use astute observational skills to monitor both accuracy of the dose and its effect on the patient.

If medication dosage is insufficient to significantly improve the patient's condition, certain *invasive techniques* may be of some benefit. Temporary transvenous pacing of the heart may restore or enhance cardiac function until such time as a permanent pacemaker can be implanted. Intraaortic balloon counterpulsation (IABC) may be necessary for the patient who would benefit from temporary assistance in decreasing the work load on the myocardium. A balloon-tipped catheter is threaded into the aorta from a femoral artery; the balloon inflates during ventricular diastole to increase coronary artery filling and deflates just prior to ventricular systole to decrease afterload and improve left ventricular ejection. Care of the patient with IABC includes critical minute-to-minute assessment of the patient's physiologic response to IABC therapy and interventions to prevent complications.

Another advanced technique of myocardial support is the left-heart assist device (LHAD). A relatively new therapy that is usually restricted to patients with severely damaged myocardiums, it is most often used to assist patients who cannot be weaned from cardiopulmonary bypass. It is a temporary assist technique in which catheters are implanted into the left atrium or left ventricle to divert oxygenated blood into a roller pump located outside of the body. The pump returns the blood directly to the aorta, thus bypassing the left ventricle and reducing the work load on the heart. The nurse caring for the patient with a LHAD must continually assess the patient's response to therapy through evaluation of hemodynamic data and must also observe for proper function of the assist device.

Table 41-3. Intravenously administered cardiac and vasoactive drugs commonly used in ICU

Drug	Method	Clinical use
Atropine sulfate	IV push (diluted or undiluted in 10 ml sterile water)	Symptomatic bradyarrhythmias
Bretylium tosylate (Bretylol)	IV push, undiluted; may be followed by infusion	Ventricular fibrillation, ventricular tachycardia unresponsive to other agents such as lidocaine
Calcium chloride	IV push	Cardiac arrest, systemic hypocalcemia
Digoxin (Lanoxin)	IV push	Congestive heart failure, atrial fibrillation, paroxysmal atrial tachycardia
Dopamine hydrochloride (Intropin)	Diluted in infusion	Shock, hypotension, to improve renal perfusion
Dobutamine hydrochloride (Dobutrex)	Diluted in infusion	Low cardiac output states, cardiogenic shock
Epinephrine hydrochloride (Adrenalin)	IV bolus; intracardiac, intratracheal, IV infusion	Asystole, ventricular fibrillation, shock/hypotension, anaphylactic reactions
Isoproterenol hydrochloride (Isuprel)	IV infusion	Heart block, bradyarrhythmias, asystole, shock/hypotension
Lidocaine hydrochloride (Xylocaine)	IV bolus followed by IV infusion	To suppress ventricular arrhythmias or resistant seizure activity (low dose)
Morphine sulfate	IV bolus, IV infusion	Pulmonary edema, congestive heart failure, pain management
Nitroglycerine (Nitro-Bid IV)	IV infusion	Hypertensive crisis, congestive heart failure associated with acute myocardial infarction, angina pectoris
Nitroprusside sodium (Nipride)	IV infusion	Hypertensive crisis, congestive heart failure
Norepinephrine (Levarterenol, Levophed)	IV infusion	Hypotension, shock
Propranolol (Inderal)	IV bolus	Supraventricular and ventricular tachyarrhythmias, angina pectoris
Sodium bicarbonate	IV bolus, IV infusion	Acidosis
Verapamil (Calan, Isoptin)	IV push	Paroxysmal supraventricular tachycardia

---

Indications and complications of IABC therapy

Indications	Complications
Cardiogenic shock with a reversible component	Ischemia of catheterized leg
Low cardiac output states	Thrombus formation with eventual embolization
Assist in removing patient from cardiopulmonary bypass	Infection
Unstable angina	Aortic damage (aortic wall dissection, intimal laceration)
Acute myocardial infarction	Balloon rupture with gas embolus (rare)
Drug-resistant lethal arrhythmias with ischemic cause	

Measures to reduce myocardial work load

Enhance oxygenation	Supplemental oxygen
	Assisted ventilation
Decrease physical exertion	Bedrest
	Passive range of motion exercises
Decrease sympathetic stimulation	Reduced environmental stimuli (noise, light)
	Rest periods
	Information and reassurance to patient and family

Nursing interventions to prevent increased ICP in critically ill patients

Maintain patent airway
Minimize arterial blood gas changes
  Oxygenate patient before and after suctioning
  Limit suctioning to 15 seconds
Elevate head of bed 30° (facilitates venous drainage without impeding arterial supply)
Maintain head and neck in straight alignment
Prevent overly tight tracheostomy ties
Prevent valsalva maneuver
  Assist patient in turning
  Prevent coughing, sneezing, constipation
Monitor hydration status intake and output

Prevention of physiologic stressors to the cardiovascular system is a continual priority of care for all ICU patients. Most preventive measures are aimed at myocardial work load reduction.

Finally, in addition to decreasing myocardial work load the myocardium must also be protected from a particular hazard of the critical care environment, *electrical microshock*. The invasive monitoring and therapeutic interventions used in critically ill patients often creates a direct pathway to the heart. Direct contact with stray or leaked current could prove fatal, particularly in critically ill patients whose resistance may be further decreased by other breaks in skin integrity and through electrolyte imbalances. Nursing staff in critical care areas are responsible for the safe and proper use of electrical equipment as well as for the implementation of appropriate electrical safety precautions.

NEUROLOGIC SYSTEM

A number of neurologic disorders, most often either the result of trauma or of intracranial neoplasms, may necessitate intensive care during an acute phase of illness. These include subdural and subarachnoid hemorrhage, direct head injuries, massive cerebral vascular accident, intracranial aneurysm rupture, and pre- and postoperative care of certain patients undergoing craniotomy for surgical repair of a structural defect.

Specialized neurologic interventions for critically ill patients are aimed at maintaining a homeokinetic state of brain metabolism and controlling elevations in intracranial pressure. Monitoring may be used to assess the extent of potentially dangerous rises in ICP. In ICP monitoring an epidural screw or intraventricular catheter is attached to a transducer and monitor, enabling continuous viewing of the pressure waveform and numerical ICP values. Meticuluous insertion site and tubing care are essential to prevent the devastating complication of intra-cranial infection. Scrupulous observations by the critical care nurse are necessary to maintain the patency of the system and to detect changes in ICP.

Removal of cerebrospinal fluid is one method of controlling rising ICP. Other interventions include osmotic diuresis to remove excess brain tissue water and mechanical hyperventilation to artificially reduce circulating carbon dioxide (CO_2) levels. Lowered CO_2 levels will cause cerebral vasoconstriction, reducing the potential for progressive interstitial cerebral edema.

Efforts to lower the overall metabolism of the brain will reduce the brain's requirements for its natural substrates, oxygen and glucose. This is especially important when transport of these elements is impaired. Interventions to reduce brain metabolism include generalized hypothermia via a cooling mattress and induction of barbiturate coma. Caring for the artificially comatose patient requires the same attentive observations and extensive nursing interventions to prevent complications as are used in the naturally comatose patient, with the addition of mechanical ventilation (see Chapter 20). In addition, complete neurologic assessment must be thoroughly performed at those times when sedation is withdrawn to evaluate patient progress. A lightened level of consciousnes at those times necessitates sensitive communication with the patient, even though the ability to comprehend may not be apparent.

Nursing interventions to prevent physiologic stressors to the neurologic system are generally aimed at preventing elevations in ICP.

RENAL SYSTEM

Acute renal failure in the critically ill patient may result from a primary intrarenal cause, such as acute glomerulonephritis or acute cortical necrosis, or to a structural defect. It may be the result of directly nephrotoxic agents such as heavy metal poisoning or pharmacologic

---

Advantages and disadvantages of hemodialysis and peritoneal dialysis

Hemodialysis

Rapid, efficient correction of severe serum abnormalities

Short time required

Expensive

Requires highly technical equipment

Poorly tolerated by patients with very unstable conditions

Risk of hemorrhage

Peritoneal dialysis

Well tolerated by even very unstable patients

Inexpensive

Technologically simple

Must be performed over several hours or days

Cannot be performed after recent abdominal surgery

Risk of peritonitis

---

agents (for example, aminoglycoside antibiotics). But most commonly acute renal failure in critically ill patients is the secondary result of any disorder that severely reduces cardiac output and renal perfusion, including cardiac arrest, left ventricular failure, or hemorrhage.

Interventions for the patient with renal failure are intended to provide the regulatory functions the kidneys can no longer maintain. The nurse keeps accurate daily weight and intake/output records so that only the exact amounts of body fluids lost plus a percentage for insensible loss, are replaced. Laboratory values are monitored carefully, with electrolyte intake limited and pharmacologic means of electrolyte removal utilized as necessary, for example, sodium polystyrene sulfonate (Kayexalate). Diuretics are given to increase marginal renal function. Nutrition is altered through restricted protein intake, because the body cannot appropriately excrete the nitrogen that is produced by amino acid breakdown. The nurse evaluates acid base balance, anticipating metabolic acidosis from the build up of acid metabolic wastes (carbonic and lactic acids). All other body systems are affected by the progression of acute renal failure, and continuous interventions are necessary to prevent altered acid base and electrolyte levels to impair cardiovascular, respiratory, and neurologic function. Therefore the nurse is alert for such things as ECG changes indicative of increased myocardial irritability and altered contractility, changes in ventilatory pattern such as Kussmaul breathing and acidotic breath, and decreased level of consciousness or altered mentation or behavior.

When renal failure has reached a level unresponsive to medical intervention, dialysis becomes necessary to mechanically remove the waste products of body metabolism. Either hemodialysis or peritoneal dialysis may be initiated in the critically ill patient.

GASTROINTESTINAL SYSTEM

The most common gastrointestinal problem seen in the critical care setting is *acute gastrointestinal bleeding*. This may be the initial sign in a newly admitted patient, or it may be a complication, such as a stress ulcer, in an already critically ill person. Interventions, such as gastric lavage with iced saline solution and administration of antacid agents are intended to control bleeding until its cause and extent are determined. A Sengstaken-Blakemore tube may be used to provide direct compression of esophageal varices in order to tamponade a serious bleed. Administration of blood components and crystalloid fluids is initiated to reverse the hypovolemia of acute hemorrhage. Vasopressor medications cannot be administered to raise systemic blood pressure until the hypovolemic state is corrected. Once the patient's condition has stabilized sufficiently and the site of bleeding has been identified, surgical intervention to repair the affected area may be performed.

The primary function of the gastrointestinal system is the ingestion and digestion of liquid and solid nutrients. For many critically ill patients this process is interrupted for a lengthy period, during which either enteral or total parenteral nutrition (TPN) may be substituted. TPN solutions contain the essential protein, carbohydrates, and fat necessary to establish a catabolic state in which positive nitrogen balance is maintained. The critical care nurse assesses the adequacy of hydration status and electrolyte balance as well as caloric intake. In addition, the nurse takes active measures to prevent the primary complication of TPN, infection.

Prevention of gastrointestinal complications such as stress ulcers in critically ill patients requires active interventions. Patients at highest risk include those who are receiving no food orally, who are receiving mechanical ventilation, have liver dysfunction, are receiving anticoagulants, and who have undergone any severe physiologic stress. In addition to the administration of local antacids and systemic anticholinergic agents (cimetidine), active interventions are required to reduce the psychologic stress inherent in the critical care environment.

MUSCULOSKELETAL/INTEGUMENTARY SYSTEM

Although few primary musculoskeletal problems necessitate intensive care, the majority of critically ill patients have severe restrictions placed on their mobility. Bedrest, weakness, and pain, as well as numerous therapeutic and monitoring devices, serve to significantly limit normal

---

Nursing interventions for prevention of pulmonary embolus

Elevation of lower extremities
Use of antiembolism stockings
Hourly active foot doorsiflexion
Active/resistive range of motion exercises
Observation for Homan's sign

Coughing and deep-breathing exercises
Administration of low-dose heparin as ordered
Inspection of intravenous sites with routine needle changes

---

motion. Preserving function of weight-bearing muscles, maintaining joint mobility, and preserving continuous skin integrity are significant challenges to critical care nurses. All of the preventive and supportive nursing care techniques used in any patient with restricted mobility are appropriate in the ICU. Progress of the ICU patient to the highest level of activity within physiologic capabilities both facilitates continued improvement in physiologic function and visually reassures the patient of an improving condition.

One of the most serious potential complications of immobility is development of a deep-vein thrombus, which can embolize and travel to the lungs. Pulmonary emboli are found at autopsy in up to 60% of all individuals. Signs and symptoms of pulmonary embolism include dyspnea, pleuritic chest pain, fever, hemoptysis, tachycardia, and pleural friction. Preventive interventions can be instrumental in reducing the risk of serious complication.

Alleviation and prevention of psychologic stressors

Despite the continuous attention that the critical care nurse must devote to the assessment of and intervention in physiologic derangements, the nurse must also focus attention on recognizing the psychologic stressors that confront the patient and family. The emotional discomfort and distress that the patient and family must endure will not only affect psychologic health but will have a direct impact on physical recovery as well.

The initial step in preventing or alleviating psychologic stress if to identify the patient's and family's perception of the critical event. Their perceptions will be affected by their individual personalities, current psychologic health, general understanding of the current situation and its projected outcome, tolerance of ambiguity, and normal patterns of coping. Initial perceptions are often significantly affected by prior exposure to previous similar events, either positive or negative, and general level of familiarity with medical interventions and the hospital environment. Five specific interventions that nurses in any setting can implement to reduce the psychologic stress of illness on the family are described on the following pages.

Acknowledge, accept, and encourage patient and family to air feelings

Because the critically ill person is alienated from familiar surrounding and daily living patterns and is dependent on others to meet the most basic needs of survival, the patient becomes partially or totally isolated from usual support systems. Feelings of helplessness, powerlessness, loneliness, and depersonalization as well as disturbances in body image are common. Modes of expressing and therefore relieving the frustration, anger, hostility, fear, and depression generated by these feelings are limited by the physical constraints of the critical care environment.

Maintaining an atmosphere of openness and acceptance that encourages expression of feelings can help to provide patients with a means of coping. Talking with patients openly and honestly decreases feelings of depersonalization and anxiety and prevents isolation and alienation. Recognizing that anger and hostility are often indicative of fear and anxiety and that depression and withdrawal may be signs of feelings of hopelessness, loneliness, powerlessness, or loss assist the nurse in accepting these feelings as normal and expected in this situation. Encouraging expression of feelings helps the patient identify reasons for feeling or behaving in a way that may seem strange or wrong. At the same time it provides protection and permission to feel and act that way. Nurses or other health team members who are helping a patient to talk about feelings must be ready to accept whatever emotionally laden information might be expressed. Nonjudgmental recognition and acceptance of the patient's feelings will help to reinforce the patient's right to the feelings.

Patients who are intubated are unable to freely express their feelings even when alert and oriented, and therefore are particularly vulnerable to psychologic stressors. It is a natural tendency to communicate less with those who cannot talk easily and the nurse must guard against this. Keeping paper and pencil or a "magic slate" within the patient's reach and providing assistance when necessary will help to reduce the sense of isolation. However, such methods are not convenient for the expression of personal feelings or involved concerns. The nurse can recognize clues to the patient's emotional state by appearance and behavior and by knowing the types of concerns the patient is most likely to experience. The nurse can verbalize the potential concerns, allowing the patient to validate them as appropriate. Being empathetic with the patient and family conveys acceptance and understanding.

Provide information and clarify misconceptions about physical status, goals of treatment, and interventions

Because it is the patient's *perception* of stress and not the stressor itself that determines the patient's reaction to the illness and the environment, it is essential that the patient and family receive adequate information and simple explanations. Without explanations the critical care environment presents a mysterious and threatening array of noxious stimuli, which may be perceived as extremely unnatural and even magical. The high degree of technical sophistication increases the patient's feelings of vulnerability, and the patient may worry that the cardiac monitor is actually keeping the heart beating, that a blood transfusion indicates hemorrhaging, or that chest physiotherapy indicates pneumonia. A very common misconception of patients after coronary artery bypass is that "open heart" surgery involved cutting the heart wide open and sewing it back together again. Such a perception can lead to a drastic alteration in body image.

Much of what patients learn about their health problems depends on what is taught, both directly and indirectly, by the health care team. Patient teaching in critical care requires establishment of short-term goals. Pain, discomfort, weakness, anxiety, and transient confusion are some of the obstacles to learning that these patients experience. Despite these obstacles, patients and families need simple, repetitive explanations of all procedures and the purpose of each intervention, as well as an introduction to rehabilitation plans and health maintenance strategies. Patients may not understand or believe what they are told the first time, or anxiety and denial may prevent recollection of it. Reinterpretation and reiteration of diagnosis, prognosis, goals of treatment, types of interventions, and expectations of the patient and family may be continually necessary during the entire ICU stay. Keeping the patient and family apprised of the patient's current status as well as of changes in plans helps them to perceive the situation accurately and plan for the future realistically, and promotes cooperation by making them members of the health team.

Encourage and support involvement of patient and family in decision making and care

The essence of crisis intervention is to help individuals cope with a major life crisis such as a critical illness might precipitate. Critical care nursing in itself is far broader in scope and more future oriented than crisis intervention alone, but specific situations within the critical care setting may require the immediacy and limited focus of crisis intervention. At that time the patient and family are directed in establishing short-term goals and are given limited choice in acceptable responses. As the crisis situation stabilizes, even though it may be no less critical, the patient and family are given additional information and further responsibility in establishing mutual goals and choosing alternative responses. When the patient and family are knowledgeable about the goals of therapy and understand the patient's diagnosis, current status, and prognosis, they can be involved in many aspects of care planning and can make decisions consistent with the treatment regimen.

Involvement of the individuals who represent the patient's significant support system decreases their feelings of powerlessness, frustration, and anxiety. In addition, when these emotionally important figures, whether family or friends, understand and support the treatment goals and are involved in the patient's care, they are better able to sustain and expand this behavior after the patient leaves the ICU and the hospital. Even when a patient is unconscious, visits by key support figures who talk to and touch the patient may have positive, if unmeasurable, effects and help to decrease the family's feelings of helplessness.

An alert patient can be directly involved in establishing goals of treatment and care planning. One specific mechanism to increase the patient's feeling of personal control is to encourage involvement in structuring the daily schedule of activities. The knowledge that patient preferences are important to the nursing staff and that the person is viewed as capable of making certain decisions will support self-esteem and reinforce the centrality of the patient role in recovery.

Promote and maintain a sensory-regulated environment

The environment of the critical care unit is a major stressor with which both the patient and family must cope. (The many sources of external stress are outlined in the first section of this chapter.) In addition, disturbed thought processes and perceptual distortions are often likely to be seen in patients receiving narcotics and sedatives, highly anxious patients, patients with multiple interrelated debilitating physical problems, patients with disturbed metabolic and respiratory function, patients deprived of sleep, and older patients. Reality reinforcement on a continuing basis is necessary for these individuals. Although some environmental factors cannot be altered, there are some specific interventions that the nurse can implement to provide a sensory regulated environment (see box on p. 1206).

Prepare the patient and family for transfer from the ICU

Transfer from the critical care unit can represent a significant stress for some patients and their families. The critical care area with its sophisticated electronic equipment and attentive, highly skilled staff represents security and protection. Patients know that transfer will be to an area where there are fewer nursing personnel per patient, less direct contact with nursing personnel, no automatic monitoring devices, and no direct observation of the bed from the nurses' station. Greater independence and higher levels of activity will be expected on the transfer unit, yet there will be loss of support of nursing

---

Interventions to minimize sensory deprivation overload

Reduce noise level

Avoid excessive conversation

Avoid raising voice to talk to persons outside conversational range

Use carpeting as feasible

Avoid droning of continuous radio or TV; turn on/off at appropriate intervals

Locate nursing lounge away from patient care area

Maintain day night orientation

Dim lights at night

Raise/lower shades or open/close window curtains in normal day/night pattern

Reinforce progress of day in relation to specific events, such as meals

Maintain time orientation

Position large-numeral clocks in easy view

Provide wall calendars

Allow wristwatches for certain patients

Provide frequent reorientation to person, place, time

Promote rest and sleep

Schedule most exerting activities before rest period

Coordinate health team activities to provide periods of uninterrupted sleep

Minimize routine cleaning or stocking at night

Provide positive tactile stimuli

Touch/hold patient's hand during conversation

Use soothing physical contact as able (backrubs, face cleansings)

Encourage family to touch patient, hold hands despite dressings

Maintain personal/social integrity

Address patient by name, identify self by name

Provide full and complete information, explanations, and instructions

Avoid discussion over the patient; include the patient in rounds

Encourage visits by family, significant others

Allow important personal belongings at bedside

Reduce pain and discomfort

Administer analgesics appropriately to relieve pain

Reposition immobile patients every two hours

Prepare patients for all potentially uncomfortable or painful procedures

Maintain future orientation

Discuss transfer plans early with both patient and family

Initiate teaching regarding rehabilitation and health maintenance strategies as appropriate

---

staff who have come to know them. Patients may have conflicting feelings about the transfer as an indicator of physical improvement if they do not feel as well or as independent as they anticipated they would be by transfer time.

The anxiety precipitated by the transfer can be prevented or reduced if the patient and family are taught to interpret particular signs and symptoms and are helped to understand the true purpose of equipment and routines. Signs that indicate progress need to be pointed out continuously, beginning when they first appear. Initiating the discussion of transfer plans with the patient and family as soon as the patient's condition begins to stabilize in the ICU will help them adjust to the idea and prepare for this eventuality. Along with the projected date of transfer, patient and family need to know what to expect on the new unit and what will be expected of them. Ideally, a nurse from the receiving unit should meet the patient and family prior to transfer. After transfer, visits from members of the ICU staff are helpful in conveying con-

tinued concern for the patient's welfare and in providing objective validation of continued progress. With careful planning and execution, transfer from the critical care unit can be a triumphant rather than a traumatic event.

Alleviation and prevention of social stressors for patient and family

In the critical care setting the patient's physiologic needs often assume priority over psychologic needs, and the patient as a social being may be at risk of virtually being ignored. Limited visiting hours, the strange technical environment, and the aura of danger in the ICU isolates patients from their supportive family and friends and prevents them from assuming their usual social roles. For the most part, a person who is critically ill is viewed by staff primarily as a patient. The more significant roles of spouse, parent, child, lover, sibling, friend, or provider may go virtually unrecognized unless nursing staff initiate interventions to provide continuity in these relationships.

Such continuity is fostered through some of the same types of interventions that were used to reduce psychologic stress: increased visiting between patient and family; inclusion of family in discussions of disease process, prognosis, and plans of care; and reporting by family of events and activities occurring in the other significant spheres of the patient's life. Relaying telephone messages between the patient and distant friends is one way of maintaining contact with the patient's external world.

One of the most effective and important ways to prevent disruption in relationships is to prepare family or friends for their first visit with the patient in the ICU. The patient's physical appearance and the critical care environment should be explained thoroughly before the visitor enters. Visitors need to understand the patient's level of consciousness, ability to communicate, and ability to comprehend communication. They need to be made aware of the importance of their presence to the patient and the patient's need for their support. When the visitor approaches the bedside a staff member should remain with them to facilitate the initial interaction with the patient. At each subsequent visit the nurse caring for the patient meets with the significant others to answer questions and apprise them of the patient's progress.

In addition to supporting the maintenance of the patient's current roles and relationships the critical care nurse must also recognize the inevitability of actual role change for some patients and families during a critical illness. Roles of provider, decision maker, employer or employee, and leader may be altered, reversed, or eliminated. At this point some of the responsibilities of the patient need to be assumed by family and friends.

During the critical phase of illness the family members will be attempting to cope with precipitous role changes and may need assistance in working through problems that arise as family members and friends assume or fail to assume these additional responsibilities. The nurse needs to be aware of how problematic this time is and may need to help the family in requesting professional guidance, such as from a social worker, in assisting the family to reorganize themselves and their resources. The nurse may help the family appoint a temporary leader from among their ranks, one who could be requested to identify the wishes of the family as a whole and who could be contacted in the event of an emergency. The nurse may also help the family to plan visiting schedules that will meet the patient's needs without preventing the family members from maintaining their own responsibilities. It is a period of great emotional stress for both patient and family.

That emotional stress may eventually climax in the death of the critically ill patient. (The reader is referred to Chapter 16 for a complete discussion of dying and death.) The following are some suggestions for the critical care nurse caring for a dying patient:

1. Examine your own feelings about death.
2. Listen, to assess the needs of the patient and family.
3. Remain available; be physically and emotionally present.
4. Help with administrative needs such as making telephone calls, obtaining permit slips.
5. Provide reassurance of the patient's continued care, even if the patient is not to be resuscitated. Provide information.
6. Respect the person-family relationship, which existed long before the patient-hospital relationship.
7. Attempt to remain nonjudgmental about family or hospital issues.
8. Include the family in care.
9. Provide for patient and family privacy.
10. Provide the opportunity for the family to exercise religious or cultural traditions.
11. Use touch in caring for the patient and family.

The critical care environment is a dynamic milieu intended to maximize the application of critical interventions for the very ill. Nursing care of the highest caliber is required to safeguard the patient from its potential hazards while promoting optimum patient outcomes.

REFERENCES*

1. *Adams, M., et al.: Psychological response in critical care units, Am. J. Nurs. **78**(9):1504-1512, 1978.
2. Aguilera, D.C., and Messick, J.M.: Crisis intervention: theory and methodology, ed. 4, St. Louis, 1982, The C.V. Mosby Co.
3. American Association of Critical Care Nurses: Standards of nursing care for the critically ill, Reston, Pa., 1979, Reston Publishing Co., Inc.
4. Andreoli, K.G., et al.: Comprehensive cardiac care, St. Louis, 1979, The C.V. Mosby Co.
5. Borg, N., et al.: Core curriculum for critical-care nursing, Philadelphia, 1981, W.B. Saunders.
6. *Brantigan, C.O.: Hemodynamic monitoring: interpreting values, Am. J. Nurs. **82**(1):86-89, 1982.
7. *Breu, C., and Dracup, K.: Helping the spouses of critically ill patients, Am. J. Nurs. **78**(1):50-53, 1978.
8. Daily, E.K., and Schroeder, J.S.: Techniques in bedside hemodynamic monitoring, St. Louis, 1981, The C.V. Mosby Co.
9. Daly, B.J., editor: Intensive care nursing, Garden City, N.Y., 1980, Medical Examination Publishing Co., Inc.
10. *Fuchs, P.L.: Understanding continuous mechanical ventilation, Nurs. 79 **9**(12):26-33, 1979.
11. *Gardner, D., et al.: The nurse's dilemma: mediating stress in critical care units, Heart Lung **9**(1):103-106, 1980.
12. *Giving cardiac care, Nursing 81 Photobook, Horsham, Pa., 1981, Intermed Communications.
13. *Giving cardiovascular drugs safely, Nursing 79 Skillbook, Horsham, Pa., 1979, Intermed Communications, Inc.
14. *Hamilton, W.P.: Common cardiovascular problems in the postoperative period, Nurs. Clin. North Am. **10**:27-41, 1975.
15. Holloway, N.M.: Nursing the critically ill adult, Menlo Park, Ca., 1979, Addison-Wesley Publishing Co., Inc.

---

*References preceded by an asterisk are particularly well suited for student reading.

16. Hudak, C.M., Lohr, T., and Gallo, B.M.: Critical care nursing, ed. 3, Philadelphia, 1982, J.B. Lippincott Co.

17. *ICU psychosis (nursing grand rounds), Nurs. 82 **12**(1):58-63, 1982.

18. Kiely, W.F., and Procci, W.R.: Psychiatric aspects of critical care. *In* Zschoche, D.A., editor: Mosby's comprehensive review of critical care, ed. 2, St. Louis, 1980, C.V. Mosby Co.

19. Kinney, M.R., editor: AACN's clinical reference for critical-care nursing, New York, 1981, McGraw-Hill Book Co.

20. *Kuenzi, S.H., and Fenton, M.V.: Crisis intervention in acute care areas, Am. J. Nurs. **75**:830-834, 1975.

21. *Lamb, J.: Intra-arterial monitoring, Nurs. 77 **7**(11):65-71, 1977.

22. *Millar, S., et al.: Methods in critical care: The AACN manual, Philadelphia, 1980, W.B. Saunders Co.

23. Mondejar, E.S.: The patient with left-heart assist device: nursing management, Heart Lung **8**(2):296-301, 1979.

24. *Murray, R.: Assessment of psychological status in the surgical ICU patient, Nurs. Clin. North Am. **10**:69-81, 1975.

25. *Nielsen, L.: Mechanical ventilation: patient assessment and nursing care, Am. J. Nurs. **80**:2191-2196, 1980.

26. *Nursing critically ill patients confidently, Horsham, Pa., 1979, Intermed Communications, Inc.

27. Phipps, W.J., Long, B.C., and Woods, N.F.: Medical-surgical nursing: concepts and clinical practice, ed. 2, St. Louis, 1983, C.V. Mosby Co.

28. *Purcell, J.A., Pippin, L., and Mitchell, M.: Intra-aortic balloon pump therapy, Am. J. Nurs. **83**(5):775-790, 1983.

29. Roberts, S.L.: Behavioral concepts and the critically ill patient, Englewood Cliffs, N.J., 1976, Prentice-Hall, Inc.

30. Roberts, S.L.: Systems approach in assessing behavioral problems of critical care patients, Heart Lung **4**:593-598, 1975.

31. Storlie, F.: Patient teaching in critical care, New York, 1975, Appleton-Century-Crofts.

32. *Stark, J.L.: How to succeed against acute renal failure, Nurs. 82 **12**(7):26-33, 1982.

33. *Stephenson, C.A.: Stress in the critically ill patient, Am. J. Nurs. **77**:1806-1809, 1977.

34. *Using monitors, Nursing 81 Photobook, Horsham, Pa., 1981, Intermed Communications, Inc.

Classic

35. *Cassem, N.H., Hackett, T., and Bascon, C.: Reactions of coronary patients to the CCU nurse, Am. J. Nurs. **70**:312-319, 1970.

36. Hay, D., and Oken, D.: The psychological stresses of intensive care nursing, Psychosom. Med. **34**:117, 1972.

37. Klein, K., Kliner, W., and Lipos, D.: Transfer from a coronary care unit: some adverse responses, Arch. Intern. Med. **122**:104-108, 1968.

38. *Obier, K., and Haywood, L.J.: Enhancing therapeutic communication with acutely ill patients, Heart Lung **2**:49-53, 1973.

39. Strauss, A.: The intensive care unit: its characteristics and social relationships, Nurs. Clin. North Am. **3**:7-15, 1968.

40. Woods, N.F., and Falk, S.A.: Noise stimuli in the acute care area, Nurs. Res. **23**:144-150, 1974.

Appendixes

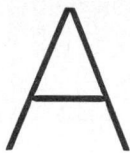

Normal Laboratory Values

Blood, plasma or serum values

Reference range

Determination	Conventional	SI
Acetoacetate plus acetone	0.3-2.0 mg/100 ml	3-20 mg/l
Aldolase	1.3-8.2 mU/ml	12-75 nmol · s⁻¹/l
Alpha amino nitrogen	3.0-5.5 mg/100 ml	2.1-3.9 mmol/l
Ammonia	80-110 μg/100 ml	47-65 μmol/l
Ascorbic acid	0.4-1.5 mg/100 ml	23-85 μmol/l
Barbiturate	0	0 μmol/l
	Coma level: phenobarbital, approximately 10 mg/100 ml; most other drugs, 1-3 mg per 100 ml	
Bilirubin (van den Bergh test)	One minute: 0.4 mg/100 ml	Up to 7 μmol/l
	Direct: 0.4 mg/100 ml	Up to 17 μmol/l
	Total: 1.0 mg/100 ml	
	Indirect is total minus direct	
Blood volume	8.5-9.0% of body weight in kg	80-85 ml/kg
Bromide	0	0 mmol/l
	Toxic level: 17 mEq/l	
Bromsulfalein (BSP)	Less than 5% retention 45 min after 5 mg/kg IV	<0.05 l
Calcium	8.5-10.5 mg/100 ml (slightly higher in children)	2.1-2.6 mmol/l
Carbon dioxide content	24-30 mEq/l	24-30 mmol/l
	20-26 mEq/l in infants (as HCO₃⁻)	
Carbon monoxide	Symptoms with over 20% saturation	0 (1)
Carotenoids	0.8-4.0 μg/ml	1.5-7.4 μmol/l
Ceruloplasmin	27-37 mg/100 ml	1.8-2.5 μmol/l
Chloride	100-106 mEq/l	100-106 mmol/l
Cholinesterase (pseudocholinesterase)	0.5 pH U or more/h	0.5 or more arb. unit
	0.7 pH U or more/h for packed cells	
Copper	Total: 100-200 μg/100 ml	16-31 μmol/l
Creatine phosphokinase (CPK)	Female 5-35 mU/ml	0.08-0.58 μmol · s⁻¹/l
	Male 5-55 mU/ml	
Creatinine	0.6-1.5 mg/100 ml	60-130 μmol/l

Modified from Kaye, D.A., and Rose, L.F.: Fundamentals of internal medicine, St. Louis, 1983, The C.V. Mosby Co. Adapted by permission from the New England Journal of Medicine, Vol. 302, pages 37-48, 1980.
Abbreviations used: SI, Système international d'Unités (The SI for the Health Professions. World Health Organization, Office of Publications, Geneva Switzerland, 1977); d, 24 hours; P, plasma; S, serum; B, blood; U, urine; l, liter; h, hour; and s, second.

Continued.

Blood, plasma or serum values—cont'd

Reference range—cont'd

Determination	Conventional	SI
Ethanol	0.3-0.4%, marked intoxication; 0.4-0.5%, alcoholic stupor; 0.5% or over, alcoholic coma	65-87 mmol/l 87-109 mmol/l >109 mmol/l
Glucose	Fasting: 70-110 mg/100 ml	3.9-5.6 mmol/l
Iron	50-150 μg/100 ml (higher in males)	9.0-26.9 μmol/l
Iron-binding capacity	250-410 μg/100 ml	44.8-73.4 μmol/l
Lactic acid	0.6-1.8 mEq/l	0.6-1.8 mmol/l
Lactic dehydrogenase	60-120 U/ml	1.00-2.00 μmol · s^{-1}/l
Lead	50 μg/100 ml or less	Up to 2.4 μmol/l
Lipase	2 U/ml or less	Up to 2 arb. unit
Lipids		
Cholesterol	120-220 mg/100 ml	3.10-5.69 mmol/l
Cholesterol esters	60-75% of cholesterol	
Phospholipids	9-16 mg/100 ml as lipid phosphorus	2.9-5.2 mmol/l
Total fatty acids	190-420 mg/100 ml	1.9-4.2 g/l
Total lipids	450-1000 mg/100 ml	4.5-10.0 g/l
Triglycerides	40-150 mg/100 ml	0.4-1.5 g/l
Lithium	Toxic level 2 mEq/l	2 mmol/l
Magnesium	1.5-2.0 mEq/l	0.8-1.3 mmol/l
5'Nucleotidase	0.3-3.2 Bodansky U	30-290 nmol · s^{-1}/l
Osmolality	285-295 mOsm/kg water	285-295 mmol/kg
Oxygen saturation (arterial)	96-100%	0.96-1.00 l
PCO_2	35-43 mm Hg	4.7-6.0 kPa
pH	7.35-7.45	Same
PO_2	75-100 mm Hg (dependent on age) while breathing room air Above 500 mm Hg while on 100% O_2	10.0-13.3 kPa
Phenylalanine	0-2 mg/100 ml	0-120 μmol/l
Phenytoin (Dilantin)	Therapeutic level, 5-20 μg/ml	19.8-79.5 μmol/l
Phosphorus (inorganic)	3.0-4.5 mg/100 ml (infants in 1st year up to 6.0 (mg/100 ml)	1.0-1.5 mmol/l

Blood, plasma or serum values—cont'd

Reference range—cont'd

Determination	Conventional	SI
Potassium	3.5-5.0 mEq/l	3.5-5.0 mmol/l
Primidone (Mysoline)	Therapeutic level 4-12 µg/ml	18-55 µmol/l
Protein: Total	6.0-8.4 g/100 ml	60-84 g/l
Albumin	3.5-5.0 g/100 ml	35-50 g/l
Globulin	2.3-3.5 g/100 ml	23-35 g/l
Electrophoresis	*% of total protein*	*Of total protein*
Albumin	52-68	0.52-0.68
Globulin:		
$Alpha_1$	4.2-7.2	0.042-0.072
$Alpha_2$	6.8-12	0.068-0.12
Beta	9.3-15	0.093-0.15
Gamma	13-23	0.13-0.23
Pyruvic acid	0-0.11 mEq/l	0-0.11 mmol/l
Quinidine	Therapeutic: 1.5-3 µg/ml	4.6-9.2 µmol/l
	Toxic: 5-6 µg/ml	15.4-18.5 µmol/l
Salicylate:	0	
Therapeutic	20-25 mg/100 ml; 25-30 mg/100 ml to age 10 yrs. 3 h post dose	1.4-1.8 mmol/l 1.8-2.2 mmol/l
Toxic	Over 30 mg/100 ml	Over 2.2 mmol/l
	Over 20 mg/100 ml after age 60	Over 1.5 mmol/l
Sodium	135-145 mEq/l	135-145 mmol/l
Sulfate	0.5-1.5 mg/100 ml	0.05-1.2 mmol/l
Sulfonamide	0 mg/100 ml	0 mmol/l
	Therapeutic: 5-15 mg/100 ml	
Transaminase (SGOT) (aspartate amino-transferase)	10-40 U/ml	$0.08\text{-}0.32 \ \mu mol \cdot s^{-1}/l$
Urea nitrogen (BUN)	8-25 mg/100 ml	2.9-8.9 mmol/l
Uric acid	3.0-7.0 mg/100 m	0.13-0.42 mmol/l
Vitamin A	0.15-0.6 µg/ml	0.5-2.1 µmol/l
Vitamin A tolerance test	Rise to twice fasting level in 3 to 5 h	

Urine values

Reference range

Determination	Conventional	SI
Acetone plus acetoacetate (quantitative)	0	0 mg/l
Alpha amino nitrogen	64-199 mg/d; not over 1.5% of total nitrogen	4.6-14.2 mmol/d
Amylase	24-76 U/ml	24-76 arb. unit
Calcium	150 mg/d or less	3.8 or less mmol/d
Catecholamines	Epinephrine: under 20 μg/d	<55 nmol/d
	Norepinephrine: under 100 μg/d	<590 nmol/d
Copper	0-100 μg/d	0-1.6 μmol/d
Coproporphyrin	50-250 μg/d	80-380 nmol/d
	Children under 80 lb 0-75 μg/d	0-115 nmol/d
Creatine	Under 100 mg/d or less than 6% of creatinine. In pregnancy: up to 12%. In children under 1 yr.: may equal creatinine. In older children: up to 30% of creatinine	<0.75 mmol/d
Cystine or cysteine	0	0
Follicle-stimulating hormone:		
Follicular phase	5-20 IU/d	Same
Mid/cycle	15-60 IU/d	
Luteal phase	5-15 IU/d	
Menopausal	50-100 IU/d	
Men	5-25 IU/d	
Hemoglobin and myoglobin	0	
5-Hydroxyindole acetic acid	2-9 mg/d (women lower than men)	10-45 μmol/d
Lead	0.08 μg/ml or 120 μg or less/d	0.39 μmol/l or less
Phenolsulfonphthalein (PSP)	At least 25% excreted by 15 min; 40% by 30 min; 60% by 120 min	0.25 l
Phosphorus (inorganic)	Varies with intake, average 1 g/d	32 mmol/d
Porphobilinogen	0	0
Protein:		
Quantitative	<150 mg/24 hr	<0.15 g/d
Steroids:		

17-Ketosteroids (per day)

Age (yr)	Male (mg)	Female (mg)	Male (μmol/d)	Female (μmol/d)
10	1-4	1-4	3-14	3-14
20	6-21	4-16	21-73	14-56
30	8-26	4-14	28-90	14-49
50	5-18	3-9	17-62	10-31
70	2-10	1-7	7-35	3-24

Determination	Conventional	SI
17-Hydroxysteroids	3-8 mg/d (women lower than men)	8-22 μmol/d as hydrocortisone
Sugar:		
Quantitative glucose	0	0 mmol/l
Identification of reducing substances		
Fructose	0	0 mmol/l
Pentose	0	0 mmol/l
Titratable acidity	20-40 mEq/d	20-40 mmol/d
Urobilinogen	Up to 1.0 Ehrlich U	To 1.0 arb. unit
Uroporphyrin	0	0 nmol/d
Vanilmandelic acid (VMA)	Up to 9 mg/24 hr	Up to 45 μmol/d

Special endocrine tests

Reference range

Determination	Conventional	SI
Steroid hormones		
Aldosterone	Excretion: 5-19 µg/24 h	14-53 nmol/d
Fasting, at rest, 210 mEq sodium diet	Supine: 48 ± 29 pg/ml	133 ± 80 pmol/l
	Upright: (2 h) 65 ± 23 pg/ml	180 ± 64 pmol/l
Fasting, at rest, 110 mEq sodium diet	Supine: 107 ± 45 pg/ml	279 ± 125 pmol/l
	Upright: (2 h) 239 ± 123 pg/ml	663 ± 341 pmol/l
Fasting, at rest, 10 mEq sodium diet	Supine: 175 ± 75 pg/ml	485 ± 208 pmol/l
	Upright: (2 h) 532 ± 228 pg/ml	1476 ± 632 pmol/l
Cortisol		
Fasting	8 a.m.: 5-25 µg/100 ml	0.14-0.69 µmol/l
At rest	8 p.m.: Below 10 µg/100 ml	0-0.28 µmol/l
20 U ACTH	4 h ACTH test: 30-45 µg/100 ml	0.83-1.24 µmol/l
Dexamethasone at midnight	Overnight suppression test: Below 5 µg/100 ml	<0.14 nmol/l
	Excretion: 20-70 µg/24 h	55-193 nmol/d
11-Deoxycortisol	Responsive: Over 7.5 µg/100 ml (after metrapone)	>0.22 µmol/l
Testosterone	Adult male: 300-1100 ng/100 ml	10.4-38.1 nmol/l
	Adolescent male: over 100 ng/100 ml	>3.5 nmol/l
	Females: 25-90 ng/100 ml	0.87-3.12 nmol/l
Unbound testosterone	Adult male: 3.06-24.0 ng/100 ml	106-832 pmol/l
	Adult female: 0.09-1.28 ng/100 ml	3.1-44.4 pmol/l
Polypeptide hormones		
Adrenocorticotropin (ACTH)	15-70 pg/ml	3.3-15.4 pmol/l
Calcitonin	Undetectable in normals	0
	>100 pg/ml in medullary carcinoma	>29.3 pmol/l
Growth hormone		
Fasting, at rest	Below 5 ng/ml	<233 pmol/l
After exercise	Children: Over 10 ng/ml	>465 pmol/l
	Male: Below 5 ng/ml	<233 pmol/l
	Female: Up to 30 ng/ml	0-1395 pmol/l
After glucose	Male: Below 5 ng/ml	<233 pmol/l
	Female: Below 10 ng/ml	0-465 pmol/l
Insulin		
Fasting	6-26 µU/ml	43-187 pmol/l
During hypoglycemia	Below 20 µU/ml	<144 pmol/l
After glucose	Up to 150 µU/ml	0-1078 pmol/l
Leuteinizing hormone	Male: 6-18 mU/ml	6-18 u/l
Pre- or postovulatory	Female: 5-22 mU/ml	5-22 u/l
Midcycle peak	30-250 mU/ml	30-250 u/l
Parathyroid hormone	<10 µl equiv/ml	<10 ml equiv/l
Prolactin	2-15 ng/ml	0.08-6.0 nmol/l
Renin activity		
Normal diet	Supine: 1.1 ± 0.8 ng/ml/h	0.9 ± 0.6 (nmol/l)h
	Upright: 1.9 ± 1.7 ng/ml/h	1.5 ± 1.3 (nmol/l)h
Low-sodium diet	Supine: 2.7 ± 1.8 ng/ml/h	2.1 ± 1.4 (nmol/l)h
	Upright: 6.6 ± 2.5 ng/ml/h	5.1 ± 1.9 (nmol/l)h
Low-sodium diet	Diuretics: 10.0 ± 3.7 ng/ml/h	7.7 ± 2.9 (nmol/l)h

Continued.

Special endocrine tests—cont'd

Reference range—cont'd

Determination	Conventional	SI
Thyroid hormones		
Thyroid-stimulating-hormone (TSH)	0.5-3.5 μU/ml	0.5-3.5 mU/l
Thyroxine-binding globulin capacity	15-25 μg T_4/100 ml	193-322 nmol/l
Total tri-iodothyronine by radioimmu-noassay (T_3)	70-190 ng/100 ml	1.08-2.92 nmol/l
Total thyroxine by RIA (T_4)	4-12 μg/100 ml	52-154 nmol/l
T_3 resin uptake	25-35%	0.25-0.35
Free thyroxine index (FT_4I)	1-4 ng/100 ml	12.8-51-2 pmol/l

Cerebrospinal fluid values

Reference range

Determination	Conventional	SI	Determination	Conventional	SI
Bilirubin	0	0 μmol/l	Glucose	50-75 mg/100 ml (30%-50% less than blood)	2.8-4.2
Chloride	120-130 mEq/l (20 mEq/l higher than serum)			70-180 mm of water	mmol/l 70-80 arb. u.
Albumin	Mean: 29.5 mg/100 ml ±2 SD: 11-48 mg/100 ml	0.295 g/l ±2 SD: 0.11-0.48	Pressure (initial) Protein: Lumbar	15-45 mg/100 ml	0.15-0.45 g/l
IgG	Mean: 4.3 mg/100 ml ±2 SD: 0-8.6 mg/100 ml	0.043 g/l ±2 SD: 0-0.086	Cisternal Ventricular	15-25 mg/100 ml 5-15 mg/100 ml	0.15-0.25 g/l 0.05-0.15 g/l

Hematologic values

Reference range

Determination	Conventional	SI
Coagulation factors:		
Factor I (fibrinogen)	0.15-0.35 g/100 ml	4.0-10.0 μmol/l
Factor II (prothrombin)	60-140%	0.60-1.40
Factor V (accelerator globulin)	60-140%	0.60-1.40
Factor VII-X (proconvertin-Stuart)	70-130%	0.70-1.30
Factor X (Stuart factor)	70-130%	0.70-1.30
Factor VIII (antihemophilic globulin)	50-200%	0.50-2.0
Factor IX (plasma thromboplastic cofactor)	60-140%	0.60-1.40
Factor XI (plasma thromboplastic antecedent)	60-140%	0.60-1.40
Factor XII (Hageman factor)	60-140%	0.60-1.40
Coagulation screening tests:		
Bleeding time (Simplate)	3-9 min	180-540 s
Prothrombin time	Less than 2-s deviation from control	Less than 2-s deviation from control
Partial thromboplastin time (activated)	25-37 s	25-37 s
Whole-blood clot lysis	No clot lysis in 24 h	O/d
Fibrinolytic studies:		
Euglobin lysis	No lysis in 2 h	0 (in 2 h)
Fibrinogen split products:	Negative reaction at greater than 1:4 dilution	0 (at >1:4 dilution)
Thrombin time	Control ± 5 s	Control ± 5 s
"Complete" blood count:		
Hematocrit	Male: 45-52%	Male: 0.42-0.52
	Female: 37-48%	Female: 0.37-0.48
Hemoglobin	Male: 13-18 g/10 ml	Male: 8.1-11.2 mmole/l
	Female: 12-16 g/100 ml	Female: 7.4-9.9 mmol/l
Leukocyte count	4300-10,800/mm^3	4.3-10.8 × 10^9/l
Erythrocyte count	4.2-5.9 million/mm^3	4.2-5.9 × 10^{12}/l
Mean corpuscular volume (MCV)	80-94 μm^3	80-94 fl
Mean corpuscular hemoglobin (MCH)	27-32 pg	1.7-2.0 fmol
Mean corpuscular hemoglobin concentration (MCHC)	32-36%	19-22.8 mmol/l
Erythrocyte sedimentation rate (Westergren method)	Male: 1-13 mm/h	Male: 1-13 mm/h
	Female: 1-20 mm/h	Female: 1-20 mm/h
Erythrocyte enzymes		
Glucose-6-phosphate dehydrogenase	5-15 U/gHb	5-15 U/g
Pyruvate kinase	13-17 U/gHb	13-17 U/g

Continued.

Hematologic values—cont'd

Reference range—cont'd

Determination	Conventional	SI
Ferritin (serum)		
Iron deficiency	0-20 ng/ml	0-20 μg/l
Iron excess	Greater than 400 ng/l	>400 μg/l
Folic acid		
Normal	Greater than 1.9 ng/ml	>4.3 mmol/l
Borderline	1.0-1.9 ng/ml	2.3-4.3 mmol/l
Haptoglobin	100-300 mg/100 ml	1.0-3.0 g/l
Hemoglobin studies:		
Electrophoresis for A_2 hemoglobin	1.5-3.5%	0.015-0.035
Hemoglobin F (fetal hemoglobin)	Less than 2%	<0.02
Hemoglobin, met- and sulf-	0	0
Serum hemoglobin	2-3 mg/100 ml	1.2-1.9 μmol/l
Thermolabile hemoglobin	0	0
L.E. (lupus erythematosus) preparation:		
Heparin as anticoagulant	0	0
Defibrinated blood	0	0
Leukocyte alkaline phosphatase:		
Quantitative method	15-40 mg of phosphorus liberated/ h/10^{10} cells	15-40 mg/h
Qualitative method	Males: 33-188 U	33-188 U
	Females (off contraceptive pill): 30-160 U	30-160 U
Muramidase	Serum, 3-7 μg/ml	3-7 mg/l
	Urine, 0-2 μg/ml	0-2 mg/l
Osmotic fragility of erythrocytes	Increased if hemolysis occurs in over 0.5% NaCl; decreased if hemolysis is incomplete in 0.3% NaCl	
Peroxide hemolysis	Less than 10%	<0.10
Platelet count	150,000-350,000/mm³	150-350 × 10^9/l
Platelet function tests:		
Clot retraction	50-100%/2 hr	0.50-1.00/2 h
Platelet aggreation	Full response to ADP, epinephrine and collagen	1.0
Platelet factor 3	33-57 s	33-57 s
Reticulocyte count	0.5-1.5% red cells	0.005-0.15
Vitamin B_{12}	90-280 pg/ml (borderline: 70-90)	66-207 pmol/l (borderline: 52-66)

Miscellaneous values

Reference range

Determination	Conventional	SI
Autoantibodies in serum		
Thyroid colloid and microsomal antigens	Absent	
Stomach parietal cells	Absent	
Smooth muscle	Absent	
Kidney mitochondria	Absent	
Rabbit renal collecting ducts	Absent	
Cytoplasm of ova, theca cells, testicular interstitial cells	Absent	
Skeletal muscle	Absent	
Adrenal gland	Absent	
Carcinoembryonic antigen (CEA) in blood	0-2.5 ng/ml, 97% healthy non-smokers	0-2.5 μg/l, 97% healthy nonsmokers
Cryoprecipitable proteins in blood	0	0 arb. unit
Digitoxin in serum	17 ± 6 ng/ml	22 ± 7.8 nmol/l
Digoxin in serum		
0.25 mg/d	1.2 ± 0.4 ng/ml	1.54 ± 0.5 nmol/l
0.5 mg/d	1.5 ± 0.4 ng/ml	1.92 ± 0.5 nmol/l
Duodenal drainage:		
pH	5.5-7.5	5.5-7.5
Amylase	Over 1200 U/total sample	>1.2 arb. u
Trypsin	Values from 35 to 160% "normal"	0.35-1.60
Viscosity	3 min or less	180 s or less
Gastric analysis	Basal:	
	Females 2.0 ± 1.8 mEq/h	0.6 ± 0.5
	Males 3.0 ± 2.0 mEq/h	0.8 ± 0.6 μmol/s
	Maximal: (after histalog or gastrin)	
	Females 16 ± 5 mEq/h	4.4 ± 1.4 μmol/s
	Males 23 ± 5 mEq/h	6.4 ± 1.4 μmol/s
Gastrin-I in blood	0-200 pg/ml	0-95 pmol/l
Immunologic tests		
Alpha-feto-globulin	Abnormal if present	
Alpha 1-antitrypsin	200-400 mg/100 ml	2.0-4.0 g/l
Antinuclear antibodies	Positive if detected with serum diluted 1:10	
Anti-DNA antibodies	Less than 15 units/ml	
Complement, total hemolytic	150-250 U/ml	
C3	Range 55-120 mg/100 ml	0.55-1.2 g/l
C4	Range 20-50 mg/100 ml	0.2-0.5 g/l

Continued.

Miscellaneous values—cont'd

Reference range—cont'd

Determination	Conventional	SI
Immunoglobulins in blood:		
IgG	1140 mg/100 ml	11.4 g/l
	Range 540-1663	5.5-16.6 g/l
IgA	214 mg/100 ml	2.14 g/l
	Range 66-344	0.66-3.44 g/l
IgM	168 mg/100 ml	1.68 g/l
	Range 39-290	0.39-2.9 g/l
Viscosity	1.4-1.8 expressed as relative viscosity of serum compared to water	
Iontophoresis	Children: 0-40 mEq sodium/liter	0-40 mmol/l
	Adults: 0-60 mEq sodium/l	0-60 mmol/l
Propranolol (includes bioactive 4-OH metabolite) in serum 4h after last dose	100-300 ng/ml	386-1158 nmol/l
Stool fat	Less than 5 g in 24 h or less than 4% of measured fat intake in 3-d period	<5 g/d
Stool nitrogen	Less than 2 g/d or 10% of urinary nitrogen	<2 g/d
Synovial fluid:		
Glucose	Not less than 20 mg/100 ml lower than simultaneously drawn blood sugar	See blood glucose mmol/l
Mucin	Type 1 or 2 Grades as: Type 1-tight clump Type 2-soft clump Type 3-soft clump that breaks up Type 4-cloudy, no clump	1-2 arb. u
D-Xylose absorption	5-8 g/5 h in urine	33-53 mmol
	40 mg per 100 ml in blood 2 h after ingestion of 25 g of D-xylose	2.7 mmol/l

B

Abbreviations in Common Usage

ā	Before	Cx	Cervix
aa	Of each	Cysto	Cystoscopy
ac	Before meals	D/C	Discontinue
ad lib	As desired	D & C	Dilation and curettage
A/G ratio	Albumin/globulin ratio	Diff	Differential white blood cell count
AK	Above knee	DIP	Distal interphalangeal joint
aPTT	Activated partial thromboplastin time	DJD	Degenerative joint disease
A/R pulse	Apical/radial pulse	DM	Diabetes mellitus
ARDS	Adult respiratory distress syndrome	DOA	Dead on arrival
ARV	Aortic valve replacement	DOE	Dyspnea on exertion
ASHD	Arteriosclerotic heart disease	DPT	Diphtheria, pertussis, tetanus toxoid
ASCVD	Arteriosclerotic cardiovascular disease	Dx	Diagnosis
BaE	Barium enema	ECG	Electrocardiogram
b.i.d.	Twice daily	EEG	Electroencephalogram
BFT	Biofeedback therapy	EENT	Eye, ear, nose, and throat
BK	Below knee	EMG	Electromyogram
BMR	Basal metabolism rate	ENT	Ear, nose and throat
BPH	Benign prostatic hypertrophy	ESR	Erythrocyte sedimentation rate
B.R.P.	Bathroom privileges	FB	Foreign body
BS	Bowel sounds	FBS	Fasting blood sugar
BSP	Bromsulphalein	FH	Family history
BUN	Blood urea nitrogen	FUO	Fever of unknown origin
Bx	Biopsy	FWB	Full weight bearing
c̄	With	Fx	Fracture
CA	Cancer	GI	Gastrointestinal
CABG	Coronary artery bypass graft	gtt	Drops
CAD	Coronary artery disease	GTT	Glucose tolerance test
CBC	Complete blood count	GU	Genitourinary
cc	Chief complaint	h	Hour
CCK	Cholecystokinin	HAV	Hepatitis A virus
C.D.	Constant drainage	HBV	Hepatitis B virus
CDC	Centers for Disease Control	Hct	Hematocrit
CHF	Congestive heart failure	HCTZ	Hydrochlorothiazide
CNS	Central nervous system	HCVD	Hypertensive cardiovascular disease
c/o	Complained of	HDL	High-density lipoproteins
COPD	Chronic obstructive pulmonary disease	Hgb	Hemoglobin
CPK	Creatine phosphokinase	HMO	Health maintenance organization
CPR	Cardiopulmonary resuscitation	HNP	Herniated nucleus pulposus
C & S	Culture and sensitivities	HPI	History of present illness
CSF	Cerebrospinal fluid	HTN	Hypertension
CT	Computed tomography	h.s.	At bedtime
CVA	Cerebrovascular accident	Hwb	Hot water bottle
CVA	Costovertebral angle	hx	History
CVP	Central venous pressure	IABP	Intraaortic balloon counterpulsation

ICP	Intracranial pressure	p.c.	After meals
ICS	Intercostal space	PCWP	Pulmonary capillary wedge pressure
ICU	Intensive care unit	P.D.	Postural drainage
IDDM	Insulin-dependent diabetes mellitus	PEEP	Positive end expiratory pressure
IHSS	Idiopathic hypertrophic subaortic stenosis	PERRLA	Pupils equal, round, reactive to light and accomodation
IM	Intramuscular	PFT	Pulmonary function test
IMB	Intermenstrual bleeding	Ph	Past history
I & O	Intake and output	PI	Present illness
IPPB	Intermittent positive pressure breathing	PIP	Proximal interphalangeal joint
ITP	Idiopathic thrombocytopenic purpura	Plt	Platelet
IV	Intravenous	PMI	Point of maximal impulse
IVC	Intravenous cholangiogram	PMNs	Polymorphonuclear leukocytes
IVP	Intravenous pyelogram	PMP	Past menstrual period
LBP	Low back pain	PND	Paroxysmal nocturnal dyspnea
LDH	Lactic dehydrogenase	PNS	Peripheral nervous system
LDL	Low-density lipoproteins	po	By mouth
L.E. prep	Lupus erythematosus prep	POD	Postoperative day
LLL	Left lower lobe	PPD	Postpartum day
LLQ	Left lower quadrant	PPD	Purified protein derivative
LMD	Local medical doctor	prn	According to necessity
LMP	Local medical physician	Pro time	Prothrombin time
LMP	Last menstrual period	PSP	Phenosulphonphthalein
LOC	Level of consciousness	PSRO	Professional standards review organization
LP	Lumbar puncture	PT	Prothrombin time
LVEDP	Left ventricular end-diastolic pressure	P.T.	Physical therapy
L & W	Living and well	PTA	Prior to admission
lytes	Electrolytes	PTT	Partial thromboplastin time
ⓜ	Murmur	PVC	Premature ventricular contraction
MCH	Mean corpuscular hemoglobin	PWB	Partial weight bearing
MCHC	Mean corpuscular hemoglobin concentration	PZI	Protamine zinc insulin
MCP	Metacarpopharangeal joint	qd	Every day
MCV	Mean corpuscular volume	qhs	At bedtime
MGW enema	Magnesium, glycerin, and water enema	qod	Every other day
MST	Mean survival time	qid	Four times a day
MTP	Metacarpophalangeal joint	qh	Every hour
MVR	Mitral valve replacement	qns	Quantity not sufficient
MWB	Minimal weight bearing	qoh	Every other hour
NAD	No acute distress	qpr	At earliest convenience
NIDDM	Noninsulin dependent diabetes mellitus	qs	As much as necessary
NMR	Nuclear magnetic resonance	qs	As much as necessary
NPH	Nonprotein Hagedorn (insulin)	RBC	Red blood cells
NPN	Nonprotein nitrogen	RLL	Right lower lobe
N.P.O.	Nothing by mouth	RLQ	Right lower quadrant
NVD	Neck vein distention	R/O	Rule out
NWB	Nonweight bearing	ROS	Review of symptoms
OD	Overdose	RSR	Regular sinus rhythm
O.D.	Right eye	Rx	Treatment
OOB	Out of bed	s̄	Without
O.R.	Operating room	SBE	Subacute bacterial endocarditis
ORIF	Open reduction internal fixation	sc	Subcutaneous
O.S.	Left eye	Sed rate	Sedimentation rate
O.T.	Occupational therapy	SGOT	Serum glutamic oxidase transaminase
O.U.	Both eyes	SGPT	Serum glutamic pyruvate transaminase
p̄	After	SLE	Sytemic lupus erythematosus
P & A	Percussion and auscultation	SLR	Straight leg raising
PAEDP	Pulmonary artery end-diastolic pressure	SOB	Short of breath
PAP	Pulmonary artery pressure	s.o.s.	Administer once if necessary
PAP	Papanicolaou smear	S/P	Status post (occurred in past)
PBI	Protein bound iodine	SR	Systems review

SSE	Soapsuds enema		TPN	Total parenteral nutrition (hyperalimentation)
stat	At once		TSP	Total serum protein
STD	Sexually transmitted disease		TSS	Toxic shock syndrome
STS	Serologic test for syphilis		TURP	Transurethral resection of prostate
T_3	Triiodothyronine		Tx	Traction
T_4	Thyroxine		ung	Ointment
tab	Tablet		URI	Upper respiratory infection
TBC	Tuberculosis		US	Ultrasound
TBG	Thyroxine binding globulin		UTI	Urinary tract infection
TENS	Transcutaneous electrical nerve stimulator		UV	Ultraviolet
THA	Total hip arthroplasty		VC	Vital capacity
THR	Total hip replacement		VDRL	Venereal disease research laboratory test
TIA	Transient ischemic attacks		VNA	Visiting nurse association
t.i.d.	Three times a day		VS	Vital signs
TKA	Total knee arthroplasty		wa	While awake
TKR	Total knee replacement		WBC	White blood count
TM	Tympanic membrane		WNL	Within normal limits
TP	Total protein			

C

Recommended Daily Dietary Allowances, Revised 1980

Mean heights and weights and recommended energy intake

Category	Age (years)	Weight		Height		Energy needs (with range)		
		kg	lb	cm	in	kcal		MJ
Infants	0.0-0.5	6	13	60	24	kg × 115	(95-145)	kg × .48
	0.5-1.0	9	20	71	28	kg × 105	(80-135)	kg × .44
Children	1-3	13	29	90	35	1300	(900-1800)	5.5
	4-6	20	44	112	44	1700	(1300-2300)	7.1
	7-10	28	62	132	52	2400	(1650-3300)	10.1
Males	11-14	45	99	157	62	2700	(2000-3700)	11.3
	15-18	66	145	176	69	2800	(2100-3900)	11.8
	19-22	70	154	177	70	2900	(2500-3300)	12.2
	23-50	70	154	178	70	2700	(2300-3100)	11.3
	51-75	70	154	178	70	2400	(2000-2800)	10.1
	76+	70	154	178	70	2050	(1650-2450)	8.6
Females	11-14	46	101	157	62	2200	(1500-3000)	9.2
	15-18	55	120	163	64	2100	(1200-3000)	8.8
	19-22	55	120	163	64	2100	(1700-2500)	8.8
	23-50	55	120	163	64	2000	(1600-2400)	8.4
	51-75	55	120	163	64	1800	(1400-2200)	7.6
	76+	55	120	163	64	1600	(1200-2000)	6.7
Pregnancy						+300		
Lactation						+500		

From Recommended Dietary Allowances, Revised 1980. Food and Nutrition Board National Academy of Sciences-National Research Council, Washington, D.C.

The data in this table have been assembled from the observed median heights and weights of children together with desirable weights for adults for the mean heights of men (70 in) and women (64 in) between the ages of 18 and 34 years as surveyed in the U.S. population (HEW/NCHS data).

The energy allowances for the young adults are for men and women doing light work. The allowances for the two older age groups represent mean energy needs over these age spans, allowing for a 2% decrease in basal (resting) metabolic rate per decade and a reduction in activity of 200 kcal per day for men and women between 51 and 75 years, 500 kcal for men over 75 years, and 400 kcal for women over 75. The customary range of daily energy output is shown for adults in parentheses and is based on a variation in energy needs of ±400 kcal at any one age, emphasizing the wide range of energy intakes appropriate for any group of people.

Energy allowances for children through age 18 are based on median energy intakes of children these ages followed in longitudinal growth studies. The values in parentheses are 10th and 90th percentiles of energy intake, to indicate the range of energy consumption among children of these ages.

Daily dietary guide—the basic four food groups

Food group	Main nutrients	Daily amounts*
Milk		
Milk, cheese, ice cream, or other products made with whole or skimmed milk	Calcium Protein Riboflavin	Children under 9: 2-3 cups Children 9-12: 3 or more cups Teen-agers: 4 or more cups Adults: 2 or more cups Pregnant women: 3 or more cups Nursing mothers: 4 or more cups (1 cup = 8 oz fluid milk or designated milk equivalent†)
Meats		

Beef, veal, lamb, pork, poultry, fish, eggs	Protein
	Iron
	Thiamin
		2 or more servings
		Count as 1 serving
		   2-3 oz of lean, boneless, cooked meat, poultry, or fish
		   2 eggs

Alternates: dry beans, dry peas, nuts, peanut butter	Niacin Riboflavin	1 cup cooked dry beans or peas 4 tbsp peanut butter
Vegetables and fruits		4 or more servings Count as 1 serving ½ cup of vegetable of fruit or a portion such 1 medium apple, banana, orange, potato, or ½ a medium grapefruit, melon Include
	Vitamin A	A dark-green or deep-yellow vegetable or fruit rich in vitamin A at least every other day
	Vitamin C (ascorbic acid)	A citrus fruit or other fruit or vegetable rich in vitamin C daily
	Smaller amounts of other vitamins and minerals	Other vegetables and fruits including potatoes
Bread and cereals		4 or more servings of whole grain, enriched or restored Count as 1 serving 1 slice of bread
	Thiamin Niacin	1 oz (1 cup) ready to eat cereal, flake or puff varieties
	Riboflavin Iron	½-¾ cup cooked cereal ½-¾ cup cooked pastes (macaroni, sphaghetti, noodles)
	Protein	Crackers: 5 saltines, 2 squares graham crackers

*Use additional amounts of these foods or added butter, margarine, oils, sugars, etc., as desired or needed.
†Milk equivalents: 1 oz cheddar cheese, 3 servings cottage cheese, 1 cup fluid skimmed milk, 1 cup buttermilk, ½ cup dry skimmed milk powder, 1 cup ice milk, 1⅔ cups ice cream, ½ cup evaporated milk.

Recommended daily dietary allowances for growth

	Age (yr)	Weight kg	Weight lb	Height cm	Height in	Energy (kcal)	Protein (g)	Fat soluble vitamins — Vit. A μg RE	Vit. A IU	Vit. D (μg*)	Vit. E (mgαTE)
Infants	Birth-0.5	6	13	60	24	kg × 115	kg × 2.2	420	1,400	10	3
	0.5-1	9	20	71	28	kg × 105	kg × 2.0	400	2,000	10	4
Children	1-3	13	29	90	35	1,300	23	400	2,000	10	5
	4-6	20	44	112	44	1,700	30	500	2,500	10	6
	7-10	28	62	132	52	2,400	34	700	3,300	10	7
Males	11-14	45	99	157	62	2,700	45	1,000	5,000	10	8
	15-18	66	145	176	69	2,800	56	1,000	5,000	10	10
Females	11-14	46	101	157	62	2,200	46	800	4,000	10	8
	15-18	55	120	163	64	2,100	46	800	4,000	10	8

*As cholecalciferol; 10 μg cholecalciferol = 400 IU vitamin D.

Recommended daily dietary allowances of some selected nutrients for pregnancy and lactation

Nutrients	Nonpregnant girl 12-14 yr 47 kg (103 lb)	Nonpregnant girl 14-18 yr 55 kg (120 lb)	Nonpregnant woman 25 yr 58 kg (128 lb)	Pregnancy Added need	Pregnancy Girl 12-14 yr	Pregnancy Girl 14-18 yr	Pregnancy Woman 25 yr	Lactation (850 ml daily) Added need	Lactation Girl 12-14 yr	Lactation Girl 14-18 yr	Lactation Woman 25 yr
Calories	2,200	2,100	2,000	300	2,500	2,400	2,300	500	2,700	2,600	2,500
Protein (g)	46	46	44	30	76	76	74	20	66	68	64
Calcium (g)	1.2	1.2	0.8	0.4	1.6	1.6	1.2	0.4	1.6	1.6	1.2
Iron (mg)	18	18	18	‡	18+	18+	18+	‡	18+	18+	18+
Vitamin A (RE)*	800	800	800	200	1,000	1,000	1,000	400	1,200	1,200	1,200
Thiamin (mg)	1.1	1.1	1.0	0.4	1.5	1.5	1.4	0.5	1.6	1.6	1.5
Riboflavin (mg)	1.3	1.3	1.2	0.3	1.6	1.6	1.5	0.5	1.8	1.8	1.7
Niacin equivalent and tryptophan (mg)	15	14	13	2	17	16	15	5	20	19	18
Ascorbic acid (mg)	50	60	60	20	70	80	80	40	90	100	100
Vitamin D (μg)†	10	10	5	5	15	15	10	5	15	15	10

*Retinol equivalents.
†Cholecalciferol; 10 μg equals 400 IU vitamin D.
‡Required iron supplement 30-60 mg.

	Water-soluble vitamins						Minerals					
Vit. C (mg)	Folacin (μg)	Niacin (mg)	Riboflavin (mg)	Thiamin (mg)	Vit. B$_6$ (mg)	Vit. B$_{12}$ (μg)	Calcium (mg)	Phosphorus (mg)	Iodine (μg)	Iron (mg)	Magnesium (mg)	Zinc (mg)
35	30	6	0.4	0.3	0.3	0.5	360	240	40	10	50	3
35	45	8	0.6	0.5	0.6	1.5	540	360	50	15	70	5
45	100	9	0.8	0.7	0.9	2.0	800	800	70	15	150	10
45	200	11	1.0	0.9	1.3	2.5	800	800	90	10	200	10
45	300	16	1.4	1.2	1.6	3.0	800	800	120	10	250	10
50	400	18	1.6	1.4	1.8	3.0	1,200	1,200	150	18	350	15
60	400	18	1.7	1.4	2.0	3.0	1,200	1,200	150	18	400	15
50	400	15	1.3	1.1	1.8	3.0	1,200	1,200	150	18	300	15
60	400	14	1.3	1.1	2.0	3.0	1,200	1,200	150	18	300	15

Index

A

A-delta fibers, 175, 177, 186
AA; *see* Alcoholics Anonymous
Ab; *see* Antibodies
Abbreviations, common, 1221-1223
ABCs of emergency assessment, 1166, 1171
Abdomen
  assessment of, 1167
    shock and, 167
  bleeding in, 1174
  changes with aging, 37
  distention of, 31, 881; *see also* Ascites
    casts and, 516
    cholecystitis and, 861
    diarrhea and, 882
    hernia repair and, 920
    postoperative, 345, 1066
    urologic surgery and, 972
  examination of, 31-32, 1167
    palpation and percussion in, 24
    radiologic, 953
  pain in, digitalis and, 670
  wounds of, 1181
Abdominal breathing
  chronic obstructive pulmonary disease and,
    601-602
Abdominoperineal resection, 930, 931
  care of patient with, 929
ABO system, 1155
Abortion, 1052
Above-knee amputation, 709
Abramson drain, 332
Abscesses, 73
  anal, 905
  brain, 410-411
Absorption, small intestine and, 878
Accessory muscles, 545
Accidents
  in home, 1164
  prevention of, 1163-1165
  young adults and, 50
Acclimatization, 546-547
Accommodation, 437, 438
Ace bandage, burns and, 1139
Acetaminophen, 182, 250, 843
  eye inflammation and, 451
  headache and, 366
  neurologic pain and, 371
Acetazolamide, 456, 463, 974
Acetic acid solution, 970
Acetoacetate plus acetone, 1211, 1214

Acetohexamide, 777
Acetylcholine, 354, 356
Acetylcysteine, 553
Acetyldigitoxin, 670
Acetylsalicylic acid; *see* Aspirin
Achalasia, 883, 884
Achilles tendon reflex, 826
Acid ash diet, 970
Acid base balance, 147, 148-150, 943
  burns and, 1133
  compensatory mechanisms in, 148-149
  shock and, 163, 166-167
Acidophilic adenoma, 798
Acidophilus culture, 1060
Acidophilus yogurt, 1060
Acidosis, 148
  renal failure and, 996, 1004
  respiratory, 148
  metabolic, 148
Acinar cells, 834
Acinetobacter species, 553, 557
Acids; *see* specific acid
  organic, 135
Acne, immunosuppressive therapy and, 1023
Acquired immune deficiency disease, 1078,
    1146
Acromegaly, 799
  sexual dysfunction and, 1034
ACTH; *see* Adrenocorticotropic hormone
Actinic keratosis, 1119
Actinomycin D, 83
Action potential, 353, 628
Activated partial thromboplastin time, 743
Active artificial immunity, 197
Active immunization, 197-198
Active range of motion, 484
Activities of daily living
  blindness and, 444
  cerebrovascular accident and, 404, 405-406
  chronic illness and, 268-269
  headache and, 366
  motor dysfunction and, 383
  paralysis and, 381
Activity
  diabetes mellitus and, 782
  elderly and, 57-58
  limitation of, chronic illness and, 259-260
  motor function disturbance and, 380-381,
    383
  musculoskeletal disorders and, 485
  postoperative, 346-347
  preoperative assessment of, 295, 296

Activity—cont'd
  vascular system and, 697
Acupuncture, 315
  pain relief and, 185
Acylanid; *see* Acetyldigitoxin
Adam's apple, 529
Adaptation, 106
Adaptic gauze, 1125
Addisonian crisis, 811
  signs of, 803
Addison's disease, 140, 807, 809
  clinical findings in, 814
  nursing care of patient with, 815
  sexual dysfunction and, 1034
Adenocarcinoma, 217
Adenohypophysis, 792
Adenoids, 529
  removal of, 531
Adenoma, 217
  anterior pituitary, 798
Adenosine triphosphate
  heart failure and, 667
  shock and, 160
ADH; *see* Antidiuretic hormone
Adipose tissue
  aging and, 58
  cortisol and, 807
ADL; *see* Activities of daily living
Adrenal crisis, 811
Adrenal gland, 794, 1219
  cortex of, 794
    deficiency, 809
    dysfunction, tests for, 811-813
    excess, 809
    hormones of, 135
    hyperplasia of, 809
    secretory disorders of, 796
    tumor of, 809
  dysfunction of, 807-816
  hormones of, 807, 808
  hypersecretion of, 807-810
  hypoplasia of, 809
  hyposecretion of, 810-811
  medulla of, 108, 796
    hypersecretion of, 796
  surgery and, 815-816
Adrenalectomy, 809
  sexual dysfunction and, 1034
Adrenalin; *see* Epinephrine
Adrenergic agents; *see also* specific drug
  chronic obstructive pulmonary disease and,
    606

Adrenergic agents—cont'd
 glaucoma and, 456
Adrenocorticosteroids, 108, 243; see also Corticosteroids
 rheumatoid arthritis and, 493
Adrenocorticotropic hormone, 108, 792, 1215
 deficiency/excess of, 797
 multiple sclerosis and, 395
 stimulation tests and, 801
Adriamycin; see Doxorubicin
Adult respiratory distress syndrome, 161, 166, 575-576, 1200
Advisory Committee on Immunization Practices, 197, 198
Aerobes, pneumonia and, 553
Aerobic exercise, 97, 98
Aerosols, chronic obstructive pulmonary disease and, 606
Affiliation needs, 11
Aflatoxin, 13
 cancer and, 219, 221
Afterload, 631, 665
Aggressive behavior, 119
Age
 adaptation to, 55
 blood pressure and, 943
 cancer and, 213, 219
 cataract and, 451
 chronic illness and, 260
 coronary artery disease and, 651
 fluid loss and, 134
 heart and, 631-632
 gastrointestinal tract and, 878
 genital system and, 1047, 1049
 glucose tolerance and, 762
 hematopoiesis and, 731
 hypertension and, 722
 musculoskeletal system and, 483
 physical changes with, 36, 37
 premature death and, 278
 renal system and, 943-944
 sexuality and, 1030-1031
 skin and, 1106-1107
 vascular system and, 696
Aging
 components of, 53
 models of, 54
Agranulocytosis, 748
AHA; see American Hospital Association
AIDS; see Acquired immune deficiency syndrome
Air conduction, 462
Air humidification, tracheostomy and, 619
Air pollution, chronic obstructive pulmonary disease and, 608
Air pressure mattress, 513
Air shields respiratory, 620
Air tonometer, 453
Airway, artificial, 327, 328
Airway
 burns and, 1134, 1136-1137
 chronic obstructive pulmonary disease and, 613-620
 respiratory insufficiency and, 612
 obstruction of, 579, 1169
 postoperative, 326, 327
 patency of, 326-328, 546, 547
Akinetic seizures, 386
Akineton; see Biperiden
Al-Anon, 124
Al-Ateen, 124
Albert Smith pessary, 1065

Albumin, 74, 1213, 1216
 fluid replacement therapy and, 168
Alcaine; see Proparacaine
Alcohol, 743; see also Alcoholism
 absolute, 424
 absorption of, 121
 cancer and, 219, 223
 diabetes mellitus and, 782
 diuretic effect of, 121
 excretion of, 121
 headache and, 366
 liver disease and, 843
 metabolism of, 121
 sexual dysfunction and, 1035
 withdrawal from, 123-124
Alcoholics Anonymous, 124
Alcoholism, 120-124
 cardiomyopathy and, 675, 677
 cirrhosis and, 846
 hepatitis and, 846
 hospitalization for, 123
 in middle age, 53
 pathophysiology of, 121
 stress and, 105
 young adults and, 50
Aldactazide; see Spironolactone-hydrochlorothiazide
Aldactone; see Spironolactone
Aldolase, 1211
Aldomet; see Spironolactone
Aldosterone, 108, 109, 135-136, 137, 1215
 deficiency/excess of, 809, 810
 functions of, 808
Aldosteronism, primary, 815
ALG; see Antilymphocyte globulin
Alka-2; see Calcium carbonate
Alkalosis, 148
Alkeran; see Melphalan
Alkylating agents, 83, 84, 242, 243
ALL; see Leukemia, acute lymphocytic
Allergy, 1059, 1149-1155
 alveolitis and, 574
 asthma and, 1150, 1151
 causes of, 1151
 contact dermatitis and, 1114
 diagnostic tests for, 1152
 rhinitis and, 529, 1150
 skin tests and, 1152
 stress and, 105
 symptoms of, 1150, 1151
 teaching and, 1153-1154
Allograft, rejection of, 1158
Allopecia; see Hair, loss of
Allopurinol, 974
Alpha-adrenergic drugs, shock and, 169
Alpha-chymotrypsin, cataract surgery and, 452
Alpha-Deri, 1113
Alpha-fetoprotein, 82
Alpha-globulins, 74
ALS; see Amyotrophic lateral sclerosis; Antilymphocytic serum
Alseroxylon fraction, 723
Aluminum acetate, 1113
Alveolar capillary membrane, 544
Alveolus, 544
Alzheimer's disease, 56, 393, 399-400
Amantadine hydrochloride, 397
Ambu bag, 618
Ambulation
 aids for, 485
 with chest tube, 590
 chronic illness and, 270

Ambulation—cont'd
 postoperative, 346, 347
Amebecides, inflammation of reproductive tract and, 1059
Amebiasis, 896
American Academy of Nursing, 263
American Annals of the Deaf, 471
American Association of Diabetes Education, 273, 781
American Association of Fitness Directors in Business and Industry, 274
American Association of Retired Persons, 273
American Cancer Society, 221, 222, 226, 228, 273
 cigarette smoking and, 548
 laryngectomy and, 539, 540, 541
 transportation program of, 1100
 uterine cancer and, 1049
American Coalition of Citizens with Disabilities, 273
American Diabetes Association, 273, 776, 786
American Federation of the Physically Handicapped, Inc., 471
American Foundation for the Blind, 783
American Heart Association, 273
American Hospital Association, 191
American Lung Association, 222, 273, 548, 570
American Nurses' Association, 270
American Parkinson Disease Association, 273
American Public Health Association, cancer screening criteria, 224
American Red Cross, disasters and, 1186
American Speech and Hearing Association, 471, 540
American Thoracic Society, 564
Ametropia, 438
Amicar; see Aminocaproic acid
Amino acids; see also Proteins
 essential, 87
Aminocaproic acid, 406
Aminophylline, 89
Amitryptyline, 371, 1035
AML; see Leukemia, acute myelogenous
Ammonia, 1211
Ammonium carbonate, 553
Ammonium chloride, 155, 553
Amphetamine, 125
 sexual function and, 1036
Amphiarthroses, 482
Amphogel, 912
Amphotericin B, 570
 nephritis and, 961
Ampicillin, 89, 559, 560, 1059
 chronic obstructive pulmonary disease and, 606
Amputation, 706-711, 1181-1182
 bandaging and, 709
 body image and, 1036
 diabetes mellitus and, 769
 types of, 706, 709
Amyl nitrite, 1036
Amylase, 1214
Amylotic enzyme, 835
Amyotrophic lateral sclerosis, 393, 398-399
 sexuality and, 1033
Anabolism, 86, 143
Anaerobes, 201
 pneumonia and, 553
Analgesia, 367
 waking-imagined, 187

Analgesics
  nonnarcotic, 182
  synthetic, 125
  trigeminal neuralgia and, 424
Anamnestic response, 79
Anaphylaxis, 159, 1150
  local, 1151
  eosinophilic chemotactic factor in, 609
  prevention of, 1153
  systemic, 1151
Anaplasia, 216
Anasarca, 141
Anastomoses, 628, 925
Anatomy and physiology
  biologic defense mechanisms and, 64, 66
  cardiovascular system and, 626-632
  of ear, 460-462
  of endocrine system, 759-761
  of eye, 436-437
  of gastrointestinal tract, 875-878
  of hematologic system, 728-731
  of musculoskeletal system, 480-483
  of neurologic system, 351-358
  of nose and throat, 527-529
  of reproductive tract, 1044-1049
  of respiratory tract, 543-548
  of skin, 1105-1107
  of urinary tract, 941-944
  of vascular system, 693-696
Androgens, 243, 808, 809, 810
Anemia, 732
  aplastic, 733, 734, 735-738
  from blood loss, 732-733, 734
  burns and, 1134
  chronic, 733, 734
  hemolytic, 734, 735, 738-741
  erythrocytosis and, 735, 742
  liver and, 841-842, 857
  megaloblastic, 735, 741
  nutritional, 735, 741-742
    iron deficiency and, 735, 741
  renal failure and, 1004
  risk factors for, 731-732
  sickle cell, 734, 738-739
Anerobic exercise, 98
Anerobic metabolism, shock and, 160
Anesthesia
  action and effect of, 314-315
  alcohol and, 121
  anxiety about, 316
  balanced, 319
  choice of, 315
  dissociative, 320
  epidural, 314
  eye disease and, 450
  general, 314, 316, 319
    stages of, 319
  induced hypothermia and, 321, 322
  general, 314
  methods of administration of, 314-315, 316-
    317
    monitoring of, 322, 323
  preparation of patient for, 316
  regional, 314
  safety and, 323
  spinal, 314
  types of, 314-315
  usage of, 315
Anesthetic agents, comparison of, 316-317
Aneurysm, 686-690
  abdominal aortic, 687, 688, 689-690
  cardiovascular syphilis and, 677
  extremities and, 701, 702

Aneurysm—cont'd
  removal of, 711, 713
Angel dust; see Phencyclidine
Angina pectoris, 652-655
  pain and, 667
  stress and, 105
  teaching and, 655
Angiography, 702; see also Arteriography
  aortic aneurysm and, 688
  cerebral, 402
  gastric hemorrhage and, 910
  renal, 954
Angiotensin, 943
Anhydron; see Cyclothiazide
Anions, 135
Ankylosis, 488, 499-500
Annuloplasty, 685
Annulus fibrosus, 504
Anorexia, 72, 94
  digitalis and, 670
  drug abuse and, 127
  factors influencing, 94
  fluids and, 142
  pain and, 106
Anosognosia, 403, 405
Ansolysen; see Pentolinium
Antacids, peptic ulcer and, 911, 912
Antabuse; see Disulfiram
Anterior chamber, 436, 437
Anterior cord syndrome, 417
Anthralin, 1112
Anthrax, 69
Antiarrhythmic agents, 639
Antibiotics, 83, 243
  broad-spectrum, 67
  burns and, 1138
  ear problems and, 463
  infection control and, 190
  nephritis and, 961
  ophthalmic, 450
  reproductive tract and, 1059
Antibodies, 66, 73, 74
  binding of, 74
  circulating, 70
  complement and, 70
  enhancement of, 82
  production of, 249
Anticholinergic agents, 553
  Parkinson's disease and, 397
  peptic ulcer and, 911
Anticoagulants; see specific agent Anticonvul-
    sants, 389
Antidepressants, sexual dysfunction and, 1035
Antidiuretic hormone, 136, 137, 140, 792, 793
  function tests of, 806
  postoperative stimulation of, 343
  secretory disorders of, 804-805
Anti-DNA antibodies, 1219
Antiemetics
  chemotherapy and, 246-247
Antifibrinolytic agents, intracranial hemor-
    rhage and, 406
Antifungal agents, reproductive tract and,
    1059
Antigen-antibody interaction, 74
Antigenic challenge, 76-77
Antigenic determinants, 73
Antigens, 73
  carcinoembryonic, 82
  histocompatibility, 83, 1158
  human leukocyte, 83
  inhalant, 1153
  live attenuated, 196

Antigens—cont'd
  oncofetal, 82
  tumor-specific, 82
Antiglobin test, 739
Antihemophilic factor, 1154
Antihistamines; see specific agent
Antihypertensive drugs; see specific agent
  sexual dysfunction and, 1035
Antiinflammatory agents
  nonsteroidal, 494
  pain relief and, 182
  rheumatoid arthritis and, 493
Antilymphocyte serum, 83, 84, 1022
Antimalarial agents, 494
Antimetabolites, 83, 84, 242, 243
Antimicrobial agents, 66-67; see also specific
    agent
  chronic obstructive pulmonary disease and,
    606-607
  preoperative, 313
Antinuclear antibodies, 1219
Antiserum, 81
Antishock trousers, 1181
Antispasmodics, sexual dysfunction and, 1035
Antithymocyte globulin, 1022
Antithyroid drugs, 828-829
Antitoxins, 198
α_1-Antitrypsin, 1219
Antitussive agents, 553
Antivenins, 198
Antivert; see Meclizine
Antivertiginous agents, 476
Antrectomy, 924
Antrum puncture, 531
Anuria, 946, 995
Anus
  lesions of, 905
  sexual dysfunction and, 1034
  surgery and, 906
Anxiety, 107, 114-116
  anesthesia and, 316
  breast cancer and, 1091, 1093
  chronic obstructive pulmonary disease and,
    609
  heart failure and, 667
  immunodeficiency and, 1148
  pain and, 187-188
  postoperative, 347
  retinal detachment and, 459
  severe, interventions for, 116
  shock and, 171
  surgery and, 293, 294, 298
Aplastic anemia, 733, 734, 735-738
Aplastic crisis, 739
Appendicitis, 896
Aorta
  aneurysm of, 687-690
  insufficiency of, 680, 681, 683
  resection of, 689
  stenosis of, 679, 681, 683
Aortic valve, 34, 628
Aortitis, 677
Aortogram, 688
Aphakia, 457
Aphasia, 403
Apnea/hyperpnea, 666-667
Appetite, lack of; see Anorexia
Apresoline; see Hydralazine
Apthous stomatitis, 894
Aquatag; see Benzthiazide
Aqueous humor, 437
Arachidonic acid, 87
Arachnoid villi, 356

Aralen; *see* Chloroquine
Aramine; *see* Metaraminol
Architectural and Transportation Barriers Compliance Board, 273
ARDS; *see* Adult respiratory distress syndrome
Areflexia, 377, 417
Arfonad; *see* Trimethaphan
Argyll Robertson pupil, 412
Aristocort; *see* Triamcinolone
Arlidin; *see* Nylidrin
Arm exercises, 590
Arousal, sexual, disorders of, 1037-1038
Arsenic
    cancer and, 219
    nephritis and, 961
Artane; *see* Trihexphenidyl
Arterial blood gases; *see* Blood gases, arterial
Arteries
    blood flow disorders of, 705
    bypass surgery and, 705-706
    carotid, 355
    disorders of, 699-713
    embolisms of, 700, 702
    excision of, 705
    or lower extremities, 694
    reconstruction of, 706
        surgery and, 705
    vertebral, 355
Arteriography, 702; *see also* Angiography
    brain tumor and, 429
Arterioles, 693
    dilators and, 699
Arteriosclerosis, 696
    aortic aneurysm and, 686, 687
Arteriovenous fistula, 701, 702, 1013, 1014
Arteriovenous graft, 1013, 1014
Arteriovenous malformations, 406
Arteriovenous shunt, 1013, 1014
Arthritis Foundation, 273
Arthrodesis, 503, 507
Arthroplasty, 496, 503
    replacement, 494-497
Arthrotomy, 496
Articular cartilage, 481
Artificial airways, 613
Artificial immunity, 197
Artificial insemination, 1057
Artificial pacemaker, 639
Artificial tears, 380, 1005
Asbestos
    cancer and, 219, 221
    lung disease and, 572-573
Aschoff bodies, 677
Ascites, 141
    assessment of, 856
    liver tumor and, 840, 842
    massive, 850
    reduction of, 857
Ascorbic acid, 1211
Asepsis, surgical, 307-310
L-Asparaginase, 750
Asphyxia, 1169, 1170
Aspiration
    biopsy and, 1088
    pneumonia and, 553, 558-560
Aspirin, 182
    and codeine, 182
    ear inflammation and, 463
    eye inflammation and, 451
    migraine and, 366
    neurologic pain and, 371
    rheumatoid arthritis and, 493
    tension headache and, 366

Assessment, *see also* Examination; specific disorder
    alcoholism and, 122
    baseline, 1199
    cancer and, 228-232
    chronic illness and, 263
    of cranial nerve function, 359
    critically ill patient and, 1193-1199
    drug abuse and, 125, 127
    emergency, 1166
    of fluid and electrolyte balance, 151-153
    of infection, 194-196
    neurologic, 359-361
    of nutrient intake, 88-90
    of pain relief, 188, 189
    postoperative, 329-334
    preoperative, 305
    surgery and, 294-297
Assessment worksheet, 1198
Association of Operating Room Nurses, 304
Asterexis, 848
Asthma, 609-612
    chronic mild, 611
    occupational, 573
Astigmatism, 438
Astrocytoma, 217, 426
Atabrine; *see* Quinacrine
Atelectasis, 339, 547
    postoperative, 340
    respiratory insufficiency and, 612
Atherosclerosis, 52, 650, 699, 701
    cholesterol and, 87-88
    diabetes mellitus and, 767
Atherosclerosis obliterans, 699, 701
Athlete's foot, 1109, 1110
Atopic dermatitis, 1115, 1150, 1151
ATP; *see* Adenosine triphosphate
Atrioventricular block, 638, 643
Atrioventricular valves, 34, 628
At-risk status, 5
Atrium, 34
    diastolic gallop and, 34
    fibrillation and, 637, 641-642
Atrophy, 775
Atropine, 301, 449, 553, 579, 639, 1173, 1201
Atropisol; *see* Atropine
Attenuated live vaccines, 81
Attire, operating room, 308-309
Attitudes
    cancer and, 212
    death and dying and, 280-281
Atypical pneumonia syndrome, 553, 558, 559
Audiography, 467
Audiologists, 469
Audiometry, 465-468
Auditory acuity, 29, 465
Auditory canal, 460
Auditory training, 470
Aura, seizures and, 387
Aural rehabilitation, 468-472
Auricle, 460
Auscultation, 24
    cardiac, 33-37
    pulmonary, 31, 33
Australian antigen, 836
Autogenic training, 110, 185
Autograft, 1123
Autoimmune diseases, 55, 82, 762, 1146, 1158, 1159
Automatic bladder, 989
Automaticity, 671
Autonomic dysreflexia, 419, 422
Autonomic hyperflexia, 418

Autonomic nervous system, 356, 631
Autonomous bladder, 417
Autonomy, 216
Autoregulation, pain control and, 185
Autotransfusion, 168
Aventyl; *see* Nortriptyline
Awareness, 24
Axillae, contact dermatitis and, 1115
Axillary crutches, 711
Axons, 352
5-Azacytidine, 247
Azapetine, 704
Azathioprine, 83, 84, 743, 1022
Azotemia, 842, 1001, 1004

B

B cells, 74, 75, 730
    deficiency of, tests for, 1147
Babinski sign, 374
Bacilli, coliform, burns and, 1138
Bacillus anthracis, 69
Bacillus Calmette-Guérin vaccine, 81, 249-250
Bacitracin, 450
Back, examination of, 31, 32
Baclofen, 381, 395
Bacteremia, 73; *see also* Septicemia
    nosocomial, 203-204
    secondary, 200
Bacteria
    arthritis and, 490, 508-509
    aspiration pneumonia and, 558
    intestinal, 878
    normal, 196
    nose and throat and, 529
    pneumonia and, 553
    pulmonary system and, 553-560
    skin infections and, 1108, 1114
Bacteroides, 201
Bactrim; *see* Trimethoprim-sulfamethoxazole
Balanitis, sexual dysfunction and, 1034
Balloon pump, 171
Balloon catheter, 658
Balnetar, 1117
Barbiturates, 88, 125
    coma and, 1211
        intracranial surgery and, 431
Barium
    enemas and, 900
    gastrointestinal series and, 908
Barrel chest, 54
Bartholin's glands
    abscess of, 1060
    cysts and, 1058
        sexual dysfunction and, 1034
    infection and, 1058
Basal cell carcinoma, 1119
Basal ganglia, 354
Basal metabolism, 826
    nutrition and, 86
Basic four food groups, 1225
Basic life support, 1170, 1171, 1172-1173
Basophilic adenoma, 798
Basophils, 69, 194
Baths, 1113
Bath oils, 1113
BCG vaccine; *see* Bacillus Calmette-Guérin
Bedside equipment, intensive care and, 1192
Beer heart, 122
Behavior, 113
    adaptive, 119
    aggressive, 119
    depressed, 119
    health promoting, 86

Behavior—cont'd
illness and, 119-120
maladaptive, 113
young adults and, 50
somatic, 120
suspicious, 120
withdrawn, 120
Behavior modification, 110
pain and, 185, 188
weight reduction and, 93
Belladonna alkaloids; see also specific drug
migraine and, 366
pain and, 182
suppositories and, 182
Bell's palsy, 425
Bellevue bridge, 1074
Bellows, 546, 547
Belonging, 11
Below-knee amputation, 706
Benadryl; see Diphenhydramine
Benign prostatic hypertrophy, 975-979
Bennett respirator, 614, 620, 621
Benperidol, 1035
Benson's relaxation response, 111, 187
Benzidine test, 900
Benzol, cancer and, 219, 221
Benzonatate, 553
Benzopyrene, cancer and, 222
Benztropine mesylate, 397
Benzquinamide, 370
Benzthiazide, 723
Beriberi, 87
Berry aneurysm, 406
Beta-adrenergic blocking agents; see also Adrenergic agents; specific drug
angina and, 655
glaucoma and, 456
shock and, 169
Beta globulins, 74
Beta-naphthylamine, 975
Betadine; see Povidone-iodine
Bethanechol, 344, 395, 887, 949
BHA, 222
BHT, 222
Bicarbonate, 135
acid-base balance and, 149
body fluids and, 147
carbonate ratio, 148
deficit, 149
excess, 149-150
normal values, 949
Bicuspid valve, 628
Bier block, 314
Bigeminy, digitalis and, 670
Biochemical defense mechanisms, 66-67
Bifocal lenses, 439
Bile, 135
Bile pigment metabolism, 841
Biliary system, 834, 835
carcinoma and, 861, 862
cirrhosis and, 845
disorders of, 861-867
diagnostic tests for, 863, 864
drainage of, 865
surgery and, 865-867
Bilirubin, 1216
metabolism and, 834
tests for, 836, 1211
Billroth procedures, 913, 914
Bilocadren; see Timolol
Biofeedback, 110
pain control and, 185
Biologic adaptation, 106

Biologic age, 53, 54
Biologic clock, 54
Biologic defense mechanisms, 62-84
concept and scope of, 62-64
Biologic health, 4
Biologic sex, 1028
Biologic valves, 686
Biopsy
of breast, 1088-1089
cancer and, 231
renal, 954-955
Biotin, 87
Biperiden, 397
Bird respirator, 614, 620
Birth control pills; see Oral contraceptives
Bisacodyl, 404, 422, 883
Bisexuality, 1031
Bitemporal hemianopsia, 798
Bivalved cast, 516
Black lung disease, 571
Bladder
automatic, 989
catheterization and, 344
exstrophy of, 956
function, evaluation of, 949
perforation of, 993
retraining of, 990-991
segmental resection of, 975
sphincter, artificial, 992
tumors of, 974-975
Blakemore-Sengstaken tube, 857, 858
Blastomyces dermatitidis, 569
Blastomycosis, 567, 568-569
Bleeding; see also Hemorrhage
external, 1174
gastrointestinal, 1203
internal, 1174
intervention for, 1175
liver disorders and, 841-842, 857
signs of, 918
Bleeding time, 743, 1217
Blenoxane; see Bleomycin
Bleomycin, 243, 247, 463
Blepharitis, 445
Blepharospasm, 442, 445
Blind spot, 374, 442
Blindness
diabetes mellitus and, 768
legal, 443
Blood; see also Hematologic system
alcohol level of, 121
cellular components of, 69, 728, 729
cooling of, 321
as defense, 68-70
differential count, infection and, 195
flow of; see Blood flow
fluid factors of, 69-70
fluid replacement, shock and, 168
glucose in; see Glucose, blood
infections of, nosocomial, 201, 203-204
loss of, monitoring during anesthesia, 322
normal laboratory values of, 1211-1213, 1217-1218
pressure of, 141
protein in, substitutes for, 155
sedimentation rate of, 72
shock and, 162
stored, 168
studies of, 656-657
volume of, 1211
Blood coagulation, 730, 731
disorders of, 742-748
laboratory values for, 1217

Blood coagulation—cont'd
tests of, 743, 1217
vitamins and, 87
Blood gases
bronchitis and, 596-600
monitoring
adult respiratory distress syndrome and, 166
anesthesia and, 322
pulmonary emphysema and, 597
respiratory failure and, 612-613
Blood groups, 1155
ulcers and, 908
Blood pressure
aging and, 943
anesthesia and, 318, 322
intracranial pressure and, 374
narcotics and, 183
renal regulation of, 943
renin-angiotensin system, 721
shock and, 162
vital function and, 183
Blood transfusion
complications of, 1156-1157
reactions to, 1155-1157
types of, 1154
Blood urea nitrogen, 951
Blow bottles, 341
Blue bloater, 597
Body boundary, 1143
Body fluids, 134, 135
Body frame, estimation of, 90
Body hair, aging and, 1107
Body heat, 134
Body image
cancer and, 231
sexuality and, 1036
skin disorders and, 1107
young adults and, 48-49
Body lice, 1111
Body position; see Positioning of patient; Posture
Body temperature; see Temperature
Body water; see Fluids and electrolyte balance
Boils, 1108
Bone marrow
aspiration of, 736-737
biopsy needle, 736
chemotherapy and, 246, 247
transplantation of, 751
Bones, 480-481
cancellous, 481
conduction and, 462
flat, 482
fracture of, 509-513
healing of, 511
irregular, 482
shaft of, 480
trauma to, 510
Bornholm's disease, 549
Bougies, 887
Bowel; see Intestines
Bowman's capsule, 941, 942
Braces, spinal cord trauma and, 422
musculoskeletal disorders and, 485-487
spinal cord trauma and, 422
Brachytherapy, 239
Bradycardia, digitalis and, 670
Bradykinin, 72
Brain; see also Neurologic disorders
abscess of, 410-411
circulation of, 355-356
edema and, 414

Brain—cont'd
  shock and, 161
Brain stem, 355-356
Breath sounds, 33
Breaker bottle, 588, 589
Breasts
  biopsy of, 1088-1089
  body image and, 1036
  cancer and, 1092-1101
    adjuvant therapy and, 1100
    examination for, 224
    incidence of, 223
    risk of, 219
  contact dermatitis and, 1115
  diagnostic test and, 1088-1089
  discomfort and
    physical activity and, 1086
    premenstrual, 1085-1086
  disorders of, 1085-1101
    benign, 1089-1092
    malignant, 1091, 1092-1101
  inspection of, 31
  prostheses and, 1096-1098
  reconstruction of, 1099, 1100
  self-examination of, 31, 224, 225, 1086-1087
  surgery and, 1093-1101
Breathing Easy, 222
Breathing exercises
  chronic obstructive pulmonary disease and, 601-602
  postoperative, 328
Bretylium tosylate, 639, 1173, 1201
Bretylol; *see* Bretylium tosylate
Broca's area, 355
Bromide, 1211
Bromocryptine mesylate, 802
Brompton's cocktail, 252
Bromsulfalein, 1211
Bronchi, clapping/vibrating and, 605
Bronchial asthma, 105
Bronchitis
  acute, 552
  chronic, 596-600
Bronchodilators, 606
Bronchogenic carcinoma, 577
Bronchopleural fistula, 590, 592
Bronchoscope, 578
Bronchoscopy, 578
  surgery and, 583
Bronchospasm, 579
Bronchus
  anterior, clapping/vibrating and, 605
  apical, 605
Bronkotabs, 612
Broviac catheter, 96
Brown lung, 574
Brown-Sequard syndrome, 383, 417
Brudzinski's sign, 409
Brufen; *see* Ibuprofen
Bruising, 1179
Bryant's traction, 517
Buck's extension, 505, 517, 520, 521
Buerger's disease, 701
Buffer systems, 147
Bulbar paralysis, 411
BUN; *see* Blood urea nitrogen
Bundle branch block, 638, 643
Bupivacaine, 317
Bureau of Health Education, 274
Burkitt's lymphoma, 219, 223
Burns, 1128, 1144, 1177
  body image and, 1036

Burns—cont'd
  classification of, 1129, 1134
  coverings and, 1139
  care of, 1136, 1137, 1138-1139
  discharge instructions for patient with, 1142
  diuretic stage of, 1133-1134
  emotional responses to, 1141
  health teaching and, 1129
  hypovolemic stage of, 1130, 1132, 1133
  open therapy for, 1138
  pathophysiology of, 1129-1134
  prehospital emergency care of, 1135-1136
  rehabilitative stage, 1134
  severity of, 1134
  team approach to care of, 1136
  topical medications and, 1138, 1139
Burrow's solution, 1113
Bursa of Fabricus, 75
Bursae, 482
Bursitis, 500
Busulfan, 243, 247
Butazolidin; *see* Phenylbutazone
Butylated hydroxyanisole, 222
Butyrophenones, Parkinson's disease and, 396
Bypass graft, 705
Byssinosis, 574

C

C fibers, 175, 177, 186
C polysaccharide, 70
C-reactive protein, 70
Cachexia, 230
Caffeine
  migraine and, 366
  sexual function and, 1036
Caged-ball valves, 686
Calan, 1201
Calcimar; *see* Calcitonin salmon
Calcitonin, 1215
Calcitonin salmon, 819
Calcium, 87, 135, 145-146, 1211, 1214
  antagonists, 669
  in blood, 145
  normal values, 949
  serum levels, 145
  young adults and, 50
Calcium carbonate, 912
Calcium channel blockers
  angina and, 655
  shock and, 170
Calcium chloride, 1173, 1201
Calcium-phosphate metabolism, 943
Caldwell-Luc surgery, 531
Calistin, nephritis and, 961
Callus, 509, 511, 1119
Calmette-Guérin vaccine, 563-564
Calor, 72
Caloric test, 477
Caloric intake
  alcohol and, 121
  cancer and, 219
Can Surmount, 227
Canal of Schlemm, 436, 437
Cancer, 211-257; *see also* Carcinoma; Neoplasia
  advanced, 254-255
  attitudes about, 212, 226
  of breast, 1092-1101
  checkups, guidelines for, 224-225
  chronic irritation and, 219, 220
  common sites of, 212-214, 225
  community services and, 227, 228
  coping skills and, 229

Cancer—cont'd
  data analysis and planning and, 232, 233-235
  diagnostic studies for, 230, 231
  early detection and treatment of, 224-225
  environment and, 220
  epidemiology of, 212-214
  etiology of, 218-224
  female reproductive tract and, 1068-1073
  of gastrointestinal tract, 920-938
  genetic factors and, 218-219
  geographic factors and, 213
  grading of, 218
  health practices and, 219, 221-223
  home care and, 253-254
  hormones and, 219, 220
  host susceptibility and, 218-219
  immunology and, 82, 219, 220
  immunotherapy and, 249-250
  interdisciplinary approach to, 253
  of lung, 576-592
  of male reproductive tract, 1075-1078
  pain and, 183, 250-252
  pathophysiology of, 214-218
  patient knowledge of diagnosis and, 228-229
  prevention and health education, 224-228
  psychologic response to, 229, 230
  psychologic support and, 252
  psychosocial factors and, 219, 223
  respiratory failure and, 612
  spread of, 216-217
  staging of, 218
  surveillance of, 78
  teaching and, 255
  of testicle, 225
  warning signals of, 225
  weight loss and, 225
Cancer Call PAC, 228
Cancer Care, Inc., 228
Cancer Clinical Research Centers, 227
Cancer Information Service, 227
Cancer Prevention Study II, 222
Cancer quackery, 226
Cancer registries, 225
Candida albicans, 201, 1057
  burns and, 1138
  nosocomial infection and, 201
  oral chemotherapy and, 246
  stoma, 933
Candidiasis, 1078, 1109
Canker sore, 894
Cannabis, 125, 126
Cantharis, 1036
Cantor tube, 891
Capillaries, 693
  dynamics of, 140-141
  Starling's law of, 140, 141
Capreomycin, 463, 566
Carbacel; *see* Carbachol
Carbachol, 456
Carbamazepine, 389, 412, 424
Carbetapentane citrate, 553
Carbidopalevodopa, 397
Carbocaine, 317
Carbohydrates, 87
  metabolism of, 833, 834
Carbon dioxide narcosis, 150, 613
Carbon tetrachloride, 843
  nephritis and, 961
Carbonic acid, 147
  deficit/excess, 150
Carbonic anhydrase inhibitors, 456
Carbuncle, 1108

Carcinoembryonic antigen, 82, 927
Carcinogenesis, 218-224, 1219
Carcinoma
  basal cell, 1119
  squamous cell, 1119, 1120
  term of, 218
Cardiac activation, 628; *see also* Cardiovascular
    system; Heart
Cardiac arrest, 1173; *see also* Cardiopulmonary
    resuscitation
Cardiac arrhythmias, 632-650
  postoperative, 328
Cardiac catheterization, 684
Cardiac cirrhosis, 845
Cardiac complex, 633, 634
Cardiac cycle, 628, 630
Cardiac index, 1195
Cardiac massage, 1172
Cardiac monitoring, 635, 1194
Cardiac muscle, 482
Cardiac output, 630-632, 1195
Cardiac rhythm, 635-639
Cardiac sphincter, 876
Cardiac tamponade, 676, 1181
Cardiac toxicity, chemotherapy and, 249
Cardiogenic shock, 158, 159, 663-665
Cardiopulmonary bypass, 659-663
Cardiopulmonary problems
    special, 1173-1174
    trauma and, 1169
Cardiopulmonary resuscitation, 165, 1170-
    1173
Cardiovascular system
    age and, 54
    critically ill patient and, 1200-1202
    digitalis toxicity and, 670
    disorders of, 650-690
    drugs and, 1201
    obesity and, 87
    problems of, 626-692
    renal failure and, 1002
    sexuality and, 1033, 1034
    shock and, 163
    syphilis and, 675, 677
Cardioversion, 639, 649
Cardrase; *see* Ethoxzolamide
Carmustine, 247
Carotinoids, 1211
Carotid vessels, 355
    endarterectomy and, 405
Carpal tunnel syndrome, 501-502
Carpopedal spasm, 145, 817
Carriers, 67, 136
Cartilage, 481
Cartridge inhalator, 606
Caseation, 562
Casts
    bivalved, 516
    care of patient with, 514-517
Castration, 1034
CAT scan; *see* Computed tomography
Catabolism, 86, 143
Catapres; *see* Clonidine
Cataract glasses, 452
Cataracts, 451-453
    diabetes mellitus and, 768
Catecholamines, 170, 1214
    excess of, 809, 810
    heart failure and, 669
Catheters
    Broviac, 96
    central venous, 165
    Condi, 979, 980

Catheters—cont'd
    distal lumen, 658
    Hickman, 96, 244, 245
    intermittent use of, 985-986
    nosocomial infection and, 202, 203
    pulmonary artery, 165, 166
    urinary, 167, 979-982
Cations, 135
Cauda equina, 417
Caudate nucleus, 354
Causalgia, 180, 367
Cavitary disease, 562
CDC; *see* Centers for Disease Control
CEA; *see* Carcinoembryonic antigen
Cedilanid; *see* Lanotoside C
Cedilanid-D; *see* Deslanoside
Cefamandole, 559
Cefazolin, 559
Cell body, 352
Cell-mediated immunity, 74
Cell-mediated response, 78
Cell membrane, 352
Cells
    fibrotic, 73
    growth of, 242
    immune response system and, 75-76
    malignant, characteristics of, 214-216
    phagocytic, 68
Cellular dehydration, 139
Cellular exudate, 72
Cellular immune response, 249
Cellular starvation, 765
Cellulitis, 73, 1108
Center for Health Promotion, 274
Centers for Disease Control, 190
    hepatitis guidelines and, 838
Central cord syndrome, 417
Central nervous system, 354-356
    depressants and, 125, 126
    disorders of, sexuality and, 1033
    drugs, hypertension and, 723-724
    ether anesthesia and, 318
    hypoglycemia and, 778
    pathways of, urinary incontinence and, 988,
        989
    stimulants and, 125, 126
Central venous catheters, 165
Central venous pressure
    anesthesia and, 322
    hypovolemia and, 595
    measurement of, 165
    shock and, 165
Centrilobular emphysema, 600
Cephalosporins, 559
Cephalothin, 559
Cerebellum, 355, 357
Cerebral arteriography, 402
Cerebral arterioles, rupture of, 406
Cerebral clouding, 988
Cerebral embolus, 401
Cerebral hemorrhage, 406
Cerebral hypoxia, 167
Cerebral perfusion, 54
Cerebral thrombosis, 401
Cerebrospinal fluid, 134
    characteristics of, 356
    laboratory values of, 1216
Cerebrovascular accident
    assessment of, 402-403
    causes of, 400-401
    data analysis and planning and, 403-404
    expected outcomes in, 404
    eye manifestations of, 442

Cerebrovascular accident—cont'd
    implementation and, 404-406
    interventions in, 405
    motor function and, 405
    nursing diagnoses in, 403-404
    pathophysiology of, 400-402
    sexuality and, 1033
    surgery and, 405
    symptoms of, 403
Cerebrum, 354-355
Ceruloplasmin, 1211
Cerumen, 462
Cervical dysplasia, 219
Cervical injury, 420
Cervical spine, 504
Cervicitis, 1057, 1058, 1078
    vaginal discharge and, 1059
Cervix
    biopsy of, 1066
    cancer of, 1045, 1069
        incidence of, 223
    cauterization of, 1060
    conization of, 1066
    polyps of, 1065, 1066
Cesium, 137, 239
CFS; *see* Cancer family syndrome
Chalazion, 445
Challenging dose, 1152
Chambers of heart, 628
Chancroid, 1078
Chapparel chamomile, 1060
Charcot's joint, 412
Chemical immunosuppressive agents,
    83
Chemical mediators, asthma and, 609
Chemical pollutants, cancer and, 219, 221
Chemosurgery, 1120-1121
Chemotaxis, 69
Chemotherapeutic agents, 242-244
    leukemia and, 750
    methods of administration of, 244-246
Chemotherapy
    adjuvant, 242
    benefits of, 241-242
    cancer and, 241-249
    combination, 244
    female reproductive tract and, 1073
    dose calculation for, 244
    induction, 750-751
    intracranial tumor and, 432
    intravenous, 244
    leukemia and, 750-751
    nursing care of patients with, 248
    oral, 244
    pathologic principles of, 242
    side effects of, 246-249
Chemstrip bG, 784
Chemodeoxycholic acid, 865
Chest
    anterior, respiratory pattern of, 31
    emergency assessment of, 1167
    percussion of, 603-604, 605
    radiographs of
        angina and, 654
        valvular heart disease and, 682
    surgery of; *see* Thoracic surgery
    trauma to, 592-595
    wounds of, 1181
        penetrating, 594-595
        pneumothorax and, 595
Chest tubes
    ambulation with, 590
    lung surgery and, 586-588

Chest tubes—cont'd
  removal of, 590
  resectional surgery and, 582
  stripping of, 586-588
Chest wall injury, 1180
Chewing gum, thirst and, 156
Cheyne-Stokes respiration, 374, 666-667
Chickenpox; *see* Herpes zoster
Chin lift, asphyxia and, 1171
Chlamydia, 1057
Chlophedianol hydrochloride, 553
Chloral hydrate, 301
Chlorambucil, 243, 750
Chloramphenicol, 83, 450, 463, 559, 733
Chlordiazepoxide, 123, 124, 1035
Chloride, 87, 135, 1211, 1216
  normal values of, 949, 1211
Chloromycetin; *see* Chloramphenicol
Chloroptic; *see* Chloramphenicol
Chloroquine, 463, 494
Chlorothiazide, 89, 671, 723
  fluid and electrolyte balance and, 154
Chlorpheniramine, 1035
Chlorprocaine, 317
Chlorpromazine, 301, 802, 843, 1035
Chlorpropamide, 777
Chlorprothixene, 1035
Chlorthalidone, 723
Chlor-Trimeton; *see* Chlorpheniramine,
  1035
Chocolate cysts, 1065
Cholangiocellular tumors, 840
Cholangiography, 863
Cholangitis, 864
Cholecystectomy, 865
Cholecystitis, 861-862
Cholecystography, 863
Cholecystogastrostomy, 865
Cholecystokinin, 834
Cholecystokinin-pancreozymin, 835
Cholecystostomy, 865
Cholecystyramine resin, 855
Choledochoduodenostomy, 865
Choledochojejunostomy, 865
Choledocholithotomy, 865
Choledochtomy, 865
Cholelithiasis, 861, 862
Cholera vaccine, 81
Cholesterol, 52, 1212
  atherosclerosis and, 87-88
  coronary artery disease and, 651
  serum levels, 826
Cholesterol esters, 1212
Choline salicylates, 493
Cholinergic drugs, multiple sclerosis and, 395
Cholinesterase, 1211
Cholinesterase inhibitors, 456
Chondroma, 217
Chondrosarcoma, 217
Chordae tendineae, 628, 679
Chordee, 956
Choriocarcinoma, 217
Choroid, 436, 437
p-Chorophenylalanine, 1036
Chromium, 87
  cancer and, 219, 221
Chromophobic adenoma, 798
Chromosomal abnormalities, cancer and, 219
Chronic illness, 258-276
Chronic infection, nosebleeds and, 534
Chronic obstructive pulmonary disease, 297,
  595-612
  incidence of, 596

Chronically ill, special needs of, 263-265
Chronologic age, 54
Chronotropic effects, 170
Chvostek's sign, 146, 817
Chyme, 835, 877
Cigarette drain, 332
Cigarette smoking
  bladder cancer and, 975
  cardiopulmonary system and, 548
  coronary artery disease and, 651
  lung cancer and, 577
Cilia, 544
Ciliary body, 437
Cimetidine, 416, 910
Circle of Willis, 406
CircOlectric bed, 186, 513, 970
Circulating antibodies, 70
Circulating nurse, 306
Circulation
  brain and, 355-356
  compromise of, 697
  fluid and electrolyte balance and, 154
  interference with, 546, 547
  postoperative, 328
  assessment of, 330, 331
    pathophysiology of, 340
  preoperative
    assessment of, 295
    tests and, 295
Circumcision, penile cancer and, 223
Circumflex coronary artery, 628
Cirrhosis, 845-847
  liver and, 122, 836, 844
  sexual dysfunction and, 1034
  types of, 845
Cis-platinum, 247
Cisternal puncture, 364
Civilian triage, 1187
Clapping, 603-604, 605
Climacteric; *see* Menopause
Clindamycin, 559, 560
Clinical laboratory tests, cancer and,
  231
Clinical unit, admission to, 329-334
*Clinician's Dictionary Guide to Bacteria and
  Fungi*, 196
Clinistix, 763, 765, 785
Clinitest, 763, 785
Clinoril; *see* Sulindac
CLL; *see* Leukemia, chronic lymphocytic
Clonazepam, 389
Clones
  lymphocytes and, 77, 78
  selection theory and, 80
Clonic convulsion, 387
Clonidine, 724
Clonopin; *see* Clonazepam
Clonus, 379
Closed drainage, 980
Closed fracture, 511
Closed-loop insulin delivery, 776
Closed manipulation of fracture, 514-517
Closed therapy for burns, 1138
Closed wounds, 1179
Closer Look National Information Center for
  the Handicapped, 273
Clostridium botulinum, 201
  food poisoning and, 1176, 1177
Clostridium tetani, 1181
Clot formation, vitamins and, 87
Clot retraction, 1218
Clothing, restrictive, cancer and, 219, 220
Clotrimazole, 1059

Clotting; *see* Blood coagulation
Clotting time, 743
Cloxacillin, 89
Cluster headache, 360
  medications for, 366
CMI; *see* Cell-mediated immunity
CML; *see* Leukemia, chronic myelogenous
CNS; *see* Central nervous system
Coagulation; *see* Blood coagulation
Coal miner's pneumoconiosis, 571
Coal tars, 1112
  cancer and, 219, 220
Cobalt 60, 239
Cobra venom, 424
Cocaine, 125, 317
  sexual dysfunction and, 1036
Coccidioidoides immitis, 569
Coccidioidomycosis, 567, 568, 569
Cochlea, 460
Codeine, 553
  headache and, 366
Cogentin; *see* Benztropine mesylate
Cognition, elderly and, 56
Coitus, pain with, 1038
Colace; *see* Docusate sodium
Colchicine, 508, 733
Cold
  injuries from, 1178
  musculoskeletal disorders and, 485
Cold packs, headache and, 366
Cold sore; *see* Herpes simplex
Cold turkey, 127
Coliform bacteria, vaginitis and, 1057
Colitis, ulcerative, 1158
Collagen, 336
Colloid osmotic pressure, 136, 140, 141
Colloids, 1113
  shock and, 168
Colly-Seal, 935
Colon; *see* Intestines
Colonization, 191
Colonoscopy, 901
Colostomy, 931, 932
  ascending, 932
  closure of, 938
  irrigation of, 934-936
  outcome criteria and, 41
Colporrhaphy, 1064
Colpostat, 1072
Coma
  cerebral edema and, 142
  hyperglycemic, 765-766
Comfort
  elderly and, 58
  postoperative, 329, 330, 345-346
  preoperative assessment of, 295, 296
  shock and, 171
Comminuted fracture, 511
Commission on Chronic Illness, 259, 270
Committee on Infectious Diseases of the
  American Academy of Pediatrics,
  197
Common cold, 530, 549
Common pneumonia, 559
Communication
  anxiety and, 115
  hearing impaired and, 471, 472
  in operating room, 305, 306
  therapeutic, 1039
Community
  accident prevention   1164
  disasters and, 1186
  emergency care in,

Community—cont'd
infection control in, 196-199
residential, drug abusers and, 127
Community health nurse, infection control and, 196
Community resources
alcoholics and, 124
blind and, 444
chronic illness and, 272, 273-274
elderly and, 56
Compazine; see Prochlorperazine
Compensation, acid-base balance and, 148
Complement, 70
hemolytic, 1219
Complement cascade, 70
Complete blood count, 1217
Complete cord injury, 417
Complete fracture, 511
Compliance, 262
Composite resection, 541
Compound fracture, 511
of skull, 413
Compression pump therapy, 606
Computed tomography
brain tumor and, 429
cancer and, 231
diagnosis of infection and, 195
headache and, 362
renal tumor and, 974
of urinary tract, 953
Concentration, pain control and, 185
The Concern for Dying, 227
Concussion, 413
Condé catheter, 979, 980
Conduction system of heart, 628, 629, 630
Conductive hearing loss, 465
Cones of retina, 436
Confidant nurse as, 283-284
Confusion, digitalis and, 670
Congenital defects, 451
Congestive heart failure; see Heart failure, congestive
Conization of cervix, 1066
Conjunctiva, 437
examination of, 29
redness of, 442
Conjunctivitis, 445
Consciousness
ether anesthesia and, 318
level of
assessment of, 1167-1168
intracranial pressure and, 372, 373
postoperative assessment of, 331
Constipation, 881
cerebrovascular accident and, 404
drug abuse and, 127
elderly and, 58
fluid intake and, 142
postoperative, 344
Contact dermatitis, 1110, 1114-1115
Contact isolation, 205
Contact lenses, 439
cataract surgery and, 452
extended wear, 440
gas-permeable, 440
Contamination, 191
Continent ileostomy, 902, 903
Continuing care
chronic illness and, 269-272
patterns and facilities for, 270-272
Continuous ambulatory peritoneal dialysis, 1020

Contraception, 1052
oral; see Oral contraceptives
Contractility, 631
Contractures, burns and, 1140
Contusion, 1179
of brain, 413
Conus medullaris syndrome, 417
Convulsions
craniocerebral trauma and, 415
edema of cerebral tissues and, 142
Cooling blanket, 321
Coombs' test, 739
Coordination, 32-33
aging and, 37
COPD; see Chronic obstructive pulmonary disease
Coping, 109-112
colostomy and, 937-938
problem solving and, 111
strategies for, 109
visual loss and, 443
Copper, 87, 1211, 1214
Coproporphyrin, 1214
Cord injury; see Spinal cord injury
Cordotomy, 371
pain control and, 184, 185
Corgard; see Nadolol
Cornea, 436, 437
examination of, 29
graft of, 488-450
ulcer and, 445
Corneal reflex, anesthesia and, 318
Corns, 1119
Coronary arteries, 628, 629
blood supply to, obstruction of, 650
bypass surgery of, 659-663
disease of
cholesterol and, 87
family history and, 651
risk factors for, 650-652
Corpus of uterus, 1045
Corrective lenses, cataract surgery and, 452-453
Corrective shoes, 486
Corsets, spinal cord trauma and, 422
Cortagen; see Cortisone acetate
Cortef; see Hydrocortisone
Cortex
lesions of, urinary incontinence and, 988-989
resection of, seizures and, 389
Cortone; see Cortisone acetate
Corticospinal tracts, 357
Corticosteroids, 83, 88
adrenal, spinal cord edema and, 421
chronic obstructive pulmonary disease and, 607
delerium tremens and, 124
intracranial pressure and, 375
multiple sclerosis and, 395
potencies of, 810
Corticotropin-releasing factor, 108
Cortisol, 1215
deficiency of, 809
excess of, 808-810
replacement of, 804
Cortisone acetate, 810
Cortisone suppression test, 801
Coryza, 530
Cosmegan; see Dactinomycin
Cosmetic surgery, 292, 1125-1127

Cough
adult respiratory distress syndrome and, 166
congestive heart failure and, 667
lung surgery and, 585
medications for, 553
persistent, 552
Cough reflex, 552
ether anesthesia and, 318
Cough syrup, 125
Coumadin, 704
Council on Mental Health of American Medical Association, 127
Counseling
of newly blind, 443
surgery and, 298-299
Counterirritants, pain relief and, 182
Counterpositioning, 381
Counterpressure wrappings, 1139
Coxsackie virus B, diabetes mellitus and, 762
Cranberry juice, urinary tract infection and, 395
Cranial nerves
assessment of, 359
I, 359
II, 359, 437
III, 359
IV, 359
V, 359, 368, 460
VI, 359
VII, 359, 411
VIII, 359, 461
IX, 359, 411
X, 359, 411, 460
XI, 359
XII, 359
Craniectomy, 431
Craniocerebral trauma, 413-417
Cranioplasty, 431
Craniotomy, 431
Creams, 111, 1112
Creatine, 135, 1211, 1214
Creatine phosphokinase, 1211
myocardial infarction and, 657
Crede method, 990
Crepitus, 492
Crescendo angina, 653
Cretinism, 821, 822
CRF; see Corticotropin-releasing factor
Cricoid cartilage, 529
Cricothyroid ligament, 529
Crisis intervention, 116
Critical care nursing, 1189-1208
Critical care unit, 1191-1208
Critical illness, interventions in, 1199-1207
Crohn's disease, 897, 898-899
Crutch walking, 710-711
Crutchfield tongs, 420
Cryoextraction, cataract and, 452
Cryoprecipitate, 746, 1154
Cryoprecipitate proteins, 1219
Cryosurgery, 456, 477, 1121
Cryptorchidism, 1055
Crystalline zinc insulin, 774
Crystalloid solutions, shock and, 168
Crystodigin; see Digitoxin
CT scan; see Computed tomography
Cuemid; see Cholestryramine resin
Cul-de-sac of Douglas, 1045
Culdoscopy, 1053, 1071
Culposcopy, 1071
Culpotomy, 1053

Culture(s)
  chronic illness and, 261
  in diagnosis of infection, 195
  sexual expression and, 1031
Cuprimine; *see* Pencillamine
Curative surgery, 292
Curet, 1120, 1121
Curettage, skin tumors and, 1120
Cushing's disease, 807, 814
  sexual dysfunction and, 1034
Cutaneous nerves, pain control and, 186
CVA; *see* Cerebrovascular accident
CVP; *see* Central venous pressure
Cyanosis, 27
Cyclamates, cancer and, 219, 221
Cyclandelate, 704
Cyclogyl; *see* Cyclopentolate
Cyclopentolate, 449
Cyclophosphamide, 83, 84, 243, 247, 750,
    1022
Cycloplegic agents, 449
Cyclopropane, 317, 319
Cycloserine, 566
Cyclospasmol; *see* Cyclandelate
Cyclosporin A, 84
Cyclosporine, 83, 84
Cyclothiazide, 723
Cyproterone acetate, 1035
Cystectomy, 975
Cystic medicinal necrosis, aortic aneurysm
    and, 687
Cystine, 87, 1214
Cystitis, 959
  bladder tumor and, 975
Cystocele, 1061, 1062
Cystography, 952
Cystometrography, 395, 949
Cystoscopy, 951, 952
  bladder tumors and, 975
Cystostomy, 973
Cytarabine, 243, 247, 750
Cytoid bodies, 497
Cytology, cancer and, 231
Cytomegalovirus, 1078
Cytomel; *see* Liothyronine sodium
Cytoreduction, 751
Cytosar; *see* Cytarabine
Cytoxan; *see* Cyclophosphamide
Cytotoxic drugs; *see also* specific agent
  hypersensitivities to, 1155-1157
  side effects of, 246-249

D

D and C; *see* Dilation and curettage
Da Nang lung, 161, 575
Dacarbazine, 247
Dacron graft, 705, 711
Dactinomycin, 243, 247
Daily dietary allowances, 1224-1227
  growth and, 1226
  pregnancy/lactation and, 1226
Daily food guide, 90, 92
Daily weight record, 152-153
Dalmane; *see* Flurazepam hydrochloride
Dandruff, 1115
Dantrium; *see* Dantrolene sodium
Dantrolene sodium, 381, 395
Daranide; *see* Dichlorphenamide
Darvon; *see* Propoxyphene
Data
  analysis of, 13-14
    emergency and, 1167-1170

Data—cont'd
  analysis of—cont'd
    nursing practice and, 10
    and planning, cancer and, 232, 233-235
  collection of, 11, 12, 13
    emergency and 1166, 1167
    methods of, 42
Datril; *see* Acetaminophen
Daunomycin, 243, 247
Daunorubicin; *see* Daunomycin
Day care centers, chronic illness and, 271
Deafness; *see* Hearing, impaired
Death
  accidents and, 50, 52
  alcohol-related, 120
  attitudes toward, 280
  and dying
    dimensions of, 286-288
    fantasies of, cancer and, 229-230
  good/bad, 279-280
  premature, age and, 278
  prolonged, 278
Debrox; *see* Hydrogen peroxide in glyceryl
Decadron; *see* Dexamethasone
Decamethonium bromide, 320
Decerebrate rigidity, 374
Decortication, 580, 582
Decubitus ulcers, prevention of, 512
Deep breathing
  lung surgery and, 585
  postoperative, 341
Defense mechanisms, 117-119
  biologic, 62-84
  external, 64
  external nonspecific, 64-67
  internal, 64
  internal nonspecific, 67-73
  scope of, 63
  specific, 73-81
Defibrillation, 639, 648-649
Degenerative disease
  of joints, 490, 502-503
    of spine, 504-505
  neurologic, 393-400
  sexual dysfunction and, 1034
Dehydration
  burns and, 1130
  cellular, 139
  diabetic ketoacidosis and, 767
  signs of, 765
Delayed healing/union of bone, 509
Delirium tremens, 123-124
Deltasone; *see* Prednisone
Demecarium bromide, 456
Dementia, presenile, 56
Demerol; *see* Meperidine hydrochloride
Dendrites, 352
Denial
  death and, 280
  stress and, 118-119
Denver shunt, 857
Dental prosthesis, 538
Dentures, 57
11-Deoxycortisol, 1215
Deoxyribonucleic acid, 215, 216
Depakene; *see* Valproic acid
Dependency, 119-120
  alcohol/drugs and, 123
Depolarization, 353
  action potentials and, 628
Depo-Medrol; *see* Methylprednisolone
Depoprovera; *see* Progestins

Depressants, 89
Depression
  behavior and, 119
  cancer and, 219
  clinical signs of, 119
  elderly and, 56
  interventions in, 119
Dermabrasion, 1125, 1126
Dermatitis, 1114-1116
Dermatitis medicamentosa, 1118-1119
Dermatology; *see* Skin
Dermatomyositis; *see* Polymyositis
Dermatophytoses, 1109, 1110
Dermis, 1105; *see also* Skin
DES; *see* Diethylstilbestrol
Desensitization, 1153
  systematic, 110
Deserpidine, 723
Desipramine, 1035
Deslanoside, 670, 671
Desoxycorticosterone, 810
Desoxyribonuclease, 553
Detoxification, 834
Development
  emotional
    elderly and, 55
    middle age and, 51-52
    young adults and, 49
  intellectual, 49
    middle age and, 51
  physical
    elderly and, 54
    young adults and, 48
  psychosocial
    elderly and, 55
    middle age and, 51
    young adults and, 48
Deviated septum, 534, 535
Dexamethasone, 395, 404, 415, 450, 810,
    1215
  intracranial pressure and, 375
Dextran, 155, 168
Dextromethorphan hydrobromide, 553
Dextrose, 135
  in Ringer's lactate solution, 155
  in saline solution, 155, 156
  in water, 155, 156
DFP; *see* Isofluorophate
Diabetes insipidus, 805-806
  dehydration and, 139
  pituitary surgery and, 804
Diabetes mellitus, 759-790
  autoimmunity and, 762
  blood tests for, 764
  cataract and, 451
  classification of, 760, 761-762
  control of, illness and, 786
  coronary artery disease and, 651
  detection of, 764-765
  education and, 781-788
  eye manifestations of, 442
  foot care and, 787
  gestational, 760, 761-762
  hygiene and, 786-787
  insulin-dependent, 760, 761
  microvascular changes and, 767-768
  neuropathy and, 768-769
  obesity and, 87
  perioperative management of, 780
  primary prevention of, 762
  psychologic adjustment to, 786
  risk factors for, 762

Diabetes mellitus—cont'd
  self-care and, 787
  sexual dysfunction and, 1034
  treatment of, 780-781
  visual impairment and, 783-784
Diabetic ketoacidosis, 765-767
  correction of, 779-780
  hypermagnesemia in, 147
Diabetic nephropathy, 968
Diabetic retinopathy, 442, 768
Diabinase; see Chlorpropamide
Diagnosis of cancer, patient knowledge of, 228-229
Diagnosis, nursing, 14
Diagnosis Related Groups, 270
Diagnostic surgery, 292
Diagnostic tests
  elderly and, 59
  intracranial pressure and, 375
Dialysis
  peritoneal, 1016-1020
    continuous ambulatory, 1020
  physiologic imbalance and, 1013-1015
  principles of, 1011-1020
Diamond fraise, 1125, 1126
Diamox; see Acetazolamide
Dianabol; see Methandrostenolone
Diaphoresis, 152, 154
Diarrhea, 882
  as defense mechanism, 66
  dehydration and, 139
  digitalis and, 670
Diarthroses, 482
Diastix, 763, 765, 785
Diastole, 630
Diathermy, 456
Diazepam, 320, 381, 389, 390, 395, 576, 579, 951, 1035
  neurologic pain and, 371
  tension headache and, 366
Diazoxide, 724
Dibenamine, 704
Dibenzyline; see Phenoxybenamine
Dibucaine, 317, 422
DIC; see Disseminated intravascular coagulation
Dichlorphenamide, 456
Dicoumarol, 704
Diencephalon, 355
Diet
  cancer and, 219, 222
  delerium tremens and, 124
  high-caloric, high-vitamin, 124
  history, assessment of, 91
  lactovegetarian, 92
  modification of, 92-93
  peptic ulcer and, 911
  planning, diabetes mellitus and, 771
  preoperative, 297
  requirements of, 771
Dietetic foods, 781-782
Diethylstilbestrol
  cancer and, 219, 221
Differential count, 194
Differential permeability, 352
Diffusion, 136, 545, 583
  dialysis and, 1011, 1012
  facilitated, 136
Digestive system, organs of, 876
Digifortis; see Digitalis
Digiglusin; see Digitalis
Digital subtraction angiography, 403

Digitalis
  confusion and, 670
  chronic obstructive pulmonary disease and, 607
  heart failure and, 670-671
  powdered, 670
  toxicity of, 144, 670
Digitalis lanata, 670
Digitalis purpurea, 670
Digitoxin, 670, 671
  in serum, 1219
Digoxin, 670, 671, 1201
  in serum, 1219
Dihydrostreptomycin, 463
Dilantin; see Phenytoin sodium
Dilation and curettage, 1066
Diltiazem, angina and, 655
Dilution syndrome, 139
Dimenhydrinate, 476
Diphenhydramine, 397, 570, 1035
Diphenoxylate, 897
Diphenoxylate-atropine, 246
Diphtheria, 197
  pertussis and tetanus, 197, 198
Disability, chronic, 261
Discharge
  from eye, 442
  vaginal, 1059
Discharge planning
  postoperative, 348, 662-663
Disaster syndrome, 1187
Disasters, 1185-1188
Discomfort, stress-related, 110
Diseases, 6-9; see also specific disease
  autoimmunity and, 1158
  exacerbation of, 259
  germ theory of, 190
  nutrition and, 86
  pathophysiology of, 7
  remission of, 259
  terminology of, 6
Disengagement, 55
Disequilibrium, dialysis and, 1015
Disopyramide, 639
Dissecting aneurysm, 687
Disseminated intravascular coagulation, 744-748
  shock and, 162, 167
Distraction, pain and, 187
Disulfiram, 124
Ditropan; see Oxybutynin chloride
Diuretics
  alcohol and, 121
  ear and, 463
  fluid and electrolytes and, 154
  heart failure and, 669, 671-672
  hypertension and, 723
  potassium-saving, 154
  sodium and, 142
Diuril; see Chlorothiazide
Diverticulitis, 898, 899
Diverticulosis, 58, 899, 968
Division of Radiological Health, 237
Dizziness, 54
DNA; see Deoxyribonucleic acid
Dobutamine, 169, 669
Dobutrex; see Dobutamine
DOCA; see Desoxycorticosterone
Docusate sodium, 395
Döderlein's bacilli, 1058
Domol, 1113
Domavac; see Desoxyribonuclease

Dolophine; see Methadone hydrochloride
Donor selection
  kidney, 1021
  transfusion and, 1021
L-Dopa, 1036
Dopamine, 169, 669, 1201
Dobutamine, 1173, 1201
Dobutrex; see Dobutamine
Doppler effect, 715
Doriden, 125
Dorsal column stimulators, 183, 184
Dorsalis pedis artery, 694
Double-barrel ostomy, 931
Double vision, 442
Douches, vinegar, 59
Dowager's hump, 483
Doxorubicin, 243, 244, 247, 750, 975
DPT; see Diphtheria, pertussis and tetanus
Drainage; see also Catheters
  duodenal, 1219
  infection control and, 208
  systems, 333
    assessment of, 331
  urologic surgery and, 972-973
Dramamine; see Dimenhydrinate
Draping, 313-314
Dressings, postoperative, 330, 331, 972
Droperidol and fentanyl, 317, 320
Drowsiness, 670
Drug holiday, 398
Drugs
  abuse of, 50, 53, 124-127
  acid unstable, 89
  cardioactive, 1200, 1201
  cell cycle, 242
  dependence on, 183
  glaucoma and, 456
  half-life, 54
  kidneys and, 943
  mind-altering, 125
  peptic ulcers and, 908
  responses to, elderly and, 59
  therapy, shock and, 170
  thrombocytopenia and, 743
  tolerance and, 183
  vasoactive, 1200, 1201
    shock and, 169
Dry drowning, 1174
Dry gangrene, 769
DSA; see Digital subtraction angiography
Duct of Wirsung, 834
Dulcolax; see Bisacodyl
Dumping syndrome, 925-926
Duodenal ulcer, 50, 906, 907, 908
Duplication of ureters, 956
Dupuytren's contracture, 502
Durabolin; see Nandrolone phenpropionate
Dura mater, 356
  trauma and, 413
Dust in the lungs; see Pneumoconioses
Dwarfism, hypopituitary, 800
Dwyer screws, 507
Dying; see also Death and dying
  knowledge of, 283
  Kubler-Ross stages of, 281-282
  nursing care of, 285-287
  person, rights of, 278-279
Dymelor; see Acetohexamide
Dynamic equilibrium, 6
Dyrenium; see Triamterene
Dysesthesia, 376
Dysmenorrhea, 1050-1051

Dyspareunia, 1038, 1061
Dyspepsia, 142
Dysphagia, 139, 885
Dysplasia
    of breast, 1090
    cervical, 219
    of kidneys, 957
Dyspnea, 666
    adult respiratory distress syndrome and, 166
Dysuria, 946

E

Ears
    aging and, 37
    contact dermatitis and, 1115
    examination of, 29
    external, 460
        inflammation of, 473
    inflammations of, 472
    problems of, 460-479
    protectors, 464
Ear drops, 473, 474
Eardrum; see Tympanic membrane
Ear plugs, 464
Ear wax; see Cerumen
Eaton-Lambert syndrome, 391
Eburnation, 503
EBV see Epstein-Barr virus
ECF see Extracellular fluid
ECG see Electrocardiogram
Echography
    cancer and, 231
    heart disease and, 682, 684
Echothiopate iodide, 456
Ectopic arrhythmia, 637, 640-643
    digitalis and, 670
Edecrin; see Ethacrynic acid
Edema, 72, 138, 140-142
    assessment of, 857
    of brain, 414
    of eye, 29
    pitting, 27, 32, 140
    reduction of, 142, 857
    of skin, 27
Ejaculation, 1038
Elase see Fibrinolysin
Elastic cartilage, 481
Elastic stockings, 717
Elavil see Amitriptyline hydrochloride
Elderly
    blood volume and, 142
    health problems of, 55
    home safety for, 1164
    physiologic changes in, 54
    surgery and, 296-297
Electric shock, 649
Electrical injuries, 1174
Electrical microshock, 1202
Electrical stimulators, pain relief and, 183-184
Electrocardiogram, 628, 632-634
    anesthesia and, 322
    angina and, 653
    lead placement in, 635
    paper for, 632
    valvular heart disease and, 682
Electrocochleography, 468
Electrodessication, 1120, 1121
Electroencephalography, 388
    biofeedback and, 185
Electrolytes; see also Fluid and electrolytes
    balance of, 135, 142-147, 943
    burns and, 1137

Electrolytes—cont'd
    craniocerebral trauma and, 415
    movement of, 136
    regulation of, 996, 1003-1004
    replacement of, 135
Electromyography, 379, 380, 477, 499, 949
Elimination
    cancer and, 255
    cerebrovascular accident and, 404
    craniocerebral trauma and, 415-416
    elderly and, 58-59
    multiple sclerosis and, 395
    paralysis and, 381
    preoperative assessment of, 295, 296
    prostatic resection and, 1077
    spinal cord trauma and, 417, 419, 422
EMB; see Ethambutol
Embolectomy, 711
Embolism, 401
Emergencies
    ABCs of assessment in, 1166, 1171
    and disasters, 1161-1188
    legal aspects of care in, 1166
Emergency aid stations, 1187
Emergency medical technicians, 1165
Emerson respirator, 620
Emerson suction machine, 589
Emete-Con; see Benzquinamide
EMG; see Electromyography
Emmetropia, 438
Emphysema, 600-609
    subcutaneous, chest surgery and, 585-586
Empyema, 73, 590, 592
    pneumonia and, 563
Encephalitis, 410, 1108
    postvaccination, 82
End stoma, 931
Endarterectomy, 705, 706, 711
Endocardium, 627
    infection of, 675, 676-677
Endocrine cells, 759, 761
Endocrine system
    functions of, in female, 1045-1047
    disorders of, 796-831
        prevention of, 796
    kidney failure and, 1002
    processes of, 792
Endolymph, 461, 475
Endometrium, 1045
    cancer and, 1069
        tissue sampling in, 224
    implants in, sites of, 1065
    infection of, 1065-1066
        sexual dysfunction and, 1034
    jet washings of, 1070
    vacuum curettage of, 1070
Endorphins, 175, 177
Endoscopic retrograde cholangiopancreatography, 865
Endoscopy, 863, 900, 901
    biliary disorders and, 863
    cancer and, 231
    reproductive tract and, 1070, 1071
Endotracheal intubation, 614, 615, 616
Endrophonium chloride, 391
Enduron; see Methychlothiazide
Enemas
    fluid and electrolyte balance and, 153
    preoperative, 297-298
Energy
    intake of, 1224
    nutrients providing, 86

Energy substrates, shock and, 171
Enflurane, 316
Engstrom respirator, 620
Enhancing antibodies, 82
Entamoeba histolytica, 839
Enteritis, 895
Enterobacter, 201, 553, 960
Enteric precautions, 207
Enterococcus, 201
Environment
    allergies and, 1153
    cancer and, 219
    chronic obstructive pulmonary disease and, 608
    fire prevention and, 1128-1129
    injuries and, 1178-1179
    sexuality and, 1036-1037
Environmental Protection Agency, 220
Enzymes
    digestive, 835
    replacement therapy, 870
Eosinophils, 69, 194
Ephedrine, 612
Epicardium, 627
Epidemic pleurodynia, 549
Epidemiology, 7
    of alcoholism, 120-121
    of cancer, 212-214
    of drug abuse, 124-125
Epidermis, 1105, 1106
Epididymitis, 1073, 1074, 1078
Epidural hematoma, 414
Epiglottis, 529
Epilepsy, 385-390
Epinephrine, 169, 456, 1173, 1201
    asthma and, 612
    functions of, 808
    heart rate and, 639
Epinephrine bitartrate, 456
Epinephryl borate, 456
Epiphyses, 481
Episiotomy, 1033
Epispadias, 956
Epistaxis, 535
Epitrate; see Epinephrine bitartrate
Eppy; see Epinephrine borate
Epstein-Barr virus, 219, 223
Equilibrium, dynamic, 106
Equipment
    cardiac surgery and, 660
    in intensive care unit, 1192
    postoperative assessment of, 330
    unsealed internal radiation and, 240, 241
Erickson's eight ages of man, 48
Ergot preparations, 366
Ergotamine tartrate, 366
Ernst applicator, 240
Erythema, 27
Erythema multiforme, 1119
Erythrocyte sedimentation rate, 1217
Erythrocytes; see Red blood cells
Erythromycin, 89, 559
Erythropheresis, 740
Erythropoietin, 943
Eschar, 1138
Escherichia coli, 201, 839
    pneumonia and, 553
    pyelonephritis and, 966
    urinary tract infection and, 960
Eserine; see Physostigmine
Esidrix; see Hydrochlorothiazide
Esophageal speech, 540

Esophagogastric tamponade, 857
Esophagogastric tube, 857
Esophagogastrostomy, 924
Esophagojejunostomy, 924
Esophagus, 875-876
  cancer and, 921
  dilation of, 887
  disorders of, 883-889
  diverticulum, 883, 884
  strictures of, 884
  surgery and, 887, 889
  tamponade and, 857-859
  ulcers and, 906
  varices and, 847
Essential amino acids, 87
Essential hypertension, 721
Estargel, 1117
Estrogens, 243, 803, 1045, 1047
  cancer and, 220
Ethacrynic acid, 463, 671, 723
  fluid and electrolyte balance and, 154
Ethambutol, 566
Ethanol, 1212
Ether, 317, 318, 319
Ethionamide, 566
Ethmoid sinus, 528
  carcinoma of, 537
Ethmoidectomy, 531
Ethnicity, chronic illness and, 261
Ethosuximide, 389
Ethoxzolamide, 456
Ethrane; *see* Enflurane
Ethyl alcohol; *see* Alcohol
Ethyl aminobenzoate, 102
Ethyl biscoumacetate, 704
Ethylene glycol, 961
Euglobin lysis, 1217
Euglycemia, 759
Eustachian tube, 460, 528
Eustress, 106
Euthroid; *see* Liotrix
Evaluation; *see also* specific diseases
  nursing process and, 10, 18
  postoperative, 305
  quality assurance and, 40
Excisional biopsy, 231
Excitability, 353
Excitement phase of sexual response, 1028,
    1029, 1030
Exercises
  amputation and, 709
  breathing, chronic obstructive pulmonary
    disease and, 602-603
  burns and, 1141
  coronary artery disease and, 652
  health promotion and, 97-100
  hypoglycemia and, 771, 773
  mastectomy and, 1094-1095
  middle age and, 52
  range-of-motion, 30, 484
  types of, 99-100
  weight control and, 93
  young adults and, 50
Exhibitionism, 1031
Exna; *see* Benzthiazide
Exophthalmos, 823
Expectorants, 553
  chronic obstructive pulmonary disease and,
    606
Expiratory reserve volume, 583
Explanations, anxiety and, 115
External beam therapy, 1100

External cardiac compression, 1172
External otitis, 472
External stabilization, paradoxical breathing
    and, 594
External surgery, 291
Extracellular fluid, 134, 139
Extracorporeal cooling, 321
Extradural space, 356
Extraocular movement, 29
Extrapyramidal system, 357
Extremities; *see also* Legs
  aging and, 37
  assessment of, 1167
  examination of, 32-33
Exudates, 134
  fluid, 72
Eye Banks for Sight Restoration, Inc., 449
Eye pads, 447
Eyedrops, 448
Eyeglasses, 439, 440
Eyelids
  contact dermatitis and, 1115
  as defense mechanism, 66
  examination of, 29
Eyes
  aging and, 37
  anatomy of, 436-437
  anterior chamber of, 436, 437
  care of, in elderly, 57
  compresses for, 446
  ether anesthesia and, 318
  examination of, 27, 29
  inflammation of, 446
  injuries of, 441
  irrigation of, 446-447
  medications for, 447-448, 449, 450
  muscles of, 437
  pain and, 442
  problems of, 436-459
  renal failure and, 1005
  safety of, 441
  surgery of, 448-449, 451

F

Face
  contact dermatitis and, 1115
  examination of, 30
Face mask, 555
Facet joint, 503
Factor deficiency, 745; *see also* Blood disorders
Fallopian tubes, inflammation of, 1058
Falls in hospitals, 1165
Familial polyposis of colon, 219
Family
  dimensions of, dying and, 284-285
  postoperative care and, 334
Farmer's lung, 574
Farsightedness; *see* Hyperopia
Fascia, 482
Fasciculations, 377
Fat, 87
  metabolism of, 833, 834
  saturated, middle age and, 52
Fat embolism, 512
Fatigue, 72
  chronic, renal failure and, 1005
  heart failure and, 667
Fatigue fracture, 509, 510
Fatty acids, 1212
  as defense mechanism, 66
Fatty streak, 650
Fears, surgery and, 293

Fecal continence; *see* Elimination; Inconti-
    nence
Fecal diversion, 931-938
Fecal impaction, 881
Federal Food, Drug, and Cosmetic Act, U.S.,
    Delaney amendment to, 222-223
Feelings, anxiety and, 115
Fellatio, 1183
Female reproductive system; *see* Reproductive
    system, female
Femoral artery, 694
Femoral hernia, 920
Femoral pulse, 703
Femoral vein catheterization, 1013, 1014
Femur, 481
  blood supply to, 513
Fenprofen calcium, 182, 493
Fentanyl and droperidol, 301
Ferritin, 1218
Ferrous sulfate, 89
Fertilization, in vitro, 1056-1057
Fetishism, 1031
α-Fetoglobulin, 1219
Fetor hepaticus, 848
FEV; *see* Forced expiratory volume
Fever, 27
  idiopathic, 549
Fever blister, 894, 1108, 1109
Fiber in diet, 87
Fiberoptic bronchoscopy, 579, 713
Fiberoptic catheter, 1196
Fibrillation, 637, 641-643
Fibrin, 70, 72, 509, 511
Fibrinogen, 715, 1217
Fibrinolysin, 704
Fibrinolytic factors, 704-705
Fibroadenoma
  of breast, 1090
  sexual dysfunction and, 1034
Fibrocystic disease of breasts, 1090
Fibroid tumor, 1065, 1066
Fibroma, 217
Fibrosarcoma, 217
Fibrous cartilage, 481
Filiform catheter, 979, 980
Filtration, 136
Finances, chronic illness and, 264
Finger coordination, 32
Fingernails; *see* Nails
Fire safety, 1165
Firearms, hearing loss and, 463, 464
First-degree burns, 1129, 1130
Fishberg concentration test, 950
Fistula
  bronchopleural, 590, 592
  closure of, 711
  draining, 153
Fistulectomy, 1064
Fixed cells, 68
Fixed-rate pacing, 646
Fixed receptors, 795
Flaccid bladder, 989
Flaccidity, 377
Flagyl, 89
Flail chest, 593, 1180
Flammable Fabrics Acts, 1128
Flap grafts, 1123, 1125
Flatulence, 881
Flavobacterium, 557
Flagyl; *see* Metronidazole
Fleet enema, 344
Floaters, 442

Flora, normal, 191
    bacterial, 196
    microbic, 67
Florafur, 247
Florinef; see Fludrocortisone
Floropryl; see Isoflurorophate
Flotation pads, 513
Flow sheet, 17, 18
    for intensive care unit, 1196-1197
Fluorocortisone, 810
Fluid and electrolyte balance, 134-135; see also
        Fluids
    assessment of, 151-153
    compartments in, 134
    electrolyte component of, 135
    elderly and, 54
    hormones and, 136-137
    impairment of, 133-157
        bowel disorders and, 903-904
        burns and, 1137
        coronary artery bypass surgery and, 662
        deficits, 138, 153
        gastrointestinal tract and, 153, 878
        liver disease and, 842
        management of, 153-156
        patient data in, 151, 152
        renal disease and, 997-998, 1103
        shock and, 167
        thirst and, 156
    mechanisms of, 134-137
    postoperative, 329, 343
Fluid lines, postoperative assessment of, 331
Fluid overload, 142
Fluids
    administration of, 156
    carbonate in, 147
    deficits of, 138, 139
        persons at risk for, 153
        shock and, 170
    excesses of, 138, 139-142
    extracellular, 134, 139
    imbalance, gastrointestinal tract and, 153
    intake of, 134, 135, 153
        oral, 155
        record of, 152
    loss of, 134, 139
        prevention of, 154
    movement of, 136
    output, record of, 152-153
    parenteral, 155-156
    pressure of, 140-141
    replacement of, 134, 154-156, 168, 779
    shift of, burns and, 1130, 1132, 1134
    third-spacing of, 141, 167
Fluorine, 87
Fluorometholone, 450
5-Fluorouracil, 243, 247, 975
Fluothane; see Halothane
Flurazepam hydrochloride, 301
Flushed face, 767
Folacin; see Folic acid
Foley catheter, 415, 422, 949
    anchoring of, 980, 981
    prostate surgery and, 977-982
Folic acid, 87, 1218
    alcohol and, 121
    deficiency of, 741
Follicle-stimulating hormone, 792, 1214
Folliculitis, 1108
Food additives, cancer and, 219, 222
Food and Drug Administration, 469
Food exchange system, 771-773

Food poisoning, 896, 1175-1176
Food care, 698
    diabetes mellitus and, 787
Foot drop, 122, 516
Footboard, 485
Food intake
    analysis of, 90
    daily guide for, 90, 92
    excessive, 53
    medications and, 88-89
Forane; see Isoflurane
Forced expiratory volume, 583, 584
Forced vital capacity, 583
Foriegn bodies
    eye and, 442
    nose and, 534
Formula, parenteral, 94
Foster bed, 186, 420, 421, 513
Foster homes, chronic illness and, 271-272
Fototar, 1117
Four-point gait, 485, 710, 712
Fovea, 437
Fowler's position
    asthma and, 612
    chronic obstructive pulmonary disease and,
        607
    heart failure and, 668-669
α-FP; see Alpha-fetoprotein
Fractures
    assessment of, 1182
    of bone, 509-513
    displacement with, 511
    of hip, 510, 513-522
    line of, 511
    management of, 1182
    of ribs, 592-593
    types of, 510, 511
Free grafts, 1123, 1124
Frequency of urination, 945, 946
Fresh-frozen plasma, 746, 1154
Frontal lobe, 354
    tumors of, 427
        sexuality and, 1033
Frontal sinus, 528
Frostbite, 1178
Frozen red cells, 1154
Fructose, 1214
Fruity breath odor, 767
FSH; see Follicle-stimulating hormone
5-FU; see 5-Fluorouracil
Full-thickness grafts, 1123, 1125
Functional residual capacity, 583
Functional splints, 486
Fundus, uterine, 1045
Fungal infection, 567, 568-570
    of skin, 1109-1110, 1114
Fungi, 201
Fungizone; see Amphotericin B
Furadantin; see Nitrofurantoin
Furosemide, 144, 463, 669, 671, 723
    fluid and electrolyte imbalance and, 154
    potassium loss and, 144
Furuncle, 1108
Fusiform aneurysm, 406, 687
Fusion, 503
FVC; see Forced vital capacity

G

G solution, 973
Gag reflex, 318, 885
Gait patterns, 710-712
Gallamine triethiodide, 320

Gallaudet College, 471
Gallbladder, 832, 833, 834
Gallium scan, 195
Gallstones, 836, 862
Gamma globulins, 74, 1147, 1154
    pooled human, 81
Gammopathies, 82, 1146, 1148-1149
Ganglia, 356
Ganglioneuroma, 217
Gantrisin; see Sulfisoxazole
Garamycin; see Gentamicin sulfate
Gardnerella vaginalis, 1057, 1078
GAS; see General adaptation syndrome
Gases
    blood; see Blood gases
    exchange, 544, 545
    movement of, 136
    transport problems, 525, 755
Gastrectomy, 924, 926
Gastric analysis, 909, 1219
Gastric bleeding, 915
Gastric crisis, 412
Gastric drainage, 925
Gastric juice as defense mechanism, 66
Gastric partitioning, 924
Gastric resection, 914
Gastric ulcers, 50, 906, 907
Gastric washings, 565
Gastrin, 835, 1219
Gastritis, 895, 896
Gastroduodenostomy, 924
Gastroenteritis, 895, 896
Gastroesophageal reflux, 883
Gastrointestinal system
    activity of, 877
    aging and, 878
    cancer and, 920-938
    chemotherapy and, 246
    critical illness and, 1203
    digitalis toxicity and, 670
    fluid loss and, 138
        record of, 152
    immobilization and, 513
    immunosuppressive agents and, 1023
    infection and, 194
    inflammatory disorders of, 893-918
    intubation of, 889-893
    liver disease and, 857
    motility of, interference with, 880-883
    problems of, 880-938
    radiation and, 237
    renal disease and, 1002
    secretions of, 134, 138
    shock and, 161, 163
Gastrointestinal tubes, 889-893
Gastrojejunostomy, 924
Gastroscopy, 910
Gastrostomy, 886, 887, 924
Gate control theory of pain, 185
Gated pool blood imaging, 657
Gateway House, 127
Gaviscon, 887
Gelusil, 912
Gender disorders, 1038
Gender identity and role, 1028
General adaptation syndrome, 107
Generality versus stagnation, 51
Genitalia
    diseases of, sexual dysfunction and, 1034
    female, 1044-1047
    herpes and, 1034
    male, 1047, 1048

Genitalia—cont'd
  warts and, 1078, 1081
Genitourinary system; *see* Genitalia; Reproductive system; Urinary system
Gentamicin, 450, 961
Gentian violet, 1060
German measles; *see* Rubella
Gestational diabetes, 760, 761-762
GH; *see* Growth hormone
Ghon tubercle, 562
Gigantism, 799
Gigli saw, 431
Gingival hyperplasia, 389
Gingivitis, 894
Gitalin, 670
Glandular changes, terms of, 795
Glasgow Coma Scale, 372-373, 374
Glaucoma, 453-457; *see also* Interocular pressure
Glaucon; *see* Epinephrine
Glioblastoma multiforme, 217
Glioma, 431
Glipizide, 777
Globa pallidus, 354
Global aphasia, 403
Globin zinc insulin, 774
Globulins
  alpha, 74, 1213
  beta, 74, 1213
  gamma; *see* Gamma globulins
Globulin fraction, 198
Glomerular filtration rate, 942, 1001
Glomerulonephritis, 961-964, 1158
Glomerulosclerosis, 968
Glomerulus, 941, 942
Glossectomy, 922
Glottis, 529
Glucocorticoids, 83, 108, 109, 808
Glucometer, 784
Glucose
  blood, 1214
    fasting, 1212
    hormonal regulation of, 759, 761
  criteria for control of, 784
  synovial fluid, 1220
  tolerance, inpaired, 760, 761
Glucose-6-phosphate dehydrogenase, 739
Glucotrol; *see* Glipizide
Gluteal exercises, 299
Glutethamide, 125
Glyburide, 777
Glycerin, 456, 462
Glycopyrrolate, 1035
Glycosuria, 763, 765
Glycosylation, 784-785
Goal setting, 14, 16
Goblet cells, 544
Goiter, 796, 821
Gold, 239
Gold salts, 494
Goldenseal, 1060
Gomco machine, 892
Gonadotropins, 792, 798, 804
Gonococcal pharyngitis, 529
Gonococci, 1057
Gonorrhea, 1078, 1081-1082
Good Samaritan laws, 1166
Gout, 490, 507-508
Grafts, 1123
Gram-negative rods, 201
Gram stain, 195
Grand mal seizures, 123, 386

Granulation tissue, 336
Granulocytes, 69
Granuloma inguinale, 1078
Graves' disease, 797, 823
Gray matter, 354
Greenstick fracture, 511
Grief
  cancer and, 229
  chronic, 264-265
Group therapy, 266
Growth
  cell population, 242
  and development; *see* Development
  nutrition and, 86, 87
Growth hormone, 792, 1215
  deficits, 797
  excess, 797-799
  suppression of, 802
G-strophanthin; *see* Ouabain
Guaiac test, 900
Guanethidine, 723, 1035
Guillain-Barré-Strohl syndrome, 411-412, 1158
Guilt, cancer and, 229
Gums, 30
Gyne-Lotrimin; *see* Clotrimozole
Gynecologic surgery, 1068

H
Haemophilus influenzae, 553, 554
Hair
  aging and, 37, 1107
  examination of, 29
  loss of, 29
    chemotherapy and, 247, 248
    drugs and, 247
    immunosuppression therapy and, 1023
    radiation and, 238
    renal disease and, 1002
    trauma and, 1122
Half-life, 235, 237
Hallucinogens, 125, 126
Haloperidol, 396
Halos, visual, 442
Halothane, 316, 319, 323
Haptens, 73
Haptoglobin, 1218
Hard lenses, 330
Hard palate, 528
Harmonyl; *see* Deserpidine
Harrington rods, 507
Harrison Narcotic Act, 127
Hashimoto's thyroiditis, 821
Hay fever, 530, 1150, 1151
Hb A$_{lc}$; *see* Hemoglobins
Hb$_s$Ag; *see* Hepatitis B surface antigen
Head
  assessment of, emergency 1167
  examination of, 27, 29-30
  sagittal section of, 793
Head coverings, 309
Head injury, 413, 416
Head lice, 1111
Head tilt, 1171
Headache, 361-367
  assessment of, 361-362
  causes of, 361, 366-367
  cerebral edema and, 142
  digitalis and, 670
  intracranial pressure and, 372
  medications for, 366
  renal failure and, 1005

Headache—cont'd
  spinal anesthesia and, 321
  stress and, 105
  types of, 360, 361
Healing, 73, 87
Health
  adaptive, 4
  adulthood and, 47-61
  behaviors in, 225-226
  definitions of, 4
  elderly and, 55-56
  environment and, 6
  middle age and, 52-53
  patient, 24
  young adulthood and, 49-50
Health care, 3
  costs of, 38
Health goals, national, 274-275
Health history; *see* Nursing history
Health promotion, 4, 85-101
Hearing
  assessment of, 465
  impaired, 464-473
  intensity of, 462
  loss of
    behavior and, 464
    fluctuant, 475, 476
  mechanism of, 462
Hearing aids, 468-470
Hearing threshold, 466
Heart
  aging and, 631-632
  disorders of; *see* Cardiovascular system, disorders of
  enlargement of, 122
  structure of, 626-628
Heart block, 638, 643-644
Heart failure
  acute, 665
  chronic, 665
  congestive
    care of patient with, 672, 673
    cough and, 667
    medications for, 668, 669
    signs and symptoms of, 666, 667
Heart rate, 631
  analysis of, 636
  control of, 631-632
  ether anesthesia and, 318
  pacemakers and, 646
Heart sounds, 31, 34-35
Heartburn, 885, 886
Heat
  injuries from, 1177, 1178
  musculoskeletal disorders and, 485
Heat cramps, 1177, 1178
Heat exhaustion, 1177, 1178
Heavy metals, 961
Height-weight tables, 89
Heimlich maneuver, 1170
Heineke-Mikulicz procedure, 292, 915
Helper T cells, 78
Hemangioma, 217
Hemangiosarcoma, 217
Hematocrit, 729, 1217
Hematogenous pneumonia, 560
Hematologic system; *see also* Blood
  assessment of, 730
  problems of, 728-755
  renal disease and, 1002
  shock and, 163, 167
Hematoma, 414, 509, 511

Hematopoietic system, 728-732
Hematuria, 946
   renal disease and, 971, 974, 975
Hemianopsia, 405, 442
Hemiglossectomy, 922
Hemilaryngectomy, 538
Hemoccult test, 900
Hemoconcentration, 1130, 1133
Hemodynamics, 163, 1194, 1195
Hemodialysis, 1012-1016
   advantages and disadvantages of, 1203
   assessment of, 1009-1010
   care plan for, 1018-1019
   patient care during, 1015-1016
Hemoglobin, 1214, 1217
   A$_{lc}$, 784-785
   disorders of, 738
   interference with, 546
   mean corpuscular, 1217
   normal values of, 729
   studies, 1218
Hemoglobinuria, 1157
Hemogram, 733
Hemolytic anemia, 738-741
Hemophilia, 744, 745-746
Hemoptysis, 579
Hemorrhage, 1174-1175; see also Blood, loss of
   cerebrovascular accident and, 401
   fluid loss and, 138
   peptic ulcer and, 914, 915
   thyroid surgery and, 829
   urologic surgery and, 972
Hemorrhoids, 905, 1034
Hemothorax, 547, 1174, 1180
Hemovac, 333
Heparin, 404, 704
Heparin-hydrocortisone succinate, 404
Hepatic cellular plates, 832
Hepatic coma, 844, 847-848, 860
Hepatic sinusoids, 832
Hepatic stomatitis, 894
Hepatic system, 832-834
Hepatitis, 127, 835-836, 843-845, 1034
Hepatitis A, 837, 838-839
Hepatitis antibodies, 838
Hepatitis antigens, 838
Hepatitis B, 201, 837, 1078
   carriers of, 192
   vaccine, 197-198, 836
Hepatitis B immune globulin, human, 199, 836
Hepatitis B surface antigen, 836
Hepatocellular tumors, 840
Hepatotoxins, 843
Herd immunity, 197
Hereditary spherocytosis, 734
Heredity, cancer and, 219
Hermaphroditism, 1038
Hernia, 920, 1033
Herniorrhaphy, 920
Heroin, 125, 1036
Herpes genitalis, 1078, 1081
Herpes simplex, 425, 894, 1057, 1108, 1109
Herpes zoster, 412, 1108, 1109
Herpesvirus, 201, 1057
Herpesvirus hominis, 219, 223, 1083
HES; see Hydroxyethyl starch
Hesitancy of urination, 945-946
Heterograft, 1123
Heterosexuality, 1031
Hexamethonium chloride, 422
Hexamethylmelamine, 247

Hexocyclium, 1035
Hiatal hernia, 884, 885
Hiccoughs, 374, 375
Hickman catheter, 244, 245, 751
High-density lipoproteins, 651
High-intensity music, hearing loss and, 463, 464
Hip, fracture of, 510, 514, 1182
Hip joint, 513
Hip prostheses, 495
Hip replacement, 496-497
Hip spica cast, 514
Histamine, 72, 609, 746, 813, 1151
Histocompatibility antigens, 83, 1155
Histiocytes, 68
Histologic grading, 218
Histoplasma capsulatum, 569
Histoplasmosis, 567, 568, 569
Hives, 1150
HLA antigens; see Histocompatibility antigens
Hoarseness, 537
Hodgen splint, 520
Hodgkin's disease, 752, 753-754
Hollihesive, 935
Holter monitor, 653
Homan's sign, 340, 714
Homatropine, 449
Home
   accidents in, 1164
   blood glucose monitoring in, 784
Home care
   chronic illness and, 270-271
   dying and, 284-285
   infectious disease and, 199
Home health aide services, 271
Homemaker services, 271
Homeostasis, 6, 106, 730
Homograft, 711, 1123
Homonymous hemianopsia, 403
Homosexuality, 1031-1032
Hordoleum, 445
Horizon House, 127
Hormones, 108, 109, 137
   activity of, 135, 795
   cancer and, 220, 1078
   fluid and electrolytes and, 136-137
   imbalance, 795, 803-804
   radioimmunoassay of, 801
   regulation of, 795
   replacement of, 803, 804, 816
   surgery and, 293
Horseshoe kidney, 957
Hospices, 253-254
Hospitals
   accident prevention in, 1164-1165
   emergency care in, 1165-1166
   federal narcotics, 127
HSV; see Herpes simplex virus
HSV-2; see *Herpesvirus hominis*
Human chorionic somatomammotropin, 762
Human immune serum, 198, 199
Human insulin, 775
Human leukocyte antigens, 83, 1155
Human needs, 11
Humerus, 481
Humidifiers, 555
Humidity, 306
Humoral immune response, 75, 77-78
Humorsol; see Demecarium bromide
Hyaline cartilage, 481
Hyaloid canal, 437
Hydatiform mole, 217

Hydralazine, 88, 669, 724
Hydration, 557
Hydrocele, 1075
Hydrocephalus, 432
Hydrochloric acid, 877
Hydrochlorothiazide, 671, 723, 973
   fluid and electrolytes and, 154
Hydrocortisone, 810
HydroDiuril; see Hydrochlorothiazide
Hydrogen peroxide in glyceryl, 462
Hydromax; see Quinethazone
Hydronephrosis, 968-969
Hydrostatic pressure, 141
Hydrotherapy, burns and, 1138
Hydroton; see Chlorthalidone
Hydroureter, 956
Hydroxychloroquine, 494
Hydroxyethyl starch, 168
5-Hydroxyindole acetic acid, 1214
Hydroxyurea, 247
Hygiene
   cancer and, 255
   diabetes mellitus and, 786-787
Hyoid bone, 529
Hyoscine; see Scopolamine
Hyoscyamine, 397
Hypaque, 702
Hyperalgesia, 367
Hyperalimentation, 96-97
   nosocomial infection and, 204
Hyperbaric oxygen, 237
Hypercalcemia, 146
Hypercapnia, 150, 615
Hyperemia, 72
Hypergammaglobulinemia, 1148-1149
Hyperglycemia, 765, 770
Hyperkalemia, 144, 145, 149, 996-997
Hyperlipidemia, 651
Hypermagnesemia, 147
Hypernatremia, 143
Hyperopia, 438
Hyperosmolality, 765
Hyperosmolar nonketotic coma, 779-780
Hyperparathyroidism, 817, 818, 819
Hyperpigmentation, 1121-1122
Hyperreflexia, 374
Hypersensitivity, 73, 82
   cell-mediated, 1157-1158
   diseases, 573-574
   type I, 1149, 1150, 1151-1155
   type II, 1150, 1155-1157
   type III, 1150, 1157
   type IV, 1150, 1157-1158
Hyperstar; see Diazoxide
Hypertension
   aortic aneurysm and, 687
   contributory factors to, 944
   coronary artery disease and, 651
   diabetes mellitus and, 768
   nosebleeds and, 534
   obesity and, 87
   stress and, 105
   World Health Organization definition of, 720
Hyperthermia, 383
Hyperthyroidism, 823-824, 827
   stress and, 105
Hypertonic fluid deficit, 138, 139
Hypertrophic arthritis, 502
Hypertrophy, 775
Hyperuricemia, 508
Hyperventilation, 139, 150

Hypesthesia, 501
Hypnosis, 315
  pain control and, 185
Hypoanesthesia, 315
Hypocalcemia, 145
Hypochondriasis, 53
Hypocoagulability, 745
Hypoglycemia, 777-778
  self-treatment of, 785-786
Hypoglycemic drugs, 743
Hypogonadism, 1034
Hypokalemia, 143, 144
  burns and, 1134
Hypomagnesemia, 146, 147
Hyponatremia, 142, 997
Hypoparathyroidism, 817
Hypopharynx, 528, 529
Hypophosphatemia, 779
Hypopigmentation, 1121-1122
Hypopituitarism, 1034
Hypoplasia, 957
Hypoproteinemia, 1130
Hypospadias, 956
  body image and, 1036
Hypostatic pneumonia, 339, 340
Hypotension
  anesthesia and, 321
  induced, 323
  orthostatic, 54
  postoperative, 328
Hypothalamus, 793-794
Hypothermia, 1178
  brain surgery and, 431
  induced, 321, 322
Hypothyroid membrane, 529
Hypothyroidism, 821, 827-828, 1034
Hypotonia, 377
Hypotonic fluid, 137, 138, 139-140
Hypoventilation, postoperative, 327, 340
Hypovitaminosis, 1134
Hypovolemia, 159
  dialysis and, 1013, 1015
  burns and, 1130, 1132
  shock and, 158, 159
Hypoxia, 547
  cerebrovascular accident and, 401
  paradoxical breathing and, 593
  pneumonia and, 563
Hysterectomy, 1066
  body image and, 1036
Hysteroscopy, 1071

I

I Can Cope, 227
Ibuprofen, 182, 493, 1051
Ice, thirst and, 156
ICF; see Intracellular fluid
Icotest, 836
ICRF-159, 247
Idiopathic thrombocytopenic purpura, 743, 744
Idoxuridine, 450
IDU; see Idoxuridine
Ig; see Immunoglobulins
Ileal pouch, 902, 903-904
Iliostomy, 931, 932
Ilidar; see Azapetine
Illness, 5-6
  acute, 259
  behavior in, 7, 119-120
  care in, 85

Illness—cont'd
  chronic, 259, 261-263
    activities of daily living and, 268, 269
    age and, 260
    community resources and, 272, 273-274
    continuing care and, 269-272
    coping and, 262, 264
    culture and, 261
    goals in, 265, 274-275
    independent living centers and, 271
    National Health Survey list of, 259
    occupational therapy and, 264, 268, 269
    outcome criteria in, 272, 274-275
    physical therapy and, 269
    prevention of, 262-263
    psychosocial considerations and, 259-261, 263-265
    rehabilitation and, 265-269
    self-care and, 269
    self-help groups and, 270
    special services and, 265-267
  diabetes and, 786
Imipramine, 1035
Immobility
  cancer and, 255
  problems of, 99, 100, 512-513
Immovable joints, 482
Immune animal serum, 198
Immune complex, hypersensitivities and, 1157
Immune globulins, 198
Immune response, 11, 74-84
  combined, 78
  components of, 249
  elderly and, 55
  heath problems of, 1145-1159
  humoral, 75
  nutrition and, 87
  primary, 76-78, 79
  secondary, 78-79
Immune serum globulin, 198, 836
Immune surveillance, 220
Immune tolerance, 80-81
Immunity
  absolute, 63
  acquired, 64, 65
  artificial, 197
  concept of, 63-64
  innate, 64
  natural, 64
  nonspecific, 64
  specific, 64
    concept of, 73
Immunization, 81
  active, 81, 197-198
  complications of, 82
  contraindications to, 199
  hepatitis and, 836, 838
  nursing responsibilities and, 199
  passive, 81, 197, 198-199
Immunization schedules, 197, 198
Immunodeficiency, 82, 1145-1148
  cancer and, 219
  diagnostic tests for, 1147
  disorders of, 1146
Immunoglobulins, 66, 74, 1147, 1216
  A, 66, 1220
  G, 78, 1220
  M, 78
Immunology
  cancer and, 82
  classification of disorders of, 1146
  problems of, 1145-1159

Immunology—cont'd
  tests and, 1219
Immunosuppression, 82, 751
  chemical agents and, 83
  induced, 1147
Immunotherapy, 249-250, 1153
  cancer and, 219
  side effects of, 1023
Impacted fracture, 511
  of hip, 514
Impedance audiometry, 468
Imperforate hymen, 1033
Impotence, 1037
Impulses, 638-644
Imuran; see Azathioprine
Inactivated vaccines, 196
Incarcerated hernia, 920
Incentive spirometer, 341
Incest, 1031
Incident reports, 43
Incise drape, 315
Incisional biopsy, 231
Incisional hernia, 920
Incisions, 299, 585-586, 1179
Incomplete antigens, 73
Incomplete cord injury, 417
Incomplete fracture, 511
Incontinence, 59, 1064
  cerebrovascular accident and, 404
  fecal, 882-883
  stress, 58
  urinary, 991-992
Incontinence urinal, 992
Incubation period, 191
Incus, 460
Independent living centers, 271
Inderal; see Propranolol
Indocin; see Indomethacin
Indomethacin, 89, 182, 493, 1051
Induction chemotherapy, 750-751
Industrial noise, 463
Infarction, 54, 656
Infection control practitioners, 191
Infection control reports, 44
Infections
  acute, 191
  alcoholism and, 122
  aortic aneurysm and, 687
  apparent, 191
  burns and, 1137-1138
  chain of, 192
  chemotherapy and, 246
  chronic, 191
  community acquired, 199
  control of, 72, 190-210
    community and, 196-199
    immunization and, 196-199
    isolation and, 209
    in operating room, 306, 307-310
  craniocerebral trauma and, 415
  diabetic ketoacidosis and, 767
  diagnostic tests and, 194-196
  generalized, 191, 194
  home care and, 199
  host susceptibility and, 193
  immunodeficiency and, 1147-1148
  inapparent, 191
  latent, 191
  liver and, 842, 856
  localized, 191, 194
  malnutrition and, 87
  nosocomial, 191

Infections—cont'd
  nosocomial—cont'd
    control of, 199-210
      CDC guidelines for, 191
    prevention of, 196
    pulmonary tract and, 549-570
    risk for, 190
    sexual dysfunction and, 1034
    signs and symptoms of, 194
    transmission of, 72, 192, 193
    urinary incontinence and, 988, 989
    white blood cell response to, 195
Infertility, 1052, 1055-1057
  male, 1158
Infiltration anesthesia, 314
Inflammations, 71
  cardiovascular system and, 647-649
  ear and, 472
  eye and, 445-451
  gastrointestinal tract and, 893-918
  musculoskeletal system and, 487-509
  nose and throat and, 529-534
  reproductive tract and, 1057-1061
    drugs and, 1059
    male, 1073-1074
  skin and, 1114
  types of, 72, 73
  urinary system and, 958-968
Inflammatory response, 71-73
Influenza, 549
  immunization and, 197, 198
Information; see Communication; Teaching
Informed consent, 293-294
Infusion pump, 245, 246
Inguinal hernia, 920
INH; see Isoniazid
Inhalation anesthesia, 314, 319-320
Inhalators, 606
Inhibition, hormonal, 793
Injection sites, 314
Injuries
  body response to, 336
  electrical, 1174
  environmental, 1178-1179
  postoperative, 329
  preoperative, 300
  shock and, 171
  tetanus prophylaxis and, 1180, 1181
Inner ear, 460-461
Innovar; see Fentanyl and droperidol
Inotropic agents, heart failure and,
    669
Inotropic effect, 170
Insomnia, 105, 1005
Inspection, physical examination and, 24
Inspiratory capacity, 583
Inspiratory reserve volume, 583
Institute for Sex Research, 1032
Institutional resources, chronic illness and,
    271
Insulin, 759-761, 773-776, 1215
  action of, 760
  administration of, 775
    self-injection of, 783
  deficit, 765, 779
  knowledge, 782-783
  needle guide for, 783
  properties of, 773-775
  resistance to, 774
  storage of, 783
  therapy, 779
Insulin pumps, 776

Insulin-dependent diabetes mellitus; see Diabetes mellitus, insulin-dependent
Insulinoma, 868
Integrity versus disgust, 55
Integument; see Skin
Intellectual development, 49
Intensive care unit, 1191-1193
  equipment in, 1192
  stressors in, 1193
  transfer from, 1205-1206
Interaction, antigen-antibody, 74
Intercourse, discomfort during, 51
Interferon, 70-71
  immunotherapy and, 250
Intermittent catheterization, 985-987
Intermittent claudication, 702-703
Intermittent coronary syndrome, 653
Intermittent mandatory ventilation, 622
Intermittent suction, 891
Internal environment, 133
Internal fixation of fracture, 509, 520-522
Internal stabilization, paradoxical breathing
    and, 594
Internal surgery, 291
International Association of Laryngectomees,
    227, 540
International Classification of Epileptic Seizures, 385
International Union Against Cancer, 218
Interstitial cell-stimulating hormone, 792
Interstitial fluid, 34, 135
Intertrigo, 1110
Intertrochanteric fracture, 514
Intervention
  alcoholism and, 123-124
  cancer pain and, 251-252
  depression and, 119
  drug abuse and, 127
  intraoperative, 303-325
  stress and, 118-119
Interviews, guidelines for, 21
Intestines, 877-878
  cancer and, 58, 921, 927
  diverticulitis and, 898, 899
  elimination and, 344
  inflammatory disorders of, 897-904
  motility of, 902
  sounds and, 31
  spinal cord injury and, 422
  surgery and, 297-298, 928
  training, 883
Intimacy versus isolation, 48
Intoxication
  mind-altering drugs and, 126
  water, 138, 139-140
Intraaortic balloon counterpulsation, 171, 664-665, 1200, 1201
Intraarterial monitoring, 162, 165, 1195
Intracavitary implant, 1071-1072
Intracellular fluid, 134
Intracerebral hemorrhage, 406-408
Intracranial pressure, 371-376
  activity and, 803
  eye and, 442
  monitoring, 1197-1199
  prevention of, 1202
Intracranial surgery, 431
Intracranial tumors, 425-433
Intradermal skin test, 1152
Intraocular lens, 452-453
Intraocular pressure, 453; see also Glaucoma
Intrapleural fluid spaces, 141

Intrapulmonary detoxification mechanism, 551
Intrauterine devices, inflammation and, 1058
Intravascular fluid, 34, 135
Intravenous anesthesia, 314, 319
Intravenous nerve block, 314
Intravenous pyelography, 953, 974
Intravenous solutions, 155
Intravertebral tumors, 433
Intropin; see Dopamine
Intussusception, 919
Inversine; see Mecamylamine
Iodine, 87
  replacement therapy, 828
Ions, 135
Iontophoresis, 1220
Ipecac, 553
Iridencleisis, 456
Iridium 192, 100, 239
Iris, 437
Iron, 87, 1212, 1218
  young adults and, 50
Iron-binding capacity, 1212
Irreducible hernia, 920
Irritability
  digitalis and, 670
Irritant contact dermatitis, 1114
Ischemia, 54, 628
  kidney and, 994
ISG; see Immune serum globulin
Islet cell tumors, 868
Ismelin; see Guanethidine
Isoetharine, 606
Isofluorophate, 456
Isoflurane, 317, 319
Isohemagglutinins, 1155
Isolation, 187
  cancer and, 229
  chemotherapy and, 246
  contact, 205
  infection control and, 204-209
Isoleucine, 87
Isometric exercises, 99-100
Isoniazid, 562, 563, 566, 843
Isoproterenol, 169, 639, 1173, 1201
Isopto-Atropine; see Atropine sulfate
Isopto-Homatropine; see Homatropine
Isopten, 1201
Isotonic exercises, 100
Isotonic fluid, 138, 139, 140-142
Isotonic solutions, 137
Isotopes, 235, 239
Isoxsuprine, 704
Isuprel; see Isoproterenol
Itch mite, 1110
Itching, 1112
  vaginal, 1059, 1061

J

Jackson tracheostomy tube, 614
Jacksonian seizures, 386
Jackson-Pratt apparatus, 333
Jaundice, 27, 840, 841
Jaw, 30
JCAH; see Joint Commission for Accreditation
    of Hospitals, 191
Jeri-Bath, 1113
Jet washings, 1070
Jock itch, 1109, 1110
The John Tracy Clinic, 471
Joint Commission on Accreditation of Hospitals, 191
  infection control and, 191

Joint Commission on Accreditation of Hospitals—cont'd
standards, 39
Joints, 482, 483
fluid spaces of, 141
mobility of, 484-485
replacement of, 503
Jugular vein
physical examination of, 30
shock and, 162, 163
Juvenile Diabetes Foundation, 786

K

Kanamycin, 463, 566, 961
Kayexalate, 145
Keloids, 1122
Kemadrin; *see* Procyclidine
Kenacort; *see* Triamcinolone
Keratitis, 445, 448, 1108
Keratoplasty, 448-450
Keratoses, 57, 1119, 1120
Kerlix, 1112, 1139
Kernig's sign, 409
Ketacoanzole, 570
Ketamine, 317, 320
Ketoacidosis, 149
diabetic; *see* Diabetic ketoacidosis
Keto-Diastix, 763
Ketosis, 765
Kidney stones, 969-970
Kidneys, 940
agenesis of, 956
anatomy of, 940-941
failure of, 996-998
functions of, 941
in elderly, 54
fluid loss and, 138
heart failure and, 665
injury and, 994
mitochondria and, 1219
physiology of, 942-944
shock and, 160-161
transplantation of, 1020-1024
trauma and, 993
Killed vaccines, 81
Killer T cells, 78
Kinins, 72
Kirschner wire, 518
Klebsiella, 201, 553, 554, 960
Knee
prostheses for, 495
replacement of, 497
Knee jerk reflex, 355
Know Your Body Project, 274
Krebiozen, 226
Krebs-Henseleit cycle, 834
Kupffer cells, 730, 833
Kussmaul breathing, 767
K-Y jelly, 892
Kyphosis, 548

L

Laboratory values, normal, 1211-1220
Labyrinth, 460, 461
disorders of, 475-478
Labyrinthectomy, 477
Labyrinthitis, 472, 473
Lacerations, 1179
of brain, 413, 414
Lactase deficiency, 917
Lactation, breast cancer and, 223
Lactic acid, 1212

Lactic acidosis, 149
Lactic dehydrogenase, 1212
myocardial infarction and, 657
Lactobacillus bulgaris, 222
Lactovegetarian diet, 92
Laennec's cirrhosis, 845, 846
Laetrile, 226
Laminar airflow unit, 246, 247
Lanatoside C, 670
Language, assessment of, 295
Lanoxin; *see* Digoxin
Laparoscopy, 1053, 1071
Large fibers, 353
Laryngeal nerve injury, 829
Laryngeal reflex, 318
Laryngectomy, 538-541
Laryngectomy tube, 539
Laryngitis, 530
Laryngofissure, 538
Laryngoscopy, 538
Laryngotracheobronchitis, 549
Larynx, 528, 529
artificial, 540, 541
carcinoma of, 537
edema of, 529, 579
thyroid surgery and, 829
LAS; *see* Local adaptation syndrome
Laser photocoagulation, 768
Lasix; *see* Furosemide
Late adulthood, 53-59; *see also* Elderly
Lateral position, 312
Laxatives, 219
Lead, 1212, 1214
nephritis and, 961
Leeching, 3
Left anterior descending artery, 628
Left ventricular failure, 666
Left-heart assist device, 1200
Legs, 694, 695-696
abduction of, 522
diabetes mellitus and, 769
exercises for, 602
Legionella pneumophila, 191, 553, 558, 559
Legionellosis, 558
Legionnaires' disease, 558
Leiomyoma, 217
Leiomyosarcoma, 217
Lens implant, 452-453
Lenses, corrective, 439-440
Lente insulin, 774
Leriche's syndrome, 1033
Lesions
motor neuron, 378
precancerous, 219, 220
of skin, 27, 28
of spinal cord, 417
of foot, diabetes mellitus and, 769
Leucine, 87
Leukapheresis, 740
Leukaran; *see* Chlorambucil
Leukemia Society of America, 227, 273
Leukemias, 748-752
acute lymphocytic, 749
chronic lymphocytic, 749, 750
lymphatic, 217
myelogenous, 749-750
sexuality and, 1033
teaching and, 751
Leukocyte alkaline phosphatase, 1218
Leukocyte-poor red cells, 1154
Leukocytes; *see also* White blood cells
differential count of, 1217

Leukocytes—cont'd
granular, 730
Leukocytosis, 72
Leukopenia, 733, 1023
radiation and, 1179
Leukoplakia, 57, 220, 1119, 1034
Leukorrhea, 1058
Levaterenol bitartrate, 169, 1173
LeVeen shunt, 857
Levin tube, 333, 889, 890
Levodopa, 397
Levophed; *see* Levaterenol bitartrate
Levopropoxyphene naphsylate, 553
Levothyroxine sodium, 828
LH; *See* Luteinizing hormone
Librium, 123
Lice, 29, 1110, 1111
Lichen planus, 1117
Lidocaine, 317, 450, 579, 639, 1173, 1201
Life change units, 53
Life island, 246
Ligaments, 481
Lingula, 605
Linoleic acid, 87
Lioresal; *see* Baclofen
Liothyronine sodium, 828
Liotrix, 828
Lipase, 877, 1212
Lipids, 1212
diabetes mellitus and, 767-768
Lipoma, 217
Lipodystrophy, 775
Lipolytic enzymes, 835
Liposarcoma, 217
Lipreading, 470-471
Lips
cancer of, 921
contact dermatitis and, 1115
physical examination of, 30
Liquefaction narcosis, 562
Listening skills, 470
Lithium, 1212
Litholapaxy, 973
Lithotomy position, 312
Lithotrite, 973
Live attenuated antigens, 197
Liver, 832, 833
abscess and, 839, 840
biopsy and, 850, 853
chemotherapy and, 249
cirrhosis and, 122, 836
disease of, 842, 848, 850-853
disorders of, 839-861
examination of, 848-851
radiography and, 852
scintography and, 852
shock and, 161
surgery and, 854
transplantation, 854
tumors of, 840
trauma and, 839-840
ventricular failure and, 667
Living/dying patterns, 282-283
Living will, 279
LMN; *see* Lower motor neuron
Lobectomy, 580, 581
Lobotomy, 185
Local adaptation syndrome, 107
Local anesthesia, 314
toxicity to, 320
Local pain, 367
Log cell kill hypothesis, 242

Lomotil; *see* Diphenoxylate and atropine
Lomustine, 247
Long-acting thyroid stimulator, 823
Long bones, 480-481
Long-term care, 263
Loop diuretics, 671
Loop of Henle, 941, 943
Loop stoma, 931
Lopressor; *see* Metoprolol
Lost Chord Club, 539
Lotions, 1111, 1112
Lou Gehrig's disease; *see* Amyotrophic lateral
    sclerosis
Low-density lipoproteins, 651
Lower airway, 543
Lower bowel, 1002
Lower esophageal sphincter, 883
Lower motor neurons, 357
    bladder and, 417
    lesions of, 988, 989
    motor function and, 377, 378
Low-molecular dextran, 155
LSD; *see* Lysergic acid diethylamide
Lugol's solution, 828
Luken's tube, 594
Lumbar injury, 421
Lumbar puncture, 363
Lumbar sympathetic block, 704, 1033
Luminal; *see* Phenobarbital
Lumpectomy, 1094
Lungs
    age and, 548
    anatomy of, 544-545
    auscultation of, 31, 33, 34
    cancer of, 576-592
        screening and, 548
    capacities and volumes of, 584
    compliance of, 584
    defense mechanisms of, 550-551
    gas exchange in, 545
    obstructive diseases of, 595-612
    restrictive diseases of, 549-595
    shock and, 161
Lupus erythematosus, 1119-1120
Luteinizing hormone, 792, 1215
Lymph nodes, 76
Lymph system, 134, 695-696
    disorders of, 752-754
    metastasis and, 217
Lymphadenitis, 72, 73
Lymphadenopathy, 752
Lymphangiography, 752
Lymphangioma, 217
Lymphangiosarcoma, 217
Lymphangitis, 73
Lymphatics; *see* Lymph system
Lymphedema, 719, 720
    mastectomy and, 1098
Lymphocytes, 69, 194, 730
    in cerebrospinal fluid, 356
    clones of, 77, 78
    normal values of, 729
Lymphocytic leukemia
    acute, 749
    chronic, 749, 750
Lymphogranuloma venereum, 1078
Lymphokines, 75
Lymphomas, 752-753
Lyophilized factor VIII concentrate,
    746
Lysergic acid diethylamide, 125, 1036
Lysine, 87

Lysis, 70
Lysozyme, 66-67

M

Maalox, 912
Macrodantin; see Trimethoprim-sulfamethox-
    azole
Macrophages, 68, 730
    immune response and, 75
Mafenide, 1139
Magnesium 87, 135, 146, 147, 1212
Mainlining, 127
Mainstream, Inc., 273
Maintenance chemotherapy, 751
Make Today Count, 227
Malabsorption syndrome, 917-918
Maladaptation, 106
Malecot catheter, 982, 983
Malignancies, 55; *see also* Neoplasms
Malignant hypertension, 722
Malignant melanoma, 1119, 1120, 1121
Malleus, 460
Malnutrition
    alcoholism and, 122
    burns and, 1134
    cirrhosis and, 122
    elderly and, 58
    essential nutrients and, 87
    obesity and, 87
Mammography, 224, 1088
Mammoplasty, 1127
Manganese, 87
Mannitol, 456
    fluid and electrolytes and, 154
    intracranial pressure and, 375
Mantoux test, 564
Manual muscle tests, 499
Marathon House, 127
Marblen, 912
Marginal ulcer, 906
Marijuana, 125, 1036
Marital choice, 49
Marshall-Marchetti operation, 990, 1064
Masks, operating room, 309
Maslow's hierarchy of needs, 48, 55
Masochism, 1031
MAST; *see* Military antishock trousers
Mastectomy
    body image and, 1036
    care of patient with, 1098
    types of, 1094
Mastication, 875
Mastitis, 1090
Mastoidectomy, 474
Mastoiditis, 472, 473
Maternal antibodies, 80
Mature cataract, 451
Maxilla, carcinoma of, 537
Maxillary sinus, 528, 529
Maxillectomy, 538
Maximal voluntary ventilation, 583, 584
McGill Pain Scale, 180
Meals-on-Wheels, 271
Mean arterial pressure, 1195
Measles vaccine, 197, 198
Meat preservatives, 219
Mecamylamine, 724, 1035
Mechanical decompression, 375
Mechanical ventilation, 620-622, 1199-1200;
    see also Ventilators
Meclizine, 476
Medical practice acts, 39

Medic-Alert jewelry, 778, 807
Mechanisms
    compensatory, 139
    defense, 117-119
    protective, 110
Medicare, 261
Medications
    angina and, 655
    cancer and, 251-252
    chronic obstructive pulmonary disease and,
        606-607
    craniocerebral trauma and, 415
    elderly and, 59
    food and, 88-89
    intracranial pressure and, 375
    myasthenia gravis and, 393
    nutrition and, 86
    pain and, 182
    paralysis and, 381, 383
    Parkinson's disease and, 397-398
    preanesthesia, 300, 301
    rheumatoid arthritis and, 493-494
    seizures and, 388-389
    skin and, 1118
Meditation, 608
Medicorten; *see* Prednisone
Medral; *see* Methylprednisone
Medroxyprogesterone, 802, 1185
Medulla, 355
Megakaryocytes, 743
Megaphen; *see* Chlorpromazine, 1035
Melanin, 26
Melanocyte-stimulating hormone, 811
Melanoma, 1121
Melphalan, 243, 247
Memory, loss of, 123
Memory cells, 78, 79
Ménière's disease, 475, 476
Meninges, 356
Meningioma, 426, 431
Meningitis, 408-410
Menopause, 50, 51, 1051-1052
The Menopause, A Positive Approach, 1053
Menstruation, 1046, 1047, 1050-1051
Menstruation and Menopause, 1053
Mental health, 4
Mental Health Materials Center, 273
Meperidine, 182, 183, 301, 346, 585, 951
Mental status
    immunosuppressive therapy and, 1023
    parameters of, 848
    shock and, 163
Mephenytoin, 733
6-Mercaptopurine, 243, 747, 750
Mercury, 961
Mescaline, 125
Mesh graft, 1124, 1125
Mesoridazine, 1035
Mestinon; *see* Pyridostigmine
Metabolic acidosis, 148, 149-150, 1004
    burns and, 1133, 1134
    shock and, 167
Metabolic cirrhosis, 845
Metabolic crisis, 779-780
Metabolic wastes, 135, 943, 996-999, 1004
Metabolism, 940
    bile pigment, 841
    burns and, 1139
    calcium phosphate, 943
    disruptions of, 1034
    heart rate and, 539
    preoperative tests of, 295

Metabolism—cont'd
  problems of, 757-871
  renal disease and, 1002
Metaproterenol, 606
Metaraminol, 169, 1173
Metastases, 216
  brain tumors and, 426
  breast cancer and, 1101
  central nervous system and, 358
  gravitational, 217
  liver and, 840
  lung cancer and, 577
Methadone, 127, 183
Methadone maintenance program, 127
Methandrostenolone, 1035
Methanol, 961
Methantheline, 1035
Methaqualone, 125
Methazolamide, 456
Methicillin, 559
Methimazole, 828
Methiodal, 952
Methionine, 87
Methotrexate, 88, 243, 247, 750
Methoxsalen, 1118
Methoxyflurane, 316
Methychlothiazide, 723
Methyl salicylate, 182
Methylcellulose, 380, 450, 1005
Methyldopa, 723
Methylenedianiline, 843
Methylprednisolone, 244, 450
Methylprednisone, 810
Metoclopramide, 887
Metocurine, 320
Metoprolol, 724
Metrizamide, 370
Microbial antagonism, 67
Micronase; see Glyburide
Micronazole, 1059
Microsomal antibodies, 1219
Midbrain, 355
Middle adulthood, 50-53
Middle ear, 460
Migraine, 360, 361
  medications for, 366
Military antishock trousers, 169, 170
Military triage, 1187
Miller-Abbott tube, 890
Milwaukee brace, 506
Mineral oil, 88, 462
Mineralocorticoids, 808
Minerals, 87
Minilaparotomy, 1053
Minipres; see Prazosin
Minute volume, 583
Miotics, 449, 456
Mithracin; see Mithramycin
Mithramycin, 243, 247
Mitomycin, 243, 247
Mitral valve, 34, 628, 679, 680, 683
Mittelschmerz, 1047
Mobile receptor model, 795
Mobility, 1140
Möerch respirator, 620
Moisture
  air passages and, 33
  skin and, 27
Mold, 219, 221
Molecules, 135, 136
Moles
  changes in, 26

Moles—cont'd
  hydatiform, 217
  pigmented, 219
Molybdenum, 87
Monilia, 1059
Monistat; *see* Micronazole
Monitoring
  cardiac, 166
  chronic obstructive pulmonary disease and,
    622
  critically ill and, 1192, 1194-1199
  intraarterial, 165
  physiologic, 305
  respiratory tract and, 167
Monoamine oxidase, 89
Monoclonal gammopathies, 1149
Monocytes, 68, 69, 194, 730
  normal values for, 729
Mononucleosis, 1034
Morbidity and Mortality Weekly Reports, 197
Morphine, 301, 579, 585, 1036, 1201
Motor aphasia, 403
Motor function, 26
  cerebrovascular accident and, 404, 405
  disturbance of, 376-382
  intracranial pressure and, 374
Motrin; *see* Ibuprofen
Mountain sickness, 546
Mouth, 875-876
  cancer and, 920-924
  care of
    elderly and, 57
    esophageal surgery and, 887
    thirst and, 156
  inflammatory disorders of, 893-895
  physical examination of, 30
  renal disease and, 1002
Mouth-to-mouth ventilation, 1172
Movement, 30, 31
6-MP; *see* 6-Mercaptopurine
MTX; *see* Methotrexate
Mucin, 1220
Mucolytic agents, 553
Mucomyst; *see* Acetylcysteine
Mucous membranes
  chemotherapy and, 246
  as defense mechanism, 66
  radiation and, 237
Mucus, 875
Multiple endocrine adenomatosis, 219
Multiple myeloma, 217, 753, 1149
Multiple sclerosis, 393-395, 1158
  environment and, 395
  eye disease and, 442
  sexuality and, 1033
Multiple spots in eye, 442
Multisystem coordination, 55
Multivalent antigens, 73, 74
Mumps, diabetes mellitus and, 762
Mumps immune globulin, human, 199
Mumps vaccine, 197
Muramidase, 1218
Murmurs, 34-35
Muscles, 481
  biopsy and, 499
  contraction of, 482
  cramping and, 1005
  flaccidity of, 377
  pump exercises, 299
  relaxants and, 300, 320
  strength, 30, 32
  tone of, 376-382

Muscles—cont'd
  wasting of, 807
  weakness of, 670
Muscular Dystrophy Association, 273
Musculoskeletal system, 480-482
  aging and, 483
  critically ill and, 1203-1204
  disorders of, 481-523
  health problems of, 487-522
  immobilization and, 513
  injuries and, 1179-1183
  trauma and, 509-522
Mushrooms, poisonous, 961
Mutamycin; *see* Mitomycin
Mutation, 216
Myasthenia gravis, 390-393
Mycobacterium tuberculosis, 564, 565
Mycoplasma pneumoniae, 553, 558, 559
Mycostatin; *see* Nystantin
Mycotic aneurysm, 406
Mydriacyl; *see* Tropicamide
Mydriatics, 449
Myelin, 353
Myelogenous leukemia, 749, 750
Myelography, 369, 370, 419
Myeloma, 1149
Mylanta, 912
Myleran; *see* Busulfan
Myocardial depressant factor, 160
Myocardial hypertrophy, 665
Myocardial infarction, 105, 652, 656-659,
  1173-1174
Myocardial ischemia, 650
  prolonged, 656
  surgery and, 659-663
Myocardial work load, 1202
Myocarditis, 675, 676
Myocardium, 627
Myochrysine; *see* Gold salts
Myoclonic seizures, 386
Myoglobin, 1214
Myoma, 1066
Myometrium, 1045
Myopia, 438
Myringotomy, 474
Mysoline; *see* Primidone
Myxedema, 821, 823

N

Nadolol, 655, 724
Nafcillin, 559, 560
Nails
  aging and, 37, 57, 1107
  inspection of, 32
  renal disease and, 1002
Nalfon; *see* Fenprofen calcium
Naloxone, 171
Nandrolone phenpropionate, 1035
Naprosyn; *see* Naproxen
Naproxen, 493, 1051
Naqua; *see* Trichlormethazide
Narcotics
  addiction and, 183
  pain and, 125, 182-183
    cancer and, 251-252
  preoperative, 301
  sexual function and, 1036
  synthetic, 182-183
  vital functions and, 183
Nardil; *see* Phenylzine sulfate
Nasal bones, 527
Nasal cannulas, 555

Nasal cavities, 527
Nasal hair, 66
Nasal packing, 531-532
Nasal polypectomy, 536
Nasal polyps, 534, 535
Nasal surgery, 531-532, 535, 536
Nasogastric intubation, 124
  fluid and electrolytes and, 153
  insertion of, 891
  laryngectomy and 539, 540
  types of, 889-891
Nasopharynx, 528-529
  carcinoma and, 537
Nasoseptoplasty, 536
National Aid to Retarded Citizens, 273
National Association of Hearing and Speech
  Agencies, 471
National Association for Visually Handi-
  capped, 273
National Asthma Center, 273
National Cancer Act (1971), 227
National Cancer Institute, 226
National Center for a Barrier-free Environ-
  ment, 274
National Center for Law and the Handi-
  capped, 274
National Clearinghouse for Drug Abuse Infor-
  mation, 127
National Clearinghouse for Smoking and
  Health, 222
National Conference on Classification of
  Nursing Diagnosis, 14, 15
National Congress of Organizations of the
  Physically Handicapped, 274
National Council on Aging, 273
National Council on Alcoholism, 122
National Health Survey, 259
National Hemophilia Foundation, 747
The National Hospice Organization,
  227
National Interagency Council on Smoking and
  Health, 222
National Kidney Foundation, 273
National Multiple Sclerosis Society, 273
National Paraplegia Foundation, 274
National Safety Act (1966), 1165
Natural tolerance, 80
Nausea, 670, 767
  postoperative, 345
Near-drowning, 1174
Nearsightedness; see Myopia
Nebulizers, 606, 607
Neck
  aging and, 37
  contact dermatitis and, 1115
  emergency assessment of, 1167
  hyperextension of, 1170, 1171
  physical examination of, 30
Neck lift, 1171
Neck vein distention, 667
Nectadon; see Noscapine
Needle sites, 775, 776
Needs
  affiliation, 11
  chronically ill and, 263-265
  Maslow's hierarchy of, 11, 48
Negative feedback, 795
Negative nitrogen balance, 293
Neisseria, 66, 72, 529, 1081
Nembutal; see Pentobarbital sodium
Neo-Hombreol; see Androgens
Neomycin, 88, 450, 463, 961, 1139

Neoplasms, 211-212
  breasts and, 1086
  characteristics of, 215
  growth of, 216
  naming and classifying of, 217, 218
  nose and throat and, 529, 537-541
  sexual function and, 1034
Neosporin; see Bacitracin
Neostigmine, 392
Neo-Synephrine; see Phenylephrine
Nephrectomy, 973, 974
Nephritis, 961
Nephrolithiasis, 969
Nephrolithotomy, 973
Nephron, 941, 942
Nephropathy, diabetic, 768, 968
Nephropexy, 993
Nephroptosis, 993
Nephrosclerosis, 968
Nephrostomy tube, 982, 983
Nephrotic syndrome, 964-966
Neptazane; see Methazolamide
Nerve block, 314, 371
  pain control and, 185
Nervous system; see also Neurologic disorders
  aging and, 54, 357-358
  alcoholism and, 122
  anatomy and physiology of, 351-358
  assessment and, 359, 361
    postoperative, 330
  critically ill and, 1202
  digitalis and, 670
  divisions of, 354-356
  functions of, 351
  health problems of, 385-433
  impulse conduction in, 142, 385-395
  metastases and, 358
  pain and, 180, 367-371
    medications and, 371
    surgery and, 371
  renal failure and, 1002
  shock and, 167
  trauma and, 358
  vascular disease and, 358
Neural shock; see Areflexia
Neuralgia, 180
Neurectomy, 371
  pain control and, 184, 185
Neuroblastoma, 217, 809
Neurocirculatory impairment, 515
Neuroendocrine response, 11
  stress and, 107-108
Neurofibroma, 426
Neurogenic bladder, 989, 990
Neurogenic polydipsia, 805
Neurogenic sarcoma, 217
Neurogenic shock, 159
Neurohypophysis, 792
Neuroleptanalgesic agents, 301
Neurologic disorders
  degenerative, 393-400
  demyelinating, 442
  infectious/inflammatory, 408-412
  manifestations of, 358-385
  neoplastic, 425-433
  prevention of, 358
  traumatic, 413-425
  vascular, 401-408
Neuroma, 217, 426
Neuromuscular blocking agents, 300, 320
Neurons, 352-354
Neurosyphilis, 412

Neutropenia, 748
Neutrophic ulcer, 769
Neutrophilia, 748
Neutrophils, 69, 729, 730
New Voice Club, 539
Niacin, 87
Nicotinic acid, 424
Nicotinyl alcohol, 704
Nifedipine, 655
Nilevar; see Norethandrolone
Nipple discharge, 1089, 1091
Nipride; see Nitroprusside
Nitrates
  angina and, 655
  cancer and, 219, 222
  heart failure and, 669
Nitrobid; see Nitroglycerin
Nitrofurantoin, 422, 960
Nitrogen, 1133, 1134, 1211, 1214
Nitrogen mustard, 244, 247, 463
Nitroglycerin, 182, 655, 1201
Nitroprusside; see Sodium nitroprusside
Nitroprusside urine test, 971
Nitrosamines, 219
Nitrous oxide, 316, 319
Nizoral; see Ketocoanzole
NMR; see Nuclear magnetic resonance imag-
  ing
Nocturia, 945, 946
Nodes of Ranvier, 353
Noise, pain and, 186-187
Noise pollution, 463-464
Nonarticular rheumatism, 500-502
Noncompliance, 6, 262
Nonelectrolytes, 135
Nongonococcal urethritis, 1078
Non-Hodgkin's lymphoma, 752, 753
Non-insulin-dependent diabetes mellitus, 760
Nonnarcotic analgesics, 182
Nonnarcotic antitussives, 553
Nonself, 62
Nonsteroidal anti-inflammatory agents, 182,
  743
Nonunion, 512
Norepinephrine, 169, 354, 431, 808, 1201
Norethandrolone, 1035
Normal saline, 155, 168
Norpace; see Disopyramide
Norpramine; see Desipramine
Nortriptyline, 1035
Noscapine, 553
Nose
  contact dermatitis and, 1115
  physical examination of, 30
  and sinuses, 527
  and throat, problems of, 527-542
Nosebleeds, 534, 535
Nosocomial infection, 199-210
Novrad; see Levopropoxyphene napsylate
NPH insulin, 774
Nuchal rigidity, 803
Nuclear magnetic resonance imaging, 231
Nucleolytic enzymes, 835
5'Nucleotidase, 1212
Nucleus pulposus, 503
Nupercaine ointment; see Dibucaine
Nurse practice acts, 39
Nurse audit, 43
Nursing care, 9; see also Nursing diagnosis;
      Nursing interventions
  action strategies in, 7, 16-17
  data collection and, 10, 12, 13

Nursing care—cont'd
 implementation of, 16-18
 priorities in, 14
 quality assurance in, 38-46
 scope of, 3
Nursing Conference Group, 802
Nursing diagnosis; 14, 92, 167, 334 *see also* Nursing care; Nursing interventions
Nursing history, 20-23
 critically ill patient and, 1193-1194
 and physical examination, 20-37
Nursing interventions, 9
 cancer and, 230, 232, 252
 chemotherapy and, 248
 death and dying and, 286-287
 elderly and, 56-59
 immunization and, 199
 in operating room, 307-315
Nursing orders, 16
Nursing process, 7, 10-19
Nutrients, 86, 741; *see also* Nutrition
 assessment of, 88-90
 essential, 87
Nutrient supplements, 88
Nutrition; *see also* Nutrients
 alcoholism and, 124
 bowel disorders and, 902, 904
 burns and, 1139-1140
 cancer and, 219, 222-223, 254
 cerebrovascular accident and, 404
 chronic obstructive pulmonary disease and, 607
 colostomy and, 936
 deficits of, 86-87
 diabetes mellitus and, 781-782
 effects of, 87
 elderly and, 54, 58
 endotracheal tube and, 619
 esophageal surgery and, 887
 excess of, 87-88
 eye disorders and, 442
 gastric surgery and, 925
 growth and, 86, 87
 health promotion and, 86-97
 history, 88
 liver disease and, 856
 middle age and, 52
 multiple sclerosis and, 395
 paralysis and, 381, 383
 parenteral, 95, 96-97
 postoperative, 343, 590
 preoperative assessment of, 295, 296
 renal failure and, 998, 1005
 vascular system and, 697
 tracheostomy and, 619
 young adults and, 50
Nutrition Foundation, Inc., 273
Nylidrin, 704
Nystagmus, 473
Nystatin, 933, 1059

O

Obesity, 52
 body image and, 1036
 coronary artery disease and, 650-652
 factors influencing, 93
 fluid loss and, 134
 malnutrition and, 87, 93
 morbid, 93
Oblique fracture, 511
Obstetric trauma, 1033

Obstructive disorders
 intestines and, 918-920
 lungs and, 549, 607
 nose and throat and, 529, 534-537
Occipital lobe, 354
 tumor of, 427
Occlusive wraps, 1117
Occultest, 900
Occupation
 asthma and, 573
 choice of, 49
 hearing loss and, 463
 lung disease and, 570-574
Occupational Safety and Health Act (1970), 463
Oculist, 438
Odors, 26
OFA; *see* Oncofetal antigens
Ohio 560 respirator, 620
Oil of cloves, 182
Oil of wintergreen, 182
Ointments, 1111, 1112
Old tuberculin, 564
Olecranon bursa, 482
Oliguria, 842, 946, 995
Omaya reservoir, 244
Oncofetal antigens, 82
Oncotic pressure, 140, 141, 142
Oncovin; *see* Vincristine
Oophorectomy, 1034, 1066
Open fracture, 511
Open reduction, 520-522
Open wounds, 1179, 1181
Open-angle glaucoma, 453- 454
Open-loop insulin delivery, 776
Operating room
 admitting procedure, 311
 attire, 308-309
 design of, 306
 nursing practice in, 303-304, 307-315
 transport to, 301
Operating team, 304
Operative positions, 312, 313
Ophthaine; *see* Proparacaine
Ophthalmic drugs, 449, 450
Ophthalmic solutions, 447, 448
Ophthalmologist, 438
Ophthetic; *see* Proparacaine
Opium alkaloids, 182
Opsonins, 70
Opthalgan; *see* Glycerin
Optic nerve, 437
Optician, 438
Optometrist, 438
OPV; *see* Poliomyelitis vaccine
Oral chemotherapy, 244
Oral contraceptives, 88
 coronary artery disease and, 652
 sexuality and, 1035
 vaginal pH and, 66
Oral hypoglycemic agents, 777
Orbital exenteration, 538
Orchidectomy, 1034
Orchitis, 1073, 1074
Oretic; *see* Hydrochlorothiazide
Organ of Corti, 461
Organic acids, 135
Organic brain syndromes, 56
Organs
 chemotherapy and, 249
 immune response and, 76
 renal failure and, 1002

Orgasm, 1028, 1029, 1030, 1038
Orinase; *see* Tolbutamide
Oropharynx, 528, 529
Orthopedic splinting, 509
Orthoplast brace, 506
Orthopnea, 666
Orthoses, 485
Orthostatic hypotension, 54
Orthotist, 487
Orthotoluidine, 900
Oscillometry, 704
Osmitrol; *see* Mannitol
Osmoglyn; *see* Glycerin
Osmolality, 136, 137, 950, 1212
Osmosis, 136, 1012
Osmotic agents, 154, 449, 456
Osmotic diuresis, 139, 765
Osmotic pressure, 136
Osteoarthritis, 87, 502, 503
Osteoarthrosis, 502
Osteoblasts, 480, 509, 511
Osteogenesis, 480
Osteoma, 217
Osteopathic flap, 531
Osteophytes, 502
Osteosarcoma, 217
Osteotomy, 503
Ostomies
 double-barrel, 931
 reasons for, 931
 self-image and, 1036
 sexual function and, 1042
OT; *see* Old tuberculin
Otitis media, 472, 473
Otologist, 469
Otosclerosis, 475
Otoscopy, 466
Ototoxic drugs, 463
Ouabain, 670, 671
Our Bodies, Our Selves, 1052
Outcome criteria, 41; *see also* Specific diseases
Ovaries, 1045
 cancer and, 1069
 cysts and, 1034, 1065
 tumors and, 1065
Overdependency, 120
Overflow incontinence, 989
Overhydration, 139, 343
Oxacillin, 559
Oxybutynin chloride, 395
Oxygen
 arterial, 1212
 chronic obstructive pulmonary disease and, 605-606, 613
 interference with, 546
 needs, 11
Oxygen saturation, 1212
Oxygen therapy, 585
 pneumonia and, 554-555
 postoperative, 328
Oxygen toxicity, 613
Oxygen transport, 1004
Oxygenation, 662, 668
Oxygen-carbon dioxide exchange, 545-548
Oxyhemoglobin dissociation curve, 599
Oxytocin, 792, 793

P

P wave, 636
Pacemakers
 electrocardiogram and, 647
 permanent, 647-648

Pacemakers—cont'd
temporary, 646-647
Pacing modes, 646
Packed red cells, 1154
Paget's disease, 219
Pain, 174-189
abdominal, 670
acute, 177, 178
narcotics and, 183
anginal, 667
anorexia and, 106
behavioral manifestations of, 181
assessment of, 180-181
cancer and, 225, 250-252
chronic, 177, 179
narcotics and, 183
team approach to, 188
coitus and, 1038
control of
neurosurgical procedures for, 184-185
nursing approaches to, 186-188
psychologic approaches to, 185
elderly and, 56
expected outcomes and, 182
experience of, 175
extremities and, 32
gate theory of, 184
local, 367
lung surgery and, 585
neurologic, 180
pelvic inflammatory disorders and, 1059,
1061
perception of, 176, 177
phantom limb, 180
physiology of, 175, 181
postoperative, 345-346
prevention of, 186
psychogenic, 180
reaction to, 177
receptors of, 367
referred, 179, 367
relief of, 188
burns and, 1137
guidelines for, 186
response to, modification of, 187-188
somatic, 179
stimulus, 175
modification of, 186-187
as stressor, 106
transmission of, 175, 176, 177
trauma and, 1167
types of, 177-180
urinary tract disorders and, 946
visceral, 179
Pain clinics, 188
Pain scales, 180, 181
Pain teams, 188
Palliative surgery, 292
Palpation, 24
Pancreas, 833, 834-835
adenomas and, 868
disorders of, 867-871
secretory, 796
surgery for, 870-871
Pancreatitis, 867-868
acute, 870
Pancuronium bromide, 320
Pancytopenia, 733
Panhypopituitarism, 803
Panic, 124
Panlobular emphysema, 600
Pannus, 487

Pantopaque, 370
Pantothenic acid, 87
Pap test; see Papanicolaou stain
Papanicolaou stain, 52, 224, 225, 1070
Papaverine, 182, 704
Paper tape urine test, 763
Papilledema, 374, 472
Papilloma, 217
Papulosquamous disorders, 1117-1118
Para-aminosalicylic acid, 566
Paracentesis, 856-857
Paradoxical breathing, 593-594
Paraldehyde, delirium tremens and,
124
Paralysis, 377
Paralytic ileus, 889-893
Paralyzed Veterans of America, 274
Paramedics, 1165
Parametrium, 1045
Paranasal sinuses, 527
Paraneoplastic syndrome, 230
Parasites, 1110, 1111, 1113, 1114
Parasympathetic nervous system, 356
innervation of, 631
Parathormone, 136-137
Parathyroid gland, 795
dysfunction of, 816-821
injury and, 829
secretory disorders of, 796
surgery and, 819, 829
Parathyroid hormone, 816-817, 1215
Parathyroidectomy, 819
Paregoric, 897
Parenteral fluids, 156
Parenthood, 49
Paresis, 377, 412
Paresthesia, 367
Pargyline, 1035
Parietal lobe, 354
tumors and, 427
Parietal pleura, 545
Parkinson's disease, 393-398
Parlodel; see Bromocryptine mesylate
Parnate, 89
Paroxysmal nocturnal dyspnea, 666
Paroxysmal tachycardia, 641
Partial laryngectomy, 538
Partial thromboplastin time, 743, 1217
PAS; see Para-aminosalicylic acid
Passive range of motion, 484
Paste, 1111
Patch graft, 705
Patch test, 1152
Pathogenicity, 191
Pathogens, 63, 191, 192
Pathologic fracture, 509, 510
Pathways
motor, 357
sensory, 356-357
Patient
knowledge of diagnosis and, 228-229
moving of, 487
safety and, 311-315, 1164, 1165
Patient data, 12, 13, 21-37
Patient satisfaction questionnaire, 43
PCP; see Phencyclidine
Pearson attachment, 519, 520, 521
Pectoralis muscle, 545
Pedal pulse, 703
Pediculosis, 1110, 1111
Pediculosis pubis, 1059, 1078
Peer review, 43

Pellagra, 87
alcoholism and, 122
Pelvic examination, 224, 1070
Pelvic exenteration, 1033, 1066
Pelvis
emergency assessment of, 1167
infection and, 1058
inflammatory disorders of, 1059, 1078
sexual function and, 1034
radiation and, 1074
Pencillamine, 494
Penectomy, 1075
sexuality and, 1033
D-Penicillamine, 733, 743
Penicillin, 88, 559
infection and, 190
Penicillin G, 89, 559, 1059
Penicillin V, 559
Penis
cancer and, 223, 1075-1076
injury to, 1033
surgery and, 1077
thrombus and, 1033
trauma to, 1034
Penile prosthetic implant, 1037
Penrose drain, 332, 931
Penthrane; see Methoxyflurane
Pentobarbital sodium, 301
Pentolinium, 724
Pentose, 1214
Pentothal sodium; see Thiopental sodium
Pepsinogen, 877
Peptic ulcer
complications of, 915-917
drug therapy and, 910-911
perforated 915-916
stress and, 105
surgery and, 913-915
types of, 906
Percussion, 24
Percutaneous biopsy, 955
Percutaneous implanted spinal cord epidural
stimulator, 183, 184
Percutaneous transluminal coronary angio-
plasty, 663
Perfusion, 545, 583
chemotherapy and, 244, 246
Perianal area, contact dermatitis and, 1115
Pericardial fluid spaces, 141
Pericardiocentesis, 595, 678
Pericarditis, 675, 676
Pericardium, 627
Perichondrium, 481
Perilymph, 460
Perineal exercises, 989-990
Perineal prostatectomy, 976, 978
Perineal resection, 1033
Periodontitis, 894
Perioperative nursing, 289-348
standards of, 304
Perioral area, contact dermatitis and, 1115
Peripheral edema, 667
Peripheral facial paralysis; see Bell's palsy
Peripheral nervous system, 356
trauma and, 422-424
Peripheral pulses, 703
Peripheral vascular disorders, 693-727
Peripheral vascular resistance, 696
Peristalsis, 877
Peritoneal dialysis, 1016-1020, 1203
Peritoneal fluid spaces, 141
Peritoneojugular shunt, 857

Peritonitis, 73
Pernicious anemia, 1158
Peroxide hemolysis, 1218
PERRLA, 29
Personality, 113
  alcoholism and, 122-123
Perspiration. 66
Pertofrane; *see* Desipramine
Pertussis immune globulin, human, 199
Pertussis vaccine, 81, 197
Pessary, 1062, 1063, 1064
Pesticides, 961
Petit mal seizures, 386
Petrolatum, 1125
Peyote, 125
Peyronie's disease, 1034
Pezzar catheter, 982, 983
pH, 135, 1212
  acid base imbalance and, 148
  in stored blood, 168
Phacoemulsion, 452
Phagocytes, 68
Phagocytosis, 69, 72
Phanacetin, 366
Phantom limb pain, 180
Phantom rectal sensations, 931
Pharyngeal reflex, 318
Pharyngitis, 530
Pharynx, 527, 528, 529
  examination of, 30
Phenacetin, 366
Phenazopyridine, 961
Phencyclidine, 125
Phenergan; *see* Promethazine hydrochloride
Phenobarbital, 366, 389
Phenolsulfonphthalein, 951, 1214
Phenothiazines
  cancer and, 252
  Parkinson's disease and, 396
Phenoxybenzamine, 704, 724, 1035
Phentolamine, 669, 724
Phenylalanine 87, 1212
Phenylbutazone, 89, 182, 493, 733, 743
Phenylephrine, 449, 535, 892
Phenylzine, 89, 1035
Phenytoin, 89, 123, 375, 389, 412, 1212
Pheochromocytoma, 807, 809, 810, 815
Pheresis, 740
Philadelphia chromosome, 750
Phimosis, 1034
pHisoHex, 618
Phlebography, 715
Phlebotomy, 674
Phoenix House, 127
Phosphate, 135
Phospholine iodide; *see* Echothiopate iodide
Phospholipids, 1212
Phosphorus, 87, 843, 1214
  inorganic, 1212
  radioactive, 239
Photophobia, 445
Photoreceptors, 436
Photosensitivity, 1118, 1119
Physical examination,
  cancer and, 231
  critically ill patient and, 1194
  head-to-toe, 24-37
  malnutrition and, 90
  modalities of, 24
Physical fitness, 98
Physical therapy, 269
Physiologic data, 295-296

Physiologic defense mechanisms, 1103-1159
Physiologic saline solution, 447
Physostigmine, 456
Pia mater, 356
Pigmented moles, 219, 1119
Pilocarpine, 453, 456
Pinkeye, 445
Pinna, 460
Pinworms, 1059
PISCES; *see* Percutaneous implanted spinal
    cord epidural stimulator
Pitressin; *see* Vasopressin
Pitting edema, 140
Pituitary gland
  anatomy of, 792
  anterior
    dysfunction of, 797-804
    pituitary-adrenocortical mechanism and,
      108
    secretory disorders of, 797, 799-800
    surgery and, 431, 802-803
  diagnostic tests and, 801-802
  endocrine system and, 798
  function tests, 801-802
  hypothalamus and, 793-794
  neurologic system and, 798
  posterior, 794
    secretory disorders of, 796
  tumors and, 426
Pituitary fossa and, 528
Pituitary hormones, 792
  tests of, 801
Pityriasis rosea, 1117
Planning
  nursing and, 10, 14, 16
  preoperative, 305
Plant alkaloids, 243
Plant poisons, 843
Plaquenil; *see* Hydroxychloroquine
Plasma, 69-70, 134, 1154
  fluid replacement therapy and, 168
  laboratory values of, 1211-1213
  pH of, 135
  proteins in, 139
Plasma cells, 77
Plasma creatinine concentration, 1001
Plasma exchange, 740
Plasma expanders, 155
Plastic strip urine test, 763
Plastic surgery, 291, 1122-1127
Plateau phase of sexual response, 1028, 1029
Platelet aggregation, 1218
Platelet concentration, 1154
Platelet count, 1218
Platelets, 69, 730
  disorders of, 742-743, 744, 745
  dysfunction of, 744
    tests of, 1218
  normal values of, 729
  pheresis of, 740
Plethysmography, 703-704
Pleura, 545
Pleural cavity, 1180, 1181
Pleural effusion, 547
  cancer and, 577
Pleural space, 586-588
PleureVac system, 586
Pleuritis, 73
PMF; *see* Progressive massive fibrosis
Pneumococcal pneumonia vaccine, 197
Pneumoconioses, 571-572
Pneumoencephalography, 428, 429

Pneumonectomy, 580-581, 590, 591
Pneumonia, 553-560
  alcoholism and, 122
  hypostatic, 339
  nosocomial, prevention of, 203
Pneumothorax, 547, 594, 595, 579, 1180
PNS; *see* Peripheral nervous system
Poison control centers, 1175
Poisoning, 1175-1177
Poldine, 1035
Poliomyelitis, 201, 411
  vaccines for, 81, 197
Polyclonal gammopathies, 1149
Polycyclic hydrocarbons, 219, 221
Polycystic disease
  kidneys and, 957-958
  ovaries and, 1065
Polydypsia, 765
Polymorphonuclear leukocytes, 69, 730
Polymyositis, 488, 498-499
Polymyxin B, 450
  and colistin, 463
Polyneuritis; *see* Guillain-Barré-Strohl syn-
    drome
Polyneuropathy, alcoholism and, 122
Polypeptide hormones, 1215
Polyphagia, 765
Polyps
  colorectal, 219
  nasal, 531
Polysaccharide C, 70
Polysporin; *see* Bacitracin
Polythiazide, 723
Polyunsaturated fat, 87
Polyuria, 765, 946
Pons, 355
Popliteal pulse, 703
Porphobilinogen, 1214
Portal hypertension, 837, 859-860
Port-wine urine, 1157
Positioning of patient, 506, 507
  airway maintenance and, 547
  burns and, 1140
  exhalation and, 601
  lung surgery and, 585
  operative, 311-313
  pneumonia and, 556
  postoperative, 327, 331, 340
  side-lying, 522
Positive end-expiratory pressure, 171, 620-622
Posterior bronchus, 605
Posterior chamber of eye, 436, 437
Posterior chest tube, 586
Posterior tibial artery, 694
Postictal period, 387-388
Postictal stupor, 123
Postnasal packing, 535, 536
Postnecrotic cirrhosis, 845
Postural drainage, 603-605
Postural hypotension, 54
Posture, 484-485; *see also* Positioning
Potassium, 87, 89, 135, 143-145, 1213
  burns and, 1133
  excretion of, 135
  imbalance, 143-145
  infusion rate, 144
  loss, 142
  normal values of, 949
  renal failure and, 144, 996-997
  serum concentration of, 143
  sources of, 144
Potassium chloride, 155

Potassium iodide, 553
Potassium nitrate, 1035
Potassium permanganate, 1113
Potassium salts, 144
Potassium-sparing diuretics, 671
  hypertension and, 723
Potential space, 141, 545
Pouches for ostomies, 934, 935
Povidone-iodine, 736, 1139
  burns and, 1138
  douches, 1060
Powders, 1111
PPD; see Purified protein derivative
Prazosin, 669, 724
Preanesthetic medication, 300, 316
Precentral gyrus tumor, 427
Precordial thump, 1172-1173
Prednisolone, 89, 350
Prednisone, 83, 395, 450, 750, 810
Preinfarction angina, 653
Preload, 631, 665
Premalignant tumors of skin, 1119
Premalignant beats, 637, 640-641
Premature ejaculation, 1038
Premedication; see Preanesthetic medication
Preoperative care, 291-302
Preresection thoracoplasty, 590
Presbycusis, 465
Presbyopia, 50, 438
Presenile dementia, 56
President's Committee on Employment of the
  Handicapped, 274
President's Council on Physical Fitness and
  Sports, 274
Pressure, normal hemodynamic, 1194
Pressure points, 1175
Pressure-cycled ventilator, 620
Priapism, 1034
Primary aldosteronism, 807
Primary complex, 562
Primary hypertension, 721, 722
Primary intention, 335
Primary tubercle, 562
Primidone, 389, 1213
Prinzmetal's angina, 653
Priorities, 14
Priscoline; see Tolazoline
Pro-Banthine; see Propantheline bromide
Problem solving, 111
Procainamide, 639
Procaine, 317, 559
Procarbazine, 247
Process criteria, 41
Prochlorperazine, 247, 370, 570, 897, 1035
Proctoscopy, 52
Procyclidine, 397
Professional standards review organizations,
  38
Profundoplasty, 705-706
Progesterone, 1047
Progestins, 243
Progressive histoplasmosis, 568
Progressive massive fibrosis, 572
Progressive pulmonary congestion, 575
Progressive relaxation, 111, 187
Prolactin, 792, 798-799, 1215
Proliferative retinopathy, 768
Promethazine, 301, 570, 1035
Prone position, 484
  surgery and, 312
Pronestyl; see Procainamide
Propacil; see Propylthiouracil

Propantheline bromide, 182, 395
Proparacaine, 450
Propoxyphene, 366, 371
Propranolol, 723, 1201, 1220
  angina and, 655
  heart rate and, 639
  migraine and, 366
Proprioception, 383
Propylthiouracil, 828
Prostate gland, 975, 1047
  cancer and, 1075
  hypertrophy of, 59, 944
    benign, 975-979
  resection of, 1077
  surgery of, 976
Prostatectomy
  impotence and, 1074
  sexuality and, 1033
Prostatitis, 1073
  sexual function and, 1034
Prosthesis, dental, 538
Prostigmine; see Neostigmine
Protamine zinc insulin, 774
Protein, 135
  burns and, 1133
  deficit, 918
  essential, 87
  metabolism of, 833, 834
  movement of, 136
  quantitative, 1214
  serum, 74
  wound healing and, 343
  total, 1213
  young adults and, 50
Protein-bound iodine, 826
Proteinuria, 768
Proteus, 201, 553, 960
Prothrombin time, 743, 1217
Protriptyline, 1035
Providencia, 201
Prune belly syndrome, 956
Pruritus, 855-856, 1112-1113
  renal failure and, 1005
Pseudocholinesterase, 1211
Pseudofolliculitis barbae, 1122
Pseudomonas, 201, 445, 960
  burns and, 1138
  nosocomial infection and, 190, 200
Psoralen; see Methoxsalen
Psoriasis, 1110, 1117
PSRO; see Professional standards review orga-
  nizations
Psychoactive drugs, 1036
Psychogenic pain, 180
Psychologic adaptation, 106
Psychologic age, 53
Psychologic health, 4
Psychologic needs, 347-348
Psychologic response, 932
Psychologic status
  chronic illness and, 263-264
  surgery and, 294, 305
Psychologic support, 305
Psychomotor seizures, 386
Psychopharmacologic agents, 607
Psychosocial needs
  chronic illness and, 264-265
  elderly and, 59
Psychosocial Counseling Service, 228
Psychotherapy
  alcoholism and, 124
  headache and, 366

PTH; see Parathyroid hormone
Ptosis, 29
Ptyalin, 875
Pubic lice, 1111
Public health, national goals for, 274-275
Public Health Service immunization sched-
  ules, 197
Pubococcygeus muscle, 1033
Pulmonary artery catheterization, 165, 166,
  657, 658
  monitoring, 1195, 1196
  pressure, 165, 166
Pulmonary auscultation, 33
Pulmonary blastomycosis, 569
Pulmonary capillary wedge pressure, 165
Pulmonary circulation, 659-660
Pulmonary disorders, 548
  postoperative, 340
  sexual dysfunction and, 1035
Pulmonary edema, 141, 673-674
Pulmonary embolus, 1204
Pulmonary emphysema, 597-598
Pulmonary function tests, 583-584
  bronchitis and, 596, 597
  emphysema and, 597
  obstructive disease and, 549
  restrictive disease and, 549
Pulmonary system
  chemotherapy and, 249
  problems of, 543-625
  renal failure and, 1002
  respiratory failure and, 612
Pulmonary vascular resistance, 1195
Pulmonary ventilation, 326-328, 545, 925
Pulmonic valve, 34, 628, 682
Pulse deficit, 670
Pulse generators, 646
Pulse rate, target, exercise and, 98
Pulsus paradoxus, 995
Pump lung, 575
Puncture wounds, 1179
Pupillary reflex, 29
Pupils, 437
  Argyll Robertson, 412
  in unconscious patient, 1168
Pure-tone audiometry, 466, 468
Purified protein derivative, 564
Purple foxglove, 670
Purpura, medications and, 1118
Pus, 72
Putamen, 354
PUVA therapy, 1118
Pyelolithotomy, 973
Pyelonephritis, 959, 966-967
Pyeloplasty, 973
Pyelostomy tube, 982
Pyloric obstructive, 916-917
Pyloroplasty, 914, 915, 924
Pyocyanea, 72
Pyrazinamide, 566
Pyridostigmine, 392
Pyrophosphate scanning, 657
Pyruvate kinase, 1217
Pyruvic acid, 1213
PZA; see Pyrazinamide

Q

QRS complex, 636
QT interval, 636
Quaalude, 125
Quadriceps drill, 299

Quality assurance, 38-46
  reviews, 39-43
Questran; *see* Cholestyramine resin
Quinacrine, 494
Quinethazone, 723
Quinidine, 463, 639, 743, 1213
Quinine, 463

R

Rabbit renal collecting ducts, 1219
Rabies, 198
Race
  cancer and, 213
  chronic illness and, 261
  coronary artery disease and, 651
Radiation
  cancer and, 235-241
    of breast, 1100
    of mouth, 922, 924
  delivery of, 235
  exposure to, 237
  external, 237-238
  hazards of, 235, 236, 237
  injury and, 1178-1179
  ionizing, cancer and, 219, 220-221
  male reproductive tract and, 1077-1078
  reactions to, 237
  sealed internal, 239
    linens and, 240, 241
  sexual dysfunction and, 1034
  shielding and, 237
  tumor and,
    of pituitary gland, 802
    intracranial, 432
  types of, 235, 236
Radiation sickness, 1179
Radical mastoidectomy, 474
Radical neck dissection, 541, 922
Radical prostatectomy, 976
Radioactive agents, 239
Radioactive iodine, 239, 837, 839, 1078
Radiography
  aortic aneurysm and, 688
  biliary disorders and, 863
  breasts and, 1088
  infection and, 195
  urinary tract and, 953-954
Radioimmunoassay, 806
Radionecrosis, 237
Radionuclide imaging, 657
Radiotherapy
  cancer and, 235-241
  external, 237-238
  Hodgkin's disease and, 754
  internal, 238-241
    unsealed, 240, 241
Radium, 226, 235, 239
Radon, 239, 240
Rales, 33, 34, 667
Range of motion
  active/passive, 484
  assessment of, 32
Rape, 1183-1185
Rape crisis centers, 1183
Rape trauma syndrome, 1183
Rapid-acting insulin pumps, 774
Rash, erythematous, medications and, 1118
Raudixin; *see* Whole root Rauwolfia
Rauwiloid; *see* Alseroxylon fraction
Rauwolfia compounds, 723
Raynaud's phenomenon, 700, 701-702
Reach to Recovery, 227, 1094

Reactors, 564
Records, problem-oriented, 18
Recovery room
  discharge from, 329
  transport to, 323-324
Recovery room notes, 334
Rectocele, 1061
Rectovaginal fistula, 1063
Rectum, digital examination of, 224
Rectus muscle, 437
Red blood cells, 729-730, 1217
  disorders of, 732-742
  enzymes and, 1217
  normal values of, 729
  osmotic fragility of, 1218
  production of, 943
The Red Book, 197
Red dye, 219
Reducible hernia, 920
Reduction of fracture, 514-522
Referred pain, 179, 367
Reflex neurogenic bladder, 417
Reflexes, 318, 355
Refraction, 437
Regional anesthesia, 314, 320-321
Regitine; *see* Phentolamine
Regression, 119
Regular insulin, 774
Regurgitation, 885
Rehabilitation
  alcoholism and, 124
  chronic illness and, 265-269
  specialized centers for, 266
  vocational, 267
Reinfection histoplasmosis, 568
Rejection, transplantation and, 1022
Relaxation
  pain and, 187
  progressive, 111
Relaxation exercises, 608
Relaxation response, Benson's, 111, 112
Relaxation techniques, 111
Releasing factor, 793
Reliaseal, 935
Remission, 259
Remodeling of bone, 509, 511
Renacidin, 970, 973
Renal artery stenosis, 967-968
Renal biopsy, 954-955
Renal calculi, 969-974
Renal colic, 971
Renal disease; *see also* Kidneys; Renal failure
  diabetes mellitus and, 768
  end-stage, 1011-1020
    fertility and, 1001, 1002
  fluid and electrolytes and, 154
  sexual dysfunction and, 1034
Renal failure
  acute, 994-1000
  chronic, 1000-1024
    coping with, 1006
    treatment goals in, 1003
Renal function
  assessment of, 944-955
  burns and, 1133
  tests of, 950-951
Renal neoplasms, 974-979
Renal stones, 971
Renal system
  aging and, 943-944
  critically ill patient and, 1202-1203
  preoperative tests of, 295

Renal system—cont'd
  shock and, 163
Renese; *see* Polythiazide
Renin, 943, 1215
Rennin, 877
Renografin, 702
Renography, 954
Repolarization, 353, 628
Reports, 43, 44
Reproduction, 1052-1057
Reproductive system
  disorders of, 1033
  health problems of, 1057-1084
  inflammation of, 1061
  organs of
    female, 1044-1047
    male, 1075
  removal of, 1061
  problems of, 1044-1084
  structural disorders of, 1061-1064
  tumors of, 1065-1068
  surgery and, 1066-1068
RES; *see* Reticuloendothelial system
Resectional surgery, 582, 590, 592
Resectoscope, 977
Reserpine, 89, 396, 723, 1035
Residual urine, 949
Residual volume, 583, 584
Resolution of sexual response, 1028, 1029
Respirations
  assessment of
    emergency and, 1167
    postoperative, 339
    preoperative, 295, 296
  Cheyne-Stokes, 374
  control of, 545
  ether anesthesia and, 318
  intracranial pressure and, 374
Respirator centers, 1191
Respirators, 620
Respiratory acidosis, 148, 150
Respiratory alkalosis, 148, 150
Respiratory centers; 546, 547-548
Respiratory isolation, 206
Respiratory system
  age and, 54, 548
  anatomy and physiology of, 543-548
  assessment of
    postoperative, 330, 331
    preoperative, 295
  chemotherapy and, 246
  clearance mechanisms of, 550
  critically ill and, 1199-1200
  disorders of, 549, 612-622
    diagnostic criteria for, 613
  failure of
    acute, 1199-1200
  health problems of, 549-622
  impairment of, fluid and electrolytes and, 154
  infection of, 194, 548-549
    nosocomial, 201, 203
  shock and, 163, 171
Rest
  elderly and, 58
  headaches and, 366
  middle age and, 52
  neurologic pain and, 371
  respiratory insufficiency and, 622
  shock and, 171
  stress management and, 110
  young adults and, 50

Resting splint, 486
Restorative surgery, 292
Restrictive lung disease, 549-595
Reticular formation, 355
Reticulocytes, 1218
Reticuloendothelial system, 68, 161, 731-732
Retina, 436, 437, 457
  blind spot of, 374
  damage to, 442
  detachment of, 442, 457-459
  edema of, hypertension and, 442
  hypertension and, 442
Retinal artery, 437
Retinal vein, 437
Retinoblastoma, 219
Retinopathy, diabetes and, 442, 768
Retrograde pyelography, 953
Retropubic prostatectomy, 976, 978
Reverse Trendelenburg position, 312
Rh blood system, 1155
Rhabdomyoma, 217
Rhabdomyosarcoma, 217
Rheumatic diseases, 488-491, 492
Rheumatic fever, 675, 677, 1158
Rheumatoid arthritis, 487, 488, 492-497
Rheumatoid factor, 492
Rhinitis, 530
Rhinopharyngitis, 807
Rhinoplasty, 530, 1125, 1126, 1127
Rhizotomy, 371
  pain control and, 184, 185
  sexuality and, 1033
Rhonchi, 33, 34
Rhythm strip, 635, 636
Rhytidoplasty, 1127
Rib fracture, 592-593, 1180
Riboflavin, 87
  young adult and, 50
Ribonucleic acid, 215, 216
Rifampin, 559, 566
Right coronary artery, 628
Right ventricular failure, 667
Rights of dying person, 278-279
Rigidity, 374
Ringer's solution, 155, 156, 168, 447
Ringworm, 1109
Riopan, 912
Risk factors, 5
RNA; *see* Ribonucleic acid
Robinson catheter, 979, 980, 982, 985
Robinul; *see* Glycopyrrolate
Rods, retinal, 436
Romilar; *see* Dextromethorphan hydrobromide
Roniacol; *see* Nicotinyl alcohol
  cataract and, 451
  diabetes mellitus and, 762
Rubella, 201
Rubella vaccine, 197
Rubor, 72
Rugae, 877
Rule of nines, 1135
Russell traction, 514, 517-518, 520

S

Sabin vaccine, 81, 411
Saccharin, 219, 221
Saccular aneurysm, 687
Saddle embolus, 702
Sadism, 1031
Safety
  Alzheimer's disease and, 400
  intraoperative, 305

Safety—cont'd
  motor function disturbance and, 380, 383
  postoperative, 329, 330, 331-334
Safety devices, 484, 485
Safety needs, 11
Salem sump tube, 889
Salibi clamp, 408
Salicylates, 743
  ear disorders and, 563
  rheumatoid arthritis and, 493
  therapeutic level, 1213
  toxic level, 1213
Saline lead test, 916
Saline solution, 155
  for eye compresses, 446
  for sputum collection, 565
Saliva, 875
  as defense mechanism, 66
Salk vaccine, 81, 411
Salmonella, 201, 1176, 1177
Salpingectomy, 1066
Salpingitis, 1057, 1058
Sandril; *see* Reserpine
Saphenous vein, 718
Saratoga sump drain, 332
Saturation, 120
Scabies, 1059, 1078, 1110, 1111
Scalene muscles, 545
Scaling papular disorders, 1117-1118
Scalp, 30
Scapula, 1115
Scar tissue, 73, 338
  body image and, 1036
Schiotz tonometer, 453, 455
Schistosoma, 960
Schistosoma haematobium, 975
Schwannoma, 426
Sclera, 436, 437
Sclerotomy, 456
Scoliosis, 490, 505-507
Scopolamine hydrobromide, 449
Scopolamine hydrochloride, 301, 397
Scratch test, 1152
Screening, 764-765
Scrotum, hernia repair and, 920
Scrub nurse, 305-306
Scurvy, 87
Seborrheic dermatitis, 1115
Seborrheic keratoses, 57, 1119
Secobarbital sodium, 301
Seconal; *see* Secobarbital sodium
Second-degree burn, 1129, 1130
Secondary bacteremia, 200
Secondary drowning, 1174
Secondary hypertension, 721, 722
Secondary immune response, 78-79
Secondary intention, 335
Secondary thrombocytopenia, 744
Secretin, 835
Secretions, gastrointestinal, 134, 135, 878
Secretory inhibitors, 449
Sedatives, 125
  asthma and, 612
  delirium tremens and, 124
  pain and, 183
  sexual function and, 1035
  shock and, 167
Sedative-hypnotics, preoperative, 301
Seeding, 217
Segmental reflux, 355
Segmental resection, 580, 581-582
Segmentectomy, 580, 581-582

Seizures, 385-390
  alcohol withdrawal and, 123
  cortical resection and, 389
  Jacksonian, 386
Selenium, 87
Self, 62-63
  perceptions of, 86
  recognition of, 73
Self-actualization, 11
Self-care
  chronic illness and, 269
  diabetes mellitus and, 781
  elderly and, 56-57
Self-control, pain and, 185
Self-esteem, 11, 86
  elderly and, 56
  young adults and, 48
Self-help devices, 381, 382
Self-help groups, chronic illness and, 270
Self-monitoring, 784
Semen, 1047
Semicircular canals, 461
Semilunar valves, 628
Semustine, 247
Senescent arthritis, 502
Senile cataracts, 442
Senile keratosis, 219, 1119
Senile kyphosis, 483
Senile vaginitis, 1034
Sensation, assessment of, 1167
Senses, preoperative assessment of, 295
Sensitized T cell lymphocytes, 78
Sensitizing dose, 1152
Sensorimotor problems, 349-523
Sensorineural hearing loss, 465
Sensory aphasia, 403
Sensory deprivation overload, 1206
Sensory nerve fibers, 368
Sensory perception, 54
Sensory system,
  function of, 383-384
  pathways of, 356-357
Septal deviation, 534, 535
Septic shock, 159
Septicemia, 73
Septum
  of heart, 628
  nasal, 527
Serentil; *see* Mesoridazine
Serology
  rheumatoid disease and, 492
  syphilis and, 1083
Serous otitis media, 472, 473
Serous secretion, 875
Serpasil; *see* Reserpine
Serratia, 201
Serratia liquefaciens, 201
Serratia marcescens, 201, 553
Serum
  amylase in, 869
  autoantibodies, 1219
  calcium in, 145
  creatinine in, 951
  electrolytes in
    normal values of, 949
    shock and, 167
  enzymes in
    myocardial infarction and, 657
    shock and, 167
    tests of, 499
  heterologous, 81
  laboratory values of, 1211-1213

Serum—cont'd
  magnesium in, 146
  potassium in, 143
    shock and, 167
  proteins in, 74
  sodium in, 142, 143
Serum sickness, 81, 1157
Seven warning signals of cancer, 225
Sex hormone preparations, 1035
Sexual assault, 1183-1185
Sexuality
  aging and, 1030-1031
  cancer and, 212, 213, 219, 223, 229
  colostomy and, 936-937
  concerns about, 1037
  coronary artery disease and, 651, 663
  counseling and, 1039
  cultural influences and, 50, 51
  desire and, 1037
  dysfunction of, 1037
  elderly and, 54
  evolution of, 1027-1028
  expression of, 1031-1032
  gender disorders and, 1036
  health and, 1027-1032
  illness and, 1032-1043
  mastectomy and, 1096
  middle age and, 50, 51
  myocardial infarction and, 658-659
  pharmacologic agents and, 1034-1036
  physiologic aspects of, 1028-1030
  problems of, 1037, 1039-1040
  spinal cord trauma and, 419, 422, 423
  therapy and, 1042
  values and, 1039
  young adults and, 48
Sexually transmitted diseases, 1078
Shaving before surgery, 313
Sheepskin pads, 513
Shelters in disasters, 1187
Shingles, 1108, 1109; see also Herpes zoster
Shock, 139, 158-173
  assessment in, 162-171
  bleeding and, 1174-1175
  cardiac support in, 171
  fluid replacement in, 168
  injuries and, 171
  irreversible, 160
  organ damage in, 160-162
  postoperative, 328
  signs of, 162, 163, 594
  stages of, 159-160
  trauma and, 1167
  vasoactive drugs and, 169
Shock lung, 161, 575
Shocking dose, 1152
Shorr regimen, 974
Short bones, 481
Shunting, 432
Sick role, 7
Sickle cell crises, 739
Sickle cell disorders, 738, 739, 1033
Sickle cell trait, 738
Side-lying position, 522
Siemen's Servo respirator, 620
Sighing of respirator, 621
Sigmoid colostomy, 932
Sigmoidoscopy, 224
Silicosis, 571
Silver nitrate, 1139
Silver sulfadiazine, 1139
Silverstone clamp, 408
Simplate test, 1217

Simple fracture, 511
Sinoatrial node, 631
Sinus arrhythmia, 637, 639-640
Sinus bradycardia, 637, 640
Sinus tachycardia, 637, 639-640
Sinuses, 73, 527, 528
  surgery of, 532
Sinusitis, 530
Skeletal muscle, 482
  ether anesthesia and, 318
Skeletal traction, 420
Skin, 1105-1127
  aging and, 37, 57, 1106-1107
  anatomy of, 1105-1106
  biopsy of, 498
  burns and, 1138
  care of
    elderly and, 57
      multiple sclerosis and, 395
      paralysis and, 380, 383
  chemotherapy and, 246, 247, 249
  color, 26-27
  as defense mechanism, 64, 66
  dermatologic problems of, 1105-1127
    in blacks, 1121-1122
  elasticity/turgor of, 27
  examination of, 26-27
  fluid loss through, 138
  function of, 1106
  health problems of, 1108-1127
  immobilization and, 512-513
  lesions of, 27, 28
  markings, removal of, 1125
  medications and, 1118
  moisture of, 27
  physiology of, 1106
  preoperative preparation of, 298, 312
  radiation and, 237
  renal failure and, 1002
  shock and, 163
  systemic diseases and, 1118-1120
  systemic, lupus erythematosus and, 498
  temperature of, 27
  tumors of, 27, 1119, 1120-1121
  vascular system and, 697-698
Skin sutures, 336
Skin grafts, 1123-1125
  burns and, 1139
Skin staples, 337
Skin tests
  infection and, 195
  intradermal, 1152
Skiodan; see Methiodal
Skull fracture, 413, 1182
SLE; see Lupus erythematosis, systemic
Sleep
  elderly and, 58
  obstructive pulmonary disease and, 608-609
  young adults and, 50
Sleeping sickness, 410
Slow-acting insulin, 774
SM; see Streptomycin
Small fibers, 353
Smallpox, 196
  immunization and, 197
Smoked foods, cancer and, 219, 222
Smoking
  cancer and, 219, 221-222
  peptic ulcer and, 908, 913
  surgery and, 297
  vascular system and, 697
Smooth muscle, 482, 1219

Sneezing, 534
Snellen chart, 438, 439
Soaks, 1113
SOAP format, 18
Social adaptation, 106
Social age, 53
Social isolation, 187
Social and Rehabilitative Service, 267, 444
Social Security Administration, 261
Social status, 264
Society of Prospective Medicine, 274
Sociologic crisis, 1183
Sociologic health, 4
Sodium, 87, 135, 142-143, 1213
  burns and, 1133, 1134
  deficit, 142
  depletion, 154
  excess, 143
  normal values of, 949
  renal failure and, 997
  resorption of, 135
  in serum, 142
Sodium bicarbonate, 244, 1173, 1201
Sodium chloride, 135, 156
Sodium iodide, 553, 828
Sodium lactate 155
Sodium nitroprusside, 169, 422, 669, 724, 1201
Sodium-restricted diet, 672-673
Soft contact lenses, 440
Soft tissue injury, 509-513
Solar keratosis, 1119
Solganol; see Gold salts
Solu-Medrol; see Methylprednisolone
Solu-B; see Vitamin B
Solu-Cortef; see Heparin and hydrocortisone succinate
Solutes, 136
Solutions
  intravenous, 155
  nutrient, 97
  osmolality of, 137
Solvents, 136, 961
Soma, 352
Somatic pain, 179
Somatotropin, 792
Somogyi phenomenon, 778
Sonography, 688
Sopor, 125
Sorbitol, 769
Sounds, 461
Specimen collection, 195
Speech, 26
  centers of, 355
  esophageal, 540
Speech audiometry, 468
Speech reading, 470-471
Speech rehabilitation, 540
Speech training, 471
Spermatic cords, 1075
Spermatocele, 1075
Sphenoid sinus, 528
Sphenoidotomy, 531
Sphincter of Oddi, 834, 865
Spina bifida, 1033
Spinal anesthesia, 314, 321
Spinal cord, 355
  decompression of, 420, 421
  injury and, 417-420
    muscle function after, 418
    sexual function and, 419, 422, 423, 1033, 1042

Spinal cord—cont'd
  tumors and, 1033
Spinal fracture, 1182-1183
Spinal fusion, 505-507
Spine
  emergency assessment of, 1167
  physical examination of, 31
Spiral fracture, 511
Spironolactone, 671, 723, 1035
  fluid and electrolytes and, 154
  hydrochlorothiazide and, 723
Splanchnic veins, 847
Spleen, 76
Splinting
  musculoskeletal disorders and, 485-487
    types of, 509
Splinting catheter, 982, 983
Split-thickness graft, 538, 1123, 1124
Spongy bone, 481
Spontaneous pneumothorax, 595
Spring-loaded braces, 485-486
Sputum, 554
  tuberculosis and, 564-565
Squamous cell carcinoma, 217, 1119
Squeeze technique, 1038
SRS; *see* Social and Rehabilitation Service
SSKI; *see* Saturated solution of potassium io-
    dide
S-T segment, 636
Stab wounds, 1179
Staff satisfaction survey, 44
Stages
  of cancer pain, 250-251
  of dying, 281-282
Standards for Advanced Life Support, 649
Standards of Nursing Practice, 39, 40-41
Stapedectomy, 475
Stapes, 460
Staphylococcus aureus, 67, 77, 201, 839, 1057
  burns and, 1138
  food poisoning and, 1176, 1177
  nosocomial infection and, 200
  penicillin-resistant, 190
  pneumonia and, 533, 554, 559
  toxic shock syndrome and, 1058
Starch, 87
Starling's law, 140, 141, 665
  of heart, 631
Stasis dermatitis, 1115
State Offices of Vocational Rehabilitation,
    471
Status asthmaticus, 611
Status epilepticus, 387
Steatorrhea, 917
Stein-Leventhal disease, 1065
Steinmann pin, 518
Stem cell differentiation, 729
Sterile fluorescein, 445
Sterility
  chemotherapy and, 249
  epididymitis and, 1073, 1078
Sterilization, 1052-1055
  informed consent and, 1054
  reversal of, 1055
Sternocleidomastoid muscles, 545
Steroid hormones, 1215
Steroids
  eye disorders and, 449, 450, 1214
  pain relief and, 182
  shock and, 170
Stethoscope, 322
Stokes-Adams syndrome, 644

Stomach, 877
  cancer and, 921, 924-926
  inflammatory disorders of, 895-897
  renal failure and, 1002
Stomahesive, 935
Stomas, 931-938
Stomatitis, 246
Stool
  fat in, 1220
  nitrogen in, 1220
  occult blood in, 900
Strangulated hernia, 920
Strep throat, 529
Streptococci, 201, 1057
Streptococcus pneumoniae, 70, 198, 553,
    559
Streptococcus pyogenes, 67, 77
Streptococcus thermophilus, 222
Streptodornase-streptokinase, 704
Streptomycin, 463, 566
Streptozotocin, 247
Stress
  adaptation and, 105
  cancer and, 219
  coronary artery disease and, 652
  disorders related to, 105
  elderly and, 55
  head injury and, 416
  management of, 110-111
  prevention of, 110
  response to, 27, 106-108, 113-129
  signs and symptoms of, 109
  ulcers and, 908, 912
  young adults and, 50
Stress incontinence, 58, 989-990
Stress index, 53
Stress testing, 653
Stressors, 106, 1199-1207
Striae, 807
Striated muscle, 482
Stroke; *see* Cerebrovascular accident
Stroke Clubs of America, 273
Stroke index, 1195
Stroke volume, 631, 639, 1195
Strophanthus gratus, 670, 671
Stryker frame, 186, 420, 421, 513
Stuart factor, 1217
Stump care, 709-710
Sty, 445
Subarachnoid space, 356
Subcapital fracture, 514
Subcutaneous emphysema, 585-586
Subcutaneous tissue, 1106
Subdural space, 356
Submucous resection, 536
Subtotal gastrectomy, 913, 914
Succinylcholine, 320
Sucralfate, 910
Suction control bottle, 588, 589
Suctioning
  postoperative, 327
  tracheostomy tube and, 617-619
  waterseal, 588-590
Suffixes, surgical, 292
Sugars, 87, 1214
Suicide
  alcohol and, 120
  middle age and, 53
  young adults and, 50
Sulfamylon; *see* Mafenide
Sulfate, 135, 1213
Sulfisoxazole, 960

Sulfonamides, 743, 1213
  anemia and, 733
  infection and, 190
Sulfonylureas, 777
Sulfur bath, 1113
Sulindac, 493
Sun, cancer and, 219, 220
Sunstroke, 1177
Superficial fascia, 482
Superficial frostbite, 1178
Superinfection, 191, 200
Supine position, 312
Support groups, 270, 786
Supportive devices, 485, 1192
Suppositories, 182
Supraglottic partial laryngectomy, 538
Suprapubic prostatectomy, 976, 977-978
Surgeon General's Reports, 221, 222
Surgeon's orders, 334
Surgery
  anxiety and, 293, 294, 298
  aortic aneurysm and, 688-690
  cancer and, 232
  cataract and, 451-453
  cerebrovascular accident and, 405
  classification of, 291-292
  comfort and, 300
  cosmetic, 292, 1125-1127
  curative, 292
  data analysis and planning and, 297
  diabetes mellitus and, 780, 781
  diagnostic, 292
  documentation, 323
  ear problems and, 448-449, 451, 474
  elderly and, 296-297
  external, 291
  fears and, 293
  informed consent for, 293-294
  intestinal obstruction and, 920
  intracranial, 406-407, 431
  intravertebral tumors and, 433
  myocardial ischemia and, 659-663
  nasal, 531-532, 535, 536
  neurologic pain and, 371
  nursing diagnosis and, 297
  palliative, 292
  Parkinson's disease and, 398
  peptic ulcer and, 913-915
  peripheral vascular disease and, 705-713
  pituitary gland and, 802-803
  postanesthetic phase of, 326-329
  postoperative phase of, 299, 323, 326-348
  preoperative phase of, 297-298, 300, 301,
    303, 313-314
  pulmonary complications of, 299
  restorative, 292
  retinal detachment and, 458, 459
  rheumatoid arthritis and, 496
  risk and, 296
  seizures and, 389
  stomach and, 924, 925-926
  trigeminal neuralgia and, 424-425
  tumors and, 1120-1121
  types of, 291-292
  valvular heart disorders and, 685-686
  venous disorders and, 716-717
  wounds and, infection and, 201, 203
Surgical asepsis, 307-308
Surgical drains, 323, 332
Surgical gloving/gowning, 310
Surgical notes, 334
Surgical personnel, 306

Surgical scrub, 309-310
Surrogate mothers, 1057
Susceptibility, 63
Suspensory ligament, 437
Suspicious behavior, 120
Suture and patch graft reconstruction, 705
Swallowing, 876-877
Swan-Ganz catheter, 165, 658, 1137, 1195, 1196
Sweat, 134
Sweeteners, 219, 221
Swing-through gait, 710, 712
Swing-to gait, 710, 712
Symmetrel; *see* Amantadine hydrochloride
Sympathectomy, 184, 185
Sympathetic nervous system, 356
  hypoglycemia and, 778
  stimulation and, 665
  surgery and, 293
Sympathetic-adrenal medullary mechanism, 107-108
Sympathomimetics, 606
Synanon, 127
Synapses, 352, 353-354
Synaptic transmission, 353
Synarthroses, 482
Synergism, 320
Synovectomy, 496
Synovial fluid, 1220
Synthetic analgesics, 125
Synthetic anticholinergic drugs, 397
Synthroid; *see* Levothyroxine sodium
Syphilis, 687, 1078-1083
Syringes, 393
Syringomyelia, 393
Systemic hypertension, 442
Systemic lupus erythematosus, 488, 497-498, 1158
Systemic vascular resistance, 1195
Systole, 630

T

T cells, 74, 75, 78, 730
  deficiency test of, 1147
T-tube, 332, 864, 865
Tabes dorsalis, 412
Tachycardia, 670
Tagamet; *see* Cimetadine
Tailoring thoracoplasty, 590
Tampons, toxic shock syndrome and, 1058
Tandem, 1072
Tapazole; *see* Methimazole
Tar baths, 1113
Taractan; *see* Chlorprothixene
Tassette, 1064
Tattooing, 1125
Teaching
  arterial disorders and, 713
  cancer and, 212, 224, 255
  cerebrovascular accident and, 406
  coronary artery bypass and, 661
  headache and, 367
  immunization and, 199
  immunodeficiency and, 1148
  inflammatory disorders and, 897-904
  leukemia and, 751
  menopause and, 1051-1052
  menstruation and, 1050
  musculoskeletal disorders and, 484-487
  myocardial infarction and, 659
  nervous system and, 358
  nose and throat and, 533

Teaching—cont'd
  nutrition and, 92-93
  pain and, 371
  Parkinson's disease, 398
  reproductive tract and, 1061
  seizures and, 390
  stoma and, 933-937
  surgery and, 294, 298-299
  ulcer and, 913
Team nursing, 265-267, 304-306
Tears
  as defense mechanism, 66
  ether anesthesia and, 318
  substitutes for, 450
Technetium-99m pyrophosphate, 657
Tedral, 612
Teeth, 30, 57
Teflon graft, 705, 711
Tegretol; *see* Carbamazepine
Telemetry, 635
Telescoped fracture, 511
Telfa dressings, 1125
Temaril; *see* Trimeprazine tartrate
Temperature
  anesthesia and, 322
  craniocerebral trauma and, 415
  operating room and, 306
  postoperative changes in, 330
  shock and, 171
  skin and, 27
Temporal lobe, 354
  tumors and, 1033
Tendons, 481
TENS; *see* Transcutaneous electrical nerve stimulator
Tensilon; *see* Endrophonium chloride
Tension headache, 360
  medications for, 366
Teratomas, 218
Terbutaline, 606, 612
Terminal respiratory unit, 545, 546, 547
Terminology, 6
Terpin hydrate, 553
Tertiary intention, 335
Tessalon; *see* Benzonatate
Tes-Tape, 415, 763, 765, 785
Testes
  cancer and, 225, 1075, 1219
  self-examination of, 1076
  torsion of, 1074
  surgery and, 1076-1077
Testosterone, 1047, 1215
Tests
  diagnostic, 59
  preoperative, 295
Tetanus, 197
Tetanus immune globulin, human, 199
Tetanus prophylaxis, 1180, 1181
Tetanus vaccine, 197
Tetany, 145, 817, 819-820
Tetracaine, 317
Tetracycline, 83, 88, 89, 559, 600, 843, 1059
Tetrahydrocannibinol, 246
Thalamotomy, 185
Theca cells, 1219
Thallium 201, 657
THC; *see* Tetrahydrocannibinol
Theophylline, 612
Therapeutic touch, 187
Thermography, 1088
Thiamin, 87, 121, 424

Thiazide, 88, 142, 144, 154, 607, 671, 743, 843
6-Thioguanine, 750
Thiopental sodium, 317, 319-320
Thioridazine, 1035
Thiotepa, 975
Thiouracil, 843
Third-degree burns, 1129, 1130
Thirst, 156
Thomas splint, 519, 520, 521
Thoracic artery aneurysm, 687-688, 689
Thoracoplasty, 590
Thoracotomy, 580
Thorax
  aging and, 37, 548
  anatomy of, 544
  injury to, 421
  surgery and, 580-591
Thorazine; *see* Chlorpromazine
Three-point gait, 485, 710, 711
Threonine, 87
Thrombin time, 1217
Thromboangitis obliterans, 700, 701
Thrombocytes, 69, 730
Thrombocytopenia, 733, 743, 744
Thrombocytopenic drug, 743
Thrombocytosis, 743, 744
Thromboembolism, 715
Thrombophlebitis, 713-717
Thromboplastin, 730
Thrombotic crisis, 739
Thrombus, 401, 712
Thrush, 894
Thymectomy, 76
Thymus, 76
Thymus-dependent lymphocytes, 74
Thyrocalcitonin, 822
Thyroid, 794-795
  dysfunction of, 820, 821-830
  scan of, 827
  surgery and, 829-830
Thyroid antibody tests, 826
Thyroid colloid antigens, 1219
Thyroid cartilage, 529
Thyroid crisis, 820, 823, 824
Thyroid function tests, 826-827
Thyroid hormone, 820, 822, 1216
  replacement therapy, 804, 820, 828
Thyroid notch, 529
Thyroid-stimulating hormone, 792, 797, 827
Thyroid storm, 823-824
Thyroid suppression test, 827
Thyroidectomy, 829
Thyroiditis, 821, 1158
Thyrolar; *see* Liotrix
Thyroxine, 821, 823, 825, 833
Thyroxine-binding globulin, 825
TIA; *see* Transient ischemic attack
Tic doloreaux, 424-425
Tidal volume, 583
Tigan; *see* Trimethobenzamide
Timolol, 456, 724
Timoptic; *see* Timolol
Tinea capitis, 1109, 1110
Tinea corporis, 1109
Tinea cruris, 1109, 1110
Tinea pedis, 1109, 1110
Tinel's sign, 502
Tinnitis, 473
Tissues
  fibrotic, 73
  immune response and, 76

Tissues—cont'd
  transplantation of, 82-84, 1157-1158
  typing of, 1158
TNM staging of cancer, 218, 1092
Tobramycin, 559
Toclase; *see* Carbetapentane
Toenails, 1107
Tolazamide, 777
Tolazoline, 704
Tolbutamide, 777
Tolectin; *see* Tolmetin sodium
Tolerance
  drugs/alcohol and, 123
  pain and, 175
Tolinase; *see* Tolazamide
Tolmetin sodium, 493
Tomography, 365
Tongue
  cancer and, 921
  physical examination of, 30
Tonic convulsions, 387
Tonicity, 137
Tonometers, 453
Tonsillectomy, 532-534
Tonsils, 528, 529
  cancer and, 537
  inflammation and, 530
Topical anesthesia, 314
  eye disorders and, 449
Topical antibiotics, 449
Topical medications, 1111
Total laryngectomy, 538-541
Total lung capacity, 583
Total parenteral nutrition, 1203
TOUCH, 228
Touching
  anxiety and, 116
  therapeutic, 187
Tourniquets, 675
Toxic hepatitis, 835, 843
Toxic injury, 994
Toxic shock syndrome, 1057, 1058
Toxigenicity, 191
Toxoids, 81
TPN; *see* Total parenteral nutrition
Trabeculae, 481
Trabeculectomy, 456
Trachea, 529
  physical examination of, 30
Tracheostomy, 613, 614, 617, 619
Tracheostomy tubes, 540, 614-619
Traction, 516-520
Traction weights, 520, 521
Tractotomy, 185
Tral; *see* Hexocyclium
Tranquilizers, 125
  delirium tremens and, 124
  pain and, 183
  preoperative, 301
  sexual function and, 1035
Transaminase, 1213
Transcendental meditation, 185
Transcervical fracture, 514
Transcutaneous electrical nerve stimulator, 183, 184
Transderm; *see* Nitroglycerin isosorbide
Transfrontal surgery, 803
Transient ischemic attack, 401-402
Transplacental immunization, 81
Transposed skin graft, 1125
Transsexualism, 1038
Transsphenoidal surgery, 802-803

Transurethral fulguration, 975
Transurethral prostatectomy, 203, 976-977
Transverse aorta, 688
Transverse colostomy, 932
Transverse fracture, 511
Transvestism, 1031, 1038
Tranylcypromine, 89, 1035
Trapezius, 545
Trauma
  aneurysm and, 587
  brain damage and, 413
  cataract and, 451
  central nervous system and, 358
  chest and, 592-595
  craniocerebral, 413-417
  interventions in, 1168-1169
  musculoskeletal system and, 509-522
  nosebleeds and, 534
  nutrient needs and, 86
  peripheral nervous system and, 422-425
  psychologic, 1169
    rape and, 1183
  spinal cord and, 417, 422
  urinary tract and, 993
Traumatic alopecia, 1122
Traumatic neuroma, 423
Traumatic wet lung, 575
Tremor, 123
Trendelenburg position, 312
Trnedelenburg test, 715
Trephine, 456
Treponema pallidum, 1082
Triage, 1186, 1187
Triamcinolone, 450, 810
Triamterene, 89, 154, 671, 723
Triazinate, 247
Trichinosis, 896
Trichlormethazide, 723
Trichomonas, 1057, 1059
Trichomoniasis, 1078
Tricuspid valve, 34, 628, 681-682, 683
Tridione; *see* Trimethadione
Trifocal lenses, 439
Trigeminal neuralgia, 424-425
Triglycerides, 87, 651, 1212
Trigone, 941
Trihexphenidyl, 397
Triiodothyronine, 821, 822, 823
Trimeprazine tartrate, 1005
Trimethadione, 389, 733
Trimethaphan, 724, 1035
Trimethobenzamide, 897
Trimethoprim-sulfamethoxazole, 89, 395, 422, 559, 956
Trionine; *see* Liothyronine sodium
Triplication of ureters, 956
Triticeous cartilage, 529
Trochanter rolls, 484
Tromaxan; *see* Ethyl miscoumacetate
Tropicamide, 449
Trousseau's sign, 145-146, 817
TRU; *see* Terminal respiratory unit
Trypsin, 704
Tryptar; *see* Trypsin
Tryptophan, 87
TSH; *see* Thyroid-stimulating hormone
TSTA; *see* Tumor-specific transplantation antigens
Tubal sterilization, 1053
Tube feeding, 94-96
Tube pedicle graft, 1125
Tubercle bacilli, 562

Tuberculin reaction, 564
Tuberculosis, 561-567
  alcoholism and, 122
  chemotherapy and, 563
  classification of, 562, 563
  drugs for, 566
  isolation and, 206
  transmission of, 567
Tuberculous meningitis, 356
Tubocurarine chloride, 320
Tubules, 941, 943
Tumors, 72, 211
  bladder and, 974-975
  cholangiocellular, 840
  feminizing, 1034
  intravertebral, 433
  liver and, 840
  malignant, 211
  pancreas and, 867, 868
  skin and, 27, 211
Tumor-specific transplantation antigens, 82
Tunica adventitia, 693
Tunica intima, 693
Tunica media, 693
Tuning fork tests, 468
Turbinates, 527, 528
  hypertrophy of, 534
Turgor of skin, 27
TURP; *see* Transurethral prostatectomy
Two-drop urine test, 763
Two-point gait, 485, 711
Tylenol; *see* Acetaminophen
Tympanic membrane, 460, 465, 466
Tympanoplasty, 474
Typhoid fever, immunization and, 81, 197
Tyramine, 89
Tyrosine, 87

U

Ulcerative colitis, 897, 898-899
  stress and, 105
  surgery and, 902
Ulceromembranous stomatitis, 894
Ulcers, 50
  medications for, 1118
Ulo; *see* Chlophedianol hydrochloride
Ultrafiltration, 1012
Ultralente insulin, 774
Ultrasound
  breasts and, 1088
  cancer and, 231
  infection and, 195
  reproductive tract and, 1070
  urinary tract and, 954
  venous disorders and, 715
Ultraviolet light, 1117
Umbilicus
  hernia and, 920
  physical examination of, 31
UMN; *see* Upper motor neurons
Unconsciousness, 1168
Underweight, 94
United Cancer Council, Inc., 227
United Ostomy Association, 227, 273, 937
University Group Diabetes Program, 777
Unstable angina, 653
Upper airway, 543, 550
Upper motor neuron bladder, 417
Upper motor neurons, 377, 378, 379, 988, 989
Upper respiratory tract infection, 50, 529
Upper throat, 527, 528, 529
Urea, 134, 135, 375, 456

Urea nitrogen, 1213
Ureaphil; *see* Urea
Urecholine; *see* Bethanechol chloride
Uremia, 995
Uremic acidosis, 149
Ureterolithotomy, 973
Ureters, 941
    catheterization and, 938, 948-949, 952
    duplication of, 956
    tearing of, 993
    triplication of, 956
Urethral sphincter, 941
Urethral strictures, 979
Urethral tearing, 993
Urethritis, 959, 1073
Urethrobladder reflex, 988, 989
Urethrography, 953
Urethroplasty, 979, 983
Urevert; *see* Urea
Urgency of urination, 945, 946
Uric acid, 1213
Uric acid stones, 974
Urinalysis, 947
Urinary drainage, 991-992, 1077
Urinary incontinence, 946, 987-993, 998
Urinary output, 946, 972, 1137
Urinary retention record of, 152, 931, 979-987
Urinary tract
    congenital disorders of, 955-958
    diagnostic tests and, 946-955
    health problems of, 955-1024
    immobilization and, 513
    infection and, 194, 959-961
        nosocomial, 201, 202-203
        postoperative, 344
        risk factors and, 959
    multiple sclerosis and, 395
    obstructive disorders of, 968-1024
    radiologic examination of, 949, 953-954
    structures of, 941
    trauma and, 993
    vascular disorders of, 967-968
Urine, 134, 946
    chemistry tests of, 950
    collection of, 947, 948
    as defense mechanism, 66
    laboratory values for, 1214
    retention of, 344, 946
    specific gravity of, 153, 950
    sugar tests and, 785
    suppression of, 946
    unsealed internal radiation and, 240, 241
Urobilinogen, 834, 1214
Urokinase, 715
Urolithiasis, 969
Uroporphyrin, 1214
Ursodeoxycholic acid, 865
Urticaria, 1150
Uterus
    cancer and, 1049-1050
    displacement of, 1061, 1062
    prolapse of, 1034, 1061, 1062
Utilization review program, 44
Uveitis, 445, 451, 1158
Uvula, 528

V

Vaccine, 197
    attenuated live, 81
    inactivated, 196
    killed, 81

Vagina, 1045
    congenital absence of, 1033
    discharge from, 1059
    infection and, 1034, 1049
    secretions from, as defense mechanism, 66
Vaginal spray/deodorant, 1034
Vaginectomy, 1033
Vaginismus, 1038
Vaginitis, 66, 1057, 1058
    alternative therapies for, 1060
    discharge and, 1059
    radiation therapy and, 1034
Vagolytic agents, 301
Vagotomy, 913-915
Vagus nerve, 529, 631, 835; *see also* Cranial
        nerve X
Valine, 87
Valium; *see* Diazepam
Valley fever; *see* Coccidioidomycosis
Valproic acid, 389
Valsalva maneuver, 99, 670
Valves of heart, 34, 628
    disease and, 670-686
    repair of, 685
    replacement of, 685-686
Valvuloplasty, 685
Valvulotomy, 685
van den Bergh test, 1211
Vancomycin, 463, 559
Vanilylmandelic acid, 1214
Vaporizers, 557
Variant angina, 653
Varicella virus, 201
Varicella zoster, 1108, 1109
Varicocele, 1075
Varicosities, 717-719
Varidase; *see* Streptodornase-streptokinase
Vas deferens, 1047
Vascular compartment, 163
Vascular embolism, 217
Vasectomy, 1053
Vasoactive drugs, 169, 170
Vasoconstriction, 320
Vasodilan; *see* Isoxsuprine
Vasodilators
    hypertension and, 724
    peripheral vascular disease and, 704
    shock and, 169
Vasogenic shock, 158, 159
Vasopressin, 807, 857
Vegan diet, 92
Vegetarian diet, 92
Velban; *see* Vinblastine
Vena cava, ligation of, 716-717
Veneral disease, 1078-1084
Veneral Disease Research Laboratory, 1083
Venography, 715
Venous disorders, 714
Venous ligation, 718-719
Venous pressure, 318
Venous stasis, 142, 299, 342
Venous thrombosis, 713-717
Ventilation, 545, 583
    mouth-to-mouth, 1172
    postoperative, 327-328, 340, 341
Ventilators, 1200
    weaning from, 622
Ventimask, 613
Ventricles, 628
Ventricular diastolic gallop, 34
Ventricular dilation, 665
Ventricular ejection, 630

Ventricular fibrillation, 637, 642-643
Ventricular pacing, 645
Ventricular standstill, 638, 644
Ventriculography, 429, 430
Venules, 693
Verapamil, 639, 655, 1201
Verruca, 1109
Vertebrae, 482
Vertebral arteries, 355
Vertigo, 474
Vesicant drugs, 244
Vesicoureteral reflux, 960
Vesicovaginal fistula, 975, 1062,
        1063
Vesicourethropexy, 990
Vestibule of ear, 461
Veterans Administration, 471
Viamycin, 463
Vinblastine, 243, 244
Vinca alkaloids, 242, 243
Vincent's angina, 894
Vincristine, 244, 247, 255, 750
Vinegar douche, 1060
Vinke tongs, 420
Vinyl chloride, 219
Viomycin, 566
Viral disease
    hepatitis and, 835, 836-839
    pneumonia and, 549
    pulmonary tract and, 549-553
    skin and, 1108-1109, 1114
Virginia tongs, 420
Viruses, 201, 529
    cancer and, 219, 223
Visceral muscle, 482
Visceral pain, 179
Visceral pleura, 545
Viscosity, 1220
Visidex, 784
Vision, 437
    acuity of, 29, 438-439
    blurred, 442
    digitalis and, 670
    eye disease and, 442
    fields of, 453
    impaired, 442, 443
    loss of, 443
Visual analog pain scales, 181
Visual stimuli, 186-187
Visually handicapped, 442-444, 445
Vital capacity, 583
Vital signs
    craniocerebral trauma and, 415
    lung surgery and, 585
    postoperative, 328, 330
    shock and, 162
Vitamin-deficient diets, 219, 222
Vitamins
    A
        deficiency, 442
        tolerance test, 1213
    B, 155
    B_6, 87
        young adults and, 50
    B_{12}, 87, 1218
        alcohol and, 123
        deficiency, 741
    B-complex, 122
    C, 87
        young adults and, 50
        wound healing and, 343, 590
    D, 87, 819, 820

Vitamins—cont'd
E, 87
sexual function and, 1036
young adults and, 50
K, 87, 534, 742
deficiency of
alcoholism and, 122
infertility and, 1056
signs of, 917
fat-soluble, 917
Vitrectomy, 768
Vitreous body, 437, 457
Vitreous hemorrhage, 442
Vitreous humor, 437
Vivactil; *see* Protriptyline
Vocal cords, 829
Vocational rehabilitation, 267
Voiding, 58
Voiding cystourethrogram, 952
Volume-controlled ventilators, 620, 621
Volunteers, 272
Volvulus, 919
Vomiting, 880, 881
as defense mechanism, 66
fluid and electrolytes and, 153
postoperative, 345
projectile, 374
unsealed internal radiation and, 240
von Economo's disease, 410
Voyeurism, 1031
VP-16-213, 247
Vulva, 1059
Vulvitis, 1057, 1058
V-Z; *see* Varicella zoster

W

Waking-imagined analgesia, 187
Wallerian degeneration, 423
Wandering macrophages, 68
Warts, 1109
Washed red cells, 1154
Water deprivation test, 806

Water intoxication, 138, 139-140, 143, 977
Water replacement, 139
Water-seal drainage, 582
Water siphon test, 885
Wedge resection, 580, 582
Weight
daily record of, 152-153
gain of, 94
burns and, 1140
loss of, 93-94
burns and, 1134
cancer and, 225
measurement of, 89
reduction of, 93-94
elderly and, 58
Weight Watchers, 93
Wernicke's area, 355
Westergren method, 1217
Wet dressings, 1112, 1139
Wet drowning, 1174
Wet gangrene, 769
Wheezes, 33, 34
Whistle-tip catheter, 979, 980, 982
White blood cells, 730
disorders of, 748-752
infection and, 195
normal values of, 729
types of, 194
White foxglove, 670
White lung, 161
White matter, 353
WHO; *see* World Health Organization
Whole blood, 1154
Wholistic Health Center, 274
Whooping cough, 197
Widow's hump, 483
Well Aware about Health, 274
Wellness Associates, 274
Wilms' tumor, 974
Withdrawal
alcohol and, 123-124
elderly and, 55

Withdrawal—cont'd
mind-altering drugs and, 126
Women's liberation movement, 49, 52
World Health Organization, 4, 125
Wounds, 1179, 1181-1182
dehiscence of, 338
drainage of, 152, 240, 332
evisceration and, 338
healing of, 335-338, 1023
separation of, 338
types of, 1179
Wound suction apparatus, 333
Wrist drop, 122

X

Xanthine compounds, 606
Xenylamine, 975
Xeroderma pigmentosa, 219, 220
Xeroradiography
breasts and, 1088, 1089
cancer and, 231
Xylocaine; *see* Lidocaine
D-Xylose, 1220
X-rays, 235, 239

Y

Y-tube, 618
Yawn, 341
Yogurt, 222
Yohimbine, 1036
Young adulthood, 47-50
Yttrium, 239
implantation of, 802

Z

Zarontin; *see* Ethosuximide
Zero loudness, 468
Zinc, 87
Zinostatin, 247
Zollinger-Ellison syndrome, 868, 909
Zoophilia, 1031
Zoster immune globulin, human, 199